Infectious Diseases Handbook

including

Antimicrobial Therapy & Diagnostic Tests/Procedures

6th Edition

Judith A. Aberg, MD
Principal Investigator, AIDS Clinical Trials Unit
Director of HIV
Bellevue Hospital Center
Associate Professor of Medicine
New York University
New York, New York

Morton P. Goldman, PharmD, BCPS, FCCP
Assistant Director, Pharmacotherapy Services
Department of Pharmacy
The Cleveland Clinic Foundation
Cleveland, Ohio

Larry D. Gray, PhD, ABMM
Director of Clinical Microbiology
TriHealth Laboratories,
Volunteer Assistant Professor
University of Cincinnati College of Medicine,
President
Clinical Microbiology Laboratory Consultants, LLC
Cincinnati, Ohio

Jennifer K. Long, PharmD, BCPS
Infectious Diseases Clinical Specialist
The Cleveland Clinic Foundation
Cleveland, Ohio

LEXI-COMP

APhA

This handbook is intended to serve the user as a handy reference and not as a complete infectious disease resource. The publication covers common diseases with empiric treatment recommendations, common microorganisms, testing procedures necessary for diagnosis, and the majority of anti-infective agents available in the United States. The individual sections of this handbook are specifically designed to present certain important aspects of the disease states, the organisms, laboratory tests, and antimicrobial therapy in a more concise format than is typically found in medical literature or infectious disease texts.

The nature of infectious diseases and their diagnosis and treatment is that it is constantly evolving because of ongoing research and clinical experience and is often subject to interpretation. While great care has been taken to ensure the accuracy of the information presented, the reader is advised that the authors, editors, reviewers, contributors, and publishers cannot be responsible for the continued currency of the information or for any errors, omissions, or the application of this information, or for any consequences arising therefrom. Therefore, the author(s) and/or the publisher shall have no liability to any person or entity with regard to claims, loss, or damage caused, or alleged to be caused, directly or indirectly, by the use of information contained herein. Because of the dynamic nature of infectious disease as a discipline, readers are advised that decisions regarding the diagnosis and treatment of specific organisms and disease states must be based on the independent judgment of the clinician, changing information regarding drug therapy (eg, as reflected in the literature and drug manufacturer's most current product information), and changing medical practices. The editors are not responsible for any inaccuracy of quotation or for any false or misleading implication that may arise due to the text or formulas used or due to the quotation of revisions no longer official.

The editors, authors, and contributors have written this book in their private capacities. No official support or endorsement by any federal or state agency or pharmaceutical company is intended or inferred.

The publishers have made every effort to trace the copyright holders for borrowed material. If they have inadvertently overlooked any, they will be pleased to make the necessary arrangements at the first opportunity.

If you have any suggestions or questions regarding any information presented in this handbook, please contact our drug information pharmacist at (330) 650-6506.

This manual was produced using the FormuLex
A complete publishing service of Lexi-Comp, Inc.

LEXI-COMP

1100 Terex Road
Hudson, Ohio 44236
(330) 650-6506

ISBN 1-59195-121-6

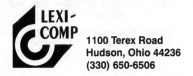

TABLE OF CONTENTS

TABLE OF CONTENTS *(Continued)*

ABOUT THE AUTHORS

Judith A. Aberg, MD

Dr Aberg received a degree in Laboratory Technology from Norfolk General Hospital in 1975 and worked in medical microbiology, where she was responsible for the Mycology Laboratory and curriculum. After 11 years of laboratory experience, Dr Aberg graduated from Millersville University of Pennsylvania, Magna Cum Laude, BSMT. Dr Aberg then graduated from Pennsylvania State University College of Medicine.

During Dr Aberg's medical school training, she was a research technologist in neuroimmunology, resulting in publication of her work with multiple sclerosis. After medical school, Dr Aberg completed her internal medicine residency at the Cleveland Clinic, during which time she worked as a limited clinical practitioner in the Emergency Department and was involved in research projects in the Department of Infectious Disease. Dr Aberg then held a joint position as both Chief Medical Resident and Clinical Associate in Immunology at the Cleveland Clinic.

Dr Aberg completed a fellowship in Infectious Disease at the Washington University School of Medicine in the Department of Infectious Disease. She then was an Assistant Professor of Medicine in the AIDS and Oncology Division at the University of California, San Francisco where she was also Co-Principal Investigator of the AIDS Clinical Trials Unit. She then became the Director of HIV Services at Washington University. She currently is an Associate Professor of Medicine and the Principal Investigator of the AIDS Clinical Trials Unit at New York University. In addition, she is the Director of HIV at Bellevue Hospital Center. She is an active member of the AIDS Clinical Trials Group, American Society for Microbiology, and Infectious Diseases Society of America.

Morton P. Goldman, PharmD

Dr Goldman received his bachelor's degree in pharmacy from the University of Pittsburgh, College of Pharmacy and his Doctor of Pharmacy degree from the University of Cincinnati, Division of Graduate Studies and Research. He completed his concurrent 2-year hospital pharmacy residency at the VA Medical Center in Cincinnati. Dr Goldman is presently the Assistant Director of Pharmacotherapy Services for the Department of Pharmacy at the Cleveland Clinic Foundation (CCF) after having spent over 4 years at CCF as an Infectious Disease pharmacist and 4 years as Clinical Manager. He holds faculty appointments from The University of Toledo, College of Pharmacy, Ohio Northern University, Raabe College of Pharmacy, and Case Western Reserve University, College of Medicine and is the Pharmacology Curriculum Coordinator for the new Cleveland Clinic Lerner College of Medicine. Dr Goldman is a Board-Certified Pharmacotherapy Specialist (BCPS) with added qualifications in infectious diseases.

In his capacity as Assistant Director of Pharmacotherapy Services at CCF, Dr Goldman remains actively involved in patient care and clinical research with the Department of Infectious Disease, as well as the continuing education of the medical and pharmacy staff. He is an editor of CCF's *Guidelines for Antibiotic Use* and participates in their annual Antimicrobial Review retreat. He is a member of the Pharmacy and Therapeutics Committee and many of its subcommittees. Dr Goldman has authored numerous journal articles and lectures locally and nationally on infectious diseases topics and current drug therapies. He is currently a reviewer for the *Annals of Pharmacotherapy* and the *Journal of the American Medical Association*, an editorial board member of the *Journal of Infectious Disease Pharmacotherapy*, and coauthor of the *Drug Information Handbook* and the *Drug Information Handbook for the Allied Health Professional* produced by Lexi-Comp, Inc. He also provides technical support to Lexi-Comp's Clinical Reference Library™ publications.

Dr Goldman is an active member of the Ohio College of Clinical Pharmacy, the Society of Infectious Disease Pharmacists, the American College of Clinical Pharmacy (and is a Fellow of the College), and the American Society of Health-Systems Pharmacists.

ABOUT THE AUTHORS *(Continued)*

Larry D. Gray, PhD, ABMM

Dr Gray received his bachelor's degree from the University of North Carolina at Chapel Hill and his master's and doctorate degrees from Wake Forest University. He received his postdoctoral training in Clinical Microbiology and Infectious Diseases at the Mayo Clinic.

Dr Gray has been the Director of the TriHealth Clinical Microbiology at Bethesda and Good Samaritan Hospitals in Cincinnati, Ohio for the last 17 years. He is a Volunteer Assistant Professor of Pathology and Laboratory Medicine and Volunteer Clinical Professor of Allied Health Sciences at the University of Cincinnati College of Medicine, and is a Diplomate of the American Board of Medical Microbiology. In addition, he is an active member of the American Society for Microbiology, the American Board of Medical Microbiology, and the South Central Association for Clinical Microbiology. Dr Gray is also the president of Clinical Microbiology Laboratory Consultants, LLC.

Dr Gray is the 2004 recipient of the Outstanding Contributor to Clinical Microbiology Award given by the South Central Association for Clinical Microbiology. Dr Gray's background includes 12 years of research in the pathogenesis of ocular and pulmonary bacterial infections and the publication of many research and clinical articles, abstracts, and book chapters.

Jennifer K. Long, PharmD, BCPS

Dr Long received her Doctor of Pharmacy degree from Purdue University. She completed a pharmacy practice residency at the Louis Stokes VAMC in Cleveland, Ohio and Infectious Diseases pharmacy residency at The Cleveland Clinic Foundation (CCF). Dr Long currently holds the position of Infectious Diseases Clinical Specialist as well as Clinical Coordinator of Pharmacotherapy Services at CCF. Dr Long is a Board-Certified Pharmacotherapy Specialist (BCPS).

Dr Long is actively involved in the clinical practice and rounds with the ID consult services. She is actively involved in clinical research with the Departments of Infectious Diseases and Microbiology. She is an editor for CCF's Guidelines for Antimicrobial Usage and coordinates the annual Antimicrobial Review retreat for CCF. In addition, she is a member of the Infection Control Committee. Dr Long is active in the education of pharmacists and medical staff. She serves as primary preceptor for the infectious diseases residency program at CCF, is a member of the Cleveland Clinic Lerner College of Medicine (CCLCM) curriculum committee, and participates in educational programs for infectious diseases fellows. Additional teaching responsibilities include lecturing for CCLCM, the Ohio College of Podiatric Medicine, and clinical precepting for University of Toledo and Ohio Northern University. Dr Long has authored journal articles and has presented locally and nationally on infectious disease topics and drug therapy.

Dr Long is an active member of the Ohio College of Clinical Pharmacy, the American College of Clinical Pharmacy, and the American Society of Health-Systems Pharmacists.

EDITORIAL ADVISORY PANEL

EDITORIAL ADVISORY PANEL *(Continued)*

Morton P. Goldman, PharmD
Assistant Director, Pharmacotherapy Services
The Cleveland Clinic Foundation
Cleveland, Ohio

Julie A. Golembiewski, PharmD
Clinical Associate Professor
Colleges of Pharmacy and Medicine
Pharmacotherapist, Anesthesia/Pain
University of Illinois
Chicago, Illinois

Jeffrey P. Gonzales, PharmD
Critical Care Pharmacy Specialist
The Cleveland Clinic Foundation
Cleveland, Ohio

Barbara L. Gracious, MD
Assistant Professor of Psychiatry and Pediatrics
Case Western Reserve University
Director of Child Psychiatry and Training & Education
University Hospitals of Cleveland
Cleveland, Ohio

Larry D. Gray, PhD, ABMM
TriHealth Clinical Microbiology Laboratory
Bethesda and Good Samaritan Hospitals
Cincinnati, Ohio

James L. Gutmann, DDS
Professor and Director of Graduate Endodontics
The Texas A & M University System
Baylor College of Dentistry
Dallas, Texas

Tracey Hagemann, PharmD
Associate Professor
College of Pharmacy
The University of Oklahoma
Oklahoma City, Oklahoma

Charles E. Hawley, DDS, PhD
Professor Emeritus
Department of Periodontics
University of Maryland
Consultant on Periodontics
Commission on Dental Accreditation of the American Dental Association

Martin D. Higbee, PharmD, CGP
Associate Professor
Department of Pharmacy Practice and Science
The University of Arizona
Tucson, Arizona

Jane Hurlburt Hodding, PharmD
Director, Pharmacy
Miller Children's Hospital
Long Beach, California

Rebecca T. Horvat, PhD
Assistant Professor of Pathology and Laboratory Medicine
University of Kansas Medical Center
Kansas City, Kansas

EDITORIAL ADVISORY PANEL *(Continued)*

Jerrold B. Leikin, MD, FACP, FACEP, FACMT, FAACT
Director, Medical Toxicology
Evanston Northwestern Healthcare-OMEGA
Glenbrook Hospital
Glenview, Illinois
Associate Director
Toxikon Consortium at Cook County Hospital
Chicago, Illinois
Professor of Medicine
Pharmacology and Health Systems Management
Rush Medical College
Chicago, Ilinois
Professor of Medicine
Feinberg School of Medicine
Northwestern University
Chicago, Ilinois

Jeffrey D. Lewis, PharmD
Pharmacotherapy Specialist
Lexi-Comp, Inc
Hudson, Ohio

Jennifer K. Long, PharmD BCPS
Infectious Diseases Clinical Specialist
The Cleveland Clinic Foundation
Cleveland, Ohio

Laurie S. Mauro, BS, PharmD
Associate Professor of Clinical Pharmacy
Department of Pharmacy Practice
College of Pharmacy
The University of Toledo
Toledo, Ohio

Vincent F. Mauro, BS, PharmD, FCCP
Professor of Clinical Pharmacy
College of Pharmacy
The University of Toledo
Adjunct Professor of Medicine
College of Medicine
Medical University of Ohio at Toledo
Toledo, Ohio

Timothy F. Meiller, DDS, PhD
Professor
Diagnostic Sciences and Pathology
Baltimore College of Dental Surgery
Professor of Oncology
Greenebaum Cancer Center
University of Maryland Baltimore
Baltimore, Maryland

Franklin A. Michota, Jr, MD
Head, Section of Hospital and Preoperative Medicine
Department of General Internal Medicine
The Cleveland Clinic Foundation
Cleveland, Ohio

Michael A. Militello, PharmD, BCPS
Clinical Cardiology Specialist
Department of Pharmacy
The Cleveland Clinic Foundation
Cleveland, Ohio

EDITORIAL ADVISORY PANEL *(Continued)*

Francis G. Serio, DMD, MS
Professor & Chairman
Department of Periodontics
University of Mississippi
Jackson, Mississippi

Dominic A. Solimando, Jr, MA
Oncology Pharmacist
President, Oncology Pharmacy Services, Inc
Arlington, VA

Joni Lombardi Stahura, BS, PharmD, RPh
Pharmacotherapy Specialist
Lexi-Comp, Inc
Hudson, Ohio

Carol K. Taketomo, PharmD
Pharmacy Manager
Children's Hospital Los Angeles
Los Angeles, California

Mary Temple, PharmD
Pediatric Clinical Research Specialist
Hillcrest Hospital
Mayfield Heights, Ohio

Liz Tomsik, PharmD, BCPS
Pharmacotherapy Specialist
Lexi-Comp, Inc
Hudson, Ohio

Beatrice B. Turkoski, RN, PhD
Associate Professor, Graduate Faculty,
Advanced Pharmacology
College of Nursing
Kent State University
Kent, Ohio

Dave Weinstein, PhD
Pharmacotherapy Specialist
Lexi-Comp, Inc.
Hudson, Ohio

Anne Marie Whelan, PharmD
College of Pharmacy
Dalhouise University
Halifax, Nova Scotia

Richard L. Wynn, PhD
Professor of Pharmacology
Baltimore College of Dental Surgery
Dental School
University of Maryland Baltimore
Baltimore, Maryland

PREFACE

"All disease is infectious disease." Although that may not be completely accurate, infectious disease crosses every discipline of medicine and surgery. With few exceptions, all physicians will diagnose and/or treat infectious diseases in their day-to-day practices. Infectious diseases are becoming more complicated to diagnose and treat. We are making many of our patients more immunocompromised and are performing more invasive procedures. There are more sophisticated diagnostic tests including serologies, probes, and polymerase chain reaction (PCR). The infecting organisms are becoming smarter - more resistant to routine therapies; and the number of antimicrobial agents available to us is staggering. Billions of dollars are spent each year on antimicrobial agents in the United States with billions more spent on office visits, hospitalization, and diagnostic procedures related to infection.

It is safe to say that infectious disease as a discipline is not easy, nor can it be made easy. This handbook is not, therefore, intended as a simplification of infectious disease. Instead, we wish to make the most pertinent aspects of infectious disease readily available to all practitioners as an aid in their infectious disease endeavors. The disease syndromes provide concise, straightforward information on the clinical presentation, differential diagnosis, and drug therapy recommended for treatment of the more common diseases. The organisms provide descriptions of the microbiology, epidemiology, diagnosis, and treatment of each organism. The diagnostic tests/procedures chapter provides information on the more commonly ordered and more useful diagnostic tests used in the laboratory diagnosis of the disease syndromes and in the detection of specific etiological agents. In addition, the section includes concise information on specimen collection and the appropriate use, limitations, and interpretations of the test/procedures. The antimicrobial therapy chapter provides what we believe are the most important facts and considerations regarding each drug product. In addition, the appendix offers a compilation of tables and guidelines which can be helpful in consideration of patient care. Finally, an alphabetical index offers convenient cross-referencing by page number to each item found in every section of the book.

A unique feature of this handbook is that entries in each of the three sections of the book (disease syndromes / organisms, diagnostic tests / procedures, and antimicrobial therapy) contain relative information and cross-referencing to one or more of the other two sections.

The authors envision this handbook to be a useful tool for physicians, residents, students, dentists, nurses, pharmacists, and anyone who has the opportunity to diagnose, treat, or care for patients with infectious diseases.

Accuracy, completeness, and timeliness of each fact or recommendation presented were major goals of the authors of this handbook. The authors hope these goals have been met. Users of the handbook, however, are strongly encouraged to offer suggestions for improvement, additional entries, and corrections to current entries. Such suggestions will be sincerely welcome and considered for future editions.

ACKNOWLEDGMENTS

The *Infectious Diseases Handbook* exists in its present form as the result of the concerted efforts of the following individuals: Robert D. Kerscher, publisher and president of Lexi-Comp Inc; Stacy S. Robinson, editorial manager; Mark F. Bonfiglio, BS, PharmD, RPh, director of pharmacotherapy resources; Barbara Kerscher, production manager; David C. Marcus, director of information systems; Darik Warnke, product manager; Tracey J. Henterly, graphic designer; Alexandra Hart, composition specialist; and Julian I. Graubart, American Pharmaceutical Association (APhA), Director of Books and Electronic Products.

Special acknowledgment to all Lexi-Comp staff for their contributions to this handbook.

Much of the material contained in this book was a result of pharmacy contributors throughout the United States and Canada. Lexi-Comp has assisted many medical institutions to develop hospital-specific formulary manuals that contain clinical drug information as well as dosing. Working with clinical pharmacists, hospital pharmacy and therapeutics committees, and hospital drug information centers, Lexi-Comp has developed an evolutionary drug database that reflects the practice of pharmacy in these major institutions.

In addition, the authors wish to thank their families, friends, and colleagues who supported them in their efforts to complete this handbook.

DESCRIPTION OF SECTIONS AND FIELDS USED IN THIS HANDBOOK

The *Infectious Diseases Handbook* is organized into three major chapters, an appendix, a Classification of Organisms Index, an alphabetical index, and an international brand names index. Information is presented in a consistent format with extensive cross-referencing between chapters. Each chapter will provide the following.

DISEASE SYNDROMES & ORGANISMS CHAPTER

DISEASE SYNDROMES

Disease Syndrome Name	Common nomenclature for the disease
Related Information	Cross-references to other pertinent information found in the Appendix and other parts of the book
Synonyms	Other names or abbreviations for the disease state
Clinical Presentation	Signs, symptoms, and findings from physical and laboratory examination
Differential Diagnosis	A wide differential diagnosis of the disease
Likely Pathogens	Possible organisms causing the disease syndrome. Organisms listed in order of probability. Cross-references provided to the organism monographs.
Diagnostic Tests/ Procedures	Appropriate tests for diagnosis. Bulleted tests are more diagnostic. Cross-references to diagnostic tests/procedures chapter.
Drug Therapy Comment	Comment about treatment
Empiric Drug Therapy	Appropriate recommended and alternative empiric therapy in the opinion of the authors. Definitive therapy should be used when microbiologic diagnosis is made. Cross-reference to antimicrobial therapy chapter.
Selected Readings	General references are provided

ORGANISMS

Organism Name	Genus and species name
Related Information	Cross-references to other pertinent information found in the Appendix and other parts of the book
Synonyms	Other names or abbreviations for the organism
Refer To	For organism class monographs. Provides a listing and cross-reference for individual organisms belonging to the classification group.
Applies To	Other organisms included in the named genus
Microbiology	A description of the organism by morphology, stain, biochemistry, serological differences, etc.
Epidemiology	May include the natural habitat and mode of transmission of the organism. May also include information on outbreaks and transmission prevention.
Clinical Syndromes	Specific disease states that can be caused by the organism
Diagnosis	Methods for determining that the organism is causing disease
Diagnostic Tests/ Procedures	Appropriate tests for diagnosis. Cross-references to diagnostic tests/procedures chapter.
Duration of Therapy	Length of treatment
Treatment	Description of treatment including nondrug therapies
Drug Therapy Comment	Comment about treatment
Drug Therapy	Recommended and alternative drug therapy in the opinion of the authors. When necessary, the drug therapy is further specified into **Pediatric** and **Adult** drug therapy. Cross-reference to antimicrobial therapy chapter.
Selected Readings	General references are provided

DIAGNOSTIC TESTS/PROCEDURES CHAPTER

Name	Common name for the test
Related Information	Cross-references to other pertinent information found in the Appendix and other parts of the book
Synonyms	Other names or abbreviations for the laboratory test/procedure
Refer To	Provides cross-references to more specific versions of the test/procedure
Applies To	Refers to various sample sites or specimen types that follow the same procedure
Test Includes	All laboratory tests or procedures that may occur when the named test is performed
Abstract	A brief description of the test and its use
Patient Preparation	Any special preparation that the patient must undergo prior to the procedure.
Aftercare	Special instructions or warnings for medical personnel for the care of the patient after the procedure is performed
Special Instructions	Specific instructions for the acquisition and handling of specimens
Complications	Problems that may arise for the patient due to testing
Equipment	All equipment needed to perform the procedure
Technique	Explanation of how the procedure is performed
Data Acquired	Data obtained from the procedure
Specimen	All possible specimens that can be used for testing
Container	Type of container that specimen must be collected in to acquire and maintain a usable specimen
Sampling Time	The time-frame a specimen should be collected
Collection	General and specific collection instructions that should be followed to obtain a proper and usable specimen
Storage Instructions	The appropriate storage of the specimen after collection but prior to testing
Causes for Rejection	Possible reasons a specimen may be rejected by the laboratory
Turnaround Time	Time it takes for test to be performed and results to be reported
Reference Range or Normal Findings	Serves as a general guideline. See specific testing facility for their ranges
Critical Values	Values that alert the medical staff that the patient has reached a value that may be hazardous to the patient
Possible Panic Range	Values that alert the medical staff to a potentially life-threatening situation
Use	Common uses for the test/procedure
Limitations	Limits of the test/procedure
Contraindications	Reasons why this test should not be performed
Methodology	Testing methodologies available
Additional Information	Additional information about the test/procedure and its uses
Selected Readings	General references are provided

DESCRIPTION OF SECTIONS AND FIELDS USED IN THIS HANDBOOK *(Continued)*

ANTIMICROBIAL THERAPY CHAPTER

Generic Name	U.S. adopted name
Pronunciation	Phonetic pronunciation guide
Related Information	Cross-references to other pertinent information found in the Appendix and other parts of the book
U.S. Brand Names	Trade names (manufacturer-specific) found in the United States
Canadian Brand Names	Trade names found in Canada
Synonyms	Other names or accepted abbreviations for the generic drug
Generic Available	Drugs available in generic form
Use	Information pertaining to appropriate FDA-approved indications of the drug
Unlabeled / Investigational Use	Information pertaining to non-FDA approved indications of the drug
Refer To	For drug class monographs. Provides a listing and cross-reference for drugs belonging to the class.
Drug of Choice or Alternate For	Cross-references to disease syndromes and organisms chapter for which this drug is indicated
Restrictions	The controlled substance classification from the Drug Enforcement Agency (DEA). U.S. schedules are I-V. Schedules vary by country and sometimes state (ie, Massachusetts uses I-VI).
Pregnancy Risk Factor	Five categories established by the FDA to indicate the potential of a systemically absorbed drug for causing birth defects
Pregnancy Implications	Information pertinent to or associated with the use of the drug as it relates to clinical effects on the fetus
Contraindications	Information pertaining to inappropriate use of the drug
Warnings/Precautions	Hazardous conditions related to use of the drug and disease states or patient populations in which the drug should be cautiously used
Adverse Reactions	Side effects are grouped by percentage of incidence
Overdosage/Toxicology	Comments and/or considerations offered when appropriate
Drug Interactions	
Cytochrome P450 Effect	If a drug has demonstrated involvement with cytochrome P450 enzymes, the initial line(s) of this field will identify the drug as an inhibitor, inducer, or substrate of specific isoenzymes (ie, CYP1A2); a bolded entry identifies that enzyme involvement as clinically significant
Increased Effect/Toxicity	Drug combinations that result in an increased or toxic therapeutic effect between the drug listed in the monograph and other drugs or drug classes.
Decreased Effect	Drug combinations that result in a decreased therapeutic effect between the drug listed in the monograph and other drugs or drug classes.
Ethanol/Nutrition/Herb Interactions	Information regarding potential interactions with food, nutritionals, herbal products, vitamins, or ethanol.
Stability	Information regarding storage and steps for reconstitution.
Mechanism of Action	How the drug works in the body to elicit a response
Pharmacodynamics/ Kinetics	Pharmacokinetics are expressed in terms of absorption, distribution (including appearance in breast milk and crossing of the placenta), metabolism, bioavailability, half-life, time to peak serum concentration, and elimination. Additional pharmacokinetic data can be found in the appendix.
Dosage	The amount of the drug to be typically given or taken during therapy
Dietary Considerations	Information is offered, when appropriate, regarding food, nutrition, and/or alcohol

Administration	Information regarding the recommended final concentrations, rates of administration for parenteral drugs, or other guidelines when giving the medication
Monitoring Parameters	Laboratory tests and patient physical parameters that should be monitored for safety and efficacy of drug therapy are listed when appropriate
Reference Range	Therapeutic and toxic serum concentrations listed when appropriate
Test Interactions	Listing of assay interferences when relevant; (B) = Blood; (S) = Serum; (U) = Urine
Patient Information	Comments and/or considerations are offered when appropriate
Additional Information	Information about sodium content and/or pertinent information about specific brands
Dosage Forms	Information with regard to form, strength, and availability of the drug
Extemporaneous Preparations	Directions for preparing liquid formulations from solid drug products. May include stability information and references.
Selected Readings	General references are provided

Appendix

The appendix offers a compilation of tables, guidelines, nomograms, and conversion information which can often be helpful when considering patient care.

Classification of Organisms Index

All organisms found in the handbook are listed according to their major classification.

Alphabetical Index

All disease syndromes, organisms, diagnostic tests/procedures, and antimicrobial therapy names, along with the brand names and synonyms are listed alphabetically with the page number on which the monograph may be found.

International Brand Names Index

Brand names listed for 76 countries.

FDA PREGNANCY CATEGORIES

Throughout this book there is a field labeled Pregnancy Risk Factor (PRF) and the letter A, B, C, D or X immediately following which signifies a category. The FDA has established these five categories to indicate the potential of a systemically absorbed drug for causing birth defects. The key differentiation among the categories rests upon the reliability of documentation and the risk:benefit ratio. Pregnancy Category X is particularly notable in that if any data exists that may implicate a drug as a teratogen and the risk:benefit ratio is clearly negative, the drug is contraindicated during pregnancy.

These categories are summarized as follows:

- A — Controlled studies in pregnant women fail to demonstrate a risk to the fetus in the first trimester with no evidence of risk in later trimesters. The possibility of fetal harm appears remote.
- B — Either animal-reproduction studies have not demonstrated a fetal risk but there are no controlled studies in pregnant women, or animal-reproduction studies have shown an adverse effect (other than a decrease in fertility) that was not confirmed in controlled studies in women in the first trimester and there is no evidence of a risk in later trimesters.
- C — Either studies in animals have revealed adverse effects on the fetus (teratogenic or embryocidal effects or other) and there are no controlled studies in women, or studies in women and animals are not available. Drugs should be given only if the potential benefits justify the potential risk to the fetus.
- D — There is positive evidence of human fetal risk, but the benefits from use in pregnant women may be acceptable despite the risk (eg, if the drug is needed in a life-threatening situation or for a serious disease for which safer drugs cannot be used or are ineffective).
- X — Studies in animals or human beings have demonstrated fetal abnormalities or there is evidence of fetal risk based on human experience, or both, and the risk of the use of the drug in pregnant women clearly outweighs any possible benefit. The drug is contraindicated in women who are or may become pregnant.

SAFE WRITING

Health professionals and their support personnel frequently produce handwritten copies of information they see in print; therefore, such information is subjected to even greater possibilities for error or misinterpretation on the part of others. Thus, particular care must be given to how drug names and strengths are expressed when creating written health-care documents.

The following are a few examples of safe writing rules suggested by the Institute for Safe Medication Practices, Inc.*

1. There should be a space between a number and its units as it is easier to read. There should be no periods after the abbreviations mg or mL.

Correct	Incorrect
10 mg	10mg
100 mg	100mg

2. Never place a decimal and a zero after a whole number (2 mg is correct and 2.0 mg is **incorrect**). If the decimal point is not seen because it falls on a line or because individuals are working from copies where the decimal point is not seen, this causes a tenfold overdose.
3. Just the opposite is true for numbers less than one. Always place a zero before a naked decimal (0.5 mL is correct, .5 mL is **incorrect**).
4. Never abbreviate the word unit. The handwritten U or u, looks like a 0 (zero), and may cause a tenfold overdose error to be made.
5. IU is not a safe abbreviation for international units. The handwritten IU looks like IV. Write out international units or use int. units.
6. Q.D. is not a safe abbreviation for once daily, as when the Q is followed by a sloppy dot, it looks like QID which means four times daily.
7. O.D. is not a safe abbreviation for once daily, as it is properly interpreted as meaning "right eye" and has caused liquid medications such as saturated solution of potassium iodide and Lugol's solution to be administered incorrectly. There is no safe abbreviation for once daily. It must be written out in full.
8. Do not use chemical names such as 6-mercaptopurine or 6-thioguanine, as sixfold overdoses have been given when these were not recognized as chemical names. The proper names of these drugs are mercaptopurine or thioguanine.
9. Do not abbreviate drug names (5FC, 6MP, 5-ASA, MTX, HCTZ, CPZ, PBZ, etc) as they are misinterpreted and cause error.
10. Do not use the apothecary system or symbols.
11. Do not abbreviate microgram as µg; instead use mcg as there is less likelihood of misinterpretation.
12. When writing an outpatient prescription, write a complete prescription. A complete prescription can prevent the prescriber, the pharmacist, and/or the patient from making a mistake and can eliminate the need for further clarification. The legible prescriptions should contain:
    a. patient's full name
    b. for pediatric or geriatric patients: their age (or weight where applicable)
    c. drug name, dosage form and strength; if a drug is new or rarely prescribed, print this information
    d. number or amount to be dispensed
    e. complete instructions for the patient, including the purpose of the medication
    f. when there are recognized contraindications for a prescribed drug, indicate to the pharmacist that you are aware of this fact (ie, when prescribing a potassium salt for a patient receiving an ACE inhibitor, write "K serum level being monitored")

*From "Safe Writing" by Davis NM, PharmD and Cohen MR, MS, Lecturers and Consultants for Safe Medication Practices, 1143 Wright Drive, Huntington Valley, PA 19006. Phone: (215) 947-7566.

FDA NAME DIFFERENTIATION PROJECT: THE USE OF TALL-MAN LETTERS

Confusion between similar drug names is an important cause of medication errors. For years, The Institute For Safe Medication Practices (ISMP), has urged generic manufacturers to use a combination of large and small letters as well as bolding (ie, chlorpro**MAZINE** and chlorpro**PAMIDE**) to help distinguish drugs with look-alike names, especially when they share similar strengths. Recently the FDA's Division of Generic Drugs began to issue recommendation letters to manufacturers suggesting this novel way to label their products to help reduce this drug name confusion. Although this project has had marginal success, the method has successfully eliminated problems with products such as diphenhydr**AMINE** and dimenhy**DRINATE**. Hospitals should also follow suit by making similar changes in their own labels, preprinted order forms, computer screens and printouts, and drug storage location labels.

Lexi-Comp Medical Publishing will begin using these "Tall-Man" letters for the drugs suggested by the FDA.

The following is a list of product names and recommended FDA revisions.

Drug Product	Recommended Revision
acetazolamide	aceta**ZOLAMIDE**
acetohexamide	aceto**HEXAMIDE**
bupropion	bu**PROP**ion
buspirone	bus**PIR**one
chlorpromazine	chlorpro**MAZINE**
chlorpropamide	chlorpro**PAMIDE**
clomiphene	clomi**PHENE**
clomipramine	clomi**PRAMINE**
cycloserine	cyclo**SERINE**
cyclosporine	cyclo**SPORINE**
daunorubicin	**DAUNO**rubicin
dimenhydrinate	dimenhy**DRINATE**
diphenhydramine	diphenhydr**AMINE**
dobutamine	**DOBUT**amine
dopamine	**DOP**amine
doxorubicin	**DOXO**rubicin
glipizide	glipi**ZIDE**
glyburide	gly**BURIDE**
hydralazine	hydr**ALAZINE**
hydroxyzine	hydr**OXY**zine
medroxyprogesterone	medroxy**PROGESTER**one
methylprednisolone	methyl**PREDNIS**olone
methyltestosterone	methyl**TESTOSTER**one
nicardipine	ni**CAR**dipine
nifedipine	**NIFE**dipine
prednisolone	predniso**LONE**
prednisone	predni**SONE**
sulfadiazine	sulfa**DIAZINE**
sulfisoxazole	sulfi**SOXAZOLE**
tolazamide	**TOLAZ**amide
tolbutamide	**TOLBUT**amide
vinblastine	vin**BLAS**tine
vincristine	vin**CRIS**tine

Institute for Safe Medication Practices. "New Tall-Man Lettering Will Reduce Mix-Ups Due to Generic Drug Name Confusion," *ISMP Medication Safety Alert*, September 19, 2001. Available at: http://www.ismp.org.

Institute for Safe Medication Practices. "Prescription Mapping, Can Improve Efficiency While Minimizing Errors With Look-Alike Products," *ISMP Medication Safety Alert*, October 6, 1999. Available at: http://www.ismp.org.

U.S. Pharmacopeia, "USP Quality Review: Use Caution-Avoid Confusion," March 2001, No. 76. Available at: http://www.usp.org.

DISEASE SYNDROMES/ORGANISMS

ABPA *see* *Aspergillus* Species *on page 38*

Abscess, Brain *see* Brain Abscess *on page 58*

Abscess, Liver *see* Liver Abscess *on page 211*

Abscess, Lung *see* Lung Abscess *on page 212*

Abscess, Pancreatic *see* Pancreatitis/Pancreatic Abscess *on page 253*

Acanthamoeba Species

Microbiology *Acanthamoeba* is a unicellular, free-living, nonparasitic ameba. There are four genera of ameba which have been identified as pathogenic for humans: *Acanthamoeba*, *Entamoeba*, *Naegleria*, and *Vahlkampfia*. *Acanthamoeba* is a small organism, about 10-40 µm in diameter. The life cycle consists of an active trophozoite and a dormant cystic stage. The trophozoites are about 40 µm in diameter and have a single nucleus and characteristic fine cytoplasmic projections called acanthapodia. The cyst forms are also uninucleate but smaller (12 µm in diameter) and have a distinctive external wall surrounding a stellate endocyst (double wall).

Epidemiology The organism is present in many geographic areas and is associated with water and soil. Data from serologic studies and nasopharyngeal cultures of soldiers suggest that environmental exposure to *Acanthamoeba* appears to be common in the normal population. The organism has also been cultured from the nares of normal individuals being studied for respiratory virus infection. It is thought that *Acanthamoeba* is inhaled in the cyst phase, but it is unclear whether this organism is a part of the normal respiratory flora. Despite this common exposure, disease is uncommon. *Acanthamoeba* keratitis (see Clinical Syndromes) is a condition seen in healthy individuals who are contact lens wearers. Disease occurs following direct corneal inoculation. Risk factors for corneal infection with *Acanthamoeba* include wearing contact lenses while swimming and use of homemade saline for contact lens cleaning and storage. In contrast, *Acanthamoeba*-associated granulomatous encephalitis occurs mainly in persons who are debilitated and immunocompromised, including persons with AIDS, diabetes, transplant recipients, and persons undergoing chemotherapy. *Acanthamoeba* granulomatous encephalitis is not associated with fresh-water exposure, unlike primary amebic encephalitis caused by *Naegleria*. Because of the limited numbers of reported cases, the epidemiology of *Acanthamoeba* in AIDS patients remains to be defined. However, it appears that persons with AIDS may be predisposed to this infection of the central nervous system since in one series, 7 of the reported 60 cases of *Acanthamoeba* encephalitis occurred in persons with AIDS. Most recently, a disseminated form of *Acanthamoeba* has been described in immunocompromised persons which appears distinct from granulomatous encephalitis.

Clinical Syndromes

- **Granulomatous amebic encephalitis:** This is a rare disease (less than 200 reported cases). It can be caused by either *Acanthamoeba* or *Naegleria*. The vast majority of patients are immunocompromised. Pathologically, there are areas of necrotizing granulomatous inflammation in the brain parenchyma, with cerebral edema. Both trophozoites and cysts are seen in areas of inflammation. Multinucleated giant cells may be present. Invasion of blood vessel walls by the trophozoites may be seen. Gross lesions tend to involve the posterior structures such as the brain stem, cerebellum, and midbrain. It is believed that this central nervous system infection is a result of hematogenous dissemination; *Acanthamoeba* organisms have been identified in other tissues outside the CNS including skin and lung. Clinically, patients present with the gradual onset of headaches, mental status changes, and focal neurologic deficits. Other symptoms reported include fever and seizures. Skin lesions have been reported in some cases and have been nodular or ulcerative. Head CT scans may show nonenhancing cortical mass lesions.
- **Disseminated *Acanthamoeba*:** This is a rare, but well-documented, form of *Acanthamoeba* infection. In general, disseminated infection is rapidly fatal although there are now several reports of successful treatment using multiple antibiotic agents. Disseminated disease has been described only in immunosuppressed patients such as these with advanced AIDS and bone marrow and renal transplant recipients. Infection is characterized by multiple nodular skin lesions although a variety of other skin lesions have been reported including plaques, papules, pustules, ulcers, and cellulitis. Organisms have been isolated from a variety of other sites including liver, gastrointestinal tract, and lung. The brain is not involved in many of the reported cases.
- ***Acanthamoeba* keratitis:** This serious infection is an important cause of corneal infection in the United States. It is associated with the use of soft contact lenses in healthy persons. Pathologically, cysts and trophozoite forms are seen in the cornea with an associated inflammatory reaction which may contain giant cells. As the infection progresses, sometimes there is a characteristic ring-shaped infiltrate in the cornea which can be seen by an ophthalmologist. Inflammation of the anterior

chamber (anterior uveitis) is also often present on ophthalmologic examination, and organisms may be present in the aqueous humor. Clinically, patients present with tearing in the eye, progressive pain and photophobia, and decreased visual acuity. The symptoms are nonspecific and often the condition is misdiagnosed as herpes or bacterial conjunctivitis/iritis for many weeks before the diagnosis of amebic keratitis is entertained.

Diagnosis *Acanthamoeba* can be detected in routine cytology preparations (eg, from corneal epithelial scrapings) and in histologic sections of tissue biopsy specimens (eg, skin, liver). Some authors have emphasized the limited sensitivity of routine laboratory methods, and in some cases, multiple tissue biopsies were required to identify the organism. In addition, specialized cytologic techniques have been described to improve the sensitivity. The organisms may also be misidentified on biopsy specimens with necrotic debris, histiocytes, and macrophages; the pathologist should be alerted to the possibility of *Acanthamoeba*. It may be difficult to distinguish *Acanthamoeba* from other pathogenic ameba solely on the basis of morphology, and culture confirmation may be necessary. The organism will not grow on routine culture media. The microbiology laboratory should be consulted prior to biopsy if *Acanthamoeba* culture is desired, since the specimen will require special media preparation (or may need to be sent to a reference laboratory). *Acanthamoeba* has been isolated from fresh tissue planted on non-nutrient agar plates (seeded with *Escherichia coli* broth to encourage the growth of *Acanthamoeba*) and cell culture systems. In general, tissue specimens submitted for *Acanthamoeba* culture should **not** be placed in any fixative (such as formalin) and should **not** be frozen. Some authors have recommended the use of Page's media for transportation of specimens to the laboratory for culture rather than sterile saline to increase the yield.

Acanthamoeba granulomatous encephalitis is difficult to diagnose antemortem, and most cases have been identified only at autopsy. This entity should be considered in immunocompromised persons presenting with a mass lesion of the brain of unknown etiology, particularly if skin lesions are present. Biopsy of concomitant skin lesions may reveal the organism. Lumbar puncture is not useful in diagnosing this infection because *Acanthamoeba* has never been identified in the CSF; the lumbar puncture may be useful in excluding other infectious etiologies. Definitive diagnosis usually requires a brain biopsy with identification of the organism in histologic sections.

Acanthamoeba keratitis: This should be considered in any patient with a persistent keratitis not responding to antibacterial or antiviral topical therapy, especially if associated with contact lens use. Early referral to an ophthalmologist is essential since dendriform epithelial changes may be identified prior to the development of the ring infiltrates in the cornea. Definitive diagnosis requires corneal scrapings and/or biopsies. Tissue material should be submitted for wet mount, cytology and histologic staining (hematoxylin-eosin, Wright-Giemsa stain, periodic acid Schiff, and others), and for specialized culture. Indirect fluorescent antibody examination of fixed slides has also been used successfully. Spray fixation is used if felt to be necessary prior to air-drying of smears to preserve the trophozoites. In many cases, culture of the contact lens solution has yielded the organism. Submit lens, case, and fluid in case to the laboratory.

Diagnostic Tests/Procedures

Brain Biopsy *on page 405*
Histopathology *on page 496*
Ocular Cytology *on page 551*
Acanthamoeba culture (performed by reference laboratories; contact laboratory for advice regarding most appropriate specimen to collect and send)

Treatment There are no established therapies for *Acanthamoeba* encephalitis or disseminated infection. The organism demonstrates *in vivo* resistance to a number of agents including amphotericin B and sulfonamides; pentamidine and related agents show activity against the organism but the clinical efficacy is unclear. In the few cases of successful therapy of disseminated infection reported thus far, multidrug antibiotic therapy has been used, including a regimen of itraconazole, pentamidine, 5-flucytosine (5-FC), and topical chlorhexidine gluconate and ketoconazole cream.

Acanthamoeba keratitis may respond to a combination of surgical debridement of abnormal epithelium and topical antimicrobial agents. The optimal medical and/or surgical regimen remains under study. Some authorities have recommended the combination of topical miconazole nitrate, propamidine isethionate, and Neosporin® ophthalmics. In a recent prospective study, propamidine isethionate 0.1% solution administered concomitantly with neomycin-polymyxin B-gramicidin ophthalmic solution (Neosporin®) resulted in an 83% success rate. Others have reported success with bacitracin and polymyxin B with or without neomycin. Oral antibiotics that have been used successfully include paromomycin, ketoconazole, and itraconazole. Experimental infections with *Acanthamoeba* have responded to sulfadiazine, but the clinical efficacy is still unclear. See references Seal, 2003 and Schuster, 2004 for

(Continued)

Acanthamoeba Species *(Continued)*

comments regarding the potentially beneficial effects of biguanides and other contemporary antiparasitic agents. Many patients may require corneal grafting; the role of keratoplasty is still controversial. Vision may remain significantly limited even with aggressive intervention.

Selected Readings

Centers for Disease Control and Prevention (CDC), "Primary Amebic Meningoencephalitis - Georgia, 2002," *MMWR*, 2003, 52(40):962-4.

Gardner LM, Mathers WD, and Folberg R, "New Technique for the Cytologic Identification of Presumed *Acanthamoeba* From Corneal Epithelial Scrapings," *Am J Ophthalmol*, 1999, 127(2):207-9.

Kumar R and Lloyd D, "Recent Advances in the Treatment of *Acanthamoeba* Keratitis," *Clin Infect Dis*, 2002, 35(4):434-41.

Marciano-Cabral F and Cabral G, "*Acanthamoeba* spp. as Agents of Disease in Humans," *Clin Microbiol Rev*, 2003, 16(2):273-307.

Namdari H, Pascucci SE, and Bottone EJ, "Well Water as a Source for *Acanthamoeba* Keratitis," *Clin Microbiol Newslett*, 2000, 22(7):53-5.

Oliva S, Jantz M, Tiernan R, et al, "Successful Treatment of Widely Disseminated Acanthamoebiasis," *South Med J*, 1999, 92(1):55-7.

Schuster FL and Visvesvara GS, "Free-Living Amoebae as Opportunistic and Non-opportunistic Pathogens of Humans and Animals," *Int J Parasitol*, 2004, 34(9):1001-27.

Schuster FL and Visvesvara GS, "Opportunistic Amoebae: Challenges in Prophylaxis and Treatment," *Drug Resist Updat*, 2004, 7(1):41-51.

Seal D, "Treatment of Acanthamoeba Keratitis," *Expert Rev Anti Infect Ther*, 2003, 1(2):205-8.

Achromobacter xylosoxidans *see Alcaligenes* Species *on page 31*

Acinetobacter Species

Microbiology *Acinetobacter* is an aerobic, gram-negative coccobacillus which is an important cause of nosocomial colonization and disease. Microbiologically, *Acinetobacter* is related to *Neisseria* and *Moraxella* and can sometimes be confused with these organisms on Gram stain. The organism is readily identified biochemically. All members of the genus *Acinetobacter* are lactose nonfermenters (ie, lactose-negative), oxidase-negative, nonmotile, and catalase-positive. The negative oxidase test is a rapid means of distinguishing *Acinetobacter* from many other gram-negative nonfermenters commonly isolated from hospitalized patients. Taxonomic systems for the classification of the genus *Acinetobacter* have undergone a number of changes over the years, in large part due to new molecular typing methods which clarify the relatedness of the various species. DNA sequencing studies have led to a new classification scheme in which several genomic species have been identified and some have been formally named. The main human pathogens are *A. calcoaceticus* and *A. baumannii*.

A. baumannii causes the majority of significant human infection and is the species most associated with nosocomial outbreaks of *Acinetobacter* spp. Other *Acinetobacter* species have sporadically been associated with nosocomial disease including *A. lwoffii*, *A. johnsonii*, and others. Recovery of the less common *Acinetobacter* spp from clinical specimens can be difficult to interpret since many of these species are natural commensals on the skin or can be environmental contaminants, and are not common causes of disease.

Epidemiology *Acinetobacter* is ubiquitous in nature and can be isolated in nearly 100% of soil and water samples tested. The organism is commensal in the human respiratory tract, skin, and urinary tract. It is estimated that up to 25% of healthy adults are colonized with *Acinetobacter* on the skin and >5% in the pharynx. Patients requiring tracheostomies for long-term mechanical ventilation have a much higher rate of respiratory colonization. Within the hospital environment, *Acinetobacter* is frequently found in areas of moisture such as humidifiers, bedside commodes, and ventilator tubing. In some series, it is the most common gram-negative organism carried on the hands of hospital workers.

Despite the prevalence of this organism in the environment, *Acinetobacter* is a relatively uncommon cause of bacteremia. The great majority of significant *Acinetobacter* infections are nosocomial and not community acquired. *Acinetobacter* species have been well described as a sporadic cause of hospital outbreaks, frequently in intensive care unit settings. However, in one of the largest studies reported, 52 episodes of *Acinetobacter* bacteremia were examined over a 6-year period and found to occur at a constant rate with no notable outbreaks or clusters.

Risk factors for hospital-acquired *Acinetobacter* bacteremia include the following.

- Malignancies: Some studies suggest a strong association with leukemia and breast cancer, in particular. Neutropenia itself does not seem to be a significant risk factor.
- Trauma patients: Particularly young men in motor vehicle accidents. The source of bacteremia in these cases is more likely from nosocomial pneumonia than from wound infection.

- Burn patients: The portal of entry for *Acinetobacter* is most likely from extensive soft tissue infection. In burn patients, *Acinetobacter* may be present as part of a polymicrobial bacteremia.
- Presence of an intravenous catheter: In some series, the presence of an indwelling central venous catheter appears to be an important risk factor for bacteremia, but in other series, the association is weak or absent. Some authors have speculated that an intravascular catheter should be regarded more as a marker of severity of illness rather than as a risk factor per se for bacteremia.

Clinical Syndromes *Acinetobacter* is an organism of relatively low virulence and is mainly a nosocomial pathogen. In the debilitated hospital patient, the severity of infection may range from mild to life-threatening. It is important to realize that many isolates of *Acinetobacter* from clinical specimens may represent benign colonization, especially when such isolates are reported from the respiratory tract in intubated patients. For this reason, the true *Acinetobacter* nosocomial infection rate is difficult to know with certainty. Surveillance studies in the United States have estimated that 0.3% to 1.4% of all nosocomial infections are caused by *Acinetobacter* spp.

Common nosocomial infections include the following.

- Pneumonia, usually ventilator-associated and multilobar. Data from the National Nosocomial Infection Study estimates that 4% of all nosocomial pneumonias are caused by *Acinetobacter* spp. Several studies have examined *Acinetobacter* infection rates in the highest risk group for nosocomial pneumonia, namely mechanically-ventilated patients in an intensive care unit. Using specimens obtained by bronchoscopy to minimize upper airway contamination, *Acinetobacter* spp were found to be the cause of ventilator-associated pneumonia in 15% to 20% of episodes. Estimates of crude mortality associated with *Acinetobacter* pneumonia varies between 30% to 75%. Some studies have suggested that the mortality associated with *Acinetobacter* pneumonia is higher than nosocomial pneumonia caused by other gram-negative organisms (55%) with the exception of *Pseudomonas aeruginosa*. Outbreaks of multidrug-resistant *Acinetobacter* pneumonias are becoming increasingly more common.
- Bacteremia, most commonly from a pulmonary focus but also secondary to intravenous catheters. Again, the most common species is *A. baumannii*. Immunocompromised patients are at highest risk. Outbreaks of bacteremia have been described in neonatal intensive care units. Bacteremias also may be polymicrobial, particularly when associated with intravascular catheter infection.
- Meningitis, following neurosurgical procedures or associated with ventricular shunt devices
- Urinary tract infections, including cystitis or pyelonephritis associated with indwelling bladder catheters or renal stones. This is a relatively uncommon *Acinetobacter* spp infection.
- Intra-abdominal sepsis, usually as part of a polymicrobial infection
- Soft tissue infections, particularly with postoperative wound dehiscence or extensive burn injuries

Community-acquired *Acinetobacter* infections are unusual but have been reported in certain situations:

- tracheobronchitis in healthy children
- community-acquired pneumonia in alcoholics

Diagnosis The diagnosis of *Acinetobacter* species infections is made by identification of the organism through Gram stain and culture in a patient with a relevant clinical syndrome. No special media or conditions are necessary to grow these organisms. Special requests to culture for *Acinetobacter* are not necessary.

Diagnostic Tests/Procedures

Aerobic Culture, Appropriate Site *on page 365*
Gram Stain *on page 473*

Treatment Since the mid 1970s, isolates of *Acinetobacter* have steadily become resistant to antibiotics of a variety of classes. Resistance to multiple antibiotics has been demonstrated by a number of mechanisms including the production of high levels of beta-lactamase enzymes, either plasmid-mediated resistance and/or chromosomally-mediated resistance; alterations in penicillin-binding proteins; alterations in cell permeability; and production of aminoglycoside-inactivating enzymes.

Resistance to β-lactam antibiotics in many isolates of *Acinetobacter* is mediated by the production of the TEM-1 and TEM-2 plasmid-mediated β-lactamases, enzymes which are involved in resistance with other gram-negative bacilli. Other mechanisms involved in penicillin resistance include cell permeability changes and alterations of penicillin-binding proteins. *A. baumannii* commonly produces cephalosporinases, which are chromosomally-mediated mutations. Cephalosporinases seem to account for most of the high level cephalosporin resistance. Carbapenemases have also been identified that afford resistance to the carbapenems. Aminoglycosides have been found to be synergistic in combination with extended-spectrum penicillins in many

(Continued)

Acinetobacter Species *(Continued)*

clinical isolates of *Acinetobacter* species. Aminoglycoside resistance of *Acinetobacter* spp has been increasing as well. Quinolone resistance has also been reported in increasing numbers. The mechanism for this resistance is probably mutation in DNA gyrase (as has been reported in other gram-negative bacilli), but this has been more difficult to prove in *Acinetobacter*. Serious infections caused by multiple-drug resistant species are often quite difficult to treat and may require the use of newer, alternative agents. Recently, the role of sulbactam in the treatment of *Acinetobacter* sp. has gained increased attention, since sulbactam has intrinsic activity against many strains of *Acinetobacter*, separate from its role as a β-lactamase inhibitor. The combination of ampicillin-sulbactam may be effective.

Acinetobacter species resistant to cephalosporins and extended-spectrum penicillins may be susceptible to either imipenem and/or ampicillin/sulbactam, but the clinician must carefully review the antibiogram. One author has described a decreasing susceptibility to ampicillin/sulbactam with only 61% of *Acinetobacter* isolates now susceptible *in vitro*. In addition, *Acinetobacter* species are no longer uniformly susceptible to imipenem. Outbreaks of imipenem-resistant *A. baumannii* have recently been described. A new β-lactamase termed ARI-1 has been identified in some imipenem-resistant isolates and has become a great concern; it appears to be plasmid-mediated and easily transferable between strains. In such cases of imipenem-resistant, β-lactam-resistant *Acinetobacter*, there may be no proven alternative therapy.

Because of these aforementioned considerations, the optimal therapy of *Acinetobacter* infection depends on the specific antibiotic-susceptibility pattern of each isolate. Empiric therapy for *Acinetobacter* infection (ie, before susceptibility data is known) is difficult and should be based on known drug-resistance patterns in the hospital.

Drug Therapy

Recommended:

Penicillins, Extended-Spectrum *on page 997*

Alternate:

Cephalosporins, 3rd Generation *on page 730*

Imipenem and Cilastatin *on page 861*

Ampicillin and Sulbactam *on page 660*

Aztreonam *on page 677*

Meropenem *on page 936*

Selected Readings

Bergogne-Berezin E and Towner KJ, "*Acinetobacter* spp. as Nosocomial Pathogens: Microbiological, Clinical, and Epidemiological Features," *Clin Microbiol Rev*, 1996, 9(2):148-65.

Chastre J and Trouillet JL, "Problem Pathogens (*Pseudomonas aeruginosa* and *Acinetobacter*)," *Semin Respir Infect*, 2000, 15(4):287-98.

Chen HP, Chen TL, Lai CH, et al, "Predictors of Mortality in *Acinetobacter baumannii* Bacteremia," *J Microbiol Immunol Infect*, 2005, 38(2):127-36.

Falagas ME, Kasiakou SK, and Michalopoulos A, "Treatment of Multidrug-Resistant *Pseudomonas aeruginosa* and *Acinetobacter baumannii* Pneumonia," *J Cyst Fibros*, 2005, 4(2):149-50.

Garnacho-Montero J, Ortiz-Leyba C, Fernandez-Hinojosa E, et al, "*Acinetobacter baumannii* Ventilator-Associated Pneumonia: Epidemiological and Clinical Findings," *Intensive Care Med*, 2005, 31(5):649-55.

Levin AS, "Multiresistant *Acinetobacter* Infections: A Role for Sulbactam Combinations in Overcoming an Emerging Worldwide Problem," *Clin Microbiol Infect*, 2002, 8(3):144-53.

Michalopoulos A, Kasiakou SK, Rosmarakis ES, et al, "Cure of Multidrug-Resistant *Acinetobacter baumannii* Bacteraemia With Continuous Intravenous Infusion of Colistin," *Scand J Infect Dis*, 2005, 37(2):142-5.

Tilley PA and Roberts FJ, "Bacteremia With *Acinetobacter* Species: Risk Factors and Prognosis in Different Clinical Settings," *Clin Infect Dis*, 1994, 18(6):896-900.

Wood GC, Hanes SD, Croce MA, et al, "Comparison of Ampicillin-Sulbactam and Imipenem-Cilastatin for the Treatment of *Acinetobacter* Ventilator-Associated Pneumonia," *Clin Infect Dis*, 2002, 34(11):1425-30.

Acne Rosacea

Synonyms Rosacea

Clinical Presentation Rosacea is a dermatologic disorder of unknown etiology, which is often referred to as adult acne. The number of individuals affected has been estimated to be 13 million people in the United States. The areas of the face, which are normally affected include the nose, cheeks, chin, and forehead. Eye involvement is also found in as many as 50% of cases. The development peaks between the ages of 40 and 50 and affects men and women equally. Lesions are characterized by erythema and telangiectasis. These lesions are vascular in origin, arising from a terminal artery or dilated capillary. The disease initially presents as episodes of blushing, which progress to permanent erythema on the cheeks and nose, and later

to pustules and papules. Finally, telangiectasis develop which may progress to hyperplasia and deformity of the nose. Exacerbating factors include alcohol, hot liquids, caffeine, spicy foods, or any factor which promotes facial flushing.

Likely Pathogens The relationship to a specific etiologic agent is unclear. *Demodex follicularum* (a mite) has been implicated and *Helicobacter pylori* has also been suspected as a cause.

Helicobacter pylori on page 162

Empiric Drug Therapy

Recommended:

Metronidazole *on page 940*

Alternate:

Doxycycline *on page 787*

Acne Vulgaris

Clinical Presentation Typical onset is early-to-late puberty and is associated with the overproduction of androgens, hyper-responsiveness of the sebaceous glands, and hypersensitivity to *Propionibacterium*, as well as its metabolic products. *Propionibacterium* colonizes an obstructed follicle, hydrolyzing triglycerides to free fatty acids, producing inflammatory responses. Acne develops in areas where sebaceous glands are most numerous, affecting the face, scalp, neck, chest, back, and upper arms and shoulders.

Some patients will be affected into their third decade of life. Males are more commonly affected than females. A higher prevalence has been noted in Caucasians. Females may experience cyclical variation (worsening prior to menses). Cases may be less severe in the summer months. Some cases are associated with androgenic steroid use.

Comedonal acne: Absence of *Propionibacterium*; primarily comedonal

Inflammatory acne: Characterized by increased extent of inflammation and popular and pustular lesions. May advance to deeper inflammatory nodule and cyst formation.

Differential Diagnosis Folliculitis; molluscum contagium

Likely Pathogens

Propionibacterium acnes

Diagnostic Tests/Procedures Serum testosterone levels may be of assistance in individuals who develop acne without a prior history. Rule out rosacea.

Drug Therapy Comment Gentle cleansing once or twice daily with mild soap is recommended. No dietary factor has been demonstrated to affect acne. Keratinolytic agents alone may be beneficial in mild cases. Topical agents may be applied to lesions and surrounding areas of skin. More severe cases may require antibiotic therapy in conjunction with a keratolytic agent. Isotretinoin (Accutane®) is generally reserved for patients with widespread cystic acne which fails to respond to systemic antibiotic therapy. Avoid the use of tetracycline in pregnant females.

Empiric Drug Therapy

Recommended:

Erythromycin *on page 807*

Clindamycin and Benzoyl Peroxide *on page 756*

Note: Above may be combined with oral antibiotic therapy.

Tretinoin (Topical) *on page 1127*

Alternate:

Oral antibiotic therapy:

Doxycycline *on page 787*

Minocycline *on page 947*

Clindamycin *on page 752*

Erythromycin *on page 807*

Sulfamethoxazole and Trimethoprim *on page 1087*

Acquired Immunodeficiency Syndrome *see* Human Immunodeficiency Virus *on page 181*

Actinomyces Species

Microbiology *Actinomyces* species are gram-positive, "higher order" bacteria and are related to *Nocardia* species. The most common *Actinomyces* species to cause disease is *Actinomyces israelii*, accounting for about 75% of all cases. These organisms are normal residents of the oral flora and are of low virulence. In the laboratory, *Actinomyces* species grow optimally under anaerobic conditions; growth may also occur in a microaerophilic environment (and sometimes aerobically). When stained, the organism appears thin, with filamentous branches, and may be difficult to distinguish from *Nocardia* species. Growth is slow even under optimal conditions, and the

(Continued)

Actinomyces Species *(Continued)*

laboratory should be notified if *Actinomyces* is suspected. If a patient receives antibiotics, the organism will only rarely grow in culture because of its susceptibility to a number of agents.

In clinical specimens, *Actinomyces israelii* is often found associated with characteristic **sulfur granules**. These granules are irregularly shaped, mineralized masses consisting of calcium phosphate, inflammatory cells, and masses of *Actinomyces* filaments. Occasionally, sulfur granules may be caused by other organisms but are most commonly associated with *Actinomyces israelii*.

Epidemiology *Actinomyces* species are commensal organisms found in the oral cavity and may be cultured from tooth cavities, gingival creases, dental plaque, tonsils, and related areas; they are harmless saprophytes and do not cause disease when mucous membranes are intact. These organisms also may be part of the normal gastrointestinal flora and can be cultured from the female genital region in the absence of disease. The majority of patients who develop *Actinomyces* infections are immunocompetent. Actinomycosis is not considered an opportunistic infection, although it has been reported occasionally with malignancies and AIDS. Infection usually results from breakdown in the normal mucosal barrier with spread of the organism into deeper sites, such as after dental extractions, trauma, etc.

Clinical Syndromes

- **Cervicofacial actinomycosis:** This is the most common syndrome produced by this organism. Also known as the "lumpy jaw syndrome", patients may present with subacute or acute soft tissue swelling in the head or neck. In chronic cases, progression of localized abscesses may lead to draining sinuses and fistulas. Often a history of a preceding dental procedure can be obtained. In some cases, cervicofacial involvement may be dramatic and rapid, with trismus.
- **Pulmonary actinomycosis:** Patients may develop pulmonary *Actinomyces* infection, usually following an aspiration event or as a complication of head and neck actinomycosis. Clinical symptoms may be mild with only a minor cough and no fever. With serious disease, lung cavitation resembling *M. tuberculosis* may be seen. Other potential chest x-ray or CT scan findings include alveolar pneumonia, upper lobe infiltrates, a lung mass with or without invasion into the chest wall, mediastinal mass, rib destruction, and others. Occasionally, a sinus tract may develop from the lung to the chest wall which is highly suggestive of this organism.
- **Abdominal actinomycosis:** Following abdominal surgery or rupture of an abdominal viscus (eg, perforated duodenal ulcer), patients may develop abdominal actinomycosis. This may be a very difficult diagnosis to establish. The development of sinus tracts is suggestive of this organism.
- **Pelvic actinomycosis:** Actinomycosis has been well-known as a potential complication of intrauterine devices (IUDs). There is a wide spectrum of presentations, including pelvic inflammatory disease. It should be noted that since *Actinomyces* species may be harmless residents of the female genital tract, positive cervical cultures or Pap smears for *Actinomyces* species may or may not represent an infectious disease.
- **Brain abscess:** This may occur as a result of direct extension from a cervicofacial site or hematogenously.
- **Human bite wounds:** Local actinomycosis may occur as a complication of a human bite.
- **Disseminated disease:** On rare occasions, *Actinomyces* can disseminate hematogenously and deposit on skin and other organs.

Diagnosis The clinician should consider *Actinomyces* in any patient presenting with a painful subcutaneous swelling in the head and neck. Draining sinus tracts are highly suggestive of actinomycosis, whether in the head and neck, or the thorax. Recurrent infections are the hallmark of this chronic infection, and patients empirically given oral antibiotics for mandibular or neck swelling may show a partial response followed by relapse.

At times, sulfur granules may be found in purulent fluid from abscesses or sinus tracts when the patient is examined at the bedside. These granules are about 2 mm in size and are hard, yellow to white in color, and round in appearance. They should be sent for histopathologic analysis and culture, since other organisms can produce similar-appearing granules. The absence of sulfur granules in no way excludes actinomycosis. Every effort should be made to isolate the organism in the Microbiology Laboratory. Since *Actinomyces* is fastidious, multiple aspirations or biopsies may be necessary.

As noted above, the finding of a positive culture for *Actinomyces* does not always indicate significant disease since it is part of the normal oral and gastrointestinal flora of many persons.

Treatment Penicillin G remains the drug of choice. For cervicofacial actinomycosis, penicillin G given at 10-20 million units daily I.V. has been effective and well tolerated by most. Surgical debridement may often be necessary in addition to antibiotics and treatment failures with antibiotics alone may occur. After several weeks of parenteral penicillin, oral penicillin at high doses may be substituted, such as penicillin V potassium up to 4 g daily. Some clinicians may use probenecid in combination with oral penicillin. For the penicillin-allergic, several antibiotics may be used including erythromycin, tetracycline, and clindamycin. Quinolones and cephalosporins should be avoided.

Drug Therapy

Recommended:

Penicillin G (Parenteral/Aqueous) *on page 993*

Ampicillin *on page 657*

Alternate:

Doxycycline *on page 787*

Selected Readings

Burden P, "Actinomycosis," *J Infect*, 1989, 19(2):95-9.

Lippes J, "Pelvic Actinomycosis: A Review and Preliminary Look at Prevalence," *Am J Obstet Gynecol*, 1999, 180(2 Pt 1):265-9.

Russo TA, "Agents of Actinomycosis," *Principles and Practice of Infectious Diseases*, 5th ed, Mandell GL, Bennett JE, and Dolin R, eds, Philadelphia, PA: Churchill Livingstone, 2000, 2645-53.

Smego RA Jr and Foglia G, "Actinomycosis," *Clin Infect Dis*, 1998, 26(6):1255-61.

Actinomycosis *see Actinomyces* Species *on page 27*

Acute Cholangitis *see* Cholangitis, Acute *on page 79*

Acute Endocarditis, I.V. Drug Abuse *see* Endocarditis, Acute, I.V. Drug Abuse *on page 123*

Acute Native Valve Infective Endocarditis *see* Endocarditis, Acute Native Valve *on page 124*

Acute Obstructive Cholangitis *see* Cholangitis, Acute *on page 79*

Acute Sinusitis, Community-Acquired *see* Sinusitis, Community-Acquired, Acute *on page 299*

Acute Suppurative Cholangitis *see* Cholangitis, Acute *on page 79*

Acute Suppurative Otitis *see* Otitis Media, Acute *on page 253*

Adenovirus

Microbiology Adenovirus is a double-stranded DNA virus which can cause several infectious syndromes in both adults and children. Exposure to this virus is common, and serologic studies suggest that by 10 years of age most children have experienced either clinical or subclinical infection. The symptoms associated with adenovirus infection are likely due to lysis of infected host cells coupled with a brisk host immune response. Most cases of symptomatic disease are associated with the initial infection in a nonimmune host. However, some evidence suggests that adenovirus can enter a latent (asymptomatic) phase in some individuals and can reactivate later in life, particularly if the host becomes immunosuppressed (organ transplantation, corticosteroids, etc).

Epidemiology With humans providing the only known reservoir for adenoviruses, 5% to 10% of all viral respiratory illnesses in civilians are caused by these viruses. Epidemics are usually restricted to the military with small outbreaks among children. Person-to-person transmission through respiratory and ocular secretions is thought to be the major route of transmission. Adenoviruses associated with infantile gastroenteritis are probably transmitted by the fecal-oral route.

Clinical Syndromes

- **Acute respiratory disease:** This is the most common manifestation of adenovirus infection and is responsible for approximately 10% of infant and childhood ambulatory respiratory infections. In boarding schools or military camps, outbreaks of influenza-like respiratory infections have been well described. Adenovirus has also been implicated as a common cause of atypical pneumonia in adults, characterized by low-grade fever, subacute onset, prominent constitutional symptoms (headache, myalgias, malaise), and an absence of purulent sputum.
- **Asymptomatic infection of the tonsils and adenoids (usually adenovirus types 1,2,5) in infants**
- **Pharyngitis in infants**
- **Infantile diarrhea**
- **Pharyngoconjunctival fever in older children:** Especially in summer camps or schools. This is manifested by the acute onset of conjunctivitis, sore throat, fever, and rhinitis, and tends to be a self-limited illness.
- **Hemorrhagic cystitis in adults:** Usually caused by types 11 and 21
- **Keratoconjunctivitis:** Adenovirus is an important cause of epidemic keratoconjunctivitis. Patients present with inflamed conjunctivae (often bilateral) with preauricular adenopathy.

(Continued)

Adenovirus *(Continued)*

- **Adenovirus and HIV infection:** Persons infected with the human immunodeficiency virus may be carriers of adenovirus. Despite this, there appears to be a very low incidence of recognized adenovirus in persons with AIDS. Case reports have described disseminated adenovirus with hepatic necrosis, adenovirus colitis, and necrotizing adenovirus infection of the renal tubules.
- **Infections in other immunosuppressed patients:** Adenovirus infections occur in 5% to 21% of patients following stem cell transplantation (SCT), with an associated mortality of up to 50%. Fatal adenovirus infections due to disseminated disease have also been described in solid organ transplant recipients, as well as other chronically immunosuppressed patients.
- **Serious infections in healthy persons:** In 2000, the CDC reported two deaths associated with disseminated adenovirus infections in U.S. military recruits.

Diagnosis Laboratory studies can confirm suspected cases of adenovirus infection, but the turnaround time can exceed 1 week. Serologic studies demonstrating a fourfold or greater rise in specific IgG titer to adenovirus strongly supports the diagnosis of recent infection. Direct cultures for the virus are available in many laboratories, but the time for viral isolation is variable and highly dependent on the amount of virus in the clinical specimen. Antigen detection is a rapid means of diagnosis especially from respiratory species. Consideration should be given to doing adenovirus surveillance by PCR in susceptible hosts such as transplant patients with severe lymphopenia.

Diagnostic Tests/Procedures

Adenovirus Antibody Titer *on page 364*

Adenovirus Culture *on page 365*

Virus Detection by DFA *on page 619*

Polymerase Chain Reaction *on page 567*

Treatment No antiviral agents have been proven to be effective in the treatment of adenovirus infections. A small series of cases have reported on limited success of ribavirin in severe cases. Cidofovir is under study for adenovirus keratoconjunctivitis. Supportive care is the treatment of choice.

Selected Readings

Altemeier WA 3rd, "The Importance of Adenoviral Infections in Pediatrics," *Pediatr Ann*, 2001, 30(8):439-40, 452.

Baum SG, "Adenovirus," *Principles and Practice of Infectious Diseases*, 5th ed, Mandell GL, Bennett JE, and Dolin R, eds, Philadelphia, PA: Churchill Livingstone, 2000, 1624-30.

Chakrabarti S, Mautner V, Osman H, et al, "Adenovirus Infections Following Allogeneic Stem Cell Transplantation: Incidence and Outcome in Relation to Graft Manipulation, Immunosuppression, and Immune Recovery," *Blood*, 2002, 100(5):1619-27.

Gavin PJ and Katz BZ, "Intravenous Ribavirin Treatment for Severe Adenovirus Disease in Immunocompromised Children," *Pediatrics*, 2002, 110(1 Pt 1):e9.

Klinger JR, Sanchez MP, Curtin LA, et al, "Multiple Cases of Life-Threatening Adenovirus Pneumonia in a Mental Health Center," *Am J Respir Crit Care Med*, 1998, 157(2):645-9.

Lukashok SA and Horwitz MS, "New Perspectives in Adenoviruses," *Curr Clin Top Infect Dis*, 1998, 18:286-305.

Runde V, Ross S, Trenschel R, et al, "Adenoviral Infection After Allogeneic Stem Cell Transplantation (SCT): Report on 130 Patients From a Single SCT Unit Involved in a Prospective Multi Center Surveillance Study," *Bone Marrow Transplant*, 2001, 28(1):51-7.

Adult Osteomyelitis *see* Osteomyelitis, Healthy Adult *on page 250*

Adult T-Cell Leukemia/Lymphoma (ALT) *see* Human T-Cell Lymphotropic Viruses *on page 192*

Aeromonas Species

Microbiology *Aeromonas* species are gram-negative bacilli which can be recovered from a variety of fresh water sources. They belong to the family Vibrionaceae and several species are important for human disease including *A. caviae* and *A. hydrophila.* The organisms can also be recovered from the stool of some healthy individuals. *Aeromonas* species are lactose-variable (either lactose-positive or lactose-negative) and oxidase-positive, which helps distinguish the organism from other enteric gram-negative bacilli found in the stool. Growth is supported on several routine solid media although special techniques are often necessary to isolate the organism from stool samples. The Microbiology Laboratory should be notified if *Aeromonas* is suspected.

Epidemiology Cases of *Aeromonas* have been reported worldwide. Since *Aeromonas* is found in fresh and brackish waters, human infections have been reported to follow injuries related to contaminated water exposure. *Aeromonas* infections have also been associated with the medical use of leeches since the organism is part of the normal flora of the leech. Cases of diarrhea secondary to *Aeromonas* have been reported from a variety of countries and tends to be sporadic. Daycare outbreaks of *Aeromonas*-associated diarrhea have been well described.

Clinical Syndromes

- **Diarrheal illness**: *Aeromonas* has recently been recognized as a cause of a nonbloody diarrhea. The illness tends to be self resolving but sometimes the patient may be ill with fever and bloody diarrhea. Occasionally, a protracted diarrhea may develop.
- **Soft tissue infection**: *Aeromonas hydrophila* is known to cause a rapidly progressive cellulitis following exposure of wounds or traumatized body areas to fresh water. Deeper infections such as myositis and osteomyelitis have been described. Necrosis with gas formation is a serious complication. Surgical site infections may be infected without a history of water exposure. *Aeromonas* soft tissue infection has recently been reported as a complication of medicinal therapy with leeches.
- **Bloodstream infection**: Mainly seen in patients with leukemia and lymphoma, although other immunosuppressed individuals are at risk. Mortality rates are high.

Diagnosis *Aeromonas* infection should be suspected in persons presenting with a soft tissue infection following exposure to water. *Vibrio* species are also in the differential diagnosis. *Aeromonas* should also be considered in persons with an acute diarrheal illness where other more common pathogens have been excluded. Laboratory confirmation of *Aeromonas* is necessary. Appropriate samples of stool, wound discharge, and/or blood should be submitted for special *Aeromonas* culture.

Diagnostic Tests/Procedures

Blood Culture, Aerobic and Anaerobic *on page 391*
Stool Culture *on page 585*
Wound Culture *on page 620*

Treatment A number of antibiotics are effective. *Aeromonas* is susceptible to third generation cephalosporins, fluoroquinolones, sulfamethoxazole and trimethoprim, gentamicin, and tobramycin. It is less susceptible or resistant to the extended-spectrum penicillins (ticarcillin, ampicillin, piperacillin). Multidrug-resistant isolates have been isolated from clinical specimens and therapy should be based on formal antibiotic susceptibility testing.

Drug Therapy

Recommended:

Cephalosporins, 3rd Generation *on page 730*
Fluoroquinolones *on page 824*
Sulfamethoxazole and Trimethoprim *on page 1087*

Selected Readings

Barillo DJ, McManus AT, Cioffi WG, et al, "*Aeromonas* Bacteraemia in Burn Patients," *Burns*, 1996, 22(1):48-52.

Deutsch SF and Wedzina W, "*Aeromonas sobria*-Associated Left-Sided Segmental Colitis," *Am J Gastroenterol*, 1997, 92(11):2104-6.

Janda JM and Abbott SL, "Evolving Concepts Regarding the Genus *Aeromonas*: An Expanding Panorama of Species, Disease Presentations, and Unanswered Questions," *Clin Infect Dis*, 1998, 27(2):332-44.

Janda JM and Abbott SL, "Unusual Food-Borne Pathogens. *Listeria monocytogenes, Aeromonas, Plesiomonas,* and *Edwardsiella* Species," *Clin Lab Med*, 1999, 19(3):553-82.

Jones BL and Wilcox MH, "*Aeromonas* Infections and Their Treatment," *J Antimicrob Chemother*, 1995, 35(4):453-61.

AIDS Virus *see* Human Immunodeficiency Virus *on page 181*

Alcaligenes Species

Synonyms *Achromobacter xylosoxidans*

Microbiology *Alcaligenes* species are aerobic, gram-negative bacilli which are increasingly important in nosocomial infections. They are considered "nonfermenters", meaning the organisms do not utilize (ferment) glucose. Growth in culture is easily supported on common solid media including blood agar plates; special culture techniques are not necessary. The organism is oxidase-positive. There are several important *Alcaligenes* species: *Alcaligenes xylosoxidans* subspecies *xylosoxidans* (also called *Achromobacter xylosoxidans*), *Alcaligenes xylosoxidans* subspecies *dentrificans*, *Alcaligenes piechaudii*, and *Alcaligenes faecalis*. These organisms may be difficult to treat in some patients because of the organisms' ability to produce several β-lactamase enzymes which inactivate commonly used antibiotics. Some strains produce very high levels of β-lactamase and may be particularly difficult to treat.

Epidemiology Like other nonfermenting gram-negative bacilli, *Alcaligenes* species may be recovered from a variety of environmental sources including water and soil. *A. xylosoxidans* also appear to be part of the normal flora of the gastrointestinal tract and of the ear. In hospitalized patients, the organism can be recovered from some additional sites including the airways of intubated patients and the skin. Contamination of hospital equipment by *Alcaligenes* has been reported, including ventilatory tubing, saline flushes, intravenous fluids, hemodialysis equipment, and others. Risk

(Continued)

Alcaligenes Species *(Continued)*

factors for infection appear to be prolonged hospitalization and perhaps underlying malignancy. Outbreaks of *Alcaligenes* may occur.

Clinical Syndromes

- **Community-acquired infection:** This remains unusual. *Alcaligenes xylosoxidans* can be a cause of recurrent otitis in some individuals. The organism has also been isolated from children with chronic otitis media. Some authors feel that *Alcaligenes* should not be considered a colonizer or contaminant if isolated from ear fluid, particularly in the presence of clinical signs and symptoms of ear infection. In addition, occasional cases of community-acquired prosthetic joint infections have been reported.
- **Nosocomial infection:** Infection with *Alcaligenes* species generally is seen in debilitated patients who have been hospitalized for a prolonged period of time. There is no single distinctive clinical syndrome characteristic of *Alcaligenes*. Some sites of infection include:

  pneumonia, especially in patients requiring mechanical ventilation; empyema may be seen as a complicating feature

  bloodstream infections, often primary infections or catheter-related. In one review of the literature (Duggan et al), 77 cases of bacteremia due to *Achromobacter xylosoxidans* were analyzed. Nosocomial bacteremia occurred in 70%, and in 36% the bacteremia was part of an outbreak or acquired from a discrete point source. The most common underlying illnesses were malignancies (30%) and cardiac disease. Primary bacteremias accounted for 19% of cases, catheter-associated bacteremia 19%, and pneumonia accounted for 16%. The case-fatality rate was 30%. The case-fatality rate of persons with primary or catheter-associated bacteremia was very low (3%), but a much higher mortality rate was found in patients with meningitis, endocarditis, and pneumonia (65%). The case-fatality rate in neonates was extremely high, almost 80%.

  postoperative wound infections, especially after gastrointestinal tract surgery

  postoperative neurosurgical infections, including meningitis.
- ***Alcaligenes* infection in persons with AIDS:** This is an uncommon infection in persons with HIV, although several series of *Alcaligenes* bloodstream infection have been reported. In one series, seven cases of *Alcaligenes xylosoxidans* bacteremia and/or respiratory disease in patients infected with HIV were described. This complication occurred during different phases of HIV infection and was associated with leukopenia in four patients and a central vascular catheter in two. Although the majority of cases were diagnosed after day 3 of hospitalization, a specific source of infection was never identified. In four patients with advanced HIV infection, *Alcaligenes* was present as part of a polymicrobial infection. *In vitro* resistance to several classes of antibiotics was present, but treatment with fluoroquinolones, piperacillin, or an aminoglycoside in combination with either ceftazidime or pefloxacin was successful in all cases.

Diagnosis Since the clinical syndromes caused by *Alcaligenes* are nonspecific and may be caused by other organisms, laboratory diagnosis is important. Routine cultures from appropriate sites are adequate for isolating *Alcaligenes*. It should be emphasized that the recovery of *Alcaligenes* from some body sites does not necessarily mean significant clinical disease. Positive cultures from respiratory secretions in intubated patients may or may not be clinically significant since colonization may occur without disease. Recovery of *Alcaligenes* from sterile body fluids such as cerebrospinal fluid, pleural fluid, and bloodstream nearly always indicates disease.

Diagnostic Tests/Procedures

Aerobic Culture, Appropriate Site *on page 365*
Blood Culture, Aerobic and Anaerobic *on page 391*

Treatment *Alcaligenes* species may become resistant to a variety of antibiotics because of the production of high levels of β-lactamase. Generally, *Alcaligenes* are susceptible to third generation cephalosporins and ureidopenicillins, and imipenem. The organisms are often less susceptible or variably susceptible to quinolones, aminoglycosides, and aztreonam. It is important to obtain antibiotic susceptibility results on clinical isolates of *Alcaligenes* to help direct appropriate therapy, particularly in patients who have been receiving antibiotics.

In the series of 77 patients with *Alcaligenes* bacteremia described above, susceptibility studies showed that all strains were resistant to aminoglycosides, most were resistant to quinolones, and all were susceptible to broad-spectrum penicillins, imipenem, ceftazidime, and trimethoprim-sulfamethoxazole. Time-kill studies showed synergy or additive effects for the combination of gentamicin and piperacillin against most strains.

Drug Therapy

Recommended:

Cephalosporins, 3rd Generation *on page 730*
Piperacillin *on page 1002*
Imipenem and Cilastatin *on page 861*
Meropenem *on page 936*

Alternate:

Fluoroquinolones *on page 824*
Aminoglycosides *on page 641*
Aztreonam *on page 677*

Selected Readings

Decre D, Arlet G, Danglot C, et al, "A Beta-Lactamase Overproducing Strain of *Alcaligenes denitrificans* Subspecies *xylosoxidans* Isolated From a Case of Meningitis," *J Antimicrob Chemother*, 1992, 30(6):769-79.
Duggan JM, Goldstein SJ, Chenoweth CE, et al, "*Achromobacter xylosoxidans* Bacteremia: Report of Four Cases and Review of the Literature," *Clin Infect Dis*, 1996, 23(3):569-76.
Mandell WF, Garvey GJ, and Neu HC, "*Achromobacter xylosoxidans* Bacteremia," *Rev Infect Dis*, 1987, 9(5):1001-5.
Manfredi R, Nanetti, Ferri M, et al, "Bacteremia and Respiratory Involvement by *Alcaligenes xylosoxidans* in Patients Infected With the Human Immunodeficiency Virus," *Eur J Clin Microbiol Infect Dis*, 1997, 16(12):933-8.
McGown J and Steinberg JP, "Other Gram-Negative Bacilli," *Principles and Practice of Infectious Diseases*, 4th ed, Mandell GL, Bennett JE, and Dolin R, eds, New York, NY: Churchill Livingstone, 1995, 2111-2.
Mensah K, Philippon A, Richard C, et al, "Susceptibility of *Alcaligenes denitrificans* Subspecies *xylosoxidans* to Beta-Lactam Antibiotics," *Eur J Clin Microbiol Infect Dis*, 1990, 9(6):405-9.
Wintermeyer SM and Nahata MC, "*Alcaligenes xylosoxidans* Subsp *xylosoxidans* in Children With Chronic Otorrhea," *Otolaryngol Head Neck Surg*, 1996, 114(2):332-4.

Allergic Bronchopulmonary Aspergillosis *see Aspergillus* Species *on page 38*

Amebiasis *see Entamoeba histolytica on page 130*

American Trypanosomiasis *see Trypanosoma cruzi on page 341*

Amnionitis

Synonyms Chorioamnionitis; IAIS; Intra-amniotic Infection Syndrome; Septic Abortion

Clinical Presentation Amnionitis is an infection of the amniotic membrane, which usually occurs following premature rupture of membranes. Amnionitis occurs in 0.5% to 1% of all pregnancies. In the case of premature rupture of membranes at term, amnionitis complicates 3% to 15% of pregnancies. The presence of amnionitis puts the fetus at great risk of sepsis, particularly if colonized by group B *Streptococcus*. Symptoms include maternal fever, maternal and/or fetal heart rate elevation, maternal leukocytosis, foul-smelling or pus-filled vaginal discharge, and uterine tenderness. In septic abortion, *Clostridium perfringens* may cause intravascular hemolysis.

Differential Diagnosis In postpartum patients with pulmonary emboli or fever without an identifiable source, consider septic pelvic vein thrombosis.

Likely Pathogens

Bacteroides and *Prevotella* Species *on page 46*
Streptococcus agalactiae on page 313
Streptococcus pyogenes on page 321
Enterobacter Species *on page 132*
Chlamydia trachomatis on page 74
Clostridium perfringens on page 88

Diagnostic Tests/Procedures

Blood Culture, Aerobic and Anaerobic *on page 391*

Drug Therapy Comment Therapy is typically initiated intrapartum. Early maternal treatment does not mask signs/symptoms of neonatal infection. Following septic abortion, treatment includes D&C of uterus.

Empiric Drug Therapy

Recommended:

Cesarean delivery and septic abortion:

One of the following:

Cefoxitin *on page 712*
Ticarcillin and Clavulanate Potassium *on page 1114*
Ampicillin and Sulbactam *on page 660*
Piperacillin and Tazobactam Sodium *on page 1003*

plus

Doxycycline *on page 787*

Alternate:

Cephalosporins, 3rd Generation *on page 730*

plus

Clindamycin *on page 752*

Anaerobic *Streptococcus* *see Streptococcus*-Related Gram-Positive Cocci *on page 325*

Ancylostoma duodenale

Synonyms Hookworm

Applies to *Necator americanus*

Microbiology *Ancylostoma duodenale* is an intestinal roundworm. Often called "Old World hookworm," this parasite is one of two common hookworms causing human disease. The second hookworm, *Necator americanus* ("New World hookworm"), is structurally related to *Ancylostoma duodenale* and differs mainly in geographic distribution. Hookworms have been estimated to infect nearly 25% of the world's population.

Like all other nematodes (roundworms), *Ancylostoma duodenale* is visible to the naked eye, although the adult tends to be only 1 cm long. The infectious cycle begins when filariform larvae penetrate intact skin of the host. The most common portal of entry is the human foot, usually associated with walking barefoot on contaminated soil. Once through the skin, the larvae are carried via the venous circulation into the right heart and pulmonary circulation. The larvae then migrate through the alveoli of the lungs, in a fashion similar to *Ascaris lumbricoides*. Later, the parasites move into the trachea and pharynx and are then swallowed by the host. Within the small bowel, the adult hookworms attach to the mucosa and can remain there for years. The worms suck blood continuously from the intestinal tissue and can ultimately cause an iron deficiency anemia, with an estimated blood loss of 0.2 mL per day. Thousands of eggs are laid each day by the adult worm and are passed into the feces of the host. When contaminated human feces are mixed into the soil, larvae are released. Under the appropriate environmental conditions, these noninfective larvae become infective (filariform larvae), and the cycle begins again.

Epidemiology Hookworm infection is most common in tropical or subtropical regions and has been reported worldwide. Warm climates favor hookworm infection, since the ova do not tolerate cold soil temperatures. Prevalence is highest in areas where sanitation is poor and human feces are mixed with topsoil. Efforts to control hookworm infection in the United States have been generally successful, although cases still occur in the southeastern states.

Clinical Syndromes

- **Iron deficiency anemia:** Caused by the adult hookworm parasitizing blood in the upper small intestine
- **Pneumonitis:** Occurring during the lung migration phase. This is characterized by wheezing, eosinophilia, and diffuse pulmonary infiltrates, resembling Löffler's syndrome.
- **Ground itch:** An allergic reaction to the hookworm localized to the area of initial skin penetration. The individual may present with erythema, pruritus, and a papular rash in the lower extremity.
- **Abdominal pain, diarrhea, weight loss, and malabsorption:** In developing countries, mental retardation can result from chronic nutritional deficiencies caused by the hookworm.

Diagnosis The clinical suspicion of hookworm infection is confirmed by direct examination of stool specimens for the presence of the characteristic eggs.

Diagnostic Tests/Procedures

Ova and Parasites, Stool *on page 551*

Treatment Mebendazole is the drug of choice with cure rates exceeding 90%. The anemia caused by *Ancylostoma duodenale* usually responds to standard iron supplementation.

Drug Therapy

Recommended:

Mebendazole *on page 928*

Alternate:

Thiabendazole *on page 1111*

Pyrantel Pamoate *on page 1021*

Selected Readings

Grencis RK and Cooper ES, "*Enterobius, Trichuris, Capillaria,* and Hookworm Including *Ancylostoma caninum*," *Gastroenterol Clin North Am*, 1996, 25(3):579-97.

Juckett G, "Common Intestinal Helminths," *Am Fam Physician*, 1995, 52(7):2039-48, 2051-2.

Loukas A and Prociv P, "Immune Responses in Hookworm Infections," *Clin Microbiol Rev*, 2001, 14(4):689-703.

Mahmoud AA, "Intestinal Nematodes (Roundworms)," *Principles and Practice of Infectious Diseases*, 4th ed, Mandell GL, Bennett JE, and Dolin R, eds, New York, NY: Churchill Livingstone, 1995, 2526-31.

Miller TA, "Hookworm Infection in Man," *Adv Parasitol*, 1979, 17:315-84.

Warren KS, "Hookworm Control," *Lancet*, 1988, 2(8616):897-8.

Anthrax *see Bacillus anthracis on page 41*

Antibiotic-Associated Colitis *see Clostridium difficile on page 85*

Appendicitis *see* Intra-abdominal Abscess *on page 194*

Arboviruses

Microbiology The group of viruses commonly known as arboviruses (arthropod-borne viruses) is composed of approximately 500 viruses which have in common the fact that the vectors which transmit these viruses to humans are arthropods (mosquitoes, ticks, and certain blood-sucking flies). Mosquitoes are the most common vectors. Arboviruses are morphologically diverse and can be either enveloped or nonenveloped, and either icosahedral or helical; however, most arboviruses are 40-110 nm and contain RNA. Some of the more commonly discussed and encountered arbovirus infections in the United States are shown in the table.

Arboviruses

Disease	Virus	Vector	Clinical Syndrome	Geographical Location	Mortality (%)
Colorado tick fever[1]	Orbivirus	Tick	F, M, H	West U.S.	<1
Congo-Crimean hemorrhagic fever	Nariovirus	Tick, infected blood	H	Africa, Europe, Asia	10-50
Dengue	Flavivirus	Mosquito	F, H	Tropical, world-wide	5 (H)
Eastern equine encephalitis[1]	Alphavirus	Mosquito	M	East U.S., Central & South America	30
LaCrosse encephalitis[1]	Bunyavirus	Mosquito	M	East U.S.	<1
Powassan encephalitis[1]	Flavivirus	Tick, mosquito	M	U.S., Russia, China, Canada	
Rift Valley fever	Phlebovirus	Mosquito, infected blood	F, M, H	Africa, Middle East	<1
St Louis encephalitis[1]	Flavivirus	Mosquito	M	North, Central, & South America	7
Tick-borne encephalitis	Flavivirus	Tick	F, M, H	Europe, Asia	1-10
Western equine encephalitis[1]	Alphavirus	Mosquito	M	West U.S., South America, Canada, Mexico	5
West Nile encephalitis	West Nile virus	Mosquito	F, M	U.S., Africa, Eastern Europe, Asia	4-99
Yellow fever	Flavivirus	Mosquito	F, H	South America, Africa	15

[1]One of the six significant arbovirus diseases in the United States.

F = febrile illness; M = meningoencephalitis; H = hemorrhagic fever.

Information in this table is adapted from the publications by Tsai TF. See Selected Readings.

Epidemiology Arboviruses are found worldwide but are more common in tropical than in temperate climates. Only about 150 of the ~500 arboviruses cause disease in humans. Generally, arboviruses are transmitted between small mammals and birds. The aforementioned arthropod vectors transmit the arboviruses from these small animals to humans who are dead-end hosts for these viruses.

Clinical Syndromes Most arbovirus infections in humans are mild viral infections which are often indistinguishable from many other viral infections. Acute arbovirus infections are often characterized by sudden onset of headache, fever, muscle and joint pain, and other constitutional symptoms. If disease progresses beyond these symptoms, the disease can be extremely serious and usually manifests as a severe febrile illness (with or without rash, with or without arthritis), meningoencephalitis, or hemorrhagic fever. In more severe cases, more than one of these three conditions can be present (see table).

Diagnosis The basis of a definitive diagnosis of an arbovirus infection is a thorough physical examination and an extremely close examination of the exposure, travel, work, and socioeconomic history of the patient. Enzyme immunoassay, immunofluorescence, and nucleic acid hybridization with or without polymerase chain reaction amplification methods can be used to detect virus antigens in throat and blood specimens and paraffin-embedded tissues. However, these tests are not widely available and are applicable to only a few arboviruses. The test of choice in the laboratory diagnosis of an arbovirus infection is serology. Acute and convalescent sera must be collected if an accurate diagnosis is sought. Immunofluorescence, enzyme immunoassay, hemagglutination inhibition, complement fixation, and antibody neutralization tests are generally available at reference laboratories and the Centers for Disease

(Continued)

Arboviruses *(Continued)*

Control and Prevention. Contact the local laboratory for details on specimen collection, availability of tests, turnaround time, and discussions regarding the most likely virus to cause the disease of a particular infection.

Diagnostic Tests/Procedures

Encephalitis Viral Serology *on page 452*

Treatment Treatment for specific arbovirus infections usually is supportive and directed toward making the patient comfortable and reducing symptoms. Ribavirin may be active against a number of these viruses (Colorado tick fever, LaCrosse, West Nile), but human data is limited. Interferon alpha-2b is active against West Nile *in vitro*, and may decrease symptoms in some patients with St Louis meningoencephalitis.

Drug Therapy Comment There is no specific antiviral agent(s) for arboviruses.

Selected Readings

Calisher CH, "Medically Important Arboviruses of the United States and Canada," *Clin Microbiol Rev*, 1994, 7(1):89-116.

Johnson RT, "Acute Encephalitis," *Clin Infect Dis*, 1996, 23(2):219-24.

Lowry PW, "Arbovirus Encephalitis in the United States and Asia," *J Lab Clin Med*, 1997, 129(4):405-11.

Nelson JA, "Tick-Borne Illnesses: United States," *Clin Microbiol Newslett*, 1992, 14(14):105-8.

Petersen LR and Marfin AA, "West Nile Virus: A Primer for the Clinician," *Ann Intern Med*, 2002, 137(3):173-9.

Tsai TF and Chandler LJ, "Arboviruses," *Manual of Clinical Microbiology*, 8th ed, Murray PR, Baron EJ, Jorgensen JH, et al, eds, Washington DC: American Society for Microbiology, 2003, 1553-69.

Tsai TF and Kuno G, "Arboviruses," *Manual of Clinical Immunology*, 5th ed, Rose NR, de Macario, Folds JD, et al, eds, Washington DC: American Society for Microbiology, 1997, 729-36.

Weaver SC and Barrett AD, "Transmission Cycles, Host Range, Evolution and Emergence of Arboviral Disease," *Nat Rev Microbiol*, 2004, 2(10):789-801.

Whitley RJ and Gnann JW, "Viral Encephalitis: Familiar Infections and Emerging Pathogens," *Lancet*, 2002, 359(9305):507-13.

Vernet G, "Diagnosis of Zoonotic Viral Encephalitis," *Arch Virol Suppl*, 2004, 18:231-44.

Arthritis, Septic

Synonyms Septic Arthritis

Clinical Presentation The onset of septic arthritis is usually abrupt. Symptoms include chills, fever, and a monarthritis with warmth, swelling, erythema, and tenderness. Ten percent of afflicted individuals present with polyarthritis. It most commonly affects large joints, especially knees, ankles, and wrists. Presentation may be more indolent in patients with rheumatoid arthritis. Gonococcus is the most common cause of septic arthritis in adults.

Differential Diagnosis Crystal induced; palindromic rheumatism; other infections (ie, tubercular, fungal, viral); tendonitis, bursitis, juvenile rheumatoid arthritis

Likely Pathogens

Neisseria gonorrhoeae on page 244

Staphylococcus aureus, Methicillin-Susceptible *on page 307*

Diagnostic Tests/Procedures

•Aerobic Culture, Body Fluid *on page 365*

•Arthrocentesis *on page 384*

•Biopsy Culture, Routine *on page 390*

•Gram Stain *on page 473*

Lyme Disease Serology *on page 527*

Mycobacteria Culture, Biopsy or Body Fluid *on page 539*

Neisseria gonorrhoeae Culture *on page 547*

Drug Therapy Comment Community-acquired MRSA infections have been reported among athletes, children, military recruits, Pacific Islanders, Alaskan natives, and prisoners. Isolates many be susceptible to sulfamethoxazole and trimethoprim, doxycycline, and/or clindamycin. Sulfamethoxazole and trimethoprim is the drug of choice in high-risk populations.

Empiric Drug Therapy

Recommended:

Oxacillin *on page 983*

If there is a high suspicion of gonococcal infection from the clinical setting:

Ceftriaxone *on page 722*

Selected Readings

Donatto KC, "Orthopedic Management of Septic Arthritis," *Rheum Dis Clin North Am*, 1998, 24(2):275-86.

Garcia-De La Torre I, "Advances in the Management of Septic Arthritis," *Rheum Dis Clin North Am*, 2003, 29(1):61-75.

Goldenberg DL, "Septic Arthritis," *Lancet*, 1998, 351(9097):197-202.

Perry CR, "Septic Arthritis," *Am J Orthop*, 1999, 28(3):168-78.

Shetty AK and Gedalia A, "Septic Arthritis in Children," *Rheum Dis Clin North Am*, 1998, 24(2):287-304.

Ascaris

Microbiology Over 4 million individuals in the United States are infected with the intestinal parasite *Ascaris lumbricoides*, commonly referred to as "the giant roundworm." Ascariasis is the term used to describe human infection with *A. lumbricoides*. With a worldwide prevalence over 1 billion, ascariasis is the single most common worm infection of humans.

Ascaris lumbricoides is a nematode (roundworm) which passes through several developmental stages: egg (ova), larva, and mature adult. The infectious cycle for the human begins with ingestion of *Ascaris* eggs by the host; these eggs are found most often in contaminated food or soil. In the small intestine, the larvae are released from the egg and penetrate through the intestinal mucosa. After entering the venous circulation. the larvae migrate into the pulmonary vessels. For a period of 10-14 days, the larvae grow within the alveoli of the lungs, the so-called "pulmonary phase." The larvae then pass up the trachea and are coughed up and swallowed by the host. The worms return to the jejunum where they mature into adult forms. During this "intestinal phase" which can last several months, the adult worm attains a length of over 15 cm. Thousands of fertilized eggs are passed into the feces of the host and eventually into the environment, where the cycle begins again.

Epidemiology *Ascaris* infections occur worldwide, although more commonly in tropical climates. In the United States, ascariasis is most prevalent in the southeastern states. Poor sanitation is a predisposing factor to infection. The eggs of *Ascaris lumbricoides* are hardy and can survive cold temperatures and dry environments. In communities where human feces contaminate both the food and water supply, ascariasis is endemic because of its fecal-oral transmission. School-age children are at particularly high risk of parasitism.

Clinical Syndromes The clinical presentation depends to some degree on the worm burden and the specific host organ involved.

- **Asymptomatic infection:** This is the most common manifestation, and usually occurs when only a small number of eggs are ingested.
- **Pneumonitis, caused by migration of large numbers of larvae through the lungs:** The individual presents with bronchospasm, pulmonary infiltrates on the chest radiograph, and peripheral blood eosinophilia. This may be mistaken for an asthmatic attack or Löffler's syndrome.
- **Intestinal obstruction, especially when the worm burden is high:** Appendicitis has also been described when a tangled mass of worms obstructs the lumen of the appendix.
- **Common bile duct obstruction, usually caused by a single adult worm:** Characteristically, the individual has nausea, vomiting, abdominal pain, and sometimes jaundice.
- **Nutritional deficiencies, particularly in children**

Diagnosis The clinical suspicion of ascariasis is confirmed by direct examination of stool specimens. Because of the enormous numbers of eggs which are shed in the feces each day, in most cases there is little difficulty identifying the fertilized and unfertilized eggs. Less commonly, the adult worm may be passed in the stool as well. In rare cases, the diagnosis of ascariasis may be suspected or confirmed by using radiographic contrast studies of the bowel or biliary tract; the outline of the worm may be seen as a filling defect.

Diagnostic Tests/Procedures

Ova and Parasites, Stool *on page 551*

Treatment Mebendazole is considered the drug of choice for intestinal ascariasis. Piperazine citrate is indicated for cases of intestinal or biliary obstruction. **Note**: In cases of dual or multiple infections with *Ascaris* and other intestinal parasites, *Ascaris* must be treated first. Some antiparasitic agents not directed toward *Ascaris* can antagonize *Ascaris* and cause the large worms to react violently to the point of damaging or even penetrating the bowel.

Drug Therapy

Recommended:

Mebendazole *on page 928*

Alternate:

Pyrantel Pamoate *on page 1021*

Selected Readings

Khuroo MS, Zargar SA, Mahajan R, et al, "Sonographic Appearances in Biliary Ascariasis," *Gastroenterology*, 1987, 93(2):267-72.

Mahmoud AA, "Intestinal Nematodes (Roundworms)," *Principles and Practice of Infectious Diseases*, 4th ed, Mandell GL, Bennett JE, and Dolin R, eds, New York, NY: Churchill Livingstone, 1995, 2526-31.

Sarinas PS and Chitkara RK, "Ascariasis and Hookworm," *Semin Respir Infect*, 1997, 12(2):130-7.

Stephenson LS, "The Contribution of *Ascaris lumbricoides* to Malnutrition in Children," *Parasitology*, 1980, 81(1):221-33.

Aspergillosis *see Aspergillus* Species *on page 38*

Aspergillus Species

Microbiology *Aspergillus* is a potentially pathogenic fungus found throughout the environment. Aspergillosis is the term used to describe human infection caused by any one of the 900 reported species of this mold. Infection with *Aspergillus* can range from benign colonization of the respiratory tract to lethal blood vessel invasion and remains a major cause of morbidity and mortality in neutropenic patients.

Aspergillus is a mold and is composed of hyphae which grow by extension and branching. The fungus is recognized in tissue specimens by its septate hyphae and its dichotomous, acute angle branching. A definitive diagnosis of *Aspergillus* is quite difficult from histopathologic sections alone unless characteristic sporulation is seen. Confirmation of *Aspergillus* requires growth of the mold on appropriate culture media, but it is well recognized clinically that fungal cultures may still be negative despite positive tissue sections.

Epidemiology *Aspergillus* is ubiquitous in the environment but is not considered part of the normal flora of humans. Although there is no specific reservoir for this fungus, it tends to grow heavily in hay, dung, soil (including the soil of potted plants), grain, and compost piles; occasionally, a history of a massive inhalational exposure can be obtained from individuals with overwhelming infection. Well-documented studies have shown that *Aspergillus* can be recovered from the air of hospital wards, and outbreaks in susceptible patients have been associated with heavily colonized hospital air-ventilation systems. *Aspergillus* outbreaks have also been reported following hospital renovation projects.

Although *Aspergillus* is universally present in the environment, it causes disease in relatively few individuals. Life-threatening acute infection is nearly always limited to immunocompromised patients. *Aspergillus* infections of a more chronic and indolent nature are often seen in individuals with less debilitating underlying diseases (eg, asthma, chronic bronchitis, sarcoidosis). Acquisition of *Aspergillus* is exclusively via inhalation of airborne spores; person-to-person transmission does not occur.

Clinical Syndromes There are three major manifestations of an *Aspergillus* infection which can overlap in an individual patient.

- **Allergic bronchopulmonary aspergillosis (ABPA):** This is a specific form of hypersensitivity pneumonitis. It is characterized by asthma, eosinophilia, immediate skin reactivity to *Aspergillus* antigen, elevated immunoglobulin E (IgE), and positive *Aspergillus* precipitins in the serum. This is considered an allergic response to *Aspergillus* and is not truly infectious in nature. Treatment is with corticosteroids in selected cases, rather than antifungal therapy.
- ***Aspergillus* colonization:** This is the most common scenario, in which *Aspergillus* exists as a fungus ball in a lung cavity such as an old tuberculosis cavity. This fungus ball is a mass of hyphal elements which elicits little inflammatory response. A patient can be colonized for years without symptoms or tissue damage, except for hemoptysis. However, serious complications can occur such as empyema or bronchopleural fistula.
- **Invasive fungal infection:** This occurs almost exclusively as an opportunistic infection in the severely immunocompromised patient. Prolonged neutropenia is a well recognized risk factor. Rarely, invasive disease has been described in otherwise healthy hosts. Systemic aspergillosis is an often lethal infection with fever, progressive pneumonitis with or without cavitation, and widespread dissemination to almost any organ system. *Aspergillus* characteristically invades blood vessels in the lungs and other tissues.
- **Miscellaneous:** Other manifestations of *Aspergillus* have been described, including cerebral infarction, endocarditis, gastrointestinal ulcerations in immunocompromised hosts, necrotizing skin ulcers, and bone lesions. Meningitis has been described rarely.

Diagnosis *Aspergillus* requires identification of the fungus in biopsy samples and/or appropriate body fluids. It should be noted that the recovery of *Aspergillus* from clinical specimens such as expectorated sputum or bronchial lavage fluid does not necessarily imply clinically significant infection. In some cases, *Aspergillus* may be present as a colonizer without damage to surrounding tissues; this does not warrant specific therapy. Demonstration of tissue invasion on histopathologic specimens is the gold standard for diagnosing invasive aspergillosis. In all cases, a positive culture for *Aspergillus* must be viewed in the context of the individual case.

Diagnostic Tests/Procedures

Cytology, Body Fluids *on page 438*
Fungus Culture, Appropriate Site *on page 461*
KOH Preparation *on page 513*

Treatment Surgical excision of sequestered foci of *Aspergillus* infection may be the treatment of choice for diseases such as brain lesions, sinus involvement, infections on prosthetic material, and some lung lesions, with subsequent drug therapy with

amphotericin B. The mainstay treatment of invasive *Aspergillus* infection has been amphotericin B, administered at doses of 1 mg/kg/day or higher. Itraconazole has been used in some centers for fungal prophylaxis in some heavily immunocompromised patients (neutropenic patients, bone marrow transplant recipients, lung transplant recipients, and others). Recently, the newer azole antifungals, such as voriconazole, have shown promise in the treatment of invasive aspergillosis, as well as fungal prophylaxis in the febrile, neutropenic patient.

Drug Therapy

Recommended:

Amphotericin B (Conventional) *on page 650*

Alternate:

Amphotericin B Cholesteryl Sulfate Complex *on page 649*
Amphotericin B (Lipid Complex) *on page 653*
Amphotericin B (Liposomal) *on page 655*
Caspofungin *on page 695*
Itraconazole *on page 895*
Voriconazole *on page 1151*

Selected Readings

Cockrill BA and Hales CA, "Allergic Bronchopulmonary Aspergillosis," *Annu Rev Med*, 1999, 50:303-16.
Herbrecht R, Denning DW, Patterson TF, et al, "Voriconazole Versus Amphotericin B for Primary Therapy of Invasive Aspergillosis," *N Engl J Med*, 2002, 347(6):408-15.
Kontoyiannis DP and Bodey GP, "Invasive Aspergillosis in 2002: An Update," *Eur J Clin Microbiol Infect Dis*, 2002, 21(3):161-72.
Latge JP, "*Aspergillus fumigatus* and Aspergillosis," *Clin Microbiol Rev*, 1999, 12(2):315-50.
Robinson LA, "*Aspergillus* and Other Fungi," *Chest Surg Clin N Am*, 1999, 9(1):193-225, x.
Soubani AO and Chandrasekar PH, "The Clinical Spectrum of Pulmonary Aspergillosis," *Chest*, 2002, 121(6):1988-99.
Talbot GH, Huang A, and Provencher M, "Invasive *Aspergillus* Rhinosinusitis in Patients With Acute Leukemia," *Rev Infect Dis*, 1991, 13(2):219-32.

Asymptomatic Bacteriuria

Synonyms Bacteriuria, Asymptomatic; Urinary Tract Infection/Colonization, Asymptomatic

Clinical Presentation Presence of significant amounts of bacteria in the urine without accompanying signs/symptoms of infection.

Likely Pathogens Typically aerobic Gram-negative bacilli (*E. coli*) - occasionally *Staphylococcus haemolyticus*

Gram-Negative Bacilli *on page 157*
Enterococcus Species *on page 134*
Streptococcus agalactiae *on page 313*

Diagnostic Tests/Procedures Note: Urine culture is recommended for the following groups: Pregnant females, men undergoing TURP, or for urological procedures in which mucosal bleeding is anticipated.

Urine Culture, Clean Catch *on page 609*

Drug Therapy Comment Treatment is based on clinical evaluation and demographics/concurrent conditions.

Empiric Drug Therapy

Recommended:

Note: Empiric therapy is generally not recommended. Treatment is initiated based on positive culture and may be guided by sensitivity. The IDSA guidelines do not provide empiric recommendations but focus on duration and whom should be screened. Typical regimens include:

Children: Treatment based on specific culture/sensitivity

Pregnant females (avoid quinolones):
Nitrofurantoin *on page 971*
Cephalosporins, 1st Generation *on page 729*
Sulfamethoxazole and Trimethoprim *on page 1087* (stop treatment 2 weeks prior to delivery)
Trimethoprim *on page 1130*

Adults, invasive procedure/catheterization:
Sulfamethoxazole and Trimethoprim *on page 1087*

Adults, neurogenic bladder: No treatment indicated

Adults, elderly without symptoms: No treatment indicated (unless adjunct to corrective surgery for obstructive uropathy)

Treatment course:
Pregnant females:

- 3-7 days
- Periodic screening for recurrent bacteriuria should be undertaken following therapy

(Continued)

Asymptomatic Bacteriuria *(Continued)*

- No recommendation regarding repeat screening of culture negative pregnancy later in pregnancy.

TURP and urological procedures:

- Initiate shortly before procedure
- Therapy should not continue beyond procedure unless catheter remains in place.

Selected Readings

Nicolle LE, Bradley S, Colgan R, et al, "Infectious Diseases Society of America Guidelines for the Diagnosis and Treatment of Asymptomatic Bacteriuria in Adults," *Clin Infect Dis*, 2005, 40:643-654.

Athlete's Foot *see* Dermatophytes *on page 114*

Babesia microti

Microbiology *Babesia microti* is an intracellular protozoan which causes a febrile illness in the northeastern United States. The illness, babesiosis, resembles malaria. *Babesia microti* primarily infects animals; humans are incidental hosts. In the United States, rodents are the primary animal reservoir, including the white-footed deer mouse, rats, and field mice. The vector for transmission of the organism from the rodent to the human is the tick *Ixodes dammini*, the hard-shelled tick also responsible for the transmission of Lyme disease. Following the bite of an infected tick, *Babesia microti* invade the human circulation and enter erythrocytes. The trophozoites of *Babesia microti* divide within erythrocytes into two or four daughter cells, sometimes forming a characteristic tetrad ring which can be recognized on a blood smear. The organisms eventually leave the red blood cells, perforating the membrane and causing asynchronous cell lysis. With the merozoites being released, other host erythrocytes are at risk for infection, and the infectious cycle is maintained.

Epidemiology Babesiosis occurs most commonly along the northeastern seaboard of the United States in states such as Massachusetts, New York, and Rhode Island. In particular, Martha's Vineyard, Cape Cod, Shelter Island, Fire Island, and Nantucket Island report a high prevalence. Infections mainly occur from May to September when the nymph form of *Ixodes dammini* is feeding. Epidemiologic studies suggest that most infections with *Babesia microti* are subclinical or asymptomatic. A seroprevalence rate of 3% to 4% was found in endemic areas, with many individuals unaware of past infection. Less commonly, babesiosis has been transmitted by transfusion from an asymptomatic donor.

Clinical Syndromes The incubation period following the bite of the infected tick is 1-3 weeks. The majority of patients are not able to recall a recent tick bite. Most infections with *Babesia microti* are either asymptomatic or mild. In severe cases, symptoms include fever up to 40°C, chills, sweats, myalgias, malaise, and headache. Some individuals may experience photophobia, sore throat, and cough. Hepatosplenomegaly may be observed less commonly, but generalized lymphadenopathy is not seen. The most fulminant cases of babesiosis occur in patients who are asplenic, emphasizing the important role of the spleen in the host defense against this protozoan.

Diagnosis The diagnosis of babesiosis is suspected when there is a characteristic clinical presentation in an individual from an endemic area. The diagnosis is confirmed microbiologically by examination of Wright-Giemsa stained thick and thin blood smears. The parasite is visualized within the erythrocytes. At times it may be difficult to distinguish *Babesia* sp from other intracellular parasites such as *Plasmodium falciparum* (one of the causative agents of malaria). The finding of intracellular merozoites in a tetrad configuration is pathognomonic for babesiosis but frequently is absent. Blood smears may be falsely negative if the level of parasitemia is very low. Other laboratory aids include the classic findings of an intravascular hemolytic anemia with hemoglobinuria, elevated reticulocyte count, and depressed haptoglobin level. Other laboratory abnormalities include thrombocytopenia, leukopenia, and mild increases in transaminases. The diagnosis can also be confirmed by using an indirect immunofluorescent antibody titer against *Babesia microti* for both IgG and IgM. PCR for *B. microti* is now commercially available.

Diagnostic Tests/Procedures

Peripheral Blood Smear, Thick and Thin *on page 563*

Treatment Many patients with babesiosis recover without specific therapy. When infection is severe or the patient is known to be asplenic, the drugs of choice are clindamycin intravenously and quinine orally. Chloroquine, which is effective in some cases of malaria, has no efficacy in treating babesiosis; thus, it is important to distinguish babesiosis from malaria on the peripheral blood smear. Life-threatening infections may respond to exchange transfusions in combination with antimicrobial therapy, in an effort to decrease the degree of parasitemia. Another regimen which has been recently studied is atovaquone in combination with azithromycin. In one

prospective clinical trial, atovaquone-azithromycin was as effective as clindamycin-quinine.

Drug Therapy

Recommended:

Clindamycin *on page 752*

plus

Quinine *on page 1030*

Alternate:

Atovaquone *on page 670*

plus

Azithromycin *on page 674*

Selected Readings

Belman AL, "Tick-Borne Diseases," *Semin Pediatr Neurol*, 1999, 6(4):249-66.
Gelfand JA and Callahan MV, "Babesiosis," *Curr Clin Top Infect Dis*, 1998, 18:201-6.
Krause PJ, "Babesiosis," *Med Clin North Am*, 2002, 86(2):361-73.

Babesiosis *see Babesia microti on page 40*

Bacillary Angiomatosis *see Bartonella* Species *on page 48*

Bacillus anthracis

Related Information

Prophylaxis for Patients Exposed to Common Communicable Diseases *on page 1309*

Microbiology *Bacillus anthracis* is an aerobic, Gram-positive bacillus with a large polypeptide capsule. Some isolates may appear gram-variable rather than Gram-positive. On Gram stain, there is a characteristic "box car" appearance to these organisms, a feature common to the genus *Bacillus*. The organism forms endospores when grown aerobically in the laboratory, but spores usually are not seen in clinical specimens (endospores in necrotic lesions). Virulence factors for this organism include anthrax toxin (made up of three components) and a capsule (which protects against host antibodies).

Epidemiology *Bacillus anthracis* causes the disease anthrax. The organism can be found in some areas of the world in soil and decaying vegetation. The endospores of the organism are hardy and survive for years under adverse conditions. These endospores can contaminate the hide of herbivores such as cattle, sheep, and goats. Animals consume the endospores and ultimately expire. In this way, anthrax is a zoonosis, with humans only incidentally exposed. Direct contact with the contaminated hides or hair of these herbivores leads to human disease sporadically. The disease has historically been more common in the Middle East than in the United States; in 1992, there was only one case of anthrax reported.

In 2001, there was a surge of bioterrorism related anthrax in the United States. As of December 2001, there were 22 cases of confirmed or suspected cases of inhalational (11 cases) and cutaneous anthrax (11 cases) reported to the Centers for Disease Control and Prevention (CDC). These cases came from a variety of states including New York, New Jersey, Florida, the District of Columbia, Connecticut, Maryland, and Pennsylvania. Nearly all cases were acquired from exposure to the endospores of *Bacillus anthracis* which was sent through the mail, although in several cases the source of inhalational anthrax has remained unclear. The majority of cases occurred in postal workers and mail handlers or sorters. Other cases occurred in several media workers, a hospital worker, a journalist, a bookkeeper, and an elderly woman in Connecticut.

Clinical Syndromes

- **Cutaneous anthrax:** This form of human infection results from direct inoculation of *Bacillus anthracis* endospores into the skin. Exposure results from handling insulation made from animal hair (usually commercial buildings), infected animal hides, clothing products, or wool. Less commonly, endospores come from contaminated soil. Endospores enter intact or exposed skin in an extremity such as the forearm. A papule develops locally at the site of inoculation of the endospores and later ulcerates and turns into a black eschar. Systemic symptoms of fever, chills, and total body edema can result from the effects of anthrax toxin. The disease is often rapidly fatal if the diagnosis and treatment are delayed.
- **Inhalation anthrax:** Also known as Woolsorter's disease, inhalational anthrax presents as a rapidly progressive pneumonitis. Widening of the mediastinum is a common finding on chest x-ray and may be a clue to the diagnosis. Meningeal involvement is common. Mortality is high.
- **Gastrointestinal anthrax:** This rare form of anthrax is characterized by fever, severe abdominal pain, and sepsis syndrome. This generally occurs after eating undercooked meat contaminated with anthrax endospores. The incubation period is estimated to be 1-7 days. Inflammation in the lower colon leads to hematemesis and bloody diarrhea. A form of GI anthrax involving the oropharynx has also been

(Continued)

Bacillus anthracis (Continued)

reported, where patients develop lesions at the base of the tongue, along with dysphagia and cervical adenopathy. The mortality of GI anthrax is approximately 50%.

- **Bioterrorism-related anthrax:** One concern has been that the presentation of bioterrorism-related anthrax may differ from the historical presentation of anthrax. The recent cases of bioterrorism-related anthrax have been studied in detail and publicly disseminated so that healthcare workers may become familiar with the presentation. For the 11 cases of inhalational anthrax, the majority presented with fever, chills, severe fatigue, and nonproductive cough. Chest discomfort or pleuritic pain was common, and some experienced nausea and vomiting with abdominal pain. Dyspnea, headache, and myalgias were also reported. Initially, WBCs were either normal or slightly elevated (7.5-13.3 x $10^3/mm^3$). An increase in the number of band forms was common. The presenting chest X-ray was abnormal in all of the cases. Abnormalities on chest X-ray and CT scan of the chest included mediastinal widening, mediastinal lymphadenopathy, paratracheal/hilar fullness, hilar fullness, and pleural effusions. Two patients had no mediastinal abnormalities but presented with pleural effusions. Effusions were hemorrhagic and in some cases required chest tube placement. Pulmonary infiltrates, often involving multiple lobes were reported in 4 patients. For the 11 cases of cutaneous anthrax, the incubation period was approximately 5 days (1-10 days). The anthrax lesions were painless and found on the forearm, neck, chest, and fingers. Patients did complain of a tingling sensation or pruritus at the skin lesion site.

Diagnosis The diagnosis of cutaneous anthrax should be suspected clinically in a patient with a nontender, nonhealing ulcerative skin lesion with necrosis, which is otherwise unexplained. The skin lesions usually present as papules, followed by vesiculation and rapid development of a deep skin ulcer, often with severe surrounding edema. Necrosis is usually present. The organism can often be identified on Gram stain of a swab or aspirate of a skin lesion. Typically, the Gram stain of a cutaneous anthrax lesion shows few or no polymorphonuclear leukocytes and sporulating Gram-positive rods.

The diagnosis of inhalational anthrax should be suspected clinically in a patient who presents with a progressive, otherwise unexplained, respiratory illness, particularly if there is mediastinal widening on radiographs. However, the early diagnosis of inhalational anthrax may be very difficult since patients early on present with nonspecific systemic symptoms which may mimic influenza and other common respiratory infections. The CDC has recommended the following laboratory criteria for the diagnosis of anthrax: (1) isolation of *B. anthracis* from a clinical specimen, or (2) other supportive laboratory tests, including (a) detection of *B. anthracis* DNA by polymerase chain reaction (PCR) from clinical specimens, (b) demonstration of *B. anthracis* in a clinical specimen by immunohistochemical staining, or (c) serologic testing.

The organism can be isolated from nasal swabs, skin lesions, cerebrospinal fluid, and induced sputum without special culture techniques. For suspected cases of anthrax, the CDC recommends at least the following specimens be obtained: (1) for inhalational anthrax, blood cultures and cerebrospinal fluid cultures if meningeal signs are present (2) cutaneous anthrax, blood cultures and vesicular fluid cultures, (3) gastrointestinal anthrax, blood cultures. In the bioterrorism-related inhalational anthrax cases, the organism was isolated in routine blood cultures in all patients who had not received prior antibiotic therapy. *B. anthracis* can also be isolated from other body fluids including pleural effusions, pleural biopsies, lymph nodes, and other tissues.

Large-scale (mass) nasal swab screening for potential exposure to *Bacillus anthracis* is neither productive nor clinically useful, and is not recommended. Such tests should be reserved for known or highly likely exposures to *Bacillus anthracis*.

Serologic tests are available to aid in the diagnosis of anthrax. Specific serum IgG to the protective antigen component of *B. anthracis* toxin can be measured by enzyme immunoassay. Demonstration of a 4-fold rise in specific antibody is confirmatory of acute anthrax. Serologic testing was used to confirm some of the bioterrorism-related cases with negative blood and tissue cultures. PCR tests to detect specific DNA sequences are also available and can be performed on blood and involved tissue specimens.

Diagnostic Tests/Procedures

Aerobic Culture, Appropriate Site *on page 365*
Aerobic Culture, Sputum *on page 367*
Gram Stain *on page 473*

Treatment In the past, penicillin was the antibiotic of choice for *B. anthracis*. The organism has traditionally been very susceptible to a number of antibiotics including penicillin, tetracyclines, quinolones, and macrolides. However, the isolates of *B. anthracis* from the bioterrorism-related cases in 2001 demonstrated *in vitro* resistance

to a number of antibiotics including vancomycin, imipenem, clarithromycin, rifampin, chloramphenicol, and clindamycin. The organisms maintained *in vitro* susceptibility to penicillin and ampicillin, but the isolates demonstrated constitutive and inducible beta-lactamases, which could lead to clinically significant penicillin and ampicillin resistance. Based on this, the CDC advised against the use of either penicillin or ampicillin as single agent therapy. Interim recommendations for treatment of inhalational anthrax and cutaneous anthrax related to bioterrorism have been published by the CDC (see tables below and on next page). The treatment of choice for inhalational anthrax is either ciprofloxacin or doxycycline, in combination with a second antibiotic. The initial treatment is with intravenous antibiotics, which may later be changed to oral antibiotics when clinically stable. The above recommendation is for empirical treatment; the antibiotic regimen may need to be altered depending on the results of antimicrobial susceptibility testing. The total recommended length of treatment (oral and intravenous) is 60 days. The treatment of choice for cutaneous anthrax is ciprofloxacin or doxycycline.

One important issue is the role of postexposure prophylaxis (ie, antibiotic treatment of individuals who have had a potential aerosol exposure to anthrax but who have no signs or symptoms of disease). The nature of the exposure is the key to determining if a person should receive postexposure prophylaxis, since there is not a completely reliable laboratory method for determining if an exposure has occurred. Nasal swabs

Inhalational Anthrax Treatment Protocol[1,2] for Cases Associated With a Bioterrorism Attack

Category	Initial Therapy (I.V.)[3,4]	Duration
Adults	Ciprofloxacin 400 mg every q12h[7] **or** Doxycycline 100 mg q12h[6] **and** 1 or 2 additional antimicrobials[4]	I.V. treatment initially[5]. Switch to oral antimicrobial therapy when clinically appropriate: Ciprofloxacin 500 mg po bid **or** Doxycycline 100 mg po bid Continue for 60 days (I.V. and oral combined)[7]
Children	Ciprofloxacin 10-15 mg/kg q12h[8,9] **or** Doxycycline:[6,10] >8 years and >45 kg: 100 mg q12h >8 years and ≤45 kg: 2.2 mg/kg q12h ≤8 years: 2.2 mg/kg q12h **and** 1 or 2 additional antimicrobials[4]	I.V. treatment initially.[5] Switch to oral antimicrobial therapy when clinically appropriate: Ciprofloxacin 10-15 mg/kg po q12h[9] **or** Doxycycline:[10] >8 years and >45 kg: 100 mg po bid >8 years and ≤45 kg: 2.2 mg/kg po bid ≤8 years: 2.2 mg/kg po bid Continue for 60 days (I.V. and oral combined)[7]
Pregnant women[11]	Same for nonpregnant adults (the high death rate from the infection outweighs the risk posed by the antimicrobial agent)	I.V. treatment initially. Switch to oral antimicrobial therapy when clinically appropriate.[2] Oral therapy regimens same for nonpregnant adults.
Immunocompromised persons	Same for nonimmunocompromised persons and children	Same for nonimmunocompromised persons and children

Reference: U.S. Department of Health and Human Services, "Update: Investigation of Bioterrorism-Related Anthrax and Interim Guidelines for Exposure Management and Antimicobial Therapy, October 2001," *MMWR Morb Mortal Wkly Rep*, 2001, 50(42):909-40.

[1]For gastrointestinal and oropharyngeal anthrax, use regimens recommended for inhalational anthrax.

[2]Ciprofloxacin or doxycycline should be considered an essential part of first-line therapy for inhalational anthrax.

[3]Steroids may be considered as an adjunct therapy for patients with severe edema and for meningitis based on experience with bacterial meningitis of other etiologies.

[4]Other agents with *in vitro* activity include rifampin, vancomycin, penicillin, ampicillin, chloramphenicol, imipenem, clindamycin, and clarithromycin. Because of concerns of constitutive and inducible beta-lactamases in *Bacillus anthracis*, penicillin and ampicillin should not be used alone. Consultation with an infectious disease specialist is advised.

[5]Initial therapy may be altered based on clinical course of patient; one or two antimicobial agents (eg, ciprofloxacin or doxycycline) may be adequate as the patient improves.

[6]If meningitis is suspected, doxycycline may be less optimal because of poor central nervous system penetration.

[7]Because of the potential persistence of spores after an aerosol exposure, antimicrobial therapy should be continued for 60 days.

[8]If I.V. ciprofloxacin is not available, oral ciprofloxacin may be acceptable because it is rapidly and well absorbed from the GI tract with no substantial loss by first-pass metabolism. Maximum serum concentrations are attained 1-2 hours after oral dosing but may not be achieved if vomiting or ileus are present.

[9]In children, ciprofloxacin dosage should not exceed 1 g/day.

[10]The American Academy of pediatrics recommends treatment of young children with tetracyclines for serious infections (eg, Rocky Mountain spotted fever).

[11]Although tetracyclines are not recommended during pregnancy, their use may be indicated for life-threatening illness. Adverse effects on developing teeth and bones are dose related; therefore, doxycycline might be used for a short time (7-14 days) before 6 months of gestation.

(Continued)

Bacillus anthracis (Continued)

were obtained in a large number of individuals who had potential exposure to anthrax in 2001, but the CDC has stressed that the sensitivity of nasal swabs may be limited. The CDC has recommended ciprofloxacin or doxycycline for adults and children who have had a suspected exposure to anthrax. The duration of antibiotic prophylaxis is 60 days. Because of the potential adverse effects of both of these drugs for children, the risks and benefits must be weighed on an individual basis.

A vaccine against anthrax is available and has been licensed in the U.S. This vaccine is not currently available to the general public but has been used to immunize the U.S. military. The vaccine is recommended only in certain groups such as laboratory workers who work directly with the organism, some persons who work with animal hides and furs, and veterinarians who work in foreign countries where anthrax is more common. The CDC has also offered the vaccine to those who are receiving anthrax postexposure prophylaxis, in addition to the antibiotic regimen.

Drug Therapy

Recommended: See tables on previous page and below.

Cutaneous Anthrax Treatment Protocol[1] for Cases Associated With a Bioterrorism Attack

Category	Initial Therapy (Oral)[2]	Duration
Adults[1]	Ciprofloxacin 500 mg bid **or** Doxycycline 100 mg bid	60 days[3]
Children[1]	Ciprofloxacin 10-15 mg/kg every 12 hours (not to exceed 1 g/day)[2] **or** Doxycycline:[4] >8 years and >45 kg: 100 mg q12h >8 years and ≤45 kg: 2.2 mg/kg q12h ≤8 years: 2.2 mg/kg q12h	60 days[3]
Pregnant women[1,5]	Ciprofloxacin 500 mg bid **or** Doxycycline 100 mg bid	60 days[3]
Immunocompromised persons[1]	Same for nonimmunocompromised persons and children	60 days[3]

Reference: U.S. Department of Health and Human Services, "Update: Investigation of Bioterrorism-Related Anthrax and Interim Guidelines for Exposure Management and Antimicobial Therapy, October 2001," *MMWR Morb Mortal Wkly Rep*, 2001, 50(42):909-40.

[1]Cutaneous anthrax with signs of systemic involvement, extensive edema, or lesions on the head or neck require I.V. therapy, and a multidrug approach is recommended.

[2]Ciprofloxacin or doxycycline should be considered first-line therapy. Amoxicillin 500 mg po tid for adults or 80 mg/kg/day divided q8h for children is an option for completion of therapy after clinical improvement. Oral amoxicillin dose is based on the need to achieve appropriate minimum inhibitory concentration levels.

[3]Previous guidelines have suggested treating cutaneous anthrax for 7-10 days, but 60 days is recommended in the setting of this attack, given the likelihood of exposure to aerosolized *B. anthracis*.

[4]The American Academy of Pediatrics recommends treatment of young children with tetracyclines for serious infections (eg, Rocky Mountain spotted fever).

[5]Although tetracyclines or ciprofloxacin are not recommended during pregnancy, their use may be indicated for life-threatening illness. Adverse effects on developing teeth and bones are dose related; therefore, doxycycline might be used for a short time (7-14 days) before 6 months gestation.

Selected Readings

Brachman PS, "Inhalation Anthrax," *Ann N Y Acad Sci*, 1980, 353:83-93.

Inglesby TV, O'Toole T, Henderson DA, et al, "Anthrax as a Biological Weapon, 2002: Updated Recommendations for Management," *JAMA*, 2002, 287(17):2236-52.

Kiratisin P, Fukuda CD, Wong A, et al, "Large-Scale Screening of Nasal Swabs for *Bacillus anthracis*: Descriptive Summary and Discussion of the National Institutes of Health's Experience," *J Clin Microbiol*, 2002, 40(8):3012-6.

Lew D, "*Bacillus anthracis* (Anthrax)," *Principles and Practice of Infectious Diseases*, 4th ed, Mandell GL, Bennett JE, and Dolin R, eds, New York, NY: Churchill Livingstone, 1995, 1885-9.

Spencer RC, "*Bacillus anthracis*," *J Clin Pathol*, 2003, 56(3):182-7.

Swartz MN, "Recognition and Management of Anthrax--An Update," *N Engl J Med*, 2001, 345(22):1621-6.

Bacillus, Calmette-Guérin *see Mycobacterium bovis on page 229*

Bacillus cereus

Related Information

Clinical Syndromes Associated With Foodborne Diseases *on page 1276*

Microbiology *Bacillus cereus* is an aerobic, gram-positive bacillus associated with a variety of disease states including food poisoning, ocular infections, bacteremia, and septicemia. *Bacillus cereus* is a spore-forming aerobe which stains gram-positive or gram-variable. It grows readily on standard laboratory media and does not need special culturing techniques.

Epidemiology *Bacillus cereus* is ubiquitous in the environment, growing readily in such diverse areas as soil, water, vegetables, decaying matter, and dust. In certain individuals, it can be part of the normal human flora, explaining in part its tendency to colonize surgical wounds and serious burn injuries. The needles and syringes of heroin addicts in the United States have also been found to be contaminated with this bacterium. *Bacillus cereus* food poisoning, caused by ingestion of a toxin elaborated by this organism, has been reported from several countries around the world, including the United States and Canada.

Clinical Syndromes

- **The "emetic form" of *Bacillus cereus* food poisoning:** This results from the ingestion of a preformed toxin produced by this organism. Nausea, vomiting, and abdominal cramping usually occur soon (1-6 hours) following the ingestion of contaminated foods. In particular, this emetic toxin has been associated with fried rice served in Chinese food restaurants. The spores of *B. cereus* can survive the process of boiling rice followed by quick frying.
- **The "diarrheal form" of *Bacillus cereus* food poisoning:** This results from ingestion of a different, heat-labile enterotoxin. The incubation period is longer than for the emetic form, usually more than 9 hours. Profuse watery diarrhea is the predominant symptom, along with abdominal cramping.
- **Ocular infection, including endophthalmitis:** *Bacillus cereus* is a leading pathogen in post-traumatic endophthalmitis. Other common settings include ophthalmitis in farm workers and intravenous drug users. In the latter case, infection can be fulminant. Several toxins have been identified which may play a role in this often rapidly destructive panophthalmitis: cereolysin, necrotic toxin, and phospholipase C.
- **Bacteremia:** Isolation of *Bacillus cereus* from the blood may have little clinical significance (as in the transient *Bacillus* bacteremia commonly seen in the intravenous drug user or in blood culture contamination) or may represent life-threatening septicemia. Clinically significant bacteremias tend to occur most often in patients with indwelling intravascular catheters and may warrant treatment.
- **Miscellaneous infections:** *Bacillus cereus* can be a cause of pneumonia in the compromised host (rare), endocarditis in the intravenous drug user, necrotizing fasciitis, acute or chronic osteomyelitis, meningitis (often in the setting of disseminated infection), ventricular shunt infection, and can be a part of a polymicrobial wound infection (eg, surgical wounds, tumor, breast prostheses).

Diagnosis *Bacillus cereus* is readily identified in the laboratory from cultures of blood and other sterile body fluids. In cases of suspected *Bacillus* food poisoning, the implicated foods should be cultured for this organism. There is little benefit in culturing the patient's stool since gastrointestinal tract colonization is not uncommon. As mentioned previously, isolation of *Bacillus cereus* from the blood need not be treated in every case, and clinical judgment is required.

Diagnostic Tests/Procedures

Aerobic Culture, Appropriate Site *on page 365*
Gram Stain *on page 473*

Treatment *Bacillus cereus* food poisoning does not respond to antimicrobial therapy. Attention should instead be focused on supportive measures such as hydration and electrolyte balance. Clinically significant infections with this organism should be treated with vancomycin intravenously. Unlike other *Bacillus* species (eg, *Bacillus alvei, B. subtilis, B. circulans*, etc), *Bacillus cereus* is often resistant to beta-lactam antibiotics such as the penicillins and cephalosporins. Vancomycin should be used until the antimicrobial susceptibility pattern is finalized; limited data suggests the addition of an aminoglycoside to vancomycin may have some minor benefit in serious infections.

Drug Therapy

Recommended:

Vancomycin *on page 1144*

Selected Readings

"*Bacillus cereus* Food Poisoning Associated With Fried Rice at Two Child Day Care Centers - Virginia, 1993," *MMWR*, 1994, 43(10):177-8.

Davey RT Jr and Tauber WB, "Post-traumatic Endophthalmitis: The Emerging Role of *Bacillus cereus* Infection," *Rev Infect Dis*, 1987, 9(1):110-23.

Schricker ME, Thompson GH, and Schreiber JR, "Osteomyelitis Due to *Bacillus cereus* in an Adolescent: Case Report and Review," *Clin Infect Dis*, 1994, 18(6):863-7.

Sliman R, Rehm S, and Shlaes DM, "Serious Infections Caused by *Bacillus* Species," *Medicine (Baltimore)*, 1987, 66(3):218-23.

Terranova W and Blake PA, "*Bacillus cereus* Food Poisoning," *N Engl J Med*, 1978, 298(3):143-4.

Bacterial Endophthalmitis *see* Endophthalmitis, Bacterial and Fungal *on page 128*

Bacterial Gastroenteritis *see* Gastroenteritis, Bacterial *on page 154*

Bacterial Keratitis *see* Keratitis, Bacterial and Fungal *on page 199*

Bacterial Vaginosis *see* Vaginosis, Bacterial *on page 347*

Bacteriuria, Asymptomatic *see* Asymptomatic Bacteriuria *on page 39*

Bacteroides and *Prevotella* Species

Synonyms *Bacteroides* Species; *Prevotella* Species

Microbiology *Bacteroides* and *Prevotella* species are important anaerobes which cause a variety of clinical syndromes. The two species are closely related, and all of the *Prevotella* species were previously classified as *Bacteroides* species (eg, *Bacteroides melaninogenicus* subsp. *melaninogenicus* has been renamed *Prevotella melaninogenica*). Both species are gram-negative, anaerobic, pleomorphic rods, some of which are aerotolerant. Gram staining is pale. The organisms stain irregularly. *B. fragilis* grows as a nonhemolytic glistening colony on blood agar. *Prevotella melaninogenica* appears as pigmented, brown-to-black colonies which fluoresce under UV light. *B. fragilis* will grow in 20% bile; *P. melaninogenica* will not. Catalase positivity and resistance to kanamycin, vancomycin, and colistin are used for preliminary speciation. Biochemical testing utilizing carbohydrate fermentation and gas-liquid chromatography (GLC) are used for definitive speciation. DNA homology has allowed clarification of the taxonomy of the *Bacteroides* species. The *Bacteroides fragilis* group is particularly important medically and is known to demonstrate relative resistance *in vitro* to a number of antimicrobial agents.

Epidemiology *Bacteroides* species are the predominant organism in the colon, where anaerobes far outnumber aerobes, and concentrations of anaerobic bacteria exceed 10^{10} organisms/gram of stool. *Prevotella* species are common colonizers of dental crevices, dental plaques, and the vagina. *Prevotella* species are considered part of the normal oral flora, whereas *Bacteroides fragilis* is very rarely found in the oral flora. Thus, *Prevotella* species are commonly found in lung abscesses associated with aspiration, but *B. fragilis* is rare.

Bacteroides species are the organisms most frequently isolated from suppurative anaerobic infections. Nosocomial colonization by virulent strains of *B. fragilis* may occur. Although *B. fragilis* makes up only a small fraction of the oral and colonic flora, it accounts for a disproportionate percentage of infections due to *Bacteroides* species.

Clinical Syndromes

- **Intra-abdominal abscess:** *Bacteroides* species infections are associated with closed abdominal abscesses and are frequently present in mixed or polymicrobic infections. The most common precipitating factors are diverticulitis, rupture of the appendix, surgical procedures, and abdominal trauma or tumor. The liver and subdiaphragmatic space are also frequent sites for abscess formation. Splenic, kidney, and perinephric abscesses are also well known. Liver abscess may occur as the result of peritoneal seeding or by spread from the portal or biliary system. *B. fragilis* may be isolated from more than 50% of intra-abdominal abscesses, despite the fact that *B. fragilis* accounts for <1% of organisms in the colon. Most intra-abdominal abscesses are mixed, with aerobic and facultative organisms also being present and likely acting synergistically with the anaerobes. Sixty percent to 70% of pelvic abscesses also involve *B. fragilis*.
- **Lung abscess and empyema:** Some cases of community-acquired aspiration pneumonia and lung abscess are caused by anaerobes, particularly *P. melaninogenica*. Since many of these cases are caused by aspiration of oral flora (particularly in patients with poor dentition), the organisms associated with the lung abscess are similar to the normal oral flora, with *P. melaninogenica* more often implicated than *B. fragilis*. In most cases, lung abscesses are polymicrobic including viridans streptococci and others.
- **Brain abscess:** Anaerobes including *Bacteroides* and *Prevotella* species are common causes of brain abscesses, often as a polymicrobic infection with oral streptococci. This is due to the fact that many brain abscesses are associated with odontogenic infections, sinusitis, and other infections which involve anaerobes.
- **Infections of the female genital tract:** *Prevotella* species have been associated with a variety of female genital tract infections, including bacterial vaginosis.
- **Bacteremia:** In some series of hospital-associated bacteremias, anaerobic bacteremias are relatively infrequent (perhaps <5%), with *B. fragilis* the most common anaerobe isolated. In most cases, the cause of the anaerobic bacteremia is an intra-abdominal abscess, but other anaerobic infections have been reported.
- **Endocarditis:** Rare, but has been observed in patients without underlying valvular disease.
- **Skin infection:** Often associated with trauma surgery, decubitus ulcers, diabetic foot ulcers, and human bites. Contamination by feces, saliva, and oropharyngeal secretions may allow anaerobic organisms to become established and cause infection.
- **Gangrene, synergistic cellulitis, necrotizing fascitis, and crepitant cellulitis:** May also be frequently attributed to infection with *Bacteroides* species.

Diagnostic Tests/Procedures

Anaerobic Culture *on page 371*
Gram Stain *on page 473*

Treatment Since anaerobic infections are commonly associated with abscess formation, it is important to consider drainage of fluid collections, whether by surgical intervention or needle drainage under CT scan or ultrasound guidance. In many cases, adequate drainage of one or more fluid collections is the single most important treatment consideration.

In the past, anaerobic infections were often categorized as "above or below the diaphragm," due to the presence of *B. fragilis* "below the diaphragm" and the observation that *B. fragilis* was the only anaerobic organism resistant to penicillin. Thus, intra-abdominal abscesses were treated with antibiotics other than penicillin, but lung abscesses "above the diaphragm" could be treated with penicillin. However, there is increasing penicillin resistance among some common oral anaerobes including *P. melaninogenica*. The mechanism of resistance is the production of β-lactamase, but other resistance mechanisms have been described. To complicate the situation, antimicrobial susceptibility testing for anaerobes is technically difficult and controversial; most centers do not routinely perform susceptibility tests on anaerobes. Thus, the selection of the antibiotic for anaerobic infection is mainly empiric.

Abscesses caused by *B. fragilis* as the sole pathogen can be treated with metronidazole or clindamycin. More commonly, intra-abdominal abscesses are caused by a number of organisms including *B. fragilis* and other mixed aerobic/anaerobic flora. Polymicrobial infections of this type can be treated with metronidazole or clindamycin in combination with other antibiotics which would cover aerobic coliforms. *B. fragilis* remains highly susceptible to metronidazole but there are a small number of *B. fragilis* strains which are resistant to clindamycin and some broad-spectrum agents such as cefoxitin. This number of resistant isolates is small but may be increasing. Combination antibiotics with beta-lactamase inhibitors such as piperacillin-tazobactam, ticarcillin-clavulanate, and others are also effective in treating polymicrobial abscesses which include *B. fragilis*. *Prevotella* species, mainly *P. melaninogenica*, are generally more susceptible to antibiotics than *B. fragilis*, but the incidence of penicillin-resistant *P. melaninogenica* may be about 15% to 30%.

Community-acquired lung abscess caused by aspiration of oral secretions often involves *Prevotella* species (not *Bacteroides* species). Treatment with clindamycin alone has been effective, and is probably superior to penicillin alone based on several studies. Metronidazole should not be used alone in this situation due to poor activity against common oral streptococci. Community-acquired aspiration is less likely to be caused by gram-negative aerobes (unlike nosocomial aspiration which commonly involves gram-negative aerobes), and these organisms usually do not need to be covered empirically.

Anaerobic infections of the female genital tract can include both *Bacteroides* and *Prevotella* species and often other organisms are involved.

Drug Therapy

Recommended:

Metronidazole *on page 940*
Clindamycin *on page 752*

Alternate:

Ampicillin and Sulbactam *on page 660*
Carbapenems *on page 693*
Cefotetan *on page 710*
Cefoxitin *on page 712*
Piperacillin and Tazobactam Sodium *on page 1003*
Ticarcillin and Clavulanate Potassium *on page 1114*

Selected Readings

Edwards R, "Resistance to Beta-Lactam Antibiotics in *Bacteroides* Spp," *J Med Microbiol*, 1997, 46(12):979-86.

Lorber B, "*Bacteroides, Prevotella, Porphyromonas*, and *Fusobacterium* Species (and Other Medically Important Anaerobic Gram-Negative Bacilli)," *Principles and Practice of Infectious Diseases*, 5th ed, Mandell GL, Bennett JE, and Dolin R, eds, New York, NY: Churchill Livingstone, 2000, 2561-70.

Patrick S, "The Virulence of *Bacteroides fragilis*," *Rev Med Microbiol*, 1993, 4:40-9.

Styrt B and Gorbach SL, "Recent Developments in the Understanding of the Pathogenesis and Treatment of Anaerobic Infections," *N Engl J Med*, 1989, 321(5):298-302.

Wexler HM, "Susceptibility Testing of Anaerobic Bacteria - State of the Art," *Clin Infect Dis*, 1993, 16(Suppl 4):S328-33.

***Bacteroides* Species** *see Bacteroides* and *Prevotella* Species *on page 46*

Balanitis

Synonyms Balanoposthitis

Clinical Presentation Inflammation of the glans penis. Balanitis involving the foreskin or prepuce is termed balanoposthitis. Patients usually present with penile discharge, inability to retract foreskin, difficulty urinating or controlling urine stream (in very severe cases), and/or tenderness/sensitivity of the glans penis. Physical examination reveals erythema and edema, inability to visualize glans penis or urethral meatus, discharge, ulceration, and/or plaques. May be complicated by phimosis. The risk of balanitis is increased in uncircumcised men with poor personal hygiene. Obesity, diabetes, or edematous conditions (renal or cardiovascular failure) are commonly associated with balanitis. In some cases, chemical irritants or penile cancer may contribute to the risk of balanitis.

Differential Diagnosis Malignancy; Reiter's syndrome

Likely Pathogens

Candida Species *on page 67* (most commonly associated with diabetes)
Human Papillomavirus *on page 191*
Gardnerella vaginalis on page 153
Treponema pallidum on page 334 (syphilis)
Trichomonas vaginalis on page 339
Streptococcus agalactiae on page 313
Borrelia vincentii

Diagnostic Tests/Procedures

Blood Culture, Aerobic and Anaerobic *on page 391*
Gram Stain *on page 473*

Empiric Drug Therapy

Recommended:

Fluconazole *on page 819*

Balanoposthitis *see* Balanitis *on page 48*

Bartonella Species

Synonyms *Rochalimaea* Species

Microbiology *Bartonella* species are small, pleomorphic gram-negative bacilli which have received considerable attention over recent years because of their role in two important diseases: cat scratch disease and bacillary angiomatosis. Until recently, *Bartonella henselae* and *Bartonella quintana* species were considered *Rochalimaea* species. *Bartonella henselae* was first isolated and described in 1992, when it was cultured from the blood of an HIV-infected individual. *Bartonella* species are slow-growing and difficult to isolate in the laboratory. The organisms have occasionally been recovered from blood cultures, skin biopsies, spleen tissue, and lymph node biopsies. However, because of the fastidious nature of these organisms, clinical specimens may often be culture-negative. Of note, *Bartonella* species are best visualized in clinical specimens (such as lymph nodes) using a Warthin-Starry stain; the finding of Warthin-Starry staining bacteria in lymph node tissue is suggestive of cat scratch disease.

Epidemiology

Cat scratch disease: For years, the cause of cat scratch disease was unknown. Although the epidemiology, clinical manifestations, and therapies of cat scratch disease have been described in the past, only within the past 2 years has *B. henselae* been implicated as the major causative agent of cat scratch disease (CSD).

The exact distribution of *Bartonella* in the environment is not known, but the organism can be found in soil. Cats appear to be an important reservoir of this organism. In the United States, there are approximately 22,000 cases of cat scratch disease diagnosed each year with about 10% requiring hospitalization. Most cases of CSD occur in children and adolescents who are otherwise healthy (ie, immunocompetent). Family outbreaks have been reported. The majority of cases seem to occur in the fall and winter. Transmission is from direct animal contact. Nearly all patients (90% to 99%) report a recent exposure to a cat, and a history of a cat scratch or bite can be elicited in many (75% to 90%). In some series, kittens appear more likely to transmit disease than older cats. Most animals who transmit CSD are otherwise healthy. Rarely, the picture of CSD has been described in individuals without an animal exposure.

Bacillary angiomatosis: Unlike cat scratch disease, bacillary angiomatosis usually is seen in the immunocompromised, particularly in persons with AIDS. This infection usually occurs late in HIV infection; in one study the average $CD4^+$ cell count was 57/µL. Both *B. henselae* and *B. quintana* can cause this disease. A history of a recent cat scratch from a patient with bacillary angiomatosis is uncommon, in some series <20%. *B. henselae* has been isolated from the blood of pet cats in some AIDS

patients with bacillary angiomatosis. Limited evidence suggests that fleas of infected cats may also become infected with *B. henselae*, although the importance of insect transmission is unknown. Since many cases of bacillary angiomatosis cannot be linked to a feline source, other modes of acquisition are likely and are currently being studied.

Clinical Syndromes

- **Cat scratch disease:** Typically, patients with CSD present with fever and painful lymphadenopathy. In 60% to 90% of cases an "inoculation lesion" is present, consisting of an erythematous pustule or papule at the site of the initial cat scratch or bite. These are most commonly found on the arms, head, and neck. The hallmark of CSD is regional adenopathy which develops within 2 weeks proximal to the initial site of the bite or inoculation lesion. Common nodes involved are the axillary, cervical, and supraclavicular nodes, but others have been described. Other symptoms include headache, malaise, arthralgias, and conjunctivitis. In 1% to 2% of cases, there may be unusual complications such as encephalopathy, Parinaud's oculoglandular syndrome, erythema nodosum, thrombocytopenic purpura, pneumonia, osteomyelitis, hepatosplenomegaly, and others.
- **Bacillary angiomatosis:** Bacillary angiomatosis can be either cutaneous or extracutaneous. Patients with cutaneous bacillary angiomatosis present with bright red round papules on the skin. Often they are multiple but occasionally may be solitary. These lesions are highly vascular and blanch on pressure. Often there are associated constitutional symptoms such as fever and malaise. The lesions may be difficult to distinguish from Kaposi's sarcoma in HIV-infected persons (see Selected Readings).

Diagnosis A variety of methods are available to help diagnose *Bartonella* infection. The organism can be recovered from blood cultures and from tissue biopsy specimens. However, since the organism is fastidious, other methods may be helpful including:

- histologic examination of tissue (ie, lymph nodes) with Warthin-Starry staining
- serologic methods - indirect fluorescence antibody for *B. henselae* or enzyme immunoassay
- cat scratch skin test (not widely available)
- polymerase chain reaction

Diagnostic Tests/Procedures

Polymerase Chain Reaction *on page 567*

Treatment Successful therapy of cat scratch disease has been reported with a variety of antimicrobial agents including erythromycin, doxycycline, sulfamethoxazole and trimethoprim, ciprofloxacin, gentamicin, and rifampin. No controlled trials are available to determine the most beneficial therapy as each of these agents has also been associated with significant failure rates. The macrolides are considered first-line agents as are the tetracyclines.

Drug Therapy

Recommended:

Erythromycin *on page 807*
Doxycycline *on page 787*

Alternate:

Sulfamethoxazole and Trimethoprim *on page 1087*

Selected Readings

Anderson BE and Neuman MA, "*Bartonella* Spp as Emerging Human Pathogens," *Clin Microbiol Rev*, 1997, 10(2):203-19.

Jacomo V and Raoult D, "Human Infections Caused by *Bartonella* spp. Part 1," *Clin Microbiol Newslett*, 2000, 22(1):1-5.

Jacomo V and Raoult D, "Human Infections Caused by *Bartonella* spp. Part 2," *Clin Microbiol Newslett*, 2000, 22(2):9-13.

Hensel DM and Slater LN, "The Genus *Bartonella*," *Clin Microbiol Newslet*, 1995, 17(2):9-13.

Margileth AM, "Antibiotic Therapy for Cat-Scratch Disease: Clinical Study of Therapeutic Outcome in 268 Patients and a Review of the Literature," *Pediatr Infect Dis J*, 1992, 11(6):474-8.

Maurin M and Raoult D, "*Bartonella* (*Rochalimaea*) *quintana* Infections," *Clin Microbiol Rev*, 1996, 9(3):273-92.

BCG *see Mycobacterium bovis on page 229*

Bilharziasis *see Schistosoma mansoni on page 294*

BK Virus *see* JC Virus and BK Virus *on page 196*

Black Molds *see* Dematiaceous Fungi *on page 112*

Black Piedra *see* Dematiaceous Fungi *on page 112*

Blastocystis hominis

Microbiology *Blastocystis hominis* is a protozoan that reproduces by binary fission. Bacteria must be present for the organisms to grow and replicate. Three morphological types have been described: ameboid, granular, and vacuolated. Its exact taxonomic position as a parasite or fungus has not been established.

(Continued)

Blastocystis hominis (Continued)

Epidemiology The role of *B. hominis* as an intestinal pathogen is unclear because it may be found in stool specimens of both asymptomatic and symptomatic persons. Although the concentration of *B. hominis* in stools of symptomatic patients tends to be higher than in asymptomatic patients, some asymptomatic patients may have larger numbers of organisms present. *B. hominis* is frequently isolated in the presence of other intestinal pathogens. Endoscopic examination has failed to reveal any intestinal injury in symptomatic patients with *B. hominis*. In addition, fecal leukocytes are not usually seen. Intestinal permeability is not altered. May be more pathogenic in children and patients with AIDS. Contaminated drinking water is thought to be the reservoir.

Clinical Syndromes Symptoms that may be associated with *B. hominis* include abdominal pain, bloating, flatus, diarrhea, constipation, anorexia, nausea, vomiting, weight loss, and fatigue. May be associated with chronic urticaria and/or eosinophilia.

Diagnosis *B. hominis* is easily detected in iodine wet mount or trichrome. May be detected on touch prep (imprint from endoscopic biopsy specimen) stained with Giemsa. Acridine orange stain differentiates the cystic and central body forms.

Diagnostic Tests/Procedures

Ova and Parasites, Stool *on page 551*

Treatment The treatment of *Blastocystis* remains controversial, and the efficacy of antibiotics is unclear. Symptomatic patients without evidence of another intestinal pathogen may be treated with metronidazole or nitazoxanide for eradication of *B. hominis*. A nonrandomized study suggests the SMX/TMP may be of benefit. An apparent therapeutic response may be related to treatment of an undetected pathogen or may be coincidental, as nearly 60% of untreated symptomatic patients will have resolution of symptoms.

Drug Therapy

Recommended:

Metronidazole *on page 940*

Selected Readings

Albrecht H, Stellbrink HJ, Koperski K, et al, "*Blastocystis hominis* in Human Immunodeficiency Virus-Related Diarrhea," *Scand J Gastroenterol*, 1995, 30(9):909-14.

Diaz E, Mondragon J, Ramirez E, et al, "Epidemiology and Control of Intestinal Parasites With Nitazoxanide in Children in Mexico," *Am J Trop Med Hyg*, 2003, 68(4):384-5.

Ok UZ, Girginkardesler N, Balcioglu C, et al, "Effect of Trimethoprim-Sulfamethaxazole in *Blastocystis hominis* Infection," *Am J Gastroenterol*, 1999, 94(11):3245-7.

Stenzel DJ and Boreham PF, "*Blastocystis hominis* Revisited," *Clin Microbiol Rev*, 1996, 9(4):563-84.

Udkow MP and Markell EK, "*Blastocystis hominis*: Prevalence in Asymptomatic Versus Symptomatic Hosts," *J Infect Dis*, 1993, 168(1):242-4.

Blastomyces dermatitidis

Microbiology *Blastomyces dermatitidis* is a dimorphic fungus uncommonly seen in the immunocompromised population. In the mold form (usually in the environment and in culture), it has round to pyriform 4-5 μm conidia attached directly on the hyphae or on short stalks. Initially, the colony appears yeast-like at room temperature, then develops hyphal projections eventually becoming a fluffy white mold. The spores are difficult to isolate from the soil or bird droppings but have been recovered from wet soil.

The yeast form (usually *in vivo*) grows as a brown, wrinkled, folded colony at 37°C. Microscopically, the yeasts appear as round, budding, thick-walled yeast cells with a daughter cell forming a single bud that has a broad base 5-15 μm in diameter and which may be found extra- or intracellular in macrophages.

Epidemiology Blastomycosis usually occurs in healthy hosts and is associated with point-source exposure; more commonly in men than women which may be secondary to more male occupational exposures. Immunosuppressed patients typically develop infection following exposure but may be secondary to reactivation. It is uncommon in the AIDS population and is not recognized as an AIDS-defining illness. When an AIDS patient does develop blastomycosis, it is usually more severe with multiple visceral involvement plus CNS infection and progresses to a fatal course rapidly.

Blastomycosis is endemic in the south-central, southeastern, and midwestern United States and the Canadian provinces bordering the Great Lakes. After inhalation of the spores, which are taken up by bronchopulmonary macrophages, there is an approximate 30- to 45-day incubation period. The initial response is suppurative and progresses to granuloma formation (also referred to as a pyogranulomatous response). *Blastomyces* most commonly infects the lungs followed by skin, bone, prostate, and CNS.

Clinical Syndromes

- **Subclinical:** Approximately 60% of people living in an endemic area with occupational exposure have laboratory evidence via immune markers of *Blastomyces* but no clinical disease.

- **Acute blastomycosis:** Typically presents as a flu-like illness with fever, malaise, fatigue, weight loss, and pulmonary involvement. Occurs more commonly in men 25-50 years of age with occupational/environmental exposure. Rarely infects children except in epidemics.
- **Acute pneumonia:** Self-limited. Presents with fever, chills, purulent sputum, and sometimes hemoptysis. Chest radiograph reveals alveolar or mass-like infiltrates. May be associated with erythema nodosum.
- **Chronic pneumonia:** Symptoms last 2-6 months, and patient presents with weight loss, night sweats, fever, chest pain, and productive cough.
- **Cutaneous:** Verrucous or ulcerative lesions. Mimics squamous cell cancer and keratoacanthoma. May be found in the brain, skeletal system, prostate, myocardium, pericardium, sinuses, pituitary, or adrenal glands. May invade the reticuloendothelial system.
- **Osteomyelitis:** Up to 25% of extrapulmonary cases. Noncaseating granulomas, suppuration or necrosis in the bone may occur. May require surgical debridement as well as antifungal treatment.
- **Genitourinary:** Prostatitis and epididymo-orchitis. Has been isolated in the urine after prostatic massage. Female tract complications have been reported, transmitted by male sexual partner with cutaneous form of disease.
- **CNS:** Five percent to 10% of disseminated disease may cause epidural or cranial abscesses, as well as meningitis.

No matter where the infection exists, always obtain a chest x-ray because there is almost always a simultaneous pulmonary infection. Infrequent complication is adult respiratory distress syndrome.

Diagnosis Skin test and serological markers are useful epidemiological tools but have too low sensitivity and specificity to be diagnostic, and should be used only as supplemental tests to culture. Diagnosis depends on direct examination of tissue or the isolation of *Blastomyces* in culture.

Diagnostic Tests/Procedures

Fungus Culture, Appropriate Site *on page 461*
Fungus Culture, Biopsy *on page 461*
Fungus Culture, Body Fluid *on page 462*
Fungus Culture, Skin *on page 464*
Fungal Serology *on page 458*

Treatment There are no randomized, blinded trials comparing the antifungal agents and there is limited data available on the treatment of blastomycosis in patients who are infected with HIV. Therapy is determined by the severity of the clinical presentation and presentation and consideration of the toxicities of the antifungal agent. Typically, mild-to-moderate pneumonia in immunocompetent patients is treated with itraconazole 200-400 mg/day orally. Amphotericin B, up to 2.5 g, is recommended in life-threatening systemic disease. There is a 97% cure rate with amphotericin B as opposed to 89% with ketoconazole. Itraconazole, 200-400 mg/day orally, is better absorbed, has enhanced antimycotic activity, and is better tolerated than ketoconazole. Ketoconazole 400-800 mg/day or fluconazole 400-800 mg/day for at least 6 months is an effective alternative therapy for nonlife-threatening disease. Neither ketoconazole nor itraconazole penetrate the blood-brain barrier so they are not recommended for CNS involvement. Fluconazole or itraconazole may be used as suppressive therapy. The IDSA guidelines recommend that all patients with HIV and blastomycosis be treated with 0.7-1 mg/kg/day amphotericin B and consideration to switch to itraconazole after patients are clinically stable in those individuals without CNS involvement. Voriconazole has activity against blastomycosis, but there is little human data demonstrating efficacy.

Drug Therapy

Recommended:

Severe infection:

Amphotericin B (Conventional) *on page 650* (total dose 1.5-2.5 g)

then switch to

Itraconazole *on page 895*

Mild to moderate infection:

Itraconazole *on page 895*

Alternate:

Ketoconazole *on page 903*
Fluconazole *on page 819*

Selected Readings

Aberg JA, "Blastomycosis and HIV," *HIV InSite Knowledge Base*, Peiperl L and Volberding PA, eds, 2003, http://hivinsite.ucsf.edu/InSite.jsp?page=kb-05&doc=kb-05-02-09.

Assaly RA, Hammersley JR, Olson DE, et al, "Disseminated Blastomycosis," *J Am Acad Dermatol*, 2003, 48(1):123-7.

Boswell E and Aziz H, "Blastomycosis: A Case Study of a Dimorphic Fungal Disease," *Clin Lab Sci*, 2004, 17(3):145-8.

(Continued)

Blastomyces dermatitidis (Continued)

Bradsher RW, "Histoplasmosis and Blastomycosis," *Clin Infect Dis*, 1996, 22(Suppl 2):S102-11.
Gray NA and Baddour LM, "Cutaneous Inoculation Blastomycosis," *Clin Infect Dis*, 2002, 34(10):E44-9.
Martynowicz MA and Prakash UB, "Pulmonary Blastomycosis: An Appraisal of Diagnostic Techniques," *Chest*, 2002, 121(3):768-73.
Pappas PG and Dismukes WE, "Blastomycosis: Gilchrist's Disease Revisited," *Curr Clin Top Infect Dis*, 2002, 22:61-77.
Sobel JD, "Practice Guidelines for the Treatment of Fungal Infections. For the Mycoses Study Group. Infectious Diseases Society of America," *Clin Infect Dis*, 2000, 30(4):652.

Blastomycosis *see Blastomyces dermatitidis on page 50*

Blennophthalmia *see* Conjunctivitis *on page 93*

Blepharitis

Synonyms Seborrheic Blepharitis

Clinical Presentation Inflammation of the eyelid margins most commonly caused by *Staphylococcus aureus*. Symptoms include redness of the lid margins and the eye, itchy or irritated lid margins, crusting, dryness, or eye fatigue. Symptoms tend to be worse upon awakening, and may vary in intensity over the course of the day. Dry eye very frequently accompanies blepharitis. Blepharitis is caused by staphylococcal colonization of the Zeis glands of eyelid margin. Risk factors include seborrheic dermatitis, acne rosacea, diabetes mellitus, and immunocompromised states.

Seborrheic blepharitis: Erythema at the lid margin, with dry flakes and oily secretions of the eyelashes or eyelid, often associated with dandruff of the scalp and/or eyebrows. Often presents as a mixed syndrome with staphylococcal infection.

Staphylococcus aureus: Severe itching, burning, and lacrimation, with symptoms worse in the morning. Ulcerations may form at the base of the eyelashes and the lower half of the cornea demonstrates a fine, epithelial keratitis. May occur in association with impetigo contagiosa, infectious eczematoid dermatitis, or scalded skin syndrome. Differentiate from squamous cell, basal cell, or sebaceous cell carcinoma, which may result in persistent inflammation and thickening of the eyelid margin. Swelling and/or inflammation which does not resolve within a month of treatment should be suspected to be an underlying carcinoma.

Likely Pathogens

Staphylococcus aureus, Methicillin-Susceptible *on page 307*

Diagnostic Tests/Procedures

Biopsy Culture, Routine *on page 390* (in atypical or unresponsive cases for suspicion of carcinoma)

Empiric Drug Therapy

Recommended:

Note: Uncomplicated blepharitis is often treated with warm compresses alone

Topical:
- Bacitracin *on page 679*
- Erythromycin *on page 807*

Systemic (in association with acne rosacea):
- Tetracycline *on page 1106*

Blood Fluke *see Schistosoma mansoni on page 294*

Boils *see* Furunculosis *on page 151*

Bordetella bronchiseptica

Synonyms Kennel Cough; Snuffles

Microbiology *B. bronchiseptica* is an aerobic gram-negative coccobacillus that distinguishes itself from *B. pertussis* by its ability to grow readily on MacConkey agar, possess peritrichous flagella for motility, reduces nitrate, and is urea-positive (see table). Although it does possess the pertussis toxin, only *B. pertussis* can elaborate the toxin. The dermonecrotic toxin of *B. bronchiseptica* is thought to contribute to inflammation and destruction of the bony and cartilaginous tissues in the upper respiratory tract of animals, but its role in human disease is unknown.

***Bordetella bronchiseptica* Properties**

Test	*B. pertussis*	*B. bronchiseptica*
Growth on MacConkey agar	No	Yes
Urease	No	Yes
Nitrate reduction	No	Yes
Oxidase	Yes	Yes
Motility	No	Yes

Epidemiology *B. bronchiseptica* is predominantly an animal pathogen that causes respiratory infections such as kennel cough in dogs, snuffles in rabbits, atrophic rhinitis in swine, and pneumonia in koala bears. Most patients have a history of exposure to animals. Immunocompromised patients are at a higher risk than immunocompetent hosts. It is recommended that patients with AIDS avoid exposure to sick animals and exposure to known environmental sources such as kennels.

Clinical Syndromes

- **Respiratory:** Most often presents as bronchitis or pneumonia characterized by fever and cough. May have paroxysmal cough similar to whooping cough.
- **Other:** Sinusitis, bacteremia, endocarditis, and meningitis have been reported.

Diagnosis Confirmatory diagnosis made by isolation of organism in infected source, most commonly respiratory cultures.

Diagnostic Tests/Procedures

Aerobic Culture, Appropriate Site *on page 365*
Gram Stain *on page 473*

Treatment May have variable susceptibility to beta-lactams, macrolides, and sulfonamides. Treatment failures are common and treatment usually requires a prolonged course of therapy to eradicate the organism. For patients with AIDS, a two-drug therapy such as antipseudomonal penicillin or fluoroquinolones with an aminoglycoside is recommended.

Drug Therapy

Recommended:

Penicillins, Extended-Spectrum *on page 997*
or
Fluoroquinolones *on page 824*
plus
Aminoglycosides *on page 641*

Alternate:

Cephalosporins, 3rd Generation *on page 730* (if susceptible)
or
Imipenem and Cilastatin *on page 861*
plus
Aminoglycosides *on page 641*

Selected Readings

Gomez L, Grazziutti M, Sumoza D, et al, "Bacterial Pneumonia Due to *Bordetella bronchiseptica* in a Patient With Acute Leukemia," *Clin Infect Dis*, 1998, 26(4):1002-3.

Lorenzo-Pajuelo B, Villanueva JL, Rodriguez-Cuesta J, et al, "Cavitary Pneumonia in an AIDS Patient Caused by an Unusual *Bordetella bronchiseptica* Variant Producing Reduced Amounts of Pertactin and Other Major Antigens," *J Clin Microbiol*, 2002, 40(9):3146-54.

Woodard DR, Cone LA, and Fostvedt K, "*Bordetella bronchiseptica* Infection in Patients With AIDS," *Clin Infect Dis*, 1995, 20(1):193-4.

Bordetella pertussis

Related Information

Prophylaxis for Patients Exposed to Common Communicable Diseases *on page 1309*

Microbiology *Bordetella pertussis* is a fastidious, nonmotile, gram-negative coccobacillus which tends to arrange itself singly and in pairs. "Pertussis" means violent cough, an appropriate name for the etiologic agent of whooping cough. *B. pertussis* is difficult to grow in culture. The starch-blood-agar medium described by Bordet and Gengou in 1900 was first used to isolate this organism *in vitro*. Some modern microbiology laboratories still use the Bordet and Gengou medium, but others have adopted a synthetic medium with growth factors which supports the growth of this fastidious organism equally well. It is important to notify the Microbiology Laboratory promptly if infection with *B. pertussis* is suspected since the organism usually cannot grow on routine agar used for planting sputum and other respiratory specimens.

Several virulence factors for *Bordetella pertussis* have been identified.

- Filamentous hemagglutinin - promotes attachment of *Bordetella* to the respiratory epithelium.
- Tracheal cytotoxin - causes ciliostasis in the respiratory epithelium and direct tracheal cell damage. This interferes with the "first line of defense".
- Adenylate cyclase toxin - causes accumulation of cyclic AMP in leukocytes leading to impairment of phagocyte functions such as chemotaxis.
- Dermonecrotic toxin - causes ischemic necrosis of the soft tissue in mice and likely causes local damage to the tracheal mucosa.
- Pertussis toxin - causes a sustained impairment in phagocytosis by a variety of different biological mechanisms and is thought to account for many of the systemic manifestations of pertussis.

Epidemiology Despite the introduction of the pertussis vaccine in many countries, there are still an estimated 51 million cases of pertussis annually worldwide with

(Continued)

Bordetella pertussis (Continued)

600,000 fatalities. In most populations, pertussis is endemic (ie, there is a relatively constant background level of disease), but superimposed epidemics occur at 3- to 4-year intervals. For example, recent peaks in pertussis in the United States occurred in 1983, 1986, and 1990.

The whole-cell pertussis vaccine became available in the United States in the early 1940s. Prior to this, pertussis was most common in children 1-5 years of age. Maternally-acquired antibodies provided passive protection in the first year of life. After the whole-cell pertussis vaccine was licensed as DTP in 1949, there was a steady decrease in the number of pertussis cases in the U.S., reaching a nadir of about 1000 cases in 1976. However, since 1976 there has been a steady increase in the number of pertussis cases in the U.S. with 1990 being a 20-year peak. In the United States in 2002, 8,296 cases of pertussis were reported to the CDC. It is not clear whether this represents a true increase in the incidence of pertussis in the community or whether there is only improved reporting of cases. In addition, there has been a shift in the population at highest risk. Infants younger than 1 year of age now account for half the reported cases; many of these infants were never vaccinated or did not receive vaccinations as recommended (2, 4, 6, and 15-18 months). Vaccination coverage in school-aged children has been relatively broad, accounting for much of the decline in pertussis in this older group.

Pertussis is a highly contagious infection with an attack rate estimated at 50% to 100%. Transmission is via the respiratory route with the organism being carried for several feet in aerosolized droplets. Humans are the only natural reservoir for *B. pertussis*. It is likely that infected adults with undiagnosed pertussis are the major (and perhaps only) reservoir for the organism, which is then transmitted by cough to a susceptible infant.

About 10% to 15% of pertussis cases now involve persons older than 15 years of age. Large outbreaks of pertussis are rare in adolescents and young adults. However, in Massachusetts during 1992, there was an unusual increase in the number of adult pertussis cases. In that year, 78% of reported cases involved people 10-19 years of age, with only 9% involving infants. Many of the cases involved an outbreak in a high school and nearby middle school. A similar outbreak was reported in a Maryland high school the same year. It is clear that vaccine immunity decreases over time and is estimated to last about 12 years. Thus, pertussis can occur in adolescents and adults, regardless of vaccination status as a child. Adults lacking immunity cannot offer passive immunity to infants, who are at the greatest risk for morbidity and mortality.

Clinical Syndromes

- **Pertussis or whooping cough:** The presentation of pertussis can be divided into three phases: catarrhal phase, paroxysmal (cough) phase, and recovery phase. The catarrhal stage of pertussis begins with symptoms of the common cold (rhinorrhea, conjunctivitis, coryza, and low-grade fever). Infants may present with apneic spells. This phase generally lasts from several days to 1 or more weeks and is indistinguishable from any other upper respiratory infection. After this, the patient develops a mild cough which escalates to severe, violent coughing, or the paroxysmal stage. The typical "whooping cough" is characterized by several brief expiratory coughs in succession followed by a rapid inspiration of air past a swollen glottis (which produces the classic "whoop"). Many patients will not present with the classic "whoop," particularly infants and adults. Vomiting after a paroxysm of coughing is common. The paroxysmal state may last for 1-4 weeks. Coughing paroxysms may continue for up to 6 months after infection. (In China, pertussis has been called the "cough of 100 days".) Potential complications of the paroxysmal state include severe vomiting with subsequent weight loss, dehydration, and malnutrition. Other complications include those related to high intrathoracic pressures (eg, subconjunctival hemorrhages, pneumothorax, hernias, etc). Secondary bacterial infections, such as aspiration pneumonia during vomiting and coughing, are the leading cause of death. Central nervous system manifestations are relatively common in pertussis. These include seizures and encephalopathy in up to 2% of hospitalized pertussis cases. During the recovery or convalescent phase, the cough and frequency of paroxysms slowly decreases. Apparent "relapses" of cough are not uncommon during the recovery phase but are most likely due to common respiratory viruses rather than relapses of *B. pertussis*.
- **"Atypical" pertussis:** The clinical picture described above may be altered in infants and in older individuals who are partially immunized. The catarrhal phase may be shortened or absent in some cases. Adults often do not have a typical "whoop", and thus, the diagnosis of pertussis is often not even considered. In HIV-infected persons, *B. pertussis* has been reported to cause a chronic, paroxysmal cough with dyspnea but otherwise negative cultures.

Diagnosis Pertussis is often difficult to diagnose, particularly if the typical whooping cough is absent. Pertussis also should be considered in the differential diagnosis of any person with prolonged upper respiratory infection and cough which fails to resolve after 2 weeks, regardless of the childhood DTP vaccination status. The laboratory diagnosis of *B. pertussis* is important, but many of the available laboratory techniques suffer from poor sensitivity, specificity, or both. Thus, a clinical case definition for pertussis has been used. For reporting purposes, the Centers for Disease Control have defined a clinical case of endemic or sporadic pertussis as any cough illness lasting 14 days or more (without apparent cause) with any of the following: paroxysms of coughing, inspiratory "whoop", or post-tussive vomiting.

In situations where an outbreak of pertussis is occurring, a clinical case has been defined as a cough illness lasting 14 days or more.

Laboratory confirmation of *B. pertussis* should be attempted in all suspected cases. Techniques include:

- Nasopharyngeal culture: This is considered the gold standard for diagnosing pertussis. If possible, a nasopharyngeal wash should be performed to maximize the yield, although a nasopharyngeal swab (calcium alginate swab) is acceptable but is much less productive. Despite careful specimen collection, *B. pertussis* may fail to grow in culture. This is considered a relatively insensitive technique.
- Direct fluorescent antibody (DFA): DFA systems for detection of *B. pertussis* are widely used but are also insensitive and have the additional problem of variable specificity. The CDC has recommended that DFA should not be used as the criterion for laboratory confirmation of pertussis.
- Serologic tests: Antibody tests for *B. pertussis* are not reliable for the diagnosis of pertussis and should not be used.
- Polymerase chain reaction (PCR) amplification tests for *B. pertussis*-specific nucleic acid sequences are extremely sensitive and specific, widely available, and highly recommended as the most appropriate laboratory test for pertussis.

Individuals with a prolonged cough and a nasopharyngeal culture positive for *B. pertussis* are considered to have a confirmed case of clinical pertussis (although *B. pertussis* can sometimes be cultured from asymptomatic contacts who never develop disease). Those with a positive DFA and cough for more than 14 days without culture confirmation still have a high likelihood of pertussis. Persons with a cough for longer than 14 days but with a negative DFA and negative culture may have pertussis to a variable degree of certainty, since other organisms can occasionally cause an acute respiratory illness followed by prolonged cough. Persons with a positive DFA, negative culture, and a cough less than 14 days have a much lower likelihood of pertussis. Persons with a cough less than 14 days and a negative DFA and culture probably do not have pertussis.

Diagnostic Tests/Procedures

Bordetella pertussis Direct Fluorescent Antibody *on page 402*
Bordetella pertussis Nasopharyngeal Culture *on page 403*
Polymerase Chain Reaction *on page 567*

Treatment Although a variety of antibiotics appear to be effective against *B. pertussis in vitro*, the drug of choice is erythromycin, given at a dose of 50 mg/kg/day, up to about 2 g/day. Erythromycin has been shown to decrease symptoms even if started after the catarrhal phase. Treatment should be at least 14 days, and longer courses may be necessary. Alternative agents include the newer macrolides such as azithromycin and clarithromycin, tetracycline, sulfamethoxazole and trimethoprim, and chloramphenicol, but the data regarding clinical efficacy of these agents is limited. Ampicillin has been associated with clinical failures and should not be used. Hospitalization of infants may be warranted to avoid complications. Adjunctive therapies such as corticosteroids and beta-adrenergic agonists are either controversial or unwarranted and should be reserved for severe disease at physician discretion.

Prevention of *B. pertussis* remains the cornerstone for containment of this infection. There are two vaccines available, the whole-cell vaccine and the acellular vaccine. The whole-cell vaccine is used most frequently throughout the world with an efficacy of >80% in most series. The main drawback of the whole-cell vaccine is its reactogenicity (local pain and swelling, systemic symptoms). The World Health Organization recommends the whole-cell vaccine as part of the diphtheria-tetanus-pertussis combination vaccine and this recommendation is followed in many countries worldwide. The acellular pertussis vaccine was developed to minimize the problems of reactogenicity of the whole-cell vaccine. In addition to relatively common local reactions to the whole-cell vaccine such as swelling and pain at the injection site, some infants will have systemic symptoms such fevers and vomiting. Serious neurologic sequelae have been reported following the use of the whole-cell pertussis vaccine, although controversy exists regarding a cause and effect relationship. The acellular pertussis vaccine has a lower rate of reactogenicity than the
(Continued)

Bordetella pertussis (Continued)

whole-cell vaccine. In 1996, the Advisory Committee on Immunization Practices (ACIP) and the Committee on Infectious Diseases, American Academy of Pediatrics, recommended that children routinely receive a series of 5 doses of vaccine against diphtheria, tetanus, and pertussis before age 7.

Two diphtheria and tetanus toxoids and acellular pertussis (DTaP) vaccines (Acel-Imune® and Tripedia®) have been licensed for several years, but originally only for administration of the fourth and fifth doses in the series to children aged 15 months to 6 years who previously had received 3 or more doses of diphtheria and tetanus toxoids and whole-cell pertussis (DTP) vaccine. The Food and Drug Administration (FDA) has recently licensed three DTaP vaccines for use among children aged 6 weeks to 6 years. Tripedia® was licensed for the initial 4 doses, and Acel-Imune® for all 5 doses of diphtheria, tetanus and pertussis vaccination series. A third DTaP vaccine (Infanrix®) was licensed in January 1997 for the initial 4 doses of the series. In 1997, the ACIP recommended Tripedia®, Acel-Imune®, and Infanrix® for routine vaccination of infants and young children, although whole-cell pertussis vaccines remain acceptable alternatives. Tripedia®, Acel-Imune®, and Infanrix® are recommended for all remaining doses in the schedule for children who have started the vaccination series with one, two, three, or four doses of whole-cell pertussis vaccines. In September 1996, the FDA licensed the use of TriHIBit® (ActHIB® reconstituted with Tripedia®) for the fourth dose in the series of vaccinations against diphtheria, tetanus, pertussis, and *Haemophilus influenzae* type b disease.

Drug Therapy

Recommended:

Prophylaxis:

Diphtheria, Tetanus Toxoids, and Acellular Pertussis Vaccine *on page 782*

Diphtheria, Tetanus Toxoids, and Acellular Pertussis Vaccine and *Haemophilus influenzae* b Conjugate Vaccine *on page 785*

Treatment:

Erythromycin *on page 807*

Alternate:

Azithromycin *on page 674*

Clarithromycin *on page 749*

Tetracycline *on page 1106*

Sulfamethoxazole and Trimethoprim *on page 1087*

Chloramphenicol *on page 733*

Selected Readings

Cherry JD, "The Science and Fiction of the "Resurgence" of Pertussis," *Pediatrics*, 2003, 112(2):405-6.

Edwards KM, "Pertussis in Older Children and Adults," *Adv Pediatr Infect Dis*, 1997, 13:49-77.

Herwaldt LA, "Pertussis in Adults. What Physicians Need to Know," *Arch Intern Med*, 1991, 151(8):1510-2.

Hewlett EL, "*Bordetella* Species," *Principles and Practice of Infectious Diseases*, 5th ed, Mandell GL, Bennett JE, and Dolin R, eds, New York, NY: Churchill Livingstone, 2000, 2414-22.

Marcon M, "Clinical and Laboratory Diagnostic Features of *Bordetella* spp - Pertussis and Beyond," *Clin Microbiol Newslett*, 1997, 19(24):185-91.

U.S. Department of Health and Human Services, "Pertussis Vaccination: Use of Acellular Pertussis Vaccine Among Infants and Young Children. Recommendations of the Advisory Committee on Immunization Practices (ACIP)," *MMWR*, 1997, 46(RR-7):1-25.

Yeh SH, "Pertussis: Persistent Pathogen, Imperfect Vaccines," *Expert Rev Vaccines*, 2003, 2(1):113-27.

Borrelia burgdorferi

Related Information

Immunization Recommendations *on page 1249*

Microbiology *Borrelia burgdorferi* is a tick-borne spirochete which causes Lyme disease. The organism is essentially a 10-25 μm gram-negative rod which spirals around a long axostyle and is entirely encased in a membrane.

Epidemiology Lyme disease (more properly, Lyme borreliosis) is the most commonly reported vector-borne illness in the United States. The spirochete is transmitted by the bite of the tick *Ixodes scapularis* (black leg tick or deer tick) in the northeast coastal regions of the U.S., the midwest, and the mid-Atlantic states and by the bite of the tick *Ixodes pacificus* (western deer tick) on the U.S. Pacific coast. Nine states account for 90% of the cases: Massachusetts, New York, New Jersey, Connecticut, Rhode Island, Pennsylvania, Minnesota, Wisconsin, and California. In very endemic areas, 30% to 75% of *Ixodes scapularis* ticks are infected with *B. burgdorferi*. Lyme disease is most common in individuals living near wooded areas with abundant deer, especially transitional zones of woods to brush. Peak seasons for Lyme disease are May to September, in particular June, July, and August.

There are two insect vectors that can transmit *B. burgdorferi*, *Ixodes scapularis* and *Ixodes pacificus*. *Ixodes scapularis* is much more efficient in transmitting the disease. The tick has three stages. The larva hatches from eggs during the spring and ingests

a blood meal from the white-footed mouse host (*Peromyscus leucopus*) later in the summer. An infected mouse then transmits the infection (*B. burgdorferi*) to the larva. The larva detach from the mouse and develop into nymphs during the following spring. The nymphal ticks feed during the late spring/summer on other white-footed mice and on human hosts. The nymphal ticks mature into adult male and female ticks and feed on white-tailed deer (*Odocoileus virginianus*) in the fall, winter, and early spring. Females lay eggs which will hatch to larva, and the cycle starts again.

Infection can be transmitted during any stage, but the nymphs are the most efficient. Since the nymph is the size of a poppy seed, it is easily missed or just brushed off. When the nymph bites, it secretes a cement-like substance to keep it attached to the host and secretes a coumarin-like substance which maintains the blood capillary feeding lesion. It feeds to engorgement over about 3 days. Approximately 10% of people bitten by infected ticks will acquire Lyme disease.

Clinical Syndromes The clinical manifestations of Lyme disease were originally divided into three stages: stage I, II, III. More recently, manifestations have been divided into early Lyme disease (stage I and II) and late (III).

Stage I: 3-32 days after the tick bite, a rash develops. A papule appears at the site of the bite followed by an annular (ring-like) rash which spreads outwardly. There is often an area of central clearing. This rash is termed erythema chronicum migrans (ECM). The rash usually resolves in time, even if untreated. Patients may complain of additional symptoms such as headache, malaise, and myalgias. In some, the infection progresses. Approximately 75% of Lyme borreliosis patients will demonstrate ECM.

Stage II: This stage involves the heart and nervous system primarily. Cardiac symptoms begin about 5 weeks after the bite (range 4 days to 7 months). Atrioventricular heart block is the most common finding and is usually self-limited. From 10% to 20% of people will develop neurologic disease weeks to months after the bite. This includes aseptic meningitis, cranial nerve palsy, peripheral radiculopathy, and Bell's palsy. Examination of the cerebrospinal fluid may show a lymphocytic pleocytosis. Intrathecal production of IgG directed against *B. burgdorferi* can be shown in some patients.

Stage III: Arthritis is the hallmark of stage III Lyme disease. The large joints are generally involved (knees, hips, etc). Joint symptoms begin from several days to over 2 years after the erythema chronicum migrans rash.

Diagnosis Lyme disease is a clinical diagnosis, not a laboratory diagnosis. Laboratory tests are not standardized and **never** should be used alone. Laboratory results should be used to support a clinical diagnosis.

Diagnostic Tests/Procedures

Lyme (*Borrelia*) C6 Peptide Immunoassay *on page 527*
Lyme Disease Serology *on page 527*
Lyme Disease Serology by Western Blot *on page 528*
Polymerase Chain Reaction *on page 567*

Treatment The treatment for Lyme disease depends in large part on the stage of the disease.

- Erythema chronicum migrans: Amoxicillin or doxycycline are the drugs of choice.
- Carditis: Ceftriaxone (penicillin or cefotaxime as alternatives)
- Neurologic: Ceftriaxone (penicillin or cefotaxime as alternatives)
- Arthritis: Ceftriaxone (penicillin or cefotaxime as alternatives)

Pediatric Drug Therapy

Recommended:

Ceftriaxone *on page 722*

Alternate:

Ampicillin *on page 657*
Penicillin G (Parenteral/Aqueous) *on page 993*
Cefotaxime *on page 708*
Cefuroxime *on page 725*

Adult Drug Therapy

Recommended:

Ceftriaxone *on page 722*
Doxycycline *on page 787*
Amoxicillin *on page 642*

Alternate:

Ampicillin *on page 657*
Penicillin G (Parenteral/Aqueous) *on page 993*
Cefuroxime *on page 725*
Cefotaxime *on page 708*

Selected Readings

Evans J, "Lyme Disease," *Curr Opin Rheumatol*, 1998, 10(4):339-46.

(Continued)

Borrelia burgdorferi (Continued)

Haass A, "Lyme Neuroborreliosis," *Curr Opin Neurol*, 1998, 11(3):253-8.
Hathaway LR, "Patient Education Series. Lyme Disease," *Nursing*, 2005, 35(4):44-5.
Hayes E and Mead P, "Lyme Disease," *Clin Evid*, 2004, (12):1115-24.
Liang FT, Steere AC, Marques AR, et al, "Sensitive and Specific Serodiagnosis of Lyme Disease by Enzyme-Linked Immunosorbent Assay With a Peptide Based on an Immunodominant Conserved Region of *Borrelia burgdorferi* vlsE," *J Clin Microbiol*, 1999, 37(12):3990-6.
Marques AR, Martin DS, and Philipp MT, "Evaluation of the C6 Peptide Enzyme-Linked Immunosorbent Assay for Individuals Vaccinated With the Recombinant OspA Vaccine," *J Clin Microbiol*, 2002, 40(7):2591-3.
Nadelman RB and Wormser GP, "Lyme Borreliosis," *Lancet*, 1998, 352(9127):557-65.
Schmidt BL, "PCR in Laboratory Diagnosis of Human *Borrelia burgdorferi* Infections," *Clin Microbiol Rev*, 1997, 10(1):185-201.
Sigal LH, "Musculoskeletal Manifestations of Lyme Arthritis," *Rheum Dis Clin North Am*, 1998, 24(2):323-51.
"Treatment of Lyme Disease," *Med Lett Drugs Ther*, 2005, 47(1209):41-3.
Wormser GP, Nadelman RB, Dattwyler RJ, et al, "Practice Guidelines for the Treatment of Lyme Disease. The Infectious Diseases Society of America," *Clin Infect Dis*, 2000, 31(Suppl 1):1-14.

Botulism *see Clostridium botulinum on page 83*

Bowel Perforation *see* Peritonitis, Secondary *on page 263*

Brain Abscess

Synonyms Abscess, Brain

Clinical Presentation Brain abscess is an uncommon, serious, life-threatening infection. May originate from a contiguous site of infection (eg, chronic otitis media, mastoiditis, sinusitis, dental infections), from hematogenous spread or trauma, or cryptogenic. Occurs more frequently in males and mid-age. Twenty-five percent of cases occur in children <15 years of age. Occurs more frequently in children with a history of cyanotic congenital heart disease. Signs and symptoms vary depending on the size and location of the abscess. Moderate-to-severe headache, frequently hemicranial is the most common complaint. Altered mental status, fever, focal neurological deficits, nausea, and vomiting occur in approximately 50% of the cases. Papilledema, nuchal rigidity, and seizures occur in 25% to 35% of the cases. Children are more likely to experience fever. Duration of symptoms is usually 2 weeks prior to diagnosis. Frontal lobe abscesses are more likely to present with headache, drowsiness, and altered mental status, whereas cerebellar abscesses are more likely to present with ataxia, nystagmus, dysmetria, and vomiting. May have leukocytosis and elevated sedimentation rate. A lumbar puncture is contraindicated due to its poor diagnostic yield and significant morbidity (eg, potential for herniation).

Differential Diagnosis Subdural empyema, epidural abscess, pyogenic meningitis, neoplasm, viral encephalitis, hemorrhagic leukoencephalopathy, CNS vasculitis, infarction, mycotic aneurysm, subdural hematoma

Likely Pathogens

Non-AIDS:

Streptococcus, Viridans Group *on page 326*
Staphylococcus aureus, Methicillin-Resistant *on page 304*
Staphylococcus aureus, Methicillin-Susceptible *on page 307*
Streptococcus pneumoniae, Drug-Susceptible *on page 319*
Gram-negative rods and/or polymicrobial infections more common postoperatively or secondary to trauma.

Immunocompromised hosts without AIDS:

Pseudomonas aeruginosa on page 282
Nocardia Species *on page 247*
Mycobacterium kansasii on page 231
Mycobacterium tuberculosis on page 234
Mycobacterium Species, not MTB or MAI *on page 232*
Mycobacterium avium-intracellulare (Complex) *on page 228*

AIDS: The most common cause of a CNS mass lesion:

Toxoplasma gondii on page 331
Trypanosoma cruzi on page 341
Other etiologies include CNS lymphoma; progressive multifocal leukoencephalopathy; HIV encephalopathy; fungal, mycobacterial, viral, other malignancies

Diagnostic Tests/Procedures

Computed Transaxial Tomography, Appropriate Site *on page 424*
Electroencephalography *on page 447*
Magnetic Resonance Scan, Brain *on page 532*

Drug Therapy Comment Antimicrobials used should have acceptable penetration into brain abscess. Penicillins, cephalosporins, and vancomycin have reasonable penetration into the CSF with inflamed meninges. Chloramphenicol, metronidazole, and sulfonamides penetrate well, with or without inflammation. This information may be moot because alteration of blood-brain barrier occurs in abscess, and brain tissue

levels have not been extensively studied. With increasing incidence of penicillin-resistant *Pneumococcus* and MRSA, vancomycin should be considered as part of initial therapy.

Empiric Drug Therapy

Recommended: Note: In immunocompetent patients, empiric therapy is based on predisposing condition.

Bacterial endocarditis:

Vancomycin *on page 1144*
plus
Gentamicin *on page 841*
Nafcillin *on page 955*
plus
Ampicillin *on page 657*
plus
Gentamicin *on page 841*

Congenital heart disease:

Cephalosporins, 3rd Generation *on page 730*

Dental sepsis:

Penicillin G (Parenteral/Aqueous) *on page 993*
plus
Metronidazole *on page 940*

Lung abscess, empyema, bronchiectasis:

Penicillin G (Parenteral/Aqueous) *on page 993*
plus
Metronidazole *on page 940*
plus (if Nocardia suspected)
Sulfamethoxazole and Trimethoprim *on page 1087*

Otitis media, mastoiditis, or sinusitis:

Cephalosporins, 3rd Generation *on page 730*
plus
Metronidazole *on page 940*
plus (if Staphylococcus aureus suspected)
Vancomycin *on page 1144*

Penetrating trauma or postneurosurgical:

Cephalosporins, 3rd Generation *on page 730*
plus
Vancomycin *on page 1144*

Unknown:

Cephalosporins, 3rd Generation *on page 730*
plus
Vancomycin *on page 1144*
plus
Metronidazole *on page 940*

AIDS patients:

The following 3 used in combination
Pyrimethamine *on page 1025*
SulfaDIAZINE *on page 1083*
Folinic Acid
The following 3 used in combination
Pyrimethamine *on page 1025*
Clindamycin *on page 752*
Folinic Acid

Selected Readings

Falcone S and Post MJ, "Encephalitis, Cerebritis, and Brain Abscess: Pathophysiology and Imaging Findings," *Neuroimaging Clin N Am*, 2000, 10(2):333-53.

Gupta RK, Vatsal DK, Husain N, et al, "Differentiation of Tuberculous From Pyogenic Brain Abscesses With *In Vivo* Proton MR Spectroscopy and Magnetization Transfer MR Imaging," *AJNR Am J Neuroradiol*, 2001, 22(8):1503-9.

Jansson AK, Enblad P, and Sjolin J, "Efficacy and Safety of Cefotaxime in Combination With Metronidazole for Empirical Treatment of Brain Abscess in Clinical Practice: A Retrospective Study of 66 Consecutive Cases," *Eur J Clin Microbiol Infect Dis*, 2004, 23(1):7-14.

Mathisen GE and Johnson JP, "Brain Abscess," *Clin Infect Dis*, 1997, 25(4):763-79.

Principles and Practice of Infectious Diseases, 6th ed, Mandell GL, Bennett JE, Dolin R, eds, New York, NY: Churchill Livingstone, 2005, 1158.

Xiao F, Tseng MY, Teng LJ, et al, "Brain Abscess: Clinical Experience and Analysis of Prognostic Factors," *Surg Neurol*, 2005, 63(5):442-9.

Branhamella catarrhalis *see Moraxella catarrhalis on page 223*

Breakbone Fever *see* Dengue Virus *on page 113*

Breast Infection *see* Mastitis *on page 214*

Bronchitis

Synonyms Tracheobronchitis

Clinical Presentation Chronic bronchitis may be present in as many as 15% of all adults. Characterized by cough, hypersecretion of mucus, and expectoration of sputum for at least 3 months of the year for more than 2 consecutive years. Acute exacerbations may be either bacterial or viral. Bacterial exacerbations are characterized by increased frequency and severity of cough, increased sputum production, purulent sputum, chest discomfort and congestion, dyspnea, and wheezing. Acute bacterial exacerbation in chronic bronchitis is the most common cause of hemoptysis. Patients may experience loss of appetite and feelings of fever and chills; however, true fever, rigors, or pleuritic pain suggest pneumonia. Physical exam may be misleading as some patients with chronic bronchitis always have abnormal breath sounds, and it is helpful to know patient's baseline lung exam.

Differential Diagnosis Chronic bronchitis; chronic obstructive pulmonary disease; emphysema; pneumonia; acute bronchitis

Likely Pathogens

Influenza Virus *on page 193*
Respiratory Syncytial Virus *on page 285*
Adenovirus *on page 29*
Parainfluenza Virus *on page 254*
Streptococcus pneumoniae, Drug-Susceptible *on page 319*
Haemophilus influenzae on page 159
Moraxella catarrhalis on page 223
Bordetella pertussis on page 53
Mycoplasma pneumoniae on page 238
Chlamydophila pneumoniae on page 78

Diagnostic Tests/Procedures

Aerobic Culture, Sputum *on page 367*
Gram Stain *on page 473*

Drug Therapy Comment The majority of acute bronchitis cases may be attributed to viral etiologies in which antibiotic therapy is not indicated. Treatment of adults with nonspecific upper respiratory tract infection does not enhance illness resolution and is not recommended. For severe exacerbations of bronchitis in hospitalized patients, intravenous forms of antimicrobial therapy should be used. For mild-to-moderate recurrent episodes, the various recommended oral antibiotics may be cycled. Symptomatic therapy should be initiated, such as cough suppressants and analgesics. Routine antibiotic treatment of uncomplicated acute bronchitis is not recommended. Patients with bronchial hyper-reactivity may benefit from bronchodilator therapy. Patients with influenza may benefit from neuraminidase inhibitors if initiated within 48 hours of symptom onset.

Empiric Drug Therapy

Recommended:

Note: Empiric therapy is recommended only in persons in whom therapy is warranted (symptoms >7 days; accompanying purulent discharge or localizing features may be considered).

Amoxicillin *on page 642*
Amoxicillin and Clavulanate Potassium *on page 645*
Cephalosporins, 2nd Generation *on page 729*
Sulfamethoxazole and Trimethoprim *on page 1087*
Doxycycline *on page 787*
Erythromycin *on page 807*
Azithromycin *on page 674*
Clarithromycin *on page 749*

Alternate:

Fluoroquinolones *on page 824*

Selected Readings

Bent S, Saint S, Vittinghoff E, et al, "Antibiotics in Acute Bronchitis: A Meta-analysis," *Am J Med*, 1999, 107(1):62-7.

Brunton S, Carmichael BP, Colgan R, et al, "Acute Exacerbation of Chronic Bronchitis: A Primary Care Consensus Guideline," *Am J Manag Care*, 2004, 10(10):689-96.

Evans AT, Husain S, Durairaj L, et al, "Azithromycin for Acute Bronchitis: A Randomised, Double-Blind, Controlled Trial," *Lancet*, 2002, 359(9318):1648-54.

Gonzales R, Bartlett JG, Besser RE, et al, "Principles of Appropriate Antibiotic Use for Treatment of Uncomplicated Acute Bronchitis: Background," *Ann Intern Med*, 2001, 134(6):521-9.

Macfarlane J, Holmes W, Gard P, et al, "Reducing Antibiotic Use for Acute Bronchitis in Primary Care: Blinded, Randomised Controlled Trial of Patient Information Leaflet," *BMJ*, 2002, 324(7329):91-4.

Stockley RA, O'Brien C, Pye A, et al, "Relationship of Sputum Color to Nature and Outpatient Management of Acute Exacerbations of COPD," *Chest*, 2000, 117(6):1638-45.

Brucella Species

Related Information

Clinical Syndromes Associated With Foodborne Diseases *on page 1276*

Microbiology *Brucella* species are small, aerobic, gram-negative coccobacilli which primarily cause disease in domestic animals. There are four species which cause human disease:

- *B. abortus* (cattle)
- *B. melitensis* (goats and sheep)
- *B. suis* (swine)
- *B. canis* (dogs)

The organism is nonmotile and does not form spores. All species tend to be slow-growing and fastidious. Supplemental carbon dioxide is required for optimal growth of *B. abortus*. The cell walls of *B. abortus*, *B. suis*, and *B. melitensis* contain endotoxin and two major surface antigens (A and M). The endotoxin is structurally and biologically different from endotoxins produced by many other enteric gram-negative bacilli.

Epidemiology Human brucellosis occurs worldwide. Approximately 500,000 cases are reported annually. The incidence has declined following mandatory pasteurization of dairy products and immunization of cattle with live-attenuated *Brucella abortus* vaccine. Endemic areas include the Mediterranean basin, South America, and Mexico. In the United States, more than half the cases of human brucellosis occur in Texas, California, Virginia, and Florida. A small number of cases (1% to 2%) are laboratory-acquired and result from exposure to *Brucella* in the clinical microbiology or research laboratory.

Transmission to humans occurs by one of three routes:

- Direct contact of infected tissue, blood, or lymph with broken skin or conjunctivae
- Ingestion of contaminated meat or dairy products
- Inhalation of infected aerosols

Clinical Syndromes *Brucella* species enter the human via breaks in the skin or mucous membranes or via inhalation. Normal human serum has good bactericidal activity against *B. abortus* but not *B. melitensis*. Organisms not killed by polymorphonuclear leukocytes travel to regional lymph nodes, then enter the circulation, and localize in organs of the reticuloendothelial system where they are ingested by macrophages. Some will survive intracellularly and multiply, but when the macrophage is activated, the intracellular organisms are killed and release endotoxin. The host response to endotoxin can result in the signs and symptoms of acute brucellosis.

The clinical manifestations depend on both the immune status of the patient and the species of *Brucella* involved.

- **Asymptomatic infection**
- **Acute brucellosis, or "Malta fever":** Acute symptoms appear 1 week to several months following exposure. Symptoms include fever, sweats, chills, weakness, malaise, headache, and anorexia. In 25% to 50% of cases, there is weight loss, myalgias, arthralgias, and back pain. Epididymis is common in some series. Splenomegaly occurs in 20% to 30% of cases and lymphadenopathy in 10% to 20%.

  A number of complications of acute brucellosis have been reported. When infection is present for more than 2 months without therapy, the complication rate can approach 30%.
- **Musculoskeletal:** Sacroiliitis, arthritis, osteomyelitis, paraspinal abscess
- **Neurologic:** Meningoencephalitis, myelitis, others
- **Genitourinary:** Epididymo-orchitis, prostatitis
- **Endocarditis**
- **Granulomatous hepatitis**
- **Caseating or noncaseating granulomatous disease**
- **Splenic abscess**
- **Nodular lung lesions; lung abscess**
- **Erythema nodosum; other skin manifestations**
- **Ocular lesions**
- **Localized disease:** Can occur in any of the sites listed above
- **Subclinical infection**

Diagnosis The clinician should suspect brucellosis in any individual presenting with fever and who has a history of travel to endemic areas; exposure to livestock; a history of consuming unpasteurized milk, cheese, or other dairy products; or suggestive occupational risk factors (veterinarians, laboratory workers, etc). Laboratory confirmation is essential since the signs and symptoms of human brucellosis may be nonspecific. The diagnosis is established by recovery of the organism from blood, fluid, or other tissues (bone, abscesses, etc). In patients with *B. melitensis* infections,

(Continued)

Brucella Species *(Continued)*

cultures of blood will be positive in 70% of cases. Bone marrow biopsy for histopathology and culture may be positive when other specimens are negative. In many laboratories, blood cultures for *Brucella* sp are processed using the Castañeda technique which utilizes biphasic media in a bottle. The Microbiology Laboratory should always be informed if *Brucella* sp are highly suspected.

Serologic techniques for diagnosing brucellosis include a standard tube agglutination test. A *Brucella* titer ≥1:160 or a fourfold rise in titer is considered presumptive evidence of recent infection with *Brucella* sp.

Diagnostic Tests/Procedures

Aerobic Culture, Appropriate Site *on page 365*
Blood Culture, *Brucella on page 394*
Gram Stain *on page 473*

Treatment The recommendation from the World Health Organization for the treatment of acute brucellosis is doxycycline 200 mg/day with rifampin 600-900 mg/day for 6 weeks. Longer courses may be required in severe infections or if focal suppurative complications are present. Single agent therapy with tetracycline, streptomycin, rifampin, or trimethoprim are associated with a high relapse rate. For relapsed infection or central nervous system infection, the suggested regimens are third generation cephalosporin and rifampin or tetracycline, streptomycin, and rifampin, in combination.

Pediatric Drug Therapy

Recommended:

Sulfamethoxazole and Trimethoprim *on page 1087*
plus
Gentamicin *on page 841*

Adult Drug Therapy

Recommended:

Doxycycline *on page 787*
plus
Rifampin *on page 1046*

Alternate:

Sulfamethoxazole and Trimethoprim *on page 1087*
plus
Gentamicin *on page 841*

Selected Readings

"Brucellosis Outbreak at a Pork Processing Plant - North Carolina, 1992," *MMWR*, 1994, 43(7):113-6.
Corbel MJ, "Brucellosis: An Overview," *Emerg Infect Dis*, 1997, 3(2):213-21.
"From the Centers for Disease Control and Prevention. Suspected Brucellosis Case Prompts Investigation of Possible Bioterrorism-Related Activity--New Hampshire and Massachusetts, 1999," *JAMA*, 2000, 284(3):300-2.
Hadjinikolaou L, Triposkiadis F, Zairis M, et al, "Successful Management of *Brucella melitensis* Endocarditis With Combined Medical and Surgical Approach," *Eur J Cardiothorac Surg*, 2001, 19(6):806-10.
Ko J and Splitter GA, "Molecular Host-Pathogen Interaction in Brucellosis: Current Understanding and Future Approaches to Vaccine Development for Mice and Humans," *Clin Microbiol Rev*, 2003, 16(1):65-78.
Mert A, Ozaras R, Tabak F, et al, "The Sensitivity and Specificity of *Brucella* Agglutination Tests," *Diagn Microbiol Infect Dis*, 2003, 46(4):241-3.
Reguera JM, Alarcon A, Miralles F, et al, "*Brucella* Endocarditis: Clinical, Diagnostic, and Therapeutic Approach," *Eur J Clin Microbiol Infect Dis*, 2003, 22(11):647-50.
Shehabi A, Shakir K, el Khateeb M, et al, "Diagnosis and Treatment of 106 Cases of Human Brucellosis," *J Infect*, 1990, 20(1):5-10.

Brucellosis *see Brucella* Species *on page 61*
Bubonic Plague *see Yersinia pestis on page 355*

Burkholderia cepacia

Related Information

Community-Acquired Pneumonia in Adults *on page 1278*

Microbiology The genus *Burkholderia* (formerly *Pseudomonas*) is composed of four species, *B. cepacia, B. galdioli, B. mallei*, and *B. pseudomallei. Burkholderia* spp are motile, gram-negative, nonspore-forming rods. *B. cepacia* is not difficult to grow and isolate in a clinical laboratory because the bacterium grows readily on most standard media. However, physicians should notify the laboratory whenever *B. cepacia* is suspected or whenever pulmonary specimens from cystic fibrosis (CF) patients are submitted for culture because *B. cepacia* can require up to 3 days of incubation before colonies of the bacterium are able to be observed on selective media, and technologists need to be especially aware of the potential presence of *B. cepacia*.

Epidemiology *Burkholderia* spp are found worldwide in water and soil, and on many plants, including vegetables and fruit. In agriculture, *B. cepacia* is most known for causing "slippery skin" rot in onions; in humans, *B. cepacia* is most known for being

an opportunistic nosocomial pathogen. *B. cepacia* was first described as an opportunistic pathogen in a cystic fibrosis patient in 1972. By the mid 1980s, up to 40% of patients who were attending cystic fibrosis clinics in the United States, Canada, and the United Kingdom were reported to be colonized with *B. cepacia*. In hospitals, *B. cepacia* has been found on equipment and in medications, lotions, and disinfectants. Highly efficient person-to-person transmission of certain molecular types of *B. cepacia* is well documented, especially among cystic fibrosis patients. This high efficiency of transmission is especially important because it occurs not only nosocomially but also in social settings such as cystic fibrosis support groups, conferences, and camps. Sadly, patients with documented *B. cepacia* colonization are often subjected to social isolation.

Clinical Syndromes

- ***Burkholderia cepacia***, in immunocompetent persons, can cause nosocomially-acquired septicemia, urinary tract infections, and respiratory tract infections. Such infections usually are not life-threatening in immunocompetent persons because *B. cepacia* is not especially virulent. However, in immunocompromised persons and persons with cystic fibrosis or chronic granulosis disease, pulmonary infections caused by *B. cepacia* can be fulminant and severe. In cystic fibrosis patients who have undergone lung transplants, *Burkholderia cepacia* can cause life-threatening pulmonary infections with a mortality rate as high as 80%.
- ***Burkholderia pseudomallei*** is the etiological agent of melioidosis, a disease with protean manifestations which range from asymptomatic infection to soft tissue abscesses to fulminant septicemia. Melioidosis is found mostly in southeast Asia and Australia.

Diagnosis In Gram-stained specimens, *Pseudomonas* spp and *Burkholderia cepacia* usually are not distinguishable. The suggestion of *B. cepacia* in a Gram-stained specimen or the growth of *B. cepacia* in culture is not automatically indicative of *B. cepacia* being an etiological agent of an infectious process. The Gram stain and culture information must be interpreted in the context of an appropriate clinical presentation (eg, cystic fibrosis or an association with a nosocomial setting). **Note:** The laboratory should be notified of the diagnosis when a pulmonary specimen (including sputum) is collected from a cystic fibrosis patient and submitted for culture.

Diagnostic Tests/Procedures

Aerobic Culture, Sputum *on page 367*
Gram Stain *on page 473*

Treatment Many strains of *B. cepacia* are resistant to multiple antibacterial agents, especially in the setting of patients with cystic fibrosis. The extended-spectrum penicillins, quinolones, carbapenems, third generation cephalosporins, tobramycin, sulfamethoxazole and trimethoprim, minocycline, and chloramphenicol have all shown activity against this organism. Susceptibility testing is imperative, especially in CF patients who have received multiple antimicrobial regimens and have exacerbations of their disease. These patients also have altered pharmacokinetics of many antibacterials including cephalosporins and aminoglycosides. This along with potentially higher MICs for infecting organisms often necessitates higher doses of standard therapies. Some authors suggest combination drug therapy that would show synergy, such as aminoglycoside/beta-lactam or ciprofloxacin/beta-lactam combinations. Other authors suggest that triple drug therapy, including an aminoglycoside and carbapenem, may be more effective than two drugs *in vitro*. There is also a suggestion that amiloride may be synergistic with tobramycin *in vitro*.

Drug Therapy

Recommended:

Tobramycin *on page 1122*
plus
Ceftazidime *on page 717*

Tobramycin *on page 1122*
plus
Penicillins, Extended-Spectrum *on page 997*

Ciprofloxacin *on page 742*
plus
Ceftazidime *on page 717*

Ciprofloxacin *on page 742*
plus
Penicillins, Extended-Spectrum *on page 997*

Alternate:

Carbapenems *on page 693*
Chloramphenicol *on page 733*
Ciprofloxacin *on page 742*
Minocycline *on page 947*
Sulfamethoxazole and Trimethoprim *on page 1087*

(Continued)

Burkholderia cepacia (Continued)

Selected Readings

Aaron SD, Ferris W, Henry DA, et al, "Multiple Combination Bactericidal Antibiotic Testing for Patients With Cystic Fibrosis Infected With *Burkholderia cepacia*," *Am J Respir Crit Care Med*, 2000, 161(4 Pt 1):1206-12.

Gibson RL, Burns JL, and Ramsey BW, "Pathophysiology and Management of Pulmonary Infections in Cystic Fibrosis," *Am J Respir Crit Care Med*, 2003, 168(8):918-51.

LiPuma JJ, "*Burholderia cepacia*, Management Issues and New Insights," *Clin Chest Med*, 1998, 19(3):473-86.

Miller MB and Gilligan PH, "Laboratory Aspects of Management of Chronic Pulmonary Infections in Patients With Cystic Fibrosis," *J Clin Microbiol*, 2003, 41(9):4009-15.

Reed R, "Community-Acquired *Burkholderia cepacia* Sepsis in Children," *Clin Microbiol Newslett*, 1998, 20(17):147-8.

Vartivarian S and Anaissie E, "*Stenotrophomonas maltophilia* and *Burkholderia cepacia*," *Principles and Practice of Infectious Diseases*, 5th ed, Mandell GL, Bennett JE, and Dolin R, eds, New York, NY: Churchill Livingstone, 2000, 2335-9.

Burkholderia mallei

Microbiology The genus *Burkholderia* (formerly *Pseudomonas*) is composed of twenty-two species including *B. mallei* and *B. pseudomallei*. *Burkholderia* spp are motile, gram-negative, nonspore-forming rods. *B. mallei* is not difficult to grow and isolate in a clinical laboratory because the bacterium grows readily on most standard media. However, physicians should notify the laboratory whenever *B. mallei* is suspected.

Epidemiology *Burkholderia* spp are found worldwide in water and soil, and on many plants, including vegetables and fruit. This high efficiency of transmission is especially important because it occurs not only nosocomially but could be used as an agent for bioterrorism. ***B. mallei* is a category B agent of bioterrorism.** Humans and animals are believed to acquire the infection by inhalation of dust, ingestion of contaminated water, and contact with contaminated soil especially through skin abrasions, and for military troops, by contamination of war wounds. Person-to-person transmission can occur.

Clinical Syndromes

- **Melioidosis:** *Burkholderia pseudomallei* is the etiological agent of melioidosis, a disease with protean manifestations which range from asymptomatic infection to soft tissue abscesses to fulminant septicemia. Melioidosis is found mostly in southeast Asia and Australia.

Diagnosis In Gram-stained specimens, *Pseudomonas* spp and *Burkholderia* species usually are not distinguishable. The suggestion of *B. mallei* in a Gram-stained specimen or the growth of *B. mallei* in culture is not automatically indicative of *B. mallei* being an etiological agent of an infectious process. The Gram stain and culture information must be interpreted in the context of an appropriate clinical presentation (eg, cystic fibrosis or an association with a nosocomial setting).

Diagnostic Tests/Procedures

Aerobic Culture, Sputum *on page 367*
Gram Stain *on page 473*

Treatment Many strains of *B. mallei* are resistant to multiple antibacterial agents. The extended-spectrum penicillins, quinolones, carbapenems, third generation cephalosporins, tobramycin, sulfamethoxazole and trimethoprim, minocycline, and chloramphenicol have all shown activity against this organism. Potentially higher MICs for infecting organisms often necessitate higher doses of standard therapies. Some authors suggest combination drug therapy that would show synergy such as aminoglycoside/beta-lactam or ciprofloxacin/beta-lactam combinations. There is also suggestion that amiloride may be synergistic with tobramycin *in vitro*.

Drug Therapy

Recommended:

Imipenem and Cilastatin *on page 861*
Penicillins, Extended-Spectrum *on page 997*
Cephalosporins, 3rd Generation *on page 730*
plus
Sulfamethoxazole and Trimethoprim *on page 1087*

Alternate:

Chloramphenicol *on page 733*
Ciprofloxacin *on page 742*
Minocycline *on page 947*
Doxycycline *on page 787*
Sulfamethoxazole and Trimethoprim *on page 1087*

Selected Readings

Aldhous P, "Tropical Medicine: Melioidosis? Never heard of it," *Nature*, 2005, 434(7034):692-3.

Kenny DJ, Russell P, Rogers D, et al, "*In vitro* Susceptibilities of *Burkholderia mallei* in Comparison to Those of Other Pathogenic *Burkholderia spp*," *Antimicrob Agents Chemother*, 1999, 43(11):2773-5.

Leelarasamee A, "Recent Development in Melioidosis," *Curr Opin Infect Dis*, 2004, 17(2):131-6.
White NJ, "Melioidosis," *Lancet*, 2003, 361(9370):1715-22.

Calymmatobacterium granulomatis

Related Information

Treatment of Sexually Transmitted Infections *on page 1311*

Microbiology *Calymmatobacterium granulomatis* is the causative agent of granuloma inguinale, a sexually transmitted disease. The organism is an encapsulated gram-negative bacillus found within vacuoles of large histiocytic cells. The bacteria multiply within these vacuoles (about 30 organisms per vacuole), mature, and eventually rupture the cell.

Epidemiology Granuloma inguinale, also referred to as donovanosis, is quite rare in the United States, but in many developing countries, it is one of the most prevalent sexually transmitted diseases. Granuloma inguinale is common in India, the Caribbean, and Africa. In 1984, an outbreak of 20 cases was recognized in Texas (Rosen et al). The epidemiology and pathogenesis of donovanosis in the United States (and endemic countries as well) are poorly characterized. The precise role of sexual transmission is unclear, but repeated anal intercourse appears to be a risk factor for rectal and penile lesions in homosexual couples. Available data suggest that the infection is only mildly contagious and repeated exposures to an infected partner are necessary for transmission.

Clinical Syndromes

- **Granuloma inguinale**: The major disease associated with *Calymmatobacterium granulomatis* is granuloma inguinale, an infection characterized by genital ulceration and regional lymphadenopathy. As such, it must be differentiated from other classic STDs which can cause genital ulceration with regional adenopathy, such as primary syphilis, genital herpes simplex virus, chancroid, and lymphogranuloma venereum.
- **Genital ulcers:** The incubation period for granuloma inguinale varies from 8-80 days. Genital lesions initially appear as subcutaneous nodules (either single or multiple) which later erode. The ulcerations that form above the nodules are painless, clean, granulomatous, and often "beefy-red" with occasional contact bleeding. The lesions are most common on the glans or prepuce of the male and labial area in the female. The ulcers progressively enlarge in a chronic, destructive fashion. The ulcerations of donovanosis may be misidentified as carcinoma of the penis, chancroid, condyloma lata of secondary syphilis (when perianal lesions are present), and others.
- **Inguinal enlargement:** Infection with *Calymmatobacterium granulomatis* does not produce true regional lymphadenopathy. Instead, the granulomatous process in the genitals may extend into the inguinal region causing further fibrosis and granulation tissue, termed "pseudobuboes." These are present in only 10% of patients with donovanosis and are variably painful.
- **Constitutional symptoms:** In most cases of granuloma inguinale, constitutional symptoms are usually absent.

Diagnosis The diagnosis of granuloma inguinale can be confirmed by finding the characteristic **"Donovan bodies"** in a crush preparation. Fresh granulation tissue from a genital ulcer is spread over a clean microscope slide, air-dried, and stained with Wright or Giemsa stain. "Donovan bodies" are multiple, darkly-staining intracytoplasmic bacteria (*Calymmatobacterium granulomatis*) found within the vacuoles of large mononuclear cells. Donovan bodies can also be identified in formal biopsy specimens using standard light microscopy.

Treatment Granuloma inguinale responds well to the following first-line oral antibiotics (used singly): doxycycline 100 mg orally twice daily or sulfamethoxazole and trimethoprim (Bactrim™ DS) one tablet twice daily. Antibiotics are continued until the lesions are completely healed, usually 21 days or more; shorter courses are associated with relapses. Alternative therapies include ciprofloxacin 750 mg orally twice daily for a minimum of 3 weeks, or erythromycin base 500 mg orally 4 times/day for a minimum of 3 weeks. In pregnancy, erythromycin 500 mg orally 4 times/day is recommended. The treatment for HIV-infected individuals with granuloma inguinale is the same. An aminoglycoside may be added for severe lesions.

Drug Therapy

Recommended:

Sulfamethoxazole and Trimethoprim *on page 1087*
Doxycycline *on page 787*

Alternate:

Erythromycin *on page 807*
Ciprofloxacin *on page 742*

Selected Readings

Holmes KK, "Donovanosis (Granuloma Inguinale)," *Harrison's Principles of Internal Medicine*, 13th ed, Isselbacher KJ, Braunwald E, Wilson JD, et al, eds, New York, NY: McGraw-Hill, 1994, 694-5.

(Continued)

Calymmatobacterium granulomatis (Continued)

Krockta WP and Barnes RC, "Sexually Transmitted Diseases. Genital Ulceration With Regional Adenopathy," *Infect Dis Clin North Am*, 1987, 1(1):217-33.

Rosen T, Tschen JA, Ramsdell W, et al, "Granuloma Inguinale," *J Am Acad Dermatol*, 1984, 11(3):433-7.

"1998 Guidelines for Treatment of Sexually Transmitted Diseases. Centers for Disease Control and Prevention," *MMWR*, 1998, 47(RR-1):1-111.

Campylobacter jejuni

Related Information

Clinical Syndromes Associated With Foodborne Diseases *on page 1276*

Microbiology *Campylobacter jejuni* is a curved, gram-negative bacillus which is the most common cause of bacterial diarrhea in the United States. On Gram stain, *Campylobacter jejuni* appears as a curved, comma-shaped, gram-negative rod which often has a distinctive "seagull wing" appearance.

Campylobacter jejuni is a microaerophilic organism and fails to grow under routine aerobic and anaerobic conditions. The laboratory should be informed that *C. jejuni* is suspected clinically and a special request made for *Campylobacter* culture. A 5% to 10% oxygen, 5% to 10% carbon dioxide, and 80% to 90% nitrogen atmosphere is generally used to facilitate growth.

Epidemiology Infection with this agent occurs worldwide. With over 2 million cases per year in the U.S., *Campylobacter*-induced enteritis is more common than *Salmonella* and *Shigella* combined. The organism is found in the gastrointestinal flora of a number of wild and domestic animals, most notably in chickens. Transmission to humans generally occurs by consumption of the meat or milk of an infected animal, consumption of water contaminated with the feces of infected animals (eg, mountain streams), or fecal-oral transmission from an infected human or household pet. Undercooked chicken is notorious for transmission of *C. jejuni*, accounting for >50% of the cases of campylobacteriosis. Outbreaks have been linked to unpasteurized goat's cheese, clams, and untreated stream water in Wyoming. Infection occurs year round but is most common in the summer months.

Clinical Syndromes

- **Acute enteritis:** The organism can cause destructive, ulcerative changes in the mucosal surfaces of the small intestine (especially jejunum and distal ileum) and colon. Invasion of the organism causes inflammation of the lamina propria, bowel wall edema, and crypt abscesses. Patients initially present with nonspecific symptoms such as fever, headache, and myalgias. One to 2 days later, there is crampy abdominal pain and diarrhea. The quality and severity of the diarrhea is variable (although usually mild), and stools may be frequent and watery or visibly bloody. Most cases resolve spontaneously without antimicrobial therapy within 1 week. Less commonly, a fulminant acute colitis may occur. Again, a nonspecific prodrome of fever and malaise precedes any gastrointestinal complaints. However, the diarrhea which follows is voluminous and bloody with large amounts of mucous. Tenesmus is common and further suggests involvement of the colon. Fevers can reach 40°C, and occasionally the patient can appear in extremis. This syndrome may be confused with bacillary dysentery from *Shigella* species, severe salmonellosis, or even the initial presentation of inflammatory bowel disease (particularly if it is in a young adult). Toxic megacolon may complicate the hospital course.
- **Appendicitis-like syndrome:** Occasionally, *C. jejuni* can cause right lower quadrant pain mimicking appendicitis, without diarrhea. This "pseudoappendicitis" has been seen in association with other enteric pathogens including *Yersinia enterocolitica*.
- **Bacteremia:** This is an unusual finding in *C. jejuni* infection (even when the patient is febrile), unlike *Campylobacter fetus* which is commonly recovered from the blood. Blood cultures may turn positive several days after a mild diarrheal illness has already resolved; in such cases, antibiotic therapy is usually unnecessary. In other cases, bacteremia may be sustained, particularly in immunocompromised hosts, and this may suggest a deep focus of infection. Consultation with an Infectious Disease specialist is appropriate in such cases since prolonged antimicrobial therapy may be necessary.
- **Septic abortion:** *C. jejuni* infection in the pregnant female may lead to this complication. However, *Campylobacter* bacteremia during pregnancy does not automatically justify a therapeutic abortion since the outcome is not uniformly poor.
- **Reactive arthritis:** Following *Campylobacter* enteritis, a reactive arthritis may be seen, particularly in patients who are HLA-B27 positive.
- **Miscellaneous:** Guillain-Barré syndrome, hepatitis, and the hemolytic-uremic syndrome have been associated with *C. jejuni*.

Diagnosis *Campylobacter jejuni* should be suspected in any case of acute gastroenteritis or fulminant colitis. The findings of fecal leukocytes and occult blood in the stool is suggestive of campylobacteriosis and other gastrointestinal infections such as

those caused by *Salmonella* sp, *Shigella* sp, enteroinvasive *E. coli*, enterohemorrhagic *E. coli* (O157:H7), Crohn's disease or ulcerative colitis, and others. The diagnosis is confirmed by a positive stool culture for *C. jejuni* or positive blood cultures for the organism.

Diagnostic Tests/Procedures

Blood Culture, Aerobic and Anaerobic *on page 391*

Stool Culture *on page 585*

Treatment The organism is sensitive *in vitro* to many common antimicrobial agents including erythromycin, ciprofloxacin, tetracyclines, aminoglycosides, and others. Ampicillin or penicillin should usually be avoided, and the susceptibility to sulfamethoxazole and trimethoprim is variable. Most patients with *Campylobacter* enteritis do not require antibiotics; they recover quickly without sequelae. Antimicrobial therapy should be targeted towards the more acutely ill patient. Limited clinical trials suggest that the following groups may benefit from the prompt use of antibiotics: children with severe dysentery, adults with severe bloody diarrhea and fever, individuals with worsening symptoms when seeking medical attention, and prolonged diarrhea (more than 1 week). Treatment with antibiotics does not prolong the fecal carriage of *C. jejuni* (as opposed to *Salmonella*). The drug of choice is erythromycin. For the toxic patient, combination therapy may be useful, but consultation should be made with an Infectious Disease specialist.

Drug Therapy

Recommended:

Erythromycin *on page 807*

Doxycycline *on page 787*

Alternate:

Fluoroquinolones *on page 824*

Selected Readings

Blaser MJ, "*Campylobacter* and Related Species," *Principles and Practice of Infectious Diseases*, 4th ed, Mandell GL, Bennett JE, and Dolin R, eds, New York, NY: Churchill Livingstone, 1995, 1948-56.

Blaser MJ, Wells JG, Feldman RA, et al, "*Campylobacter* enteritis in the United States. A Multicenter Study," *Ann Intern Med*, 1983, 98(3):360-5.

Johnson RJ, Nolan C, Wang SP, et al, "Persistent *Campylobacter jejuni* Infection in an Immunocompromised Patient," *Ann Intern Med*, 1984, 100(6):832-4.

Peterson MC, Farr RW, and Castiglia M, "Prosthetic Hip Infection and Bacteremia Due to *Campylobacter jejuni* in a Patient With AIDS," *Clin Infect Dis*, 1993, 16(3):439-40.

Sorvillo FJ, Lieb LE, and Waterman SH, "Incidence of Campylobacteriosis Among Patients With AIDS in Los Angeles County," *J Acquir Immune Defic Syndr*, 1991, 4(6):598-602.

Campylobacter pylori *see Helicobacter pylori on page 162*

Candida Species

Related Information

Treatment of Sexually Transmitted Infections *on page 1311*

USPHS / IDSA Guidelines for the Prevention of Opportunistic Infections in Persons Infected With HIV *on page 1237*

Microbiology *Candida* species are normal host saprophyte yeasts found commonly in the gastrointestinal tract, genitourinary tract, and oropharynx. On direct mounts of infected material, they appear as small, oval, thin-walled, budding cells 2-5 μm in diameter with or without the presence of pseudohyphae. They stain gram-positive.

C. albicans is identified by the ability to produce germ tubes and/or chlamydospores in cornmeal agar. All *Candida* species may be identified to species by sugar fermentation and assimilation tests.

Epidemiology *Candida* species are found worldwide. Seventy percent of nosocomial candidal infections are due to *Candida albicans*. The other 30% are due to *C. glabrata*, *C. guilliermondii*, *C. krusei*, *C. pseudotropicalis*, *C. stellatoidea*, and *C. tropicalis*. According to the National Nosocomial Infections Surveillance System, *Candida* is now the fifth most common blood pathogen isolated from hospitalized patients and the fourth most common in ICU patients.

Risk factors for candidiasis include age extremes, central venous catheters, TPN, burns, exogenous hormone therapy, prosthetic devices, malnourishment, metabolic disease, concurrent infections with other pathogens, antibiotic therapy, uncontrolled diabetes mellitus, GI surgery, AIDS, mechanical disruption of epithelial surfaces, and physiological impairment of epithelial barrier function.

Clinical Syndromes

- **Cutaneous:** Intertriginous infection occurs most commonly in diabetes and obesity. Patients present with pain, burning, and/or itching. Skin appears uniformly erythematous and inflamed with small papules and pustules. Satellites distal to the border of the lesion may be present. Follicular candidiasis usually occurs in areas that are occluded (ie, under bandages). Paronychial infection is characterized by swelling, tenderness, and redness around the nail.

(Continued)

Candida Species *(Continued)*

- **Oral candidiasis:** Early premonitory sign of HIV. Presents as pseudomembranous, hyperplastic, atrophic, or angular cheilitis. Most commonly appears as erythematous patches with white discharge on the buccal mucosa with complaints of burning. The most efficient and cost-effective method of diagnosis is direct microscopic detection of *Candida* in a scraped sample of the oral lesion.
- **Candiduria:** Significance and natural history of progression are not known. Colony count is not predictive of severity of infection or location. Treatment is based on clinical judgment of severity of illness and risk factors. Symptoms include nocturia, frequency, and dysuria. Candiduria is associated with urethritis, cystitis, and primary renal candidiasis.
- **Disseminated:** Requires pathological identification of organism (yeast) in tissues and growth of the yeast in culture. Thirty percent of patients with fungemia have endophthalmitis. Rarely occurs early postoperatively. It is indistinguishable from bacterial sepsis and can occur simultaneously with bacterial pathogens. Only 25% of patients with extensive invasive organ infection will have positive blood cultures. Mortality exceeds 80%. Ten percent to 13% will have cutaneous manifestations. Other foci include septic arthritis, osteomyelitis, pericarditis (especially status post-open heart surgery), suppurative phlebitis, and abscesses. Dissemination is likely if three or more colonized sites are present. *Candida* meningitis should be in the differential in patients with a history of intravenous drug abuse especially in the setting of HIV infection.
- **Vulvovaginitis:** Second most common cause of vaginal infections. Seventy-five percent of childbearing age women will acquire this infection, and 40% will have a second occurrence. Less than 5% will experience recurrent disease defined as more than four infections in a 12-month period. Eighty-five percent of occurrences are due to *C. albicans*. Associated with pregnancy, high estrogen oral contraceptives, uncontrolled diabetes mellitus, tight-fitting clothes, antibiotic therapy, dietary factors, intestinal colonization, and sexually-transmitted disease. The relationship between HIV infection and the risk of vulvovaginitis remains unclear. Human to human transmission is questionable, although male sexual partners may experience a transient rash, erythema, pruritus, or burning sensation of the penis minutes to hours after unprotected sexual intercourse. May cause balanitis. Present with marked itching, watery to cottage cheese thick discharge, vaginal erythema with adherent white discharge, dyspareunia, external dysuria, erythema, and swelling of labia and vulva with discrete pustulopapular peripheral lesions. Cervix appears normal. Symptoms exacerbate the week preceding menses with some relief once menstrual flow begins.

Diagnosis Diagnosis is dependent on visualization of budding yeast with or without pseudohypha and the presence of clinical symptoms. If wet mounts, KOH, or histological stains are negative, culture is needed. Direct staining (ie, fungal staining) of oral mucosal scrapings which show yeasts is diagnostic for thrush. Endophthalmitis is diagnosed by vitrectomy or anterior chamber aspiration (presumptive diagnosis by indirect fundoscopic exam). Serological tests such as nonspecific antigen tests vary in sensitivity and specificity. Serological detection of mannan, beta-1,3-glucan, and enolase are still investigational.

Diagnostic Tests/Procedures

Fungus Culture, Appropriate Site *on page 461*
Gram Stain *on page 473*
KOH Preparation *on page 513*
Skin Biopsy *on page 580*

Treatment Note: Antifungal susceptibility testing should be considered for all non-*Candida albicans* isolates from normally sterile specimens. Such isolates do not have predictable susceptibilities to common antifungal agents.

- **Cutaneous:** Requires drying. Nystatin powder or imidazole (butoconazole, clotrimazole, miconazole, tioconazole) powder. Topical steroids may be used to reduce inflammation for the first 5-7 days of therapy. Paronychia infections may require topical imidazole up to 3 months.
- **Oral candidiasis**: Nystatin 100,000 units 3-5 times/day for 14 days versus azoles topically (eg, clotrimazole troches) or orally (eg, fluconazole). Amphotericin products, voriconazole, or caspofungin may be considered for refractory cases. Micafungin has also recently been approved for the treatment of oral candidiasis.
- **Candiduria:** Remove predisposing factors such as Foley catheters. Asymptomatic patients probably do not require therapy. Symptomatic patients should be treated with fluconazole (200 mg/day for 7-14 days), amphotericin B, or oral flucytosine (flucytosine should not be used in patients with renal insufficiency; emergence of flucytosine resistance is not uncommon). Amphotericin bladder irrigation is rarely indicated.

- **Disseminated candidiasis:** Azoles (fluconazole, voriconazole), amphotericin B formulations, or caspofungin have all been used successfully in the treatment of disseminated candidiasis. With few exceptions, *Candida* species are susceptible to amphotericin B and caspofungin. Susceptibility testing should be performed for azoles particularly when considering the treatment of non-*Candida albicans*. For candidemia, therapy should continue for at least 2 weeks after the last positive culture. Amphotericin ± flucytosine should be administered for at least 4 weeks in the treatment of *Candida* meningitis. Although fluconazole penetrates the CNS, limited data is available on its use for this disease. *Candida* endophthalmitis should be treated aggressively. Amphotericin B ± flucytosine has been most commonly employed with fluconazole as an alternative. No data is available on the use of voriconazole for this syndrome. Intravitreal injections of amphotericin B may also be required.
- **Vulvovaginitis:** For uncomplicated vaginal candidiasis, short courses of topical agents including imidazoles, triazoles (such as nystatin), or oral fluconazole or itraconazole are quite effective, For complicated vaginal candidiasis, longer courses (at least 7 days of topical or two doses of fluconazole >2 hours apart) are required. For recurrent vaginitis, 2 weeks of topical followed by oral azole therapy for 6 months (various regimens) can be effective.

Drug Therapy

Recommended:

Amphotericin B (Conventional) *on page 650*
Fluconazole *on page 819*
Antifungal, Topical *on page 666*

Alternate:

Itraconazole *on page 895*
Ketoconazole *on page 903*
Amphotericin B (Lipid Complex) *on page 653*
Amphotericin B (Liposomal) *on page 655*
Caspofungin *on page 695*
Micafungin *on page 944*
Flucytosine *on page 822*
Voriconazole *on page 1151*

Selected Readings

Ally R, Schurmann D, Kreisel W, et al, "A Randomized, Double-Blind, Double-Dummy, Multicenter Trial of Voriconazole and Fluconazole in the Treatment of Esophageal Candidiasis in Immunocompromised Patients," *Clin Infect Dis*, 2001, 33(9):1447-54.

Arathoon EG, Gotuzzo E, Noriega LM, et al, "Randomized, Double-Blind, Multicenter Study of Caspofungin Versus Amphotericin B for Treatment of Oropharyngeal and Esophageal Candidiases," *Antimicrob Agents Chemother*, 2002, 46(2):451-7.

Casado JL, Quereda C, Oliva J, et al, "Candidal Meningitis in HIV-Infected Patients: Analysis of 14 Cases," *Clin Infect Dis*, 1997, 25(3):673-6.

Ellepola AN and Morrison CJ, "Laboratory Diagnosis of Invasive Candidiasis," *J Microbiol*, 2005, 43 Spec No:65-84.

Espinel-Ingroff A, "Clinical Relevance of Fungal Susceptibility Testing and Antifungal Resistance," *Microbiol Newslett*, 2000, 22(18):137-9.

Fichtenbaum CJ and Aberg JA, "Candidiasis and HIV," *A Textbook on HIV Disease From the University of California, San Francisco and the San Francisco General Hospital*, Peiperl L and Volberding P, eds, 2002, http://hivinsite.ucsf.edu/InSite.jsp?page=kb-05&doc=kb-050203.

Pappas PG, Rex JH, Sobel JD, et al, "Guidelines for Treatment of Candidiasis," *Clin Infect Dis*, 2004, 38(2):161-89.

Randhawa GK and Sharma G, "Echinocandins: A Promising New Antifungal Group," *Indian J Pharmacol*, 2004, 36(2):65-71.

Saiman L, "Neonatal Candidiasis," *Clin Microbiol Newslett*, 1998, 20(18):149-52.

Vazquez JA and Sobel JD, "Mucosal Candidiasis," *Infect Dis Clin North Am*, 2002, 16(4):793-820.

Candidiasis *see Candida* Species *on page 67*

CAP *see* Pneumonia, Community-Acquired *on page 270*

CAPD-Associated Peritonitis *see* Peritonitis, CAPD-Associated *on page 262*

Capnocytophaga Species

Synonyms DF-2

Microbiology *Capnocytophaga* is a thin, fusiform gram-negative rod. The long fusiform appearance of this organism is characteristic and helps to distinguish it from other gram-negative organisms. It is a pleomorphic organism and is facultatively anaerobic. There are three species that colonize the oral cavity of normal adults: *C. ochracea, C. sputigena, C. gingivalis.* Two species colonize the oral flora of dogs (the "dog bite" organism): *C. canimorsus* and *C. cynodegmi.* Growth of *Capnocytophaga* is supported by routine media such as blood agar. However, the organism may be fastidious and optimal growth requires 5% to 10% CO_2. The Microbiology Laboratory should be notified if *Capnocytophaga* is being considered (such as after a dog bite).

Epidemiology The species of *Capnocytophaga* that are part of the oral flora of adults have been recently recognized as a cause of disease in immunocompromised individuals, especially patients with neutropenia and mucositis. A wide spectrum of illness
(Continued)

Capnocytophaga Species *(Continued)*

has also been described in otherwise healthy individuals, mainly infections in the oral cavity but also keratoconjunctivitis, lung abscess, osteomyelitis, and others. Other species of *Capnocytophaga* are part of the oral flora of canines (and some other animals including cats). Serious human infections including sepsis have been well described following dog-bite injuries. Cases of *C. canimorsus* tend to occur in older men.

Clinical Syndromes

- **"Dog bite sepsis":** *C. canimorsus* has caused a fulminant, life-threatening infection after a dog bite injury in immunocompromised patients. Patients present with septic shock, disseminated intravascular coagulopathy, and local necrosis at the site of inoculation. Pneumonitis, meningitis, and endocarditis may occur. Most notably, fulminant disease occurs in patients who are asplenic. Other groups at risk for the sepsis syndrome include alcoholics and other immunocompromised individuals. Not all patients with sepsis have a history of a recent dog exposure. Rapid diagnosis is essential because there is a high fatality rate of this syndrome.
- **Localized infection following dog bites:** A mild form of *Capnocytophaga* infection can occur in both healthy and immunocompromised persons.
- **Sepsis in immunocompromised patients:** This can result from those *Capnocytophaga* species normally inhabiting the oral cavity of humans. Patients tend to be neutropenic and blood cultures are often positive. The portal of entry is presumed to be odontogenic or via defects in the oral mucosa especially in patients with mucositis.
- **Miscellaneous:** Wound infections, abdominal abscesses, lung disease, and others have been reported.

Diagnosis *Capnocytophaga* infection should be considered in any patient who has a dog bite injury, especially if the person is asplenic or otherwise immunocompromised. It should also be considered in neutropenic patients with fever. Laboratory confirmation is required and cultures of appropriate wound sites, blood, or other appropriate body fluids should be submitted.

Diagnostic Tests/Procedures

Aerobic Culture, Appropriate Site *on page 365*
Gram Stain *on page 473*
Wound Culture *on page 620*

Treatment Most isolates of *Capnocytophaga* are susceptible to penicillin and this is considered the antibiotic of choice. For asplenic patients with sepsis, consultation with an Infectious Disease specialist is strongly recommended. Recommended drug therapy in immunocompromised hosts includes clindamycin, erythromycin, ciprofloxacin, or imipenem.

Drug Therapy

Recommended:

Penicillin V Potassium *on page 998*

Alternate:

Amoxicillin and Clavulanate Potassium *on page 645*

Catheter-Associated Urinary Tract Infection *see* Urinary Tract Infection, Catheter-Associated *on page 345*

Catheter Infection, Intravascular

Synonyms Intravascular Catheter Infection; Line Sepsis

Clinical Presentation Catheter-related infection refers to an obvious sign of infection at the catheter site such as erythema, induration, or purulence. Catheter-related bacteremia refers to isolation of an organism in a catheter segment culture and in the peripheral blood without any clinical signs of sepsis. Less than 1% of patients go on to develop sepsis; however, if sepsis occurs, there is a 10% to 20% mortality rate. Use of triple-lumen central venous catheters coated with chlorhexidine and silver sulfadiazine appear to offer no benefit over uncoated catheters. For patients with removable peripheral or central venous catheters, the catheter should be removed and the tip sent for culture. Consider antibiotic lock therapy if device cannot be removed. All patients with infection due to *Candida* species should have the device removed and should receive antifungal therapy for 14 days after fungemia has cleared. For patients with tunneled or surgically implanted devices, it may be prudent to try to salvage the device and treat with antibiotics for 10-14 days for uncomplicated infections, due to coagulase-negative staphylococci, *Staphylococcus aureus*, or gram-negative bacilli. Complicated infections (eg, septic thrombosis, endocarditis, osteomyelitis) require antimicrobial therapy for 4-8 weeks.

Likely Pathogens

Staphylococcus aureus, Methicillin-Susceptible *on page 307*
Staphylococcus aureus, Methicillin-Resistant *on page 304*

Staphylococcus epidermidis, Methicillin-Susceptible *on page 310*
Gram-Negative Bacilli *on page 157*
Enterococcus Species *on page 134*
Candida Species *on page 67*

Diagnostic Tests/Procedures

- Blood Culture, Aerobic and Anaerobic *on page 391*
- Blood Culture, Fungus *on page 395*
- Gram Stain *on page 473*
- Intravenous Line Culture *on page 511*

Empiric Drug Therapy

Recommended:

Vancomycin *on page 1144*
plus one of the following
Cephalosporins, 3rd Generation *on page 730*
Penicillins, Extended-Spectrum *on page 997*

Alternate:

Cefazolin *on page 700*
Penicillins, Penicillinase-Resistant *on page 997*

Alternative for gram-negative coverage (in combination with vancomycin):
Fluoroquinolones *on page 824*

Selected Readings

Cook D, Randolph A, Kernerman P, et al, "Central Venous Catheter Replacement Strategies: A Systematic Review of the Literature," *Crit Care Med*, 1997, 25(8):1417-24.
Heard SO, Wagle M, Vijayakumar E, et al, "Influence of Triple-Lumen Central Venous Catheters Coated With Chlorhexidine and Silver Sulfadiazine on the Incidence of Catheter-Related Bacteremia," *Arch Intern Med*, 1998, 158(1):81-7.
Mermel LA, Farr BM, Sherertz RJ, et al, "Guidelines for the Management of Intravascular Catheter-Related Infections," *Clin Infect Dis*, 2001, 32(9):1249-72.
O'Grady NP, Alexander M, Dellinger EP, et al, "Guidelines for the Prevention of Intravascular Catheter-Related Infections. Centers for Disease Control and Prevention," *MMWR*, 2002, 51(RR-10):1-29.
Raad I, "Intravascular-Catheter-Related Infections," *Lancet*, 1998, 351(9106):893-8.
Rubin LG, Shih S, Shende A, et al, "Cure of Implantable Venous Port-Associated Bloodstream Infections in Pediatric Hematology-Oncology Patients Without Catheter Removal," *Clin Infect Dis*, 1999, 29(1):102-5.

Cat Scratch Disease *see* *Bartonella* Species *on page 48*

Cellulitis *see* Skin and Soft Tissue *on page 300*

Cervicitis

Synonyms Mucopurulent Cervicitis

Clinical Presentation The most common symptoms of cervicitis include purulent vaginal discharge, pelvic pain, backache, and/or urinary tract symptoms. Cervical inflammation may lead to cervical erosion/ulceration. Infectious cervicitis is a sexually transmitted disease, and may be caused by any of the implicated organisms (see Likely Pathogens).

Differential Diagnosis Although considerably less common, noninfectious cervicitis can be caused by local trauma, radiation, or malignancy.

Likely Pathogens

Chlamydia trachomatis on page 74
Neisseria gonorrhoeae on page 244
Human Papillomavirus *on page 191*

Note: See individual monographs for a discussion of specific organisms.

Diagnostic Tests/Procedures

Gram Stain *on page 473*
Genital Culture *on page 470*
Polymerase Chain Reaction *on page 567*
Trichomonas Preparation *on page 600*
To rule out concurrent syphilis:
VDRL, Cerebrospinal Fluid *on page 613*
RPR *on page 574*

Drug Therapy Comment Specific dosing of antibiotics: Ceftriaxone 125 mg I.M. as a single dose with doxycycline 100 mg twice daily for 7 days. Alternatively, azithromycin 1 g as a single dose may be used.

Note: An increase in fluoroquinolone-resistant *Neisseria gonorrhoeae* has been noted among homosexual men.

Empiric Drug Therapy

Recommended:

Suspected infectious cervicitis (Coverage for both *N. gonorrhoeae* and *Chlamydia* is recommended. Partners should also be treated):
Ceftriaxone *on page 722*
followed by

(Continued)

Cervicitis *(Continued)*

Doxycycline *on page 787*

or

Azithromycin *on page 674*

Alternate:

Ofloxacin *on page 977*

Chlamydia in pregnancy:

Erythromycin *on page 807*

Amoxicillin *on page 642*

Gonococcal treatment:

Oral route:

Cefixime *on page 707*

Penicillin-allergic:

Ciprofloxacin *on page 742*

Ofloxacin *on page 977*

Levofloxacin *on page 908*

Selected Readings

Centers for Disease Control and Prevention (CDC), "Sexually Transmitted Diseases Treatment Guidelines, 2002," *MMWR*, 51(RR-6):1-78.

Hollier LM and Workowski K, "Treatment of Sexually Transmitted Diseases in Women," *Obstet Gynecol Clin North Am*, 2003, 30(4):751-75.

"Increases in Fluoroquinolone-Resistant *Neisseria gonorrhoeae* Among Men Who Have Sex with Men - United States, 2003, and Revised Recommendations for Gonorrhea Treatment, 2004," *MMWR*, 2004, 53(16):335-338.

Cestodes

Synonyms Tapeworms

Microbiology Cestodes (tapeworms; segmented worms) are intestinal and tissue parasites of mammals and some fish and are found worldwide. Cestodes have complex life cycles which involve intermediate hosts, in which the worms develop into only a larvae, and definitive hosts, in which worms have sexual reproduction and develop into adults. Humans can serve as both kinds of hosts. Cestodes can be divided into two groups according to the common sites they infect in humans, intestinal and tissue cestodes (see table). Cestodes cause illness in humans in two stages of their life cycles, larvae and adults. If larvae are ingested, the larvae mature into adults which attach by their heads to the intestinal mucosa, grow, lay eggs, and usually produce only minimal damage and discomfort to the host. If eggs are ingested, stomach acid releases larvae from eggs, larvae migrate to specific organs, and encyst. Cysts can grow and damage surrounding tissue. The form of the cyst (cysticercus, coenurus, hydatid cyst, etc) depends on the type of cestode.

Cestodes

Cestode	Ingested Infectious Form and Source
Intestinal	
Diphyllobothrium latum	Larvae in freshwater fish
Taenia solium	Larvae in undercooked pork or eggs in soil or feces
Taenia saginata	Larvae in undercooked beef or eggs in soil or feces
Hymenolepis nana	Larvae in arthropods or eggs in human feces
Hymenolepis diminuta	Larvae in arthropods or eggs in human feces
Dipylidium caninum	Larvae in dog fleas
Tissue	
Echinococcus granulosus	Eggs in dog feces
Echinococcus multilocularis	Eggs in fox and cat feces
Spirometra mansonoides	Larvae in freshwater fish
Diphyllobothrium latum	Larvae in freshwater fish
Multiceps sp	Eggs in dog fleas

Epidemiology Cestodes are parasites of humans, wild animals, domestic animals, and fish. Cestodes and cestode diseases have been recognized since the time of Hippocrates and continue to occur worldwide. Infections occur almost invariably because of poor sanitation habits, carelessness, ingestion of poorly cooked meat, or letting infected animals lick oral membranes (eg, child being licked by dog or cat which has crushed infected fleas in its mouth).

Clinical Syndromes The presentation of someone infected with cestodes is astonishingly varied and includes but is not limited to the following: unusual "things" in stools, "uncomfortable" intestinal symptoms, change in mental status, abdominal cramps, "hunger pains", etc. In addition CNS symptoms (headache, hemiparesis, altered vision, seizures, etc) can suggest cystic disease.

Diagnosis Diagnosis is most commonly made by ova and parasite examination (for eggs and proglottids) of stool. Cystic disease is visualized best by CT or MRI of suspected infected organs (often, brain and liver). Sensitive and specific serological tests (enzyme immunoassay and Western blot) are available for detecting antibody to *Echinococcus*.

Diagnostic Tests/Procedures

Brain Biopsy *on page 405*
Computed Transaxial Tomography, Appropriate Site *on page 424*
Magnetic Resonance Scan, Brain *on page 532*
Ova and Parasites, Stool *on page 551*

Drug Therapy

Recommended:

Praziquantel *on page 1017*
Albendazole *on page 635*

Selected Readings

Garcia LS and Bruckner DA, *Diagnostic Medical Parasitology*, Washington DC: American Society for Microbiology, 1993, 266-301.
King CH, "Cestodes (Tapeworms)," *Principles and Practice of Infectious Diseases*, 4th ed, Mandell GL, Bennett JE, and Dolin R, eds, New York, NY: Churchill Livingstone, 1995, 2544-53.
Maddison SE, "Serodiagnosis of Parasitic Diseases," *Clin Microbiol Rev*, 1991, 4(4):457-69.

CFS *see* Chronic Fatigue Syndrome *on page 81*
Chagas' Disease *see Trypanosoma cruzi on page 341*
Chancroid *see Haemophilus ducreyi on page 158*
Chickenpox *see* Varicella-Zoster Virus *on page 347*
Chlamydia pneumoniae *see Chlamydophila pneumoniae on page 78*

Chlamydia psittaci

Microbiology *Chlamydia psittaci* is an obligate intracellular bacterium and is the causative agent of psittacosis, or parrot fever. In the past, *Chlamydia* was classified as a virus, in part because of its nature as a cellular parasite. However, the organism also has many bacteria-like characteristics and is now regarded as a specialized bacterium. *Chlamydia psittaci* is one of three distinct species within the genus *Chlamydia. Chlamydia pneumoniae* (also called *Chlamydia* TWAR) and *Chlamydia trachomatis*, the cause of trachoma (an eye infection) and a cause of urethritis, are the other two. All *Chlamydia* species are obligate parasites of eukaryotic cells and are unable to replicate extracellularly. *Chlamydia* species are unique in having two separate forms with separate functions; the elementary body (EB), which is well-suited for extracellular life but lacks the ability to replicate, and the reticulate body (RB), which is adapted to intracellular life and can divide by binary fission.

Epidemiology Infections from *C. psittaci* occur sporadically. Approximately 50 cases are reported annually in the United States, with 50% occurring in individuals who own pet birds. High risk groups include pigeon collectors, employees of pet shops, and veterinarians. Outbreaks of psittacosis have been reported in turkey processing plants. Psittacosis has been traditionally associated with psittacine birds such as parrots, and this group remains an important reservoir for infection. However, it is clear that many other bird species can act as reservoirs, such as pigeons, turkeys, canaries, cockatiels, ducks, and many others. *C. psittaci* can be harbored in several sites within an infected bird including the bloodstream, feathers, liver, spleen, and feces. The organisms remain viable for prolonged periods of time within bird excreta. Some infected birds appear only mildly ill (anorexia, diarrhea), and the sympathetic pet owner may deliberately increase the amount of physical contact and time spent with the bird. Transmission can take place by several routes such as inhalation of dried, infected bird feces (this appears to be the most common route of human infection), touching contaminated bird feathers, physical intimacy with a highly infected bird, and person-to-person spread (very rare).

Prolonged, intimate contact with an infected bird is not necessary for transmission. Cases have been reported following brief avian contact. Birds can also be infected but show no signs of clinical disease; viable organisms continue to be shed in the feces for weeks.

Clinical Syndromes

- **Psittacosis (parrot fever):** Infection occurs in two stages. In the first stage, the organisms enter the host via the respiratory tract and travel to the liver and spleen. The organisms replicate in these sites. In the second stage, the organisms disseminate via the bloodstream to various sites, especially the lungs. Patients present with the sudden onset of high fevers and a severe headache. The presence of a severe headache, although nonspecific, is important in suggesting psittacosis and is highly characteristic of this infection. A variable number of days into the illness, patients frequently develop a nonproductive cough which can be paroxysmal and severe. Other symptoms include chills, muscle aches, gastrointestinal upset, and

(Continued)

Chlamydia psittaci (Continued)

anorexia. On physical examination, the patient presentation can range from comfortable to acutely ill. As with other infections from intracellular pathogens, there may be a pulse-temperature dissociation (ie, the pulse is slow relative to the degree of fever). Lung examination usually shows localized inspiratory rales. Signs of lung consolidation can occur with severe disease. An important physical finding is the presence of hepatomegaly and/or splenomegaly which frequently develop in psittacosis. Routine laboratory studies are usually not helpful and Gram stain of sputum reveals no predominant microorganisms and few polymorphonuclear leukocytes. A variety of chest x-ray findings have been reported including a patchy interstitial lower lobe infiltrate (most common), a miliary pattern resembling tuberculosis, and occasionally a densely consolidated lobar pneumonia.

- **Endocarditis:** *C. psittaci* is a rare but reported cause of endocarditis. The diagnosis may be entertained in difficult cases of "culture-negative endocarditis" where multiple blood cultures properly collected are negative for pathogens. An Infectious Disease specialist may be useful in approaching this problem.

Diagnosis *Chlamydia pneumoniae* should be suspected in any case of atypical pneumonia, particularly if there is pharyngitis and hoarseness. The other diagnostic considerations for atypical pneumonia should include *Mycoplasma pneumoniae*, *Legionella* infections, viral lower respiratory infections, and others. The diagnosis can be confirmed primarily with serologic studies. The two major antigens which are used for antibody tests are lipopolysaccharide antigens and major outer membrane protein antigen. Lipopolysaccharide antigen, which is common to all members of the *Chlamydia* genus. This antigen is measured using complement fixation. Thus, positive studies are not specific for *C. pneumoniae* and can be positive during *C. trachomatis* and *C. psittaci*. Major outer membrane proteins (MOMPs), which are specific for the different species of *Chlamydia*. These proteins are the basis for microimmunofluorescence (MIF) studies.

There are two patterns of antibody response with chlamydial infections. Primary infection: Early, complement fixation antibody is positive; 10 days to 1 month, MIF IgM is positive; 6 weeks, IgG is positive. Secondary infection: Complement fixation antibody is negative; IgM is positive in low titer; IgG response is more prompt. *C. pneumoniae* also can be isolated in cell culture systems, but can be difficult. The organism grows in HeLa cell culture and identification has been enhanced by development of monoclonal antibodies specific for *C. pneumoniae*.

Diagnostic Tests/Procedures

Chlamydophila psittaci Serology *on page 417*

Treatment Large controlled studies comparing different antimicrobial agents have not been performed. Available data suggest that tetracycline and erythromycin are clinically effective. Failure with erythromycin have been reported. Therapy is usually continued for 10-14 days.

Pediatric Drug Therapy

Recommended:

Erythromycin *on page 807*

Adult Drug Therapy

Recommended:

Doxycycline *on page 787*

Alternate:

Erythromycin *on page 807*

Selected Readings

Barnes RC, "Laboratory Diagnosis of Human Chlamydial Infections," *Clin Microbiol Rev*, 1989, 2(2):119-36.

Kuritsky JN, Schmid GP, Potter ME, et al, "Psittacosis. A Diagnostic Challenge," *J Occup Med*, 1984, 26(10):731-3.

Potter ME, Kaufmann AK, and Plikaytis BD, "Psittacosis in the United States 1979," *MMWR CDC Surveill Summ*, 1983, 32(1):27SS-31SS.

Schlossberg D, "*Chlamydia psittaci* (Psittacosis)," *Principles and Practice of Infectious Diseases*, 4th ed, Mandell GL, Bennett JE, and Dolin R, eds, New York, NY: Churchill Livingstone, 1995, 1693-6.

Yung AP and Grayson ML, "Psittacosis - A Review of 135 Cases," *Med J Aust*, 1988, 148(5):228-33.

Chlamydia trachomatis

Related Information

Treatment of Sexually Transmitted Infections *on page 1311*

Microbiology *Chlamydia trachomatis* is a bacterium-like obligate intracellular organism. There are at least 15 recognized serotypes (immunotypes, serovars, biovars) of *C. trachomatis* which can be distinguished by immunofluorescent techniques. Certain serotypes are highly associated with disease syndromes. *C. trachomatis* types L1, L2, and L3 are found only in patients with the disease lymphogranuloma venereum; types A, B, B_a, and C are associated with trachoma, an infection of the eye and the most common preventable cause of blindness; and types D, E, F, G, H, I, J, and K are

associated with nongonococcal urethritis, pelvic inflammatory disease, mucopurulent cervicitis, and prostatitis.

C. trachomatis is closely related to two other species within the family Chlamydiaceae: *Chlamydophila psittaci* (the cause of psittacosis) and *Chlamydophila pneumoniae* (a cause of community-acquired tracheobronchitis and pneumonia). *Chlamydia* species are unique in having two separate forms with separate functions: the **elementary body (EB)**, which is well-suited for extracellular life but lacks the ability to replicate and the **reticulate body (RB)**, which is adapted to intracellular life and can divide by binary fission.

The life cycle of *Chlamydia trachomatis* is as follows:

1. Elementary bodies attach to the host cell,
2. EBs enter the cell by inducing their own phagocytosis,
3. EBs transform into larger reticulate bodies,
4. the RBs grow and replicate by binary fission within vacuoles; these vacuoles become filled with EBs and appear as inclusion bodies in the host cytoplasm,
5. vacuoles rupture and release infectious organisms, and the cycle begins again.

C. trachomatis is difficult to identify on a Gram stain. The Giemsa stain can be used for staining elementary bodies, reticulate bodies, and intracellular inclusion bodies but should not be trusted for definitive diagnosis.

Epidemiology Is specific for each disease state and clinical syndrome for which it is responsible. This information is included below.

Clinical Syndromes

Infections in Adults:

- **Nongonococcal urethritis (NGU) in men:** *Chlamydia trachomatis* accounts for about 50% of the cases of NGU. The organism is usually sexually acquired and is harbored in the urethra. About 25% of infected men are asymptomatic but are still able to transmit the organism. When symptoms such as dysuria and/or penile discharge occur, they tend to be mild. This is in contrast to gonococcal urethritis, which tends to be more severe. The characteristic watery or mucoid urethral discharge should be examined under Gram stain to rule out *Neisseria gonorrhoeae*. Serious complications from chlamydial NGU are rare in males.
- **Mucopurulent cervicitis:** This is the female counterpart of NGU in the male. *Chlamydia trachomatis* is an important cause of mucopurulent cervicitis, usually acquired through sexual intercourse. The differential diagnosis of acute cervicitis includes *C. trachomatis*, *Neisseria gonorrhoeae*, herpes simplex virus, and others, making accurate diagnosis important. Many patients with chlamydial infections of the cervix remain asymptomatic. The diagnosis is further suggested by a positive "swab test" (ie, endocervical mucous appearing yellow-green when collected on a white cotton-tipped swab). Gram staining of endocervical secretions is essential to confirm the presence of inflammatory cells (>10 polymorphonuclear cells per high power field correlates well with infectious cervicitis) and to exclude *Neisseria gonorrhoeae*. Complications of chlamydial cervicitis include pelvic inflammatory disease.
- **Pelvic inflammatory disease (PID):** This is probably the most important manifestation of *C. trachomatis* infection with respect to morbidity, permanent sequelae, and cost. In some women, chlamydial infection ascends from the cervix to the upper reproductive tract. The incidence and predisposing factors for this are unclear. Symptoms may be mild, with only nonspecific abdominal discomfort, but at laparoscopy, inflammation can be severe. Salpingitis, endometritis, and peritonitis can occur. Perihepatitis due to *C. trachomatis* has been described (the **Fitz-Hugh Curtis syndrome**).

  Complications of PID include involuntary infertility, chronic and recurrent pelvicoabdominal pain, and ectopic pregnancy. PID is also commonly caused by *Neisseria gonorrhoeae*. The number of cases due to either *Neisseria* or *Chlamydia* varies widely depending on the population studied.
- **Lymphogranuloma venereum (LGV):** Several serotypes of *C. trachomatis* cause LGV, a rare sexually transmitted disease in the United States (170 cases reported in the U.S. in 1984). LGV is an important cause of the syndrome of genital lesions with regional adenopathy. The incubation period for LGV ranges from 3-21 days. The LGV genital lesion is not striking and may be missed by the patient or the physician. The lesion is usually single and painless; it may be a papule, vesicle, or an ulcer. It resolves within several days. The key to the diagnosis of LGV is the nature of the regional adenopathy, not the genital lesion. The inguinal nodes in LGV develop 2-6 weeks after the primary lesion. The nodes are matted, fluctuant, and large. They tend to be unilateral (66% of the cases) and painful. Fistulas have been described, especially after diagnostic needle aspiration. Constitutional symptoms are very prominent, with complaints of fever, headache, myalgias, and malaise.

(Continued)

Chlamydia trachomatis (Continued)

- **Acute urethral syndrome:** *C. trachomatis* may play an important role in a subgroup of young women who present with recurrent dysuria and pyuria but who have repeatedly sterile urine cultures.
- **Ocular infections:** Worldwide, *C. trachomatis* is one of the leading causes of blindness. Over 400 million people suffer from trachoma, a chronic keratoconjunctivitis caused by *C. trachomatis*. Trachoma is an ancient disease described thousands of years ago. Initial infection occurs in childhood: a gradual onset of epithelial keratitis, infiltrates in the subepithelium, and invasion of blood vessels into the cornea (pannus formation). Bacterial coinfection and scarring of the conjunctiva are common. Trachoma is endemic in Africa, Asia, and the Mediterranean basin. Sporadic cases still occur in the U.S.

  C. trachomatis can also cause inclusion conjunctivitis, an ocular infection different from trachoma (but possibly related). This is most commonly seen in sexually active young adults. The pathogenesis of this ocular infection is either self-inoculation with infected genital secretions or exposure of the eye to infected secretions during orogenital contact.
- **Proctocolitis:** An acute proctocolitis can be caused by *C. trachomatis*, particularly in homosexual males who practice receptive anal intercourse. Symptoms include tenesmus, watery rectal discharge, and rectal pain, but many patients remain asymptomatic.
- **Epididymitis:** *C. trachomatis* accounts for nearly 50% of cases of epididymitis in adolescents and young adults. *Neisseria gonorrhoeae* usually makes up the remainder of cases in this age group.
- **Reiter's syndrome (conjunctivitis, reactive arthritis, and urethritis):** The majority of cases of Reiter's syndrome appear to be related to *C. trachomatis*, although a "postdiarrheal" Reiter's syndrome is well recognized. *C. trachomatis* can be cultured from the urethra in the majority of cases of Reiter's syndrome. Untreated chlamydial urethritis appears to be a risk factor. Although *C. trachomatis* has not been isolated from synovial fluid from patients with Reiter's syndrome, elementary bodies suggestive of *Chlamydia* have been found in joint fluid.

Infections in infants: Newborns acquire *C. trachomatis* infection usually during passage through an infected birth canal. About 66% of those exposed during vaginal delivery ultimately become infected.

- **Pneumonia in infants:** *C. trachomatis* is one of the leading causes of pneumonia in infants 1-6 months of age. About 16% of neonates exposed to *C. trachomatis* during delivery will develop pneumonia. Infants present subacutely with rhinitis and a characteristic "staccato cough" followed by tachypnea and inspiratory rales. Fever is absent. Many have had a preceding conjunctivitis or will develop it during the course of the pneumonia. Chest radiographs show a diffuse interstitial pneumonitis. There is an increased incidence of pulmonary function test abnormalities later in childhood.
- **Conjunctivitis in infants:** Approximately 25% of newborns exposed to *C. trachomatis* during delivery will develop *Chlamydia* conjunctivitis. *C. trachomatis* remains the most common cause of neonatal conjunctivitis, despite prophylaxis with ophthalmic silver nitrate. Newborns present with a mucopurulent ocular discharge and inflamed conjunctivae 2 days to 3 weeks after birth. Most cases resolve spontaneously within several months without long-term sequelae, but some may develop a chronic ocular infection resembling a mild case of trachoma.

Diagnosis Recommendations by the Centers for Disease Control (1998) have emphasized the importance of more aggressive testing for the confirmation of *Chlamydia*. A variety of newer, more accurate tests are available, and the CDC recommends laboratory testing of clinically-suspected cases, sex partners of known or suspected cases, and certain asymptomatic individuals in high risk groups (sexually active women younger than 20 year of age, women 20-24 years of age who do not use barrier contraceptives and who have a new sex partner in the previous 3 months, and others).

Diagnostic tests can be classified as follows:

1. Cell culture
2. Nonculture tests:
   - Direct fluorescent antibody (DFA) tests
   - Enzyme immunoassays (EIA) tests
   - Nucleic hybridization (DNA probe) tests (both amplified and nonamplified)

For additional information regarding the different tests, see the Laboratory Diagnosis section and the referenced article by the Centers for Disease Control and Prevention.

For the diagnosis of lymphogranuloma venereum (LGV), a very rare disease, serologic titers for LGV may be useful. The complement fixation (CF) test is positive in most cases of active LGV at titers ≥1:64. Such titers become positive between 1 and 3 weeks postinfection. Occasionally, high CF titers have been found in individuals with other chlamydial infections and in asymptomatic patients. Titers <1:64 are suggestive but not diagnostic of LGV. It is difficult to demonstrate a classical fourfold rise in specific antibody titer in LGV due to the late presentation of many patients. Microimmunofluorescent tests are more sensitive than CF for the detection of LGV-producing *C. trachomatis* strains. However, the microimmunofluorescent antibody test is available only in a select number of research laboratories. Finally, *Chlamydia* species can be isolated in cell culture systems in some laboratories. The rate of recovery of LGV *Chlamydia* from buboes or genital lesions is about 30% or less.

Diagnostic Tests/Procedures

Chlamydia Culture *on page 413*
Chlamydia trachomatis by Molecular Probe *on page 415*
Ocular Cytology *on page 551*

Treatment

Urethritis or cervicitis in the adult: There are several benefits for treatment of genital chlamydial infection: (1) the risk of transmission to sex partners is reduced; (2) if the infected individual is pregnant, therapy potentially may decrease the transmission of *C. trachomatis* to infants; (3) antibiotic treatment may help to prevent reinfection if both partners are infected.

Recommended drug therapy, adult:
- Azithromycin 1 g orally in a single dose, or
- Doxycycline 100 mg orally twice daily for 7 days

Alternate drug therapy, adult:
- Erythromycin base 500 mg orally 4 times/day for 7 days, or
- Erythromycin ethylsuccinate 800 mg orally 4 times/day for 7 days, or
- Ofloxacin 300 mg orally twice daily for 7 days
- Levofloxacin 500 mg orally for 7 days

For pregnant women with cervicitis, treatment options are more limited since the quinolones and tetracyclines, and erythromycin estolate stearate should be avoided in pregnancy. The safety of azithromycin in pregnant and lactating women has not been fully established, and is recommended as an alternative choice. The CDC recommends repeat testing for *C. trachomatis*, preferably by culture, 3 weeks after completion of therapy in pregnant women for several reasons: (1) the antibiotic regimens in pregnancy are not as effective as standard therapy and (2) gastrointestinal side effects of erythromycin may lead to noncompliance.

Recommended drug therapy, pregnant women:
- Erythromycin base 500 mg orally 4 times/day for 7 days, or
- Amoxicillin 500 mg orally 3 times/day for 7 days

Alternative drug therapy, pregnant women:
- Erythromycin base 250 mg orally 4 times/day for 14 days, or
- Erythromycin ethylsuccinate 800 mg orally 4 times/day for 7 days, or
- Erythromycin ethylsuccinate 400 mg orally 4 times/day for 14 days, or
- Azithromycin 1 g orally in a single dose

Lymphogranuloma venereum:

Recommended drug therapy, adult, not pregnant:
- Doxycycline 100 mg orally twice daily for 21 days

Alternate drug therapy, adult, including pregnant women:
- Erythromycin base 500 mg orally 4 times/day for 21 days

Pediatric drug therapy:

For ophthalmia neonatorum, the recommended therapy is erythromycin 50 mg/kg/day orally divided into 4 doses daily for 10-14 days. Topical antibiotics are not necessary when oral erythromycin is administered. Some infants require a second course of treatment.

For infant pneumonia caused by *C. trachomatis*, the recommended drug therapy is erythromycin base 50 mg/kg/day orally divided into 4 doses daily for 10-14 days.

For older children with *C. trachomatis* infection, the recommended drug therapy is as follows:

Children <45 kg: Erythromycin base 50 mg/kg/day orally divided into 4 doses daily for 10-14 days.

Children ≥45 kg, but <8 years of age: Azithromycin 1 g orally in a single dose.

Children ≥8 years of age:

Azithromycin 1 g orally in a single dose, or

Doxycycline 100 mg orally twice a day for 7 days.

Selected Readings

Caliendo AM, "Diagnosis of *Chlamydia trachomatis* Infection Using Amplification Methods: Can We Afford It?" *Clin Microbiol Newslett*, 1998, 20(9):75-8.

(Continued)

Chlamydia trachomatis (Continued)

Centers for Disease Control and Prevention, "Sexually Transmitted Diseases Treatment Guidelines 2002," *MMWR*, 2002, 51(RR-6):1-78.

Hu D, Hook EW 3rd, and Goldie SJ, "Screening for *Chlamydia trachomatis* in Women 15 to 29 Years of Age: A Cost-Effectiveness Analysis," *Ann Intern Med*, 2004, 141(7):501-13.

Mabey D and Fraser-Hurt N, "Trachoma," *Clin Evid*, 2004, (11):880-91.

Miller WC, "Screening for Chlamydial Infection: Are We Doing Enough," *Lancet*, 2005, 365(9458):456-8.

Peeling RW and Brunham RC, "Chlamydiae as Pathogens: New Species and New Issues," *Emerg Infect Dis*, 1996, 2(4):307-19.

Chlamydophila pneumoniae

Synonyms *Chlamydia pneumoniae*; TWAR

Microbiology *Chlamydophila pneumoniae*, like all *Chlamydia*, is an obligate intracellular bacterium. *Chlamydophila pneumoniae* is often discussed in association with two other species: *C. psittaci* (the cause of psittacosis) and *Chlamydia trachomatis* (a cause of nongonococcal urethritis and the eye infection called trachoma). *C. pneumoniae* shares 5% to 10% DNA sequence homology with these two species. *Chlamydophila pneumoniae* has two separate morphological forms with separate functions: the elementary body (EB), which is well-suited for extracellular life but lacks the ability to replicate and the reticulate body (RB), which is adapted to intracellular life and divides by binary fission.

The life cycle of *C. pneumoniae* is as follows:

1. EBs attach to the host cell.
2. EBs enter the cell by inducing their own phagocytosis.
3. EBs transform into larger RBs.
4. RBs grow and replicate by binary fission within vacuoles, which become filled with EBs and appear as inclusion bodies in the host cytoplasm.
5. Vacuoles rupture and release EBs, and the cycle begins again.

Epidemiology There is no known animal reservoir for *C. pneumoniae*, unlike *C. psittaci* which is highly associated with birds. Transmission is person-to-person, usually by a respiratory route. Seroprevalence studies have shown that infection is uncommon in early childhood and increases during the teenage years (prevalence 25% to 50%). By young adulthood about 50% are seropositive for *C. pneumoniae*. The organism is an unusual cause of serious respiratory tract infections in infants, but is an important pathogen in older school-age children. Approximately 10% of adult cases of community-acquired pneumonia requiring hospitalization are caused by *C. pneumoniae*. Most cases of *C. pneumoniae* are sporadic cases in the community, but occasionally outbreaks have been reported.

Clinical Syndromes

- **Community-acquired pneumonia (atypical pneumonia):** *C. pneumoniae* has been recognized as an important cause of community-acquired pneumonia. Approximately 10% of both outpatient and inpatient pneumonias are caused by this agent. Patients present with subacute malaise, cough, and low-grade fever. Hoarseness and pharyngitis are prominent. In some patients, there may be two distinct phases of the illness. The first phase is characterized by prominent upper respiratory symptoms which later resolve, followed by a second phase characterized only by cough. In many patients, fever is minimal and may be absent altogether. Chest x-ray shows a single subsegmental infiltrate in most cases. Other radiographic findings have been reported recently including lobar consolidation and pleural effusions. There is no distinctive radiographic pattern of *C. pneumoniae* infection. The pneumonia is usually mild to moderate in severity, but symptoms may be prolonged for several weeks.
- **Bronchitis:** *C. pneumoniae* is also a frequent cause of bronchitis, accounting for about 45% of bronchitis cases in young adults. Typically, patients present with pharyngitis followed by dry cough. Chest x-rays are clear.
- **Pharyngitis:** Cases may be quite severe, with prolonged hoarseness. Some cases progress to lower respiratory tract infections.
- **Sinusitis:** The spectrum of *C. pneumoniae* sinusitis is becoming better recognized. In young adults, about 5% of cases of primary sinusitis are due to *C. pneumoniae*.
- **Relationship with atherosclerotic heart disease:** In recent years, there has been increasing evidence that *C. pneumoniae* might play a role in the pathogenesis of atherosclerosis. This suggested role is based on several lines of evidence including: (1) seroepidemiologic studies showing a higher seropositivity rate for *C. pneumoniae* in patients with coronary artery disease and cerebrovascular disease; (2) detection of the organism in atheromatous plaques from patients with coronary artery disease; (3) animal studies; and (4) several prospective antibiotic trials using macrolides for patients with known coronary artery disease who were seropositive for *C. pneumoniae*. Currently, a cause-and-effect relationship has not been established although this is an area of active research.
- **Other:** Fever of unknown origin, influenza-like illness

Diagnosis *Chlamydophila pneumoniae* should be suspected in any case of atypical pneumonia, particularly if there is pharyngitis and hoarseness. Other diagnostic considerations for atypical pneumonia should include *Mycoplasma pneumoniae*, *Legionella* infections, viral lower respiratory infections, and others.

The diagnosis of *C. pneumoniae* infection can be confirmed primarily with serologic studies. The antigens which are used for antibody tests include lipopolysaccharide antigens and major outer membrane protein antigens. Lipopolysaccharide antigen is common to most members of the *Chlamydia* and *Chlamydophila* genus. Thus, positive studies are not specific for *C. pneumoniae* and can be positive during *C. trachomatis* and *C. psittaci* infections. Contact the testing laboratory to determine the cross-reactivity of the particular chosen test.

There are two patterns of antibody response with *C. pneumoniae* infections. Primary infection: Early on, complement fixation antibody is positive; 10 days to 1 month, MIF IgM is positive; 6 weeks, IgG is positive. Secondary infection: Complement fixation antibody is negative, IgM is positive in low titer; IgG response is more prompt.

Diagnostic Tests/Procedures

Chlamydia Culture *on page 413*
Chlamydophila pneumoniae Serology *on page 416*
Chlamydia and *Chlamydophila* Species Serology *on page 413*
Polymerase Chain Reaction *on page 567*

Treatment Large controlled studies comparing different antimicrobial agents have not been performed. Available data suggest that tetracycline and doxycycline are clinically effective, and the most experience is with these agents (which are also inexpensive). Erythromycin is also effective in many cases, although occasional treatment failures have been described. The newer macrolides are effective *in vitro* and have performed well in a limited number of clinical trials. The fluoroquinolones also appear effective in some trials of adult community-acquired pneumonia. Therapy is usually continued for 10-14 days.

Pediatric Drug Therapy

Recommended:

Erythromycin *on page 807*

Adult Drug Therapy

Recommended:

Doxycycline *on page 787*
Tetracycline *on page 1106*
Erythromycin *on page 807*
Azithromycin *on page 674*
Clarithromycin *on page 749*
Fluoroquinolones *on page 824*

Selected Readings

Boman J, Gaydos CA, and Quinn TC, "Molecular Diagnosis of *Chlamydia pneumoniae* Infection," *J Clin Microbiol*, 1999, 37(12):3791-9.

Ewald PW and Cochran GM, "*Chlamydia pneumoniae* and Cardiovascular Disease: An Evolutionary Perspective on Infectious Causation and Antibiotic Treatment," *J Infect Dis*, 2000, 181(Suppl 3):S394-401.

Kauppinen M and Saikku P, "Pneumonia Due to *Chlamydia pneumoniae*: Prevalence, Clinical Features, Diagnosis, and Treatment," *Clin Infect Dis*, 1995, 21:S244-52.

Marrie TJ, "Empiric Treatment of Ambulatory Community-Acquired Pneumonia: Always Include Treatment for Atypical Agents," *Infect Dis Clin North Am*, 2004, 18(4):829-41.

Marrie TJ, Poulin-Costello M, Beecroft MD, et al, "Etiology of Community-Acquired Pneumonia Treated in an Ambulatory Setting," *Respir Med*, 2005, 99(1):60-5.

Rosenfeld ME, Blessing E, Lin TM, et al, "*Chlamydia*, Inflammation, and Atherogenesis," *J Infect Dis*, 2000, 181(Suppl 3):S492-7.

Schmidt SM, Muller CE, Gurtler L, et al, "*Chlamydophila pneumoniae* Respiratory Tract Infection Aggravates Therapy Refractory Bronchitis or Pneumonia in Childhood," *Klin Padiatr*, 2005, 217(1):9-14.

Cholangitis, Acute

Synonyms Acute Cholangitis; Acute Obstructive Cholangitis; Acute Suppurative Cholangitis; Toxic Cholangitis

Clinical Presentation Caused by infection in an obstructed (most frequently by stones) biliary system. Fifty percent to 100% of patients present with Charcot's triad; fever and chills, right upper quadrant pain, and jaundice. Less than 14% present with Reynolds pentad; Charcot's triad plus altered mental status and shock. Fever occurs in 90%, jaundice >60%, abdominal pain >70%, and peritoneal signs in 14% to 45%. Majority of patients have leukocytosis and abnormal liver function tests consistent with cholestasis (elevated bilirubin, 2-5 times normal alkaline phosphatase, and mildly elevated transaminases). Bacteremia is common.

Differential Diagnosis Cholecystitis, recurrent cholangitis, AIDS cholangiopathy, sclerosing cholangitis, pancreatitis, right pyelonephritis, right lower lobe pneumonia, perforated duodenal ulcer, pulmonary infarcts

(Continued)

Cholangitis, Acute *(Continued)*

Likely Pathogens

Escherichia coli on page 142
Klebsiella Species *on page 200*
Enterococcus Species *on page 134*
Candida Species *on page 67*

Most often polymicrobial including anaerobes especially:
Bacteroides and *Prevotella* Species *on page 46*
Clostridium perfringens on page 88

Diagnostic Tests/Procedures

Computed Transaxial Tomography, Abdomen Studies *on page 423*
Ultrasound, Abdomen *on page 604*

Laboratory tests should include complete blood count with differential, liver function tests, and coagulation studies. Plain film radiograph of abdomen is abnormal in approximately 15% of patients. Abdominal ultrasound should be performed initially. If cause or site of obstruction is not seen on ultrasound, abdominal CT scan is warranted. If no dilated ducts are noted on ultrasound, then a cholescintigraphy may be needed.

Drug Therapy Comment Given the significant mortality seen in cholangitis, surgery and gastroenterology should be consulted especially if the patient has not responded to medical management within the first 24 hours. Approximately 45% patients will not respond to medical management of I.V. hydration and antibiotics. Percutaneous drainage, endoscopic retrograde cholangiopancreatography for possible endoscopic sphincterotomy, stone extraction and/or placement of indwelling prosthesis, or surgical intervention may be needed.

Empiric Drug Therapy

Recommended:

The following 3 used in combination
Piperacillin *on page 1002*
Aminoglycosides *on page 641*
Metronidazole *on page 940*

Ampicillin and Sulbactam *on page 660*
with or without
Aminoglycosides *on page 641*

Ticarcillin and Clavulanate Potassium *on page 1114*
with or without
Aminoglycosides *on page 641*

Piperacillin and Tazobactam Sodium *on page 1003*
with or without
Aminoglycosides *on page 641*

Alternate:

One of the following
Cephalosporins, 2nd Generation *on page 729*
Cephalosporins, 3rd Generation *on page 730*
Ertapenem *on page 805*
Moxifloxacin *on page 949*
plus
Aminoglycosides *on page 641*
with or without
Metronidazole *on page 940*

The following 3 used in combination
Ciprofloxacin *on page 742*
Aminoglycosides *on page 641*
Metronidazole *on page 940*

Selected Readings

Bornman PC, van Beljon JI, and Krige JE, "Management of Cholangitis," *J Hepatobiliary Pancreat Surg*, 2003, 10(6):406-14.
Carpenter HA, "Bacterial and Parasitic Cholangitis," *Mayo Clin Proc*, 1998, 73(5):473-8.
Hanau LH and Steigbigel NH, "Cholangitis: Pathogenesis, Diagnosis, and Treatment," *Curr Clin Topics Infect Dis*, 1995, 15:153-78.
van den Hazel SJ, Speelman P, Tytgat GN, et al, "Role of Antibiotics in the Treatment and Prevention of Acute and Recurrent Cholangitis," *Clin Infect Dis*, 1994, 19(2):279-86.

Cholera *see Vibrio cholerae on page 351*

Chorioamnionitis *see* Amnionitis *on page 33*

Chromoblastomycosis *see* Dematiaceous Fungi *on page 112*

Chromomycosis *see* Dematiaceous Fungi *on page 112*

Chronic Fatigue Syndrome

Synonyms CFS

Clinical Presentation In 1994, a consensus of CFS experts agreed to the following criteria:

(1) Have severe chronic fatigue of 6 months or longer in duration with other known medical conditions excluded by clinical diagnosis; *and*

(2) Concurrently have four or more of the following symptoms: Substantial impairment in short-term memory or concentration; sore throat; tender lymph nodes; muscle pain; multi-joint pain without swelling or redness; headaches of a new type, pattern, or severity; unrefreshing sleep; and postexertional malaise lasting >24 hours.

Symptoms must have persisted or recurred during 6 or more consecutive months of illness and must not have predated the fatigue (http://www.cdc.gov/ncidod/diseases/cfs/).

The relationship between chronic fatigue syndrome and defined neuropsychiatric syndromes is particularly important. Anxiety disorders, somatoform disorders, major depression, and other symptomatically defined syndromes are characterized by profound fatigue. Some of the features of chronic fatigue may represent deconditioning due to physical inactivity associated commonly with a diverse group of illnesses.

Whether chronic fatigue syndrome is viral, postviral, immune, allergic, psychological, or idiopathic remains to be determined. The high incidence of concurrent psychiatric symptoms compounds the difficulties encountered in the diagnosis and management of CFS.

The diagnosis of chronic fatigue syndrome is one of exclusion. It is established only after other medical and psychiatric causes of chronic fatigue illness have been ruled out.

Diagnostic Tests/Procedures No specific tests or pathognomonic signs for CFS have been validated. Bates et al observed statistically significant differences from control populations for the following analytes.

- Immune complexes ≥0.23 g/L
- Immunoglobulin G ≥12.5 g/L
- Antinuclear antibody titer ≥1:40
- Alkaline phosphatase ≥89 units/L
- Cholesterol ≥200 mg/dL (≥5.17 mmol/L)
- Lactic dehydrogenase ≥196 units/L
- Atypical lymphocyte count ≥2%

Other tests which are commonly performed include ALT, AST, CBC, sedimentation rate, and TSH. The immunologic abnormalities are consistent with the concept that a chronic low level activation of the immune system is a common finding in CFS. Pursuit of both objective physical and laboratory abnormalities in more loosely defined cases of fatigue has been relatively nonrewarding.

Drug Therapy Comment No specific therapy has been defined for CFS. Clinical care integrating medical and psychological management concepts, as well as symptomatic management, may prevent significant secondary impairment.

Selected Readings

Bates DW, Buchwald D, Lee J, et al, "A Comparison of Case Definitions of Chronic Fatigue Syndrome," *Clin Infect Dis*, 1994, 18(Suppl 1):S11-5.

Bates DW, Buchwald D, Lee J, et al, "Clinical Laboratory Test Findings in Patients With Chronic Fatigue Syndrome," *Arch Intern Med*, 1995, 155(1):97-103.

Bentler SE, Hartz AJ, and Kuhn EM, "Prospective Observational Study of Treatments for Unexplained Chronic Fatigue," *J Clin Psychiatry*, 2005, 66(5):625-32.

Fukuda K, Straus SE, Hickie I, et al, "The Chronic Fatigue Syndrome: A Comprehensive Approach to Its Definition and Study," *Ann Intern Med*, 1994, 121(12):953-9.

Lange G, Steffener J, Cook DB, et al, "Objective Evidence of Cognitive Complaints in Chronic Fatigue Syndrome: A BOLD fMRI Study of Verbal Working Memory," *Neuroimage*, 2005, 26(2):513-24.

Lapp CW and Cheney PR, "The Chronic Fatigue Syndrome," *Ann Intern Med*, 1995, 123(1):74-5.

Moss-Morris R, Sharon C, Tobin R, et al, "A Randomized Controlled Graded Exercise Trial for Chronic Fatigue Syndrome: Outcomes and Mechanisms of Change," *J Health Psychol*, 2005, 10(2):245-59.

Straus SE, Komaroff AL, and Wedner HJ, "Chronic Fatigue Syndrome: Point and Counterpoint," *J Infect Dis*, 1994, 170(1):1-6.

Wilson A, Hickie I, Lloyd A, et al, "The Treatment of Chronic Fatigue Syndrome: Science and Speculation," *Am J Med*, 1994, 96(6):544-50.

Chronic Sinusitis, Community-Acquired *see* Sinusitis, Community-Acquired, Chronic *on page 299*

Citrobacter Species

Microbiology *Citrobacter* species are gram-negative rods which are important causes of nosocomial infection and are only rarely associated with community-acquired infections in normal hosts. *Citrobacter* species are moderate-sized, aerobic,

(Continued)

Citrobacter Species *(Continued)*

gram-negative bacilli which belong to the large family Enterobacteriaceae. The organism is morphologically indistinguishable from other members of Enterobacteriaceae. *Citrobacter* species are closely related to such gram-negative bacilli as *Klebsiella*, *Serratia*, *Salmonella*, and *E. coli*. Currently recognized *Citrobacter* species are *C. diversus*, *C. freundii*, and *C. amalonaticus*, all of which are potential human pathogens. Laboratory identification is generally straightforward. Special requests for isolation of *Citrobacter* are not necessary.

Citrobacter shares several potential virulence factors with other members of Enterobacteriaceae, including endotoxin, the lipopolysaccharide (LPS) associated with the outer membrane of the bacteria. When cell lysis occurs (as with antibiotic therapy), the LPS is released into the host and can lead to such inflammatory responses as fever, leukopenia or leukocytosis, hypotension, and disseminated intravascular coagulation. Thus, LPS is regarded as an important mediator of the sepsis syndrome.

Epidemiology Because *Citrobacter* commonly inhabits the human gastrointestinal tract, it is considered one of the members of Enterobacteriaceae (enteric bacteria). In hospitalized patients, *Citrobacter* can asymptomatically colonize the urine, respiratory tract, abdominal wounds, decubitus ulcers, and others. Community-acquired infection is rare.

Clinical Syndromes

- **Lower respiratory tract infection:** Nosocomial *Citrobacter* infections are often seen in debilitated and ventilator-dependent patients. It should be noted that *Citrobacter* and other gram-negative bacilli can asymptomatically colonize the upper respiratory tract of hospitalized patients. Thus, the recovery of *Citrobacter* in a sputum or tracheal aspirate culture does not necessarily indicate a significant infectious disease. The diagnosis of a pneumonia still rests on standard criteria such as the presence of purulence (many leukocytes) on the Gram stain of sputum, the presence of a pulmonary infiltrate, and signs of systemic inflammation in the patient. A positive sputum culture alone is not sufficient justification for initiating antimicrobial therapy.
- **Urinary tract infection:** Seen in hospitalized patients, often in those with indwelling Foley catheters. However, *Citrobacter* may harmlessly colonize the urine of patients with chronic bladder catheters without causing disease. The decision to initiate antibiotics in such patients should be based on the clinical situation (the presence of pyuria on urinalysis, suprapubic pain, fever, etc). Even the finding of large numbers of *Citrobacter* in a urine culture (>10^5 colony-forming units/mL) by itself does not automatically indicate antibiotic therapy.
- **Hospital-associated bacteremias:** *Citrobacter* may be recovered from blood cultures in association with a known focus of infection (eg, pneumonia or catheter infection) or may be a "primary bacteremia" with no clear source. *Citrobacter* may also be cultured as part of a polymicrobial bacteremia, usually from an intravascular catheter or intra-abdominal sepsis. Endocarditis has rarely been reported.
- **Neonatal central nervous system infections:** *Citrobacter diversus* is a recognized cause of meningitis and brain abscesses in this age group.

Diagnosis The clinical presentations of the various nosocomial infections caused by *Citrobacter* are not distinctive, and laboratory isolation is necessary.

Diagnostic Tests/Procedures

Aerobic Culture, Appropriate Site *on page 365*
Gram Stain *on page 473*

Treatment *Citrobacter* species present a challenging therapeutic problem, especially with nosocomial infection. Appropriate treatment of patients infected with *Citrobacter* depends on antimicrobial susceptibility testing of individual isolates.

High level drug resistance has been described in some isolates. Preliminary data suggest that the popular third generation cephalosporins may act to select mutants of *Citrobacter* that are resistant to a wide variety of antibiotics, including both cephalosporins and extended-spectrum penicillins. Susceptibility to these organisms is not predictable. Consultation with an Infectious Disease specialist may be useful in such cases.

Drug Therapy

Recommended:

Penicillins, Extended-Spectrum *on page 997*

Alternate:

Cephalosporins, 3rd Generation *on page 730*
Imipenem and Cilastatin *on page 861*
Meropenem *on page 936*
Fluoroquinolones *on page 824*

Selected Readings

Aller SC and Chusid MJ, "*Citrobacter koseri* Pneumonia and Meningitis in an Infant," *J Infect*, 2002, 45(1):65-7.

Chen YS, Wong WW, Fung CP, et al, "Clinical Features and Antimicrobial Susceptibility Trends in *Citrobacter freundii* Bacteremia," *J Microbiol Immunol Infect*, 2002, 35(2):109-14.

Drelichman V and Band JD, "Bacteremia Due to *Citrobacter diversus* and *Citrobacter freundii*: Incidence, Risk Factors, and Clinical Outcome," *Arch Intern Med*, 1985, 145(10):1808-10.

Kim PW, Harris AD, Roghmann MC, et al, "Epidemiological Risk Factors for Isolation of Ceftriaxone-Resistant Versus -Susceptible *Citrobacter freundii* in Hospitalized Patients," *Antimicrob Agents Chemother*, 2003 47(9):2882-7.

Pepperell C, Kus JV, Gardam MA, et al, "Low-Virulence *Citrobacter* Species Encode Resistance to Multiple Antimicrobials," *Antimicrob Agents Chemother*, 2002, 46(11):3555-60.

Clostridium botulinum

Related Information

Clinical Syndromes Associated With Foodborne Diseases *on page 1276*

Microbiology The etiologic agent of botulism is *Clostridium botulinum*. The organism is a gram-positive, anaerobic bacillus. The natural reservoir is soil and sediment where the organism survives by forming spores. Most food-borne epidemics are associated with home canned foods. Restaurants and commercially canned products are also the source of outbreaks.

Deliberate contamination of food or beverages with botulinum toxin is the most likely route of dissemination for bioterroristic attack. As the bacteria grow and undergo autolysis, a powerful polypeptide neurotoxin is released. The toxin is heat labile and thus, is destroyed by appropriate heating in commercial canning processes. An acidic pH inhibits spore germination. This is the basis for adding ascorbic acid to home-canned products. Ingestion of even a small amount of contaminated food may cause severe clinical symptoms. Dispersion of aerosolized toxin is also possible. Aerosolized particles of botulinum toxin are approximately 0.1-0.3 micrometer in size and experts have estimated that 1 g of aerosolized botulinum toxin could kill up to 1.5 million people.

Epidemiology *Clostridium botulinum* is found in soil worldwide. Incidence of reported botulism is increasing. Most cases are individual or occur as a small cluster. If the outbreak is the result of contaminated commercially distributed food, the cases may occur in a widespread area. Early consultation with the State Health Department in conjunction with the Center for Disease Control is imperative for case management and epidemic control. Botulism is almost always caused by *C. botulinum* types A, B, and E in the western U.S., eastern U.S., and Alaska, respectively.

Clinical Syndromes

- **Infant botulism:** The most commonly reported form of botulism in the United States is infant botulism. *C. botulinum* toxin is released from organisms colonizing the intestinal tract. The toxin binds to synaptic membranes of cholinergic nerves and prevents the release of acetylcholine. Transmission of nerve fiber impulses to muscle is interrupted with resultant autonomic nerve dysfunction which progresses to motor weakness (flaccid paralysis).

  Subsequently, cranial and peripheral nerve weakness, constipation, and autonomic instability is the result of toxin effect on the ganglionic and postganglionic parasympathetic synapses. Typically, infants 1 week to 1 year of age present with progressive descending weakness following a period of constipation. Weak suck and poor feeding are frequent complaints. The pathogenesis of intestinal botulism in adults is similar to that of infant botulism.
- **Inhalational botulism:** Disease is caused by inhalation of aerosolized preformed botulinum toxin with subsequent absorption through the lungs into the circulation.
- **Food-borne botulism:** Symptoms of botulism begin as descending paralysis or weakness within a few hours to 1-2 days following ingestion of contaminated food. Symptoms may commence as late as 1 week. Dizziness, lassitude, and weakness are common. Nausea and vomiting are less common. Blockage of autonomic nerve impulse transmission causes dry tongue, mouth, and pharynx which is unrelieved by fluids. Urinary retention, ileus, and constipation frequently follow. Paralysis descends from cranial nerves to extremities and the respiratory muscles. Speech and vision are often impaired. Key clinical observations include the fact that the patients are oriented, alert, or easily roused and afebrile. They may demonstrate postural hypotension and dilated unreactive pupils.
- **Wound botulism:** Botulism may result from germination of spores contaminating traumatic wounds. Wounds caused by intravenous drug and nasal cocaine abuse have also been reported as sources. The clinical syndrome resembles that of foodborne botulism. Toxin can be recovered from the serum and wound drainage of affected patients. *C. botulinum* may be recovered from debrided tissue and drainage.

Diagnosis Outbreaks of botulism may be documented by identifying toxin in the stool or serum of symptomatic patients or from suspected food. Isolation of *C. botulinum*

(Continued)

Clostridium botulinum (Continued)

from stool or demonstration of the toxin by the mouse neutralization test establishes the diagnosis. Toxin is difficult to recover from serum; therefore, toxin recovery from stool may be more productive, but acquiring a stool specimen may be difficult because of the constipation. A low volume, normal saline, colonic irrigation may yield a useful specimen. Electromyography and repetitive nerve stimulation may yield corroborative evidence. The electromyographer should be alerted to the suspicion of botulism so that the study can be directed toward the diagnosis. A cerebrospinal fluid analysis to exclude meningitis, poliomyelitis, and Fisher Guillain-Barré syndrome is a useful part of the work-up.

Diagnostic Tests/Procedures Samples collected for botulism testing should be handled using Standard Precautions. *C. botulinum* toxin detection should be performed only by trained individuals at level C or higher LRN laboratories. Sodium hypochlorite (0.1%) or sodium hydroxide (0.1 N) inactivate the toxin and are recommended by the CDC for decontaminating work surfaces and spills of cultures or toxin. The mouse bioassay is currently the only diagnostic method used for detection and identification of botulinum toxin.

Botulism, Diagnostic Procedure *on page 405*
Cerebrospinal Fluid Analysis *on page 408*
Polymerase Chain Reaction *on page 567*

Treatment

Infant botulism: The primary modes of treatment for infant botulism are supportive involving rehydration, nutritional supplementation, and respiratory support. Nasogastric tube feedings have been used relatively early in the course; however, the patients should be monitored for ileus. Oral feeding should not be reinstituted until ileus is gone, a gag reflex is present, and swallowing is normal. Intubation is required in the majority of cases for airway protection and, in about 25%, for ventilation. These patients have a significant risk of atelectasis and aspiration. Antitoxin is usually not used because the level of circulating toxin available to be bound is very low. In addition, there are significant complications of antitoxin therapy which include serum sickness, anaphylaxis, and life-long sensitivity to horse serum. Aminoglycoside antimicrobial therapy is contraindicated because aminoglycosides can cause neuromuscular blockade. Since sepsis is a key differential diagnosis, alternatives to aminoglycosides such as third generation cephalosporins should be considered in cases where botulism is in the differential. Therapy directed at eradication of *C. botulinum* toxin from the bowel has not been shown to produce objective clinical benefit.

Hospitalizations have a mean of about 50 days with complications including atelectasis, inappropriate antidiuretic hormone, autonomic instability, urinary tract infection, pneumonia sepsis, seizures, and subglottic stenosis as a complication of intubation. Despite the complications, mortality is very low (<3%), and prognosis for complete recovery is good.

Food-borne botulism: In cases of foodborne botulism, administration of equine antitoxin should be considered. In conjunction with the State Department of Health, consultation with the Foodborne Diseases branch of the Center for Disease Control is available, (404) 639-2206. The electromyogram, cerebrospinal fluid analysis, summary of the clinical syndrome, and chronology of the patient's illness should be available to facilitate the consultation. The main principle of therapy for botulism is respiratory support. Botulism antitoxin also can be administered and is most effective if given early in the clinical course. Although antitoxin will not reverse existing paralysis, it will prevent additional nerve damage if given before all circulating toxin is bound at the neuromuscular junction. If the type of botulinum toxin is not known, all three types of antitoxin should be administered. If the toxin type is known, then either bivalent AB antitoxin or type E antitoxin should be administered on the basis of the identified toxin type.

Wound botulism: Treatment is similar to the therapy for foodborne botulism. Incision and debridement of the wound should also be considered.

Drug Therapy

Recommended:

Botulinum Pentavalent (ABCDE) Toxoid *on page 689*
Botulism Immune Globulin (Intravenous-Human) *on page 690*

Selected Readings

Arnon SS, Schechter R, Inglesby TV, et al, "Botulinum Toxin as a Biological Weapon: Medical and Public Health Management," *JAMA*, 2001, 285(8):1059-70.

"Biological and Chemical Terrorism: Strategic Plan for Preparedness and Response. Recommendations of the CDC Strategic Planning Workgroup," *MMWR Recomm Rep*, 2000, 49(RR-4):1-14.

Craven KE, Ferreira JL, Harrison MA, et al, "Specific Detection of *Clostridium botulinum* Types A, B, E, and F Using the Polymerase Chain Reaction," *J AOAC Int*, 2002, 85(5):1025-8.

Shapiro RL, Hatheway C, and Swerdlow DL, "Botulism in the United States: A Clinical and Epidemiologic Review," *Ann Intern Med*, 1998, 129(3):221-8.

Clostridium difficile

Microbiology *Clostridium difficile* is a gram-positive, spore-forming, anaerobic rod which causes millions of human infections each year, with an increasing incidence in recent years. It is the most frequent cause of antibiotic-associated colitis. This organism is difficult to isolate in culture (hence the name *C. difficile*) and requires anaerobic conditions and special media for growth in the laboratory. Under the proper environmental conditions, the majority of strains are capable of elaborating toxins within the intestinal lumen (ie, toxigenic); the most common being toxin A (an *in vivo* enterotoxin) and B (an *in vitro* cytopathic toxin). The majority of strains causing diarrheal disease produce both toxin A and B, but there are rare clinical isolates which elaborate only one of the two toxins. This observation has potential clinical relevance since many laboratory methods for the detection of *C. difficile* detect only toxin B. Toxins A and B cause necrosis and inflammation of intestinal cells. Some strains of *C. difficile* elaborate other toxins which similarly damage the intestinal mucosa and cause secretion of fluid into the intestinal lumen. A variable number of *C. difficile* strains lack the gene for toxin A and B; these nontoxigenic strains do not cause diarrheal disease.

The organism can exist in a vegetative form or in a spore form, with the vegetative form being more common. The vegetative form is very sensitive to oxygen and can be killed by even a brief exposure to oxygen. The spore form, in contrast, is heat-stable and very hardy. The spore form can survive a number of adverse environmental conditions including gastric acidity and some commercial disinfectants.

Epidemiology Colonization with *C. difficile* can be seen at all ages, and may or may not be associated with clinical disease. The organism can be cultured from the stool of about 3% to 5% of healthy adults. The percentage of hospitalized adult patients who are colonized with this agent is higher, approximately 10% to 30%. The organism is acquired while in the hospital, and some studies suggest a 37% incidence of diarrhea at the time of infection. The rates of stool colonization with toxigenic *C. difficile* is highest in neonates, with greater than 50% of neonates harboring the organism. Despite these high rates of colonization with toxin-producing strains, the majority of patients colonized with *C. difficile* remain free of diarrhea. Thus, the finding of *C. difficile* in a stool culture can be difficult to interpret, and does not necessarily mean that the organism is the cause of diarrhea for a given individual.

Similarly, clinical disease (*C. difficile* colitis) can be seen in all age groups, but is most frequent in elderly persons and in hospitalized patients. The overwhelming risk factor for the development of *C. difficile* diarrhea is recent treatment with antibacterial agents. In some epidemiologic studies, the use of cancer chemotherapy has been associated with *C. difficile* diarrhea without exposure to antibiotics, but this is rare. Several factors need to be present for the development of diarrhea: (1) the patient needs to receive a sufficient amount of antibiotic to alter the normal intestinal flora; (2) the individual needs to be infected with *C. difficile*, which usually occurs as an acute infection by the fecal-oral route while in the hospital; (3) the *C. difficile* strain must be a toxin-producer. It is well known that heat-resistant spores of *C. difficile* commonly contaminate hospital environments, and up to 90% of *C. difficile* infections occur in hospitals with ≤5% coming from the community. In addition to contamination of the stool, clothing, and immediate bedspace of the infected hospital patient, *C. difficile* has been isolated from a number of sources, including the hands of healthcare workers, fomites such as hospital toilet seats and sinks, endoscopy equipment, and other instruments. Asymptomatically-infected hospital patients serve as an important reservoir for the organism. Transmission occurs by the fecal-oral route, from patient to patient or from healthcare worker to patient; transmission from an inanimate surface to a patient can also occur. Recent models of the pathogenesis of *C. difficile* colitis emphasize the importance of the initial infection with *C. difficile*, and help explain the various epidemiologic findings. The initial infection is felt to be similar to infection with other bacteria which cause acute enteric disease; in some studies, about one-third of those acquiring *C. difficile* developed some degree of diarrhea. However, it is the unique interaction of antibiotics and *C. difficile* which determines both whether the patient becomes colonized after acute infection and whether a patient will develop diarrhea and/or colitis later. Antibiotics cause suppression of the normal intestinal flora, which permit both initial infection and later overgrowth of *C. difficile*, with resultant high levels of toxin production. Without the selective pressure of the antibiotics, the acute infection with *C. difficile* is self-limited and the patient remains asymptomatic afterwards.

C. difficile colitis can occur as sporadic cases within a hospital or as a nosocomial outbreak. Such outbreaks are relatively frequent in hospitals, and can occur in

(Continued)

Clostridium difficile (Continued)

nursing homes as well. Infection control measures such as handwashing with chlorhexidine (or other effective disinfectant), use of disposable gloves, avoidance of rectal thermometers, and careful cleaning of contaminated rooms have been shown to be effective to varying degrees. However, outbreaks have been reported to persist despite strict infection control measures.

Clinical Syndromes The range of severity of symptoms is broad, ranging from asymptomatic carriage to a fulminant, life-threatening colitis. In general, symptoms begin several days after receiving antibiotics, but can occur 2 months after antibiotic exposure. The antibiotics most commonly associated with *C. difficile* are the cephalosporins, clindamycin, broad-spectrum penicillins, and ampicillin. Nearly every antibacterial agent has been associated with *C. difficile* diarrhea. Cases have been described after a single dose of antibiotics given for surgical prophylaxis. It is important to realize that not all cases of antibiotic-associated colitis are caused by *C. difficile*. In fact, probably only 20% of AAC is caused by this organism, with the remainder caused by a variety of factors including direct antibiotic toxicity. The various clinical manifestations of *C. difficile* are as follows:

- **Asymptomatic carriage:** As noted above, about 3% to 5% of adults and over 50% of neonates are asymptomatically infected with *C. difficile*. About 25% to 30% of hospitalized adults are *C. difficile* carriers, most of whom acquire infection in the hospital and remain asymptomatic. The factors predisposing to carriage have not been fully determined.
- **Mild to moderate diarrhea:** This is one of the most common presentations of *C. difficile*. Patients complain of mild to moderate watery diarrhea, usually nonbloody, along with abdominal cramping in some cases. Patients are not systemically ill from the diarrhea, and are nontoxic in appearance. Sigmoidoscopy usually shows no significant abnormalities and thus is not routinely indicated.
- ***C. difficile* colitis without pseudomembranes:** A more severe manifestation of *C. difficile* is characterized by fever, malaise, high volume diarrhea, and moderate to severe abdominal pain. Stools may have trace blood but rectal bleeding is rare. Leukocytosis is common, and can be a clue to the diagnosis. The colitis is patchy and moderate in degree on sigmoidoscopy, but no pseudomembranes are present.
- **Pseudomembranous colitis (PMC):** Patients who develop PMC are systemically ill, with abdominal pain and tenderness, fever, and severe diarrhea. Diarrhea may be bloody. Marked elevations of the WBC to 30-50 x 10^9/L can be seen and can be a clue to the diagnosis. Abdominal imaging such as a KUB or CAT scan may show thickening of the bowel wall, and other abnormalities such as pneumatosis or "thumbprinting," the latter finding a result of severe colonic wall edema. Lower GI endoscopy shows the presence of pseudomembranes, which represent a coalescence of yellow inflammatory plaques. Most severe cases of PMC are a pancolitis and pseudomembranes can be seen with sigmoidoscopy alone. About 10% of cases are right-sided only, and are associated with ileus and no diarrhea. These cases will have a negative sigmoidoscopic exam and require full colonoscopy to identify pseudomembranes.
- **Acute abdomen with sepsis syndrome:** In rare instances, *C. difficile* can present with a "sepsis syndrome" characterized by fever, hypotension, and an acute abdomen. Distention and rebound tenderness may be seen, and the presentation may be indistinguishable from an abdominal perforation. Patients with the *C. difficile* "sepsis syndrome" usually have no diarrhea. Typically there is ileus, dilation of the colon on abdominal radiographs, and even megacolon, all of which prevent the development of diarrhea. Severe leukocytosis is common. Some patients may demonstrate a marked serositis, with large pleural and peritoneal effusions. Because of the risk of perforation, sigmoidoscopy or colonoscopy are relatively contraindicated. Some authors feel that proctoscopy is safe in this situation (with minimal air insufflation), and can lead to the diagnosis quickly. Patients with this most severe form of disease often require combined medical therapy and surgical intervention.
- **Recurrent *C. difficile* diarrhea:** Most cases of *C. difficile* diarrhea are successfully treated with medical therapy alone, but about 10% to 20% of cases relapse. Treatment of first-time relapsed patients is usually successful. A small number of persons relapse repeatedly. This may be due to several factors including resistance to metronidazole (rare but reported), reinfections from the environment, and persistence of spores in the GI tract after treatment of the vegetative forms.

Diagnosis *C. difficile*-associated diarrhea should be suspected in hospitalized patients with diarrhea concurrent with, or soon after, the administration of antibiotics. It should

also be suspected in individuals with acute diarrhea who are receiving oral or parenteral antibiotics at home or in a nursing home. Since *C. difficile* diarrhea and associated symptoms are nonspecific, laboratory confirmation is essential.

There are several laboratory methods available:

(1) Isolation of *C. difficile* in stool culture (special culture media required)
(2) Cytotoxin assay (cell culture facilities required)
(3) Enzyme immunoassay for the toxin of *C. difficile*

Isolation of the organism in stool culture requires specialized laboratory techniques and should not be routinely ordered. Since the organism is present in a substantial number of patients in the hospital, with or without disease, interpretation of a positive culture is problematic. In addition, diarrhea is caused by the toxin, and the mere presence of the organism on a stool culture does not necessarily imply cause and effect (some strains do not produce toxin). Thus, the emphasis is on the laboratory detection of the toxin.

A cytotoxin assay based on detection of toxin B in cell culture was the standard for laboratory detection in the past. The assay is still considered the reference standard since it is highly sensitive and specific, but like other tissue-culture systems, it is expensive and labor intensive. Many laboratories have changed from the cytotoxin assay to the enzyme immunoassay (EIA). These EIA tests are rapid, commercially available, and usually less expensive than the cytotoxin assay. In general, the EIA has good sensitivity and excellent specificity for detecting toxin A and/or B. Since no assay is 100% sensitive, submitting a repeat stool specimen for one of the toxin assays is reasonable if the first specimen was negative but the clinical suspicion for *C. difficile* remains high. Occasionally, cases of *C. difficile* may remain toxin-negative on repeated testing and the diagnosis only established by colonoscopy. Follow-up testing as a test-of-cure does not yield clinically relevant or useful results and is not recommended.

Fecal leukocyte testing is of limited value in the diagnosis of *C. difficile*-associated diarrhea. The presence of fecal leukocytes is associated with a positive toxin in some studies, but by itself fecal leukocytes lack specificity for *C. difficile*. Assay for the toxin is recommended.

Diagnostic Tests/Procedures

Clostridium difficile Toxin Assay *on page 418*

Fecal Leukocyte Stain *on page 455*

Treatment The initial step in the treatment for *C. difficile*-associated diarrhea is discontinuation of the offending antibiotic(s), whenever feasible. Metronidazole is the drug of choice when treatment is indicated. Oral vancomycin is very effective also, but its cost is high and the development of vancomycin-resistant enterococci remains a growing concern. Treatment may differ somewhat according to the clinical manifestation.

Asymptomatic carriage: Neither metronidazole nor oral vancomycin has been proven effective in reducing the carriage state and treatment is not indicated in asymptomatic persons.

Mild to moderate *C. difficile*-associated diarrhea: Metronidazole at 250 mg orally 4 times/day for 10 days is the regimen of choice. For patients intolerant of metronidazole, vancomycin 125 mg orally 4 times/day is equally effective, but at over 20 times the cost of metronidazole. Both are about 95% effective, and vancomycin has not been shown to be superior to metronidazole.

***C. difficile* colitis, with or without pseudomembranes:** Oral metronidazole or oral vancomycin are still the preferred agents for more severe *C. difficile* cases. Some authors feel that oral vancomycin has theoretic advantages over oral metronidazole in severe cases, but superiority has not yet been proven in clinical trials. Ileus can often complicate moderate to severe cases and adequate delivery of the antibiotic to the colon is an issue. A nasogastric tube can be used in such cases to deliver oral metronidazole or vancomycin. The concomitant administration of intravenous metronidazole has been proposed in patients with ileus because its hepatobiliary secretion leads to high levels of drug in the stool. Other methods for delivery of vancomycin have been used in persons with severe ileus, including vancomycin retention enemas and surgical creation of a "blow-hole" in the transverse colon, allowing for the direct administration of a vancomycin solution into the colon. There is not a clear role for intravenous vancomycin even in severe cases.

***C. difficile* toxic megacolon:** This severe manifestation of *C. difficile* usually does not respond to medical management alone and often requires surgical resection, including total colectomy in some cases.

Recurrent *C. difficile*: Since mild relapses often resolve without specific treatment the use of metronidazole or vancomycin therapy is optional. More severe relapses should be treated with a second course of metronidazole, and a switch to oral

(Continued)

Clostridium difficile (Continued)

vancomycin is not clearly better. This approach is very effective and over 90% will not have another relapse. Some persons, however, experience multiple relapses and for those individuals the optimal treatment strategy is undefined. A number of salvage regimens have been reported for persons with multiple relapses, but none is clearly superior. Reported salvage regimens include vancomycin in combination with rifampin, bacitracin, cholestyramine, vancomycin enema, fecal enemas, ingestion of nontoxigenic *C. difficile* strains, *Lactobacillus* GG, *Saccharomyces boulardii* (a so-called probiotic agent), and others. Some clinicians recommend a longer course (4-6 weeks) of tapering doses of oral vancomycin or metronidazole. The best approach remains unknown.

Drug Therapy

Recommended:

Metronidazole *on page 940*

Alternate:

Vancomycin *on page 1144*

Selected Readings

Bartlett JG, "Clinical Practice. Antibiotic-Associated Diarrhea," *N Engl J Med*, 2002, 346(5):334-9.

Fedorko DP, "Controversies in *Clostridium difficile* Testing," *Clin Microbiol Newslett*, 2002, 24(10):76-9.

Fekety R, "Guidelines for the Diagnosis and Management of *Clostridium difficile*-Associated Diarrhea and Colitis. American College of Gastroenterology, Practice Parameters Committee," *Am J Gastroenterol*, 1997, 92(5):739-50.

Johnson S and Gerding DN, "*Clostridium difficile*-Associated Diarrhea," *Clin Infect Dis*, 1998, 26(5):1027-36.

Malnick SD and Zimhony O, "Treatment of *Clostridium difficile*-Associated Diarrhea," *Ann Pharmacother*, 2002, 36(11):1767-75.

Mylonakis E, Ryan ET, and Calderwood SB, "*Clostridium difficile*-Associated Diarrhea: A Review," *Arch Intern Med*, 2001, 161(4):525-33.

McGowan KL and Kader HA, "*Clostridium difficile* Infection in Children," *Clin Microbiol Newslett*, 1999, 21(7):49-53.

Stoddart B and Wilcox MH, "*Clostridium difficile*," *Curr Opin Infect Dis*, 2002, 15(5):513-8.

Wilkins TD and Lyerly DM, "*Clostridium difficile* Testing: After 20 years, Still Challenging," *J Clin Microbiol*, 2003, 41(2):531-4.

Clostridium perfringens

Related Information

Clinical Syndromes Associated With Foodborne Diseases *on page 1276*

Microbiology *Clostridium perfringens* is an anaerobic gram-positive rod; occasionally it can appear gram-negative or gram-variable. It is a spore-forming organism, but the spores are not usually seen on Gram stain. It has been termed "aerotolerant" because of its ability to survive when exposed to oxygen for limited periods of time.

The organism produces 12 toxins active in tissues and several enterotoxins which cause severe diarrhea. Four toxins can be lethal. The toxins separate the species into five types, A-E.

- Alpha toxin: A lecithinase which damages cell membranes. It is produced by *C. perfringens* type A. It is the major factor causing tissue damage in *C. perfringens*-induced gas gangrene (myonecrosis). The toxin is a phospholipase which hydrolyzes phosphatidylcholine and sphingomyelin and leads to increased vascular permeability, myocardial depression, hypotension, bradycardia, and shock.
- Enterotoxin: Produced mainly by *C. perfringens* type A but also by types C and D. This toxin is responsible for the diarrheal syndromes classically ascribed to this organism. The enterotoxin binds to intestinal epithelial cells after the human ingests food contaminated with *C. perfringens*. The small bowel (ileum) is primarily involved. The toxin inhibits glucose transport and causes protein loss.
- Beta toxin: Produced by *C. perfringens* type B and C. This toxin causes enteritis necroticans or pigbel. This disease is seen in New Guinea where some natives ingest massive amounts of pork at feasts after first gorging on sweet potatoes. The sweet potatoes have protease inhibitors which prevent the person from degrading the beta toxin which is ingested in the contaminated pork.

Epidemiology *C. perfringens* is ubiquitous in the environment, being found in soil and decaying vegetation. The organism has been isolated from nearly every soil sample ever examined except in the sand of the Sahara desert. In the human, *C. perfringens* is common in the human gastrointestinal tract. In one study, it was found in 28 of 40 adults. It can also be commonly recovered from many mammals including cats, dogs, whales, and others.

Clinical Syndromes The organism can be pathogenic, commensal, or symbiotic. Important diseases caused by *C. perfringens* include the following.

- **Food poisoning:** *C. perfringens* is one of the most common causes of food poisoning in the United States. Foods commonly contaminated with *C. perfringens* are meat, poultry, and meat products such as gravies, hash, and stew.

Human disease is caused by ingestion of heat-labile toxin. The highest risk comes from meats which are partially cooked, cooled, then reheated. Spores present in the food germinate during the reheating process. Symptoms include watery diarrhea and abdominal cramps, which occur about 12 hours after the meal. Fever is generally not part of this illness. Vomiting is unusual. Duration of symptoms is about 24 hours. The diagnosis is made by culturing the stools and, for epidemiological purposes, the food.

- **Pigbel:** See description under Microbiology. This follows massive ingestion of contaminated pork and sweet potatoes. Incubation period is 24 hours. There is intense abdominal pain, bloody diarrhea, vomiting, shock, and intestinal perforation in some cases. A vaccine is available for travelers.
- **Gynecologic infections:** *C. perfringens* has been isolated in association with septic abortions, tubo-ovarian abscesses, and uterine gas gangrene. Interestingly, *C. perfringens* has been isolated from the blood of healthy females in the immediate postnatal period; the organism appeared to be a commensal in the blood since the patients remained well without antibiotic therapy. This underscores the often enigmatic nature of *C. perfringens.*
- **Skin and soft tissue infection colonization:** Many wounds can be contaminated with *C. perfringens*, particularly when there is an open wound exposed to soil. The organism may or may not be causing disease, and its relevance should be based on clinical findings; a superficial wound growing *C. perfringens* can often be treated using local care alone.
- **Anaerobic cellulitis:** *C. perfringens* alone or in a mixed infection causes a local tissue invasion with some necrosis. Patients are afebrile, and there is little pain or swelling. Gas may be quite noticeable in the infected tissues. Anaerobic cellulitis is seen in patients with infected diabetic foot ulcers and patients with perirectal abscesses. Localized infection can spread if not appropriately treated.
- **Fasciitis:** Patients with *C. perfringens* fasciitis present with rapidly progressive infection through soft tissue planes. **This is a medical emergency.** Anaerobic organisms cause pain, swelling, and gas formation; and patients frequently present in a florid sepsis syndrome. The classic setting for this is the patient with known colonic cancer with presumed abdominal fascial metastases; this is the nidus for colonic contamination, followed by rapid movement along the fascial planes. Although the muscle is not involved, the mortality of anaerobic cellulitis remains very high even with early surgical intervention.
- **Clostridial myonecrosis:** This entity has been described after traumatic wounds, especially during war time when wounds are grossly contaminated with soil. In World War II, 30% of battlefield wounds were associated with this, but in Vietnam only 0.02%. Clostridial myonecrosis can also be seen with crush injury, colon resections, septic abortions, and other conditions. Clinically, there is systemic toxicity, with tissue hypoxia and vascular insufficiency. The involved muscles appear black and gangrenous. Often there is abundant gas felt as crepitance in the wound. Treatment is surgical removal of devitalized tissue and, often, amputation.

Diagnosis The diagnosis of infection by *C. perfringens* begins with a high index of suspicion when a patient presents with one of the clinical syndromes described above. One important caveat is that the laboratory isolation of *C. perfringens* from a necrotic wound does not necessarily imply disease from this organism; many wounds can be colonized. In the right clinical setting, however, a positive *C. perfringens* culture and a compatible clinical presentation are highly suggestive of disease caused by this agent. Gram stain preparations of wound material, uterine tissue, cervical discharge, muscle tissues, and other relevant materials should be made; a predominance of gram-positive rods should bring anaerobic infection, including *C. perfringens*, to mind.

In patients with clostridial septicemia, accompanying abnormalities may be a clue to clostridial disease before culture confirmation is made. Patients may have disseminated intravascular coagulation with a brisk hemolysis, hemoglobinuria, and proteinuria. X-rays of diseased areas may reveal the presence of gas in muscle or soft tissue; this is suggestive of clostridial infection, although other anaerobes (and aerobes) can cause gas formation. If clostridial myonecrosis is suspected, a muscle biopsy usually performed at the time of tissue debridement, can be diagnostic.

Diagnostic Tests/Procedures

Anaerobic Culture *on page 371*
Gram Stain *on page 473*
Skin Biopsy *on page 580*

Treatment In general, the treatment of clostridial infection is high-dose penicillin G, to which the organism has remained susceptible. For skin and soft tissue infections, the extent of infection determines the need for surgical debridement. When wounds are

(Continued)

Clostridium perfringens (Continued)

simply colonized with clostridia, neither antibiotics nor surgery are indicated. Localized soft tissue infections can often be managed by surgical debridement alone, without antibiotics. When systemic symptoms are present and there is extension of infection into deeper tissues, antibiotics and surgical intervention are required. In fulminant cases of gas gangrene with myonecrosis, immediate surgical intervention (debridement, amputation) is the primary treatment of choice, and antibiotics have little effect.

Drug Therapy

Recommended:

Penicillin G (Parenteral/Aqueous) *on page 993*

Metronidazole *on page 940*

Alternate:

Carbapenems *on page 693*

Clindamycin *on page 752*

Selected Readings

Greenfield RA, Brown BR, Hutchins JB, et al, "Microbiological, Biological, and Chemical Weapons of Warfare and Terrorism," *Am J Med Sci*, 2002, 323(6):326-40.

McClane BA, "The Complex Interactions Between *Clostridium perfringens* Enterotoxin and Epithelial Tight Junctions," *Toxicon*, 2001, 39(11):1781-91.

Tweten RK, "*Clostridium perfringens* Beta Toxin and *Clostridium septicum* Alpha Toxin: Their Mechanisms and Possible Role in Pathogenesis," *Vet Microbiol*, 2001, 82(1):1-9.

Clostridium tetani

Microbiology *Clostridium tetani* is a strictly anaerobic, gram-positive, motile, spore-forming rod. Bacteria in very young or very old cultures can be gram-negative. Under adverse conditions, vegetative cells form polar ("drumstick" or "tennis racquet" appearance) spores which are extremely resistant to drying, boiling for 1 hour, and chemical disinfectants; the spores are killed by autoclaving. *C. tetani* is the etiological agent of tetanus, a strikingly dramatic infectious disease which has been recognized for many centuries. *C. tetani* was first isolated in pure culture in 1889 by Kirtasato, and the tetanus toxoid was first prepared the following year.

Epidemiology *Clostridium tetani* and its spores are found in the soil (especially manured soil) worldwide; the spores can survive in soil for many years. Sometimes *C. tetani* is also found in the lower intestinal tracts of humans and animals. In the United States since the mid 1970s, the number of cases of tetanus per year has remained at about 0.5 per 100,000 persons. Tetanus is most prevalent in the older age group (>60 years of age) and, in all populations, is directly related to an absence of immunization or to inadequate immunization. Tetanus is not uncommon (1 million cases per year) in developing countries, where mortality rates are high, probably because of a lack of intensive and proper supportive care. In developing countries, most cases occur in mothers with incompletely removed and subsequently infected placentas and in their newborns with unclean and infected umbilical cord stumps.

The portal of entry of *C. tetani* is usually a traumatized site (eg, piercing wound, burn, parenteral drug abuse, implantation of infected soil, war, and traumatic motor vehicle accident). Predisposing wounds often are quite small (eg, prick of a rose thorn or small splinter) and not recognized. Resulting traumatized or deep necrotic tissue environment is conducive to germination of implanted spores and the subsequent production of tetanospasmin, the potent neurotoxin of *C. tetani*. The vegetative cells produce the neurotoxin at the site of trauma and do not invade. Tetanospasmin circulates through the blood and lymphatic systems, attaches strongly to ganglioside receptors of presynaptic inhibitory neuron synapses, and inhibits the release of glycine, an inhibitory transmitter. The result of this binding and inhibition is simultaneous contraction of opposing flexor and extensor muscle groups and subsequent, often extremely violent, local and generalized muscle spasms.

Clinical Syndromes

- **Tetanus:** The incubation period for tetanus can be from a few days to several months. Shorter incubation periods are associated with more severe disease. The initial presentation of tetanus usually is characterized by general weakness, cramping, stiffness, and/or difficulty swallowing or chewing. "Lockjaw" can be an early sign. During the first week, spasms occur more frequently and become more generalized. Later, spasms can become intensely painful and more severe to the point of affecting breathing, speech, swallowing, and cardiac function. Cardiac, respiratory, and renal failure are the major causes of death. Mortality rates for mild, moderate, severe, and neonatal tetanus have been reported to be 0%, 9%, 44%, and 75%, respectively.

Diagnosis The diagnosis of tetanus is made by clinical judgment and patient history. Culture of specimens is not productive and not clinically useful. A history of appropriate immunization against tetanus almost always eliminates the possibility of

tetanus. A differential diagnosis can include rabies, meningitis, peritonitis, antipsychotic drugs, poisoning, and epilepsy.

Treatment Supportive therapy with emphasis on appropriate ventilation should be the major consideration in the treatment of patients with tetanus. The neuromuscular symptoms and spasms from tetanus may be managed with benzodiazepines. Additional sedation may also be necessary. Tetanus immune globulin (TIG) should be administered immediately in a dose of 500-3000 units. Intrathecal TIG (250 units) may be administered, but its use is still investigational. Equine antiserum has also been used but is associated with significantly more adverse reactions than TIG.

Patients should also be treated with antimicrobial therapy. Although intravenous penicillin is often used, metronidazole is at least as effective. Theoretically, TIG should be administered prior to antibiotic therapy to abate any increase in toxin release caused by antibiotic administration. Local wound care is also important.

Tetanus Prophylaxis in Wound Management

Number of Prior Tetanus Toxoid Doses	Clean, Minor Wounds		All Other Wounds	
	Td[1]	TIG[2]	Td[1]	TIG[2]
Unknown or fewer than 3	Yes	No	Yes	Yes
3 or more[3]	No[4]	No	No[5]	No

[1]Adult tetanus and diphtheria toxoids; use pediatric preparations (DT or DTP) if the patient is younger than 7 years old.

[2]Tetanus immune globulin.

[3]If only three doses of fluid tetanus toxoid have been received, a fourth dose of toxoid, preferably an adsorbed toxoid, should be given.

[4]Yes, if more than 10 years since last dose.

[5]Yes, if more than 5 years since last dose.

Adapted from Report of the Committee on Infectious Diseases, American Academy of Pediatrics, Elk Grove Village, IL: © American Academy of Pediatrics, 1986.

Other clinical manifestations that may require therapeutic intervention include autonomic instability, increased risk of pulmonary embolus, increased risk of stress ulceration, decubitus ulcers, fluid and electrolyte imbalance, and nutritional imbalance.

Tetanus can be prevented by appropriate immunization. Immunization guidelines can be found in the Appendix *on page 1249.*

Drug Therapy

Recommended:

Tetanus Immune Globulin (Human) *on page 1103*
plus
Metronidazole *on page 940*

Tetanus Immune Globulin (Human) *on page 1103*
plus
Penicillin G (Parenteral/Aqueous) *on page 993*

Selected Readings

Bleck TP, "*Clostridium tetani*," *Principles and Practice of Infectious Diseases*, 4th ed, Mandell GL, Bennett JE, and Dolin R, eds, New York, NY: Churchill Livingstone, 1995, 2173-8.
"Tetanus Fatality - Ohio, 1991," *MMWR*, 1993, 42(8):148-9.

CMV *see* Cytomegalovirus *on page 107*

Coccidioides immitis

Related Information

USPHS / IDSA Guidelines for the Prevention of Opportunistic Infections in Persons Infected With HIV *on page 1237*

Microbiology *Coccidioides immitis* is a dimorphic fungus. In the mycelial form on culture, the mold grows relatively fast producing a flat, moist, gray colony in 3-5 days and then developing fluffy white aerial mycelium. Wet mount reveals branching septate hyphae and chains of thick-walled, barrel-shaped arthrospores (up to 10 µm) separated by "ghost" spaces (remnants of empty cells). **Arthrospores are highly infectious to laboratory workers.** The yeast form can be seen on direct examination of infected material as round, thick-walled spherules 20-80 µm with many small endospores.

Epidemiology *Coccidioides immitis* is a normal inhabitant of the sandy, salty, dry soil of the lower Sonora Desert. It is found only in the western hemisphere and has been isolated in specific areas of Argentina and Central America, as well as the southwestern United States. The warm, dry environment facilitates the growth of arthroconidia that break from the parent mycelium and become airborne. The infectious arthroconidia are inhaled and within the pulmonary acinus convert to spherules and reproduce by endosporulation.

(Continued)

Coccidioides immitis (*Continued*)

Coccidioides infects more than 50,000 people each year and is increasing in incidence. In 1991, there was a threefold increase followed by a tenfold increase in 1992 in California as compared to the previous 5 years. Most cases occur in late childhood and early middle age. Epidemics are typically associated with dust storms, construction, archaeological digs, and exploration for oil. Infections in persons residing outside endemic areas arise from travel exposure, laboratory exposure, or inhalation of contaminated fomites.

Impaired T-cell immunity is associated with severe pulmonary and disseminated disease. Approximately 33% of AIDS patients have no focal lesion or only focal pulmonary lesions despite evidence of systemic disease. *Coccidioides* is an AIDS-defining illness.

Risk factors for dissemination include infants and elderly, male sex, race (Filipinos > Blacks > Native Americans > Hispanic > Oriental), negative skin test, serum complement fixation >1:64, immunosuppression, second half of pregnancy, and postpartum.

Clinical Syndromes

- **Asymptomatic:** Subclinical infection. Positive skin test without clinical evidence of disease. Occurs in approximately 60% of cases.
- **Primary pulmonary:** Acute respiratory illness characterized by fever, cough, headache; often associated with malaise, myalgias, and fatigue. Self-limited. Approximately 25% develop more severe disease associated with pleuritic chest pain, yet very few will progress. May have erythema nodosum or erythema multiforme. May develop arthritis, most commonly in the knee, which is an immune complex reaction and not dissemination (referred to as Desert Rheumatism).
- **Pulmonary sequelae:** Characterized by pulmonary infiltrates that are frequently subpleural with overlying pleural effusions (12%), which is usually self-limited. Hilar adenopathy is common, but paratracheal or superior-mediastinal adenopathy suggests dissemination as does diffuse miliary infiltrates. Five percent develop persistent cavities or thin-walled coccidioidal abscesses or nodules (coccidioidoma). Thirty-three percent of the cavities will close within 2 years while the rest may rupture, bleed, or develop secondary infections which may require surgical excision.
- **Chronic persistent fibrocavitary disease:** Associated with pre-existing bronchopulmonary disease.
- **Disseminated disease:** In approximately 1% of infected individuals. Spreads beyond pulmonary parenchyma or hilar nodes. Found in every organ except GI. Most common site of spread is the skin (granulomas) followed by subcutaneous abscesses, synovitis, and osteomyelitis. Majority of deaths secondary to meningitis which occurs 2-3 weeks to years after initial infection. Hydrocephalus is frequent and is a severe complication. Direct cranial nerve involvement is secondary to a vasculitis that may present as a stroke-like syndrome or transverse myelitis.

Diagnosis Skin tests and serological markers are useful epidemiologic, as well as prognostic tools. More than 50% of the population in endemic areas are skin test positive. The presence of substantial or prolonged infection in the presence of negative skin test is a poor prognostic marker. Similarly, high complement fixation titers (>1:64) are associated with extrapulmonic spread and poor prognosis. Serial rising titers are significant.

Diagnosis is made by biopsy material revealing granulomatous response with characteristic spherules with evidence of endosporulation or isolation in culture.

Diagnostic Tests/Procedures

Fungal Serology *on page 458*
Fungus Culture, Appropriate Site *on page 461*
KOH Preparation *on page 513*

Treatment Severe infection requires 1-3 g amphotericin B. First-line therapy for the treatment of nonmeningeal coccidioidomycosis is fluconazole 400 mg daily or itraconazole 200 mg twice daily. Nonimmunocompromised patients with nonmeningeal disease may be treated with ketoconazole 400 mg daily. There is approximately a 15% to 30% relapse when treated with azoles. Primary asymptomatic disease in immunocompetent hosts typically requires no treatment. Mounting clinical evidence indicates that fluconazole is at least as effective as amphotericin B independent of whether patients are HIV-infected or not. Given the practical difficulties of administering amphotericin B intrathecally and the high frequency of associated adverse effects, initiation of fluconazole treatment (800-1000 mg/day orally) in patients with coccidioidal meningitis has become the preferred initial treatment. Itraconazole 400-600 mg/day may also be effective. Only in patients who do not respond clinically after 1-2 months of therapy should intrathecal amphotericin B be considered. As with other forms of disseminated disease, life-long therapy may be

necessary in patients with meningitis. The efficacy of lipid formulations of amphotericin B and caspofungin is unknown.

Drug Therapy

Recommended:

Amphotericin B (Conventional) *on page 650*
Fluconazole *on page 819*

Alternate:

Itraconazole *on page 895*
Ketoconazole *on page 903*

Selected Readings

Aberg JA, "Coccidioidomycosis and HIV," *HIV InSite Knowledge Base*, Peiperl L and Volberding PA, eds, 2003, http://hivinsite.ucsf.edu/InSite.jsp?page=kb-05-02-04.

Galgiani JN, Ampel NM, Catanzaro A, et al, "Practice Guideline for the Treatment of Coccidioidomycosis," *Clin Infect Dis*, 2000, 30(4):658-61.

Galgiani JN, Catanzaro A, Cloud GA, et al, "Comparison of Oral Fluconazole and Itraconazole for Progressive, Nonmeningeal Coccidioidomycosis. A Randomized, Double-Blind Trial. Mycoses Study Group," *Ann Intern Med*, 2000, 133(9):676-86.

Galgiani JN, Catanzaro A, Cloud GA, et al, "Fluconazole Therapy for Coccidioidal Meningitis. The NIAID-Mycoses Study Group," *Ann Intern Med*, 1993, 119(1):28-35.

Singh VR, Smith DK, Lawerence J, et al, "Coccidioidomycosis in Patients Infected With Human Immunodeficiency Virus: Review of 91 Cases at a Single Institution," *Clin Infect Dis*, 1996, 23(3):563-8.

Stevens DA, "Coccidioidomycosis," *N Engl J Med*, 1995, 332(16):1077-82.

Stevens DA and Shatsky SA, "Intrathecal Amphotericin in the Management of Coccidioidal Meningitis," *Semin Respir Infect*, 2001, 16(4):263-9.

Woods CW, McRill C, Plikaytis BD, et al, "Coccidioidomycosis in Human Immunodeficiency Virus-Infected Persons in Arizona, 1994-1997: Incidence, Risk Factors, and Prevention," *J Infect Dis*, 2000, 181(4):1428-34.

Coccidioidomycosis *see Coccidioides immitis on page 91*

Colorado Tick Fever *see* Arboviruses *on page 35*

Community-Acquired Meningitis, Adult *see* Meningitis, Community-Acquired, Adult *on page 216*

Community-Acquired Pneumonia *see* Pneumonia, Community-Acquired *on page 270*

Community-Acquired Sinusitis, Acute *see* Sinusitis, Community-Acquired, Acute *on page 299*

Community-Acquired Sinusitis, Chronic *see* Sinusitis, Community-Acquired, Chronic *on page 299*

Congo-Crimean Hemorrhagic Fever *see* Arboviruses *on page 35*

Conjunctivitis

Synonyms Blennophthalmia; Koch-Weeks; Pink Eye; Red Eye

Clinical Presentation Inflammation of the conjunctiva associated with marked hyperemia and mucopurulent or watery discharge. The hyperemia is less intense in the perilimbal region as compared to ciliary flush.

Differential Diagnosis Conjunctivitis - allergic, viral, bacterial, granulomatous; iritis/iridocyclitis; herpes simplex keratitis; acute angle-closure glaucoma; episcleritis; scleritis; subconjunctival hemorrhage; pterygium; foreign body/abrasions

Likely Pathogens

Adenovirus *on page 29*
Chlamydia trachomatis on page 74
Herpes Simplex Virus *on page 172*
Staphylococcus aureus, Methicillin-Susceptible *on page 307*
Neisseria gonorrhoeae on page 244
Haemophilus influenzae on page 159
Streptococcus pneumoniae, Drug-Susceptible *on page 319*

Diagnostic Tests/Procedures

Aerobic Culture, Appropriate Site *on page 365*
Adenovirus Culture *on page 365*
Chlamydia Culture *on page 413*
Gram Stain *on page 473*
Herpes Simplex Virus Culture *on page 494*
Ocular Cytology *on page 551*

Drug Therapy Comment Treatment should be based on suspected organism diagnosed. Many of the ophthalmic anti-infective agents are combined with steroids for their anti-inflammatory activity. Antibiotics are not indicated for allergic conjunctivitis.

Selected Readings

Bielory L, Lien KW, and Bigelsen S, "Efficacy and Tolerability of Newer Antihistamines in the Treatment of Allergic Conjunctivitis," *Drugs*, 2005, 65(2):215-28.

McGill JI, "A Review of the Use of Olopatadine in Allergic Conjunctivitis," *Int Ophthalmol*, 2004, 25(3):171-9.

Robert PY and Adenis JP, "Comparative Review of Topical Ophthalmic Antibacterial Preparations," *Drugs*, 2001, 61(2):175-85.

(Continued)

Conjunctivitis *(Continued)*

Weber CM and Eichenbaum JW, "Acute Red Eye. Differentiating Viral Conjunctivitis From Other, Less Common Causes," *Postgrad Med*, 1997, 101(5):185-6, 189-92, 195-6.

Coronaviridae (Including SARS)

Related Information

Community-Acquired Pneumonia in Adults *on page 1278*

Synonyms HCoV; SARS Virus

Microbiology Coronavirus particles contain RNA, are irregularly-shaped, are approximately 60-220 nm in diameter, and have an outer envelope bearing distinctive, "club-shaped" peplomers approximately 20 nm long x 10 nm wide. The name Coronavirus (Corona = crown in Latin) refers to the projection of these peplomers around the virus. When viewed with electron microscopy, the projections give the appearance of a "corona" around the virus. First isolated from chickens in 1937, Coronaviruses cause a large proportion of cold-like illnesses in humans. More recently, a severe, acute respiratory syndrome (SARS) with significant mortality has been attributed to a member of this family.

The Coronavirus envelope contains two glycoproteins, a spike glycoprotein (S) which participates in receptor binding and cell fusion, and a membrane glycoprotein (M) which participates in budding and envelope formation. Genetic material of Coronaviruses consists of a single-stranded (+) sense RNA, approximately 27-31 kb in length. The entire 29,736 nucleotide sequence has been identified. The genome is associated with a basic phosphoprotein (N). The polymerase gene is the most highly conserved portion of the Coronavirus genome. Analysis of the genome by PCR and sequencing has demonstrated that the recently recognized (in 2003) severe acute respiratory syndrome (SARS) is caused by a novel Coronavirus which has not been previously identified in humans.

Clinically, most Coronavirus infections cause a mild, self-limited disease (classical "cold" symptoms) in which growth appears to be localized to the epithelium of the upper respiratory tract. However, SARS infection encompasses the lower respiratory tract, and results in a much higher severity of symptoms.

The prototype strains HCoV 229E and HCoV OC43 are primarily associated with common cold syndrome. Reinfections with Coronaviruses appear to occur throughout life, implying multiple serotypes (at least four are known) and/or antigenic variation, which may limit the possibility of successful vaccine development.

Epidemiology Coronaviruses are transmitted by aerosols of respiratory secretions, by the fecal-oral route, and by mechanical transmission. Viral replication occurs primarily in epithelial cells; however, infection of other cell types, including macrophage, liver, kidneys, and heart have been described. Coronavirus infection is very common and occurs worldwide. A strong seasonal relationship (greatest incidence in children during the winter months) is present for most Coronavirus infections.

In March 2003, the World Health Organization reported a multicountry outbreak of an atypical pneumonia referred to as severe acute respiratory syndrome (SARS) which has since caused significant morbidity and mortality. SARS has been described in patients in Asia, North America, and Europe. As of March 21, 2003, the majority of patients identified as having SARS have been previously healthy adults between 25 and 70 years of age. Few suspected cases of SARS have been reported among children. The SARS outbreak is believed to have originated in February 2003 in the Guangdong province of China, where 300 people became ill, and at least five died. The Coronavirus responsible for SARS has several unusual properties, including growth in cell culture (most Coronaviruses cannot be cultivated). Global case counts are available at http://www.who.int.

Clinical Syndromes In humans, Coronaviruses may cause a variety of clinical syndromes, including respiratory infections (primarily cold-type illnesses), enteric infections (primarily in infants), and rare neurological syndromes. These are generally self-limiting. New attention has focused on this family following the description of severe lower respiratory tract infections (SARS).

- **Severe Acute Respiratory Syndrome (SARS):** The incubation period for SARS is typically 2-7 days and may be as long as 10 days. A prodrome has been described, consisting of high fever [>100.4°F (>38.0°C)], possibly associated with chills, rigors, and other flu-like symptoms (headache, myalgia, malaise). Mild respiratory symptoms may be present at the onset of illness. Rash, neurologic symptoms, or gastrointestinal disturbances are typically absent, although diarrhea during the febrile prodrome has been reported.

  After 3-7 days, a second phase involving the lower respiratory tract begins. Symptoms include a dry, nonproductive cough and/or dyspnea, which may progress to hypoxemia. The severity of illness appears to be highly variable,

ranging from mild illness to death. Respiratory compromise requiring intubation and mechanical ventilation may occur in 10% to 20% of cases. The case-fatality rate among persons with illness meeting the current WHO case definition of SARS is approximately 3%. Some close contacts, including healthcare workers, have developed similar illnesses.

In a substantial proportion of patients, the respiratory phase is characterized by early focal interstitial infiltrates. These frequently progress to generalized, patchy, interstitial infiltrates. Consolidation may be observed in some patients during the late stages of SARS. In some cases, chest radiographs remain normal during the prodrome and throughout the course of the illness. Laboratory findings may include thrombocytopenia and leukopenia. Early in the respiratory phase, elevated creatine phosphokinase levels (as high as 3000 IU/L) and elevated hepatic transaminases have been noted.

Diagnosis The CDC has provided the following SARS case definition criteria (as of December 2003):

Revised CST SARS Surveillance Case Definition (Summary of Criteria) (available at http://www.cdc.gov/mmwr/preview/mmwrhtml/mm5249a2.htm)

Clinical criteria:

Early illness:

- Two or more of the following: Fever, chills, rigors, myalgia, headache, sore throat, rhinorrhea

Mild-to-moderate respiratory illness:

- Temperature >100.4°F, *and*
- One or more clinical findings of LRT illness (eg, cough, SOB, difficulty breathing)

Severe respiratory illness:

- Meets clinical criteria of mild-to-moderate respiratory illness, *and*
  - radiographic evidence of pneumonia
  - acute respiratory distress syndrome
  - autopsy findings consistent with pneumonia or acute respiratory distress syndrome

Epidemiological evidence:

Possible exposure to SARS-associated coronavirus (SARS-CoV): One of more of the following in the 10 days before symptoms:

- Travel to a location with recent transmissions of SARS, *or*
- Close contact with a person with LRT illness and the aforementioned travel history

Likely exposure to SARS-CoV: One or more of the following in the 10 days before symptoms:

- Close contact with a confirmed case of SARS-CoV disease, *or*
- Close contact with a person with LRT illness for whom a chain of transmission can be linked to a case of SARS-CoV in the 10 days prior to symptoms

Laboratory criteria (not completely established):

- Detection of antibody to SARS-CoV, *or*
- Isolation of SARS-CoV in cell culture, *or*
- Detection of SARS-CoV RNA molecular methods and subsequent confirmation

Diagnostic Tests/Procedures Consult the clinical microbiology laboratory for advice and information regarding specimen selection, collection, and transport **before** selecting, collecting, and transporting specimens for the laboratory diagnosis of SARS.

CDC-Recommended Specimens for Evaluation of Potential Cases of SARS

Specimen	Outpatient	Inpatient	Fatal
Blood	• Serum (acute and convalescent >28 days postonset) • Plasma	• Serum (acute and convalescent >28 days postonset)	• Serum • Plasma
Upper respiratory	• N/P wash/aspirate • N/P or O/P swabs	• N/P wash/aspirate • N/P or O/P swabs	• N/P wash/aspirate • N/P or O/P swabs
Lower respiratory	• Sputum	• Bronchoalveolar lavage, tracheal aspirate, pleural fluid • Sputum	• Bronchoalveolar lavage, tracheal aspirate, pleural fluid
Stool	Yes	Yes	Yes
Tissue			• Fixed from all major organs • Frozen from lung and upper airway

Source: www.cdc/gov/ncidod/sars/guidance/f/app4.htm

(Continued)

Coronaviridae (Including SARS) *(Continued)*

Treatment Generally involves supportive treatment only, including hemodynamic and ventilatory support. A variety of antiviral agents are currently being evaluated.

In some cases, antiviral agents such as oseltamivir or ribavirin have been given empirically without known efficacy. In addition, steroids have been administered orally or intravenously in combination with ribavirin. The efficacy of these agents has not been confirmed.

In the United States, clinicians who suspect cases of SARS are requested to report such cases to their state health departments. CDC requests that reports of suspected cases from state health departments, international airlines, cruise ships, or cargo carriers be directed to the SARS Investigative Team at the CDC Emergency Operations Center, telephone 770-488-7100. Outside the United States, clinicians who suspect cases of SARS are requested to report such cases to their local public health authorities. Additional information about SARS (eg, infection control guidance and procedures for reporting suspected cases) is available at http://www.cdc.gov/ncidod/sars.

Selected Readings

Centers for Disease Control, "Guidelines for Collection of Specimens From Potential Cases of SARS," www.cdc.gov/ncidod/sars/specimen_collection_sars2.htm, last accessed April 23, 2003.

Centers for Disease Control, "Update: Outbreak of Severe Acute Respiratory Syndrome - Worldwide, 2003," *MMWR*, 2003, 52(13).

Ksiazek TG, Erdman D, Goldsmith C, et al, "A Novel Coronavirus Associated With Severe Acute Respiratory Syndrome," *N Engl J Med*, 2003, April 10 [epub ahead of print].

Oxford JS, Balasingam S, Chan C, et al, "New Antiviral Drugs, Vaccines, and Classic Public Health Interventions Against SARS Coronavirus," *Antivir Chem Chemother*, 2005, 16(1):13-21.

Skowronski DM, Astell C, Brunham RC, et al, "Severe Acute Respiratory Syndrome (SARS): A Year in Review," *Annu Rev Med*, 2005, 56:357-81.

Srikantiah P, Charles MD, Reagan S, et al, "SARS Clinical Features, United States, 2003," *Emerg Infect Dis*, 2005, 11(1):135-8.

Corynebacterium diphtheriae

Microbiology *Corynebacterium diphtheriae* is the causative agent of the once common disease human diphtheria. On Gram stain, the organism appears as a pleomorphic, gram-positive rod (bacillus) and has a characteristic appearance resembling "Chinese characters" or "Chinese letters". The organism has a clubbed appearance at both ends and does not form spores. Although it can be grown in culture using a variety of solid media, optimal isolation of *C. diphtheriae* from clinical specimens requires special selective media which inhibits the growth of other bacterial species; this is especially true if the specimen is submitted from the throat which is often colonized with other nonpathogenic bacteria. Thus, the laboratory should be notified if diphtheria is suspected. The organism itself is not considered highly virulent, despite its ability to cause lethal disease. An asymptomatic carrier state was recognized as far back as the late 19th century. Even in patients with diphtheria, the organism generally does not invade the host tissues and does not cause local tissue destruction. Instead, the virulence of *C. diphtheriae* comes from the ability of some strains to elaborate a potent exotoxin. These strains carry a lysogenic β-phage which is integrated into the bacterial DNA. The mechanism of action of this important toxin has been well studied. Diphtheria toxin binds to the membrane of the host cell, enters the cytoplasm, inactivates elongation factor 2, which ultimately leads to termination of polypeptide production within the host cell. The diphtheria toxin is a potent cardio- and neurotoxin although damage to almost any organ can be seen.

Epidemiology Diphtheria was once a leading cause of death in children. Over the past 75 years there has been a relatively steady decline in the number of cases in the United States and is considered a rare disease. No significant outbreaks have been reported in the U.S. in the 1990s but sporadic cases continue. Worldwide, the incidence of diphtheria has also generally decreased although less consistently, and the disease remains endemic in some developing countries and in some urban areas in Eastern Europe. The epidemiology of diphtheria has changed. Diphtheria was thought to be primarily a disease of childhood but more contemporary epidemics have involved adults. Groups at risk include the urban poor, injection drug users, and minority groups. Cases usually involve persons who have not been adequately immunized with the diphtheria vaccine, although diphtheria has been reported in fully immunized individuals.

Transmission of *C. diphtheriae* occurs primarily person-to-person by the respiratory route. Some cases have been reported transmitted by other routes such as ingestion of milk. Skin disease due to *C. diphtheriae* can occur, and spread via exposure to infected skin has been well described.

Clinical Syndromes

- **Asymptomatic infection:** Asymptomatic carriage of *C. diphtheriae* is rare in the U.S. but occurs in a low percentage of the population in endemic areas. The organism usually colonizes the upper respiratory tract. This is felt to be the main reservoir of the organism in the community since there are no recognized animal sources.
- **Respiratory tract:** *C. diphtheriae* causes local inflammation in a variety of areas in the upper respiratory tract, including the nares, pharynx, larynx, and/or tracheobronchial tree. Disease of the pharynx is the most common manifestation and is characterized by a thick "pseudomembrane" covering the tonsils, uvula, palate, and other areas of the pharynx. The membrane is usually gray often with areas of necrosis. It consists of respiratory epithelium, fibrin, inflammatory cells, and organisms. The membrane can also involve the nasopharynx, and there may be purulent discharge from the nares. Although the pharyngeal membrane is the hallmark of diphtheria, it may be absent in 50% of culture-proven cases. Regional adenopathy in the cervical area is common, and in severe cases, the patient may present with a "bull neck". The voice may be hoarse. The spectrum of disease is wide and patients may present with localized pharyngeal disease without fever, and others may have significant constitutional symptoms with respiratory compromise with stridor.
- **Systemic disease:** Diphtheria toxin is an extremely potent peptide and can cause a wide range of systemic disease. Studies have shown that these systemic complications are unusual when the local respiratory tract disease is mild and are much more likely to occur when the local disease is advanced, diagnosis is delayed, and diphtheria antitoxin is given late. Complications include myocarditis, both subclinical and fulminant cardiac involvement; cranial nerve palsies, especially paralysis of the palate; motor neuron dysfunction, ranging from mild weakness to paralysis; renal failure with acute tubular necrosis.
- **Skin disease:** *C. diphtheriae* has been associated with nonhealing cutaneous ulcers, sometimes associated with a membrane on the skin lesion. This form of diphtheria has been primarily seen in tropical climates but has recently been described in homeless and indigent adults in the United States. Individuals with chronic skin ulcers caused by *C. diphtheriae* represent another reservoir for the organism in the population and transmission from an infected skin lesion can occur. However, some controversy exists regarding the significance of isolating *C. diphtheriae* from a chronic skin lesion; some experts feel it may sometimes be a harmless colonizer and should not be automatically considered the cause of the lesion.

Diagnosis The diagnosis of diphtheria may be quite difficult in the United States due to the rarity of the disease and lack of clinical experience. Clearly, there are a number of etiologies of tonsillitis and pharyngitis, but the unusual case of diphtheria should be considered if a membrane is seen on examination (although the membrane may be absent in many cases). Other clues include the presence of toxin-mediated complications such as neuropathies or myocarditis, and the presence of stridor in an adult. Laboratory diagnosis is important for confirmation. Throat swabs and membrane material should be planted on selective culture media. It should be noted that other diseases may cause tonsillar membranes, including infectious mononucleosis.

Diagnostic Tests/Procedures

Throat Culture for *Corynebacterium diphtheriae* *on page 593*

Treatment Diphtheria antitoxin is recommended for pharyngeal and laryngeal diphtheria. This neutralizing agent has been shown to improve outcome and is derived from horse antiserum. Thus, a hypersensitivity reaction to horse-derived products may be seen. Antitoxin should be administered as soon as feasible (within 48 hours if possible) since it does not act on toxin which has already entered the cells. Antibiotic therapy against *C. diphtheriae* is also recommended to decrease the organism burden (and thus decrease toxin production) and improve local disease such as pharyngitis. The organism is sensitive to a variety of agents but generally procaine penicillin G or erythromycin is recommended.

The cornerstone of disease control remains the use of the diphtheria vaccine (diphtheria toxoid). This is included in the standard recommendations for vaccination issued by the Centers for Disease Control and Prevention, both as part of the diphtheria-pertussis-tetanus (DPT) vaccine for children and the tetanus-diphtheria (Td) toxoid in older children and adults.

Drug Therapy

Recommended:

Treatment:

Penicillin G Procaine *on page 995*

Erythromycin *on page 807*

(Continued)

Corynebacterium diphtheriae (Continued)

Prophylaxis:

Diphtheria and Tetanus Toxoid *on page 778*

Diphtheria, Tetanus Toxoids, and Acellular Pertussis Vaccine *on page 782*

Diphtheria, Tetanus Toxoids, and Acellular Pertussis Vaccine and *Haemophilus influenzae* b Conjugate Vaccine *on page 785*

Selected Readings

Harnisch JP, Tronca E, Nolan CM, et al, "Diphtheria Among Alcoholic Urban Adults. A Decade of Experience in Seattle," *Ann Intern Med*, 1989, 111(1):71-82.

Janda WM, "The Corynebacteria Revisited: New Species, Identification Kits, and Antimicrobial Susceptibility Testing," *Clin Microbiol Newslett*, 1999, 21(22):175-80.

MacGregor RR, "*Corynebacterium diphtheriae*," *Principles and Practice of Infectious Diseases*, 4th ed, Mandell GL, Bennett JE, and Dolin R, eds, New York, NY: Churchill Livingstone, 1995, 1865-72.

Millar OS, Cooper On, Kakkar VV, et al, "Invasive Infection With *Corynebacterium diphtheriae* Among Drug Users," *Lancet*, 1992, 339(8805):1359-63.

Wilson AP, Efstratiou A, Weaver E, et al, "Unusual Non-Toxigenic *Corynebacterium diphtheriae* in Homosexual Men," *Lancet*, 1992, 339(8799):998.

Corynebacterium equi *see Rhodococcus* Species *on page 288*

***Corynebacterium* Group JK** *see Corynebacterium jeikeium on page 98*

Corynebacterium jeikeium

Synonyms *Corynebacterium* Group JK

Microbiology *Corynebacterium jeikeium* was described as a human pathogen in 1976. Like other *Corynebacterium* species, it is a gram-positive, aerobic bacterium but tends to have a more coccobacillary (rather than bacillary) appearance and must be distinguished from streptococci. It is considered one of the "diphtheroids," a term which encompasses several similarly-appearing gram-positive bacilli or coccobacilli which morphologically resemble and are in the same genus as *Corynebacterium diphtheriae.*

Epidemiology *Corynebacterium jeikeium* can colonize the skin of many hospitalized patients. *Corynebacterium jeikeium* has been cultured from the skin of 50% of hospitalized oncology patients. Sites of colonization include the rectum, axilla, and inguinal areas. Healthy individuals living in the community are less likely to be colonized with this organism.

Clinical Syndromes

- **Septicemia:** *Corynebacterium jeikeium* has been increasingly recognized as a cause of bloodstream infections, particularly in those with underlying malignancies. There are also reports of bacteremias in cardiac surgery patients. In many cases, the portal of entry appears to be a skin defect, and often a bloodstream infection is associated with an indwelling vascular catheter. Risk factors also include neutropenia, lengthy hospitalization, and multiple prior antibiotics.
- **Endocarditis:** Several cases of early prosthetic valve endocarditis from *Corynebacterium jeikeium* have been described.
- **Other infections:** Infected peritoneal dialysis catheters, intravascular catheters, prosthetic central nervous system shunt infections, prosthetic orthopedic implant infections, pneumonitis, and others.

Diagnosis *Corynebacterium jeikeium* diagnosis is made by identification of the organism by Gram stain and culture in a patient with a relevant clinical syndrome. No special media or conditions are necessary for growth. **Any *Corynebacterium* isolated from multiple blood cultures or the catheter of an immunocompromised patient should be examined to determine if the isolate is *Corynebacterium jeikeium*.**

Diagnostic Tests/Procedures

Aerobic Culture, Appropriate Site *on page 365*

Anaerobic Culture *on page 371*

Gram Stain *on page 473*

Treatment *Corynebacterium jeikeium* is unique in that it is highly resistant to antimicrobial therapy. The clinically-isolated strains of JK tend to be resistant to cephalosporins and penicillins; some data suggest that antibiotic-susceptible strains of *C. jeikeium* are replaced by resistant strains during prolonged hospitalization. The antibiotic of choice is vancomycin.

Drug Therapy

Recommended:

Vancomycin *on page 1144*

Alternate:

Penicillin G (Parenteral/Aqueous) *on page 993*

plus

Gentamicin *on page 841*

Selected Readings

Balci I, Eksi F, and Bayram A, "Coryneform Bacteria Isolated From Blood Cultures and Their Antibiotic Susceptibilities," *J Int Med Res*, 2002, 30(4):422-7.

Janda WM, "The Corynebacteria Revisited: New Species, Identification Kits, and Antimicrobial Susceptibility Testing," *Clin Microbiol Newslett*, 1999, 21(22):175-80.

Rozdzinski E, Kern W, Schmeister T, et al, "*Corynebacterium jeikeium* Bacteremia at a Tertiary Care Center," *Infection*, 1991, 19(4):201-4.

Schiffl H, Mucke C, and Lang SM, "Exit-Site Infections by Non-diphtheria Corynebacteria in CAPD," *Perit Dial Int*, 2004, 24(5):454-9.

Spach DH, Opp DR, and Gabre-Kidan T, "Bacteremia Due to *Corynebacterium jeikeium* in a Patient With AIDS," *Rev Infect Dis*, 1991, 13(2):342-3.

Tleyjeh IM, Qutub MO, Bakleh M, et al, "*Corynebacterium jeikeium* Prosthetic Joint Infection: Case Report and Literature Review," *Scand J Infect Dis*, 2005, 37(2):151-3.

Corynebacterium Species, Other Than *C. jeikeium*

Microbiology *Corynebacterium* species are gram-positive bacteria which are part of the normal flora of humans. They are important members of a larger group of loosely related organisms referred to as "coryneform bacteria" or "diphtheroids" because they morphologically resemble the organism *Corynebacterium diphtheriae*. All members of the diphtheroid group (including *Corynebacterium* species) are aerobic, gram-positive bacilli or coccobacilli that often appear pleomorphic in clinical samples. Medically important coryneform bacteria include *Corynebacterium jeikeium* (see entry *Corynebacterium jeikeium on page 98*), *Corynebacterium* CDC group D-2, *Corynebacterium ulcerans*, *Arcanobacterium haemolyticum* (formerly *Corynebacterium haemolyticum*), and *Corynebacterium minutissimum*. A number of additional *Corynebacterium* species are potential pathogens.

Epidemiology Many *Corynebacterium* species are part of the normal flora of humans and are thus common isolates in a clinical microbiology laboratory. Various sites that are commonly colonized by *Corynebacterium* species include the skin of healthy persons (eg, *C. pseudodiphtheriticum*, *C. xerosis*), the skin of hospitalized patients (eg, *Corynebacterium* CDC group D-2), and the nasopharynx (several species). It may be difficult to determine the significance of a single isolate of *Corynebacterium* from a clinical specimen since it may represent colonization, skin contamination, or true disease.

Clinical Syndromes As noted above, the isolation of *Corynebacterium* species from a clinical specimen (eg, wound culture, vascular catheter culture, blood culture) requires careful interpretation by the physician. Serious disease has been associated with some *Corynebacterium* species, and the finding of a positive culture does not necessarily imply skin contamination or colonization. *Corynebacterium* species are considered organisms of low pathogenicity, and patients may present with a mild or chronic illness. Some species have been associated with specific illnesses as follows:

- **Urinary tract infections:** *Corynebacterium* CDC group D-2 has recently been recognized as a potential cause of urinary tract infections. This organism is similar to *Proteus mirabilis* in its ability to use the enzyme urease to hydrolyze urea; this leads to alkalinization of the urine and formation of struvite kidney stones which can become chronically infected. Complications include chronic cystitis secondary to infected stones and pyelonephritis. Again, the finding of a positive urine culture for "diphtheroids" or corynebacteria should be interpreted cautiously since this could also represent contamination of the urine sample from normal flora in the urethral region.
- **Erythrasma:** This common infection of the skin has been associated with *Corynebacterium minutissimum*, although the precise etiology of erythrasma is still unknown. Patients with erythrasma present with a patchy, erythematous rash often in the groin region. Under the fluorescent light of a Wood's lamp, the rash of erythrasma characteristically appears coral red. Cultures for *C. minutissimum* from patients with suspected erythrasma are not usually necessary since the diagnosis can usually be made clinically.
- **Pharyngitis:** *Arcanobacterium haemolyticum* (formerly *Corynebacterium haemolyticum*) can cause a pharyngitis associated with a scarlatiniform skin rash, particularly in young adults. The organism *C. ulcerans* (part of the flora of cows and horses) has occasionally been associated with a diphtheria-like pharyngitis in humans.
- **Pneumonia:** *Corynebacterium* species only rarely have been associated with pneumonia. There are case reports describing pneumonia in AIDS patients from *C. pseudodiphtheriticum*.
- **Bacteremia:** Since many *Corynebacterium* species are part of the normal skin flora, they may contaminate blood cultures (reported as "diphtheroids" in many laboratories). However, these organisms have been reported to cause both true bacteremia and endocarditis.

(Continued)

Corynebacterium Species, Other Than *C. jeikeium* (*Continued*)

Diagnosis Most of the clinical manifestations of *Corynebacterium* species (with the exception of erythrasma) are nonspecific and isolation of the organism in the laboratory is necessary. The organisms, in general, grow readily on standard media. At times, *Corynebacterium* CDC group D-2 may be more difficult to grow from urine cultures, and the laboratory should be notified that this organism is suspected (alkaline urine, gram-positive bacilli on Gram stain, presence of stones, etc).

Diagnostic Tests/Procedures

Aerobic Culture, Appropriate Site *on page 365*
Anaerobic Culture *on page 371*
Gram Stain *on page 473*

Treatment Treatment of *Corynebacterium* depends on the severity of the infection and to some extent on the species involved. *Corynebacterium* CDC Group D-2 tends to be somewhat more antibiotic resistant than other species, and some isolates are resistant to the quinolones, which are commonly used for urinary tract infections. *Corynebacterium* species are generally susceptible to erythromycin, vancomycin, and to most beta-lactam antibiotics. If serious infections are documented, full susceptibility testing of the organism should be performed. Note that *Corynebacterium jeikeium* (see entry *on page 98*) is often resistant to multiple antibiotics.

Drug Therapy

Recommended:

Erythromycin *on page 807*

Alternate:

Penicillin G (Parenteral/Aqueous) *on page 993*

Selected Readings

Cohen Y, Force G, Gros I, et al, "*Corynebacterium pseudodiphtheriticum* Pulmonary Infection in AIDS Patients," *Lancet*, 1992, 340(8811):114-5.
Coyle MB and Lipsky BA, "Coryneform Bacteria in Infectious Diseases: Clinical and Laboratory Aspects," *Clin Microbiol Rev*, 1990, 3(3):227-46.
George MJ, "Clinical Significance and Characterization of *Corynebacterium* Species," *Clin Microbiol Newslett*, 1995, 17(23):177-180.
Holmes RK, "Diphtheria, Other Corynebacterial Infections, and Anthrax," *Harrison's Principles of Internal Medicine*, 13th ed, Isselbacher KJ, Braunwald E, Wilson JD, et al, eds, New York, NY: McGraw-Hill, 1994, 623-30.
Janda WM, "The Corynebacteria Revisited: New Species, Identification Kits, and Antimicrobial Susceptibility Testing," *Clin Microbiol Newslett*, 1999, 21(22):175-80.
Soriano F, Aguado JM, Ponte C, et al, "Urinary Tract Infection Caused by *Corynebacterium* Group D-2: Report of 82 Cases and Review," *Rev Infect Dis*, 1990, 12(6):1019-34.

Coxiella burnetii

Related Information

Community-Acquired Pneumonia in Adults *on page 1278*

Microbiology *Coxiella burnetii* is an obligately intracellular, gram-negative coccobacillus and a member of the group of organisms known as Rickettsiae (*Rickettsia*, *Ehrlichia*, *Rochalimaea*, and *Coxiella*). *C. burnetii* survives extracellularly probably in spore form and can survive weeks to years as such in adverse environmental conditions. *C. burnetii* exists in two antigenic forms or "phases". Phase I organisms are avirulent, exist in nature and in laboratory animals, and react serologically with convalescent sera. Phase II organisms are virulent and react with acute sera. If phase I organisms are passed through chicken eggs, the phase I organisms become phase II organisms. ***C. burnetii* is extremely infectious to humans; a single organism can cause infection.**

Epidemiology Q fever, first described in Australia in 1937 (Q: "query"), occurs worldwide and is not uncommon. Cattle, goats, sheep, and ticks are natural reservoirs. Persons at high risk for Q fever are persons associated with slaughter houses, persons who work with the aforementioned animals, persons who work with hides and wool, farmers, veterinarians, and researchers. The most common causes of infection are inhalation of organisms, handling of infected birth products (especially cat and cattle placentas), skinning infected animals, and transport of infected animals. *C. burnetii* is not transmitted person-to-person and only rarely by blood products.

Clinical Syndromes Humans are the only known animals who regularly develop infection with *C. burnetii*. The incubation period is 2-4 weeks. The most common form of Q fever is a self-limited febrile illness. Q fever can also present as a rapidly progressive disease or as a secondary finding in someone with fever of unknown origin. Endocarditis, hepatitis, and atypical pneumonia are the most common manifestations of nonself-limiting disease. Endocarditis is the primary manifestation of chronic Q fever. The hepatitis form can present as infectious hepatitis.

Diagnosis Typical signs and symptoms include headache, unusually high fever, chills, fatigue, and myalgia. Other symptoms depend on which organ is affected. A rash can occur in the chronic endocarditis form of Q fever; a rash occurs only rarely in acute Q

fever. Isolation of *C. burnetii* is an extremely dangerous laboratory procedure and is not practical. The most practical and clinically relevant method is serology. Complement fixation (CF) and immunofluorescence (IF) are the two most commonly used serological methods. CF is widely available and can demonstrate a fourfold rise in titer; however, CF does not separate IgG from IgM. Immunofluorescence uses separate phase I and II antigens and is more clinically useful. Phase II and I antibody titers are usually high in acute and convalescent disease, respectively. IgM antibody can persist for more than a year in some cases, but this is not a common finding. Some laboratories offer enzyme immunoassay (EIA) serology. EIA is probably the most sensitive of the three tests.

Diagnostic Tests/Procedures

Q Fever Serology *on page 569*

Drug Therapy Comment Infections due to *C. burnetii* are usually mild and self-limiting, and do not necessarily require antibiotic therapy. Typically, antibiotics only decrease duration of symptoms by 1-3 days. Doxycycline is probably the most active agent against this organism. Fluoroquinolones and chloramphenicol are reasonable alternatives. Recent data suggests that macrolides are also active.

Pediatric Drug Therapy

Recommended:

Chloramphenicol *on page 733*

Adult Drug Therapy

Recommended:

Doxycycline *on page 787*
plus
Hydroxychloroquine *on page 859*
Doxycycline *on page 787*
plus
Fluoroquinolones *on page 824*

Alternate:

Fluoroquinolones *on page 824*
Chloramphenicol *on page 733*
Macrolides *on page 924*
During pregnancy:
Sulfamethoxazole and Trimethoprim *on page 1087*

Selected Readings

Alarcon A, Villanueva JL, Viciana P, et al, "Q Fever: Epidemiology, Clinical Features and Prognosis. A Study From 1983 to 1999 in the South of Spain," *J Infect*, 2003, 47(2):110-6.

Brennan RE and Samuel JE, "Evaluation of *Coxiella burnetii* Antibiotic Susceptibilities by Real-Time PCR Assay," *J Clin Microbiol*, 2003, 41(5):1869-74.

Gikas A, Kofteridis DP, Manios A, et al, "Newer Macrolides as Empiric Treatment for Acute Q Fever Infection," *Antimicrob Agents Chemother*, 2001, 45(12):3644-6.

Houpikian P, Habib G, Mesana T, et al, "Changing Clinical Presentation of Q Fever Endocarditis," *Clin Infect Dis*, 2002, 34(5):E28-31.

Marrie TJ and Raoult D, "Update on Q Fever, Including Q Fever Endocarditis," *Curr Clin Top Infect Dis*, 2002, 22:97-124.

Nicholson WL, McQuiston J, Vannieuwenhoven TJ, et al, "Rapid Deployment and Operation of a Q Fever Field Laboratory in Bosnia and Herzegovina," *Ann N Y Acad Sci*, 2003, 990:320-6.

Scola BL, "Current Laboratory Diagnosis of Q Fever," *Semin Pediatr Infect Dis*, 2002, 13(4):257-62.

Coxsackieviruses

Microbiology The name "Coxsackievirus" is derived from the town where this agent was first isolated: Coxsackie, New York. These viruses are composed of single-stranded RNA and have a positive-sense linear genome. They belong to the genus Enterovirus and the family Picornaviridae. The name "Picornaviridae" summarizes the nature of the family: pico (small), -rna (ribonucleic acid), -viruses. Coxsackieviruses are related to poliovirus, echovirus, and rhinovirus. There are two major types of Coxsackieviruses, types A and B. These are further subdivided into numbered serotypes.

Epidemiology Coxsackieviruses can infect all age groups. The virus is found worldwide and predominantly during the summer months. Transmission is mainly by the fecal-oral route, but droplet infection by the respiratory route is also possible. Infection rates are higher in communities with poor sanitation and crowding.

Clinical Syndromes

Diseases caused by Coxsackieviruses, group A:

- **Herpangina:** Patients present with sore throat, fever, and sometimes nausea and vomiting. On examination, there are vesicles present on the soft palate, a location unusual for other agents. Lesions are also seen on the uvula, and less commonly on the hard palate. Cultures of active ulcerating vesicles will yield the organism. Symptoms resolve spontaneously over several days.
- **Hand-foot-and-mouth syndrome**
- **Epidemic conjunctivitis**
- **Pharyngitis**

(Continued)

Coxsackieviruses *(Continued)*

Diseases caused mainly by Coxsackieviruses, group B:

- **Epidemic pleurodynia:** Group B Coxsackieviruses cause this syndrome of fever, sharp pleuritic pain in the rib cage or upper abdomen. Patients describe this as a "stitch" in the side and is caused by disease of the muscle (not pleura or ribs). The pain is spasmodic in nearly all cases. The diagnosis can be confirmed by obtaining cultures of the throat and/or stool for this virus, or by demonstrating a rise in antibody titer.
- **Myocarditis, pericarditis**
- **Overwhelming infection of the newborn, congenital neurodevelopmental delays**

Diseases caused by either group A or B Coxsackieviruses:

- **Acute aseptic meningitis**
- **Undifferentiated febrile illness**
- **Fever with upper respiratory infection**
- **Encephalitis**
- **Asymptomatic infection**

In addition, the Coxsackieviruses have been linked with such diverse diseases as the Guillain-Barré syndrome, hemolytic uremic syndrome, diarrheal illnesses, myositis, Reye's syndrome, and a syndrome similar to infectious mononucleosis.

Diagnosis Coxsackievirus infection is suspected when an individual presents with one of the syndromes mentioned above. The differential diagnosis of these syndromes is wide, and laboratory confirmation is often necessary. Appropriate specimens of cerebrospinal fluid, rectal swabs, conjunctival swabs, or throat swabs should be promptly submitted to the Microbiology Laboratory. A special request for a Coxsackievirus (or enterovirus) culture should be made.

Diagnostic Tests/Procedures

Coxsackie A Virus Serology *on page 427*
Coxsackie B Virus Serology *on page 428*
Enterovirus Culture *on page 453*

Drug Therapy Comment

No antiviral agents have been proven effective.

Selected Readings

Cree BC, Bernardini GL, Hays AP, et al, "A Fatal Case of Coxsackievirus B4 Meningoencephalitis," *Arch Neurol*, 2003, 60(1):107-12.
Euscher E, Davis J, Holzman I, et al, "Coxsackie Virus Infection of the Placenta Associated With Neurodevelopmental Delays in the Newborn," *Obstet Gynecol*, 2001, 98(6):1019-26.
Modlin JF, "Coxsackieviruses, Echoviruses, and Newer Enteroviruses," *Principles and Practice of Infectious Diseases*, 4th ed, Mandell GL, Bennett JE, and Dolin R, eds, New York, NY: Churchill Livingstone, 1995, 1620-36.

Creutzfeldt-Jacob Disease *see* Spongiform Encephalopathy *on page 301*

Croup *see* Parainfluenza Virus *on page 254*

Cryptococcosis *see Cryptococcus neoformans on page 102*

Cryptococcus neoformans

Related Information

USPHS / IDSA Guidelines for the Prevention of Opportunistic Infections in Persons Infected With HIV *on page 1237*

Microbiology *Cryptococcus neoformans* is an encapsulated round to oval yeast 4-6 µm with a surrounding polysaccharide capsule ranging in size (when found *in vivo*) from 1 to over 30 µm. In its natural environment, it is smaller and poorly encapsulated.

It is distinguished from other yeasts by its ability to assimilate urea and possesses membrane-bound phenoloxidase enzymes that convert phenolic compounds to melanin as easily demonstrated on certain agars (ie, birdseed agars).

Epidemiology There are four serotypes designated A, B, C, and D. Serotypes A and D (*C. neoformans* var *neoformans*) is the most common cause of infection and usually occurs in immunocompromised hosts. Serotypes B and C (*C. neoformans* var *gattii*) is typically seen in normal hosts and has a predilection for CNS invasion.

Cryptococcus is found worldwide. *C. neoformans var gattii* is endemic in the tropical and subtropical regions (Southern California, Australia, Southeast Asia, Brazil, Central America), particularly in the soils under eucalyptus trees. *Cryptococcus* grows readily from soil contaminated with avian excreta, particularly pigeon droppings but also has been isolated from nonavian sources such as fruits, vegetables, and dairy products. There have been no outbreaks attributable to environmental sources.

Cryptococcosis is the etiological agent of the most common life-threatening meningitis in AIDS. Prior to the introduction of potent antiretroviral therapy, 5% to 8% of AIDS patients developed a cryptococcal infection. The incidence of AIDS-related

cryptococcal disease is decreasing presumably due to the use of potent antiretroviral therapy and the increased use of azoles. Prior to AIDS, 50% of patients had no known underlying immune defect. Risk factors prior to AIDS include diabetes, rheumatoid arthritis, cirrhosis, leukopenia, and malignancy. It was rarely seen in children, and the incidence in men was three times that of women.

Mortality risk factors include positive India ink, increased opening CSF pressure, decreased CSF glucose, CSF leukocyte count <20 cells/µL, extraneural site, absent *Cryptococcus* antibody, *Cryptococcus* antigen >1:32, and steroids or lymphoreticular malignancy. Good prognostic indications include headache as a symptom, normal mental status, and CSF leukocytes >20 cells/µL. Most important prognostic factor is patient's underlying disease process. Morbidity, mortality, and relapse are all increased in immunocompromised hosts.

Clinical Syndromes

- **Asymptomatic:** Solitary or multiple nodules found on plain chest x-ray.
- **Pulmonary cryptococcosis:** Most common infection. Present with cough, fever, and lobar infiltrates or mass. May see diffuse interstitial pattern or pleural effusion. If positive serum *Cryptococcus* antigen, look for disseminated disease.
- **CNS:** Second most common site of infection. Presents as either acute (headache, fever, nuchal rigidity) or chronic (headache, altered mental status) meningitis. May see cryptococcomas on CT or MRI. Usually secondary to lung but may represent reactivation similar to *Histoplasma* and tuberculosis.
- **Cutaneous:** Wide variation, may appear as papules, tumors, vesicles, plaques, abscesses, cellulitis, purpura, draining sinus, ulcers, bullae, or subcutaneous swelling. Usually a sign of dissemination.
- **Other:** Rarely invades eyes, bones, joints, liver, kidneys, or adrenal glands.

Diagnosis Diagnosis is confirmed by isolation from sterile body fluids including blood or histopathology revealing encapsulated yeast cells by alcian blue or mucicarmine. The India ink stain is positive only approximately 50% of the time in normal hosts and >80% of the time in AIDS patients. Specificity of the India ink test is low.

Cryptococcal antigen has >95% sensitivity and specificity but does cross react with *Trichosporon beigelii* and can be inhibited by rheumatic fever. It is difficult to interpret a persistently high titer even though high titers have been associated with poor prognosis. Cryptococcal antigen in the CSF is produced locally in the subarachnoid space by the invading yeast and not by passive or active diffusion from serum into the CNS. **Serial monitoring of serum cryptococcal antigen in patients with AIDS-related cryptococcal disease on treatment does not provide any useful clinical data and should not be repeated after the initial diagnosis is made.** On the other hand, serial monitoring of titers in immunocompetent patients can be clinically useful. CSF findings include a pleocytosis lasting 6-12 months, low glucose concentrations, and high protein concentrations.

All AIDS patients with a positive serum cryptococcal antigen **must** have a lumbar puncture performed to exclude CNS disease.

Diagnostic Tests/Procedures

Cryptococcal Antigen Serology, Serum or Cerebrospinal Fluid *on page 431*
Cryptococcus Serology *on page 431*
Fungus Culture, Appropriate Site *on page 461*
India Ink Preparation *on page 507*
KOH Preparation *on page 513*

Treatment Current practice guidelines for the treatment of *Cryptococcus neoformans* meningitis in patients with or without AIDS is amphotericin B, 0.7-1 mg/kg/day given in combination with flucytosine, 100 mg/kg/day, for 2 weeks, followed by fluconazole 400-800 mg/day for 10 weeks. In HIV patients, this is followed by lifelong maintenance with fluconazole until or unless the patient has a sustained immunologic response to antiretroviral therapy.

In patients with mild to moderate pulmonary disease, patients may be treated with fluconazole, 200-400 mg/day for 6-12 months. Moderate to severe disease should be treated as disseminated disease with amphotericin B.

Drug Therapy

Recommended:

Amphotericin B (Conventional) *on page 650*
plus
Flucytosine *on page 822*
Fluconazole *on page 819*

Alternate:

Fluconazole *on page 819*
Itraconazole *on page 895*
Amphotericin B (Lipid Complex) *on page 653*

(Continued)

Cryptococcus neoformans (Continued)

Selected Readings

Aberg JA, Mundy LM, and Powderly WG, "Pulmonary Cryptococcosis in Patients Without HIV Infection," *Chest*, 1999, 115(3):734-40.

Aberg JA and Powderly WG, "Cryptococcosis and HIV," *A Textbook on HIV Disease From the University of California, San Francisco and the San Francisco General Hospital*, Peiperl L and Volberding P, eds, 2002, http://hivinsite.ucsf.edu/InSite.jsp?page=kb-05&doc=kb-05-02-05.

Aberg JA, Watson J, Segal M, et al, "Clinical Utility of Monitoring Serum Cryptococcal Antigen (sCRAG) in Patients With AIDS-Related Cryptococcal Disease," *HIV Clinical Trials*, 2000, 1(1):1-6.

Adeyemi OM, Pulvirenti J, Perumal S, et al, "Cryptococcosis in HIV-Infected Individuals," *AIDS*, 2004, 18(16):2218-9.

Bicanic T and Harrison TS, "Cryptococcal Meningitis," *Br Med Bull*, 2005, 72:99-118.

Saag MS, J Graybill R, Larsen RA, et al, "Practice Guidelines for the Management of Cryptococcal Disease," *Clin Infect Dis*, 2000, 30(4):710-8.

Sobel JD, "Practice Guidelines for the Treatment of Fungal Infections. For the Mycoses Study Group. Infectious Diseases Society of America," *Clin Infect Dis*, 2000, 30(4):652.

van der Horst CM, Saag MS, Cloud GA, et al, "Treatment of Cryptococcal Meningitis Associated With the Acquired Immunodeficiency Syndrome. The National Institute of Allergy and Infectious Diseases Mycoses Study Group and the AIDS Clinical Trials Group," *N Engl J Med*, 1997, 337(1):15-21.

Cryptosporidiosis *see Cryptosporidium on page 104*

Cryptosporidium

Microbiology Although *Cryptosporidium* was identified as early as 1907, it was not recognized as a human pathogen until 1976. *Cryptosporidium* is classified as a protozoan and is structurally related to *Toxoplasma gondii* and *Cyclospora cayetanensis*. Several species of *Cryptosporidium* have been found; the species most associated with human disease is *C. parvum*. The organism is approximately 2.5 µm in diameter and is about the same size and shape as many yeasts. *Cryptosporidium* can be identified by use of an acid-fast stain or an immunofluorescence test of a fresh stool specimen.

The parasite has four spores (sporozoites) within an oocyst. Its life cycle occurs within a single host. Human infection begins when the mature oocyst form of *Cryptosporidium* is ingested or perhaps inhaled. The four sporozoites excyst and divide asexually into meronts which release merozoites which can either reinvade the human or develop sexually into meronts. The sexual cycle ends in the formation of oocysts. The oocysts can then exit the body of the host through the feces to begin the infectious cycle in a new human or in the same host (autoinfection).

Epidemiology Cryptosporidial infections occur worldwide. In the United States, the organism is most prevalent in persons with AIDS, with infection rates ranging from 3% to 20%. In such countries as Africa and Haiti, *Cryptosporidium* can infect over 50% of the AIDS population. The organism is also a cause of sporadic diarrheal illness in normal individuals. Outbreaks of cryptosporidiosis have been well-described in the U.S. and include a recent outbreak in Wisconsin related to a contaminated metropolitan water supply.

The modes of transmission are as follows:

- Person-to-person (more common): Accounts for spread of infection within daycare centers, households, and hospitals. Transmission is usually by a fecal-oral route.
- Environmental contamination (more common): The oocyst can be found in rivers and other natural water supplies, and thus, the traveler and camper is at risk. *Cryptosporidium* resists standard chlorination procedures in many areas and thus, can initiate major outbreaks of diarrheal illness when water supplies are contaminated.
- Animal-to-human (less common)
- Food-borne illness (less common)

Clinical Syndromes

- **Acute diarrhea in the normal host:** The most common manifestation of human cryptosporidiosis is a syndrome characterized by profuse, watery diarrhea, malaise, and abdominal cramping or pain. Fevers to the 39°C to 40°C range have occurred even in immunologically competent individuals. The incubation period is estimated to be 2-14 days following exposure to the parasite. The diarrhea often has an acute onset and symptoms can last 2 weeks or more.
- **Acute diarrhea in the immunocompromised host:** Cryptosporidiosis can be more subacute in onset. However, it is still characterized by voluminous diarrhea and weight loss over a several-week period can occur.
- **Cryptosporidial cholecystitis:** This has been described in immunocompromised patients. Symptoms include right upper quadrant abdominal pain, nausea, vomiting, and fever. There can be a concomitant diarrheal illness.

Diagnosis The symptoms of human cryptosporidiosis are nonspecific and cannot be distinguished from other causes of acute diarrheal illnesses. A high level of suspicion

must be maintained because the organism cannot be readily identified using standard fecal smears.

Standard laboratory blood tests are not helpful in establishing the diagnosis. The leukocyte count may be normal, and usually there is not a peripheral blood eosinophilia to suggest a parasitic disease. Abnormalities in radiographic studies such as barium enemas and small bowel series have been described but again are not diagnostic of the organism.

The only reliable means of detecting *Cryptosporidium* in stool in the laboratory is to perform a direct exam (acid-fast stain, direct fluorescence test) or enzyme immunoassay of a stool sample. Real-time PCR tests for *Cryptosporidium parvum* are available in some reference and research laboratories. Because excretion of the parasite in the feces may be intermittent, it is recommended that two or more separate samples be submitted to the laboratory.

Physicians must specifically order tests for *Cryptosporidium* if this organism is suspected because routine tests ("O and P") for parasites in stool do not include examination for *Cryptosporidium.*

Diagnostic Tests/Procedures

Acid-Fast Stain *on page 361*

Cryptosporidium Diagnostic Procedures, Stool *on page 432*

Treatment At present, there is no widely accepted antimicrobial agent is effective against *Cryptosporidium.* Some initial reports suggested that the extended-spectrum macrolides, such as clarithromycin and azithromycin, may have some use, but further studies are needed. There has also been some evidence of the activity of protease inhibitors either alone or in conjunction with paromomycin. This has not been confirmed with clinical trials.

Drug Therapy Comment

Supportive care as treatment of choice.

Selected Readings

Allam AF and Shehab AY, "Efficacy of Azithromycin, Praziquantel and Mirazid in Treatment of Cryptosporidiosis in School Children," *J Egypt Soc Parasitol*, 2002, 32(3):969-78.

Bissuel F, Cotte L, Rabodonirina M, et al, "Paromomycin: An Effective Treatment for Crytosporidial Diarrhea in Patients With AIDS," *Clin Infect Dis*, 1994, 18(3):447-9.

Chen XM, Keithly JS, Paya CV, et al, "Cryptosporidiosis," *N Engl J Med*, 2002, 346(22):1723-31.

Goodgame RW, "Understanding Intestinal Spore-Forming Protozoa: Cryptosporidia, Microsporidia, *Isospora*, and *Cyclospora*," *Ann Intern Med*, 1996, 124(4):429-41.

Gradus MS, "*Cryptosporidium* and Public Health: From Watershed to Water Glass," *Clin Microbiol Newslett*, 2000, 22(4):25-32.

Hommer V, Eichholz J, and Petry F, "Effect of Antiretroviral Protease Inhibitors Alone, and in Combination With Paromycin, on the Excystation, Invasion, and In Vitro Development of *Cryptosporidium pavum*," *J Antimicrob Chemother*, 2003, 52(3):359-64.

Johnston SP, Ballard MM, Beach MJ, et al, "Evaluation of Three Commercial Assays for Detection of *Giardia* and *Cryptosporidium* Organisms in Fecal Specimens," *J Clin Microbiol*, 2003, 41(2):623-6.

Leav BA, Mackay M, and Ward HD, "*Cryptosporidium* Species: New Insights and Old Challenges," *Clin Infect Dis*, 2003, 36(7):903-8.

Limor JR, Lal AA, and Xiao L, "Detection and Differentiation of *Cryptosporidium* Parasites That Are Pathogenic for Humans by Real-Time PCR," *J Clin Microbiol*, 2002, 40(7):2335-8.

Mele R, Gomez Morales MA, Tosini F, et al, "Indinavir Reduces *Cryptosporidium parvum* Infection in Both In Vitro and In Vivo Models," *Int J Parasitol*, 2003, 33(7):757-64.

Cyanobacterium-Like Body *see Cyclospora cayetanensis on page 105*

Cyclospora cayetanensis

Synonyms Cyanobacterium-Like Body

Microbiology *Cyclospora cayetanensis* is a protozoal parasitic organism which can cause prolonged diarrhea in both immunocompromised and healthy individuals. Originally it was thought to be similar to blue-green algae and thus referred to as "Cyanobacteria-like bodies"; later the organism was found to be distinct from any known Cyanobacteria type. Based on characteristics such as excystation and sporulation, *Cyclospora* is now classified in the coccidian genus. *Cyclospora* is similar to but distinct from *Cryptosporidium* species, a related protozoal organism which causes infectious diarrhea. In the past, *Cyclospora* has been referred to as "big cryptosporidia". The oocysts of *Cyclospora* are 8-10 μm in diameter, approximately twice as large as *Cryptosporidium* species, an important distinguishing feature. After excretion in human feces, the oocysts are not immediately infectious and require some days to weeks under the proper conditions to sporulate.

Cyclospora is difficult to identify by conventional means. It cannot be recovered on routine stool culture and cannot be seen with a variety of stains including Gram stain, hematoxylin-eosin (H & E), Giemsa, methylene blue, silver stain, and others. The organism can be identified by several techniques.

1. Modified acid-fast stain of stool, in which organisms often stain deep red or pink.
2. Ultraviolet microscopy of either fresh or preserved stool (*Cyclospora* autofluoresce under ultraviolet light).

(Continued)

Cyclospora cayetanensis (Continued)

Although the modified acid-fast stain is rapid and can establish the diagnosis in many cases, some *Cyclospora* oocysts are not acid-fast and may be missed. Some techniques may not be available in all laboratories and stool specimens in suspected cases can be referred to reference laboratories.

Epidemiology *Cyclospora* has only recently been recognized as a cause of human disease, with the first case diagnosed in 1977. Cases have been reported worldwide, particularly in Nepal during the rainy season. In one study, 11% of travelers and residents in Nepal who had gastrointestinal symptoms had *Cyclospora* in stool specimens as compared with 1% of healthy controls. Children from slum areas in Lima, Peru had a high rate of *Cyclospora* infection (up to 18%), although most were asymptomatic. Other at-risk areas include Mexico, Morocco, India, and Pakistan. Disease has been reported in U.S. travelers returning from all of these areas. The true prevalence of this disease globally is unknown and is under study. Transmission is by the fecal-oral route, with human to human transmission unlikely. Disease is primarily water-borne and usually follows ingestion of contaminated food or water. Cases are clustered in the spring and summer.

The first outbreak of *Cyclospora* in the United States was reported in 1995 from 11 persons working in a Chicago hospital. The source of the *Cyclospora* was identified as tap water from a physicians' dormitory, probably as a result of stagnant water in a storage tank. Since then, three other outbreaks have been reported in the United States. The most recent outbreak occurred in May, 1996 in Charlestown, South Carolina where 37 of 64 persons attending a luncheon developed *Cyclospora* infection. The offending food items were identified as raspberries and possibly strawberries. Cases have since been reported from 10 states associated with consumption of fresh fruits at social functions.

Clinical Syndromes

- **Asymptomatic infection**: Studies have suggested that *Cyclospora* may be identified in the stool of persons with no diarrheal symptoms.
- **Diarrhea in immunocompetent persons**: *Cyclospora* causes a nonspecific diarrheal illness characterized by cycles of exacerbations and remissions. The primary area of pathology appears to be the small bowel. The average incubation period is 1 week. Disease is characterized mainly by frequent watery stools; other symptoms include abdominal cramping, muscle aches, anorexia, fever, nausea, and vomiting. Symptoms may be prolonged, with an average of 6 weeks in some studies, although the diarrhea is usually self-limited.
- **Diarrhea in immunocompromised persons**: *Cyclospora* is a potential cause of prolonged diarrhea in persons with AIDS. The clinical course is similar to diarrhea in immunocompetent persons and is essentially the same as diarrhea caused by Cryptosporidia or *Isospora belli.* There appears to be a high recurrence rate for *Cyclospora* diarrhea and antibiotic prophylaxis has been suggested.

Diagnosis *Cyclospora* is still infrequently identified but should be considered in the differential diagnosis of prolonged diarrhea in persons traveling to high risk areas, patients with AIDS and diarrhea of unknown origin, and in outbreak settings which appear to be food- or water-borne. Stool specimens should be submitted in suspected cases. The organism has also been identified in duodenal aspirates and small bowel biopsy. This organism may be missed on routine stool studies and thus should be considered in culture-negative and stain-negative cases. Specialized laboratory techniques are necessary for optimal identification (see Microbiology above). It is important to establish a proper diagnosis since treatment for *Cyclospora* is available.

Diagnostic Tests/Procedures

Acid-Fast Stain *on page 361*

Note: Tests for both *Cyclospora* and *Cryptosporidium* must be specifically ordered, and are not included in routine bacterial or parasitic examinations of stool.

Treatment The drug of choice is sulfamethoxazole and trimethoprim. Although only limited data is available concerning treatment options, sulfamethoxazole and trimethoprim for 7 days administered orally proved superior to placebo both in clinical symptoms and eradication of the organism from the stools. In persons with AIDS and *Cyclospora* infection, some authorities have recommended chronic prophylaxis with sulfamethoxazole and trimethoprim, given the high relapse rate. Alternative agents for persons who are sulfa-allergic are as yet unknown; ciprofloxacin has been studied in a small trial and was moderately effective for secondary prophylaxis, but less effective than sulfamethoxazole and trimethoprim. Rehydration, electrolyte replacement, and supportive care remain important features of treatment.

Drug Therapy

Recommended:

Sulfamethoxazole and Trimethoprim *on page 1087*

Selected Readings

Eberhard ML, Pieniazek NJ, and Arrowood MJ, "Laboratory Diagnosis of *Cyclospora* Infections," *Arch Pathol Lab Med*, 1997, 121(8):792-7.

Goodgame RW, "Understanding Intestinal Spore-Forming Protozoa: Cryptosporidia, Microsporidia, *Isospora*, and *Cyclospora*," *Ann Intern Med*, 1996, 124(4):429-41.

Hoge CW, Shlim DR, Ghimire M, et al, "Placebo-Controlled Trial of Co-Trimoxazole for *Cyclospora* Infections Among Travelers and Foreign Residents in Nepal," *Lancet*, 1995, 345:691-3.

Huang P, Weber JT, Sosin DM, et al, "The First Reported Outbreak of Diarrheal Illness Associated With *Cyclospora* in the United States," *Ann Intern Med*, 1995, 123(6):409-14.

Mansfield LS and Gajadhar AA, "*Cyclospora cayetanensis*, a Food- and Waterborne Coccidian Parasite," *Vet Parasitol*, 2004, 126(1-2):73-90.

Ochoa TJ, Salazar-Lindo E, and Cleary TG, "Management of Children With Infection-Associated Persistent Diarrhea," *Semin Pediatr Infect Dis*, 2004, 15(4):229-36.

Ortega YR and Sterling CR, "*Cyclospora cayetanensis*: Epidemiology and Diagnosis," *Clin Microbiol Newslett*, 1996, 18(22):169-72.

Sivapalasingam S, Friedman CR, Cohen L, et al, "Fresh Produce: A Growing Cause of Outbreaks of Food-Borne Illness in the United States, 1973 Through 1997," *J Food Prot*, 2004, 67(10):2342-53.

Verdier RI, Fitzgerald DW, Johnson WD Jr, et al, "Trimethoprim-Sulfamethoxazole Compared With Ciprofloxacin for Treatment and Prophylaxis of *Isospora belli* and *Cyclospora cayetanensis* Infection in HIV-Infected Patients. A Randomized, Controlled Trial," *Ann Intern Med*, 2000, 132(11):885-8.

Yazar S, Yalcln S, and Sahin I, "Human Cyclosporiosis in Turkey," *World J Gastroenterol*, 2004, 10(12):1844-7.

Cystitis *see* Urinary Tract Infection, Uncomplicated *on page 346*

Cytomegalovirus

Related Information

USPHS / IDSA Guidelines for the Prevention of Opportunistic Infections in Persons Infected With HIV *on page 1237*

Synonyms CMV; hCMV; Human CMV

Microbiology As a member of the herpesvirus family, human CMV is a double-stranded DNA virus consisting of a nucleoprotein capsid surrounded by a lipid-containing envelope. Like other herpesviruses, CMV replicates in the cell nucleus. Infected cells are often destroyed by the CMV with release of infective virions. The virus can also establish a state of latency within an infected cell. A number of different organs can harbor latent infection, but CMV appears to be restricted to certain cell types especially granulocytes, monocytes, CD4 and $CD8^+$ T-cells, and endothelial cells. In particular, the polymorphonuclear leukocyte fraction of granulocytes appears to harbor CMV (some assays for CMV only test the polymorphonuclear fraction of cells). Latent CMV can exist in both the nucleus and cytoplasm. Infected epithelial cells may demonstrate characteristic CMV inclusions within the nucleus called "owl's eye" inclusions. Strains of human CMV are antigenically heterogeneous with differences expressed through endonuclease mapping. No serological distinctions are made. Although difficult to grow in experimental animals, it can be cultured (1-4 weeks) in human fibroblasts.

Epidemiology CMV infections occur worldwide. Infection is uncommon in the newborn but is common throughout childhood, in part because the virus is present in saliva, feces, and urine and spread from child to child. Transmission generally requires repeated, prolonged contact. Spread is known to occur in daycare centers. In young adults, CMV can also be a sexually transmitted disease, with asymptomatic carriage in the semen and cervical secretions. Infected children can cause CMV infection in a susceptible parent, and there is a second peak in incidence of CMV in adults 20-30 years old due to sexual activity and parenting. About 50% of the general population is seropositive by the third decade of life. The incidence of CMV infection is more common in underdeveloped countries, lower socioeconomic groups, and in individuals with multiple sexual partners. The rate of CMV infection approaches 100% in homosexually active men. CMV may also be acquired from blood transfusions or organ transplantation. In general, CMV infection is latent and asymptomatic throughout life. Reactivations of latent CMV occur in immunocompetent persons but are usually asymptomatic. Individuals at risk for symptomatic CMV infection are those with deficits in T-cell immunity, such as persons with HIV with low $CD4^+$ T-cells, organ transplant recipients, and persons receiving high dose corticosteroids.

Clinical Syndromes

- **Congenital CMV infection:** The fetus may become infected with CMV in two ways, primary CMV infection of the mother during pregnancy or reactivation of latent CMV in the mother during pregnancy. Primary maternal infection is much more likely to cause significant fetal infection. The manifestations of disease in the fetus are quite variable. Severe CMV disease is seen in only a small percentage of infected fetuses (5%). At birth, infants have hepatosplenomegaly, jaundice, microcephaly, and other abnormalities. Prognosis depends on the severity of the disease. The majority of congenitally-infected neonates appear healthy at birth. Up to 25% of these asymptomatically infected infants will show developmental disorders later in childhood, such as deafness and mental retardation. Severe CMV infections are associated with a mortality approaching 30%.

(Continued)

Cytomegalovirus *(Continued)*

- **Perinatal infection:** These infants are not infected *in utero* but instead acquire CMV during delivery. Seropositive mothers may shed virus into the birth canal due to CMV reactivation. Many infants infected in this manner remain healthy. In a small number of cases, neonates may develop pneumonia, lymphadenopathy, and rash. Infants excrete CMV for months. Neonatal infection can also be transmitted by breast milk.
- **CMV mononucleosis syndrome:** In normal adults, primary infection with CMV is usually asymptomatic. The most common form of clinically apparent disease in previously healthy adults is a febrile illness resembling Epstein-Barr virus mononucleosis. Typically, the patient presents with fever, chills, myalgias, and headache. Examination reveals an enlarged spleen and liver, but unlike EBV infection, adenopathy and pharyngitis are minimal. Most patients recover without incident but occasionally symptoms may persist for weeks. Laboratory studies show elevated liver function tests and circulating atypical lymphocytes on blood smear. Heterophil antibody tests for Epstein-Barr virus are negative. CMV can be recovered in urine and saliva for an extended period of time. The physician must rely on laboratory tests to distinguish CMV mononucleosis from similar syndromes caused by either EBV, human herpesvirus 6, or *Toxoplasma gondii*.
- **CMV in the transplant recipient:** One of the most feared complications of transplantation is CMV infection, particularly pneumonia. The highest risk for symptomatic CMV infection is an organ donor who is CMV IgG positive and the recipient is CMV IgG negative, a "CMV mismatch." CMV disease can also occur if either or both the donor and recipient are CMV IgG positive, but the risk of disease and disease severity is less. The peak time for CMV disease occurs several weeks post-transplantation, the so-called "40-day fever". CMV pneumonitis carries a high morbidity. Patients present with dyspnea, fever, cough, and interstitial infiltrates on chest x-ray. Bronchoscopy is usually necessary for both culture and lung biopsy. The diagnosis of CMV pneumonia has been somewhat controversial; it is apparent that a bronchial lavage culture positive for CMV is not necessarily diagnostic of pneumonia. Many clinicians prefer to see the characteristic CMV "owl's eye" inclusion bodies on lung biopsy before diagnosing true pneumonia. Treatment of CMV pneumonia is with ganciclovir intravenously, but failures still occur. Some researchers advocate the use of CMV hyperimmune globulin (concentrated CMV immunoglobulins) in conjunction with ganciclovir, but results of such use have been mixed. A number of other organ systems can be infected with CMV, including the liver, gastrointestinal tract, brain and spinal cord, and kidneys. A "CMV syndrome" is well-recognized in both bone marrow and solid organ transplant recipients. This is characterized by fever, myalgias, and leukopenia which is nonspecific but at times may be severe and prolonged. The CMV syndrome requires detection of CMV in the blood, exclusion of other causes of a nonspecific "viral syndrome" and may respond to antiviral therapy.
- **CMV retinitis in AIDS:** Several different organs may be infected with CMV in individuals with AIDS. Prior to the widespread use of highly active antiretroviral therapy (HAART) against HIV, CMV retinitis was the most common manifestation of CMV in AIDS occurring in 30% of persons with CD4 <50 cells/mm^3. Patients typically complain of altered vision or "floaters" in one or both eyes. Examination reveals white exudates involving the retina, with or without retinal hemorrhages ("cottage cheese and catsup" appearance). Vitritis is usually minimal. Retinal involvement is classified by zones as follows:

  Zone 1: <3000 µm from the center of the fovea
  Zone 2: From zone 1 (vascular arcades) to the vortex veins
  Zone 3: Most peripheral

  Complications of CMV retinitis include (1) loss of central visual acuity, particularly if the optic nerve and macula are involved, and (2) retinal detachment. In some persons, the retina breaks along the margin; treatment consists of vitrectomy and silicone oil, and laser photocoagulation.

  Patients with advanced AIDS and very low CD4 counts require prolonged antiviral therapy. Progression of retinitis is common despite adequate therapy, although the retinitis can be suppressed for extended periods of time. Since 1996, the widespread use of combination antiretroviral therapy in the U.S. has significantly decreased the incidence of CMV retinitis. The incidence has declined dramatically with perhaps an 80% decline in new cases. CMV retinitis is still seen in persons with newly diagnosed AIDS who have not received HAART, individuals who have failed HAART, and in countries where HAART is not available.

  An "immune reconstitution syndrome" has been described in a limited number of patients with inactive CMV retinitis who have responded well to HAART therapy.

These individuals develop acute visual loss several months after discontinuing CMV maintenance therapy and have sight-threatening uveitis, optic disc edema, macular edema, and other visual symptoms, but no active CMV. The etiology of this is unclear but the syndrome is postulated as being immune mediated, possibly against residual CMV antigens.

- **Extraocular CMV:** A number of visceral organs can develop CMV disease. Prior to the advent of HAART, extraocular CMV was present in nearly 10% of persons with AIDS with a CD4 count <50 cells/mm^3. CMV colitis, adrenalitis, and esophagitis were frequently seen. The incidence of CMV pneumonia in AIDS is unclear, but is probably much less common than in transplant recipients. Neurologic manifestations of CMV in AIDS include CMV radiculopathy, encephalopathy, and myelopathy. With the advent of HAART, the incidence of extraocular CMV has declined precipitously. Similarly, organ transplant recipients can develop visceral CMV (see above), the most dreaded complication being CMV pneumonia. CMV retinitis is rare in transplant recipients.

Diagnosis Cytomegalovirus-associated disease can be difficult to diagnose because CMV can sometimes be detected in normal patients without the presence of any clinical disease. Diagnosis of active infection depends on clinical symptoms consistent with CMV disease along with laboratory confirmation of CMV presence, since many of the manifestations of CMV are indistinguishable from other causes of infection on the basis of clinical presentation alone. The detection of CMV from specimens such as blood or bronchial lavage fluid can be helpful in the presumptive diagnosis of CMV disease, but is not definitive. The presence of CMV inclusion bodies from biopsy material of appropriate sites is considered the gold standard for diagnosis of visceral infection, and the most definitive method of diagnosis. For example, a transplant patient with an interstitial pulmonary infiltrate and detectable CMV DNA in the blood does not necessarily have CMV pneumonitis. Most would consider this a "possible" or "probable" case of CMV but would not consider this a definite case without pathologic evidence of CMV inclusions on lung biopsy.

Several assays are available for the rapid detection of CMV in blood. These antigen-based or sequence-based assays are more rapid than traditional cell culture for CMV, which can take days to weeks to complete. These assays can be used in several ways:

(1) To determine if the cause of a mononucleosis-like syndrome is from CMV (fever, myalgias, leukopenia, reactive lymphocytosis, pharyngitis, splenomegaly). CMV-related infectious mononucleosis may be indistinguishable from Epstein-Barr virus on clinical grounds alone.

(2) To determine if CMV infection is the cause of fever in an immunocompromised host who has no identifiable focus of infection (ie, the "CMV syndrome"). Laboratory testing in this setting must be interpreted cautiously since some patients may asymptomatically shed CMV in the blood during febrile episodes.

(3) To determine if CMV may be the cause of disease in a patient with an identified source of infection (ie, the transplant patient with a new pulmonary infiltrate of unknown etiology). Again, a positive DNA result must be interpreted carefully.

(4) To identify high-risk patients early in the course of CMV infection (ie, "pre-emptive therapy").

The CMV antigenemia test identifies the virus in polymorphonuclear leukocytes (PMNs) from venous blood. The antigenemia assay detects the lower matrix protein pp65 of CMV (the UL83 gene product) in CMV-infected leukocytes. The pp65 protein is a specific marker for active CMV infection and is present early in infection. The assay is performed by preparing a direct smear of PMNs on a slide, adding a monoclonal antibody specific for pp65, immunostaining (either immunofluorescence or immunoperoxidase), and counting the number of CMV-infected cells. The assay has also been used to quantify the presence of CMV in the blood (ie, to determine the CMV "viral load.") The CMV antigenemia test is one of several assays for CMV that has become popular for identifying patients at highest risk for serious CMV disease. The assay is the key element of a "**pre-emptive approach**" for management of CMV infection in many transplant centers. This therapeutic strategy is based on the identification of early subclinical disease by the use of a reliable laboratory test which can identify a subgroup of patients at the highest risk for clinical disease. CMV dissemination in the blood is now understood to be an important early step in the pathogenesis of CMV disease, and the early detection of circulating antigen-positive PMNs can hopefully identify infection before the development of disease. Pre-emptive therapy differs from prophylactic therapy in that pre-emptive therapy is based on a specific marker for disease (usually a positive laboratory test) which has sufficient predictive power to justify starting antimicrobial therapy. In general, the higher the degree of CMV antigenemia, or the higher the CMV viral load, the better the positive predictive value for the development of clinical disease. In contrast, prophylactic therapy is

(Continued)

Cytomegalovirus *(Continued)*

started before there is evidence of infection and involves treating larger numbers of people than the pre-emptive approach.

CMV hybrid capture (HC) is a new molecular hybridization assay designed for the direct detection of CMV nucleic acid in white blood cells. This assay differs from polymerase chain reaction (PCR) assays since there are no viral amplification steps with HC. In the United States, the assay is commercially available as the Digene CMV Hybrid Capture System™ (Digene Corp, Silver Spring, MD). HC is relatively simple to perform, rapid (6 hours), and does not require tissue culture techniques or molecular amplification steps. HC technology uses a CMV RNA probe which is capable of binding to a 40,000 base pair segment of the CMV genome. When the probe binds with the target CMV DNA, a "hybrid" of RNA-DNA is formed. The hybrids are then "captured" or immobilized within a special tube coated with antibodies specifically directed against the hybrids. The assay has been approved for qualitative determinations of CMV (virus absent or present), but can be used for quantitative measurements of CMV (eg, copies/mL of whole blood).

Some laboratories offer polymerase chain reaction (PCR) techniques to detect CMV DNA directly in specimens (most commonly, peripheral blood mononuclear cells). The test is extremely sensitive and specific but does not yield clinically-relevant results in all situations and is neither cost-effective enough nor practical enough to be used routinely. PCR can detect the onset of CMV viremia 1-2 weeks earlier than culture or antigenemia tests and can detect CMV DNA in 30% of specimens which are culture- and antigenemia-negative. The clinical significance of such extreme sensitivity and early detection of CMV in asymptomatic patients who are not culture positive and who do not show antigenemia has not been demonstrated. In addition, such results in these patients do not correlate with an indication for antiviral therapy. For most patients, PCR for CMV DNA appears to correlate best with seropositivity rather than active infection; however, the CMV viral load is frequently used as a marker for the initiation of pre-emptive therapy.

Diagnostic Tests/Procedures

Cytomegalovirus Culture *on page 438*
Cytomegalovirus Culture, Blood *on page 439*
Cytomegalovirus DNA Hybrid Capture *on page 440*
Cytomegalovirus Isolation, Rapid *on page 442*
Cytomegalovirus Serology *on page 442*
Immunofluorescent Studies, Biopsy *on page 507*
Polymerase Chain Reaction *on page 567*

Treatment Oral valganciclovir, intravenous ganciclovir, intravenous ganciclovir followed by oral valganciclovir, intravenous foscarnet, intravenous cidofovir, and in the case of CMV retinitis, the ganciclovir intraocular implant with oral valganciclovir are all effective treatments. Intravenous ganciclovir or oral valganciclovir is the treatment of choice for all CMV diseases including "CMV syndrome", retinitis, colitis, pneumonitis, and hepatitis. For treatment of colitis, pneumonitis, and hepatitis, a defined 2- to 3-week course is usually sufficient, even in patients with AIDS. For patients receiving high doses of immunosuppressive agents, decreasing the amount of immunosuppressant may be as critical as starting an antiviral agent. An alternative agent in failures or those patients who are intolerant to ganciclovir is foscarnet. Foscarnet is at least as active as ganciclovir against CMV but is more toxic. The addition of cytomegalovirus immune globulin (CMVIG) has not been proven to be any more effective than either of the antiviral agents alone. Acyclovir, which is not effective in treating CMV disease, has also been shown to be an effective prophylactic agent, but controversy remains.

A number of treatment regimens are available for CMV retinitis in AIDS. In general, these regimens are effective in slowing or even reversing CMV retinitis initially, but all eventually fail without some degree of immune reconstitution with HAART. The choice of initial therapy for CMV retinitis depends on the location and severity of the disease. Progression of retinitis occurs after about 2 months for intravenous ganciclovir, and other regimens have used this for comparison. In the early SOCA trials (Studies of the Ocular Complications of AIDS), intravenous ganciclovir and foscarnet were equally efficacious although foscarnet was associated with greater toxicity but improved survival. For years, the treatment of choice for CMV retinitis was intravenous ganciclovir. A number of options are now available for primary therapy including:

1. Ganciclovir intravenously
2. Ganciclovir implant (Vitrasert®) in combination with oral valganciclovir
3. Ganciclovir implant only and initiation of antiretroviral therapy with or without valganciclovir
4. Foscarnet intravenously (potential renal failure and metabolic abnormalities)
5. Cidofovir intravenously (associated with uveitis and other direct ocular toxicities)

6. Intravitreal injections of ganciclovir or foscarnet
7. Intravitreal fomivirsen
8. Ganciclovir orally (poor bioavailability)
9. Valganciclovir orally

Of the various treatment regimens, the ganciclovir implant in combination with oral ganciclovir has given the longest time to progression of 200 days or greater. Valganciclovir is now preferred over oral ganciclovir given its better bioavailability and less pill burden. In patients who can tolerate oral medications, oral valganciclovir is preferred over intravenous antivirals given the potential for line-related complications. Since none of these regimens can cure CMV retinitis, chronic maintenance is necessary after the retinitis becomes inactive (secondary prophylaxis) usually by continuing the same regimen used for induction. Antiretroviral therapy is the most effective treatment for CMV retinitis in patients with AIDS. It is recommended that patients with neurological disease be treated with both intravenous ganciclovir and foscarnet.

Prophylaxis: A number of different CMV prophylaxis regimens are in use, and these regimens vary from one organ system to another and from center to center. CMV-seronegative recipients of transplants from CMV-seronegative donors should receive only leukocyte-reduced or CMV-seronegative RBCs and/or leukocyte-reduced platelets to prevent transfusion-associated CMV infection. Some transplant centers do not use CMV prophylaxis and instead use a pre-emptive therapy approach (see above). One published regimen for CMV prophylaxis in heart transplant patients consists of 4 weeks of therapy with intravenous ganciclovir at full doses (induction) (5 mg/kg twice daily) for the first 2 weeks and lower doses (maintenance) (5-6 mg/kg/day) for the last 2 weeks. A number of other prophylactic regimens are in use for heart transplant recipients. Prophylaxis in allogeneic BMTs is also variable with one regimen consisting of 100 consecutive days of intravenous ganciclovir therapy. The field of CMV prophylaxis is under intense study in organ transplant recipients with regimens generally comparing intravenous ganciclovir, oral ganciclovir, acyclovir, and the valine esters. Valganciclovir and valacyclovir are now the preferred oral agents.

Primary CMV prophylaxis has also been studied in persons with AIDS. Two large studies using oral ganciclovir have been reported, with conflicting results. Oral ganciclovir appeared to have a protective effect on the development of CMV retinitis in AIDS (0.49 relative risk), but a similar study showed no benefit. Frequent ophthalmologic monitoring may be more cost effective and less toxic than prophylaxis. Oral ganciclovir is not often used by clinicians for primary prophylaxis of CMV for several reasons: (1) the widespread use of HAART has dramatically decreased the incidence of CMV in AIDS, (2) the number of additional pills required is large (12 pills), (3) the cost of oral ganciclovir is relatively high, and (4) about 75% of patients do not need prophylaxis.

Drug Therapy Comment Ganciclovir, valganciclovir, cidofovir, and foscarnet are limited by their toxicities. Resistance has been reported to all of these drugs. Occasionally, it may be necessary to use the combination of two drugs to minimize toxicity and improve efficacy in patients failing single-drug therapy. Ganciclovir and valganciclovir commonly cause leukopenia to a variable degree and often require filgrastim (G-CSF) to elevate the WBC. Patients require close monitoring while receiving these medications.

The greatest impact on the therapy of CMV retinitis has been the use of HAART. In 1999, the U.S. Public Health Service addressed the issue of discontinuing chronic maintenance therapy for CMV retinitis in patients who have responded to HAART. For persons with a sustained (>3-6 months) increase in CD4 T-cell counts to >100-150 cells/μL, the USPHS felt secondary prophylaxis could be safely stopped.

Drug Therapy

Recommended:

Ganciclovir *on page 834*
Valganciclovir *on page 1143*

Alternate:

Cidofovir *on page 740*
Foscarnet *on page 829*
Fomivirsen *on page 826*

Prophylaxis:

Valganciclovir *on page 1143*
Valacyclovir *on page 1140*

Selected Readings

Centers for Disease Control and Prevention; Infectious Disease Society of America; American Society of Blood and Marrow Transplantation, "Guidelines for Preventing Opportunistic Infections Among Hematopoietic Stem Cell Transplant Recipients," *MMWR Recomm Rep*, 2000, 49(RR-10):1-125.

(Continued)

Cytomegalovirus *(Continued)*

"Immunocompromised Host Society Consensus Conference on Epidemiology, Prevention, Diagnosis, and Management of Infections in Solid-Organ Transplant Patients. Davos, Switzerland, 23 June 1998, Fully Updated Summer 2000," *Clin Infect Dis*, 2001, 33 (Suppl 1):S1-65.

Ljungman P, de La Camara R, Milpied N, et al, "Randomized Study of Valacyclovir as Prophylaxis Against Cytomegalovirus Reactivation in Recipients of Allogeneic Bone Marrow Transplants," *Blood*, 2002, 99(8):3050-6.

Martin DF, Kuppermann BD, Wolitz RA, et al, "Oral Ganciclovir for Patients With Cytomegalovirus Retinitis Treated With a Ganciclovir Implant. Roche Ganciclovir Study Group," *N Engl J Med*, 1999, 340(14):1063-70.

Martin DF, Sierra-Madero J, Walmsley S, et al, "A Controlled Trial of Valganciclovir as Induction Therapy for Cytomegalovirus Retinitis," *N Engl J Med*, 2002, 346(15):1119-26.

Nokta MA, Holland F, De Gruttola V, et al, "Cytomegalovirus (CMV) Polymerase Chain Reaction Profiles in Individuals With Advanced Human Immunodeficiency Virus Infection: Relationship to CMV Disease," *J Infect Dis*, 2002, 185(12):1717-22.

Reusser P, "Oral Valganciclovir: A New Option for Treatment of Cytomegalovirus Infection and Disease in Immunocompromised Hosts," *Expert Opin Investig Drugs*, 2001, 10(9):1745-53.

Studies of Ocular Complications of AIDS Research Group and The AIDS Clinical Trials Group, "The Ganciclovir Implant Plus Oral Ganciclovir Versus Parenteral Cidofovir for the Treatment of Cytomegalovirus Retinitis in Patients With Acquired Immunodeficiency Syndrome: The Ganciclovir Cidofovir Cytomegalovirus Retinitis Trial," *Am J Ophthalmol*, 2001, 131(4):457-67.

Zaia JA, "Prevention of Cytomegalovirus Disease in Hematopoietic Stem Cell Transplantation," *Clin Infect Dis*, 2002, 35(8):999-1004.

Darling's Disease *see Histoplasma capsulatum on page 177*

Dematiaceous Fungi

Synonyms Black Molds; Black Piedra; Madura Foot; Phaeomycotic Cyst; Tinea Nigra

Microbiology There are over 100 species of dematiaceous fungi that are pathogenic. Dematiaceous fungi are those fungi that are darkly pigmented due to the presence of melanin in their cell wall. The McGinnis classification divides the dematiaceous fungi into two major distinct clinical entities: chromoblastomycosis and phaeohyphomycosis. Chromoblastomycosis is a cutaneous and subcutaneous infection characterized by hyperkeratosis and epidermal hyperplasia, intraepidermal microabscess formation, granulomatous inflammation in the dermis. and presence of sclerotic bodies. Sclerotic bodies probably represent vegetative forms intermediate between yeast and hyphae. Yeast and hyphae are not seen. Phaeohyphomycosis is a group of diseases in which the involved tissue contains yeast forms, hyphae, and/or pseudohyphae. Sclerotic bodies are not seen. Phaeohyphomycosis is further subdivided into superficial, cutaneous and corneal, subcutaneous, and systemic phaeohyphomycosis. The most common dematiaceous fungi isolated are *Phialophora* species, *Fosecaea* species, *Cladosporium* species, *Exophilia* species, *Exserohilum* species, *Curvularia* species, *Alternaria* species, and *Bipolaris* species. Isolation of fungi may take 4-6 weeks of incubation at 25°C to 30°C. Species are distinguished from one another by morphology, biochemical properties, and DNA analysis.

Epidemiology The dematiaceous fungi are ubiquitous organisms found in the soil and vegetation. *Phialophora* species are common contaminants of wood and cause bluing of wood and paper products. The mode of acquisition is usually inoculation with subsequent formation of a subcutaneous granuloma or abscess. Invasive disease is unusual and most often seen in immunocompromised patients. The majority of patients cannot recall the inciting trauma probably due to the prolonged period after an inoculation injury to development of infection. Soils of cultivated indoor plants may serve as reservoirs of conidia within the hospital environment. Although the organisms may be dispersed throughout the environment by insects and animals, there have been no reported cases of insect or animal transmission to humans.

Clinical Syndromes

- **Chromoblastomycosis:** Most commonly seen in males secondary to occupational exposure in the tropical/subtropical regions of the Americas and Africa. Presents as chronic infection of skin and soft tissue. Initially may appear as scaly, pink to violaceous papule at site of traumatic inoculation. Lesions may appear as nodular, tumorous, verrucous, plaque-like, or cicatricial. May develop deformity at anatomic site.
- **Phaeohyphomycosis:** Systemic phaeohyphomycosis may present as either progressive localized disease or dissemination secondary to lower respiratory tract infection. Sinusitis is the most common invasive manifestation reported in immunocompromised hosts. Sinusitis due to dematiaceous fungi does not appear to be as aggressive as sinusitis caused by the more common opportunistic fungi such as *Aspergillus* species and *Mucor* species. Sinusitis due to the dematiaceous fungi presents as an indolent process in immunocompetent hosts that have a history of allergic rhinitis, nasal polyps, or recurrent bacterial infections. CNS lesions are most often secondary to a traumatic injury with inoculation of contaminated material; however *Cladosporium* species, *Xylohypha* species, and *Dactylaria* species have a predilection for CNS invasion with primary infection being the lung. Patients present with signs and symptoms of intracranial mass lesion such as headache, seizure,

and focal neurological deficits without fever. The fungal abscess is usually limited to the cerebrum and rarely found invading the cerebellum or brainstem. Meningitis has been reported.

- **Phaeohyphomycotic cyst:** A distinct type of subcutaneous phaeohyphomycosis which presents as a solitary, well-encapsulated subcutaneous granuloma with necrosis. The overlying skin is normal. There is no regional lymphadenopathy. Usually secondary to subcutaneous inoculation with contaminated materials. It is associated with malnutrition, malignancy, hematologic or lymphoreticular malignancy, tuberculosis, leprosy, filariasis, syphilis, schistosomiasis, chronic renal failure, steroids, and diabetes mellitus. Lesions vary in size from 1-7 cm. May be present for months to years. *Exophilia* species and *Philophora* species predominate in normal hosts.
- **Mycetoma:** Chronic disease of the skin and underlying structures caused by a variety of actinomycetes and fungi including dematiaceous fungi. Most commonly occurs in feet secondary to inoculation trauma. Most often seen in farm workers in tropical/subtropical environment. Presents as a nodular mass with abscess or sinus tract formation draining seropurulent exudate containing granules or grains. The granules form a compact mass of organized hyphae.

Diagnosis Histopathology may be confused with other molds unless melanin-specific stain such as Fontanna-Masson is performed. Definitive diagnosis is made by identification of mold from culture of tissue.

Diagnostic Tests/Procedures

Fungus Culture, Biopsy *on page 461*

Treatment Flucytosine with or without amphotericin B plus surgical excision or incision and drainage is treatment of choice for chromoblastomycosis and mycetomas. Alternative therapy includes ketoconazole, itraconazole, voriconazole, or fluconazole. Flucytosine plus an azole may be effective. Phaeohyphomycotic cysts usually respond to excision alone. Phaeohyphomycosis responds best to itraconazole, however, the other azoles or amphotericin B may be effective. Antifungal susceptibility testing lacks correlation with clinical response.

Drug Therapy

Recommended:

Flucytosine *on page 822*
with or without
Amphotericin B (Conventional) *on page 650*

Alternate:

Ketoconazole *on page 903*
Itraconazole *on page 895*
Fluconazole *on page 819*
Voriconazole *on page 1151*
Terbinafine *on page 1097*

Selected Readings

Garg P, Gopinathan U, Choudhary K, et al, "Keratomycosis: Clinical and Microbiologic Experience With Dematiaceous Fungi," *Ophthalmology*, 2000 107(3):574-80.

Howden BP, Slavin MA, Schwarer AP, et al, "Successful Control of Disseminated *Scedosporium prolificans* Infection With a Combination of Voriconazole and Terbinafine," *Eur J Clin Microbiol Infect Dis*, 2003, 22(2):111-3.

Nucci M, Akiti T, Barreiros G, et al, "Nosocomial Fungemia Due to *Exophiala jeanselmei var. jeanselmei* and a *Rhinocladiella* Species: Newly Described Causes of Bloodstream Infection," *J Clin Microbiol*, 2001, 39(2):514-8.

Sharkey PK, Graybill JR, Rinaldi MG, et al, "Itraconazole Treatment of Phaeohyphomycosis," *J Am Acad Dermatol*, 1990, 23(3 Pt 2):577-86.

Stracher AR and White MH, "Dematiaceous Fungal Infections in Patients With Cancer," *Infect Med*, 1995, 12(7):303-8.

Sutton DA, Slifkin M, Yakulis R, et al, "U.S. Case Report of Cerebral Phaeohyphomycosis Caused by *Ramichloridium obovoideum* (*R. mackenziei*): Criteria for Identification, Therapy, and Review of Other Known Dematiaceous Neurotropic Taxa," *J Clin Microbiol*, 1998, 36(3):708-15.

Tintelnot K, "Therapy of Infections Caused by Dematiaceous Fungi," *Mycoses*, 1997, 40(Suppl 1):91-6.

Dengue *see* Arboviruses *on page 35*

Dengue Fever *see* Dengue Virus *on page 113*

Dengue Virus

Microbiology Dengue virus is a member (species) of the genus *Flavivirus* which is a member of the family Flaviridiae. Dengue virions are 45-55 nm viruses which exist as a single strand of RNA enclosed in a protein capsid which is enclosed in a host cell membrane-derived envelope. There are four serologically distinct types of dengue virus.

Epidemiology Dengue fever is essentially an urban disease of most tropical countries, especially southeast Asia, India, and the American tropics. In the 1950's, dengue was recognized and reported in only 9 countries. Today, dengue is reported worldwide in over 100 countries. WHO estimates over 2.5 billion persons are at risk for developing dengue infections. Dengue fever has been well documented to be
(Continued)

Dengue Virus *(Continued)*

occurring in epidemics for the last 200 years. Taken together, two factors suggest the distinct possibility that dengue fever can easily occur in epidemic form in the United States: increasing numbers of cases have been reported in the Caribbean, northern Mexico, and southern Texas, and vectors of dengue virus (*Aedes aegypti* and *A. albopictus* mosquitoes) have been found in southern Texas and other Gulf Coast areas. The natural reservoirs of dengue virus are humans. The distribution of dengue fever is equivalent to that of malaria. As of 1995, dengue fever was the most important mosquito-borne disease in the world. Dengue virus infects and causes disease (often life-threatening) in millions of people worldwide each year.

Clinical Syndromes

- **Dengue fever ("breakbone fever"):** An acute febrile viral disease characterized by sudden onset, fever of less than 1 week, intense headache, myalgia, retro-orbital pain, arthralgia, anorexia, GI disturbances, and development of a general maculopapular rash as the fever subsides. Recovery is extremely gradual, and fatalities are rare.
- **Dengue hemorrhagic fever/shock syndrome:** The most severe form of dengue disease, characterized by hypovolemia, dramatic internal and cutaneous bleeding disorders, and shock. The mortality rate of this severe form of dengue disease is ≥10%.

Diagnosis Dengue disease is difficult to distinguish from many arthropod-borne and/or febrile diseases (eg, malaria, bacterial sepsis, numerous viral infections, and many viral hemorrhagic viral fevers). A complete and well-studied history of the patient's travel and lifestyle is imperative in the preparation of a differential diagnosis.

Diagnostic Tests/Procedures

- Specific serological tests for anti-dengue IgG and IgM antibodies; contact clinical laboratory for details.
- Molecular methods (eg, reverse transcription of specific RNA sequences and subsequent PCR amplification and detection by probes and nucleic acid sequencing); such molecular tests for dengue are available only in reference laboratories; contact the clinical laboratory for details.

Treatment Treatment for typical dengue fever is symptomatic and supportive. Treatment of dengue hemorrhagic fever/shock syndrome should be directed toward extremely early supportive care, intensive monitoring of vital signs, hydration, and control of bleeding.

Drug Therapy Comment No specific drugs or antiviral agents are available.

Selected Readings

Guha-Sapir D and Schimmer B, "Dengue Fever: New Paradigms for a Changing Epidemiology," *Emerg Themes Epidemiol*, 2005, 2(1):1.

Kao CL, King CC, Chao DY, et al, "Laboratory Diagnosis of Dengue Virus Infection: Current and Future Perspectives in Clinical Diagnosis and Public Health," *J Microbiol Immunol Infect*, 2005, 38(1):5-16.

Ligon BL, "Dengue Fever and Dengue Hemorrhagic Fever: A Review of the History, Transmission, Treatment, and Prevention," *Semin Pediatr Infect Dis*, 2005, 16(1):60-5.

Teles FR, Prazeres DM, and Lima-Filho JL, "Trends in Dengue Diagnosis," *Rev Med Virol*, 2005, Jan 25; [Epub ahead of print].

Tsai TF, "Flaviviruses (Yellow Fever, Dengue, Dengue Hemorrhagic Fever, Japanese Encephalitis, St Louis Encephalitis, Tick-Borne Encephalitis)," *Principles and Practice of Infectious Diseases*, 5th ed, Mandell GL, Bennett JE, and Dolin R, eds, New York, NY: Churchill Livingstone, 2000, 1714-36.

Wichmann O and Jelinek T, "Dengue in Travelers: A Review," *J Travel Med*, 2004, 11(3):161-70.

Dermatomycoses *see* Dermatophytes *on page 114*

Dermatophytes

Microbiology Dermatophytes are fungi that invade the keratinized areas of the body (hair, nails, and skin) and are members of the genera *Epidermophyton*, *Microsporon*, or *Trichophyton*. Dermatophytes may be classified by the organism's name, their ecology (anthropophilic, geophilic, or zoophilic), or anatomical location of invasion.

They are differentiated by their colonial morphology, microscopic appearance of conidia, hair perforation or fluorescence, and biochemical/nutritional requirements.

Epidemiology Dermatophytes are the most common fungal infections in humans. They are found worldwide with some species limited geographically. They colonize nonviable structures. Invasion occurs when the role of penetration of the dermatophyte into the keratin exceeds the role of keratin growth and shedding. Local trauma-altered primary host defenses and impaired cell-mediated immunity contribute to infection. *E. floccosum* is the only species of *Epidermophyton* that infects man. It only invades the skin and nails and not hair. *Microsporon* and *Trichophyton* have many species that infect humans. *M. gypseum* is the most important geophilic dermatophyte and typically causes infections secondary to occupational exposure from direct contact with the soil. *M. canis* may be transmitted from animals to their owners and handlers. *T. tonsurans* is the most common cause of tinea capitis worldwide.

Clinical Syndromes

- **Tinea barbae:** Occurs on the bearded areas of face and neck. Most frequently seen in farm workers. May occur as circinate spreading type, vesiculopustular border with central scaling or superficial type characterized by perifollicular involvement with fever, malaise, and regional adenopathy. Most common organism is *T. mentagrophytes*.
- **Tinea capitis:** More common in pediatrics. Present with erythema, marked scaling, and hair loss. Severe form associated with large, boggy pustules, fever, leukocytosis, and regional lymphadenopathy. Associated with erythema nodosum. Transmitted person to person. *T. mentagrophytes* is the most common organism, previously *M. audouinii*.
- **Tinea corporis:** Infection of the skin except groin, palms, scalp, or soles. Affects all ages and sexes. More frequent in hot, humid, tropical areas. Transmitted from other humans, animals, fomites, and, rarely, soil. Presents as erythematous papules with a red, pruritic, raised scaling border with central cleaning.
- **Tinea cruris:** Pruritic, erythematous eruption with circumscribed inflammatory margins that begins on the inner thigh and spreads to groin, perineum, and perianal regions. Risk factors include obesity, diabetes, intertrigo, humidity, and tight-fitting clothes. Arthroconidia may survive for years, necessitating sterilization of clothes and linens.
- **Tinea pedis:** May occur as intertriginous involvement of toe webs or chronic hyperkeratotic form with minimal inflammation of soles and sides of feet or acutely as erythematous, clear vesicles which may become secondarily infected. Twenty-five percent to 75% of the normal population are culture positive and asymptomatic. Incidence increases with age. Most common organism is *T. rubrum*.
- **Tinea unguium:** Invasion of the nail; must be differentiated from onychomycosis which is a general term for any nail infection.
- **Deep local invasion:** Dissemination; uncommon; seen in immunosuppressed population.

Diagnosis Diagnosis is made by KOH examination of infected material or identification of characteristic macroconidia in culture. Up to 50% of KOH-positive samples may be culture-negative. Some of the organisms may be fluorescent under a Wood's lamp (ie, *M. canis* yellow and green, *T. schoenleinii* dull bluish white). Erythrasma caused by *Corynebacterium minutissimum* will be coral red under Wood's lamp. Other diagnostic tests employed are the hair perforation test and DTM (dermatophyte test media).

Diagnostic Tests/Procedures

Fungus Culture, Skin *on page 464*
KOH Preparation *on page 513*
Skin Biopsy *on page 580*

Treatment The most important aspect of therapy is educating patients for the need to continue therapy for a period of time after the infection appears resolved. Therapy is directed at anatomical location. Although comparative randomized trials are lacking, oral azoles and terbinafine have largely replaced the use of the more toxic agent griseofulvin.

- **Tinea barbae:** Griseofulvin or terbinafine for 4-6 weeks
- **Tinea capitis:** Griseofulvin for 1-2 weeks after lesion cleared for a total of 4-8 weeks. Alternative therapy is ketoconazole or terbinafine.
- **Tinea corporis:** Imidazole creams or topical keratolytics. In severe infection, griseofulvin, or ketoconazole.
- **Tinea cruris:** Topical imidazole 3-4 weeks
- **Tinea pedis:** Topical imidazole 3-4 weeks. Chronic form requires griseofulvin, however, *T. rubrum* may develop resistance.
- **Tinea unguium:** Terbinafine 250 mg/day for 12 weeks. Alternate therapy:
  Itraconazole: Oral: 200 mg twice daily for 1 week every month for 4 months or 200 mg/day for 3 months
  Fluconazole: Oral: 150-300 mg 1 day a week for 3 months (non-FDA approved indication)
  Griseofulvin ultramicrosize: Oral: 330-750 mg/day for 3-6 months. Not recommended due to adverse drug effects especially hepatotoxicity.
- **Deep or disseminated:** Amphotericin B

Drug Therapy

Recommended:

Superficial infection:
Antifungal, Topical *on page 666*
Terbinafine *on page 1097*
Itraconazole *on page 895*
Fluconazole *on page 819*
Griseofulvin *on page 845*
Ketoconazole *on page 903*

(Continued)

Dermatophytes *(Continued)*

Disseminated infection:

Amphotericin B (Conventional) *on page 650*

Selected Readings

De Backer M, De Vroey C, Lesaffre E, et al, "Twelve Weeks of Continuous Oral Therapy for Toenail Onychomycosis Caused by Dermatophytes: A Double-Blind Comparative Trial of Terbinafine 250 mg/day Versus Itraconazole 200 mg/day," *J Am Acad Dermatol*, 1998, 38(5 Pt 3):S57-63.
Elewski BE, "Treatment of Tinea Capitis: Beyond Griseofulvin," *J Am Acad Dermatol*, 1999, 40(6 Pt 2):S27-30.
Fuller LC, Child FJ, Midgley G, et al, "Diagnosis and Management of Scalp Ringworm," *BMJ*, 2003, 326(7388):539-41.
Gupta AK, Einarson TR, Summerbell RC, et al, "An Overview of Topical Antifungal Therapy in Dermatomycoses. A North American Perspective," *Drugs*, 1998, 55(5):645-74.
Hainer BL, "Dermatophyte Infections," *Am Fam Physician*, 2003, 67(1):101-8.
McClellan KJ, Wiseman LR, and Markham A, "Terbinafine. An Update of Its Use in Superficial Mycoses," *Drugs*, 1999, 58(1):179-202.
Scher RK, "Onychomycosis: Therapeutic Update," *J Am Acad Dermatol*, 1999, 40(6 Pt 2):S21-6.

Desert Rheumatism *see Coccidioides immitis on page 91*
DF-2 *see Capnocytophaga* Species *on page 69*
Diabetic Foot Osteomyelitis *see* Osteomyelitis, Diabetic Foot *on page 249*
Diarrheagenic *E. coli* *see Escherichia coli*, Diarrheagenic *on page 143*
Diphtheria *see Corynebacterium diphtheriae on page 96*
Diphyllobothrium latum *see* Cestodes *on page 72*
Dipylidium caninum *see* Cestodes *on page 72*

Diverticulitis

Clinical Presentation Diverticulitis is an inflammation around a diverticular sac, usually caused by a small mass of undigested food and bacteria (fecalith) which is retained in a pre-existing colonic diverticula. The thin diverticular sac becomes inflamed due to a diminished blood supply, and the innumerable colonic bacteria in the area infect the sac. In addition to local inflammation, small perforations of inflamed diverticula are common. At times, diverticulitis can be very mild and the attack resolves without treatment. Patients with more symptomatic acute diverticulitis characteristically present with fever and left lower quadrant abdominal pain. In addition to the characteristic left lower quadrant pain, there may be other associated symptoms such as constipation, pelvic or scrotal pain, and dysuria and urinary frequency (if the inflamed segment of colon rests on the urinary bladder). Physical examination is significant for tenderness in the left lower quadrant, and at times, a palpable mass may be present on digital rectal examination. Stools are often positive for microscopic blood, but massive lower GI bleeding with acute diverticulitis is unusual. In cases where there is free diverticular perforation, pain and tenderness are no longer limited to the left lower quadrant, and typical signs of generalized peritonitis develop with rebound tenderness. Occasionally, patients may present with diverticulitis on the right side of the abdomen since diverticula are potentially found throughout the length of colon. Although there are a number of imaging studies available to confirm a clinical suspicion of diverticulitis, CAT scan is a safe and effective means of establishing the diagnosis. Typical CAT scan findings include inflammation of fat around the colon, the presence of one or more diverticula, thickened bowel wall, or even small peridiverticular abscesses. Ultrasound may also be helpful in acute diverticulitis, which may show a thickening of the colon in a localized area, and a hypoechoic segment. During acute diverticulitis, barium enema and sigmoidoscopy carry a risk of free perforation, and these procedures are generally postponed until after the acute episode has resolved.

Differential Diagnosis Appendicitis; Crohn's disease; ulcerative colitis; colon cancer

Likely Pathogens Most cases of diverticulitis are caused by a mixture of bowel flora, which includes a wide range of anaerobic organisms, particularly *Bacteroides* species since these are present in large numbers in stool. Other anaerobic and aerobic bacteria are invariably present, but in most cases, no specific microbiologic diagnosis is made unless a peridiverticular abscess is drained and cultured.

Bacteroides and *Prevotella* Species *on page 46*
Streptococcus-Related Gram-Positive Cocci *on page 325*
Escherichia coli on page 142
Gram-Negative Bacilli *on page 157*
Enterococcus Species *on page 134*

Diagnostic Tests/Procedures

Computed Transaxial Tomography, Abdomen Studies *on page 423*
Ultrasound, Abdomen *on page 604*
Blood Culture, Aerobic and Anaerobic *on page 391*

Drug Therapy Comment Acute diverticulitis is usually managed with immediate empiric treatment with oral antibiotics if the episode is mild and the patient is not

systemically ill, along with a liquid diet. Since antibiotic treatment is usually empiric, a number of oral antibiotic regimens would be effective as long as the antibiotic(s) cover a broad-spectrum of bacterial pathogens. Typical outpatient regimens include the combination of ciprofloxacin and metronidazole, or amoxicillin-clavulanate alone. Other oral antibiotic combinations are likely effective. If the severity of the diverticulitis is moderate to severe, or if oral intake is limited, then hospital admission is indicated. A number of parenteral antibiotic regimens would be effective. One of the more common combination regimens is ampicillin, gentamicin, and metronidazole intravenously. Monotherapy with broad-spectrum antibiotics is also effective and none clearly superior to the others. Piperacillin-tazobactam, ticarcillin-clavulanate, and imipenem each can be used as monotherapy. If a peridiverticular abscess is present, CAT scan guided drainage, along with parenteral antibiotics, is warranted. Surgical evaluation is indicated in patients with an acute abdomen.

Empiric Drug Therapy

Recommended:

The following 3 used in combination
- Ampicillin *on page 657*
- Metronidazole *on page 940*
- Aminoglycosides *on page 641*

Ticarcillin and Clavulanate Potassium *on page 1114*
with or without
- Aminoglycosides *on page 641*

Piperacillin and Tazobactam Sodium *on page 1003*
with or without
- Aminoglycosides *on page 641*

Ampicillin and Sulbactam *on page 660*
with or without
- Aminoglycosides *on page 641*

Alternate:

Choice of one of the following
- Cephalosporins, 2nd Generation *on page 729*
- Cephalosporins, 3rd Generation *on page 730*

plus
- Aminoglycosides *on page 641*

with or without
- Metronidazole *on page 940*

The following 3 used in combination
- Fluoroquinolones *on page 824*
- Aminoglycosides *on page 641*
- Metronidazole *on page 940*

Selected Readings

Ferzoco LB, Raptopoulos V, and Silen W, "Acute Diverticulitis," *N Engl J Med*, 1998, 338(21):1521-6.

Stollman NH and Raskin JB, "Diagnosis and Management of Diverticular Disease of the Colon in Adults. Ad Hoc Practice Parameters Committee of the American College of Gastroenterology," *Am J Gastroenterol*, 1999, 94(11):3110-21.

"Surgical Treatment of Diverticulitis, Patient Care Committee of the Society for Surgery of the Alimentary Tract (SSAT)," *J Gastrointest Surg*, 1999, 3(2):212-3.

Wong WD, Wexner SD, Lowry A, et al, "Practice Parameters for the Treatment of Sigmoid Diverticulitis - Supporting Documentation. The Standards Task Force. The American Society of Colon and Rectal Surgeons," *Dis Colon Rectum*, 2000, 43(3):290-7.

Dog Bite Sepsis *see Capnocytophaga* Species *on page 69*

Donovanosis *see Calymmatobacterium granulomatis on page 65*

DRSP *see Streptococcus pneumoniae*, Drug-Resistant *on page 316*

Dysentery *see Shigella* Species *on page 297*

Early Infection Joint Replacement *see* Joint Replacement, Early Infection *on page 197*

Eastern Equine Encephalitis *see* Arboviruses *on page 35*

Eaton's Agent *see Mycoplasma pneumoniae on page 238*

Ebola Virus

Applies to Marburg Virus

Microbiology Members of the Filoviridae, these viruses are stable, highly infective particles, approximately 80-100 nm in diameter. They are filamentous, elongated, flexible, and enveloped, with genetic material composed of a single nonsense, nonsegmented RNA strand. Four subtypes of Ebola virus have been identified, in addition to two forms of the Marburg virus. Although some cross reactivity has been demonstrated between Ebola subtypes, no cross reactivity have been demonstrated between the Marburg and Ebola viruses. Viruses may be antigenically differentiated (Continued)

Ebola Virus *(Continued)*

by their transmembrane spike protein. The spike protein is highly glycosylated, which has been speculated to inhibit immune recognition and response.

Epidemiology Initially isolated in Primates (monkeys and macaques), epidemics in humans have occurred in several African countries including Zaire, Sudan, and the Ivory Coast. In addition, isolated cases have been associated with monkey importation (including the original Marburg, Germany importation). Blood exposure is a consistent factor in the development of epidemics.

The mode of transmission appears to involve close contact with blood and/or tissue from an infected individual or host. Airborne transmission does not appear to be a significant route of human infection, although experimental evidence suggests that this route is a possible source of infection. The reservoir for this virus has not been adequately characterized. During African epidemics, it has been noted that interhuman spread among hospital workers may be greatly reduced with the implementation of standard barrier infection control procedures (glove-gown-mask).

Clinical Syndromes

- **Hemorrhagic fever:** Following an incubation period of 5-10 days, the onset of hemorrhagic fever begins with an abrupt fever, headache, and myalgia (particularly in the lumbar area). After 1-3 days, additional gastrointestinal symptoms develop, which may include nausea, vomiting, watery diarrhea, abdominal cramping and pain. Chest pain, cough, and pharyngitis may also be present. Conjunctivitis is present in nearly 50% of cases. Photophobia, conjunctival injection, lymphadenopathy, jaundice, pancreatitis, as well as central nervous system involvement (somnolence, delirium, and coma) may occur.

  The disease progresses rapidly over a 5-7 day interval, as hemorrhagic manifestations assume higher degree of prominence. Petechiae, ecchymoses, and mucous membrane hemorrhages occur in approximately 50% of cases. A prominent maculopapular rash frequently develops on the trunk. Fine desquamation of the palms and soles may be apparent.

  The second week of infection may be accompanied by defervescence; however, this is frequently followed by a second febrile interval. Splenomegaly and hepatomegaly, as well as complications including orchitis, myocarditis, and pancreatitis commonly accompany this phase. A small number of patients will not progress and a protracted convalescence may begin. However, mortality associated with Ebola has been as high as 90%.

Diagnosis Due to its characteristic course and epidemiology, a history of exposure in an endemic area (ie, sub-Saharan Africa) may prompt clinical suspicion. Culture is positive during the acute stages, and laboratory confirmation via polymerase chain amplification and/or antigen detection may be used.

Treatment Generally involves supportive treatment only, including replacement of depleted coagulation factors, hemodynamic and ventilatory support. Vaccines are in development.

Selected Readings

Casillas AM, Nyamathi AM, Sosa A, et al, "A Current Review of Ebola Virus: Pathogenesis, Clinical Presentation, and Diagnostic Assessment," *Biol Res Nurs*, 2003, 4(4):268-75.

Polesky A and Bhatia G, "Ebola Hemorrhagic Fever in the Era of Bioterrorism," *Semin Respir Infect*, 2003, 18(3):206-15.

Sullivan N, Yang ZY, and Nabel GJ, "Ebola Virus Pathogenesis: Implications for Vaccines and Therapies," *J Virol*, 2003, 77(18):9733-7.

Sullivan NJ, Geisbert TW, Geisbert JB, et al, "Accelerated Vaccination for Ebola Virus Haemorrhagic Fever in Non-Human Primates," *Nature*, 2003, 424(6949):681-4.

Takada A and Kawaoka Y, "The Pathogenesis of Ebola Hemorrhagic Fever," *Trends Microbiol*, 2001, 9(10):506-11.

EBV *see* Epstein-Barr Virus *on page 139*

Echinococcus granulosus *see* Cestodes *on page 72*

Echinococcus multilocularis *see* Cestodes *on page 72*

Echovirus

Microbiology Echoviruses are very small, single-stranded RNA viruses belonging to the family Picornaviridae which has recently been reclassified to comprise four groups based on genomic sequence information. One of these groups is the Enterovirus in which echoviruses are a subclass. The other subclasses are polioviruses, Coxsackieviruses, and newer enteroviruses. (See Poliovirus *on page 275*, Coxsackievirus *on page 101*, and Enterovirus *on page 136*.) When these viruses were first isolated from stool specimens from children, they were noted to produce cytopathic effects in primate cell cultures but were nonpathogenic in mice and the primate central nervous system; hence they were called enteric cytopathic human orphan viruses or Echoviruses. There are now 31 serotypes of echoviruses recognized.

Epidemiology Infection rates vary with the season, geography, age, and socioeconomic status. In temperate climates, infections occur more frequently in the summer and autumn. The majority of echovirus infections occur in children younger than 15 years of age with the highest frequency occurring in infants younger than 1 year. An estimated 30 million nonpolio enterovirus infections occur annually in the United States. Of more than 3000 cerebrospinal fluid, nasopharyngeal swab, or stool isolates obtained from 1993 to 1996, echovirus 9 was the predominant serotype reported. Echoviruses 6, 7, 11, and 30 are among the most frequently detected serotypes associated with aseptic meningitis, encephalitis, and pneumonia. Echovirus 9 was the etiologic agent responsible for the aseptic meningitis outbreak that occurred in Whiteside County, Illinois in 1995. Although transmission of echoviruses usually is person-to-person, either through fecal-oral or oral-oral routes or communal contamination such as a swimming facility, no point source contamination could be located in the Whiteside outbreak.

Clinical Syndromes

- **Acute aseptic meningitis:** Characterized by fever, headache, stiff neck and photophobia in the presence of cerebrospinal fluid pleocytosis and negative bacteria/fungal cultures. Pharyngitis and upper respiratory tract symptoms are common. The illness may be biphasic with fever and myalgias initially present for a few days followed by no symptoms for 2-10 days and then development of a sudden reappearance of headache and fever. Five percent to 10% of children may develop seizures, lethargy, coma, or other neurological disorders.
- **Encephalitis:** May or may not be associated with meningitis. Usually a generalized encephalitis characterized by lethargy but may occur more localized characterized by partial motor seizures or ataxia or paresis.
- **Exanthems:** Associated with little morbidity. Can present as rubelliform, roseoliform, vesicular or petechial.
- **Respiratory disease:** Characterized by sore throat, cough, and coryza. Echovirus 11 is the most common cause of upper respiratory tract disease and is associated with croup.
- **Myopericarditis:** More associated with Coxsackieviruses than echoviruses. Predilection for adolescents and young adults. An upper respiratory tract infection precedes the onset of cardiac manifestations by 1-2 weeks. Patients present with dyspnea, dull precordial pain, fever, and malaise. Sharp pleuritic pain may accompany pericarditis. Approximately 50% will have evidence of a pericardial effusion or cardiac dilatation on chest radiograph. Congestive heart failure occurs in 20%. EKG may show evidence of pericarditis, arrhythmias, or heart block.
- **Neonatal infections:** Echovirus 6 and 11 have been associated with fatal disease in the newborn. Mild and nonspecific symptoms such as listlessness and anorexia usually occur within the first 3-7 days of life. Fever may or may not be present. Approximately 33% will have a biphasic illness. While Coxsackieviruses are more associated with myocarditis, the echoviruses cause a fulminant hepatitis associated with hypotension, hemorrhage, and multiple organ failure. There are reports of fatal pneumonia secondary to echoviruses occurring within the first few days of life. Echoviruses particularly serotype 22 has been associated with gastroenteritis.

Diagnosis Isolation of virus in cell culture from infected source.

Diagnostic Tests/Procedures

Viral Culture, Central Nervous System Symptoms *on page 614*
Viral Culture, Stool *on page 616*
Viral Culture, Throat *on page 617*

Treatment Supportive care for symptoms. No known effective antivirals. Immunoglobulin prophylaxis may be useful during neonatal outbreaks. Avoidance of transmission via good handwashing and personal hygiene.

Selected Readings

"Nonpolio Enterovirus Surveillance - United States, 1993-1996," *MMWR*, 1997, 46(32):748-50.
"Outbreak of Aseptic Meningitis - Whiteside County, Illinois, 1995," *MMWR*, 1997, 46(10):221-4.
Ventura KC, Hawkins H, Smith MB, et al, "Fatal Neonatal Echovirus 6 Infection: Autopsy Case Report and Review of the Literature," *Mod Pathol*, 2001, 14(2):85-90.

***E. coli* O157:H7** *see Escherichia coli*, Enterohemorrhagic *on page 145*
EHEC *see Escherichia coli*, Enterohemorrhagic *on page 145*

Ehrlichia Species

Microbiology *Ehrlichia* species are small gram-negative bacteria (0.5 μm) which can cause fever and pancytopenia in several mammalian hosts. The genus *Ehrlichia* contains several species which are primarily pathogenic for animals (eg, dogs, horses, jackals, and others). *Ehrlichia canis* was first identified as the agent of ehrlichiosis in dogs in the 1930s and was found to be transmitted to the dog by a tick vector. Infection in humans was not identified in the United States until 1986. Although human ehrlichiosis was originally thought to be caused by *E. canis*, it is later became

(Continued)

Ehrlichia Species *(Continued)*

apparent that human disease is caused by a genetically distinct species which has recently been named *Ehrlichia chaffeensis*.

Ehrlichia species are aerobic, gram-negative bacilli which are related to *Rickettsia* in terms of DNA content, geographic distribution, and clinical disease. *Ehrlichia* are obligate intracellular organisms which cluster within vacuoles of the infected cell; these intracellular inclusion bodies have been identified on light and electron microscopy and are called morulae (meaning mulberry-like). *Ehrlichia chaffeensis* infects the cytoplasm of macrophages. A newly described species of *Ehrlichia* distinct from *E. chaffeensis* (as yet unnamed) has recently been found to infect human granulocytes instead of macrophages. It has been called the agent of "human granulocytic ehrlichiosis". Morulae from *E. chaffeensis* can sometimes be identified on careful examination of peripheral blood smears (buffy coats) of infected patients using a Giemsa stain, but the sensitivity of this technique is very low. In contrast, the agent of human granulocytic ehrlichiosis is frequently seen as morulae in circulating leukocytes. The organisms do not grow on routine blood cultures. Special culture techniques utilizing cell culture systems have been occasionally successful in isolating the organism, but the sensitivity of culture is low.

Epidemiology *Ehrlichia* is spread to humans by the bite of a tick. The precise insect vector is still under study but *Dermacentor variabilis* (dog tick) and *Amblyomma americanum* (Lone Star tick) have been implicated, as have others. The peak incidence is from May to July. Infection is four times more common in men then women and cases are reported most commonly from rural areas. Geographic areas at highest risk are in the southern and south-central regions, as follows:

- South: South Carolina, North Carolina, Florida, Alabama, Kentucky, Tennessee, Georgia, Virginia, Maryland
- South-central/central: Arkansas, Oklahoma, Missouri, Texas, Louisiana
- Others: New Jersey, Wyoming, Vermont, Washington.

Over 300 cases of human ehrlichiosis have been reported to date, but this is likely an underestimate of the true prevalence of the disease.

Clinical Syndromes

- **Asymptomatic infection**: Studies have shown that many individuals with a demonstrable seroconversion to *E. chaffeensis* develop no symptoms.
- **Human ehrlichiosis**: The spectrum of human ehrlichiosis is very broad, ranging from a mild illness in many patients to a multiorgan system failure with protracted fever. After the tick bite, the organisms enter a number of host cells including the macrophage system. The incubation period between the tick bite and the onset of clinical symptoms is about 1 week. Infected persons typically present with the acute onset of nonspecific symptoms such as malaise, fever, headache and muscle pains. More severely ill persons may have additional symptoms such as nausea and vomiting, diarrhea, dyspnea, and cough. Serious complications have been reported in 40% of hospitalized patients. These include hypotension, neurologic abnormalities (ie, encephalitis, cerebrospinal fluid pleocytosis), coagulopathies, acute renal failure, hepatocellular necrosis, and death. It is important to note that a rash is present in only 33% of patients. Ehrlichiosis has been nicknamed "Rocky Mountain **spotless** fever" because of the similarities between ehrlichiosis and this common rickettsial illness. In general, the symptoms of ehrlichiosis are not unique and may be seen in a variety of other illnesses.

Diagnosis Laboratory abnormalities are common in ehrlichiosis and may be important clues to the disease. A mild leukopenia and thrombocytopenia are common. Elevated liver function tests are also common during the acute phase of the illness. The chest X-ray may show transient infiltrates. Anemia is seen after about 1 week of illness.

Human ehrlichiosis should be suspected in any patient with an unexplained febrile illness who resides in or has traveled to an area endemic for this disease. A history of a tick bite is useful but not necessary. The disease may be difficult to distinguish from Rocky Mountain spotted fever (RMSF) which has a similar geographic distribution. Several characteristics may be used to separate the two diseases: skin rash is less common in ehrlichiosis; when a skin rash is present in ehrlichiosis, it is less often petechial, as is the case with RMSF; leukopenia is more common in ehrlichiosis.

Laboratory confirmation of ehrlichiosis rests primarily on serologic studies. Indirect immunofluorescence assays (IFA) for *E. chaffeensis* are available from some specialty laboratories. A fourfold rise in titer between acute and convalescent samples is diagnostic. Although the direct visualization of ehrlicial morulae in host white blood cells has been reported in some cases, this appears to be a rare finding and is insensitive for the diagnosis of *E. chaffeensis*. Neither *E. chaffeensis* nor the agent of human granulocytic ehrlichiosis can be cultured on routine aerobic blood culture media.

The differential diagnosis of human ehrlichiosis includes RMSF, viral syndromes, and bacterial septicemia. Because of the variable clinical presentation, consultation with an Infectious Diseases specialist may be useful if this infection is suspected.

Diagnostic Tests/Procedures

Ehrlichia Serology *on page 446*

Polymerase Chain Reaction *on page 567*

Treatment Tetracycline and doxycycline appear to be useful. Intravenous chloramphenicol also has been used successfully.

Pediatric Drug Therapy

Recommended:

Chloramphenicol *on page 733*

Adult Drug Therapy

Recommended:

Tetracycline *on page 1106*

Doxycycline *on page 787*

Chloramphenicol *on page 733*

Selected Readings

Belman AL, "Tick-Borne Diseases," *Semin Pediatr Neurol*, 1999, 6(4):249-66.

Dumler JS, "Laboratory Diagnosis of Human Rickettsial and Ehrlichial Infections," *Clin Microbiol Newslet*, 1996, 18(8):57-61.

Eng TR, Harkess JR, Fishbein DB, et al, "Epidemiologic, Clinical, and Laboratory Findings of Human Ehrlichiosis in the United States, 1988," *JAMA*, 1990, 264(17):2251-8.

Everett ED, Evans KA, Henry RB, "Human Ehrlichiosis in Adults After Tick Exposure. Diagnosis Using Polymerase Chain Reaction," *Ann Intern Med*, 1994, 120(9):730-5.

Fishbein DB, Dawson JE, and Robinson LE, "Human Ehrlichiosis in the United States, 1985 to 1990," *Ann Intern Med*, 1994, 120(9):736-43.

"Human Ehrlichiosis - United States," *MMWR*, 1988, 37(17):270, 275-7.

Magnarelli LA and Dumler JS, "Ehrlichiosis: Emerging Infectious Diseases in Tick-Infested Areas," *Clin Microbiol Newslett*, 1996, 18(11):81-3.

McDade JE, "Ehrlichiosis - A Disease of Animals and Humans," *J Infect Dis*, 1990, 161(4):609-17.

Rikihisa Y, "The Tribe Ehrlichieae and Ehrlichial Diseases," *Clin Microbiol Rev*, 1991, 4(3):286-308.

Walker DH and Dumler JS, "Emergence of the Ehrlichioses as Human Health Problems," *Emerg Infect Dis*, 1996, 2(1):18-29.

Walker DH and Dumler JS, "Human Monocytic and Granulocytic Ehrlichiosis. Discovery and Diagnosis of Emerging Tick-Borne Infections and the Critical Role of the Pathologist," *Arch Pathol Lab Med*, 1997, 121(8):785-91.

Ehrlichiosis *see Ehrlichia* Species *on page 119*

Encephalitis, Viral

Synonyms Viral Encephalitis

Clinical Presentation The term encephalitis refers to inflammation of the brain parenchyma, as opposed to the term meningitis which refers to inflammation mainly confined to the meninges. There is some overlap between these two important syndromes and a number of organisms can cause either encephalitis or meningitis. Encephalitis can have both infectious and noninfectious etiologies. The most common etiology of encephalitis is from viral infection, with about 20,000 cases of viral encephalitis in the United States per year. Important epidemiologic clues to evaluate include the seasonality and exposure history (animal bites, rodent exposure, tick bites). Patients with viral encephalitis have variable degrees of fever and the presentation is usually acute or subacute. The hallmark of encephalitis is an altered level of consciousness, which can vary from mild lethargy to coma. Typically, patients are confused and delirious, and bizarre behavior is not uncommon (eg, hallucinations, psychosis, and personality change). On examination, common focal neurologic findings include ataxia and aphasia, hemiparesis (often with increased deep tendon reflexes and extensor plantar responses), and cranial nerve deficits such as ocular and facial palsies. Because of the disruption of the hypothalamic-pituitary axis in viral encephalitis, fever, diabetes insipidus, and the syndrome of inappropriate ADH (SIADH) can accompany the mental status changes. In general, it is not possible to distinguish one type of viral encephalitis from other forms of encephalitis on clinical grounds alone, despite the pathologic evidence that different viruses injure different areas of the brain. The CSF profile in viral encephalitis is similar to viral meningitis and consists of a modest elevation in the CSF WBCs, mainly lymphocytic. In over 95% of cases, the CSF contains >5 cells/μL. More marked CSF pleocytosis is unusual and in only 10% of the time, the CSF WBCs will be >500 cells/μL. The CSF WBCs are usually lymphocytes. If the CSF WBCs are mainly polymorphonuclear leukocytes, this is more suggestive of bacterial etiologies, leptospirosis, and noninfectious causes (acute hemorrhagic leukoencephalitis). Occasionally, viral encephalitis from Eastern equine encephalitis or enteroviruses can give polymorphonuclear leukocytes in CSF. There is usually a mild increase in CSF protein, and CSF glucose is usually normal.

Differential Diagnosis Infectious causes of encephalitis (nonviral): *Listeria* rhomboencephalitis; *Mycoplasma pneumoniae* (especially if a pulmonary infiltrate is

(Continued)

Encephalitis, Viral *(Continued)*

present); *Legionella*; abscess and subdural empyema; *Mycobacterium* tuberculosis; fungal (*Cryptococcus*, others); *Rickettsia*; *Bartonella* (cat scratch encephalitis)

Noninfectious "mimics" of encephalitis: Vascular diseases; toxic encephalopathy; subdural hematoma; Rasmussen's encephalitis; Reye's syndrome; systemic lupus erythematosus

Likely Pathogens The most common cause of community-acquired encephalitis is herpes simplex virus encephalitis (HSV-1). Other common causes of viral encephalitis include arboviruses, which are a diverse group of viruses that cause encephalitis via an arthropod vector, and enteroviruses. Mumps virus is a potential cause of encephalitis, but the number of cases has decreased as the disease has become less common due to routine vaccination. Less common causes of viral encephalitis are HIV, Epstein-Barr virus, cytomegalovirus, varicella-zoster virus, measles virus, and adenoviruses. There are a number of other viruses which can cause encephalitis, but these are rare. One important rare cause is rabies.

Herpes Simplex Virus *on page 172*
Arboviruses *on page 35*
Enterovirus *on page 136*
Human Immunodeficiency Virus *on page 181*
Measles Virus *on page 215*
Epstein-Barr Virus *on page 139*
Cytomegalovirus *on page 107*
Varicella-Zoster Virus *on page 347*
West Nile Virus *on page 353*
Rabies Virus *on page 283*
Influenza Virus *on page 193*

Diagnostic Tests/Procedures Since it is nearly impossible to establish a specific etiology of viral encephalitis on the basis of clinical presentation alone, laboratory diagnosis remains essential. In many cases, however, a specific viral (or nonviral) etiology of encephalitis cannot be determined, due in part to limitations in laboratory diagnostics. Cultures of cerebrospinal fluid in viral encephalitis are invariably negative, due to poor sensitivity. Polymerase chain reaction (PCR) is considered the diagnostic procedure of choice for CSF analysis. The most commonly ordered diagnostic test on CSF in cases of encephalitis is the herpes simplex virus PCR since (1) it is the most common cause of encephalitis, (2) HSV culture and antigen are insensitive, (3) findings on MRI and EEG can be highly suggestive of HSV encephalitis but are not always present, and (4) the sensitivity and specificity of CSF PCR is equivalent to brain biopsy for the diagnosis of HSV encephalitis. For other viruses, CSF PCR is available but less studied than HSV PCR. There is growing literature on the utility of enteroviral CSF PCR. Acute and convalescent serum titers for arboviruses are necessary to establish the diagnosis of arboviral encephalitis.

CAT scan or MRI of the brain should be performed on patients with encephalitis to rule out a structural brain lesion. The finding of a focal area of encephalitis in the temporal-parietal area suggests HSV encephalitis, although this finding is not entirely specific. EEG may show focal spikes on a background of slow activity in the temporal area in HSV encephalitis. The need for brain biopsy in the diagnosis of viral encephalitis has declined in recent years due to the sensitivity and specificity of HSV CSF PCR.

Cerebrospinal Fluid Analysis *on page 408*
Polymerase Chain Reaction *on page 567*
Encephalitis Viral Serology *on page 452* (Arbovirus serology)
Computed Transaxial Tomography, Head Studies *on page 424*
Magnetic Resonance Scan, Brain *on page 532*
Lumbar Puncture *on page 524*
Electroencephalography *on page 447*

Drug Therapy Comment Of the many potential etiologies of viral encephalitis, few are treatable. Establishing a diagnosis of HSV encephalitis is important since this is potentially treatable. Acyclovir is the drug of choice for HSV encephalitis given at a dose of 10 mg/kg every 8 hours I.V. for at least 14 days. HIV encephalitis is usually a manifestation of advanced AIDS, although occasionally has been reported in individuals with early disease; this may or may not respond to antiretroviral agents. Ganciclovir and/or foscarnet should be given for CMV encephalitis. An investigational antiviral agent (pleconaril) is being studied for enteroviral meningitis and encephalitis, but no agents are currently approved for enterovirus. There is no therapy available for arboviral encephalitis at this time. Corticosteroids as an adjunct treatment are not generally recommended. A neurosurgical consult is indicated for increased intracranial pressure refractory to medical management or for suspicion of impending herniation.

Herpes B virus may also cause encephalitis. It is rare, usually transmitted to laboratory workers from animals, especially monkeys. It is usually fatal; however, ganciclovir is often given when CNS symptoms are present.

Empiric Drug Therapy

Recommended:

Acyclovir *on page 629*

Selected Readings

Hinson VK and Tyor WR, "Update on Viral Encephalitis," *Curr Opin Neurol*, 2001, 14(3):369-74.

http://aidsinfo.nih.gov/guidelines/op_infections/TOI_AA.pdf

Marfin AA and Gubler DJ, "West Nile Encephalitis: An Emerging Disease in the United States," *Clin Infect Dis*, 2001, 33(10):1713-9.

Steiner I, Budka H, Chaudhuri A, et al, "Viral Encephalitis: A Review of Diagnostic Methods and Guidelines for Management," *Eur J Neurol*, 2005, 12(5):331-43.

Straumanis JP, Tapia MD, and King JC, "Influenza B Infection Associated With Encephalitis: Treatment With Oseltamivir," *Pediatr Infect Dis J*, 2002, 21(2):173-5.

Endocarditis, Acute, I.V. Drug Abuse

Related Information

Antibiotic Treatment of Adults With Infective Endocarditis *on page 1271*
Prevention of Bacterial Endocarditis *on page 1302*

Synonyms Acute Endocarditis, I.V. Drug Abuse

Clinical Presentation In acute left-side bacterial endocarditis, patients typically present with high fever and rapid valvular dysfunction resulting in congestive heart failure or arrhythmias. In acute right-sided endocarditis, patients appear ill with fever, have pulmonary infiltrates, and have the murmur of tricuspid or pulmonary insufficiency. Patients that "wash" needles with fresh lemon are at risk of *Candida* endocarditis.

Likely Pathogens

Pseudomonas aeruginosa on page 282
Staphylococcus aureus, Methicillin-Susceptible *on page 307*
Staphylococcus aureus, Methicillin-Resistant *on page 304*
Candida Species *on page 67*

Diagnostic Tests/Procedures

•Blood Culture, Aerobic and Anaerobic *on page 391*
•Chest Films *on page 412*
•Gram Stain *on page 473*
Blood Culture, Fungus *on page 395*
C-Reactive Protein *on page 428*
Echocardiography, M-Mode *on page 445*
Sedimentation Rate, Erythrocyte *on page 576*
Serum Bactericidal Test *on page 578*
Transesophageal Echocardiography *on page 598*

Drug Therapy Comment Short-term treatment (eg, 2 weeks) may be considered for *Staphylococcus aureus* right-sided endocarditis without complications (cannot have renal failure, extrapulmonary metastatic infectious complications, aortic or mitral involvement, meningitis, or MRSA) in I.V. heroin users known to be HIV-negative. Alternatively, a 28-day course of oral ciprofloxacin plus rifampin may also be considered for the patient population described above. Patients must be followed very closely for possible recurrence. Cardiology and Cardiothoracic Surgery should be consulted to alert for potential complications if intervention is warranted.

Empiric Drug Therapy

Recommended:

Vancomycin *on page 1144*
plus
Rifampin *on page 1046*

Alternate:

If *Pseudomonas* is suspected:
One of the following
Ceftazidime *on page 717*
Piperacillin and Tazobactam Sodium *on page 1003*
plus
Gentamicin *on page 841*

Selected Readings

Baddour LM, Wilson WR, Bayer AS, et al, "Infective Endocarditis: Diagnosis, Antimicrobial Therapy, and Management of Complications: A Statement for Healthcare Professionals From the Committee on Rheumatic Fever, Endocarditis, and Kawasaki Disease, Council on Cardiovascular Disease in the Young, and the Councils on Clinical Cardiology, Stroke, and Cardiovascular Surgery and Anesthesia, American Heart Association - Executive Summary: Endorsed by the Infectious Diseases Society of America," *Circulation*, 2005, 111(23):3167-84.

Chambers HF, "Short-Course Combination and Oral Therapies of *Staphylococcus aureus* Endocarditis," *Infect Dis Clin North Am*, 1993, 7(1):69-80.

(Continued)

Endocarditis, Acute, I.V. Drug Abuse *(Continued)*

Cherubin CE and Sapira JD, "The Medical Complications of Drug Addiction and the Medical Assessment of the Intravenous Drug User: 25 Years Later," *Ann Intern Med*, 1993, 119(10):1017-28.

Heldman AW, Hartert TV, Ray SC, et al, "Oral Antibiotic Treatment of Right-Sided Staphylococcal Endocarditis in Injection Drug Users: Prospective Randomized Comparison With Parenteral Therapy," *Am J Med*, 1996, 101(1):68-76.

Endocarditis, Acute Native Valve

Related Information

Antibiotic Treatment of Adults With Infective Endocarditis *on page 1271*
Prevention of Bacterial Endocarditis *on page 1302*

Synonyms Acute Native Valve Infective Endocarditis

Clinical Presentation Between 60% and 80% of patients have a pre-existing cardiac lesion such as rheumatic valvular disease, congenital heart disease, or degenerative heart disease.

In acute left-side bacterial endocarditis, patients typically present with high fever and rapid valvular dysfunction resulting in congestive heart failure or arrhythmias. In acute right-sided endocarditis, patients appear ill with fever, have pulmonary infiltrates, and have the murmur of tricuspid or pulmonary insufficiency.

Likely Pathogens

Staphylococcus aureus, Methicillin-Susceptible *on page 307*
Streptococcus pneumoniae, Drug-Susceptible *on page 319*
Neisseria gonorrhoeae on page 244

Diagnostic Tests/Procedures

•Blood Culture, Aerobic and Anaerobic *on page 391*
•Echocardiography, M-Mode *on page 445*
•Gram Stain *on page 473*
C-Reactive Protein *on page 428*
Sedimentation Rate, Erythrocyte *on page 576*
Serum Bactericidal Test *on page 578*
Transesophageal Echocardiography *on page 598*

Drug Therapy Comment Linezolid may be considered for patients who may be intolerant to vancomycin and/or specific organisms (VISA/GISA, VRSA, VRE). Cardiology and Cardiothoracic Surgery should be consulted to alert for potential complications if intervention is warranted.

Empiric Drug Therapy

Recommended:

Vancomycin *on page 1144*
plus
Gentamicin *on page 841*

Alternate:

Ampicillin and Sulbactam *on page 660*
plus
Gentamicin *on page 841*

Selected Readings

Baddour LM, Wilson WR, Bayer AS, et al, "Infective Endocarditis: Diagnosis, Antimicrobial Therapy, and Management of Complications: A Statement for Healthcare Professionals From the Committee on Rheumatic Fever, Endocarditis, and Kawasaki Disease, Council on Cardiovascular Disease in the Young, and the Councils on Clinical Cardiology, Stroke, and Cardiovascular Surgery and Anesthesia, American Heart Association - Executive Summary: Endorsed by the Infectious Diseases Society of America," *Circulation*, 2005, 111(23):3167-84.

Bansal RC, "Infective Endocarditis," *Med Clin North Am*, 1995, 79(5):1205-40.

Bayer AS, Bolger AF, Taubert KA, et al, "Diagnosis and Management of Infective Endocarditis and its Complications," *Circulation*, 1998, 98(25):2936-48.

Dajani AS, Taubert KA, Wilson W, et al, "Prevention of Bacterial Endocarditis. Recommendations by the American Heart Association," *JAMA*, 1997, 277(22):1794-801.

Durack DT, Lukes AS, and Bright DK, "New Criteria for Diagnosis of Infective Endocarditis: Utilization of Specific Echocardiographic Findings. Duke Endocarditis Service," *Am J Med*, 1994, 96(3):200-9.

Lamas CC and Eykyn SJ, "Suggested Modifications to the Duke Criteria for the Clinical Diagnosis of Native Valve and Prosthetic Valve Endocarditis: Analysis of 118 Pathologically Proven Cases," *Clin Infect Dis*, 1997, 25(3):713-9.

Olaison L and Pettersson G, "Current Best Practices and Guidelines. Indications for Surgical Intervention in Infective Endocarditis," *Cardiol Clin*, 2003, 21(2):235-51.

Wilson WR, Karchmer AW, Dajani AS, et al, "Antibiotic Treatment of Adults With Infective Endocarditis Due to Streptococci, Enterococci, Staphylococci and HACEK Microorganisms. American Heart Association," *JAMA*, 1995, 274(21):1706-13.

Endocarditis, Prosthetic Valve, Early

Related Information

Antibiotic Treatment of Adults With Infective Endocarditis *on page 1271*
Prevention of Bacterial Endocarditis *on page 1302*

Synonyms Prosthetic Valve Endocarditis, Early; PVE, Early

Clinical Presentation Occurs within 60 days of surgery and is a consequence of valve contamination or bacteremia perioperatively. This usually presents as an acute event. In left-sided early prosthetic valve endocarditis, patients typically present with high fever and rapid valvular dysfunction resulting in congestive heart failure or arrhythmias. In right-sided disease, patients appear ill with fever, have pulmonary infiltrates, and have insufficiency murmurs.

Likely Pathogens

Staphylococcus epidermidis, Methicillin-Susceptible *on page 310*
Staphylococcus epidermidis, Methicillin-Resistant *on page 309*
Staphylococcus aureus, Methicillin-Susceptible *on page 307*
Staphylococcus aureus, Methicillin-Resistant *on page 304*
Gram-Negative Bacilli *on page 157*
Candida Species *on page 67*

Diagnostic Tests/Procedures

•Blood Culture, Aerobic and Anaerobic *on page 391*
•Gram Stain *on page 473*
Blood Culture, Fungus *on page 395*
C-Reactive Protein *on page 428*
Echocardiography, M-Mode *on page 445*
Sedimentation Rate, Erythrocyte *on page 576*
Serum Bactericidal Test *on page 578*
Transesophageal Echocardiography *on page 598*

Drug Therapy Comment Linezolid may be considered for patients who may be intolerant to vancomycin and/or specific organisms (VISA/GISA, VRSA, VRE). Cardiology and cardio-thoracic surgery should be consulted to alert for potential complications if intervention is warranted.

Empiric Drug Therapy

Recommended:

Vancomycin *on page 1144*
plus
Gentamicin *on page 841*
plus
Rifampin *on page 1046*

Alternate:

If *Candida* suspected:
Amphotericin B (Conventional) *on page 650*
Fluconazole *on page 819*

Selected Readings

Baddour LM, Wilson WR, Bayer AS, et al, "Infective Endocarditis: Diagnosis, Antimicrobial Therapy, and Management of Complications: A Statement for Healthcare Professionals From the Committee on Rheumatic Fever, Endocarditis, and Kawasaki Disease, Council on Cardiovascular Disease in the Young, and the Councils on Clinical Cardiology, Stroke, and Cardiovascular Surgery and Anesthesia, American Heart Association - Executive Summary: Endorsed by the Infectious Diseases Society of America," *Circulation*, 2005, 111(23):3167-84.

Bansal RC, "Infective Endocarditis," *Med Clin North Am*, 1995, 79(5):1205-40.

Lamas CC and Eykyn SJ, "Suggested Modifications to the Duke Criteria for the Clinical Diagnosis of Native Valve and Prosthetic Valve Endocarditis: Analysis of 118 Pathologically Proven Cases," *Clin Infect Dis*, 1997, 25(3):713-9.

Nottin R, Al-Attar N, Ramadan R, et al, "Aortic Valve Translocation for Severe Prosthetic Valve Endocarditis: Early Results and Long-Term Follow-up," *Ann Thorac Surg*, 2005, 79(5):1486-90.

Wilson WR, Karchmer AW, Dajani AS, et al, "Antibiotic Treatment of Adults With Infective Endocarditis Due to Streptococci, Enterococci, Staphylococci, and HACEK Microorganisms. American Heart Association," *JAMA*, 1995, 274(21):1706-13.

Endocarditis, Prosthetic Valve, Late

Related Information

Antibiotic Treatment of Adults With Infective Endocarditis *on page 1271*
Prevention of Bacterial Endocarditis *on page 1302*

Synonyms Prosthetic Valve Endocarditis, Late; PVE, Late

Clinical Presentation Occurs more than 60 days after valve surgery. This usually presents as an acute event. In left-sided late prosthetic valve endocarditis, patients typically present with high fever and rapid valvular dysfunction resulting in congestive heart failure or arrhythmias. In right-sided disease, patients appear ill with fever, have pulmonary infiltrates, and have insufficiency murmurs.

Likely Pathogens

Streptococcus, Viridans Group *on page 326*
Staphylococcus epidermidis, Methicillin-Susceptible *on page 310*
Staphylococcus epidermidis, Methicillin-Resistant *on page 309*

Diagnostic Tests/Procedures

•Blood Culture, Aerobic and Anaerobic *on page 391*

(Continued)

Endocarditis, Prosthetic Valve, Late *(Continued)*

•Gram Stain *on page 473*
C-Reactive Protein *on page 428*
Echocardiography, M-Mode *on page 445*
Sedimentation Rate, Erythrocyte *on page 576*
Serum Bactericidal Test *on page 578*
Transesophageal Echocardiography *on page 598*

Drug Therapy Comment Linezolid may be considered for patients who may be intolerant to vancomycin and/or specific organisms (VISA/GISA, VRSA, VRE). Cardiology and Cardiothoracic Surgery should be consulted to alert for potential complications if intervention is warranted.

Empiric Drug Therapy

Recommended:

Vancomycin *on page 1144*
plus
Gentamicin *on page 841*
plus
Rifampin *on page 1046*

Alternate:

If *Candida* suspected:
Amphotericin B (Conventional) *on page 650*
Fluconazole *on page 819*

Selected Readings

Baddour LM, Wilson WR, Bayer AS, et al, "Infective Endocarditis: Diagnosis, Antimicrobial Therapy, and Management of Complications: A Statement for Healthcare Professionals From the Committee on Rheumatic Fever, Endocarditis, and Kawasaki Disease, Council on Cardiovascular Disease in the Young, and the Councils on Clinical Cardiology, Stroke, and Cardiovascular Surgery and Anesthesia, American Heart Association - Executive Summary: Endorsed by the Infectious Diseases Society of America," *Circulation*, 2005, 111(23):3167-84.

Bansal RC, "Infective Endocarditis," *Med Clin North Am*, 1995, 79(5):1205-40.

Lamas CC and Eykyn SJ, "Suggested Modifications to the Duke Criteria for the Clinical Diagnosis of Native Valve and Prosthetic Valve Endocarditis: Analysis of 118 Pathologically Proven Cases," *Clin Infect Dis*, 1997, 25(3):713-9.

Nottin R, Al-Attar N, Ramadan R, et al, "Aortic Valve Translocation for Severe Prosthetic Valve Endocarditis: Early Results and Long-Term Follow-up," *Ann Thorac Surg*, 2005, 79(5):1486-90.

Wilson WR, Karchmer AW, Dajani AS, et al, "Antibiotic Treatment of Adults With Infective Endocarditis Due to Streptococci, Enterococci, Staphylococci, and HACEK Microorganisms. American Heart Association," *JAMA*, 1995, 274(21):1706-13.

Endocarditis, Subacute Native Valve

Related Information

Antibiotic Treatment of Adults With Infective Endocarditis *on page 1271*
Prevention of Bacterial Endocarditis *on page 1302*

Synonyms Subacute Native Valve Endocarditis

Clinical Presentation Symptoms generally begin approximately 2 weeks after precipitating event. Onset is gradual with low-grade fever, malaise, and arthralgias. Cardiac murmur is usually present. May present with splenomegaly, petechia, splinter hemorrhages, Roth spots, Osler nodes, Janeway lesions, and clubbing. Embolic events, mycotic aneurysms, brain abscesses, meningitis, and renal disease may occur.

Differential Diagnosis Acute rheumatic fever; lupus erythematosus and other collagen vascular diseases; sickle cell; nonbacterial thrombotic endocarditis; malignancy; tuberculosis

Likely Pathogens

Streptococcus, Viridans Group *on page 326*
Enterococcus Species *on page 134*
HACEK Group *on page 158*
Streptococcus bovis *on page 315*

Diagnostic Tests/Procedures

•Blood Culture, Aerobic and Anaerobic *on page 391*
•Gram Stain *on page 473*
Chest Films *on page 412*
C-Reactive Protein *on page 428*
Echocardiography, M-Mode *on page 445*
Q Fever Serology *on page 569*
Sedimentation Rate, Erythrocyte *on page 576*
Serum Bactericidal Test *on page 578*
Transesophageal Echocardiography *on page 598*

Drug Therapy Comment Among patients with a clinical syndrome consistent with infectious endocarditis who have recently received antibiotics, empiric antimicrobial therapy may be delayed if they do not have a toxic appearance and have no clinical or echocardiographic evidence of severe or progressive valve regurgitation or of

congestive heart failure. In patients who have not previously been treated, therapy for patients with subacute infectious endocarditis may be delayed for up to 6 hours while cultures are obtained and should not be delayed in the setting of acute infectious endocarditis. At least 2 sets of blood cultures should be obtained every 24-48 hours until bloodstream infection is cleared.

Linezolid may be considered for patients who may be intolerant to vancomycin and/or specific organisms (VISA/GISA, VRSA, VRE).

Empiric Drug Therapy

Recommended:

Vancomycin *on page 1144*

plus

Gentamicin *on page 841*

Alternate:

Ampicillin and Sulbactam *on page 660*

plus

Gentamicin *on page 841*

Selected Readings

Ayres NA, Miller-Hance W, Fyfe DA, et al, "Indications and Guidelines for Performance of Transesophageal Echocardiography in the Patient With Pediatric Acquired or Congenital Heart Disease: Report From the Task Force of the Pediatric Council of the American Society of Echocardiography," *J Am Soc Echocardiogr*, 2005, 18(1):91-8.

Baddour LM, Wilson WR, Bayer AS, et al, "Infective Endocarditis: Diagnosis, Antimicrobial Therapy, and Management of Complications: A Statement for Healthcare Professionals From the Committee on Rheumatic Fever, Endocarditis, and Kawasaki Disease, Council on Cardiovascular Disease in the Young, and the Councils on Clinical Cardiology, Stroke, and Cardiovascular Surgery and Anesthesia, American Heart Association - Executive Summary: Endorsed by the Infectious Diseases Society of America," *Circulation*, 2005, 111(23):3167-84.

Dajani AS, Taubert KA, Wilson W, et al, "Prevention of Bacterial Endocarditis. Recommendations by the American Heart Association," *JAMA*, 1997, 277(22):1794-801.

Durack DT, Lukes AS, and Bright DK, "New Criteria for Diagnosis of Infective Endocarditis: Utilization of Specific Echocardiographic Findings. Duke Endocarditis Service," *Am J Med*, 1994, 96(3):200-9.

Elliott TS, Foweraker J, Gould FK, et al, "Guidelines for the Antibiotic Treatment of Endocarditis in Adults: Report of the Working Party of the British Society for Antimicrobial Chemotherapy," *J Antimicrob Chemother*, 2004, 54(6):971-81.

Lamas CC and Eykyn SJ, "Suggested Modifications to the Duke Criteria for the Clinical Diagnosis of Native Valve and Prosthetic Valve Endocarditis: Analysis of 118 Pathologically Proven Cases," *Clin Infect Dis*, 1997, 25(3):713-9.

Endometritis

Synonyms Postabortal Endometritis; Postpartum Endometritis (PPE)

Clinical Presentation More common following cesarean section than vaginal delivery. Associated with premature rupture of membranes (PROM) and the duration of PROM before delivery. *Chlamydia trachomatis* is associated with a late form of postpartum endometritis (PPE) which occurs 2 days to 6 weeks postpartum. PPE generally occurs 1-2 days following delivery and the hallmark sign is fever defined as temperature ≥38.5°C in the first 24 hours or for at least 4 consecutive hours >24 hours postdelivery. Other findings include lower abdominal pain, uterine tenderness, and leukocytosis. Prophylactic antibiotics are given per standard of care in any patient who requires a cesarean section after labor or rupture of membranes. Preoperative vaginal scrub with povidone-iodine decreases the incidence of postcesarean endometritis.

Differential Diagnosis Pelvic abscess; puerperal ovarian vein thrombosis; noninfectious source of fever (eg, breast engorgement)

Likely Pathogens

Polymicrobial including:

Streptococcus agalactiae on page 313

Enterococcus Species *on page 134*

Streptococcus Species *on page 326*

Gardnerella vaginalis on page 153

Escherichia coli on page 142

Bacteroides and *Prevotella* Species *on page 46*

Bacteroides and *Prevotella* Species *on page 46*

Other vaginal flora

Diagnostic Tests/Procedures

Blood Culture, Aerobic and Anaerobic *on page 391*

Transvaginal Cultures

Drug Therapy Comment Women with subacute endometritis may benefit from short-course antibiotic therapy with cefixime or azithromycin plus metronidazole.

Empiric Drug Therapy

Recommended:

Monotherapy:

Cefotetan *on page 710*

(Continued)

Endometritis *(Continued)*

Ticarcillin and Clavulanate Potassium *on page 1114*
Piperacillin and Tazobactam Sodium *on page 1003*
Cefoxitin *on page 712*
Ampicillin and Sulbactam *on page 660*

Combination therapy:
Clindamycin *on page 752*
plus
Gentamicin *on page 841*

Alternate:
Fluoroquinolones *on page 824*
plus
Metronidazole *on page 940*
Clindamycin *on page 752*
plus
Ciprofloxacin *on page 742*

The following 3 used in combination
Ciprofloxacin *on page 742*
Doxycycline *on page 787*
Metronidazole *on page 940*

Selected Readings

Brumfield CG, Hauth JC, and Andrews WW, "Puerperal Infection After Cesarean Delivery: Evaluation of a Standardized Protocol," *Am J Obstet Gynecol*, 2000, 182(5):1147-51.
Eckert LO, Thwin SS, Hillier SL, et al, "The Antimicrobial Treatment of Subacute Endometritis: A Proof of Concept Study," *Am J Obstet Gynecol*, 2004, 190(2):305-13.
Edwards RK, Locksmith GJ, and Duff P, "Expanded-Spectrum Antibiotics With Preterm Premature Rupture of Membranes," *Obstet Gynecol*, 2000 96(1):60-4.
Hartmann KE, Barrett KE, Reid VC, et al, "Clinical Usefulness of White Blood Cell Count After Cesarean Delivery," *Obstet Gynecol*, 2000, 96(2):295-300.
Starr RV, Zurawski J, and Ismail M, "Preoperative Vaginal Preparation With Povidone-Iodine and the Risk of Postcesarean Endometritis," *Obstet Gynecol*, 2005, 105(5 Pt 1):1024-9.

Endophthalmitis, Bacterial and Fungal

Synonyms Bacterial Endophthalmitis; Fungal Endophthalmitis

Clinical Presentation Bacterial and fungal endophthalmitis is inflammation within the fluid-filled chambers of the eye, specifically, involving the vitreous and aqueous chambers. Ocular inflammation is manifested usually 1-5 days after surgery or nonsurgical trauma. Bacterial endophthalmitis is characterized by increasingly acute pain, blurred vision, and headache. Other symptoms can include lid edema, corneal haze, conjunctival hyperemia, and cells in the anterior chamber. Fungal endophthalmitis is characterized by slowly progressing loss of vision with little or no pain. Onset is typically a week to months after surgery or nonsurgical trauma. As the disease progresses, an increasingly larger number of whitish lesions can appear around the retinal vessel. With time, these lesions (seen by the patient as floaters) appear to extend ("puff/fluff") into the vitreous fluid.

Note: Bacterial and fungal endophthalmitis is a medical emergency, which can be fulminant and can lead to severe visual impairment, blindness, and/or loss of the eye. If the disease and accompanying corneal ulceration are severe or extensive enough, the patient should be hospitalized because (1) the risk of corneal perforation is high and (2) the frequency of, and intense need for therapy requires qualified medical personnel.

Differential Diagnosis Bacterial endophthalmitis; fungal endophthalmitis; viral endophthalmitis; parasitic endophthalmitis

Likely Pathogens

Bacterial:
Staphylococcus aureus, Methicillin-Resistant *on page 304*
Staphylococcus aureus, Methicillin-Susceptible *on page 307*
Staphylococcus epidermidis, Methicillin-Resistant *on page 309*
Staphylococcus epidermidis, Methicillin-Susceptible *on page 310*
Streptococcus pneumoniae, Drug-Susceptible *on page 319*
Streptococcus, Viridans Group *on page 326*
Bacillus cereus on page 44
Enterobacter Species *on page 132*
Pseudomonas aeruginosa on page 282
Propionibacterium acnes
Haemophilus influenzae on page 159
Neisseria meningitidis on page 245

Fungal:
Yeast:
Candida Species *on page 67*
Cryptococcus Species

Zygomycetes:
Rhizopus Species
Mucor Species *on page 225*
Dematiaceous Fungi *on page 112*
Curvularia
Cephalosporium
Many others
Hyaline molds:
Aspergillus Species *on page 38*
Pseudallescherichia
Fusarium Species *on page 151*
Many others
Dimorphic fungi:
Histoplasma capsulatum on page 177
Blastomyces dermatitidis on page 50
Coccidioides immitis on page 91

Diagnostic Tests/Procedures Note: Contact the testing laboratory prior to collecting specimen for (1) special instructions regarding ocular cultures, (2) special media for bacterial and fungal cultures, and (3) special procedures for culturing and transporting extremely small volumes of ocular fluids.

Gram Stain *on page 473*
Methenamine Silver Stain *on page 534*
Periodic Acid-Schiff Stain *on page 563*
Aerobic Culture, Body Fluid *on page 365*
Anaerobic Culture *on page 371*
Fungus Culture, Body Fluid *on page 462*

Drug Therapy Comment Antimicrobial therapy is empiric until the specific etiological agent is isolated and identified. However, specific therapy directed toward a specific or suspected bacterial or fungal pathogen(s) should be given as soon as possible. Initial therapy can, wholly or in part, be based on the results of the Gram or fungal stain. Determination of intraocular administration should be made through ophthalmologic consultation.

Empiric Drug Therapy

Recommended:

Note: This is an ophthalmological emergency.

Bacterial:
Vancomycin *on page 1144*
plus
Ceftazidime *on page 717*

Fungal:
Amphotericin B (Conventional) *on page 650*

Alternate:

Bacterial:
Vancomycin *on page 1144*
plus one of the following:
Gentamicin *on page 841*
Tobramycin *on page 1122*
Amikacin *on page 639*
Fungal:
Caspofungin *on page 695*
Voriconazole *on page 1151*

Selected Readings

Baum J, "Infections of the Eye," *Clin Infect Dis*, 1995, 21(3):479-86.
Ciulla TA, "Update on Acute and Chronic Endophthalmitis," *Ophthalmology*, 1999, 106(12):2237-8.
Fahey DK, Fenton S, Cahill M, et al, "*Candida* Endophthalmitis: A Diagnostic Dilemma," *Eye*, 1999, 13(Pt 4):596-8.
Garzozi HJ and Harris A, "Intraocular Lens Implants and Risk of Endophthalmitis," *Br J Ophthalmol*, 2000, 84(5):554.
Kunimoto DY, Das T, Sharma S, et al, "Microbiologic Spectrum and Susceptibility of Isolates: Part II. Post-traumatic Endophthalmitis. Endophthalmitis Research Group," *Am J Ophthalmol*, 1999, 128(2):242-4.
Lohmann CP, Linde HJ, Reischl U, "Improved Detection of Microorganisms by Polymerase Chain Reaction in Delayed Endophthalmitis After Cataract Surgery," *Ophthalmology*, 2000, 107(6):1047-51; discussion 1051-2.
Ng JQ, Morlet N, Pearman JW, et al, "Management and Outcomes of Postoperative Endophthalmitis Since the Endophthalmitis Vitrectomy Study: The Endophthalmitis Population Study of Western Australia (EPSWA)'s Fifth Report," *Ophthalmology*, 2005, 112(7):1199-206.
Pavan PR, Oteiza EE, Hughes BA, et al, "Exogenous Endophthalmitis Initially Treated Without Systemic Antibiotics," *Ophthalmology*, 1994, 101(7):1289-96; discussion 1296-7.

(Continued)

Endophthalmitis, Bacterial and Fungal *(Continued)*

West ES, Behrens A, McDonnell PJ, et al, "The Incidence of Endophthalmitis After Cataract Surgery Among the U.S. Medicare Population Increased Between 1994 and 2001," *Ophthalmology*, 2005, 112(8):1388-94.

Entamoeba histolytica

Microbiology *Entamoeba histolytica* is an enteric protozoan that exists in two forms, cyst and trophozoite. The cyst ranges in size from 5-20 μm and contains one to four nuclei. The trophozoite is an ameba, ranges in size from 12-60 μm, and contains a single nucleus with a centrally-located nucleolus with a uniformly distributed peripheral chromatin. Although all strains of *E. histolytica* are morphologically identical, there is epidemiological and biological evidence that there are pathogenic and nonpathogenic strains. Isoenzyme analysis reveals that there are four distinct zymodemes which appear to correlate with the virulence of the ameba.

Epidemiology It is estimated that 10% of the world is infected with *E. histolytica*, with 50,000-100,000 *E. histolytica*-associated deaths per year, making amebiasis the third leading parasitic cause of death in the world. It is endemic in Mexico, India, West and South Africa, and portions of Central and South America. It appears to be most virulent in the tropics. The vast majority (90%) of patients remain asymptomatic. High risk factors for invasive diseases in the United States include recent immigration, institutionalization, and homosexuality, although 30% to 40% of male homosexuals harbor a nonpathogenic strain. It is imperative to exclude other etiologies of diarrhea in patients with AIDS given the large number of asymptomatic carriers. Infection with *E. histolytica* begins with ingestion of the cyst via contaminated food or water or fecal-oral route. The ingested mature cyst excysts in the lower ileum and multiplies by binary fission producing eight trophozoites. The trophozoites may remain in the lumen of the colon and multiply or invade the wall of the colon and spread hematogenously. Trophozoites encyst in the colon, and both mature and immature cysts are excreted in the feces.

Clinical Syndromes

Intestinal:

- **Asymptomatic colonization:** Affects 90% of those infected. Also referred to as cyst passage.
- **Acute amebic colitis:** Present with lower abdominal pain and explosive bloody diarrhea. Approximately 30% to 40% will have fever. Onset over 7-10 days with a 1- to 4-week duration. More severe in children, pregnant women, and immunosuppressed individuals, especially those on steroids. Toxic megacolon associated with steroid use. Almost all patients will have heme-positive stools but few or no leukocytes presumably due to ability of ameba to lyse leukocytes hence the name "histolytica". Chronic colitis must be differentiated from inflammatory bowel disease.
- **Fulminant colitis:** More common in children. Diffuse abdominal pain and profuse bloody diarrhea. Seventy-five percent of children may develop colonic perforation.
- **Ameboma:** Develops in 1% of patients with colitis. Localized chronic amebic infection usually in cecum or ascending colon. Presents as a tender mass.

Extraintestinal:

- **Hepatic abscess:** Acute hepatic abscess presents with dull, pleuritic, right upper quadrant pain and fever. Subacute less likely to have fever. Ten percent to 15% may present with fever and no pain. Fifty percent acute presentations will have multiple hepatic lesions, whereas 80% subacute will have a single lesion located in the right lobe liver. Fifty percent will have no history of antecedent dysentery. Laboratory reveals leukocytosis without eosinophilia, alkaline phosphatase elevated >75%, transaminase elevated >50%.

  Other rare complications of hepatic abscess include genitourinary, skin, adrenal, and kidney invasion.
- **Pleuropulmonary:** Most common complication of hepatic abscess, occurring 20% to 35%. Typically associated with lesion from left lobe liver. Presents with pleuritic pain, cough. May have serous effusions, consolidation, empyema, or hepatobronchial fistula.
- **Peritoneal:** Second most common complication of hepatic abscess is intraperitoneal rupture in 2% to 7.5%. Indolent leaks much more common than rupture or abscess.
- **Pericardial:** Most serious complication of hepatic abscess. Perforation of abscess into the pericardium usually results in tamponade and/or shock. Greater than 60% have abscesses in left lobe liver. Mortality is 40%.
- **CNS:** Brain abscesses occur where intestinal amebiasis is endemic. Aggressive, multifocal disease known as secondary cerebral amebiasis (SCA). Must be differentiated from *Naegleria* and *Acanthamoeba* as treatment differs. Rapidly

progressive disease with spreading abscesses with internal necrosis of gray-white junction of cerebral cortex. SCA occurs in 0.6% to 0.8% patients with hepatic abscess. Extremely rare without hepatic invasion. Presentation depends on size, location, and number of lesions. May present as chronic infection with fever, weight loss, hepatomegaly, abdominal pain, dyspnea, and pleuritic pain. Diarrhea may be absent. Less than 33% will have positive ova and parasite fecal exam. Incubation period is typically 2-5 months. Male to female ratio is 5:1. CSF examination reveals mononuclear cells with normal and low glucose. CT scan reveals ring enhancing lesions.

Diagnosis Eighty percent to 90% of patients with acute dysentery will have cysts or trophozoites on fecal examination after examining three samples. Trophozoites rapidly die after passage; therefore, feces must be examined within 20 minutes of collection. Serology titers are positive in 60% to 90% of the cases after 7 days, however, 6% to 20% of patients in endemic areas will have positive serologies which may persist for years after acute infection. Sigmoidoscopy or colonoscopy with biopsy is recommended for patients with chronic colitis to differentiate between inflammatory bowel versus amebiasis. Extraintestinal disease should be diagnosed by aspiration of abscess or biopsies. Liver abscess aspirate is classically chocolate colored or has an anchovy paste appearance. More than 90% will have positive serology. Absence of serology titer is strong evidence against amebiasis.

Entamoeba dispar is morphologically identical to *E. histolytica*, and most laboratories do not have the ability to distinguish them apart. Therefore, it is imperative that one consider the risk factors and likelihood that the organism reported is in fact *E. histolytica*. *E. dispar* is a gut commensal and is not associated with dysentery.

Diagnostic Tests/Procedures

Entamoeba histolytica Serology *on page 452*
Ova and Parasites, Stool *on page 551*
Ova and Parasites, Urine or Aspirates *on page 554*

Treatment Note: Treatment varies by site and severity of infection. Luminal therapy alone may be appropriate in asymptomatic cases, while tissue agent (systemic therapy) is required in most infections. When systemic/tissue therapy is appropriate, treatment with a systemic agent should be followed by a full treatment course of a luminal amebicide (iodoquinol, diloxanide furoate, or paromomycin as listed above for asymptomatic infection). Some clinicians initiate luminal treatment concurrently with tissue (systemic) agent.

Asymptomatic intestinal infection (luminal therapy): Iodoquinol 650 mg 3 times/day for 20 days, diloxanide furoate (from CDC) for 10 days, or paromomycin 25-35 mg/kg in three divided doses for 7 days.

Mild to moderate to intestinal disease (dysentery): Metronidazole 500-750 mg 3 times/day for 7-10 days; tinidazole 2 g once daily for 3 days may be used in place of metronidazole. Fluid electrolyte support. May need surgical decompression if mega-colon. Also see "**Note**" above concerning luminal therapy.

Severe intestinal disease or extraintestinal disease (hepatic): Metronidazole 750 mg 3 times/day for 10 days. May need percutaneous draining. Tinidazole 2 g once daily for 5 days may be used in place of metronidazole. Also see "**Note**" above concerning luminal therapy.

CNS: Metronidazole plus surgical drainage. If no surgical drainage, metronidazole 500 mg 4 times/day for 4 weeks. Also see "**Note**" above concerning luminal therapy.

Prevention: Boiling is only means of eradicating *E. histolytica* cysts in water. Vegetables must be cleansed in strong detergent soap and soaked in acetic acid or vinegar for 10-15 minutes. Travelers to endemic areas should be advised to avoid uncooked vegetables, salads, fruits that cannot be peeled, and ice cubes.

Drug Therapy

Recommended:

Asymptomatic (cyst passers):
Diloxanide Furoate *on page 778*
Paromomycin *on page 989*

Invasive infection:
Metronidazole *on page 940*
followed by
Diloxanide Furoate *on page 778*

Alternate:

Invasive infection:
Metronidazole *on page 940*
followed by one of the following
Paromomycin *on page 989*
Iodoquinol *on page 891*

(Continued)

Entamoeba histolytica (Continued)

Selected Readings

Campbell S, "Amebic Brain Abscess and Meningoencephalitis," *Semin Neurol*, 1993, 13(2):153-60.

Haque R, Huston CD, Hughes M, et al, "Amebiasis," *N Engl J Med*, 2003, 348(16):1565-73.

Jackson TF, "*Entamoeba histolytica* and *Entamoeba dispar* Are Distinct Species; Clinical, Epidemiological, and Serological Evidence," *Int J Parasitol*, 1998, 28(1):181-6.

Petri WA Jr and Singh U, "Diagnosis and Management of Amebiasis," *Clin Infect Dis*, 1999, 29(5):1117-25.

Rossignol JF, Ayoub A, and Ayers MS, "Treatment of Diarrhea Caused by *Giardia intestinalis* and *Entamoeba histolytica* or *E. dispar*. A Randomized, Double-Blind, Placebo-Controlled Study of Nitazoxanide," *J Infect Dis* 2001, 184(3):381-4.

Yau YC, Crandall I, Kain KC, et al, "Development of Monoclonal Antibodies Which Specifically Recognize *Entamoeba histolytica* in Preserved Stool Samples," *J Clin Microbiol*, 2001, 39(2):716-9.

Enterobacter Species

Microbiology *Enterobacter* species are gram-negative rods which are increasingly important causes of nosocomial infection, particularly because of the emergence of highly antibiotic-resistant isolates. *Enterobacter* species are aerobic gram-negative bacilli which normally colonize the intestinal tract. The genus name "*Enterobacter*" should not be confused with the broader family name "Enterobacteriaceae;" the latter designation refers to many gram-negative bacteria including *Enterobacter* species, *E. coli*, *Klebsiella*, *Serratia*, and others. Based on studies of DNA relatedness, *Enterobacter* is most closely related to *Klebsiella*, with >50% DNA sequence homology. The organism cannot be distinguished from other related GNBs on the basis of Gram stain alone, and identification by culture is necessary. The major species of *Enterobacter* which are pathogenic for humans include *E. cloacae*, *E. aerogenes*, and *E. agglomerans*.

Enterobacter produces endotoxin, the lipopolysaccharide (LPS) component which is associated with the outer membrane of the bacteria. When cell lysis occurs (as with antibiotic therapy) the LPS is released into the host and can lead to such inflammatory responses as fever, leukopenia or leukocytosis, hypotension, and disseminated intravascular coagulation. Thus, LPS is regarded as an important mediator of the sepsis syndrome.

Enterobacter species have become increasingly recognized as producers of extremely important and clinically-relevant extended-spectrum beta-lactamases (ESBL). See Treatment.

Epidemiology Because *Enterobacter* commonly inhabits the human gastrointestinal tract, it is considered one of the "enteric bacteria." In hospitalized patients, it often asymptomatically colonizes the urine, respiratory tract, abdominal wounds, decubitus ulcers, and other sites. Community-acquired infection is rare, and *Enterobacter* is generally considered an opportunist of the hospitalized, debilitated individual.

Clinical Syndromes

- **Lower respiratory tract infection:** Nosocomial *Enterobacter* infections are seen in patients with extended hospitalizations, particularly those who are ventilator-dependent. Patients who have been on prolonged broad-spectrum antibiotics seem at particular risk for *Enterobacter* infection. Lengthy courses of broad-spectrum antibiotics do not "protect" the patient from opportunistic *Enterobacter* infections. It should be noted that *Enterobacter* and other gram-negative bacilli can asymptomatically colonize the upper respiratory tract of hospitalized patients. Thus, the recovery of a sputum or tracheal aspirate culture for *Enterobacter* does not necessarily indicate a significant infectious disease. The diagnosis of a pneumonia still rests on standard criteria such as the presence of purulence (many leukocytes) on the Gram stain of sputum, the presence of a pulmonary infiltrate, and signs of systemic inflammation in the patient. A positive sputum culture alone is not sufficient justification for initiating antibiotic therapy.
- **Burn wound infections:** Outbreaks of serious *Enterobacter* infections (primarily septicemias) have been reported in burn units.
- **Urinary tract infection:** Seen in hospitalized patients, often those with indwelling Foley catheters. However, *Enterobacter* may harmlessly colonize the urine of patients with chronic bladder catheters without causing disease. The decision to initiate antibiotics in such patients should be based on the clinical situation (the presence of pyuria on urinalysis, suprapubic pain, fever, etc). Even the finding of large numbers of *Enterobacter* in a urine culture (>10^5 colony forming units/mL) by itself does not automatically indicate antimicrobial therapy.
- **Hospital-associated bacteremias:** In 1975, *Enterobacter* strains were associated with a national epidemic of contaminated intravenous products. The organisms were found to grow in commercially available fluids used for intravenous infusions and were the cause of rapid-onset septicemia. There have been no nationwide *Enterobacter* outbreaks since then, but the organism is still recovered periodically from blood cultures.

Diagnosis The clinical presentations of the various nosocomial infections caused by *Enterobacter* are not distinctive, and laboratory isolation is necessary.

Diagnostic Tests/Procedures

Aerobic Culture, Appropriate Site *on page 365*
Gram Stain *on page 473*

Treatment Increasing resistance of Enterobacteriaceae to beta-lactam antimicrobial agents has been recognized for several years. This resistance has made infections caused by these resistant bacteria increasingly more difficult to treat.

A major mechanism of bacterial resistance to beta-lactam antimicrobial agents is the natural production of beta-lactamases. Mutations of these enzymes over the years have resulted in plasmid-encoded beta-lactamases with extended-spectra that now include newer and commonly used antimicrobial agents such as the monobactam aztreonam and the newer oxyimino-cephalosporins such as cefotaxime, ceftriaxone, ceftazidime, and cefpodoxime. These enzymes are known as extended-spectrum beta-lactamases (ESBL) and occur more commonly in *Escherichia coli* and *Klebsiella* species and are becoming more commonly detected in other genera of Enterobacteriaceae, such as *Enterobacter*, *Serratia*, *Citrobacter*, *Salmonella*, and *Proteus*.

ESBL-producing bacteria species usually test susceptible to beta-lactams *in vitro* in the clinical lab. However, susceptibilities to all beta-lactams (except imipenem and beta-lactam combinations) are reported as resistant because the agents will not be effective *in vivo*.

Enterobacter species present a challenging therapeutic problem, especially when isolates exhibit high level antibiotic resistance. Preliminary data suggest that the popular third generation cephalosporins may act to select naturally-occurring mutants of *Enterobacter* that are resistant to a wide variety of antibiotics. In the typical case, the cephalosporin is able to eradicate the vast majority of sensitive *Enterobacter* species. However, when the bacterial load is high (as in an abscess), these mutants may be present in small numbers along with the normally susceptible bacteria and continue to divide in the face of selective antibiotic pressure. In time, this resistant strain will dominate and often demonstrates complete resistance to all cephalosporins and all penicillins, even if penicillins were not given. This disturbing trend is particularly common in intensive care units, where prolonged courses of antibiotics are given empirically for fever without a clear focus of infection. Infectious disease consultation may be helpful since imipenem resistance can develop rapidly as well.

Drug Therapy

Recommended:

Piperacillin and Tazobactam Sodium *on page 1003*
Ticarcillin and Clavulanate Potassium *on page 1114*

Alternate:

Cefepime *on page 705*
Cephalosporins, 3rd Generation *on page 730*
Imipenem and Cilastatin *on page 861*
Meropenem *on page 936*
Fluoroquinolones *on page 824*

Selected Readings

Bradford PA, "Extended-Spectrum Beta-Lactamases in the 21st Century: Characterization, Epidemiology, and Detection of This Important Resistance Threat," *Clin Microbiol Rev*, 2001, 14(4):933-51
Chow JW, Fine MJ, Shlaes DM, et al, "*Enterobacter* Bacteremia: Clinical Features and Emergence of Antibiotic Resistance During Therapy," *Ann Intern Med*, 1991, 115(8):585-90.
Colodner R, "Extended-Spectrum Beta-Lactamases: A Challenge for Clinical Microbiologists and Infection Control Specialists," *Am J Infect Control*, 2005, 33(2):104-7.

Enterobius vermicularis

Synonyms Pinworm

Microbiology *Enterobius vermicularis*, or pinworm, causes a form of perianal pruritus called enterobiasis, often seen in children. *Enterobius vermicularis* is a nematode, or roundworm, and is thus related to such parasites as *Ascaris lumbricoides*, *Ancylostoma duodenale* (hookworm), and *Strongyloides stercoralis*. *E. vermicularis* is a small, white worm with a cylindric unsegmented body. It is visible to the naked eye. The infectious cycle begins when the human host ingests the embryonated egg, which is infective within hours. The eggs hatch in the small intestine, and the emerging larval forms migrate to the large intestine. There, the larvae penetrate and develop within the mucosa and mature into male and female adult forms over a 2- to 6-week period. Fertilization takes place and the gravid female migrates to the perianal region of the host at night and lays its eggs in the perianal folds. The eggs mature rapidly and are infectious within hours.

Epidemiology Pinworm infection is most common in school children, although infection may occur at all ages. Infection is favored by close living conditions and is typically seen in institutions, schools, and daycare centers. Cases frequently are

(Continued)

Enterobius vermicularis (Continued)

clustered in families. All socioeconomic groups are at risk. Over 500 million cases occur worldwide, with about 40 million individual infections in the United States. Humans are the only known reservoir. Transmission occurs primarily via direct person-to-person spread. Eggs of the parasite frequently are carried beneath the fingernails of children who have been scratching the irritated perianal area. *E. vermicularis* eggs are relatively hardy and remain viable in dust, clothing, day care toys, furniture, and other fomites; infection can occur from inhalation of the eggs contained in infested dust.

Clinical Syndromes

- **Asymptomatic carriage:** Many infected individuals experience no symptoms from *E. vermicularis* but are still capable of spreading the worm.
- **Perianal pruritus:** This is the most common manifestation of pinworm infestation. Often there is severe local pruritus, interfering with sleep. Excessive scratching of the perianal region may lead to bacterial infection in severe cases.
- **Miscellaneous:** Unusual complications include appendicitis, salpingitis, granuloma formation, penetration through the intestinal wall, and bowel lesions.

Diagnosis Pinworm infestation is usually suspected in the individual who presents with refractory itching in the perianal area, particularly in children. The "Scotch tape test" is an accurate and inexpensive means of confirming the diagnosis. Clear adhesive tape is pressed to the perianal region early in the morning, prior to bathing or bowel movement . The eggs deposited overnight by the migrating adult readily adhere to the cellophane tape. This tape may be brought in later for examination by the physician. The thin-walled eggs are easily seen at low power under the microscope. Several examinations over consecutive days may be necessary since a single test may be falsely negative in 50% of cases. Commercial kits may be used in place of the less formal Scotch tape method; these kits utilize an adhesive paddle and follow the same general principles. Stool examinations are rarely diagnostic for pinworm. Peripheral eosinophilia is not characteristically seen.

Diagnostic Tests/Procedures

Pinworm Preparation *on page 565*

Treatment The drug of choice is mebendazole (Vermox®), which leads to a cure in >90% of the cases. Retreatment may be necessary in some cases, especially if reinfection occurs. Family members should be tested, even if asymptomatic, and treated as necessary.

Drug Therapy

Recommended:

Mebendazole *on page 928*

Pyrantel Pamoate *on page 1021*

Selected Readings

Mahmoud AA, "Intestinal Nematodes (Roundworms)," *Principles and Practice of Infectious Diseases*, 4th ed, Mandell GL, Bennett JE, and Dolin R, eds, New York, NY: Churchill Livingstone, 1995, 2526-31.

Wagner ED and Eby WC, "Pinworm Prevalence in California Elementary School Children, and Diagnostic Methods," *Am J Trop Med Hyg*, 1983, 32(5):998-1001.

Enterococcus Species

Related Information

Antibiotic Treatment of Adults With Infective Endocarditis *on page 1271*

Microbiology Historically, the term *Enterococcus* was used to describe hardy, nonfastidious streptococci usually found in the gastrointestinal tract; thus, the name *entero*cocci. The enterococci, *Streptococcus bovis* and *Streptococcus equinus* were classified as group D streptococci. Subsequently in 1984, the genus streptococci was divided into three genera, *Streptococcus*, *Lactococcus*, and the totally separate genus *Enterococcus*. Enterococci, on Gram stain, are gram-positive, catalase-negative cocci that occur in pairs or short chains. In culture, they can grow in 6.5% NaCl broth at 10°C to 45°C, can hydrolyze esculin in the presence of bile, and hydrolyze L-pyrholidonyl β-napththylamide.

Typically, enterococci have low level resistance to aminoglycosides. High level aminoglycoside resistance mediated by plasmids and transposons has become an increasing problem. *E. faecalis* frequently exhibits high level resistance to all currently available aminoglycosides. In serious infections, high level synergy testing is recommended for gentamicin and streptomycin. Because of β-lactamase production by some strains, β-lactamase testing (nitrocefin) also is performed by some laboratories. Vancomycin resistance is emerging; therefore, susceptibility testing for vancomycin is also indicated.

The resistance determinants of the enterococci reside on highly mobile genetic elements (plasmids and transposons) which have the potential to spread within the genus as well as to other gram-positive cocci. Thus, recognition, appropriate therapy, and awareness of the potential for nosocomial spread are of particular importance.

Epidemiology In the human host, the main reservoir for *Enterococcus* species is the intestinal tract. They are also commonly found in the oral cavity, urethra, and vagina. Infections may arise from endogenous flora and may be spread as nosocomial infections by hand and environmental contamination. *E. faecalis* and *E. faecium* are the species recovered in 80% to 90% of enterococcal infections. Isolates of enterococci from blood are generally considered pathogenic because 85% of these patients have clinical infections. Broad-spectrum antibiotic therapy may suppress normal flora and allow enterococcal overgrowth of the intestinal flora. Wound colonization is common and superinfection in compromised hosts and those on antimicrobial therapy also occurs frequently. The organism is considered to have low intrinsic virulence and is considered to be primarily an opportunistic pathogen.

Vancomycin-resistant enterococci (VRE) were first reported in Europe in 1986, and in the United States in 1988. Since that time, VRE has become increasingly detected in essentially all hospitals. Virtually all VRE are *E. faecium*, and most isolates of *E. faecium* in hospitals are VRE. Virtually all isolates of *E. faecalis* are susceptible to vancomycin.

Clinical Syndromes The enterococci are recognized as causes of urinary tract infections, bacteremia, endocarditis, intra-abdominal infections, and osteomyelitis primarily in diabetic patients. Pneumonia and meningitis due to *Enterococcus* are rare in adult patients. Fifteen percent to 20% of bacterial endocarditis is caused by enterococci. *Streptococcus viridans* and *Staphylococcus* are the only organisms more frequently isolated. Enterococcal endocarditis occurs in the elderly more in association with urinary tract manipulation (ie, cystoscopy and catheterization); in young women associated with childbirth, cesarean sections, intrauterine devices (IUDs), curettage (D & Cs), and abortions. Intravenous drug abusers have a high incidence of enterococcal endocarditis which most frequently affects the mitral and/or aortic valves. Bacteremia is frequently detected in patients with serious underlying medical conditions including recent surgery, trauma, or burns. Enterococcal bacteremia is frequently nosocomial and often represents superinfection. Polymicrobic infections are frequently more fulminant with a higher incidence of shock, thrombocytopenia, and disseminated intravascular coagulation (DIC) than infections where enterococci are the sole pathogens. Gram-negative bacilli are the most frequently encountered copathogens. Prior antimicrobial therapy and long hospital stays are risk factors. The urinary tract is a frequent source of enterococcal bacteremia; however, because these cases are almost always associated with host factors, enterococcal urinary tract infections (UTIs) are rarely encountered in office patients who are healthy otherwise. In intra-abdominal infections, enterococci are frequently present in part of a mixed infection where they may act synergistically with other bacteria. Neonatal meningitis may occur as nosocomial epidemics associated with prematurely low birth weight, previous antimicrobial therapy, arterial or venous catheterization, and nasogastric intubation.

Diagnostic Tests/Procedures

Aerobic Culture, Appropriate Site *on page 365*

Antimicrobial Susceptibility Testing, Aerobic and Facultatively Anaerobic Organisms *on page 379*

Blood Culture, Aerobic and Anaerobic *on page 391*

Gram Stain *on page 473*

Duration of Therapy Enterococcal endocarditis is commonly treated with combination therapy for 4-6 weeks. Therapy for other enterococcal infections ranges from 7-14 days.

Treatment Appropriate therapy for serious enterococcal infections includes a cell wall-acting agent such as penicillin, ampicillin, or vancomycin plus an aminoglycoside (gentamicin or streptomycin). For urinary tract infections, a single cell wall agent may be appropriate. Some urinary tract infections can be treated with nitrofurantoin or fosfomycin depending on susceptibilities. If high-level aminoglycoside resistance is present, the addition of the aminoglycoside is not useful.

Treatment of serious infections with vancomycin-resistant enterococci may include linezolid, quinupristin/dalfopristin, doxycycline, or chloramphenicol. Susceptibility testing should be performed to determine resistance patterns for these agents. For example, quinupristin/dalfopristin is typically active against *Enterococcus faecium*, but resistant to *Enterococcus faecalis*. Although daptomycin is often active against these organisms, some resistance is being seen. Combination therapy with newer agents requires more data.

Treatment of enterococcal endocarditis depends on the susceptibility of the organism and whether there is the presence of prosthetic material. For native valve endocarditis susceptible to all the agents, it is recommended that penicillin or ampicillin plus gentamicin (low-dose) be administered for 4-6 weeks or vancomycin plus gentamicin

(Continued)

Enterococcus Species *(Continued)*

(low-dose) for 6 weeks. For prosthetic valve endocarditis, streptomycin is recommended to be substituted for gentamicin. For vancomycin resistant *E. faecium* infections, linezolid or quinupristin/dalfopristin are the recommended drugs of choice administered for at least 8 weeks. Vancomycin-resistant *E. faecalis* is much less common and the recommendations include imipenem plus ampicillin or ceftriaxone plus ampicillin for at least 8 weeks.

Drug Therapy

Recommended:

Penicillin G (Parenteral/Aqueous) *on page 993*
plus one of the following
Gentamicin *on page 841*
Streptomycin *on page 1078*

Ampicillin *on page 657*
plus one of the following
Gentamicin *on page 841*
Streptomycin *on page 1078*

Vancomycin-resistant *Enterococcus:*
Linezolid *on page 914*
Quinupristin and Dalfopristin *on page 1032*
Doxycycline *on page 787*
Chloramphenicol *on page 733*

Alternate:

Vancomycin *on page 1144*
plus
Gentamicin *on page 841*

Penicillin G (Parenteral/Aqueous) *on page 993*
plus
Streptomycin *on page 1078*

Ampicillin *on page 657*
plus
Streptomycin *on page 1078*

Selected Readings

Alder JD, "Daptomycin: A New Drug Class for the Treatment of Gram-Positive Infections," *Drugs Today (Barc)*, 2005, 41(2):81-90.

Baddour LM, Wilson WR, Bayer AS, et al, "Infective Endocarditis: Diagnosis, Antimicrobial Therapy, and Management of Complications: A Statement for Healthcare Professionals From the Committee on Rheumatic Fever, Endocarditis, and Kawasaki Disease, Council on Cardiovascular Disease in the Young, and the Councils on Clinical Cardiology, Stroke, and Cardiovascular Surgery and Anesthesia, American Heart Association - Executive Summary: Endorsed by the Infectious Diseases Society of America," *Circulation*, 2005, 111(23):3167-84.

Donskey CJ and Rice LB, "The Influence of Antibiotics on Spread of Vancomycin-Resistant Enterococci: The Potential Role of Selective Use of Antibiotics as a Control Measure," *Clin Microbiol Newslett*, 1999, 21(8):57-65.

Goldrick BA, "MRSA, VRE, and VRSA: How Do We Control Them in Nursing Homes?" *Am J Nurs*, 2004, 104(8):50-1.

Kauffman CA, "Therapeutic and Preventative Options for the Management of Vancomycin-Resistant Enterococcal Infections," *J Antimicrob Chemother*, 2003, 51(Suppl 3):iii23-30.

Leclercq R and Courvalin P, "Resistance to Glycopeptides in Enterococci," *Clin Infect Dis*, 1997, 24(4):545-56.

Linden PK and Miller CB, "Vancomycin-Resistant Enterococci: The Clinical Effect of a Common Nosocomial Pathogen," *Diagn Microbiol Infect Dis*, 1999, 33(2):113-20.

Linden PK, "Treatment Options for Vancomycin-Resistant Enterococcal Infections," *Drugs*, 2002, 62(3):425-41.

Megran DW, "Enterococcal Endocarditis," *Clin Infect Dis*, 1992, 15(1):63-71.

Menichetti F, "Current and Emerging Serious Gram-Positive Infections," *Clin Microbiol Infect*, 2005, 11(Suppl 3):22-8.

Moellering RC Jr, "Vancomycin-Resistant Enterococci," *Clin Infect Dis*, 1998, 26(5):1196-9.

Raghavan M and Linden PK, "Newer Treatment Options for Skin and Soft Tissue Infections," *Drugs*, 2004, 64(15):1621-42.

Rand KH and Houck H, "Daptomycin Synergy With Rifampicin and Ampicillin Against Vancomycin-Resistant Enterococci," *J Antimicrob Chemother*, 2004, 53(3):530-2.

Weber DJ, Raasch R, and Rutala WA, "Nosocomial Infections in the ICU: The Growing Importance of Antibiotic-Resistant Pathogens," *Chest*, 1999, 115(3 Suppl):34S-41S.

Yeh KM, Siu LK, Chang JC, et al, "Vancomycin-Resistant *Enterococcus* (VRE) Carriage and Infection in Intensive Care Units," *Microb Drug Resist*, 2004, 10(2):177-83.

Enterovirus

Microbiology Enteroviruses are small, single-stranded RNA viruses belonging to the family Picornaviridae. The term "enterovirus" may be a source of confusion since it may refer to either the genus Enterovirus (which includes echovirus, Coxsackieviruses A and B, poliovirus, and enterovirus) or the species enterovirus. The following discussion applies to the species enterovirus, which is further classified into

enterovirus serotypes 68-71. These agents are sometimes referred to as the "newer enteroviruses" because of their recent recognition as agents of disease. The enteroviruses lack a lipid envelope. Important biophysical properties include the ability to survive in conditions of low pH and relatively high temperatures, and resistance to chlorine and alcohol decontamination. Enteroviruses grow best at body temperature. They replicate well in the upper respiratory and gastrointestinal tracts and can survive the acid environment of the stomach.

Epidemiology The newer enteroviruses are widely distributed throughout the world. Enteroviruses 70 and 71 are the two serotypes best characterized from an epidemiological and clinical standpoint. Enterovirus serotype 70 was first reported as a pathogen in 1969 during an outbreak of hemorrhagic conjunctivitis in Indonesia. This previously unrecognized virus has since spread throughout the globe and has been linked to millions of cases of hemorrhagic conjunctivitis. Pandemics are reported almost yearly. The majority of cases occur in the Far East, India, and Africa, generally in crowded urban areas with tropical climates. In the western hemisphere, most cases have been reported from Central America and the Caribbean, although an outbreak was reported from Florida in 1981 in an indigent population.

Enterovirus 71 was first isolated in 1969 from the stools of an infant in California with encephalitis. Over the next 10 years, a total of 8 epidemics were reported globally. The largest outbreak occurred in 1973 in Japan with over 3000 cases with hand-foot-and-mouth disease and aseptic meningitis. In 1975, an epidemic in Bulgaria involving 700 persons received worldwide attention. Over 20% of cases, mostly children, developed a polio-like paralysis with a significant number of fatalities; this was the first time a virus other than poliovirus was found to cause an epidemic paralytic disease. Small clusters of cases have been reported in the United States including a 1972 New York State outbreak characterized by meningitis and encephalitis in 11 cases and a similar small outbreak in 1977 in Rochester, New York, with two patients developing a self-resolving paralysis. An additional 5 children developed a polio-like paralysis in the summer of 1987 in Philadelphia, which remains the largest series of Enterovirus 71-associated paralysis reported in the United States.

Infections caused by the genus Enterovirus most commonly involve infants and younger children. Although specific data regarding Enterovirus 71 is somewhat limited, infants and younger children are at highest risk for infection with this serotype, based on data derived from the major epidemics of Enterovirus 71. In addition, most of the serious complications of Enterovirus 71, such as muscle paralysis and encephalitis, were reported in young children. Infections caused by Enterovirus 70 seem to involve all age groups equally.

Less is known about the transmission of the newer enteroviruses than related Enteroviruses such as poliovirus or Coxsackievirus. In general, the fecal-oral route is felt to be the major route of spread for the genus Enterovirus. Live virus may be shed from the oropharynx for weeks after acute infection, and there may be persistent shedding of virus in the stools for months. Direct person-to-person spread via the fecal-oral route is likely in this setting. Enterovirus 70 is an exception to this rule in that spread most likely occurs directly from hand-to-eye or indirectly from fomites to the eye.

Clinical Syndromes Infections caused by the newer enteroviruses have a diverse clinical spectrum but tend to be neurovirulent. There is also some overlap in the types of illnesses caused by the newer enteroviruses, poliovirus, Coxsackievirus A and B, and Echovirus.

- **Asymptomatic infection:** Many of the infections caused by viruses of the genus Enterovirus are asymptomatic, with an estimated 90% or more of enteroviral infections resulting in a nonspecific febrile illness. This likely holds true for the newer enteroviruses.
- **Poliomyelitis-like paralysis:** As noted above, Enterovirus 71 is a potential cause of an epidemic, lower motor neuron paralysis similar to polio. Anterior horn cells in the spinal cord are involved, as in poliomyelitis. The disease is acute in onset and usually involves children. Patients present with asymmetric flaccid paralysis of the extremities with absent reflexes in the involved extremity. The sensory system is typically intact. This clinical syndrome is still rare in the United States but should be considered in the differential diagnosis of a child presenting with an unexplained paralytic disease.
- **Acute hemorrhagic conjunctivitis:** This disease, caused by Enterovirus serotype 70, tends to occur in an epidemic fashion and is highly contagious. Patients present with acute onset of a hemorrhagic conjunctivitis, with pain in the eye, photophobia, and periorbital swelling. Some may have constitutional symptoms such as fever and malaise. Nearly all will have subconjunctival bleeding, and this is distinctive. Complications include keratitis and occasionally neurologic complications such as motor paralysis have been reported following the conjunctivitis. Since only a limited number of cases have been reported from the western

(Continued)

Enterovirus *(Continued)*

hemisphere, this diagnosis is unlikely in the United States but should be considered in immigrants or travelers.

- **Aseptic meningitis:** Like other enteroviruses, Enterovirus 71 has been associated with the syndrome of aseptic meningitis. Patients present with headache, neck stiffness, and a lymphocytic pleocytosis in the spinal fluid. Enterovirus 71 is a relatively uncommon cause of this syndrome, with many studies demonstrating Coxsackievirus as the major etiologic agent.
- **Hand-foot-and-mouth syndrome:** Like Coxsackievirus A16, Enterovirus 71 can cause this syndrome of vesicular lesions in the palms of the hands (exanthem) and the mucous membranes of the mouth (enanthem). This is a self-limited disease.

Diagnosis The clinical suspicion of enteroviral infection needs to be confirmed by viral culture. It is less important to differentiate the newer enteroviruses from Coxsackievirus or echovirus, than it is to differentiate it from bacterial causes of infection. The virus can be isolated in cell culture, particularly from rectal swabs or from throat secretions. In addition, it can be grown in cell culture from clinical specimens such as cerebrospinal fluid, skin lesions, or pericardial fluid.

Serologic studies are available to look for specific antibody responses to enterovirus. IgG antibody and IgM antibody against enteroviruses are available, and the finding of a fourfold increase in IgG or the presence of IgM antibody is helpful in establishing the diagnosis. However, it should be noted that recovery of enterovirus from a throat swab or a rectal swab does not necessarily establish enterovirus as the cause of an illness, since asymptomatic viral shedding may persist for periods of time. However, recovery of enterovirus from a site such as spinal fluid or a swab of a conjunctival lesion is confirmatory.

Diagnostic Tests/Procedures

Enterovirus Culture *on page 453*
Polymerase Chain Reaction *on page 567*

Drug Therapy Comment Currently, there are no antiviral agents available which are active *in vivo* against enterovirus.

Selected Readings

Huang CC, Liu CC, Chang YC, et al, "Neurologic Complications in Children With Enterovirus 71 Infection," *N Engl J Med*, 1999, 341(13):936-42.
Kupila L, Vuorinen T, Vainionpaa R, et al, "Diagnosis of Enteroviral Meningitis by Use of Polymerase Chain Reaction of Cerebrospinal Fluid, Stool, and Serum Specimens," *Clin Infect Dis*, 2005, 40(7):982-7.
Petersson K, Norbeck O, Westgren M, et al, "Detection of Parvovirus B19, Cytomegalovirus and Enterovirus Infections in Cases of Intrauterine Fetal Death," *J Perinat Med*, 2004, 32(6):516-21.
Rittichier KR, Bryan PA, Bassett KE, et al, "Diagnosis and Outcomes of Enterovirus Infections in Young Infants," *Pediatr Infect Dis J*, 2005, 24(6):546-50.
Steiner I, Budka H, Chaudhuri A, et al, "Viral Encephalitis: A Review of Diagnostic Methods and Guidelines for Management," *Eur J Neurol*, 2005, 12(5):331-43.

Epidemic Pleurodynia *see* Coxsackieviruses *on page 101*

Epididymitis/Orchitis

Related Information

Treatment of Sexually Transmitted Infections *on page 1311*

Clinical Presentation An inflammatory condition of the epididymis, presenting with pain, swelling, and induration of the epididymis and scrotum. May extend to involve both testicles. Pain may extend to the groin region. Urinary tract symptoms and/or penile discharge may be present. In addition, fever and chills may be present in severe infections. Usually occurs in younger sexually active males, less commonly in prepubertal males. May also occur in older males as a complication of urinary tract infections.

Differential Diagnosis Noninfectious epididymitis; epididymitis secondary to vasectomy, testicular torsion, mumps orchitis, testicular carcinoma, trauma, cyst, hydrocele, varicocele; sterile urine reflux (after TURP); granulomatous reaction following BCG intravesical therapy

Likely Pathogens Varies with age:

Younger sexually active males:

Chlamydia trachomatis on page 74
Neisseria gonorrhoeae on page 244

Older males: Usually coliforms (urinary tract pathogens):

Escherichia coli on page 142
Staphylococcus aureus, Methicillin-Resistant *on page 304*
Staphylococcus aureus, Methicillin-Susceptible *on page 307*
Mycobacterium tuberculosis on page 234 (sterile pyuria, vas deferens nodularity)

Diagnostic Tests/Procedures

Testicular Ultrasound
Neisseria gonorrhoeae Culture *on page 547*

Drug Therapy Comment Treatment varies based on demographic characteristics and likely pathogens. Younger sexually active males likely to involve sexually transmitted organisms, including *Chlamydia* (serious urethral discharge) and *Neisseria* (purulent discharge).

Empiric Drug Therapy

Recommended:

Monotherapy:
- Ofloxacin *on page 977*

Combination therapy:
- Ceftriaxone *on page 722*
  plus
  Doxycycline *on page 787*

Sexually active males: Septic/toxic:
- Fluoroquinolones *on page 824*
- Ampicillin and Sulbactam *on page 660*
- Piperacillin and Tazobactam Sodium *on page 1003*

Alternate:

If *Staphylococcus aureus* is suspected:
- Rifampin *on page 1046*
- Vancomycin *on page 1144*

Tuberculosis: See *Mycobacterium tuberculosis on page 234*

Selected Readings

Hagley M, "Epididymo-orchitis and Epididymitis: A Review of Causes and Management of Unusual Forms," *Int J STD AIDS*, 2003, 14(6):372-7.

Epiglottitis

Synonyms Supraglottitis

Clinical Presentation Acute epiglottitis is a rapidly progressive inflammation/cellulitis of the epiglottis which may cause airway obstruction. Small children typically present with fever and dysphagia, while older children and adults complain of sore throat. Inspiratory stridor and hoarseness occur frequently, and patients may present with drooling. Diagnosis is confirmed by the presence of an edematous "cherry red" epiglottis which should be visualized in a controlled environment in which one should be able to secure the airway.

Differential Diagnosis Croup; diphtheria; allergic laryngeal edema; foreign body aspiration; abscess - retropharyngeal, peritonsillar

Likely Pathogens

Children:
- *Haemophilus influenzae on page 159*

Adults:
- *Streptococcus pyogenes on page 321*

Diagnostic Tests/Procedures

- Aerobic Culture, Appropriate Site *on page 365*
- Group A *Streptococcus* Antigen Test *on page 475*
- Throat Culture for Group A Beta-Hemolytic *Streptococcus on page 594*

Empiric Drug Therapy

Recommended:

Children:
- Cephalosporins, 2nd Generation *on page 729*
- Cephalosporins, 3rd Generation *on page 730*

Adults:
- Cephalosporins, 2nd Generation *on page 729*

Epstein-Barr Virus

Synonyms EBV

Microbiology EBV is a DNA virus and a member of the herpesvirus family (the other three members are herpesvirus, varicella-zoster virus, and cytomegalovirus). Two strains of EBV, differing in their B-lymphocyte transformation and in viral gene sequence expression, infect humans. The structure of the viral DNA of EBV is unique as compared to other herpesvirus. The virus selectively infects human B lymphocytes and produces "immortalized" cell lives and usually causes latent infection.

Epidemiology Infection with EBV is common, with about 95% of the population demonstrating specific antibodies to this virus. In the U.S., the first peak of EBV infection occurs in children, with nearly 50% of 5 year olds seroconverting. There is a second peak of infection in the 20-30 year old age group.

EBV is transmitted by exchange of saliva containing live virus. EBV often persists for months in the throat of acutely infected individuals. Periodic asymptomatic shedding

(Continued)

Epstein-Barr Virus *(Continued)*

of virus is common. EBV may be cultured from the throat of 10% to 20% of healthy adults. Many with acute EBV are not aware of a sick contact who may have transmitted the disease. Prolonged intimate contact is necessary for spread. In general, the data suggest that EBV is widespread but is a virus of relatively low pathogenicity. Following the initial exposure to the virus, there is a 1- to 2-month incubation period prior to clinical disease. During this time, the virus disseminates through the reticuloendothelial system (liver, spleen, lymph nodes).

Clinical Syndromes

- **Infectious mononucleosis:** In the United States, "mono" occurs most commonly in individuals between 15-25 years of age. Characteristically, the patient presents with the "classic triad" of fever, sore throat, and lymphadenopathy. Rash is seen in only 5% of cases, but the rash is seen in nearly 100% of patients who mistakenly receive ampicillin for their symptoms. The tonsils are enlarged and the pharynx is inflamed, often with petechiae. Splenomegaly is an important physical finding in this setting and is present in nearly 50% of cases. Liver enlargement may also occur and liver function tests are frequently elevated. In many cases, the clinician must rely heavily on laboratory confirmation of suspected infectious mononucleosis, since both toxoplasmosis and cytomegalovirus can cause a similar syndrome. A compatible clinical syndrome, a positive heterophil test, and atypical lymphocytosis on blood smear are usually enough to establish the diagnosis of EBV mononucleosis. However, many cases may lack one or more of these findings; children are particularly prone to have heterophil-negative EBV mononucleosis. More detailed serologic testing is often necessary to confirm the diagnosis. Most patients recover completely from infectious mononucleosis over 2-3 weeks. However, a variety of complications have been reported: splenic rupture, hemolytic anemia, airway obstruction, profound thrombocytopenia, encephalitis, and the Guillain-Barré syndrome. Rare patients demonstrate objective evidence of ongoing EBV infection, with leukopenia, pulmonary infiltrates, and progressive neurologic disorders; this is in distinction to the "chronic EBV syndrome" described below. Although acyclovir inhibits EBV *in vitro* and probably *in vivo* as well, it appears to have minimal benefit in acute EBV mononucleosis. In large part, this is likely due to the observation that the clinical events in EBV mononucleosis result from the host's immune response rather than from direct viral invasion. Case reports have described the benefit of acyclovir in life-threatening EBV, but data are limited. The use of corticosteroids is controversial. Some have advocated corticosteroids only in complicated EBV infection (airway obstruction, thrombocytopenia, etc), but the benefits are unclear.
- **Possible relationship with the chronic fatigue syndrome (CFS):** Persistent EBV infection has been theorized to cause CFS. This controversial syndrome is characterized by overwhelming fatigue, muscle aches, poor concentration, low grade fevers, and minor lymphadenopathy. Initially, this symptom complex was termed the "chronic mononucleosis syndrome" due to its similarities with the prodromal symptoms of infectious mononucleosis. EBV was further implicated as an etiologic cause of "chronic mono" because many such individuals demonstrated high titers of EBV-specific antibody. Carefully controlled studies later showed that EBV titers were equivalent in patients with CFS and matched normal controls. In addition, clinical trials using acyclovir in CFS demonstrated no benefit. Currently, there is little objective evidence to link CFS and EBV.
- **EBV and malignancies:** EBV has been implicated as a cofactor in the development of Burkitt lymphoma, a malignancy common in Africa. A direct causal relationship is suspected but has yet to be proven. EBV DNA sequences and virions have been identified in biopsy samples of Burkitt lymphoma. EBV has also been strongly associated with nasopharyngeal carcinoma, a neoplasm most common in the Orient. Again, EBV nucleic acid has been found within malignant tissues. It has also been implicated as a potential cofactor or etiology in Hodgkin lymphoma.
- **EBV in transplant recipients:** In patients who have undergone solid organ or bone marrow transplantation, EBV has been reported to cause an unusual lymphoma-like syndrome called "post-transplantation lymphoproliferative disorder." Patients receiving cyclosporin A, a medication used to prevent organ rejection, appear to be at increased risk. Biopsies of involved organs reveal a B-cell lymphoproliferative malignancy with identifiable EBV nucleic acid sequences. The spectrum of this disorder is still under study. In general, and unlike cytomegalovirus or herpes simplex virus, EBV is an unusual opportunistic pathogen in the transplant population.
- **EBV infection in patients with AIDS:** An EBV-related lymphoproliferative syndrome has also been reported in patients with advanced HIV infection. Another disease associated with EBV infection is oral hairy leukoplakia. This disease is a commonly seen lesion of the tongue and is frequently noted in advanced AIDS.

EBV has been implicated as a possible etiologic cause (or cofactor) in this disorder and in non-Hodgkin lymphoma including primary CNS lymphoma.

Diagnostic Tests/Procedures

Epstein-Barr Virus Serology *on page 454*
Immunofluorescent Studies, Biopsy *on page 507*
Infectious Mononucleosis Serology *on page 509*
Polymerase Chain Reaction *on page 567*

Drug Therapy Comment No antiviral agents have been proven to be effective in the treatment of Epstein-Barr virus infections. Supportive care is the treatment of choice.

Selected Readings

Auwaerter PG, "Infectious Mononucleosis: Return to Play," *Clin Sports Med*, 2004, 23(3):485-97.
Cohen JI, "Epstein-Barr Virus infection," *N Engl J Med*, 2000, 343(7):481-92.
Ellen Rimsza M and Kirk GM, "Common Medical Problems of the College Student," *Pediatr Clin North Am*, 2005, 52(1):9-24.
Fafi-Kremer S, Morand P, Brion JP, et al, "Long-Term Shedding of Infectious Epstein-Barr Virus After Infectious Mononucleosis," *J Infect Dis*, 2005, 191(6):985-9.
"Information From Your Family Doctor. Things to Know About Infectious Mononucleosis," *Am Fam Physician*, 2004, 70(7):1289-90.
Jenson HB, "Virologic Diagnosis, Viral Monitoring, and Treatment of Epstein-Barr Virus Infectious Mononucleosis," *Curr Infect Dis Rep*, 2004, 6(3):200-7.

Erysipelas

Clinical Presentation Acute inflammatory process involving superficial skin and lymphatics. Differentiated from cellulitis by prominent lymphatic involvement and more clearly demarcated margins. Occurs most frequently on the lower legs, ears, and face. Typically, the face (especially the nasal area) and ears are involved. Usually occurs in infants or in adults >40 years of age. Highest incidence in adults >75 years of age. May be more common in individuals with fissured or inflamed skin (trauma or abrasion), immunocompromised, or chronic diseases such as diabetes. Prodromal symptoms include headache, malaise, chills, and fever. Vomiting is a frequent manifestation. Begins as an acute onset of facial erythema and pruritus, initially forming an erythematous patch with a sharp border. The patch spreads outward as the central area clears. Vesicles may form and followed by desquamation.

Differential Diagnosis Contact dermatitis; angioneurotic edema; scarlet fever; systemic lupus erythematosus

Likely Pathogens

Streptococcus pyogenes *on page 321*
Staphylococcus aureus, Methicillin-Susceptible *on page 307*
Streptococcus agalactiae *on page 313*

Diagnostic Tests/Procedures

Blood Culture, Aerobic and Anaerobic *on page 391*

Empiric Drug Therapy

Recommended:

Penicillin V Potassium *on page 998*

If *Staphylococcus* is suspected (uncommon):
Cephalosporins, 1st Generation *on page 729*
Amoxicillin and Clavulanate Potassium *on page 645*
Dicloxacillin *on page 773*

Alternate:

Azithromycin *on page 674*
Clarithromycin *on page 749*
Cephalosporins, 1st Generation *on page 729*

Erysipeloid *see Erysipelothrix rhusiopathiae on page 141*

Erysipelothrix rhusiopathiae

Microbiology *Erysipelothrix rhusiopathiae* is a thin, gram-positive rod that has been known to be an important animal pathogen since the late 1800s. More recently it has been recognized as a potentially serious cause of human disease. The organism is an aerobic bacillus (or facultatively anaerobic) that sometimes can appear as long nonbranching filaments. The organism can appear pleomorphic. *E. rhusiopathiae* can be distinguished from *Bacillus* species (another gram-positive rod) by the lack of spore formation in the former. *E. rhusiopathiae* grows on routine culture media where it has two distinctive forms on solid agar, one smooth and pinpoint, the other flat and rough and does not require specialized techniques for recovery from the blood.

Epidemiology The organism is ubiquitous in the environment and has a predilection for dead or decomposing nitrogenous substances. It can be found worldwide primarily as a colonizer of animals. The major reservoir of *E. rhusiopathiae* is probably domestic pigs, although the organism can be recovered from several species including birds, rats, and fowl. The slime that covers various species of fish also harbors the organism where it acts as a harmless commensal. Human infection

(Continued)

Erysipelothrix rhusiopathiae (Continued)

generally occurs by direct inoculation from an infected animal to a human. The highest incidence of human disease occurs in those individuals with frequent exposures to animals, fish, poultry, grease, and fertilizer. Occupations at highest risk for *E. rhusiopathiae* infection are fish handlers, butchers, slaughterhouse workers, fisherman, and veterinarians.

Clinical Syndromes

- **Erysipeloid ("erysipelas-like"):** This is the most common clinical syndrome. Erysipeloid is a localized cellulitis which occurs as a result of cuts or abrasions to the hand followed by inoculation of the organism into the wounds from infected fish or animal meat. Clinically, patients present with severe pain, itching, and swelling of the finger or hand, often with discrete purplish erythema in the skin. These violaceous lesions are elevated and demarcated. Joint involvement may occur in the fingers. Left untreated, the infection often spreads proximally, and axillary adenopathy may develop. Vesicles are relatively uncommon, unlike true erysipelas caused by streptococci. This syndrome has been called the erysipeloid of Rosenbach, whale finger, seal finger, or fish poisoning. A more diffuse form of skin infection has also been described but is much less common; the violaceous skin lesions are more severe and progressive, and patients are more systemically ill.
- **Bacteremia and endocarditis:** This is a serious but uncommon complication, with about 60 reported cases. Skin lesions were seen in approximately 33% of bacteremic cases. Endocarditis has developed on previously normal valves and has a poorly understood tropism for the aortic valve. There is still a strong correlation with specific occupations. Mortality is high.

Diagnosis *Erysipelothrix* infection should be considered in any individual who presents with a significant hand or digital pain or swelling, particularly if there are occupational risk factors. Other considerations include staphylococcal or streptococcal infections, *Sporothrix* infection, mycobacterial infection, and lymphangitis. The violaceous lesions are distinctive for *Erysipelothrix* but are not always present. Laboratory confirmation is essential. The organism is best identified by deep soft tissue biopsy submitted for histopathology and culture. Blood cultures are negative in the erysipeloid form of the disease.

Diagnostic Tests/Procedures

Biopsy Culture, Routine *on page 390*
Blood Culture, Aerobic and Anaerobic *on page 391*
Gram Stain *on page 473*
Histopathology *on page 496*
Skin Biopsy *on page 580*

Treatment *E. rhusiopathiae* is highly susceptible to penicillin but resistant to vancomycin. Other agents highly active against the organism *in vitro* include imipenem and the cephalosporins. Most authorities consider penicillin the drug of choice. It is important to note that the organism is resistant to vancomycin, an agent commonly used for empiric therapy of serious soft tissue infections. *E. rhusiopathiae* is also relatively resistant to trimethoprim-sulfamethoxazole and aminoglycosides and is only variably susceptible to erythromycin and tetracyclines.

Drug Therapy

Recommended:

Penicillin V Potassium *on page 998*
Penicillin G (Parenteral/Aqueous) *on page 993*

Alternate:

Imipenem and Cilastatin *on page 861*
Cephalosporins, 1st Generation *on page 729*

Erythema Infectiosum *see* Parvovirus B19 *on page 255*

Escherichia coli

Related Information

Clinical Syndromes Associated With Foodborne Diseases *on page 1276*

Microbiology *Escherichia coli* is a lactose-positive, gram-negative, facultative bacillus with variable motility. A member of the Enterobacteriaceae family, *E. coli* is probably the most widely studied free-living organism. Most *E. coli* are nonpigmented, produce lysine decarboxylase, utilize acetate as a carbon source, and hydrolyze tryptophan to indole. Serologic typing is based on three surface antigens (O, H, K). The lipopolysaccharide of the cell wall is known as endotoxin and is a factor in sepsis and septic shock in infected individuals.

Epidemiology *E. coli*, as well as other members of Enterobacteriaceae, are normal colonizers of the human and animal gastrointestinal tract. It is often considered an opportunistic pathogen in hospitalized or debilitated patients but is the most common cause of urinary tract infections among "normal" hosts.

Clinical Syndromes

- **Urinary tract infections:** In the United States, *E. coli* is the most common cause of urinary tract infections both in normal hosts and immunocompromised or hospitalized patients. Although most common in sexually active young women, *E. coli* urinary tract infections occur in patients who are at increased risk of urinary tract infections in general (catheterized, obstructed, diabetic, prostatitis, etc).
- **Lower respiratory infections:** *E. coli* causes a significant number of nosocomial pneumonias in the United States and is an uncommon cause of community-acquired pneumonia or bronchitis. *E. coli* may also colonize the respiratory tract of hospitalized patients without causing disease, and its treatment in the absence of clinically-relevant findings is usually unwarranted.
- **Neonatal meningitis:** Although uncommon in older populations, *E. coli* is a rare but important cause of meningitis and subsequent mortality in neonates.
- **Peritonitis:** *E. coli* is a major pathogen in polymicrobial intra-abdominal infections.
- **Sepsis and other infections:** *E. coli* is one of the leading causes of bacteremia, sepsis, and septic shock. It can also cause a variety of other infections including wound infections, cellulitis, and diarrhea.

Diagnosis *E. coli* infection diagnosis can be made by identification through Gram stain and culture of clinically-appropriate specimens from patients with relevant clinical syndromes. Special media or conditions are not necessary to grow this organism. *E. coli* should always be one of several suspected organisms in patients with peritonitis.

Diagnostic Tests/Procedures

Aerobic Culture, Appropriate Site *on page 365*
Gram Stain *on page 473*

Treatment Although the majority of *E. coli* are still sensitive to ampicillin, amoxicillin, first generation cephalosporins, and sulfamethoxazole and trimethoprim, increasing resistance is being noted, especially in nosocomial isolates. Most mild to moderate urinary tract infections can be treated with amoxicillin or sulfamethoxazole and trimethoprim until susceptibility confirmation. In more serious or nosocomial infections, more broad-spectrum antibiotics, such as third generation cephalosporins, should be initiated until susceptibility data is available. In patients who are septic, supportive care will also be necessary along with appropriate antibiotics. Fluoroquinolones are routinely active against this organism. Piperacillin is less active than piperacillin and tazobactam against most strains.

Drug Therapy

Recommended:

Severe infection:
Cephalosporins, 3rd Generation *on page 730*

Mild to moderate infection:
Ampicillin *on page 657*
Sulfamethoxazole and Trimethoprim *on page 1087*

Alternate:

Carbapenems *on page 693*
Cephalosporins, 1st Generation *on page 729*
Cephalosporins, 2nd Generation *on page 729*
Fluoroquinolones *on page 824*

Selected Readings

Eisenstein BI, "Enterobacteriaceae," *Principles and Practice of Infectious Diseases*, 5th ed, Mandell GL, Bennett JE, and Dolin R, eds, New York, NY: Churchill Livingstone, 2000, 2294-310.

Escherichia coli, Diarrheagenic

Synonyms Diarrheagenic *E. coli*

Applies to *Escherichia coli*, Enterhemorrhagic (EHEC); *Escherichia coli*, Enteroaggregative (EAEC); *Escherichia coli*, Enteroinvasive (EIEC); *Escherichia coli*, Enteropathogenic (EPEC); *Escherichia coli*, Enterotoxigenic (ETEC)

Microbiology Diarrheagenic *E. coli* include the following: Enterohemorrhagic *E. coli* (EHEC), enteroinvasive *E. coli* (EIEC), enteropathogenic *E. coli* (EPEC), enteroaggregative *E. coli* (EAEC), and enterotoxigenic *E. coli* (ETEC). See table on next page.

Nondiarrheagenic *E. coli*: Nondiarrheagenic (typical or common) *E. coli* is a facultative gram-negative rod and is the most common gram-negative bacterium isolated in the clinical microbiology laboratory and causes numerous types of extraintestinal infections.

Diarrheagenic *E. coli*: Like the typical *E. coli*, the five aforementioned diarrheagenic *E. coli* grow extremely well on commonly used laboratory media and are easily identified as *E. coli* by commonly used biochemical tests. In most cases, typical *E. coli* and diarrheagenic *E. coli* usually are indistinguishable when observed grossly on solid laboratory media and microscopically when stained with the Gram stain. EHEC, ETEC, EIEC, EPEC, and EAEC have characteristic virulence factors which define each as a specific type of diarrheagenic *E. coli*.

(Continued)

Properties of *E. coli* Strains That Cause Enteric Infections

Diarrheagenic *E. coli*	Pathogenic Mechanisms	Enteric Infection(s)	Common Clinical Presentations	Common Age Group	Common Risk Factor	Diagnostic Tests[1]
Enterotoxigenic *E. coli* (ETEC)	Heat-stable enterotoxin; Heat-labile enterotoxin	Diarrhea; traveler's diarrhea	Profuse watery diarrhea, cramps, nausea, dehydration	Children, adults	Foreign travel (usually Mexico)	EIA for enterotoxins; cell culture for cytotoxicity
Enteropathogenic *E. coli* (EPEC)	Adherence factor; attachment to and effacement of intestinal epithelium	Acute diarrhea	Watery diarrhea, fever, vomiting, mucus in stool	Children <2 years of age, adults	<2 years of age	Adherence to HEp-2 cell cultures
Enteroinvasive *E. coli* (EIEC)	Invasion and destruction of intestinal mucosal epithelium; enterotoxin?	Diarrhea; rarely dysentery similar to *Shigella* dysentery	Watery diarrhea; dysentery: scant stool, blood, mucus, and leukocytes in stool; fever; cramps	Adults	Foreign travel (usually Mexico)	Cytopathic effect of HeLa cell cultures
Enterohemorrhagic *E. coli* (EHEC)	Shiga-like toxins	Diarrhea; hemorrhagic colitis	Diarrhea (no leukocytes); abdominal cramps; blood in stool; fever, HUS[2], and TTP[3] may or may not be present	Children, elderly	Consumption of undercooked ground beef	Isolation in culture; EIA for toxin in stool
Enteroaggregative *E. coli* (EAEC)	Characteristic histopathologic lesion; cytotoxin?	Chronic and acute diarrheas	Watery diarrhea, vomiting	All ages	Unknown	Adherence pattern to HEp-2 cell cultures

[1]Many of the tests to confirm the identification of ETEC, EIEC, EPEC, and EAEC as etiological agents are relatively difficult to perform and are usually performed only in specialized reference laboratories.

[2]HUS: hemolytic uremic syndrome

[3]TTP: thrombotic thrombocytopenic purpura

Adapted from Larry D. Gray, "*Escherichia*, *Salmonella*, *Shigella*, and *Yersinia*," *Manual of Clinical Microbiology*, 6th ed, Murray PR, Baron EJ, Pfaller MA, et al, eds, Washington, DC: American Society for Microbiology, 1995, 451, with permission.

Epidemiology The diarrheagenic *E. coli* are enteric pathogens which are found in different environments throughout the world: bowels of cattle, areas of poor sanitation, contaminated water supplies, slaughter houses where fresh meat contacts cattle fecal material, and agricultural areas where fresh vegetables and fruits contact cattle fecal material. The portal of entry for diarrheagenic *E. coli* is oral/ingestion. The organisms (and, thus, the diseases) are transmitted person-to-person extremely efficiently by hand contact. See table.

Clinical Syndromes Some strains of *E. coli* (the diarrheagenic strains) can cause severe and life-threatening diarrhea. There are five distinct groups of diarrheagenic *E. coli* which cause gastrointestinal illnesses ranging from mild diarrhea to cholera-like diarrhea to potentially fatal complications such as hemolytic uremic syndrome. These groups are EHEC, ETEC, EIEC, EPEC, and EAEC.

- EHEC causes (often bloody) diarrhea and hemorrhagic colitis usually in children and the elderly and is associated with contaminated beef (usually hamburger). In addition, EHEC can cause hemolytic uremic syndrome, for which children are at particularly high risk.
- ETEC causes a profuse watery diarrhea most commonly known as "traveler's diarrhea" (also tourista, deli belly, Montezuma's revenge, the hot galloping screamo's, etc).
- EPEC causes an acute diarrhea in children usually <2 years of age.
- EIEC causes diarrhea which, in some (rare) cases, is similar to the dysentery caused by *Shigella*.
- EAEC is not well characterized but has been reported to cause both chronic and acute watery diarrhea in all age groups. See table.

Diagnosis Attribution of diarrhea to one of the diarrheagenic *E. coli* depends on evaluation of the type of diarrhea, age of the patient, travel history, blood/mucus in the stool, duration of diarrhea, and the consideration that the diarrhea might be caused by more common causes of diarrhea (viruses, *Giardia*, *Salmonella*, *Shigella*, and *Campylobacter*). Diagnosis is confirmed by isolation of the particular pathogen and biochemical proof that the isolate is *E. coli*, and then subsequent demonstration of characteristic surface antigens by serologic agglutination with specific antisera (eg, EPEC and EIEC), the production of characteristic enterotoxins in culture (eg, ETEC), the ability to invade mammalian cell cultures (eg, EIEC), or the ability to adhere to certain mammalian cell cultures (eg, EAEC).

Diagnostic Tests/Procedures Many of the tests to confirm the identification of EHEC, ETEC, EIEC, EPEC, and EAEC as etiological agents are relatively difficult to perform and are usually performed only in specialized reference laboratories. Some of the tests/reagents/kits used to detect these *E. coli* are commercially available to standard clinical microbiology laboratories, and, therefore, are available to physicians locally. Contact the Microbiology Laboratory for advice regarding collection of specimens, isolation of the *E. coli*, which tests are available, the analyte (antigen, toxin, organism, etc) detected by each test, and which tests can and should be ordered. See table.

Shiga Toxin Test, Direct *on page 579*
Stool Culture, Diarrheagenic *E. coli on page 587*

Treatment Treatment is supportive.

Selected Readings

Boyce TG, Swerdlow DL, and Griffin PM, "*Escherichia coli* O157:H7 and Hemolytic Uremic Syndrome," *N Engl J Med*, 1995, 333(6):364-8.

Gray LG, "*Escherichia*, *Salmonella*, *Shigella*, and *Yersinia*," *Manual of Clinical Microbiology*, 6th ed, Murray PR, Baron EJ, Pfaller, et al, eds, Washington DC: American Society for Microbiology, 1995, 450-6.

Nataro JP and Kaper JB, "Diarrheagenic *Escherichia coli*," *Clin Microbiol Rev*, 1998, 11(1):142-201.

Raj P, "Pathogenesis and Laboratory Diagnosis of *Escherichia coli*-Associated Enteritis," *Clin Microbiol Newslett*, 1993, 15(3):89-93.

Slutsker L, Ries AA, Greene KD, et al, "*Escherichia coli* O157:H7 Diarrhea in the United States: Clinical and Epidemiologic Features," *Ann Intern Med*, 1997, 126(7):505-13.

***Escherichia coli*, Enterhemorrhagic (EHEC)** *see Escherichia coli*, Diarrheagenic *on page 143*

***Escherichia coli*, Enteroaggregative (EAEC)** *see Escherichia coli*, Diarrheagenic *on page 143*

Escherichia coli, Enterohemorrhagic

Related Information

Clinical Syndromes Associated With Foodborne Diseases *on page 1276*

Synonyms *E. coli* O157:H7; EHEC; Shiga Toxin *E. coli*; STEC

Microbiology Enterohemorrhagic *E. coli* causes a distinct form of hemorrhagic colitis in humans. Like all *E. coli* strains, enterohemorrhagic *E. coli* (EHEC or STEC) is a facultative, gram-negative bacillus. There are many serotypes of EHEC, each of which can cause hemorrhagic colitis and each of which is defined by a somatic (O)
(Continued)

Escherichia coli, Enterohemorrhagic *(Continued)*

antigen and a flagellar (H) antigen (eg, O38:H21, O103:H2, and O157:H7). The most common serotype is O157:H7. Essentially, all published information regarding enterohemorrhagic *E. coli* refers only to this serotype.

Epidemiology In 1982, the first large-scale outbreak of *E. coli* O157:H7 colitis was described. Multiple cases of severe bloody diarrhea were found to be epidemiologically linked to ingestion of contaminated undercooked hamburger meat. Since then, the organism has been recognized as an important cause of bloody diarrhea and the hemolytic uremic syndrome (HUS). Over 12 major outbreaks have been reported, along with numerous sporadic cases. The majority of cases have been traced to contaminated ground beef, although other potential sources have been cited, including unpasteurized milk, apple cider, municipal water, and roast beef. The organism inhabits the gastrointestinal tract of some healthy cattle and is thought to contaminate meat during slaughter and the processing of ground beef ("internal contamination"). If the ground beef is undercooked, the organism remains viable. Undercooking of hamburger patties has proven important in several outbreaks.

In 1993, a well-publicized multistate outbreak of *E. coli* O157:H7 took place in the western United States (Washington, California, Idaho, and Nevada). Over 500 infections and four deaths were documented. The vast majority of cases were ultimately linked to contaminated hamburger meat from a particular restaurant chain. Further investigation by the Centers for Disease Control identified several slaughter plants in the United States and one in Canada as the probable source. Thousands of contaminated patties not yet consumed were discovered. In March, 1994, the USDA Food Safety and Inspection Service recommended that all raw meat should be cooked thoroughly, with an increase in the internal temperature for cooked hamburgers to 155°F.

A 2-year nationwide surveillance study by the Centers for Disease Control has found *E. coli* O157:H7 to be the most commonly identified pathogen associated with bloody diarrhea. In many parts of the U.S., *E. coli* O157:H7 is the second most common cause of bacterial diarrhea.

Acquisition of disease is usually by ingestion of contaminated food, but person-to-person transmission has been documented, especially in daycare centers. Children and elderly individuals are at highest risk for severe infections. Simple and careful hand washing essentially eliminates the probability of person-to-person transmission.

Clinical Syndromes

- **Hemorrhagic colitis:** *E. coli* O157:H7 and many other serotypes of EHEC cause a bloody diarrhea associated with abdominal cramps. Pathologically, there is no invasion or inflammation of the intestinal mucosa, and thus fever is often absent. The diarrhea is caused by Shiga-like toxins. In most cases, the illness resolves within 7 days, but death can occur in the elderly.
- **Hemolytic uremic syndrome:** 5% to 10% of patients with *E. coli* O157:H7 diarrhea develop a syndrome characterized by acute renal failure, thrombocytopenia, and evidence of hemolysis on a peripheral blood smear. Children are at particularly high risk for this syndrome. The patient may be toxic-appearing, and the presentation may be confused with a variety of diseases including sepsis with disseminated intravascular coagulation, vasculitis, thrombotic thrombocytopenia purpura, and others. The estimated mortality is 3% to 5%.

Diagnosis Enterohemorrhagic *E. coli* should be strongly considered in any patient presenting with bloody diarrhea, whether or not hemolytic uremic syndrome is present. It is likely that many sporadic cases of *E. coli* O157:H7 diarrhea occur in the community and go unrecognized for two reasons: Many clinicians do not order stool cultures for stable patients with diarrhea; and many microbiology laboratories do not routinely culture stools for EHEC or the Shiga toxin produced by EHEC unless there is a specific order for EHEC from the physician.

Laboratory diagnosis is made by (1) isolation of EHEC from stool specimens and subsequent serological confirmation or (2) detection of the EHEC Shiga toxin in the stool. Both of these tests require special media for culture and techniques for detection of Shiga toxin. Most clinical laboratories culture only the O157:H7 serotype. The disadvantage of such a practice is that serotypes other than O157:H7 (although rare) will not be detected.

Diagnostic Tests/Procedures

Shiga Toxin Test, Direct *on page 579*
Stool Culture, Diarrheagenic *E. coli on page 587*

Treatment Treatment is supportive. Patients should be monitored for signs and symptoms of hemolytic uremic syndrome. O157:H7 serotypes of *E. coli* are susceptible *in vitro* to most common antimicrobial agents; however, the agents should be avoided

clinically because the bacterium is not susceptible to these agents *in vivo*. A recent prospective study found that patients treated with antimicrobial agents had a higher incidence of HUS than those who did not receive antibiotics. Antimotility agents are always contraindicated in patients with bloody diarrhea.

Drug Therapy Comment No antibiotics proven effective; in fact, antibiotics may increase the risk of developing HUS.

Selected Readings

Acheson DWK and Jaegar JL, "Shiga Toxin-Producing *Escherichia coli*," *Clin Microbiol Newslett*, 1999, 21(23):183-8.

Bender JB, Hedberg CW, Besser JM, et al, "Surveillance by Molecular Subtype for *Escherichia coli* O157:H7 Infections in Minnesota by Molecular Subtyping," *N Engl J Med*, 1997, 337(6):388-94.

Boyce TG, Pemberton AG, Wells JG, et al, "Screening for *Escherichia coli* O157:H7 - A Nationwide Survey of Clinical Laboratories," *J Clin Microbiol*, 1995, 33(12):3275-7.

Ina K, Kusugami K, and Ohta M, "Bacterial Hemorrhagic Enterocolitis," *J Gastroenterol*, 2003, 38(2):111-20.

Kehl SC, "Role of the Laboratory in the Diagnosis of Enterohemorrhagic *Escherichia coli* Infections," *J Clin Microbiol*, 2002, 40(8):2711-5.

Mahon BE, Griffin PM, Mead PS, et al, "Hemolytic Uremic Syndrome Surveillance to Monitor Trends in Infection With *Escherichia coli* O157:H7 and Other Shiga Toxin-Producing *E. coli*," *Emerg Infect Dis*, 1997, 3(3):409-12.

Mead PS and Griffin PM, "*Escherichia coli* O157:H7," *Lancet*, 1998, 352(9135):1207-12.

Nataro JP and Kaper JB, "Diarrheagenic *Escherichia coli*," *Clin Microbiol Rev*, 1998, 11(1):142-201.

Slutsker L, Ries AA, Greene KD, et al, "*Escherichia coli* O157:H7 Diarrhea in the United States: Clinical and Epidemiologic Features," *Ann Intern Med*, 1997, 126(7):505-13.

Vallance BA, Chan C, Robertson ML, et al, "Enteropathogenic and Enterohemorrhagic *Escherichia coli* Infections: Emerging Themes in Pathogenesis and Prevention," *Can J Gastroenterol*, 2002, 16(11):771-8.

Wong CS, Jelacic S, Habeeb RL, et al, "The Risk of the Hemolytic-Uremic Syndrome After Antibiotic Treatment of *Escherichia coli* O157:H7 Infections," *N Engl J Med*, 2000, 342(26):1930-6.

***Escherichia coli*, Enteroinvasive (EIEC)** *see Escherichia coli,* Diarrheagenic *on page 143*

***Escherichia coli*, Enteropathogenic (EPEC)** *see Escherichia coli,* Diarrheagenic *on page 143*

***Escherichia coli*, Enterotoxigenic (ETEC)** *see Escherichia coli,* Diarrheagenic *on page 143*

Esophagitis

Clinical Presentation Patients present with odynophagia worse with acidic foods or dysphagia more commonly associated with solids than liquids. Infectious esophagitis is more commonly seen in immunosuppressed patients. Mucositis from chemotherapy may predispose patients to *Candida* infections. Esophageal candidiasis almost always occurs in the setting of refractory mucocutaneous candidiasis. Oral HSV may progress to esophagitis. Pain may precede development of vesicles followed by ulceration. Primary event is usually the most painful and may be associated with constitutional symptoms such as fever, malaise, and localized lymphadenopathy. Ulcers typically resolve in 7-14 days. CMV esophagitis most commonly seen in patients with AIDS.

Differential Diagnosis Noninfectious etiologies including: Aphthous ulcers; drug-induced mucositis; peptic esophagitis; malignancy

Likely Pathogens

Herpes Simplex Virus *on page 172*
Cytomegalovirus *on page 107*
Candida Species *on page 67*
Less likely other fungal or mycobacterial diseases

Diagnostic Tests/Procedures

Double-Contrast Esophagography
Endoscopy With Pathogen-Specific Cultures and Special Stains
Polymerase Chain Reaction *on page 567*

Empiric Drug Therapy

Recommended:

Therapy should be directed at suspected pathogen:

Candida:
- Fluconazole *on page 819*
- Itraconazole *on page 895*

HSV:
- Acyclovir *on page 629*
- Valacyclovir *on page 1140*
- Famciclovir *on page 815*

CMV:
- Ganciclovir *on page 834*
- Valganciclovir *on page 1143*

(Continued)

Esophagitis *(Continued)*

Alternate:

Candida:

Voriconazole *on page 1151*

Caspofungin *on page 695*

Amphotericin B (Conventional) *on page 650*

CMV:

Foscarnet *on page 829*

Cidofovir *on page 740*

Selected Readings

Ally R, Schurmann D, Kreisel W, et al, "A Randomized, Double-Blind, Double-Dummy, Multicenter Trial of Voriconazole and Fluconazole in the Treatment of Esophageal Candidiasis in Immunocompromised Patients," *Clin Infect Dis*, 2001, 33(9):1447-54.

Monkemuller KE and Wilcox CM, "Diagnosis of Esophageal Ulcers in Acquired Immunodeficiency Syndrome," *Semin Gastrointest Dis*, 1999, 10(3):85-92.

Pappas PG, Rex JH, Sobel JD, et al, "Guidelines for Treatment of Candidiasis," *Clin Infect Dis*, 2004, 38(2):161-89.

Parente F and Bianchi Porro G, "Treatment of Cytomegalovirus Esophagitis in Patients With Acquired Immune Deficiency Syndrome: A Randomized Controlled Study of Foscarnet Versus Ganciclovir. The Italian Cytomegalovirus Study Group," *Am J Gastroenterol*, 1998, 93(3):317-22.

Vazquez JA, "Options for the Management of Mucosal Candidiasis in Patients With AIDS and HIV Infection," *Pharmacotherapy*, 1999, 19(1):76-87.

Villanueva A, Arathoon EG, Gotuzzo E, et al, "A Randomized Double-Blind Study of Caspofungin Versus Amphotericin for the Treatment of Candidal Esophagitis," *Clin Infect Dis*, 2001, 33(9):1529-35.

European Blastomycosis *see Cryptococcus neoformans on page 102*

Exanthem Subitum *see* Human Herpesvirus-6 *on page 180*

Fasciitis *see* Skin and Soft Tissue *on page 300*

Fasciitis, Necrotizing *see* Necrotizing Fasciitis *on page 243*

Fever, Neutropenic

Related Information

Neutropenic Fever Guidelines *on page 1295*

Synonyms Neutropenic Fever

Clinical Presentation Classically, patients present with absolute neutropenia and fever without evidence of source either by history or physical examination. Generally lack symptoms of sweats and rigors.

Differential Diagnosis Infections - bacterial, viral, fungal, parasitic; drug associated; malignancy, especially lymphoma, leukemia

Likely Pathogens

Gram-Negative Bacilli *on page 157*

Staphylococcus aureus, Methicillin-Susceptible *on page 307*

Staphylococcus epidermidis, Methicillin-Susceptible *on page 310*

Candida Species *on page 67*

Streptococcus Species *on page 326*

Enterococcus Species *on page 134*

Diagnostic Tests/Procedures

•Aerobic Culture, Sputum *on page 367*

•Blood Culture, Aerobic and Anaerobic *on page 391*

•Blood Culture, Fungus *on page 395*

•Intravenous Line Culture *on page 511*

•Gram Stain *on page 473*

•Urine Culture, Clean Catch *on page 609*

Drug Therapy Comment See Neutropenic Fever Guidelines *on page 1295* in the Appendix.

Empiric Drug Therapy

Recommended:

Low-risk individuals: Oral:

Ciprofloxacin *on page 742*

plus

Amoxicillin and Clavulanate Potassium *on page 645*

High-risk individuals:

If vancomycin is **not** needed:

Monotherapy:

Cefepime *on page 705*

Ceftazidime *on page 717*

Imipenem and Cilastatin *on page 861*

Meropenem *on page 936*

Ertapenem *on page 805*

Combination therapy: **Note:** Any drug listed above as monotherapy may be combined with an aminoglycoside:

Penicillins, Extended-Spectrum *on page 997*

plus

Aminoglycosides *on page 641*

If vancomycin is needed:

Vancomycin *on page 1144*

plus one of the following

Ceftazidime *on page 717*

Cefepime *on page 705*

plus optional combination with

Aminoglycosides *on page 641*

Vancomycin *on page 1144*

plus

Penicillins, Extended-Spectrum *on page 997*

plus

Aminoglycosides *on page 641*

Selected Readings

Hughes WT, Armstrong D, Bodey GP, et al, "1997 Guidelines for the Use of Antimicrobial Agents in Neutropenic Patients With Unexplained Fever. Infectious Diseases Society of America," *Clin Infect Dis*, 1997, 25(3):551-73.

Hughes WT, Armstrong D, Bodey GP, et al, "2002 Guidelines for the Use of Antimicrobial Agents in Neutropenic Patients With Cancer," *Clin Infect Dis*, 2002, 34(6):730-51.

Fifth Disease *see* Parvovirus B19 *on page 255*

Fitz-Hugh Curtis Syndrome *see Chlamydia trachomatis on page 74*

Follicular Abscess *see* Furunculosis *on page 151*

Francisella tularensis

Related Information

Community-Acquired Pneumonia in Adults *on page 1278*

Microbiology *Francisella tularensis* is a nonmotile, pleomorphic, strictly aerobic, gram-negative rod. The bacterium possesses a lipid capsule which is a virulence factor and which might be responsible, at least in part, for the ability of the bacterium to survive weeks to months in adverse environmental conditions such as water, mud, and decaying animal carcasses. The bacterium is biochemically inert when grown (for identification purposes) *in vitro* on sugars or other substrates. The bacterium exists as two clinically significant biogroups. Biogroup *F. tularensis* (type A, mortality rate 5%) is found in North America and produces the most severe form of tularemia. Biogroup *palearctica* (type B, extremely low mortality) is found only in the northern hemisphere (particularly Asia and Europe) and produces a milder form of tularemia. Biogroup *Francisella tularensis* causes tularemia (rabbit fever, deer fly fever), a zoonosis of wild animals and the third most common human tick-borne illness in the United States.

Epidemiology *Francisella tularensis* is found throughout the United States (except the southeast, the northeast, and the Great Lakes areas). Tularemia is endemic in Missouri, Arkansas, and Oklahoma (together, 50% of all United States cases). The bacterium is strikingly absent from the United Kingdom, Africa, South America, and Australia. Hundreds of wild animal species and common house pets are hosts of the bacterium which is perpetuated freely and often in nature as it is passed from wild animal to wild animal by ectoparasites, poor environmental conditions, and less-than-respectable eating and culinary habits. The most common vectors which transmit *F. tularensis* to humans (incidental and dead-end hosts) are ticks and biting flies. In addition, humans who handle hides, woodland water, and animal carcasses can acquire the bacterium by the respiratory route. Occupations associated with a higher risk for tularemia are laboratory worker, veterinarian, sheep worker, hunter, trapper, and meat handler. Since 1965, the number of cases of tularemia in the United States has remained between 0.05 and 0.15 per 100,000. Person-to-person transmission of tularemia has not been documented.

Clinical Syndromes The severity of tularemia depends on the virulence of the biotype, portal of entry, inoculation dose, extent of dissemination, and immunocompetence of the host. After an incubation period of 2-10 days, flu-like symptoms usually occur. These symptoms can be chronic and debilitating. A nonhealing skin ulcer or lesion can develop at the cutaneous portal of entry and last for months. Tularemia usually presents in one or more of the following forms.

- **Ulceroglandular**: 21% to 87% of cases; obvious nonhealing, erythematous, eroding ulcers
- **Glandular**: 3% to 20% of cases; cutaneous ulcers are not found
- **Oculoglandular**: 0% to 5% of cases; severely painful, yellow, pinpoint conjunctival ulcers
- **Esophageal**: Severely painful sore throat; enlarged tonsils; white pseudomembrane

(Continued)

Francisella tularensis (Continued)

- **Systemic**: 5% to 30% of cases; "typhoidal form"; acute septicemia; classic ulcers and lymphadenopathy usually not present
- **Gastrointestinal**: consumption of contaminated food and water; persistent diarrhea; fulminating and often fatal
- **Pulmonary**: 7% to 20% of cases; usually presents as a nonproductive pneumonia which is observed radiographically but not clinically

The most common complaints of these forms of tularemia are lymphadenopathy and necrosis of infected lymph nodes (even with appropriate treatment). Severe cases of tularemia are complicated - dissemination of the bacterium, toxemia, DIC, renal failure, and hepatitis. The most likely form of intentional release of *F. tularensis* organisms would be via infectious aerosols. In 1969, the World Health Organization estimated that an aerosol dispersal of 50 kg of virulent *F. tularensis* over a metropolitan area with 5 million inhabitants in a developed country would result in 250,000 illnesses, including 19,000 deaths. Most of the cases would be primary pneumonic tularemia; however, some would present with either nonspecific febrile illness of varying severity or oculoglandular tularemia from eye contamination or glandular/ulceroglandular disease through exposure of broken skin to infectious aerosol or esophageal disease through inhalation of organisms. The incubation period in this case could be as little as one day to 14 days after exposure.

Diagnosis Physicians must take a complete physical, occupational, recreational, and travel history, and, preferably, be suspicious of tularemia. Cultures of blood, tissue, gastric washings, and sputum are possible and can yield the bacterium; however, culture is extremely nonproductive. Physicians must notify laboratory personnel when culture for *F. tularensis* is ordered because the bacterium is an extreme health hazard to laboratory workers. The most recommended, useful, and productive tests to help diagnose tularemia are serological methods (standard tube agglutination, hemagglutination, and enzyme immunoassay [the most sensitive tests]). Antibodies in sera from infected persons are detectable and are highest 2-5 weeks postinfection, respectively. A single titer ≥160 and a fourfold rise in titer are presumptive and diagnostic for tularemia, respectively. Titers ≥1024 are common late in the acute stage of disease. Both IgG and IgM titers of 20-80 can persist for years.

Diagnostic Tests/Procedures

Tularemia Serology *on page 603*
Gram Stain *on page 473*
Polymerase Chain Reaction *on page 567*

Treatment Treatment is directed toward the symptoms associated with gram-negative bacterial infection and, if present, septicemia.

Commercially available bleach or a 1:10 dilution of household bleach and water is considered adequate for cleaning contaminated surfaces. After 10 minutes, a 70% solution of alcohol can be used to further clean the area and reduce the corrosive action of the bleach

Drug Therapy Comment Antimicrobial susceptibility testing cannot be performed with *F. tularensis* because the bacterium is too fastidious to be tested by standardized, reliable methods. Aminoglycosides (especially streptomycin) are the antimicrobial agents of choice. Doxycycline, fluoroquinolones, and chloramphenicol are alternatives. Generally, tetracycline, beta-lactams (except for imipenem), sulfonamides, and macrolides are not as effective as aminoglycosides. Relapses are more common with both tetracycline and chloramphenicol than the aminoglycosides probably due to its bacteriostatic action rather than cidal activity. Tetracycline should be administered at a minimum dose of 2 g/day to be effective. Chloramphenicol should be added to the aminoglycosides in the treatment of meningitis secondary to this organism. Tetracycline has also been used with some success in the treatment of tularemia. Erythromycin is also active but little clinical experience is available.

Drug Therapy

Recommended:

Streptomycin *on page 1078*
Gentamicin *on page 841*

For meningitis:

Chloramphenicol *on page 733*

Postexposure prophylaxis in setting of bioterrorism: Postexposure vaccination is under investigation. Because of the long time to develop immunity postvaccination and the relatively short incubation period, vaccination does not appear to be effective.

Doxycycline *on page 787*
Ciprofloxacin *on page 742*

Alternate:

Doxycycline *on page 787*
Chloramphenicol *on page 733*
Ciprofloxacin *on page 742*

Selected Readings

Cross JT and Penn RL, "*Francisella tularensis* (Tularemia)," *Principals and Practice of Infectious Diseases*, 5th ed, Mandell GL, Bennett JE, and Dolin R, eds, New York, NY: Churchill Livingstone, 2000, 2393-402.

Dennis DT, Inglesby TV, Henderson DA, et al, "Tularemia as a Biological Weapon: Medical and Public Health Management," *JAMA*, 2001, 285(21):2763-73.

Ellis J, Oyston PC, Green M, et al, "Tularemia," *Clin Microbiol Rev*, 2002, 15(4):631-46.

Feldman KA, Enscore RE, Lathrop SL, et al, "An Outbreak of Primary Pneumonic Tularemia on Martha's Vineyard," *N Engl J Med*, 2001, 345(22):1601-6.

Grunow R, Splettstoesser W, McDonald S, et al, "Detection of *Francisella tularensis* in Biological Specimens Using a Capture Enzyme-Linked Immunosorbent Assay, an Immunochromatographic Handheld Assay, and a PCR," *Clin Diagn Lab Immunol*, 2000, 7(1):86-90.

Johansson A, Berglund L, Gothefors L, et al, "Ciprofloxacin for Treatment of Tularemia in Children," *Pediatr Infect Dis J*, 2000, 19(5):449-53.

Tarnvik A and Berglund L, "Tularaemia," *Eur Respir J*, 2003, 21(2):361-73.

Wong JD and Shapiro DS, "*Francisella*," *Manual of Clinical Microbiology*, 7th ed, Murray PR, Baron EJ, Pfaller MA, et al, eds, Washington, DC: American Society for Microbiology, 1999, 647-51.

Fungal Endophthalmitis *see* Endophthalmitis, Bacterial and Fungal *on page 128*

Fungal Keratitis *see* Keratitis, Bacterial and Fungal *on page 199*

Furunculosis

Synonyms Boils; Follicular Abscess

Clinical Presentation Infection of a hair follicle, which may spread to adjacent dermal layers. Incidence increases in adolescents and young adults. Results in formation of painful pustular nodules with marked erythema and tenderness. They are not accompanied by fever and may be multiple. The process typically results in spontaneous drainage of pus.

Differential Diagnosis Folliculitis; carbuncles; ruptured epidermal cyst; hidradenitis suppurativa

Likely Pathogens

Staphylococcus aureus, Methicillin-Susceptible *on page 307*

Diagnostic Tests/Procedures Immunoglobulin levels may be helpful (in rare cases) to determine immunodeficiency state.

Drug Therapy Comment Drug therapy may be necessary in cases of multiple abscesses, immunocompromised patients, marked inflammation, or extension. Treatment should be continued for at least 14 days. Treat close contacts to eliminate reservoir.

Community-acquired MRSA infections have been reported among athletes, children, military recruits, Pacific Islanders, Alaskan natives, and prisoners. Isolates many be susceptible to sulfamethoxazole and trimethoprim, doxycycline, and/or clindamycin. Sulfamethoxazole and trimethoprim is the drug of choice in high-risk populations. Incision and drainage is usually necessary for adequate treatment.

Empiric Drug Therapy

Recommended:

Dicloxacillin *on page 773*

Note: Treatment varies with affected location, severity, and suspected organisms

Note: Furuncles associated with hot tub use may involve *Pseudomonas* sp. and not respond to antibiotics.

Alternate:

Cephalosporins, 1st Generation *on page 729*
Clindamycin *on page 752*
Sulfamethoxazole and Trimethoprim *on page 1087*

Fusarium Species

Microbiology *Fusarium* is a member of the hyalohyphomycosis, molds that are light-colored with branched or unbranched hyphae with nonpigmented cell walls. There are several different classification systems based on the morphology of the macroconidia, microconidia, and chlamydospores. *F. solani*, *F. oxysporum*, *F. chlamydosporum*, and *F. moniliforme* are the common species pathogenic to humans. *F. sporotrichioides* produce the mycotoxin T-2 resulting in toxic alimentary aleukia which was attributed to the poisoning of approximately 1 million people during World War II after ingesting contaminated grain. Other *Fusarium* species may produce similar fumonisins which cause significant morbidity and mortality to grazing animals. Its adherence properties, especially to plastic catheters and contact lenses, may enhance its pathogenicity. *Fusarium* grows readily on potato dextrose agar and blood culture medium. Identification is based on the conidia characteristics.

(Continued)

Fusarium Species *(Continued)*

Epidemiology *Fusarium* species are ubiquitous soil organisms that are pathogenic to plants. Human infection most commonly results from traumatic inoculation of contaminated material; however, disseminated disease is becoming more common in neutropenic patients without clear evidence of inoculation. Disseminated disease in a normal healthy human host is exceedingly rare. More than 60% of the reported cases of invasive fusariosis have occurred in the United States; however, the organism has been found worldwide. The geographic discrepancy is unclear and may have to do with host factors and/or laboratory investigation rather than climatic differences.

Clinical Syndromes

- **Cutaneous:** Cutaneous lesions most often secondary to traumatic inoculation; may cause mycetoma. Also seen secondary to dissemination which initially appear as a maculopapular to vesicular rash, then develop into lesions with necrotic centers with surrounding induration. May present as cellulitis, onychomycosis, and keratitis.
- **Pulmonary:** *Fusarium* species may colonize the upper airway or cause an upper respiratory infection, particularly sinusitis. Approximately 40% of disseminated disease is attributed to a lower respiratory tract infection. Clinical presentation is similar to aspergillosis in that patients may develop a fungal ball or pneumonia. Allergic bronchopulmonary fusariosis has been described similarly to that seen with aspergillosis.
- **Gastrointestinal:** Alimentary toxic aleukia is caused by mycotoxins in infected grains. Presents as gastrointestinal illness characterized by nausea, vomiting, diarrhea, fever, and chills. Patients may develop headache, stomatitis, dermatitis, CNS disease, and suppression of the bone marrow leading to aplastic anemia and hemorrhaging. Urov or Kashin-Beck disease is also probably related to mycotoxins in infected grain resulting in a chronic, disabling, deforming, dystrophic osteoarthritis. Akakabi-byo is a disease of various grains in Japan that may cause gastrointestinal upset in humans.
- **Disseminated:** Most commonly seen in neutropenic patients secondary to cytotoxic therapy for hematologic malignancies. Most often presents as fever, myalgias, disseminated cutaneous lesions, and fungemia with multiorgan system failure although may present as neutropenic fever without localizing signs or symptoms. A mycotoxin may play a role in prolonging the aplasia initially induced by chemotherapy. Also seen in severe burn victims. Portals of entry include central-venous catheters, respiratory tract, gastrointestinal tract, and onychomycosis or cutaneous lesions. Blood cultures are positive in approximately 60% to 80%. Without recovery of neutrophils, mortality is essentially 100% except in cases of vascular catheter-related infections in which the catheter can be removed.
- **Miscellaneous:** Septic arthritis, catheter-related peritonitis, cystitis, endophthalmitis, and CNS lesions have been reported.

Diagnosis Histopathology may be confused with other molds especially aspergillosis given its propensity for vascular invasion. Definitive diagnosis is made by identification of the mold from tissue or blood culture.

Diagnostic Tests/Procedures

Blood Culture, Fungus *on page 395*
Fungus Culture, Biopsy *on page 461*
KOH Preparation *on page 513*

Treatment Treatment of disseminated disease is targeted at treatment of the underlying illness. Antifungal therapy including amphotericin B has remained ineffective without recovery of the neutrophils. Investigational agents are being studied. Surgical excision is warranted in localized infections. Catheter-related infections should have all catheters removed. Localized infections such as septic arthritis or osteomyelitis secondary to trauma may respond to amphotericin B.

Drug Therapy Comment Azoles are typically ineffective against *Fusarium.*

Drug Therapy

Recommended:

Amphotericin B (Conventional) *on page 650*

Alternate:

Amphotericin B Cholesteryl Sulfate Complex *on page 649*
Amphotericin B (Lipid Complex) *on page 653*
Amphotericin B (Liposomal) *on page 655*
Voriconazole *on page 1151*

Selected Readings

Anaissie E, Nelson P, Beremand M, et al, "*Fusarium*-Caused Hyalohyphomycosis: An Overview," *Curr Top Med Mycol*, 1992, 4:231-49.

Boutati EI and Anaissie EJ, "*Fusarium*, a Significant Emerging Pathogen in Patients With Hematologic Malignancy: Ten Years' Experience at a Cancer Center and Implications for Management," *Blood*, 1997, 90(3):999-1008.

Martino P, Gastaldi R, Raccah R, et al, "Clinical Patterns of *Fusarium* Infections in Immunocompromised Patients," *J Infect*, 1994, 28(Suppl 1):7-15.

Nelson PE, Dignani MC, and Anaissie EJ, "Taxonomy, Biology, and Clinical Aspects of *Fusarium* Species," *Clin Microbiol Rev*, 1994, 7(4):479-504.

Rombaux P, Eloy P, Bertrand B, et al, "Lethal Disseminated *Fusarium* Infection With Sinus Involvement in the Immunocompromised Host: Case Report and Review of the Literature," *Rhinology*, 1996, 34(4):237-41.

GABHS *see Streptococcus pyogenes on page 321*

Gangrene *see* Necrotizing Fasciitis *on page 243*

Gangrene, Gas *see* Myositis *on page 242*

Gardener's Disease *see Sporothrix schenckii on page 302*

Gardnerella vaginalis

Microbiology *Gardnerella vaginalis* is a small gram-negative rod which is part of the normal vaginal flora in many healthy women. It has been implicated as the cause of bacterial vaginosis, a common superficial infection of the vaginal mucosa. The organism is a nonmotile, pleomorphic, gram-negative (or gram-variable) rod. It lacks a capsule and does not form spores. Although *Gardnerella vaginalis* stains gram-negative in clinical specimens, the cell wall is morphologically more characteristic of gram-positive bacteria. Most isolates are facultatively anaerobic, and the organism can be isolated in the laboratory without anaerobic culture techniques. The organism tends to be fastidious in its growth and nutritional requirements. Specific enrichment media may be used in the laboratory to optimize its recovery in culture; these media are combinations of Columbia agar base and human blood.

Epidemiology *Gardnerella vaginalis* can be recovered from the vagina in up to 60% of asymptomatic females. In the condition called bacterial vaginosis, it can be cultured in 95% to 100% of women. Its role as the causative agent of bacterial vaginosis is controversial, since it is so frequently found in healthy individuals. Other organisms comprising the normal vaginal flora can also significantly increase in women with bacterial vaginosis, including the obligate anaerobes *Peptococcus*, *Eubacterium*, and *Mobiluncus*. Some believe these other bacteria work in combination with *Gardnerella* to alter the physiologic environment within the vagina which ultimately leads to bacterial vaginosis. This is not a sexually transmitted disease. Although *Gardnerella* may at times be cultured from the urethra of the male sexual partner of a woman with bacterial vaginosis, there is no clinical counterpart of this condition in men.

Clinical Syndromes

- **Bacterial vaginosis:** As noted above, the precise role of *Gardnerella vaginalis* in the pathogenesis of this condition is not known. In bacterial vaginosis, there is characteristically a new vaginal discharge with a "fishy odor." The woman may be otherwise asymptomatic or may have mild vaginal irritation. Vaginal pruritus or severe burning are not seen. Bacterial vaginosis may be diagnosed clinically if the following are present: (1) a thin, homogeneous vaginal discharge is present on pelvic examination; (2) the pH of the vaginal mucosa/discharge is >4.5 (normal is <4); (3) the vaginal discharge has a "fishy odor" when a drop of 10% KOH is added to the discharge on a microscope slide ("whiff test"); (4) "clue cells" are seen on a wet mount of the vaginal discharge. These distinctive cells are actually the normal large vaginal epithelial cells which have been covered by sheets of gram-negative *Gardnerella* organisms. Generally, the presence of three of these four criteria is sufficient to establish bacterial vaginosis and to separate this condition from the two other common causes of vaginitis, namely *Candida albicans* and *Trichomonas vaginalis*.
- **Urinary tract infections:** *Gardnerella* is a rare (<1%) cause of either lower or upper urinary tract infections. Since the organism so often colonizes the normal vaginal flora, it is often difficult to determine if a positive urine culture for *Gardnerella* represents vaginal contamination. However, case reports have argued that it may be truly pathogenic in the urinary tract in a small number of patients, particularly young women and men with underlying renal disease.
- **Bacteremia:** Isolation of *Gardnerella* in blood cultures has been reported following various obstetric and gynecologic manipulations, including septic abortion and postpartum endometritis. It has also been reported in men following transurethral resection of the prostate (TURP).
- **Miscellaneous infections:** Less commonly, *Gardnerella* has also been associated with salpingitis, vaginal abscesses, and infection following cesarean section. Preliminary studies have implicated bacterial vaginosis as a potential cause of premature delivery and premature rupture of membranes in pregnant women. It is hypothesized that *Gardnerella* has phospholipase A_2 activity which may initiate labor. This relationship is still under study.

Diagnosis The diagnosis of bacterial vaginosis is made clinically, based on the criteria outlined above. Routine laboratory studies such as the complete blood count or electrolyte panel are not necessary. The Gram stain of vaginal discharge is helpful in identifying clue cells, which are pathognomonic for bacterial vaginosis. A striking decrease in the number of lactobacilli (gram-positive rods) normally dominant in the

(Continued)

Gardnerella vaginalis (Continued)

vaginal flora is also characteristic of bacterial vaginosis. A direct wet mount of vaginal secretions is useful in identifying clue cells and ruling out the presence of trichomonads (as seen in vaginal trichomoniasis) or yeast cells (as seen in candidal vaginitis). Although often obtained, cultures of the vagina for *Gardnerella* do little to establish the presence of bacterial vaginosis and are not indicated in the majority of cases. Vaginal Gram stains have been shown to be as sensitive as vaginal cultures (including semiquantitative culture techniques), with greater specificity and positive predictive value. Cultures for *Gardnerella vaginalis* from extravaginal sites (such as blood) are appropriate in the proper clinical setting. *Gardnerella* can be grown in blood culture media which is free of sodium polyanetholsulfonate (SPS).

Diagnostic Tests/Procedures

Gram Stain *on page 473*
KOH Preparation *on page 513*
Trichomonas Preparation *on page 600*

Treatment Unlike other gram-negative bacilli, *Gardnerella vaginalis* is susceptible to penicillin, ampicillin, vancomycin, and clindamycin. Most strains are resistant to nalidixic acid, sulfadiazine, and neomycin. The organism is resistant to metronidazole *in vitro*, but is effective *in vivo*, probably due to an active metabolite of metronidazole. Treatment guidelines are as follows:

1. For nonpregnant women with bacterial vaginosis, metronidazole (Flagyl®) is the drug of choice, 500 mg orally 2 times a day for 7 days. As an alternative, clindamycin may be used, 300 mg orally 2 times a day for 7 days. Since bacterial vaginosis is not a sexually transmitted disease, there is no need to routinely treat the male sexual partner.
2. For the pregnant female, treatment is at the physician's discretion. Limited data has linked bacterial vaginosis with premature delivery, but the benefits of antibiotic therapy, if any, are presently unknown. Metronidazole is contraindicated in the first trimester of pregnancy. The Centers for Disease Control have recommended clindamycin in this situation, should treatment be initiated.
3. For bacteremia with *Gardnerella*, a variety of antibiotics may be used including ampicillin.

Drug Therapy

Recommended:

Metronidazole *on page 940*

Alternate:

Ampicillin *on page 657*
Clindamycin *on page 752*

Selected Readings

Josephson S, Thomason J, Sturino K, et al, "*Gardnerella vaginalis* in the Urinary Tract: Incidence and Significance in a Hospital Population," *Obstet Gynecol*, 1988, 71(2):245-50.
Spiegel CA, "*Gardnerella vaginalis* and *Mobiluncus* Species," *Principles and Practice of Infectious Diseases*, 4th ed, Mandell GL, Bennett JE, and Dolin R, eds, New York, NY: Churchill Livingstone, 1995, 2050-3.
"1998 Guidelines for Treatment of Sexually Transmitted Diseases. Centers for Disease Control and Prevention," *MMWR*, 1998, 47(RR-1):1-111.

GAS *see Streptococcus pyogenes on page 321*
Gas Gangrene *see* Myositis *on page 242*

Gastroenteritis, Bacterial

Synonyms Bacterial Gastroenteritis

Clinical Presentation Patients with bacterial gastroenteritis frequently present with lower gastrointestinal symptoms (diarrhea) with or without fever. Patients less likely present with primary upper gastrointestinal symptoms (ie, vomiting). The presence of bloody diarrhea suggests a bacterial pathogen, although *C. difficile* is usually nonhemorrhagic. It is impossible to separate different pathogens based on clinical diagnosis alone.

Differential Diagnosis Gastroenteritis, viral; drug toxicity; inflammatory bowel disease; parasitic gastroenteritis (eg, *Giardia*, cryptosporidia, microsporidia)

Likely Pathogens

Campylobacter jejuni *on page 66*
Salmonella Species *on page 291*
Shigella Species *on page 297*
Escherichia coli, Enterohemorrhagic *on page 145*

Diagnostic Tests/Procedures

Stool Culture *on page 585*
Stool Culture, Diarrheagenic *E. coli* *on page 587*
Stool Culture, Uncommon Organisms *on page 588*
Clostridium difficile Toxin Assay *on page 418*

Drug Therapy Comment Rehydration is the key to management. Empiric antimicrobial therapy should be offered in the setting of traveler's diarrhea, otherwise it is imperative for one to consider the risks vs benefits of empiric therapy. Drug therapy based on identification of the causative agent.

Empiric Drug Therapy

Recommended:

Ciprofloxacin *on page 742*

Sulfamethoxazole and Trimethoprim *on page 1087*

Selected Readings

Altekruse SF, Stern NJ, Fields PI, et al, "*Campylobacter jejuni* - An Emerging Food-Borne Pathogen," *Emerg Infect Dis*, 1999, 5(1):28-35.
Boone JH and Carman RJ, "*Clostridium perfringens*: Food Poisoning and Antibiotic-Associated Diarrhea," *Clin Microbiol Newslett*, 1997, 19(9):65-7.
Guerrant RL, Van Gilder T, Steiner TS, et al, "Practice Guidelines for the Management of Infectious Diarrhea," *Clin Infect Dis*, 2001, 32(3):331-51.
Kaspar CW and Weiss R, "Bacterial Food-Borne Illness - The Unwanted Dinner Guest," *Clin Microbiol Newslett*, 1998, 20(19):161-4.
Novak SM, "Food-Borne Illness - Chemical Fish and Shellfish Poisoning," *Clin Microbiol Newslett*, 1998, 20(3).
Siegel DL, Edelstein PH, Nachamkin I, "Inappropriate Testing for Diarrheal Diseases in the Hospital," *JAMA*, 1990, 263(7):979-82.
Thielman NM and Guerrant RL, "Clinical Practice. Acute Infectious Diarrhea," *N Engl J Med*, 2004, 350(1):38-47.

Gastroenteritis, Viral

Synonyms Viral Gastroenteritis

Clinical Presentation Patients with viral gastroenteritis may present with upper gastrointestinal symptoms (vomiting), lower gastrointestinal symptoms (diarrhea), or both. Stools tend to be nonhemorrhagic. Viral gastroenteritis is much more common than bacterial gastroenteritis.

Differential Diagnosis Gastroenteritis, bacterial; drug toxicity; inflammatory bowel disease; parasitic gastroenteritis (eg, *Giardia*, cryptosporidia, microsporidia)

Likely Pathogens

Rotavirus *on page 290*

Diagnostic Tests/Procedures

Viral Culture, Stool *on page 616*

Rotavirus, Direct Detection *on page 573*

Enterovirus Culture *on page 453*

Drug Therapy Comment No antiviral agents have been proven to be effective in the treatment of rotavirus infections. Supportive therapy is recommended.

Selected Readings

Atmar RL and Estes MK, "Nonculturable Agents of Viral Gastroenteritis," *Clin Microbiol Newslett*, 1997, 19(23):177-82.
Gastanaduy AS and Begue RE, "Acute Gastroenteritis," *Clin Pediatr (Phila)*, 1999, 38(1):1-12.
Guerrant RL, Shields DA, Thorson SM, et al, "Evaluation and Diagnosis of Acute Infectious Diarrhea," *Am J Med*, 1985, 78(6B):91-8.
Hedberg CW and Osterholm MT, "Outbreaks of Food-Borne and Waterborne Viral Gastroenteritis," *Clin Microbiol Rev*, 1993, 6(3):199-210.
Kapikian AZ, "Overview of Viral Gastroenteritis," *Arch Virol*, 1996, 12:7-19.
Lifschitz CH, "Treatment of Acute Diarrhea in Children," *Curr Opin Pediatr*, 1997, 9(5):498-501.
Siegel DL, Edelstein PH, Nachamkin I, "Inappropriate Testing for Diarrheal Diseases in the Hospital," *JAMA*, 1990, 263(7):979-82.

Genital Herpes *see* Herpes Simplex Virus *on page 172*

Genital HSV *see* Herpes Simplex Virus *on page 172*

Giardia lamblia

Microbiology *Giardia lamblia* is an important intestinal parasite classified as a protozoan flagellate. It is related to other clinically-relevant protozoans such as *Trichomonas vaginalis* and *Dientamoeba fragilis*. The organism exists as either a trophozoite or a cyst, and both can be detected in stool samples. Microscopically, *G. lamblia* trophozoites are characterized by long flagella at one end (which provide motility in fluid environments), a ventral adhesive disk (which attaches to the intestinal villi of humans), and two parabasal bodies located near the nucleus. These paired bodies give a characteristic and easily identifiable appearance of "two eyes" looking at the examiner. The cyst form of *Giardia* is somewhat smaller than the trophozoite and is considered the infective form of *Giardia*.

The infectious cycle for humans begins with ingestion of *Giardia lamblia* cysts (eg, from contaminated water or food). As few as 10 organisms can initiate human disease. In the stomach, excystation is promoted by gastric acid, and trophozoites are released in the duodenum and multiply by longitudinal binary fission. The trophozoites attach to the intestinal villi by means of the ventral sucking disk. Histologically, there is a mild to moderate inflammation of the small bowel mucosa. Both the cyst and trophozoite are passed into the human feces.

(Continued)

Giardia lamblia (Continued)

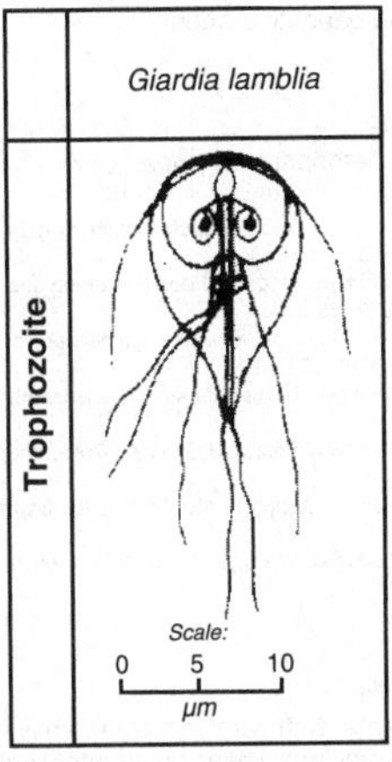

From Brooks MM and Melvin DM, *Morphology of Diagnostic Stages of Intestinal Parasites of Humans,* 2nd ed, Atlanta, GA: U.S. Department of Health and Human Services, Publication No. 84-8116, Centers for Disease Control, 1984, with permission.

Epidemiology Infection with *Giardia* occurs worldwide. In particular, it can be found in wilderness streams, lakes, and mountainous areas. Beavers, muskrats, and other wild animals serve as another reservoir for this organism. Common means of acquisition include:

- Ingestion of contaminated water. Outbreaks from contaminated water in mountain resorts have been described. *Giardia lamblia* cysts are not killed by the chlorine concentrations used in many water treatment facilities. It is important to obtain a travel history (including recent camping) in patients with acute giardiasis.
- Ingestion of contaminated food.
- Oral-anal sexual contact. This is an important means of person-to-person spread, particularly among male homosexuals.
- Fecal-oral spread, especially in children attending daycare centers.

Clinical Syndromes

- **Asymptomatic carriage:** In almost 50% of cases, infection with *Giardia lamblia* occurs in the absence of symptoms. This state of carriage can persist indefinitely in some individuals.
- **Gastrointestinal disease:** The spectrum of symptomatic giardiasis is variable and ranges from a mild nonspecific diarrheal illness to a more severe illness characterized by abdominal pain, bloating, and profuse diarrhea. A chronic malabsorption syndrome has been described. The diarrhea tends to be watery and associated with abdominal cramping; stools are almost always guaiac-negative since *Giardia* does not invade the mucosal tissues. Patients at particular risk for severe or relapsing giardiasis are individuals with an underlying IgA deficiency or diverticulosis.

Diagnosis Preserved stool (formalin or PVA) can be stained with trichrome or iron hematoxylin. Diagnosis is commonly made by (1) staining preserved stool and examining for *Giardia* cysts or trophs or (2) testing stool for the presence of *Giardia*-specific antigen.

Diagnostic Tests/Procedures

Giardia Specific Antigen (GSA65) *on page 473*

Ova and Parasites, Stool *on page 551*

Treatment A 5- to 7-day course of metronidazole or a single 2 g dose of tinidazole are probably the most effective agents in the treatment of giardiasis. Both drugs are contraindicated in the first trimester of pregnancy, in which case, paromomycin for 5-10 days should be used. Other agents that have been shown to be effective include

albendazole and bacitracin administered orally. Two other drugs that are widely used outside of the United States, quinacrine and furazolidone, are not available in the U.S.

Drug Therapy

Recommended:

Metronidazole *on page 940*
Tinidazole *on page 1118*

Alternate:

Albendazole *on page 635*
Paromomycin *on page 989*

Selected Readings

Adam RD, "The Biology of *Giardia* spp," *Microbiol Rev*, 1991, 55(4):706-32.
Centers for Disease Control and Prevention, "Cryptosporidiosis Surveillance - United States 1999-2002 and Giardiasis Surveillance - United States, 1998-2002," *MMWR*, 2005, 54(SS-1).
Gardner TB and Hill DR, "Treatment of Giardiasis," *Clin Microbiol Rev*, 2001, 14(1):114-28.
Harp JA, "Parasitic Infections of the Gastrointestinal Tract," *Curr Opin Gastroenterol*, 2003, 19(1):31-6.
Hlavsa MC, Watson JC, and Beach MJ, "Giardiasis Surveillance - United States, 1998-2002," *MMWR Surveill Summ*, 2005, 54(1):9-16.
Lengerich EJ, Addiss DG, and Juranek DD, "Severe Giardiasis in the United States," *Clin Infect Dis*, 1994, 18(5):760-3.
Ortega YR and Adam RD, "*Giardia*: Overview and Update," *Clin Infect Dis*, 1997, 25(3):545-50.
Overturf GD, "Endemic Giardiasis in the United States - Role of the Day Care Center," *Clin Infect Dis*, 1994, 18(5):764-5.

Giardiasis *see Giardia lamblia on page 155*

Gilchrist's Disease *see Blastomyces dermatitidis on page 50*

Glanders *see Burkholderia mallei on page 64*

GNB *see* Gram-Negative Bacilli *on page 157*

Gonorrhea *see Neisseria gonorrhoeae on page 244*

Gram-Negative Bacilli

Synonyms GNB

Refer to

Acinetobacter Species *on page 24*
Aeromonas Species *on page 30*
Alcaligenes Species *on page 31*
Bartonella Species *on page 48*
Bordetella bronchiseptica on page 52
Bordetella pertussis on page 53
Brucella Species *on page 61*
Burkholderia cepacia on page 62
Calymmatobacterium granulomatis on page 65
Campylobacter jejuni on page 66
Capnocytophaga Species *on page 69*
Citrobacter Species *on page 81*
Enterobacter Species *on page 132*
Escherichia coli on page 142
Escherichia coli, Diarrheagenic *on page 143*
Escherichia coli, Enterohemorrhagic *on page 145*
Francisella tularensis on page 149
Gardnerella vaginalis on page 153
HACEK Group *on page 158*
Haemophilus ducreyi on page 158
Haemophilus influenzae on page 159
Helicobacter pylori on page 162
Klebsiella Species *on page 200*
Legionella pneumophila on page 202
Pasteurella multocida on page 258
Proteus Species *on page 278*
Providencia Species *on page 281*
Pseudomonas aeruginosa on page 282
Salmonella Species *on page 291*
Serratia Species *on page 296*
Shigella Species *on page 297*
Stenotrophomonas maltophilia on page 312
Vibrio cholerae on page 351
Yersinia enterocolitica on page 354
Yersinia pestis on page 355

Ground Itch *see Ancylostoma duodenale on page 34*

Group D *Streptococcus* *see Streptococcus bovis on page 315*

Group A β-Hemolytic *Streptococcus* *see Streptococcus pyogenes on page 321*

Group A *Streptococcus* *see Streptococcus pyogenes on page 321*

Group B *Streptococcus* *see Streptococcus agalactiae on page 313*

HACEK Group

Related Information

Antibiotic Treatment of Adults With Infective Endocarditis *on page 1271*

Microbiology HACEK is a pneumonic which includes:

- *Haemophilus aphrophilus*
- *Actinobacillus actinomycetemcomitans*
- *Cardiobacterium hominis*
- *Eikenella corrodens*
- *Kingella kingae*

These organisms are pleomorphic, coccobacilli, and bacilli and occur as chains or filamentous forms. These organisms are all fastidious, gram-negative bacteria which require specific types of growth conditions. These conditions include enhanced CO_2, specific growth factors (*Haemophilus*), growth only on chocolate and/or blood agar, and often increased time for incubation. Organisms in this group may be differentiated by reaction to oxidase and catalase, cell shape, indole positivity, nitrate to nitrite, and fermentation of carbohydrates. In a microbiology laboratory, these five bacteria are identified and reported separately.

Epidemiology Members of the HACEK group are normal flora of the mouth and respiratory tract and are opportunistic organisms that cause infections in patients with oral cavity disease or trauma and in immunocompromised hosts. *Eikenella* infections are often associated with other mouth flora organisms.

Clinical Syndromes Although many of the HACEK organisms have been know to cause disease in several organ systems and clinical settings, endocarditis is by far the most common and most significant. Endocarditis is usually subacute with a very insidious onset, often in patients with previously damaged or prosthetic valves. Although medical treatment is often successful, reporting bias must be considered.

Diagnosis The diagnosis of a HACEK group infection can only be made by identification of the specific pathogen through culture in a patient with a relevant clinical syndrome. Patients with seemingly culture-negative endocarditis can have their blood cultures incubated for an extended time to increase the chances of growing HACEK bacteria. However, with most modern automated blood culture instruments and excellent blood culture media, extended incubation is usually not necessary to grow and detect HACEK bacteria from blood.

Physicians should inform the laboratory if a HACEK bacterium is suspected of causing an infection.

Diagnostic Tests/Procedures

Blood Culture, Aerobic and Anaerobic *on page 391*
Gram Stain *on page 473*

Treatment Empiric therapy with a third generation cephalosporin should be considered if a HACEK organism is suspected in patients with endocarditis. There are a large number of strains of these organism which have been shown to produce beta-lactamases that inactivate ampicillin. The final therapeutic decision should be based on clinical condition of the patient (especially while cultures are pending or negative) and sensitivity testing. Treatment should be maintained for 4-6 weeks.

Drug Therapy

Recommended:

Cephalosporins, 3rd Generation *on page 730*

Selected Readings

Baron EJ and Finegold SM, eds, "Gram-Negative Facultatively Anaerobic Bacilli and Aerobic Coccobacilli," *Bailey & Scott's Diagnostic Microbiology*, St Louis, MO: CV Mosby Co, 1990, 408-30.

Berbari EF, Cockerill FR 3d, and Steckelberg JM, "Infective Endocarditis Due to Unusual or Fastidious Microorganisms," *Mayo Clin Proc*, 1997, 72(6):532-42.

Das M, Badley AD, Cockerill FR, et al, "Infective Endocarditis Caused by HACEK Microorganisms," *Annu Rev Med*, 1997, 48:25-33.

Feder HM Jr, Roberts JC, Salazar JC, et al, "HACEK Endocarditis in Infants and Children: Two Cases and a Literature Review," *Pediatr Infect Dis J*, 2003, 22(6):557-62.

Kugler KC, Biedenbach DJ, and Jones RN, "Determination of the Antimicrobial Activity of 29 Clinically Important Compounds Tested Against Fastidious HACEK Group Organisms," *Diagn Microbiol Infect Dis*, 1999, 34(1):73-6.

Meyer DJ and Gerding DN, "Favorable Prognosis of Patients With Prosthetic Valve Endocarditis Caused by Gram-Negative Bacilli of the HACEK Group," *Am J Med*, 1988, 85(1):104-7.

Haemophilus ducreyi

Related Information

Treatment of Sexually Transmitted Infections *on page 1311*

Microbiology *Haemophilus ducreyi* is a gram-negative coccobacillus which causes a sexually transmitted disease called chancroid. It is indistinguishable on Gram stain from other *Haemophilus* species (eg, *H. influenzae*).

Epidemiology In 1838, chancroid (soft chancre) was first differentiated from syphilis (or hard chancre) by the French microbiologist Ricord. Although chancroid has remained an uncommon sexually transmitted disease in the U.S., its worldwide incidence may exceed that of syphilis. In 1986, there were 3418 cases reported, the largest number since the 1950s.

From 1981 to 1987, nine major outbreaks of chancroid were reported in the U.S. Chancroid was seen mainly in Hispanic and black heterosexual men who patronized prostitutes. In Florida, chancroid was seen in highly sexually active men without clear prostitute exposure. In Boston, the outbreak may have been related to individuals who had been originally infected in endemic foreign countries, such as Haiti and the Dominican Republic.

Clinical Syndromes *H. ducreyi* is an important cause of the syndrome of **genital ulceration with regional adenopathy**. Other sexually transmitted diseases that can cause this syndrome include primary syphilis, genital herpes simplex virus, lymphogranuloma venereum, and others. The incubation period for *H. ducreyi* is 1-21 days with an average of 7 days. Chancroid ulcers are painful, deep, shaggy and friable. The borders of the ulcer are undermined. In men, ulcers are more commonly single, but in women, the ulcers are multiple. Regional adenopathy occurs simultaneously with the ulcer and is seen in 50% to 65% of cases. The nodes are quite tender and tend to be unilateral. In addition, they tend to be fluctuant and can easily fistulize. Constitutional symptoms are uncommon.

Diagnosis Isolation of *Haemophilus ducreyi* from an active genital ulcer is the only accurate means of confirming a case of chancroid. However, special media and culture techniques are required to culture this fastidious organism, and the Microbiology Laboratory must be alerted to the possibility of *H. ducreyi*. Cotton or calcium alginate swabs should be rolled over a purulent ulcer base. The Gram stain of an ulcer specimen may be misleading because of the presence of polymicrobial flora colonizing genital ulcers. Isolation of *H. ducreyi* from active genital ulcers is variable (50% to 80% depending on the culture medium). *H. ducreyi* is almost never isolated from aspiration of inguinal buboes.

Unfortunately, it is difficult to diagnose chancroid on the basis of clinical suspicion alone. Chancroid is presumptively diagnosed in patients presenting with genital ulcers with a negative RPR/VDRL, darkfield-negative for *T. pallidum*, and negative for HSV (by clinical appearance). However, as pointed out by Salzman et al, many such presumptive cases are ultimately found not to be chancroid.

Treatment Chancroid is an unusual disease in the U.S., and consultation with an Infectious Disease specialist is appropriate. Azithromycin, ceftriaxone, ciprofloxacin, and erythromycin are all effective. Ciprofloxacin is contraindicated in pregnancy and the safety of azithromycin in pregnancy is unclear. Drug resistance has been reported in some areas of the world. Chancroid may be more difficult to treat in persons with HIV infection. Although direct comparison trials are not available, some recommend the 7-day erythromycin course for HIV-infected persons.

Recommended therapy:

Azithromycin 1 g orally in a single dose, or
Ceftriaxone 250 mg I.M. in a single dose, or
Ciprofloxacin 500 mg orally twice daily for 3 days, or
Erythromycin base 500 mg orally 4 times/day for 7 days

Drug Therapy

Recommended:

Azithromycin *on page 674*
Ceftriaxone *on page 722*
Ciprofloxacin *on page 742*
Erythromycin *on page 807*

Selected Readings

Hammond GW, Slutchuk M, Scatliff J, et al, "Epidemiologic, Clinical, Laboratory, and Therapeutic Features of an Urban Outbreak of Chancroid in North America," *Rev Infect Dis*, 1980, 2(6):867-79.
Ronald AR and Plummer FA, "Chancroid and *Haemophilus ducreyi*," *Ann Intern Med*, 1985, 102(5):705-7.
Schmid GP, Sanders LL Jr, Blount JH, et al, "Chancroid in the United States. Re-establishment of an Old Disease," *JAMA*, 1987, 258(22):3265-8.
"1998 Guidelines for Treatment of Sexually Transmitted Diseases. Centers for Disease Control and Prevention," *MMWR*, 1998, 47(RR-1):1-111.

Haemophilus influenzae

Related Information

Community-Acquired Pneumonia in Adults *on page 1278*
Immunization Recommendations *on page 1249*
Prophylaxis for Patients Exposed to Common Communicable Diseases *on page 1309*

Microbiology *Haemophilus influenzae* are typically gram-negative, aerobic (facultatively anaerobic), coccobacilli; however, they are often pleomorphic, gram-variable,

(Continued)

Haemophilus influenzae (Continued)

and filamentous. There are six types (a-f) based on polysaccharide capsular properties; type b is the most invasive. There are also nonencapsulated, nontypable *Haemophilus influenzae*. There are eight different biotypes (with different biochemical properties) of which biotype 1 is most prevalent as a pathogen.

Haemophilus influenzae grows on chocolate agar which has X and V factors necessary for growth. It can also grow on Levinthal and Fildes enriched agar which are useful in determining encapsulation properties.

Epidemiology The epidemiology of *Haemophilus influenzae* changed in the 1990s because of successful early childhood immunization, which is dramatically decreasing the incidence of invasive disease caused by *Haemophilus influenzae* b. *Haemophilus influenzae* is often found in the nasopharynx of normal asymptomatic individuals. Most *Haemophilus influenzae* isolates in the United States are nonencapsulated and rarely are pathogenic. Historically, the frequency of invasive disease was based on age with meningitis most common in children 2 month to 2 years of age, epiglottitis in the 3-5 years of age range, and other infections having an increasing incidence in older adults. The total increase incidence over the past two decades may have been due in part to improved laboratory identification of organisms.

Clinical Syndromes Early *Haemophilus influenzae* b vaccination has decreased the incidence of serious *Haemophilus influenzae* b disease dramatically over the past few years. *Haemophilus influenzae* can cause a variety of clinical syndromes including meningitis, epiglottitis, cellulitis, otitis, respiratory tract infection, and other infections.

- **Meningitis:** Although not a high mortality when diagnosed early, *Haemophilus influenzae* meningitis often causes permanent neurologic sequelae even when "successfully" treated. Meningitis characteristically occurred in infants up to 2 years of age.
- **Epiglottitis (ages 3-5 years):** Is a medical emergency which often requires ventilatory support if not managed promptly.
- ***Haemophilus influenzae* otitis:** Common in children of various ages.
- **Respiratory tract infections:** More common in adults, especially those with chronic obstructive pulmonary disease and smokers.

Diagnosis Diagnosis can be made by Gram stain and culture of specimens from appropriate sites. Gram stain will reveal gram-negative coccobacilli but is neither sensitive nor specific enough to be diagnostic. *Haemophilus influenzae* grows well on chocolate agar supplemented by growth factors V and X. These factors differentiate it from other *Haemophilus* species. Satellite colonies may appear around *S. aureus* species. Antigen detection for the polyribophosphate capsule is available but is no more sensitive than Gram stain or culture. Subgrouping may be performed for epidemiologic purposes.

Diagnostic Tests/Procedures

Aerobic Culture, Appropriate Site *on page 365*
Gram Stain *on page 473*

Treatment Meningitis and epiglottitis should be treated with a third generation cephalosporin when *Haemophilus influenzae* is suspected, as these are medical emergencies. Up to 30% of *Haemophilus influenzae* b strains are resistant to ampicillin. Less serious infections may be treated with ampicillin or amoxicillin (when susceptible), sulfamethoxazole and trimethoprim, or a second generation cephalosporin. Most strains are also susceptible to chloramphenicol and quinolones (not first line agents). *Haemophilus influenzae* b vaccine is now a part of routine vaccinations administered in the first few months of life.

Prophylaxis may be desirable in *H. influenzae* outbreaks or in close contacts with invasive disease. Rifampin is the recommended agent for prophylaxis in a 4-day regimen of 600 mg daily for adults and 20 mg/kg daily for infants and children.

Drug Therapy

Recommended:

Severe infection:
Cephalosporins, 3rd Generation *on page 730*

Mild infection:
Sulfamethoxazole and Trimethoprim *on page 1087*

Alternate:

Severe infection:
Cephalosporins, 2nd Generation *on page 729*
Chloramphenicol *on page 733*
Fluoroquinolones *on page 824*

Mild infection:
Ampicillin *on page 657*
Amoxicillin and Clavulanate Potassium *on page 645*
Cefaclor *on page 697*
Amoxicillin *on page 642*

Selected Readings

Adams WG, Deaver KA, Cochi SL, et al, "Decline of Childhood *Haemophilus influenzae* Type b (Hib) Disease in the Hib Vaccine Era," *JAMA*, 1993, 269(2):221-6.

Baron EJ and Finegold SM, eds, "Gram-Negative Facultatively Anaerobic Bacilli and Aerobic Coccobacilli," *Bailey & Scott's Diagnostic Microbiology*, St Louis, MO: CV Mosby Co, 1990, 408-30.

Mohammadkhani M and Ruoff KL, "A 29-Year-Old Man With *Haemophilus influenzae* in the Cerebrospinal Fluid: Case Report and Review of the Organism," *Clin Microbiol Newslett*, 1998, 20(5):36-9.

Neumann MA and Thompson KD, "Acute Bacterial Meningitis: Prevention and Treatment," *Clin Microbiol Newslett*, 1998, 20(22):181-4.

Quagliarello V and Scheld WM, "Bacterial Meningitis: Pathogenesis, Pathophysiology, and Progress," *N Engl J Med*, 1992, 327(12):864-72.

Hantavirus

Microbiology The virus family Bunyaviridae is composed of more than 200 mostly arthropod-borne RNA viruses (arboviruses) such as California encephalitis virus, LaCrosse virus, Rift Valley fever virus, Congo-Crimean hemorrhagic fever virus, Hantaan virus, and the genus Hantavirus. Hantavirus is composed of several (hantaviruses) which usually cause one of two severe clinical syndromes: hemorrhagic fever with renal syndrome (HFRS) and hantavirus pulmonary syndrome (HPS). Hantavirus, as the term is being used in the United States, most commonly refers to Muerto Canyon/Sin Nombre virus and to Black Creek Canal virus, both of which cause HPS. Muerto Canyon virus is the virus which was responsible for the infamous outbreak of HPS in the Four Corners area (the intersection of New Mexico, Utah, Arizona, and Colorado) of the southwest United States in May, 1993. Hantaviruses are single-strand RNA, 80-120 nm, spherical, pleomorphic, enveloped viruses which are susceptible to most disinfectants.

Epidemiology Hantaviruses occur almost worldwide (see table). Human infection by hantavirus became a public health concern in the United States in the 1950s when U.S. soldiers who served in the Korean War developed Korean hemorrhagic fever (Hantaan virus). Muerto Canyon virus has been found only in North America. As of July 27, 1994, 83 cases of HPS (54% mortality) had been reported to the CDC, including the cases in the 1993 Four Corners outbreak, during which the natural history of Muerto Canyon virus was elucidated. The reservoir of the virus is *Peromyscus maniculatus*, the deer mouse, which always remains asymptomatic. If high populations of *Peromyscus* experience times of drought, scarce food, and reduced natural cover, the mice will seek food and shelter in human dwellings and outbuildings and drastically increase their contact with humans. Muerto Canyon virus is easily transmitted to humans by inhalation of aerosolized droplets of mouse urine and feces and by saliva from the bites of mice. The virus can be acquired in a laboratory setting; however, the virus is not transmitted human to human.

Hantavirus

Hantavirus	Geographical Location	Disease	Mortality (%)
Hantaan (prototype) and Seoul	Asia	HFRS	1-15
Puumala	Scandinavia, Western Europe	HFRS	Rare
Belgrade/Dobrava	Central and Eastern Europe	HFRS	5-35
Prospect Hill	Eastern and Midwest United States	None	?
Muerto Canyon and Black Creek Canal	North America	HPS	50-70

Clinical Syndromes HPS usually occurs in healthy young adults, and the presentation of HPS can be considered to be similar to that of acute respiratory distress syndrome (ARDS). The incubation period of HPS is 10-30 days. HPS usually begins with a short period of general myalgia and fever which is followed by 1-10 days of fever, cough, tachycardia, and tachypnea. Mild pulmonary edema can follow. In some cases, fulminating severe pulmonary edema manifested as ARDS can develop and can lead to shock and death in only a few hours. The mortality rate of HPS is extremely high (56% to 70%); however, successful respiratory therapy is possible, and complete recovery can occur in a few days. Histopathologically, lung tissue from patients with HPS show interstitial infiltration of lymphocytes and severe alveolar edema. Necrosis and polymorphonuclear infiltration is not present. The complete pathogenesis of HPS has not been completely established. HPS should be considered in any healthy adult who presents with unexplained ARDS.

Diagnosis The diagnosis of HPS is clinical and depends on careful examination of the patient's travel, work, and social history, on the patients living conditions, and on timely recognition of ARDS. The laboratory diagnosis of HPS caused by Muerto Canyon virus can be accomplished by viral culture and serology. Culture is not practical and not widely available. Almost all patients with HPS will have anti-Muerto

(Continued)

Hantavirus *(Continued)*

Canyon IgG and IgM antibodies at the time of presentation and acute disease. Therefore, serological methods (enzyme immunoassay, hemagglutination inhibition, indirect immunofluorescence, complement fixation, and antibody neutralization) are the methods of choice. Both acute and convalescent sera must be tested if an accurate diagnosis of HPS is sought. Polymerase chain reaction and nucleic acid hybridization have been used to amplify and detect, respectively, Muerto Canyon virus DNA in fixed and sectioned tissue from infected patients.

Diagnostic Tests/Procedures

Hantavirus Serology *on page 477*

Polymerase Chain Reaction *on page 567*

Treatment Treatment is supportive and should be given in an intensive care unit.

Drug Therapy Comment Ribavirin has been used to treat HPS; however, reproducible success has not been documented. Ribavirin used for this purpose can be obtained from the CDC.

Selected Readings

Beebe JL, "Emerging Infections: Hantavirus Disease Outbreak," *Clin Microbiol Newslett*, 1994, 16(10): 73-6.

Butler JC and Peters CJ, "Hantaviruses and Hantavirus Pulmonary Syndrome," *Clin Infect Dis*, 1994, 19(3):387-95.

Peters CJ and Khan AS, "Hantavirus Pulmonary Syndrome: The New American Hemorrhagic Fever," *Clin Infect Dis*, 2002, 34(9):1224-31.

Yablonski T, "The Mystery of the Hantavirus," *Laboratory Medicine*, 1994, 25:557-60.

Zhao X, "The Epidemiology of Hantavirus Infections," *Clin Microbiol Newslett*, 1997, 19(7):49-52.

Hantavirus Pulmonary Syndrome (HPS) *see* Hantavirus *on page 161*

HAV *see* Hepatitis A Virus *on page 164*

HBV *see* Hepatitis B Virus *on page 165*

hCMV *see* Cytomegalovirus *on page 107*

HCoV *see Coronaviridae* (Including SARS) *on page 94*

HCV *see* Hepatitis C Virus *on page 167*

HDV *see* Hepatitis D Virus *on page 170*

Helicobacter pylori

Related Information

Helicobacter pylori Treatment *on page 1288*

Synonyms *Campylobacter pylori*

Microbiology Controversy surrounds *Helicobacter pylori*, a gram-negative bacillus recently implicated as a cause of duodenal and gastric ulcers and a potential cause of the nonulcer dyspepsia syndrome. Originally named *Campylobacter pyloridis*, then *Campylobacter pylori*, this organism was renamed *Helicobacter pylori* in 1989. It is a spiral-shaped gram-negative bacillus which is susceptible *in vitro* to a variety of antimicrobial agents including tetracycline, metronidazole, amoxicillin, and clarithromycin. Resistance to these antibiotics has been described in some isolates, including metronidazole-resistant strains which have been associated with treatment failures. The organism is unique in its ability to survive the acidic pH of gastric fluids, which is otherwise sterile in healthy individuals. *H. pylori* is most commonly recognized in histologic analysis of gastric biopsies. Cultures for the organism are available in some laboratories but the sensitivity of culture varies greatly.

Epidemiology *H. pylori* has been associated with infection in adults over the age of 20 years, with an increased incidence with aging. The natural reservoir appears to be in humans, although the precise source is unknown. Transmission has been theorized to be fecal-oral. In some studies, *H. pylori* has been recovered from nearly 100% of patients with duodenal ulcers and has thus stimulated much research concerning its role as a possible etiologic agent of peptic ulcer disease.

Clinical Syndromes

- **Duodenal ulcers:** *H. pylori* has been implicated as a cause of duodenal ulcers in patients who are not receiving nonsteroidal anti-inflammatory agents. This is based on a number of lines of evidence. The prevalence of *H. pylori* in duodenal ulcer cases is nearly 100%. Eradication of *H. pylori* decreases the relapse rate of duodenal ulcers when compared with patients with duodenal ulcers who have persistent infection with *H. pylori*. Other experts have strongly disagreed with these findings and conclusions and suggest that *H. pylori* is only a cofactor in causation of duodenal ulcers.
- **Gastric ulcers:** Again, epidemiologic evidence suggests a relationship between *H. pylori* and gastric ulcers. Studies have suggested a weaker relationship with gastric ulcers than with duodenal ulcers, with 60% of gastric ulcer cases positive for *H. pylori*. (Some studies have shown a higher rate of recovery, approaching 100%.) Relapse rates in patients who have been successfully treated for *H. pylori* have been close to 0% at 1 year, as compared with 60% in controls.

- **Nonulcer dyspepsia:** In this difficult to define entity, individuals complain of chronic symptoms of abdominal pain similar to peptic ulcer disease but have no objective disease on upper endoscopy. *H. pylori* has also been associated with this condition. The results of studies eradicating *H. pylori* in nonulcer dyspepsia have been inconclusive to date. The data suggest a subgroup of patients may in fact benefit from eradication of the organism, but the difficulty has been identifying such individuals prior to therapy.
- **Gastric carcinoma:** Limited evidence has linked chronic *H. pylori* infection with some individuals with gastric cancer. Recent evidence suggests that *H. pylori* is likely associated with gastric cancer. In fact, the International Agency for Cancer Research has reached the conclusion that infection with *H. pylori* is carcinogenic to humans.

Diagnostic Tests/Procedures

Helicobacter pylori Antigen, Direct *on page 478*
Helicobacter pylori Culture and Urease Test *on page 479*
Helicobacter pylori Culture, Gastric Biopsy *on page 480*
Helicobacter pylori Serology *on page 480*
Helicobacter pylori Urea Breath Test (UBT) *on page 481*

Treatment An increasing body of literature is supporting the practice of treating individuals diagnosed with *H. pylori* infection. Patients who appear to benefit the most from therapy are those with recurrent duodenal ulcers (endoscopically proven), duodenal ulcers resistant to conventional therapy, or perforated duodenal ulcers. The data do not suggest that all patients with peptic ulcer disease will benefit from antibiotics. Only patients who have chronic *H. pylori* infection associated with peptic ulcer disease benefit from therapy; those with other mechanisms to produce ulcers (such as nonsteroidal-induced ulcers or Zollinger-Ellison syndrome) are not likely to benefit. There is a significant incidence of minor side effects such as nausea, vomiting, and diarrhea with these oral regimens. Patient compliance may be low, and close monitoring and encouragement is necessary. There are a number of regimens available for successful treatment of peptic ulcer disease with *H. pylori.* Increases in resistance of *H. pylori* to the common antibiotics utilized have been documented. This should be taken into consideration in the treatment of recurrences where 4-drug therapy should be considered.

Drug Therapy

Recommended:

See *Helicobacter pylori* Treatment *on page 1288* for a complete listing of treatment regimens in the appendix. All regimens include PPI, H_2 antagonist, or bismuth product.

Amoxicillin *on page 642*
Tetracycline *on page 1106*
Metronidazole *on page 940*

Alternate:

Bismuth *on page 686*

Selected Readings

Correa P, "New Strategies for the Prevention of Gastric Cancer: *Helicobacter pylori* and Genetic Susceptibility," *J Surg Oncol*, 2005, 90(3):134-8.
Dunn BE, Cohen H, and Blaser MJ, "*Helicobacter pylori*," *Clin Microbiol Rev*, 1997, 10(4):720-41.
Ford CA, Delaney BC, Forman D, et al, "Eradication Therapy in *Helicobacter pylori* Positive Peptic Ulcer Disease: Systematic Review and Economic Analysis," *Am J Gastroenterol*, 2004, 99(9):1833-55.
Gisbert JP, Gonzalez L, and Calvet X, "Systematic Review and Meta-analysis: Proton Pump Inhibitor vs Ranitidine Bismuth Citrate Plus Two Antibiotics in *Helicobacter pylori* Eradication," *Helicobacter*, 2005, 10(3):157-71.
Hirschl AM and Makristathis A, "Non-invasive *Helicobacter pylori* Diagnosis: Stool or Breath Tests?" *Dig Liver Dis*, 2005, May 27; [Epub ahead of print].
Pathak CM, Bhasin DK, and Khanduja KL, "Urea Breath Test for *Helicobacter pylori* Detection: Present Status," *Trop Gastroenterol*, 2004, 25(4):156-61.
Versalovic J, "Intestinal *Helicobacters*," *Clin Microbiol Newslett*, 2002, 24(13):97-101.

Hemorrhagic Fever With Renal Syndrome (HFRS) *see* Hantavirus *on page 161*
Hepatic Abscess *see* Liver Abscess *on page 211*

Hepatitis

Clinical Presentation See individual organisms for clinical presentation information.

Likely Pathogens

Hepatitis A Virus *on page 164*
Hepatitis B Virus *on page 165*
Hepatitis C Virus *on page 167*
Hepatitis D Virus *on page 170*
Hepatitis E Virus *on page 171*
Epstein-Barr Virus *on page 139*
Cytomegalovirus *on page 107*
(Continued)

Hepatitis *(Continued)*

Diagnostic Tests/Procedures

Hepatitis A Profile *on page 482*
Hepatitis B Profile *on page 483*
Hepatitis C Serology *on page 484*
Hepatitis D Serology *on page 489*
Epstein-Barr Virus Serology *on page 454*
Cytomegalovirus Serology *on page 442*

Drug Therapy Comment Drug therapy based on identification of the causative agent.

Selected Readings

Dienstag JL, Schiff ER, Wright TL, et al, "Lamivudine as Initial Treatment for Chronic Hepatitis B in the United States," *N Engl J Med*, 1999, 341(17):1256-63.
Heathcote EJ, Shiffman ML, Cooksley WG, et al, "Peginterferon Alfa-2a in Patients With Chronic Hepatitis C and Cirrhosis," *N Engl J Med*, 2000, 343(23):1673-80.
Jaeckel E, Cornberg M, Wedemeyer H, et al, "Treatment of Acute Hepatitis C With Interferon Alfa-2b," *N Engl J Med*, 2001, 345(20):1452-7.
Saab S and Martin P, "Tests for Acute and Chronic Viral Hepatitis. Finding Your Way Through the Alphabet Soup of Infection and Superinfection," *Postgrad Med*, 2000, 107(2):123-6, 129-30.
Zeuzem S, Feinman SV, Rasenack J, et al, "Peginterferon Alfa-2a in Patients With Chronic Hepatitis C," *N Engl J Med*, 2000, 343(23):1666-72.

Hepatitis A Virus

Related Information

Hepatitis Laboratory Diagnosis and Management *on page 1201*
Immunization Recommendations *on page 1249*
Prophylaxis for Patients Exposed to Common Communicable Diseases *on page 1309*
USPHS / IDSA Guidelines for the Prevention of Opportunistic Infections in Persons Infected With HIV *on page 1237*

Synonyms HAV

Microbiology Hepatitis A virus (HAV; enterovirus 72) is a member of the Picovirus family (poliovirus, Coxsackievirus, echovirus). Mature HAV virions are nonenveloped, have icosahedral capsids, and contain single-stranded RNA.

Epidemiology HAV caused "infectious" hepatitis which was observed and recorded by Hippocrates. Epidemics of infectious hepatitis have been recorded throughout modern history, especially during World Wars I and II. Today, infectious hepatitis occurs worldwide and is very common in areas with poor sanitation and in institutional settings such as facilities for the developmentally disabled, the military, prisons, and daycare centers. In developing countries, almost all persons become infected with HAV (or at least become HAV antibody-positive) during childhood. In developed countries, the number of HAV antibody-positive persons is age-dependent and increases sharply with adulthood. The natural reservoir for HAV is humans. HAV is spread by the oral-fecal route. Transmission of HAV by blood and blood products occurs, but it is a rare event. Chronic excretion of HAV has not been documented.

Clinical Syndromes HAV causes acute infectious hepatitis which is usually mild in children and young patients, more severe in adults, and almost impossible to distinguish from acute hepatitis caused by other viruses. The incubation period for infectious hepatitis is about 30 days (range, 10-50 days). Typically, infectious hepatitis is characterized by a 1- to 7-day prodrome phase (fever, headache, fatigue, vomiting, abdominal pain, elevated serum ALT and AST levels [especially ALT]). (In all types of hepatitis, ALT levels are higher than AST levels.) Subsequently, more specific characteristics develop (dark urine, light-colored stool, jaundice, right upper quadrant pain, enlarged liver and spleen). Infectious hepatitis usually is acute and self-limiting. Infectious hepatitis is not chronic.

Diagnosis Infectious hepatitis is diagnosed clinically and serologically. The most useful methods for the laboratory diagnosis of infectious hepatitis are enzyme immunoassays for HAV-specific antibody (total and IgM). Almost all patients have anti-HAV IgM by the time symptoms are observed; IgM levels usually are not detectable 3-6 months after infection.

Diagnostic Tests/Procedures

Hepatitis A Profile *on page 482*

Drug Therapy Comment

No antiviral agents active against hepatitis A, but for pre-exposure and postexposure, prophylaxis intravenous immunoglobulins may be appropriate.

Drug Therapy

Recommended:

Immune Globulin (Intramuscular) *on page 866*
plus
Hepatitis A Vaccine *on page 853*

Selected Readings

Battegay M, Gust ID, and Feinstone SM, "Hepatitis A Virus," *Principles and Practice of Infectious Diseases*, 4th ed, Mandell GL, Bennett JE, and Dolin R, eds, New York, NY: Churchill Livingstone, 1995, 1636-56.

Hojvat SA, "Diagnostic Tests for Viral Hepatitis," *Clin Microbiol Newslett*, 1989, 11:33-9.

Hepatitis B Virus

Related Information

Hepatitis Laboratory Diagnosis and Management *on page 1201*

Immunization Recommendations *on page 1249*

Management of Healthcare Worker Exposures to HBV, HCV, and HIV *on page 1227*

Prophylaxis for Patients Exposed to Common Communicable Diseases *on page 1309*

Synonyms HBV

Microbiology Hepatitis B virus (HBV) is the etiological agent of serum hepatitis. HBV (archaic term, Dane particle) is a nonenveloped, partially double-stranded DNA virus which is trophic for liver cells. HBV is composed of a surface protein coat, a nucleocapsid, and internal proteins and nucleic acid. HBV usually is referred to as being composed of three antigens, surface (HB_sAg), core (HB_cAg), and e (HB_eAg). The surface of HBV is a complex antigen with many determinants/epitopes. The amount of HB_sAg produced during an infection usually is excessive, extremely large, and out of proportion to the amount needed to assemble mature, complete circulating HBV virions produced during infection. The HB_cAg (nucleocapsid) is found in the blood only as an internal part of the complete HBV virion; HB_cAg has not been detected free in blood. The HB_eAg is always associated with complete infectious HBV particles and, therefore, with infectivity.

Epidemiology Serum hepatitis is a common and serious endemic disease throughout the world. The prevalence of serum hepatitis depends on age and socioeconomic situation. At least 280 million cases and 1 million persons are chronic carriers of HBV worldwide and in the United States, respectively. The carrier rate in some parts of Asia is 15%. The natural reservoirs of HBV are humans and probably a few other Primates, such as chimps and monkeys. HBV is transmitted parenterally by needles and intravenous equipment, sexually, in unscreened blood products, and perinatally. HBV is not transmitted by the fecal-oral route. One of the sequelae of HBV infection, hepatocellular carcinoma, is a major public health problem worldwide. HBV probably is the cause of 80% of all cases of hepatocellular carcinoma worldwide. HBV has been found in almost all body secretions, but only blood, serum, semen, and vaginal fluids have been shown to be infectious. Perinatal transmission in developing countries is believed to be the main reason HBV is so prevalent worldwide. Perinatal infection has a high incidence resulting in chronic hepatitis, cirrhosis, and hepatocellular carcinoma.

Clinical Syndromes Most primary HBV infections are subclinical, self-limiting, and resolve within 3-6 months. HBV can produce mild to fulminant acute hepatitis, chronic persistent hepatitis, chronic active hepatitis, and hepatocellular carcinoma. The incubation period for serum hepatitis is 4-28 weeks. Signs and symptoms of acute serum hepatitis are quite variable and often include insidious onset of serum sickness-like illness, rash, and fever for several days to weeks. Subsequently, liver disease and joint involvement become clinically apparent. The presence of jaundice and abdominal pain are variable. This clinical condition usually is not distinguishable from that of acute disease caused by hepatitis A virus. Several variant forms of serum hepatitis have been described.

Diagnosis Diagnosis usually is made clinically, and determination of the specific etiological agent is made by serological and specific viral tests. Serological tests for several HBV antigens (surface and core) and antibodies to those antigens (antisurface, anticore, and anti-e) are widely available and clinically useful. Results of these tests are interpreted by consulting widely available charts which correlate various results (antigen and antibody patterns) with stages of infection. See the following tables.

Diagnostic Tests/Procedures

Hepatitis B Profile *on page 483*

Drug Therapy Comment

Both alpha interferon and lamivudine are approved for chronic active hepatitis. No drug therapy for acute hepatitis B. Hepatitis B immune globulin for prophylaxis.

Drug Therapy

Recommended:

Interferon Alfa-2b *on page 881*

Lamivudine *on page 905*

Prophylaxis:

Hepatitis B Immune Globulin *on page 855*

Hepatitis B Vaccine *on page 856*

(Continued)

Hepatitis B Virus *(Continued)*

Hepatitis B Serological Profile

Core Window Identification

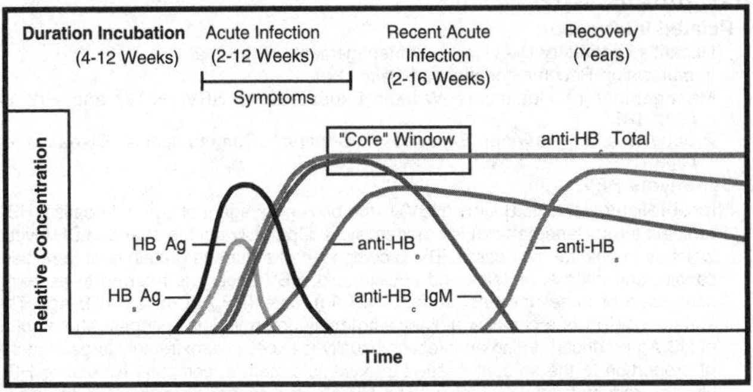

Hepatitis B Chronic Carrier

No Seroconversion

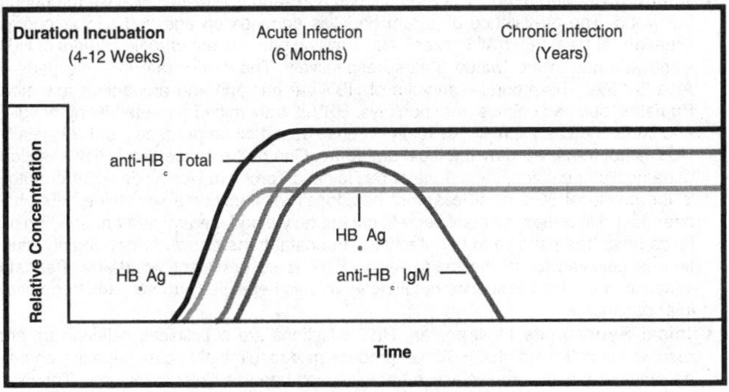

Hepatitis B Chronic Carrier

Late Seroconversion

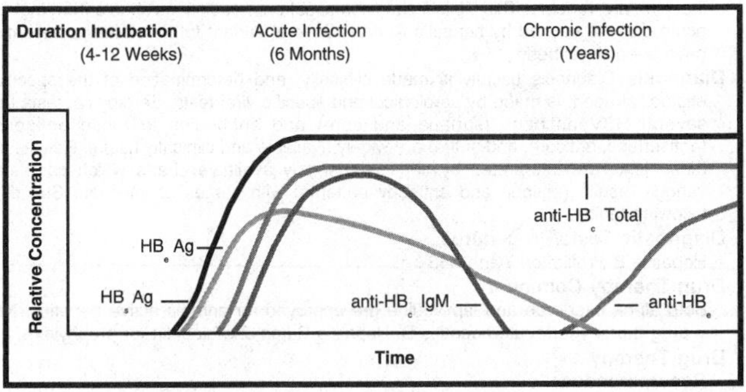

Selected Readings

Hojvat SA, "Diagnostic Tests for Viral Hepatitis," *Clin Microbiol Newslett*, 1989, 11:33-9.

Robinson WS, "Hepatitis B Virus and Hepatitis D Virus," *Principles and Practice of Infectious Diseases*, 4th ed, Mandell GL, Bennett JE, and Dolin R, eds, New York, NY: Churchill Livingstone, 1995, 1406-39.

Hepatitis C Virus

Related Information

Hepatitis Laboratory Diagnosis and Management *on page 1201*

Management of Healthcare Worker Exposures to HBV, HCV, and HIV *on page 1227*

Synonyms HCV

Microbiology Hepatitis C virus (HCV) is a small, lipid-enveloped, single-stranded RNA virus belonging to the family Flaviviridae. There are approximately 10,000 nucleotides in the viral genome arranged in a single large open reading frame. A large polyprotein is encoded which is later processed into a number of smaller proteins. There are now six viral genotypes and more than 80 subtypes of HCV based on genetic relatedness. This has been determined by direct sequence analysis. Genotypes 1, 2, and 3 have a worldwide distribution, whereas genotypes 4, 5, and 6 are more localized. In the United States, about 66% of hepatitis C cases are due to genotype 1 (1a and 1b). The clinical significance of the various genotypes and subtypes is still under study, and it is not clear whether the natural history of the liver disease differs from one genotype to the other. However, response to antiviral therapy has been shown to be genotype-dependent.

During viral replication, a number of mutations occur which leads to substantial heterogeneity of the viral population. The RNA polymerase introduces random nucleotide errors at a high rate as it copies the viral RNA, particularly within the hypervariable region (HVR1) of one of the envelope proteins. For an individual patient infected with HCV, there exist a number of closely related, but heterogeneous, genome sequences termed "quasispecies". During the course of infection, antibodies develop against HVR1; but over a period of time, some of the evolving quasispecies may not be recognized by these neutralizing antibodies. This is one mechanism by which the virus can elude the immune system.

Epidemiology In the United States, HCV is the most common chronic blood-borne infection, according to the Centers for Disease Control and Prevention (CDC). Approximately 3.9 million Americans are infected with HCV, an incidence of 1.8%. The majority of these individuals are 30-50 years of age, asymptomatic, and unaware of their infection. The number of new cases of HCV in the U.S. has fallen considerably over the past decade, from 230,000 new cases per year in the late 1980s to 28,000 in 1998, an almost 90% decline. A number of factors have probably contributed to this decline, including the availability of laboratory assays for routine screening for HCV in blood donors, a decrease in the use of shared needles amongst injection drug users (primarily due to concerns for HIV transmission), and a decrease in the use of blood from paid donors. However, despite this recent decline in new cases, there is a large population who were infected during the HCV epidemic 10-20 years ago and this will lead to a "cohort effect" in which the clinical impact of an epidemic 10-20 years ago will become apparent in the near future.

Routes of transmission:

Blood transfusions: HCV is the most common cause of transfusion-related hepatitis. Formerly termed non-A, non-B hepatitis, it is now clear that HCV is responsible for the majority of these cases. However, blood transfusion is not the most common route of transmission of HCV; in 1990, transfusions accounted for only 6% of new HCV cases. Aggressive screening of blood donors has helped decrease the incidence of HCV infection.

Intravenous drug use: Is the most commonly identified means of transmission. Up to 85% of I.V. drug users have serologic evidence of HCV infection. In 1990, about 40% of HCV cases appeared to be related to I.V. drug use.

Sexual transmission: Current data suggests that sexual transmission of HCV is inefficient. Some studies have shown no increased risk of HCV transmission between sex partners in a stable and monogamous relationship. Hepatitis B virus and HIV are much more easily acquired sexually.

Sporadic hepatitis: A number of individuals with serologic evidence of HCV infection have no obvious risk factor for acquisition. The extent of these "sporadic" cases has been debated with some estimates around 20% of all acute cases.

Miscellaneous: Other higher risk groups include healthcare workers, hemodialysis patients, individuals requiring multiple transfusions (hemophiliacs), and others.

Based on these considerations of the epidemiology of HCV, the CDC has made the following recommendations for screening for HCV.

Group 1: Patients who should be routinely tested for HCV (risk history - lifetime)

- Persons who injected illegal drugs, including those who injected even once many years ago and do not consider themselves as drug users

(Continued)

Hepatitis C Virus *(Continued)*

- Clotting factor recipients (before 1987)
- Transfusion or solid organ recipients (before July, 1992)
- Persons notified that they received blood from a donor who later tested HCV-positive
- Long-term dialysis patients
- Persons with evidence of liver disease
- Healthcare workers exposed to anti-HCV antibody-positive blood
- Infants older than 12 months of age born to HCV-positive women

Group 2: Uncertain need for HCV testing

- Intranasal cocaine and other noninjection illegal drug users
- Persons with history of tattooing and body piercing
- Recipients of transplanted tissue (eg, corneal, musculoskeletal, skin, ova, sperm)
- Persons with a history of multiple sex partners or sexually transmitted diseases
- Long-term steady sexual partners of HCV-positive persons

Group 3: Routine HCV testing not recommended (risk history - lifetime)

- Men who have sex with men
- Healthcare, emergency medical, and public safety workers
- Pregnant women
- Household (nonsexual) contacts of HCV-infected persons

Clinical Syndromes

- **Asymptomatic infection:** The majority of cases (~75%) of HCV infection are asymptomatic. Some individuals are identified by serologic testing (eg, blood donor screening programs), but many remain undetected. This is particularly problematic for several reasons. The virus can be unknowingly transmitted to others, liver damage occurs despite the absence of symptoms, and >50% will develop a chronic hepatopathy.
- **Acute HCV infection:** Following an initial incubation period (2 weeks to 6 months), the patient enters a "preicteric" phase. Symptoms tend to be nonspecific, with malaise and anorexia. In some cases, there is also right upper quadrant pain, nausea, and vomiting. This is followed by the "icteric" phase, where the patient presents with jaundice and dark urine. Systemic symptoms usually improve during the icteric phase. Several points should be noted: Infection with HCV cannot be accurately distinguished from other causes of viral hepatitis (including hepatitis B) on the basis of clinical presentation alone; the course of acute HCV tends to be more indolent than hepatitis B; clinical symptoms may be quite variable; a high clinical suspicion should be maintained since serologic tests for HCV may be negative early on. Fulminant hepatic failure secondary to acute HCV infection is a rare but important complication.

  Although a serum sickness-like illness with fever, arthritis, and skin rash has been well recognized in acute hepatitis B infection, only rarely has this been reported with hepatitis C infection. Other extrahepatic complications of acute HCV include aplastic anemia and pancreatitis.
- **Chronic HCV infection:** Over 50% of individuals infected with HCV develop chronic liver disease (hepatitis B, 5% to 10%). Symptoms are usually mild and nonspecific, with the main complaint being fatigue. The diagnosis is often difficult since liver function tests may be normal or only minimally elevated much of the time. Liver abnormalities include chronic persistent hepatitis, chronic active hepatitis, and cirrhosis.

  Chronic HCV infection has been associated with several syndromes, including membranoproliferative glomerulonephritis, type II cryoglobulinemia, hepatocellular carcinoma; growing evidence supports an epidemiologic link between chronic HCV and hepatocellular carcinoma, independent of hepatitis B infection or alcoholic liver disease.

Diagnosis As noted above, the diagnosis of HCV infection is quite difficult on clinical grounds alone and routine liver function tests may intermittently be normal. Thus, laboratory confirmation is essential.

Serologic tests: These assays are designed to detect or confirm host antibodies to recombinant HCV antigens. Several caveats: Antibodies to HCV remain undetectable until weeks or months after the initial infection; serologic studies may be needed at 6

months (90% of seroconverters identified) and possibly 12 months; in a few individuals, antibodies to HCV fail to develop for unclear reasons at any time postinfection. Available tests include:

- Enzyme-linked immunosorbent assay (ELISA) is used for the detection of antibody (generally IgG) against the C1OO-3 protein and other HCV-specific antigens.
- Radioimmunoblot assay (RIBA) is used as a supplemental or confirmatory test for patients who are anti-HCV positive by ELISA. Currently, the RIBA is designed to detect distinct antibodies to four different HCV proteins, including protein C1OO-3. The RIBA is used to confirm positive results of patients who are in low (<10%) HCV prevalence populations. In 2003, the CDC issued guidelines which allowed laboratories to confirm only those results which were below a certain signal to cut-off ratio. This action will result in the elimination of much unnecessary laboratory testing and in the savings of many healthcare dollars for laboratories, which routinely confirmed all positive results.

Molecular detection methods:

Nucleic acid testing can play an important role in the diagnosis and treatment of HCV infections. Qualitative molecular methods (amplification by polymerase chain reaction [PCR]) can be used to confirm positive antibody screening test results. Quantitative molecular methods (real-time PCR and branched chain DNA) can be used as important tests to relate the viral load of an infected person to the liklihood of a favorable response to treatment. Quantitative tests are recommended for patients before and during treatment, and are used to monitor a decline in viral load, which is associated with a favorable response.

Molecular genotyping of circulation HCV particles is used to determine which type (1a, 1b, 2, 3, 4, 5, or 6) of HCV is infecting the patient and to determine the liklihood of a patient's response to treatment. Patients with types 1a, 2, 3, and 5 are more likely to have favorable outcomes.

Diagnostic Tests/Procedures

Hepatitis C Serology *on page 484*
Hepatitis C Viral RNA Genotyping *on page 486*
Hepatitis C Viral RNA, Quantitative bDNA *on page 487*
Hepatitis C Viral RNA, Quantitative PCR *on page 488*

Treatment The treatment of HCV infection is rapidly evolving and changes in recommended therapies occur often. A specialist in hepatology or infectious diseases should be consulted if therapy is being considered.

In 1991, interferon (IFN-alpha2b) became the first drug approved for use in hepatitis C. This was administered at 3 million units 3 times/week for a 6-month period. The sustained response rate was low, about 10% to 20%. (In clinical trials, a "sustained response" is defined as having normal ALT tests and undetectable HCV by PCR 6 months after discontinuing the therapy. Relapses after therapy usually occur within 6 months). Although the number of patients who demonstrated a sustained response was low, 90% of those who did respond were still in remission 5 years later, with undetectable HCV, normal ALTs, and improvements in liver biopsy histology. Later, it was shown that treating for a longer period of time, 12-18 months, with IFN-alpha2b led to a modest increase in the sustained response rate.

More recently, studies have shown that the combination of IFN-alpha2b given in combination with ribavirin is about three times greater than monotherapy with IFN-alpha2b alone. Ribavirin as monotherapy is ineffective. The IFN-alpha2b and ribavirin combination has led to a 40% sustained response rate in clinical trials. The success of this combination depends in large part on the HCV genotype of the individual patient. Persons with genotype 1 (the most common in the United States) have a 28% sustained response compared with 66% of persons infected with genotypes 2 and 3. There are a number of side effects seen with this regimen including flu-like symptoms, psychiatric manifestations, and hemolytic anemia.

In one study, predictors of a sustained response with initial IFN-alpha2b/ribavirin therapy included:

- HCV genotype 2 or 3
- HCV RNA <2 x 10^4 copies/mL
- liver fibrosis stage 0-1
- female sex
- age <40 years

The risks and benefits of combination therapy are under study in several groups with HCV infection including:

- Patients with normal liver function tests - earlier studies suggested that treatment might exacerbate liver disease and cause increased ALT (at least with IFN monotherapy)

(Continued)

Hepatitis C Virus *(Continued)*

- Persons with hemophilia - there has been a concern that IFN would stimulate antifactor VIII antibody production
- Persons with renal disease - IFN may be poorly tolerated in this group with high dropout rates
- Persons with HIV and HCV

In 1997, the National Institutes of Health (NIH) consensus statement on management of HCV recommended the following:

Persons Recommended for Treatment (greatest risk for progression to cirrhosis):
- Patients with persistently elevated ALT levels,
- Detectable HCV RNA, *and*
- A liver biopsy indicating either portal or bridging fibrosis and at least moderate degrees of inflammation and necrosis.

Persons for Whom Treatment Is Unclear:
- Patients with compensated cirrhosis (without jaundice, ascites, variceal hemorrhage, or encephalopathy)
- Patients with persistent ALT elevations but with less severe histologic changes (ie, no fibrosis and minimal necroinflammatory changes). In these patients, progression to cirrhosis is likely to be slow, if at all. Therefore, observation and serial measurements of ALT and liver biopsy every 3-5 years are an acceptable alternative to treatment with interferon.
- Patients <18 years or >60 years of age

Persons for Whom Treatment Is Not Recommended:
- Patients with persistently normal ALT values
- Patients with advanced cirrhosis who might be at risk for decompensation with therapy
- Patients who are currently drinking excessive amounts of alcohol or who are injecting illegal drugs (treatment should be delayed until these behaviors have been discontinued for >6 months)
- Persons with major depressive illness, cytopenias, hyperthyroidism, renal transplantation, evidence of autoimmune disease, or who are pregnant

Drug Therapy
Recommended:
Interferon Alfa-2b *on page 881*
Interferon Alfa-2b and Ribavirin *on page 884*

Selected Readings

Alter MJ, Kuhnert WL, and Finelli L, "Guidelines for Laboratory Testing and Result Reporting of Antibody to Hepatitis C Virus," *MMWR*, 2003, 52(RR-3):1-13, 15.
Alter MJ, Mast EE, Moyer LA, et al, "Hepatitis C," *Infect Dis Clin North Am*, 1998, 12(1):13-26.
Camma C, Licata A, Cabibbo G, et al, "Treatment of Hepatitis C: Critical Appraisal of the Evidence," *Expert Opin Pharmacother*, 2005, 6(3):399-408.
Clanon KA, Johannes Mueller J, and Harank M, "Integrating Treatment for Hepatitis C Virus Infection Into an HIV Clinic," *Clin Infect Dis*, 2005, 40(Suppl 5):S362-6.
Cook L, "Hepatitis C Virus Diagnosis and Therapeutic Monitoring: Methods and Interpretation," *Clin Microbiol Newslett*, 1999, 21(9):67-72.
Davis GL, Esteban-Mur R, Rustgi V, et al, "Interferon Alfa-2b Alone or in Combination With Ribavirin for the Treatment of Relapse of Chronic Hepatitis C. International Hepatitis Interventional Therapy Group," *N Engl J Med*, 1998, 339(21):1493-9.
Fleming CA, Tumilty S, Murray JE, et al, "Challenges in the Treatment of Patients Coinfected With HIV and Hepatitis C Virus: Need for Team Care," *Clin Infect Dis*, 2005, 40(Suppl 5):S349-54.
Liang TJ, "Combination Therapy for Hepatitis C Infection," *N Engl J Med*, 1998, 339(21):1549-50.
"Recommendations for Prevention and Control of Hepatitis C (HCV) Infection and HCV-Related Chronic Disease. Centers for Disease Control and Prevention," *MMWR*, 1998, 47(RR-19):1-39.
Spiegel BM, Younossi ZM, Hays RD, et al, "Impact of Hepatitis C on Health Related Quality of Life: A Systematic Review and Quantitative Assessment," *Hepatology*, 2005, 41(4):790-800.

Hepatitis D Virus

Related Information
Hepatitis Laboratory Diagnosis and Management *on page 1201*

Synonyms HDV

Microbiology Hepatitis D virus (HDV) is the etiological agent of delta hepatitis. HDV was first recognized in an Amazon tribe in 1969 and was first described in 1977. HDV is a small (35-40 nm) virus composed of only a circular single-strand RNA genome and a two-protein complex (the delta antigen) which surrounds and is intimately associated with the RNA. The RNA genome is the smallest of any animal virus. HDV can replicate on its own but requires the presence of HBV for transmission. Therefore, HDV is a defective/incomplete virus and invariably is found only in persons with acute or chronic HBV infection. During coinfection and when HBV and HDV are within the same cell, the HDV acquires a protein coat (envelope) composed of HBV surface antigen. This coat allows HDV to infect other cells. HDV will not be found in a HBV surface antigen-negative person.

Epidemiology HDV is present in extremely high numbers in circulating blood and usually is transmitted parenterally in ways similar to those of HBV (eg, by blood, blood products, and contaminated needles). In general, delta hepatitis is most prevalent in populations at high risk for hepatitis B (eg, multiply infused patients, intravenous drug users, hemophiliacs, inhabitants of underdeveloped countries, etc). Sexual transmission of HDV has been reported. Hepatitis D is a worldwide problem because the many millions of worldwide carriers of HBV surface antigen are potentially susceptible to HDV. Worldwide, HDV is present in about 5% of HBV carriers. Many epidemics of hepatitis D outside of the United States have been described, particularly in Africa and South America. In the United States, hepatitis B is a reportable disease, but hepatitis D is not reportable. This is probably because hepatitis D is not easy to diagnose, it is not common in the United States, and it is not yet a public health problem. HDV causes <1% of all viral hepatitis diseases.

Clinical Syndromes Acute viral hepatitis is a distinct clinical entity and usually is not too difficult to diagnose. In general, the diseases produced by hepatitis A, B, C, D, and E viruses are clinically indistinguishable. The clinical presentations of the diseases vary drastically from asymptomatic infections to icteric hepatitis to fulminant and fatal hepatitis.

Acute delta hepatitis occurs either as a coinfection at the same time as acute hepatitis B or as a superinfection during chronic hepatitis B. In both cases, the resulting disease is more severe than hepatitis B alone. A third type of hepatitis D has been suggested, a latent HDV infection which is active only after a subsequent HBV infection. Hepatitis D coinfection usually is clinically indistinguishable from acute hepatitis B, except the course is more severe. Less than 5% of patients with acute HDV coinfection develop chronic hepatitis D; however, most patients with hepatitis D acquired as a superinfection develop chronic hepatitis D. Patients who experience a superinfection can deteriorate rapidly and experience abrupt liver failure. Both acute and chronic hepatitis D are usually severe. Mortality rates for acute hepatitis D are 2% to 20%. Sixty percent to 70% of patients with chronic hepatitis D develop cirrhosis; most of these patients die of liver disease.

Diagnosis Viral hepatitis usually is diagnosed clinically, and determination of the specific etiological agent is made by serological and specific viral tests. Serological tests for anti-HDV IgG and IgM antibodies are widely available and clinically useful. Results of these tests are interpreted by consulting widely available charts which correlate various results (antigen and antibody patterns) with stages of infection. Tests for HDV antigen are available but are technically demanding and are not particularly diagnostically useful. Hepatitis A, B, C, D, and E viruses produce somewhat characteristic, but essentially indistinguishable, lesions in the liver. Polymerase chain reaction and associated nucleic acid probe tests for HDV RNA and HDV antigen have been reported.

Diagnostic Tests/Procedures

Hepatitis D Serology *on page 489*

Drug Therapy Comment Currently, no antiviral therapy effective against hepatitis D.

Selected Readings

Gupta S, Govindarajan S, Cassidy WM, et al, "Acute Delta Hepatitis: Serological Diagnosis With Particular Reference to Hepatitis Delta Virus RNA," *Am J Gastroenterol*, 1991, 86(9):1227-31.

Holt DA, Baran DA, Oehler RL, et al, "Delta Hepatitis: A Diagnostic Algorithm," *Infect Med*, 1993, 10:23-9.

Hsu HH, Feinstone SM, and Hoofnagle JH, "Acute Viral Hepatitis," *Principles and Practice of Infectious Diseases*, 4th ed, Mandell GL, Bennett JE, and Dolin R, eds, New York, NY: Churchill Livingstone, 1995, 1136-53.

Modahl LE and Lai MM, "Hepatitis Delta Virus: The Molecular Basis of Laboratory Diagnosis," *Crit Rev Clin Lab Sci*, 2000, 37(1):45-92.

Polish LB, Gallagher M, Fields HA, et al, "Delta Hepatitis: Molecular Biology and Clinical and Epidemiological Features," *Clin Microbiol Rev*, 1993, 6(3):211-29.

Hepatitis E Virus

Related Information

Hepatitis Laboratory Diagnosis and Management *on page 1201*

Synonyms HEV

Microbiology Hepatitis E virus (HEV) is an unenveloped single-strand RNA virus, is structurally similar to calicivirus, and is found in the stool of hepatitis E patients during incubation and early acute phase of the disease. HEV is the etiological agent of "epidemic" or "enterically transmitted" non-A, non-B hepatitis and is associated with epidemics and contaminated water. ("Classic" non-A, non-B hepatitis is caused by hepatitis C virus and is associated with parenteral exposure.)

Epidemiology HEV causes <1% of all viral hepatitis diseases. Hepatitis E is transmitted by the fecal-oral route, is found in stool, and has been reported to be the cause of several large outbreaks of hepatitis in India, China, Peru, Russia, Africa, and Mexico. None of these epidemics were associated with either HAV or HBV; most of these outbreaks were associated with fecally contaminated water supplies and poor sanitation. Hepatitis E is very rare in the United States. HEV has not caused

(Continued)

Hepatitis E Virus *(Continued)*

outbreaks in the United States and western Europe. Hepatitis E occurs only rarely in the United States, where persons with hepatitis E are almost always immigrants from endemic areas. Mortality rates of pregnant females who acquire hepatitis E are very high (15% to 30%), and fetal wastage is common.

Clinical Syndromes Clinically, hepatitis E is similar to hepatitis A except for the following: early presentations tend to include pruritus and joint pain; cholestasis is common; concentrations of serum aminotransferase and alkaline phosphatase tend to be lower and higher, respectively.

Diagnosis Hepatitis E is diagnosed clinically. Antibody to HEV develops early in the disease. Laboratory tests to detect antibody to HEV (immune electron microscopy and inhibition of immunofluorescence) are available in only a few (usually research) laboratories.

Diagnostic Tests/Procedures

Hepatitis E Serology *on page 490*

Drug Therapy Comment Currently, no antiviral therapy effective against hepatitis E.

Selected Readings

"Hepatitis E Among U.S. Travelers, 1989-1992," *MMWR*, 1993, 42(1):1-4.

Hsu HH, Feinstone SM, and Hoofnagle JH, "Acute Viral Hepatitis," *Principles and Practice of Infectious Diseases*, 4th ed, Mandell GL, Bennett JE, and Dolin R, eds, New York, NY: Churchill Livingstone, 1995, 1136-53.

Yarbough PO, "Hepatitis E: Diagnosis of Infection," *Clin Microbiol Newslett*, 1993, 15(15):113-5.

Herpangina *see* Coxsackieviruses *on page 101*

Herpes Simplex Virus

Related Information

Treatment of Sexually Transmitted Infections *on page 1311*

USPHS / IDSA Guidelines for the Prevention of Opportunistic Infections in Persons Infected With HIV *on page 1237*

Synonyms HSV

Microbiology Herpes simplex virus (HSV) is a double-stranded DNA virus. There are two subtypes of herpes simplex virus, HSV-1 and HSV-2, which have about 50% sequence homology and are known to have somewhat different clinical manifestations. HSV-1 and HSV-2 can be differentiated by serologic tests that detect antibodies directed to unique surface proteins, particularly the epitopes glycoprotein G1 and G2.

The virus is composed of several components: (1) an inner capsid which contains the viral DNA, (2) the tegument, which surrounds the capsid "shell," and (3) a lipid bilayer surrounding the tegument called the envelope. When a host cell is infected by HSV, the first step is attachment and fusion of the viral envelope with the cell membrane of the host. The capsid, which contains the viral genome, enters the host cell cytoplasm, regulatory proteins are released from the nucleocapsid which initiate transcription of the virus. The "early genes" of HSV produce proteins required for synthesis of important "late" polypeptides, such as DNA polymerase, allowing viral DNA synthesis to take place. This cascade continues, structural proteins are synthesized, and both the viral DNA and structural proteins enter the host nucleus. The host cell may die as a result of infection, but can also become latently infected. In some neurons, HSV can exist indefinitely in the host cell, and the cell is able to carry out its metabolic functions normally. The virus is not truly "latent" and has been shown to maintain some transcriptional activity, albeit at a very low level. Latent virus can periodically reactivate in neurons, and become transcriptionally active. Viral replication begins again with the same steps of protein synthesis. The factors that control the latent phase remain unknown.

Epidemiology Herpes simplex virus (HSV) infections occur worldwide. HSV-1 infection is common in childhood. By the fourth decade, approximately 90% of individuals will be seropositive for HSV-1. In lower socioeconomic groups, the incidence is even higher. HSV-2 is less common than HSV-1, and primary infections tend to occur in an older age group. The seroprevalence of HSV-2 in the U.S. is increasing and over 20% of the general population demonstrates serologic evidence of past HSV-2 infection. It is important to note that only a minority of individuals seropositive for HSV-2 report having had genital lesions. Clearly, there are thousands of asymptomatic carriers of HSV-2 who are potential transmitters of HSV-2. Seroprevalence correlates well with increasing sexual activity. The general rule that HSV-1 causes "above the waist" infections and HSV-2 causes "below the waist" infections holds true for the most part, but cross infections are increasingly common.

The incubation period following exposure to the virus is about 1 week, although prolonged incubation periods up to 3-4 weeks have been described. HSV transmission is most efficient in individuals with active ulcerations of the mucous membranes or genitalia but can occur when virus is shed asymptomatically. HSV-1 can be

cultured from the oropharynx of 2% to 9% of healthy adults and 5% to 8% of healthy children, indicating that asymptomatic shedding of HSV-1 is common. Similarly, HSV-2 can be recovered from the genital tracts of asymptomatic, sexually active patients. Based on several studies, some HSV-infected women asymptomatically shed virus from the genital tract on 2% to 6% of the days a viral culture was performed. The precise rate of asymptomatic shedding in infected women is not known, but it is likely greater than 2% to 6% since viral culture for HSV is not overly sensitive and has a false negative rate of 20% to 30%. HSV detection by polymerase chain reaction (PCR) is at least 3 times more sensitive than culture. Recent studies in infected women have found much higher rates of viral shedding using HSV PCR. Asymptomatic viral shedding in men is less common, and in one study occurred on 2% of days cultured.

HSV is spread by direct contact. The virus can enter through small breaks in the skin but can also penetrate intact mucosa in the mouth or genitals. Replication occurs in epithelial cells then follows peripheral sensory neurons where latent infection is established in the ganglia.

Clinical Syndromes

- **Primary genital herpes:** Herpes genitalis is more commonly caused by HSV 2 (70% to 90% of cases), although there are a sizeable number of cases caused by HSV 1 (10% to 30%). In the U.S., HSV is the most common cause of genital ulcer. Young adults and adolescents are most commonly infected. In males, vesicular lesions occur on the penile shaft or glans. In the female, similar lesions are seen in a variety of areas, including the cervix, perineum, vulva, and vagina. Primary infection with HSV (initial infection) may vary in severity from a mild or subclinical illness to a more severe disease. Symptoms are more severe during the first episode of genital herpes, then during recurrences. Symptoms tend to be more severe in persons who have not previously been exposed to either HSV-1 or HSV-2 and lack antibody. Persons who have had past oral HSV infection and have either HSV-1 or HSV-2 generally have milder primary genital HSV. Primary infection with HSV-1 and HSV-2 are similar in severity and clinical presentation. In moderate to severe cases of primary infection, patients may display fever, headache, malaise, and inguinal lymph node enlargement. The characteristic genital lesions are grouped vesicles which are typically tender and have an erythematous base. The finding of grouped vesicles in the genital region is highly characteristic of HSV and few other diseases cause this. Lesions may persist for weeks with severe primary infections but eventually crust over. The vesicles typically ulcerate and crust after a period of time, but often a combination of vesicles, ulcers, and crusting lesions can be seen at the same time. When the vesicles ulcerate, the lesions are difficult to distinguish from ulcers caused by a number of other sexually transmitted diseases (eg, syphilis, chancroid). More severe cases of primary HSV may be complicated by sacral radiculomyelitis with shooting neuralgic pains, obstipation and urinary retention, aseptic meningitis, or abdominal pain.
- **Recurrent genital herpes:** After primary HSV infection, recurrent genital lesions can occur in both sexes, and in one study almost 90% of persons with HSV-2 infection had one or more recurrences over a median observation period of 418 days. This cohort experienced a median of four HSV recurrences per year, but 20% experienced over 10 recurrences per year. Patients with severe and/or prolonged primary HSV infection had more recurrences. Recurrence rates are much lower in those with genital HSV-1 than HSV-2. Some individuals will have a decrease in the number of recurrences per year after several years, but it appears that this may be a minority of individuals. The systemic symptoms and severity of the lesions are diminished in comparison with primary infection. Patients will often complain of a prodrome of burning 1-2 days prior to an outbreak. Lesions typical for HSV develop during recurrences and heal over 7-10 days even without therapy. Factors which appear to initiate recurrences include sun exposure, menstruation, stress, and sexual intercourse.
- **Oral HSV infections:** Primary herpes gingivostomatitis is seen mainly in children and is caused by HSV 1 in 90% of cases. Less commonly, primary infection occurs in the young adult; in such cases infection may be from either HSV 1 or 2. The incubation period following exposure is 2-12 days. Vesicles develop in the oral cavity, including the pharynx, palate, buccal mucosa, and/or tongue. The vesicles rapidly break down into small ulcers and are covered with an exudate. Lesions may extend to involve the lips and cheek. Severe primary lesions can be accompanied by high fevers, malaise, cervical lymphadenopathy, and dehydration. However, it is known that primary oral HSV infections are most commonly asymptomatic or mild. The lesions generally resolve without therapy in 2 weeks. HSV pharyngitis is probably under-recognized in the college-aged population, where it may be misdiagnosed as "strep throat." Recurrent HSV labialis (lip lesions) is problematic in some adults. Recent data suggest that chronic daily acyclovir may have some minor benefit in this group. In patients who are immunosuppressed, recurrences of

(Continued)

Herpes Simplex Virus *(Continued)*

HSV labialis can be quite severe. Persons with underlying atopic eczema may develop eczema herpeticum, characterized by recurrent episodes of severe HSV-1 gingivostomatitis and often extensive skin lesions.

- **Herpetic keratitis:** HSV 1 is one of the most common causes of corneal blindness. Patients typically present with unilateral eye pain, lacrimation, conjunctivitis, and blurred vision. It is important to identify HSV because topical corticosteroids can worsen the condition. Recurrences are common. Permanent visual damage may occur if there is significant corneal scarring. Other eye diseases associated with HSV infection include chorioretinitis (seen in HIV-infected individuals as a result of disseminated HSV) and the acute retinal necrosis syndrome (a rare cause of visual loss seen in healthy adults).
- **Herpetic whitlow:** This is the term used for HSV infection of the finger. It may result from occupational exposure, as in a respiratory technologist whose finger is inoculated with virus from a patient excreting the virus orally. Characteristically, there are vesicular lesions on the finger, with redness and edema. Recurrences are common. The lesions may be mistaken for bacterial pustules, especially when the patient presents with fever and regional lymphadenopathy. Many physicians mistake these lesions as being filled with pus and, subsequently, lance the lesions. The lesion can then develop a secondary bacterial infection.
- **HSV infections of the central nervous system:** HSV 1 is the most common cause of sporadic encephalitis in the United States. Encephalitis may result from primary HSV 1 infection, reactivation, or reinfection. It is theorized that the virus travels along the olfactory nerve of a susceptible host and reaches the temporal lobe of the brain. Patients present with the subacute onset of confusion. Other features include fever, headache, focal seizures, and olfactory hallucinations. It is difficult to distinguish encephalitis caused by HSV from other etiologies of encephalitis (such as arboviruses, tuberculosis, fungal infections, etc). Cerebrospinal fluid findings are usually nondiagnostic, and HSV 1 is only rarely isolated from spinal fluid culture, but can be reliably detected using the polymerase chain reaction (PCR). Electroencephalography (EEG) is helpful in localizing the area of inflammation to the temporal lobe. CT scan or MRI scan of the brain can reveal necrosis of the temporal lobe in some cases, a finding highly suggestive of HSV encephalitis. The definitive diagnostic test is the brain biopsy, with viral culture and histopathology. However, the use of HSV PCR detection in cerebrospinal fluid has essentially replaced the brain biopsy as the initial diagnostic procedure of choice in suspected cases, given the sensitivity and specificity of HSV PCR.
- **HSV and AIDS:** Severe and recurrent HSV infections are seen in persons with AIDS, although this may be declining with the widespread use of combination antiretroviral therapy and immune system reconstitution in many HIV-infected persons. In patients with low $CD4^+$ T cell counts, HSV can cause disease in the genital and/or anal regions (proctocolitis), and other visceral organs. Progressive perianal ulcerations with proctitis may be due to either HSV 1 or 2. This infection may be quite debilitating, with anorectal pain, bloody stools, tenesmus, and fever. Such patients usually respond to I.V. or oral acyclovir. Since recurrences are the rule in persons with low $CD4^+$ T cell counts, these patients are often placed on chronic acyclovir suppression. This has led to sporadic cases of acyclovir-resistant HSV mutants and progressive rectal infection. In addition, HSV esophagitis may result from direct extension of oral HSV lesions into the esophagus or from reactivation of HSV in the vagus nerve which innervates the esophagus. The clinical presentation is indistinguishable from *Candida* esophagitis, another common condition in AIDS. Unfortunately, HSV esophageal lesions have a nonspecific appearance both on barium swallow and upper endoscopy, and tissue biopsy is required to rule out *Candida* (or cytomegalovirus) esophagitis.
- **HSV pneumonia:** This unusual manifestation of HSV is seen in the immunosuppressed. Cases have also been reported in burn unit patients. The pathogenesis is direct extension of herpetic tracheobronchitis into the lungs. A necrotizing pneumonia results, and bronchoscopy is usually required to confirm the diagnosis.
- **Neonatal infection:** HSV infection in newborns (younger than 6 weeks of age) is frequently devastating. Visceral dissemination of the virus and central nervous system infection are common. Untreated, the mortality exceeds 65%. Many who survive exhibit developmental disabilities. Infection occurs most commonly during delivery as the neonate passes through an infected birth canal. Most cases are due to HSV-2. *In utero* infection, while reported, is much less common.
- **Urethritis:** HSV is a known cause of urethritis, although uncommon. Women presenting with the acute urethral syndrome with episodic dysuria and negative bacterial urine cultures should be examined for HSV.
- **Other:** HSV can cause a variety of infections of the skin and mucous membranes. One example is herpes gladiatorum, a condition described in male wrestlers. In this

condition, wrestlers spread HSV to a variety of cutaneous and mucous membrane sites through areas of minor trauma.

Diagnosis The diagnosis of genital, rectal, or oral HSV is usually suspected when a patient presents with typical grouped vesicles involving skin or a mucous membrane. As previously mentioned, this finding is not always present and laboratory confirmation may be necessary. HSV encephalitis should be considered in the differential diagnosis of any person presenting with community-acquired encephalitis. Diagnostic procedures usually obtained for suspected HSV encephalitis include the CT scan or MRI scan of the brain, electroencephalography, and lumbar puncture. Some of the other manifestations of HSV may be more difficult to diagnose clinically. There are a variety of laboratory tests available. The simplest is the Tzanck test which is performed by scraping a suspected lesion, usually an exposed vesicle or ulcer on the genitals. The scrapings are placed on a microscope slide, stained with a Wright-Giemsa stain (or other stains), and the slide examined for the presence of multinucleated giant cells with characteristic intranuclear inclusions. The Tzanck test is positive for herpesviruses in general, and is not specific for HSV (ie, vesicular lesions caused by varicella zoster virus can have the same appearance).

HSV culture is performed using standard tissue culture techniques, with cytopathic effects visible in the cell monolayer as early as 24-48 hours after inoculation. Monoclonal antibodies are used by most laboratories to confirm the presence of HSV growing in tissue culture. The rate of false-negative cultures can be as high as 20% to 30%, and this relates to the age of the lesion cultured, the adequacy of the specimen collected, transportation, and laboratory handling. Many laboratories offer a shell vial assay for HSV which is a rapid, tissue-culture based detection system. Another common rapid technique is direct fluorescent antibody (DFA) staining, which involves collecting a swab specimen from an active vesicular lesion and directly staining for the presence of HSV within cellular material, without culturing for the virus. Other rapid tests for HSV include enzyme immunoassays (EIA), antigen capture assays, and immunofluorescence. A number of assays are available to distinguish HSV 1 from HSV 2, but some clinical laboratories will not distinguish the subtypes (due in part to the added expense) unless specifically requested by the clinician. Subtype analysis may be helpful in evaluation of the person with primary genital HSV for prognostic reasons, since the number of recurrences with HSV 1 genital infection is low. A number of clinical laboratories offer polymerase chain reaction (PCR) for the detection of HSV DNA directly in body fluids, most commonly from cerebrospinal fluid. PCR is significantly more sensitive than culture and enzyme immunoassays. Unlike culture methods, PCR can detect viral DNA in herpetic lesions and body secretions several days after symptoms subside and after lesions no longer yield culturable virions. The clinical relevance of this ability to detect prolonged presence and shedding of virus is not known. PCR is very sensitive and specific for the detection of HSV DNA in CSF from patients with HSV meningitis and/or encephalitis, and is considered the initial diagnostic procedure of choice for persons with suspected HSV encephalitis.

Diagnostic Tests/Procedures

Electroencephalography *on page 447*
Herpes Cytology *on page 491*
Herpes Simplex Antibody *on page 492*
Herpes Simplex Virus Culture *on page 494*
Herpes Simplex Virus by Direct Immunofluorescence *on page 493*
Herpes Simplex Virus Isolation, Rapid *on page 495*
Polymerase Chain Reaction *on page 567*
Skin Biopsy *on page 580*

Treatment Acyclovir was the first antiviral drug approved for infections caused by HSV-1 and HSV-2. Recently several other antiviral drugs have been approved for HSV, mainly with somewhat different pharmacokinetic profiles.

Genital Infection: For the treatment of primary genital HSV infection, recommended regimens are: Acyclovir 200 mg orally 5 times/day for 7-10 days, or 400 mg orally 3 times/day for 7-10 days. For persons unable to tolerate oral drugs, acyclovir 5% ointment can be applied topically every 6 hours for 7 days but this is substantially less efficacious. For severe primary infections, acyclovir can be given 5 mg/kg intravenously every 8 hours for 5-7 days or until resolution.

Also effective for primary genital infection is famciclovir given 250 mg orally 3 times/day for 7-10 days, or valacyclovir given 1 g twice daily for 7-10 days. There is no significant difference in efficacy between acyclovir, valacyclovir, or famciclovir in primary HSV and all are considered first-line therapy. Treatment of primary infection does not seem to influence the frequency of later recurrences.

Recurrent genital HSV is common and several strategies are available: (1) observation without antivirals, (2) episodic treatment of recurrences, and (3) suppressive
(Continued)

Herpes Simplex Virus *(Continued)*

therapy. Some individuals will have infrequent and mild recurrences and do not require antiviral therapy. For those with more severe recurrences, starting antiviral therapy with the first symptom of a recurrence (eg, with burning sensation, prior to the vesicle) may reduce the duration of symptoms and viral shedding. Acyclovir, famciclovir, and valacyclovir have all been used in this manner, and appear equivalent. However, the overall benefit of episodic treatment of recurrences is modest at best and many patients will not experience a significant improvement. Regimens include: (1) acyclovir 200 mg orally 5 times/day for 5 days, (2) acyclovir 400 mg orally 3 times/day for 5 days, (3) acyclovir 800 mg orally twice daily for 5 days, (4) famciclovir 125-250 mg orally twice daily for 5 days, or (5) valacyclovir 500 mg orally twice daily for 5 days.

Suppressive therapy of recurrent genital HSV is a strategy that is effective in persons with frequent recurrences. The original studies of suppressive therapy were conducted in persons experiencing ≥6 outbreaks per year and were randomized to daily acyclovir versus placebo. A decrease in the number of episodes per year by 80% to 90% was demonstrated, with few side effects. However, individuals still experience some outbreaks each year, asymptomatic viral shedding still occurs intermittently, and transmission to a susceptible partner is possible. Acyclovir appears safe in persons on daily treatment over 6 years; the safety of valacyclovir and famciclovir after 1 year is still under study. The frequency of acyclovir-resistant HSV in immunocompetent persons receiving suppression therapy appears to be extremely low. The use of daily suppression does not appear to alter the rate of recurrences and individuals may or may not return to their baseline rate of recurrences once the suppression is stopped. It is recommended to reassess suppressive therapy at 1-2 years. Regimens for daily suppression include: (1) acyclovir 400 mg orally twice daily, (2) famciclovir 250 mg orally twice daily, (3) valacyclovir 500 mg orally once daily if <10 recurrences per year, (4) valacyclovir 1000 mg orally once daily if ≥10 recurrences per year.

Oral-Labial HSV: For symptomatic primary oral HSV, acyclovir can be of benefit. The usual dose is 200 mg orally 5 times/day. For recurrences of oral HSV, episodic treatment with oral acyclovir has minimal or no benefit. Topical acyclovir ointment also has no significant benefit. Topical penciclovir cream may have a modest effect. For those with frequent, moderate to severe recurrences of oral-labial HSV, oral acyclovir suppression may be helpful. In those with reactivation associated with sun exposure, acyclovir can be given 400 mg orally twice daily starting before the exposure and continued about 5 days.

Proctitis: In persons with AIDS, severe episodes of HSV proctitis should be treated with intravenous acyclovir. Less severe infections can be treated with oral acyclovir. There is less experience using famciclovir and valacyclovir in this setting but both would likely be effective.

Esophagitis: HSV esophagitis in persons with AIDS is usually treated with acyclovir 5 mg/kg intravenously every 8 hours. Mild cases can be treated with oral acyclovir, famciclovir, or valacyclovir.

Hepatic Keratitis: Herpes keratitis is often treated with topical ophthalmics such as idoxuridine, trifluridine, and acyclovir. An ophthalmologist should be consulted.

Herpes Simplex Encephalitis: This life-threatening condition requires high doses of intravenous acyclovir, 10 mg/kg every 8 hours for a minimum of 10 days. Oral antiviral agents are not recommended. Prompt initiation of intravenous acyclovir has decreased the mortality rate but almost one-third of individuals will still have neurologic deficits even after appropriate therapy. Many recommend early initiation of empiric acyclovir if HSV encephalitis is suspected prior to laboratory confirmation.

Acyclovir-Resistant HSV: Immunocompromised persons on long-term acyclovir suppression may develop progressive disease due to strains of HSV which are resistant to acyclovir. Progressive disease due to acyclovir resistant HSV has been described particularly in AIDS patients. HSV strains resistant to acyclovir are also resistant to valacyclovir, famciclovir, and ganciclovir. Most remain susceptible to foscarnet and to cidofovir.

Neonatal HSV: Because of the high morbidity and mortality associated with neonatal HSV, high doses of intravenous acyclovir is indicated, usually 45-60 mg/kg/day for at least 3 weeks. Despite high dose therapy, morbidity remains high in the neonate.

Prevention in HIV-infected persons: The following is a statement from the Centers for Disease Control and Prevention (CDC) regarding the prevention of HSV infection in persons with HIV infection:

Prevention of Exposure: HIV-infected persons should use latex condoms during every act of sexual intercourse to reduce the risk for exposure to herpes simplex virus (HSV) and to other sexually-transmitted pathogens. They should specifically avoid sexual contact when herpetic lesions (genital or orolabial) are evident.

Prevention of Disease: Prophylaxis of initial episodes of HSV disease is not recommended.

Prevention of Recurrence: Because acute episodes of HSV infection can be treated successfully, chronic therapy with acyclovir is not required after lesions resolve. However, persons who have frequent or severe recurrences can be administered daily suppressive therapy with oral acyclovir or famciclovir. Valacyclovir is also an option. Intravenous foscarnet or cidofovir can be used to treat infection due to acyclovir-resistant isolates of HSV, which are routinely resistant to ganciclovir as well.

Special Considerations:

Children: The recommendations for preventing initial disease and recurrence among adults and adolescents apply to children as well.

Pregnant Women: Oral acyclovir prophylaxis during late pregnancy is a controversial strategy recommended by some experts to prevent neonatal herpes transmission. However, such prophylaxis is not routinely recommended. For patients who have frequent, severe recurrences of genital HSV disease, acyclovir prophylaxis might be indicated. No pattern of adverse pregnancy outcomes has been reported after acyclovir exposures.

Drug Therapy

Recommended:

Acyclovir *on page 629*
Valacyclovir *on page 1140*
Famciclovir *on page 815*

Alternate:

Cidofovir *on page 740*
Foscarnet *on page 829*
Ganciclovir *on page 834*
Valganciclovir *on page 1143*

Selected Readings

Arao Y, Schmid DS, Pellett PE, et al, "Herpesviruses Beyond HSV-1 and -2," *Clin Microbiol Newslett*, 1999, 21(19):153-9.

Corey L, "Herpes Simplex Viruses," *Harrison's Principles of Internal Medicine*, 14th ed, Fauci AS, Braumwald E, Isselbacher KJ, et al, eds, New York, NY: McGraw-Hill, 1998, 1080-6.

Erlich KS, Mills J, Chatis P, et al, "Acyclovir-Resistant Herpes Simplex Virus Infections in Patients With the Acquired Immunodeficiency Syndrome," *N Engl J Med*, 1989, 320(5):293-6.

Field AK and Biron KK, ""The End of Innocence" Revisited: Resistance of Herpesvirus to Antiviral Drugs," *Clin Microbiol Rev*, 1994, 7(1):1-13.

Geers TA and Isada CM, "Update on Antiviral Therapy for Genital Herpes Infection," *Cleve Clin J Med*, 2000, 67(8):567-73.

Marcon MJ and Salamon D, "Traditional and Newer Approaches to Laboratory Diagnosis of Herpes Simplex Virus Infections," *Clin Microbiol Newslett*, 1997, 19(2):9-14.

"1999 USPHS/IDSA Guidelines for the Prevention of Opportunistic Infections in Persons Infected With Human Immunodeficiency Virus," *MMWR*, 1999, 48(RR-10):28-9.

Whitley RJ, Kimberlin DW, and Roizman B, "Herpes Simplex Viruses," *Clin Infect Dis*, 1998, 26(3):541-55.

Herpes Zoster *see* Varicella-Zoster Virus *on page 347*

Herpetic Keratitis *see* Herpes Simplex Virus *on page 172*

Herpetic Whitlow *see* Herpes Simplex Virus *on page 172*

HEV *see* Hepatitis E Virus *on page 171*

HHV-6 *see* Human Herpesvirus-6 *on page 180*

Histoplasma capsulatum

Related Information

Community-Acquired Pneumonia in Adults *on page 1278*
USPHS / IDSA Guidelines for the Prevention of Opportunistic Infections in Persons Infected With HIV *on page 1237*

Microbiology *Histoplasma capsulatum* is a dimorphic fungus. It differs from other pathogenic fungi in that it is primarily a parasite of the reticuloendothelial system and is rarely found extracellular.

In the mold form (usually in the environment and in laboratory culture), it has microconidia (2-6 μm) on short lateral branches or sessile on the sides of hyphae and large round to pyriform tuberculate macroconidia (8-14 μm). This mold form is found in the

(Continued)

Histoplasma capsulatum (Continued)

soil and grows best in humid, shady environments at modest temperatures. Bird droppings and bat guano facilitate its growth. The spores become airborne and are inhaled.

The yeast form (usually *in vivo*) may be seen in human infections by direct examination. The cells are ovoid, 1-2 μm by 3-3.5 μm, and proliferate in macrophages (and occasionally neutrophils) which can be seen intracellularly throughout the reticuloendothelial system including lymph nodes, bone marrow, spleen, liver, and adrenal glands.

Epidemiology Histoplasmosis is the most frequently diagnosed systemic fungal disease with approximately 500,000 cases per year in the United States. Endemic areas include the Mississippi and Ohio River Valleys, as well as some parts of Central America. Environmental sources include caves, chicken coops, bamboo canebrakes, bird roosts, school yards, prison grounds, decayed wood piles, dead trees, chimneys, and old buildings. Epidemics typically occur where contaminated soil is disturbed causing the spores to become airborne.

Clinical Syndromes

- **Asymptomatic:** Approximately 99% of all cases of histoplasmosis are asymptomatic and an incidental finding on autopsy or are seen as calcification on plain films of the lungs or spleen or noted as lymphadenopathy.
- **Acute histoplasmosis:** Typically presents as a flu-like syndrome with fever (95%), anorexia (85%), nonproductive cough (75%), and chest pain (75%). Retrosternal pain is a prominent feature and may be related to mediastinal adenopathy. Skin and joint involvement are more common in women. Physical exam is typically normal except for pulmonary crackles and adenopathy. Chest x-ray may reveal hilar and mediastinal adenopathy with or without patchy or diffuse infiltrates. Rarely, patients present with pericarditis with or without tamponade. This syndrome is typically self-limited, lasting approximately 2 weeks.
- **Histoplasmomas:** Granulomatous nodules form on the lungs, usually in the lower lobes and <3 cm. Usually associated with hilar lymph node calcification, and 75% are found to be solitary lesions.
- **Acute pulmonary histoplasmosis:** Self-limited interstitial pneumonitis.
- **Chronic histoplasmosis:** Chronic pulmonary disorder that typically occurs in older patients with emphysema. Mimics tuberculosis. Referred to as the "marching cavity" because, in >50% of the cases, the walls of the lung cavity gradually enlarge.
- **Mediastinal histoplasmosis:** Approximately 25% of patients who develop this syndrome present with SVC syndrome, pulmonary vessel or esophageal or large airway obstruction, which may require surgical intervention. Rarely, associated with fibrosing mediastinitis.
- **Disseminated:** Defined as extrapulmonic spread with progressive clinical illness (ie, intestinal or oral ulcers, endocarditis, adrenal involvement). Both reactivation of previously acquired infections and newly acquired infections can occur in immunocompromised individuals. Classified as an AIDS-defining illness. Ten percent to 20% of all HIV-infected patients with disseminated histoplasmosis experience a rapid, fulminant course of the infection with findings of hypotension, respiratory insufficiency, multiple end-organ failure, disseminated intravascular coagulation, and mental status changes. In the remainder of patients, the disease can be more chronic, manifesting as fever, weight loss, dry cough, hepatomegaly, splenomegaly, and lymphadenopathy. Approximately 10% of AIDS patients with disseminated histoplasmosis have nonspecific skin manifestations. The chest radiographic findings of disseminated histoplasmosis in AIDS patients are varied and nonspecific. Over 50% of AIDS patients with disseminated histoplasmosis will have normal chest radiographs. Unusual manifestations of disseminated histoplasmosis including chorioretinitis, meningitis, and brain abscesses have been observed in patients with HIV disease. Since the presence of CNS disease may influence the choice of antifungal therapy, a brain imaging study should be performed in AIDS patients with disseminated histoplasmosis and symptoms indicating possible CNS involvement.

Diagnosis Direct examination and isolation in culture is the preferred diagnostic procedure.

A *Histoplasma* antigen test (enzyme immunoassay) is an extremely useful clinical laboratory test offered by MiraVista Diagnostics (Indianapolis, IN; 866-647-2847) and should be considered in cases of suspected histoplasmosis.

Skin tests are usually not helpful. Over 50% of the population in endemic areas may have positive skin tests. Approximately 50% of patients that have disseminated diseases may have negative skin tests secondary to impaired immunity. False-positive skin tests may occur secondary to other systemic fungal diseases.

Similar results are found with the complement fixation tests, however, a fourfold rise in titer is significant.

Diagnostic Tests/Procedures

Fungal Serology *on page 458*
Fungus Culture, Appropriate Site *on page 461*
Histoplasma capsulatum Antigen Assay *on page 497*
Histoplasmosis Serology *on page 498*
KOH Preparation *on page 513*

Treatment No antifungal treatment is necessary for mild or asymptomatic histoplasmosis. Acute, nondisseminated disease is self-limited and requires only symptomatic care unless it persists for more than one month, at which time itraconazole may be initiated. Heavy exposure, acute diffuse pulmonary involvement with respiratory insufficiency, and disseminated disease require treatment with amphotericin B.

AIDS patients with moderate to severe disseminated histoplasmosis should be treated with a 12-week "induction" of antifungal therapy. If the patient is hospitalized, an amphotericin B product should be initiated followed by itraconazole when tolerated. Outpatients can receive an itraconazole induction with itraconazole 300 mg twice daily for 3 days then 200 mg twice daily for 12 weeks followed by chronic suppressive therapy with itraconazole 200-400 mg/day.

High-dose fluconazole, 800 mg/day, is associated with a higher relapse rate compared with itraconazole.

Life-long suppressive therapy is recommended in HIV-infected individuals due to the high frequency of relapse. Relapse rates of 50% to 90% have been reported in AIDS patients with disseminated histoplasmosis who have not received any maintenance therapy. Infusions of amphotericin B (50-80 mg weekly or biweekly) prevent relapse. Oral itraconazole is the preferred drug of choice for chronic suppressive therapy for histoplasmosis. Fluconazole 200-400 mg/day orally appears to be somewhat less effective than itraconazole as long-term suppressive therapy but may be used in patients who are unable to tolerate or absorb itraconazole.

Drug Therapy

Recommended:

Severe infection:

Amphotericin B (Conventional) *on page 650*

Chronic pulmonary infection in immunocompetent hosts:

Ketoconazole *on page 903*
Itraconazole *on page 895*

Alternate:

Mild infection:

Fluconazole *on page 819*

Severe infection:

Amphotericin B (Lipid Complex) *on page 653*

Selected Readings

Kahi CJ, Wheat LJ, Allen SD, et al, "Gastrointestinal Histoplasmosis," *Am J Gastroenterol*, 2005, 100(1):220-31.
Moser SA, "Laboratory Diagnosis of Histoplasmosis," *Clin Microbiol Newslett*, 1999, 21(12):95-100.
Sobel JD, "Practice Guidelines for the Treatment of Fungal Infections. For the Mycoses Study Group. Infectious Diseases Society of America," *Clin Infect Dis*, 2000, 30(4):652.
Thompson GR 3rd, LaValle CE 3rd, and Everett ED, "Unusual Manifestations of Histoplasmosis," *Diagn Microbiol Infect Dis*, 2004, 50(1):33-41.
Tom S and Dharmadhikari A, "Disseminated Histoplasmosis," *Am J Hematol*, 2002, 71(3):223.
Wheat J, Hafner R, Korzun AH, et al, "Itraconazole Treatment of Disseminated Histoplasmosis in Patients With the Acquired Immunodeficiency Syndrome. AIDS Clinical Trial Group," *Am J Med*, 1995, 98(4):336-42.
Wheat JL, "Current Diagnosis of Histoplasmosis," *Trends Microbiol*, 2003, 11(10):488-94.
Wheat J, Sarosi G, McKinsey D, et al, "Practice Guidelines for the Management of Patients With Histoplasmosis," *Clin Infect Dis*, 2000, 30(4):688-95.
Wheat LJ and Kauffman CA, "Histoplasmosis," *Infect Dis Clin North Am*, 2003, 17(1):1-19.
Wheat LJ, Musial CE, and Jenny-Avital E, "Diagnosis and Management of Central Nervous System Histoplasmosis," *Clin Infect Dis*, 2005, 40(6):844-52.

Histoplasmosis *see Histoplasma capsulatum on page 177*
HIV *see* Human Immunodeficiency Virus *on page 181*
HLTV-I *see* Human T-Cell Lymphotropic Viruses *on page 192*
Hookworm *see Ancylostoma duodenale on page 34*
Hospital-Acquired Pneumonia *see* Pneumonia, Hospital-Acquired *on page 272*
Hospital-Acquired Sinusitis *see* Sinusitis, Hospital-Acquired *on page 300*
HPV *see* Human Papillomavirus *on page 191*
HSV *see* Herpes Simplex Virus *on page 172*
HTLV-II *see* Human T-Cell Lymphotropic Viruses *on page 192*
HTLV-III *see* Human Immunodeficiency Virus *on page 181*

Human CMV *see* Cytomegalovirus *on page 107*

Human Herpesvirus-6

Synonyms HHV-6

Microbiology In 1986, a novel cytopathic virus was isolated from peripheral blood cells from patients with lymphoproliferative disease. The virus was originally named human β-lymphotropic virus because of its ability to infect B cells *in vitro* but later was found to be tropic for primarily T lymphocytes. It has since been classified as one of the human herpesviruses. It is a double-stranded DNA virus with an icosahedral capsid and outer envelope. HHV-6 is indistinguishable from other herpesviruses by electron microscopy, with the same morphology and size. In addition to its T-lymphocyte tropism, HHV-6 can infect B cells, monocytes, macrophages, and other cell lines. $CD4^+$ T cells, in particular, are targets for viral infection. The genome has been analyzed and sequenced for research purposes. A close homology between HHV-6 DNA and cytomegalovirus DNA has been found. The degree of relatedness of these two viruses remains to be seen since the gene products of HHV-6 are still being studied. There appear to be two general types of HHV-6, types A and B. The clinical significance of these two types is unknown, although most clinical isolates are type B.

Epidemiology Knowledge of the epidemiology of HHV-6 is still evolving. Much of the epidemiologic data for this virus will rest on the use of specific serologic tests. Unfortunately, serologic techniques are still being developed and have yet to be standardized. Earlier use of an immunofluorescence assay for antibody detection has been criticized on technical grounds and is probably too insensitive. To date there is no accepted gold standard for serologic tests and "borderline" positive specimens are difficult to interpret.

Available data indicate that HHV-6 infection occurs at an early age, between 6 months and 3 years most commonly. The seroprevalence is about 80% in the general population. It is likely to be as common as other herpesvirus infections. Newborns have a high level of antibody, probably from passive transfer from the mother. The titer of antibody rapidly decreases in the neonate as maternal antibody is lost; this is followed later by a second peak of antibody signifying primary infection in childhood.

Preliminary data suggest that asymptomatic HHV-6 shedding occurs in seropositive individuals. The virus has been isolated from the saliva of healthy children and adults who have had prior HHV-6 infection. Asymptomatic salivary excretion in the general population has been hypothesized as the main reservoir of the virus in the community and potentially could explain the large number of children who become infected. Initial studies reported very high salivary excretion rates, but later studies failed to confirm these results. Some experts have been critical of the methodologies employed in the earlier studies, suggesting that some of the viral isolates could have been HHV-7 rather than HHV-6. At the present time, it is clear that salivary excretion does take place, but the precise incidence is still debatable.

The mechanism(s) of HHV-6 transmission have not been definitively established. It is also unclear whether the virus can be transmitted by transfusion of blood products or by transplantation of organs.

Clinical Syndromes

- **Exanthem subitum (roseola):** Also known as roseola infantum, exanthem subitum is a benign disease of childhood that is caused by HHV-6. The disease is most common in children aged 6 months to 3 years old. In typical cases, there is an abrupt onset of high fever (often 40°C), and in a variable number of cases there may be additional symptoms such as sore throat, otitis, or cervical adenopathy. After 3-5 days, the fever resolves completely. This is followed 24-48 hours later by a maculopapular rash involving the trunk and neck. Although the rash itself is nonspecific in appearance, the timing of the rash is distinctive for roseola. The rash also resolves spontaneously after several days. Roseola is nearly always a benign disease. More serious complications of acute HHV-6 infection have been described (meningoencephalitis, hepatitis). During the febrile phase of exanthem subitum, HHV-6 can be cultured from peripheral blood mononuclear cells. Seroconversion can also be documented.
- **Undifferentiated febrile illness:** Primary HHV-6 infection appears to be a common, identifiable cause of high fevers in children. In a recent study, 14% of children who presented to an emergency room for evaluation of fever were found to have HHV-6 viremia. Of note, the rash of classic roseola was absent in many children, and the most common presentation was irritability, inflamed tympanic membranes, and temperatures higher than 40°C. Although the full range of HHV-6 infection has yet to be determined, it is likely that many primary infections are either nonspecific, febrile syndromes or entirely asymptomatic.
- **HHV-6 in adults:** Primary infection with HHV-6 is probably uncommon in adults. The clinical course of such infections have been described in small numbers of adults with documented seroconversion. Symptoms included fever, headache, and

fever lasting over 1 week. Cervical lymphadenopathy was noted in several cases and was persistent for months. Laboratory abnormalities included a minor elevation in liver function tests, leukopenia, and atypical lymphocytosis. Latent HHV-6 infection appears to take place following primary infection, as with other herpesviruses. Reactivation has also been reported in adults. Little is known about the incidence or mechanisms underlying either latency or reactivation.

- **HHV-6 in immunocompromised hosts:** The role of HHV-6 in transplant recipients is still largely unknown. The following observations have been made: (1) Many individuals are seropositive for HHV-6 prior to transplantation. (2) An increase in specific antibody against HHV-6 is commonly seen after transplantation. Viremia with HHV-6 also appears to be common at 2-3 weeks post-transplantation, earlier than the peak for cytomegalovirus. The importance of these findings has yet to be determined. (3) Primary infection with cytomegalovirus in the transplant patient is often associated with a significant rise in HHV-6 antibodies. The significance of this simultaneous seroconversion is unclear. (4) Some kidney biopsy specimens which have demonstrated acute rejection have stained positive for HHV-6. The relationship between HHV-6 and acute rejection is unknown.

HHV-6 has also been implicated by some as a possible cofactor in HIV infection. This is based on several observations, including the mutual tropism for the host's $CD4^+$ T lymphocytes. Whether HHV-6 alters the natural course of HIV infection is still under study.

Diagnosis Viral isolation can be performed in specialized laboratories. HHV-6 can be cultured in peripheral blood mononuclear cells (with or without the addition of donor cells). Standard tissue culture used for isolation of other viruses is suboptimal for HHV-6. Even under optimal conditions, the cytopathic effect of HHV-6 in peripheral blood mononuclear cells can be subtle; multiple passages of the virus in culture may be necessary. Detection methods are then necessary to confirm the presence of this virus.

HHV-6 has been isolated from clinical samples of saliva and blood. Antigen detection methods, while still being perfected, have been used to identify the virus directly from biopsy samples. Polymerase chain reaction has been used successfully in limited reports. A serologic test has recently become available.

Diagnostic Tests/Procedures

Human Herpesvirus 6, IgG and IgM Antibodies, Quantitative *on page 506*

Treatment Most infections caused by HHV-6 are mild and self-limiting. Susceptibility to antiviral agents are probably similar to CMV, where acyclovir only inhibits the organism at high concentrations. Ganciclovir has been shown to inhibit HHV-6 at achievable concentrations, although this data is inconsistent.

Drug Therapy Comment No drug therapy is recommended.

Selected Readings

Agbede O, "Human Herpesvirus 6: A Virus in Search of a Disease," *Clin Microbiol Newslett*, 1993, 15(4):25-28.

Chou S, "Human Herpesvirus 6 Infection and Associated Disease," *J Lab Clin Med*, 1993, 121(3):388-93.

Pruksananonda P, Hall CB, Insel RA, et al, "Primary Human Herpesvirus-6 Infection in Young Children," *N Engl J Med*, 1992, 326(22):1445-50.

Rathore MH, "Human Herpesvirus 6," *South Med J*, 1993, 1197-1205.

Yamanishi K, "Pathogenesis of Human Herpesvirus 6 (HHV-6)," *Infect Agents Dis*, 1992, 1(3):149-55.

Human Immunodeficiency Virus

Related Information

Antiretroviral Agents *on page 1206*

Antiretroviral Therapy for HIV Infection *on page 1219*

Management of Healthcare Worker Exposures to HBV, HCV, and HIV *on page 1227*

Prevention of Perinatal HIV-1 Transmission *on page 1235*

Synonyms AIDS Virus; HIV; HTLV-III; Human T-Cell Lymphotropic Virus

Microbiology HIV is a human retrovirus composed of two copies of single-stranded RNA (SSRNA). There are two human immunodeficiency viruses, HIV-1 and HIV-2. The predominant cause of AIDS is from HIV-1. HIV-2 is less common and is more restricted to West Africa. The virus particle consists of (1) a core particle containing the SSRNA genome and other important viral proteins, and (2) an outer lipid envelope containing the important glycoproteins gp120 (which forms "spikes" and has an affinity for the $CD4^+$ molecule) and the transmembrane gp41. The life cycle of HIV begins when the gp120 protein on the virus envelope binds to the CD4 molecule found on the surface of a human host cell. This CD4 molecule is a protein found mainly on a group of T-lymphocytes called "T-helper" cells. The CD4 molecule is also found on other cells including some macrophages and monocytes.

Recent research has uncovered the role of at least 2 coreceptors for HIV-1 on the host cell surface that are necessary for the fusion and entry of the viral RNA. Normally

(Continued)

Human Immunodeficiency Virus *(Continued)*

these coreceptors function as receptors for chemoattractant cytokines and thus have been called chemokines. These include:

- CCR-5, which is expressed by monocytes and lymphocytes. This chemokine allows entry of certain strains of HIV called nonsyncytium-inducing (NSI) strains.
- CXCR-4, also known as Fusin. This is found only on T-lymphocytes and allows entry of syncytium-inducing (SI) strains of HIV.

The identification of these chemokines has helped explain why some individuals at high risk for HIV infection remain uninfected despite multiple sexual exposures to HIV. About 13% of individuals of Northern European descent have a mutation in one of their two CCR-5 genes; this results in a missing 32 amino acid segment from half of their CCR-5 receptors. Approximately 1% to 2% of Caucasians are homozygous for this deletion. *In vitro*, the peripheral blood mononuclear cells of those persons with the homozygous allele resist entry of NSI strains of HIV.

After binding of the viral gp120 to CD4 and to either CCR5 or CXCR4, the viral gp41 fuses to the host cell membrane, and the viral RNA is injected into the cell's cytoplasm. The next step, reverse transcription, is critical for infection and is the site where several drugs act. The enzyme reverse transcriptase (contained in the original viral particle) transcribes the single-stranded viral RNA into double-stranded DNA. This HIV DNA is then transported into the nucleus of the host cell where it is incorporated into the host chromosome in a process ordinated by the viral integrase enzyme and thus is aptly termed integration. This integrated DNA is called a provirus, and remains there for the life of the cell. Over the course of the life of the cell, the provirus may remain latent (does not produce any products) or may produce high levels of active virus. The factors that mediate the transcription of the provirus are complex. When transcription of the proviral DNA occurs in an activated cell, the products are either genomic RNA or messenger RNA (mRNA). The mRNA is translated into the HIV structural proteins and enzymes. The gag gene codes for the structural proteins in the viral core (eg, p24 antigen); the pol gene codes for the three enzymes that serve as targets for clinical therapeutic strategies: reverse transcriptase, protease, and integrase enzymes. The env gene codes for the envelope glycoproteins (eg, gp120 and gp41). A number of other genes are present which are important in HIV expression. The protease enzyme cuts and modifies the other translated HIV proteins into mature and functioning structural proteins and enzymes. The HIV genomic RNA, along with the translated proteins, and enzymes are packaged into the viral core and envelope and begin exiting the host cell in a process called budding.

Epidemiology HIV is now the fifth leading cause of death of men aged 25-40, the first leading cause of death among African-American men aged 25-40, and the third leading cause of death in African-American women 25-44 years of age. It is estimated that over 2.4 million residents in the Americas including 1 million U.S. residents are HIV infected. The Carribean is the second most highly affected region in the world after sub-Saharan Africa. As of 2001, over 60 million individuals have been infected with HIV and approximately 3 million died in the year 2001 alone. There are approximately 40 million individuals in the world living with HIV/AIDS currently. It is estimated that in the years 2000-2020, 68 million individuals will die prematurely due to AIDS.

Approximately 50% of newly diagnosed cases of HIV in the U.S. are transmitted via men who have sex with men. HIV secondary to I.V. drug use and heterosexual transmission continues to rise in the United States. Since 1985, the proportion of all AIDS cases reported among adult and adolescent women has more than tripled, from 7% in 1985 to 25% in 1999. Minorities account for a disproportionate amount of AIDS as expected by population statistics.

Clinical Syndromes Infection with HIV results in a decline in the $CD4^+$ group of T-lymphocytes, the main targets of viral infection. These $CD4^+$-bearing T-lymphocytes are also called T-helper or T-inducer cells. Many other cells besides T-helper cells have the CD4 molecule and these are also at risk for HIV binding and infection. The $CD4^+$ T-cells decrease in total number but it is clear that the remaining cells are also dysfunctional. The precise mechanism(s) which cause $CD4^+$ T-cell depletion are still under study. When the number of $CD4^+$ cells declines below a certain level, the patient becomes at risk for unusual (opportunistic) infections and certain neoplasms which are the hallmark of AIDS.

The clinical course of an HIV-infected individual is divided into two phases: (1) Primary or acute infection and (2) chronic or established infection which can be divided into two categories: asymptomatic and symptomatic.

Primary infection: This refers to the time when an individual is initially infected with HIV. In many cases, the primary infection is asymptomatic, and others may experience a mild fever. In up to 50% of individuals, the primary infection is more dramatic and referred to as the acute HIV syndrome and resembles infectious

mononucleosis. This occurs 3-6 weeks after exposure, and is associated with fevers, lymphadenopathy, malaise, and reactive lymphocytosis. Approximately 10% with have thrush. This correlates well with viremia. During primary infection, there is likely circulating virus which seeds a variety of organ systems, including the lymph nodes. The degree of viremia varies from person to person and the amount of virus present, the viral load, is very important in determining the course of events in later years. Since this is very early in the course of infection, the CD4 cell counts are normal (500-1000 cells/µL).

The immune responses following primary infection (and thereafter) are under intense study. It is known that following primary infection the amount of the virus in the blood begins to decline even before neutralizing antibodies develop. Thus, it is thought that some other immunologic mechanism other than neutralizing antibody brings about the initial control of viral infection. Several immunologic mechanisms play a role including the development of CD8 cytotoxic T-lymphocyte activity (CTL), and antibody-dependent cellular cytotoxicity (ADCC). Both CTL and ADCC appear early, before neutralizing antibody. There also appears to be a role for HIV-specific cell-mediated immunity early on, mediated by CD4 lymphocytes.

Chronic infection: Eventually a host immune response develops which helps to contain the virus and symptoms of primary infection (if any) resolve. The patient then enters the so-called "clinical latent phase," where the patient generally feels well and the majority of patients have little or no symptoms (thus the term "latent phase"). In the 1980s and early 1990s, this (erroneous) notion of a latent viral infection was based on several observations including an inability to culture HIV from the blood, negative p24 antigen tests, and stable CD4 counts for years. It was assumed that few cells produce HIV and that viral replication was restricted during the period of clinical latency (a theory later proven false). Only very few cells contain the HIV provirus (about 1 in 10,000 cells) and even fewer are expressing HIV mRNA. Nevertheless, in the majority of patients there is a progressive decrease in the number of $CD4^+$ T-cells, which occurs at a variable rate. Patients can be divided into an early asymptomatic phase with T-cells >500 and an intermediate stage with T-cells between 200 and 500. The length of the asymptomatic stage is variable, but on the average is about 10 years. Some individuals with high levels of circulating virus progress more quickly (rapid progressors), with development of AIDS within 18 months. A small number of patients do not appear to progress (long-term nonprogressors) and maintain CD4 lymphocyte counts in the normal range for 15 or more years. The precise reason for this is unclear and appears to be related to genetic factors of the host and/or variations in the HIV strains. For the majority of patients, the CD4 T-cells decline from 500-1000 cells/µL to 200 cells over a number of years.

Symptomatic disease: When the CD4 cells are ≤200, the risk for opportunistic infections and AIDS-related cancers increases significantly and the well-known complications such as *Pneumocystis jiroveci* (formerly *carinii*) pneumonia, cytomegalovirus retinitis, etc, become more common.

New research has led to advances in the understanding of viral dynamics during all phases of HIV infection. Several factors led to the abandonment of a "latent virus" model, including the development of quantitative HIV PCR which showed that HIV replicates at all stages of the infection. Using a mathematical model, the life span of HIV appears quite short, with a viral half-life of around 6 hours. Even at a normal CD4 cell count up to 10 billion new virus particles are produced each day. Over 50% of the viral population in plasma is turned over within hours. About 99% of HIV viremia is sustained by ongoing infection of CD4 cells and subsequent release of new viral particles. These findings have important implications for drug therapy, since HIV has a strong tendency to mutate with each replicative cycle; thus, this can lead to many "quasi species" and to drug resistant mutants. Similarly, the half-life of CD4 cells which are infected is also very short, 1.5 days. Several billion CD4 cells are destroyed each day. This occurs even if the measurable CD4 count appears to be stable in a given patient. This is at a high cost, since the body has to make up a tremendous number of new CD4 cells per day.

With the advent of quantitative HIV PCR and branched-chain assay (HIV-1 RNA Quantitative bDNA) for HIV, the amount of circulating virus, or viral load, can now be measured directly from plasma. One caveat is that lymphocytes in the peripheral blood represent only a small fraction (about 2%) of all the lymphocytes in the body. Recent studies have looked carefully at the viral load of patients immediately following their primary infection with HIV. Within days of infection, HIV replication is enormous with plasma HIV levels of ≥1,000,000 copies/mL. Within 3-6 weeks, the immune system partially contains the infection and reduces viral replication to a set point. At the set point, the amount of virus produced equals

(Continued)

Human Immunodeficiency Virus *(Continued)*

the amount which is cleared. This appears to be a unique number for each individual, but ranges widely from person to person. Commonly, the set point ranges between 10^2-10^5 copies/mL. Data from the Multicenter AIDS Cohort Study (MACS) has shown that the level of the set point determines the rate of disease progression. Patients with a high set point progress to an AIDS-defining event more quickly than those with a low set point. Patients with a viral load <5000 copies/mL had the lowest risk of progression; those with a viral load of 30,000-50,000 had the highest risk of progression. The viral load is an independent predictor of HIV disease progression, independent of CD4. The plasma HIV RNA levels indicate the magnitude of HIV replication and its associated rate of CD4 T-cell destruction, while the CD4 count indicates the extent of immune system damage.

The plasma viral load reflects the extent of total virus replication with reasonable accuracy. It correlates with RNA levels in lymph nodes (the major sites of viral replication) and correlates with the number of acutely infected cells. Virus is released from lymph nodes (the major reservoir) into the peripheral circulation where it is measurable by the assay, but it is unclear if other compartments have significant communication with the plasma (such as the central nervous system). "Ultrasensitive" viral load assays are now available and can detect down to 50 copies/mL of virus.

There is also a dynamic associated with CD4 T-cells, in that there is heightened production and destruction of cells even though the numeric level appears constant. The majority of CD4 T-cells are in lymphoid organs, not peripheral blood lymphocytes. A subclass of CD4 cells called memory CD4 cells are known to be preferential targets of the virus. These cells are lost even before there is a measurable fall in the total CD4 counts. Studies have shown that the greater the baseline viral load, the greater the rate of decline of the CD4 count depending on the fitness of the virus.

Please see the Treatment of AIDS Wasting *on page 1205* and USPHS/IDSA Guidelines for the Prevention of Opportunistic Infections in Persons Infected With HIV *on page 1237* in the Appendix for further information.

Prognostic Value of Viral RNA Counts

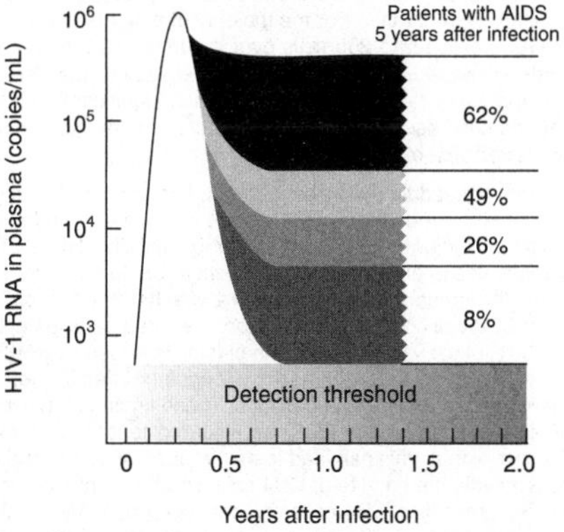

From Ho DD, "Viral Counts Count in HIV Infection," *Science*, 272 (5265):1124-5.

Diagnosis Is made serologically. Detection of HIV antibody by ELISA must be confirmed by Western blot. Alternate diagnosis may be made by viral culture, antigen detection, or HIV by polymerase chain reaction (PCR). Maternal antibodies may persist in infants until 18 months of age; therefore, CD4 counts, viral culture, and/or PCR followed by antibody detection after 18 months must be performed in order to diagnose HIV in infants.

Serial plasma HIV RNA testing is now a standard of care, both for patients receiving antiretroviral therapy and those who are being observed off therapy. See table 1 on page 188.

Note: Tables 1-3 are adapted from "Guidelines for Using Antiretroviral Agents Among HIV-1-Infected Adults and Adolescents. Recommendations of the Panel on Clinical Practices for Treatment of HIV," April 7, 2005, available at www.aidsinfo.nih.gov.

Surrogate End Points Reflect Clinical Course

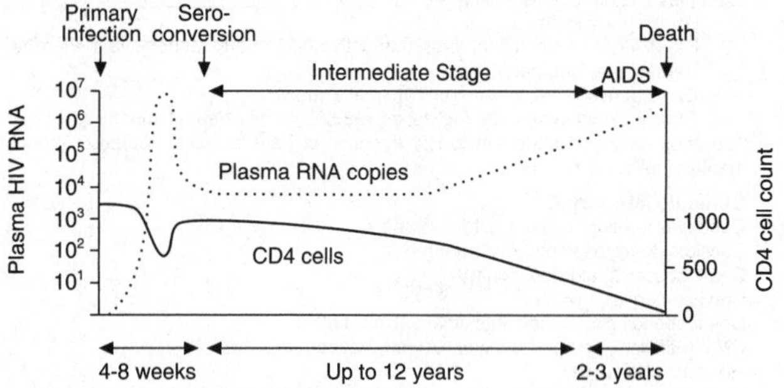

Adapted from Piatak M Jr, et al, *Science*, 1993, 259:1749-53 and Weiss RA, *Science*, 1993, 260:1273-9.

1993 Revised CDC HIV Classification System and Expanded AIDS Surveillance Definition for Adolescents and Adults (*MMWR Morb Mortal Wkly Rep*, 1992, 41:RR-17.)

The revised system emphasizes the importance of CD4-lymphocyte testing in clinical management of HIV-infected persons. The system is based on three ranges of CD4 counts and four clinical categories giving a matrix of nine exclusive categories. The system replaces the 1986 classification.

Criteria for HIV Infection

Persons 13 years of age or older with repeatedly (2 or more) reactive screening tests (ELISA) plus specific antibodies identified by a supplemental test, eg, Western blot ["reactive" pattern = positive for any two of p24, gp41, or gp120/160 (*MMWR*,1991, 40:681)]. Other specific methods of diagnosis of HIV-1 include virus isolation, antigen detection, and detection of HIV genetic material by PCR.

Classification System

CD4 Cell[2] Category	Clinical Category[1]		
	A	B	C
≥500/mm^3	A1	B1	*C1*
200-499/mm^3	A2	B2	*C2*
<200/mm^3	*A3*	*B3*	*C3*

[1]See following clinical definitions. Italics indicate expansion of AIDS surveillance definition. Category C currently "reportable." Categories A3 and B3 are "reportable" as AIDS effective January 1, 1993.

[2]There is a diurnal variation in CD4 counts averaging 60/mm^3 higher in the afternoon in HIV-positive individuals and 500/mm^3 in HIV-negative persons. Blood for sequential CD4 counts should be drawn at about the same time of day each time (*J AIDS*, 1990, 3:144). The equivalence between CD4 counts and CD4 % of total lymphocytes: ≥500 = ≥29%, 200-499 = 14%-28%, <200 = <14%.

Diagnostic Tests/Procedures

HIV Genotyping *on page 503*
HIV-1 RNA, Quantitative bDNA, 3rd Generation *on page 499*
HIV-1 RNA, Quantitative PCR, 2nd Generation *on page 500*
HIV-1 Serology *on page 501*
Human Immunodeficiency Virus Culture *on page 506*
p24 Antigen *on page 555*
T4/T8 Ratio *on page 590*
Lymphocyte Subset Panels *on page 531*
(Continued)

Human Immunodeficiency Virus *(Continued)*

Clinical Category A
Asymptomatic HIV infection
Persistent generalized lymphadenopathy (PGL)[1]
Acute (primary) HIV illness

Clinical Category B
Symptomatic, not A or C conditions
Examples include but not limited to:
- Bacillary angiomatosis
- Candidiasis, vulvovaginal: persistent >1 month, poorly responsive to therapy
- Candidiasis, oropharyngeal
- Cervical dysplasia, severe, or carcinoma *in situ*
- Constitutional symptoms (eg, fever >38.5°C or diarrhea >1 month)

The above must be attributed to HIV infection or have aclinical course or management complicated by HIV.

Clinical Category C[2]
Candidiasis: esophageal, trachea, bronchi
Coccidioidomycosis, extrapulmonary
Cryptococcosis, extrapulmonary
Cervical cancer, invasive[2]
Cryptosporidiosis, chronic intestinal (>1 month)
CMV retinitis, or other than liver, spleen, nodes
HIV encephalopathy
Herpes simplex with mucocutaneous ulcer >1 month, bronchitis, pneumonia
Histoplasmosis: disseminated, extrapulmonary
Isosporiasis, chronic (>1 month)
Kaposi's sarcoma
Lymphoma: Burkitt's, immunoblastic, primary in brain
M. avium or *M. kansasii*, extrapulmonary
M. tuberculosis,[2] pulmonary or extrapulmonary
Mycobacterium, other species disseminated or extrapulmonary
Pneumocystis jiroveci (formerly *carinii*) pneumonia
Pneumonia,[2] recurrent (≥2 episodes in 1 year)
Progressive multifocal leukoencephalopathy
Salmonella bacteremia, recurrent
Toxoplasmosis, cerebral
Wasting syndrome due to HIV

[1]Nodes in two more extrainguinal sites, at least 1 cm in diameter for ≥3 months.
[2]These are the 1987 CDC case definitions (*MMWR*, 1987, 36:15). The 1993 CDC *Expanded Surveillance Case Definition* includes all conditions contained in the 1987 definition (above) plus persons with documented HIV infection and any of the following: (1) CD4 T-lymphocyte count <200/mm^3 (or CD4 <14%), (2) pulmonary-tuberculosis, (3) recurrent pneumonia (≥2 episodes within 1 year) or, (4) invasive cervical carcinoma.

Treatment Current drugs only prevent infection of new cells and do not alter already infected cells.

There are 4 major classes of antiretrovirals: Nucleoside and nucleotide reverse transcriptase inhibitors (NRTIs), non-nucleoside RTIs (NNRTIs), protease inhibitors (PIs), and fusion inhibitors (investigational).

Drug-drug interactions: There are a number of important drug-drug interactions between antiretroviral agents and other medications. See Antiretroviral Agents *on page 1206* in the Appendix for further information.

When to initiate antiretroviral therapy: The issue of when to begin HAART remains controversial. Some feel that all patients with HIV deserve antiviral therapy regardless of stage of disease and viral load, where others feel there may be a group in whom therapy may be delayed. Potential benefits for early treatment include easier control of viral replication and mutations, preservation of immune function, delayed progression to AIDS, and possibly less risk of drug toxicity. Risks of early therapy include earlier development of drug resistance, unknown long-term drug toxicities, limited choices of future antiretrovirals, and reduced quality of life. See table 2 on page 188.

Initial treatment regimens: See table 3 on page 189.

Clinical response to HAART and drug failure: Although dramatic responses have been reported with HAART, it is clear that not all patients respond virologically. Several recent studies have shown a variable success rate; in general, 30% to 60% of patients have still shown a detectable viral load after 12 months of combination antiretrovirals. It also appears that the durability of response to drug therapy can be predicted by the viral load nadir; that is, the time to viral rebound in patients who have been undetectable is markedly longer than in patients who failed to achieve undetectable viral loads on HAART. Studies also show that decreases in HIV viral load as a result of therapy predict a better clinical outcome. One study showed that each 0.5 log reduction in HIV RNA from HAART was associated with a decrease in the risk of progression to AIDS by about 33%. Each 10% increase from baseline of the CD4 cells reduced the risk of progression by 18%, even accounting for the effects of the baseline plasma viral load and CD4 count.

However, not all failures are due to drug resistance. In one study by Mayers in 1997, a cross-section of patients failing therapy with high viral load and falling CD4 count were studied. Antiviral resistance studies showed that 21% of these drug failures had no mutation in either reverse transcriptase or protease. Additional observational studies of this nature are underway, but it appears that there is more wild type virus present than expected in patients with high viral loads while on HAART. Most, but not all, treatment failure is associated with drug resistance and perhaps 50% to 80% of drug failure is due to drug-resistant mutants.

There appears to be a number of reasons for drug failure including: (1) limited potency of available therapies, even in combination; (2) development of resistant variants; (3) subinhibitory drug levels, including nonadherence to therapy, poor absorption, rapid clearing, nonactivation within cells; and (4) host immune factors, especially CD4 function, cytotoxic T-lymphocyte activity, chemokines, and others. All of these factors lead to persistent viral replication, with evolution of drug resistance, which feeds back to more viral replication, in a vicious cycle.

When should therapy be changed?

The goal of antiretroviral therapy is suppression below detectable levels (currently <50 copies/mL) early enough to preserve immune function. Specific criteria for failure include reduction of <0.5 log in viral load at 4 weeks after initiation of HAART, or <1 log reduction by 8 weeks, or also, failure to suppress plasma viral load to undetectable within 4-6 months of initiating therapy. If a patient has been initially detectable, repeated detection of virus in the plasma is suggestive of resistance (although not necessarily drug resistance). The NIH consensus panel suggests a break through of 500-5000 copies/mL in a previously undetectable individual should be followed closely and their regimen not necessarily changed, although most often the plasma viremia continues to increase. Other criteria for considering a change in therapy include persistently declining CD4 counts and clinical deterioration.

Drug regimens for patients in whom antiretroviral therapy has failed are limited. In general, it is important to distinguish whether a regimen needs to be changed because of drug intolerance or virologic failure. If failure is due to drug intolerance, a one-for-one switch in medications may be considered. Otherwise, one principle of drug therapy is to always use at least 2 new drugs for a failing regimen, and if possible 3 new drugs.

Antiviral resistance: Resistance of HIV to antiretroviral agents is a complex and evolving field. Recent advances in understanding viral dynamics has shed new light on the factors influencing drug resistance. It is now known that the replication rate of HIV is about 10 billion new virions/day, even when patients are asymptomatic. Mutation rates are high, and with chronic antiretroviral therapy now the standard of care, there is tremendous selective pressure for the development of drug-resistant mutants. Factors which lead to drug resistance in HIV-infected persons include:

- high rates of viral production and turnover
- high spontaneous mutation rates
- mixed populations of virus
- multiple body compartments serving as reservoirs for virus
- relatively low antiviral efficacy of some drugs leading to suboptimal viral suppression
- need for continuous antiviral therapy
- immunosuppressed state of the host

A number of HIV genotype assays are commercially available for the detection of drug resistance. Please see HIV genotyping *on page 503* for further information.

(Continued)

Human Immunodeficiency Virus *(Continued)*

Table 1: Indications for Plasma HIV RNA Testing[1]

Clinical Indication	Information	Use
Syndrome consistent with acute HIV infection	Establishes diagnosis when HIV antibody test is negative or indeterminate	Diagnosis[2]
Initial evaluation of newly diagnosed HIV infection	Baseline viral load "set point"	Decision to start or defer therapy (in conjunction with $CD4^+$ T-cell counts)
Every 3-4 months in patients not on therapy	Changes in viral load	Decision to start therapy (in conjunction with $CD4^+$ T-cell counts)
2-8 weeks after initiation or change in antiretroviral therapy	Initial assessment of drug efficacy	Decision to continue or change therapy
3-4 months after start of therapy	Virologic effect of therapy	Decision to continue or change therapy
Every 3-4 months in patients on therapy	Durability of antiretroviral effect	Decision to continue or change therapy
Clinical event or significant decline in $CD4^+$ T cells	Association with changing or stable viral load	Decision to continue, initiate, or change therapy

[1]Acute illness (eg, bacterial pneumonia, tuberculosis, HSV, PCP) and immunizations can cause increases in plasma HIV RNA for 2-4 weeks; viral load testing should not be performed during this time. Plasma HIV RNA results should usually be verified with a repeat determination before starting or making changes in therapy.

[2]Diagnosis of HIV infection determined by HIV RNA testing should be confirmed by standard methods (eg, Western blot serology) performed 2-4 months after the initial indeterminate or negative test.

Table 2: Indications for the Initiation of Antiretroviral Therapy in the Chronically HIV-1 Infected Patient

Clinical Category	$CD4^+$ T-Cell Count	Plasma HIV RNA	Recommendation
AIDS-defining illness or severe symptoms[1]	Any value	Any value	Treat
Asymptomatic[2]	$CD4^+$ T cells $<200/mm^3$	Any value	Treat
Asymptomatic	$CD4^+$ T cells $>200/mm^3$ but $\leq 350/mm^3$	Any value	Treatment should be offered following full discussion of pros and cons with each patient
Asymptomatic	$CD4^+$ T cells $>350/mm^3$	$\geq 100,000$ copies/mL	Most clinicians recommend deferring therapy, but some clinicians will treat
Asymptomatic	$CD4^+$ T cells $>350/mm^3$	$<100,000$ copies/mL	Defer therapy

[1]AIDS-defining illness per Centers for Disease Control, 1993. Severe symptoms include unexplained fever or diarrhea >2-4 weeks, oral candidiasis, or >10% unexplained weight loss.

[2]Clinical benefit has been demonstrated in controlled trials only for patients with $CD4^+$ T cells $<200/mm^3$; however, the majority of clinicians would offer therapy at a $CD4^+$ T-cell threshold $<350/mm^3$. A collaborative analysis of data from 13 cohort studies from Europe and North America found that lower CD4 count, higher HIV viral load, injection drug use, and age >50 were all predictors of progression to AIDS or death in antiretroviral naive patients beginning combination antiretroviral therapy. These data indicate that the prognosis is better for patients who initiate therapy at >200 cells/mm^3, but risk after initiation of therapy does not vary considerably at >200 cells/mm^3.

Acute Retroviral Syndrome: Associated Signs and Symptoms (Expected Frequency)

- Fever (96%)
- Lymphadenopathy (74%)
- Pharyngitis (70%)
- Rash (70%)
  - Erythematous maculopapular with lesions on face and trunk and sometimes extremities, including palms and soles.
  - Mucocutaneous ulceration involving mouth, esophagus, or genitals.
- Myalgia or arthralgia (54%)
- Diarrhea (32%)
- Headache (32%)
- Nausea and vomiting (27%)
- Hepatosplenomegaly (14%)
- Weight loss (13%)

- Thrush (12%)
- Neurologic symptoms (12%)
  - Meningoencephalitis or aseptic meningitis
  - Peripheral neuropathy or radiculopathy
  - Facial palsy
  - Guillain-Barré syndrome
  - Brachial neuritis
  - Cognitive impairment or psychosis

Table 3: Antiretroviral Regimens Recommended for Treatment of HIV-1 Infection in Antiretroviral Naive Patients

Regimens should be individualized based on the advantages and disadvantages of each combination such as pill burden, dosing frequency, toxicities, drug-drug interaction potential, comorbid conditions, and level of plasma HIV-RNA. Preferred regimens are in bold type; regimens are designated as "preferred" for use in treatment-naive patients when clinical trial data suggest optimal and durable efficacy with acceptable tolerability and ease of use. Alternative regimens are those where clinical trial data show efficacy, but it is considered alternative due to disadvantages compared to the preferred agent, such as antiviral activity, durability, tolerability, drug interaction potential, or ease of use. In some cases, based on individual patient characteristics, a regimen listed as an alternative regimen in this table may actually be the preferred regimen for a selected patient. Clinicians initiating antiretroviral regimens in the HIV-1-infected pregnant patient should refer to "Recommendations for Use of Antiretroviral Drugs in Pregnant HIV-1-Infected Women for Maternal Health and Interventions to Reduce Perinatal HIV-1 Transmission in the United States," at **http://aidsinfo.nih.gov/guidelines**.

	Preferred Regimens
NNRTI-Based	**Efavirenz + (lamivudine or emtricitabine) + (zidovudine or tenofovir DF) [Note:** Efavirenz is not recommended for use in first trimester of pregnancy or in women with high pregnancy potential[1]]
PI-Based	**Lopinavir/ritonavir (coformulation) + (lamivudine or emtricitabine) + zidovudine**
	Alternative Regimens
NNRTI-Based	**Efavirenz** + (lamivudine or emtricitabine) + (abacavir or didanosine or stavudine) [**Note:** Efavirenz is not recommended for use in first trimester of pregnancy or in women with high pregnancy potential[1]]
	Nevirapine + (lamivudine or emtricitabine) + (zidovudine or stavudine or didanosine or abacavir or tenofovir) [**Note:** High incidence (11%) of symptomatic hepatic events was observed in women with pre-nevirapine $CD4^+$ T-cell counts >250 cells/mm^3 and men with $CD4^+$ T-cell counts >400 cells/mm^3 (6.3%). Nevirapine should not be initiated in these patients unless the benefit clearly outweighs the risk.]
PI-Based	**Atazanavir** + (lamivudine or emtricitabine) + (zidovudine or stavudine or abacavir or didanosine) or (tenofovir + ritonavir 100 mg/d)
	Fosamprenavir + (lamivudine or emtricitabine) + (zidovudine or stavudine or abacavir or tenofovir or didanosine)
	Fosamprenavir/ritonavir[2] + (lamivudine or emtricitabine) + (zidovudine or stavudine or abacavir or tenofovir or didanosine)
	Indinavir/ritonavir[2] + (lamivudine or emtricitabine) + (zidovudine or stavudine or abacavir or tenofovir or didanosine)
	Lopinavir/ritonavir + (lamivudine or emtricitabine) + (stavudine or abacavir or tenofovir or didanosine)
	Nelfinavir + (lamivudine or emtricitabine) + (zidovudine or stavudine or abacavir or tenofovir or didanosine)
	Saquinavir (soft or hard gel capsule or tablets)/**ritonavir**[2] + (lamivudine or emtricitabine) + (zidovudine or stavudine or abacavir or tenofovir or didanosine)
3 NRTI-Based	**Abacavir** + zidovudine + lamivudine – **only when a preferred or an alternative NNRTI- or a PI-based regimen cannot or should not be used**

[1]Women with childbearing potential implies women who want to conceive or those who are not using effective contraception.

[2]Low-dose (100-400 mg) ritonavir per day.

(Continued)

Human Immunodeficiency Virus *(Continued)*

Summary of Guidelines for Changing an Antiretroviral Regimen for Suspected Treatment Regimen Failure

Patient Assessment

- Review antiretroviral treatment history.
- Assess for evidence of clinical progression (eg, physical exam, laboratory and/or radiologic tests).
- Assess adherence, tolerability, and pharmacokinetic issues.
- Distinguish between limited, intermediate, and extensive prior therapy and drug resistance.
- Perform resistance testing while patient is taking therapy (or within 4 weeks after regimen discontinuation).
- Identify active drugs and drug classes to use in designing new regimen.

Patient Management: Specific Clinical Scenarios

- **Limited or intermediate prior treatment with low (but not suppressed) HIV RNA level (eg, <5000 copies/mL):** The goal of treatment is to resuppress HIV RNA to below level of assay detection. Consider intensifying with one drug (eg, tenofovir) or pharmacokinetic enhancement (use of ritonavir boosting of a protease inhibitor), perform resistance testing if possible, or most aggressively, change two or more drugs in the regimen. If continuing the same treatment regimen, HIV RNA levels should be followed closely because ongoing viral replication will lead to accumulation of additional resistance mutations.
- **Limited or intermediate prior treatment with resistance to one drug:** Consider changing the one drug, pharmacokinetic enhancement (few data available), or, most aggressively, change two or more drugs in the regimen.
- **Limited of intermediate prior treatment with resistance to more than one drug:** The goal of treatment is to suppress viremia to prevent further selection of resistance mutations. Consider optimizing the regimen by changing classes (eg, PI-based to NNRTI-based and vice versa) and/or adding new active drugs.
- **Prior treatment with no resistance identified:** Consider the timing of the drug resistance test (eg, was the patient off antiretroviral medications?) and/or nonadherence. Consider resuming the same regimen or starting a new regimen and then repeating genotypic testing early (eg, 2-4 weeks) to determine if a resistant virus becomes evident.
- **Extensive prior treatment and drug resistance:** It is reasonable to continue the same antiretroviral regimen if there are few or no treatment options. In general, avoid adding a single active drug because of the risk for the rapid development of resistance to that drug. In advanced HIV disease with a high likelihood of clinical progression (eg, CD4 cell count <100 cells/mm^3), adding a single drug may reduce the risk of immediate clinical progression. In this complicated scenario, expert advice should be sought.

Drug Therapy

Recommended:

Fusion inhibitor:
- Enfuvirtide *on page 802*

Protease inhibitor:
- Amprenavir *on page 662*
- Atazanavir *on page 668*
- Fosamprenavir *on page 827*
- Indinavir *on page 872*
- Lopinavir and Ritonavir *on page 919*
- Nelfinavir *on page 960*
- Ritonavir *on page 1055*
- Saquinavir *on page 1060*
- Tipranavir *on page 1120*

Reverse transcriptase inhibitor (non-nucleoside):
- Delavirdine *on page 769*
- Efavirenz *on page 795*
- Nevirapine *on page 967*

Reverse transcriptase inhibitor (nucleoside):
- Abacavir *on page 624*
- Abacavir, Lamivudine, and Zidovudine *on page 627*
- Didanosine *on page 774*
- Emtricitabine *on page 799*
- Emtricitabine and Tenofovir *on page 801*
- Lamivudine *on page 905*

Stavudine *on page 1076*
Zalcitabine *on page 1155*
Zidovudine *on page 1159*
Zidovudine and Lamivudine *on page 1162*

Reverse transcriptase inhibitor (nucleotide):
Tenofovir *on page 1095*

Selected Readings

Greene WC and Peterlin BM, "Charting HIV's Remarkable Voyage Through the Cell: Basic Science as a Passport to Future Therapy," *Nat Med*, 2002, 8(7):673-80.

"Guidelines for Using Antiretroviral Agents Among HIV-1-Infected Adults and Adolescents," updated April 7, 2005, available at www.aidsinfo.nih.gov.

"Guidelines for the Use of Antiretroviral Agents in Pediatric HIV Infection," available at www.aidsinfo.nih.gov.

Kaplan JE, Masur H, and Holmes KK, "Guidelines for Preventing Opportunistic Infections Among HIV-Infected Persons 2002. Recommendations of the U.S. Public Health Service and the Infectious Diseases Society of America," *MMWR Recomm Rep*, 2002, 51(RR-8):1-52.

"Public Health Service Task Force Recommendations for the Use of Antiretroviral Drugs in Pregnant HIV-1 Infected Women for Maternal Health and Interventions to Reduce Perinatal HIV-1 Transmission in the United States," available at www.aidsinfo.nih.gov.

Human Papillomavirus

Related Information

Treatment of Sexually Transmitted Infections *on page 1311*

Synonyms HPV

Microbiology Papillomaviruses are nonenveloped, 45-55 nm in diameter with an icosahedral capsid. The genetic material of papillomavirus consists of a double-stranded circular DNA genome of approximately 7900 bp. Over 77 types of papillomavirus have been identified based on DNA characterizations.

Epidemiology Close personal contact appears to be required for transmission, and minor trauma (such as cuts or abrasions) may be necessary at the site of inoculation. Anogenital infections are believed to be sexually transmitted, although young children may acquire genital warts from nongenital lesions via hand contact. Respiratory disease in neonates usually appears to be acquired during passage during delivery through the birth canal of an infected individual. However, some cases may be acquired in utero, leading to an early appearance of the disease.

Clinical Syndromes

- **Cutaneous:** Viral replication is associated with an excessive proliferation of epidermal cells, with the exception of the basal layer, resulting in the formation of hyperkeratotic papules with a rough surface.

  Cutaneous lesions occur most frequently on keratinized skin on the hands or feet, typically as a solitary lesion. Following excision, they rarely recur. They may reach a diameter of 1 cm. Cutaneous lesions are categorized into two broad types: Flat (superficial) or plantar (deep). These lesions may occur at a prevalence of between 4% and 20% among school-aged children. Spontaneous resolution over several years is common.

  Plantar warts are often painful, raised lesions affecting adolescents and young adults, often affecting the palms of the hands or soles of the feet. Shaving of the lesion reveals punctuate blood vessels, which distinguishes these lesions from callus.

  Juvenile, plane, or flat warts are papules which may be slightly elevated with a smooth surface and irregular contour, generally occurring on the face or neck. Laryngeal lesions are less common and are generally benign, except when they occur in children, since the growth may compromise airway function.
- **Anogenital (condyloma acuminatum):** Hyperkeratotic papules which are flesh or gray-colored and may vary from 1 millimeter to plaques covering several square centimeters (following merging of individual papules). Papules may have smooth surfaces or jagged growths. These lesions typically affect the squamous epithelia of the external genitalia. Involvement of the perianal area may occur, depending on sexual practices.

  Approximately 75% of patients are asymptomatic, although less commonly itching, burning, or pain may be reported. Condyloma acuminatum is the most common sexually transmitted disease in the United States.
- **Cervical dysplasia and neoplasia:** Although rare, neoplasia is the greatest concern for papillomavirus infection. Cervical cancer is greatly increased in the presence of high-risk papilloma lesions. The natural history of intraepithelial neoplasias has been established in cervical tissues, progressing from cervical epithelial neoplasia (CIN) grades I to III over a period of 1-4 years.

Diagnosis Clinical examination and, when appropriate colposcopy with acetic acid application. Molecular probes may be used to detect HPV DNA in cervical swabs/ tissues. Consensus guidelines on the terminology for reporting cervical cytology
(Continued)

Human Papillomavirus *(Continued)*

results as well as the management of women with cervical cytological abnormalities have been published (see Selected Readings).

Diagnostic Tests/Procedures

Pap smear

Treatment Cutaneous lesions may be removed by electrocautery, surgical cryotherapy, or chemical means. Vaccines are currently under investigation.

Selected Readings

Bosch FX, Lorincz A, Munoz N, et al, "The Causal Relation Between Human Papillomavirus and Cervical Cancer," *J Clin Pathol*, 2002, 55(4):244-65.

Jenkins D, "Diagnosing Human Papillomaviruses: Recent Advances," *Curr Opin Infect Dis*, 2001, 14(1):53-62.

Solomon D, Davey D, Kurman R, et al, "The 2001 Bethesda System: Terminology for Reporting Results of Cervical Cytology," *JAMA*, 2002, 287(16):2114-9.

Unger ER and Duarte-Franco E, "Human Papillomaviruses: Into the New Millennium," *Obstet Gynecol Clin North Am*, 2001, 28(4):653-66.

Wright TC Jr, Cox JT, Massad LS, et al, "2001 Consensus Guidelines for the Management of Women with Cervical Cytological Abnormalities," *JAMA*, 2002, 287(16):2120-9.

Human T-Cell Lymphotropic Virus *see* Human Immunodeficiency Virus *on page 181*

Human T-Cell Lymphotropic Viruses

Synonyms HLTV-I; HTLV-II

Microbiology Human retroviruses are members of the family Retroviridae: 100 nm, enveloped, single-strand RNA viruses which contain a reverse transcriptase used by the viruses to transcribe viral RNA into DNA. The newly formed DNA can integrate into host cell genome DNA. The family Retroviridae is composed of three genera: *Oncovirinae* (HTLV-I and -II), Lentivirinae (HIV-1 and HIV-2), and Spumavirinae (syncytial foamy viruses of cattle and cats). HTLV-I and -II are not related genetically, medically, or antigenically to HIV-1 and -2. However, the four viruses have similar routes of transmission and can have extremely long periods of latency prior to manifestation of disease. In addition, blood is screened for the presence of each of the four viruses.

Epidemiology HTLV-I is endemic in southern Japan (3% to 20%), the Carribean (2% to 5%), the U.S. Gulf Coast, and many other scattered populations throughout the world. Most of the persons infected with HTLV-I are asymptomatic. HTLV-II is endemic in some Native American populations in Florida and New Mexico but is detected mostly in intravenous drug users and their sexual partners. In the United States, seroprevalence of anti-HTLV in asymptomatic blood donors, and intravenous drug users and prostitutes is ~0.05% and 7% to 49%, respectively. Specific testing for separate antibodies to HTLV-I and HTLV-II is not routinely available, especially for large scale screening and epidemiological studies. HTLV-I and (probably) HTLV-II are transmitted transplacentally (extremely effective), parenterally (almost exclusively by sharing needles), by sexual contact (especially male to female), and by receipt of infected blood products.

Clinical Syndromes

- **Adult T-cell leukemia/lymphoma (ALT):** HTLV-I is the etiological agent of adult T-cell leukemia/lymphoma (ATL), a malignant proliferation of infected T cells. ATL can be extremely slow progressing or it can be fulminant and lead to death in a few months. ATL commonly is characterized by skin lesions, lymphadenopathy, splenomegaly, and hepatomegaly.
- **Tropical spastic paraparesis (TSP):** HTLV-I also causes most of the cases of tropical spastic paraparesis (TSP), more recently known as **HTLV-I-associated myelopathy (HAM)**. TSP/HAM is characterized by deficits such as weakness in the legs which progresses to spastic paraparesis and incontinence, in many ways not unlike the characteristics of multiple sclerosis. Approximately 5% and 0.25% of carriers of HTLV-I will develop ATL and HAM, respectively.
- HTLV-II has been detected in some patients with T-cell malignancies and in some patients with TSP/HAM-like illnesses, and it probably causes illnesses similar to those caused by HTLV-I. However, HTLV-II has not been conclusively shown to be the etiological agent of any specific disease.

CDC Guidelines for patients: The following advice from the CDC should be given to all patients who are seropositive for HTLV.

- HTLV is not HIV and does not cause AIDS.
- Inform your physician of your positive status if the physician does not know.
- Do not donate blood, semen, organs, or any other tissues.
- Do not share needles or syringes.
- Do not breast feed.
- Use latex condoms during sex (practice safe sex) if your monogamous partner is HTLV-negative or if you have multiple sex partners.

Diagnosis The diagnosis of HTLV-I and -II infections is a clinical diagnosis supported by laboratory diagnosis. HTLV nucleic acid in peripheral lymphocytes can be detected directly by Southern blot restriction mapping and by polymerase chain reaction amplification and subsequent nucleic acid hybridization. Peripheral leukocytes from persons suspected of having HTLV can be cultured *in vitro*, but culture is extremely specialized and not widely available. Serology is the routine method of choice. In the serological diagnosis of HTLV infection, most laboratories follow an algorithm to assure maximum sensitivity and specificity. Sera are screened for HTLV by use of an enzyme immunoassay which is repeated if a positive result is obtained. A second positive screen result is followed by confirmation by some combination of immunofluorescence, immunoblotting, and radioimmunoprecipitation methods.

Diagnostic Tests/Procedures

HTLV-I/II Antibody *on page 505*

Selected Readings

Dobkin JF, "Update on HIV's Distant Cousins: HTLV-I and -II," *Infect Med*, 1993, 10(11).

Lee H, Burczak JD, and Shih J, "Human T-Cell Lymphotropic Virus Type I and II," *Manual of Clinical Microhiology*, 6th ed, Murray PR, Baron EJ, Pfaller MA, et al, eds, Washington, DC: American Society for Microbiology, 1995, 1115-20, Progressive Multifocal.

Recommendations for Counseling Persons Infected With Human T-Lymphotropic Virus, Types I and II. Centers for Disease Control and Prevention and U.S. Public Health Service Working Group, *MMWR*, 1993, 42(RR-9):1-13.

Stoeckle W, "Introduction-Type C Oncoviruses Including Human T-Cell Lymphotropic Viruses Types I and II," *Principals and Practice of Infectious Diseases*, 4th ed, Mandell GL, Bennett JE, and Dolin R, eds, New York, NY: Churchill Livingstone, 1995, 1579-84.

Hymenolepis diminuta *see* Cestodes *on page 72*

Hymenolepis nana *see* Cestodes *on page 72*

IAIS *see* Amnionitis *on page 33*

Impetigo

Clinical Presentation Impetigo is a contagious superficial pyoderma caused by staphylococci and/or streptococci that typically begins as a solitary vesicle ruptures and forms a thick, yellow, honey-colored crust. Patients usually present after multiple lesions occur, most frequently on the face. A superficial glistening base is seen under the crust and no ulcerations are present.

Differential Diagnosis Secondary bacterial infection; ecthyma; herpes simplex, late stage; inflammatory fungal infections

Likely Pathogens

Streptococcus pyogenes on page 321

Staphylococcus aureus, Methicillin-Susceptible *on page 307*

Diagnostic Tests/Procedures

Aerobic Culture, Appropriate Site *on page 365*

Drug Therapy Comment Although mupirocin may be effective in the treatment of limited impetigo, multiple studies have demonstrated that systemic antimicrobial therapy is more efficacious than topical and is preferred over topical.

Community-acquired MRSA infections have been reported among athletes, children, military recruits, Pacific Islanders, Alaskan natives, and prisoners. Isolates many be susceptible to sulfamethoxazole and trimethoprim, doxycycline, and/or clindamycin. Sulfamethoxazole and trimethoprim is the drug of choice in high-risk populations.

Empiric Drug Therapy

Recommended:

Penicillin V Potassium *on page 998*

Erythromycin *on page 807*

Cephalosporins, 1st Generation *on page 729*

Mupirocin *on page 953*

Alternate:

Clindamycin *on page 752*

Doxycycline *on page 787*

Influenza *see* Influenza Virus *on page 193*

Influenza Virus

Related Information

USPHS / IDSA Guidelines for the Prevention of Opportunistic Infections in Persons Infected With HIV *on page 1237*

Microbiology Influenza virus is the etiological agent of influenza, is an enveloped, double-stranded (multisegmented) RNA virus, and is the only member of the Orthomyxovirus family. Influenza virus is broadly classified into three groups (A, B, and C) which are based primarily on antigenic (serological) differences in internal proteins. The envelope of influenza virus contains transmembrane proteins H (three types) and N (two types) which are associated with hemagglutination and neuraminidase activities, respectively. Gradual and continual antigenic changes in the H and N proteins (Continued)

Influenza Virus *(Continued)*

(usually the H) are called "antigenic drift" and are responsible for bypassing human immunity year to year. Sudden and major antigenic changes in the H and N proteins are called "antigenic shift" and are responsible for worldwide epidemics (pandemics) of influenza every 10-20 years or so. Strains of influenza are designated by the type of internal protein, host species (human if not designated), strain number, year of isolation, and H/N types (eg, A/California/10/78/H1N2). The natural reservoirs of influenza virus are as follows: type A, humans and many types of animals; type B, humans; type C, swine. Type A is by far the most prominent and important because of its association with pandemics of influenza.

Epidemiology Influenza virus causes influenza and is an important cause of worldwide respiratory disease. Recurrent episodes of influenza (due to antigenic drift and usually in isolated countries or regions of the world) have been observed every 1-3 years for the last 400 years. Worldwide pandemics of influenza occur every 10-20 years and have been responsible for an estimated 21 million deaths. Influenza virus is spread person to person by inhalation of the virus in aerosolized droplets and possibly by contaminated fomites.

Clinical Syndromes Signs and symptoms of influenza vary greatly and can range from a mild upper respiratory tract illness to rapidly fatal pneumonia. There are three basic clinical presentations of influenza virus infection.

1. **Uncomplicated rhinotracheitis:** Abrupt onset of headache, myalgia, malaise, runny nose, chills, and cough. The course of this disease is usually 7-10 days.
2. **Rhinotracheitis and subsequent bacterial pneumonia:** Typical rhinotracheitis, a brief period of feeling well, and subsequent secondary bacterial pneumonia typically caused by *Streptococcus pneumoniae*, *Staphylococcus*, or *Haemophilus influenzae*.
3. **Frank viral pneumonia:** Can be fulminating and can lead to hypoxia and death in only a few days.

Diagnosis Influenza usually is diagnosed clinically, but laboratory diagnosis and confirmation is highly recommended because symptoms of influenza are not often readily distinguishable from those caused by other respiratory pathogens. Influenza virus is rather easily grown in cell culture, and positive cultures can be observed within 4 days. Some laboratories offer direct detection of influenza-infected cells obtained from nasopharyngeal aspirates or swabs, or from sputum. Serological tests for antibodies for influenza virus are easy to perform and are cost-efficient. Influenza-specific antibodies can often be detected as soon as 4-7 days after the onset of symptoms and can reach peak titers at 14-21 days after symptoms. However, serological tests are retrospective, and acute and convalescent sera must be examined for a fourfold rise in titer.

Diagnostic Tests/Procedures

Influenza A and B Serology *on page 509*
Influenza Virus Culture *on page 510*
Viral Culture, Throat *on page 617*
Virus Detection by DFA *on page 619*

Drug Therapy Comment

Use amantadine or rimantadine for influenza A infections only. No antiviral therapy for influenza B infections.

Drug Therapy

Recommended:

Amantadine *on page 636*
Rimantadine *on page 1054*

Alternate:

Oseltamivir *on page 981*
Zanamivir *on page 1157*

Selected Readings

Centers for Disease Control, "Update: Influenza Activity - United States, 2004-04 Season," *MMWR*, 53(13):284-7.

Shaw MW, Arden NH, and Maassab HF, "New Aspects of Influenza Viruses," *Clin Microbiol Rev*, 1992, 5(1):74-92.

Treanor JJ, "Influenza Virus," *Principles and Practice of Infectious Diseases*, 5th ed, Mandell GL, Bennett JE, and Dolin R, eds, New York, NY: Churchill Livingstone, 2000, 1823-49

Intra-abdominal Abscess

Synonyms Appendicitis; Intra-abdominal Infection

Clinical Presentation Includes infections that extend beyond the hollow viscus of origin into the peritoneal space and that are associated either with abscess formation or peritonitis (also see Peritonitis, Secondary and Peritonitis, Spontaneous Bacterial). Patients typically present with abrupt onset of fever, abdominal pain, nausea, vomiting, diarrhea, abdominal tenderness, rebound tenderness, and hypoactive or absent bowel sounds. The diagnosis of acute abdominal infection is often suspected

based upon the history and the physical examination. These infections require either operative or percutaneous intervention to resolve.

Differential Diagnosis Pneumonia; sickle cell anemia; herpes zoster; diabetic ketoacidosis; tabes dorsalis; porphyria; familial Mediterranean fever; plumbism; lupus erythematosus; uremia; peritonitis, cholangitis

Likely Pathogens

Community-acquired: Gram-negative aerobes including:

Escherichia coli on page 142
Klebsiella Species *on page 200*
Bacteroides and *Prevotella* Species *on page 46*

Nosocomial:

Enterobacter Species *on page 132*
Enterococcus Species *on page 134*
Proteus Species *on page 278*
Pseudomonas aeruginosa on page 282
Staphylococcus aureus, Methicillin-Resistant *on page 304*
Candida Species *on page 67*

Diagnostic Tests/Procedures

Blood Culture, Aerobic and Anaerobic *on page 391*
Paracentesis *on page 555*
Ultrasound, Abdomen *on page 604*
Computed Transaxial Tomography, Abdomen Studies *on page 423*

Drug Therapy Comment Likely pathogens are determined by site of acquisition, community-acquired or healthcare-associated. Infections are frequently polymicrobial. Infection past the proximal small bowel may involve facultative and aerobic gram-negative organisms while infections beyond the proximal ileum may be caused by a variety of anaerobic bacteria. Nosocomial intra-abdominal infections are generally complications of previous intra-abdominal surgery and/or invasive procedures. As such, these may be influenced by local pathogen and resistance profiles.

Current guidelines do not address intraparenchymal abscesses of the liver or spleen, infections arising in the genitourinary system, or infections of the retroperitoneum, with the exception of pancreatic infections. In addition, the current guidelines do not address primary peritonitis or infections occurring in children <18 years of age.

Empiric Drug Therapy

Recommended:

Mild-to-moderate severity:

Ampicillin and Sulbactam *on page 660*
Ticarcillin and Clavulanate Potassium *on page 1114*
Ertapenem *on page 805*
One of the following
Cefazolin *on page 700*
Cefuroxime *on page 725*
plus
Metronidazole *on page 940*
Fluoroquinolones *on page 824*
plus
Metronidazole *on page 940*

More severe infections:

Piperacillin and Tazobactam Sodium *on page 1003*
Meropenem *on page 936*
Imipenem and Cilastatin *on page 861*
One of the following
Cefotaxime *on page 708*
Ceftriaxone *on page 722*
Ceftizoxime *on page 720*
Ceftazidime *on page 717*
Cefepime *on page 705*
plus
Metronidazole *on page 940*
Ciprofloxacin *on page 742*
plus
Metronidazole *on page 940*
Aztreonam *on page 677*
plus
Metronidazole *on page 940*

Selected Readings

Solomkin JS, Mazuski JE, Baron EJ, et al, "Guidelines for the Selection of Anti-infective Agents for Complicated Intra-abdominal Infections," *Clin Infect Dis*, 2003, 37:997-1005.

Intra-abdominal Infection *see* Intra-abdominal Abscess *on page 194*

Intra-amniotic Infection Syndrome *see* Amnionitis *on page 33*

Intravascular Catheter Infection *see* Catheter Infection, Intravascular *on page 70*

Isospora belli

Microbiology *Isospora belli* is a host-specific coccidian protozoan parasite. Both the asexual and sexual stages occur within the host's small intestine which results in the passage of an environmentally resistant cyst stage, the oocyst. The oocysts mature within a few days. Infections are acquired by the ingestion of infective oocysts in contaminated food or water.

Epidemiology Occurs more commonly in tropical and subtropical climates. In the United States, it is more commonly seen in patients with AIDS. Has been implicated in institutional outbreaks and as a cause of traveler's diarrhea.

Clinical Syndromes

- **Immunocompetent hosts:** Presents as a self-limiting diarrheal illness characterized by watery diarrhea without blood or fecal leukocytes, crampy abdominal pain, anorexia, weight loss, and occasionally fever.
- **Immunocompromised hosts including AIDS:** Symptoms as above but much more severe with profuse watery diarrhea resulting in dehydration. The disease is often chronic with detectable organisms in the stool or biopsy specimen for several months to years. Relapse is common. Rare cases of dissemination have been reported. May have peripheral eosinophilia.

Diagnosis Diagnosis is dependent on the identification of oocysts by wet mount or acid-fast stains in fecal material. Histopathologic examination of the small intestine reveals atrophic mucosa, shortened villi, hypertrophic cysts, and inflammation of the lamina propria including eosinophils.

Diagnostic Tests/Procedures

Ova and Parasites, Stool *on page 551*

Treatment Sulfamethoxazole and trimethoprim DS 4 times/day usually results in rapid clearance of *I. belli.* Immunocompromised hosts frequently require a long course such as 8 weeks and may require life-long suppression with either low-dose Sulfamethoxazole and trimethoprim or sulfadoxine and pyrimethamine. Although not as effective as sulfamethoxazole and trimethoprim, ciprofloxacin may be used as an alternative for those patients intolerant of sulfa.

Drug Therapy

Recommended:

Sulfamethoxazole and Trimethoprim *on page 1087*

Alternate:

Sulfadoxine and Pyrimethamine *on page 1085*

Ciprofloxacin *on page 742*

Selected Readings

Lindsay DS, Dubey JP, and Blagburn BL, "Biology of *Isospora* spp From Humans, Nonhuman Primates, and Domestic Animals," *Clin Microbiol Rev*, 1997, 10(1):19-34.

Verdier RI, Fitzgerald DW, Johnson WD Jr, et al, "Trimethoprim-sulfamethoxazole Compared With Ciprofloxacin for Treatment and Prophylaxis of *Isospara belli* and *Cyclospora cayetanensis* Infection in HIV-infected Patients. A Randomized, Controlled Trial," *Ann Intern Med*, 2000, 132(11):885-8.

JC Virus and BK Virus

Synonyms BK Virus

Microbiology The virus family Papovaviridae is composed of two genera: Polyomavirus (JC and BK viruses) and Papillomavirus (wart viruses). JC virus (JCV) and BK virus (BKV) are nonenveloped, slowly growing, icosahedral, 40 nm, double-stranded DNA viruses. JCV and BKV can be cultured *in vitro*; however, culture is not routinely performed in most clinical virology laboratories because the viruses grow slowly (weeks to months) and because susceptible cells are not readily available. JCV and BKV are serologically distinct. Little is known about the portal of entry, transmission, and primary infection of these viruses.

Epidemiology JCV and BKV are found worldwide. Humans appear to be the only animal reservoir for these viruses. Eighty percent of humans develop antibodies to JCV and BKV by the age of 8. Throughout their lives, many persons maintain detectable levels of antibodies to one or both viruses. Ten percent to 25% of healthy adults excrete BKV in their urine.

Clinical Syndromes The majority of JCV and BKV infections are asymptomatic. Most JCV and BKV infections occur in immunocompromised persons and probably are reactivations of latent infections. Asymptomatic shedding of JCV and/or BKV in the urine of transplant patients and pregnant females is common. JCV is associated with progressive multifocal leukoencephalopathy (PML). In PML, JCV infects oligodendrocytes in the brain, and elicits plaques of demyelination in the white matter. The clinical manifestations of PML are motor dysfunction, visual deficits, and progressive dementia or cognitive impairment. PML occurs in ~5% of AIDS patients. BKV is

associated with renal infections, hemorrhagic cystitis, and ureteral stricture in bone marrow and renal transplant patients. The presence of BKV does not always predict poor prognosis or clinical illness of the transplant patients.

Diagnosis Before submitting a specimen, consult the Microbiology Laboratory to determine the availability of reference laboratory tests for JCV and BKV. Routine culture for the viruses is not practical and not routinely available. The results of serological tests for the viruses are not clinically relevant because of the high prevalence in infection and antibody in the population. Antigen detection and DNA hybridization tests are the most useful tests for the laboratory diagnosis of JCV and BKV infections. Immunofluorescence methods to detect JCV and BKV antigens in excreted renal cells and in brain (JCV), kidney (JCV and BKV), and bone marrow (JCV) are the methods of choice. DNA hybridization tests to detect JCV and BKV DNA in the aforementioned four specimens are reported to be more sensitive and specific than are immunofluorescence tests to detect antigen.

Diagnostic Tests/Procedures

Polymerase Chain Reaction *on page 567*

Treatment Most JCV and BKV infections are asymptomatic and do not require treatment. Cytosine arabinoside, interferon, 5-iodo-2′-deoxyuridine, and zidovudine have been anecdotally reported to improve the clinical progress of PML. However, a commonly accepted treatment for symptomatic JCV and BKV infections does not exist.

Selected Readings

Demeter LM, "JK, BK, and Other *Polyomaviruses*: Progressive Multifocal Leukoencephalopathy," *Principals and Practice of Infectious Diseases,* 4th ed, Mandell GL, Bennett JE, and Dolin R, eds, New York, NY: Churchill Livingstone, 1995, 1400-4.

Major EO, "*Polyomaviruses*," *Manual of Clinical Microbiology,* 6th ed, Muffay PR, Baron EJ, Pfaller MA, et al, eds, Washington DC: American Society for Microbiology, 1995, 1090-6.

Jock Itch *see* Dermatophytes *on page 114*

Joint Replacement, Early Infection

Synonyms Early Infection Joint Replacement

Clinical Presentation Most patients present with a progressive increase in joint pain and occasional draining sinuses. May present with acute joint sepsis characterized by high fever, severe joint pain with localized warmth, swelling, and edema.

Differential Diagnosis Hemarthrosis; gout; bland loosening; dislocation

Likely Pathogens

Staphylococcus aureus, Methicillin-Susceptible *on page 307*
Staphylococcus epidermidis, Methicillin-Resistant *on page 309*
Staphylococcus epidermidis, Methicillin-Susceptible *on page 310*
Pseudomonas aeruginosa on page 282

Diagnostic Tests/Procedures

- Aerobic Culture, Body Fluid *on page 365*
- Arthrocentesis *on page 384*
- Biopsy Culture, Routine *on page 390*
- Blood Culture, Aerobic and Anaerobic *on page 391*
- Gram Stain *on page 473*

Arthrogram *on page 387*
C-Reactive Protein *on page 428*
Sedimentation Rate, Erythrocyte *on page 576*

Drug Therapy Comment Optimum therapy may require the removal of the prosthetic joint if appropriate with treatment for a minimum of 6 weeks prior to replacement. Confounding factors include limitations of removing prosthetic device completely, vascular supply, and operative risks vs benefits.

Empiric Drug Therapy

Recommended:

Vancomycin *on page 1144*
plus (if device not able to be removed)
Rifampin *on page 1046*

If *Pseudomonas* suspected:
Ciprofloxacin *on page 742*
Piperacillin and Tazobactam Sodium *on page 1002*

Alternate:

Penicillins, Penicillinase-Resistant *on page 997*
Ceftazidime *on page 717*

Selected Readings

Berbari EF, Hanssen AD, Duffy MC, et al, "Prosthetic Joint Infection Due to *Mycobacterium tuberculosis*: A Case Series and Review of the Literature," *Am J Orthop,* 1998, 27(3):219-27.

Berbari EF, Hanssen AD, Duffy MC, et al, "Risk Factors for Prosthetic Joint Infection: Case-Control Study," *Clin Infect Dis,* 1998, 27(5):1247-54.

(Continued)

Joint Replacement, Early Infection *(Continued)*

Fisman DN, Reilly DT, Karchmer AW, et al, "Clinical Effectiveness and Cost-Effectiveness of 2 Management Strategies for Infected Total Hip Arthroplasty in the Elderly," *Clin Infect Dis*, 2001, 32(3):419-30.

Gillespie WJ, "Prevention and Management of Infection After Total Joint Replacement," *Clin Infect Dis*, 1997, 25(6):1310-7.

Murdoch DR, Roberts SA, Fowler Jr VG Jr, et al, "Infection of Orthopedic Prostheses After *Staphylococcus aureus* Bacteremia," *Clin Infect Dis*, 2001, 32(4):647-9.

Joint Replacement, Late Infection

Synonyms Late Infection Joint Replacement

Clinical Presentation Most patients present with a long indolent course characterized by progressive increase in joint pain and occasional draining sinuses. May present with acute joint sepsis characterized by high fever, severe joint pain with localized warmth, swelling, and edema.

Differential Diagnosis Hemarthrosis; gout; bland loosening; dislocation

Likely Pathogens

Staphylococcus epidermidis, Methicillin-Resistant *on page 309*
Staphylococcus epidermidis, Methicillin-Susceptible *on page 310*
Staphylococcus aureus, Methicillin-Susceptible *on page 307*

Diagnostic Tests/Procedures

•Aerobic Culture, Body Fluid *on page 365*
•Arthrocentesis *on page 384*
•Biopsy Culture, Routine *on page 390*
•Blood Culture, Aerobic and Anaerobic *on page 391*
•Gram Stain *on page 473*
Arthrogram *on page 387*
C-Reactive Protein *on page 428*
Sedimentation Rate, Erythrocyte *on page 576*

Drug Therapy Comment Optimum therapy may require the removal of the prosthetic joint if appropriate with treatment for a minimum of 6 weeks prior to replacement. Confounding factors include limitations of removing prosthetic device completely, vascular supply, and operative risks vs benefits.

Empiric Drug Therapy

Recommended:

Vancomycin *on page 1144*
plus
Rifampin *on page 1046*

Alternate:

Penicillins, Penicillinase-Resistant *on page 997*
Cefazolin *on page 700*
Ceftriaxone *on page 722*
Clindamycin *on page 752*

Selected Readings

Berbari EF, Hanssen AD, Duffy MC, et al, "Prosthetic Joint Infection Due to *Mycobacterium tuberculosis*: A Case Series and Review of the Literature," *Am J Orthop*, 1998, 27(3):219-27.

Berbari EF, Hanssen AD, Duffy MC, et al, "Risk Factors for Prosthetic Joint Infection: Case-Control Study," *Clin Infect Dis*, 1998, 27(5):1247-54.

Gillespie WJ, "Prevention and Management of Infection After Total Joint Replacement," *Clin Infect Dis*, 1997, 25(6):1310-7.

Murdoch DR, Roberts SA, Fowler VG Jr, et al, "Infection of Orthopedic Prostheses After *Staphylococcus aureus* Bacteremia," *Clin Infect Dis*, 2001, 32(4):647-9.

Kawasaki Syndrome

Synonyms Mucocutaneous Lymph Node Syndrome

Clinical Presentation A rare illness that typically affects children <5 years of age. The cause is currently unknown, although relationship to some bacteria has been suspected (*Staphylococcus* or *Streptococcus* spp.). There has been no confirmation that Kawasaki syndrome can be transmitted via contact. Kawasaki syndrome involves widespread systemic inflammation, which may include myocarditis, pericarditis, valvulitis, meningitis, or produce inflammation in the skin, eyes, lungs, lymph nodes, joints, and mouth. Vasculitis is the most dangerous manifestation, particularly with coronary artery involvement, due to the possible development of aneurysms along the length of these vessels. In rare cases, the vasculitic changes may lead to myocardial infarction.

Symptoms include a persistently high fever (usually 104°F or above) for at least 5 days in conjunction with at least four of the following: Bilateral conjunctivitis, oral erythema/inflammation (involving the mouth, throat, lips, or tongue), hand or foot inflammation, including palmar or plantar erythema/edema; rash (primarily localized to the trunk area), and lymph node swelling in the neck. Additional symptoms may include arthralgia, diarrhea, vomiting, abdominal pain, cough, earache, rhinitis, irritability, seizures, asthenia, cardiac arrhythmia, or heart failure.

Kawasaki syndrome progresses through three distinct stages over a period of several weeks. The acute phase lasts for 1-2 weeks and is associated with the most intense symptomatology. This is followed by the subacute phase which begins when the child's fever, rash, and lymphadenopathy resolve. It may include irritability, a poor appetite, and slight eye redness. The skin of the fingers and toes may peel. This stage usually ends 3-4 weeks after the onset of fever. The convalescent stage begins when clinical symptoms are resolved, but laboratory evidence of inflammation remains, including a persistent elevation of the erythrocyte sedimentation rate (ESR). Normalization usually requires 6-8 weeks after the onset of fever.

Differential Diagnosis Kawasaki syndrome is a diagnosis of exclusion. Drug reaction, scarlet fever, measles, and Rocky Mountain spotted fever should be excluded.

Diagnostic Tests/Procedures Echocardiogram and/or coronary arteriogram to evaluate coronary artery involvement.

Drug Therapy Comment Without proper treatment, 20% to 25% of patients with Kawasaki syndrome develop coronary abnormalities. With treatment, this is reduced to between 2% and 4%. In general, the risk of death due to cardiac complications is about 1% to 2%, with the greatest risk within the first 12 weeks.

Empiric Drug Therapy

Recommended: Intravenous gamma-globulin, together with orally administered aspirin. Gamma globulin infusion may be repeated over several days. Aspirin is continued for 6-8 weeks after the acute symptoms of Kawasaki syndrome subside.

Alternate: Other treatments, including corticosteroids or immunosuppressants are of uncertain benefit, but may be used in some cases where standard therapy is ineffective.

Kennel Cough *see Bordetella bronchiseptica on page 52*

Keratitis, Bacterial and Fungal

Synonyms Bacterial Keratitis; Fungal Keratitis

Clinical Presentation Bacterial keratitis is characterized by pain and inflamed cornea accompanied by various combinations of corneal opacification and/or ulceration, photophobia, and tearing. In severe cases of bacterial keratitis and in some cases of fungal keratitis, an accumulation of pus (hypopyon) in the anterior chamber can be observed. Fungal keratitis is characterized by slow (over weeks) progression of corneal inflammation of the epithelium, which can be intact or ulcerated. If present, the ulcerated areas usually show feathery edges, heaped margins, and satellite lesions.

Note: Bacterial and fungal keratitis are medically urgent situations, which can lead to severe visual impairment, blindness, and/or loss of the eye. If the disease and accompanying corneal ulceration are severe or extensive enough, the patient should be hospitalized because (1) the risk of corneal perforation is high and (2) the frequency of, and intense need for therapy requires qualified medical personnel.

Differential Diagnosis Fungal keratitis; viral keratitis; parasitic keratitis; trachoma corneal opacification, which resembles infectious keratitis

Likely Pathogens

Approximately 82% of the cases of keratitis are caused by bacteria:

- *Staphylococcus aureus*, Methicillin-Resistant *on page 304*
- *Staphylococcus aureus*, Methicillin-Susceptible *on page 307*
- *Staphylococcus epidermidis*, Methicillin-Resistant *on page 309*
- *Staphylococcus epidermidis*, Methicillin-Susceptible *on page 310*
- *Streptococcus* Species *on page 326*
- *Pseudomonas aeruginosa on page 282*
- *Haemophilus influenzae on page 159*
- Enteric Gram-Negative Rods:
  - *Escherichia coli on page 142*
  - *Klebsiella* Species *on page 200*
  - *Citrobacter* Species *on page 81*
  - *Serratia* Species
  - *Enterobacter* Species *on page 132*
- Anaerobic bacteria and mycobacteria are infrequent causes

Approximately 16% of the cases of keratitis are caused by fungi:

- *Fusarium* Species *on page 151*
- *Candida* Species *on page 67*
- *Aspergillus* Species *on page 38*
- *Alternaria* Species
- *Curvularia* Species
- *Penicillium marneffei on page 260*

Diagnostic Tests/Procedures Note: Contact the testing laboratory prior to collecting specimen for (1) special instructions regarding ocular cultures, (2) special

(Continued)

Keratitis, Bacterial and Fungal *(Continued)*

media for bacterial and fungal cultures, and (3) special procedures for culturing and transporting extremely small amounts of corneal specimen.

Gram Stain *on page 473*
Methenamine Silver Stain *on page 534*
Periodic Acid-Schiff Stain *on page 563*
Corneal Culture, Bacterial and Fungal *on page 426*

Drug Therapy Comment Antimicrobial therapy is empiric until the specific etiological agent is isolated and identified. However, specific therapy directed toward a specific or suspected bacterial or fungal pathogen(s) should be given as soon as possible. Initial therapy can, wholly or in part, be based on the results of the Gram or fungal stain.

Note: Fluoroquinolone monotherapy is not recommended in severe bacterial keratitis. Such therapy should be specifically directed to the etiological agent. See Forster (1998) reference in Selected Readings.

Empiric Drug Therapy

Recommended:

Note: Regimens are based on causative agent.

Broad-Spectrum:

Bacterial:
Cephalosporins, 1st Generation *on page 729*
plus
Aminoglycosides *on page 641*

Fungal:
Amphotericin B (Conventional) *on page 650*

Pathogen-Specific: Bacterial:

Staphylococcus Species/Gram-Positive Bacteria:
Cephalosporins, 1st Generation *on page 729*
plus
Vancomycin *on page 1144*

Streptococcus pneumoniae:
Penicillin G (Parenteral/Aqueous) *on page 993*

Gram-Negative Rod:
Aminoglycosides *on page 641*
Fluoroquinolones *on page 824*

Pseudomonas aeruginosa:
One of the following
Fluoroquinolones *on page 824*
Aminoglycosides *on page 641*
plus one of the following
Ticarcillin *on page 1113*
Piperacillin *on page 1002*

Proteus Species:
Aminoglycosides *on page 641*
plus one of the following
Ticarcillin *on page 1113*
Piperacillin *on page 1002*

Selected Readings

Forster RK, "Conrad Berens Lecture. The Management of Infectious Keratitis as We Approach the 21st Century," *CLAO J*, 1998, 24(3):175-80.

Gangopadhyay N, Daniell M, Weih L, et al, "Fluoroquinolone and Fortified Antibiotics for Treating Bacterial Corneal Ulcers," *Br J Ophthalmol*, 2000, 84(4):378-84.

Levey SB, Katz HR, Abrams DA, et al, "The Role of Cultures in the Management of Ulcerative Keratitis," *Cornea*, 1997, 16(4):383-6.

O'Brien TP, "Keratitis," *Principles and Practices of Infectious Diseases*, 5th ed, Mandell GL, et al, eds, New York, NY: Churchill Livingstone, 2000, 1257-67.

Klebsiella Species

Microbiology *Klebsiella* species are aerobic gram-negative bacilli belonging to the family Enterobacteriaceae. The main species causing human disease are *K. pneumoniae* and *K. oxytoca*. A distinctive characteristic of most isolates of *Klebsiella* is the polysaccharide capsule which imparts a mucoid appearance of the organisms when growing on solid media. The prominent capsule also makes the organism appear relatively large on Gram stain. The presence of the capsule is a virulence factor. As with other gram-negative bacilli of this family, *Klebsiella* produces endotoxin, a mediator of the sepsis syndrome.

Epidemiology *Klebsiella* sp are primarily nosocomial pathogens. However, the organism is associated with one important community-acquired infection, primary lobar pneumonia.

Clinical Syndromes

- **Primary lobar pneumonia:** This infection is community-acquired and is seen in alcoholics and other patients with chronic debilitating underlying illnesses (such as chronic obstructive pulmonary disease). It is rarely seen in the otherwise healthy individual and is considered a type of opportunistic infection. Characteristically, a patient with underlying alcoholism presents with the acute onset of fever, purulent sputum with a "currant jelly" appearance (reflecting lung necrosis and blood), and dyspnea. The classic x-ray finding is the "bowed fissure;" the lobe is swollen and the fissure appears to be sagging and widened. Complications include lung abscess, empyema, cavity formation, and progressive infiltrates. This form of pneumonitis is severe with extensive necrosis. Many patients expire, in part due to their comorbidity conditions.
- **Bronchitis and bronchopneumonia:** Not all forms of *Klebsiella* lung infection lead to the severe form of necrotizing pneumonia described above. Community-acquired *Klebsiella* bronchitis and bronchopneumonia do occur but are much less frequently seen than hospital-acquired respiratory infections.
- **Nosocomial pneumonia:** Hospital-acquired *Klebsiella* lower respiratory infections are seen in debilitated, ventilator-dependent patients. *Klebsiella* and other gram-negative bacilli can asymptomatically colonize the upper respiratory tract of hospitalized patients. Thus, the recovery of *Klebsiella* from a sputum or tracheal aspirate culture does not necessarily indicate a significant infection. The diagnosis of a nosocomial pneumonia still rests on standard criteria such as the presence of purulence (many leukocytes) on the Gram stain of sputum, the presence of a pulmonary infiltrate, and signs of systemic inflammation in the patient. **A positive sputum culture alone is not sufficient justification for initiating antibiotic therapy.**
- **Nosocomial urinary tract infections:** Hospitalized patients with indwelling Foley catheters are at risk for cystitis or pyelonephritis from *Klebsiella. Klebsiella* may be recovered more frequently from the urine than from any other site, including the respiratory tract. However, the organism may also harmlessly colonize the urine of patients with chronic bladder catheters without causing disease. The decision to initiate antibiotics in such patients should be based on the clinical situation (the presence of pyuria on urinalysis, suprapubic pain, fever, etc). Even the finding of large quantity of *Klebsiella* in a urine culture ($>10^5$ colony-forming units/mL) by itself does not automatically indicate antibiotic therapy.
- **Hospital-associated bacteremias:** *Klebsiella* is a common cause of primary bacteremia. In some series, it approaches *E. coli* as one of the most frequently recovered gram-negative bacillus from the bloodstream.
- **Surgical wound infections.**
- **Biliary tract infections, especially following instrumentation.**

Diagnosis The diagnosis of lobar pneumonia secondary to *Klebsiella* should be considered in any debilitated patient who presents with a necrotizing pneumonia. The history of "currant jelly" sputum and the finding of a "bowed fissure" on chest x-ray are highly suggestive but are not always present. The differential diagnosis of such cases should include anaerobic lung abscess, tuberculosis, *Pseudomonas* and other gram-negative bacilli, and mixed aspiration pneumonitis, among others. The presentation of nosocomial *Klebsiella* infections are more nonspecific and can be due to a variety of pathogenic gram-negative bacilli. Culture and Gram stain of appropriate clinical specimens (sputum, urine, blood, catheter tips, etc) is necessary to make the diagnosis.

Diagnostic Tests/Procedures

Aerobic Culture, Appropriate Site *on page 365*
Gram Stain *on page 473*

Treatment Increasing resistance of Enterobacteriaceae to beta-lactam antimicrobial agents has been recognized for several years. This resistance has made infections caused by these resistant bacteria increasingly more difficult to treat.

A major mechanism of bacterial resistance to beta-lactam antimicrobial agents is the natural production of beta-lactamases. Mutations of these enzymes over the years have resulted in plasmid-encoded beta-lactamases with extended-spectra that now include newer and commonly used antimicrobial agents such as the monobactam aztreonam and the newer oxyimino-cephalosporins such as cefotaxime, ceftriaxone, ceftazidime, and cefpodoxime. These enzymes are known as extended-spectrum beta-lactamases (ESBL) and occur more commonly in *Escherichia coli* and *Klebsiella* species and are becoming more commonly detected in other genera of Enterobacteriaceae, such as *Enterobacter*, *Serratia*, *Citrobacter*, *Salmonella*, and *Proteus*.

Like many other nosocomial pathogens, *Klebsiella* sp may be difficult to treat because of antimicrobial resistance. Although the organisms have been traditionally susceptible to cephalosporins, including the first generation agents, increasing problems with resistance are emerging. Isolates of *Klebsiella* which are resistant to

(Continued)

Klebsiella Species *(Continued)*

cephalosporins and aminoglycosides have emerged because of widespread use of these antimicrobial agents. In institutions where ESBL-related resistance is prevalent, cephalosporins should be avoided as empiric therapy. In all cases, the final selection of antibiotics must be based on the susceptibility pattern of the particular isolate because the organism is no longer predictably sensitive to all agents.

Drug Therapy

Recommended:

Cephalosporins, 1st Generation *on page 729*
Cephalosporins, 2nd Generation *on page 729*
Cephalosporins, 3rd Generation *on page 730*

Alternate:

Penicillins, Extended-Spectrum *on page 997*
Imipenem and Cilastatin *on page 861*
Aztreonam *on page 677*
Fluoroquinolones *on page 824*
Meropenem *on page 936*

Selected Readings

Bradford PA, "Extended-Spectrum Beta-Lactamases in the 21st Century: Characterization, Epidemiology, and Detection of This Important Resistance Threat," *Clin Microbiol Rev*, 2001, 14(4):933-51.

Carpenter JL, "*Klebsiella* Pulmonary Infections: Occurrence at One Medical Center and Review," *Rev Infect Dis*, 1990, 12(4):672-80.

Colodner R, "Extended-Spectrum Beta-Lactamases: A Challenge for Clinical Microbiologists and Infection Control Specialists," *Am J Infect Control*, 2005, 33(2):104-7.

Kang CI, Kim SH, Park WB, et al, "Bloodstream Infections Due to Extended-Spectrum Beta-Lactamase-Producing *Escherichia coli* and *Klebsiella pneumoniae*: Risk Factors for Mortality and Treatment Outcome, With Special Emphasis on Antimicrobial Therapy," *Antimicrob Agents Chemother*, 2004, 48(12):4574-81

Koch-Weeks *see* Conjunctivitis *on page 93*

LaCrosse Encephalitis *see* Arboviruses *on page 35*

Late Infection Joint Replacement *see* Joint Replacement, Late Infection *on page 198*

Legionella pneumophila

Related Information

Community-Acquired Pneumonia in Adults *on page 1278*

Microbiology *Legionella pneumophila* is an aerobic, gram-negative rod which was first isolated in 1947 and which causes a pneumonia called Legionnaires' disease (or legionellosis), as well as a distinct febrile illness called Pontiac fever. There are over 30 *Legionella* species, with *L. pneumophila* accounting for about 90% of human infections. There are 15 serotypes of *L. pneumophila*; serotype 1 is responsible for most cases of legionellosis. The organism is very difficult to visualize on Gram stain of clinical specimens. Other (and less commonly used) stains are more effective in identifying the organism, such as the silver stain (Dieterle or Warthin-Starry stains), Gimenez stain, and others. The organism also requires special medium for growth and cannot be cultured using standard bacteriologic media. Buffered charcoal yeast extract (BCYE) is the medium most commonly used for culture isolation.

In vivo, *L. pneumophila* is an intracellular pathogen and is taken up by the monocyte system of the human host. The alveolar macrophages phagocytose the organism after initial entry into the respiratory tract. The organism can survive and multiply within the cell, eventually leading to cell rupture and further spread. *L. pneumophila* also replicates well in water cooling systems that also contain organisms, such as protozoans, in which the *L. pneumophila* can enter and live intracellularly.

Epidemiology The importance of this organism was recognized in 1976 following an outbreak of pneumonia involving an American Legion convention in Philadelphia, Pennsylvania. The cause of this well-publicized outbreak which involved over 200 individuals was initially unknown. Only later was the bacterium *Legionella pneumophila* isolated from lung autopsy specimens by the Centers for Disease Control. Another epidemic of Legionnaires' disease had been described in 1965, where the diagnosis was established using serologic studies rather than identification of the organism. Since then, prospective studies have shown *L. pneumophila* to be one of the three more common causes of community-acquired pneumonia. The prevalence of *L. pneumophila* varies geographically. In some areas of the United States, it is the most common cause of community-acquired pneumonia.

The organism typically inhabits lakes, rivers, ponds, and polluted waters where it exists in small numbers. The organism is relatively hardy and can survive chlorination systems and water temperatures ranging from 0°C to 60°C. From naturally-occurring bodies of water, the organism can pass into water storage and distribution systems. Under the correct environmental conditions, the organism can proliferate within the

water storage systems. Transmission of *Legionella* can occur by one of several routes, including aspiration of contaminated water, aerosolization of infected organisms with airborne spread, and direct inoculation by means of contaminated respiratory care equipment or contaminated water used to irrigate wounds. Aerosol spread from air conditioning towers, mist machines, and possibly showerheads has been implicated in some cases. Person-to-person transmission does not occur and individuals hospitalized with *Legionella* pneumonia do not require isolation.

Risk factors for *L. pneumophila* infection include chronic obstructive pulmonary disease, history of cigarette smoking, advanced age, and alcoholism. Pediatric legionellosis is becoming increasingly recognized. Adults with hairy cell leukemia are at particularly high risk of infection, probably from the monocyte dysfunction. Organ transplant recipients are at risk for nosocomial legionellosis. Although cell-mediated immunity is important in the control of *L. pneumophila*, infection is uncommon in persons with AIDS.

Clinical Syndromes

- **Community-acquired pneumonia:** The incidence of *L. pneumophila* as a cause of community-acquired pneumonia has ranged from 1% to 15%. It is a common cause of severe community-acquired pneumonia requiring admission to an intensive care unit, often second only to pneumococcal pneumonia. *L. pneumophilia* pneumonia is significantly underdiagnosed with one study suggesting only 3% of cases are recognized correctly. There is a well-described, broad-spectrum of clinical symptoms. Patients may present with a minor cough or with a progressive five-lobe pneumonia with shock. Fever is almost always present, and often over 40°C. Typically, the cough is nonproductive although pleuritic chest pain may occur. Other accompanying features are shaking, chills, relative bradycardia, diarrhea and other gastrointestinal symptoms (up to 50% of cases), and hyponatremia. No single symptom or constellation of symptoms is diagnostic of legionellosis. In one study, the extrapulmonary symptoms, such as diarrhea and neurologic findings, were not found more frequently with Legionnaires' disease in comparison with other forms of pneumonia. Expectorated sputum usually shows numerous polymorphonuclear leukocytes, but no significant organisms on Gram stain. The chest radiograph classically shows unilateral patchy infiltrates early on, which progress over several days to consolidation. However, a very wide variety of x-ray abnormalities has been described with this infection including nodular lesions and cavitary lung lesions. Pleural effusions are common. Hilar adenopathy is very unusual in legionellosis and should bring to mind other pulmonary diseases such as sarcoidosis, histoplasmosis, tuberculosis, and others.
- **Nosocomial pneumonia:** *L. pneumophila* is a sporadic cause of hospital-acquired pneumonias. The clinical presentation is also variable, although it tends to be a rapidly progressive pneumonia involving multiple lobes.
- **Pontiac fever:** This is a febrile illness caused by *L. pneumophila* which tends to be self-resolving without antibiotics. Patients present with fever, myalgias, headache, and malaise, mimicking the flu, however, pneumonia is not present.
- **Miscellaneous:** *L. pneumophila* has been described rarely as a cause of endocarditis, sinusitis, pericarditis, peritonitis, pancreatitis, encephalopathy, and wound infections.

Diagnosis A high level of suspicion must be maintained by the clinician since the presentation of Legionnaires' disease is varied and nonspecific. Laboratory testing is essential in making the diagnosis. As mentioned above, Gram stain of respiratory secretions, such as expectorated or induced sputum, bronchial wash specimens, and bronchoalveolar lavage (BAL) fluid, usually reveals many PMN cells, but no organisms. This is a useful clue to the diagnosis of *L. pneumophila*, but is a nonspecific finding that can be seen in a variety of other "atypical" pneumonias including *Mycoplasma* and viral respiratory infections. Respiratory specimens submitted to the laboratory for routine culture will not grow *L. pneumophila* and a special request to rule-out *Legionella* must be made. Culture of respiratory specimens on special BCYE is 70% to 90% sensitive, but requires a variable number of days of incubation and can be strongly influenced by prior or current antibiotics. Direct fluorescent antibody testing on respiratory specimens is more rapid than culture, but the sensitivity is variable (50% to 70%) and usually is lower than that of culture. The *Legionella* urinary antigen test has come into common use in recent years, because of its availability, comparable sensitivity (70%), and ease of specimen collection. The *Legionella* urinary antigen detects the lipopolysaccharides of *L. pneumophila* serogroup 1 only, but this serogroup is the cause of the majority of cases of legionellosis. Results of this serological test can remain positive for months after the initial infection. Specific IgG and IgM serological tests for anti-*L. pneumophila* antibodies are available but are only about 50% sensitive for diagnosing legionellosis. Demonstration of a fourfold rise in IgG titer from acute to convalescent phase is virtually diagnostic of recent *L. pneumophila* infection, but is of limited value to the clinician managing the acute disease. In addition, a fourfold increase in IgG may be difficult to demonstrate even in

(Continued)

Legionella pneumophila (Continued)

culture-proven cases. Some authors feel a single high titer in a low prevalence area is highly suggestive of acute infection. A positive *L. pneumophila* IgM titer is also highly suggestive of acute infection, but many consider this a presumptive diagnosis only, with culture identification of the organism the only definitive laboratory method. Polymerase chain reaction (PCR) for *L. pneumophila* is available in some reference laboratories and can detect the organism in sputum, BAL fluid, and blood. However, PCR is not more sensitive than standard methods described above and remains investigational.

Legionella species are not detected in routine cultures. Physicians should specifically request culture for *Legionella* if legionellosis is suspected.

Diagnostic Tests/Procedures

Legionella Antigen, Urine *on page 514*
Legionella DNA Probe *on page 515*
Legionella pneumophila Culture *on page 516*
Legionella pneumophila Smear *on page 517*
Legionella Serology *on page 518*
Polymerase Chain Reaction *on page 567*

Treatment Although highly active against *L. pneumophila*, erythromycin has become less attractive in the last decade due to the development of susceptibility assays for intracellular organisms, and the development of newer macrolides and quinolones. A fair amount of clinical experience with erythromycin has been accumulated, but the limitations of the drug are also known. Erythromycin has significant drawbacks including gastrointestinal side effects, high fluid volume for infusions, and local phlebitis, especially at the high doses used for legionellosis. Newer macrolides, such as azithromycin, are in general better tolerated than erythromycin with less nausea and vomiting at high doses, once-daily intravenous doses, and oral doses. In addition, the organism is an intracellular pathogen, and antibacterials which achieve high intracellular levels are more likely to be clinically effective. Newer macrolides have greater intracellular and lung concentrations than erythromycin and appear more effective *in vitro* and in animal studies. The quinolones also achieve superior intracellular levels and are highly active *in vitro* against *L. pneumophila*. Direct comparison of azithromycin, erythromycin, and quinolones in a randomized clinical trial has not been performed. According to most recent guidelines, the newer macrolides and fluoroquinolones are considered among the first-line agents against *L. pneumophila*. Some experts advocate the addition of rifampin to a macrolide for severe cases, although randomized trials with and without rifampin are lacking.

Drug Therapy

Recommended:

Azithromycin *on page 674*
individually or plus
Rifampin *on page 1046*

Erythromycin *on page 807*
individually or plus
Rifampin *on page 1046*

Alternate:

Clarithromycin *on page 749*
Fluoroquinolones *on page 824*

Selected Readings

Baltch AL, Smith RP, Ritz WJ, et al, "Antibacterial Effect of Telithromycin (HMR 3647) and Comparative Antibiotics Against Intracellular *Legionella pneumophila*," *J Antimicrob Chemother*, 2000, 46(1):51-5.

Blatt SP, Dolan MJ, Hendrix CW, et al, "Legionnaires' Disease in Human Immunodeficiency Virus-Infected Patients: Eight Cases and Review," *Clin Infect Dis*, 1994, 18(2):227-32.

Critchley IA, Jones ME, Heinze PD, et al, "In vitro Activity of Levofloxacin Against Contemporary Clinical Isolates of *Legionella pneumophila, Mycoplasma pneumoniae*, and *Chlamydia pneumoniae* From North America and Europe," *Clin Microbiol Infect*, 2002, 8(4):214-21.

Edelstein PH, "Legionnaires' Disease," *Clin Infect Dis*, 1993, 16(6):741-7.

Fields BS, Benson RF, and Besser RE, "*Legionella* and Legionnaires' Disease: 25 Years of Investigation," *Clin Microbiol Rev*, 2002, 15(3):506-26.

Kunishima H, Takemura H, Yamamoto H, et al, "Evaluation of the Activity of Antimicrobial Agents Against *Legionella pneumophila* Multiplying in a Human Monocytic Cell Line, THP-1, and an Alveolar Epithelial Cell Line, A549," *J Infect Chemother*, 2000, 6(4):206-10.

Mandell LA, Bartlett JG, Dowell SF, et al, "Update of Practice Guidelines for the Management of Community-Acquired Pneumonia in Immunocompetent Adults," *Clin Infect Dis*, 2003, 37(11):1405-33.

Murdoch DR, "Diagnosis of *Legionella* Infection," *Clin Infect Dis*, 2003, 36(1):64-9.

Nguyen MH, Stout JE, and Yu VL, "Legionellosis," *Infect Dis Clin North Am*, 1991, 5(3):561-84.

Pasculle W, "Update on *Legionella*," *Clin Microbiol Newslett*, 2000, 22(13):97-101.

Roig J and Rello J, "Legionnaires' Disease: A Rational Approach to Therapy," *J Antimicrob Chemother*, 2003, 51(5):1119-29.

Yu, VL, "*Legionella pneumophila* (Legionnaires Disease)," *Principles and Practice of Infectious Diseases*, 5th ed, Mandell GL, Bennett JE, and Dolin R, eds, New York, NY: Churchill Livingstone, 2000, 2424-35.

Yu VL, Greenberg RN, Zadeikis N, et al, "Levofloxacin Efficacy in the Treatment of Community-Acquired Legionellosis," *Chest*, 2004, 125(6):2135-9.

Legionellosis *see Legionella pneumophila on page 202*

Legionnaires' Disease *see Legionella pneumophila on page 202*

Leptospira interrogans

Microbiology *Leptospira interrogans* is an aerobic spirochete which causes the febrile human disease leptospirosis. *L. interrogans* is the main pathogenic species of the genus *Leptospira*, which is divided into 170 serotypes. A second species, *L. biflexa*, is saprophytic. The organism is a finely coiled, motile, helical rod 0.1 μm in width and 6-20 μm in length. One or both ends of the rod are usually hooked, giving the appearance of a question mark (thus the name *L. interrogans*).

Epidemiology Leptospirosis is an unusual disease in the U.S., with 50-100 cases reported annually. It is primarily a disease of wild and domestic mammals. Infected animals excrete the organism in urine, amniotic fluid, and other tissues, which contaminate soil and water. Leptospires can remain viable in the environment for months. Humans are considered accidental hosts and become infected only occasionally through direct animal contact or through indirect contact with contaminated soil or water. Transmission occurs when the organism enters the human host through mucous membranes, cuts, abrasions, or inhalation of aerosolized infected water. Groups at risk include farmers, veterinarians, abattoir workers, and sewer workers. Cases associated with recreational activities such as kayaking, wading in shallow water, swimming, and canoeing have been reported. Worldwide, rats are the most common source of human infection with a 90% carriage rate. In the U.S., the most important sources of infection are dogs, livestock, rodents, wild mammals, and cats. Person-to-person transmission is extremely rare. Most cases of leptospirosis occur in young adult men, and the peak incidence is in the summer and early fall.

Clinical Syndromes The organisms are capable of penetrating intact mucous membranes or abraded skin of the host. The leptospires enter the bloodstream and are rapidly disseminated even to "sequestered sites" such as the cerebrospinal fluid and the eye. The primary pathologic lesion is damage to the endothelium of small blood vessels.

- **Subclinical leptospirosis:** Some individuals may have minimal symptoms after infection with *L. interrogans*. This occurs most commonly in those who are frequently exposed to infected animals. Leptospires can establish a symbiotic relationship with many animal hosts, persisting for long periods in the renal tubules without producing disease or pathologic changes in the kidney.
- **Anicteric leptospirosis:** Among patients ill with leptospirosis, 90% experience a mild anicteric disease. The incubation period is usually 7-12 days. The illness is usually biphasic. In the acute phase, infected individuals experience the abrupt onset of remitting fever, headache, abdominal pain, nausea and vomiting, severe myalgias, and malaise. Ocular symptoms during the acute septicemic phase may be an important clue to the diagnosis of leptospirosis. Suffusion of the bulbar conjunctiva with conjunctival petechiae and/or hemorrhage is characteristic of leptospirosis and seen in few other diseases. Prostration may persist for 4-7 days. Meningeal symptoms are absent at this time. Other symptoms include: pain with nausea and vomiting; myalgias; splenomegaly (15% to 25% of cases); lymphadenopathy; and rash with raised 1-5 cm erythematous lesions in the pretibial area (so-called Fort Bragg fever caused by *L. autumnalis*). Following this initial flu-like illness, the patient is then afebrile for several days. The second phase, called the "immune phase" occurs in some, but not all, patients and is characterized by low grade fever, severe throbbing headaches, and sometimes delirium without encephalitis. Up to 90% will have evidence of meningitis, with a cerebrospinal fluid lymphocytic pleocytosis (usually <500 WBC/mm^3 in CSF). Although the CSF pressure is normal, characteristically the spinal tap will improve the headaches. Conjunctival suffusion and hemorrhages remain prominent clinical features, along with ocular pain and photophobia, myalgias, and adenopathy.
- **Icteric leptospirosis:** The severe form of leptospirosis is characterized by hepatic dysfunction, jaundice, impaired renal function, hemorrhage, vascular collapse, and severe mental status changes. Mortality is 5% to 40%. Weil's syndrome is one of several manifestations of severe leptospirosis; this syndrome is characterized by hepatic and renal failure. Jaundice is due to damage to hepatic capillaries, which results in hepatocellular damage without necrosis. Marked elevation of the serum creatine phosphokinase (all MM fraction), with only modest elevations of transaminases is an important clue for the diagnosis of leptospirosis. Severely jaundiced patients are the ones most likely to exhibit renal failure and subsequent loss of intravascular volume. Renal failure is primarily the result of tubular damage, with the leptospires visible in the tubular lumen. Acute interstitial nephritis and/or immune complex glomerulonephritis may be seen on

(Continued)

Leptospira interrogans (Continued)

kidney biopsy. Urinalysis shows proteinuria, hematuria, and casts. Other manifestations of severe leptospirosis include atrial arrhythmias, congestive heart failure, coronary arteritis, and hemorrhagic myocarditis. The adult respiratory distress syndrome (ARDS) has been described along with pneumonitis.

Diagnosis Definitive diagnosis can only be made by isolation of the organism from a sterile body site. During the first 10 days of the illness, the organism can be isolated from blood, urine, or cerebrospinal fluid. Culture of the organism requires special media (eg, Fletcher's or Stuart's media) and requires 6 or more weeks of incubation. The microbiology laboratory should be notified in suspected cases of leptospirosis and specimen collection and handling details should be reviewed. After 10 days, the organism can no longer be isolated from blood and some laboratories will not accept blood cultures for *Leptospira* if clinical symptoms have been present for more than 10 days. During the second and third week of illness, the urine culture may still be positive for the organism. In general, cultures for *Leptospira* are considered the gold standard for diagnosis but have a low yield.

Serologic diagnosis is important since cultures for *Leptospira* have low sensitivity. A presumptive diagnosis of leptospirosis can be made by demonstrating a seroconversion (greater than 4-fold rise in serologic titer). There are a variety of serological tests available including a macroscopic slide agglutination test (killed antigen), microscopic agglutination test (live antigen), indirect hemagglutination test, and an ELISA assay for *Leptospira* IgM. A urine dipstick test for *Leptospira* detection has also recently been described.

Direct detection of the organism can be performed using darkfield microscopy. Since *Leptospira* is a spirochete, it can be visualized on occasion using the same type of darkfield microscopy as with syphilis. This test is relatively difficult to perform and not offered in many laboratories. Other techniques include PCR and immunohistochemical staining; techniques which are still under study.

Diagnostic Tests/Procedures

Darkfield Examination, Leptospirosis *on page 443*

Leptospira Culture *on page 518*

Leptospira Serology *on page 519*

Treatment Early studies suggested that penicillin or tetracycline might shorten the duration of fever and reduce the incidence of renal, hepatic, meningeal, and hemorrhagic complications, but only if therapy was started by the fourth day of illness. Recently, it was found that therapy may be effective in severe disease even when treatment was delayed. Administration of a single dose of doxycycline, 200 mg once a week, prevented infection in soldiers in Panama.

Treatment recommendations for moderate to severe leptospirosis are penicillin G, 1.5 million units every 6 hours or ampicillin, 1000 mg I.V. every 6 hours. In mild to moderate disease, oral therapy with doxycycline, 100 mg orally twice daily or ampicillin, 500-750 mg orally every 6 hours for 5-7 days.

In the U.S., there is no licensed human vaccine, but in other countries, human vaccine against leptospirosis has been reported to be useful.

Pediatric Drug Therapy

Recommended:

Penicillin G (Parenteral/Aqueous) *on page 993*

Ampicillin *on page 657*

Adult Drug Therapy

Recommended:

Penicillin G (Parenteral/Aqueous) *on page 993*

Ampicillin *on page 657*

Alternate:

Tetracycline *on page 1106*

Doxycycline *on page 787*

Selected Readings

Emmanouilides CE, Kohn OF, and Garibaldi R, "Leptospirosis Complicated by a Jarisch-Herxheimer Reaction and Adult Respiratory Distress Syndrome," *Clin Infect Dis*, 1994, 18(6):1004-6.

O'Neil KM, Rickman LS, and Lazarus AA, "Pulmonary Manifestations of Leptospirosis," *Rev Infect Dis*, 1991, 13(4):705-9.

Tappero JW, Ashford DA, and Perkins BA, "*Leptospira* Species (Leptospirosis)," *Principles and Practice of Infectious Diseases*, 5th ed, Mandell GL, Bennett JE, and Dolin R, eds, New York, NY: Churchill Livingstone, 2000, 2495-500.

Leptospirosis *see Leptospira interrogans on page 205*

Lice

Synonyms *Pediculus humanus*; *Phthirus pubis*

Microbiology Human lice are ectoparasites and thus tend to live on or in the skin of the host. They belong to the insect class *Hexapoda*. There are three species important in human infection. *Pediculus humanus* var *corporis* is the human body louse, *Pediculus humanus* var *capitis* is the human head louse, and *Phthirus pubis* is the crab louse. The body and head louse have similar appearances and are about 4 mm long. The pubic louse is much wider and has a crab-like appearance from which its name is derived. The eggs adhere to human hair and to clothing and are termed nits.

Epidemiology Humans are the reservoir for lice. Infestations have been described worldwide especially in areas of overcrowding. The incubation period is about 1-4 weeks following exposure. Individuals are communicable until all the lice and eggs have been treated and destroyed. Pediculosis capitis is a particular problem with school-aged children, where the practice of sharing combs or brushes facilitates epidemic transmission. All socioeconomic backgrounds are at risk for head lice. In contrast, pediculosis corporis is seen mainly in areas of poor sanitation. The body louse resides almost exclusively in soiled clothing, rather than the skin, and only leaves the clothing for a blood meal from the host. Pediculosis corporis also transmits the rickettsial infection epidemic typhus, as well a several others. *Phthirus pubis* is usually sexually transmitted, although spread via infested bedding or clothing can occur.

Clinical Syndromes

- **Pediculosis corporis:** Typically, the patient complains of severe pruritus, and small, erythematous papules are found on the body. Often extensive self-induced excoriations across the trunk are noted. If left untreated for long periods, hyperpigmentation and scarring may occur, called "vagabond's disease."
- **Pediculosis capitis:** The most common presentation is intractable scalp pruritus. On examination there may be evidence of secondary bacterial infection of the scalp from excoriations. At times, an "id reaction" occurs, characterized by a dramatic skin eruption over the arms and trunk, felt to be a hypersensitivity reaction.
- **Pediculosis pubis:** Most patients present with pruritus in the region of the pubic hairs, but other areas may be involved including the eyelashes and hairs in the axilla. Secondary bacterial infections are less common.

Diagnosis The diagnosis of pediculosis is often suspected when an individual presents with severe pruritus. On some occasions, the patient may have identified lice themselves or have had a recent contact history. The diagnosis is confirmed by finding lice (1-4 mm long, depending on species) and/or the "nits" (usually 1 mm or less, attached to hairs).

Diagnostic Tests/Procedures

Arthropod Identification *on page 387*

Treatment General principles of treating pediculosis include discarding or carefully laundering clothing, discarding infested combs or hats, and laundering bedsheets. In general, clothes and bedsheets can be effectively decontaminated by dry cleaning or by machine washing and drying in a hot cycle. Secondary bacterial infections of the skin are common and generally respond to antibiotics effective against *Staphylococcus aureus* (dicloxacillin, erythromycin, and others). Pruritus is typically quite severe and may be alleviated by hydroxyzine (Atarax®), diphenhydramine (Benadryl®), and/or topical steroid creams. Treatment guidelines are as follows:

1. Pediculosis corporis: Since the louse resides mainly in the creases of clothes and not on the host, the infection can often be eradicated by delousing contaminated items and maintaining careful hygiene.
2. Pediculosis capitis. Several agents are effective: 1% lindane (Kwell®) shampoo to the scalp, pyrethrin liquid (RID), or permethrin creme rinse (Nix®). These insecticides are probably equal in efficacy. Recently permethrin resistance in head lice was reported from Israel and the Czech republic, but not from the United States. Only lindane requires a prescription. **Caution:** Lindane has been associated with seizures and other nervous system toxicities. However, the risk of serious adverse effects during treatment for pediculosis is small due to its minimal systemic absorption. Nevertheless, lindane should be avoided in pregnancy and in lactating women.
3. Pediculosis pubis. The treatment recommendations are the same as for pediculosis capitis. In addition, sexual partners should be identified and treated in the same manner. Pediculosis involving the eyelashes should **not** be treated with insecticides. Instead, occlusive ophthalmic ointment should be applied to the eyelashes twice daily for at least 8 days in an attempt to smother the parasites.

Patients should be seen in follow-up if symptoms persist 1 week after treatment. A second application may be necessary. Some clinicians routinely instruct patients to reapply the insecticide at the 1 week point.

(Continued)

Lice *(Continued)*

Drug Therapy

Recommended:

Lindane *on page 913*

Pyrethrins and Piperonyl Butoxide *on page 1023*

Permethrin *on page 1001*

Selected Readings

DiLiddo AP and Schachner LA, "Scabies and Lice Infestations," *Dermatol Thera*, 1997, 2:41-50.

Hogan DJ, Schachner LA, and Tanglertsampan C, "Diagnosis and Treatment of Childhood Scabies and Pediculosis," *Pediatr Clin North Am*, 1991, 38(4):941-57.

Line Sepsis *see* Catheter Infection, Intravascular *on page 70*

Listeria monocytogenes

Related Information

Clinical Syndromes Associated With Foodborne Diseases *on page 1276*

Microbiology *Listeria monocytogenes* is a gram-positive bacillus which causes sporadic cases of meningitis, septicemia, brain stem encephalitis, and several less common syndromes. It is an important cause of meningitis in the elderly, neonates, and other immunocompromised individuals, particularly organ transplant patients.

The organism is an aerobic, gram-positive rod which does not produce spores. At times it may assume a more coccoid appearance on Gram stain of clinical samples (eg, cerebrospinal fluid) and may thus be mistaken for gram-positive cocci. *Listeria* can also be confused morphologically with the more commonly seen *Corynebacterium* species, which are also gram-positive bacilli (but are often contaminants). *Listeria* is primarily an intracellular pathogen, and tends to reside within mononuclear phagocytes of the host. This feature is thought to contribute to its pathogenicity, since the organism can spread from cell to cell in a somewhat protected fashion.

When *Listeria monocytogenes* meningitis is suspected, the clinician should try to submit at least 10 mL of cerebrospinal fluid for bacterial culture, since only a few *Listeria* organisms may be present. The organism generally grows well on most routine media used in the laboratory. Special requests for selective or enrichment cultures for *Listeria* are usually not necessary for culturing the organism from normally sterile body fluids such as cerebrospinal fluid, joint fluid, or blood. For isolation of the organism from nonsterile body sites, such as stool, selective media may be helpful (the Microbiology Laboratory should be notified in advance). It is important for the clinician not to automatically dismiss a report of a "gram-positive rod" isolated from blood cultures or a sterile body site as a contaminant, particularly in an immunocompromised host or elderly patient in whom *Listeria* infection is possible.

Epidemiology *L. monocytogenes* is ubiquitous in the environment, being present in soil, contaminated water, and in the feces of many animals. In addition to being widespread in soil and animal products, the organism grows very well at a wide range of temperatures from 4°C to 37°C. Because of these factors, the organism can multiply readily in contaminated foods kept in standard refrigerators. Studies from the Centers for Disease Control and Prevention (CDC) demonstrated that many foods harbor significant numbers of *Listeria* despite being refrigerated, with an overall rate of 10% contamination of raw foods such as vegetables, chicken, beef, and milk. Delicatessen food appears to be particularly vulnerable to contamination.

It is estimated that there are about 1000 cases of listeriosis annually in the U.S., despite increased agricultural and food processing regulations. It is clear that the number of cases of listeriosis is quite relative to the repeated exposures to the organism in the general population. Asymptomatic carriage of *Listeria* in stools is relatively frequent; some studies suggest a fecal excretion rate of 5% or more in healthy humans. In addition to food-borne acquisition, which is by far the most common, humans may occasionally be exposed to *Listeria* by one of several other routes: Infection of the neonate *in utero* or during delivery, direct exposure to infected animals, or exposure to environmental reservoirs (soil, water, etc).

Cases of listeriosis tend to be sporadic and difficult to predict. Most infections occur in the summer months and are more common in urban than rural settings, despite its reputation as a zoonotic infection. Often, the source of the *Listeria* remains unknown. In addition to occasional sporadic cases, outbreaks of listeriosis continue to be reported on a regular basis, implicating a number of foods including Mexican-style cheese, ice cream, coleslaw, alfalfa sprouts, undercooked chicken, hot dogs, dairy products, and a number of other foods.

Infection with *Listeria* usually occurs in definable groups in the community. Cell-mediated immunity is critically important in defense against *Listeria*, whereas neutropenia is not clearly a risk factor. Those at highest risk include patients with solid

organ transplants, malignancies (particularly lymphoma), and patients receiving corticosteroids. Pregnant females, neonates, and alcoholics are additional groups at risk for infection. It is important to note that elderly patients are at increased risk of listeriosis, and in a number of serious cases, advanced age is the sole predisposing factor. Interestingly, listeriosis does not appear to be a common pathogen in patients with AIDS, despite the deficiencies in T-cell function. This may be due to the routine use of trimethoprim-sulfamethoxazole for *Pneumocystis* prophylaxis, which also has activity against *L. monocytogenes.* Although uncommon, serious infections with *Listeria* have been described in otherwise healthy individuals.

Clinical Syndromes

- **Adult meningitis:** *Listeria* is an increasingly important cause of community-acquired meningitis in immunocompetent adults. In some series, *Listeria* is the second or third most common cause of community-acquired bacterial meningitis in adults, following *Streptococcus pneumoniae.* In immunocompromised persons, such as organ transplant recipients, patients with lymphoma, or patients receiving corticosteroids, *Listeria* is one of the most common etiologies of bacterial meningitis. *Listeria* meningitis can be quite variable in its presentation and can range from a subacute course to a rapid and fulminant one. In some cases, the diagnosis may be quite difficult when high fevers and nuchal rigidity are absent. There are no pathognomonic features of *Listeria* meningitis which allow diagnosis on clinical grounds alone. However, *Listeria* meningitis tends to have a somewhat higher incidence of ataxia, cranial palsies, and seizures than other causes of bacterial meningitis. Routine laboratory studies are not helpful. There is usually not a monocytosis on the peripheral blood smear despite the name of the organism (a misnomer). CSF chemical analysis is variable and frequently nondiagnostic. The degree of CSF pleocytosis can range from several cells to >12,000 cells/mm^3. Differential cell counts vary from nearly 100% polymorphonuclear cells to 100% mononuclear cells. Often a modest elevation of CSF protein is seen, along with a minor decrease in CSF glucose. The organism is visible on Gram stain in less than half of the cases. The differential diagnosis of a subacute meningitis in an immunosuppressed host must also include *Cryptococcus neoformans.* The finding of focal brain lesions by CT scan or MRI broadens the differential to include toxoplasmosis, *Nocardia asteroides,* bacterial brain abscess, fungal meningitis, and others.
- **Meningoencephalitis of the neonate:** This is a "late-onset" neonatal disease, occurring several days to weeks postpartum. As with adult cases, isolated neonatal meningitis from *Listeria* can be variable in its presentation. Fever may be low grade or absent, and irritability and failure to thrive may be the only clues. CSF findings in the neonate are similar to those in the adult. It is important to review the Gram stain of CSF carefully to avoid confusing *Listeria* with Group B streptococci, a common cause of neonatal meningitis.
- **Rhomboencephalitis:** This form of central nervous system infection is gaining increased recognition. This manifestation of *Listeria* differs from meningitis in that the primary site of infection is in the brain stem, not the meninges. Patients may complain of fever, cephalgia, and hemiparesis. This form of listeriosis may be mistaken for a stroke, vasculitis, brain tumor, or abscess. CT and MRI scans suggest focal inflammation without a discrete abscess or ring enhancement. Cerebrospinal fluid is usually normal and CSF cultures are negative for *Listeria.* The diagnosis is usually made when *Listeria* is isolated from blood cultures.
- **Listeriosis in pregnancy:** Unfortunately, this is often difficult to diagnose, since the woman may be asymptomatic or complain of only a mild fever and malaise. Other symptoms variably present include diarrhea and flank pain. The differential diagnosis is usually broad and listeriosis may be mistaken for pyelonephritis, lower urinary tract infection, and viral syndromes (eg, influenza). Blood cultures may be positive and should be performed. Complications include premature delivery, septic abortion, and *in utero* fetal infection.
- **Granulomatosis infantiseptica:** This unique, transplacentally acquired infection is severe and often lethal. It is an "early onset" neonatal infection apparent within hours of birth. Typically, the infants are seriously ill. There are widespread abscesses involving visceral organs such as the liver, spleen, lungs, intestinal tract, and brain. The lesions are usually abscesses with polymorphonuclear leukocytes, but granulomas have also been seen (referred to as "miliary granulomatosis"). Dark papular skin lesions may be present on the trunk and lower extremities, suggesting the diagnosis. Gram stain and culture of meconium, amniotic fluid, conjunctival exudates, CSF, throat, blood, or skin lesions are frequently positive for *L. monocytogenes.* Antibiotic therapy should be started immediately if this diagnosis is suspected, since death may occur if treatment is withheld until cultures are finalized.
- **Septicemia:** *Listeria* can be isolated from the blood of adults and neonates who present from the community with nonspecific fever and chills. Bacteremias are

(Continued)

Listeria monocytogenes (Continued)

more likely in profoundly immunosuppressed hosts but have been seen in alcoholics, diabetics, pregnancy, and normal healthy individuals. The clinical presentation can be indistinguishable from gram-negative sepsis, with high fevers and hypotension (so-called "typhoidal *Listeria*"). On rare occasion, the diagnosis is suggested by the finding of a monocytosis on the peripheral blood smear, but blood cultures remain the highest yield.

- **Gastroenteritis:** *Listeria* has recently been shown to be a cause of fever and diarrhea, which appears to be a self-resolving illness. The incidence of this febrile gastroenteritis is unknown, but has been shown convincingly in some studies of *Listeria* outbreaks.
- **Miscellaneous:** Endocarditis, ocular infections, lymphadenitis, osteomyelitis, brain abscess, peritonitis, and other focal infections have been rarely reported.

Diagnosis Except for granulomatosis infantiseptica, the clinical presentations of listeriosis are not unique and microbiological confirmation is necessary. Depending on the clinical site of infection, specimens of blood and body fluids should be sent, as described above. Agglutination studies for antibodies directed against *L. monocytogenes* have little value. It is very helpful to the clinical microbiology laboratory when a physician notifies the lab that *Listeria* is suspected in a culture.

Diagnostic Tests/Procedures

Aerobic Culture, Cerebrospinal Fluid *on page 366*
Blood Culture, Aerobic and Anaerobic *on page 391*
Cerebrospinal Fluid Analysis *on page 408*
Gram Stain *on page 473*
Lumbar Puncture *on page 524*

Treatment No randomized comparison trials have been performed to determine the drug(s) of choice for listeriosis. *In vitro* data show the organism is susceptible to many antibiotics. The most clinical experience has been limited to penicillin and ampicillin, and they are probably equivalent. Occasionally, penicillin-resistant strains of *Listeria* have been reported. There is some *in vitro* evidence to suggest the combination of penicillin (or ampicillin) with an aminoglycoside may be synergistic against *Listeria*, and this combination has been used in serious, life-threatening infections. The combination of ampicillin and gentamicin has also been advocated for bacteremia and/or meningitis in immunocompromised hosts. It is important to know that the cephalosporins, as a group, are not active against this organism and should not be used for cases of *Listeria* meningitis.

In 2005, the Clinical and Laboratory Standards Institute published a standardized method to perform antimicrobial susceptibility testing on *Listeria* species (publication M100-515, 2005). This publication provides the breakpoints for ampicillin (≤2 mcg/mL = susceptible) and penicillin (≤2 mcg/mL = susceptible).

Consultation with an Infectious Disease specialist is appropriate in complicated cases or in the patient with a penicillin allergy.

Drug Therapy

Recommended:

Monotherapy:
Ampicillin *on page 657*
Penicillin G (Parenteral/Aqueous) *on page 993*
Combination therapy:
Ampicillin *on page 657*
plus
Gentamicin *on page 841*
Penicillin G (Parenteral/Aqueous) *on page 993*
plus
Gentamicin *on page 841*

Alternate:

Sulfamethoxazole and Trimethoprim *on page 1087*

Selected Readings

Jamal WY, Al-Shomari S, Boland F, et al, "*Listeria monocytogenes* Meningitis in an Immunocompetent Adult Patient," *Med Princ Pract*, 2005, 14(1):55-7.

"*Listeria monocytogenes* - Questions and Answers," *J Environ Health*, 2004, 67(2):41, 45.

Lorber B, "*Listeria monocytogenes*," *Principles and Practice of Infectious Diseases*, 5th ed, Mandell GL, Bennett JE, and Dolin R, eds, New York, NY: Churchill Livingstone, 2000, 2208-15.

Lorber B, "Listeriosis," *Clin Infect Dis*, 1997, 24(1):1-11.

Ooi ST and Lorber B, "Gastroenteritis due to *Listeria monocytogenes*," *Clin Infect Dis*, 2005, 40(9):1327-32.

Listeriosis *see Listeria monocytogenes on page 208*

Liver Abscess

Synonyms Abscess, Liver; Hepatic Abscess

Clinical Presentation Pyogenic abscesses are most frequently secondary to biliary disease. May be infectious complication following liver transplant. Bacterial abscess more common than amebic in the USA. Patients present with fever and chills they have had for several days to weeks. Right upper quadrant pain may radiate to right shoulder and patient may have have pleural rub. Jaundice is unusual unless ascending cholangitis present. Differentiation of amebic from pyogenic is difficult. Patients with amebic abscess may report history of diarrhea. Serum alkaline phosphatase is frequently elevated. Blood cultures positive in >50% of pyogenic cases. Endoscopic sphincterotomy and local antibiotic lavage may be an effective treatment. Surgery and GI consult indicated.

Differential Diagnosis Hepatocellular carcinoma; echinococcal cyst

Likely Pathogens

Pyogenic:
- Mixed gram-negative aerobic and anaerobic flora
- *Streptococcus* Species *on page 326*
- *Staphylococcus aureus*, Methicillin-Susceptible *on page 307*

Ameba:
- *Entamoeba histolytica on page 130*

Diagnostic Tests/Procedures

Ultrasound, Abdomen *on page 604*
Computed Transaxial Tomography, Abdomen Studies *on page 423*
Entamoeba histolytica Serology *on page 452*
MRI
Ultrasound-Guided Aspirate for Culture and Special Stains

Empiric Drug Therapy

Recommended:

Pyogenic:
- Cefotaxime *on page 708*
- Ceftriaxone *on page 722*

Ameba:
- Asymptomatic (cyst passers):
  - Diloxanide Furoate *on page 778*
- Invasive infection:
  - Metronidazole *on page 940*
    - *followed by*
      - Diloxanide Furoate *on page 778*

Alternate:

Pyogenic:
- Cefoxitin *on page 712*
- Cefotetan *on page 710*
- Piperacillin and Tazobactam Sodium *on page 1003*
- Ticarcillin and Clavulanate Potassium *on page 1114*
- Ampicillin and Sulbactam *on page 660*
- Imipenem and Cilastatin *on page 861*
- Meropenem *on page 936*
- Ertapenem *on page 805*
- Tigecycline *on page 1116*
- Combination therapy:
  - Ciprofloxacin *on page 742*
    - *plus*
      - Metronidazole *on page 940*

Ameba: Invasive infection:
- Metronidazole *on page 940*
  - *followed by one of the following*
    - Paromomycin *on page 989*
    - Iodoquinol *on page 891*

Selected Readings

Dull JS, Topa L, Balgha V, et al, "Nonsurgical Treatment of Biliary Liver Abscesses: Efficacy of Endoscopic Drainage and Local Antibiotic Lavage With Nasobiliary Catheter," *Gastrointest Endosc*, 2000, 51(1):55-9.
Lam YH, Wong SK, Lee DW, et al, "ERCP and Pyogenic Liver Abscess," *Gastrointest Endosc*, 1999, 50(3):340-4.
Rustgi AK and Richter JM, "Pyogenic and Amebic Liver Abscess," *Med Clin North Am*, 1989, 73(4):847-58.
Seeto RK and Rockey DC, "Amebic Liver Abscess: Epidemiology, Clinical Features, and Outcome," *West J Med*, 1999, 170(2):104-9.

Lumpy Jaw Syndrome *see Actinomyces* Species *on page 27*

Lung Abscess

Synonyms Abscess, Lung

Clinical Presentation The predisposing factors for lung abscess are aspiration (most common) and periodontal disease or gingivitis (less common). Patients with a lung abscess usually present after experiencing the following symptoms for several days to weeks: low-grade fever, malaise, fatigue, and a productive cough. Pleural pain and hemoptysis may or may not be present. Radiographic and CT examination typically show infiltrates and cavitary lesions with air-fluid levels.

Differential Diagnosis Bacterial, fungal, parasitic, and mycobacterial necrotizing pneumonia; cavitary infarction; septic embolism; vasculitis; neoplasm (cavitary carcinoma); empyema; bronchiectasis

Likely Pathogens

Aerobic Bacteria (usually involved in mixed infections with anaerobic bacteria):

- *Staphylococcus aureus*, Methicillin-Resistant *on page 304*
- *Staphylococcus aureus*, Methicillin-Susceptible *on page 307*
- *Enterobacter* Species *on page 132*
- *Streptococcus pneumoniae*, Drug-Susceptible *on page 319*
- *Streptococcus*, Viridans group *on page 326*
- *Actinomyces* Species *on page 27*

Anaerobic Bacteria (typically involved in lung abscesses):

- *Streptococcus*-Related Gram-Positive Cocci *on page 325*
- *Fusobacterium* Species
- *Bacteroides* and *Prevotella* Species *on page 46*
- *Prevotella* Species
- *Clostridium perfringens on page 88*

Diagnostic Tests/Procedures

- Gram Stain *on page 473*
- Abscess Aerobic and Anaerobic Culture *on page 360*
- Chest Films *on page 412*
- Blood Culture, Aerobic and Anaerobic *on page 391*

Drug Therapy Comment The use of antimicrobial agents is the primary method of therapy. Treatment might be needed for weeks to months. Radiographic or CT examinations, fever, and culture/examination of sputum can be monitored during treatment.

Empiric Drug Therapy

Recommended:

One of the following

- Clindamycin *on page 752*
- Metronidazole *on page 940*
  - *plus*
    - Penicillin G (Parenteral/Aqueous) *on page 993*

Alternate:

- Piperacillin and Tazobactam Sodium *on page 1003*
- Ampicillin and Sulbactam *on page 660*
- Ticarcillin and Clavulanate Potassium *on page 1114*

Selected Readings

Civen R, Jousimies-Somer H, Marina M, et al, "A Retrospective Review of Cases of Anaerobic Empyema and Update of Bacteriology," *Clin Infect Dis*, 1995, 20 (Suppl 2):S224-9.

Davis B and Systrom DM, "Lung Abscess: Pathogenesis, Diagnosis and Treatment," *Curr Clin Top Infect Dis*, 1998, 18:252-73.

Mwandumba HC and Beeching NJ, "Pyogenic Lung Infections: Factors for Predicting Clinical Outcomes of Lung Abscess and Thoracic Empyeme ," *Curr Opin Pulm Med*, 2000, 151-6.

Wu MH, Tseng YL, Lin MY, et al, "Surgical Treatment of Pediatric Lung Abscess," *Pediatr Surg Int*, 1997, 12(4):293-5.

Lyme Borreliosis *see Borrelia burgdorferi on page 56*

Lyme Disease *see Borrelia burgdorferi on page 56*

Lymphadenitis

Clinical Presentation Can be regional or diffuse depending on the causative organism. Lymph nodes are usually swollen and tender.

Differential Diagnosis Depends on the site of the enlarged node.

Generalized lymphadenopathy: HIV; scarlet fever (group A *Streptococcus*); miliary tuberculosis; brucellosis; syphilis; cat scratch disease; histoplasmosis; lymphogranuloma venereum (LGV); virus (CMV, EBV); toxoplasmosis; Whipple's disease; lymphoma

Inguinal adenopathy: Syphilis; LGV; chancroid; bacterial

Cervical adenopathy: Bacterial (*Streptococcus*); *Staphylococcus aureus*; tuberculosis; MAI; cat scratch disease; lymphoma; Kawasaki syndrome; sarcoidosis kikuchi's; others

Likely Pathogens

Toxoplasma gondii on page 331
Mycobacterium Species, not MTB or MAI *on page 232*
Bartonella Species *on page 48*
Human Immunodeficiency Virus *on page 181*
Staphylococcus aureus, Methicillin-Susceptible *on page 307*
Epstein-Barr Virus *on page 139*

Diagnostic Tests/Procedures Diagnostic tests should be obtained based on clinical suspicion since not all tests are necessary.

Abscess Aerobic and Anaerobic Culture *on page 360*
Epstein-Barr Virus Serology *on page 454*
HIV-1 Serology *on page 501*
Lymph Node Biopsy *on page 529*
Mycobacteria Culture, Biopsy or Body Fluid *on page 539*
Toxoplasma Serology *on page 596*

Drug Therapy Comment Drug therapy based on identification of the causative agent.

Lymphogranuloma Venereum (LGV) *see Chlamydia trachomatis on page 74*
MAC *see Mycobacterium avium-intracellulare* (Complex) *on page 228*
Mad-Hatter Disease *see Bacillus anthracis on page 41*
Madura Foot *see* Dematiaceous Fungi *on page 112*
Maduromycosis *see* Dematiaceous Fungi *on page 112*
MAI *see Mycobacterium avium-intracellulare* (Complex) *on page 228*
Malaria *see Plasmodium* Species *on page 265*

Malassezia furfur

Synonyms Pityriasis (Tinea) Versicolor; *Pityrosporum orbiculare*; *Pityrosporum ovale*

Microbiology The genus *Malassezia* contains three species: *M. furfur*, *M. sympodialis*, and *M. pachydermatis*. All are lipophilic yeasts found as indigenous flora of human skin. The distribution of *Malassezia* correlates with the oily areas of the skin, most notably the scalp, chest, and back. Adolescents have the greatest colonization correlating with the increased activity of the sebaceous glands. The Microbiology Laboratory should be notified if *M. furfur* is suspected because growth is dependent on the presence of an exogenous source of fatty acids. This is accomplished by overlaying the medium with olive oil. Histopathologic stains reveal filamentous structures; however in culture, *Malassezia* grows as oval yeast cells measuring up to 6 µm. The colonies are smooth, cream to yellowish brown, and glistening. Optimal growth occurs between 35°C and 37°C.

Epidemiology Although *M. furfur* is mostly implicated as the etiologic agent of various dermal infections, hematogenous infections especially in debilitated or immunosuppressed patients and neonates occur. Nosocomial outbreaks of both *M. furfur* and *M. pachydermatis* bacteremia in neonatal intensive care units attributed to person to person transmission via the hands of medical personnel have been reported. There is a strong correlation of increased risk of *Malassezia* bacteremia in neonates receiving lipid emulsions through a central venous catheter. The lipids are thought to provide nutrients to the yeasts that have colonized the catheters; however, *Malassezia* has been reported to cause bacteremias in debilitated adults not receiving any parenteral nutrition.

Clinical Syndromes

- **Cutaneous manifestations:** Folliculitis must be distinguished from other infectious etiologies (eg, bacterial, systemic candidiasis, cryptococcosis, atypical mycobacteria). Biopsy and culture of the skin should be performed. Lesions are usually multiple and distributed over the shoulders, back, and chest. Disseminated candidiasis has a higher predilection for the extremities. *Candida* folliculitis frequently involves the face. *Malassezia* folliculitis initially presents as a papulonodular eruption on an erythematous base varying in size from 2-6 mm. Lesions may become pustule or associated with hair follicles. Patients typically complain of intense pruritus.

  Tinea versicolor is a common asymptomatic superficial infection seen in young adults, particularly in warm, humid environments towards the end of summer. It appears as hypo- or hyperpigmented annular lesions of various sizes and shapes. The eruption is asymmetrical occurring on the back, chest, and neck. May go into remission without treatment.

  The role of *M. furfur* in seborrhoeic dermatitis in HIV-infected individuals is unclear, although some comparative studies have shown efficacy in combined antifungal and steroid therapy. In addition, *M. furfur* may play a role in atopic dermatitis and seborrhoeic dermatitis in non-HIV infected individuals.

(Continued)

Malassezia furfur (Continued)

- **Intravenous line sepsis:** Colonization of the central venous catheter occurs prior to *Malassezia* fungemia. Most of the cases of fungemia have been reported in premature infants receiving lipid infusions. Fever is the sole manifestation in approximately 20% of infected infants. May present with aphea, bradycardia or tachycardia, lethargy, cyanosis, tachypnea, and/or hepatosplenomegaly. Plain radiographs of the chest reveal interstitial pneumonitis in 50% to 60% of infants. Leukocytosis and thrombocytopenia occur in 50%. Lipid deposits containing *M. furfur* have been found in the pulmonary arterial walls postmortem. Adults with a history of inflammatory bowel disease or recent abdominal surgery requiring parenteral nutrition are at increased risk of *Malassezia* line sepsis. Most cases are rather indolent with fever being the most common complaint. Peripheral blood cultures are positive in only 25% of cases, which may be due to the low level of fungemia, difficulty in laboratory isolation techniques, adherence to the central venous catheter, or rapid removal of the organism by the pulmonary vasculature.

Diagnosis Gram stain of the buffy coat should be done in suspected cases of line-associated sepsis. Budding yeast cells can be seen on Gram, Giemsa, PAS, or silver stains. Suspected cases should be cultured on media overlaid with olive oil. *M. furfur* folliculitis biopsy reveals unipolar budding yeast confined to the epidermis, predominantly near the hair follicles. No pseudohyphae or hyphae are seen. Occasionally, dermal abscess formation in the perifollicular dermis and granulomatous perifolliculitis may be observed. Potassium hydroxide (KOH) preps of skin scrapings of tinea versicolor reveal the characteristic "spaghetti and meatballs" which are strands of filamentous hyphae and yeast cells.

Diagnostic Tests/Procedures

Fungus Culture, Appropriate Site *on page 461*
KOH Preparation *on page 513*

Treatment Treatment of *M. furfur* fungemia requires removal of the central venous catheter with or without systemic antifungal therapy (eg, ketoconazole, itraconazole, fluconazole, or amphotericin B). Folliculitis usually responds to clotrimazole, ketoconazole, or miconazole creams. Diffuse follicular involvement may be treated with any of the systemic azoles. Antipruritics should be prescribed to avoid excoriation and superimposed bacterial infection. Tinea versicolor responds to topical treatment of propylene glycol (50%), selenium sulfide, or azole creams. Systemic azoles are not usually indicated but may be used in refractory cases. Relapse occurs in 60% after 1 year and 80% by 2 years. Seborrhea dermatitis in AIDS may need combination therapy of an azole plus either topical or systemic steroids.

Drug Therapy

Recommended:

Line-Associated:

Amphotericin B (Conventional) *on page 650*
Fluconazole *on page 819*
Itraconazole *on page 895*
Ketoconazole *on page 903*

Dermatitides:

Clotrimazole *on page 758*
Ketoconazole *on page 903*
Miconazole *on page 945*
Selenium Sulfide *on page 1063*
Fluconazole *on page 819*
Itraconazole *on page 895*
Terbinafine *on page 1097* (1% solution)

Selected Readings

Marcon MJ and Powell DA, "Human Infections Due to *Malassezia* Species," *Clin Microbiol Rev*, 1992, 5(2):101-19.

Rhie S, Turcios R, Buckley H, et al, "Clinical Features and Treatment of Malassezia Folliculitis With Fluconazole in Orthotopic Heart Transplant Recipients," *J Heart Lung Transplant*, 2000, 19(2):215-9.

Teglia O, Schoch PE, and Cunha BA, "*Malassezia furfur* Infections," *Infect Control Hosp Epidemiol*, 1991, 12(11):676-81.

Welbel SF, McNeil MM, Pramanik A, et al, "Nosocomial *Malassezia pachydermatis* Bloodstream Infections in a Neonatal Intensive Care Unit," *Pediatr Infect Dis J*, 1994, 13(2):104-8.

Malta Fever *see Brucella* Species *on page 61*

Marburg Virus *see* Ebola Virus *on page 117*

Mastitis

Synonyms Breast Infection

Clinical Presentation Inflammation of the breast involving either the ductal tissue (adenitis) or the connective tissue (cellulitis). Symptoms include localized tenderness, redness, and heat, usually associated with systemic symptoms of fever and malaise.

May be associated with nausea and vomiting. Infections occur most frequently in postpartum females in association with breast-feeding and are typically unilateral. Risk is increased by disruptions in the skin integrity (cracked or fissured skin) or obstructed ducts. Abnormalities in the breast (such as postsurgical scarring), irregular feeding patterns, or any other factor which may lead to obstruction of the ducts can increase the risk of mastitis. In cases not associated with breast-feeding, an abscess which forms below the areola commonly involves anaerobic organisms, while an abscess above the areola is frequently caused by *Staphylococcus aureus*.

Likely Pathogens

Staphylococcus aureus, Methicillin-Resistant *on page 304*
Staphylococcus aureus, Methicillin-Susceptible *on page 307*
Bacteroides and *Prevotella* Species *on page 46*
Streptococcus-Related Gram-Positive Cocci *on page 325*

Drug Therapy Comment Generally, unless an abscess is present, breast-feeding is continued during treatment and may improve response. Abscess drainage is usually required.

Empiric Drug Therapy

Recommended:

Postpartum:
Cefazolin *on page 700*
Dicloxacillin *on page 773*

If abscess is present:
Nafcillin *on page 955*
Oxacillin *on page 983*
Vancomycin *on page 1144*

Other abscess:
Clindamycin *on page 752*
Ampicillin and Sulbactam *on page 660*
Amoxicillin and Clavulanate Potassium *on page 645*

Alternate:

Postpartum:
Clindamycin *on page 752*
Abscess:
Cefazolin *on page 700*
plus
Metronidazole *on page 940*

Measles *see* Measles Virus *on page 215*

Measles Virus

Related Information

Immunization Recommendations *on page 1249*
Prophylaxis for Patients Exposed to Common Communicable Diseases *on page 1309*

Synonyms Rubeola Virus

Microbiology Measles virus is a member of the Paramyxoviridae family (measles virus, mumps virus, parainfluenza virus, canine distemper virus, respiratory syncytial virus, and others). Measles virus is enveloped and contains single-stranded RNA. Measles virus has specific envelope proteins H and F which are responsible for adsorption/hemagglutination and cell penetration/fusion, respectively. Measles virus is extremely labile and is sensitive to light, drying, and naturally occurring enzymes and acids. Measles virus remains extremely infective for several hours as long as it remains moist and in aerosolized droplets. The fact that measles virus is easily spread by inhalation of such droplets and by direct contact with nasal secretions explains why measles virus causes one of the most contagious of all infectious diseases, measles. Measles virus exists in two forms, wild type and vaccine form. The wild type is extremely genetically stable; the same genotype and phenotype exists worldwide.

Epidemiology Measles (archaic term, rubeola) has been observed and recorded for over 2000 years and occurs today in every country. In developing countries, measles affects almost all children younger than 5 years of age and causes 1-2 million deaths per year in children. In the United States, in 1990, there were ~27,000 reported cases of measles. More than 80% of the persons who represented these cases had previously received measles vaccine, and approximately 50% of these cases were represented by poor, inner-city preschool children. Humans are the natural reservoir and, for all practical purposes, the only hosts of measles virus.

Clinical Syndromes Measles is an infection of the respiratory tract and central nervous system and can present in at least three syndromes.
(Continued)

Measles Virus *(Continued)*

- **Conventional measles:** Incubation period, 10-14 days; prodrome of "flu"-like symptoms, conjunctivitis, and other upper respiratory tract symptoms; Koplik spots; typically a 5-day rash which spreads from head to trunk to extremities to palms and soles. Most patients are not contagious after the rash reaches its peak.
- **Mild measles:** Usually observed in infants younger than 1 year of age; similar to conventional measles but is milder and usually is not characterized by all of the typical signs and symptoms of conventional measles.
- **Atypical measles:** More severe and lasts longer than conventional measles; rash usually begins peripherally and progresses toward the trunk; can be confused with chickenpox or Rocky Mountain spotted fever; antibody titers to measles virus often are extremely high.

Diagnosis Measles is usually diagnosed clinically. Measles virus can be isolated in cell culture, but this method is somewhat difficult and usually not practical. The specimens of choice are throat and nasopharyngeal washings. Serology is the diagnostic method of choice. As with most viral serology, diagnosis is made by demonstration of a fourfold rise in measles virus-specific antibody; however, the most widely used tests are immunofluorescence antibody and enzyme immunoassays for measles-specific IgM. A minimal protective IgG antibody level has not been determined. Some laboratories offer direct detection of measles virus-infected cells from nasopharyngeal washings and nasal swabs.

Diagnostic Tests/Procedures

Measles Antibody *on page 534*
Virus Detection by DFA *on page 619*

Drug Therapy Comment

No antiviral agents active against measles, but for immune suppressed patients, intravenous immunoglobulins may be indicated.

Drug Therapy

Recommended:

Immune Globulin (Intramuscular) *on page 866*

Prophylaxis:

Measles, Mumps, and Rubella Vaccines (Combined) *on page 926*
Measles Virus Vaccine (Live) *on page 927*

Selected Readings

Gershon AA, "Measles Virus (Rubeola)," *Principles and Practice of Infectious Diseases*, 4th ed, Mandell GL, Bennett JE, and Dolin R, eds, New York, NY: Churchill Livingstone, 1995, 1519-26.
"Measles - United States, First 26 Weeks, 1993," *MMWR*, 1993, 42(42):813-6.
Schlenker T, "Measles Resurgent," *Clin Microbiol Newslett*, 1991, 13:156-7.
Siegel CS, "Measles - A Review of the Virological and Serological Methods for Early Detection," *Clin Microbiol Newslett*, 1991, 13:177-9.

Melioidosis *see Burkholderia mallei on page 64*

Meningitis, Community-Acquired, Adult

Synonyms Community-Acquired Meningitis, Adult

Clinical Presentation Patients present with fever, headache, nausea, vomiting, and nuchal rigidity. Focal neurologic abnormalities and papilledema are uncommon. In a prospective study by Thomas KE, et al, the 3 classic meningeal signs (Kernig's sign, Brudzinski's sign, and nuchal rigidity) were of limited clinical diagnostic value for adults with suspected meningitis. None of these meningeal signs were able to accurately discriminate patients with meningitis from those without it.

Differential Diagnosis Bacterial, viral, or other infectious agents; drug-induced; neoplastic; granulomatous; infectious endocarditis; collagen-vascular diseases; subdural hemorrhage; subarachnoid hemorrhage

Likely Pathogens

Haemophilus influenzae on page 159
Neisseria meningitidis on page 245
Streptococcus pneumoniae, Drug-Resistant *on page 316*
Streptococcus pneumoniae, Drug-Susceptible *on page 319*
Listeria monocytogenes on page 208 (elderly, immunocompromised)

Diagnostic Tests/Procedures

•Blood Culture, Aerobic and Anaerobic *on page 391*
•Cerebrospinal Fluid Analysis *on page 408*
•Gram Stain *on page 473*
•Lumbar Puncture *on page 524*
Computed Transaxial Tomography, Head Studies *on page 424*
Cryptococcal Antigen Serology, Serum or Cerebrospinal Fluid *on page 431*
Enterovirus Culture *on page 453*
Magnetic Resonance Scan, Brain *on page 532*

Drug Therapy Comment For suspected or proven pneumococcal meningitis, consider dexamethasone 0.15 mg/kg every 6 hours for 2-4 days. First dose administered 10-20 minutes before or at least concomitant with first dose of antibiotic.

Empiric Drug Therapy

Recommended:

Note: Empiric coverage based on likely organism (preliminary CSF exam, Gram stain, and/or patient factors). Adequate dosing and coverage of all likely pathogens is essential. Treatment duration typically is 2-3 weeks.

Haemophilus influenzae, *Neisseria meningitidis*, or *Streptococcus pneumoniae*:
Choice of one of the following
Ceftriaxone *on page 722*
Cefotaxime *on page 708*
plus
Vancomycin *on page 1144*
plus (if Listeria is suspected such as in elderly or immunocompromised)
Ampicillin *on page 657*

Alternate:

Chloramphenicol *on page 733*

Alternative for *Listeria* coverage:
Sulfamethoxazole and Trimethoprim *on page 1087*

Selected Readings

Askari S and Cartwright CP, "The Changing Epidemiology of Bacterial Meningitis: Implications for the Clinical Laboratory," *Clin Microbiol Newslett*, 1998, 20(5):33-6.
Butler JC, Hofmann J, Cetron MS, et al, "The Continued Emergence of Drug-Resistant *Streptococcus pneumoniae* in the United States: An Update From the Centers for Disease Control and Prevention Pneumococcal Sentinel Surveillance System," *J Infect Dis*, 1996, 174(5):986-93.
Cabellos C, Viladrich PF, Corredoira J, et al, "Streptococcal Meningitis in Adult Patients: Current Epidemiology and Clinical Spectrum," *Clin Infect Dis*, 1999, 28(5):1104-8.
Thomas KE, Hasbun R, Jekel J, et al, "The Diagnostic Accuracy of Kernig's Sign, Brudzinski's Sign, and Nuchal Rigidity in Adults With Suspected Meningitis," *Clin Infect Dis*, 2002, 35(1):46-52.
Tunkel AR and Scheld WM, "Acute Bacterial Meningitis," *Lancet*, 1995, 346(8991-8992):1675-80.
Tunkel AR and Scheld WM, "Acute Bacterial Meningitis in Adults," *Curr Clin Topics Infect Dis*, 1996, 16:215-39.
Tunkel AR, Hartman BJ, Kaplan SL, et al, "Practice Guidelines for the Management of Bacterial Meningitis," *Clin Infect Dis*, 2004, 39:1267-1284.

Meningitis, Neonatal (<1 month of age)

Synonyms Neonatal Meningitis

Clinical Presentation Baby is feeding poorly, has fever or is hypothermic, has seizure, sleepiness, irritability, or any other unusual behavior. A full fontanelle indicates progressive disease.

Differential Diagnosis Bacterial, viral, or other infectious agents; neoplasm; metabolic disorders; central nervous system hemorrhage

Likely Pathogens

Escherichia coli, Enterohemorrhagic *on page 145*
Klebsiella Species *on page 200*
Listeria monocytogenes on page 208
Streptococcus agalactiae on page 313

Diagnostic Tests/Procedures

•Blood Culture, Aerobic and Anaerobic *on page 391*
•Cerebrospinal Fluid Analysis *on page 408*
•Gram Stain *on page 473*
•Lumbar Puncture *on page 524*
Computed Transaxial Tomography, Head Studies *on page 424*
Cryptococcal Antigen Serology, Serum or Cerebrospinal Fluid *on page 431*
Enterovirus Culture *on page 453*
Magnetic Resonance Scan, Brain *on page 532*

Empiric Drug Therapy

Recommended:

Ampicillin *on page 657*
plus
Gentamicin *on page 841*
Ampicillin *on page 657*
plus
Cefotaxime *on page 708*
if hospital acquired add
Vancomycin *on page 1144*

Alternate:

Chloramphenicol *on page 733*

(Continued)

Meningitis, Neonatal (<1 month of age) *(Continued)*

plus
Gentamicin *on page 841*
if hospital acquired add
Vancomycin *on page 1144*

Selected Readings

Arango CA and Rathore MH, "Neonatal Meningococcal Meningitis: Case Reports and Review of Literature," *Pediatr Infect Dis J*, 1996, 15(12):1134-6.

Pong A and Bradley JS, "Bacterial Meningitis and the Newborn Infant," *Infect Dis Clin North Am*, 1999, 13(3):711-33.

Roos KL, Tunkel AR, Scheld WM, "Acute Bacterial Meningitis in Children and Adults," *Infections of the Central Nervous System*, Scheld WM, Whitley RJ, and Durack DT, eds, New York, NY: Raven Press, 1991, 335-410.

Tunkel AR, Hartman BJ, Kaplan SL, et al, "Practice Guidelines for the Management of Bacterial Meningitis," *Clin Infect Dis*, 2004, 39:1267-1284.

Meningitis, Pediatric (>1 month of age)

Synonyms Pediatric Meningitis

Clinical Presentation Patients present with fever or hypothermia, seizure, sleepiness, irritability, full fontanelle, and stiff neck. Focal neurologic abnormalities and papilledema are uncommon. The incidence of *H. influenzae* has markedly decreased due to the recommended vaccination of all children.

Differential Diagnosis Bacterial, viral, or other infectious agents; neoplasm; metabolic disorders; central nervous system hemorrhage

Likely Pathogens

Haemophilus influenzae on page 159
Neisseria meningitidis on page 245
Streptococcus pneumoniae, Drug-Susceptible *on page 319*

Diagnostic Tests/Procedures

•Blood Culture, Aerobic and Anaerobic *on page 391*
•Cerebrospinal Fluid Analysis *on page 408*
•Gram Stain *on page 473*
•Lumbar Puncture *on page 524*
Bacterial Antigens, Rapid Detection Methods *on page 388*
Computed Transaxial Tomography, Head Studies *on page 424*
Cryptococcal Antigen Serology, Serum or Cerebrospinal Fluid *on page 431*
Enterovirus Culture *on page 453*
Magnetic Resonance Scan, Brain *on page 532*

Empiric Drug Therapy

Recommended:

One of the following
Ceftriaxone *on page 722*
Cefotaxime *on page 708*
plus
Vancomycin *on page 1144*

Alternate:

Monotherapy:
Meropenem *on page 936*

Combination therapy:
Chloramphenicol *on page 733*
plus
Vancomycin *on page 1144*

Selected Readings

Booy R and Kroll JS, "Bacterial Meningitis and Meningococcal Infection," *Curr Opin Pediatr*, 1998, 10(1):13-8.

Odio CM, Faingezicht I, Paris M, et al, "The Beneficial Effects of Early Dexamethasone Administration in Infants and Children With Bacterial Meningitis," *N Engl J Med*, 1991, 324(22):1525-31.

Roos KL, Tunkel AR, Scheld WM, "Acute Bacterial Meningitis in Children and Adults," *Infections of the Central Nervous System*, Scheld WM, Whitley RJ, and Durack DT, eds, New York, NY: Raven Press, 1991, 335-410.

Tunkel AR, Hartman BJ, Kaplan SL, et al, "Practice Guidelines for the Management of Bacterial Meningitis," *Clin Infect Dis*, 2004, 39:1267-1284.

Meningitis, Postsurgical

Synonyms Postsurgical Meningitis

Clinical Presentation Patients present with fever, headache, nausea, vomiting, and nuchal rigidity. Focal neurologic abnormalities and papilledema are uncommon.

Differential Diagnosis Bacterial, viral, or other infectious agents; drug-induced; neoplastic; granulomatous; infectious endocarditis; collagen-vascular diseases; subdural hemorrhage; subarachnoid hemorrhage

Likely Pathogens

Pseudomonas aeruginosa on page 282
Gram-Negative Bacilli *on page 157*
Staphylococcus aureus, Methicillin-Susceptible *on page 307*
Staphylococcus epidermidis, Methicillin-Susceptible *on page 310*
Candida Species *on page 67*
Streptococcus Species *on page 326*
Propionibacterium acnes

Diagnostic Tests/Procedures

•Blood Culture, Aerobic and Anaerobic *on page 391*
•Gram Stain *on page 473*
•Lumbar Puncture *on page 524*
Computed Transaxial Tomography, Head Studies *on page 424*
Magnetic Resonance Scan, Brain *on page 532*
Wound Culture *on page 620*

Drug Therapy Comment If *Candida* is identified or suspected, therapy should include amphotericin B (conventional) plus flucytosine.

Empiric Drug Therapy

Recommended:

Vancomycin *on page 1144*
plus one of the following
Ceftazidime *on page 717*
Cefepime *on page 705*
Meropenem *on page 936*
with or without
Aminoglycoside *on page 641*

Alternate:

Vancomycin *on page 1144*
plus
Penicillins, Extended-Spectrum *on page 997*
with or without
Tobramycin *on page 1122*

Selected Readings

Cabellos C, Viladrich PF, Corredoira J, et al, "Streptococcal Meningitis in Adult Patients: Current Epidemiology and Clinical Spectrum," *Clin Infect Dis*, 1999, 28(5):1104-8.
Nazzaro JM and Craven DE, "Successful Treatment of Postoperative Meningitis Due to *Haemophilus influenzae* Without Removal of an Expanded Polytetrafluoroethylene Dural Graft," *Clin Infect Dis*, 1998, 26(2):516-8.
Nguyen MH and Yu VL, "Meningitis Caused by *Candida* Species: An Emerging Problem in Neurosurgical Patients," *Clin Infect Dis*, 1995, 21(2):323-7.
Tunkel AR, Hartman BJ, Kaplan SL, et al, "Practice Guidelines for the Management of Bacterial Meningitis," *Clin Infect Dis*, 2004, 39:1267-1284.
van Aken MO, de Marie S, van der Lely AJ, et al, "Risk Factors for Meningitis After Transsphenoidal Surgery," *Clin Infect Dis*, 1997, 25(4):852-6.
Venes JL, "Infections of CSF Shunts and Intracranial Pressure Monitoring Devices," *Infect Dis Clin North Am*, 1989, 3(2):289-99.

Meningitis, Post-traumatic

Synonyms Post-traumatic Meningitis

Clinical Presentation Patients present with fever, headache, nausea, vomiting, and nuchal rigidity. Focal neurologic abnormalities and papilledema are uncommon.

Differential Diagnosis Bacterial, viral, or other infectious agents; drug-induced; neoplastic; granulomatous; infectious endocarditis; collagen-vascular diseases; subdural hemorrhage; subarachnoid hemorrhage

Likely Pathogens

Haemophilus influenzae on page 159
Staphylococcus aureus, Methicillin-Susceptible *on page 307*
Streptococcus pneumoniae, Drug-Susceptible *on page 319*

Diagnostic Tests/Procedures

•Aerobic Culture, Cerebrospinal Fluid *on page 366*
•Blood Culture, Aerobic and Anaerobic *on page 391*
•Computed Transaxial Tomography, Head Studies *on page 424*
•Gram Stain *on page 473*
•Lumbar Puncture *on page 524*
•Magnetic Resonance Scan, Brain *on page 532*

Empiric Drug Therapy

Recommended:

Vancomycin *on page 1144*
plus one of the following
Ceftriaxone *on page 722*
Cefotaxime *on page 708*
Meropenem *on page 936*

Note: For penetrating trauma, see treatment for Meningitis, Postsurgical.

(Continued)

Meningitis, Post-traumatic *(Continued)*

Alternate:

Vancomycin *on page 1144*

plus

Penicillins, Extended-Spectrum *on page 997*

Selected Readings

Tunkel AR, Hartman BJ, Kaplan SL, et al, "Practice Guidelines for the Management of Bacterial Meningitis," *Clin Infect Dis*, 2004, 39:1267-1284.

Microaerophilic Streptococci *see Streptococcus*-Related Gram-Positive Cocci *on page 325*

Microsporidia

Microbiology Microsporidia are single-cell obligate intracellular parasites which can form spores under extracellular (adverse) environmental conditions. Microsporidia spores are oval to spherical and are 1-20 μm long, depending on the species; however, the spores typically are only 1-5 μm long when found in humans and other mammals. In Gram-stained stool preparations, the spores appear as large, fat, gram-negative rods and often have a central and darkly stained band or dot. There are many genera of microsporidia; however, only seven genera have been associated with human disease, *Enterocytozoon, Encephalitozoon, Nosema, Pleistophora, Trachipleistophora, Brachiola*, and *Septata*.

Epidemiology Microsporidia are found in many animal species, particularly invertebrates. Microsporidia have been isolated from many human specimens, including stool (by far the most common clinical source), intestine (only the jejunum and duodenum), urine, CSF, liver, skin, sinus/nasal mucosa, cornea, conjunctiva, kidney, and lungs. Microsporidia in the intestines are usually found as complete organisms in the enterocytes and as spores in the stool. Microsporidia, particularly *Enterocytozoon* and *Septata*, probably are pathogens in AIDS patients and probably are responsible for 10% to 20% of the cases of chronic diarrhea in AIDS patients. Less than 20 of the approximately 400 reported cases of microsporidia-associated diarrhea were reported from non-AIDS cases; the remainder were AIDS cases. Most cases have been associated with male homosexuals with AIDS and extremely low CD4 cell counts.

Clinical Syndromes

- **Microsporidia-associated diarrhea:** The most common clinical presentation of microsporidia-associated diarrhea in AIDS patients is gradual onset (eventually chronic) of diarrhea (no blood or mucus), weight loss, nausea, abdominal cramps, and anorexia.

Diagnosis Diagnosis is made by clinical impression and a few laboratory tests. (1) D-xylose and fat malabsorption frequently are present. (2) Histological examination of jejunal and duodenal biopsies can be helpful if pathologists are notified of a suspected case, use appropriate stains, and are familiar with the characteristic morphology of the organism and histological alterations elicited by the organism. The staining characteristics of microsporidia in sections of tissue are variable and unpredictable, and microsporidia are often difficult to recognize in paraffin sections; they are more easily recognized in plastic sections. (3) Microsporidia are easily and reproducibly stained and recognized outside of tissue, specifically in tissue imprint preparations and direct stool smears. Stool is the most commonly submitted specimen for the laboratory diagnosis of microsporidia. Stool specimens (smears) are best stained by a modified trichrome stain such as that described by Weber (see Selected Readings). Less commonly used stains are Giemsa and calcofluor white.

Diagnostic Tests/Procedures

Microsporidia Diagnostic Procedures *on page 536*

Note: Contact laboratory for availability of tests and special instructions.

Treatment Microsporidia-induced diarrhea should be managed with supportive fluid and electrolyte replacement. Although a variety of antiprotozoals have been utilized in the treatment of this infection, success has been limited. Albendazole may have the most clinical success. Metronidazole may also be a useful therapy especially in non-HIV infected patients.

Drug Therapy

Recommended:

Metronidazole *on page 940*

Albendazole *on page 635*

Selected Readings

Didier ES, "Microsporidiosis," *Clin Infect Dis*, 1998, 27(1):1-8.

Garcia LS, "Laboratory Identification of the Microsporidia," *J Clin Microbiol*, 2002, 40(6):1892-901.

Goodgame RW, "Understanding Intestinal Spore-Forming Protozoa: Cryptospordia, Microsporidia, *Isospora*, and *Clyclospora*," *Ann Intern Med*, 1996, 124(4):429-41.

Lecuit M, Oksenhendler E, and Sarfati C, "Use of Albendazole for Disseminated Microsporidian Infections in a Patient With AIDS," *Clin Infect Dis*, 1994, 19(2):332-3.
Shadduck JA and Greeley E, "Microsporidia and Human Infections," *Clin Microbiol Rev*, 1989, 2(2):158-65.
Weber R and Bryan RT, "Microsporidial Infections in Immunodeficient and Immunocompetent Patients," *Clin Infect Dis*, 1994, 19(3):517-21.
Weber R, Bryan RT, Owen RL, et al, "Improved Light-Microscopical Detection of Microsporidia Spores in Stool and Duodenal Aspirates. The Enteric Opportunistic Infections Working Group," *N Engl J Med*, 1992, 326(3):161-6.
Weber R, Bryan RT, Schwartz DA, et al, "Human Microsporidial Infections," *Clin Microbiol Rev*, 1994, 7(4):426-61.

Microsporidiosis *see* Microsporidia *on page 220*

Middle Ear Infection *see* Otitis Media, Acute *on page 253*

Mobiluncus Species

Microbiology *Mobiluncus* species are anaerobic, curved bacteria which are gram-variable (either gram-positive or gram-negative). The organism is highly motile due to its multiple flagella. There are two species, *M. curtisii* and *M. mulieris*. *Mobiluncus* requires enriched media for optimal growth. The organism easily adheres to squamous epithelial cells of the human vagina.

Epidemiology The organism is one of the organisms associated with bacterial vaginosis (see Vaginosis, Bacterial *on page 347*). It has been isolated from the vagina of about 5% of healthy women but in nearly all patients meeting criteria for bacterial vaginosis. The main habitat of *Mobiluncus* is the vagina, but it has been isolated from the urethra of male partners of women with bacterial vaginosis and in rectal cultures of homosexual males.

Clinical Syndromes

- **Bacterial vaginosis:** *Mobiluncus* is one of several organisms associated with bacterial vaginosis. Other purported etiologic agents have included *Gardnerella vaginalis* and the genital *Mycoplasma*. *Mobiluncus* is usually isolated in culture with other anaerobic organisms. Patients present with vaginal discharge which is typically malodorous and white or gray in appearance. The discharge is homogeneous and coats the vaginal mucosa, with little or no inflammation of the vulva or introitus. There is a fish-like odor to the discharge and the pH of the fluid is usually >4.6. Bacterial vaginosis is associated with "clue cells" which are vaginal epithelial cells coated with mixed organisms, including many gram-negative bacilli.
- **Upper genitourinary infections:** Occasional case reports.
- **Miscellaneous:** Breast abscesses and mastectomy wound infections have been rarely described.

Diagnosis *Mobiluncus* species may be suspected in a woman presenting with bacterial vaginosis, as described in Clinical Syndromes.

Diagnostic Tests/Procedures

Anaerobic Culture *on page 371*
Gram Stain *on page 473*
(Physician **must** consult the Microbiology Laboratory before any anaerobic vaginal culture is ordered.)

Treatment *Mobiluncus* species are susceptible *in vitro* to a variety of antibiotics, including penicillin. However, most cases of bacterial vaginosis are treated successfully with metronidazole. Formal susceptibility testing is usually not performed.

Drug Therapy

Recommended:

Metronidazole *on page 940*

Selected Readings

Spiegel CA, "*Gardnerella vaginalis* and *Mobiluncus* Species," *Principles and Practice of Infectious Diseases*, 5th ed, Mandell GL, Bennett JE, and Dolin R, eds, New York, NY: Churchill Livingstone, 2000, 2383-6.

Moniliasis *see Candida* Species *on page 67*

Monkeypox Virus

Microbiology Monkeypox is an orthopoxvirus, a member of the family poxviridae. Other orthopoxviruses include smallpox and cowpox. Orthopoxviruses are large (200-250 nM), enveloped viruses with a genome of linear, double-stranded DNA. Monkeypox virus was first isolated in 1958 from primate source, leading to its name. However, the virus is also known to infect a number of rodent species, including squirrels and prairie dogs. Monkeypox has a clinical presentation in humans similar to smallpox, but milder and is recognized as a cause of sporadic disease outbreaks, primarily in Africa. Significant cross-immunity following vaccination against smallpox has been noted. The WHO has previously noted that the termination of smallpox vaccination programs could lead to an increased susceptibility to monkeypox. Children born after 1980, who were not vaccinated against smallpox, are more likely to be infected by monkeypox.

(Continued)

Monkeypox Virus *(Continued)*

Epidemiology Monkeypox is a sporadic zoonotic disease. Cases generally occur in Central and West Africa, particularly in remote villages where contact with potentially infected animals (squirrels and primates) is increased. Monkeypox is usually transmitted via contact with the animal's blood or through an animal bite. In recent outbreaks, it has been noted that monkeypox disease has demonstrated a higher rate of person-to-person transmission. However, monkeypox is less infectious than smallpox. In addition, several generations of transmission may be observed, with outbreaks persisting for up to a year. Primary cases are believed to be infected through contact with an infected animal. Secondary attack rates have been estimated in the range of 4% to 12%. A 2% to 10% mortality rate has been reported during outbreaks, with deaths occurring primarily in younger patients.

In the Spring of 2003, the first monkeypox outbreak in the Western Hemisphere was reported in the United States. Cases or suspected cases were identified in several states including Indiana, Wisconsin, Illinois, and New Jersey. The cases were associated with monkeypox-infected prairie dogs distributed from a single supplier in Illinois. These animals may have been sold to buyers in as many as 15 states.

Clinical Syndromes Following an incubation period of 10-14 days, the patient typically develops fever, malaise, and fatigue. A papular rash typically develops after 1-3 days. Unlike smallpox, lymphadenopathy may be observed. Initial lesions frequently appear on the face and typically generalize across the body. The lesions progress through several stages during eruption, with subsequent crusting and healing. Resolution from the onset of fever is 2-4 weeks.

Diagnosis CDC has published criteria for the diagnosis of monkeypox, including clinical, epidemiologic, and laboratory criteria (summarized below). Consult the CDC website (www.cdc.gov/ncidod/monkeypox/index.htm) for current criteria/case definitions.

Clinical criteria:

- Rash (macular, papular, vesicular, or pustular; generalized or localized; discrete or confluent) along with other signs and symptoms including:
  - Temperature >99.3°F (>37.4°C)
  - Headache
  - Backache
  - Lymphadenopathy
  - Sore throat
  - Cough
  - Shortness of breath

Epidemiological criteria:

Exposure[1] to an exotic mammalian pet[2] obtained on or after April 15, 2003, with clinical signs of illness (eg, conjunctivitis, respiratory symptoms, and/or rash)

Exposure[1] to an exotic mammalian pet[2] with or without clinical signs of illness that has been in contact with a case of monkeypox either in a mammalian pet[3] or a human

Exposure to a suspect, probable, or confirmed human case

Laboratory criteria:

Isolation of monkeypox virus in culture

Demonstration of monkeypox virus DNA by polymerase chain reaction testing in a clinical specimen

Demonstration of virus morphologically consistent with an orthopoxvirus by electron microscopy in the absence of exposure to another orthopoxvirus

Demonstration of presence of orthopox virus in tissue using immunohistochemical testing methods in the absence of exposure to another orthopoxvirus.

[1]Exposure includes living in a household, petting or handling, or visiting a pet holding facility (eg, pet store, veterinary clinic, pet distributor)

[2]Exotic or wild mammalian pets include prairie dogs, Gambian giant rats, and rope squirrels. Exposure to other exotic or nonexotic mammalian pets with be considered on a case-by-case basis; assessment should include the likelihood of contact with a mammal with monkeypox and the compatibility of clinical illness with monkeypox.

[3]Contact between mammalian pets includes living in a household, or originating from the same pet holding facility as another animal with monkeypox

Diagnostic Tests/Procedures

Viral Culture

Polymerase Chain Reaction *on page 567*

Electron Microscopy

Immunohistochemical Testing

Treatment Generally involves supportive treatment only. Smallpox vaccine is estimated to be 85% effective against monkeypox. More than 37,000 healthcare workers in the United States have been vaccinated against smallpox. The CDC recommends healthcare workers, veterinarians, and family members who have cared for or had close contact with infected people or animals should receive smallpox vaccination. Cidofovir has not been evaluated as treatment for monkeypox. CDC recommends reserving this treatment for life-threatening cases of monkeypox.

Selected Readings

Centers for Disease Control, www.cdc.gov/ncidod/monkeypox/index.htm, last accessed June 18, 2003.

Mononucleosis

Likely Pathogens

Epstein-Barr Virus *on page 139*
Cytomegalovirus *on page 107*
Toxoplasma gondii on page 331

Moraxella catarrhalis

Related Information

Community-Acquired Pneumonia in Adults *on page 1278*

Synonyms *Branhamella catarrhalis*

Microbiology *Moraxella catarrhalis* (*Branhamella*) is an aerobic, gram-negative diplococcus which resembles *Neisseria* species in its Gram stain appearance. Although generally considered an organism of low pathogenicity, *M. catarrhalis* has gained increasing attention as a common pathogen of the upper and lower respiratory tract, particularly in individuals with chronic bronchitis. The organism has an outer membrane that contains lipo-oligosaccharides (LOS) and proteins (outer membrane proteins, OMP). On a molecular level, the LOS is different from the lipopolysaccharides seen in enteric gram-negative bacilli, but LOS is also likely a virulence factor. The various patterns of OMP were under study recently as part of an antigenic target for future *M. catarrhalis* vaccines.

In the medical literature this organism has been variously named *Neisseria catarrhalis*, *Branhamella catarrhalis*, and most recently *Moraxella catarrhalis*. *M. catarrhalis* belongs to the family Neisseriaceae. *M. catarrhalis* is a kidney bean shaped coccus 0.6-1.0 μm in diameter, often appearing in pairs or tetrads. During active infection, the organisms can sometimes be seen within the cytoplasm of polymorphonuclear cells, where they appear as gram-negative intracellular diplococci. In the laboratory, the organism readily grows on routine media such as blood agar and can often grow on ordinary media without blood.

Epidemiology *Moraxella catarrhalis* is considered part of the normal flora of the human respiratory tract, particularly in the nasal cavity which is considered the main natural reservoir for this organism. Thus the isolation of *M. catarrhalis* in a respiratory culture does not necessarily imply clinical disease. It can be isolated from the oropharynx of otherwise healthy infants (30% to 60%), children, and adults (5%), although these colonization rates vary significantly among different published studies. Higher carriage rates are seen in patients with chronic bronchitis, and there is an increase in colonization during the winter months.

Clinical Syndromes

- **Exacerbations of chronic obstructive pulmonary disease (COPD):** *M. catarrhalis* has recently been recognized as an important cause of purulent exacerbations of chronic bronchitis, almost as common as *Streptococcus pneumoniae* and nontypeable *Haemophilus influenzae* in some studies. Patients with acute exacerbations of chronic bronchitis typically present with increased sputum production, worsened cough, and dyspnea, with or without fever or chills. Purulent exacerbations of COPD are usually mucosal infections and less commonly involve infection of the lower respiratory tract (see below). The clinical presentation of COPD exacerbations caused by *M. catarrhalis* is no different from other common respiratory organisms. Gram stain of the sputum typically shows gram-negative diplococci as the predominant organism along with numerous polymorphonuclear leukocytes.
- **Community-acquired pneumonia:** *M. catarrhalis* can cause acute lower respiratory tract infection in adults. This is seen most commonly in persons with underlying COPD, but has also been seen in elderly persons without predisposing lung conditions.
- **Respiratory tract infections in infants and children, particularly in asthmatics.**
- **Acute otitis media.** *M. catarrhalis* is the third leading cause of acute otitis media in children, behind *Streptococcus pneumoniae* and nontypeable *Haemophilus influenzae*. Based on studies of children with otitis media undergoing tympanocentesis, *M. catarrhalis* can be isolated from middle ear fluid in about 20% of cases, with the highest incidence in the winter months. It is felt that children with otitis media are likely colonized with the organism in the nasopharynx, and then the organism gains

(Continued)

Moraxella catarrhalis (Continued)

access to the middle ear by way of the eustachian tube. The specific factor(s) that cause a benign colonization of the nasopharynx mucosa to progress to symptomatic middle ear disease are unknown.

- **Sinusitis:** *M. catarrhalis* can be a cause of acute sinusitis in both children and adults. It is usually found with other organisms and can be recovered from properly performed sinus aspirates.
- **Acute urethritis:** This organism is occasionally a saprophyte of the genital tract and has been reported to be a rare cause of the urethral syndrome.
- **Other invasive diseases:** Cases of meningitis, endocarditis, septicemia, and peritonitis have been reported, usually in immunosuppressed patients.

Diagnosis The laboratory is easily able to separate it from related *Neisseria* species biochemically. Rapid tests used to speciate *Neisseria* do not react with *Moraxella*. *Moraxella* is frequently recovered from sputum cultures along with a variety of other organisms. Every attempt should be made to obtain a high quality sputum specimen in order to minimize contamination of samples with commensal mouth organisms, which may include *Moraxella*. The finding of many gram-negative diplococci within polymorphonuclear leukocytes on a Gram stain of expectorated sputum is suggestive of true infection, rather than colonization.

Serologic studies looking for a fourfold rise in antibody titer against *M. catarrhalis* play a limited role for most patients and remain primarily epidemiologic or investigational tools.

Diagnostic Tests/Procedures

Aerobic Culture, Sputum *on page 367*
Blood Culture, Aerobic and Anaerobic *on page 391*
Gram Stain *on page 473*

Treatment In past years, *Moraxella catarrhalis* was exquisitely sensitive to penicillin. However, in the early 1980s, an increasing number of community isolates were found to produce a beta-lactamase enzyme, which could be either plasmid or chromosomally mediated. It is now estimated that 75% to 85% of strains of *M. catarrhalis* produce beta-lactamase. Such strains generally remain susceptible to oral erythromycin and tetracycline, with only 1% to 2% *in vitro* resistance. Sulfamethoxazole and trimethoprim is active against most strains of *M. catarrhalis*, which is particularly helpful when empirically treating a patient with an exacerbation of chronic bronchitis. Ampicillin alone is ineffective in treating beta-lactamase producing *M. catarrhalis* and should not be used even if such an organism appears sensitive to ampicillin *in vitro*. The combination of ampicillin or amoxicillin with a beta-lactamase inhibitor such as clavulanate (Augmentin®) is effective against most beta-lactamase positive strains. Finally, the cephalosporins in general appear more stable than penicillins in the presence of *M. catarrhalis* beta-lactamase; however, the results of *in vitro* susceptibility testing remain important in management. No one agent is clearly superior to others, and the decision regarding choice of antibiotic should also be based on antibiotic side effects, cost, and dosing schedules. Since the majority of infections caused by *M. catarrhalis* are limited to the respiratory mucosa, oral antibiotics are usually sufficient. Only the occasional case of pneumonia or bacteremia requires parenteral antibiotics.

Drug Therapy

Recommended:

Sulfamethoxazole and Trimethoprim *on page 1087*
Amoxicillin and Clavulanate Potassium *on page 645*
Cephalosporins, 2nd Generation *on page 729*
Cephalosporins, 3rd Generation *on page 730*
Clarithromycin *on page 749*
Azithromycin *on page 674*
Fluoroquinolones *on page 824*

Selected Readings

Catlin BW, "*Branhamella catarrhalis*: An Organism Gaining Respect as a Pathogen," *Clin Microbiol Rev*, 1990, 3(4):293-320.

Garcia-Garrote F, Menasalvas A, Martínez-Sánchez L, et al, "*Moraxella catarrhalis* Bacteremia," *Clin Microbiol Newslett*, 1997, 19(23):183-4.

Murphy TF, "*Moraxella (Branhamella) catarrhalis* and Other Gram-Negative Cocci," *Principles and Practice of Infectious Diseases*, 5th ed, Mandell GL, Bennett JE, and Dolin R, eds, New York, NY: Churchill Livingstone, 2000, 2259-2266.

Verghese A, Berk SL, "*Branhamella catarrhalis*: A Microbiologic and Clinical Update," *Am J Med*, 1990, 88(Suppl 5A):1S-56S.

Verghese A, Berk SL, "*Moraxella (Branhamella) catarrhalis*," *Infect Dis Clin North Am*, 1991, 5(3):523-38.

MRSA *see Staphylococcus aureus*, Methicillin-Resistant *on page 304*

MRSE *see Staphylococcus epidermidis*, Methicillin-Resistant *on page 309*

MSSA *see Staphylococcus aureus*, Methicillin-Susceptible *on page 307*

MSSE *see Staphylococcus epidermidis*, Methicillin-Susceptible *on page 310*

Mucocutaneous Lymph Node Syndrome *see* Kawasaki Syndrome *on page 198*
Mucopurulent Cervicitis *see* Cervicitis *on page 71*
Mucormycosis *see Mucor* Species *on page 225*

Mucor Species

Microbiology Mucormycosis refers to opportunistic fungal infections caused by the mold order *Mucorales*, class Zygomycetes. Contrary to the name, *Mucor* species are rarely implicated in human disease. The most frequent fungi isolated are *Rhizopus*, *Rhizomucor*, and *Absidia*. *Mucorales* are ubiquitous organisms found worldwide in soil, dust, spoiled fruit, and bread products. They initiate and facilitate decay of organic material.

KOH preparation of infected material reveals sparsely septate mycelia 6-50 μm wide, up to 200 μm long, and rounded sporangia. Growth in culture is rapid at temperatures 25°C to 55°C (optimum temperature 28°C to 30°C) and usually begins as a cottony white mold turning gray to yellow to brown in 3-5 days. Wet mounts reveal sporangiophores arising off clusters of rhizoids (*Mucor* species lack rhizoids). H & E stains typically reveal an abundance of irregular shaped, broad hyphae with right angle branching in the midst of polymorphonuclear infiltrate and round blood vessel walls with or without invasion into the vessel wall.

Epidemiology Mucormycosis is one of the most acute and fulminant fungal infections. It has a distinct predilection for invasion of blood vessel walls with resultant ischemia and necrosis of the adjacent tissue, commonly referred to as "black pus". There are no associations with age, sex, race, or geography. Most frequently seen in poorly controlled diabetics and hematologic malignancies. Infection is secondary to direct inoculation cutaneously or inhalation of spores into the respiratory tract and taken up by alveolar macrophages.

Clinical Syndromes

- **Rhinocerebral:** Generally seen in diabetics, predilection for acidosis. Present with facial pain, headache, and fever. May see black necrotic eschar on palate or nasal mucosa. May involve orbit leading to orbital cellulitis, proptosis, chemosis, cranial nerve involvement, and eventual CNS involvement. Two-thirds develop orbital cellulitis, and 33% develop internal carotid artery thrombosis or cavernous sinus thrombosis. Overall mortality is 80% to 90%.
- **Pulmonary:** Most commonly seen in hematologic malignancies particularly with neutropenia. Present with fever, dyspnea, and chest pain. Typically, no infiltrates seen on chest radiograph secondary to absence of leukocytes. Chest radiograph may reveal necrosis and hemorrhage.
- **Cutaneous:** Usually secondary to direct inoculation from trauma burns. May be secondary to dissemination.
- **Gastrointestinal:** Present with nonspecific signs and symptoms of intra-abdominal abscess. Associated with severe malnutrition, kwashiorkor. Usually diagnosed at autopsy.
- **CNS:** Direct extension from nose or paranasal sinuses. Direct inoculation via intravenous drug abuse. Disseminated disease associated with deferoxamine therapy.
- **Miscellaneous:** Rarely affects bones, kidneys, or mediastinum. Cardiac invasion associated with myocardial infarction, congestive heart failure, valvular incompetence, and pericarditis.

Diagnosis CT scans are useful in delineating extent of rhinocerebral disease. Definitive diagnosis depends on direct examination of infected material revealing characteristic histopathology as cultures of biopsied material frequently do not grow.

Diagnostic Tests/Procedures

Fungus Culture, Biopsy *on page 461*
Fungus Culture, Bronchial Aspirate *on page 463*
KOH Preparation *on page 513*

Treatment Treatment requires extensive surgical debridement, amphotericin B 1-1.5 mg/kg per day and, if possible, correction of the underlying illness. Azoles are still under investigation. Unproven therapies include rifampin, tetracycline, and hyperbaric oxygen.

Drug Therapy

Recommended:

Amphotericin B (Conventional) *on page 650*

Alternate:

Amphotericin B (Lipid Complex) *on page 653*
Amphotericin B (Liposomal) *on page 655*
Voriconazole *on page 1151*

Selected Readings

Lee FY, Mossad SB, and Adal KA, "Pulmonary Mucormycosis: The Last 30 Years," *Arch Intern Med*, 1999, 159(12):1301-9.

(Continued)

Mucor Species *(Continued)*

Morrison VA and McGlave PB, "Mucormycosis in the BMT Population," *Bone Marrow Transplant*, 1993, 11(5):383-8.
Rinaldi MG, "Zygomycosis," *Infect Dis Clin North Am*, 1989, 3(1):19-41.
Sugar AM, "Mucormycosis," *Clin Infect Dis*, 1992, 14(Suppl 1):S126-9.
Weitzman I, "Emerging Zygomycotic Agents," *Clin Microbiol Newslett*, 1997, 19(11):81-5.

***Multiceps* species** *see* Cestodes *on page 72*

Mumps *see* Mumps Virus *on page 226*

Mumps Virus

Microbiology Mumps virus is the cause of an acute, nonsuppurative infection of the parotid glands (viral parotitis) which is primarily seen in children and adolescents. Mumps infection can also lead to serious systemic diseases including encephalitis and orchitis.

Mumps virus is an RNA virus of intermediate size (120-200 nm diameter), and belongs to the family Paramyxoviridae. It has two antigens (S and V) which can fix complement. Mumps virus can be grown in cell culture in a diagnostic virology laboratory.

Epidemiology Mumps occurs worldwide and throughout the year, with a peak in the spring (April and May). Humans are the only known reservoir. Epidemics are limited to groups where people live in close quarters, such as military barracks, institutions, or prisons. The incidence of mumps in the United States has declined by over 99% since the institution of the mumps vaccine in the late 1960s. However, a significant rise in the number of mumps cases was reported in 1986 and 1987. The incidence of mumps in the United States continues to fall with 633 cases in 1998 and 338 cases in 1999.

The virus has a reputation as being "less contagious" than other childhood illnesses such as measles or chickenpox, but this may not accurately reflect the many mumps infections which are asymptomatic or subclinical. Over 90% of adults are seropositive for mumps, indicating widespread exposure. The infection is rare in children younger than 2 years of age, and peak incidence is typically between 5 and 9 years of age. Interestingly, since the widespread use of the vaccine in the United States, new cases are occurring in an older age group, with almost one-third of mumps cases in 1996 reported in persons >15 years of age.

Transmission is by direct person-to-person spread of infected salivary secretions. An individual may be infectious for up to 1 week prior to the onset of clinical parotitis, with a peak infectivity 1-2 days before salivary gland swelling. Thus, control of spread is difficult. Mumps has also been isolated from the urine, and this remains a less important but potential route of spread (viruria may persist for weeks). After exposure, the incubation period is 2-4 weeks.

Immunity is life-long. One episode of mumps (even if subclinical) confers protection in almost all cases, and reinfections with mumps have only rarely been reported.

Clinical Syndromes During the several-week incubation period, the virus replicates in the upper respiratory tract and the cervical lymph nodes. Following this period of asymptomatic localized infection, the virus disseminates hematogenously to other organs, including the parotid glands, testes, central nervous system, ovaries, inner ear, and others. Common clinical manifestations include:

- **Acute salivary adenitis:** The salivary glands are thought to be infected during the phase of viremia, although direct extension from the respiratory tract has also been postulated. Typically, there is an abrupt onset of fever and swelling of the salivary glands. The patient may complain of earache, difficulty chewing, and swallowing. Systemic symptoms (ie, malaise, headache, sore throat, chills) may sometimes precede the acute adenitis, or may follow the onset of parotid swelling. Of the salivary glands, the parotid gland is most commonly involved and is bilateral in two-thirds. The submaxillary and/or the sublingual glands may be infected, alone or in combination with the parotids. In most (but not all) cases, the gland is exquisitely tender to palpation for several days and has a "gelatinous" texture. The ostium of Stensen's duct appears erythematous but frank pus is not expressible, as in bacterial parotitis. Inflammation of the parotid leads to release of salivary amylase, which can be detected in the serum. Most cases resolve in about 1 week without specific intervention.
- **Mumps meningitis:** It is estimated that the mumps virus involves the central nervous system in 50% of cases, although only 10% or less of patients with mumps parotitis develop clinical meningitis. Over 50% of cases of mumps meningitis will have no evidence of parotitis. Patients typically present with an "aseptic meningitis" picture, with headache, photophobia, fever, and stiff neck. Cerebrospinal fluid (CSF) reveals a lymphocytic pleocytosis, sometimes >2000 cells/mm^3, but up to 25% of patients will have a predominance of polymorphonuclear

leukocytes, leading to confusion with bacterial meningitis. CSF protein levels are modestly elevated. Hypoglycorrhachia (low CSF glucose) is common with mumps meningitis, again potentially causing confusion with bacterial meningitis. Mumps meningitis is self-resolving and benign, and comprises about 1% of aseptic meningitis cases.

- **Mumps encephalitis:** This is a more serious infection than mumps meningitis. Encephalitis may be either "early", occurring at the time of onset of parotitis, or "late", occurring 1-2 weeks later. The "early" cases may be due to direct viral invasion of brain tissue, whereas the "late" cases may be due to an autoimmune, postinfectious demyelinating syndrome (similar to Guillain-Barré). Patients typically present with marked personality changes, decreased sensorium, and high fevers; seizures and aphasia have also been reported. CSF findings are similar to mumps meningitis. Mortality is about 1% to 2%. In the absence of active parotitis, mumps encephalitis is almost impossible to distinguish from herpes simplex encephalitis on clinical grounds. Of all viral encephalitides, mumps is etiologic in <1% due to the success of the mumps vaccine.
- **Epididymoorchitis:** Most cases occur within the first 1-2 weeks following the onset of parotid symptoms, but in some cases, orchitis may occur prior to or without salivary gland involvement. About 25% of mumps cases in postpubertal males are complicated by orchitis. Characteristically, this is part of a biphasic illness, with a dramatic return of systemic symptoms (fever to 40°C, chills, vomiting, headache) accompanied by acute pain and swelling in the testicle. In most cases, there is unilateral testicular pain. Epididymitis is present in the majority of cases. Symptoms usually begin to resolve within 1 week. Sterility is unusual unless there is bilateral testicular involvement complicated by testicular atrophy.
- **Miscellaneous:** Mumps has been reported to cause pancreatitis, oophoritis (5% of postpubertal women), migratory polyarthritis, electrocardiographic abnormalities, myocarditis (rare), and others.

Diagnosis The diagnosis of mumps infection is usually made on clinical grounds, particularly if the characteristic parotid gland inflammation is present. The WBC count is often normal but may show a leukopenia, lymphocytosis, or leukocytosis (with extrasalivary involvement). The serum amylase level stays elevated for several weeks in many cases, even without obvious parotid swelling, and may be useful when mumps encephalitis is suspected.

Laboratory confirmation of the mumps virus is usually not necessary. However, culture or serologic confirmation may be important when mumps encephalitis is a reasonable possibility, extrasalivary mumps is suspected but no parotitis is present, or parotitis is unusually fulminant or prolonged. Laboratory techniques include:

1. Viral culture in cell culture systems. Appropriate specimens include viral swabs of Stensen's duct, saliva, CSF, biopsy material, and sometimes urine. Blood cultures for mumps virus are low yield. The virus grows well in monkey kidney cells and demonstrates a distinctive cytopathic effect.
2. Serologic studies. Detection of mumps specific IgM antibody is presumptive evidence of recent infection. A fourfold rise in specific IgG titer is also diagnostic.

Diagnostic Tests/Procedures

Mumps Serology *on page 537*
Mumps Virus Culture *on page 538*
Virus Detection by DFA *on page 619*

Treatment There are no antiviral agents proven effective in mumps infection. Mumps immune globulin has been used prophylactically in susceptible individuals during outbreaks but without benefit. A live-attenuated vaccine has been in use in the United States since 1967 and is part of routine pediatric immunizations. The first dose is given around 15 months of age along with the vaccines for measles and rubella, the MMR. The live attenuated vaccine should not be administered to patients with severe immunodeficiencies, including AIDS, and pregnant women. An inactivated vaccine is available in such instances.

Drug Therapy Comment

No antiviral agents proven effective.

Drug Therapy Recommended:

Prophylaxis:

Measles, Mumps, and Rubella Vaccines (Combined) *on page 926*
Mumps Virus Vaccine (Live/Attenuated) *on page 952*

Selected Readings

Baum G and Litman N, "Mumps Virus," *Principles and Practice of Infectious Diseases*, 5th ed, Mandell GL, Bennett JE, and Dolin R, eds, New York, NY: Churchill Livingstone, 2000, 1776-81.
Hersh BS, Fine PE, Kent WK, et al, "Mumps Outbreak in a Highly Vaccinated Population," *J Pediatr*, 1991, 119(2):187-93.

(Continued)

Mumps Virus *(Continued)*

Ray CG, "Mumps," *Harrison's Principles of Internal Medicine*, 13th ed, Isselbacher KJ, Braunwald E, Wilson JD, et al, eds, New York, NY: McGraw-Hill, 1994, 830-2.

***Mycobacterium avium* Complex** *see Mycobacterium avium-intracellulare* (Complex) *on page 228*

Mycobacterium avium-intracellulare (Complex)

Related Information

USPHS / IDSA Guidelines for the Prevention of Opportunistic Infections in Persons Infected With HIV *on page 1237*

Synonyms MAC; MAI; *Mycobacterium avium* Complex

Microbiology MAC is an acid-fast bacillus that grows best at 37°C after 10-21 days incubation on selective agar media. The MAC consists of the closely-related species *Mycobacterium avium* and *M. intracellularae*; for practical and clinical purposes, they are usually considered *M. avium-intracellularae.*

Epidemiology Prior to the AIDS epidemic, MAC was extremely rare. Approximately 40% of patients will develop MAC within 2 years of the diagnosis of AIDS if no prophylaxis is given. Median survival was approximately 8-9 months prior to the introduction of potent antiretroviral therapy era. MAC is associated with CD4 counts <50 cells/µL. The incidence of MAC has decreased since the introduction of MAC prophylaxis and potent antiretroviral therapy. MAC disease may start with colonization of the gastrointestinal or respiratory tract and then establish a localized infection with intermittent MAC bacteremia leading to seeding of other organs (primarily to the reticuloendothelial system (RES)). This is followed by an unknown period of proliferation in these extravascular sites until the increasing organism burden results in sustained symptoms and "spillover" sustained bacteremia.

Clinical Syndromes

- **Asymptomatic:** Normal hosts may have colonization in the respiratory or gastrointestinal tracts. Duration of asymptomatic to dissemination in HIV is unknown.
- **Localized:** Focal pneumonia, skin, endophthalmitis, and CNS infections are rare. Localized infection of the GI tract is more common with infection in the duodenum most common. Patients present with nausea, diarrhea, abdominal pain, and, less commonly, biliary obstruction secondary to lymphadenopathy. Atypical manifestations are associated with immune reconstitution following potent antiretroviral therapy.
- **Disseminated:** Patients present with fever, weight loss, night sweats, anemia, and elevated alkaline phosphatase. Diarrhea (more than three unformed stools daily) is common. Factors associated with MAC include time since diagnosis of AIDS, presence of significant anemia (hemoglobin <8 g/dL), previous opportunistic infection, and interruption of antiretroviral therapy. Pathology of infected organs reveal organomegaly, organs which may be yellow secondary to color of organism, histiocytes filled with acid-fast bacilli, and poorly formed granulomas.

Diagnosis Dependent on isolation of MAC from sterile body source. MAC isolated from sputum or GI source may represent colonization, and clinical correlation is recommended. Bone marrow cultures may be more sensitive than blood cultures due to higher organism burden and earlier infection. Acid-fast bacillus (AFB) stains of the bone marrow may be postive in up to 40% of disseminated MAC. Caution should be used when interpreting results of AFB stains as they may represent other mycobacterial disease such as disseminated tuberculosis.

Diagnostic Tests/Procedures

Acid-Fast Stain *on page 361*
Blood Culture, Mycobacteria *on page 395*
Mycobacteria Culture, Biopsy or Body Fluid *on page 539*
Mycobacteria Culture, Sputum *on page 542*

Treatment Disseminated MAC: Macrolide-based therapy is associated with improved survival and decreased relapse rates. Azithromycin 500 mg/day or clarithromycin 500 mg twice daily plus ethambutol 25 mg/kg/day is the regimen of choice. Some clinicians recommend the addition of rifabutin to this regimen as there is evidence of improved survival and decreased resistance. If rifabutin cannot be used, the addition of a fluoroquinolone or amikacin may be warranted. Antiretroviral therapy should be initiated if it is not already utilized. Patients should remain on therapy for at least 12 months with no symptoms for six months and a rise in CD4 count to >100 cells/microliter. At this point, drug therapy may be discontinued.

Relapse: Should add two drugs not previously used to treat patient. If on macrolide plus ethambutol, add rifabutin and ciprofloxacin. If on macrolide plus rifabutin, add ethambutol and ciprofloxacin. If on macrolide plus ethambutol plus rifabutin, add either ciprofloxacin or amikacin. Amikacin is available in parenteral form only and will require long-term indwelling catheter.

Prophylaxis: Azithromycin 1200 mg orally weekly or clarithromycin 500 mg orally twice weekly is recommended in all patients with a CD4 nadir <50 cells/μL. Rifabutin 300 mg/day may be used as an alternative. Caution should be used when starting macrolide prophylaxis to assure MAC is not present. Initiation of macrolide monotherapy in the setting of MAC infection may result in macrolide resistance. If the patient cannot tolerate macrolides, rifabutin is an effective alternative.

It appears safe to withdraw primary prophylaxis in AIDS patients receiving potent antiretroviral therapy whose CD4 T-cell counts are >100 cells/μL.

Some of the antibiotics used to treat MAC interact with antiretroviral agents. See Antiretroviral Agents *on page 1206* in the Appendix for further information.

Drug Therapy

Recommended:

Clarithromycin *on page 749*
plus the following
Ethambutol *on page 812*

Azithromycin *on page 674*
plus the following
Ethambutol *on page 812*

Alternate:

Amikacin *on page 639*
Ciprofloxacin *on page 742*
Rifabutin *on page 1045*

Selected Readings

Aberg JA, Yajko DM, and Jacobson MA, "Eradication of AIDS-Related Disseminated *Mycobacterium avium* Complex Infection After 12 Months of Antimycobacterial Therapy Combined With Highly Active Antiretroviral Therapy," *J Infect Dis*, 1998, 178(5):1446-9.

Batt MD, "Update on Mycobacterial Issues for the Acquired Immune Deficiency Syndrome Era," *J Intraven Nurs*, 1994, 17(4):217-9.

Benson CA, Kaplan JE, Masur H, et al, "Treating Opportunistic Infections Among HIV-Exposed and Infected Children: Recommendations From CDC, the National Institutes of Health, and the Infectious Diseases Society of America," *MMWR*, 2004, 53(RR-15):1-112.

Benson CA, Williams PL, Cohn DL, et al, "Clarithromycin or Rifabutin Alone or in Combination for Primary Prophylaxis of *Mycobacterium avium* Complex Disease in Patients With AIDS: A Randomized, Double-Blind, Placebo-Controlled Trial. The AIDS Clinical Trials Group 196/Terry Beirn Community Programs for Clinical Research on AIDS 009 Protocol Team," *J Infect Dis*, 2000, 181(4):1289-97.

El-Sadr WM, Burman WJ, Grant LB, et al, "Discontinuation of Prophylaxis for *Mycobacterium avium* Complex Disease in HIV-Infected Patients Who Have a Response to Antiretroviral Therapy. Terry Beirn Community Programs for Clinical Research on AIDS," *N Engl J Med*, 2000, 342(15):1085-92.

Gordin FM, Sullam PM, Shafran SD, et al, "A Randomized, Placebo-Controlled Study of Rifabutin Added to a Regimen of Clarithromycin and Ethambutol for Treatment of Disseminated Infection With *Mycobacterium avium* Complex. Clin Infect Dis 1999, 28(5):1080-5

Ioannidis J and Wilkinson D, "HIV: Prevention of Opportunistic Infections," *Clin Evid*, 2003, (10):809-30.

Lange CG, Woolley IJ, and Brodt RH, "Disseminated *Mycobacterium avium-intracellulare* Complex (MAC) Infection in the Era of Effective Antiretroviral Therapy: Is Prophylaxis Still Indicated?" *Drugs*, 2004, 64(7):679-92.

Nightingale SD, Cameron DW, Gordin FM, et al, "Two Controlled Trials of Rifabutin Prophylaxis Against *Mycobacterium avium* Complex Infections in AIDS," *N Engl J Med*, 1993, 329(12):828-33.

Paul SM, "Opportunistic Infections in HIV-AIDS," *N J Med*, 2004, 101(11):25-31.

Tartaglione TA, "Therapeutic Options for the Management and Prevention of *Mycobacterium avium* Complex Infection in Patients With the Acquired Immunodeficiency Syndrome," *Pharmacotherapy*, 1996, 16(2):171-82.

"2001 USPHS/IDSA Guidelines for the Prevention of Opportunistic Infections in Persons Infected with Human Immunodeficiency Virus. USPHS/IDSA Prevention of Opportunistic Infections Working Group," available at www.aidsinfo.noh.gov.

Mycobacterium bovis

Synonyms Bacillus, Calmette-Guérin; BCG

Microbiology *Mycobacterium bovis* is an acid-fast bacillus, often shorter and plumper than *M. tuberculosis* (MTB). *M. bovis* grows more slowly than most mycobacterial species and growth can be inhibited by the presence of glycerol in the media. It is biochemically differentiated from MTB by niacin and nitrate reduction tests (*M. bovis* is usually negative for both tests where MTB is generally positive). Unlike MTB, *M. bovis* is microaerophilic, sensitive to thiopin-2-carboxylic acid, and resistant to pyrazinamide. *M. bovis* grows only at 35°C and appears as tiny translucent, smooth, pyramidal colonies. These organisms grow well on most media commonly used for the culture of MTB, including the Lowenstein-Jensen and 7H11. BCG is an attenuated mutant of *M. bovis*.

Epidemiology *Mycobacterium bovis* is known as the agent of bovine tuberculosis. *M. bovis* was a significant cause of "tuberculosis" worldwide in the early 1900s and before. Destruction of animals infected with *M. bovis* and subsequent pasteurization procedures for milk decreased the human infection rate by *M. bovis* dramatically. *M. bovis* was thought to be transmitted not only by ingestion of infected milk but also aerogenously by cow to human transmission. Human to human transmission, which
(Continued)

Mycobacterium bovis (Continued)

undoubtedly occurs, is quite controversial. The potential for human to cow transmission also may occur through the aerogenous route, as well as through urine of farmers with genitourinary *M. bovis* disease, where feeding areas are contaminated by infectious urine, which is either aerosolized or ingested by cattle. Other animal reservoirs may include pigs, goats, deer, cats, dogs, foxes, badgers, marsupials, rabbits, sheep, and horses.

BCG, which has been used in many parts of the world to immunize individuals against tuberculosis, has also been used to boost immune response and treat carcinoma of the bladder. There are significant numbers of reports of systemic BCG infection developing in these treated or immunized patients. Most cases of serious "BCG" infection are associated with bloodstream absorption of the agent. BCG should not be given to patients until at least 1 week after any surgical manipulation of the bladder or tumor resection.

Clinical Syndromes Unlike tuberculosis, much of the primary disease caused by *M. bovis* occur in the cervical lymph nodes and the GI tract with its related lymphatics; however, *M. bovis* may cause pulmonary disease and cause disease in other extrapulmonary sites in a similar manner to MTB. The most common sites of *M. bovis* infection in children are involvement of the cervical lymph nodes and intra-abdominal organs as reflected in the oral portal of entry. (Incidence is extremely rare since eradication of infected cattle and widespread pasteurization of milk). Disease can occur, however, in any organ system similar to MTB. In adults, extrapulmonary *M. bovis* infection is often a reactivation of disease. The lung is still the most common organ involved when transmission is through bovine contact. *M. bovis* can cause gastric TB, tuberculous meningitis, miliary disease, epidural abscess and spinal tuberculosis, bone and joint infections, and genitourinary infection.

Systemic infection caused by administration of BCG can cause pneumonitis, hepatitis, systemic BCG infection, including life-threatening sepsis, arthritis and arthralgias, skin rash, and genitourinary tract infections. Granulomatous hepatitis may be more of a hypersensitivity reaction than infection. Sepsis following intravesical BCG installation can be lethal. The attenuation of this organism has not rendered it completely harmless. Patients may present with classic symptoms of sepsis including shock, acute respiratory distress, and disseminated intravascular coagulopathy.

Diagnosis Diagnosis should be based on appropriate history of animal exposure, occupational contact, or receipt of BCG vaccination or chemotherapy. The tuberculin skin test may be useful, except in patients with known exposure to BCG. Appropriate specimen retrieval from suspected infected sites is necessary, with subsequent acid-fast staining and cultures. *M. bovis* will grow in a routine mycobacterial culture.

Diagnostic Tests/Procedures

Acid-Fast Stain *on page 361*
Mycobacteria Culture, Biopsy or Body Fluid *on page 539*
Mycobacteria Culture, Sputum *on page 542*
Tuberculin Skin Testing, Intracutaneous *on page 601*

Treatment Manifestations of *M. bovis* disease should be treated in a similar manner as tuberculosis, with the exception that all strains are inherently resistant to pyrazinamide. Six month regimens with isoniazid and rifampin (plus ethambutol for the first 2 months) may be adequate. Typical TB treatment courses may be followed. This is also true for disseminated BCG. Organisms are routinely susceptible to all the first and second line antituberculous agents (except pyrazinamide). Susceptibility testing should be performed on all organisms cultured, as mycobacterial infections resistant to one or more drugs have been reported.

Drug Therapy

Recommended:

Combinations of 2 or more of the following:

Isoniazid *on page 893*
Rifampin *on page 1046*
Ethambutol *on page 812*
Streptomycin *on page 1078*

Alternate:

If intolerant of a first line antitubercular agent or if multidrug resistance is present, one or more of the alternate antitubercular agents should be substituted:

Antituberculars *on page 667*

Selected Readings

Bass JB Jr, Farer LS, Hopewell PC, et al, "Treatment of Tuberculosis and Tuberculosis Infections in Adults and Children. American Thoracic Society and the Centers for Disease Control and Prevention," *Am J Respir Crit Care Med*, 1994, 149(5):1359-74.

Berlin OG, "Mycobacteria," *Bailey & Scott's Diagnostic Microbiology*, St. Louis, MO: CV Mosby Co, 1990, 597-640.

Dankner WM, Waecker NJ, Essey MA, et al, "*Mycobacterium bovis* Infections in San Diego: A Clinicoepidemiologic Study of 73 Patients and a Historical Review of a Forgotten Pathogen," *Medicine*, 1993, 72(1):11-37.

"Initial Therapy for Tuberculosis in the Era of Multidrug Resistance. Recommendations of the Advisory Council for the Elimination of Tuberculosis," *MMWR*, 1993, 42(RR-7):1-8.

Lamm DL, van der Meijden PM, Morales A, et al, "Incidence and Treatment of Complications of Bacillus Calmette-Guérin Intravesical Therapy in Superficial Bladder Cancer," *J Urol*, 1992, 147(3):596-600.

Willett HP, "*Mycobacterium*," *Zinsser Microbiology*, 20th ed, Joklik WK, Willett HP, Amos DB, et al, eds, Norwalk, CT: Appleton & Lange, 1988, 423-48.

Mycobacterium kansasii

Microbiology *Mycobacterium kansasii* is an acid-fast bacillus that is a "nontuberculous" *Mycobacterium.* It is a photochromogen and appears as a long, thick bacillus on clinical specimens. The organism is not well visualized using the Gram stain and an acid-fast stain is necessary. Similarly, the organism does not grow well on routine bacteriologic media and requires appropriate media for acid-fast bacilli.

Epidemiology *M. kansasii* has been reported to cause disease worldwide. The highest incidence of disease in the United States has been reported in the southern and midwest regions, in a so-called inverted-T distribution. This type of geographic distribution suggests the organism is present in specific environments, but the precise reservoir of the organism is not clear since *M. kansasii* does not seem to be prevalent in soil, water, or other sources. Transmission is felt to be from an environmental source to the susceptible individual, and not person-to-person. Infection in children is unusual, with most cases reported in the fifth decade of life. Occupational groups at increased risk for *M. kansasii* infection include miners, welders, and painters, among others. There is also an increased incidence of chronic obstructive pulmonary disease in individuals infected with *M. kansasii.* Occasionally, healthy individuals with no underlying lung disease can develop symptomatic infection with this organism. The incidence of this is not clear although in one report 40% of non-HIV infected persons with *M. kansasii* had no known predisposing condition. Population-based studies have shown higher rates of infection in urban areas, particularly in impoverished areas.

The epidemiology of *M. kansasii* infections has undergone a change in the past two decades. Prior to the AIDS epidemic, *M. kansasii* infections were relatively uncommon with an incidence of 0.52 cases/100,000 in 1980. Since the late 1980s, there has been an increase in the number of cases of *M. kansasii*, both in persons with and without HIV coinfection. In a recent population-based study in northern California (considered a nonendemic area), the rate of *M. kansasii* infection in persons seronegative for HIV was similar to population data in the early 1980s. For persons with HIV infection, the incidence was 150 times higher and for persons with AIDS, the incidence was 900 times higher than the general population.

Clinical Syndromes

- **Pulmonary infection:** Infection by *M. kansasii* frequently causes a subacute pneumonia that is clinically very similar to that caused by *Mycobacterium tuberculosis.* Patients present with subacute onset of cough, low grade fevers, weight loss, and malaise. Routine blood studies are not helpful. A variety of radiographic abnormalities have been reported including upper lobe infiltrates, cavitary lung disease, pleural effusions, and a miliary pattern. In many cases it is difficult to distinguish the chest radiographic findings from tuberculosis. Some individuals are chronically colonized with this organism, making the clinical interpretation of a positive respiratory culture difficult. The interpretation of a single positive sputum culture for *M. kansasii* has been the source of considerable debate. The American Thoracic Society (ATS) published guidelines in 1990 requiring two or more positive respiratory cultures for the diagnosis of pulmonary disease caused by *M. kansasii.* These guidelines have been criticized by some as being too strict, particularly for AIDS patients. More recent guidelines by the ATS in 1997 have recommended that persons with symptomatic pulmonary disease and multifocal bronchiectasis and/or small nodules on high resolution CT scan could be diagnosed with pulmonary infection if the patient also met one of the following microbiologic criteria: (1) two positive sputum/bronchial wash cultures within 12 months if one or both specimens is AFB smear positive; (2) three positive sputum/bronchial wash cultures within 12 months if none of the specimens is AFB smear positive, (3) one positive bronchial wash culture with ≥2+ AFB on smear and/or growth on solid media (for persons unable to produce sputum), or (4) transbronchial or lung biopsy yielding the organism or a biopsy showing mycobacterial histopathologically (ie, granulomatous inflammation and/or AFB) and one or more respiratory cultures positive for *M. kansasii.*
- **Disseminated *M. kansasii* in persons with HIV infection:** Although the full disease spectrum of *M. kansasii* in HIV-infected persons is not known, a fulminant form of *M. kansasii* has been reported. This is still characterized mainly by fevers and pulmonary symptoms, with pulmonary infiltrates. Interestingly, *M. kansasii* in

(Continued)

Mycobacterium kansasii (Continued)

HIV-infected persons may have a relatively low incidence of cavitary lung lesions (<50%). Extrapulmonary *M. kansasii* has been reported in a variety of sites. The infection can be disseminated with positive blood cultures for AFB, although mycobacteremia appears to be relatively uncommon even in persons with advanced AIDS.

- **Extrapulmonary infection:** In non-HIV infected persons, *M. kansasii* has been reported to cause a variety of skin lesions (from local inoculation), osteomyelitis, soft tissue infection, tenosynovitis, and renal pelvis obstruction. It is a rare cause of cervical adenitis and other mycobacteria are much more common.

Diagnosis Pulmonary infection from *M. kansasii* is the most common manifestation of this organism and mimics tuberculosis both clinically and radiographically. Culture confirmation is essential. Most commonly the diagnosis is established by sending respiratory samples (sputum, bronchoscopy specimens) for acid-fast bacilli (AFB) stain and culture. In cases of extrapulmonary disease, the appropriate body fluid or tissue (skin biopsy, bone biopsy, etc) should be specified for AFB stain and culture.

Diagnostic Tests/Procedures

Acid-Fast Stain *on page 361*
Mycobacteria Culture, Biopsy or Body Fluid *on page 539*

Treatment In general, *M. kansasii* responds well to antimicrobial therapy. The role of isoniazid has been somewhat controversial since this agent has only minimal efficacy against *M. kansasii in vitro*. The American Thoracic Society (ATS) currently recommends the combination of isoniazid 600 mg orally once daily, rifampin 300 mg orally once daily, and ethambutol 15 mg/kg for initial therapy. In the United Kingdom, the recommended regimen is rifampin and ethambutol, without the isoniazid. Treatment courses are typically 18 months or more for either regimen.

For HIV-positive persons infected with *M. kansasii*, drug interactions between rifampin and the protease inhibitors, and some of the non-nucleoside reverse transcriptase inhibitors, are critical. Rifampin substantially lowers plasma levels of the protease inhibitors. Rifabutin can be used in place of rifampin for patients on the following protease inhibitors: indinavir, amprenavir, saquinavir (soft-gel capsules), and nelfinavir. For those already receiving ritonavir or saquinavir (hard-gel caps), the interaction with rifabutin may still be significant. In such cases, clarithromycin can be used in place of rifampin although only limited data is available. Similarly, patients who are on delavirdine should be on a regimen of isoniazid, ethambutol, and clarithromycin due to drug interactions with both rifampin and rifabutin.

Drug Therapy

Recommended:

The following 3 used in combination

Isoniazid *on page 893*
Rifampin *on page 1046*
Ethambutol *on page 812*

Alternate:

Rifabutin *on page 1045*
Clarithromycin *on page 749*

Selected Readings

Bamberger DM, Driks MR, Gupta MR, et al, "*Mycobacterium kansasii* Among Patients Infected With Human Immunodeficiency Virus in Kansas City," *Clin Infect Dis*, 1994, 18(3):395-400.

Bernard L, Vincent V, Lortholary O, et al, "*Mycobacterium kansasii* Septic Arthritis: French Retrospective Study of 5 Years and Review," *Clin Infect Dis*, 1999, 29(6):1455-60.

Bloch KC, Zwerling L, Pletcher MJ, et al, "Incidence and Clinical Implications of Isolation of *Mycobacterium kansasii*: Results of a 5-Year, Population-Based Study," *Ann Intern Med*, 1998, 129(9):698-704.

Brown BA and Wallace RJ, "Infections due to Nontuberculous Mycobacteria," *Principles and Practice of Infectious Diseases*, 5th ed, Mandell GL, Bennett JE, and Dolin R, eds, New York, NY: Churchill Livingstone, 2000, 2630-6.

Jacobson KL, Teira R, Libshitz HI, et al, "*Mycobacterium kansasii* Infections in Patients With Cancer," *Clin Infect Dis*, 2000, 30(6):965-9.

Pintado V, Gomez-Mampaso E, Martin-Davila P, et al, "*Mycobacterium kansasii* Infection in Patients Infected With the Human Immunodeficiency Virus," *Eur J Clin Microbiol Infect Dis*, 1999, 18(8):582-6.

Mycobacterium Species, not MTB or MAI

Microbiology Mycobacteria other than *M. tuberculosis* (MTB) and *M. avium-intracellulare* (MAI) (hereafter called "other" mycobacteria) are acid-fast bacilli which have cell walls with high lipid content and which are morphologically similar to MTB and MAI. Other mycobacteria are different from MTB and MAI in biochemical reactions, pigmentation, growth rates, natural reservoirs, pathogenesis, manifestations of disease, and susceptibilities to antimicrobial agents. Like MTB, other mycobacteria tend to cause chronic diseases and lesions. There are many species of other mycobacteria, the most commonly isolated are the following: *M. kansasii*, *M. marinum*, *M. gordonae*, *M. ulcerans*, *M. fortuitum*, *M. chelonae* subsp *chelonae*, *M. chelonae* subsp *abscessus*, and *M. scrofulaceum*. *M. genavense* and *M.*

haemophilum are recently recognized other mycobacteria with which most physicians are not familiar. These other mycobacteria are pathogens to humans (usually immunocompromised hosts), grow in blood culture broth but require special growth media for subculture, and can require 4-9 weeks to grow on solid culture media. *M. haemophilum* can require up to 12 weeks to grow and requires special chocolate medium for optimal chances of growth in culture.

Epidemiology Other mycobacteria are ubiquitous in nature. Natural reservoirs include soil, cattle and other domestic livestock, fish, water, milk and other foods, wild animals, and nonhuman Primates. The CDC has reported that other mycobacteria accounted for 35% of non-MTB mycobacteria clinical isolates. Humans become infected with other mycobacteria by inhalation of the mycobacteria through the mouth and nose and by direct inoculation into breaks in the skin. Other mycobacteria generally are not transmitted person to person.

Clinical Syndromes Other mycobacteria can cause numerous clinical syndromes, the most common of which are presented in the following table.

Clinical Syndromes of Mycobacteria

***Mycobacterium* Infection**	**Relatively Common Cause**
Chronic pulmonary	*M. kansasii, M. fortuitum*
Cervical lymphadenitis	*M. kansasii, M. scrofulaceum*
Soft tissue	*M. marinum, M. abscessus*
Disseminated	*M. kansasii*
Surgical wound	*M. fortuitum, M. chelonae* subsp
Skeletal, joint	*M. kansasii, M. fortuitum, M. ulcerans*
Skin, ulcer, abscess	*M. marinum, M. fortuitum, M. abscessus, M. ulcerans, M. chelonae* subsp

Mycobacterium fortuitum and *M. chelonae* are two important Runyon group IV "rapid growers", so-named because of their ability to grow in several days when subcultured (initial isolation of the organism may require 1 or more weeks). Both healthy and immunocompromised persons may develop infection with these agents. Skin and soft tissue infections are relatively common manifestations of these organisms and are usually associated with trauma or the presence of a foreign body; this includes infection of postoperative wounds (eg, sternal wounds after cardiac surgery), infections of orthopedic devices such as arthroplasties, breast implant infections, post-traumatic wound infections, and others. Pulmonary infection from inhalation may occur with microabscess formation in the lungs (granuloma formation is less common). Other manifestations include endocarditis, osteomyelitis, and lymphadenitis, but visceral dissemination outside of the lungs is rare. Although disseminated disease has been reported in immunocompromised individuals, a recent review suggests this is an unusual occurrence.

Mycobacterium marinum is the cause of "fishtank granuloma." Infections are characterized by multiple ulcerative skin lesions on an extremity that spread proximally along the lymphatics. The organism grows well in fresh and salt water and is associated with fishtanks, pools, and aquariums. Human disease occurs usually through direct inoculation through a break in the skin. Patients with this clinical syndrome should be asked about exposure to aquarium water or other aquatic activities. Other mycobacteria besides *M. marinum* can cause a similar syndrome, as can infection with *Sporothrix schenckii.*

Mycobacterium scrofulaceum is an important cause of cervical lymphadenitis in children. The disease remains localized, but cure often requires both antimicrobial therapy and surgery.

Mycobacterium ulcerans is pathogenic mainly in tropical countries such as Africa. It characteristically causes a necrotic ulcer on the extremities.

M. abscessus soft tissue infections of an extremity can resemble sporotrichosis.

Diagnosis The aforementioned diseases are diagnosed by culture of tissues (**not** swab specimens). Most other mycobacteria will grow in culture in 2-4 weeks. However, growth rates depend on the species and range from 3-60 days.

Diagnostic Tests/Procedures

Acid-Fast Stain *on page 361*

Mycobacteria Culture, Biopsy or Body Fluid *on page 539*

(Continued)

Mycobacterium Species, not MTB or MAI *(Continued)*

Treatment

M. fortuitum: Typically resistant to all common antitubercular agents. Amikacin and cefoxitin can be administered for 2-6 weeks followed by oral therapy with sulfamethoxazole and trimethoprim or doxycycline for 2-6 months. Clarithromycin plus doxycycline or trimethoprim and sulfamethoxazole or a fluoroquinolone (levofloxacin, moxifloxacin, gatifloxacin) are also options

M. scrofulaceum: Treatment of choice is usually surgical excision. If necessary, drug therapy regimen should include isoniazid, rifampin, and streptomycin. This organism is also sensitive *in vitro* to the macrolides and cycloserine.

M. marinum: Ethambutol plus rifampin or monotherapy with clarithromycin, trimethoprim and sulfamethoxazole, minocycline, or doxycycline for at least 3 months. Monotherapy agents can also be used in combination with ethambutol. Surgical excision may also be required.

M. chelonae: Sensitive to amikacin and the macrolides. A 6-month course of clarithromycin may be the regimen of choice.

M. ulcerans: A useful regimen includes a 6-week course of either rifampin in combination with amikacin or ethambutol in combination with sulfamethoxazole and trimethoprim.

Treatment regimens remain controversial for some of these mycobacterial agents due to a lack of formal clinical trials. Combination therapy is of use with severe infections, but even less data is available concerning the optimal agents to be used. **Antibiotic susceptibility testing is strongly recommended since the drug-susceptibility patterns are not reliably predictable.** Consultation with an Infectious Disease specialist should also be considered.

Selected Readings

Bartralot R, Garcia-Patos V, Sitjas D, et al, "Clinical Patterns of Cutaneous Nontuberculous Mycobacterial Infections," *Br J Dermatol*, 2005, 152(4):727-34.

Horowitz EA and Sanders WE Jr, "Other *Mycobacterium* Species," *Principles and Practice of Infectious Diseases*, 4th ed, Mandell GL, Bennett JE, and Dolin R, eds, New York, NY: Churchill Livingstone, 1995, 2264-73.

Falkinham JO 3d, "Epidemiology of Infection by Nontuberculous Mycobacteria," *Clin Microbiol Rev*, 1996, 9(2):177-215.

Martin-Casabona N, Bahrmand AR, Bennedsen J, et al, "Non-tuberculous *Mycobacteria:* Patterns of Isolation. A Multi-country Retrospective Survey," *Int J Tuberc Lung Dis*, 2004, 8(10):1186-93.

Salfinger M and Wallace RJ, "Susceptibility Testing for Nontuberculosis Mycobacteria: Should It Be Performed?" *Clin Microbiol Newslett*, 1997, 19(9):68-71.

Wagner D and Young LS, "Nontuberculous Mycobacterial Infections: A Clinical Review," *Infection*, 2004, 32(5):257-70.

Mycobacterium tuberculosis

Related Information

Community-Acquired Pneumonia in Adults *on page 1278*

Prophylaxis for Patients Exposed to Common Communicable Diseases *on page 1309*

Tuberculosis *on page 1315*

USPHS / IDSA Guidelines for the Prevention of Opportunistic Infections in Persons Infected With HIV *on page 1237*

Clinically Relevant Major Species of *Mycobacterium*

Group	Strict Human Pathogens	Occasional Potential Human Pathogens	Usually Environmental or Rarely Human Pathogens in the U.S.
M. tuberculosis complex	*M. tuberculosis* *M. leprae* *M. africanum* *M. ulcerans*	*M. bovis*	
Photochromogens		*M. kansasii* *M. marinum*	*M. simiae* *M. asiaticum*
Scotochromogens		*M. szulgai* *M. xenopi*	*M. gordonae* *M. flavescens* *M. scrofulaceum*
Nonchromogens	*M. genavense*	*M. avium* *M. intracellulare* *M. hemophilum*	*M. malmoense*
Rapid growers		*M. fortuitum* *M. chelonei*	*M. smegmatis*

Synonyms Tubercle Bacillus

Microbiology *Mycobacterium tuberculosis* (MTB) is a fastidious, slowly-growing, aerobic bacterium with a complex cell wall composed of peptidoglycans and many complex, long-chain lipids. The free lipids on the outer layer make *M. tuberculosis* relatively hydrophobic and resistant to many stains used in the laboratory including Gram stain and Giemsa stain. It is an acid-fast bacillus, meaning once the organism is stained, it cannot be decolorized by acid solutions.

Mycobacteria can be isolated on solid agar media or in broth cultures (which can be read by automated devices). Growth in broth is usually much more rapid than on agar.

See table on previous page for listing of important and major species of the genus *Mycobacterium* and the pathogenic potential of each species.

Epidemiology Tuberculosis remains one of the most common and deadly diseases throughout the world. It is estimated that 33% of the world's population has been infected with *M. tuberculosis*. There are approximately 30 million active cases of tuberculosis at any time.

In the past 10 years there has been a resurgence of tuberculosis in the United States. In prior years, the number of new cases of tuberculosis had been declining at a rate of about 5% per year, but since the mid 1980s, the case rate began to rise at a rate of about 3% per year; this disturbing reversal has been attributed in large part to the AIDS epidemic. In the United States, over 10 million individuals in the U.S. have been infected with MTB at some point in their lives based on the results of tuberculin skin testing. The majority of active cases of tuberculosis come from this large pool of individuals who have been exposed to MTB in the past and later present with reactivation of latent infection. A smaller number of active cases are attributable to recent exposure of a healthy individual to a person with active tuberculosis.

In the United States, there are many defined groups at high risk for MTB infection:

- individuals with HIV infection
- close contacts (ie, family members and others) of infectious TB cases
- persons with underlying medical conditions which increase the risk of TB (see below)
- persons from foreign countries with a high prevalence of TB
- indigent populations
- alcoholics and persons who use intravenous drugs
- persons residing in nursing homes, prisons, and other long-term care facilities
- healthcare workers

Certain medical conditions predispose a person to the development of active tuberculosis once a person has been infected with the organism:

- HIV infection
- silicosis
- chest x-ray which shows fibrotic lesions, consistent with prior TB
- diabetes
- steroids or other immunosuppressive medications
- lymphomas and other hematologic diseases
- end-stage renal disease, especially those on chronic dialysis
- intestinal bypass
- postgastrectomy
- chronic malabsorption syndromes
- head and neck malignancies
- weight loss of 10% below ideal body weight, from any cause

MTB is transmitted via the respiratory route when an infected individual comes in close contact with a susceptible person. The organism is carried in droplets of respiratory secretions ("airborne droplets") during coughing, sneezing, and speaking; the organism can remain airborne and infectious for a period of time. Person-to-person transmission occurs when a susceptible individual inhales the infectious droplet nuclei. Close household contacts of infected individuals puts others at risk for acquiring infection, although typically several months of exposure may be needed. The degree of contagiousness of a given patient depends on a variety of factors including the number of organisms in the sputum, presence or absence of cavitary lung disease, amount of coughing, length of time on antituberculous therapy, and others.

Clinical Syndromes

- **Primary tuberculosis:** Primary infection, or first exposure to *M. tuberculosis*, often is asymptomatic. Typically, there is a pulmonary infiltrate in the mid or lower lung fields with or without hilar adenopathy. The infiltrates are nonspecific in appearance and are not cavitary. In most cases, the pneumonitis clears without specific therapy

(Continued)

Mycobacterium tuberculosis (Continued)

and latent infection is established. In some cases, the primary infection progresses and mimics reactivation disease.

- **Latent infection:** Many individuals remain asymptomatic following the primary infection with *M. tuberculosis*. The organism remains latent within macrophages indefinitely. The tuberculin skin test is extremely important in identifying these individuals. Approximately 1 in 10 persons with infection from *M. tuberculosis* will develop clinical disease at some time in their life unless given preventative therapy.
- **Reactivation tuberculosis:** Patients with reactivation tuberculosis present with weight loss, fever, constitutional symptoms, and a generalized wasting syndrome. Drenching night sweats are common. Often, these individuals are diagnostic dilemmas since pulmonary symptoms may be very mild or absent.
- **Pulmonary tuberculosis:** The majority of cases of active pulmonary tuberculosis are due to reactivation of the latent organism. Reactivation is likely to occur in the upper lobes and the superior segments of the lower lobes due to the oxygen-rich environment. However, disease can involve any area of the lung, especially in diabetics, elderly persons, and persons with AIDS. The absence of apical infiltrates should not be used to exclude tuberculosis; and for practical purposes, TB should be included in the differential diagnosis of any undiagnosed pneumonia. The extent of disease is also variable, ranging from subtle infiltrates in chest x-ray with minimal cough to the classic cavitary tuberculosis with hemoptysis. If untreated, the pulmonary lesions develop areas of caseation or central necrosis with partial liquefaction.
- **Extrapulmonary tuberculosis:** (See Selected Readings). Tuberculous disease outside the lung parenchyma can be even more difficult to diagnose. Extrapulmonary TB can become clinically apparent during the phase of primary infection, particularly in children. More commonly, extrapulmonary TB represents reactivation of latent infection. It is important to note that a pulmonary lesion of any type will be absent in 50% or more cases of extrapulmonary TB; it is even more uncommon to have a chest x-ray showing active pulmonary infiltrates or cavities. Extrapulmonary TB includes:
  - pleural disease with effusion; the most common form of extrapulmonary TB
  - tuberculous meningitis; often a difficult diagnosis to confirm. Classically, patients present with a chronic meningitis, but a more fulminant variety resembling pyogenic meningitis is well recognized. Because there is often a basilar meningitis, patients frequently develop cranial nerve signs; tuberculous meningitis should be strongly considered in any patient with signs or symptoms of meningitis with cranial nerve deficits. The spinal fluid typically has an elevated protein, low glucose, and a lymphocytic pleocytosis, but this pattern can be seen in a number of other disease entities. Often repeated lumbar punctures with high volumes of spinal fluid submitted for mycobacterial culture are required to confirm the diagnosis. However, if the clinical suspicion for tuberculous meningitis is high (ie, positive tuberculin skin test, lymphocytic pleocytosis, etc), antituberculous therapy should be initiated.
  - pericarditis
  - peritonitis
  - tuberculous adenitis or "scrofula" (chronic tuberculous infection of the cervical lymph nodes)
  - osteomyelitis including tuberculosis of the spine (Pott's disease)
  - genitourinary tuberculosis
  - ocular infections including chorioretinitis
  - gastrointestinal tuberculosis
  - cutaneous tuberculosis (lupus vulgaris)
  - miliary tuberculosis; *M. tuberculosis* can disseminate into the lymphohematogenous system either during primary tuberculous infection or during reactivation (more common). This can be a difficult diagnosis to establish, and the chest x-ray can be normal early on.

Diagnosis A high index of suspicion must be maintained for tuberculosis. Laboratory confirmation of suspected cases is essential since the manifestations of MTB are protean. The tuberculin skin test is an important first step in identifying infected patients. Laboratory techniques for identifying *M. tuberculosis* include:

- acid-fast smears and cultures of respiratory secretions
- acid-fast smears and cultures of other potentially infected body fluids or tissues (cerebrospinal fluid, gastric fluid, urine, bone marrow biopsies, joint fluids, and many others)
- rapid methods - amplification of nucleic acid of MTB by the polymerase chain reaction (PCR) and subsequent detection by nucleic acid probes

Diagnostic Tests/Procedures

Acid-Fast Stain *on page 361*

Lumbar Puncture *on page 524*
Mycobacteria Culture, Biopsy or Body Fluid *on page 539*
Mycobacteria Culture, Sputum *on page 542*
Polymerase Chain Reaction *on page 567*
Tuberculin Skin Testing, Intracutaneous *on page 601*

Treatment The treatment of tuberculosis is based on the following principles.

- *M. tuberculosis* becomes resistant to drugs through random, spontaneous genetic mutations. For isoniazid, the proportion of naturally-occurring resistant bacteria has been established as 1 in 10^6, and for rifampin, the ratio is 1 bacterium in 10^8. This occurs particularly efficiently if only single drugs are utilized and in patients who are noncompliant.
- A regimen containing multiple drugs to which the organisms are susceptible should be used; susceptibility testing should be done on all isolates.
- Both isoniazid-resistant MTB and multidrug-resistant MTB are becoming increasing problems (see Selected Readings).
- When patient compliance is poor, directly observed therapy given twice weekly in an outpatient setting should be strongly considered.
- Failures of therapy are often due to noncompliance with the regimen. The emergence of multidrug therapy is partly due to noncompliance as well.
- Physicians must take into account the immune status of the patient.

Drug Therapy

Recommended:

Note: See Treatment for appropriate regimen.
Isoniazid *on page 893*
Rifampin *on page 1046*
Rifampin and Isoniazid *on page 1050*
Pyrazinamide *on page 1022*
Ethambutol *on page 812*
Streptomycin *on page 1078*

Alternate:

If intolerant of a first-line antitubercular agent or if multidrug resistant and TB is present, one or more of the alternative antitubercular agents should be substituted.
Antituberculars *on page 667*

Selected Readings

Barnes PF and Barrows SA, "Tuberculosis in the 1990s," *Ann Intern Med*, 1993, 119(5):400-10.
Brodie D and Schluger NW, "The Diagnosis of Tuberculosis," *Clin Chest Med*, 2005, 26(2):247-71.
Burman WJ, "Issues in the Management of HIV-Related Tuberculosis," *Clin Chest Med*, 2005, 26(2):283-94, vi-vii.
Goble M, Iseman MD, Madsen LA, et al, "Treatment of 171 Patients With Pulmonary Tuberculosis Resistant to Isoniazid and Rifampin," *N Engl J Med*, 1993, 328(8):527-32.
"Initial Therapy for Tuberculosis in the Era of Multidrug Resistance," *MMWR*, 1993, 42(RR-7):1-8.
Kunimoto D and Long R, "Tuberculosis: Still Overlooked as a Cause of Community-Acquired Pneumonia - How Not to Miss It," *Respir Care Clin N Am*, 2005, 11(1):25-34.
Myers JP, "New Recommendations for the Treatment of Tuberculosis," *Curr Opin Infect Dis*, 2005, 18(2):133-40.
Saglam L, Akgun M, and Aktas E, "Usefulness of Induced Sputum and Fibreoptic Bronchoscopy Specimens in the Diagnosis of Pulmonary Tuberculosis," *J Int Med Res*, 2005, 33(2):260-5.
Snider DE Jr and Roper WL, "A New Tuberculosis," *N Engl J Med*, 1992, 326(10):703-5.
"Treatment of Tuberculosis. American Thoracic Society, Centers for Disease Control and Prevention, and Infectious Diseases Society of America," *MMWR*, 2003, (52(RR-11):1-80.
"Treatment of Tuberculosis and Tuberculosis Infection in Adults and Children. American Thoracic Society and the Centers for Disease Control and Prevention," *Am J Respir Crit Care Med*, 1994, 149(5):1359-74.
"Trends in Tuberculosis - United States, 2004," *MMWR*, 2005, 54(10):245-9.

Mycoplasma hominis and *Mycoplasma genitalium*

Microbiology *Mycoplasma hominis* and *M. genitalium* belong to the organism class called Mollicutes. The class Mollicutes is composed of approximately 160 named species of *Mycoplasma*. The *Mycoplasmas* (including *M. hominis* and *M. genitalium*) are the smallest organisms known to be capable of being free-living and self-replicating, are only 150-250 nm in diameter, do not have cell walls, have deformable membranes, have extremely fastidious growth requirements, and appear as "fried egg" colonies on special growth media.

Epidemiology *Mycoplasmas* are ubiquitous and are commonly found in the mouths, upper respiratory tracts, and lower urogenital tracts of both healthy and diseased humans and animals. In addition, many *Mycoplasmas* are found in plants and insects. *Mycoplasmas* have long been known to cause significant health problems in domestic, commercial, and laboratory animals. Only four of the 13 species of *Mycoplasmas* which have been isolated from humans are associated with human disease: *M. pneumoniae*, *M. hominis*, *M. genitalium*, and *Ureaplasma urealyticum*.
(Continued)

Mycoplasma hominis and *Mycoplasma genitalium* (Continued)

Clinical Syndromes Overwhelming and convincing evidence that *M. hominis* and *M. genitalium* cause disease does not exist. However, evidence does support the idea that *M. hominis* probably causes some cases of pyelonephritis, pelvic inflammatory disease, and postabortion fever; is strongly associated with bacterial vaginosis; causes many cases of postpartum fever; and is associated with various conditions (including arthritis) in immunocompromised persons. The only disease with which *M. genitalium* has been strongly associated is nongonococcal urethritis.

Diagnosis Diseases potentially caused by *M. hominis* and *M. genitalium* are diagnosed clinically and supported by culture results. Consult the clinical laboratory for advice regarding appropriate specimens to collect and appropriate collection procedures and transport medium. **Note:** Special transport medium and conditions are essential for transportation and culture of all *Mycoplasmas*.

Diagnostic Tests/Procedures

Mycoplasma/Ureaplasma Culture *on page 545*

Note: Physicians should contact their laboratory for advice on how to collect and transport specimens to be cultured for *Mycoplasma* and *Ureaplasma* species. Special transport media are required.

Treatment Although both organisms are in the same genus, their susceptibility patterns are quite different. *Mycoplasma genitalium* mimics *M. pneumoniae*, both of which are susceptible to macrolides, tetracyclines, and fluoroquinolones. *M. hominis* strains resistant to tetracyclines have been appearing more frequently. Susceptibility testing should be performed. Clindamycin can be used in patients with tetracycline-resistant *M. hominis*.

Drug Therapy

Recommended:

Mycoplasma hominis:

Clindamycin *on page 752*

Tetracycline *on page 1106*

Mycoplasma genitalium:

Macrolides *on page 924*

Tetracycline *on page 1106*

Fluoroquinolones *on page 824*

Selected Readings

Deguchi T and Maeda S, "*Mycoplasma genitalium*: Another Important Pathogen of Nongonococcal Urethritis," *J Urol*, 2002, 167(3):1210-7.

McCormack WM, "Susceptibility of *Mycoplasma* to Antimicrobial Agents: Clinical Implications," *Clin Infect Dis*, 1993, 17(Suppl 1):S200-1.

Rosengarten R, Citti C, Much P, et al, "The Changing Image of Mycoplasmas: From Innocent Bystanders to Emerging and Reemerging Pathogens in Human and Animal Diseases" *Contrib Microbiol*, 2001, 8:166-85.

Taylor-Robinson D, "Infections Due to Species of *Mycoplasma* and *Ureaplasma*: An Update," *Clin Infect Dis*, 1996, 23(4):671-82.

Taylor-Robinson D, "*Ureaplasma urealyticum, Mycoplasma hominis*, and *Mycoplasma genitalium*" *Principles and Practice of Infectious Diseases*, 5th ed, Mandell GL, Bennett JE, and Dolin R, eds, New York, NY: Churchill Livingstone, 2000, 2027-32.

Mycoplasma pneumoniae

Synonyms Eaton's Agent

Microbiology *Mycoplasma pneumoniae* is the smallest and simplest prokaryote capable of self-replication. Originally, this free-living, strictly aerobic organism was thought to be a virus but later determined to be a bacterium. The diameter of *M. pneumoniae* is 0.2-0.8 μm, and the organism is highly pleomorphic. The organism lacks a cell wall and has only a trilaminar membrane (similar to the structure of the trilaminar membrane which surrounds all bacterial and mammalian cells) enclosing the cell cytoplasm. Although *M. pneumoniae* is classified as a gram-negative bacterium, it retains the Gram stain poorly and, thus, cannot be reliably seen on routine Gram stain of clinical specimens such as sputum.

Growth of *M. pneumoniae* in culture requires special laboratory techniques, and a special request for *Mycoplasma* culture must be made. The organism does not grow on routine culture media used for isolating common bacterial respiratory pathogens. *Mycoplasma pneumoniae* requires an exogenous supply of cholesterol and other sterols for membrane synthesis; these nutrients can be supplied by animal sera added to the culture medium, and an exogenous supply of nucleic acids, for synthesis of purines and pyrimidines; this can be supplied by yeast extracts. An artificial, cell-free, selective culture medium is used in many laboratories. This diphasic medium is composed of broth (liquid medium) overlying agar. A pH indicator in the agar is used to detect acid produced by *Mycoplasma* as it ferments glucose; a visible

color change in the agar is presumptive evidence of *M. pneumoniae*. The colonies of *M. pneumoniae* in culture are 50-100 μm in diameter and have a unique "fried egg" colonial morphology.

Epidemiology *Mycoplasma pneumoniae* infections occur worldwide, with a tendency towards temperate climates. Epidemics of mycoplasmal infections seem to occur every 4-6 years, although outbreaks of epidemic proportions can occur in small communities at any time. Infections with *M. pneumoniae* do not follow a seasonal pattern, unlike many other respiratory pathogens which cause bronchitis and/or pneumonia in the winter and spring months (*Streptococcus pneumoniae*, respiratory syncytial virus, influenza A and B, and others). Thus, during summer months, the proportion of respiratory infections due to *Mycoplasma pneumoniae* increases (up to 50% of pneumonia cases), although the actual number of cases stays constant month to month.

One important characteristic of *Mycoplasma* infection is its tendency to spread within a family in a stepwise fashion. Spread within the family is slow (often 2-3 weeks from one family member to the next), but many, if not all, members become infected. Often the point source for infection in a family can be identified. Clustered cases also occur in military barracks, institutionalized settings, daycare centers, and college dormitories but tend to be slower and less complete than spread within families.

The highest rates of infection are in the young; school-aged children and young adults are statistically at highest risk. Although mycoplasmal infections are less common in children younger than 5 years of age, some studies have shown this organism to be a frequent cause of mild, but symptomatic, respiratory infections in this age group. Similarly, the incidence of mycoplasmal infection decreases with advancing age but still remains a sporadic cause of pneumonia in the older adult, which may be overlooked. Transmission of *M. pneumoniae* is via infected respiratory secretions such as nasal discharge. Close contact appears to be necessary for the infection to be spread. The incubation period between exposure to the infection and the first clinical symptoms is about 2-3 weeks.

Clinical Syndromes *Mycoplasma pneumoniae* is pathogenic for the lower respiratory tract and is able to adhere to respiratory epithelium by means of a special protein called P1. This attachment factor is contained in surface projections of the organism which bind to a receptor protein on the surface of the respiratory epithelial cells. Cellular injury takes place probably by several mechanisms including the production of superoxides. In severe cases, there is likely an immunologic component of cellular destruction as well. The organism remains extracellular during infection.

- **Community-acquired pneumonia:** Also known as "walking pneumonia" or "primary atypical pneumonia", this form of *Mycoplasma* infection is seen mainly between 5 and 20 years of age. *Mycoplasma pneumoniae* is the most common cause of pneumonia in this age group. The disease tends to be mild to moderate in severity but is characteristically very slow to resolve. Hospitalization is usually not necessary, and patients remain ambulatory (hence the term "walking pneumonia").

  Patients present with prominent constitutional symptoms: persistent headache, malaise, low grade fevers, and muscle aches. Sore throat and ear pain are also present in some cases. The onset of symptoms is gradual and subacute. Respiratory symptoms usually appear after several days of malaise. Patients develop a persistent, nonproductive cough. Purulent sputum, rigors, chest pain, and gross hemoptysis are not prominent features of this infection (although each has been rarely reported). Examination of the lungs may show wheezing, localized rales and/or rhonchi. In some cases, the lungs may be completely clear. Physical findings suggestive of lung consolidation (such as egophony, bronchial breathing, and dullness to percussion) are uncommon and suggestive of other bacterial pathogens. Examination of the head and neck often shows a mild injection of the tympanic membranes, mild pharyngeal erythema, and cervical adenopathy. More severe ear inflammation may be seen in about 15% of cases, with bullous myringitis being classically associated with mycoplasmal pneumonia. However, hemorrhagic bullous myringitis is uncommon, and its absence should not exclude the diagnosis. A nonspecific maculopapular rash is seen in some patients. Chest x-rays typically reveal patchy areas of bronchopneumonia with peribronchial cuffing. Most often the lower lung fields on one side are involved, but multilobar disease can occur. At times, the chest radiograph can be more impressive than the clinical findings, and this may be a clue to infection with *M. pneumoniae*. Radiographic findings of lobar consolidation are uncommon and large pleural effusions are distinctly unusual, both findings suggestive of respiratory pathogens such as *Streptococcus pneumoniae*. The course of atypical pneumonia tends to be protracted, with or without antibiotic treatment. Most patients recover completely, although life-threatening pneumonia with the adult respiratory distress syndrome (ARDS) has been reported.

(Continued)

Mycoplasma pneumoniae (Continued)

Complications of *M. pneumoniae* respiratory infection are statistically uncommon. However, unusual and potentially lethal complications have been well-recognized, and the incidence may exceed 10% in hospitalized patients. Respiratory complications include ARDS, pleural effusions, bronchiolitis obliterans, cavitary lung lesions, and bronchiectasis. Nonrespiratory complications include: (1) Mycoplasmal encephalitis, which can be seen when respiratory complaints are minor. Patients present with variable degrees of fever, confusion, and/or personality changes. Mycoplasmal encephalitis is indistinguishable from other forms of infectious encephalitis such as herpes simplex virus encephalitis. This entity should be considered in the differential diagnosis of any patient who presents with encephalitis and a pulmonary infiltrate. Other neurologic complications: transverse myelitis, stroke, postinfectious leukoencephalitis, optic neuritis, polymyositis syndrome, and others. (2) Autoimmune hemolytic anemia, which at times can be quite severe, such patients have high titers of cold-reacting autoantibodies (cold agglutinins). (3) Erythema multiforme, erythema nodosum. (4) Myocarditis, and pericarditis.

- **Tracheobronchitis:** The majority of *M. pneumoniae* infections do not lead to pneumonia. Tracheobronchitis accounts for 70% to 80% of all infections with *M. pneumoniae*, with only about 33% progressing to pneumonia. The clinical presentation of tracheobronchitis is similar to pneumonia, with prominent constitutional symptoms followed by a dry, persistent cough. The chest x-ray in tracheobronchitis remains clear because inflammation is limited primarily to the bronchi. Overall, the disease course is milder than with pneumonia, although the disease course may be slow to resolve completely.
- **Pharyngitis:** *M. pneumoniae* can cause a primary pharyngitis, or mycoplasmal pharyngitis may develop in association with tracheobronchitis or pneumonia. Again, school-aged children and young adults are most commonly involved. Constitutional symptoms (fever, headache, malaise) are prominent. Patients complain of a severe sore throat and often have difficulty swallowing. On examination, there is tonsillar enlargement, inflammatory exudate, and pharyngeal edema and erythema. Cervical lymphadenopathy is common. The clinical presentation may be confused with streptococcal pharyngitis or primary infectious mononucleosis (from Epstein-Barr virus). Mycoplasmal pharyngitis is probably underdiagnosed.

Diagnosis Diagnosis of *M. pneumoniae* respiratory infection is usually made on a clinical basis as described above, particularly since the majority of cases are upper respiratory infections which resolve rapidly, with or without treatment. In addition, definitive diagnosis of this organism is somewhat difficult and requires special culture techniques (see Microbiology section above) which add extra expense, require several days for completion, and usually add little to patient care. Thus, most clinicians do not attempt culture or serologic confirmation of bronchitis or other upper respiratory infections if *M. pneumoniae* is suspected. Definitive laboratory diagnosis of *M. pneumoniae* may be warranted in the following circumstances: (1) the pneumonia is severe or has a protracted course; (2) the patient is immunocompromised; (3) the patient is hospitalized with community-acquired pneumonia and confirmation of a specific pathogen such as *M. pneumoniae* would allow other antibiotics to be discontinued; or (4) there are extrapulmonary manifestations which may be secondary to *M. pneumoniae* (eg, encephalitis in a patient with a bronchopneumonia). A definitive diagnosis of *M. pneumoniae* infection can be made by isolation of the organism from a respiratory site such as expectorated sputum, bronchial alveolar lavage, or lung biopsy. Swab specimens are not productive. The organism can occasionally be isolated from sterile body sites, such as pleural fluid or cerebrospinal fluid, but this is very rare.

A significant rise in antibody titer between acute and convalescent *M. pneumoniae* IgG titers is also essentially diagnostic of recent infection and may be useful in persons unable to produce an adequate respiratory specimen. Both specific IgG and IgM titers are available. A single positive *M. pneumoniae* IgM is suggestive of active or very recent infection but false positives can occur.

Diagnostic Tests/Procedures

Mycoplasma Serology *on page 545*

Mycoplasma/Ureaplasma Culture *on page 545* (of lower respiratory tract specimens)

Polymerase Chain Reaction *on page 567* (of lower respiratory tract specimens) and subsequent detection of amplified products with molecular probes

Duration of Therapy 2-3 weeks

Treatment Macrolides are the most active agents against *M. pneumoniae*. Quinolones and doxycycline also have excellent activity. The newer respiratory quinolones (gatifloxacin, levofloxacin, moxifloxacin) may have lower MICs than ciprofloxacin, and

therefore, may be more active. Macrolides, quinolones, ketolides, and doxycycline are all mong the drugs recommended for empiric therapy for community-acquired pneumonia when suspecting "atypical" pathogens such as *Mycoplasma*. Macrolides remain the drugs of choice for treatment of *M. pneumoniae*, particularly in children. Most patients can be treated as outpatient, however, more complicated or severe disease may require hospitalization and supportive care, in addition to appropriate antibiotics.

Pediatric Drug Therapy

Recommended:

Erythromycin *on page 807*
Clarithromycin *on page 749*
Azithromycin *on page 674*

Adult Drug Therapy

Recommended:

Erythromycin *on page 807*
Clarithromycin *on page 749*
Azithromycin *on page 674*

Alternate:

Doxycycline *on page 787*
Fluoroquinolones *on page 824*
Telithromycin *on page 1093*

Selected Readings

Marrie TJ, "*Mycoplasma pneumoniae* Pneumonia Requiring Hospitalization, With Emphasis on Infection in the Elderly," *Arch Intern Med*, 1993, 153(4):488-94.

Marrie TJ, Poulin-Costello M, Beecroft MD, et al, "Etiology of Community-Acquired Pneumonia Treated in an Ambulatory Setting," *Respir Med*, 2005, 99(1):60-5.

Raty R, Ronkko E, and Kleemola M, "Sample Type Is Crucial to the Diagnosis of *Mycoplasma pneumoniae* Pneumonia by PCR," *J Med Microbiol*, 2005, 54(Pt 3):287-91.

Waites KB, Bébéar C, Robertson JA, et al, "Laboratory Diagnosis of Mycoplasmal and Ureaplasmal Infections," *Clin Microbiol Newslett*, 1996, 18(14):105-11.

Waites KB and Talkington DF, "*Mycoplasma pneumoniae* and Its Role as a Human Pathogen," *Clin Microbiol Rev*, 2004, 17(4):697-728,

Mycotic Vulvovaginitis *see Candida* Species *on page 67*

Myocarditis

Clinical Presentation May be acute or chronic. Most commonly is the result of an infectious process but may be secondary to rheumatologic diseases, toxins, radiation, and drugs. Almost all infectious agents are capable of causing myocarditis, the vast majority of acute myocarditis in the United States is secondary to a viral infection. Patients typically present with an antecedent upper respiratory tract infection 1-2 weeks prior to the development of dyspnea and chest pain with fever. Approximately 50% will have evidence of a pericardial effusion or cardiac dilatation on chest radiograph. Congestive heart failure occurs in 20%. EKG may show evidence of pericarditis, arrhythmias, or heart block. May develop dilated cardiomyopathy.

Differential Diagnosis The differential diagnosis for chest pain is quite exhaustive and for this text will be broken into four major systems: cardiovascular, pulmonary, gastrointestinal, and skeletal-muscular.

Likely Pathogens

Viruses:

Coxsackieviruses *on page 101*
Echovirus *on page 118*
Influenza Virus *on page 193*
Measles Virus *on page 215*
Rubella
Poliovirus *on page 275*
Adenovirus *on page 29*
HIV-associated Pathogens
Human Immunodeficiency Virus *on page 181*

Pyogenic: (usually a complication from endocarditis)

Staphylococcus aureus, Methicillin-Resistant *on page 304*
Staphylococcus aureus, Methicillin-Susceptible *on page 307*
Cryptococcus neoformans on page 102
Mycobacterium tuberculosis on page 234

Parasitic:

Trypanosoma cruzi on page 341
Toxoplasma gondii on page 331
Borrelia burgdorferi on page 56

Diagnostic Tests/Procedures Clinically diagnosed. Pathogens may be implicated by specific cultures or serological tests.

(Continued)

Myocarditis *(Continued)*

Drug Therapy Comment Recommended drug therapy is antimicrobial therapy directed against specific pathogen and supportive care. Most viral myocarditis is self-limiting.

Selected Readings

Anandasabapathy S and Frishman WH, "Innovative Drug Treatments for Viral and Autoimmune Myocarditis," *J Clin Pharmacol*, 1998, 38(4):295-308.

Brown CA and O'Connell JB, "Implications of the Myocarditis Treatment Trial for Clinical Practice," *Curr Opin Cardiol*, 1996, 11(3):332-6.

Caforio AL and McKenna WJ, "Recognition and Optimum Management of Myocarditis," *Drugs*, 1996, 52(4):515-25.

Pawsat DE and Lee JY, "Inflammatory Disorders of the Heart. Pericarditis, Myocarditis, and Endocarditis," *Emerg Med Clin North Am*, 1998, 16(3):665-81.

Myositis

Synonyms Gangrene, Gas; Gas Gangrene; Pyomyositis; Streptococcal Necrotizing Myositis

Clinical Presentation Muscle involvement in infection may occur with a variety of etiologic agents, ranging from myalgia to direct cytotoxic effects on muscle cells. Severe muscle pain is commonly associated with bacterial infections and trichinosis. Acute rhabdomyolysis may occur with *Clostridium* and *Streptococcus pyogenes*, and may be less commonly associated with *Legionella* or some viral infections (influenza, Echovirus, Coxsackie virus, Epstein-Barré). Primary myositis from *Streptococcus pyogenes* may result in necrotizing myositis associated with severe systemic symptomatology, and occurs, in approximately half of the cases, along with necrotizing fasciitis. Pyomyositis refers to a localized *Staphylococcus* infection of the muscle tissue where the point of bacterial entry is unknown. This occurs commonly in tropical regions and generally remains a localized infection, although toxic shock may develop. Gas gangrene usually occurs as a result of penetrating trauma and damage to vascular supply. The injury introduces soil flora along with *Clostridium* species.

Likely Pathogens

Staphylococcus aureus, Methicillin-Susceptible *on page 307*
Clostridium perfringens *on page 88*
Streptococcus pyogenes *on page 321*

Diagnostic Tests/Procedures

Blood Culture, Aerobic and Anaerobic *on page 391*
Gram Stain *on page 473*
Skin Biopsy *on page 580*

Drug Therapy Comment Surgical debridement is first line treatment. As with necrotizing fasciitis, deep surgical exploration and debridement of the muscle is required. Gram stain and culture of removed material is useful to establish causative microbiology.

Note: Listed empiric therapy does not include coverage for methicillin-resistant *Staphylococcus aureus*. In clinical settings where a high prevalence of resistant stains has been encountered, empiric therapy may require coverage for MRSA.

Empiric Drug Therapy

Recommended:

Penicillin G (Parenteral/Aqueous) *on page 993*
plus
Clindamycin *on page 752*

Naegleria fowleri

Microbiology *Naegleria fowleri* is a free-living ameba. It is related to *Acanthamoeba*, another protozoan which is pathogenic for humans. *Naegleria* exists in a trophozoite form (10-30 μm in diameter) and a flagellate form. The trophozoite form can encyst into a smaller spherical cyst (10 μm). The organism is aerobic, and the trophozoite form grows well in a variety of conditions including temperatures up to 45°C which allow it to proliferate in fresh water in temperate climates.

Epidemiology *N. fowleri* is a ubiquitous organism, being isolated in many geographic areas from a variety of environmental sources including fresh water, soil, artificially heated waters, man-made thermal waters, and air. The organism is highly associated with polluted lake or river water, as well as fresh water bodies in warm climates such as Florida. Millions of individuals have been exposed to water contaminated with this ameba, but disease develops only rarely. To date, only about 80 cases of *N. fowleri* infection have been reported in the United States. The immunologic factors that determine disease progression are not known. The major clinical manifestation of *N. fowleri* is primary amebic meningoencephalitis. This disease is seen in otherwise healthy adults and children and is highly associated with swimming in freshwater areas. In the United States, cases have been reported in the southern and central states.

Clinical Syndromes

- **Primary amebic meningoencephalitis:** This rapidly fatal disease usually occurs several days after exposure to freshwater ponds, rivers, or lakes. Patients develop headache, fever, and nuchal rigidity. Severe confusion is common. Death occurs within days. The ameba are likely inhaled through the nose during swimming and penetrate through the olfactory plate into the brain. The gray matter of the brain and the meninges develop extensive hemorrhage and necrosis. The trophozoite forms alone are seen in inflammatory tissue. Myocarditis is also present in many patients at autopsy.

Diagnosis Primary amebic meningoencephalitis should be considered in a young adult who presents with a fulminant encephalitis following fresh water exposure. The diagnosis may be difficult to establish. Head CT scans do not show mass lesions, but there may be contrast enhancement of gray matter and cisterns. Cerebrospinal fluid is usually inflammatory with a variable number of polymorphonuclear leukocytes present and numerous RBCs. Hypoglycorrhachia is usually present, and the CSF protein is elevated. A wet mount of CSF should be performed in addition to Gram stain if this disease is even remotely considered because the trophozoites can be disrupted during Gram stain. In one series of patients, the *Naegleria* trophozoites were visible on nearly all wet mounts of CSF performed.

Diagnostic Tests/Procedures

Cerebrospinal Fluid Analysis *on page 408*
Computed Transaxial Tomography, Head Studies *on page 424*
Cytology, Body Fluids *on page 438*
Gram Stain *on page 473*

Treatment Primary amebic encephalitis is rapidly fatal in 95% of cases, although several survivors have been well-described, having responded successfully to intravenous and intrathecal amphotericin B, but the optimal regimen is unknown. Immunoglobulin therapy is being investigated as adjunctive therapy due to the poor prognosis of this infection. A number of antimicrobials have been tested against this organism *in vitro* and in animal models with discouraging success, including amphotericin B, quinupristin and dalfopristin, azithromycin, and ketoconazole. It is unclear whether the addition of miconazole or rifampin to amphotericin B improves the outcome. Consultation with an Infectious Disease specialist is strongly recommended if primary amebic meningoencephalitis is even remotely considered.

Selected Readings

Centers for Disease Control and Prevention (CDC), "Primary Amebic Meningoencephalitis - Georgia, 2002," *MMWR*, 2003, 52(40):962-4.
Schuster FL and Visvesvara GS, "Free-Living Amoebae as Opportunistic and Non-opportunistic Pathogens of Humans and Animals," *Int J Parasitol*, 2004, 34(9):1001-27.
Schuster FL and Visvesvara GS, "Opportunistic Amoebae: Challenges in Prophylaxis and Treatment," *Drug Resist Updat*, 2004, 7(1):41-51.
Singh U and Petri WA, "Free-Living Amebas," *Principles and Practice of Infectious Diseases*, 5th ed, Mandell GL, Bennett JE, and Dolin R, eds, New York, NY: Churchill Livingstone, 2000, 2811-7.

Necator americanus *see Ancylostoma duodenale on page 34*

Necrotizing Fasciitis

Synonyms Fasciitis, Necrotizing; Gangrene

Clinical Presentation Early pain and fever followed by inflammation, edema, and tenderness. Infection progresses to deep red, indurated epidermis along with bullae filled with dark blue or purple fluid. The epidermis becomes friable and becomes discolored to a blue, black, or maroon color. Extensive thrombosis of the dermal papillae is associated with this stage. The infection extends along fascial planes, through the lymphatics, and through venous communications. Late dissemination may produce systemic inflammatory symptoms, shock, and multisystem organ failure. Infection frequently begins at a site of nonpenetrating minor trauma. The site may be seeded by transient bacteremia or a cutaneous infection. Myositis is frequently associated, and CPK may be markedly elevated. Infection may occur in otherwise healthy individuals; however, predisposing factors include immunodeficiency, diabetes, and peripheral vascular disease. Of note, in recent years, streptococcal disease has increased in frequency and severity.

Likely Pathogens

Streptococcus pyogenes on page 321
Clostridium perfringens on page 88
Group C *Streptococcus*
Group G *Streptococcus*

Diagnostic Tests/Procedures

Blood Culture, Aerobic and Anaerobic *on page 391*
Gram Stain *on page 473*
Skin Biopsy *on page 580*

Drug Therapy Comment Surgical debridement is first-line treatment. Deep surgical exploration of the fascia and muscle is required to remove necrotic tissue.

(Continued)

Necrotizing Fasciitis *(Continued)*

Empiric Drug Therapy

Recommended:

Penicillin G (Parenteral/Aqueous) *on page 993*

plus

Clindamycin *on page 752*

Alternate:

Ceftriaxone *on page 722*

plus

Clindamycin *on page 752*

Neisseria gonorrhoeae

Related Information

Treatment of Sexually Transmitted Infections *on page 1311*

Microbiology *Neisseria gonorrhoeae* is an oxidase- and catalase-positive, gram-negative diplococcus. *N. meningitidis* produces acid from only glucose which differentiates it from the other *Neisseria* species. Typing for different strains of *N. gonorrhoeae* can be performed but is useful only for epidemiologic studies. The organism readily grows on Thayer-Martin or chocolate media and grows best in the presence of CO_2. Growth is more fastidious than that of *N. meningitidis*.

Epidemiology Humans are the only natural reservoir for *N. gonorrhoeae*. The estimate that 1 million new cases of gonorrhea have occurred each year since the early 1960s is most likely a severe underestimate. Transmission is primarily by sexual contact, with the major reservoir in asymptomatically infected persons. The organism and disease is most commonly found in individuals 20-24 years of age. Fifty percent of women will become infected after a single exposure to an infected male while only 20% of men become infected after a single exposure to an infected female.

Clinical Syndromes In men, gonorrhea is usually limited to burning on urination and a purulent urethral discharge. Ten percent of men will be asymptomatic with 1% or less developing the complications of prostatitis, urethral stricture, or epididymitis. Approximately 50% of women are asymptomatic; when symptoms occur they include dysuria, frequency, vaginal discharge, fever, and abdominal pain. Up to 15% of women with gonorrhea develop pelvic inflammatory disease (PID), with fallopian scarring or subsequent chronic PID, sterility, or ectopic pregnancies. Rectal and pharyngeal colonization and disease may also occur in women and homosexual men.

Disseminated disease may include sepsis, peritonitis, or meningitis, but most commonly causes septic arthritis in patients otherwise asymptomatic. Disseminated disease may be accompanied by petechial or papular lesions. In children, the most common form of gonococcal disease is gonorrhea ophthalmia from contamination through an infected birth canal. This is easily prevented with 1% silver nitrate aqueous drops.

Diagnosis In men with urethral symptoms, Gram stain of the purulent material is highly sensitive and specific. Gram stain is less diagnostic in asymptomatic men and clinically useless in diagnosing cervicitis in women because intracellular gram-negative diplococci could be any of the many *Neisseria* (non-*gonorrhoeae*) species which are normal vaginal flora. A positive Gram stain is usually characterized by the presence of gram-negative cocci within or closely associated with polymorphonuclear leukocytes. The Gram stain of joint fluid can detect organisms in early septic arthritis but is not particularly sensitive for skin lesions or rectal or pharyngeal disease. Specimens from appropriate sites may be inoculated on Thayer-Martin medium when contaminating organisms are present and on chocolate agar if the specimen is from a normally sterile body site. When asymptomatic or cervical disease is expected, the rectum may yield the only positive specimen. Growth is enhanced by CO_2 inoculated media. Blood cultures are positive in early disseminated disease. Infected joint fluid cultures are also usually positive.

Best culture results occur when specimens are inoculated on-site to **room temperature** Thayer-Martin medium, immediately into a CO_2-generating transport device, and transported to the laboratory **ASAP** at **room temperature**.

Diagnostic Tests/Procedures

Gram Stain *on page 473*

Neisseria gonorrhoeae Culture *on page 547*

Neisseria gonorrhoeae by Nucleic Acid Probe *on page 546*

Treatment Patients infected with *Neisseria gonorrhoeae* are often coinfected with *C. trachomatis* and should be treated for both.

Uncomplicated gonococcal infections of the cervix, urethra, and rectum: The drugs of choice for these infections include single doses of cefixime 400 mg orally, ceftriaxone 125 mg I.M., ciprofloxacin 500 mg, ofloxacin 400 mg, or levofloxacin. Alternative regimens include single doses of spectinomycin I.M., other

cephalosporins such as ceftizoxime, cefotaxime, cefotetan, or cefoxitin (probenecid 1 g orally should be added to cefoxitin therapy), gatifloxacin, lomefloxacin, or norfloxacin.

Uncomplicated gonococcal infection of the pharynx: The drugs of choice include single doses of ceftriaxone 125 mg I.M., ciprofloxacin 500 mg orally, or ofloxacin 400 mg orally.

If symptoms persist, other organisms should be considered. Also consider reinfection rather than treatment failure, however, culture and sensitivity should be performed. Patients should refer sex partners for evaluation and treatment.

Patients who are intolerant/allergic to cephalosporins, penicillins, and quinolones should be treated with spectinomycin. Pregnant women with cephalosporin intolerance/allergy should be treated with spectinomycin. Careful follow-up is necessary to assure clinical cure.

Disseminated gonococcal infection: The treatment of choice is ceftriaxone 1 g I.M. or I.V. every 24 hours. Alternative regimens include full courses of cefotaxime, ceftizoxime, ciprofloxacin, ofloxacin, levofloxacin, or spectinomycin. Patients can then be switched to oral therapy (cefixime, ciprofloxacin, ofloxacin, or levofloxacin) when improvement begins. Patients should be treated for a full week.

Gonococcal conjunctivitis in adults: Ceftriaxone 1 g I.M. one time

Gonococcal meningitis or endocarditis: Ceftriaxone 1-2 g every 12 hours. Meningitis should be treated for 10-14 days; endocarditis for 4 weeks.

Gonococcal Infections in Infants:

Ophthalmia neonatorum prophylaxis: Instillation of a prophylactic agent into the eyes of all newborns is recommended to prevent gonococcal ophthalmia neonatorum. (Required by law in most states.) Recommended regimens include single application of silver nitrate 1% aqueous, erythromycin 0.5% ophthalmic ointment, or tetracycline 1% ophthalmic ointment.

Ophthalmia neonatorum treatment: Ceftriaxone 25-50 mg/kg I.V. or I.M. in a single dose, not to exceed 125 mg. Topical therapy is inadequate and unnecessary.

Disseminated gonococcal infection and gonococcal scalp abscess in newborns: Conjunctival exudate should be cultured. The drugs of choice include ceftriaxone 25-50 mg/kg/day or cefotaxime 25 mg/kg every 12 hours for 7 days (14 days if meningitis is present).

In children, similar recommendations apply regarding the drugs of choice; doses may vary. Avoid quinolones and tetracyclines.

Pediatric Drug Therapy

Recommended:

Ceftriaxone *on page 722*

Adult Drug Therapy

Recommended:

Cefixime *on page 707*
Ceftriaxone *on page 722*
Ciprofloxacin *on page 742*
Ofloxacin *on page 977*
Levofloxacin *on page 908*

Alternate:

Monotherapy:
Ceftizoxime *on page 720*
Cefotaxime *on page 708*
Norfloxacin *on page 973*
Spectinomycin *on page 1075*

Selected Readings

Centers for Disease Control and Prevention (CDC), "Sexually Transmitted Diseases Treatment Guidelines, 2002," *MMWR*, 2002, 41(RR-6):1-78.

Knapp JS, "Antimicrobial Resistance in *Neisseria gonorhoeae* in the United States," *Clin Microbiol Newslett*, 1999, 21(1):1-7.

Moran J, "Gonorrhoea," *Clin Evid*, 2004, (11):2104-12.

Sparling PF and Hansfield HH, "*Neisseria gonorrhoeae*," *Principles and Practice of Infectious Diseases*, 5th ed, Mandell GL, Bennett JE, and Dolin R, eds, New York, NY: Churchill Livingstone, 2000, 2242-58.

Neisseria meningitidis

Related Information

Prophylaxis for Patients Exposed to Common Communicable Diseases *on page 1309*

Microbiology *Neisseria meningitidis* is an oxidase- and catalase-positive, gram-negative diplococcus. *N. meningitidis* produces acid from glucose and maltose (Continued)

Neisseria meningitidis (Continued)

but not from sucrose or lactose, which differentiates it from the other *Neisseria* species. At least nine different serogroups of *N. meningitidis* have been identified on the basis of their polysaccharide capsules. More than 20 serotypes have been identified. Serogroups A, B, C, Y, and W135 are most commonly associated with clinical diseases.

The organism grows on Thayer-Martin or chocolate media and grows best in the presence of CO_2.

Epidemiology *N. meningitidis* is exclusively a human pathogen and causes 3000-4000 cases of meningitis yearly in the United States. *N. meningitidis* is transmitted by droplets among persons with prolonged close contact and who are in direct contact with respiratory secretions. Carriage occurs in 10% to 30% of healthy adults, but disease is rare. Most disease occurs in children 6 months to 5 years of age. Outbreaks occur in other close contact populations such as the military.

Serogroups B and C account for over 75% of cases, and groups W135, Y, and A account for the rest. The last urban epidemic occurred in Brazil in 1971 (serogroups C and A), and the last United States epidemic occurred in 1946 (serogroup A).

Clinical Syndromes *N. meningitidis* causes a wide spectrum of clinical illness which ranges from a mild nonspecific febrile illness to meningitis and sepsis.

- **Meningitis:** Usually abrupt onset with fever, headache, and meningismus, although the syndrome may be less specific in young children. Mortality is 100% if untreated; 15% if treated appropriately. In meningococcemia, signs and symptoms of sepsis may be seen accompanied by characteristic meningococcal emboli (vasculitic purpura). This syndrome is occasionally preceded by petechial skin lesions. Disseminated intravascular coagulopathy and shock may follow, along with adrenal gland destruction (Waterhouse-Friderichsen syndrome).
- Can also be responsible for urethritis, pneumonias, and arthritis.

Diagnosis Diagnosis is made by Gram stain and culture of cerebrospinal fluid, blood, etc. Occasionally, the organism can be observed on Gram stain of the petechial lesions or detected in buffy coat smears. *N. meningitidis* will grow on blood or chocolate agar (best growth with increased CO_2 concentration) or in Thayer-Martin media when multiple organisms are suspected.

Rapid identification can be performed by several laboratory tests, but definitive identification must be made biochemically.

Diagnostic Tests/Procedures

Aerobic Culture, Cerebrospinal Fluid *on page 366*
Bacterial Antigens, Rapid Detection Methods *on page 388*
Gram Stain *on page 473*
Skin Biopsy *on page 580*

Treatment The treatment of choice for *N. meningitidis* meningitis that are highly penicillin susceptible (MIC <0.1 mcg/mL) is high-dose penicillin G or ampicillin with ceftriaxone, cefotaxime, or chloramphenicol as an alternative. For less susceptible organisms, ceftriaxone or cefotaxime are the drugs of choice with chloramphenicol, meropenem, or a fluoroquinolone as alternative agents.

Chemoprophylaxis is indicated for close contacts of patients with meningococcal meningitis who include household members, daycare center contacts, and anyone directly exposed to the patient's oral secretions. Recommended prophylaxis includes one of the following: A 2-day course of rifampin (600 mg every 12 hours for adults, 10 mg/kg every 12 hours for children ≥1 month of age, 5 mg/kg every 12 hours for children <1 month of age), a single dose of ciprofloxacin 500 mg, or a single dose of I.M. ceftriaxone (250 mg in adults, 125 mg in children <15 years of age).

Vaccination with the tetravalent meningococcal polysaccharide protein conjugate vaccine (MCV4; Menactra™) is recommended for all children age 11-12 years or at high school entry (~15 years of age). MCV4 is also recommended for patients between the age of 11-55 years with the following risk factors: College freshmen living in dormatories, travelers to endemic areas, microbiologists, certain outbreak settings, and patients with increased susceptibility (eg, who have terminal complement component deficiencies or asplenia). Vaccination with the tetravalent meningococcal polysaccharide vaccine (MPSV4; Menomune®-A/C/Y/W-135) is recommended for patients between the ages of 2-10 years and >55 years with the risk factors listed above.

Drug Therapy

Recommended:

Cefotaxime *on page 708*
Ceftriaxone *on page 722*
Penicillin G (Parenteral/Aqueous) *on page 993*

Prophylaxis:

Meningococcal Polysaccharide Vaccine (Groups A / C / Y and W-135) *on page 935*

Meningococcal Polysaccharide (Groups A / C / Y and W-135) Diphtheria Toxoid Conjugate Vaccine *on page 933*

Alternate:

Chloramphenicol *on page 733*

Fluoroquinolones *on page 824*

Meropenem *on page 936*

Selected Readings

Apicella MA, "*Neisseria meningitidis*," *Principles and Practices of Infectious Diseases*, 5th ed, Mandell GL, Bennett JE, and Dolin R, eds, New York, NY: Churchill Livingstone, 2000, 2228-41.

Baron EJ and Finegold SM, eds, "Aerobic Gram-Negative Cocci (*Neisseria* and *Branhamella*)," *Bailey & Scott's Diagnostic Microbiology*, St Louis, MO: CV Mosby Co, 1990, 353-62.

Bilukha OO and Rosenstein N, "Prevention and Control of Meningococcal Disease. Recommendations of the Advisory Committee on Immunization Practices (ACIP)," *MMWR*, 2005, 54(RR-7):1-21.

Campos-Outcalt D, "Meningococcal Vaccine: New Product, New Recommendations," *J Fam Pract*, 2005, 54(4):324-6.

Danzig L, "Meningococcal Vaccines," *Pediatr Infect Dis J*, 2004, 23(12 Suppl):S285-92.

Fraser A, Gafter-Gvili A, Paul M, et al, "Antibiotics for Preventing Meningococcal Infection," *Cochrane Database Syst Rev*, 2005, (1):CD004785.

Kalil AC, "The Use of Dexamethasone in Bacterial Meningitis," *Clin Infect Dis*, 2005, 40(7):1061-2.

Mitka M, "New Vaccine Should Ease Meningitis Fears," *JAMA*, 2005, 293(12):1433-4.

Ostergaard C, "Prognostic Factors in Adults With Bacterial Meningitis," *N Engl J Med*, 2005, 352(5):512-5.

Quagliarello V and Scheld WM, "Bacterial Meningitis: Pathogenesis, Pathophysiology, and Progress," *N Engl J Med*, 1992, 327(12):864-72.

Tunkel AR, Hartman BJ, Kaplan SL, et al, "Practice Guidelines for the Management of Bacterial Meningitis," *Clin Infect Dis*, 2004, 39(9):1267-84.

Neonatal Meningitis *see* Meningitis, Neonatal (<1 month of age) *on page 217*

Neutropenic Fever *see* Fever, Neutropenic *on page 148*

NGU *see* Urethritis, Nongonococcal *on page 344*

Nocardia Species

Microbiology *Nocardia* species are variably acid-fast, "higher order," aerobic bacteria. They belong to the family Nocardiaceae. There are several species of *Nocardia* which are pathogenic for humans, the most common being *Nocardia asteroides* followed by *N. brasiliensis*. Other species occasionally cause human disease such as *N. otitidiscaviarum* (formerly *N. caviae*) and the newly recognized *N. transvalensis*.

Nocardia species have a delicate, branching appearance and may appear fragmented in clinical specimens. The organisms are weakly gram-positive and have a characteristic "beaded" appearance; if present, these characteristics allow rapid preliminary identification. The organisms may be more easily visualized on an acid-fast stain rather than Gram stain. Most (but not all) strains of *Nocardia* are acid-fast and retain carbol fuchsin when decolorized with a weaker alcohol than the acid alcohol commonly used for staining mycobacterial species. It is important to realize that the acid-fast staining properties of *Nocardia* species differ from those of other acid-fast organisms such as *Mycobacterium tuberculosis*. Laboratories use a **modified** acid-fast stain (eg, a modified Ziehl-Neelsen stain and others) to optimally detect *Nocardia* in direct specimens. In most institutions, the clinician must specifically request a modified acid-fast stain for *Nocardia* if this organism is suspected. In some institutions, a *Nocardia* stain may be part of a routine protocol for processing certain clinical specimens, such as bronchoalveolar lavage fluid from immunocompromised patients.

Nocardia species grow on a variety of standard media employed in microbiology laboratories, including blood agar and Sabouraud's dextrose agar. Growth also occurs on media used for isolation of mycobacteria such as the Lowenstein-Jensen medium. Usually 4-10 days are required before growth of the organism is apparent. When *Nocardia* species are present along with other aerobic bacteria, isolation of *Nocardia* may be delayed for several weeks. *Nocardia* species are most frequently isolated from respiratory specimens; only rarely can they be isolated from standard blood cultures.

Epidemiology *Nocardia* species are distributed worldwide, and there appears to be no geographic clustering of cases. The organisms are ubiquitous in soil and areas of plant decay. Approximately 500-1000 cases are reported in the United States annually. The most common age range is 20-50 years, with several series demonstrating a male predominance. Nocardial infections occur mainly in individuals with defective T-cell immunity (cell-mediated immunity), such as organ transplant recipients, patients with malignancies (lymphoma), those receiving corticosteroids or cytotoxic agents, and persons with AIDS. A 13% incidence was once described in one cardiac transplant center, but other institutions have consistently reported much lower rates. Persons with neutrophil dysfunction also appear at increased risk, and nocardiosis has been well-described in children with chronic granulomatous disease. A large

(Continued)

Nocardia Species *(Continued)*

number of other diseases have been associated with nocardiosis including tuberculosis, alcoholism with cirrhosis, inflammatory bowel disease, various forms of vasculitis, pulmonary alveolar proteinosis, sarcoidosis, bronchiectasis, and immunoglobulin deficiencies. Nontuberculous mycobacteria has also been reported as a predisposing condition for nocardial infection. Clinically, significant nocardiosis also may occur in otherwise healthy persons, although the incidence of this has been highly variable.

Although occasional clusters of *Nocardia* infection have been described, most experts feel that the organism is not transmitted person-to-person.

Outside the United States, *Nocardia* species are commonly associated with mycetoma (see Clinical Syndromes). Individuals with frequent contact with soil and other plant matter are at risk for this form of nocardiosis.

Clinical Syndromes Disease usually results from inhalation of the organism leading to colonization in the lung. The organisms may resist local pulmonary defenses including macrophages and immunoglobulins. Infections with *Nocardia* species classically result in abscess formation, with numerous polymorphonuclear leukocytes and only a thin abscess wall.

- **Colonization in healthy persons:** Occasionally, immunocompetent persons with no significant lung disease may have positive sputum cultures for *Nocardia.* Clinical evaluation is important in deciding on the role of antibiotics.
- **Respiratory colonization in individuals with chronic obstructive pulmonary disease (COPD):** Several series have reported positive sputum cultures from asymptomatic COPD patients; in most cases, there is no active pneumonia and repeat sputum cultures were negative. Repeated isolation of *Nocardia* in these individuals is more worrisome for active disease, and consultation with an Infectious Disease specialist should be considered.
- **Pneumonia:** Immunosuppressed individuals may develop an isolated pneumonia most commonly from *N. asteroides.* The presentation may be subacute or acute. Symptoms are similar to other bacterial pneumonias with fever, purulent sputum, cough, and dyspnea. Some may have pleuritic chest pain mimicking pneumococcal pneumonia. Since *Nocardia* tends to cause suppurative disease, lung cavitation and empyema are common. Chest x-rays may show a nodular infiltrate, cavities, or a lobar pattern. Direct extension of purulent nocardial infections may occur into the pericardium and other mediastinal structures. Disease outside the lungs may be present in up to 50% of cases.
- **Brain abscess:** *Nocardia* commonly disseminates to the brain in immunosuppressed persons. Multiple brain lesions can occur, and the presentation may be subacute. Nocardial infection should be considered in a patient presenting with pneumonia and brain abscess. Meningitis from *Nocardia* is uncommon.
- **Disseminated nocardial infection:** Approximately 20% of patients with nocardiosis have no apparent lung involvement and instead present with extrapulmonary nocardiosis. The most common presentation is brain abscess. A number of other sites may be involved such as bone, skin, abdomen, and others.
- **Mycetoma:** This is usually seen in persons from tropical or subtropical regions. The pathogenesis of mycetoma is from direct inoculation of the organism into the skin rather than inhalation. The feet and/or hands are the most frequent sites. Chronic nocardial infection may develop with disfiguring skin and soft tissue changes and multiple sinus tracts.
- **Cellulitis and lymphocutaneous nodules:** These forms of direct inoculation are more common in the United States than mycetoma. The cellulitis caused by *Nocardia* species may be difficult to distinguish from other forms of bacterial cellulitis. *Nocardia brasiliensis* may cause subcutaneous nodules that spread on an arm or leg following lymphatic drainage. This may mimic infections caused by *Sporothrix schenckii.*
- **Keratitis:** Occasionally, *Nocardia asteroides* is directly inoculated into the eye following trauma.

Diagnosis *Nocardia* infection should be in the differential diagnosis of any immunocompromised patient presenting with an unexplained pneumonia. The clinical suspicion should be high if there is evidence of extrapulmonary involvement as well, particularly the presence of a central nervous system lesion. Respiratory specimens should be submitted for nocardial stain and culture. The organism may be recovered from induced sputum, but bronchoscopy may be necessary in many cases. It is difficult to isolate *Nocardia* species from blood cultures or cerebrospinal fluid but is readily identified from brain abscesses (if the patient has not received prior antibiotics). Serologic studies for *Nocardia* are not clinically helpful at present.

Diagnostic Tests/Procedures

Acid-Fast Stain, Modified, *Nocardia* Species *on page 362*
Nocardia Culture, All Sites *on page 550*

Treatment The optimal regimen for treating *Nocardia* is still controversial and under study. Sulfonamides have been the cornerstone of therapy and appear to be effective in many cases as monotherapy, even in immunocompromised persons. Sulfisoxazole at high doses (≥6 g/day) has been effective in several studies, as has sulfadiazine. Blood levels may be obtained in serious cases. Sulfamethoxazole and trimethoprim has also been used with success (given at doses up to 20 mg/kg/day of the trimethoprim component). Some experts have been concerned that the commercially available preparations of sulfamethoxazole and trimethoprim, such as Bactrim™, may not have enough trimethoprim synergistic activity against *Nocardia*. Other problems with sulfamethoxazole and trimethoprim include a somewhat higher incidence of drug toxicity than sulfonamides alone, occasional treatment failures, and relapses. However, sulfamethoxazole and trimethoprim is considered by some to be the treatment of choice.

Minocycline is effective *in vitro* and *in vivo* and can be used if patients develop hypersensitivity to one of the sulfonamides. Other tetracyclines may be less active. A number of other agents have been reported effective in clinical situations including amikacin and imipenem. Many clinicians use combination therapy in life-threatening or refractory cases, although clinical data is very limited. It is still unclear whether combination therapy (eg, sulfisoxazole and amikacin) is superior to a sulfonamide used as monotherapy.

Since *Nocardia* species tend to form abscesses, surgical drainage may be extremely important, particularly with empyema and brain abscess.

Drug Therapy

Recommended:

Sulfamethoxazole and Trimethoprim *on page 1087*
SulfiSOXAZOLE *on page 1091*
SulfaDIAZINE *on page 1083*

Alternate:

Minocycline *on page 947*

Selected Readings

Lerner PI, "*Nocardia* Species," *Principles and Practice of Infectious Diseases*, 4th ed, Mandell GL, Bennett JE, and Dolin R, eds, New York, NY: Churchill Livingstone, 1995, 2273-80.

Nocardiosis *see Nocardia* Species *on page 247*
Nongonococcal Urethritis *see* Urethritis, Nongonococcal *on page 344*
Nonspecific Vaginosis *see* Vaginosis, Bacterial *on page 347*

Osteomyelitis, Diabetic Foot

Synonyms Diabetic Foot Osteomyelitis

Clinical Presentation Usually involves small bones of the feet and toes. Patients present with pain, swelling, and/or erythema of the involved bones with or without presence of ulcer. Most common x-ray finding is mottled lytic lesions. Podiatry or surgical consult recommended.

Differential Diagnosis Charcot foot; fracture; cellulitis

Likely Pathogens

Staphylococcus aureus, Methicillin-Susceptible *on page 307*
Streptococcus-Related Gram-Positive Cocci *on page 325*
Gram-Negative Bacilli *on page 157*

Diagnostic Tests/Procedures

•Bone Films *on page 396*
•Bone Scan *on page 401*
•C-Reactive Protein *on page 428*
•Gram Stain *on page 473*
•Sedimentation Rate, Erythrocyte *on page 576*
•Biopsy Culture, Routine *on page 390*
Anaerobic Culture *on page 371*
Bone Biopsy *on page 396*
Gallium Scan *on page 469*
Indium Leukocyte Scan *on page 508*

Drug Therapy Comment If possible, a bone biopsy with culture should be obtained for definitive diagnosis and pathogen-specific antibiotic therapy should be given for a minimum of 6 weeks. Duration of therapy may be extended pending clinical examination and improvement of the WBC and ESR.

For mild infection, oral is the advised route for drug therapy. Oral or parenteral, based on organism and clinical situation, is the advised route of drug therapy for moderate infections. The advised route for severe infection is intravenous (at least initially).
(Continued)

Osteomyelitis, Diabetic Foot *(Continued)*

Empiric Drug Therapy

Recommended:

Mild:

Dicloxacillin *on page 773*
Clindamycin *on page 752*
Cephalexin *on page 727*
Sulfamethoxazole and Trimethoprim *on page 1087*
Amoxicillin and Clavulanate Potassium *on page 645*
Levofloxacin *on page 908*

Moderate:

Sulfamethoxazole and Trimethoprim *on page 1087*
Amoxicillin and Clavulanate Potassium *on page 645*
Levofloxacin *on page 908*
Cefoxitin *on page 712*
Ceftriaxone *on page 722*
Ampicillin and Sulbactam *on page 660*
Linezolid *on page 914*
with or without
Aztreonam *on page 677*
Daptomycin *on page 768*
with or without
Aztreonam *on page 677*
Ertapenem *on page 805*
Cefuroxime *on page 725*
with or without
Metronidazole *on page 940*
Ticarcillin and Clavulanate Potassium *on page 1114*
Piperacillin and Tazobactam Sodium *on page 1003*
One for the following
Levofloxacin *on page 908*
Ciprofloxacin *on page 742*
with
Clindamycin *on page 752*

Severe:

Piperacillin and Tazobactam Sodium *on page 1003*
One for the following
Levofloxacin *on page 908*
Ciprofloxacin *on page 742*
with
Clindamycin *on page 752*
Imipenem and Cilastatin *on page 861*
The following two in combination
Vancomycin *on page 1144*
Ceftazidime *on page 717*
with or without
Metronidazole *on page 940*

Selected Readings

Bamberger DM, Daus GP, and Gerding DN, "Osteomyelitis in the Feet of Diabetic Patients: Long-Term Results, Prognostic Factors, and the Role of Antimicrobial and Surgical Therapy," *Am J Med*, 1987, 83(4):653-60.

Brem H, Balledux J, Bloom T, et al, "Healing of Diabetic Foot Ulcers and Pressure Ulcers With Human Skin Equivalent: A New Paradigm in Wound Healing," *Arch Surg*, 2000, 135(6):627-34.

Kaleta JL, Fleischli JW, and Reilly CH, "The Diagnosis of Osteomyelitis in Diabetes Using Erythrocyte Sedimentation Rate: A Pilot Study," *J Am Podiatry Med Assoc*, 2001, 91(9):445-50.

Lipsky BA, Berendt AR, Deery HG, et al, "Diagnosis and Treatment of Diabetic Foot Infections," *Clin Infect Dis*, 2004, 39:885-910.

Lipsky BA, "Osteomyelitis of the Foot in Diabetic Patients," *Clin Infect Dis*, 1997, 25(6):1318-26.

Tomas MB, Patel M, Marwin SE, et al, "The Diabetic Foot," *Br J Radiol*, 2000, 73(868):443-50.

Osteomyelitis, Healthy Adult

Synonyms Adult Osteomyelitis

Clinical Presentation Usually occurs in the face of trauma with surrounding cellulitis; may be hematogenously spread in the face of bacteremia with or without endocarditis (often vertebral) osteomyelitis. Presents with point tenderness, fever, mild leukocytosis, and increased C-reactive protein and erythrocyte sedimentation rate. May be acute or chronic. Podiatry or orthopedic consult should be considered.

Differential Diagnosis Septic arthritis; skin/soft tissue infections; bursitis; tendonitis; fracture; malignancy; diskitis; epidural abscess

Likely Pathogens

Staphylococcus aureus, Methicillin-Susceptible *on page 307*

Diagnostic Tests/Procedures

- •Biopsy Culture, Routine *on page 390*
- •Bone Films *on page 396*
- •Bone Scan *on page 401*
- •C-Reactive Protein *on page 428*
- •Gram Stain *on page 473*
- •Sedimentation Rate, Erythrocyte *on page 576*
- Anaerobic Culture *on page 371*
- Bone Biopsy *on page 396*
- Gallium Scan *on page 469*
- Indium Leukocyte Scan *on page 508*
- Teichoic Acid Antibody *on page 590*

Drug Therapy Comment Linezolid or daptomycin may be reserved for patients who may be intolerant to vancomycin and/or specific organisms (VISA/GISA, VRSA, VRE).

Empiric Drug Therapy

Recommended:

Penicillins, Penicillinase-Resistant *on page 997*

Alternate:

Fluoroquinolones *on page 824* (except ciprofloxacin)
Vancomycin *on page 1144*
Cephalosporins, 1st Generation *on page 729*
Clindamycin *on page 752*

Selected Readings

Hass DW and McAndrew MP, "Bacterial Osteomyelitis in Adults: Evolving Considerations in Diagnosis and Treatment," *Am J Med*, 1996, 101(5):550-61.

Laughlin RT, Wright DG, Mader JT, et al, "Osteomyelitis," *Curr Opin Rheumatol*, 1995, 7(4):315-21.

McHenry MC, Easley KA, and Locker GA, "Vertebral Osteomyelitis: Long-Term Outcome for 253 Patients From 7 Cleveland-Area Hospitals," *Clin Infect Dis*, 2002, 34(10):1342-50.

Melzer M, Goldsmith D, and Gransden W, "Successful Treatment of Vertebral Osteomyelitis With Linezolid in a Patient Receiving Hemodialysis and With Persistent Methicillin-Resistant *Staphylococcus aureus* and Vancomycin-Resistant *Enterococcus* Bacteremias," *Clin Infect Dis*, 2000 31(1):208-9.

Rissing JP, "Antimicrobial Therapy for Chronic Osteomyelitis in Adults: Role of the Quinolones," *Clin Infect Dis*, 1997, 25(6):1327-33.

Tetsworth K and Cierny G 3rd, "Osteomyelitis Debridement Techniques," *Clin Orthop*, 1999, (360):87-96.

Osteomyelitis, Pediatric

Synonyms Pediatric Osteomyelitis

Clinical Presentation The child will not be using that extremity, may be limping, etc. Pain, fever, leukocytosis, and increased C-reactive protein and erythrocyte sedimentation rate. Is often hematogenously spread but can also be traumatic. May be acute or chronic.

Differential Diagnosis Septic arthritis; skin/soft tissue infections; bursitis; tendonitis; fracture; malignancy; diskitis; epidural abscess

Likely Pathogens

Staphylococcus aureus, Methicillin-Susceptible *on page 307*
Streptococcus pyogenes on page 321
<2 years old:
Haemophilus influenzae on page 159
HACEK Group *on page 158 (Kingella* in particular)

Diagnostic Tests/Procedures

- •Bone Films *on page 396*
- •Bone Scan *on page 401*
- •C-Reactive Protein *on page 428*
- •Gram Stain *on page 473*
- •Sedimentation Rate, Erythrocyte *on page 576*
- Biopsy Culture, Routine *on page 390*
- Bone Biopsy *on page 396*
- Gallium Scan *on page 469*
- Indium Leukocyte Scan *on page 508*
- Teichoic Acid Antibody *on page 590*

Empiric Drug Therapy

Recommended:

Penicillins, Penicillinase-Resistant *on page 997*

Alternate:

Vancomycin *on page 1144*
Cephalosporins, 1st Generation *on page 729*
Clindamycin *on page 752*

(Continued)

Osteomyelitis, Pediatric *(Continued)*

Selected Readings

Birgisson H, Steingrimsson O, and Gudnason T, "*Kingella kingae* Infections in Paediatric Patients: 5 Cases of Septic Arthritis, Osteomyelitis and Bacteremia," *Scand J Infect Dis*, 1997, 29(5):495-8.

Wall EJ, "Childhood Osteomyelitis and Septic Arthritis," *Curr Opin Pediatr*, 1998, 10(1):73-6.

Otitis Externa, Mild

Synonyms Swimmer's Ear

Clinical Presentation Acute localized otitis externa may present as a pustule, furuncle, or cellulitis within the external auditory canal. Hemorrhagic bullae may be present, as well as localized adenopathy. Gram-positive cocci are usually responsible.

Acute diffuse otitis externa (swimmer's ear) initially presents with itching and becomes painful as the canal swells and reddens. Gram-negative bacilli, particularly *Pseudomonas aeruginosa*, are the most likely pathogens.

Chronic otitis externa is characterized by intense itching secondary to the chronic irritation of drainage from chronic otitis media or granulomatous infections.

Malignant otitis externa is a severe necrotizing infection that spreads to adjacent tissue and bone. Associated with intense pain, tenderness, and pus in the canal.

Likely Pathogens

Pseudomonas aeruginosa on page 282

Diagnostic Tests/Procedures

Aerobic Culture, Appropriate Site *on page 365*

Gram Stain *on page 473*

Empiric Drug Therapy

Recommended:

Neomycin *on page 962*

Polymyxin B *on page 1012*

Ciprofloxacin *on page 742*

Otitis Externa, Severe (Malignant)

Clinical Presentation Acute localized otitis externa may present as a pustule, furuncle, or cellulitis within the external auditory canal. Hemorrhagic bullae may be present, as well as localized adenopathy. Gram-positive cocci are usually responsible.

Acute diffuse otitis externa (swimmer's ear) initially presents with itching and becomes painful as the canal swells and reddens. Gram-negative bacilli, particularly *Pseudomonas aeruginosa*, are the most likely pathogens.

Chronic otitis externa is characterized by intense itching secondary to the chronic irritation of drainage from chronic otitis media or granulomatous infections.

Malignant otitis externa is a severe necrotizing infection that spreads to adjacent tissue and bone. Associated with intense pain, tenderness, and pus in the canal.

Likely Pathogens

Pseudomonas aeruginosa on page 282

Diagnostic Tests/Procedures

Aerobic Culture, Appropriate Site *on page 365*

Computed Transaxial Tomography, Paranasal Sinuses *on page 425*

Gram Stain *on page 473*

Drug Therapy Comment Topical otic suspensions or solutions may also be indicated. Ciprofloxacin may be used as I.V. or oral therapy.

Empiric Drug Therapy

Recommended:

One of the following

- Ciprofloxacin *on page 742*
- Ceftazidime *on page 717*
- Penicillins, Extended-Spectrum *on page 997*
  - *with or without*
    - Aminoglycosides *on page 641*

Alternate:

Ciprofloxacin *on page 742*

Otitis Media, Acute

Synonyms Acute Suppurative Otitis; Middle Ear Infection

Clinical Presentation Most commonly occurs in children. Present with otalgia and fever with or without purulent discharge. Infants may present with irritability. Diagnosis is confirmed by examination of the tympanic membrane which is full or bulging, opaque, and has little or no mobility.

Likely Pathogens

Streptococcus pneumoniae, Drug-Susceptible *on page 319*
Haemophilus influenzae on page 159
Moraxella catarrhalis on page 223
Staphylococcus aureus, Methicillin-Susceptible *on page 307*

Diagnostic Tests/Procedures

Aerobic Culture, Body Fluid *on page 365*
Gram Stain *on page 473*

Drug Therapy Comment In areas where incidence of beta-lactamase-producing organisms is high, consider amoxicillin-clavulanate.

Once daily prophylaxis with amoxicillin or sulfisoxazole should be considered in children who have had either 2 episodes in the first year of life or in older children with >4 episodes/year. Referral should be made to an otolaryngologist for evaluation of possible myringotomy, adenoidectomy, and placement of tympanostomy tubes if indicated in children with recurrent disease.

Empiric Drug Therapy

Recommended:

Amoxicillin *on page 642*
Sulfamethoxazole and Trimethoprim *on page 1087*
Cephalosporins, 2nd Generation *on page 729*

Alternate:

Erythromycin and Sulfisoxazole *on page 811*
Amoxicillin and Clavulanate Potassium *on page 645*

Selected Readings

American Academy of Pediatrics Subcommittee on Management of Acute Otitis Media, "Diagnosis and Management of Acute Otitis Media," *Pediatrics*, 2004, 113(5):1451-65.
Bluestone CD, "Epidemiology and Pathogenesis of Chronic Suppurative Otitis Media: Implications for Prevention and Treatment," *Int J Pediatr Otorhinolaryngol*, 1998, 42(3):207-23.
Conrad DA, "Should Acute Otitis Media Ever Be Treated With Antibiotics?" *Pediatr Ann*, 1998, 27(2):66-7, 70-4.
Heikkinen T and Ruuskanen O, "Otitis Media," *Curr Opin Pediatr*, 1998, 10(1):9-12.

Pancreatitis/Pancreatic Abscess

Synonyms Abscess, Pancreatic

Clinical Presentation Abscess develops in <10% of patients with acute pancreatitis. Patients present with abdominal pain, which typically radiates to the back, accompanied by nausea and vomiting. Fever usually present. May have generalized peritonitis. Prognosis linked to Ranson's criteria (age, leukocytosis, hyperglycemia, elevated LDH and AST). The role of antibiotic prophylaxis in acute pancreatitis is controversial but appears indicated in severe cases. For patients with abscess, percutaneous drainage may not be effective. Surgery and GI consults are recommended.

Differential Diagnosis Extensive list not limited to the following: Peptic ulcer disease; intestinal obstruction; cholecystitis; mesenteric ischemia; myocardial infarction dissecting aortic aneurysm

Likely Pathogens

Escherichia coli on page 142
Enterobacter Species *on page 132*
Anaerobes

Diagnostic Tests/Procedures

Computed Transaxial Tomography, Abdomen Studies *on page 423*
Ultrasound, Abdomen *on page 604*

Empiric Drug Therapy

Recommended:

Imipenem and Cilastatin *on page 861*
Ampicillin and Sulbactam *on page 660*
Cefoxitin *on page 712*

Alternate:

Cefotetan *on page 710*
Piperacillin and Tazobactam Sodium *on page 1003*
Ticarcillin and Clavulanate Potassium *on page 1114*
Meropenem *on page 936*
Ertapenem *on page 805*

(Continued)

Pancreatitis/Pancreatic Abscess *(Continued)*

Selected Readings

Baril NB, Ralls PW, Wren SM, et al, "Does an Infected Peripancreatic Fluid Collection or Abscess Mandate Operation?" *Ann Surg*, 2000, 231(3):361-7.

Ho HS and Frey CF, "The Role of Antibiotic Prophylaxis in Severe Acute Pancreatitis," *Arch Surg*, 1997, 132(5):487-92.

Powell JJ, Miles R, and Siriwardena AK, "Antibiotic Prophylaxis in the Initial Management of Severe Acute Pancreatitis," *Br J Surg*, 1998, 85(5):582-7.

Runzi M and Layer P, "Nonsurgical Management of Acute Pancreatitis. Use of Antibiotics," *Surg Clin North Am*, 1999, 79(4):759-65.

Wyncoll DL, "The Management of Severe Acute Necrotising Pancreatitis: An Evidence-Based Review of the Literature," *Intensive Care Med*, 1999, 25(2):146-56.

Paraflu *see* Parainfluenza Virus *on page 254*

Parainfluenza Virus

Synonyms Paraflu

Microbiology Parainfluenza viruses are RNA viruses which frequently cause lower respiratory infections in children and are the most common cause of croup (laryngotracheobronchitis). Parainfluenza viruses are single-stranded RNA viruses with an envelope derived from the host. The virus belongs to the family Paramyxoviridae and is thus related to the mumps virus and respiratory syncytial virus. Isolates causing human disease have been divided into four serotypes, parainfluenza 1-4. Two glycoproteins are found in the envelope, with hemagglutinin and neuraminidase activity associated with one of the two glycoproteins.

Epidemiology The virus is distributed worldwide. Parainfluenza type 4 is the least common of the serotypes isolated clinically, but this may be due to difficulties in culturing *in vitro*. Parainfluenza viruses are usually considered pathogenic in the pediatric population with antibodies to types 1-3 detectable in almost all children by 8 years of age. Longitudinal studies have shown an interesting pattern; outbreaks of parainfluenza types 1 and 2 tend to occur every other year (usually odd-numbered years) and during fall months, whereas outbreaks of type 3 occur during consecutive years most commonly during the spring. Parainfluenza viruses are a common cause of lower respiratory infections in children, second only to respiratory syncytial virus. Parainfluenza type 3 virus can infect infants in the first month of life. Types 1 and 2 tend to infect children and are important causes of croup. Transmission of the virus is by either direct person-to-person contact or by large droplets (eg, sneezing). The incubation period following exposure is about 3-6 days.

Clinical Syndromes

- **Upper respiratory tract infection:** This occurs particularly in children and is manifested by fever (in >50% of cases), coryza, sore throat, and cough.
- **Croup or laryngotracheobronchitis:** Parainfluenza type 1 is the most common cause of this type of lower respiratory infection. Croup is characterized by a distinctive cough like a "barking seal." A hoarse voice is common. In severe cases, the airway may be compromised secondary to subglottal edema, with stridor and respiratory failure. Most cases of croup recover uneventfully within several days. The differential diagnosis includes epiglottitis from *Haemophilus influenzae* or influenza A.
- **Bronchiolitis or pneumonia:** These forms of lower respiratory infection are associated with parainfluenza types 2 and 3 and are characterized by progressive cough with wheezing, dyspnea, and intercostal retractions. The chest radiograph may demonstrate air trapping and interstitial infiltrates.
- **Infection in adults:** Parainfluenza usually causes a mild respiratory infection in adults and is one cause of the common cold. Approximately 5% to 10% of respiratory infections in adults may be attributable to parainfluenza virus. Often adults experience hoarseness along with rhinorrhea, sore throat, and cough. Less commonly, tracheobronchitis occurs in adults with underlying chronic bronchitis, as well as otherwise healthy individuals. Pneumonia has also been reported in the elderly, although parainfluenza is still an uncommon respiratory pathogen in this age group accounting for probably <5% of respiratory infections.
- **Infection in immunocompromised hosts:** Parainfluenza virus has recently been recognized as a significant cause of disease in pediatric and adult transplant recipients. The infection tends to have a more fulminant course in this population. In one outbreak involving a cohort of bone marrow transplant recipients, over half of those with parainfluenza infection went on to develop pneumonia and this was associated with a mortality over 35%. The precise incidence of parainfluenza infections in transplant recipients has not been fully defined.

Diagnosis Infection with parainfluenza is usually suspected when a patient presents with a "barking seal" cough. However, other than a croup-like cough, the clinical presentation of parainfluenza is very nonspecific and cannot be distinguished from other common respiratory viruses, such as respiratory syncytial virus. In mild upper

respiratory infections, virologic confirmation is optional. Microbiologic confirmation is indicated in severe cases (eg, bronchiolitis or pneumonia), atypical cases, infection in immunocompromised hosts, or suspected parainfluenza in the adult. In severe cases, it may also be important to rule out respiratory syncytial virus, for which treatment is available. Rapid identification techniques are offered in many virology laboratories, and the identification of the infecting virus may avoid unnecessary antibacterial agents or invasive diagnostic procedures.

The best respiratory sample for detecting parainfluenza virus is the nasopharyngeal wash. This is performed at the bedside by gently administering saline into the nares with a standard syringe then aspirating the fluid back into the syringe, capturing saline, mucous, and respiratory epithelial cells. Alternatively, a viral swab may be inserted into the nasopharynx, but fewer respiratory cells are obtained with this technique and the sensitivity is lower. A "respiratory panel" is offered in some microbiology laboratories, whereby a single nasopharyngeal wash (or swab) may be sent for detection of multiple viruses, such as parainfluenza, influenza, respiratory syncytial virus, and others. Laboratory detection methods include:

1. Cell culture, where the clinical specimen is inoculated onto a monolayer of cells. If parainfluenza virus is present, a characteristic change in the appearance of the monolayer is seen, called cytopathic effect (CPE). The turnaround time is variable, and may be over several days, depending on the quality of the specimen and the amount of virus present.
2. Immunofluorescence. This is a rapid technique designed to detect viral presence without culture. Results may be available within hours of sample submission, if necessary.
3. Direct viral antigen detection. This is another early detection method but is still under study.
4. Serologic studies. A fourfold or greater rise in parainfluenza IgG between paired acute and convalescent specimens is diagnostic of parainfluenza infection. This knowledge may be useful for epidemiologic purposes or for studies of parainfluenza outbreaks, but contributes little to the immediate management of a case.

Diagnostic Tests/Procedures

Parainfluenza Virus Antigen by Direct Fluorescent Antibody *on page 558*
Parainfluenza Virus Culture *on page 558*
Parainfluenza Virus Serology *on page 559*

Treatment There are no antiviral agents currently approved for parainfluenza virus, although several are being studied. Bacterial superinfection is always possible and should be considered as a potentially reversible complication in difficult cases. Severe parainfluenza infections in bone marrow and solid organ transplant recipients have been described. Some success with ribavirin was reported, but the data is mainly anecdotal and no comparative trials have been done. Most cases of croup respond to supportive therapy alone, but severe cases may require intubation.

Drug Therapy Comment

No antiviral agents proven effective.

Selected Readings

Heilman CA, "Respiratory Syncytial and Parainfluenza Viruses," *J Infect Dis*, 1990, 161(3):402-6.
Rosekrans JA, "Viral Croup: Current Diagnosis and Treatment," *Mayo Clin Proc*, 1998, 73(11):1102-6; discussion 1107.
Vainionpää R and Hyypiä T, "Biology of Parainfluenza Viruses," *Clin Microbiol Rev*, 1994, 7(2):265-75.
Wright PF, "Parainfluenza Viruses," *Principles and Practice of Infectious Diseases*, 5th ed, Mandell GL, Bennett JE, and Dolin R, eds, New York, NY: Churchill Livingstone, 2000, 1771-6.

Parrot Fever *see Chlamydia psittaci on page 73*

Parvovirus B19

Microbiology Parvovirus B19 is a small DNA virus which has received increasing attention in recent years. It is the cause of the childhood rash erythema infectiosum ("fifth disease" because it represents the "fifth" (of six) common infectious rashes of childhood). Parvovirus B19 is the cause of chronic symmetrical arthritis in some adults, transient aplastic anemia, and chronic anemia in AIDS patients.

Parvovirus B19 is a single-stranded, encapsulated DNA virus which belongs to the family Parvoviridae. There are several other parvoviruses in the same genus as B19, including the common canine parvovirus. However, B19 is a strictly human pathogen and does not cause disease in animals. Parvovirus B19 is not transmitted from dogs to humans (a common misconception); animal parvoviruses have not been shown to cause human disease. The virus predominantly infects erythrocyte precursors in the bone marrow and causes cell lysis. Myeloid precursors in the marrow appear to be spared, although the virus has occasionally been found in peripheral leukocytes. Although parvovirus B19 has been cultured *in vitro* in erythropoietin-stimulated marrow cells, such techniques are not available in clinical virology laboratories. Instead, detection of viral presence is mainly achieved through detection of either
(Continued)

Parvovirus B19 *(Continued)*

specific B19 antibody, viral antigens, or nucleic acid (using polymerase chain reaction).

Epidemiology Infection with parvovirus B19 is common in the United States, beginning in early childhood. Over 50% of the adult population has serologic evidence of prior infection. Many cases are asymptomatic or mild. The primary mode of transmission is most likely respiratory. Outbreaks within families or schools can occur because of a high secondary attack rate which sometimes exceeds 50%. Spread of the virus is facilitated by subclinically infected individuals shedding the virus unknowingly in respiratory secretions. In addition, the individual is infective for several weeks before the characteristic parvovirus rash appears. Based on human volunteer studies, the period of incubation is approximately 1 week (4-14 days).

Clinical Syndromes

- **Erythema infectiosum (slapped cheek):** This is a childhood exanthem caused exclusively by parvovirus B19, also referred to as "fifth disease." Typically, a school-aged child develops a nonspecific febrile illness (low grade fever, malaise, and myalgias), which resolves over several days. Days to weeks later, when the child is feeling well, a brightly erythematous rash develops on the face. This is the characteristic "slapped cheek" rash of erythema infectiosum and is considered benign. Mild constitutional symptoms may accompany the rash (malaise, headache, etc), but the child is usually not infectious at this point. Erythema infectiosum has also been described in the adult and is frequently accompanied by joint symptoms.
- **Adult polyarthropathy:** Parvovirus B19 has been associated with a sudden onset, symmetrical polyarthritis syndrome. The great majority of cases have been reported in previously healthy women. Patients initially experience a nonspecific viral prodrome, probably corresponding to the period of viremia (B19 nucleic acid has been detected in the serum of some individuals). Several days to weeks later, an acute arthropathy develops, symmetrically involving the small joints of the hands, feet, and knees. Other joints may be involved less commonly (spine, costochondral joints). In addition to these arthralgias, there is often evidence of arthritis and synovitis, with joint stiffness, inflammation, and joint effusions. Arthrocentesis typically shows a mild elevation in WBCs around 3000-6000 cells/mm^3, mostly mononuclear. This acute arthropathy can mimic acute rheumatoid arthritis and some individuals will have detectable rheumatoid factor transiently. It is not clear whether B19 arthropathy is due to autoimmune mechanisms or direct viral infection. B19 nucleic acid has been found in the synovial fluid of a single patient (suggesting direct infection) but is generally undetectable in the blood during the arthropathy phase (suggesting an autoimmune etiology). Less than 50% of the cases are accompanied by a rash. When present, the rash appears macular in men and "lace-like" in women. The distribution of the rash is variable but tends to include the arms and legs. In some cases, there is marked involvement of the soles of the feet and the palms (somewhat unusual locations for an exanthem). The typical "slapped cheek" rash of erythema infectiosum is uncommon in the adult. The majority of cases of B19 arthropathy resolve completely with observation alone. Occasionally, the polyarthropathy may persist or recur over a period of years, and recent studies have linked parvovirus B19 to a chronic fibromyalgia syndrome. Neither the acute nor the chronic forms of parvovirus B19 arthropathy is associated with joint destruction. Of note, there are many variations in the presentation of this syndrome, including symmetrical arthritis without a flu-like illness or rash.
- **Transient aplastic crisis:** Parvovirus B19 can cause a severe erythropoietic arrest in patients with a previous underlying blood disorder, especially sickle cell disease, hereditary spherocytosis, thalassemia, hemoglobin SC, and other chronic hemolytic states. The virus can also cause red blood cell aplastic crisis in healthy individuals who do not have an underlying hematologic disorder. In general, individuals present with profound fatigue and lethargy, dyspnea, and may or may not have a history of a preceding flu-like illness. Rash and arthralgias are usually not present. Blood counts reveal a severely decreased hemoglobin with absent reticulocytes. Urgent transfusion may be necessary. Examination of the bone marrow shows erythroid hypoplasia with other cell lines usually intact. The finding of giant pronormoblasts in the bone marrow is considered pathognomonic for this infection. B19 viremia has been demonstrated during this time, and patients are potentially still infectious. The aplastic crisis usually resolves within 1-2 weeks.
- **Transient pancytopenia:** Other cells besides the erythrocytes can be involved with an acute parvovirus B19 infection. Potentially life-threatening declines in the neutrophil and/or platelet counts have been reported. In addition, a mild and transient pancytopenia was commonly observed in human volunteers experimentally infected with B19 and likely occurs in natural infections.

- **Red cell aplasia in the immunocompromised host:** In some immunocompromised patients, parvovirus B19 may be incompletely cleared after the initial infection, resulting in a waxing and waning, persistent infection. Chronic bone marrow suppression may be seen, as the virus causes continued lysis of RBC progenitor cells. Pure red blood cell aplasia may develop. Patients may be otherwise asymptomatic despite the chronicity of infection. Cases have been reported in acute leukemia, severe combined immunodeficiency syndrome, bone marrow transplant recipients, and persons with AIDS. The host antibody response to chronic B19 infection is highly variable, and viremia has been seen in patients with a negative parvovirus IgG and IgM. Diagnosis may require demonstration of B19 DNA in the serum by polymerase chain reaction. It is important to recognize this form of chronic anemia because it may respond to immunoglobulin therapy. In 1990, persistent B19 infection was found in a group of HIV-infected patients with red cell aplasia. All patients had giant pronormoblasts in the bone marrow. In later studies, bone marrow examination in HIV-infected patients with red cell aplasia appeared more variable and giant pronormoblasts often were not present.
- **Perinatal infections: The developing fetus is at particular risk for complications related to perinatal parvovirus infection.** This is due to several factors including the immaturity of the fetal immune system, delayed and incomplete transfer of protective maternal antibody across the placenta, and the need for brisk erythrocyte production in the fetus. Maternal infections with B19 during pregnancy may lead to hydrops fetalis or fetal death. The precise risk of intrauterine transmission to the fetus is unknown, as is the risk of fetal death once transmission has taken place. However, the data available suggest that the majority of pregnant women with acute B19 infections deliver healthy infants. However, fetal demise has been reported following asymptomatic maternal B19 infections. The cause of death in the fetus has been attributed to destruction of erythroid precursors in the liver and bone marrow, followed by edema and congestive heart failure; however, virus has also been identified in tissues such as the heart. Perinatal parvovirus B19 infection has not been associated with congenital abnormalities. Thus, maternal infection is not an indication for an abortion. Although the epidemiology of perinatal parvovirus infections is still evolving, this virus is still an uncommon cause of stillbirths or spontaneous abortions in the general U.S. population (by some estimates, approximately 1% of cases of fetal loss). The Centers for Disease Control has addressed the growing public concern regarding B19 and fetal death by estimating the risks of B19 infection in pregnant women following different exposures to the virus (see Selected Readings). The risk of fetal death in susceptible women exposed to B19 during epidemic outbreaks (school, daycare centers) is roughly 1% to 2%.

Diagnosis In the absence of classic erythema infectiosum, parvovirus infection may be difficult to diagnose. The clinician must maintain a high level of suspicion for B19 in patients with unusual skin rashes, arthritis-arthralgia syndromes, aplastic anemia of unknown etiology, and chronic anemia. Laboratory studies are necessary to confirm the diagnosis, but no culture-based techniques are available. These consist of:

1. IgG and IgM antibodies for parvovirus B19. The presence of IgM antibody in the patient (or in cord blood of the fetus) confirms acute infection. A significant rise in parvovirus IgG during acute and convalescent periods is also diagnostic. A single positive IgG only suggests past infection and over half of the general population will have a positive parvovirus B19 IgG. Thus, paired samples showing seroconversion or a significant rise in titer are necessary for proper interpretation. Chronic B19 infection in immunosuppressed patients with pure RBC aplasia typically have no detectable parvovirus IgG or IgM antibodies. PCR is the method of choice in this situation.
2. Detection of viral antigen is still a research tool and not commercially available as yet.
3. Polymerase chain reaction (PCR), the most sensitive technique, has been employed successfully in many studies, with viral DNA being detected in the serum of individuals with acute viremia as well as in a variety of tissues, such as bone marrow and synovium. Patients with transient aplastic crisis from B19 frequently have high levels of circulating virus which is easily detectable by PCR. Immunocompromised persons with pure RBC aplasia have lower levels of viremia, and detection by PCR is more variable. PCR is usually negative in healthy children presenting with erythema infectiosum. Immunocompetent adults with acute B19 infection may have a persistently positive PCR from serum for many months, and a positive PCR in other tissues (eg, synovium) for years. PCR is now commercially available in a number of reference laboratories as well as from the Centers for Disease Control and Prevention (Division of Viral Diseases).
4. Electron microscopy for parvovirus-like particles (only rarely used).
5. Histologic specimens, looking for eosinophilic nuclear inclusions (not pathognomonic for B19).

(Continued)

Parvovirus B19 *(Continued)*

6. Bone marrow aspiration and biopsy. The finding of giant pronormoblasts in Wright-Giemsa stained marrow is characteristic of parvoviral infection.

B19 cannot be detected using the common cell culture systems available in clinical virology laboratories.

Diagnostic Tests/Procedures

Bone Marrow Aspiration and Biopsy *on page 397*
Parvovirus B19 DNA, Qualitative PCR *on page 559*
Parvovirus B19 Serology *on page 560*

Treatment Currently, there is no antiviral agent with significant clinical activity against the B19 virus itself. However, in some cases, the chronic anemia of B19 infection in immunosuppressed patients has been shown to respond dramatically to infusions of intravenous immunoglobulin. This important finding has also been shown in a small cohort of HIV-1 infected individuals with B19-induced anemia.

Drug Therapy Comment

No antiviral agents proven effective.

Selected Readings

Dollard S, Nasello M, and Menegus M, "Serodiagnosis of Parvovirus Infections: Problems and Pitfalls," *Clin Microbiol Newslett*, 1998, 20(3):21-3.

Frickhofen N, Abkowitz JL, Safford M, et al, "Persistent B19 Parvovirus Infection in Patients Infected With Human Immunodeficiency Virus Type 1 (HIV-1): A Treatable Cause of Anemia in AIDS," *Ann Intern Med*, 1990, 113(12):926-33.

Kurtzman GJ, Cohen B, Meyers P, et al, "Persistent B19 Parvovirus Infection as a Cause of Severe Chronic Anemia in Children With Acute Lymphocytic Leukaemia," *Lancet*, 1988, 2(8621):1159-62.

Mishra B, Malhotra P, Ratho RK, et al, "Human Parvovirus B19 in Patients With Aplastic Anemia," *Am J Hematol*, 2005, 79(2):166-7.

Petersson K, Norbeck O, Westgren M, et al, "Detection of Parvovirus B19, Cytomegalovirus, and Enterovirus Infections in Cases of Intrauterine Fetal Death," *Obstet Gynecol Surv*, 2005, 60(5):284-6.

Young NS and Brown KE, "Parvovirus B19," *N Engl J Med*, 2004, 350(6):586-97.

Pasteurella multocida

Microbiology *Pasteurella multocida* is a gram-negative rod which is primarily a pathogen in wild and domestic animals but is also an important cause of sporadic human diseases such as animal bite infection, osteomyelitis, and sepsis. *P. multocida* is a gram-negative coccobacillus which grows best as a facultative anaerobe but does not form spores. It belongs to the family Pasteurellaceae, and is related to *Haemophilus* and *Actinobacillus* species. There are six distinct species of *Pasteurella*, but the most common to cause human disease is *Pasteurella multocida*. Special requests for identification for this organism are helpful for the Microbiology Laboratory but are usually not necessary; the organism grows readily on several standard culture media such as blood agar or chocolate agar.

Epidemiology *P. multocida*is a normal commensal of the oropharynx and the gastrointestinal tract of several animal species. However, it is only rarely recovered from the respiratory tract of humans and has been found to be part of the normal oral flora only in individuals with significant animal contact (eg, veterinarians). The frequency of recovery of this organism from a healthy animal depends on the particular animal species, as follows: cats, 50% to 75%; dogs, 10% to 60%; pigs, 50%, and rats, 15%.

Pasteurella has been reported in all age groups. Human infection usually occurs following an animal bite or scratch. One study found that up to 17% of patients being treated in an emergency room for an animal bite ultimately developed a *Pasteurella* infection. Cat scratches or bites cause the majority of *Pasteurella* infections (about 65% of cases). Dog bites are responsible for about 35% of cases. A smaller number of cases of *Pasteurella* infections are due to animal exposures without a clear history of an animal bite or scratch. The patient tends to be frequently exposed to animals (such as a veterinarian, livestock handler, pet shop worker), and the infections are generally in the respiratory tract, although cases of intra-abdominal infection have also been described. A small percentage of patients are infected with *P. multocida* without any significant animal exposure.

Clinical Syndromes

- **Animal bite-wound infections:** Patients who have *Pasteurella* inoculated via a bite wound develop rapid onset of pain, erythema, and edema locally. This may occur within hours of the bite or may be delayed by several days. Common sites include the upper extremities (in particular, hands), legs, and the head and neck region. An important complication is the development of regional lymphadenopathy. Occasionally, *Pasteurella* infection may be the cause of lymph node enlargement of unknown etiology; such patients should be questioned about seemingly minor animal scratches as well. Bite-wound infections are often limited to soft tissue cellulitis or focal abscesses. At times, the course may be complicated by tenosynovitis, septic arthritis, and osteomyelitis, any of which can be particularly difficult to treat when the infection involves the hand. Note that the specific entity known as

"cat scratch disease" is caused by *Bartonella* species and not caused by *Pasteurella multocida*.

- **Upper and lower respiratory infections:** This unusual presentation of *Pasteurella* infection may be seen in patients who have had a significant exposure to animals but lack a history of an animal bite. These individuals presumably are colonized with the organism beforehand and then develop respiratory infection later. *Pasteurella* has been implicated as a rare cause of bronchitis, sinusitis, and pneumonia in both healthy individuals and those with underlying chronic bronchitis.
- **Infection in the immunocompromised host:** Serious and life-threatening *Pasteurella* infections have been reported in patients with underlying malignancies, organ transplantations, and HIV infection.
- **Miscellaneous infections:** Meningitis, peritonitis (particularly patients undergoing peritoneal dialysis), corneal ulcers, ophthalmitis, and urinary tract infections are rarely reported.

Diagnosis *P. multocida* infection should be considered in any wound infection resulting from an animal bite or deep scratch. The diagnosis is even more likely if local inflammation develops within 3-24 hours of the bite and if the animal involved was a cat. Longer periods of incubation are more suggestive of streptococcal or staphylococcal infection, although certainly cases of pasteurellosis may have a delayed onset. The diagnosis is more difficult for nonbite *Pasteurella* infections; the clinician must carefully inquire about unusual or prolonged animal exposures in the workplace and at home.

Diagnostic Tests/Procedures

Blood Culture, Aerobic and Anaerobic *on page 391*

Gram Stain *on page 473*

Wound Culture *on page 620*

Treatment The drug of choice for pasteurellosis is penicillin. If the infection is minor and limited to soft tissue, a trial of oral penicillin may be attempted (eg, penicillin V, 500 mg orally every 6 hours) when *Pasteurella* is isolated from a wound in pure culture. Antistaphylococcal penicillins such as oxacillin and dicloxacillin are less active and should be avoided. If the infection is more serious, parenteral penicillin G should be used. This includes deep wound infections of the extremities, osteomyelitis, septic arthritic, tenosynovitis, and pneumonia. Consultation with an Infectious Disease specialist may be useful in complicated cases, where therapy may be prolonged and surgical debridement necessary.

One important principle of animal bite management is that many bite wound infections are polymicrobial. In one recent study of animal bites, the average number of organisms isolated from a clinically infected wound was 3-4. Some of the common dog and cat-bite pathogens are resistant to common penicillin preparations (penicillin VK, penicillin G) and thus empiric therapy is usually more broad and includes a beta-lactamase inhibitor such as amoxicillin-clavulanate. Infection of bite wounds with *Pasteurella* as the sole pathogen is uncommon, and penicillin should be considered only if there are no other organisms are seen on Gram stain and culture.

Other antimicrobial agents are probably effective but the clinical experience is more limited: tetracycline, quinolones (ciprofloxacin, levofloxacin, and others) and the cephalosporins. Agents which are not effective include clindamycin, erythromycin, and aminoglycosides. Newer macrolides such as azithromycin and clarithromycin have better *in vitro* activity against *Pasteurella* than erythromycin but there is little clinical experience with these agents. Infectious disease consultation may be helpful in the penicillin-allergic patient to select an alternate antibiotic.

Drug Therapy

Recommended:

Penicillin G (Parenteral/Aqueous) *on page 993*

Penicillin V Potassium *on page 998*

Alternate:

Amoxicillin and Clavulanate Potassium *on page 645*

Ampicillin and Sulbactam *on page 660*

Selected Readings

Turner DPJ, Garvey M, and Donald FE, "*Pasteurella multocida* Infection - Apparent Failure of Ampicillin Treatment," *Clin Microbiol Newslett*, 1999, 21(20):167-8.

Weber DJ, Wolfson JS, Swartz M, et al, "*Pasteurella multocida* Infections. Report of 34 Cases and Review of the Literature," *Medicine (Baltimore)*, 1984, 63(3):133-154.

PCP *see Pneumocystis jiroveci on page 266*

Pediatric Meningitis *see* Meningitis, Pediatric (>1 month of age) *on page 218*

Pediatric Osteomyelitis *see* Osteomyelitis, Pediatric *on page 251*

Pediculus humanus *see* Lice *on page 207*

Pelvic Inflammatory Disease

Related Information

Treatment of Sexually Transmitted Infections *on page 1311*

Synonyms PID; Salpingitis; Tubo-Ovarian Abscess

Clinical Presentation Pelvic inflammatory disease (PID) is an infection of the pelvic organs usually by bacteria and its associated inflammatory response. Typically begins as an ascending infection from the vagina or cervix but may occur via hematogenous or lymphatic spread. Patients present with fever, chills, nausea, vomiting, anorexia, vaginal bleeding, and mucopurulent vaginal discharge. Endometritis usually develops postpartum or postabortal, whereas, salpingo-oophoritis with or without abscess is most associated with sexually transmitted diseases.

Differential Diagnosis Intestinal tract disease; urinary systems disease

Likely Pathogens

Chlamydia trachomatis on page 74
Neisseria gonorrhoeae on page 244
Escherichia coli on page 142
Streptococcus, Viridans Group *on page 326*
Bacteroides and *Prevotella* Species *on page 46*

Diagnostic Tests/Procedures

Abscess Aerobic and Anaerobic Culture *on page 360*
Aerobic Culture, Body Fluid *on page 365*
Anaerobic Culture *on page 371*
Gram Stain *on page 473*

Empiric Drug Therapy

Recommended:

One of the following
Cefotetan *on page 710*
Cefoxitin *on page 712*
plus
Doxycycline *on page 787*

Clindamycin *on page 752*
plus
Gentamicin *on page 841*

Alternate:

Fluoroquinolones *on page 824*
with or without
Metronidazole *on page 940*

Ampicillin and Sulbactam *on page 660*
plus
Doxycycline *on page 787*

The following 3 used in combination
Ciprofloxacin *on page 742*
Doxycycline *on page 787*
Metronidazole *on page 940*

Selected Readings

Center for Disease Control and Prevention (CDC), "Sexually Transmitted Diseases Treatment Guidelines 2002," *MMWR*, 2002, 51(RR-6).
Hensell DL, Little BB, Faro S, et al, "Comparison of Three Regimens Recommended by the Centers for Disease Control and Prevention for the Treatment of Women Hospitalized With Acute Pelvic Inflammatory Disease," *Clin Infect Dis*, 1994, 19(4):720-7.
Walker CK, Workowski KA, Washington AE, et al, "Anaerobes in Pelvic Inflammatory Disease: Implications for the Centers for Disease Control and Prevention's Guidelines for Treatment of Sexually Transmitted Diseases," *Clin Infect Dis*, 1999, 28 Suppl 1:S29-36.

Penicillin-Resistant *S. pneumoniae* *see Streptococcus pneumoniae*, Drug-Resistant *on page 316*

Penicillium marneffei

Microbiology *Penicillium marneffei* is the only dimorphic fungus of the genus *Penicillium* and is the only true pathogen in the *Penicillium* genus. In the mycelial form on culture, the mold grows relatively fast producing a grayish white and downy or woolly colony in 2-3 days. The underneath of the fungus appears either pink or red due to the production of a soluble red pigment that diffuses into the agar. A few other *Penicillium* species produce an obvious red diffusable pigment into solid culture media, but these species are not dimorphic. Over time, the colony becomes more rugose while the aerial mycelia becomes pink. The color of the colony changes from white to light brown to light green after 10 days. Microscopically, it appears as a typical *Penicillium* species characterized by short, branched, septated hyphae with brush-like conidiophores located laterally and terminally. The yeast form grows rapidly appearing as light tan colonies of various textures ranging from smooth to

cerebriform. Microscopically, the yeast cells are unicellular 3-6 x 1.5-2 mm in size and vary from round, ellipsoidal, and rectangular shapes. The yeast form may be mixed with hyphal elements. The yeast cells may be distinguished from other yeast by the presence of a white central septum and reproduction by fission, not budding.

Epidemiology The ecological characteristics and geographic distribution are still largely unknown. *P. marneffei* has been isolated from bamboo rats in southeast Asia but is also endemic in the southern part of China. Almost all reported cases have indicated that the infected patients have lived or traveled in southeast Asia particularly Vietnam, Laos, Singapore, Malaysia, Burma, Thailand, Indonesia, Guangxi, or Hong Kong. It occurs more commonly in males.

Although the majority of patients who acquire penicilliosis are immunocompromised, there are reports of cases occurring in patients with intact immune systems. *P. marneffei* is the third most common opportunistic infection, following tuberculosis and cryptococcosis, in patients with AIDS living in northern Thailand, southern China, and other parts of southeast Asia. It is classified as an AIDS-defining illness by several southeast Asian countries. There is a 20% mortality in AIDS patients with disseminated disease. Without chronic suppressive therapy, the relapse rate exceeds 50%. The route of transmission is believed to be either from inhalation or ingestion. Autoinoculation in a research laboratory environment has been reported.

Clinical Syndromes

- **Localized disease:** May occur from autoinoculation. Forms a cutaneous lesion and may cause localized lymphadenopathy.
- **Disseminated disease:** Clinically similar to disseminated histoplasmosis and cryptococcosis. Patients present with constitutional symptoms such as fever and weight loss. Various forms of cutaneous lesions are common and are present on the face, upper torso, pinnae, and arms. Patients often have respiratory symptoms including cough and pleuritic pain. Chest radiographs are frequently abnormal revealing infiltrates, nodules, abscesses, or even cavitation. Anemia is commonly seen. Peripheral blood cultures are frequently positive and bone marrow involvement occurs in >25%. Uncommon manifestations include pericarditis, genital ulcers, osteomyelitis, and arthritis.

Diagnosis Diagnosis is dependent on identification of the organism by histopathology and culture. Must be distinguished from *H. capsulatum* as both appear as intracellular organisms; however, *H. capsulatum* reproduces by budding whereas *P. marneffei* reproduces by fission. Immunologic assays and PCR remain investigational.

Diagnostic Tests/Procedures

Fungus Culture, Appropriate Site *on page 461*
KOH Preparation *on page 513*
Methenamine Silver Stain *on page 534*

Treatment

Non-AIDS: Amphotericin B 0.6 mg/kg/day 1-3 g total dose depending on the severity of the disease

AIDS: Amphotericin B 0.6 mg/kg/day for 2 weeks followed by itraconazole 200 mg twice daily for 10 weeks followed by itraconazole 200 mg/day for life.

Drug Therapy

Recommended:

Non-AIDS:
Amphotericin B (Conventional) *on page 650*

AIDS:
Amphotericin B (Conventional) *on page 650*
followed by
Itraconazole *on page 895*

Alternate:

Itraconazole *on page 895*

Selected Readings

Nelson KE and Sirisanthana T, "Images in Clinical Medicine. Disseminated *Penicillium marneffei* Infection in a Patient With AIDS," *N Engl J Med*, 2001, 344(23):1763.
Sirisanthana T, "*Penicillium marneffei* Infection in Patients With AIDS," *Emerg Infect Dis*, 2001, 7(3 Suppl):561.
Skoulidis F, Morgan MS, and MacLeod KM, "*Penicillium marneffei*: A Pathogen on Our Doorstep?" *J R Soc Med*, 2004, 97(8):394-6.
Ungpakorn R, "Cutaneous Manifestations of *Penicillium marneffei* Infection," *Curr Opin Infect Dis*, 2000, 13(2):129-34.

Peptic Ulcer Disease *see Helicobacter pylori on page 162*
Peptostreptococcus *see Streptococcus*-Related Gram-Positive Cocci *on page 325*

Pericarditis

Clinical Presentation Acute: Pleuritic pain may vary from a slow progressive pain to a sharp inspiratory pain to a more subtle deep ache which radiates down the arms. (Continued)

Pericarditis *(Continued)*

Characteristically, the pain is alleviated by sitting up and leaning forward. Dyspnea is common. The pericardial friction rub is the cardinal feature. The EKG typically reveals widespread elevation of the ST segments. The presence of a paradoxical pulse should alert the physician for possible cardiac tamponade although a paradoxical pulse may be seen in other diseases. Viral pericarditis occurs more frequently in young adults and is characterized by an antecedent upper respiratory tract infection by about 1-2 weeks. Patients typically have constitutional symptoms including fever. Clinical classification is defined by duration of symptoms; acute is <6 weeks, subacute is 6 weeks to 6 months, and chronic is >6 months. It is further classified by either fibrinous, effusive, or constrictive. It may also be classified according to the etiology such as infectious, autoimmune including rheumatic fever, collagen-vascular diseases, drug-induced, and postcardiac injury, and a broad category of noninfectious which includes neoplasia, uremia, acute myocardial infarction, cholesterol, myxedema, trauma, structural cardiac defects, and others.

Differential Diagnosis The differential diagnosis for chest pain is quite exhaustive and for this text will be broken into four major systems: cardiovascular, pulmonary, gastrointestinal, and skeletal-muscular.

Likely Pathogens

Viruses:
- Coxsackieviruses *on page 101*
- Echovirus *on page 118*
- Herpes Simplex Virus *on page 172*
- Adenovirus *on page 29*

Pyogenic

Mycobacterial:
- *Mycobacterium tuberculosis on page 234*
- *Mycobacterium avium-intracellulare* (Complex) *on page 228*

Fungal:
- *Histoplasma capsulatum on page 177*
- *Blastomyces dermatitidis on page 50*
- *Aspergillus* Species *on page 38*

Treponema pallidum on page 334

Parasitic
- Amebiasis
- *Toxoplasma gondii on page 331*
- *Echinococcus*
- *Trichinella spiralis on page 338*

Diagnostic Tests/Procedures

Culture (see specific organisms)
EKG
Echocardiography, M-Mode *on page 445*
Pericardiocentesis

Drug Therapy Comment Recommended drug therapy is antimicrobial therapy directed against specific pathogen and supportive care. Anti-inflammatory drugs such as NSAIDs and prednisone may be helpful.

Selected Readings

Pawsat DE and Lee JY, "Inflammatory Disorders of the Heart. Pericarditis, Myocarditis, and Endocarditis," *Emerg Med Clin North Am*, 1998, 16(3):665-81.

Perinephric Abscess *see* Urinary Tract Infection, Perinephric Abscess *on page 345*

Peritonitis, CAPD-Associated

Synonyms CAPD-Associated Peritonitis

Clinical Presentation Patients typically present with abdominal pain or tenderness, and occasionally nausea and vomiting. Fever is not a consistent finding. Cloudy dialysate fluid or drainage problems may be the first signs of peritonitis. Although gram-positive bacteria are the most common pathogens, gram-negatives, fungi, and other unusual organisms have been reported causes of CAPD-associated peritonitis.

Differential Diagnosis Perforated ulcer; intra-abdominal abscess; appendicitis; cholecystitis; pancreatitis; salpingitis; diverticulitis; neoplasm; small bowel obstruction; mesenteric ischemia

Likely Pathogens

- *Staphylococcus aureus*, Methicillin-Resistant *on page 304*
- *Staphylococcus aureus*, Methicillin-Susceptible *on page 307*
- *Staphylococcus epidermidis*, Methicillin-Resistant *on page 309*
- *Staphylococcus epidermidis*, Methicillin-Susceptible *on page 310*
- *Streptococcus* Species *on page 326*
- Gram-Negative Bacilli *on page 157*
- *Pseudomonas aeruginosa on page 282*
- *Candida* Species *on page 67*

Diagnostic Tests/Procedures
Gram Stain *on page 473*, peritoneal fluid
WBC, peritoneal fluid
Blood Culture, Aerobic and Anaerobic *on page 391*

Drug Therapy Comment Both ceftazidime and cefazolin may be administered directly into the dialysate at a dosage of 1 g daily in the long dwell. Both may be administered in the same bag.

Empiric Drug Therapy

Recommended:

Note: Selection may be influenced by initial Gram stain.
If Gram-positive:
Cefazolin *on page 700*
If Gram-negative:
Ceftazidime *on page 717*
If no Gram stain or indeterminate:
Piperacillin and Tazobactam Sodium *on page 1003*

Alternate:
Cefazolin *on page 700*
plus
Aminoglycosides *on page 641*
Vancomycin *on page 1144*
plus
Ceftazidime *on page 717*

If fungal suspected:
Amphotericin B (Conventional) *on page 650*
Fluconazole *on page 819*

Selected Readings
Keane WF, Bailie GR, Boeschoten E, et al, "Adult Peritoneal Dialysis-Related Peritonitis Treatment Recommendations: 2000 Update," *Perit Dial Int*, 2000, 20(4):396-411.

Peritonitis, Secondary

Synonyms Bowel Perforation; Secondary Peritonitis

Clinical Presentation Peritoneal inflammation results in abdominal distension, fever, chills, anorexia, nausea, and vomiting. The common findings are abdominal pain, rebound tenderness, which may be localized, elevated WBC, and loss of bowel sounds. Tachycardia and hypotension may occur, and the syndrome may rapidly progress to septic shock with multiorgan failure.

Risk factors for secondary peritonitis include diverticulitis, appendicitis, pancreatitis, inflammatory bowel disease, peptic ulcer disease, bowel obstruction, pelvic inflammatory disease, or trauma. Secondary peritonitis often involves multiple organisms, both aerobes and anaerobes, typically *E. coli* and *Bacteroides fragilis*.

Likely Pathogens
Escherichia coli on page 142
Bacteroides and *Prevotella* Species *on page 46*

Diagnostic Tests/Procedures
Paracentesis *on page 555*
Blood Culture, Aerobic and Anaerobic *on page 391*

Drug Therapy Comment The management of secondary peritonitis involves elimination of the source of infection, reduction of bacterial contamination of the peritoneal cavity, and prevention of persistent or recurrent intra-abdominal infections. Recurrent infection prevented by the use of drains, planned reoperations, and leaving the wound open. Ultrasound or CT scan may localize collections and often allows for percutaneous drainage.

Ideally guided by culture and sensitivity results, blood-culture positive peritonitis should be treated for 14 days.

Empiric Drug Therapy

Recommended:
Ampicillin and Sulbactam *on page 660*
Piperacillin and Tazobactam Sodium *on page 1003*

Alternate:
Imipenem and Cilastatin *on page 861*
Meropenem *on page 936*
Ertapenem *on page 805*
Tigecycline *on page 1116*

Fluoroquinolones *on page 824*
with or without
Metronidazole *on page 940*

Peritonitis, Spontaneous Bacterial

Synonyms Spontaneous Bacterial Peritonitis

Clinical Presentation Patients with primary peritonitis present with abrupt onset of fever, abdominal pain, nausea, vomiting, diarrhea, diffuse abdominal tenderness, rebound tenderness, and hypoactive or absent bowel sounds. Patients with cirrhosis may have an atypical presentation with an insidious onset and lack of peritoneal signs. Most cirrhotics present with fever. Patients with secondary peritonitis present as the primary process with peritoneal signs being the most prominent. More than 60% of the cases of spontaneous bacterial peritonitis (SBP) are caused by gram-negative enteric bacteria. Gram-positive cocci, predominantly streptococcal species, are implicated in approximately 25% of the cases of SBP.

Differential Diagnosis Pneumonia; sickle cell anemia; herpes zoster; diabetic ketoacidosis; tabes dorsalis; porphyria; familial Mediterranean fever; plumbism; lupus erythematosus; uremia; other intra-abdominal infections

Likely Pathogens

Klebsiella Species *on page 200*
Escherichia coli on page 142
Streptococcus Species *on page 326*

Diagnostic Tests/Procedures

Paracentesis *on page 555*
Abscess Aerobic and Anaerobic Culture *on page 360*
Aerobic Culture, Body Fluid *on page 365*
Anaerobic Culture *on page 371*
Gram Stain *on page 473*

Empiric Drug Therapy

Recommended:

Monotherapy:
Ampicillin and Sulbactam *on page 660*
Piperacillin and Tazobactam Sodium *on page 1002*
Moxifloxacin *on page 949*
Cefotaxime *on page 708*
Ceftriaxone *on page 722*
Ceftizoxime *on page 720*
Cefotaxime *on page 708*
Cefepime *on page 705*

Combination therapy:
Ciprofloxacin *on page 742*
plus
Metronidazole *on page 940*

Alternate:

Cefoxitin *on page 712*
Cefotetan *on page 710*
Ticarcillin and Clavulanate Potassium *on page 1114*
Imipenem and Cilastatin *on page 861*
Meropenem *on page 936*
Ertapenem *on page 805*
Tigecycline *on page 1116*

Selected Readings

Johnson CC, Baldessarre J, and Levison ME, "Peritonitis: Update on Pathophysiology, Clinical Manifestations, and Management," *Clin Infect Dis*, 1997, 24(6):1035-47.
McClean KL, Sheehan GJ and Harding GK, "Intra-abdominal Infection: A Review," *Clin Infect Dis*, 1994, 19(1):100-16.
Such J and Runyon BA, "Spontaneous Bacterial Peritonitis," *Clin Infect Dis*, 1998, 27(4):669-74.

Pertussis *see Bordetella pertussis on page 53*
Phaeohyphomycosis *see* Dematiaceous Fungi *on page 112*
Phaeomycotic Cyst *see* Dematiaceous Fungi *on page 112*

Pharyngitis

Synonyms Strep Throat

Clinical Presentation Acute pharyngitis is an inflammatory syndrome of the pharynx caused by multiple organisms, predominantly viral. Patients complain of soreness, scratching, or irritation of the throat along with signs of congestion, malaise, and headaches. Patients with EBV or strep typically present with fever and an exudative pharyngitis.

Differential Diagnosis Retropharyngeal abscess; epiglottitis; Lemierre's disease

Likely Pathogens

Streptococcus pyogenes on page 321
Respiratory Syncytial Virus *on page 285*
Influenza Virus *on page 193*

Parainfluenza Virus *on page 254*
Adenovirus *on page 29*
Epstein-Barr Virus *on page 139*

Diagnostic Tests/Procedures Viral detection studies indicated for severe or unusual cases and are not routine.

Group A *Streptococcus* Antigen Test *on page 475*
Throat Culture for Group A Beta-Hemolytic *Streptococcus on page 594*
Virus Detection by DFA *on page 619*
Viral Culture, Throat *on page 617*
Infectious Mononucleosis Serology *on page 509*

Drug Therapy Comment Drug therapy indicated is for *Streptococcus pyogenes* infections only.

Empiric Drug Therapy

Recommended:

Penicillin V Potassium *on page 998*
Penicillin G Benzathine *on page 991*
Penicillin G Benzathine and Penicillin G Procaine *on page 992*
Amoxicillin *on page 642*

Alternate:

Erythromycin *on page 807*
Cephalosporins, 1st Generation *on page 729*
Amoxicillin *on page 642*

Selected Readings

Bisno AL, Gerber MA, Gwaltney JM Jr, et al, "Practice Guidelines for the Diagnosis and Management of Group A Streptococcal Pharyngitis. Infectious Diseases Society of America," *Clin Infect Dis*, 2002, 35(2):113-25.

Phthirus pubis *see* Lice *on page 207*
Phycomycosis *see Mucor* Species *on page 225*
PID *see* Pelvic Inflammatory Disease *on page 260*
Pigbel *see Clostridium perfringens on page 88*
Pink Eye *see* Conjunctivitis *on page 93*
Pinworm *see Enterobius vermicularis on page 133*
Pityriasis (Tinea) Versicolor *see Malassezia furfur on page 213*
Pityrosporum orbiculare *see Malassezia furfur on page 213*
Pityrosporum ovale *see Malassezia furfur on page 213*
Plague *see Yersinia pestis on page 355*

Plasmodium Species

Related Information

Immunization Recommendations *on page 1249*
Malaria Treatment *on page 1292*

Microbiology *Plasmodium* sp are obligate intracellular protozoa related to *Babesia* and *Toxoplasma. Plasmodium* sp reproduce sexually in mosquitoes. Mosquitoes transmit the resulting sporozoites into humans where the organisms reproduce asexually. The sporozoites multiply within the liver; resulting merozoites invade erythrocytes where the merozoites multiply or mature into male and female gametocytes which eventually will be taken up by a mosquito during a blood meal.

Plasmodium sp stain well with Giemsa or Wright-Giemsa and are easily observed in stained peripheral blood smears if parasitemia is heavy enough. There are many species of *Plasmodium*; however, only the following four species infect humans: *P. falciparum*, *P. vivax*, *P. ovale*, and *P. malariae*.

Epidemiology *P. falciparum* is found in tropical areas; *P. vivax* is found throughout many tropical and subtropical parts of the world; *P. ovale* is found in central and west Africa and in some Pacific islands; and *P. malariae* is found sporadically throughout the world. *P. falciparum* and *P. vivax* cause approximately 80% and 15%, respectively, of all cases of malaria. Malaria is the most severe infectious disease of tropical and subtropical areas of the world. One-half of the world's population live in areas where malaria is endemic. Each year approximately 270 million persons become infected with *Plasmodium* sp, approximately 110 million persons develop clinical disease, and 7 million Americans visit areas where malaria is endemic.

Clinical Syndromes After experiencing a prodrome phase of constitutional "flu"-like symptoms, most persons with malaria will experience the hallmark of classic malaria, the paroxysm. A paroxysm is a 3- to 6-hour period of high fever, chills, and rigors. Paroxysms correspond to periodic release of *Plasmodium* merozoites from erythrocytes and the beginning of another life cycle of the organism within erythrocytes. Fever patterns are often irregular, but the paroxysm often occurs regularly (eg, every 2 days). Often, patients are asymptomatic between paroxysms. Patients with malaria (Continued)

Plasmodium Species *(Continued)*

can experience severe splenomegaly and hepatomegaly. Rupture of the spleen is not uncommon. Anemia is a common complication. Malaria caused by *P. falciparum* is a medically urgent situation and requires immediate diagnosis and medical intervention. Fulminant complications of malaria include renal failure, pulmonary edema, cerebral involvement, and severe reduction of the flow of blood through capillaries.

Diagnosis Smears of peripheral blood must be stained with Giemsa or Wright-Giemsa stains and examined for parasites. Blood should be collected no less than twice per day (preferably, several times a day) until malaria is ruled out or until parasites are observed and identified. The most important and immediate concerns in the management of malaria are to determine if the patient is infected with *Plasmodium* and, if so, to determine if the parasite is *P. falciparum*.

Diagnostic Tests/Procedures

Peripheral Blood Smear, Thick and Thin *on page 563*

Drug Therapy Comment A variety of regimens are available for travelers to endemic areas. These must be determined on an individual basis, depending upon region where travel is planned.

Drug Therapy

Recommended:

Chloroquine-susceptible:

Chloroquine *on page 737*
Quinidine *on page 1027*

Chloroquine-resistant:

Atovaquone and Proguanil *on page 672*
Mefloquine *on page 929*
Halofantrine *on page 850*

Alternate:

Chloroquine-resistant:

Sulfadoxine and Pyrimethamine *on page 1085*
Halofantrine *on page 850*

Selected Readings

Garcia LS, "Update on Malaria," *Clin Microbiol Newslett*, 1992, 14:65-9.
Krogstad DJ, "*Plasmodium* Species (Malaria)," *Principles and Practice of Infectious Diseases*, 4th ed, Mandell GL, Bennett JE, and Dolin R, eds, New York, NY: Churchill Livingstone, 1995, 2415-27.
Smith JH, "Malaria: Clinical Laboratory Features," *Clin Microbiol Newslett*, 1995, 17(24):185-8.

Pneumococcus, Drug-Resistant *see Streptococcus pneumoniae*, Drug-Resistant *on page 316*

Pneumocystis jiroveci

Related Information

Community-Acquired Pneumonia in Adults *on page 1278*
USPHS / IDSA Guidelines for the Prevention of Opportunistic Infections in Persons Infected With HIV *on page 1237*

Microbiology In the past, *Pneumocystis jiroveci* was classified as a protozoan, but recent gene sequencing evidence demonstrates the organism is more closely related to fungi. Studies using molecular techniques have shown a close homology between *P. jiroveci* and fungi such as *Saccharomyces* than other protozoans such as *Plasmodium* (the cause of malaria). The organism is unicellular and has three stages: trophozoite, precyst, and cyst. In clinical specimens, the trophozoites are most predominant. The life cycle of *P. jiroveci* has yet to be fully defined. The organism cannot be cultured reliably in the laboratory, even in research settings. The organism requires special staining to be visible in clinical specimens. Several stains will selectively stain the organism (methenamine-silver, toluidine blue, Wright-Giemsa, and others).

Epidemiology *P. jiroveci* is distributed worldwide and in animals. Serologic data suggests that infection with this organism is common. Most children show serologic evidence of infection by 4 years of age. Most of these primary infections with *Pneumocystis* in the normal child are insignificant, with either mild or no clinical disease. Individuals with normal immune systems generally are asymptomatic; reactivation or significant reinfection occurs only when the immune system is compromised. The precise reservoir for the organism in nature is not clear. Although an environmental source has been postulated, it is not known if the organism can exist outside of a living host. In humans and animals, the natural reservoir is the lung. The route of transmission is also unclear. Animal studies have suggested that the spread is airborne, but this remains unclear. Human to human transmission has been raised as a possible explanation of occasional outbreaks, but this remains controversial and respiratory isolation for persons with active *Pneumocystis jiroveci* pneumonia (PCP) does not appear necessary.

P. jiroveci causes an opportunistic infection in immunocompromised hosts. Early on, cases of *Pneumocystis jiroveci* pneumonia (PCP) were described in premature and debilitated infants, institutionalized children, patients with primary immunodeficiency disorders, and adults receiving immunosuppressive medications such as corticosteroids. A defect in the host cell-mediated immunity is the major risk factor for PCP. Thus patients at risk for PCP include persons with AIDS, organ transplant recipients, and persons receiving long-term corticosteroids.

Persons with AIDS are at particularly high risk for PCP and is an important AIDS-defining opportunistic infection. Before the advent of preventative therapy for PCP, about 60% to 80% of AIDS patients developed PCP. Infection with *P. jiroveci* rarely occurs when the CD4 count is >200 cells/µL, with most cases occurring when the CD4 count is <100 cells/µL.

Clinical Syndromes

- ***Pneumocystis jiroveci* pneumonia (PCP):** The initial event of PCP is probably attachment of the trophozoite to type I alveolar pneumocytes. Typically there is no tissue invasion. The organism multiplies in the alveoli and the air space becomes filled with organisms and debris. Patients classically present with fever, dyspnea on exertion, and dry cough. AIDS patients often have a very indolent presentation with symptoms present for several weeks. Other symptoms include chills, chest pain, and sputum production. On examination, patients with PCP have tachypnea and tachycardia, but the auscultation of the lungs may be completely normal. Useful laboratory tests include the arterial blood gas, which shows hypoxia, increased alveolar-arterial oxygen gradient, and respiratory alkalosis in most, but not all, patients. An increase in the serum LDH is also frequently seen. The diffusing capacity of the lung (DLCO) at rest or with exercise is decreased in many cases. The chest radiograph usually shows bilateral, symmetrical interstitial pulmonary infiltrates. A variety of unusual chest x-ray findings have been reported including nodules and cavities. It is important to realize that the chest radiograph may be completely normal in some persons. Pneumothorax is a well-recognized complication in persons with AIDS. In some patients, both the lung examination, arterial blood gas, and chest x-ray are normal.
- **Extrapulmonary pneumocystosis:** Although *P. jiroveci* most commonly involves the lung, cases of *P. jiroveci* infection outside the lung have been reported, particularly in AIDS patients receiving aerosolized pentamidine for PCP prophylaxis. These include retinal infection, lymph nodes, liver and spleen, thyroid, ear lesions, skin lesions, and mastoiditis.

Diagnosis The manifestations of *P. jiroveci* infection in the AIDS patient can be very subtle, and a high index of suspicion must be maintained. Similarly, the non-AIDS patient with PCP may present only with fever and malaise without prominent respiratory symptoms. Laboratory confirmation includes:

- Induced sputum for *P. jiroveci* (usually productive only in immunocompromised patients): Stains for *P. jiroveci* include toluidine blue, methenamine-silver, Giemsa, immunofluorescence, and Calcofluor staining procedures. The sensitivity of induced sputum for *P. jiroveci* in persons with AIDS is widely variable in the literature, ranging from 30% to 90%. This has led to some degree of controversy as to the role of induced sputum for this organism. In some centers with low rates of *P. jiroveci* identification by sputum, the microbiology laboratory will not accept induced sputum for the diagnosis of PCP, and encourage clinicians to obtain bronchoscopic lavage fluid instead. This is meant to avoid misinterpretation of a negative induced sputum. Other institutions readily accept induced sputum specimens.
- Bronchoscopy with or without transbronchial biopsy: Bronchoscopy with lavage (BAL) alone is 98% to 100% sensitive for the detection of *P. jiroveci* in AIDS. The sensitivity is lower in organ transplant recipients. BAL with transbronchial biopsy may be slightly more sensitive than BAL alone but many pulmonologists avoid biopsy given the high sensitivity of BAL.
- Open lung biopsy (infrequently required): This is usually reserved for unusual cases, BAL-negative cases where the diagnosis of PCP is still strong, and in persons who have had "partial prophylaxis" for PCP (ie, the patient intermittently taking PCP prophylaxis).

Diagnostic Tests/Procedures

Methenamine Silver Stain *on page 534*
Pneumocystis jiroveci Test *on page 566*

Treatment The mainstays of therapy for active *P. jiroveci* pneumonia remain sulfamethoxazole and trimethoprim or intravenous pentamidine. Comparison studies have shown these agents are equally efficacious but fewer adverse reactions have been noted with sulfamethoxazole and trimethoprim. Thus, sulfamethoxazole and trimethoprim is considered the agent of choice, usually administered intravenously in serious cases. The standard dose is 15 mg/kg/day in three divided doses intravenously. In
(Continued)

Pneumocystis jiroveci (Continued)

mild cases, oral sulfamethoxazole and trimethoprim may be utilized initially. The standard dose is sulfamethoxazole and trimethoprim DS 2 tablets 3-4 times/day orally. The oral route achieves excellent serum concentrations of the drug with several caveats: (1) the patient must be able to tolerate the number and size of the pills, which is a significant problem for some; (2) the gastrointestinal tract must be functional (ie, no ileus present); (3) there are no problems with malabsorption. Treatment is continued for 21 days. Studies have shown an unacceptable relapse rate at 14 days.

There is still a high incidence of adverse reactions with sulfamethoxazole and trimethoprim in AIDS patients with PCP. Adverse reactions include rash, life-threatening Stevens-Johnson syndrome, neutropenia, increased hepatic enzymes, vomiting, and diarrhea. Over 50% of persons being treated for PCP experience an adverse reaction which is treatment-limiting and necessitates change to another antibiotic. The incidence of adverse reactions is much lower in non-AIDS patients with PCP. Pentamidine is also effective at 4 mg/kg/day I.V. for 21 days. The side effect profile of pentamidine in AIDS-related PCP is even more significant than sulfamethoxazole and trimethoprim, and includes renal failure, hypotension, severe hypoglycemia, cardiac arrhythmias, and diabetes.

Alternative regimens for AIDS-related PCP have been reported including trimethoprim-dapsone, clindamycin-primaquine, atovaquone (well-tolerated but probably less efficacious than the first-line therapies), and trimetrexate with leucovorin.

Administration of corticosteroids has proven effective for the adjunctive treatment of AIDS-related PCP. The rationale for this is based on the observation that morbidity from PCP is related to the host inflammatory response as well as from the organism itself. Patients will often appear "worse before getting better" when appropriate therapy for PCP is initiated. Many will not improve or will actually deteriorate in the first 72 hours. In a randomized clinical trial of AIDS-related PCP, the combination of sulfamethoxazole and trimethoprim and corticosteroid was more effective than sulfamethoxazole and trimethoprim alone for moderate cases. Adjunctive corticosteroids are recommended for patients with PCP who have an alveolar-arterial (A-a) gradient >35 mm Hg or a pO_2 <70 mm Hg on room air. The recommended regimen is prednisone 40 mg oral twice daily for 5 days, then 40 mg oral once daily for 5 days, and 20 mg oral once daily for the rest of the course for a total of 21 days.

Because of the high rate of PCP in persons with AIDS, primary prophylaxis is routine (ie, preventive therapy in persons who have not previously had an episode of PCP). In persons with HIV infection primary prophylaxis for PCP is indicated if any of the following is true:

1. $CD4^+$ T-cell count <200 cells/mm^3 or $CD4^+$ percentage <13%, or
2. thrush, or
3. unexplained fever >100°F for over 2 weeks

The preferred regimen for primary PCP prophylaxis according to the U.S. Public Health Service (USPHS) recommendations in 1999 is:

1. sulfamethoxazole and trimethoprim DS 1 tablet daily, or
2. sulfamethoxazole and trimethoprim SS 1 tablet daily

Alternative regimens for primary PCP prophylaxis include:

1. sulfamethoxazole and trimethoprim DS 1 tablet 3 times/week
2. aerosolized pentamidine 300 mg monthly
3. dapsone 50 mg oral twice daily or 100 mg oral daily
4. dapsone and pyrimethamine (in combination), or
5. atovaquone 1500 mg oral daily

Adverse drug reactions with PCP prophylaxis are common, as with treatment of active PCP. About 25% to 50% of HIV patients discontinue PCP prophylaxis due to adverse reactions and need to be changed to an alternative regimen. Common problems include rash, pruritus, drug fever, leukopenia, diarrhea, and abnormal liver function studies. Strategies used to minimize these problems include graduated dosing of sulfamethoxazole and trimethoprim, "drug holidays" for 2 weeks, thrice weekly dosing (possibly less side effects than daily doses of sulfamethoxazole and trimethoprim), and use of aerosolized pentamidine (2% adverse event rate, but does not prevent extrapulmonary *P. jiroveci* infections). Limited information is available regarding the efficacy of these alternative strategies.

Recently, considerable attention has been paid to the possibility of stopping primary PCP prophylaxis in persons with AIDS who have responded to highly active antiretroviral therapy (HAART). Several studies have been published examining AIDS patients who had a sustained rise in $CD4^+$ T-cell count from <200/µL to >200/µL while on HAART. The incidence of PCP in these studies is extremely low. The USPHS

recommends considering discontinuing primary and secondary PCP prophylaxis when the CD4+ T-cell count was >200 cells/μL for 3-6 months.

Drug Therapy

Recommended:

Sulfamethoxazole and Trimethoprim *on page 1087*

Alternate:

Monotherapy:

Pentamidine *on page 999*
Atovaquone *on page 670*

Combination therapy:

Trimethoprim *on page 1130*
plus
Dapsone *on page 766*

Selected Readings

Bozzette SA, Sattler FR, Chiu J, et al, "A Controlled Trial of Early Adjunctive Treatment With Corticosteroids for *Pneumocystis carinii* Pneumonia in the Acquired Immunodeficiency Syndrome. California Collaborative Treatment Group," *N Engl J Med*, 1990, 323(21):1451-7.

Caliendo AM, "Enhanced Diagnosis of *Pneumocystis carinii*: Promises and Problems," *Clin Microbiol Newslett*, 1996, 18(15):113-6.

Davey RT Jr, Masur H, "Recent Advances in the Diagnosis, Treatment, and Prevention of *Pneumocystis carinii* Pneumonia," *Antimicrob Agents Chemother*, 1990, 34(4):499-504.

Furrer H, Egger M, Opravil M, et al, "Discontinuation of Primary Prophylaxis Against *Pneumocystis carinii* Pneumonia in HIV-1-Infected Adults Treated With Combination Antiretroviral Therapy. Swiss HIV Cohort Study," *N Engl J Med*, 1999, 340(17):1301-6.

National Institutes of Health - University of California Expert Panel for Corticosteroids as Adjunctive Therapy for *Pneumocystis* Pneumonia, "Consensus Statement on the Use of Corticosteroids as Adjunctive Therapy for *Pneumocystis* Pneumonia in the Acquired Immunodeficiency Syndrome," *N Engl J Med*, 1990, 323(21):1500-4.

Phair J, Munoz A Detels R, et al, "The Risk of *Pneumocystis carinii* Pneumonia Among Men Infected With Human Immunodeficiency Virus Type 1," *N Engl J Med*, 1990, 322(3):161-5.

Telzak EE, Cote RJ, Gold JW, et al, "Extrapulmonary *Pneumocystis carinii* Infections," *Rev Infect Dis*, 1990, 12(3):380-6.

U.S. Public Health Service and the Infectious Diseases Society of America, "2001 USPHS/IDSA Guidelines for the Prevention of Opportunistic Infections in Persons Infected With Human Immunodeficiency Virus," www.hivatis.org.

Wachter RM, Russi MB, Bloch DA, et al, "*Pneumocystis carinii* Pneumonia and Respiratory Failure in AIDS," *Am Rev Respir Dis*, 1991, 143(2):251-6.

***Pneumocystis jiroveci* Pneumonia** *see Pneumocystis jiroveci on page 266*

Pneumonia, Aspiration, Community-Acquired

Clinical Presentation Major symptoms are cough, fever, production of sputum, chest pain, and dyspnea. Although aspiration is a common cause of community-acquired pneumonia, it classically occurs in patients who have difficulty swallowing, no gag reflex, who are at high risk for aspirating. Pulmonary consult indicated for diagnostic bronchoscopy.

Differential Diagnosis Congestive heart failure; pulmonary embolism; aspiration of gastric contents; neoplasm; adult respiratory distress syndrome; hypersensitivity pneumonitis; radiation pneumonitis; drug reactions

Likely Pathogens

Streptococcus-Related Gram-Positive Cocci *on page 325*
Streptococcus pneumoniae, Drug-Susceptible *on page 319*
Bacteroides and *Prevotella* Species *on page 46*

Diagnostic Tests/Procedures

•Aerobic Culture, Sputum *on page 367*
•Blood Culture, Aerobic and Anaerobic *on page 391*
•Chest Films *on page 412*
•Gram Stain *on page 473*
Computed Transaxial Tomography, Thorax *on page 426*

Empiric Drug Therapy

Recommended:

Ampicillin and Sulbactam *on page 660*
Clindamycin *on page 752*

Alternate:

Amoxicillin and Clavulanate Potassium *on page 645*

Selected Readings

Bartlett JG, "Anaerobic Bacterial Infections of the Lung," *Chest*, 1987, 91(6):901-9.

Bartlett JG, Dowell SF, Mandell LA, et al, "Practice Guidelines for the Management of Community-Acquired Pneumonia in Adults. Infectious Diseases Society of America," *Clin Infect Dis*, 2000, 31(2):347-82.

Mandell LA, Bartlett JG, Dowell SF, et al, "Update of Practice Guidelines for the Management of Community-Acquired Pneumonia in Immunocompetent Adults," *Clin Infect Dis*, 2003, 37:1405-33.

Croce MA, "Diagnosis of Acute Respiratory Distress Syndrome and Differentiation From Ventilator-associated Pneumonia," *Am J Surg*, 2000 179(2 Suppl 1):26-9.

(Continued)

Pneumonia, Aspiration, Community-Acquired *(Continued)*

Leroy O, Vandenbussche C, Coffinier C, et al, "Community-Acquired Aspiration Pneumonia in Intensive Care Units. Epidemiological and Prognosis Data," *Am J Respir Crit Care Med*, 1997, 156(6):1922-9.
Morehead RS and Pinto SJ, "Ventilator-Associated Pneumonia," *Arch Intern Med*, 2000, 160(13):1926-36.

Pneumonia, Community-Acquired

Related Information

Community-Acquired Pneumonia in Adults *on page 1278*

Synonyms CAP; Community-Acquired Pneumonia; Pneumonia, Primary Atypical; Primary Atypical Pneumonia

Clinical Presentation Major symptoms are cough, fever, production of sputum, chest pain, and dyspnea. Viral or *Mycoplasma* pneumonia typically has prodromal upper respiratory tract phase associated with malaise, headache, sore throat, and nonproductive cough.

Differential Diagnosis Congestive heart failure; pulmonary embolism; aspiration of gastric contents; neoplasm; adult respiratory distress syndrome; hypersensitivity pneumonitis; radiation pneumonitis; drug reactions

Likely Pathogens

Streptococcus pneumoniae, Drug-Susceptible *on page 319*
Mycoplasma pneumoniae on page 238
Legionella pneumophila on page 202
Chlamydophila pneumoniae on page 78
Haemophilus influenzae on page 159

Immunocompromised
  Pneumocystis jiroveci on page 266

Diagnostic Tests/Procedures

Severe Infection
- •Aerobic Culture, Sputum *on page 367*
- •Blood Culture, Aerobic and Anaerobic *on page 391*
- •Chest Films *on page 412*
- •Gram Stain *on page 473*
- *Legionella* Serology *on page 518*
- *Mycoplasma* Serology *on page 545*
- *Mycoplasma*/*Ureaplasma* Culture *on page 545*

Mild Infection
- •Aerobic Culture, Sputum *on page 367*
- •Gram Stain *on page 473*

Drug Therapy Comment Therapy should be directed at the specific pathogen when the pathogen is detected. Empiric treatment and in the setting when no etiologic agent is identified, the recommendations for outpatient care are a macrolide, a fluoroquinolone with good activity against *S. pneumoniae*, or doxycycline. The recommendation for the hospitalized patient is a β-lactam with or without a macrolide or a fluoroquinolone with good activity against *S. pneumoniae*.

Empiric Drug Therapy

Recommended:

Note: When noted below, antipneumococcal fluoroquinolones include gatifloxacin, gemifloxacin, levofloxacin, moxifloxacin, and ofloxacin.

Outpatient:

Previously healthy:
- No recent antibiotic therapy:
  - Macrolides *on page 924*
  - Doxycycline *on page 787*
- Recent antibiotic therapy:
  - Fluoroquinolones *on page 824* (except Ciprofloxacin)
  - *Choice of one of the following*
    - Azithromycin *on page 674*
    - Clarithromycin *on page 749*
    - *plus one of the following*
      - Amoxicillin *on page 642*
      - Amoxicillin and Clavulanate Potassium *on page 645*

Comorbidities (COPD, diabetes, renal or congestive heart failure, malignancy):
- No recent antibiotic therapy:
  - Macrolides *on page 924*
  - Azithromycin *on page 674*
  - Clarithromycin *on page 749*
- Recent antibiotic therapy:
  - Fluoroquinolones *on page 824*
  - *Choice of one of the following*

Azithromycin *on page 674*
Clarithromycin *on page 749*
plus one of the following
Amoxicillin *on page 642*
Amoxicillin and Clavulanate Potassium *on page 645*
Cefpodoxime *on page 714*
Cefprozil *on page 716*
Cefuroxime *on page 725*

Suspected aspiration with infection:
Amoxicillin and Clavulanate Potassium *on page 645*
Clindamycin *on page 752*

Influenza with bacterial superinfection:
Amoxicillin *on page 642*
Amoxicillin and Clavulanate Potassium *on page 645*
Cefpodoxime *on page 714*
Cefprozil *on page 716*
Cefuroxime *on page 725*
Fluoroquinolones *on page 824*

Inpatient:

Medical ward:
No recent antibiotic therapy:
Fluoroquinolones *on page 824*
Choice of one of the following
Azithromycin *on page 674*
Clarithromycin *on page 749*
plus one of the following
Cefotaxime *on page 708*
Ceftriaxone *on page 722*
Ampicillin and Sulbactam *on page 660*
Ertapenem *on page 805*

Recent Antibiotic Therapy:
Choice of one of the following
Azithromycin *on page 674*
Clarithromycin *on page 749*
plus one of the following
Cefotaxime *on page 708*
Ceftriaxone *on page 722*
Ampicillin and Sulbactam *on page 660*
Ertapenem *on page 805*
Fluoroquinolones *on page 824*

ICU:
Pseudomonas infection is not an issue:
One of the following
Cefotaxime *on page 708*
Ceftriaxone *on page 722*
Ampicillin and Sulbactam *on page 660*
Ertapenem *on page 805*
plus one of the following
Azithromycin *on page 674*
Clarithromycin *on page 749*
Fluoroquinolones *on page 824*

Pseudomonas infection is not an issue, but patient is β-lactam allergic:
Fluoroquinolones *on page 824*
with or without
Clindamycin *on page 752*

Pseudomonas infection is an issue:
One of the following
Piperacillin *on page 1002*
Piperacillin and Tazobactam Sodium *on page 1003*
Imipenem and Cilastatin *on page 861*
Meropenem *on page 936*
Cefepime *on page 705*
plus
Ciprofloxacin *on page 742*
One of the following
Piperacillin *on page 1002*
Piperacillin and Tazobactam Sodium *on page 1003*
Imipenem and Cilastatin *on page 861*
Meropenem *on page 936*
Cefepime *on page 705*
plus

(Continued)

Pneumonia, Community-Acquired *(Continued)*

Aminoglycosides *on page 641*
plus one of the following
Fluoroquinolones *on page 824*
Macrolides *on page 924*
Pseudomonas infection is an issue, but patient is β-lactam allergic:
Aztreonam *on page 677*
plus
Levofloxacin *on page 908*
Aztreonam *on page 677*
plus one of the following
Moxifloxacin *on page 949*
Gatifloxacin *on page 837*
with or without
Aminoglycosides *on page 641*
Nursing home:
Receiving treatment in nursing home:
Fluoroquinolones *on page 824*
Amoxicillin and Clavulanate Potassium *on page 645*
plus one of the following
Azithromycin *on page 674*
Clarithromycin *on page 749*
Hospitalized - See treatment for medical ward and ICU.

Selected Readings

Bartlett J, "Treatment of Community-Acquired Pneumonia," *Chemotherapy*, 2000, 46 (Suppl 1): 24-31.

Bartlett JG, Dowell SF, Mandell LA, et al, "Practice Guidelines for the Management of Community-Acquired Pneumonia in Adults. Infectious Diseases Society of America," *Clin Infect Dis*, 2000, 31(2):347-82.

Fein AM, "Pneumonia in the Elderly: Overview of Diagnostic and Therapeutic Approaches," *Clin Infect Dis*, 1999, 28(4):726-9.

Fine MJ, Smith MA, Carson CA, et al, "Prognosis and Outcomes of Patients With Community Acquired Pneumonia. A Meta-Analysis," *JAMA*, 1995, 275(2):134-41.

Heffelfinger JD, Dowell SF, Jorgensen JH, et al, "Management of Community-Acquired Pneumonia in the Era of Pneumococcal Resistance: A Report From the Drug-Resistant *Streptococcus pneumoniae* Therapeutic Working Group," *Arch Intern Med*, 2000, 160(10):1399-408.

Mandell LA, Bartlett JG, Dowell SF, et al, "Update of Practice Guidelines for the Management of Community-Acquired Pneumonia in Immunocompetent Adults," *Clin Infect Dis*, 2003, 37:1405-33.

McCracken GH Jr, "Etiology and Treatment of Pneumonia," *Pediatr Infect Dis J*, 2000, 19(4):373-7.

Niederman MS, Mandell LA, Anzueto A, et al, "Guidelines for the Management of Adults With Community-Acquired Pneumonia. Diagnosis, Assessment of Severity, Antimicrobial Therapy, and Prevention," *Am J Respir Crit Care Med*, 2001, 163(7):1730-54.

Pneumonia, Hospital-Acquired

Synonyms Hospital-Acquired Pneumonia

Clinical Presentation Major symptoms are cough, fever, production of sputum, chest pain, and dyspnea. Although aspiration is a common cause of community-acquired pneumonia, it classically occurs in patients who have difficulty swallowing, no gag reflex, and who are at high risk for aspirating. Pulmonary consult indicated for diagnostic bronchoscopy.

Differential Diagnosis Congestive heart failure; pulmonary embolism; aspiration of gastric contents; neoplasm; adult respiratory distress syndrome; hypersensitivity pneumonitis; radiation pneumonitis; drug reactions

Likely Pathogens

Pseudomonas aeruginosa on page 282
Enterobacter Species *on page 132*
Klebsiella Species *on page 200*
Serratia Species *on page 296*
Staphylococcus aureus, Methicillin-Susceptible *on page 307*

Diagnostic Tests/Procedures

•Aerobic Culture, Sputum *on page 367*
•Chest Films *on page 412*
•Gram Stain *on page 473*
Clinical Pulmonary Infection Score (CPIS)

Drug Therapy Comment

Vancomycin added only if evidence of gram-positive infection.

Empiric Drug Therapy

Recommended:

Patients with no known risk factors for multidrug-resistant pathogens, early onset, and any disease severity:

Streptococcus pneumoniae, *Haemophilus influenzae*, methicillin-sensitive *Staphylococcus aureus*, antibiotic-sensitive enteric gram-negative bacilli:

Ceftriaxone *on page 722*
Levofloxacin *on page 908*
Moxifloxacin *on page 949*
Ciprofloxacin *on page 742*
Ampicillin and Sulbactam *on page 660*
Ertapenem *on page 805*

Patients with risk factors for multidrug-resistant pathogens, late-onset disease, and all disease severity:

Streptococcus pneumoniae, *Haemophilus influenzae*, methicillin-sensitive *Staphylococcus aureus*, antibiotic-sensitive enteric gram-negative bacilli, MDR pathogens, MRSA:

One of the following

Cefepime *on page 705*
Ceftazidime *on page 717*
Imipenem and Cilastatin *on page 861*
Meropenem *on page 936*
Piperacillin and Tazobactam Sodium *on page 1002*

plus one of the following

Ciprofloxacin *on page 742*
Levofloxacin *on page 908*
Amikacin *on page 639*
Gentamicin *on page 841*
Tobramycin *on page 1122*

plus one of the following

Linezolid *on page 914*
Vancomycin *on page 1144*

Selected Readings

American Thoracic Society and Infectious Diseases Society of America, "Guidelines for the Management of Adults With Hospital-Acquired, Ventilator-Associated, and Healthcare-Associated Pneumonia," *Am J Respir Crit Care Med*, 2005, 171(4):388-416.

Chastre J, Fagon JY, and Trouillet JL, "Diagnosis and Treatment of Nosocomial Pneumonia in Patients in Intensive Care Units," *Clin Infect Dis*, 1995, 21(Suppl 3):S226-37.

Croce MA, "Diagnosis of Acute Respiratory Distress Syndrome and Differentiation From Ventilator-associated Pneumonia," *Am J Surg*, 2000, 179(2 Suppl 1):26-9.

"Guidelines for the Management of Adults With Hospital-Acquired, Ventilator-Associated, and Healthcare-Associated Pneumonia," *Am J Respir Crit Care Med*, 2005, 171:388-416.

Joshi N, Localio AR, Hamory BH, "A Predictive Risk Index for Nosocomial Pneumonia in the Intensive Care Unit," *Am J Med*, 1992, 93(2):135-42.

Mandell LA and Campbell GD Jr, "Nosocomial Pneumonia Guidelines, an International Perspective," *Chest*, 1998, 113(3 Suppl):188S-93S.

Morehead RS and Pinto SJ, "Ventilator-associated Pneumonia," *Arch Intern Med*, 2000, 160(13):1926-36.

Pneumonia, Primary Atypical *see* Pneumonia, Community-Acquired *on page 270*

Pneumonia, Ventilator-Associated

Synonyms VAP; Ventilator-Associated Pneumonia

Clinical Presentation Ventilator-associated pneumonia (VAP) is defined as nosocomial pneumonia in a patient on mechanical ventilatory support for ≥48 hours. Development of pneumonia typically follows a progression from colonization with aspiration of upper airway secretions and is greatly facilitated by the mechanical interruption of normal airway defenses. Repeat intubation, nasogastric tubes, supine position, therapeutic immobilization/paralytic agent use, and neurological disease are all risk factors for the development of pneumonia. In addition, immune compromise (due to disease or drug therapy) increases the risk of ventilator-associated pneumonias. Contaminated equipment or aerosolization of hospital flora (including *Legionella*) have also been described as contributors to the development of specific outbreaks.

Colonization of the oropharynx by nosocomial species occurs rapidly in the hospitalized patient, often within 48 hours of admission. Due to the interruption of mechanical and immunologic defenses, intubated patients are at increased risk for organisms to gain access to the lower respiratory tract. Endotracheal intubation has been associated with a risk for the development of pneumonia at a rate of approximately 1% to 3% per day. Overall, between 10% and 50% of endotracheally intubated patients develop pneumonia. Mortality in patients with ventilator-associated pneumonia is extremely high, generally between 25% and 50%, and may approach 80% in high-risk groups.

(Continued)

Pneumonia, Ventilator-Associated *(Continued)*

Diagnosis of pneumonia in ventilated patients is difficult. Typical clinical symptoms (leukocytosis, new pulmonary infiltrate, purulent sputum) are nonspecific in critically ill patients, and are unreliable as the sole basis for diagnosis of VAP. Diminished efficiency of gas exchange, decreased pulmonary compliance or increased FiO_2 requirements may signal the development of pneumonia, but are also consistent with many other disease processes. Endotracheal aspirate cultures are sensitive, but have a low specificity and are of very limited value as a means to establish the cause of VAP. Protected specimen brush and bronchoalveolar lavage provide improved specificity. Quantitative culture and microscopic examination of lower respiratory tract secretions improve specificity.

Concurrent isolation of identical organisms from respiratory specimens along with blood or pleural fluid culture may be of particular value, but this applies to only a small number of cases.

Differential Diagnosis Fever in mechanically ventilated patients may be caused by extrapulmonary infection, inflammation, transfusion, or drug reaction. Pulmonary infiltrates may be due to chemical aspiration, pleural effusion, congestive heart failure, tumor, or hemorrhage. Both fever and pulmonary infiltrates occur in pulmonary embolism, atelectasis, and late acute respiratory distress syndrome (fibroproliferative stage).

Likely Pathogens Note: Infections are frequently polymicrobial.

Staphylococcus aureus, Methicillin-Resistant *on page 304*
Pseudomonas aeruginosa on page 282
Enterobacter Species *on page 132*
Klebsiella Species *on page 200*
Acinetobacter Species *on page 24*
Citrobacter Species *on page 81*
Escherichia coli on page 142
Stenotrophomonas maltophilia on page 312
Anaerobes in obstruction
Aspergillus Species *on page 38* (fungal infections)

Diagnostic Tests/Procedures

Culture, Protected Brush Catheter *on page 433*
Culture, Quantitative, Lower Respiratory Tract *on page 434*

Drug Therapy Comment Ventilator-associated pneumonia may be cause by pathogens associated with community acquired pneumonias, as well as a far greater percentage of gram-negative pathogens. Development of pneumonia has been associated with suppression of gastrointestinal acidity from stress ulcer prophylaxis; however, the risk resulting from this therapeutic intervention remains controversial. Implementation of appropriate therapy at the earliest stage is of critical importance. Empiric therapy must be instituted/adjusted with an awareness of local pathogens and susceptibilities.

Empiric Drug Therapy

Recommended:

Patients with no known risk factors for multidrug-resistant pathogens, early onset, and any disease severity:

Streptococcus pneumoniae, *Haemophilus influenzae*, methicillin-sensitive *Staphylococcus aureus*, antibiotic-sensitive enteric gram-negative bacilli:

Ceftriaxone *on page 722*
Levofloxacin *on page 908*
Moxifloxacin *on page 949*
Ciprofloxacin *on page 742*
Ampicillin and Sulbactam *on page 660*
Ertapenem *on page 805*

Patients with risk factors for multidrug-resistant pathogens, late-onset disease, and all disease severity:

Streptococcus pneumoniae, *Haemophilus influenzae*, methicillin-sensitive *Staphylococcus aureus*, antibiotic-sensitive enteric gram-negative bacilli, MDR pathogens, MRSA:

One of the following

Cefepime *on page 705*
Ceftazidime *on page 717*
Imipenem and Cilastatin *on page 861*
Meropenem *on page 936*
Piperacillin and Tazobactam Sodium *on page 1002*

plus one of the following

Ciprofloxacin *on page 742*
Levofloxacin *on page 908*

Amikacin *on page 639*
Gentamicin *on page 841*
Tobramycin *on page 1122*
plus one of the following
Linezolid *on page 914*
Vancomycin *on page 1144*

Selected Readings

Chastre J and Fagon JY, "Ventilator-Associated Pneumonia," *Am J Respir Crit Care Med*, 2002, 165(7):867-903.

"Guidelines for the Management of Adults With Hospital-Acquired, Ventilator-Associated, and Health-care-Associated Pneumonia," *Am J Respir Crit Care Med*, 2005, 171:388-416.

Iregui M, Ward S, Sherman G, et al, "Clinical Importance of Delays in the Initiation of Appropriate Antibiotic Treatment for Ventilator-Associated Pneumonia," *Chest*, 2002, 122(1):262-8.

Mayhall CG, "Ventilator-Associated Pneumonia or Not? Contemporary Diagnosis," *Emerg Infect Dis*, 2001, 7(2):200-4.

Pneumonic Plague *see Yersinia pestis on page 355*
Poliomyelitis *see* Poliovirus *on page 275*

Poliovirus

Microbiology Polioviruses are single-stranded RNA viruses which cause poliomyelitis, a central nervous system disease of once epidemic proportions. They belong to the family Picornaviridae (pico-, very small; rna-, ribonucleic acid; -viruses) and the genus Enterovirus. Thus, polioviruses are closely related to such agents as Coxsackieviruses, Enteroviruses, and ECHO viruses. Polioviruses have three distinct serotypes (types 1-3). Infection with one serotype (either natural or vaccine-related) confers serotype-specific immunity; reinfection with a different serotype has been reported.

The virus is tropic for neural tissue. Polioviruses have a narrow tissue tropism in comparison with other Enteroviruses. Polioviruses attach to anterior horn cells of spinal cord gray matter, motor neurons, and dorsal root ganglia by means of a specific receptor (cellular adhesion molecules). The neurovirulence of "wild-type" strains (ie, strains present in the general population) varies enormously. The viral strains used in the polio vaccines are of low neurovirulence and can be distinguished from wild-type strains by means of genomic sequencing and other molecular techniques.

Epidemiology Poliovirus infections were epidemic in the United States in the first half of the twentieth century. In the 1950s, epidemics occurred on a regular basis with an attack rate of 17 cases per 100,000. The introduction of the inactivated polio vaccine (IPV) by Jonas Salk in 1955 was one of the great advances in modern medicine. This introduction was followed soon afterwards by the live-attenuated oral polio vaccine (OPV) developed by Albert Sabin. A striking decline in paralytic and nonparalytic polio cases followed. With the extensive use of the OPV in both North and South America, wild-type strains of polio have nearly disappeared in the Western hemisphere, despite the large number of children who are inadequately immunized. The year 1979 marked the last reported case of endemic, wild-type poliomyelitis in the United States. The most recent case of wild-type paralytic poliomyelitis in either North or South America came from Peru in August 1991. Cases of acute flaccid paralysis continue to be screened by aggressive surveillance programs, but additional wild-type cases have not been recognized through 1992 and the first half of 1993.

Although naturally-occurring cases have been eliminated in this country, rare cases of vaccine-related poliomyelitis still occur. Each of the 5-10 annual cases in the United States can be directly linked to the OPV vaccine. Vaccine-related infections have been reported in recipients of the OPV (usually children), as well as close contacts of vaccine recipients (usually adults). Some experts believe that wild-type polioviruses have essentially been replaced with Sabin vaccine strains; these vaccine strains now circulate widely in the population, presumably causing asymptomatic or mild infections. Poliomyelitis still occurs with some frequency in developing countries outside North and South America. About 120,000 cases were recognized in 1992, mainly in sub-Saharan Africa and the Indian subcontinent. Global eradication of this infection is still possible, although there are multiple factors which account for the persistence of disease. Reintroduction of wild-type polioviruses into the United States from foreign visitors or travelers to endemic areas remains a concern, and justifies continued immunization programs.

Although infection can be induced in experimental animals, humans are believed to be the only natural host of the virus. The infectious cycle begins when the host ingests materials which contain contaminated feces (ie, a fecal-oral route of transmission). Active viral replication takes place in the oropharynx (particularly the tonsils) and in the distal portion of the small bowel (Peyer's patches, intestinal mucosa). This replication is followed by a transient phase of "minor viremia" where virus particles spread hematogenously to various organs and lymph nodes. In the majority of cases,

(Continued)

Poliovirus *(Continued)*

the infection is aborted at this stage by the host immune system; only subclinical or asymptomatic infection results ("abortive poliomyelitis"). Less commonly, viral replication is not controlled by immunologic mechanisms, and virus proliferates in the liver, spleen, marrow, and nodes. This is followed by a "major viremia" in which visceral organs are again seeded hematogenously, including the brain and spinal cord. This "major viremia" corresponds with the prodromal symptoms of poliomyelitis (fever, malaise). The incubation period between exposure and the onset of symptoms has been estimated at 5-35 days.

Clinical Syndromes

- **Asymptomatic illness:** As with other enteroviral infections, the vast majority of infections with poliovirus are asymptomatic, and never go on to develop clinical illness.
- **Aseptic meningitis:** Patients present with fever, headache, and nuchal rigidity. Cerebrospinal fluid characteristically reveals a mild lymphocytic (predominantly polymorphonuclear leukocytes early on, the lymphocytic) with elevated protein in the 40-50 mg/dL range. In some cases the virus may be directly cultured from CSF with cytopathic effect in cell culture in 1 week. There is a rapid clinical recovery within 2-10 days. Poliovirus is a relatively rare cause of the syndrome of aseptic meningitis is indistinguishable from the aseptic meningitis caused by other, more common viruses.
- **Abortive poliomyelitis:** This occurs in <10% of polio cases. Patients develop a nonspecific viral syndrome with fever, sore throat, malaise, and abdominal discomfort. Symptoms resolve quickly and there is no progression to paralytic polio.
- **Bulbar poliomyelitis:** In this form of polio, patients initially present with dysphagia and a change in speech due to paralysis of the muscles of the pharynx. Most commonly there is involvement of cranial nerves IX and X, although others may be involved.
- **Polioencephalitis:** Infants are most susceptible to this uncommon manifestation of poliovirus infection. There is alteration in the level of consciousness and seizures are common.
- **Paralytic poliomyelitis:** This is the most feared complication of poliovirus infection and occurs in less that 1 in 1000 cases. Risk factors for this syndrome include prior tonsillectomy, trauma, immunodeficiency, pregnancy, and others. Following an incubation period of 1-5 weeks, patients typically enter a period of "minor illness" (corresponding to viremia), consisting of a flu-like illness with fever, nausea, malaise, headache, sore throat, and vomiting. This nonspecific illness lasts several days then resolves completely. The "major illness" occurs about 1 week later. Patients develop a meningitic syndrome with fever and neck stiffness, along with severe muscle pain often involving the limbs and back. This is followed by the onset of muscle paralysis and weakness. The extent of muscle involvement is highly variable. In mild cases, an isolated muscle group may develop weakness. In severe cases, there may be complete quadriplegia with flaccid paralysis and loss of reflexes. The most common presentation is weakness of one leg or one arm. An important clue to the diagnosis of polio is asymmetric flaccid paralysis. The deficit is purely motor in nearly all cases. Loss of sensation is not part of paralytic poliomyelitis and should bring to mind other diagnoses such as Guillain-Barré syndrome. Following this initial attack, there may be a period of recovery of strength, but this is variable. This is followed by a long period of stability and many persons are able to function at a nearly normal level.
- **Postpolio syndrome:** This syndrome has received much attention in both the medical and lay press. There are roughly 300,000 persons who survived the last epidemic of poliomyelitis in the 1950s, and it appears that all are at risk for the postpolio syndrome. About 30 years after the initial bout of paralytic polio, some individuals have developed fatigue, muscle weakness, and sometimes pain. Most commonly the same muscle group(s) originally involved years ago are once again involved, but in some cases "new" muscle groups also develop weakness. This phenomenon was initially dismissed as being nonorganic, but recent evidence strongly suggests it is a disorder of the motor unit, with objective evidence of ongoing denervation by electromyogram and muscle biopsy even in asymptomatic patients. Although many persons may potentially develop this syndrome, the degree of muscle weakness is not as severe as the original bout of polio and it tends not to progress.
- **Vaccine-related paralytic polio:** Approximately 8-10 cases of vaccine-related poliomyelitis occur in the U.S. annually. This is caused by the OPV which is a live-attenuated vaccine. Most cases have been reported in infants <6 months of age; many of whom have an underlying B-cell immunodeficiency. Contacts of children can also develop vaccine-related polio, and this tends to be in an older age group. The risk of vaccine-related polio is very low, estimated at 1 case in 2 million.

The clinical course is similar to infection caused by wild-type polio. Vaccine-related polio appears to be declining in the U.S. due to the use of IPV in routine vaccinations since 1997.

Diagnosis Polioviruses are readily isolated in tissue culture. The highest yield for the virus is from the pharynx early in the illness. Later, virus remains viable in the stool for up to 1 month. The virus is difficult to isolate from cerebrospinal fluid.

Diagnostic Tests/Procedures

Poliovirus Serology *on page 567*
Viral Culture, Central Nervous System Symptoms *on page 614*
Viral Culture, Stool *on page 616*
Viral Culture, Throat *on page 617*

Drug Therapy Comment No antiviral agents proven effective, and the focus remains on prevention. From 1963 to 1997, the OPV was used in the U.S. for routine polio immunization and during this time period polio infection was successfully eradicated. In part, the OPV was initially chosen over the IPV because the latter was less potent and breakthrough cases of polio were known to have occurred in the 1950s despite three immunizations with the IPV. However, although wild-type polio had been eradicated in the U.S. and the potential for imported cases decreasing dramatically, the focus shifted from imported cases to the few devastating cases of vaccine-related polio each year. In addition, recent formulations of IPV became more effective and immunogenic than in the past, with seroconversion rates at least equal to the OPV. Efforts were made in the past decade to switch to the IPV for routine administration. The American Academy of Pediatrics in 1999 and the Centers for Disease Control Advisory Committee on Immunization Practices (ACIP) recommended the exclusive use of IPV for routine immunization of children. The OPV is reserved for occasional travelers to a polio-endemic area. In developing countries, the OPV is routinely used due to the higher cost of the IPV.

Selected Readings

Centers for Disease Control and Prevention, "Poliomyelitis Prevention in the United States: Updated Recommendation of the Advisory Committee on Immunization Practices (ACIP)," *MMWR*, 2000, 49(RR-5):1-38.

Colecraft CM, "An Update on Polio," *Clin Microbiol Newslett*, 1998, 20(8):67-72.

Foege WH, "A World Without Polio," *JAMA*, 1993, 270(15):1859-60.

Melnick JL, "Current Status of Poliovirus Infections," *Clin Microbiol Rev*, 1996, 9(3):293-300.

Modlin JF, "Poliovirus," *Principles and Practice of Infectious Diseases*, 5th ed, Mandell GL, Bennett JE, and Dolin R, eds, New York, NY: Churchill Livingstone, 2000, 1895-1903.

Munsat TL, "Poliomyelitis - New Problems With an Old Disease," *N Engl J Med*, 1991, 324(17):1206-7.

Pontiac Fever *see Legionella pneumophila on page 202*

Posadas-Wernicke's Disease *see Coccidioides immitis on page 91*

Postabortal Endometritis *see* Endometritis *on page 127*

Postpartum Endometritis (PPE) *see* Endometritis *on page 127*

Postsurgical Meningitis *see* Meningitis, Postsurgical *on page 218*

Post-traumatic Meningitis *see* Meningitis, Post-traumatic *on page 219*

Powassan Encephalitis *see* Arboviruses *on page 35*

***Prevotella* Species** *see Bacteroides* and *Prevotella* Species *on page 46*

Primary Atypical Pneumonia *see* Pneumonia, Community-Acquired *on page 270*

Primary Genital Herpes *see* Herpes Simplex Virus *on page 172*

Prostatitis

Clinical Presentation Acute prostatitis typically occurs in young males but may be associated with indwelling urethral catheters. Characterized by fever, chills, dysuria, and a tense or extremely tender prostate on palpation. Chronic form may present as asymptomatic bacteriuria with a normal palpable prostate. May have intermittent symptoms of frequency, urgency, and dysuria.

Prostatitis is a common syndrome which has been estimated to account for up to 25% of office visits by young and middle-age males presenting with genitourinary symptoms. Prostatitis encompasses four distinct syndromes:

Acute bacterial prostatitis: Acute presentation with chills, fever, lower back pain, genital pain, urinary frequency, nocturia, dysuria, myalgia, and usually a tense or extremely tender prostate on palpitation with a confirmed urinary tract infection.

Chronic bacterial prostatitis: Symptoms of acute prostatitis associated with an underlying structural abnormality of the prostate, which acts as a nidus for bacterial persistence. **Note:** Chills, fever, and myalgia are often absent in chronic prostatitis.

Chronic prostatitis/chronic pelvic pain syndrome: Common but poorly understood form of prostatitis. May occur in males of any age; often associated with intermittent symptomatology. Typically characterized as inflammatory or noninflammatory. In the inflammatory form, urine, semen, and other fluids from the prostate show evidence of inflammatory response/infection without an identifiable

(Continued)

Prostatitis *(Continued)*

organism. White blood cells and other indications of inflammation are absent in the noninflammatory form.

Asymptomatic inflammatory prostatitis: Seminal fluid contains inflammatory cells but the patient does not complain of typical symptoms. Usually identified during an evaluation of infertility or prostate cancer testing.

Differential Diagnosis Bacterial; nonbacterial; prostatodynia; malignancy; BPH; STD

Likely Pathogens

Candida Species *on page 67*
Borrelia vincentii
Streptococcus Species *on page 326*

Acute:
Neisseria gonorrhoeae *on page 244*
Chlamydia trachomatis *on page 74*
Escherichia coli *on page 142*

Chronic: May be nonbacterial. Bacterial species may include:
Enterococcus Species *on page 134*
Pseudomonas aeruginosa *on page 282*

Diagnostic Tests/Procedures

- Genital Culture *on page 470*
- Gram Stain *on page 473*
- *Neisseria gonorrhoeae* Culture *on page 547*
- Urine Culture, Clean Catch *on page 609*

Drug Therapy Comment Alpha-blockers may be helpful in the setting of chronic prostatitis.

Acute prostatitis should be treated for 4 weeks to prevent the development of chronic prostates. Only approximately 50% of chronic prostatitis will respond to a 1-3 month course of antimicrobial therapy. Patients should be referred to urology for evaluation for possible surgical intervention.

Empiric Drug Therapy

Recommended:

Antimicrobial treatment depends on organism identified or suspected pathogens.

Younger males: Typically treated for gonorrhea or *Chlamydia*:
One of the following:
Ofloxacin *on page 977*
Ceftriaxone *on page 722*
plus
Doxycycline *on page 787*

Older males:
Ciprofloxacin *on page 742*
Sulfamethoxazole and Trimethoprim *on page 1087*

Chronic prostatitis may require up to 3 months of treatment:
Fluoroquinolones *on page 824*
Sulfamethoxazole and Trimethoprim *on page 1087*

Selected Readings

Barbalias GA, Nikiforidis G, and Liatsikos EN, "Alpha-Blockers for the Treatment of Chronic Prostatitis in Combination With Antibiotics," *J Urol*, 1998, 159(3):883-7.

"National Guideline for the Management of Prostatitis. Clinical Effectiveness Group (Association of Genitourinary Medicine and the Medical Society for the Study of Venereal Diseases)," *Sex Transm Infect*, 1999, 75 Suppl 1:S46-50.

Pewitt EB and Schaeffer AJ, "Urinary Tract Infection in Urology, Including Acute and Chronic Prostatitis," *Infect Dis Clin North Am*, 1997, 11(3):623-46.

Roberts RO, Lieber MM, Rhodes T, et al, "Prevalence of a Physician-Assigned Diagnosis of Prostatitis: The Olmsted County Study of Urinary Symptoms and Health Status Among Men," *Urology*, 1998, 51(4):578-84.

Stevermer JJ and Easley SK, "Treatment of Prostatitis," *Am Fam Physician*, 2000, 61(10):3015-22, 3025-6.

Prosthetic Valve Endocarditis, Early *see* Endocarditis, Prosthetic Valve, Early *on page 124*

Prosthetic Valve Endocarditis, Late *see* Endocarditis, Prosthetic Valve, Late *on page 125*

Proteus Species

Microbiology *Proteus* species are facultative, gram-negative bacilli which belong to the large family Enterobacteriaceae. These organisms are considered "enteric bacilli" because they commonly inhabit the gastrointestinal tract. The two most clinically important *Proteus* species are *Proteus mirabilis* and *Proteus vulgaris*. Biochemically, nearly all strains of *P. mirabilis* are indole-positive; all other clinically relevant *Proteus*

species such as *Proteus vulgaris* are indole-negative. *Proteus* species characteristically "swarm" (spread) over the surface of a moist agar plate. The organisms have several features that promote urinary tract infections including fimbriae which facilitate colonization of the organism in the urinary tract and flagella which facilitate motility in the urinary system. In addition, *Proteus* species have the unique ability to produce urease to hydrolyze urea (found in urine of the human host) to ammonium hydroxide which can lead to renal calculi formation and urinary tract infections.

Epidemiology *Proteus* species are found in soil, water, and fecally contaminated materials. They are found in human feces and are considered part of the normal fecal flora. *Proteus* species are some of the most frequently isolated and clinically significant Enterobacteriaceae. In some studies, *Proteus mirabilis* is the second leading cause of community-acquired urinary tract infections, second only to *E. coli*. Aside from urinary tract infections, *Proteus* species rarely cause serious disease in otherwise healthy individuals. However, they are an important cause of hospital-acquired infections in debilitated patients and account for up to 10% to 15% of nosocomial infections in the United States.

Clinical Syndromes

- **Urinary tract infections:** The ability of *P. mirabilis* to hydrolyze urea to ammonia causes a rise in the urine pH. This alkaline urine leads to precipitation of magnesium, calcium, and ammonium and ultimately forms a type of kidney stone called struvite or triple phosphate stones. These stones act as obstructing foreign bodies and can lead to hydronephrosis, chronic and recurrent *Proteus mirabilis* urinary tract infections, pyelonephritis, and renal abscess. As a rule, it is difficult to treat urinary tract infections in the presence of a renal stone; medical therapy with antibiotics alone is often unsuccessful and patients are at risk for urosepsis if the stone is not removed.
- **Pneumonia:** Like other gram-negative bacilli, *Proteus* species can cause serious nosocomial pneumonia particularly in debilitated, ventilator-dependent individuals.
- **Surgical wound infections:** *Proteus* species can cause serious postoperative wound infections, either alone or as part of a polymicrobial infection, particularly in contaminated abdominal wounds.
- **Chronic destructive ear infections:** These organisms have been recovered in patients with a chronic, destructive otitis media similar to necrotizing otitis caused by *Pseudomonas aeruginosa*. This entity can involve the mastoids and central nervous system.
- **Septicemia:** Debilitated hospitalized patients can develop a life-threatening *Proteus* septicemia, most often from a urinary source. Other common origins include biliary tract sepsis (*Proteus* sp are part of the normal fecal flora), abdominal abscesses, catheter-associated bacteremia, and others.

Diagnosis The diagnosis of *P. mirabilis* infection is made by isolation of the organism from appropriate body fluids (urine, sputum, blood, etc). No special culture isolation methods are necessary; *Proteus* species grow readily in standard blood cultures and on solid media. The finding of chronic urinary tract infection in the setting of struvite stones is highly suggestive of *Proteus mirabilis* infection; particularly if there is a consistently high urinary pH.

Diagnostic Tests/Procedures

Aerobic Culture, Appropriate Site *on page 365*
Gram Stain *on page 473*

Treatment The treatment of *Proteus* infections depends in part on the species involved. *Proteus mirabilis* (indole-negative *Proteus*) was once generally susceptible to most beta-lactams, cephalosporins, and aminoglycosides, but increasing numbers of community-acquired isolates are becoming resistant to these agents. Final antimicrobial selection should be based on antibiotic susceptibility tests. Indole-positive *Proteus* species (including *Proteus vulgaris*) are more commonly hospital-acquired strains and tend to be more antibiotic-resistant than *P. mirabilis*. Multiple beta-lactam resistant *Proteus* strains are becoming more common, as are aminoglycoside-resistant strains; antimicrobial susceptibility testing is crucial in the proper selection of treatment for hospital-acquired *Proteus* infections.

Drug Therapy

Recommended:

Cephalosporins, 3rd Generation *on page 730*
Cephalosporins, 1st Generation *on page 729*
Cephalosporins, 2nd Generation *on page 729*

Alternate:

Carbapenems *on page 693*
Fluoroquinolones *on page 824*
Penicillins, Extended-Spectrum *on page 997*

Selected Readings

Bonnet R, De Champs C, Sirot D, et al, "Diversity of TEM Mutants in *Proteus mirabilis*," *Antimicrob Agents Chemother*, 1999, 43(11):2671-7

(Continued)

Proteus Species *(Continued)*

Coudron PE, Moland ES, and Thomson KS, "Occurrence and Detection of AmpC Beta-Lactamases among *Escherichia coli*, *Klebsiella pneumoniae*, and *Proteus mirabilis* Isolates at a Veterans Medical Center," *J Clin Microbiol*, 2000, 38(5):1791-6.

de Champs C, Bonnet R, Sirot D, et al, "Clinical Relevance of *Proteus mirabilis* in Hospital Patients: A Two Year Survey," *J Antimicrob Chemother*, 2000, 45(4):537-9.

Eisenstein BI, "Diseases Caused by Gram-Negative Enteric Bacilli," *Harrison's Principles of Internal Medicine*, 13th ed, Isselbacher KJ, Braumwald E, Wilson JD, et al, eds, New York, NY: McGraw-Hill Inc, 1994, 664.

Mobley HL and Belas R, "Swarming and Pathogenicity of *Proteus mirabilis* in the Urinary Tract," *Trends Microbiol*, 1995, 3(7):280-4.

Prototheca Species

Microbiology *Prototheca* species are unicellular algae which are becoming increasingly recognized as a cause of opportunistic infection. Presently there are three recognized species: *Prototheca wickerhamii*, *P. zopfii*, and *P. stagnora*. These organisms are fungus-like saprophytes which are spherical and about 3-30 µm in size. *Prototheca* lack chlorophyll and reproduce asexually by endosporulation; the presence of endospores helps identify the organism on wet mounts. The organism grows well on Sabaroud-dextrose agar.

Epidemiology *Prototheca* is ubiquitous in the environment (fresh water, soil, trees, and sewage). Human protothecal infections are unusual, with about 60 cases reported in the literature. These cases are distributed worldwide. Approximately 50% of the reported cases have been in immunocompromised individuals, such as organ transplant recipients, diabetics, and persons with malignancies. Rare cases have been reported in otherwise healthy hosts.

Clinical Syndromes Because of the low incidence of this infection, generalizations about clinical syndromes is difficult. Case reports have included the following.

- **Skin and soft tissue infection:** This appears to be the most common presentation and may be associated with some form of trauma. Patients develop single, usually painless lesion in the skin or subcutaneous tissue which fails to heal spontaneously. Cases of postoperative soft-tissue infection and cutaneous infections in the absence of surgery or other trauma have been reported. The skin lesion may be indurated, plaque-like, nodular, ulcerated, or even vesicular.
- **Olecranon bursitis:** Some cases reported after trauma.
- **Infection of continuous ambulatory peritoneal dialysis (CAPD) catheters.**
- **Nasopharyngeal ulceration:** Single case report following prolonged endotracheal intubation
- **Meningitis:** Single case report in a patient with AIDS.
- **Disseminated protothecosis:** Two cases have been reported in immunocompetent persons who presented with abdominal pain.

Diagnosis Laboratory confirmation is necessary to make a diagnosis of protothecosis since the clinical syndromes are nonspecific. The organisms may be seen on wet mounts of infected material and can be identified by its characteristic size, morphology, and endospores. Isolation of the organism on fungal media is confirmatory.

Biopsy specimens of infected soft tissue typically show granulomatous inflammation, necrosis, giant cells and chronic inflammation. Microabscesses may also be present. Numerous organisms are typically seen in tissue specimens and stain well with Gomori methenamine silver.

Diagnostic Tests/Procedures

Fungus Culture, Appropriate Site *on page 461*
Methenamine Silver Stain *on page 534*

Treatment The treatment of human protothecosis is controversial, in part due to the limited number of cases. Serious infections have been treated with amphotericin B. Surgical debridement has been used in many of the reported cases of skin and soft tissue infections; adjunctive amphotericin B has been suggested for deeper soft tissue lesions. Bursectomy has been performed in several patients with olecranon bursitis. All patients who developed CAPD catheter infection with prototheca were treated with catheter removal and antifungal agents. *Prototheca* is resistant to flucytosine, and this agent should be avoided. The role of imidazole antifungal agents is not clear. Some cases have responded to fluconazole and ketoconazole, but available data is limited.

Drug Therapy

Recommended:

Amphotericin B (Conventional) *on page 650*

Alternate:

Fluconazole *on page 819*
Ketoconazole *on page 903*

Selected Readings

Iacoviello VR, De Girolami PC, Lucarini J, et al, "Protothecosis Complicating Prolonged Endotracheal Intubation: Case Report and Literature Review," *Clin Infect Dis*, 1992, 15(6):959-67.

Kaminski ZC, Kapila R, Sharer LR, et al, "Meningitis Due to *Prototheca wickerhamii* in a Patient With AIDS," *Clin Infect Dis*, 1992, 15(4):704-6.

Providencia Species

Microbiology The *Providencia* species are members of the Enterobacteriaceae family. The genus *Providencia* consists of four species, *Providencia rettgeri*, *Providencia alcalifaciens*, *Providencia stuartii*, and *Providencia rustiganii*. These organisms can be differentiated by biochemical and cultural differences. These organisms are considered "enteric bacilli" because they commonly inhabit the gastrointestinal tract. All *Providencia* species are indole-positive, and *P. rettgeri* and some strains of *P. stuartii* are urease-positive. All members of the tribe have O, H, and K antigens. The most important human pathogen species is *P. stuartii*.

Epidemiology Members of the family Enterobacteriaceae can be found as normal colonizers of human and animal intestinal tracts and are commonly found in soil and on plants. *Providencia* species, as well as others in the tribe, are common sources of nosocomial infections, particularly in the urinary tract. Although other members of the family have higher incidences of nosocomial infections and increased antibacterial resistance, *P. stuartii* in particular remains an important and difficult pathogen in this regard.

Clinical Syndromes

- **Urinary tract infections:** Although typically not a cause of community-acquired urinary tract infections, *P. stuartii* is an important pathogen in nosocomial urinary tract infections. Patients particularly at risk are those with catheters, underlying urologic disorders, paraplegia, or advanced age.
- **Pneumonia:** Like other gram-negative bacilli, *Providencia* species can cause serious nosocomial pneumonia, particularly in debilitated, ventilator dependent individuals. Other Enterobacteriaceae cause nosocomial pneumonia more commonly.
- **Septicemia:** Debilitated hospitalized patients can develop life-threatening *Providencia* septicemia, most commonly from a urinary tract source. Other Enterobacteriaceae cause septicemia more often.
- **Gastrointestinal disease:** *P. alcalifaciens* has been associated with outbreaks of gastroenteritis and may have a possible role in the etiology of infectious diarrhea. *P. stuartii* may also be implicated.

Diagnosis The diagnosis of *Providencia* species infections is made by isolation of the organism from the appropriate body fluid (urine, sputum, blood, etc). No special culture isolation methods are necessary; *Providencia* species grow readily in standard blood cultures and on solid media.

Diagnostic Tests/Procedures

Aerobic Culture, Appropriate Site *on page 365*
Blood Culture, Aerobic and Anaerobic *on page 391*
Gram Stain *on page 473*

Treatment *Providencia* species are typically sensitive to second and third generation cephalosporins, extended-spectrum penicillins, carbapenems, quinolones, and aminoglycosides, although increased resistance to all of these drugs has occurred. Gentamicin susceptibility is often variable. Antimicrobial susceptibility testing is crucial in the proper selection of treatment for hospital-acquired *Providencia* infections, with final selection based on susceptibility tests. Sulfamethoxazole and trimethoprim is also active, particularly in patients with urinary tract infections.

Drug Therapy

Recommended:

Cephalosporins, 2nd Generation *on page 729*
Cephalosporins, 3rd Generation *on page 730*
Sulfamethoxazole and Trimethoprim *on page 1087*

Alternate:

Carbapenems *on page 693*
Penicillins, Extended-Spectrum *on page 997*

Selected Readings

Cornaglia G, Frugoni S, Mazzariol A, et al, "Activities of Oral Antibiotics on *Providencia* Strains Isolated From Institutionalized Elderly Patients With Urinary Tract Infections," *Antimicrob Agents Chemother*, 1995, 39(12):2819-21.

"Enterobacteriaceae," *Bailey & Scott's Diagnostic Microbiology*, Chapter 27, St Louis, MO: CV Mosby Co, 1990, 363-85.

Hawkey BM, "*Providencia stuartii*: A Review of a Multiple Antibiotic Resistant Bacterium," *J Antimicrob Chemother*, 1984, 13:209-26.

Mandell GL, Bennett JE, and Dolin R, *Principles and Practice of Infectious Diseases*, 4th ed, Chapter 196, New York, NY: Churchill Livingstone, 1995.

"Opportunistic Enterobacteriaceae," *Zinsser Microbiology*, 20th ed, Chapter 36, Joklik WK, Willett HP, Amos DB, et al, eds, Norwalk, CT: Appleton & Lange, 1992, 469-70.

Pseudomembraneous Colitis (PMC) *see Clostridium difficile on page 85*

Pseudomonas aeruginosa

Related Information

Community-Acquired Pneumonia in Adults *on page 1278*

Microbiology *Pseudomonas aeruginosa* is a lactose-negative, oxidase-positive, nonfermenting, aerobic, gram-negative bacillus with a single flagellum (usually). Strains that produce polysaccharide capsules (glycocalyx) are mucoid in colony appearance, with some strains producing diffusible blue, yellow, or brown pigments (pyocyanin, fluorescein, pyorubin, respectively). *Pseudomonas aeruginosa* can grow on almost all laboratory media at temperatures from 10°C to 40°C. (Optimal growth is at 35°C.)

Epidemiology *Pseudomonas aeruginosa* is ubiquitous; therefore, isolation of the organism on hospital equipment, sinks, etc, is not unexpected and by itself not meaningful. *Pseudomonas aeruginosa* is often considered an opportunistic pathogen because disease occurs most often in patients with neutropenia or neutrophil dysfunction, tissue damage, or other altered host defenses. Presence of *Pseudomonas aeruginosa* in clinical specimens may be contamination or colonization unless accompanied by a correlating clinical scenario.

In the hospital setting, up to 90% of patients staying in intensive care units for more than 7 days may become colonized with *P. aeruginosa*. In some burn centers, up to 30% of infections can be attributed to *P. aeruginosa*. *Pseudomonas aeruginosa* is also responsible for approximately 10% of nosocomial infections.

Clinical Syndromes *Pseudomonas aeruginosa* can infect any tissue or organ system including blood, lung, heart, ear, eye, urinary tract, gastrointestinal tract, or musculoskeletal system. Syndromes caused by *Pseudomonas aeruginosa* are usually indistinguishable from those caused by the Enterobacteriaceae with several exceptions. Patients with bacteremia or pneumonia caused by *Pseudomonas aeruginosa* have a higher mortality rate that when caused by the Enterobacteriaceae. *Pseudomonas aeruginosa* is the second most common organism infecting burn patients. Malignant otitis externa is characteristically caused by *P. aeruginosa*.

Diagnosis The only way a diagnosis of *Pseudomonas aeruginosa* infection can be made is by identification of the organism through culture in a patient with a relevant clinical syndrome. No special media or conditions are necessary to grow this organism.

Diagnostic Tests/Procedures

Aerobic Culture, Appropriate Site *on page 365*
Gram Stain *on page 473*

Treatment Combination of an antipseudomonal penicillin or ceftazidime plus an aminoglycoside is the standard therapy. Combination therapy is necessary for additive or synergistic affects as well as potentially decreasing the emergence of resistant pseudomonal strains. Combination therapy improves outcome in patients with *Pseudomonas aeruginosa* bacteremia. Quinolones and imipenem are active against *Pseudomonas aeruginosa* and should also be used in combination with aminoglycosides in the treatment of serious infection. Quinolones may be used with an antipseudomonal beta-lactam in the treatment of serious *Pseudomonas aeruginosa* infections; in theory, the different mechanisms of action of the two drug classes should be at least additive. Double beta-lactam therapy should be avoided.

Pediatric Drug Therapy

Recommended:

Urinary tract infection:
- Ceftazidime *on page 717*
- Penicillins, Extended-Spectrum *on page 997*

Adult Drug Therapy

Recommended:

Severe infection:
- Ceftazidime *on page 717*
  plus
  Aminoglycosides *on page 641*
- Penicillins, Extended-Spectrum *on page 997*
  plus
  Aminoglycosides *on page 641*
- Cefepime *on page 705*
  plus
  Aminoglycosides *on page 641*

Alternate:

Urinary tract infection:
- Ceftazidime *on page 717*
- Penicillins, Extended-Spectrum *on page 997*
- Fluoroquinolones *on page 824*

Severe infection:

Imipenem and Cilastatin *on page 861*

or

Meropenem *on page 936*

plus

Aminoglycosides *on page 641*

Ciprofloxacin *on page 742*

plus

Penicillins, Extended-Spectrum *on page 997*

Selected Readings

Bhandary S, Karki P, and Sinha BK, "Malignant Otitis Externa: A Review," *Pac Health Dialog*, 2002, 9(1):64-7.

Davies JC, "*Pseudomonas aeruginosa* in Cystic Fibrosis: Pathogenesis and Persistence," *Paediatr Respir Rev*, 2002, 3(2):128-34.

Fleiszig SM and Evans DJ, "The Pathogenesis of Bacterial Keratitis: Studies With *Pseudomonas aeruginosa*," *Clin Exp Optom*, 2002, 85(5):271-8.

Garau J and Gomez L, "*Pseudomonas aeruginosa* Pneumonia," *Curr Opin Infect Dis*, 2003, 16(2):135-43.

Kang CI, Kim SH, Kim HB, et al, "*Pseudomonas aeruginosa* Bacteremia: Risk Factors for Mortality and Influence of Delayed Receipt of Effective Antimicrobial Therapy on Clinical Outcome," *Clin Infect Dis*, 2003, 37(6):745-51.

Mendelson MH, Gurtman A, Szabo S, et al, "*Pseudomonas aeruginosa* Bacteremia in Patients With AIDS," *Clin Infect Dis*, 1994, 18(6):886-95.

Pollack M, "*Pseudomonas aeruginosa*," *Principles and Practice of Infectious Diseases*, 5th ed, Mandell GL, Bennett JE, and Dolin R, eds, New York, NY: Churchill Livingstone 2000, 3210-335.

Wilson R and Dowling RB, "Lung Infections. 3. *Pseudomonas aeruginosa* and Other Related Species," *Thorax*, 1998, 53(3):213-9.

Psittacosis *see Chlamydia psittaci on page 73*

PVE, Early *see* Endocarditis, Prosthetic Valve, Early *on page 124*

PVE, Late *see* Endocarditis, Prosthetic Valve, Late *on page 125*

Pyelonephritis *see* Urinary Tract Infection, Pyelonephritis *on page 346*

Pyomyositis *see* Myositis *on page 242*

Q Fever *see Coxiella burnetii on page 100*

Rabies *see* Rabies Virus *on page 283*

Rabies Virus

Microbiology Rabies virus is a bullet-shaped single-stranded RNA virus which belongs to the family Rhabdoviridae. A number of important viral proteins have been identified such as viral polymerase, nucleocapsid protein, glycoprotein, and others. Some of these proteins have been used to develop specific diagnostic monoclonal antibodies. Rabies virus can be isolated under the proper conditions in tissue culture. During active rabies infection, the virus can be cultured from a variety of human (and animal) tissues including saliva, brain tissue, respiratory secretions, and urine; the virus is most easily recovered from brain tissue.

The virus is highly neurotropic. When a human is inoculated with rabies virus, the viral glycoprotein attaches to the plasma membrane of cells, possibly the nicotinic acetylcholine receptor. The virus then replicates in skeletal muscle, and when the titer is high enough, it invades nearby sensory and motor nerves and enters the nervous system. It travels along the axon at speeds up to 20 mm/day and eventually reaches the spinal cord. From there, dissemination through the central nervous system occurs rapidly and encephalitis ensues. Other peripheral nerves become involved; the organism can be recovered from the saliva due to infection of nerves in the salivary glands.

Epidemiology Rabies remains primarily a disease of animals, not humans. In many areas of Asia, Africa, and Latin America, canine rabies is poorly controlled, and dogs account for up to 90% of animal rabies cases. In contrast, in Europe and the United States, dogs account for a much lower percentage of cases. In the United States, different species of animals are involved in well-defined geographic areas. For example, raccoons are important in two regions, the eastern seaboard states (New York, New Jersey, Delaware, Maryland, Virginia) and some southeastern states (Florida, South Carolina, Georgia, Alabama). Skunks predominate in the north central states and California, gray foxes in Texas and Arizona, and coyotes in southern Texas. A total of 10 distinct geographic areas in the United States have been identified; one terrestrial animal predominates and one antigenic variant of the rabies virus predominates. Bats remain an important reservoir of rabies and cause sporadic cases.

Human rabies is distinctly unusual in the United States although it is still problematic in some areas worldwide. In large part, this is due to the control of canine rabies in this country. Between 1980 and 1993, there were 18 reported cases of rabies in the United States with 10 of these acquired outside the country. Of the rabies cases reported since 1960, the great majority involved males younger than 16 years of age

(Continued)

Rabies Virus *(Continued)*

or older than 50 years of age. Most cases in the United States are now reported from the following groups:

- U.S. travelers to foreign countries who sustain a dog bite in a rabies-endemic region
- persons bitten by wild animals in the U.S.
- persons with unknown exposure history

A few cases of "nonbite rabies" have been reported. These include:

- laboratory exposure to rabies virus (aerosolized virus)
- rabies contracted from corneal transplant from an infected donor (4 cases)
- inhalation of aerosolized virus in caves with high concentrations of bat secretions (rare)
- contact of virus on mucous membranes, scratches, or eyes (rare)

Clinical Syndromes

- **Clinical rabies:** There is a variable period of incubation before the onset of symptoms (4 days to 19 years), but most cases occur within 1 year of exposure. The initial prodrome of rabies is nonspecific with malaise, fatigue, and fever. In many patients, there may be pain at the initial exposure site. After about 10 days, the patient enters an acute neurologic phase, characterized by bizarre behavior, hyperactivity, and confusion. A small stimulus can elicit short periods of thrashing, biting, and other behaviors. Many patients will display hydrophobia (fear of water); there is often severe laryngospasm and choking when trying to drink water. This will progress to paralysis, which dominates the clinical picture for some days. Patients typically lapse into coma and develop respiratory failure or arrhythmias, leading to death in most cases despite full support in intensive care units. Occasional cases of recovery from rabies have been reported.

Diagnosis Currently, there are no tests available to detect rabies prior to the development of symptoms. The virus is felt to be immunologically "protected" in the muscle cells or nerve cells near the inoculation site, and antibody production occurs late in infection. Rabies encephalitis may be difficult to distinguish from other forms of viral encephalitis. Laboratory tests available include:

- rabies neutralizing antibody
- rabies viral culture of saliva, cerebrospinal fluid, urine, respiratory secretions
- brain biopsy - specimens may be submitted for rabies viral culture; immunofluorescent rabies antibody staining of brain cells; and pathologic examination for Negri bodies, which are cytoplasmic inculsions characteristic of rabies encephalitis seen in 20% to 30% of cases.

Diagnostic Tests/Procedures

Brain Biopsy *on page 405*
Rabies Detection *on page 569*

Treatment There is currently no treatment for rabies once it has become clinically established. Mortality approaches 100%. Thus, the main treatment issues involve rabies prevention, particularly postexposure prophylaxis. The physician deciding whether or not to initiate rabies treatment (rabies vaccine, rabies immunoglobulin) must answer the following questions: Has a significant exposure occurred, and what is the risk that an animal is rabid?

A significant exposure includes the following.

- An animal bite, defined as penetration of the person's skin by teeth with contamination of the wound with saliva
- Contamination of the mucous membranes with saliva or other potentially infectious tissue from an infected animal
- Certain nonbite exposures, including contamination of scratches, scrapes, wounds, or mucous membranes with saliva or other infectious tissues. The risk of rabies after nonbite exposures is extremely rare, although scattered cases have been reported.

Petting a rabid animal or contacting its blood or body fluids is not an exposure. If it appears that a significant exposure has taken place, the physician must determine whether or not the animal was rabid. As outlined by Fishbein and Robinson, this depends on the percentage of animals found to be rabid in the species in the particular geographical area.

Group 1: Rabies is endemic in animal species involved in exposure. This includes:

- bats - anywhere in the United States (3% to 20% positive for rabies)
- terrestrial animals - skunks, raccoons, foxes in areas of United States where rabies is endemic
- dogs in developing countries
- dogs in the United States along the Mexican border.

For Group 1 exposure, treatment should be initiated for both bite and nonbite exposures.

Group 2: Rabies is not endemic in species involved but is endemic in other wild animals in the area. The risk of rabies is about 10 times lower in these animals compared with the predominant species. These animals include:

- wild carnivores such as wolves, bobcats, bears, and groundhogs. Up to 20% may have rabies. Bite exposures from these should be treated. Nonbite exposures should either be treated or the local health department consulted.
- rodents (squirrels, hamsters, guinea pigs, gerbils, rats, mice) have a low incidence of rabies, 0.01%. Bite exposures should not be treated (or in exceptional cases, the local health department could be consulted). Nonbite exposures should not be treated.
- dogs and cats - in the United States, the risk of rabies in dogs is <1% (except along the Mexican border) in areas where rabies is common in other land animals. In addition, dogs almost always show signs of clinical rabies shortly after the virus is present in saliva. Bite exposure should not be treated if a healthy dog (or cat) is captured; the animal should be observed for 10 days. If the animal develops signs of rabies, treatment in the human should be commenced immediately. If the animal is a stray, it should be sacrificed immediately and the head removed and shipped to an appropriate laboratory. Treatment is delayed pending laboratory testing. The same approach is recommended for nonbite exposures.

Group 3: Rabies is not endemic in the animal species involved in the exposure and is uncommon in other wild animals in the region. This incudes most domestic cats and dogs and wild land animals in Idaho, Washington, Utah, Nevada, and Colorado, where the proportion of rabid animals is very low. For bite or nonbite exposures from Group 3 animals, either consult the local health department or do not treat.

Postexposure treatment consists of:

1. Vigorous wound cleaning - this has been shown to decrease the risk of rabies.
2. Administration or rabies vaccine, either human diploid-cell rabies vaccine or rabies vaccine adsorbed. For persons not previously vaccinated, rabies vaccine should be given 1 mL I.M. on days 0, 3, 7, 14, and 28. Abbreviated regimens have been described. For persons previously vaccinated, the rabies vaccine should be given 1 mL I.M. on days 0 and 3.
3. Administration of rabies immunoglobulin. For persons not previously vaccinated, this should be given at 20 IU/kg of body weight. If possible, one-half the dose should be injected locally near the original wound and the rest given I.M. (using a new needle). For persons previously vaccinated, rabies immunoglobulin is not recommended.

Drug Therapy

Recommended:

Rabies Virus Vaccine *on page 1034*

Rabies Immune Globulin (Human) *on page 1034*

Selected Readings

Bleck TP and Rupprecht CE, "Rabies Virus," *Principles and Practice of Infectious Diseases*, 5th ed, Mandell GL, Bennett JE, and Dolin R, eds, New York, NY: Churchill Livingstone, 2000, 1811-20.

Centers for Disease Control and Prevention, "Compendium of Animal Rabies Prevention and Control, 2000," July 14, 2000, 49(RR08):19-30.

Fishbein DB and Robinson LE, "Rabies," *N Engl J Med*, 1993, 329(22):1632-8.

Smith JS, "New Aspects of Rabies With Emphasis on Epidemiology, Diagnosis, and Prevention of the Disease in the United States," *Clin Microbiol Rev*, 1996, 9(2):166-76.

Smith JS, "Rabies," *Clin Microbiol Newslett*, 1999, 21(3):17-23.

Recurrent Genital Herpes *see* Herpes Simplex Virus *on page 172*

Red Eye *see* Conjunctivitis *on page 93*

Respiratory Syncytial Virus

Synonyms RSV

Microbiology Respiratory syncytial virus (RSV) is the most common cause of bronchiolitis and pneumonia in infants and children. It is also emerging as a pathogen of the elderly and the immunosuppressed.

RSV is a single-stranded, enveloped RNA virus belonging to the family Paramyxoviridae, and comprises its own genus, *Pneumovirus*. The viral genome codes for at least 10 separate genes. The virus lacks neuraminidase or hemagglutinating activity, which differentiates it from other paramyxoviruses, such as parainfluenza and mumps virus. There are two major subgroups of RSV, group A or B, based on the presence of different surface glycoprotein antigens. The clinical significance of this strain variation is still unknown. RSV is rarely isolated from asymptomatic children and is thus not part of the normal flora.

As with other pathogenic viruses, RSV requires a tissue culture system in the laboratory to support its growth. Clinical specimens can be successfully inoculated onto a

(Continued)

Respiratory Syncytial Virus *(Continued)*

variety of cell lines. Of note, live virus from patient secretions can survive for a period of time on environmental surfaces. On a nonporous surface such as a countertop, the virus is still viable up to 7 hours. On a porous surface such as tissue paper or clothing, survival is decreased to about 1 hour.

Epidemiology Infections with RSV are common worldwide, regardless of climate. There is a definite seasonal occurrence to RSV infections, tending to occur almost exclusively in the winter and spring in temperate climates; in temperate climates there is a sharp peak in colder months. In many communities, RSV outbreaks occur every year without fail and often in a very predictable pattern, and at its peak in a season, RSV dominates influenza and other respiratory viruses. Based on studies to determine the prevalence of specific RSV antibody, it appears that nearly all children have been infected with RSV before entering school. Estimates of the attack rates vary according to age. In children younger than 2 years of age, the attack rate for lower respiratory infections was from 9-23 out of 1000, from 2-3 years old it was 7-15 out of 1000, and in the 4-5 year age group, it was 5-8 out of 1000. However, the attack rate for all forms of infection including mild infections is probably much higher based on prospective studies, with some studies estimating 6 per 100. The attack rate is extremely high in daycare centers, approaching 100%.

Recurrent infections with RSV are the rule. With each episode of clinical illness, progressively milder forms of infection are seen. Specific neutralizing antibodies develop (IgG, IgM, and secretory IgA) but are not protective. The reason for this is unclear and is not explained by differences in RSV serotypes.

Transmission can be by several routes: self-inoculation of the eyes or nares following contact with contaminated secretions; self-inoculation following contact with contaminated fomites; or aerosol spread, when infected individuals are coughing or sneezing (large droplet spread only).

Clinical Syndromes

In children, the major manifestations of RSV include:

- **Upper respiratory infection:** This often mimics the common cold, along with significant fever and profuse rhinorrhea. Typically, lower respiratory infections are preceded by several days of upper tract symptoms.
- **Bronchiolitis:** This is one of the most common manifestations of RSV and is particularly prevalent in infants 2-6 months of age. It is characterized by wheezing, cough, and tachypnea (sometimes 80 breaths per minute) reflecting the hallmark inspiratory and expiratory obstruction of the lower respiratory tract in bronchiolitis. Fever of 38°C to 40°C is common. Chest radiographs may reveal infiltrates, but these are felt to be due to atelectasis and not alveolar consolidation. Most recover spontaneously or with supportive care only, although 1% to 2% may require hospitalization. Bronchiolitis is difficult to separate from pneumonia, and some may have both.
- **Pneumonia:** The presentation of RSV pneumonia is similar to bronchiolitis. Lower respiratory infection in young children is estimated to complicate up to 70% of RSV infections. Chest radiograph abnormalities vary from interstitial infiltrates to consolidation (usually upper and/or middle lobes). Hyperinflation is common. The radiographic findings, however, are not distinctive enough to differentiate RSV pneumonia from other infectious causes of pneumonia, including bacterial pathogens. Fatalities are still uncommon with the notable exception of children with underlying congenital heart disease, pulmonary disease, or compromised immune system.
- **Croup:** RSV is an uncommon cause of croup, accounting for about 5% to 10% of croup cases.
- **Otitis media:** This is quite common in infants. Otitis media may be either primary infection (with symptoms localized to the ear only) or may be secondary to RSV infection elsewhere (usually in the lower respiratory tract).
- **Apnea and the sudden infant death syndrome (SIDS):** Infants with lower respiratory tract infections with RSV have frequent apneic episodes but are self-resolving. Although the cause of SIDS is still unknown, RSV and other respiratory viruses have been implicated due to the frequent recovery of these pathogens from the lungs of infants with SIDS.

Infections in adults:

- **Upper respiratory tract infections:** In adults, RSV commonly causes an upper respiratory infection somewhat more severe than the common cold. Nasal congestion and cough are prominent, and symptoms may be prolonged, lasting over 1 week. Otalgia is less common in adults. Episodes are self-resolving, but the severity of the URI may cause some to be bedridden for several days.
- **Lower respiratory tract infection:** Tracheobronchitis and pneumonia are relatively uncommon in the otherwise healthy adult. In the elderly patient or the

individual with chronic bronchitis, pneumonia can be quite fulminant and clinically mimics the disease as seen in infants. Outbreaks of RSV in the elderly are associated with a high incidence of pneumonia, perhaps up to 50%.

- **Nosocomial infection:** RSV is an important cause of nosocomial viral respiratory infections, both in adults and children. This is particularly problematic in pediatric wards where children are hospitalized during an outbreak of RSV; the virus spreads efficiently to the adult staff with nearly 50% infected.

Diagnosis RSV infection is suspected when there is a compatible clinical presentation, particularly in the setting of a known community outbreak. In the infant and young child, the diagnosis is often made clinically during an outbreak, with microbiologic confirmation reserved for serious or atypical cases. In the adult, RSV infection mimics other viral and bacterial causes of respiratory illness. Routine laboratory studies such as the complete blood count and electrolyte panel are not helpful in making the diagnosis. Microbiological confirmation of RSV is generally unnecessary for mild upper respiratory infections but may be useful in suspected lower respiratory infections or infections in the immunocompromised host. Potentially this may avoid unnecessary antibiotics or invasive diagnostic testing.

There are several laboratory methods available:

1. Viral culture: RSV grows best in continuous cell lines of human origin, such as HEp-2 cells. The virus causes a characteristic cytopathic effect in the cell lines (syncytial formation) from which its name is derived. Culture results may not be available for several days and not considered as sensitive as EIA (see below).
2. Direct fluorescent antibody (DFA) detection: This rapid method can detect the presence of RSV in specimens within hours but requires a specimen with cellular material.
3. Enzyme immunoassays (EIA): Another rapid test with results available on the same day. This test is considered the test of choice.
4. Serologic studies: A fourfold rise in titer of specific antibody to RSV is diagnostic but not useful for immediate diagnosis or treatment.

Diagnostic Tests/Procedures

Respiratory Syncytial Virus Antigen by EIA *on page 571*
Respiratory Syncytial Virus Culture *on page 572*
Respiratory Syncytial Virus Serology *on page 572*

Treatment Treatment is generally supportive, with supplemental oxygen and fluid replacement as needed. Most mild to moderate cases are self-resolving. Severe cases in infants have been treated with the antiviral agent ribavirin, administered as an aerosol. Ribavirin has been shown to improve arterial blood gas values in hypoxic infants, but improvement in mortality or duration of hospitalization has not been demonstrated. Corticosteroids are also not recommended for routine management of bronchiolitis caused by RSV.

Prophylaxis with palivizumab is very effective in preventing RSV infections and is recommended for high-risk patients, including those with prematurity, bronchopulmonary dysplasia, and congenital heart disease.

Drug Therapy

Recommended:

Ribavirin *on page 1040*

Selected Readings

Baker KA and Ryan ME, "RSV Infection in Infants and Young Children. What's New in Diagnosis, Treatment, and Prevention?" *Postgrad Med*, 1999, 106(7):97-9, 103-4, 107-8 passim.
Bonnet D, Schmaltz AA, and Feltes TF, "Infection by the Respiratory Syncytial Virus in Infants and Young Children at High Risk," *Cardiol Young*, 2005, 15(3):256-65.
Chavez-Bueno S, Mejias A, Jafri HS, et al, "Respiratory Syncytial Virus: Old Challenges and New Approaches," *Pediatr Ann*, 2005, 34(1):62-8.
Ebbert JO and Limper AH, "Respiratory Syncytial Virus Pneumonitis in Immunocompromised Adults: Clinical Features and Outcome," *Respiration*, 2005, 72(3):263-9.
Falsey AR and Walsh EE, "Respiratory Syncytial Virus Infection in Adults," *Clin Microbiol Rev*, 2000, 13(3):371-84.
Falsey AR, Hennessey PA, Formica MA, et al, "Respiratory Syncytial Virus Infection in Elderly and High-Risk Adults," *N Engl J Med*, 2005, 352(17):1749-59.
Moscona A, "Management of Respiratory Syncytial Virus Infections in the Immunocompromised Child," *Pediatr Infect Dis J*, 2000, 19(3):253-4.
Simoes EA, "Respiratory Syncytial Virus Infection," *Lancet*, 1999, 354(9181):847-52.
Smith DW, Frankel LR, Mathers LH, et al, "A Controlled Trial of Aerosolized Ribavirin in Infants Receiving Mechanical Ventilation for Severe Respiratory Syncytial Virus Infection," *N Engl J Med*, 1991, 325(1):24-9.
Vega R, "Rapid Viral Testing in the Evaluation of the Febrile Infant and Child," *Curr Opin Pediatr*, 2005, 17(3):363-7.

Reticuloendotheliosis *see Histoplasma capsulatum on page 177*

Rheumatic Fever *see Streptococcus pyogenes on page 321*

Rheumatic Fever Criteria (Jones Criteria) *see Streptococcus pyogenes on page 321*

Rhodococcus equi *see Rhodococcus* Species *on page 288*

Rhodococcus Species

Applies to *Corynebacterium equi*; *Rhodococcus equi*

Microbiology *Rhodococcus* species are gram-positive, aerobic organisms that may appear as cocci or pleomorphic short or long rods with branching. They are partially acid-fast due to the presence of mycolic acid in their cell walls. There are 16 species of *Rhodococcus* with four species known to be pathogenic in humans. *Rhodococcus equi* is the most common human pathogen and is most typically seen in immunocompromised hosts, particularly in patients with AIDS, lymphoreticular malignancies, and renal transplants. *Rhodococcus* species are members of the informal phylogenetic group actinomycetes.

Although *Rhodococcus* species grows well on routine nonselective media at 35°C, it may be difficult to isolate and identify. They may be misidentified as colonizing diphtheroids, especially in respiratory specimens. It may also be misdiagnosed as a mycobacterial infection given its clinical presentation of cavitary lung lesions with granuloma formation and positive acid-fast stains. They appear on agar as small as 1-3 mm, round, raised, buff to salmon colored colonies. The red-orange pigment that is produced seems to correlate with its ability to produce plasmid-mediated beta-lactamase. *R. equi* is catalase-positive, nonspore-forming, and nonmotile. The various species are differentiated by colonial morphology, biochemical analysis, and DNA analysis.

Epidemiology *Rhodococcus* species are ubiquitous in the environment. *R. equi* can be found widespread in domestic animals and their environment. *R. equi* causes suppurative bronchopneumonia, lymphadenitis, and enteritis in foals less than 6 months of age. The role of animals or soil in transmission is unclear, however, 30% to 50% of infected patients report an exposure to farm animals. It is believed that the primary lesion develops in the lung following inhalation of the soilborne organisms and disseminated hematogenously. Cutaneous inoculation from trauma is the most common mode of transmission in skin, soft tissue, and bone infections.

Clinical Syndromes

- **Pulmonary:** Onset of illness is insidious and the disease progresses slowly. Patients initially present with fever and cough. Chest pain, dyspnea, and weight loss occur over time. Pleural effusions and consolidation may occur but cavitary pneumonia is the most common presentation. Unilobar involvement of one of the lower lobes is most commonly seen on chest radiograph. Associated with cavitary lung lesions in HIV-infected individuals. Pneumonia may be chronic or relapsing. Bacteremia is present in approximately 33%. Mortality is approximately 25%.
- **Skin and soft tissue:** Approximately 50% occurs in immunocompetent hosts. May present as cellulitis, wound infection, subcutaneous nodules, or abscess.
- **CNS:** Has been identified as cause of lymphocytic meningitis in normal host. Meningitis and brain abscess are uncommon manifestations.
- **Endophthalmitis:** Associated with penetrating ocular injuries.
- **Other:** Has been implicated as cause of lymphadenitis, osteomyelitis, paraspinal abscess, pericarditis, peritonitis, pelvic abscesses, and enteritis.

Diagnosis Recovery of organism from sputum may be difficult because the morphology of the organism is similar to that of diphtheroids. Respiratory specimens collected via bronchoscopy, percutaneous drainage, or biopsy may be necessary. Morphological stains including acid-fast are helpful, but isolation and identification of organism is mandatory. Histopathology reveals inflammatory reaction with formation of granulomas which may be caseating. Organisms may be seen intracellular in macrophages. Infected histiocytes are strongly PAS-positive with coarsely granular cytoplasmic inclusions similar to those found in Whipple's disease.

Diagnostic Tests/Procedures

Acid-Fast Stain *on page 361*
Aerobic Culture, Appropriate Site *on page 365*
(Notify laboratory to look for *Rhodococcus*)
Histopathology *on page 496*
Periodic Acid-Schiff Stain *on page 563*

Treatment The best medical management for *Rhodococcus* species is unknown. Relapses are common; therefore, a prolonged course of antibiotics is recommended. Two to 6 weeks of parenteral antibiotics followed by 4-6 weeks of oral antibiotics that achieve high intracellular concentrations are recommended. Penicillins, ampicillin, and first-generation cephalosporins are not recommended due to frequently reported resistance that emerges during therapy with these agents. Erythromycin, sulfamethoxazole and trimethoprim, clarithromycin, and azithromycin all achieve high intracellular concentrations. Clindamycin and chloramphenicol may also be effective. Erythromycin is known to be synergistic with rifampin and are the drugs of choice in veterinary medicine Although vancomycin has poor intracellular penetration, it is very active against *R. equi in vitro*. Imipenem appears to be very effective as well.

Drug Therapy Comment Erythromycin (I.V.) and rifampin (I.V. or oral) can be used initially; rifampin (oral) absorption is excellent in patients with functional GI tract.

Drug Therapy

Recommended:

Erythromycin *on page 807*
plus
Rifampin *on page 1046*

Alternate:

Vancomycin *on page 1144*
Imipenem and Cilastatin *on page 861*

Selected Readings

Capdevila JA, Buján S, Gavaldà J, et al, "*Rhodococcus equi* Pneumonia in Patients Infected With the Human Immunodeficiency Virus. Report of 2 Cases and Review of the Literature," *Scand J Infect Dis*, 1997, 29(6):535-41.

De Marais PL and Kocka FE, "*Rhodococcus* Meningitis in an Immunocompetent Host," *Clin Infect Dis*, 1995, 20(1):167-9.

Frame BC and Petkus AF, "*Rhodococcus equi* Pneumonia: Case Report and Literature Review," *Ann Pharmacother*, 1993, 27(11):1340-2.

Scott MA, Graham BS, Verrall R, et al, "*Rhodococcus equi* - An Increasingly Recognized Opportunistic Pathogen," *Am J Clin Pathol*, 1995, 103(5):649-55.

Rickettsia rickettsii

Microbiology *Rickettsia rickettsii* is the etiologic agent of Rocky Mountain spotted fever (RMSF). The organism is a small coccobacillus measuring 0.2-0.5 μm by 0.3-2.0 μm. It is an obligate intracellular bacteria. The organism can be identified in smears of infected tissue using the Gimenez method, by acridine orange, or by immunofluorescence in tissue sections. The organism does not stain well by Gram stain. The spotted fever group includes other rickettsial species that are human pathogens, specifically *R. sibirica*, the etiologic agent of North Asian tick typhus, *R. conorii*, the etiologic agent of boutonneuse fever, *R. akari*, the etiologic agent of rickettsialpox, and *R. australis*, the etiologic agent of Queensland tick typhus. The cell walls of these organisms contain lipopolysaccharide and ultrastructurally resemble those of gram-negative rods. They cannot be grown in a cell-free medium but can be isolated in cell culture.

Epidemiology Rocky Mountain spotted fever is transmitted by a tick bite. The tick serves as both vector and main reservoir for the disease. *Dermacentor andersoni* (Rocky Mountain wood tick) and *D. variabilis* (American dog tick) are the main vectors in the United States. The tick transmits *Rickettsia* to humans during feeding. The initial bite may not be symptomatic and is frequently not recommended. Infection may occur as the organisms are released from the ticks salivary gland after 4-6 hours of feeding or when the tick is crushed in an attempt to remove it from the skin. The disease is seen primarily in late spring and summer. In the southeast, most cases are observed in children; while in the western states, adults who work in forestry and related industry have the highest incidence of infection. Incidence is related to tick exposure. There have been few western cases in recent years.

Clinical Syndromes The symptoms of Rocky Mountain spotted fever (RMSF) appear 2-14 days after exposure. There is sudden onset of moderate to high fever, myalgia, severe headache, chills, and conjunctival injection. Abdominal symptoms which may include nausea, pain, vomiting, diarrhea, and tenderness are sometimes present. Young patients may not complain of pain. The hallmark rash is maculopapular, appearing on the extremities by the third day and involving the palms and soles of the feet thereafter. Frequently the rash is generalized. Ultimately >90% of patients develop a rash. Late onset or "spotless" fever may delay diagnosis. RMSF without a rash occurs more frequently in blacks and adult patients. The cases are more frequently fatal in blacks than whites, in males, and in adults. Age, glucose-6-phosphate dehydrogenase deficiency, and alcoholism are predispositions to fatal outcome. The organisms target the vascular endothelium. The damaged endothelial cells increase vascular permeability with resultant edema, hypovolemia, hypoalbuminemia, and hypotension. The local vascular injuries consume platelets with resultant thrombocytopenia, although clinical DIC is rare. Lung, kidney, CNS, GI tract, pancreas, and skeletal muscle may be symptomatically involved. The case fatality rate is 15% to 20% if specific therapy is not instituted. Overall reported mortality has been about 4% in recent years.

Diagnosis Diagnosis is based on clinical signs and symptoms. Cutaneous biopsy direct immunofluorescence to identify *R. rickettsii* in tissue is available in some institutions. Specific serologic tests confirm the diagnosis. The Weil-Felix test which relies upon cross reaction with the *Proteus* OX-19 and OX-2 antigens is nonspecific and not reliable. Culture is usually not attempted because of technical demands and the extreme infection risk to laboratory workers.

Diagnostic Tests/Procedures

Polymerase Chain Reaction *on page 567*

(Continued)

Rickettsia rickettsii (Continued)

Rocky Mountain Spotted Fever Serology *on page 573*
Skin Biopsy, Immunofluorescence *on page 583*

Duration of Therapy 7 days or at least 2 days after the patient becomes afebrile

Treatment Patients with severe systemic symptoms should receive supportive therapy. Pulmonary edema caused by extravasation of fluid into the alveolar spaces requires careful management as does overall fluid volume. Doxycycline and tetracycline are considered the drugs of choice. Chloramphenicol is used in pregnant women to avoid the effects of tetracycline on fetal teeth and bones. Chloramphenicol is also favored for children younger than 7 years of age.

The use of erythromycin, β-lactams, aminoglycosides, and sulfamethoxazole and trimethoprim is not indicated.

Pediatric Drug Therapy

Recommended:

<7 years:
Chloramphenicol *on page 733*

>7 years:
Doxycycline *on page 787*
Tetracycline *on page 1106*

Alternate:

>7 years:
Chloramphenicol *on page 733*

Adult Drug Therapy

Recommended:

Doxycycline *on page 787*
Tetracycline *on page 1106*

Alternate:

Chloramphenicol *on page 733*
Ciprofloxacin *on page 742*

Selected Readings

Dumler JS, "Laboratory Diagnosis of Human Rickettsial and Ehrlichial Infections," *Clin Microbiol Newslett*, 1996, 18(8):57-61.
Salgo MP, Telzak EE, Currie B, et al, "A Focus of Rocky Mountain Spotted Fever Within New York City," *N Engl J Med*, 1988, 318(21):1345-8.
Woodward TE, "Rickettsial Diseases," *Harrison's Principles and Practice of Internal Medicine*, 13th ed, Isselbacher KJ, Braunwald E, Wilson JD, et al, eds, New York, NY: McGraw-Hill, 1994, 747-57.

Rift Valley Fever *see* Arboviruses *on page 35*
Ringworm *see* Dermatophytes *on page 114*
RMSF *see Rickettsia rickettsii on page 289*
***Rochalimaea* Species** *see Bartonella* Species *on page 48*
Rocky Mountain Spotted Fever *see Rickettsia rickettsii on page 289*
Rosacea *see* Acne Rosacea *on page 26*
Roseola Infantum *see* Human Herpesvirus-6 *on page 180*

Rotavirus

Microbiology Rotavirus is a double-stranded, nonenveloped RNA virus with two icosahedral capsids which make the virus appear as a wheel (Latin: rota) when viewed with an electron microscope. Rotavirus can be cultured but only in special cell cultures and only by special procedures. Therefore, routine culture of rotavirus is not practical. The traditional rotavirus ("typical" rotavirus) occurs worldwide, usually produces disease in young children, has a common group inner capsid antigen (VP6), and is called group A rotavirus. Nongroup A rotaviruses (groups G through F; "atypical" rotavirus) are newly described. Group B rotavirus is clinically important only in China; group C rotavirus in swine.

Epidemiology Rotaviruses are ubiquitous and are found in all parts of the world. Rotaviruses occur year round in tropical climates and mostly in the winter months in temperate climates. Rotaviruses infect humans and most animals. The most common age group affected by rotaviruses is 6 months to 2 years. Most rotaviruses which are clinically important are members of group A. Rotaviruses primarily are spread by the fecal-oral route. The incubation period for rotaviruses is less than 2 days in infants and 2-4 days in adults. Maximum shedding of rotaviruses occurs 2-5 days after the onset of diarrhea. Infant mortality due to rotavirus infection in developing countries is extremely high; in developed countries, mortality is rare. Rotavirus usually does not cause chronic disease.

Clinical Syndromes Rotavirus can cause asymptomatic to fatal disease. The most common form of rotavirus infection is sudden onset of vomiting and diarrhea. Common clinical presentations include vomiting, abdominal pain, diarrhea, and dehydration. Fever is present in ~50% of the cases. Rotavirus disease usually lasts 3-9

days, and hospitalization often is required. Nosocomial infections and epidemics are not uncommon.

Diagnosis Rotavirus should be in the differential diagnosis of any newborn or young child with the aforementioned clinical presentations or other form of gastroenteritis. Visualization of rotavirus by electron microscopy is considered by many experts to be the standard method of laboratory diagnosis, but the method is expensive and not widely available. Enzyme immunoassay (EIA) and latex agglutination (LA) are much more widely available and used. Detection of rotavirus antigen by EIA is by far the most practical and cost-efficient method. EIA probably is at least as sensitive as electron microscopy and is a highly recommended method.

Diagnostic Tests/Procedures

Rotavirus, Direct Detection *on page 573*

Drug Therapy Comment No antiviral agents proven effective. Treatment is directed at symptom relief and prevention/treatment of dehydration. Oral immune globulin has been administered with variable success.

Selected Readings

Dennehy PH, "Rotavirus Vaccines: An Update," *Curr Opin Pediatr*, 2005, 17(1):88-92.

Denno DM, Stapp JR, Boster DR, et al, "Etiology of Diarrhea in Pediatric Outpatient Settings," *Pediatr Infect Dis J*, 2005, 24(2):142-8.

Gray LG, "Novel Viruses Associated With Gastroenteritis," *Clin Microbiol Newslett*, 1991, 13:137-40.

Offit PA and Clark HF, "Rotavirus," *Principles and Practice of Infectious Diseases*, 5th ed, Mandell GL, Bennett JE, and Dolin R, eds, New York, NY: Churchill Livingstone, 2000, 1696-703.

Widdowson MA, Bresee JS, Gentsch JR, et al, "Rotavirus Disease and Its Prevention," *Curr Opin Gastroenterol*, 2005, 21(1):26-31.

RSV *see* Respiratory Syncytial Virus *on page 285*

Rubeola *see* Measles Virus *on page 215*

Rubeola Virus *see* Measles Virus *on page 215*

Salmonella Species

Related Information

Clinical Syndromes Associated With Foodborne Diseases *on page 1276*

USPHS / IDSA Guidelines for the Prevention of Opportunistic Infections in Persons Infected With HIV *on page 1237*

Microbiology *Salmonella* species are gram-negative bacilli which are important causes of bacterial gastroenteritis, septicemia, and a nonspecific febrile illness called typhoid fever. Unfortunately, the classification system for the different *Salmonella* species is complex and confusing to most clinicians. Over 2000 separate serotypes have been identified, and, in the past and currently, each is named as if it was a species. Most experts agree that there are seven distinct subgroups of *Salmonella* (1, 2, 3a, 3b, 4, 5, and 6) each of which contain many serotypes ("species"). The main pathogens in humans are serotypes, *S. choleraesuis*, *S. typhi*, and *S. paratyphi* (all in subgroup 1).

Salmonella is an aerobic gram-negative bacillus in the family Enterobacteriaceae. It is almost always associated with disease when isolated from humans and is not considered part of the normal human flora. As with other members of this family, *Salmonella* carries the endotoxin lipopolysaccharide on its outer membrane, which is released upon cell lysis.

Epidemiology It is estimated that about 3 million new cases of salmonellosis occur each year. *Salmonella* species are found worldwide. Many are easily recovered from animals such as chickens, birds, livestock, rodents, and reptiles (turtles). Some serotypes cause disease almost exclusively in man (*S. typhi*) while others are primarily seen in animals but can cause severe disease when infecting humans (*S. choleraesuis*). Transmission is via ingestion of contaminated materials, particularly raw fruits and vegetables, oysters and other shellfish, and contaminated water. Eggs, poultry, and other dairy products are important sources. Outbreaks have been described in the summer months where children consume contaminated egg salad. Other outbreaks have been associated with pet turtles, other pets, marijuana, and, rarely, food handlers. The incubation period is about 1-3 weeks. The period of communicability lasts until all *Salmonella* have been eradicated from the stool or urine.

Clinical infection is favored when there is a high inoculum of bacteria in the ingested food, since experimental models suggest that 10^6 bacteria are needed for clinical disease. Contaminated food improperly refrigerated will allow such multiplication. Host factors are important and disease is more likely in immunocompromised individuals, sickle cell disease, or achlorhydria (gastric acid decreases the viable bacterial inoculum). Although salmonellosis can occur at any age, children are most commonly infected.

Clinical Syndromes The following are the major syndromes associated with salmonellosis. It should be emphasized that these syndromes are often overlapping.

(Continued)

Salmonella Species *(Continued)*

- **Gastroenteritis:** The most common manifestation of *Salmonella* infection. After ingestion of contaminated food, the bacteria are absorbed in the terminal portion of the small intestine. The organisms then penetrate into the lamina propria of the ileocecal area. Following this, there is reticuloendothelial hypertrophy with usually a brisk host immune response. As the organisms multiply in the lymphoid follicles, polymorphonuclear leukocytes attempt to limit the infection. There is release of prostaglandins and other mediators, which stimulates cyclic AMP. This results in intestinal fluid secretion which is nonbloody. Clinically, the patient complains of nausea, vomiting, and diarrhea from several hours to several days after consumption of contaminated food. Other symptoms include fever, malaise, muscle aches, and abdominal pain. Symptoms usually resolve from several days to 1 week, even without antibiotics.
- **Sepsis syndrome:** Patients may present in flora sepsis, indistinguishable from other forms of gram-negative sepsis. Fever, confusion, hypotension, end-organ damage, and poor perfusion may all be seen. *Salmonella* bacteremia may lead to multiple metastatic foci, such as liver abscess, osteomyelitis (particularly with sickle cell disease), septic arthritis, and endocarditis. Mycotic aneurysms may develop following bacteremia, and *Salmonella* is a leading cause of infected aortic aneurysms. Bacteremia is also common in AIDS and repeated relapses with *Salmonella* are common, despite prolonged antibiotics.
- **Typhoid fever:** Also known as enteric fever, this febrile illness is caused classically by *S. typhi*. Following ingestion of the bacteria, the organisms pass into the ileocecal area where intraluminal multiplication occurs. There is a mononuclear host cell response, but the organisms remain viable within the macrophages. The bacteria are carried to the organs of the reticuloendothelial system (spleen, liver, bone marrow) by the macrophages and clinical signs of infection become apparent. Patients complain of insidious onset of fever, myalgias, headache, malaise, and constipation, corresponding to this phase of bacteremia. A pulse-temperature dissociation may be present. A characteristic rash may be seen in about 50% of patients, called "rose spots", which are 2-4 mm pink maculopapular lesions that blanch with pressure, usually on the trunk. Symptoms last for 1 or more weeks. During this time, bacteria multiply in the mesenteric lymphoid tissue, and these areas eventually exhibit necrosis and bleeding. There are microperforations of the abdominal wall. *Salmonella* spreads from the liver through the gallbladder and eventually back into the intestines. This phase of intestinal reinfection is characterized by prominent gastrointestinal symptoms including diarrhea. Overall, fatality with treatment is <2%. A similar, but milder syndrome, can occur with *S. paratyphi*, called paratyphoid fever.
- **Chronic carrier state:** Following infection with *S. typhi*, up to 5% of patients will excrete the bacteria for over 1 year. Such patients are termed chronic carriers and are asymptomatic. Millions of viable bacteria are present in the biliary tree and are shed into the bile and into the feces. Urinary carriage can also occur, particularly in patients who are coinfected with *Schistosoma haematobium*. The chronic carrier state is less important for other *Salmonella* species, where the carriage rate is <1%.

Diagnosis Laboratory confirmation is generally required, since the major syndromes are seldom distinctive enough to be diagnosed solely on clinical criteria. *Salmonella* grows readily on most media under standard aerobic conditions. Cultures from blood, joint aspirations, and cerebrospinal fluid can be plated on routine media. Specimens which are likely to contain other organisms, such as stool or sputum, require selective media, and the laboratory should be appropriately notified. Recovery of *Salmonella* from the stool is the most common means of establishing the diagnosis, and enrichment media are available to maximize the yield. Other laboratory findings may suggest salmonellosis, including a profound leukopenia often seen with typhoid fever.

Recent antimicrobial therapy may render blood and stool cultures negative. In such cases, proctoscopy with biopsy and culture of ulcerations may establish the diagnosis in the enterocolitis syndrome. Serologic tests are not particularly useful in this instance. When typhoid fever is suspected but the patient has already received antimicrobial agents, bone marrow biopsies, as well as skin biopsies of any rose spots, may yield *Salmonella typhi* in culture. Serologic studies are more helpful in diagnosing typhoid fever, but >50% of patients will fail to show the expected rise in agglutinins against the typhoid O antigen.

Diagnostic Tests/Procedures

Blood Culture, Aerobic and Anaerobic *on page 391*

Bone Marrow Culture, Routine *on page 400*

Stool Culture *on page 585*

Treatment *Salmonella* species resistant to multiple antimicrobials are increasing in frequency. *In vitro* susceptibility studies should be performed, particularly in severe cases. Treatment guidelines vary with the type of syndrome, as follows:

- Enterocolitis: The majority of cases are self-resolving and do not need antibiotics. Clinical trials have demonstrated that a variety of antibiotics fail to influence the course of mild infections and may prolong excretion of the organisms. For severe cases, or in the immunosuppressed host, a number of antibiotics are usually effective, including ampicillin, chloramphenicol, sulfamethoxazole and trimethoprim, and third generation cephalosporins.
- Typhoid fever: Cases should be treated promptly. Chloramphenicol and ampicillin are effective and have been the most extensively studied. Recent studies show that ciprofloxacin is highly active. Third generation cephalosporins and sulfamethoxazole and trimethoprim is useful in organisms that are resistant to standard agents.
- Bacteremia: Ampicillin, chloramphenicol, sulfamethoxazole and trimethoprim, and third generation cephalosporins are all effective. However, chloramphenicol should be avoided in endocarditis or mycotic aneurysms. Ciprofloxacin is effective in treating recurrent *Salmonella* bacteremia in AIDS.
- Chronic carriage: Ampicillin or amoxicillin for 6 weeks, although elapses are common if there is underlying gallbladder disease cholecystectomy may be an option with repeated relapses. Ciprofloxacin may also be effective.

Drug Therapy

Recommended:

Cephalosporins, 3rd Generation *on page 730*

Alternate:

Ampicillin *on page 657*

Sulfamethoxazole and Trimethoprim *on page 1087*

Chloramphenicol *on page 733*

Ciprofloxacin *on page 742*

Selected Readings

Edwards BH, "*Salmonella* and *Shigella* Species," *Clin Lab Med*, 1999, 19(3):469-87.

Santos RL, Tsolis RM, Baumler AJ, et al, "Pathogenesis of *Salmonella*-Induced Enteritis," *Braz J Med Biol Res*, 2003, 36(1):3-12.

Zhang S, Kingsley RA, Santos RL, et al, "Molecular Pathogenesis of *Salmonella enterica* Serotype *typhimurium*-Induced Diarrhea," *Infect Immun*, 2003, 71(1):1-12.

Salmonellosis *see Salmonella* Species *on page 291*

Salpingitis *see* Pelvic Inflammatory Disease *on page 260*

San Joaquin Fever *see Coccidioides immitis on page 91*

Sarcoptes scabiei

Microbiology *Sarcoptes scabiei*, or the human mite, is the causative agent of scabies, a common parasitic infestation of the skin. *Sarcoptes scabiei* is an ectoparasite of humans belonging to the class *Arachnida*. It tends to form skin "burrows" several millimeters wide within the stratum corneum of the epidermis. The fertilized female deposits its eggs in these skin burrows, and the larvae exit after several days to become adults weeks later. The adult is about 0.3 mm long.

Epidemiology Scabies is distributed worldwide. The incidence in the United States has been increasing since the 1970s. The reservoir resides in humans, although animal mites can sometimes cause brief human disease. Transmission is person to person by direct contact. Occasionally, transmission may occur when there is contact with heavily contaminated clothing or bedsheets. The incubation period varies from several days to weeks. Infected individuals remain communicable until all the ova and mites are eradicated from the skin.

Clinical Syndromes

- **Human scabies:** Patients present with intense itching, usually in the interdigital web spaces, along the "belt line," the genital region, the periumbilical area, and also on the wrists, elbows, knees, and feet. Additional areas are common in children, including the hands and face. On physical examination, the characteristic burrows may be seen, appearing linear and several millimeters wide, often in the interdigital spaces. Atypical presentations of scabies may occur, including vesicles and bullae in infants, eczematous eruptions, and urticaria. A variant known as "nodular scabies" has been described in which there are small, brown, intensely pruritic nodules usually on the penis and scrotum. An unusual manifestation of severe scabies called "Norwegian scabies" has been seen in immunocompromised individuals and patients with Down syndrome. The skin is diffusely scaling and thickened as a result of infestation of thousands of mites. Secondary bacterial infections of the skin may occur in all forms of scabies.
- **Animal scabies:** This is due to *Sarcoptes scabiei* var *canis*, carried on some dogs. The clinical presentation is similar to human scabies although burrows are not present.

(Continued)

Sarcoptes scabiei (Continued)

Diagnosis Infestation with scabies is often suspected when an individual presents with pruritic papules, or an otherwise compatible clinical history. Some patients may present because of a recent history of contact. It should be noted that scabies often imitates other skin lesions, and thus a broad differential diagnosis should be entertained if the linear burrows are not demonstrated. Other diagnostic considerations include impetigo, insect bites, drug eruptions, varicella, eczema, and others.

The linear burrows of the mite can be further demonstrated by applying blue ink over a possible burrow. The ink is drawn into the defect and when excess ink is wiped off with an alcohol pad, the ink within the burrow remains. This and other suspicious areas should covered with oil, the area should be scraped with a sterile blade, the scrapings should be placed into oil on a microscope slide, and the preparation should be examined with a microscope.

Diagnostic Tests/Procedures

Arthropod Identification *on page 387*

Treatment For adults and older children: Lindane 1% lotion or cream is applied to all skin areas from the neck to the toes then washed off after 8-12 hours. During the treatment period, the medication should be reapplied to the hands after routine handwashing; failure to do so may result in treatment failure since the hands are often infected. Lindane is contraindicated for pregnant or lactating women. Of note, lindane has been associated with central nervous system toxicity, particularly when an underlying skin disorder was present to allow greater than normal systemic absorption of drug. The regimen described here is generally safe. The alternative regimen is crotamiton (10%) applied as a thin smear from the neck down and left on for 1 day. A second application is done the following day, then washed off 24 hours later. Crotamiton should be used in individuals with extensive dermatitis.

For children younger than 2 years of age, infants, and pregnant women, crotamiton should be used instead of lindane. Treatment should be administered to sexual partners and close contacts in the same house. Other principles of management include cleaning all potentially contaminated clothes (dry cleaning or machine washing and drying in the hot cycle), prescribing medications for pruritus (Atarax®, diphenhydramine, topical corticosteroids, and others), and treating secondary bacterial infections of the skin with antistaphylococcal antibiotics.

Drug Therapy

Recommended:

Lindane *on page 913*
Permethrin *on page 1001*
Crotamiton *on page 762*

SARS Virus *see Coronaviridae* (Including SARS) *on page 94*
Scabies *see Sarcoptes scabiei on page 293*
Scarlet Fever *see Streptococcus pyogenes on page 321*

Schistosoma mansoni

Synonyms Blood Fluke

Microbiology *Schistosoma mansoni* also known as the blood fluke, is a common parasite in South America, the Caribbean, and Africa. The organism causes schistosomiasis (bilharziasis) with diverse clinical manifestations ranging from a mild dermatitis to a fulminant dysentery with bloody stools.

S. mansoni is a parasite classified as a trematode (fluke). As with other trematodes, it appears flat, fleshy, and has a leaf shape. There are two muscular suckers, the oral type being the beginning of an incomplete digestive system and the ventral sucker being an organ of attachment. Unlike other trematodes, *S. mansoni* is not a hermaphrodite and there are separate male and female worms. The intermediate host of *S. mansoni* is the snail, which is necessary for the parasite to complete its life cycle.

The life cycle of the organism begins when the infective forms called cercariae are liberated from the snail. These ciliated, free-swimming organisms travel through fresh water until they reach the human host. The cercariae are able to penetrate intact skin. Following this they enter the circulation and mature in the intrahepatic porta blood. During this developmental period, the parasites coat themselves with a substance that prevents the host from recognizing them immunologically. This remarkable defense explains the mechanism whereby cases of chronic infection have lasted for decades. After 3 weeks of maturation the adult migrates to the mesenteric veins, specifically the small branches of the inferior mesenteric vein near the lower colon. Fertilization occurs in these vessels and eventually eggs are released into the environment, to begin the cycle again.

Epidemiology *S. mansoni* is common in South America (Brazil, Venezuela), the Caribbean (West Indies, Puerto Rico), and Africa. Travelers or immigrants from these

areas are the main source for cases seen in the United States. The reservoir for *S. mansoni* is the human, although Primates, marsupials, and rodents can also serve as hosts. As noted, transmission occurs when there is skin penetration of the parasite larvae in stool-contaminated waters. The incubation period is 4-6 weeks after skin penetration. There is no defined period of communicability since the parasite is not transmitted person to person. However, ova may be recovered from stools for years.

Clinical Syndromes

- **Asymptomatic infection:** Occurs commonly.
- **Dermatitis:** Following skin penetration by the larvae, a brisk local allergic reaction may be seen, with pruritus, maculopapular lesions, and edema.
- **Cough:** When migrating worms reach the lungs.
- **Mesenteric adenitis:** When the adults begin to lay eggs in the mesenteric vessels, a febrile illness often results. There is abdominal pain, liver tenderness, and malaise. Eventually, the area may become walled off in a foreign-body type reaction, and fibrosis and abscess formation may be seen. Characteristically, there is bloody diarrhea.
- **Chronic infection:** After infection has become established, the patient over time may develop ascites, massive hepatosplenomegaly, lymphadenopathy, white granulomas on the liver called pseudotubercles. Extraintestinal infections may be seen, eggs may be recovered from the spinal cord, lungs, and other areas. Fibrosis is also seen at these other sites. Severe neurologic disease results from the presence of eggs in the spinal cord and brain.

Diagnosis Schistosomiasis is suspected in an individual who resides in an endemic area, or a traveler who has recently returned from such an area who presents with a compatible clinical history. Routine laboratory studies may be helpful, with elevated liver function tests and peripheral blood eosinophilia seen.

The stool examination is critical in confirming the diagnosis. Large eggs 115-175 μm long are seen in established cases. Rectal biopsy may also be considered if serial stool exams are negative but clinical suspicion remains high. The biopsy may reveal the egg tracks laid by the worms in the rectal vessels.

Diagnostic Tests/Procedures

Ova and Parasites, Stool *on page 551*
Ova and Parasites, Urine or Aspirates *on page 554*

Treatment Asymptomatic cases do not necessarily require treatment. The drugs used have potential toxicities and the situation must be weighed by the physician. The same applies to mild infections; the nature of the patient's immune status must be considered also. Moderate or severe cases respond to praziquantel.

Drug Therapy

Recommended:

Praziquantel *on page 1017*

Selected Readings

Mahmoud AA, "Trematodes (Schistosomiasis) and Other Flukes," *Principles and Practice of Infectious Diseases*, 4th ed, Mandell GL, Bennett JE, and Dolin R, eds, New York, NY: Churchill Livingstone, 1995, 2538-44.
Ross AG, Bartley PB, Sleigh AC, et al, "Schistosomiasis," *N Engl J Med*, 2002, 346(16):1212-20.
"Schistosomiasis in U.S. Peace Corps Volunteers - Malawi, 1992," *MMWR*, 1993, 42(29):565-70.
Scrimgeour EM and Gajdusek DC, "Involvement of the Central Nervous System in *Schistosoma mansoni* and *S. haematobium* Infection: A Review," *Brain*, 1985, 108(Pt 4):1023-38.
Tsang VC and Wilkins PP, "Immunodiagnosis of Schistosomiasis: Screen With FAST-ELISA and Confirm With Immunoblot," *Clin Lab Med*, 1991, 11(4):1029-39.

Schistosomiasis *see Schistosoma mansoni on page 294*
Seborrheic Blepharitis *see* Blepharitis *on page 52*
Secondary Peritonitis *see* Peritonitis, Secondary *on page 263*

Sepsis

Clinical Presentation The patient may have fever or hypothermia, may be tachycardiac and tachypneic, may have altered mental status, hypoxia, increased plasma lactate levels, oliguria, or coagulopathy. Sepsis is defined as clinical evidence of infection plus systemic response manifested by at least two of the following: temperature >38°C or <36°C, tachycardia, tachypnea, or abnormal white blood count. Sepsis syndrome is defined as sepsis plus evidence of altered organ perfusion with at least one of the following: hypoxemia, hyperlactemia, oliguria, or altered mental status. Septic shock is defined as sepsis with hypotension despite fluid resuscitation.

Likely Pathogens

Gram-Negative Bacilli *on page 157*
Staphylococcus aureus, Methicillin-Susceptible *on page 307*
Candida Species *on page 67*
Enterococcus Species *on page 134*

Diagnostic Tests/Procedures

•Aerobic Culture, Sputum *on page 367*
(Continued)

Sepsis *(Continued)*

- •Blood Culture, Aerobic and Anaerobic *on page 391*
- •Gram Stain *on page 473*
- •Intravenous Line Culture *on page 511*
- •Urine Culture, Clean Catch *on page 609*
- Computed Transaxial Tomography, Abdomen Studies *on page 423*

Empiric Drug Therapy

Recommended:

The following 3 used in combination

Ceftazidime *on page 717*
Aminoglycosides *on page 641*
Vancomycin *on page 1144*

The following 3 used in combination

Penicillins, Extended-Spectrum *on page 997*
Aminoglycosides *on page 641*
Vancomycin *on page 1144*

Consideration in adults with severe sepsis and high risk of mortality

Drotrecogin Alfa *on page 793*

Selected Readings

Bernard GR, Vincent JL, Laterre PF, et al, "Efficacy and Safety of Recombinant Human Activated Protein C for Severe Sepsis," *N Engl J Med*, 2001, 344(10):699-709.

Brun-Buisson C, "The Epidemiology of the Systemic Inflammatory Response," *Intensive Care Med*, 2000, 26 (Suppl 1):S64-74.

"Practice Parameters for Hemodynamic Support of Sepsis in Adult Patients in Sepsis. Task Force of the American College of Critical Care Medicine, Society of Critical Care Medicine," *Crit Care Med*, 1999, 27(3):639-60.

Vincent JL, Sun Q, and Dubois MJ, "Clinical Trials of Immunomodulatory Therapies in Severe Sepsis and Septic Shock," *Clin Infect Dis*, 2002, 34(8):1084-93.

Septic Abortion *see* Amnionitis *on page 33*

Septic Arthritis *see* Arthritis, Septic *on page 36*

Septic Thrombophlebitis *see* Thrombophlebitis, Suppurative *on page 330*

Serratia Species

Microbiology *Serratia* species are gram-negative rods which are important causes of nosocomial infection and are only rarely associated with community-acquired infections in normal hosts.

Serratia species are moderate-sized aerobic gram-negative bacilli which belong to the large family Enterobacteriaceae ("enteric bacteria"). The organisms cannot be identified on the basis of morphologic appearance on Gram stain alone and are indistinguishable from other members of Enterobacteriaceae. *Serratia* species are related to such gram-negative bacilli as *Klebsiella*, *Enterobacter*, and *Hafnia* (all belonging to the tribe Klebsielleae). There are several distinct species of *Serratia*, but most human disease is caused by *Serratia marcescens*. Rarely, *Serratia liquefaciens* has been isolated in serious infections. Laboratory identification is generally straightforward. It is unique in that it is the only member of Enterobacteriaceae to produce extracellular DNase. Special requests for isolation of *Serratia* are not necessary because the organism is not fastidious in its growth requirements. Most clinical isolates will exhibit growth after overnight incubation. The appearance of colonies may be delayed (or completely inhibited) if the patient is receiving antibiotic therapy. *Serratia marcescens* shares several potential virulence factors with other members of Enterobacteriaceae, including endotoxin, the lipopolysaccharide associated with the outer membrane of the bacteria. When cell lysis occurs (as with antibiotic therapy), the LPS is released into the host and can lead to such inflammatory responses as fever, leukopenia or leukocytosis, hypotension, and disseminated intravascular coagulation. Thus, LPS is regarded as an important mediator of the sepsis syndrome.

Epidemiology In contrast to the other members of the Enterobacteriaceae family, *Serratia* tends to colonize the respiratory and urinary tracts of hospitalized adults more so than the gastrointestinal tract. This colonization probably does not hold true for neonates, in whom the gastrointestinal tract is an important source of the organism. An outbreak of *Serratia marcescens* was reported in a neonatal intensive care unit in 1982; a gastrointestinal reservoir was found to be important. Nosocomial transmission can occur by several routes; the most frequent being hand-to-hand spread via nurses, physicians, and other healthcare workers. *Serratia marcescens* has also been associated with hospital outbreaks caused by contaminated respiratory equipment used for inhalational therapy, bronchoscopes, antiseptic fluids, intravenous fluids, scalp-vein needles, peritoneal dialysis catheters, and others. Community-acquired infections with *Serratia* are unusual, and the organism is mainly a nosocomial pathogen.

Clinical Syndromes

- **Lower respiratory tract infection:** Nosocomial *Serratia* infections are seen in debilitated, ventilator-dependent patients. *Serratia* and other gram-negative bacilli can asymptomatically colonize the upper respiratory tract of hospitalized patients. Thus, the recovery of *Serratia* from a sputum or tracheal aspirate culture does not necessarily indicate a significant infection. The diagnosis of a nosocomial pneumonia still rests on standard criteria such as the presence of purulence (many leukocytes) on the Gram stain of sputum, the presence of a pulmonary infiltrate, and signs of systemic inflammation in the patient. **A positive sputum culture alone is not sufficient justification for initiating antibiotic therapy**.
- **Urinary tract infection:** This infection is also seen in hospitalized patients, often with indwelling Foley catheters. However, *Serratia* may also harmlessly colonize the urine of patients with chronic bladder catheters without causing disease. The decision to initiate antibiotics in such patients should be based on the clinical situation (the presence of pyuria on urinalysis, suprapubic pain, fever, etc). Even the finding of large quantity of *Serratia* in a urine culture ($>10^5$ colony-forming units/mL) by itself does not automatically indicate the need for antibiotic therapy.
- **Hospital-associated bacteremias:** *Serratia* may be recovered from blood cultures in association with a known focus of infection (eg, catheter infection) or may be a "primary bacteremia" with no clear source. Bacteremia may follow instrumentation of the gastrointestinal or urinary tracts.
- **Surgical wound infections**

Diagnosis The clinical presentations of the various nosocomial infections caused by *Serratia marcescens* are not distinctive, and laboratory isolation of the organism is necessary.

Diagnostic Tests/Procedures

Aerobic Culture, Appropriate Site *on page 365*
Gram Stain *on page 473*

Treatment *Serratia* species present a challenging therapeutic problem. High level drug resistance has been described in some hospital isolates. Preliminary data suggest that the popular third generation cephalosporins may act to select mutants of *Serratia* that are resistant to a wide variety of antibiotics, including both cephalosporins and extended-spectrum penicillins. Susceptibility to these drugs is not uniform and appropriate treatment of patients with true *Serratia* infection depends on antimicrobial susceptibility testing of individual isolates. Consultation with an Infectious Disease specialist may be useful in such cases.

Drug Therapy

Recommended:

Penicillins, Extended-Spectrum *on page 997*
Cephalosporins, 3rd Generation *on page 730*

Alternate:

Imipenem and Cilastatin *on page 861*
Aztreonam *on page 677*
Meropenem *on page 936*
Fluoroquinolones *on page 824*

Selected Readings

Campbell JR, Diacovo T, and Baker CJ, "*Serratia marcescens* Meningitis in Neonates," *Pediatr Infect Dis J*, 1992, 11(10):881-6.

Choi SH, Kim YS, Chung JW, et al, "*Serratia* Bacteremia in a Large University Hospital: Trends in Antibiotic Resistance During 10 Years and Implications for Antibiotic Use," *Infect Control Hosp Epidemiol*, 2002, 23(12):740-7.

Dhawan B, Bonnet R, Shukla NK, et al, "Infection With an Extended-Spectrum Beta-Lactamase-Producing Strain of *Serratia marcescens* Following Tongue Reconstruction," *J Clin Microbiol*, 2003, 41(5):2233-4.

Munoz JM and Macias AE, "Nosocomial Outbreak of *Serratia marcescens* in a Neonatal Intensive Care Unit," *Infect Control Hosp Epidemiol*, 2003, 24(5):312.

van der Vorm ER and Woldring-Zwaan C, "Source, Carriers, and Management of a *Serratia marcescens* Outbreak on a Pulmonary Unit," *J Hosp Infect*, 2002, 52(4):263-7.

Shiga Toxin *E. coli* *see Escherichia coli*, Enterohemorrhagic *on page 145*

Shigella Species

Related Information

Clinical Syndromes Associated With Foodborne Diseases *on page 1276*

Microbiology *Shigella* species are gram-negative rods which cause a severe diarrheal syndrome, called shigellosis or bacillary dysentery. *Shigella* species belong to the family Enterobacteriaceae and is, for all practical purposes, biochemically and genetically identical to *E. coli*. There are 4 serogroups of *Shigella* (A, B, C, and D) which, historically, have been treated as "species:" *S. dysenteriae*, *S. flexneri*, *S. boydii*, and *S. sonnei*, respectively. There are approximately 40 serotypes within these 4 groups. *Shigella sonnei* is most common in the industrial world and accounts for about 64% of the cases in the United States. *S. flexneri* is seen primarily in

(Continued)

Shigella Species *(Continued)*

underdeveloped countries. Shigellosis can be seen following ingestion of as few as 200 organisms.

Epidemiology Infection with *Shigella* sp is primarily a problem in the pediatric population, with most infections in the 1- to 4-year age group. Outbreaks of epidemic proportions have been described in daycare centers and nurseries. The reservoir for the bacteria is in humans. Transmission is by direct or indirect fecal-oral transmission from patient or carrier. Hand transmission is important. Less commonly, transmission occurs by consumption of contaminated water, milk, and food. The organism is able to produce outbreaks in areas of poor sanitation, in part due to the low number of organisms required to produce disease. Shigellosis is the most communicable of the bacterial diarrheas.

Clinical Syndromes *Shigella* species invade the intestinal mucosa wherein they multiply and cause local tissue damage. The organisms rarely penetrate beyond the mucosa, and thus the isolation in blood cultures is unusual, even with the toxic patient. Mucosal ulcerations are common. Some strains are known to elaborate a toxin (the Shiga-toxin), which contributes to mucosal destruction and probably causes the watery diarrhea seen initially.

- **Dysentery:** Initially, the patient complains of acute onset of fever, abdominal cramping, and large volumes of very watery diarrhea. This phase is enterotoxin-mediated and reflects small bowel involvement. Within 24-48 hours, the fever resolves but the diarrhea turns frankly bloody, with mucous and pus in the stools as well. Fecal urgency and tenesmus are common. This phase reflects direct colonic invasion. This two-phased "descending infection" is suggestive of dysentery. Diarrhea and abdominal pain are almost universally present, but the other symptoms may be absent. Physical examination is variable, and patients may be comfortable or frankly toxic. Rectal examination is often painful due to friable and inflamed rectal mucosa. The course may be complicated from dehydration from diarrhea and vomiting, particularly in the elderly and in infants. Normally, the infection is self limited and resolves within about 1 week even without antibiotics. Complications are unusual and include febrile seizures (particularly in infants), septicemia, and the hemolytic uremic syndrome (usually from the Shiga-toxin from *S. dysenteriae* 1).
- **Reactive arthritis:** Following dysentery from *Shigella*, a postinfectious arthropathy resembling Reiter's syndrome has been described, particularly in patients who are HLA-B27 positive.

Diagnosis Dysentery from *Shigella* should be suspected in any patient presenting with fever and bloody diarrhea. A history of a "descending infection" as described above is further suggestive. However, the differential diagnosis of fever with bloody diarrhea is broad and includes salmonellosis, *Campylobacter* enteritis, infection with *E. coli* O157:H7, and inflammatory bowel disease. The WBC count may show either a leukocytosis, leukopenia, or be normal.

There are two important laboratory tests indicated in suspected cases.

1. Stool exam for fecal leukocytes: Numerous white blood cells will be present during the colonic phase of the infection. Note that this is not a specific test and is not diagnostic for *Shigella* infections; it indicates that the colonic mucosa is inflamed, from whatever cause. The finding of sheets of fecal leukocytes on smear narrows the differential diagnosis of infectious diarrheas considerably.
2. Stool culture for *Shigella*: Recovery of the organism from stool is more easily performed early in the illness when the concentration in the stool is highest. Samples should be brought to the laboratory as soon as possible to maximize viability, and specific culture for *Shigella* sp should be requested.

Diagnostic Tests/Procedures

Fecal Leukocyte Stain *on page 455*
Stool Culture *on page 585*

Treatment Many cases of *Shigella* dysentery are self-resolving. Some have suggested that antibiotics be reserved for severe cases, but this does not eliminate the reservoir for infection in the community. Antibiotics have been shown to shorten the period of excretion of the organism in the feces, as well as decreasing morbidity. The antibiotic of choice is sulfamethoxazole and trimethoprim for both children and adults. However, some strains are resistant to sulfamethoxazole and trimethoprim, particularly in Africa and Southeast Asia, and *in vitro* susceptibility testing should be performed on all isolates. The quinolones have been effective for shigellosis in clinical trials and are useful alternatives. Antimotility agents such as opiates, paregoric, and diphenoxylate (Lomotil®) should be avoided because of the potential for worsening the dysentery and for predisposing to toxic megacolon.

Pediatric Drug Therapy

Recommended:

Sulfamethoxazole and Trimethoprim *on page 1087*

Alternate:

Ampicillin *on page 657*
Cephalosporins, 3rd Generation *on page 730*

Adult Drug Therapy

Recommended:

Ciprofloxacin *on page 742*
Sulfamethoxazole and Trimethoprim *on page 1087*

Alternate:

Ampicillin *on page 657*
Cephalosporins, 3rd Generation *on page 730*
Fluoroquinolones *on page 824*

Selected Readings

Ahmetagic S, Jusufovic E, Petrovic J, et al, "Acute Infectious Diarrhea in Children," *Med Arh*, 2003, 57(2):87-92.
Edwards BH, "*Salmonella* and *Shigella* Species," *Clin Lab Med*, 1999, 19(3):469-87.
Fernandez MI and Sansonetti PJ, "*Shigella* Interaction With Intestinal Epithelial Cells Determines the Innate Immune Response in Shigellosis," *Int J Med Microbiol*, 2003, 293(1):55-67.
Tauxe RV, Puhr ND, Wells JG, et al, "Antimicrobial Resistance of *Shigella* Isolates in the USA: The Importance of International Travelers," *J Infect Dis*, 1990, 162(5):1107-11.

Shigellosis *see Shigella* Species *on page 297*

Shingles *see* Varicella-Zoster Virus *on page 347*

Sinusitis, Community-Acquired, Acute

Synonyms Acute Sinusitis, Community-Acquired; Community-Acquired Sinusitis, Acute

Clinical Presentation Symptoms depend on the site of involvement. Patients with maxillary sinusitis typically have pain over the canine/molar teeth and malar area. Patients with anterior ethmoid sinusitis present with temporal or retro-orbital headaches. Posterior ethmoid sinusitis presents with pain in the distribution of the trigeminal nerve and sphenoid sinusitis typically causes pain in the frontal, retro-orbital, or facial area. Patients usually complain of nasal congestion rhinitis, as most often acute sinusitis follows a viral upper respiratory tract infection. Initial treatment should consist of symptomatic relief with analgesia, topical, or systemic decongestants and steam inhalation.

Likely Pathogens

Streptococcus pneumoniae, Drug-Susceptible *on page 319*
Haemophilus influenzae on page 159
Moraxella catarrhalis on page 223
Note: Unusual organisms should be considered in immunosuppressed patients.

Diagnostic Tests/Procedures

Aerobic Culture, Appropriate Site *on page 365*
Gram Stain *on page 473*

Empiric Drug Therapy

Recommended:

Sulfamethoxazole and Trimethoprim *on page 1087*
Cephalosporins, 2nd Generation *on page 729*
Amoxicillin *on page 642*

Alternate:

Amoxicillin and Clavulanate Potassium *on page 645*
Fluoroquinolones *on page 824*
Macrolides *on page 924*

Selected Readings

Evans KL, "Recognition and Management of Sinusitis," *Drugs*, 1998, 56(1):59-71.
Gwaltney JM Jr, "Acute Community-Acquired Sinusitis," *Clin Infect Dis*, 1996, 23(6):1209-23.
Kaliner MA, Osguthorpe JD, Fireman P, et al, "Sinusitis: Bench to Bedside. Current Findings, Future Directions," *J Allergy Clin Immunol*, 1997, 99(6 Pt 3):S829-48.
Low DE, Desrosiers M, McSherry J, et al, "A Practical Guide for the Diagnosis and Treatment of Acute Sinusitis," *CMAJ*, 1997, 156(Suppl 6):S1-14.

Sinusitis, Community-Acquired, Chronic

Synonyms Chronic Sinusitis, Community-Acquired; Community-Acquired Sinusitis, Chronic

Clinical Presentation Patients generally complain of intermittent pain, nasal congestion, and rhinitis. Patients frequently have a chronic cough secondary to postnasal drip.

Differential Diagnosis Granulomatous disease

Likely Pathogens

Bacteroides and *Prevotella* Species *on page 46*
Streptococcus-Related Gram-Positive Cocci *on page 325*
(Continued)

Sinusitis, Community-Acquired, Chronic *(Continued)*

Diagnostic Tests/Procedures

Aerobic Culture, Appropriate Site *on page 365*
Anaerobic Culture *on page 371*
Gram Stain *on page 473*

Drug Therapy Comment Antibiotics are usually not effective. Use of decongestant and steroid nasal spray recommended.

Empiric Drug Therapy

Recommended:

Clindamycin *on page 752*

Alternate:

Macrolides *on page 924*

Selected Readings

Evans KL, "Recognition and Management of Sinusitis," *Drugs*, 1998, 56(1):59-71.
Kaliner MA, Osguthorpe JD, Fireman P, et al, "Sinusitis: Bench to Bedside. Current Findings, Future Directions," *J Allergy Clin Immunol*, 1997, 99(6 Pt 3):S829-48.
Orlandi RR and Kennedy DW, "Surgical Management of Rhinosinusitis," *Am J Med Sci*, 1998, 316(1):29-38.

Sinusitis, Hospital-Acquired

Synonyms Hospital-Acquired Sinusitis

Clinical Presentation Common nosocomial infection in the intensive care units secondary to prolonged intubation with a nasal tracheal or nasal gastric tube. Patients may present with fever and/or leukocytosis. Unexplained fever or leukocytosis with a nasal tube warrants simple CT of the sinuses.

Likely Pathogens

Staphylococcus aureus, Methicillin-Resistant *on page 304*
Staphylococcus aureus, Methicillin-Susceptible *on page 307*
Pseudomonas aeruginosa on page 282

Diagnostic Tests/Procedures

Aerobic Culture, Appropriate Site *on page 365*
Gram Stain *on page 473*
Computed Transaxial Tomography, Paranasal Sinuses *on page 425*

Drug Therapy Comment Fungal sinusitis should be considered in immunocompromised patients including diabetics. Empiric antifungal therapy is amphotericin B (conventional).

Empiric Drug Therapy

Recommended:

The following 3 used in combination
Vancomycin *on page 1144*
Gentamicin *on page 841*
Ceftazidime *on page 717*

The following 3 used in combination
Vancomycin *on page 1144*
Gentamicin *on page 841*
Penicillins, Extended-Spectrum *on page 997*

Alternate:

Macrolides *on page 924*

Selected Readings

Kaliner MA, Osguthorpe JD, Fireman P, et al, "Sinusitis: Bench to Bedside. Current Findings, Future Directions," *J Allergy Clin Immunol*, 1997, 99(6 Pt 3):S829-48.
Talmor M, Li P, and Barie PS, "Acute Paranasal Sinusitis in Critically Ill Patients: Guidelines for Prevention, Diagnosis, and Treatment," *Clin Infect Dis*, 1997, 25(6):1441-6.
Westergren V, Lundblad L, Hellquist HB, et al, "Ventilator-Associated Sinusitis: A Review," *Clin Infect Dis*, 1998, 27(4):851-64.

Skin and Soft Tissue

Synonyms Cellulitis; Fasciitis

Clinical Presentation Erythema, warmth, and edema around the involved area. Patient may be febrile with leukocytosis. In patients with cellulitis of the extremities, deeper infections must be ruled out. (Patients with necrotizing fasciitis experience hyperesthesia in the face of an unimpressive lesion. Necrotizing disease is a surgical emergency; broad-spectrum antimicrobial coverage including anaerobic must be administered.)

Differential Diagnosis Malignancy; osteomyelitis

Likely Pathogens

Staphylococcus aureus, Methicillin-Resistant *on page 304*
Staphylococcus aureus, Methicillin-Susceptible *on page 307*
Streptococcus Species *on page 326*
Clostridium perfringens on page 88

Diagnostic Tests/Procedures
Anaerobic Culture *on page 371*
Biopsy Culture, Routine *on page 390*
Blood Culture, Aerobic and Anaerobic *on page 391*
Gram Stain *on page 473*
Skin Biopsy *on page 580*

Drug Therapy Comment Community-acquired MRSA infections have been reported among athletes, children, military recruits, Pacific Islanders, Alaskan natives, and prisoners. Isolates many be susceptible to sulfamethoxazole and trimethoprim, doxycycline, and/or clindamycin. Sulfamethoxazole and trimethoprim is the drug of choice in high-risk populations. Incision and drainage is usually necessary for adequate treatment.

Empiric Drug Therapy

Recommended:
Penicillins, Penicillinase-Resistant *on page 997*
Cephalosporins, 1st Generation *on page 729*

Alternate:
Clindamycin *on page 752*
Vancomycin *on page 1144*

Selected Readings

Fontes RA Jr, Ogilvie CM, and Miclau T, "Necrotizing Soft-Tissue Infections," *J Am Acad Orthop Surg*, 2000, 8(3):151-8.
Nichols RL and Florman S, "Clinical Presentations of Soft-Tissue Infections and Surgical Site Infections," *Clin Infect Dis*, 2001, 33 (Suppl 2):S84-93.

Slapped Cheek *see* Parvovirus B19 *on page 255*
Smallpox *see* Variola *on page 350*
Snuffles *see Bordetella bronchiseptica on page 52*
Spirometra mansonoides *see* Cestodes *on page 72*

Spongiform Encephalopathy

Synonyms Creutzfeldt-Jacob Disease

Clinical Presentation A rare, but fatal disease of the central nervous system characterized by progressive dementia and neuromuscular dysfunction. The onset is usually between 50 and 75 years of age; however, a syndrome has been described (new variant, nvCJD) which affects younger individuals. Initially, symptoms may include insomnia, depression, confusion, memory changes, incoordination, paresthesia, and visual disturbances. Personality and behavioral changes may be observed. Disease progression is associated with a rapid progression to dementia and increasing myoclonus, resulting in severe impairment of mental and physical function.

The worldwide incidence is between 0.5-1.0 cases/million/year. Four forms of CJD have been described; all are currently incurable. Inherited forms account for 10% to 15% of cases. Higher rates are reported in selected populations (Czechoslovakia and Chile, Libyan-born Jews).

The only proven manner for contracting CJD from an infected person has been through iatrogenic transmission for material contaminated by neural tissue of an infected individual. Infection has been reported from corneal transplants, implantation of electrodes in the brain, dura mater grafts, contaminated surgical instruments and the injection of cadaveric human growth hormone. The spouses and family members who live with CJD patients do not appear to be at increased risk.

Exposure to diseased animals (for example, bovine spongiform encephalopathy or BSE) has been linked to the development of sporadic CJD. A British outbreak was correlated to the consumption of beef from diseased cattle before 1989. Following this outbreak, regulations were adopted which have subsequently reduced the risk of exposure, including disposal of potentially infectious cattle offal (including neural tissues) and a cessation of the use of sheep entrails in feeds.

Differential Diagnosis Alzheimer's disease; Pick's Disease; Huntington's Disease; cerebral hematomas and vascular irregularities

Likely Pathogens Not established: Prions, *Spiroplasma* sp., and virions have been suspected. The causative agent has not been determined. However, the disease is transmissible.

Diagnostic Tests/Procedures A definitive diagnosis of CJD has traditionally required a brain biopsy or autopsy. Pathologic specimens reveal the characteristic changes in the brain tissue. Brain biopsy may produce a false-negative result if the biopsied area was unaffected by the disease.

An important advance has been the identification of a novel spinal fluid test, the 14-3-3 assay, which appears to accurately detect sporadic CJD. Additional tests proposed to confirm a diagnosis of CJD include identifying the presence of the deadly prion protein, identifying the prion gene mutation, and transmitting the disease from

(Continued)

Spongiform Encephalopathy *(Continued)*

the human patient to animals. Magnetic brain scanning may be used to diagnose sporadic CJD. No presymptomatic screening test is available.

Empiric Drug Therapy

Recommended: No empiric treatment. Supportive treatment only.

Spontaneous Bacterial Peritonitis *see* Peritonitis, Spontaneous Bacterial *on page 264*

Sporothrix schenckii

Microbiology *Sporothrix schenckii* is a saprophytic fungus widely dispersed in the soil, on the surface of many plants, and in decaying vegetable matter. The organism is a thermally dimorphic fungus, meaning that it exists in either a yeast or a mold form depending on the temperature. At room temperature, it exists in a mold form, but at warmer temperatures, it grows as a budding yeast. In clinical specimens such as biopsies of skin lesions, *Sporothrix schenckii* appears as a round or oval budding yeast; organisms may be difficult to find in clinical specimens and when present, may have variable size and shape. Thus, culture confirmation of *Sporothrix schenckii* is important. The organism grows relatively well on a variety of fungal media used routinely in microbiology laboratories.

Epidemiology *Sporothrix schenckii* is the causative agent of sporotrichosis or "gardener's disease". Typically, the organism is inoculated directly into the hand or face of a person handling plants or soil containing the organism. *S. schenckii* can be cultured from rose thorns, hay, compost material, mulch, and other decaying plant matter. It is important to obtain a detailed occupational and recreational history in suspected cases of sporotrichosis; individuals at risk include gardeners (particularly those handling roses), florists, landscapers, farmers, loggers, and others. Individuals who are infected with *S. schenckii* generally have a normal immune system. Although zoonotic transmission has been reported, it is much rarer then traumatic implantation of the organism. Several cases have been reported of veterinarians acquiring sporotrichosis from infected cats even without an associated penetrating injury.

The largest documented U.S. outbreak of sporotrichosis occurred in 1988. The outbreak was linked to Wisconsin-grown sphagnum moss used in packing evergreen tree seedlings; 84 individuals from 15 states developed cutaneous sporotrichosis. The attack rate was 17% in New York State, where 13 cases were reported from 109 forestry workers who had handled evergreen seedlings and moss. As expected, the attack rates were highest in those workers spending more time directly exposed to the moss. Although cultures of sphagnum moss from the Wisconsin supplier were negative for *Sporothrix schenckii*, the organism was cultured from multiple samples of the moss obtained from the tree nursery in Pennsylvania thought to be the main source of the outbreak. Several tree-handling procedures at this nursery may have contributed to the outbreak, such as the use of 3-year-old moss to pack seedlings, use of a pond water system to keep the moss wet, use of a polymer gel on the root system of the seedlings, and lengthy storage of moss-packed seedlings prior to shipping. This outbreak emphasized the need for wearing protective gloves and long-sleeved shirts in persons handling evergreens and similar plants.

Clinical Syndromes Sporotrichosis is divided into cutaneous and extracutaneous forms.

- **Cutaneous sporotrichosis:** This occurs when the organism is inoculated into the subcutaneous tissues following a minor trauma to the extremities or face. The incubation period is variable, from 1 week to several months. Cutaneous sporotrichosis can be classified as either plaque sporotrichosis or lymphocutaneous sporotrichosis. In plaque sporotrichosis, a small red plaque develops on the extremity at the original site of inoculation of the organism. The plaque is nontender and may increase in size but no additional lesions develop. In lymphocutaneous sporotrichosis, the disease begins with a single papular lesion, but in time, multiple similar lesions appear more proximally following the path of lymphatic drainage. These lesions often change from painless papules to ulcers which drain pus or serosanguinous fluid. Interestingly, although new lesions form by lymphangitic spread, axillary (or inguinal) lymph nodes are seldom involved. Both forms of cutaneous sporotrichosis tend to be very chronic if left untreated.

  When examined by light microscopy, the skin lesions in cutaneous sporotrichosis show multinucleated giant cells and epithelioid cells consistent with granulomas; thus, sporotrichosis should be considered in the differential diagnosis of any granulomatous process on an extremity or the face. It is important to note that organisms may not be seen on a single skin biopsy and additional biopsies may be necessary. The finding of an "asteroid body" on histologic section of a skin biopsy is highly suggestive of sporotrichosis but is not reliably present in all biopsies. The asteroid is a fungal organism surrounded by several "rays" that

stain with periodic acid-Schiff (PAS). A recent study using electron microscopy suggested that an asteroid body is composed of crystalline products of disintegrated host cells deposited around a central fungal cell.

A number of clinical entities should be considered in the differential diagnosis of cutaneous sporotrichosis. Some can be eliminated on the basis of epidemiology alone. Diseases to consider include:

- *Mycobacterium marinum*
- *Mycobacterium kansasii*
- pyoderma gangrenosum
- *Nocardia brasiliensis*
- *Leishmania* species
- foreign body granulomas
- blastomycosis
- dermatologic diseases (especially with plaque sporotrichosis)

- **Extracutaneous sporotrichosis:** A variety of rare, extracutaneous forms have been described. The most common is osteoarticular sporotrichosis which involves the knee, elbow, wrist, or ankle. There is rarely a history of a plant or thorn injury and typically no skin lesions are present. Patients may present with either single joint involvement or a polyarticular syndrome. The onset is indolent, and the joint develops tenderness, warmth, effusions, and sometimes draining sinuses. Osteoarticular sporotrichosis is a very difficult diagnosis to make; one study reported that it usually took over 2 years to make the correct diagnosis. Other forms of sporotrichosis include:
  - Pulmonary sporotrichosis: Only a few cases have been reported. Patients present with a chronic cavitary pneumonia, usually in an upper lobe. The disease mimics tuberculosis and histoplasmosis. One recent report suggested that the Papanicolaou stain of sputum may be helpful in making this rare diagnosis.
  - Ocular disease: This usually results from penetrating ocular injury to the conjunctiva or surrounding tissues. Eighteen cases of sporotrichoid endophthalmitis have been reported, with only two cases associated with trauma; most have required enucleation.
  - Meningitis: This rare complication has been reported in a few immunocompetent individuals. In one study of meningeal sporotrichosis in 7 patients, the cerebrospinal fluid was frequently negative on both stain and fungal culture initially; repeated lumbar punctures were necessary over a 3- to 11-month period before the organism was cultured.
  - Disseminated sporotrichosis: Patients present with multiple skin lesions involving two or more extremities. Blood cultures using the lysis-centrifugation method have been reported positive for *Sporothrix schenckii* in some cases.
- **Sporotrichosis and AIDS:** Systemic sporotrichosis has been reported in patients with advanced HIV infection but remains an infrequent complication. A number of sites of infection have been reported including the lung, liver, spleen, intestine, bone, eye, joints, and disseminated cutaneous lesions. Recently, a case of meningitis was reported in a patient with known cutaneous sporotrichosis and a CD4 cell count of 56/μL. Again, the cerebrospinal fluid was sterile over a 5-month period. The skin lesions responded to a prolonged course of amphotericin B and fluconazole, but the meningeal symptoms worsened on therapy, and on autopsy, *S. schenckii* was found infiltrating into the meninges and brain parenchyma.

Diagnosis The clinical suspicion of sporotrichosis should be confirmed microbiologically because of the number of conditions which can mimic the cutaneous lesions. Cultures of appropriate specimens such as skin biopsies, joint fluid, and bursal fluid will frequently recover the organism. *S. schenckii* is difficult to identify on fungal stains of biopsy specimens or KOH preparations since the organism burden is often low. Cultures of exudates from ulcerative skin lesions are often low-yield. Blood cultures, urine cultures, and sputum are only rarely positive. As noted earlier, cerebrospinal fluid is frequently negative in meningeal sporotrichosis, and multiple samples over time are necessary.

Specific IgG antibodies to *S. schenckii* are available at specialty laboratories but are of limited usefulness. Demonstration of IgG synthesis against the organism in cerebrospinal fluid may be a useful means of diagnosing meningeal sporotrichosis when routine cultures are negative (see Penn et al reference).

Diagnostic Tests/Procedures

Fungus Culture, Body Fluid *on page 462*
Fungus Culture, Cerebrospinal Fluid *on page 464*
Fungus Culture, Skin *on page 464*

Treatment Recently, antifungal susceptibility of *Sporothrix schenckii* to several agents has become available in specialized centers (eg, Dr. Michael Rinaldi, Fungus Testing Laboratory, University Health Science Center, San Antonio, TX). This may be useful

(Continued)

Sporothrix schenckii (Continued)

in severe or refractory cases. The treatment of choice for cutaneous sporotrichosis is a saturated solution of potassium iodide (SSKI). The mechanism of action of SSKI is obscure. The dose is initiated at 5 drops of SSKI 3 times/day in juice and steadily increased to 40 drops 3 times/day. Toxicity of the medication is common and includes gastrointestinal distress and lacrimation; the dose should be lowered if these symptoms occur. Drug rash is also relatively common, but the medication can usually be continued safely. Local heat is useful in cutaneous disease and can be used either as an adjunctive measure or in patients intolerant of SSKI. The azole antifungal agents may have some activity against *S. schenckii*. Ketoconazole and fluconazole have limited or no activity; itraconazole has *in vitro* activity although the *in vivo* experience is limited.

Extracutaneous sporotrichosis is best treated with amphotericin B. Prolonged courses are usually necessary, and osteoarticular sporotrichosis often requires over 2 g amphotericin. Pulmonary and meningeal sporotrichosis are even more difficult to treat, and a specialist in Infectious Disease should be consulted.

Drug Therapy

Recommended:

Cutaneous sporotrichosis:

Potassium Iodide *on page 1014*

Extracutaneous sporotrichosis:

Amphotericin B (Conventional) *on page 650*

Selected Readings

Coles FB, Schuchat A, Hibbs JR, et al, "A Multistate Outbreak of Sporotrichosis Associated With Sphagnum Moss," *Am J Epidemiol*, 1992, 136(4):475-87.

Keiser P and Whittle D, "Sporotrichosis in Human Immunodeficiency Virus-Infected Patients: Report of a Case," *Rev Infect Dis*, 1991, 13(5):1027-8.

Penn CC, Goldstein E, and Bartholomew WR, "*Sporothrix schenckii* Meningitis in a Patient With AIDS," *Clin Infect Dis*, 1992, 15(4):741-3.

Rex JH, "*Sporothrix schenckii*," *Principles and Practice of Infectious Diseases*, 4th ed, Mandell GL, Bennett JE, and Dolin R, eds, New York, NY: Churchill Livingstone, 1995, 2321-4.

Roberts GD and Larsh HW, "The Serologic Diagnosis of Extracutaneous Sporotrichosis," *Am J Clin Pathol*, 1971, 56(5):597-600.

Sporotrichosis *see Sporothrix schenckii on page 302*

SRGPC *see Streptococcus*-Related Gram-Positive Cocci *on page 325*

SSSS *see Staphylococcus aureus*, Methicillin-Resistant *on page 304*

Staphylococcal Scalded Skin Syndrome (SSSS) *see Staphylococcus aureus*, Methicillin-Resistant *on page 304*

Staphylococcus aureus, Methicillin-Resistant

Related Information

Antibiotic Treatment of Adults With Infective Endocarditis *on page 1271*

Synonyms MRSA

Microbiology *Staphylococcus* derives its name from the Greek word staphyle meaning "bunch of grapes". On Gram stain, staphylococci are gram-positive cocci, 0.7-1.2 μm, nonspore-forming, occurring singly, in pairs, in short 4-5 cocci chains or clusters. Staphylococci grow rapidly both as aerobes and anaerobes on blood agar. The colonies are sharply defined, smooth, and 1-4 mm in diameter. Staphylococci are catalase-positive. *Staphylococcus aureus* often has a light golden pigmentation secondary to carotenoid and produces β-hemolysis on horse, sheep, or human blood agar after an incubation of 24-48 hours.

For identification purposes, staphylococci are divided into those species which do and those which do not produce coagulase, coagulase-positive and -negative, respectively. *S. aureus* is essentially the only coagulase-positive *Staphylococcus. S. epidermidis* is by far the most commonly encountered coagulase-negative *Staphylococcus.*

Epidemiology Colonization of healthcare workers with MRSA is uncommon. The two major modes of transmission of MRSA is via an infected or colonized patient, or dissemination through an infected or colonized healthcare worker; typically MRSA is transmitted on the hands of a healthcare worker after contact with an infected patient.

MRSA is not a marker for virulence nor spreading, and MRSA has not been shown to spontaneously evolve from methicillin-resistant *S. aureus* (MSSA) to MRSA during the course of antibiotic therapy. Resistance to methicillin occurs predominantly by intrinsic resistance (penicillin-binding proteins) which is transmitted chromosomally. Five percent to 20% are also resistant to erythromycin, lincomycin, and clindamycin. Rifampin cannot be used alone secondary to a high one-step mutation rate to resistance.

Although universal precautions have been adopted and must be followed by all healthcare personnel, incidence of MRSA continues to rise. The goal of all facilities is ablation of widespread colonization and is difficult to achieve. Contact isolation is recommended.

Since 2001, MRSA have become dramatically and increasingly more recognized as pathogens which are emerging from healthcare settings into the community, where they cause primary infections. These community-associated MRSA (CA-MRSA) differ in several ways from typical nosocomial MRSA. In contrast to the typical nosocomial MRSA, CA-MRSA are genetically distinct, usually resistant only to beta-lactams, are not as multiply resistant as typical MRSA, usually cause only skin and soft tissue infections, and have been associated with infections in specific populations (inmates, Native Americans, children in daycare centers, military recruits, homeless youth, and competitive athletes). The fact that community-acquired skin and soft tissue infections are now being caused by MRSA has led physicians to reconsider the way patients with such infections are treated empirically. To view images of CA-MRSA skin infections, go to www.lapublichealth.org/acd/docs/MRSA_ColorEnhanced.pdf.

Clinical Syndromes

- **Localized:** Most common type of infection usually secondary to poor personal hygiene, minor trauma, or diminished skin integrity (ie, eczema, psoriasis).

  Folliculitis - Typically clears with local antiseptic.

  Furuncle - Deep seated infection around a hair follicle beginning as a painful, red nodule then becoming a hot, painful, raised indurated lesion 1-2 cm long, over several days. Predilection for the face, neck, axillae, and buttocks.

  Carbuncle - Deep seated infection of multiple hair follicles that coalesce and spread into the subcutaneous tissue, frequently associated with sinus tracts. Need to exclude septicemia and/or septic thrombophlebitis. If recurrent, should evaluate for underlying phagocytic or metabolic dysfunction.

  Impetigo - Typically affects children on exposed areas. Approximately 10% due to *Streptococcus pyogenes* and 10% due to combined staph/strep infections. Begins as a red macule which progresses to a vesicle then to crust. May be confused with HSV and varicella. The bullous form may respond to topical mupirocin or oral antistaphylococcal agents. Nonbullous form usually responds to oral or intramuscular penicillin.

  Hydradenitis suppurative - Recurrent pyogenic abscess of apocrine sweat glands, especially axillary, perineal, and genital. Mimics LGV. Usually requires incision and drainage, as well as oral antibiotics.

  Mastitis - Occurs in 1% to 3% of nursing mothers. Requires oral antibiotics. Continued nursing is controversial.

  Wound infections - Usually occurs 2 days after surgery. May need to explore wound. Requires oral antibiotics 7-10 days. May need I.V. antibiotics 4-6 weeks for underlying prosthesis.

  Spreading pyodermas - Surgical intervention needed if necrotizing fascitis.
- **Pneumonia:** Most frequently occurs a few days after influenza; mortality is 30% to 50%. Acquired via inhalation or hematogenous route. Approximately 33% develop empyemas. Patients present with chest pain, fever, shortness of breath, tachypnea, and a pleural effusion which requires drainage. May be associated with bronchiectasis or obstructive bronchogenic cancer. Hematogenous route usually secondary to right-sided endocarditis, infected intravascular device, or septic phlebitis.
- **Toxic shock syndrome caused by TSST 1 (toxin 1):** Typically occurs in young women ages 15-25 using tampons. Starts abruptly during menses. Presents with fever, profound refractory hypotension, erythroderma with desquamation, multi-organ involvement with profuse diarrhea, and mental confusion. Approximately 50% will have elevated creatine kinase, decreased platelets, and leukocytosis. May be seen secondary to surgical wound packages, as well as associated with disseminated staph infections. Mortality is approximately 3%.
- **Staphylococcal scalded skin syndrome (SSSS):** Most commonly occurs in children and neonates; epidemics in neonatal nurseries and daycare centers. Usually caused by phage type 2. Starts abruptly with perioral erythema with sunburn-like rash rapidly turning bright red then spreading to bullae in 2-3 days and desquamating within 5 days. Positive Nikolsky sign. Recovery in 10 days. Need to exclude toxic epidermal neurolysis and Kawasaki mucocutaneous disease (culture-negative, Nikolsky-negative).
- **Food poisoning:** Usually caused by ingestion of heat stable enterotoxin B. Second most common cause of acute food poisoning. May occur by

(Continued)

Staphylococcus aureus, Methicillin-Resistant *(Continued)*

person-to-person transmission. Incubation within 2-6 hours after ingestion of toxin contained in custard filled bakery goods, canned foods, processed meats, potato salads, and ice cream. Patients present with acute salivation, nausea, vomiting progressing to abdominal cramps, and watery, nonbloody diarrhea (risk of dehydration).

- **Musculoskeletal:** Frequent cause of osteomyelitis, septic arthritis, septic bursitis, and, less frequently, pyomyositis. Blood cultures positive in approximately 50% of these cases of osteomyelitis. Need bone biopsy for definitive diagnosis. Typically hematogenous or secondary to local trauma with contiguous infection. Sternoclavicular joint usually follows septic thrombosis of upper limb and often associated with IVDA. Septic arthritis usually secondary to complication of septicemia, rheumatoid arthritis, or prepubertal trauma. (Knee > hip > elbow > shoulder.)
- **Septicemia/endocarditis:** Associated with age extremes, cardiovascular disease, decompensated diabetes, and heroin addicts. Mortality remains high (40% to 60%) despite antimicrobial therapy. Thirty-three percent of patients have no focus for infection. Overall incidence of endocarditis with *S. aureus* infection is 10%. *S. aureus* is the second most common cause of native valve endocarditis and continues to rise in incidence in bacteremias thought secondary to IVDA and use of long-term indwelling catheters.

Diagnosis It is not possible to distinguish MRSA from MSSA clinically. Susceptibility testing should be performed on all *S. aureus* isolates. Isolation of *S. aureus* from a patient with suspected toxic shock syndrome (TSS) neither confirms the diagnosis nor proves that the isolate is the etiological agent of the disease. The isolate must be shown to be capable of producing toxic shock syndrome toxin type 1 (TSST-1). Most isolates of *S. aureus* cultured from patients with clinically proven TSS produce TSST-1. Suspect isolates can be tested for the production of TSST-1 by immunodiffusion, isoelectric focusing, Western blot, and immunoblot techniques. The immunoblot technique is extremely sensitive, specific, rapid, and reliable and is the test of choice. However, the test is not widely available.

Diagnostic Tests/Procedures

Aerobic Culture, Appropriate Site *on page 365*
Gram Stain *on page 473*

Treatment MRSA is characteristically resistant to all beta-lactam antibiotics, including penicillins, cephalosporins, and carbapenems. MRSA acquired in the healthcare setting are typically multidrug resistant, whereas community-acquired MRSA are often susceptible to clindamycin and erythromycin. Doxycycline and trimethoprim/sulfamethoxazole are often active against MRSA, but usually reserved for less serious infections if susceptible *in vitro*.

Vancomycin has been the mainstay of MRSA therapy for decades. Newer agents, such as daptomycin, linezolid, and quinupristin/dalfopristin, are also quite active and may be at least as effective as vancomycin against serious MRSA infections. Rifampin and gentamicin are used along with vancomycin for synergy, particularly in life-threatening infections such as prosthetic valve endocarditis. Use of combination therapy with the newer agents has not been established.

There have been few cases of vancomycin-resistant or intermediate *S. aureus* reported. Most of these agents are susceptible to at least one of the newer agents. Susceptibility testing must be performed. New guidelines for hospital-acquired pneumonia recommend linezolid or vancomycin for empiric therapy for MRSA pneumonia.

Drug Therapy

Recommended:

Vancomycin *on page 1144*

Alternate:

Daptomycin *on page 768*
Doxycycline *on page 787*
Linezolid *on page 914*
Quinupristin and Dalfopristin *on page 1032*
Sulfamethoxazole and Trimethoprim *on page 1087*

Selected Readings

American Thoracic Society and Infectious Diseases Society of America, "Guidelines for the Management of Adults With Hospital-Acquired, Ventilator-Associated, and Healthcare-Associated Pneumonia," *Am J Respir Crit Care Med*, 2005, 171(4):388-416.

Anstead GM and Owens AD, "Recent Advances in the Treatment of Infections Due to Resistant *Staphylococcus aureus*," *Curr Opin Infect Dis*, 2004, 17(6):549-55.

Deresinski S, "Methicillin-Resistant *Staphylococcus aureus*: An Evolutionary, Epidemiologic, and Therapeutic Odyssey," *Clin Infect Dis*, 2005, 40(4):562-73.

Mounzer KC and diNubile MJ, "Clinical Presentation and Management of Methicillin-Resistant *Staphylococcus aureus* (MRSA) Infections," *Antibiotics for Clinicians*, 1998, 2(Suppl 1):15-20.

Mulligan ME, Murray-Leisure KA, Ribner BS, et al, "Methicillin-Resistant *Staphylococcus aureus*: A Consensus Review of the Microbiology, Pathogenesis, and Epidemiology With Implications for Prevention and Management," *Am J Med*, 1993, 94(3):313-28.

Regev-Yochay G, Rubinstein E, Barzilai A, et al, "Methicillin-Resistant *Staphylococcus aureus* in Neonatal Intensive Care Unit," *Emerg Infect Dis*, 2005, 11(3):453-6.

Rybak MJ, "Community-Associated Methicillin-Resistant *Staphylococcus aureus*: A Review," *Pharmacotherapy*, 2005, 25(1):74-85.

Tenover FC, "VRSA, VISA, and GISA: The Dilemma Behind the Name Game," *Clin Microbiol Newslett*, 2000, 22(7):49-53.

Staphylococcus aureus, Methicillin-Susceptible

Related Information

Antibiotic Treatment of Adults With Infective Endocarditis *on page 1271*

Synonyms MSSA

Microbiology Staphylococci derives its name from the Greek word staphyle meaning "bunch of grapes". On Gram stain, staphylococci are gram-positive cocci, 0.7-1.2 μm, nonspore-forming, occurring singly, in pairs, in short 4-5 cocci chains or clusters. Staphylococci grow rapidly both as an aerobe and anaerobe on blood agar. The colonies are sharply defined, smooth, and 1-4 mm in diameter. Staphylococci are catalase-positive and differ from micrococci by the following: anaerobic acid production from glucose, sensitivity <200 mg/mL lysostaphin, and production of acid from glycerol in the presence of 0.4 mg/mL erythromycin.

Staphylococcus aureus may have a golden pigmentation secondary to carotenoid and produce β-hemolysis on horse, sheep, or human blood agar after an incubation of 24-48 hours. *Staphylococcus epidermidis* and coagulase-negative staph (CNS) are often used interchangeably but recognize that there are over 30 species of CNS of which *S. epidermidis* is the most common. It is important to distinguish three clinically relevant species: *S. aureus*, *S. epidermidis*, and *S. saprophyticus*.

Epidemiology It is estimated that 20% to 40% of the population are persistent asymptomatic nasal carriers. The carrier state is clinically relevant in that carriers have a higher rate of staphylococci infections as compared to noncarriers. Neonates may be colonized in the perianal area, umbilical stumps, skin, and gastrointestinal tract. Adults are colonized in the anterior nares, skin, and less frequently, vagina. There is an increase carrier rate among hospital personnel, diabetics receiving insulin, hemodialysis patients, and I.V. drug users.

The portal of entry is typically the skin. Patients with chemotaxis defects (ie, Chédiak-Higashi, Wiskott-Aldrich), opsonization defects (ie, complement deficiencies), and staphylocidal defects of polymorphonuclear cells (ie, chronic granulomatous disease) are at increased risk.

Eighty percent to 90% of community-acquired staphylococci are resistant to penicillin. One of the more common forms of resistance is through the production of beta-lactamase, an extracellular enzyme coded for by plasmids that inactivate penicillin by interrupting the β-lactam ring. These organisms are still susceptible to antistaphylococcal penicillins and first generation cephalosporins.

Clinical Syndromes

- **Localized:** Most common type of infection usually secondary to poor personal hygiene, minor trauma, or diminished skin integrity (ie, eczema, psoriasis)

  Folliculitis - Typically clears with local antiseptic.

  Furuncle - Deep seated infection around a hair follicle beginning as a painful, red nodule then becoming a hot, painful, raised indurated lesion 1-2 cm long, over several days. Predilection for the face, neck, axillae, and buttocks.

  Carbuncle - Deep seated infection of multiple hair follicles that coalesce and spread into the subcutaneous tissue, frequently associated with sinus tracts. Need to exclude septicemia and/or septic thrombophlebitis. If recurrent, should evaluate for underlying phagocytic or metabolic dysfunction.

  Impetigo - Typically affects children on exposed areas. Approximately 10% due to *Streptococcus pyogenes* and 10% due to combined staph/strep infections. Begins as a red macule which progresses to a vesicle then to crust. May be confused with HSV and varicella. The bullous form may respond to topical mupirocin or oral antistaphylococcal agents. Nonbullous form usually responds to oral or intramuscular penicillin.

  Hydradenitis suppurative - Recurrent pyogenic abscess of apocrine sweat glands, especially axillary, perineal, and genital. Mimics LGV. Usually requires incision and drainage, as well as oral antibiotics.

  Mastitis - Occurs in 1% to 3% of nursing mothers. Requires oral antibiotics. Continued nursing is controversial.

(Continued)

Staphylococcus aureus, Methicillin-Susceptible *(Continued)*

Wound infections - Usually occurs 2 days after surgery. May need to explore wound. Requires oral antibiotics 7-10 days. May need I.V. antibiotics 4-6 weeks for underlying prosthesis.

Spreading pyodermas - Surgical intervention needed if necrotizing fascitis.

- **Pneumonia:** Most frequently occurs a few days after influenza; mortality is 30% to 50%. Acquired via inhalation or hematogenous route. Approximately 33% develop empyemas. Patients present with chest pain, fever, shortness of breath, tachypnea, and a pleural effusion which requires drainage. May be associated with bronchiectasis or obstructive bronchogenic cancer. Hematogenous route usually secondary to right-sided endocarditis, infected intravascular device, or septic phlebitis.
- **Toxic shock syndrome caused by TSST 1 (toxin 1):** Typically occurs in young woman ages 15-25 using tampons. Starts abruptly during menses. Present with fever, profound refractory hypotension, erythroderma with desquamation, multi-organ involvement with profuse diarrhea, mental confusion. Approximately 50% will have elevated creatine kinase, decreased platelets, and leukocytosis. May be seen secondary to surgical wound packages, as well as associated with disseminated staph infections. Mortality is approximately 3%.
- **Staphylococcal scalded skin syndrome (SSSS):** Most commonly occurs in children and neonates; epidemics in neonatal nurseries and daycare centers. Usually caused by phage type 2. Starts abruptly with perioral erythema with sunburn-like rash rapidly turning bright red spreading to bullae in 2-3 days and desquamating within 5 days. Positive Nikolsky sign. Recovery in 10 days. Need to exclude toxic epidermal neurolysis and Kawasaki mucocutaneous disease (culture-negative, Nikolsky-negative).
- **Food poisoning:** Usually caused by ingestion of heat stable enterotoxin B. Second most common cause of acute food poisoning. May occur by person-to-person transmission. Incubation 2-6 hours after ingestion of toxin contained in custard filled bakery goods, canned foods, processed meats, potato salads, and ice cream. Patients present with acute salivation, nausea, vomiting progressing to abdominal cramps, and watery, nonbloody diarrhea (risk of dehydration).
- **Musculoskeletal:** Frequent cause of osteomyelitis, septic arthritis, septic bursitis and less frequently pyomyositis. Blood cultures positive in approximately 50% of these cases of osteomyelitis. Need bone biopsy for definitive diagnosis. Typically hematogenous or secondary to local trauma with contiguous infection. Sternoclavicular joint usually follows septic thrombosis of upper limb and often associated with IVDA. Septic arthritis usually secondary to complication of septicemia, rheumatoid arthritis, or prepubertal trauma. (Knee > hip > elbow > shoulder.)
- **Septicemia/endocarditis:** Associated with age extremes, cardiovascular disease, decompensated diabetes, heroin addicts. Mortality remains high (40% to 60%) despite antimicrobial therapy. Thirty-three percent of patients have no focus for infection. Overall incidence of endocarditis with *S. aureus* infection is 10%. *S. aureus* is the second most common cause of native valve endocarditis and continues to rise in incidence in bacteremias thought secondary to IVDA and use of long-term indwelling catheters.

Diagnosis Diagnosis is made by Gram stain and culture of appropriate site. Phage typing is a useful epidemiological tool. Antiteichoic antibodies by CIE or RIA are positive in approximately 90% of patients with endocarditis, 20% to 40% positive with bacteremia, and 0% to 60% positive with localized infections. Isolation of *S. aureus* from a patient with suspected toxic shock syndrome (TSS) neither confirms the diagnosis nor proves that the isolate is the etiological agent of the disease. The isolate must be shown to be capable of producing toxic shock syndrome toxin type 1 (TSST-1). Most isolates of *S. aureus* cultured from patients with clinically proven TSS produce TSST-1. Suspect isolates can be tested for the production of TSST-1 by immunodiffusion, isoelectric focusing, Western blot, and immunoblot techniques. The immunoblot technique is extremely sensitive, specific, rapid, and reliable and is the test of choice. However, the test is not widely available.

Diagnostic Tests/Procedures

Aerobic Culture, Appropriate Site *on page 365*

Gram Stain *on page 473*

Teichoic Acid Antibody *on page 590*

Treatment Topical mupirocin may be useful in eradicating carrier states. Most localized infections will respond to penicillins or antistaphylococcal penicillins or first

generation cephalosporins. Deep-seated infections usually require surgical intervention. Penicillin-allergic individuals may be given erythromycin, clindamycin, or tetracycline. Patients with line sepsis without septicemia usually require 5-7 days parenteral antibiotics, whereas therapy is extended 10-14 days with septicemia. Controversy exists as to the removal of the intravascular device, but most authors recommend removing the catheter. Beta-lactam regimens for at least 4-6 weeks plus an aminoglycoside during the first to second week of treatment remains the treatment of choice for left-sided *S. aureus* endocarditis. Patients with β-lactam allergies or failed therapy should be treated with vancomycin plus rifampin. Patients with right-sided endocarditis are typically treated with the same regimens, however, there have been some studies suggesting the efficiency of quinolones. Two-week parenteral regimens are currently being investigated for the treatment of uncomplicated MSSA endocarditis.

Drug Therapy Comment Methicillin-susceptible *Staphylococcus aureus* is sensitive to a wide array of antibiotics including the penicillinase-resistant penicillins, 1st and most 2nd generation cephalosporins (also, *in vitro*, some 3rd generation cephalosporins), macrolides, clindamycin, tetracyclines, sulfonamides, and vancomycin. Although also often susceptible, the quinolones should not be used to treat this organism secondary to the risk of acquired resistance while on therapy. When choosing among these agents for the treatment of serious systemic infections, the penicillinase-resistant penicillins (nafcillin, oxacillin) are the drugs of choice. Organisms typically have higher MICs to vancomycin than to the penicillinase-resistant penicillins. If the organism happens to be penicillin-susceptible, penicillin would be the drug of choice.

Drug Therapy

Recommended:

Penicillins, Penicillinase-Resistant *on page 997*

Alternate:

Cephalosporins, 1st Generation *on page 729*

Clindamycin *on page 752*

Linezolid *on page 914*

Quinupristin and Dalfopristin *on page 1032*

Vancomycin *on page 1144*

Selected Readings

Archer GL, "*Staphylococcus aureus*: A Well-Armed Pathogen," *Clin Infect Dis*, 1998, 26(5):1179-81.

Chambers MD, "Short-Course Combination and Oral Therapies of *Staphylococcus aureus* Endocarditis," *Infect Dis Clin North Am*, 1993, 7(1):69-80.

Jensen AG, Espersen F, Skinhoj P, et al "Bacteremic *Staphylococcus aureus* Spondylitis," *Arch Intern Med*, 1998, 158(5):509-17.

Mortara LA and Bayer AS, "*Staphylococcus aureus*, Bacteremia and Endocarditis. New Diagnostic and Therapeutic Concepts," *Infect Dis Clin North Am*, 1993, 7(1):53-68.

Tenover FC, "VRSA, VISA, and GISA: The Dilemma Behind the Name Game," *Clin Microbiol Newslett*, 2000, 22(7):49-53.

Turnidge J and Grayson L, "Optimum Treatment of Staphylococcal Infections," *Drugs*, 1993, 45(3):353-66.

Waldvogel FA, "*Staphylococcus aureus* (Including Toxic Shock Syndrome)," *Principles and Practice of Infectious Diseases*, 4th ed, Mandell GL, Bennett JE, and Dolin R, eds, New York, NY: Churchill Livingstone, 1995, 1754-77.

Weckbach LS, Thompson MR, Staneck JL, et al, "Rapid Screening Assay for Toxic Shock Syndrome Toxin Production by *Staphylococcus aureus*," *J Clin Microbiol*, 1984, 20(1):18-22.

Williams RE and MacKie RM, "The Staphylococci - Importance of Their Control in the Management of Skin Disease," *Dermatol Clin*, 1993, 11(1):201-6.

Staphylococcus epidermidis, Methicillin-Resistant

Synonyms MRSE

Microbiology *Staphylococcus* derives its name from the Greek word staphyle meaning "bunch of grapes". On Gram stain, staphylococci are gram-positive cocci, 0.7-1.2 μm, nonspore-forming, occurring singly, in pairs, in short 4-5 cocci chains or clusters. Staphylococci grow rapidly both as aerobes and anaerobes on blood agar. The colonies are sharply defined, smooth, and 1-4 mm in diameter. Staphylococci are catalase-positive.

For identification purposes, staphylococci are divided into those species which do and those which do not produce coagulase, coagulase-positive and -negative, respectively. *S. aureus* is essentially the only coagulase-positive *Staphylococcus*. *S. epidermidis* is by far the most commonly encountered coagulase-negative *Staphylococcus*.

Epidemiology Over the past 10 years, methicillin-susceptible *S. epidermidis* (MSSE) has continued to be the major cause of nosocomial bacteremia and sepsis with a mortality approaching 30%. MSSE is a normal inhabitant of the skin. It synthesizes an extracellular polysaccharide which is associated with persistence of infection, resistance to antibiotics, and a predilection for medical devices. Approximately 24,000 patients annually develop device-related MSSE septicemia with the most common being related to insertion site infections.

(Continued)

Staphylococcus epidermidis, Methicillin-Resistant *(Continued)*

Typically, community-acquired infections are beta-lactam sensitive, whereas most hospital-acquired infections are multiply resistant. Resistance to antistaphylococcal beta-lactams is mediated by the mec gene which confers resistance by encoding a unique penicillin binding protein with low affinity for beta-lactam antibiotics.

Clinical Syndromes

- **Foreign body infections:** Common sites of infection with MSSE include intravascular catheters, pacemakers, prosthetic cardiac valves, vascular grafts, orthopedic appliances, artificial joints, CSF shunts, dialysis catheters, and breast implants.
- **Osteomyelitis:** Most commonly associated with sternal wound infections status post cardiac surgery, although overall frequently rare. Other mode of transmission is via hematogenous spread.
- **Native valve endocarditis:** Less common than PVE; occurs in approximately 5%.
- **Urinary tract infection:** Hospital acquired secondary to manipulation or catheter placement.
- **Endophthalmitis:** Increasing significantly status postintraocular lens placement.

Diagnosis Diagnosis is made by Gram stain, culture, and antimicrobial susceptibility if the isolate is from an appropriate site. Semiquantitation is useful in suggesting a true intravascular catheter sepsis when both blood culture grows MSSE and the count is >15 CFU on blood agar plate.

Diagnostic Tests/Procedures

Aerobic Culture, Appropriate Site *on page 365*
Gram Stain *on page 473*

Treatment Vancomycin remains the drug of choice for MRSE. More than 50% of all isolates are resistant to tetracycline, chloramphenicol, clindamycin, and erythromycin. MRSE is usually sensitive to rifampin and gentamicin, but resistance develops quickly and neither drug can be used as a sole agent. Although not available in the U.S., teicoplanin may be of benefit. Antimicrobial therapy for PVE should consist of vancomycin, rifampin, and/or gentamicin for 4-6 weeks. Infections secondary to MRSE may be treated with sulfamethoxazole and trimethoprim if susceptible. Other agents such as daptomycin, linezolid, or quinupristin/dalfopristin have activity against strains of MRSE. Susceptibility testing should direct therapy; limited data is available in treatment of MRSE infections with these agents.

Drug Therapy

Recommended:

Monotherapy:
Vancomycin *on page 1144*

Combination therapy:
Vancomycin *on page 1144*
plus
Gentamicin *on page 841*
Vancomycin *on page 1144*
plus
Rifampin *on page 1046*

Alternate:

The following drug may be used only if susceptible:
Sulfamethoxazole and Trimethoprim *on page 1087*

Selected Readings

Christensen GD, "The 'Sticky' Problem of *Staphylococcus epidermidis* Sepsis," *Hosp Pract (Off Ed)*, 1993, 28(9A):27-36, 38.
Hachem RY and Raad I, "Clinical Presentation and Management of Methicillin-Resistant *Staphylococcus epidermidis* (MRSE) Bloodstream Infections," *Antibiotics for Clinicians*, 1998, 2(Suppl 1):21-4.
Lai KK and Fontecchio SA, "Infections Associated With Implantable Cardioverter Defibrillators Placed Transvenously and Via Thoracotomies: Epidemiology, Infection Control, and Management," *Clin Infect Dis*, 1998, 27(2):265-9.
Rupp ME and Archer GL, "Coagulase-Negative Staphylococci: Pathogens Associated With Medical Progress," *Clin Infect Dis*, 1994, 19(2):231-43.
Whitener C, Caputo GM, Weitekamp MR, et al, "Endocarditis Due to Coagulase-Negative Staphylococci," *Infect Dis Clin North Am*, 1993, 7(1):81-96.

Staphylococcus epidermidis, Methicillin-Susceptible

Synonyms MSSE

Microbiology Staphylococci derives its name from the Greek word staphyle meaning "bunch of grapes". On Gram stain, staphylococci are gram-positive cocci, 0.7-1.2 μm, nonspore-forming, occurring singly, in pairs, in short 4-5 cocci chains or clusters. Staphylococci grow rapidly both as an aerobe and anaerobe on blood agar. The colonies are sharply defined, smooth, and 1-4 mm in diameter. Staphylococci are

catalase-positive and differ from micrococci by the following: anaerobic acid production from glucose, sensitivity <200 mg/mL lysostaphin, and production of acid from glycerol in the presence of 0.4 mg/mL erythromycin.

Staphylococcus aureus may have a golden pigmentation secondary to carotenoid and produce β-hemolysis on horse, sheep, or human blood agar after an incubation of 24-48 hours. *Staphylococcus epidermidis* and coagulase-negative staph (CNS) are often used interchangeably but recognize that there are over 30 species of CNS of which *S. epidermidis* is the most common. It is important to distinguish three clinically relevant species: *S. aureus*, *S. epidermidis*, and *S. saprophyticus*.

Epidemiology Over the past 10 years, MSSE has continued to be the major cause of nosocomial bacteremia and sepsis with a mortality approaching 30%. MSSE is a normal inhabitant of the skin. It synthesizes an extracellular polysaccharide which is associated with persistence of infection, resistance to antibiotics, and a predilection for medical devices. Approximately 24,000 patients annually develop device-related septicemia with the most common being related to insertion site infections.

Thirty percent to 40% of prosthetic valve endocarditis (PVE) is due to CNS compared to 14% due to MSSA. Hickman/Broviac infections are 54% CNS as compared to 20% MSSA. Less than 6% of all pacemaker insertions result in infections, yet 40% to 50% are due to CNS secondary to contamination at the time of insertion. Similar findings are seen in prosthetic joint infections.

Typically, community-acquired infections are beta-lactam sensitive, whereas most hospital-acquired infections are multiply resistant. Resistance to antistaphylococcal beta-lactams is mediated by the mec gene which confers resistance by encoding a unique penicillin binding protein with low affinity for beta-lactam antibiotics.

Clinical Syndromes

- **Foreign body infections:** Common sites of infection with MSSE include intravascular catheters, pacemakers, prosthetic cardiac valves, vascular grafts, orthopedic appliances, artificial joints, CSF shunts, dialysis catheters, and breast implants.
- **Osteomyelitis:** Most commonly associated with sternal wound infections status post cardiac surgery, although overall frequently rare. Other mode of transmission is via hematogenous spread.
- **Native valve endocarditis:** Less common than PVE; occurs in approximately 5%.
- **Urinary tract infection:** Hospital acquired secondary to manipulation or catheter placement.
- **Endophthalmitis:** Increasing significantly status post intraocular lens placement.

Diagnosis Diagnosis is made by Gram stain and culture with sensitivities of appropriate site. Semiquantitation roll technique by Dennis Maki in which catheter is rolled over surface of blood agar plate is useful in suggesting a true intravascular catheter sepsis when both blood culture grows MSSE and count >15 colonies on a blood agar plate.

Diagnostic Tests/Procedures

Aerobic Culture, Appropriate Site *on page 365*
Gram Stain *on page 473*

Treatment First choice antibiotic in MSSE infections are penicillins or antistaphylococcal penicillins (penicillinase-resistant). For most medical device infections, the medical device must be removed. Current recommendations for pacemaker infection is to remove the pacer during the second week of parenteral antibiotics before reimplantation. Sixty-seven percent of prosthetic joint infection occur during the first 2 years. If the joint is not loose, 6 weeks of parenteral antibiotics are recommended. If the joint is loose, then removal of the joint plus parenteral antibiotics for 6 weeks is recommended. For nonlife-threatening infections with MSSE, a first generation cephalosporin may be used. For penicillin allergic individuals, clindamycin, vancomycin, doxycycline or sulfamethoxazole and trimethoprim based on susceptibility testing may be used.

Drug Therapy

Recommended:

Penicillins, Penicillinase-Resistant *on page 997*

Alternate:

Cephalosporins, 1st Generation *on page 729*
Clindamycin *on page 752*
Vancomycin *on page 1144*

Selected Readings

Christensen GD, "The 'Sticky' Problem of *Staphylococcus epidermidis* Sepsis," *Hosp Pract (Off Ed)*, 1993, 28(9A):27-36, 38.

Lai KK and Fontecchio SA, "Infections Associated With Implantable Cardioverter Defibrillators Placed Transvenously and Via Thoracotomies: Epidemiology, Infection Control, and Management," *Clin Infect Dis*, 1998, 27(2):265-9.

Raad I, Alrahwan A, and Rolston K, "*Staphylococcus epidermidis*: Emerging Resistance and Need for Alternative Agents," *Clin Infect Dis*, 1998, 26(5):1182-7.

(Continued)

Staphylococcus epidermidis, Methicillin-Susceptible *(Continued)*

Rupp ME and Archer GL, "Coagulase-Negative Staphylococci: Pathogens Associated With Medical Progress," *Clin Infect Dis,* 1994, 19(2):231-43.
Whitener C, Caputo GM, Weitekamp MR, et al, "Endocarditis Due to Coagulase-Negative Staphylococci," *Infect Dis Clin North Am,* 1993, 7(1):81-96.

Staphylococcus saprophyticus

Microbiology Staphylococci derives its name from the Greek word staphyle meaning "bunch of grapes". On Gram stain, staphylococci are gram-positive cocci, 0.7-1.2 μm, nonspore-forming, occurring singly, in pairs, in short 4-5 cocci chains or clusters. Staphylococci grow rapidly both as an aerobe and anaerobe on blood agar. The colonies are sharply defined, smooth, and 1-4 mm in diameter. Staphylococci are catalase-positive and differ from micrococci by the following: anaerobic acid production from glucose, sensitivity <200 mg/mL lysostaphin, and production of acid from glycerol in the presence of 0.4 mg/mL erythromycin.

Staphylococcus aureus may have a golden pigmentation secondary to carotenoid and produce β-hemolysis on horse, sheep, or human blood agar after an incubation of 24-48 hours. *Staphylococcus epidermidis* and coagulase-negative staph (CNS) are often used interchangeably but recognize that there are over 30 species of CNS of which *S. epidermidis* is the most common. It is important to distinguish three clinically relevant species: *S. aureus, S. epidermidis,* and *S. saprophyticus.*

Epidemiology *Staphylococcus saprophyticus* is a common cause of urinary tract infections (UTIs) in sexually active young women, elderly men, and children. The use of spermicide-coated condoms has been associated with an increase risk of UTI in young women. Highest frequency occurs during late summer and early autumn; reasons unclear.

Clinical Syndromes

- **Urinary tract infection (UTI):** Present with acute dysuria, back or flank pain, and temperature <38.5°C. Hematuria and pyuria are usually present.

Diagnosis Diagnosis depends on isolation of organism from urine. Counts as low as 10^2 CFU/mL in young women with symptoms is considered significant.

Diagnostic Tests/Procedures

Urine Culture, Clean Catch *on page 609*

Treatment First choice therapy is sulfamethoxazole and trimethoprim. Controversy exists whether single dose, 3-day, 7-day, or 10-day course are equally effective. Studies suggest that for women, a 3-day course is equally effective to a 7-day course. Alternative therapies include nitrofurantoin, ampicillin, first generation cephalosporin, or quinolone based on susceptibility testing.

Drug Therapy

Recommended:

Sulfamethoxazole and Trimethoprim *on page 1087*

Alternate:

Nitrofurantoin *on page 971*
Ampicillin *on page 657*
Cephalosporins, 1st Generation *on page 729*
Fluoroquinolones *on page 824*

Selected Readings

Abrahamsson K, Hansson S, Jodal U, et al, "*Staphylococcus saprophyticus* Urinary Tract Infections in Children," *Eur J Pediatr,* 1993, 152(1):69-71.
Elder NC, "Acute Urinary Tract Infection in Women. What Kind of Antibiotic Therapy Is Optimal?" *Postgrad Med,* 1992, 92(6):159-62, 165-6, 172.
Fihn SD, Boyko EJ, Chen CL, et al, "Use of Spermicide-Coated Condoms and Other Risk Factors for Urinary Tract Infection Caused by *Staphylococcus saprophyticus,*" *Arch Intern Med,* 1998, 158(3):281-7.

STEC *see Escherichia coli,* Enterohemorrhagic *on page 145*

Stenotrophomonas maltophilia

Synonyms *Xanthomonas maltophilia*

Microbiology *Stenotrophomonas maltophilia* is a lactose-negative, oxidase-negative, nonfermenting, aerobic, gram-negative bacillus with polar flagella. *S. maltophilia* is an obligate aerobe with optimal growth at 35°C. The organism grows well on common laboratory media as smooth, glistening, gray/light yellow, nonhemolytic colonies.

Epidemiology *Stenotrophomonas maltophilia* is ubiquitous and is considered an opportunistic pathogen. It can be isolated from natural water sources, sewage, soil, and a variety of plant environments. It can also be found in human feces and a wide range of nosocomial sources including fomites. The increasing presence of this organism is most likely due to antimicrobial selective pressure and the increase in

debilitated patients. Virulence factors for *Stenotrophomonas maltophilia* have not been extensively investigated.

Clinical Syndromes *Stenotrophomonas maltophilia* can infect any tissue or organ system including blood, lung, heart, skin, soft tissue, bone and joint, ophthalmologic, gastrointestinal tract, urinary tract, or musculoskeletal system. Syndromes caused by *Stenotrophomonas maltophilia* are usually indistinguishable from those caused by the other members of Enterobacteriaceae. Organisms are often grown as part of mixed cultures; therefore, distinguishing colonization from true infection is often difficult. Risk factors associated with *S. maltophilia* infections include prior antibiotic therapy, central lines, immunosuppression, prolonged hospitalization, intensive care admissions, mechanical ventilation, and burns.

Diagnosis The only way a diagnosis of *Stenotrophomonas maltophilia* infection can be made is by identification of the organism through culture in a patient with a relevant clinical syndrome. No special media or conditions are necessary to grow this organism.

Diagnostic Tests/Procedures

Aerobic Culture, Appropriate Site *on page 365*
Blood Culture, Aerobic and Anaerobic *on page 391*
Gram Stain *on page 473*

Treatment *Stenotrophomonas maltophilia* is resistant to a wide variety of antimicrobial agents. The organism is almost always resistant to imipenem, and often resistant to extended-spectrum penicillins, cephalosporins, and the fluoroquinolones. Although *Stenotrophomonas maltophilia* has typically been susceptible to sulfamethoxazole and trimethoprim, resistance rates are increasing. Alternative therapies should only be considered after susceptibility testing or based on hospital-specific epidemiology. Synergy may exist with sulfamethoxazole and trimethoprim with a number of other agents including tetracyclines, quinolones, and beta-lactam/beta-lactamase inhibitor combinations. Other synergistic combinations including ciprofloxacin/Zosyn®, ciprofloxacin/Timentin®, doxycycline/Timentin®, and colistin/rifampin have also been studied.

Drug Therapy

Recommended:

Sulfamethoxazole and Trimethoprim *on page 1087*

Alternate:

Note: Consider alternate agents only if susceptible.

Fluoroquinolones *on page 824*
Ticarcillin and Clavulanate Potassium *on page 1114*
Ceftazidime *on page 717*
Doxycycline *on page 787*
Minocycline *on page 947*

Selected Readings

Dalamaga M, Karmaniolas K, Chavelas C, et al, "*Stenotrophomonas maltophilia*: A Serious and Rare Complication in Patients Suffering From Burns," *Burns*, 2003, 29(7):711-3.

Denton M and Kerr KG, "Microbiological and Clinical Aspects of Infection Associated With *Stenotrophomonas maltophilia*," *Clin Microbiol Rev*, 1998, 11(1):57-80.

Giamarellos-Bourboulis EJ, Karnesis L, and Giamarellou H, "Synergy of Colistin With Rifampin and Trimethoprim/Sulfamethoxazole on Multidrug-Resistant *Stenotrophomonas maltophilia*," *Diagn Microbiol Infect Dis*, 2002, 44(3):259-63.

Marshall WF, Keating MR, Anhalt JP, et al, "*Xanthomonas maltophilia*: An Emerging Nosocomial Pathogen," *Mayo Clin Proc*, 1989, 64(9):1097-104.

Penzak SR and Abate BJ, "*Stenotrophomonas (Xanthomonas) maltophilia*: A Multidrug-Resistant Nosocomial Pathogen," *Pharmacotherapy*, 1997, 17(2):293-301.

San Gabriel P, Zhou J, Tabibi S, et al, "Antimicrobial Susceptibility and Synergy Studies of *Stenotrophomonas maltophilia* Isolates From Patients With Cystic Fibrosis," *Antimicrob Agents Chemother*, 2004, 48(1):168-71.

St Louis Encephalitis *see* Arboviruses *on page 35*

Strep Throat *see* Pharyngitis *on page 264*

Streptococcal Necrotizing Myositis *see* Myositis *on page 242*

Streptococcus agalactiae

Synonyms Group B *Streptococcus*

Microbiology *Streptococcus agalactiae* is a β-hemolytic *Streptococcus* first recognized in 1938 as a cause of puerperal sepsis ("childbed fever"). By the Lancefield serogroup classification of β-hemolytic streptococci, *S. agalactiae* is also known as Group B *Streptococcus*. Like other streptococci, *S. agalactiae* are gram-positive cocci that appear to form chains when grown in broth. When the organism is growing on a blood agar plate, there is an area of complete hemolysis surrounding the colony, a finding called β-hemolysis. Several streptococci are β-hemolytic including Group A streptococci (*Streptococcus pyogenes*), and Groups B, C, and G streptococci. *S. agalactiae* does not require special media for growth and is readily isolated from clinical specimens.

(Continued)

Streptococcus agalactiae (Continued)

Epidemiology The spectrum of Group B streptococcal infections has been changing over the past years. In the 1970s, this organism was a leading cause of neonatal meningitis and sepsis and was an important cause of maternal peripartum infections, such as postpartum endometritis and bacteremia. More recently, surveillance studies in the 1990s have shown an incidence of 3-4 cases of invasive *S. agalactiae* infections per 100,000 adults. The majority of these infections have appeared in nonpregnant adults. A recent report in 1993 suggested an increasing incidence of invasive Group B infections in nonpregnant adults, but the reasons for this increase were unclear.

Adult groups at risk for serious Group B disease include persons with AIDS, diabetes mellitus, and cancer. Newborns are also at high risk for infection, although the presence of maternal IgG antibodies to the organism correlates with protection from serious infection in the neonate. Serious *S. agalactiae* infections are uncommon in infants older than 3 months of age, even though specific antibodies usually are not present.

Women who are colonized with *S. agalactiae* (and are not treated at delivery) are >25 times more likely to deliver infants with early-onset Group B disease than are women who have negative prenatal cultures.

Clinical Syndromes

- **Asymptomatic carriage in pregnant females:** It is estimated that 10% to 30% of women are asymptomatic carriers of Group B streptococci. Many such women who are carriers of Group B streptococci during pregnancy can be identified by special culture of the rectum and/or vagina at approximately 26 weeks of gestation. However, the presence of Group B *Streptococcus* at this time (26 weeks) does **not** predict the presence of Group B *Streptococcus* **at birth**, the time when detection of the bacterium is most clinically significant. Of this group, those women who have risk factors for infant infection are candidates for preventative therapy during delivery (see Treatment). These risk factors include premature labor, fever, premature or prolonged rupture of membranes, multiple gestations, or a history of prior Group B infection in a previous neonate. Prevention of Group B neonatal infections in this manner is recommended by the American College of Obstetricians and Gynecologists, and the American Academy of Pediatrics.
- **Invasive infections in neonates:** Infection is acquired during passage through a colonized birth canal. "Early onset" infections occur within 1 week and often less than 1 day. Approximately 50% of infants born to mothers with vaginal and rectal carriage of Group B streptococci will themselves become colonized; however, only a small percentage will develop symptomatic infection. In general, neonates are bacteremic with this organism, and many develop pneumonia with a respiratory distress syndrome. "Late-onset" infections occur between 1 week and 3 months, and meningitis is most frequently seen.
- **Invasive infections in the adult:** Pregnancy-related *S. agalactiae* infections include peripartum fever, endometritis, chorioamnionitis, often with bacteremia. In nonpregnant adults, common infections include cellulitis, diabetic ulcer infections, urinary tract infections, septic arthritis, and pneumonias. A variety of serious complications have been seen including endocarditis, pelvic abscesses, meningitis, and others.

Diagnostic Tests/Procedures

Aerobic Culture, Appropriate Site *on page 365*

Group B *Streptococcus* Antigen Test *on page 476*

Note: Physicians who screen pregnant women for *S. agalactiae* must inform the laboratory of such so the laboratory can use special procedures to enrich and isolate the bacterium.

Treatment Group B streptococci are susceptible to penicillins, although they exhibit less *in vitro* sensitivity than Group A streptococci. Adults with invasive, localized infections such as pyelonephritis or infected joint spaces should be treated with relatively high doses of penicillin G, approximately 12 million units daily. Patients with life-threatening infections such as endocarditis should receive 18 (or more) million units of penicillin G daily.

Neonates with Group B bloodstream infections should also receive penicillin G. Some limited data suggest *in vitro* synergy between penicillin and gentamicin, and many pediatricians will use this combination. Therapy is usually continued 10-14 days or more due to the risk of relapse in such conditions as meningitis.

As described above, pregnant women who are found to be carriers of Group B streptococci in the vagina or rectum **at the time of birth** may be candidates for antibiotic prophylaxis if an additional risk factor to the infant is identified. Prophylactic administration of ampicillin to the mother at the time of delivery has been shown to

decrease the rate of infection of the newborn. Indiscriminate prophylaxis of all pregnant women who are carriers of Group B streptococci is not recommended.

Drug Therapy

Recommended:

Penicillin G (Parenteral/Aqueous) *on page 993*
Amoxicillin *on page 642*
Ampicillin *on page 657*

Alternate:

Cephalosporins, 1st Generation *on page 729*
Erythromycin *on page 807*
Vancomycin *on page 1144*

Selected Readings

American College of Obstetricians and Gynecologists, "Prevention of Early-Onset Group B Streptococcal Disease in Newborns," *Int J Gynaecol Obstet*, 2003, 81(1):115-22.
Kanto WP Jr and Baker CJ, "New Recommendations for Prevention of Early-Onset Group B Streptococcal Disease in Newborns," *Pediatr Rev*, 2003, 24(7):219-21.
Schrag S, Gorwitz R, Fultz-Butts K, et al, "Prevention of Perinatal Group B Streptococcal Disease. Revised Guidelines From CDC," *MMWR Recomm Rep*, 2002, 51(RR-11):1-22.
Stiller RJ, Padilla L, Choudhary R, et al, "Group B Streptococcal Antibiotic Resistance Patterns in Pregnant Women," *Conn Med*, 2003, 67(6):323-6.

***Streptococcus*, Anaerobic** *see Streptococcus*-Related Gram-Positive Cocci *on page 325*

Streptococcus anginosus *see Streptococcus*, Viridans Group *on page 326*

Streptococcus bovis

Related Information

Antibiotic Treatment of Adults With Infective Endocarditis *on page 1271*

Synonyms Group D *Streptococcus*

Applies to *Streptococcus equinus*

Microbiology *Streptococcus bovis* and *Streptococcus equinus* possess the Group D lipoteichoic acid antigen in their cell walls. Since 1984, the enterococci have been classified in a separate genus (*Enterococcus*). *S. bovis* is associated with human infections while *S. equinus* is found predominantly in the alimentary tract of horses. These organisms are gram-positive cocci which appear in chains. They are β-hemolytic on rabbit blood, α-hemolytic or nonhemolytic on sheep blood. The ability to cause hemolysis on laboratory media does not correlate with clinical virulence.

Epidemiology *Streptococcus bovis* is a minor part of the normal flora of man where it is found in the genital and intestinal tracts. In sheep and cows, it inhabits the intestinal tract. Infection with *Streptococcus bovis* is correlated with colon and rectal carcinoma and hepatic dysfunction. These organisms have low intrinsic virulence.

Clinical Syndromes *Streptococcus bovis* is a cause of endocarditis and bacteremia primarily in the elderly. Eighty percent of cases occur in patients 60 years of age or older. The association with colon carcinoma is attributed to production by the tumor of transferrin-like chelators that facilitate bacterial growth. One-third of patients with *S. bovis* endocarditis are found to have an adenocarcinoma, villous adenoma, or colonic polyp. The association with liver disease may be the result of altered hepatic secretion of bile salts or immunoglobulins and compromise of the hepatic reticuloendothelial system. Bacteremia associated with *S. bovis* is polymicrobial in approximately 20% of cases.

Diagnosis The diagnosis of *S. bovis* endocarditis is established by positive blood culture in a patient with mild fever and malaise. The disease onset is usually gradual. Low grade fever, arthralgia and cardiac murmurs, splenomegaly, splinter hemorrhages, Roth spots, Osler nodes, and embolic phenomenon may also be presenting features. If *S. bovis* is recovered, a thorough search for adenocarcinoma of the colon or rectum should be undertaken.

Diagnostic Tests/Procedures

Aerobic Culture, Appropriate Site *on page 365*
Blood Culture, Aerobic and Anaerobic *on page 391*

Duration of Therapy Endocarditis: 4 weeks; nonendocarditis: 7-10 days

Treatment Differentiation between nonenterococcal Group D streptococci (primarily *S. bovis*) and enterococci (now classified in separate genus *Enterococcus* including *E. faecalis, E. faecium*, and *E. durans*) is important in regard to antimicrobial susceptibility. *S. bovis* is sensitive to penicillin (90% have penicillin MIC <0.2 mcg/mL), ampicillin, cephalothin, and clindamycin. Endocarditis due to *S. bovis* is frequently treated with parenteral penicillin G as monotherapy. *Enterococcus* species generally have much higher MICs, usually 2-4 mcg/mL and are resistant to achievable levels of cephalosporins and clindamycin. Therapy for enterococci requires use of a penicillin or vancomycin in combination with an aminoglycoside. See also *Enterococcus* Species *on page 134* and *Streptococcus* Viridans Group *on page 326*.

(Continued)

Streptococcus bovis (Continued)

Penicillin G, 10-20 million units/day I.V. in divided doses every 4 hours for 4 weeks for organism with an MIC ≤0.1 mcg/mL. Addition of gentamicin or streptomycin may result in more rapid cure. Streptomycin dosage 7.5 mg/kg I.M. every 12 hours or gentamicin 1 mg/kg I.V. every 8 hours for the first 2 weeks of therapy with penicillin being continued for the full 4 weeks. An additional alternative in cefazolin 1-2 g I.V. or I.M. every 6-8 hours for 4 weeks.

Vancomycin, 15 mcg/kg I.V. every 12 hours for 4 weeks.

Drug Therapy

Recommended:

Penicillin G (Parenteral/Aqueous) *on page 993*

Alternate:

Vancomycin *on page 1144*

Selected Readings

Zarkin BA, Lillemoe KD, Cameron JL, et al, "The Triad of *Streptococcus bovis* Bacteremia, Colonic Pathology, and Liver Disease," *Ann Surg*, 1990, 211(6):786-92.

Streptococcus constellatus *see Streptococcus*, Viridans Group *on page 326*

Streptococcus equinus *see Streptococcus bovis on page 315*

Streptococcus intermedius *see Streptococcus*, Viridans Group *on page 326*

Streptococcus milleri *see Streptococcus*, Viridans Group *on page 326*

Streptococcus mitis *see Streptococcus*, Viridans Group *on page 326*

Streptococcus mutans *see Streptococcus*, Viridans Group *on page 326*

Streptococcus oralis *see Streptococcus*, Viridans Group *on page 326*

Streptococcus pneumoniae, Drug-Resistant

Synonyms DRSP; Penicillin-Resistant *S. pneumoniae*; Pneumococcus, Drug-Resistant

Microbiology *Streptococcus pneumoniae* is a gram-positive coccus which has a lancet-shaped appearance. Nearly all clinical isolates have a polysaccharide capsule in addition to the pneumococcal cell wall. The pneumococcal cell wall consists of mainly teichoic acid and peptidoglycan. β-lactam antibiotics such as penicillin act at the level of the cell wall by covalently binding to key enzymes in the cell wall which mediate cell wall integrity and synthesis. Enzymes such as endo-, trans- and carboxypeptidases cross-link the many peptide side chains of the cell wall and are called "penicillin-binding proteins (PBPs)." The importance of PBPs has come to the forefront recently due to the emergence of penicillin-resistant strains of pneumococci which result from alterations in these enzymes.

In the past 20 years, the number of drug-resistant *S. pneumoniae* (DRSP) isolates has increased from scattered case reports from Australia and Africa to a global problem involving all countries including the United States. DRSP results from stepwise mutations of the bacterial genes which encode for PBPs. These genes are considered "mosaic genes" in that the coding region includes segments of genetic material derived from other related streptococcal species. It is postulated that the DNA sequences encoding these altered PBPs originally came from other streptococcal species which already exhibited varying degrees of penicillin resistance (eg, viridans streptococci). Multiple alterations in PBPs decrease the binding affinity of penicillin and other β-lactam antibiotics for these proteins, decreasing their efficacy. These mutations are chromosomally mediated and do not appear to alter the virulence of the organism; that is, penicillin-resistant pneumococci are neither more or less virulent than penicillin-sensitive isolates.

The altered PBP genes appear to spread readily to other strains of *S. pneumoniae* in a horizontal fashion, and these mutations appear to be stable. Of the 90 known serotypes of *S. pneumoniae*, the majority of penicillin-resistant isolates belong to serotypes 6, 9, 14, 19, and 23. As with penicillin-susceptible strains of *S. pneumoniae*, the organism is spread via a respiratory route from person to person such that some individuals become colonized in the nasopharynx. This state of colonization generally lasts from weeks to months. Nasopharyngeal colonization is felt to precede more invasive disease such as pneumonia or meningitis. The proportion of persons colonized with DRSP who develop invasive disease is currently under study. Clones of DRSP have been documented to spread horizontally, and this tendency has certainly contributed to the rapid dissemination of resistant isolates across the world.

Resistance of *S. pneumoniae* to other β-lactam antibiotics, such as the cephalosporins, is also mediated by PBPs. The *in vitro* susceptibility of penicillin-resistant *S. pneumoniae* to the various cephalosporins is variable, with the third-generation cephalosporins being more predictably active (see Treatment). *S. pneumoniae* can also be resistant to antibiotics other than the β-lactam antibiotics,

through mechanisms other than alterations in PBPs. Resistance can be acquired through conjugation with other related streptococci such that there is a change in the antimicrobial target, as with the macrolides (eg, erythromycin), fluoroquinolones (eg, ciprofloxacin), trimethoprim, and others. This phenomenon of multidrug resistance in *S. pneumoniae* (resistance to two or more antibiotics) is seen more commonly in isolates which are resistant to penicillin. It is unusual to see resistance to non-β-lactam antibiotics in penicillin-sensitive *S. pneumoniae*.

Epidemiology Until recently, nearly all clinical isolates of *S. pneumoniae* were exquisitely susceptible to penicillin. Testing for resistance was not necessary and serious pneumococcal infections could be treated confidently with penicillin without awaiting antibiotic susceptibility testing. The first report of a penicillin-resistant isolate causing disease came from Australia in 1967. Since then, reports from countries such as New Guinea, Australia, and South Africa have shown an increase in DRSP from 12% in the 1970s to >30% in the 1980. DRSP is now reported globally and in some regions, >50% of pneumococcal isolates have either intermediate or high level penicillin resistance. This rapid spread of DRSP is due to at least two factors, horizontal spread of resistant clones and emergence of new clones of DRSP due to heavy use of antibiotics.

In the United States, several recent epidemiologic studies have shown that about 25% to 30% of pneumococcal isolates are now resistant to penicillin (either intermediate or high-level resistance). This increase has mainly taken place over the last decade. However, not all communities have this high a rate; penicillin-resistance appears quite variable across the United States, with some regions having <5% DRSP (usually rural) compared with rates >30% in some urban areas. Surveillance studies have shown that rates of DRSP can vary markedly within the same community, from hospital to hospital, and from adults to children. One problem regarding accurate surveillance of resistance trends is that DRSP is not a mandatory reportable illness. To address this, the Centers for Disease Control has launched an initiative to track resistant isolates nationwide.

Several risk factors have been identified for the development of DRSP:

- age younger than 6 years of age
- recent treatment with antibiotics
- multiple comorbid diseases
- child attending daycare (and family members of same)
- the elderly
- HIV infection and other immunodeficiency states
- recent hospitalization
- residence in a nursing home or prison

Much of the development and spread of DRSP is due to the heavy use of antimicrobial agents for children in day care centers. Common conditions such as acute otitis media and other upper respiratory infections in these populations have led to the empiric and often inappropriate use of antimicrobial agents in children with the emergence of new DRSP clones.

Clinical Syndromes

- **Meningitis caused by DRSP**: A number of case series have described *S. pneumoniae* meningitis caused by strains that were either intermediate or highly resistant to penicillin. The clinical features of meningitis due to DRSP are the same as with penicillin-susceptible pneumococci, a finding consistent with the fact that drug-resistant isolates are not more virulent. The therapy of meningitis caused by DRSP is complex although a general consensus has been reached (see Treatment).
- **Pneumonia caused by DRSP**: Only a limited amount of information is available concerning the clinical course and outcomes of pneumonia caused by DRSP. In one study of children in South Africa with pneumococcal pneumonia, the clinical presentation of children with penicillin-resistant and penicillin-susceptible strains was equivalent. A similar finding was noted in a large U.S. pediatric multicenter pneumococcal surveillance study. Interestingly, a number of cases of pneumonia caused by DRSP have been treated successfully with penicillin, in contrast with the treatment of meningitis (see Treatment).
- **Others**: Bacteremia, acute otitis media, and sinusitis have all been reported to be caused by DRSP. Only a limited amount of information is available for clinical presentations and outcomes of these conditions.

Diagnosis The finding of lancet-shaped gram-positive cocci in ordinarily sterile body fluids such as cerebrospinal fluid, blood, sinus aspirates, or pleural fluid is virtually diagnostic of *S. pneumoniae* infection. However, such a finding is not necessarily diagnostic when found in expectorated sputum since respiratory colonization is common (particularly in chronic bronchitics). With respiratory secretions, it is important to note the presence of both polymorphonuclear leukocytes, as well as numerous

(Continued)

Streptococcus pneumoniae, Drug-Resistant *(Continued)*

pneumococci on Gram stain; this combination is suggestive of true infection, but physician judgment is critical.

Gram stain and cultures are by far the most sensitive and specific laboratory tests to detect *S. pneumoniae* infection.

Latex agglutination tests to detect *S. pneumoniae* antigens in CSF are often ordered by physicians and widely offered by laboratories. However, these tests are neither sensitive nor specific.

Infections caused by penicillin-resistant *S. pneumoniae* are indistinguishable at the bedside from those caused by penicillin-susceptible isolates, and laboratory determination of drug resistance is essential. However, although infection with *S. pneumoniae* may be suspected early on because of a Gram stain of a clinical specimen (lancet-shaped diplococci), or on the basis of the clinical presentation alone, results of *in vitro* susceptibility testing is not generally available for 24 hours or more. Rapid assays to detect DRSP in 6 hours or less are being developed at this time but remain research tools.

The Clinical and Laboratory Standards Institute (CLSI) has recommended that all isolates of *S. pneumoniae* obtained from usually sterile sites undergo testing for penicillin resistance. This is accomplished by screening isolates using a 1 mcg oxacillin disk. If the oxacillin disk results in a zone of inhibition of bacterial growth ≥20 mm, the isolate is considered penicillin-susceptible, and further laboratory testing is not necessary. If the oxacillin zone diameter is ≤19 mm, then penicillin resistance is considered probable. Screening with the oxacillin disk is 99% sensitive and fairly specific (80% to 90%) and should detect almost all isolates resistant to penicillin and extended-spectrum cephalosporins (eg, ceftriaxone or cefotaxime). Those isolates that appear nonsusceptible by oxacillin disk should then undergo further testing using standard quantitative minimal inhibitory concentration (MIC) tests against penicillin, extended-spectrum cephalosporin(s), chloramphenicol, vancomycin, and other drugs. MIC testing should be performed by established methods such as the broth microdilution procedure (using Mueller-Hinton broth with 3% lysed horse blood), agar dilution, disk diffusion, or antimicrobial gradient strips (eg, E-test), but not by automated methods.

The CLSI has defined the following MIC breakpoints for interpreting the susceptibility of *S. pneumoniae* to penicillin:

Susceptible: MIC of penicillin ≤0.06 mcg/mL
Intermediate: MIC of penicillin 0.12-1.0 mcg/mL
Resistant: MIC of penicillin ≥2.0 mcg/mL

These breakpoints of susceptible, intermediate, and resistant are based on several factors including available data on clinical response to antibiotic therapy and on achievable levels of penicillin in blood. The CLSI has defined interpretive standards for *S. pneumoniae* MIC breakpoints for a number of other antibiotics, including non-β-lactam antibiotics.

Diagnostic Tests/Procedures

Aerobic Culture, Appropriate Site *on page 365*
Bacterial Antigens, Rapid Detection Methods *on page 388*
Gram Stain *on page 473*

Treatment It is important to note that recommendations for treatment of penicillin-intermediate and penicillin-resistant *S. pneumoniae* are evolving. Only a limited amount of information is available to correlate clinical failure with the interpretive MIC breakpoints (ie, to determine if an isolate of *S. pneumoniae* that is penicillin-resistant *in vitro* actually fails to respond to therapy with penicillin). To complicate matters, it is likely that the significance of penicillin resistance is not the same for meningitis, pneumonia, bacteremia, and upper respiratory infections, given varying concentrations of the drug at each site. The following recommendations are based on current data, which is likely to change. An infectious disease consultation should be considered in difficult cases.

Meningitis due to DRSP: Clinical failures have been reported when penicillin has been used to treat intermediate and high level resistant strains. Extended-spectrum cephalosporins, such as ceftriaxone, are useful for treating intermediately resistant strains as long as the MIC was <2.0 mcg/mL, since treatment failures have been reported with use of the cephalosporins above this level. For high level resistant strains of *S. pneumoniae* to penicillin, treatment with vancomycin and an extended-spectrum cephalosporin is indicated due to some animal data suggesting the combination is synergistic in this setting. Some authors recommend adding vancomycin to an extended-spectrum cephalosporin even when the isolate is only

intermediately resistant to cephalosporins (ie, MIC for ceftriaxone = 1 mcg/mL), but other authors do not. No vancomycin-resistant isolates of *S. pneumoniae* have been described to date, but the liberal use of vancomycin is not advised due to concerns about potential resistance developing in the future. Rifampin may have some potential role for highly penicillin- and cephalosporin-resistant isolates, but little clinical data is available. Recommendations are as follows.

Recommended Treatment for Meningitis Due to DRSP

Penicillin MIC	Ceftriaxone or Cefotaxime MIC	Recommended Therapy
<0.1 mcg/mL	≤0.5 mcg/mL	Penicillin I.V. (high dose)
0.1-1.0 mcg/mL	≤0.5 mcg/mL	Ceftriaxone
	1.0 mcg/mL	Ceftriaxone ± vancomycin
	≥2.0 mcg/mL	Ceftriaxone + vancomycin
≥2.0 mcg/mL	any MIC value	Ceftriaxone + vancomycin, ± rifampin

Pneumonia due to DRSP: A variety of regimens have been proposed in recent years. Several large clinical studies suggest that *in vitro* penicillin resistance is not as significant with pneumococcal pneumonia when compared with meningitis, and some authorities feel that penicillin can still be used when the isolate is intermediately resistant to penicillin, up to and including an MIC of 2 mcg/mL. In part this has been justified by the significantly higher concentrations of drug in respiratory tissue than in cerebrospinal fluid, along with other immunologic and host defense factors which influence clinical outcome. Ceftriaxone or cefotaxime are the drugs of choice for the treatment of pneumonia caused by intermediate or resistant *S. pneumoniae*. The gram-positive fluoroquinolones are also very effective in the treatment of DRSP. Resistance to macrolides and clindamycin is very common in these organisms and should only be utilized upon confirmation of susceptibility.

Drug Therapy

Recommended:

Meningitis:

Ceftriaxone *on page 722*

plus

Vancomycin *on page 1144*

with or without

Rifampin *on page 1046*

Pneumonia:

Ceftriaxone *on page 722*

Cefotaxime *on page 708*

Alternate:

Pneumonia:

Levofloxacin *on page 908*

Gatifloxacin *on page 837*

Moxifloxacin *on page 949*

Selected Readings

Banning M, "Infections and Their Treatment in Older People," *Nurs Older People*, 2005, 17(2):25-9.

Campbell GD and Silberman R, "Drug-Resistant *Streptococcus pneumoniae*," *Clin Infect Dis*, 1998, 26(5):1188-95.

"Defining the Public Health Impact of Drug-Resistant *Streptococcus pneumoniae*: Report of a Working Group," *MMWR*, 1996, 45(RR-1):1-20.

Kaplan SL, "*Streptococcus pneumoniae*: Impact of Antibiotic Resistance in Pediatrics," *Curr Probl Pediatr*, 1997, 27(5):187-95.

Klugman KP and Feldman C, "The Clinical Relevance of Antibiotic Resistance in the Management of Pneumococcal Pneumonia," *Infect Dis Clin Pract*, 1998, 7:180-4.

Mandell LA, "Antimicrobial Resistance and Treatment of Community-Acquired Pneumonia," *Clin Chest Med*, 2005, 26(1):57-64.

Mera RM, Miller LA, Daniels JJ, et al, "Increasing Prevalence of Multidrug-Resistant *Streptococcus pneumoniae* in the United States Over a 10-Year Period: Alexander Project," *Diagn Microbiol Infect Dis*, 2005, 51(3):195-200.

Tomasz A, "Antibiotic Resistance in *Streptococcus pneumoniae*," *Clin Infect Dis*, 1997, 24(Suppl 1):S85-8.

Streptococcus pneumoniae, Drug-Susceptible

Microbiology *Streptococcus pneumoniae* was called "the captain of the men of death" by Sir William Osler because of its lethality. It remains a leading cause of acute lobar pneumonia, otitis media, and meningitis. *Streptococcus pneumoniae* is an encapsulated gram-positive coccus. Classically, the organism appears lancet-shaped and commonly in pairs or short chains. Colonies appear circular, dimpled or mucoid, flat, and "penny-like." They cause α-hemolysis when grown aerobically on blood agar. There are several determinants of pathogenicity:

(Continued)

Streptococcus pneumoniae, Drug-Susceptible *(Continued)*

- the polysaccharide capsule, which protects the organism from phagocytosis
- adherence, which allows colonization of epithelial cells
- enzymes, such as neuraminidase (which allow growth in mucous secretions) and proteases (which degrade IgA and facilitate colonization)
- toxins, such as pneumolysis O, which directly inhibit phagocytic activity

Epidemiology *S. pneumoniae* is a common colonizer of the nasopharynx of healthy individuals. Estimates of this carriage state range from 5% to >70% and appears more common in children. Carriage seems highest in the winter and spring months, which is also the most common period for infection. New serotypes of *Streptococcus pneumoniae* are acquired throughout the year. When infection occurs, it is often with a new serotype rather than the serotype associated with years of carriage. Patients with chronic bronchitis are frequently colonized in the nasopharynx and respiratory tree with pneumococcus, and purulent exacerbations of bronchitis are often associated with this organism.

Clinical Syndromes

- **Pneumonia:** Typically, pneumococcal pneumonia begins abruptly with sudden fever and shaking chills, which resolve. Pleuritic pain may be quite severe. The patient often develops a cough productive of "rusty" mucopurulent sputum. Complications include parapneumonic effusion, empyema, bacteremia, and meningitis. *Streptococcus pneumoniae* is still the most common cause of community-acquired pneumonia in adults.
- **Otitis media:** *S. pneumoniae* is a leading cause, accounting for 35% to 50% of the cases.
- **Meningitis:** *S. pneumoniae* is the most common etiology for community-acquired meningitis in adults. Often, this is preceded by pulmonary infection or a mild upper respiratory infection. Predisposing factors include alcoholism, sickle cell disease, multiple myeloma, and general debility.
- **Bacteremia:** This may occur in 25% or more of patients with pneumococcal pneumonia and >80% of patients with meningitis. Endocarditis has also been described.

Diagnosis The finding of lancet-shaped gram-positive cocci in ordinarily sterile body fluids such as cerebrospinal fluid, blood, sinus aspirates, or pleural fluid is virtually diagnostic of *S. pneumoniae* infection. However, such a finding is not necessarily diagnostic when found in expectorated sputum since respiratory colonization is common (particularly in chronic bronchitics). With respiratory secretions, it is important to note the presence of both polymorphonuclear leukocytes, as well as numerous pneumococci on Gram stain; this combination is suggestive of true infection, but physician judgment is critical.

Gram stain and cultures are by far the most sensitive and specific laboratory tests to detect *S. pneumoniae* infection.

Latex agglutination tests to detect *S. pneumoniae* antigens in CSF are often ordered by physicians and widely offered by laboratories. However, these tests are neither sensitive nor specific.

Diagnostic Tests/Procedures

Aerobic Culture, Appropriate Site *on page 365*
Bacterial Antigens, Rapid Detection Methods *on page 388*
Gram Stain *on page 473*

Treatment Penicillin is the drug of choice for *Streptococcus pneumoniae* infections caused by penicillin-susceptible strains. It is important for the clinician to review the antibiotic susceptibility pattern of clinical isolates because drug resistance is rapidly increasing, both intermediate and high-level resistance to penicillin. For additional information, see *Streptococcus pneumoniae*, Drug-Resistant *on page 316*.

For mild-to-moderate (nonmeningeal) infections, oral therapy with amoxicillin or a macrolide can be used. Fluoroquinolones and ceftriaxone are also highly active against penicillin-susceptible *Streptococcus pneumoniae*, but may be reserved to treat more resistant organisms.

Drug Therapy

Recommended:

Meningitis:

Penicillin G (Parenteral/Aqueous) *on page 993*

Nonmeningitis:

Penicillin G (Parenteral/Aqueous) *on page 993*
Amoxicillin *on page 642*
Macrolides *on page 924*

Alternate:

Meningitis:

Vancomycin *on page 1144*

Chloramphenicol *on page 733*

Nonmeningitis:

Vancomycin *on page 1144*

Cephalosporins, 1st Generation *on page 729*

Selected Readings

Banning M, "Infections and Their Treatment in Older People," *Nurs Older People*, 2005, 17(2):25-9.

Janssens JP, "Pneumonia in the Elderly (Geriatric) Population," *Curr Opin Pulm Med*, 2005, 11(3):226-30.

Keam SJ, Croom KF, and Keating GM, "Gatifloxacin: A Review of Its Use in the Treatment of Bacterial Infections in the U.S.," *Drugs*, 2005, 65(5):695-724.

Mandell LA, "Antimicrobial Resistance and Treatment of Community-Acquired Pneumonia," *Clin Chest Med*, 2005, 26(1):57-64.

Mera RM, Miller LA, Daniels JJ, et al, "Increasing Prevalence of Multidrug-Resistant *Streptococcus pneumoniae* in the United States Over a 10-Year Period: Alexander Project," *Diagn Microbiol Infect Dis*, 2005, 51(3):195-200.

Musher DM, "Infections Caused by *Streptococcus pneumoniae*: Clinical Spectrum, Pathogenesis, Immunity, and Treatment," *Clin Infect Dis*, 1992, 14(4):801-7.

van der Eerden MM, Vlaspolder F, de Graaff CS, et al, "Value of Intensive Diagnostic Microbiological Investigation in Low- and High-Risk Patients With Community-Acquired Pneumonia," *Eur J Clin Microbiol Infect Dis*, 2005, Apr 19; [Epub ahead of print].

Streptococcus pyogenes

Related Information

Community-Acquired Pneumonia in Adults *on page 1278*

Synonyms GABHS; GAS; Group A β-Hemolytic *Streptococcus*; Group A *Streptococcus*

Microbiology *Streptococcus pyogenes* are gram-positive cocci, which are frequently encountered in clinical microbiology laboratories. Group A refers to a specific carbohydrate (Lancefield) antigen which is part of the cell wall and is used for serogrouping streptococcal species. The M-protein in the cell wall, of which there are more than 100 serotypes, is associated with resistance to phagocytosis by polymorphonuclear leukocytes. M-protein acts by decreasing alternative complement pathway activation and thereby limiting deposition of C3 on the surface of the bacteria. Immunity results from the development of type specific antibodies to the M-protein. Serum antibodies are thought to be protective against invasive infection but do not prevent the carrier state. Lipoteichoic acid on the surface of group A streptococci is responsible for binding the bacteria to the epithelial cell membranes of the oropharynx initiating colonization which is the first stage in infection. The hyaluronic acid capsule also is an additional virulence factor. Extracellular products produced by group A streptococci include streptolysin O, deoxyribonuclease B (DNase B), and hyaluronidase. These antigens evoke the formation of antibodies which (when detected in serum) confirm recent streptococcal infection in cases of acute glomerulonephritis or acute rheumatic fever. In addition, DNases A, C, and D; streptolysin S; proteinase; nicotinamide adenine deaminase; streptokinase; and the pyrogenic exotoxins A, B, C, and D are produced. These exotoxins cause the rash of scarlet fever, alter the blood-brain barrier, damage organs and may cause shock, block the reticuloendothelial system, and alter T-cell function. The effects of these toxins are thought to be mediated by hypersensitivity of the host to the toxins, as well as the direct toxic effect. In culture at 35°C, *Streptococcus pyogenes* is β-hemolytic on blood agar. Streptococci are catalase-negative. Presumptive diagnosis can be made by bacitracin susceptibility followed by confirmation using agglutination or coagglutination or other rapid antigen-antibody specific tests.

Epidemiology Infections due to *Streptococcus pyogenes* are ubiquitous in temperate and semitropical areas. They are less common in the tropics. Inapparent infections are as frequent as clinical infections. Serotypes associated with acute glomerulonephritis include 1, 3, 4, 12, and 25 in association with throat infections and 2, 4, 9, 55, 57, 58, 59, and 60 in association with skin infections. M types associated with rheumatic fever include 1, 3, 5, 6,14, 18, 19, and 24. The lists are not comprehensive.

Rheumatic fever remains a major public health concern in developing countries. Strep throat occurs with a peak incidence in late winter and spring. Children and adolescents are most often affected. Outbreaks occur in school and military recruit populations. Food-borne epidemics may occur during any season. The outbreaks are most frequently associated with milk, milk products, deviled eggs, and egg salad. The reservoir for *Streptococcus pyogenes* is man; transmission is by direct or intimate contact. Transmission by hand contact or objects is rare. Nasal carriers are particularly prone to transmit the disease. Eradication of the carrier state may require several courses of antimicrobials and is difficult.

Clinical Syndromes *Streptococcus pyogenes* is ubiquitous and is an extremely important, well recognized pathogen commonly encountered in clinical specimens. (Continued)

Streptococcus pyogenes (Continued)

Acute pharyngitis ("strep throat") and impetigo or pyoderma are the most common clinical presentations. Other manifestations include septicemia, otitis, sinusitis, cellulitis, peritonsillar and retropharyngeal abscess, pneumonia, lymphangitis, gangrene, myositis, vaginitis, peripheral sepsis, perianal cellulitis, and scarlet fever. Group A streptococcal infections are associated with important nonsuppurative sequelae specifically acute glomerulonephritis, acute rheumatic fever, and rarely toxic shock-like syndrome.

Patients with streptococcal sore throat may have minimal symptoms or may develop fever, painful sore throat, exudative tonsillitis and/or pharyngitis, and anterior cervical adenopathy. The pharynx, tonsillar pillars, and soft palate may exhibit petechiae against a background of edema and erythema. Otitis media and peritonsillar abscess often complicate severe cases. Acute glomerulonephritis may follow with a mean time of 10 days. Acute rheumatic fever may follow in 7-35 days with a mean of 19 days.

Scarlet fever is characterized by a fine erythematosus rash which blanches on pressure. It has a sandpaper-like touch and is commonly seen over the neck, chest, folds of the axilla, groin, elbow, and inner thigh. It is the result of infection by a strain-producing erythrogenic toxin to which the patient is sensitive but not immune. Acute glomerulonephritis and rheumatic fever can follow.

The American Heart Association (AHA) guidelines for the diagnosis of initial attack of rheumatic fever (Jones Criteria, 1992 Update). See table.

Guidelines for the Diagnosis of Initial Attack of Rheumatic Fever (Jones Criteria, 1992 Update)[1]

Major Manifestations
Carditis
Polyarthritis
Chorea
Erythema marginatum
Subcutaneous nodules
Minor Manifestations
Clinical findings
Arthralgia
Fever
Laboratory findings
Elevated acute phase reactants
Erythrocyte sedimentation rate
C-reactive protein
Prolonged PR interval
Supporting Evidence of Antecedent Group A Streptococcal Infection
Positive throat culture or rapid streptococcal antigen test
Elevated or rising streptococcal antibody titer

[1]If supported by evidence of preceding group A streptococcal infection, the presence of two major manifestations or of one major and two minor manifestations indicates a high probability of acute rheumatic fever.

From Diagnosis of Rheumatic Fever " Special Writing Group, "Guidelines for the Diagnosis of Rheumatic Fever," *JAMA*, 1992, 268(15):2069-73.

A case definition has been developed for Group A streptococcal toxic shock syndrome (TSS) which should facilitate diagnosis and may lead to the evolution of prevention strategies and more effective therapy. See Tables 1 and 2 on next page.

Diagnosis Clinical diagnosis of "strep throat" is only 30% to 60% sensitive. Throat culture is the gold standard for the diagnosis of streptococcal pharyngitis. Culture obtained during an active infection in an untreated patient is almost always positive. The culture does not distinguish between acute streptococcal infection and streptococcal carriers with viral infections. The vast majority of symptomatic sore throat patients have viral sore throat. Rapid tests for the detection of group A streptococcal antigen are specific (~95%), but sensitivity varies widely from 60% to 90%. Their sensitivity is less than that of throat culture. **A negative antigen test should be confirmed by a culture.** The organism is readily recovered by routine aerobic culture from other sites.

Diagnostic Tests/Procedures

Aerobic Culture, Appropriate Site *on page 365*

Antideoxyribonuclease-B Titer, Serum *on page 376*

Antistreptolysin O Titer, Serum *on page 383*

Gram Stain *on page 473*

Group A *Streptococcus* Antigen Test *on page 475*

Streptozyme *on page 589*

Throat Culture for Group A Beta-Hemolytic *Streptococcus on page 594*

Table 1. Proposed Case Definition for the Streptococcal Toxic Shock Syndrome[1]

I. Isolation of group A streptococci (*Streptococcus pyogenes*)

A. From a normally sterile site (eg, blood, cerebrospinal, pleural, or peritoneal fluid, tissue biopsy, surgical wound, etc)

B. From a nonsterile site (eg, throat, sputum, vagina, superficial skin lesion, etc)

II. Clinical signs of severity

A. Hypotension: Systolic blood pressure ≤90 mm Hg in adults or <5th percentile for age in children

and

B. Two or more of the following signs:

- Renal impairment: Creatinine ≥177 µmol/L (≥2 mg/dL) for adults or greater than or equal to twice the upper limit of normal for age. In patients with pre-existing renal disease, a twofold or greater elevation over the baseline level.
- Coagulopathy: Platelets ≤100 x 10^9/L (≤100,000/mm^3) or disseminated intravascular coagulation defined by prolonged clotting times, low fibrinogen level, and the presence of fibrin degradation products
- Liver involvement: Alanine aminotransferase (ALT), aspartate aminotransferase (AST), or total bilirubin levels greater than or equal to twice the upper limit of normal for age. In patients with pre-existing liver disease, a twofold or greater elevation over the baseline level.
- Adult respiratory distress syndrome defined by acute onset of diffuse pulmonary infiltrates and hypoxemia in the absence of cardiac failure, or evidence of diffuse capillary leak manifested by acute onset of generalized edema, or pleural or peritoneal effusions with hypoalbuminemia
- A generalized erythematous macular rash that may desquamate
- Soft-tissue necrosis, including necrotizing fascitis or myositis, or gangrene

[1]An illness fulfilling criteria IA and II (A and B) can be defined as a **definite** case. An illness fulfilling criteria IB and II (A and B) can be defined as a **probable** case if no other etiology for the illness is identified.

Table 2. Classification of Group A Streptococcal Infection[1]

I. **Streptococcal toxic shock syndrome (streptococcal TSS):** Defined by criteria in Table 1

II. **Other invasive infections:** Defined by isolation of group A streptococci from a **normally sterile site** in patients not meeting criteria for streptococcal TSS

A. Bacteremia with no identified focus

B. Focal infections with or without bacteremia. Includes meningitis, pneumonia, peritonitis, puerperal sepsis, osteomyelitis, septic arthritis, necrotizing fascitis, surgical wound infections, erysipeas, and cellulitis

III. **Scarlet fever:** Defined by a scarlatina rash with evidence of group A streptococcal infection, most commonly pharyngotonsillitis

IV. **Noninvasive infections:** Defined by the isolation of group A streptococci from a nonsterile site

A. Mucous membrane: Includes pharyngitis, tonsillitis, otitis media, sinusitis, vaginitis

B. Cutaneous: Includes impetigo

V. **Nonsuppurative sequelae:** Defined by specific clinical findings with evidence of a recent group A streptococcal infection

A. Acute rheumatic fever

B. Acute glomerulonephritis

[1]Examples of conditions in each category are not inclusive.

From Streptococcal Toxic Shock Syndrome Case Definition Working Group, "Defining the Group A Streptococcal Toxic Shock Syndrome," *JAMA*, 1993, 269(3):390-1.

(Continued)

Streptococcus pyogenes (Continued)

Treatment Patients who have had rheumatic fever are at high risk of suffering recurrent attacks if they develop streptococcal upper respiratory infections. Even asymptomatic infections can cause recurrence, and recurrence can occur in optimally-treated symptomatic infections. Thus, continuous prophylaxis with antimicrobials is recommended. This therapy should be continued into the patient's early 20s and for at least 5 years after the last recurrence. Patients who have had carditis are at relatively high risk for recurrences of carditis. Discontinuance of prophylaxis should not be undertaken without consideration of the epidemiological risk factors for the particular patient (ie, likelihood of exposure to school children, daycare, military recruit, college student, etc). The American Heart Association (AHA) has recommended the following therapy.

Primary Prevention of Rheumatic Fever (Treatment of Streptococcal Tonsillopharyngitis)

Agent	Dose	Mode	Duration
Benzathine penicillin G	600,000 units for patients <60 lb 1,200,000 units for patients >60 lb	I.M.	Once
	or		
Penicillin V (phenoxymethyl penicillin)	250 mg 3 times/day	P.O.	10 days
	For individuals allergic to penicillin:		
Erythromycin estolate	20-40 mg/kg/day 2-4 times/day (maximum: 1 g/day)	P.O.	10 days
	or		
Erythromycin ethylsuccinate	40 mg/kg/day 2-4 times/day (maximum: 1 g/day)	P.O.	10 days

The following agents are acceptable but usually not recommended: amoxicillin, dicloxacillin, oral cephalosporins, and clindamycin.

The following are not acceptable: sulfonamides, trimethoprim, tetracyclines, and chloramphenicol.

From Dajani AS, Bisno AL, and Chung KJ, "Prevention of Rheumatic Fever," *Circulation,* American Heart Association, 1988, 78:1082-6.

Secondary Prevention of Rheumatic Fever (Prevention of Recurrent Attacks)

Agent	Dose	Mode
Benzathine penicillin G	1,200,000 units	I.M., every 4 weeks[1]
	or	
Penicillin V	250 mg twice daily	P.O.
	or	
Sulfadiazine	0.5 g once daily for patients <60 lb 1 g once daily for patients >60 lb	P.O.
	For individuals allergic to penicillin and sulfadiazine:	
Erythromycin	250 mg twice daily	P.O.

[1]In high-risk situations, administration every 3 weeks is advised.

From Dajani AS, Bisno AL, and Chung KJ, "Prevention of Rheumatic Fever," *Circulation,* 1988, 78:1082-6.

Drug Therapy

Recommended:

Penicillin G (Parenteral/Aqueous) *on page 993*

Alternate:

Erythromycin *on page 807*

Vancomycin *on page 1144*

Cephalosporins, 1st Generation *on page 729*

Selected Readings

Bisno AL, "Group A Streptococcal Infections and Acute Rheumatic Fever," *N Engl J Med,* 1991, 325(11):783-93.

Bisno AL, Gerber MA, Gwaltney JM, et al, "Diagnosis and Management of Group A Streptococcal Pharyngitis: A Practice Guideline. Infectious Diseases Society of America," *Clin Infect Dis,* 1997, 25(3):574-83.

Campos JM, "Laboratory Diagnosis of Group A Streptococcal Pharyngitis," *Infect Dis Clin Pract,* 1993, 2:303-7.

Chuang YY, Huang YC, and Lin TY, "Toxic Shock Syndrome in Children: Epidemiology, Pathogenesis, and Management," *Paediatr Drugs*, 2005, 7(1):11-25.
Crum NF, Russell KL, Kaplan EL, et al, "Pneumonia Outbreak Associated With Group A *Streptococcus* Species at a Military Training Facility," *Clin Infect Dis*, 2005, 40(4):511-8.
Hoge CW, Schwartz B, Talkington DF, et al, "The Changing Epidemiology of Invasive Group A Streptococcal Infections and the Emergence of Streptococcal Toxic-Shock Like Syndrome," *JAMA*, 1993, 269(3):384-9.
"Invasive Group A Streptococcal Infections - United Kingdom, 1994," *MMWR*, 1994, 43(21):401-2.
Leung AK and Kellner JD, "Group A Beta-Hemolytic Streptococcal Pharyngitis in Children," *Adv Ther*, 2004, 21(5):277-87.
Musher DM, Hamill RJ, Wright CE, et al, "Trends in Bacteremic Infection Due to *Streptococcus pyogenes* (Group A *Streptococcus*), 1986-1995," *Emerg Infect Dis*, 1996, 2(1):54-6.
Nimishikavi S and Stead L, "Images in Clinical Medicine. Streptococcal Pharyngitis," *N Engl J Med*, 2005, 352(11):e10.
Stevens DL, "Streptococcal Toxic-Shock Syndrome: Spectrum of Disease, Pathogenesis, and New Concepts in Treatment," *Emerg Infect Dis*, 1995, 1(3):69-78.

Streptococcus-Related Gram-Positive Cocci

Synonyms Anaerobic *Streptococcus*; SRGPC; *Streptococcus*, Anaerobic

Applies to *Peptostreptococcus*; Microaerophilic Streptococci

Microbiology *Streptococcus*-related gram-positive cocci (SRGPC) which are clinically important include species of the genera *Peptostreptococcus*, *Streptococcus*, and *Gemella*. SRGPC which rarely cause clinical infections include species of the genera *Peptococcus*, *Coprococcus*, *Ruminococcus*, *Sarcina*, and *Staphylococcus saccharolyticus*. *Peptostreptococcus* is the most significant pathogen and is recovered almost as frequently (~25%) as *Bacteroides fragilis* from clinical specimens. *Peptostreptococcus* and *Bacteroides* species are frequently recovered together and in combination with aerobic bacteria in abscess cavities throughout the body. The *Peptostreptococcus* species most frequently recovered include *P. magnus*, *P. asaccharolyticus*, *P. prevotii*, and *P. anaerobius*. SRGPC are speciated by biochemical and chromatographic methods in the laboratory. Reclassification of these species utilizing modern DNA, ribosomal RNA, and cell wall polysaccharide content analyses will continue.

Epidemiology SRGPC comprise a large portion of the normal flora of the mouth, intestinal tract, and vagina. Infections in humans are often the result of contamination from normal flora sites or contiguous extension of infection from colonized sites onto adjacent tissues.

Clinical Syndromes SRGPC are often recovered from abscesses, frequently in polymicrobial infections, at virtually any site in the body. More often than not, SRGPC are contaminants if isolated with other bacteria, and clinical interpretation of their presence is often difficult. Head and neck infections include infection of paranasal sinuses, brain abscess, dental abscess, lateral (pharyngomaxillary) and retropharyngeal space infections, and in Ludwig's angina (bilateral submandibular and sublingual cellulitis often, 50% to 90%, of dental origin). Thoracic infections include lung abscess and empyema. Abdominal infections include liver abscess, visceral abscess, and pelvic and perirectal abscesses. Skin and subcutaneous tissue infections often involve devitalized or necrotic skin, muscle, and subcutaneous tissue. Specific examples include anaerobic streptococcal myositis, a fulminant disease characterized by pain, marked edema, crepitant myositis, and a purulent or seropurulent exudate that on Gram stain reveals gram-positive cocci in chains. Progressive synergistic gangrene is caused by polymicrobic infection with *Staphylococcus aureus* and microaerophilic or anaerobic streptococci. The infection occurs around surgical incisions as an ulcerated lesion with surrounding gangrenous tissue. Chronic burrowing ulcer is an infection of deep soft tissue. It erodes (burrows) through subcutaneous tissue to erupt as an ulcer at a distant site.

Diagnosis Documentation of the diagnosis of infection with SRGPC requires that potentially contaminating normal flora be excluded from the cultures. Needle aspiration of loculated pus by the percutaneous route is a frequently good approach. Often Gram stain yields more information than culture because of the fastidious nature of the organisms (difficult to recover by usual laboratory methods) and the frequent polymicrobial nature of the infections.

Diagnostic Tests/Procedures

Anaerobic Culture *on page 371*
Gram Stain *on page 473*

Duration of Therapy 7-10 days

Treatment Successful therapy for anaerobic and microaerophilic streptococcal infections usually involves debridement or drainage of involved area or abscess and intravenous antimicrobial therapy usually with intravenous penicillin.

Drug Therapy

Recommended:

Penicillin G (Parenteral/Aqueous) *on page 993*

(Continued)

Streptococcus-Related Gram-Positive Cocci *(Continued)*

Alternate:

Ampicillin and Sulbactam *on page 660*
Amoxicillin and Clavulanate Potassium *on page 645*
Cephalosporins, 1st Generation *on page 729*
Clindamycin *on page 752*
Vancomycin *on page 1144*

Streptococcus salivarius *see Streptococcus*, Viridans Group *on page 326*
***Streptococcus sanguis* I** *see Streptococcus*, Viridans Group *on page 326*

Streptococcus Species

Refer to

Streptococcus agalactiae on page 313
Streptococcus bovis on page 315
Streptococcus pneumoniae, Drug-Susceptible *on page 319*
Streptococcus pyogenes on page 321
Streptococcus-Related Gram-Positive Cocci *on page 325*
Streptococcus, Viridans Group *on page 326*

Streptococcus, Viridans Group

Related Information

Antibiotic Treatment of Adults With Infective Endocarditis *on page 1271*
Streptococcus bovis on page 315

Synonyms Viridans Streptococci

Applies to *Streptococcus anginosus*; *Streptococcus constellatus*; *Streptococcus intermedius*; *Streptococcus milleri*; *Streptococcus mitis*; *Streptococcus mutans*; *Streptococcus oralis*; *Streptococcus salivarius*; *Streptococcus sanguis* I

Microbiology Viridans streptococci are normal inhabitants of the oral cavity, gastrointestinal tract, and female genital tract. Historically "viridans" or green streptococci were separated from other "β-hemolytic" strains of streptococci by their ability to produce α-hemolysis ("greening") on blood agar, although many strains produce γ-hemolysis (nonhemolytic). More recently, antigenic, physiological, biochemical, and DNA homology techniques have resulted in more precise characterization of these organisms. The Lancefield serogroup (eg, A, B, C, D, etc) cross species lines. New species are being described and many reclassifications have been made. *S. bovis* and *S. pneumoniae* are α-hemolytic. Upon isolation of α, β, or nonhemolytic streptococci on blood agar, presumptive identification of nongroup A, B, or D can be made by resistance to bacitracin, negative hippurate or CAMP test, negative or weakly reactive bile esculin hydrolysis, negative PYR test, negative pyruvate, and failure to grow in 6.5% NaCl.

Some of these organisms are nutritionally fastidious and can require complex supplemented media. CO_2 may enhance growth. There is no correlation between serogroup and biochemical speciation. Speciation can be accomplished by biochemical testing. *S. morbillorum* has been transferred to the genus *Gemella*.

Clinical Syndromes Clinically, viridans streptococci are associated primarily with endocarditis, although infection of all tissues has been reported. *S. sanguis* I, *S. sanguis* II, and *S. mitis* are most frequently implicated in endocarditis, while *S. intermedius* is associated with noncardiac suppurative infections. *S. anginosus* and *S. constellatus* are closely related and are sometimes classified together with *S. intermedius* and *Streptococcus* MG as *Streptococcus milleri* or *S. milleri* group.

Viridans streptococci often pose a problem as they may be detected in blood culture as the result of transient insignificant bacteremia or may represent insignificant contaminants. Fifty percent of all bacterial endocarditis is due to viridans streptococci which is often diagnosed in patients with valvular heart disease. The course is subacute with cure rates in excess of 90%. Transient seeding of the blood by viridans streptococci is regarded as a commonplace occurrence. The organism has low intrinsic virulence. See table on next page.

Diagnosis Diagnosis is usually accomplished by repeated positive blood culture or recovery of the organism in cultures from the affected site.

Diagnostic Tests/Procedures

Aerobic Culture, Appropriate Site *on page 365*
Blood Culture, Aerobic and Anaerobic *on page 391*
Gram Stain *on page 473*

Treatment Susceptibility testing has not been standardized for fastidious CO_2-requiring *Streptococcus* species. Most isolates are reported to be susceptible to penicillin with MICs $\leq$0.12 mcg/mL. Rare isolates have penicillin MICs $\geq$1.0 mcg/mL.

Streptococcus Viridans Group

Species	Viridans Group	Lancefield Groups	Normal Human Habitat	Normal Veterinary Habitat	Human Disease	Veterinary Disease
S. acidominimus		NG, E, F		Milk, genital and intestinal tracts	Rare	—
S. anginosus, S. constellatus, S. intermedius	*Anginosus group*	NG, A, C, F, G, K	Oropharynx, teeth surface, skin, intestinal tract		Endocarditis, suppurative infections, abcesses, bacteremia	—
S. bovis	Bovis group	D	Genital and intestinal tracts	Bovine and sheep — intestinal tracts	Endocarditis, bacteremia	Endocarditis
S. cremoris		N	Oropharynx	Milk	Rare	Mastitis
S. dysgalactiae		A, C, G, L	Upper respiratory tract, skin, vagina	Bovine and sheep	—	Mastitis
S. lactis		N	Oropharynx	Milk	Rare	Mastitis
S. mitis S. sanguis S. ovalis	Mitis group	NG, A, C, F, G, H, K, M, O	Oropharynx, intestinal tract		Endocarditis, caries	—
S. morbillorum	*Gemella morbillorum*	NG	Intestinal and urogenital tracts		Endocarditis, suppurative infections	—
S. mutans	Mutans group	NG, E, F, K	Teeth surface, intestinal tract		Endocarditis, caries	—
S. pneumoniae		—	Upper respiratory tract		Common	—
S. salivarius	Salivarius group	NG, F, H, K	Oropharynx, intestinal tract		Endocarditis	—
S. suis		D (R, S, T)		Swine	Rare	Bacteremia, bone and joint infections
S. uberis		NG, E, F, K		Milk, oropharynx, skin, intestinal tract	Rare	Mastitis

NG = nongroupable.

Adapted from Gallis HA, "Viridans and B-Hemolytic (Non-Group A, B, and D) Streptococci," *Principles and Practice of Infectious Diseases*, Mandell GL, Douglas RG Jr, and Bennett JE, eds, New York, NY: Churchill Livingstone, 1990, 1563-72, with permission.

Streptococcus, Viridans Group *(Continued)*

Other effective agents include cephalosporins (first and second generation), cefotaxime, clindamycin, erythromycin, and vancomycin. *In vitro* resistance to aminoglycosides is observed; however, synergy is observed *in vitro* with cell wall active agents.

For treatment of highly penicillin susceptible viridans streptococcal native valve endocarditis, penicillin G 12-18 million units/day in divided doses or ceftriaxone 2 g every 24 hours are the recommended drugs of choice. An alternative regimen of penicillin or ceftriaxone plus low-dose gentamicin can be used for a 2-week duration (only if there is no abscess, normal renal function, and no impaired 8th cranial nerve function). Vancomycin may be used in patients unable to tolerate recommended regimens. If organisms are relatively resistant (MIC >0.12 mcg/mL to ≤0.5 mcg/mL), penicillin 24 million units/day in divided doses or ceftriaxone 2 g/day should be administered for 4 weeks along with low-dose gentamicin for 2 weeks.

In patients with prosthetic valve endocarditis and highly susceptible organisms, the higher dose of penicillin or ceftriaxone should be administered for 6 weeks with or without 2 weeks of low-dose gentamicin. In patients with relatively resistant strains, the gentamicin should be administered with the beta-lactam for the entire 6-week period. Vancomycin remains an alternate.

Drug Therapy

Recommended:

Endocarditis:

Penicillin G (Parenteral/Aqueous) *on page 993*

individually or plus

Gentamicin *on page 841*

Ceftriaxone *on page 722*

individually or plus

Gentamicin *on page 841*

Nonendocarditis:

Penicillin G (Parenteral/Aqueous) *on page 993*

Alternate:

Endocarditis:

Vancomycin *on page 1144*

Nonendocarditis:

Cephalosporins, 1st Generation *on page 729*

Vancomycin *on page 1144*

Selected Readings

Baddour LM, Wilson WR, Bayer AS, et al, "Infective Endocarditis: Diagnosis, Antimicrobial Therapy, and Management of Complications: A Statement for Healthcare Professionals From the Committee on Rheumatic Fever, Endocarditis, and Kawasaki Disease, Council on Cardiovascular Disease in the Young, and the Councils on Clinical Cardiology, Stroke, and Cardiovascular Surgery and Anesthesia, American Heart Association - Executive Summary: Endorsed by the Infectious Diseases Society of America," *Circulation*, 2005, 111(23):3167-84.

Blanco-Carrion A, "Bacterial Endocarditis Prophylaxis," *Med Oral Patol Oral Cir Bucal*, 2004, 9(Suppl):44-51; 37-43.

Bochud PY, Eggiman P, Calandra T, et al, "Bacteremia Due to Viridans *Streptococcus* in Neutropenic Patients With Cancer: Clinical Spectrum and Risk Factors," *Clin Infect Dis*, 1994, 18(1):25-31.

Elting LS, Bodey GP, and Keefe BH, "Septicemia and Shock Syndrome Due to Viridans Streptococci: A Case-Control Study of Predisposing Factors," *Clin Infect Dis*, 1992, 14(6):1201-7.

Johnson CC and Tunkel AR, "Viridans Streptococci and Group C and G Streptococci," *Principles and Practice of Infectious Diseases*, 5th ed, Mandell GL, Bennett JE, and Dolin R, eds, New York, NY: Churchill Livingstone, 2000, 2167-83.

Prabhu RM, Piper KE, Baddour LM, et al, "Antimicrobial Susceptibility Patterns Among Viridans Group Streptococcal Isolates From Infective Endocarditis Patients From 1971 to 1986 and 1994 to 2002," *Antimicrob Agents Chemother*, 2004, 48(11):4463-5.

Strongyloides stercoralis

Microbiology *Strongyloides stercoralis* is a small roundworm (nematode) which can cause human disease in several ways. The "direct" cycle of infection begins when the human comes in contact with soil containing the worm in its infective (filariform) larval stage. *Strongyloides* penetrates the skin and enters the circulation of the host. When the worms reach the alveolar capillaries, a pulmonary phase begins in which the parasites enter the alveoli and ascend the respiratory tract. Once in the pharynx, the organisms are swallowed. Maturation and reproduction occur in the small intestine. The fertilized adult female burrows into the mucosa of the upper small intestine and begins to lay eggs. The larvae which hatch are in a noninfectious (rhabditiform) stage; they eventually bore through the intestinal epithelium to reach the bowel lumen and are passed in the feces. The rhabditiform larvae can transform to infective filariform larvae in soil, thus completing the cycle.

In addition to this direct cycle, *Strongyloides* can also reproduce without a human host. In this "**indirect cycle**," larvae are passed into the soil, as described above. If proper environmental conditions are present, larvae mature into adult helminths capable of reproduction. After copulation, large numbers of new larvae are produced, potentially infectious to humans.

A less common but clinically important aspect of *Strongyloides* is its "**autoinfection cycle**." Instead of being passed in the stool, noninfectious larvae transform into infectious larvae in the lumen of the intestine. They can then reenter the host circulation either by boring through the intestinal wall or penetrating the perianal skin. This "autoinfection" can cause repeated infections over the years and at times can be life-threatening because of the associated heavy worm burden ("hyperinfection syndrome").

Epidemiology *Strongyloides* infections occur worldwide. Infections are common in the tropics where the prevalence may approach 50% in some areas. In the United States, the disease is much less common, even in the southern states where the most number of cases are reported (prevalence <4%). In addition to the direct penetration of the skin, *Strongyloides* can be sexually transmitted.

Clinical Syndromes

- **Asymptomatic infection:** About 33% of infected individuals have no symptoms.
- **Abdominal pain and diarrhea (sometimes bloody):** This usually occurs as the larvae hatch in the intestinal mucosa and are passed through the lumen. Complications include ileus, weight loss, and malabsorption syndromes. Important clues to the diagnosis are concomitant peripheral eosinophilia and an urticarial skin rash.
- **Eosinophilic pneumonitis, a Löffler's-type syndrome:** This is similar to other hookworm infections which have a prominent pulmonary phase. Patients present with fever, cough, and wheezing as the larvae migrate through the pulmonary circulation and alveoli. A pruritic rash may be seen.
- **Autoinfection** (see Microbiology): Chronic and recurrent *Strongyloides* infections can occur over months or years because of the organism's ability to autoinfect the host. These patients can present with a wide variety of symptoms, either gastrointestinal (nausea, vomiting, abdominal pain, explosive diarrhea) and/or pulmonary (wheezing, cough) depending on the phase of the parasite's life cycle. Immunocompromised individuals are at risk for life-threatening, disseminated hyperinfections with massive worm burdens. The majority of cases have been reported in organ transplant recipients and in patients with lymphoma or leukemia; in some cases, hyperinfection occurs in otherwise healthy individuals. An overwhelming pneumonitis is characteristically seen with cough, dyspnea, bronchospasm, and sputum production. Peripheral eosinophilia is common but may be absent. Other complications include bacterial sepsis, respiratory failure, bacterial meningitis, and death. The hyperinfection syndrome is an uncommon manifestation of strongyloidiasis.
- ***Strongyloides* in AIDS:** In the past, disseminated *Strongyloides* has been regarded as an AIDS-defining condition in people who are seropositive for HIV. However, it has proven a relatively uncommon occurrence even in patients from endemic areas.

Diagnosis Strongyloidiasis should be suspected in travelers or immigrants from an endemic area and presenting with diarrhea and eosinophilia. It should also be considered in the differential diagnosis of eosinophilic pneumonia (Löffler's-type syndrome) or unexplained diarrhea in an immunocompromised patient. Peripheral eosinophilia, while important, may be absent. In all cases, laboratory confirmation is essential and includes:

- Stool examination to identify the characteristic larval forms (rather than the eggs, which are rarely found). A single negative fecal exam does not rule out strongyloidiasis.
- Duodenal aspiration to identify the organism in the upper intestinal tract. This can be done as part of an upper endoscopic procedure.

Diagnostic Tests/Procedures

Ova and Parasites, Stool *on page 551*
Ova and Parasites, Urine or Aspirates *on page 554*

Treatment The drug of choice for strongyloidiasis is thiabendazole. However, it is well known that treatment failures occur with the standard drug doses for unclear reasons. A recent report has suggested that ivermectin may also be effective in people with AIDS.

Since disseminated *Strongyloides* is seen in organ transplant recipients, individuals from endemic areas awaiting transplantation should be carefully screened and treated if positive.

Drug Therapy

Recommended:

Thiabendazole *on page 1111*
Ivermectin *on page 899*
(Continued)

Strongyloides stercoralis (Continued)

Selected Readings

Gompels MM, Todd J, Peters BS, et al, "Disseminated Strongyloidiasis in AIDS: Uncommon but Important," *AIDS*, 1991, 5(3):329-32.

Longworth DL and Weller PF, "Hyperinfection Syndrome With Strongyloidiasis," *Curr Clin Top Infect Dis*, 1986, 10:1-26.

Torres JR, Isturiz R, Murillo J, et al, "Efficacy of Ivermectin in the Treatment of Strongyloidiasis Complicating AIDS," *Clin Infect Dis*, 1993, 17(5):900-2.

Strongyloidiasis *see Strongyloides stercoralis on page 328*

Subacute Native Valve Endocarditis *see* Endocarditis, Subacute Native Valve *on page 126*

Suppurative Thrombophlebitis *see* Thrombophlebitis, Suppurative *on page 330*

Supraglottitis *see* Epiglottitis *on page 139*

Surgical Wound Infection *see* Wound Infection, Surgical *on page 354*

Swimmer's Ear *see* Otitis Externa, Mild *on page 252*

Syphilis *see Treponema pallidum on page 334*

Taenia saginata *see* Cestodes *on page 72*

Taenia solium *see* Cestodes *on page 72*

Tapeworms *see* Cestodes *on page 72*

Tetanus *see Clostridium tetani on page 90*

Thrombophlebitis, Septic *see* Thrombophlebitis, Suppurative *on page 330*

Thrombophlebitis, Suppurative

Synonyms Septic Thrombophlebitis; Suppurative Thrombophlebitis; Thrombophlebitis, Septic

Clinical Presentation Frequently associated with thrombosis and bacteremia. Upper extremity suppurative thrombophlebitis usually shows signs of local inflammation and fever. The majority of patients have an implicated catheter left in place for ≥5 days. Local inflammation is less prominent in lower extremity disease. Pelvic suppurative thrombophlebitis typically develops 1-2 weeks postpartum or postoperatively presenting with fever, chills, anorexia, nausea, vomiting, and abdominal pain. Majority of pelvic suppurative thrombophlebitis occurs unilaterally. Vascular surgery consult is indicated to evaluate for possible vein excision.

Lemierre's syndrome is a suppurative thrombophlebitis of the internal jugular vein in the presence of oropharyngeal infection more commonly seen in children. Other causes include deep neck infections and central venous catheterization. Usually associated with gram-negative anaerobic organisms such as *Fusobacterium necrophorum*.

Differential Diagnosis Septic nonsuppurative thrombophlebitis

Likely Pathogens

Staphylococcus epidermidis, Methicillin-Susceptible *on page 310*
Staphylococcus aureus, Methicillin-Susceptible *on page 307*
Staphylococcus epidermidis, Methicillin-Resistant *on page 309*
Staphylococcus aureus, Methicillin-Resistant *on page 304*
Candida Species *on page 67*

Diagnostic Tests/Procedures

Blood Culture, Aerobic and Anaerobic *on page 391*
If deep venous thrombosis is suspected:
Ultrasound, Peripheral Arteries and Veins *on page 605*

Empiric Drug Therapy

Recommended:

Penicillins, Penicillinase-Resistant *on page 997*
Vancomycin *on page 1144*

If *Candida* is suspected:
Amphotericin B (Conventional) *on page 650*
Fluconazole *on page 819*

Selected Readings

Armstrong AW, Spooner K, and Sanders JW, "Lemierre's Syndrome," *Curr Infect Dis Rep*, 2000, 2(2):168-173.

Benoit D, Decruyenaere J, Vandewoude K, et al, "Management of Candidal Thrombophlebitis of the Central Veins: Case Report and Review," *Clin Infect Dis*, 1998, 26(2):393-7.

Khan EA, Correa AG, and Baker CJ, "Suppurative Thrombophlebitis in Children: A Ten-year Experience," *Pediatr Infect Dis J*, 1997, 16(1):63-7.

Thrush *see Candida* Species *on page 67*

Tick-Borne Encephalitis *see* Arboviruses *on page 35*

Tinea *see* Dermatophytes *on page 114*

Tinea Nigra *see* Dematiaceous Fungi *on page 112*

T-*Mycoplasma* *see Ureaplasma urealyticum on page 342*
Toxic Cholangitis *see* Cholangitis, Acute *on page 79*

Toxic Shock Syndrome

Clinical Presentation See individual organisms for clinical presentation information.

Likely Pathogens

Staphylococcus aureus, Methicillin-Resistant *on page 304*
Staphylococcus aureus, Methicillin-Susceptible *on page 307*
Streptococcus pyogenes on page 321

Diagnostic Tests/Procedures

Blood Culture, Aerobic and Anaerobic *on page 391*

Empiric Drug Therapy

Recommended:

Vancomycin *on page 1144*
Penicillins, Penicillinase-Resistant *on page 997*

Selected Readings

Davis D, Gash-Kim TL, and Heffernan EJ, "Toxic Shock Syndrome: Case Report of a Postpartum Female and a Literature Review," *J Emerg Med*, 1998, 16(4):607-14.
Holm C and Mühlbauer W, "Toxic Shock Syndrome in Plastic Surgery Patients: Case Report and Review of the Literature," *Aesthetic Plast Surg*, 1998, 22(3):180-4.
Kiska DL, "Staphylococcal and Streptococcal Toxic Shock Syndrome," *Clin Microbiol Newslett*, 1997, 19(5):33-7.
Stevens DL, "Streptococcal Toxic-Shock Syndrome: Spectrum of Disease, Pathogenesis, and New Concepts in Treatment," *Emerg Infect Dis*, 1995, 1(3):69-78.

Toxo *see Toxoplasma gondii on page 331*

Toxoplasma gondii

Related Information

USPHS / IDSA Guidelines for the Prevention of Opportunistic Infections in Persons Infected With HIV *on page 1237*

Synonyms Toxo

Microbiology *Toxoplasma gondii* is a sporozoan of the order *Coccidia* and suborder *Eimeria*. The three forms of *T. gondii* are trophozoites (previously referred as tachyzoites), tissue cysts, and oocysts. The trophozoite is crescent to oval shape, 4 x 8 µm in size, and stains with both Wright and Giemsa stains. The trophozoite invades all nucleated cells, resides in vacuoles, and reproduces to form cysts. Tissue cysts measure 10-200 µm and may contain up to 3000 organisms. These cysts may remain dormant for years and can become reactivated. The organisms stain PAS-positive, but the cyst wall itself stains very weakly positive. The oocysts measure 10-12 µm and are produced only in cats. All three forms are pathogenic to humans.

Epidemiology *Toxoplasma* infects nearly all animals and birds. It is the most widely distributed of all intracellular parasites. Prior to the AIDS epidemic, the majority of cases were benign and self-limited. There are still approximately 3000 cases of congenital toxoplasmosis reported per year with an average of 0.6 cases per 1000 pregnancies in the United States. Toxoplasmosis is the most common focal CNS infection in AIDS. It is estimated that 5% to 10% of AIDS patients have toxoplasmosis although 25% to 50% of AIDS patients will have positive IgG serology indicating previous exposure suggesting that reactivation plays an important role. In heart, but not renal or liver, transplantation, 50% of the seronegative recipients who receive seropositive donor hearts develop toxoplasmosis with a mortality rate exceeding 75%. Bone marrow transplant patients appear to be at increased risk of reactivation.

Humans become infected by ingesting the cysts either through contamination with cat feces or undercooked meat, especially pork and lamb, or through direct inoculation via blood transfusions, laboratory accidents, or congenital transmission. After ingestion of the cysts, digestive enzymes disrupt the cyst wall and release viable organisms that invade the mucosa and disseminate.

Clinical Syndromes

- **Asymptomatic lymphadenitis:** Eighty percent to 90% of patients present with asymptomatic cervical lymphadenitis.
- **Mononucleosis syndrome:** Some patients may present with fever, malaise, myalgias, sore throat, maculopapular rash, and hepatosplenomegaly which is self-limited and often confused with viral illnesses such as EBV. Rarely, patients develop myocarditis or pneumonitis.
- **Congenital:** Pregnant women who acquire toxoplasmosis during the first trimester have a 25% risk of fetal transmission resulting in spontaneous abortions, stillborns, or severe disease. Sixty-five percent of infants born to women infected during the third trimester have subclinical infection with ultimately 85% developing chorioretinitis or neurological sequelae. The number of congenital cases continues to decline probably because of increased awareness of food and cat hygiene during pregnancy.

(Continued)

Toxoplasma gondii (Continued)

- **Ocular:** Vast majority of chorioretinitis is due to congenital toxoplasmosis. Patients in their second or third decade of life present with blurred vision, scotoma, eye pain, and photophobia. Fundoscopic examination reveals characteristic exudative retinal lesions. Typically bilateral in congenital toxoplasmosis and unilateral in acquired infection.
- **Pulmonary:** Second most common site after the brain in AIDS patients with CD4 T-cell counts <50 cells/µL. Present with fever, nonproductive cough, and dyspnea. Chest x-ray usually reveals bilateral interstitial infiltrates.
- **Encephalitis:** Increased incidence in homosexual AIDS patients. Patients present with headache, seizures, disorientation, fever, and focal neurological deficits depending on size, location, and number of lesions. MRI is more sensitive than CT. *Toxoplasma* typically appears as multiple small lesions with predilection for corticomedullary junction and basal ganglia, whereas lymphoma usually presents with a large solitary lesion with subependymal spread or ventricular encasement. Differential diagnosis of CNS mass lesions in AIDS is toxoplasmosis 50% to 70%, primary CNS lymphoma 20% to 30%, progressive multifocal leukoencephalopathy 10% to 20%, and, less frequently, Kaposi sarcoma, tuberculosis, fungal, or herpes. Serological test may be of limited value given 3% false-negative and increased seropositivity in AIDS.

Diagnosis Diagnosis depends on serological tests and biopsy. Ocular *Toxoplasma* is diagnosed by clinical examination. Biopsy material reveals trophozoites. Several reference laboratories offer molecular amplification (eg, PCR) and subsequent detection of *T. gondii* in clinical specimens.

Standard serology tests for IgG and IgM antibodies against *Toxoplasma gondii* are offered by several reference laboratories. A specialized IgG avidity test is offered by the Palo Alto Medical Foundation (Research Institute - (650)853-4828). The test can provide results ("high avidity") which can exclude a recent infection during the first four months of pregnancy. Serum samples for this test should be obtained within the first 4 months of pregnancy.

Diagnostic Tests/Procedures

Brain Biopsy *on page 405*
Lymph Node Biopsy *on page 529*
Muscle Biopsy *on page 538*
Polymerase Chain Reaction *on page 567*
Toxoplasma Serology by ELISA *on page 597*
Toxoplasma Serology *on page 596*

Treatment

Acute infection: Treatment should consist of sulfadiazine 1-1.5 g every 6 hours plus pyrimethamine 50-100 mg every day plus leucovorin. Sulfamethoxazole and trimethoprim (based on TMP 10 mg/kg/day) every 12 hours may be as efficacious as sulfadiazine/pyrimethamine. If intolerant of sulfa, may substitute sulfadiazine with clindamycin 450-600 mg every 6 hours. In patients intolerant of either sulfadiazine or clindamycin, the following may be substituted: azithromycin 1200 mg orally daily, clarithromycin 1 g orally twice daily, or atovaquone 750 mg orally 4 times/day plus pyrimethamine and folinic acid. Induction therapy should be given for at least 6 weeks until the lesions have resolved or stabilized at a reduced size. Ninety percent of patients will show clinical or radiographic improvement within 10-14 days of therapy. Patients without either clinical or radiographic improvement should have brain biopsy to confirm diagnosis.

A commonly employed presumptive diagnostic method is to empirically treat all AIDS patients with mass lesions for 2 weeks with antitoxoplasmosis agents and then re-evaluate clinically and radiographically. However, in patients with a negative toxoplasmosis IgG and the absence of the characteristic toxoplasmosis lesions on MRI or presence of lesions suggestive of lymphoma, the likelihood of toxoplasmosis is significantly <1%, and it is recommended that the patient undergo an immediate brain biopsy for definitive diagnosis and prompt appropriate intervention.

Maintenance (chronic suppression): Patients must be continued on suppressive therapy to avoid reactivation. Sulfadiazine 500-1000 mg orally every 6 hours plus pyrimethamine 25-75 mg orally daily plus folinic acid 10 mg orally daily (A 3 times/week regimen of sulfadiazine 1 g twice daily plus pyrimethamine 50 mg plus folinic acid 10 mg revealed similar efficacy in a small study.) or sulfamethoxazole and trimethoprim (based on 5 mg/kg TMP) orally every 12 hours. Alternate: Clindamycin 300-450 mg orally every 6 hours plus pyrimethamine 25-75 mg orally daily and folinic acid 10 mg orally daily.

In patients intolerant of either sulfadiazine or clindamycin, the following may be substituted (unknown efficacy): atovaquone, azithromycin, clarithromycin, or

dapsone. Dapsone should not be used for acute infection as it has no effect on tissue cysts but may be used as an alternate for chronic suppressive therapy.

Prophylaxis: Preventive measures include avoidance of cat feces and freezing at -20°C, thawing, and heating to >60°C to destroy cysts in contaminated meats.

Chemoprophylaxis should be initiated if a patient has a CD4 count <100 cells/μL and is seropositive for IgG antibody to *T. gondii* and is not already receiving a regimen for PCP prophylaxis that is also effective for toxoplasmosis.

Current recommended prophylaxis: Sulfamethoxazole and trimethoprim DS orally daily; dapsone 50-100 mg orally daily plus pyrimethamine 50 mg and leucovorin 25 mg/week; or dapsone 200 mg plus pyrimethamine 75 mg and leucovorin 25 mg/week. Efficacy of clindamycin/pyrimethamine, macrolides, or atovaquone for prophylaxis is unknown. Primary prophylaxis may be discontinued in AIDS patients who have had presumed immune restoration following potent antiretroviral therapy. Preliminary evidence suggests that secondary prophylaxis may be withdrawn; however, larger studies are needed before recommending such.

Drug Therapy

Recommended:

Monotherapy:

Sulfamethoxazole and Trimethoprim *on page 1087*

Combination therapy:

Pyrimethamine *on page 1025* (plus folinic acid)

plus

SulfaDIAZINE *on page 1083*

Alternate:

Clindamycin *on page 752*

plus

Pyrimethamine *on page 1025* (plus folinic acid)

Selected Readings

Abdel Hameed DM and Helmy H, "Avidity IgG: Diagnosis of Primary *Toxoplasma gondii* Infection by Indirect Immunofluorescent Test," *J Egypt Soc Parasitol*, 2004, 34(3):893-902.

Boyer KM, Holfels E, Roizen N, et al, "Risk Factors for *Toxoplasma gondii* Infection in Mothers of Infants With Congenital Toxoplasmosis: Implications for Prenatal Management and Screening," *Am J Obstet Gynecol*, 2005, 192(2):564-71.

Campagna AC, "Pulmonary Toxoplasmosis," *Semin Respir Infect*, 1997, 12(2):98-105.

Franzen C, Altfeld M, Hegener P, et al, "Limited Value of PCR for Detection of *Toxoplasma gondii* in Blood From Human Immunodeficiency Virus-Infected Patients," *J Clin Microbiol*, 1997, 35(10):2639-41.

Joiner KA and Dubremetz JF, "*Toxoplasma gondii*: A Protozoan for the Nineties," *Infect Immun*, 1993, 61(4):1169-72.

Kravetz JD and Federman DG, "Toxoplasmosis in Pregnancy," *Am J Med*, 2005, 118(3):212-6.

Lopez A, Dietz VJ, Wilson M, et al, "Preventing Congenital Toxoplasmosis," *MMWR*, 2000, 49(RR-2):59-68.

McCabe R and Chirurgi V, "Issues in Toxoplasmosis," *Infect Dis Clin North Am*, 1993, 7(3):587-604.

Torre D, Casari S, Speranza F, et al, "Randomized Trial of Trimethoprim-Sulfamethoxazole Versus Pyrimethamine-Sulfadiazine for Therapy of Toxoplasmic Encephalitis in Patients With AIDS. Italian Collaborative Study Group," *Antimicrob Agents Chemother*, 1998, 42(6):1346-9.

Wong SY and Remington JS, "Toxoplasmosis in Pregnancy," *Clin Infect Dis*, 1994, 18(6):853-61.

Toxoplasmosis *see Toxoplasma gondii on page 331*

Tracheobronchitis *see* Bronchitis *on page 60*

Trachoma *see Chlamydia trachomatis on page 74*

Traveler's Diarrhea

Clinical Presentation The onset is typically acute, often explosive may be watery or bloody. Often not accompanied by fever, but may be associated with severe systemic symptoms, including fever, abdominal cramping, diaphoresis, and central nervous complaints (headache, dizziness, lightheadedness, confusion).

As many as 60% of travelers to developing nations experience diarrhea, which tends to resolve in 5-10 days after the onset of symptoms. This is most often due to bacterial pathogens and less likely parasites and viruses. Parasites, however, are the most common causes of chronic diarrhea in travelers. Traveler's should check with a travel medicine expert or travel agency for the most common causes of diarrhea in that particular geographic region. This information may also be obtained at the CDC web site: http://www.cdc.gov/travel/.

Differential Diagnosis Appendicitis

Likely Pathogens

Escherichia coli, Diarrheagenic *on page 143*

Shigella Species *on page 297*

Campylobacter jejuni on page 66

Salmonella Species *on page 291*

Cyclospora cayetanensis on page 105

Cryptosporidium on page 104

(Continued)

Traveler's Diarrhea *(Continued)*

Giardia lamblia on page 155
Viruses

Epidemiology As many as 60% of travelers to developing nations experience diarrhea and tends to resolve in 5-10 days after the onset of symptoms. Most often due to bacterial pathogens and less likely parasites and viruses. Parasites, however, are the most common causes of chronic diarrhea in travelers. Traveler's should check with a travel medicine expert or travel agency for the most common causes of diarrhea in that particular geographic region. This information may also be obtained at the CDC web site: http://www.cdc.gov/travel/.

Diagnostic Tests/Procedures

Fecal Leukocyte Stain *on page 455*
Stool Culture *on page 585*

Drug Therapy Comment Travelers should be instructed to avoid uncooked foods, nonbottled beverages, or unpasteurized dairy products. Bottled water should be used for all purposes where ingestion is possible, including ice cubes and brushing of teeth.

Prophylaxis is rarely necessary, although travelers are often encouraged to carry a supply of antibiotics to initiate treatment. Fluoroquinolone resistance is increasing for many causative organisms. Loperamide may be used to control diarrhea unless patient is <2 years of age, experiences fever, or bloody stools are noted. Typically, three- to four-day antibiotic regimens are prescribed. Avoid fluoroquinolone use in pregnancy or in children. Single dose azithromycin (1000 mg in adults or 10-15 mg/kg in children) may be considered as a convenient alternative.

Empiric Drug Therapy

Recommended:

Ciprofloxacin *on page 742*
Ofloxacin *on page 977*
Levofloxacin *on page 908*
Azithromycin *on page 674*

Alternate:

Sulfamethoxazole and Trimethoprim *on page 1087*
Doxycycline *on page 787*

Selected Readings

Adachi JA, Ostrosky-Zeichner L, DuPont HL, et al, "Empirical Antimicrobial Therapy for Traveler's Diarrhea," *Clin Infect Dis*, 2000, 31(4):1079-83.
Okhuysen PC, "Traveler's Diarrhea Due to Intestinal Protozoa," *Clin Infect Dis*, 2001, 33(1):110-4.
Ramzan NN, "Traveler's Diarrhea," *Gastroenterol Clin North Am*, 2001, 30(3):665-78.

Treponema pallidum

Related Information

Treatment of Sexually Transmitted Infections *on page 1311*

Microbiology *Treponema pallidum* (subspecies *pallidum*) is a thin, gram-negative bacterium which belongs to the order Spirochaetales. It is one of the clinically-important spirochetes and is thus related to such agents as *Borrelia burgdorferi* (the cause of Lyme disease) and *Leptospira* (the cause of leptospirosis). *T. pallidum* is the etiologic agent of syphilis. The organism is thin, long, helical, and coiled and is difficult to see by light microscopy. Visualization of the organism in clinical specimens requires special techniques other than Gram stain or Giemsa stain. There are no clinically-available culture systems for *T. pallidum*, and microbiologic identification of the organism depends on such techniques as darkfield microscopy, direct fluorescent antibody stains, silver stains, and serologic tests.

Epidemiology Syphilis occurs exclusively in humans. The vast majority of cases are acquired via sexual contact with an infected person. Other modes of acquisition include congenital transmission to the newborn and blood transfusion, but these are much less common.

Despite public health measures, the incidence of syphilis has continued to increase to epidemic proportions. In the United States, the number of syphilis cases increased dramatically in the late 1980s, with a near doubling of total reported cases. In 1992, there were over 120,000 reported cases of syphilis (at all stages), but this number grossly underestimates the true number of infections since many cases are undiagnosed. In many urban areas in the U.S., the number of syphilis cases has increased dramatically despite a lower incidence in the homosexual community, the population previously at highest risk. In large part, this change in the at-risk population is due to the increased use of crack cocaine and the exchange of sex for drugs. Sex partners are almost impossible to locate in some urban areas and a substantial number of crack users have undiagnosed syphilis. Currently, the groups at highest risk for syphilis are black, heterosexual men and black, heterosexual women. There has also

been an increase in the number of cases of congenital syphilis corresponding roughly to the increase in primary and secondary syphilis in heterosexual women.

Sexual partner notification remains an important part of infection control measures. About 50% of partners named by an actively infected individual will also have syphilis; many partners will either be actively infected themselves or will have incubating syphilis.

Clinical Syndromes Syphilis commonly presents in one of several stages: primary, secondary, latent (early latent and late latent), or tertiary syphilis. However, it should be remembered that syphilis has been called "the great mimic" in medical literature because of its protean manifestations and tendency to mimic other diseases.

- **Primary syphilis:** This is an important cause of the common clinical syndrome of "genital ulceration with regional lymphadenopathy". This syndrome is caused by syphilis, primary herpes simplex virus infection, lymphogranuloma venereum, donovanosis, and chancroid. It may be difficult for the clinician to diagnose this on the basis of clinical findings alone. The hallmark of primary syphilis is the genital chancre. The syphilitic chancre is typically a single, painless ulcer with raised and indurated borders. The base of the ulcer is clean, usually without purulence. Up to 33% of syphilitic ulcers, however, may be mildly painful. The chancre can be found on the penis, rectum, anal verge, mouth, labia, or cervix. In the absence of treatment, chancres persist for up to 6 weeks. In addition, inguinal lymphadenopathy is present in the majority of cases of primary syphilis (about 80%). The onset of adenopathy usually occurs at the same time as the genital lesion. Characteristically, the adenopathy is painless (like the chancre), and the nodes are firm. In 70% of cases, the adenopathy is bilateral. Constitutional symptoms are usually absent in primary syphilis. In some individuals, primary syphilis goes unnoticed, especially if the chancre is small and painless. The chancre is teeming with live and active organisms and is an excellent source of material (serum and lymphatic fluid) for a darkfield examination.
- **Secondary syphilis:** In the absence of specific therapy for primary syphilis, further clinical manifestations may develop. Secondary syphilis may occur up to 2 years after initial infection. In secondary syphilis, there is evidence of a systemic illness and often the diagnosis may be difficult to make. The manifestations of secondary syphilis are protean. The most common finding is a skin rash, which is present in about 90% of cases. This rash may be macular, papular, papulosquamous, pustular, or nonspecific. The rash of secondary syphilis is somewhat unique in that it often involves the palms of the hands and soles of the feet; only a limited number of infectious and noninfectious conditions cause a rash in this distribution. In secondary syphilis, mouth or throat lesions are present in about 33% of cases, and the original genital chancre may still be present in some (15% to 20%). Hair loss can be an important clue to diagnosis; involvement of hair follicles (follicular syphilides) causes areas of alopecia. Condylomata lata are large fleshy papular lesions that may form in the perianal and genital areas and are characteristic of secondary syphilis. Constitutional symptoms such as fever, myalgias, and weight loss are also common. There may be evidence of central nervous system involvement in a number of cases; about 1% to 2% may present with acute meningitis, both clinically and by cerebrospinal fluid analysis. A larger number (up to 40%) may have asymptomatic abnormalities in the spinal fluid. The Centers for Disease Control has stated that a routine lumbar puncture in secondary lues is not indicated. However, if there is evidence of auditory, cranial nerve, meningeal, or ocular manifestations of syphilis, a lumbar puncture and careful ophthalmologic exam (including slit-lamp) should be performed.

  A variety of unusual manifestations of secondary syphilis have been well-described including nephropathy, hepatitis, arthritis, colitis, and others.
- **Latent syphilis:** The natural history of untreated secondary syphilis is that the illness resolves spontaneously after 3-12 weeks, although viable organisms persist. In the absence of specific treatment, patients enter a stage of "latency". These patients have no symptoms related to syphilis, and the only clue for the diagnosis of latent infection is a positive serologic test for syphilis. It is important for the physician to perform a careful history and physical examination looking for signs and symptoms of tertiary syphilis; only then should patients be classified as truly "latent". Patients are classified as having "early latent" disease if they are asymptomatic and have acquired infection within the past year. Those with no symptoms and infection of longer than 1-year duration are said to have "late latent" syphilis. In the asymptomatic patient with a positive serology, it may sometimes be difficult to distinguish early from late latent disease.

(Continued)

Treponema pallidum (Continued)

The role of lumbar puncture in latent syphilis has recently been addressed by the Centers for Disease Control. The yield of spinal fluid analysis in detecting unsuspected tertiary syphilis in a patient who appears to have only latent syphilis is low. Lumbar puncture should be considered in the following situations:
- patients with neurologic abnormalities
- evidence of other syphilitic disease, such as aortitis, gummas, iritis
- treatment failure
- concomitant HIV infection
- RPR or VDRL titer >1:32, unless infected <1 year
- if treatment with antibiotics other than penicillin is anticipated

- **Tertiary syphilis:** This includes the following:
  - asymptomatic neurosyphilis
  - symptomatic neurosyphilis, or tabes dorsalis
  - cardiovascular syphilis
  - syphilitic uveitis
  - late benign syphilis (gummas)
- **Syphilis and AIDS:** Syphilis in the HIV-infected individual can be highly aggressive. Patients progress from primary to tertiary syphilis over several years, as opposed to several decades in the non-HIV infected individual. When the clinical findings suggest syphilis (at any stage) but the standard serologic tests are negative, the diagnosis should be pursued with a biopsy, darkfield exam, or DFA antibody staining. Treatment of syphilis in the AIDS patient is no different; penicillin should be used if at all possible. A lumbar puncture should be considered in any patient with HIV and syphilis. A VDRL or RPR should be obtained at 1, 2, 3, 6, 9, and 12 months. If the titers fail to decrease fourfold, retreat with penicillin and perform a lumbar puncture.

Diagnosis The definitive methods for diagnosing early syphilis are darkfield examination (of active lesions) and direct fluorescent antibody tests on active lesions or tissue biopsies. Serologic tests for syphilis, while commonly used, are not diagnostic. A presumptive diagnosis of active syphilis can be made using one of various serologic tests, which are classified as follows.

Nontreponemal tests: The Venereal Disease Research Laboratory (VDRL) test and the rapid plasma reagin (RPR) test

Treponemal: Fluorescent treponemal antibody absorbed test (FTA-ABS) and the microhemagglutination assay for antibody to *Treponema pallidum* (MHA-TP)

Both a treponemal and nontreponemal test are generally necessary to presumptively diagnose primary syphilis. As a rule, the treponemal tests are specific but not particularly sensitive, and stay positive for life following the initial infection, whether or not appropriate therapy has been administered. Since treponemal tests do not correlate with disease activity, they are usually reported as either positive or negative. In contrast, nontreponemal tests are sensitive but are not specific. In addition, they correlate with the activity of disease, reaching high titers with primary infection or recent reinfection and falling over time following appropriate therapy. Nontreponemal tests are reported as semiquantitative titers. The adequacy of therapy can be determined using serial RPR (or VDRL) tests; ideally the same test in the same laboratory should be followed sequentially.

In primary syphilis, the sensitivity of the VDRL and RPR tests is about 70% and 80%, respectively. Thus, it is important to realize that a substantial number of patients with a typical syphilitic chancre may have a negative nontreponemal test. In contrast, the sensitivities of the VDRL and RPR tests in patients with secondary syphilis are almost 100% and 100%, respectively.

The sensitivities of the nontreponemal tests are 65% to 85% in primary syphilis and almost 100% in secondary syphilis.

The sensitivity of the diagnostic tests for syphilis are summarized in the following table.

Diagnostic Tests in Syphilis

Test	Primary[1]	Secondary[1]	Late[2]
Nontreponemal			
VDRL	70	100	1
RPR	80	100	0
Treponemal			
FTA-ABS	85	100	98
MHA	65	100	95

[1]Treated or untreated

[2]Treated

The only nontreponemal test which should be used is on cerebrospinal fluid in the VDRL.

Diagnostic Tests/Procedures

Darkfield Examination, Syphilis *on page 444*
FTA-ABS, Cerebrospinal Fluid *on page 457*
FTA-ABS, Serum *on page 457*
MHA-TP *on page 535*
RPR *on page 574*
VDRL, Cerebrospinal Fluid *on page 613*

Treatment The proper treatment of syphilis depends on the stage of infection. Primary, secondary, and early latent syphilis (defined as syphilis <1-year duration) are treated with benzathine penicillin G, 2.4 million units I.M. (one dose). For the penicillin-allergic patient, the alternative is doxycycline or tetracycline. The treatment of neurosyphilis in the penicillin-allergic patient is very problematic since the efficacy of other regimens is unknown; formal penicillin skin testing and/or penicillin desensitization should be considered.

The recommended therapy for the respective stages of syphilis are summarized in the table.

Syphilis Therapy

Stage	Adult, Recommended	Adult, Alternative	Children
Primary Secondary Early latent <1 year	Benzathine penicillin G I.M.: 2.4 million units x 1	Doxycycline P.O.: 100 mg twice daily for 2 weeks,[1] Tetracycline P.O.: 500 mg twice daily for 2 weeks[1] Ceftriaxone I.M. or I.V.: 1 g once daily for 7-10 days	Benzathine penicillin G I.M.: 50 thousand units/kg up to 2.4 million units x 1
Latent >1 year Tertiary (gummas and cardiovascular only)	Benzathine penicillin G I.M.: 2.4 million units every week x 3	Doxycycline P.O.: 100 mg twice daily for 4 weeks,[1] or Tetracycline P.O.: 500 mg twice daily for 4 weeks[1]	Benzathine penicillin G I.M.: 50 thousand units/kg up to 2.4 million units x 3
Neurosyphilis	Aqueous penicillin G I.V.: 18-24 million units/day in divided doses for 10-14 days	Procaine penicillin I.M.: 2-4 million units/day and probenecid 500 mg 4 times/day for 10-14 days Ceftriaxone I.M. or I.V.: 2 g once daily for 10-14 days	

[1]Avoid tetracyclines during pregnancy and in children.

From U.S. Public Health Service Recommendations, "1998 Guidelines for Treatment of Sexually Transmitted Diseases. Centers for Disease Control and Prevention," *MMWR*, 1998, 47(RR-1):1-111.

Although syphilis in HIV-infected persons can have a more aggressive clinical course, with more neurologic manifestations, drug treatment recommendations are generally the same as for HIV-negative persons with syphilis. Some authorities recommend more aggressive treatment of primary and secondary syphilis in HIV-infected persons (eg, benzathine penicillin G 2.4 million units I.M. for 3 weekly doses) but no controlled data is available. Most are in agreement, however, that HIV-infected persons require close follow-up with serologic tests drawn at 3, 6, 9, 12, and 24 months after therapy.

Drug Therapy

Recommended:

Primary, secondary, latent syphilis:

Penicillin G Benzathine *on page 991*

Neurosyphilis:

Penicillin G (Parenteral/Aqueous) *on page 993*

Alternate:

Primary, secondary, latent syphilis:

Doxycycline *on page 787*
Ceftriaxone *on page 722*

Neurosyphilis:

Penicillin G Procaine *on page 995*
Ceftriaxone *on page 722*

(Continued)

Treponema pallidum (Continued)

Selected Readings

Baughn RE and Musher DM, "Secondary Syphilitic Lesions," *Clin Microbiol Rev*, 2005, 18(1):205-16.

Centers for Disease Control and Prevention, "Sexually Transmitted Diseases Treatment Guidelines 2002," *MMWR*, 2002, 51(RR-6):1-78.

Hook EW 3d, "Diagnosing Neurosyphilis," *Clin Infect Dis*, 1994, 18(3):295-7.

Hook EW 3d and Marra CM, "Acquired Syphilis in Adults," *N Engl J Med*, 1992, 326(16):1060-9.

Marra CM, Maxwell CL, Smith SL, et al, "Cerebrospinal Fluid Abnormalities in Patients With Syphilis: Association With Clinical and Laboratory Features," *J Infect Dis*, 2004, 189(3):369-76.

Musher DM "Syphilis," *Infect Dis Clin North Am*, 1987, 1(1):83-95.

Peeling RW and Mabey DC, "Syphilis," *Nat Rev Microbiol*, 2004, 2(6):448-9.

Wendel GD Jr, Sheffield JS, Hollier LM, et al, "Treatment of Syphilis in Pregnancy and Prevention of Congenital Syphilis," *Clin Infect Dis*, 2002, 35(Suppl 2):S200-9.

Trichinella spiralis

Related Information

Clinical Syndromes Associated With Foodborne Diseases *on page 1276*

Microbiology *Trichinella spiralis*, a nematode, is the infectious agent of human trichinosis. The adult male worm measures 1.5 mm in length and the adult female measures 2-4 mm. The average lifespan is 4 months. Identification is made by demonstration of the characteristic encapsulated larvae in biopsy specimens of infected muscles. The cyst wall is derived from the host cell muscle. The larva may incite an inflammatory reaction characterized by surrounding lymphocytes and eosinophils and eventual larval calcification.

Epidemiology *Trichinella* is found worldwide except Australia and several Pacific islands. Trichinosis results from consumption of undercooked pork, unsanitary cooking practices, and contaminated meats. Its reservoirs include pigs, horses, bears, and Arctic mammals. The three subspecies reflect three sylvatic cycles - arctic, temperate, and tropical.

The incidence in the United States continues to decline probably because of increased public awareness, commercial freezing, and legislature prohibiting feeding of raw garbage to swine. From 1982-1986, approximately 57 cases per year were reported with three associated deaths. From 1987-1990, 206 cases were reported to the CDC. Most of the cases reported in the U.S. are associated with improperly cooked game animals and travel to Mexico, Asia, and other endemic areas.

Trichinosis results from ingestion of encysted larvae in the contaminated meat. The acid-pepsin environment in the stomach digest the cyst wall, releasing the infectious larvae which burrow and attach to the mucosa at the base of the villi. Over a 6-10 day period, the larvae molt four times to become sexually mature adult worms which attach to the duodenal and jejunal mucosa producing between 200-1500 larvae over the next 2 weeks. The newborn or first stage larvae penetrate the gut mucosa into the lamina propria. An immunologic reaction partially mediated by IgE-mast cell system results in release of vasoactive substances that promote intestinal motility and secretion (diarrhea). The larvae then migrate into the draining lymphatics and blood vessels and have a high predilection to invade muscles of increased use and blood flow (ie, diaphragm, extraocular muscles, masseters, tongue, deltoids, and gastrocnemius). Once penetrated into the skeletal muscle, the larvae elicit a host inflammatory response which surrounds the larvae and creates granulomas and calcifications. Only larvae that encyst mature. Larvae may remain viable and infective for many years even in calcified cysts.

The severity of the symptoms is directly related to the larvae load. Patients usually remain asymptomatic with 1-10 larvae per gram muscle and systemic illness occurs with 50-100 larvae per gram.

Clinical Syndromes

- **Asymptomatic:** Ninety percent to 95% infections are asymptomatic.
- **Self-limited:** 1-2 weeks after ingestion, patients experience enteric phase associated with nonbloody diarrhea and abdominal cramps. Approximately 2-4 weeks later, patients experience fever, intense myalgia especially extraocular and masseters, periorbital edema, conjunctivitis, headache, and/or subconjunctival and subungual petechia. Ninety percent will have peripheral eosinophilia which peaks at 3-4 weeks. Absence of eosinophilia is a poor prognostic sign. Approximately 50% will have elevated CK and LDH enzymes.
- **Arctic trichinosis:** Described in northern Canada and Alaska in which patients have eaten contaminated walruses or seals. Associated with diarrhea lasting up to 14 weeks, mild and transitory myalgia without fever, peripheral eosinophilia, and no pathogens isolated in stools to explain etiology.
- **Myocarditis:** Incidence of approximately 5% of symptomatic patients. Typically occurs 3 weeks after larvae migration and presents with tachycardia and chest pain mimicking infarction. Patients have myocardium invasion without encystment. EKG reveals benign, reversible nonspecific EKG changes. May develop nonspecific

inflammatory myocarditis predominantly eosinophilic and sometimes associated with pericarditis. Fewer than 0.1% patients die from cardiac complications (ie, congestive heart failure).

- **Pulmonary:** Up to 6% symptomatic patients may develop cough and dyspnea on exertion presumed secondary to larvae migration associated with infiltrates, hemorrhage, and allergic granulomatous reactions.
- **CNS:** Prevalence of 10% to 24% in symptomatic patients. In the first 2 weeks when larvae migration is maximal, CNS invasion can occur which appears as meningoencephalitis with delirium and confusion. Larvae encystment may result in focal neurological deficits, anal/urinary sphincter dysfunction, cranial nerve palsies especially VI and VII, seizures, vertigo, anisocoria, tinnitus, diminished auditory acuity, or ataxia. Papilledema, hemianopia, aphasia, and paresis have been reported. CNS and peripheral nerve deficits generally resolve in 4-6 months but may persist up to 10 years. May also cause eosinophilic meningitis. CT scan is usually normal but may see multiple nodular or ring enhancing lesions 3-8 mm and calcification. EEG reveals nonspecific abnormalities consistent with diffuse encephalopathy.

Diagnosis CDC case definition must fit one of two criteria:

1. Positive muscle biopsy or positive serology titer in a patient with clinical symptoms compatible with trichinosis including eosinophilia, fever, myalgias, or periorbital edema.
2. In an outbreak (at least one person must fit above criteria), must have either a positive serology titer or clinical symptoms compatible with trichinosis in a person who shared the implicated meat source.

IgM and IgE serology tests are helpful in distinguishing active from previous infection.

Diagnostic Tests/Procedures

Ova and Parasites, Stool *on page 551*
Trichinella Serology *on page 599*

Treatment Majority of symptomatic patients need supportive care only as infection is self-limited. Benzimidazole carbonates may be given. Mebendazole 200-400 mg three times/day for 3 days followed by 400-500 mg three times/day for 10 days is active against both invasive and encystment stages. Mebendazole does not cross the blood-brain barrier. Thiabendazole 25 mg/kg twice daily for 7 days is indicated to eliminate gut-dwelling adult worms. It is not effective against larval stages in tissue. Not well tolerated secondary to increased gastrointestinal side effects. Albendazole is still under investigation. Steroids (prednisone 40-60 mg daily) may reduce inflammation and is recommended in serious infections.

Overall prognosis is related to severity and intensity of initial infection as well as effectiveness of antiparasitic agents, anti-inflammatory agents, patients immune status, and whether any end-organ damage was rendered. Mortality related to pulmonary, cardiac, and CNS involvement.

All patients traveling outside the United States should receive pretravel counseling. Smoking, microwaving, and freezing contaminated meats are not reliable means of eliminating trichinosis.

Drug Therapy Comment

Steroids used in combination with mebendazole in serious infections.

Drug Therapy

Recommended:

Mebendazole *on page 928*

Alternate:

Thiabendazole *on page 1111*

Selected Readings

Capó V and Despommier DD, "Clinical Aspects of Infection With *Trichinella* spp," *Clin Microbiol Rev*, 1996, 9(1):47-54.
McAuley JB, Michelson MK, and Schantz PM, "*Trichinella* Infection in Travelers," *J Infect Dis*, 1991, 164(5):1013-6.
Watt G, Saisorn S, Jongsakul K, et al, "Blinded, Placebo-Controlled Trial of Antiparasitic Drugs for Trichinosis Myositis." *J Infect Dis*, 2000, 182(1):371-4.

Trichinosis *see Trichinella spiralis on page 338*

Trichomonas vaginalis

Related Information

Treatment of Sexually Transmitted Infections *on page 1311*

Microbiology *Trichomonas vaginalis* is the causative agent of trichomoniasis, a sexually transmitted vaginal infection. *Trichomonas vaginalis* is a flagellated protozoan which exists only in the trophozoite stage. It is easily visualized on wet mount slides under low power and high dry (40x).

Epidemiology The organism is transmitted by sexual intercourse, and the only known reservoir is humans. Occasional transmission can be indirect via contact with

(Continued)

Trichomonas vaginalis (Continued)

contaminated articles. The incubation period is 4-20 days. The period of communicability lasts the duration of the infection. Asymptomatic infections are common.

Clinical Syndromes

- **Vaginitis:** *Trichomonas* is a common cause of vaginitis and must be distinguished from other causes of vaginitis, such as *Candida* and *Gardnerella vaginalis* (the cause of bacterial vaginosis). Typically, there is a vaginal discharge accompanied by vulvar pruritus, dyspareunia, and dysuria. The vaginal discharge is often profuse, thin, frothy, and gray to yellow in color. On pelvic exam, there may be mild erythema of the vaginal walls and endocervix. In severe cases, there are vaginal erosions and petechiae, and occasionally a "strawberry cervix" may be seen where the endocervix is erythematous, granular, and friable. Addition of 10% KOH to the vaginal discharge liberates a fishy odor, as with bacterial vaginosis. On wet prep or Gram stain, there are many polymorphonuclear cells seen, reflecting the inflammatory nature of this form of vaginitis (as opposed to bacterial vaginosis). On wet prep, the motile trichomonads can be seen under low power and high dry, establishing the diagnosis. Asymptomatic infection is very common, and it is estimated that 50% of women carrying *Trichomonas* are asymptomatic.
- **Urethritis in males:** Infection with *Trichomonas* accounts for about 5% of cases of nongonococcal urethritis in males. This is characterized by persistent dysuria with a nonpurulent urethral discharge and may be suspected in patients who have failed the usual tetracycline regimens.
- **Prostatitis:** *Trichomonas* is a rare but reported cause of prostatitis in males.

Diagnosis The symptoms of vaginitis are not specific enough to distinguish infection with *Trichomonas* from other causes. In addition, patients may present following exposure to a sexual partner with *Trichomonas* and have no symptoms. Pelvic examination is mandatory in the female, as is a wet prep of any vaginal discharge. The finding of motile trichomonads is diagnostic. Negative wet mounts may be seen in asymptomatic women or in women who have recently douched. Gram-stained smears are useful in diagnosing bacterial vaginosis but add little to the yield for *Trichomonas* detection. Occasionally, forms resembling *Trichomonas* are incidentally found on Papanicolaou smears of the cervix. Since the cytologic smear is not the ideal procedure for identifying this organism, the patient should be promptly re-examined and a fresh wet mount obtained to confirm the presence of the protozoan. Culture techniques for *Trichomonas* are available in some specialized laboratories but is not usually necessary.

Prostatic and urethral secretions may similarly be examined for motile trichomonads. This may be a reasonable procedure in symptomatic males with persistent symptoms of urethritis where gonorrhea and *Chlamydia* have been excluded. Occasionally, the organism can be visualized in spun urine sediment.

Diagnostic Tests/Procedures

Trichomonas Preparation *on page 600*

Treatment Both symptomatic and asymptomatic individuals should be treated, the latter to decrease the incidence of reinfection from a sexual partner. The recommended regimen is metronidazole 2 g orally as a single dose. Alternatively, metronidazole can be given as 500 mg orally twice daily for 7 days. If failure occurs on the single dose regimen, the patient should be given the full 7-day regimen. In refractory cases, a patient may be given up to 2 g orally daily for 3-5 consecutive days. Such cases warrant consultation with an Infectious Disease specialist and *in vitro* testing of the isolate in culture for metronidazole resistance.

The sexual partners should be treated with either the 2 g single dose regimen or the 500 mg twice daily regimen for 7 days. During pregnancy, metronidazole is contraindicated based on data suggesting the drug is mutagenic in rodents. No other agent is reliable, although some authors have suggested clotrimazole intravaginally if necessary in the first trimester. During the second or third trimester of pregnancy, severe cases may be treated with a single 2 g dose at the discretion of the physician.

Drug Therapy Comment

Treat sexual partners as well.

Drug Therapy

Recommended:

Metronidazole *on page 940*

Selected Readings

"1998 Guidelines for Treatment of Sexually Transmitted Diseases. Centers for Disease Control and Prevention," *MMWR*, 1998, 47(RR-1):1-111.

Krieger JN, Tam MR, Stevens CE, et al, "Diagnosis of Trichomoniasis. Comparison of Conventional Wet-Mount Examination With Cytologic Studies, Cultures, and Monoclonal Antibody Staining of Direct Specimens," *JAMA*, 1988, 259(8):1223-7.

Lossick JG, "The Diagnosis of Trichomoniasis," *JAMA*, 1988, 259(8):1230.

Lossick JG and Kent HL, "Trichomoniasis: Trends in Diagnosis and Management," *Am J Obstet Gynecol*, 1991, 165(4):1217-22.

Sears SD and O'Hare J, "*In Vitro* Susceptibility of *Trichomonas vaginalis* to 50 Antimicrobial Agents," *Antimicrob Agents Chemother*, 1988, 32(1):144-6.

Sugarman B and Mummaw N, "Effects of Antimicrobial Agents on Growth and Chemotaxis of *Trichomonas vaginalis*," *Antimicrob Agents Chemother*, 1988, 32(9):1323-6.

Wolner-Hanssen P, Krieger JN, Stevens CE, et al, "Clinical Manifestations of Vaginal Trichomoniasis," *JAMA*, 1989, 261(4):571-6.

Trichomoniasis *see Trichomonas vaginalis on page 339*

Tropical Spastic Paraparesis (TSP) *see* Human T-Cell Lymphotropic Viruses *on page 192*

Trypanosoma cruzi

Microbiology *Trypanosoma cruzi* is a flagellated, single-celled parasitic organism. The body is approximately 20 µm in length, while the flagellum is between 15 and 30 µm. The body contains a posteriorly located kinetoplast in which the DNA is localized. The kinetoplast is contained within a large, solitary mitochondrion. This organelle is associated with the organism's single flagellum, which connects to the body by a thin membrane and undulates on movement. The flagellum extends beyond the body as a thread-like structure. *T. cruzi* often appears as a C-shaped structure in fixed preparations.

Trypanosoma cruzi is capable of infecting a large number (>150) of mammalian species, and humans are not required to complete its life cycle. Insects become infected by feeding on the blood of an infected host. The ingested trypomastigotes multiply within the midgut of the insect as a distinct morphologic subtype, the epimastogote. These transform in the insect hindgut into the infective metacyclic trypomastigote form, which is discharged in the feces. Transmission to the vertebrate host occurs by contamination of mucous membranes, conjunctivae, or broken skin. Upon entry, the parasites enter host cells, with a tendency to occupy muscle cells, where they transform into the amastigote stage and replicate in the cytoplasm. When the host cell is filled, the organisms differentiate into the trypomastigote stage and are released on rupture of the host cell to repeat the process of cellular entry, replication, and rupture.

Transmission may also occur through contaminated blood supplies from asymptomatic donors in countries where the disease may be prevalent, and procedures/supplies for testing are inadequate. In addition, accidental infection in laboratory workers has been described.

Epidemiology Triatomid insects are the arthropod vector for *T. cruzi* and are found throughout the southern portion of the United States, throughout Central America and in most of South America. Up to 18 million people are estimated to be infected with *T. cruzi*, but only 10% to 30% of infected persons will develop symptomatic chronic Chagas' disease. Increased infection rates are associated with poor housing standards, where the vector may live in close proximity with humans. Although rates of autochthonous infection are low within the United States, a sizeable number of persons with chronic *T. cruzi* infection are encountered as a result of emigration from endemic areas.

Clinical Syndromes

- **Acute Chagas' disease:** Usually occurs in children, but may occur at any age. The symptoms are generally nonspecific. A chagoma, or initial entry lesion may form where the organism enters through a break in the skin. The lesion consists of local inflammation and edema, along with parasitism of muscle cells. When the conjunctiva serves as the site of entry, a classic sign of Chagas' disease, the Romana sign, may form. This is characterized by local painless edema of the periocular tissues. Local symptoms occur after approximately 1 week following initial entry, and are typically followed by fever, anorexia, malaise, and facial or lower extremity edema. Lymphadenopathy and mild hepatosplenomegaly may be noted. Meningoencephalitis may occur in some patients, and acute myocarditis may develop in a small number of patients. Development of acute CNS infection or congestive heart failure may lead to mortality in the acute stage of the disease, but spontaneous resolution after several weeks is common. Following the acute phase, patients may enter the indeterminate phase of Chagas' disease, which is characterized by a lack of symptoms, but continued parasitemia.
- **Chronic Chagas' disease:** Symptoms of chronic disease may not occur for up to 10 years following initial infection. The two organ systems which are predominantly affected include the heart and the gastrointestinal tract.
- **Myocarditis:** The most common manifestation of chronic Chagas' disease, a pronounced bilateral ventricular enlargement is commonly noted, but the enlargement often occurs to a greater degree on the right side. Thinning of the ventricular walls, apical aneurysm, and mural thrombosis are common. Microscopically, the myocardium demonstrates marked lymphocytic infiltration, myocardial atrophy, and

(Continued)

Trypanosoma cruzi (Continued)

interstitial fibrosis. The conduction system may be affected by fibrosis and inflammatory lesions. These often correlate to premortem dysrhythmias. In contrast to acute myocarditis, dysrhythmia is common in chronic disease.

- **Gastrointestinal:** Dilation and muscular hypertrophy are striking manifestations of Chagas' disease in the gastrointestinal tract. Parasympathetic denervation may occur, most frequently involving the esophagus or colon (megaesophagus and megacolon).
- **Reactivation:** Reactivation of acute infection may occur in HIV-infected patients or in patients receiving therapeutic immunosuppression, such as in transplantation. The severity of reactivation disease may exceed the initial acute infection.

Diagnosis A history of exposure in an endemic area may assist in the diagnosis of acute infection. However, visualization of parasites in wet preparations of anticoagulated blood or buffy coat are pivotal to the diagnosis of *T. cruzi* infection. Microscopic examination of lymph node aspirates, pericardial fluid, CSF, or bone marrow aspirates may also be useful in immunocompromised patients. Culture and/or xenodiagnosis may also be used in selected circumstances. IgM assays have not been standardized. Chronic infection is usually diagnosed by IgG assay. Serodiagnostic techniques may yield a high number of false-positives. PCR-based testing is under development.

Treatment *T. cruzi* is not sensitive to drugs which are effective against African trypanosomiasis and/or other parasitic diseases. Nifurtimox has been used in some South American countries for over 20 years, but parasitic cure rates are only 70%. The long duration of therapy (90-120 days) and complicated dosing (4 doses daily), along with a high frequency of gastrointestinal and neurological effects may contribute to limited efficacy. Benznidazole is a second agent which has a similar rate of efficacy. In the United States, both agents may be obtained through the CDC. In immunocompromized patients, the use of recombinant interferon-gamma has been used to supplement antiparasitic medications.

Selected Readings

Prata A, "Clinical and Epidemiological Aspects of Chagas Disease," *Lancet Infect Dis*, 2001, 1(2):92-100.

Rassi A Jr, Rassi A, and Little WC, "Chagas' Heart Disease," *Clin Cardiol*, 2000, 23(12):883-9.

Urbina JA, "Specific Treatment of Chagas Disease: Current Status and New Developments," *Curr Opin Infect Dis*, 2001, 14(6):733-41.

Tubercle Bacillus *see Mycobacterium tuberculosis on page 234*

Tuberculosis *see Mycobacterium tuberculosis on page 234*

Tubo-Ovarian Abscess *see* Pelvic Inflammatory Disease *on page 260*

Tularemia *see Francisella tularensis on page 149*

TWAR *see Chlamydophila pneumoniae on page 78*

Typhoid Fever *see Salmonella* Species *on page 291*

Uncomplicated Urinary Tract Infection *see* Urinary Tract Infection, Uncomplicated *on page 346*

Upper Urinary Tract Infection *see* Urinary Tract Infection, Pyelonephritis *on page 346*

Ureaplasma urealyticum

Synonyms T-*Mycoplasma*

Microbiology *Ureaplasma urealyticum* is a potential human pathogen formerly known as T-*Mycoplasma* (the "T" standing for tiny). The organism belongs to the *Mycoplasma* group (class: Mollicutes; order: Mycoplasmatales, family: Mycoplasmataceae, genus: *Ureaplasma*). As with other *Mycoplasma*, *Ureaplasma* is one of the smallest free-living organisms in existence, intermediate in size between viruses and bacteria. Important points regarding its microbiology include: The organism is very difficult to see using standard light microscopy, the organism does not stain with Gram stain, the lack of a cell wall makes the organism resistant to beta-lactam antibiotics, and *Ureaplasma* demonstrates complex nutritional requirements necessitating special medium for optimal growth in culture.

Because of the fastidious nature of *Ureaplasma*, it is important to consult with the microbiology laboratory prior to obtaining cultures, particularly if important body fluids are sent (such as blood cultures, cerebrospinal fluid, synovial fluid, etc). Specimen collection is important; both the proper transport media (consult the clinical laboratory for proper transport medium) and proper swabs must be used. The organism can occasionally grow in routine blood culture media and blood agar plates, but the yield is low.

Epidemiology

Infants: *Ureaplasma* is a common colonizer of the urogenital tract in infants. The organism can be cultured from the genital tract of roughly 33% of female infants. In most cases, the organism is acquired from the mother as the newborn passes

through an infected birth canal. Male infants are colonized less frequently. After 2 years, the rate of colonization for both sexes decreases significantly, but some children have persistently positive genital tract cultures. Colonization rates are higher in sexually abused children.

Adults: Colonization of the adult urogenital tract is also quite common, but the pathogenesis is usually from sexual contact. Studies have shown that *Ureaplasma* can be cultured from the cervix and vagina in 40% to 80% of sexually active women, nearly all being asymptomatic. Risk factors for colonization include multiple sexual partners, lower socioeconomic status, and perhaps black race. Adults who are sexually inexperienced have low rates of colonization. Thus, the finding of a positive urogenital culture for *Ureaplasma* must be interpreted cautiously since, in many cases, the organism is a harmless commensal.

Clinical Syndromes *Ureaplasma* has been associated with a variety of diseases, but many of these associations are supported only at the case report level and remain controversial. The evidence for causality can be divided as follows.

Good evidence supporting the role of *Ureaplasma urealyticum*:

- **Nongonococcal urethritis (NGU) in the adult male:** The etiologic role of *Ureaplasma* in this common syndrome is supported by evidence from animal models and human volunteer studies. In addition, a small number of placebo-controlled antibiotic trials in males with urethritis has demonstrated improvement in urethral symptoms in the group receiving tetracyclines. The number of NGU cases caused by *Ureaplasma* is unknown.
- **Postpartum bacteremia:** *Ureaplasma* has been isolated from blood cultures in case reports of women with postpartum fever following vaginal delivery. Bloodstream infections with *Ureaplasma* have also been reported following abortions. The role of this organism in postpartum or postabortal fever is still unclear since blood cultures for *Ureaplasma* are rarely obtained.
- **Urethroprostatitis:** *Ureaplasma* appears to be a cause of acute urethroprostatitis in rare cases. There is no evidence to date proving *Ureaplasma* as a cause of chronic urethroprostatitis.
- **Epididymitis:** A single case report has shown *Ureaplasma* to be a likely causative pathogen in an acute case of epididymitis.
- **Septic arthritis:** An unusual septic arthritis due to *Ureaplasma urealyticum* has been described in patients with underlying hypogammaglobulinemia. Joint aspirations have yielded the organism in pure culture. Other clinical features that have accompanied the septic arthritis include subcutaneous abscesses and chronic cystitis. Septic arthritis due to *Ureaplasma* has also been reported in renal transplant patients. Important clinical clues to this syndrome include an immunocompromised host, synovial fluid on arthrocentesis that is "culture-negative" on routine testing, evidence of joint destruction without macroscopic purulence in the joint, and lack of improvement on conventional antibiotic therapy.
- **Chorioamnionitis:** Women who carry *Ureaplasma* in the urogenital tract chronically may potentially develop colonization of the endometrium during pregnancy. Cases have been described where *U. urealyticum* has been repeatedly isolated from amniotic fluid containing inflammatory cells. Symptoms may or may not be present. A low-grade chronic amnionitis has been described and may be associated with premature spontaneous labor and delivery.
- **Respiratory infection in newborns:** Increasing evidence has shown that *Ureaplasma* is a potential cause of congenital pneumonia, probably from acquisition *in utero*. Premature, low-birth weight infants appear to be at risk. The clinical spectrum of respiratory infection has ranged from asymptomatic colonization of the airways to overwhelming pneumonia with acute respiratory distress syndrome. In some cases, endotracheal aspirates, lung biopsies, and lung tissue at autopsy have all yielded pure cultures of *Ureaplasma* with histologic evidence of pneumonia. Blood cultures and cerebrospinal fluid may also be positive for *Ureaplasma*. However, it is important to note that *Ureaplasma* is frequently a harmless colonizer of the airways, and the diagnosis of ureaplasmal pneumonia must be made cautiously.
- **Chronic respiratory disease in neonates:** *Ureaplasma* has been implicated as a risk factor for bronchopulmonary dysplasia, based on limited evidence.
- **Newborn meningitis:** Several studies suggest that *Ureaplasma* may be an important but under-recognized cause of meningitis in premature infants. A fulminant meningitis with intraventricular hemorrhage has been described, but there may also be a more chronic and indolent form. This remains a controversial topic.

Limited evidence supporting the role of *Ureaplasma urealyticum*:

- **Pelvic inflammatory disease**
- **Renal calculi**
- **Reiter's syndrome**

(Continued)

Ureaplasma urealyticum (Continued)

- **Infertility**
- **Repeated spontaneous abortions**
- **Pyelonephritis**

Diagnosis Isolation of the organism from the appropriate site or body fluid is essential for confirming the diagnosis, since the clinical syndromes described above are not specific for *Ureaplasma*. The main errors in diagnosis are failure to consider this organism in the differential diagnosis of a disease syndrome, improper specimen collection, and failure to ask the laboratory to specifically culture for *Ureaplasma* (or *Mycoplasma*). Routine culturing techniques can occasionally yield the organism, but this is not recommended. Serologic testing has limited usefulness. The polymerase chain reaction using the 16S rRNA gene sequence has been described but is currently only a research tool.

Another potential error is confusing colonization of *Ureaplasma* at a body site with true disease. Several of the clinical syndromes described above are only loosely associated with the particular disease entity. There is a risk for overdiagnosis and overtreatment.

Diagnostic Tests/Procedures Some reference laboratories offer molecular detection methods for research purposes.

Genital Culture for *Ureaplasma urealyticum* *on page 471*

Treatment Because *Ureaplasma* has no cell wall, it is resistant to penicillins, cephalosporins, sulfonamides, and other cell wall-active antibiotics. The organism is often resistant *in vitro* to aminoglycosides, clindamycin, and chloramphenicol. About 90% of *Ureaplasma* strains are sensitive to the tetracyclines, and these are the drugs of choice. Tetracycline resistance has been described and is likely to increase; many strains of tetracycline-resistant *Ureaplasma* remain sensitive to erythromycin. Recent *in vitro* studies have shown a potential role for the quinolones (particularly sparfloxacin), but little clinical data is available yet.

A difficult situation arises when there is life-threatening *Ureaplasma* infection in the newborn. Tetracyclines are generally contraindicated in this age group, but some have reported the use of intravenous doxycycline in severe neonatal meningitis. Erythromycin is the drug of choice in patients younger than 8 years of age, but the penetration into the spinal fluid is poor. Consultation with an Infectious Disease specialist may be warranted in these cases.

Pediatric Drug Therapy

Recommended:

Erythromycin *on page 807*

Alternate:

>7 years:

Tetracycline *on page 1106*

Adult Drug Therapy

Recommended:

Erythromycin *on page 807*

Tetracycline *on page 1106*

Doxycycline *on page 787*

Alternate:

Clarithromycin *on page 749*

Azithromycin *on page 674*

Selected Readings

Mallard K, Schopfer K, and Bodmer T, "Development of Real-Time PCR for the Differential Detection and Quantification of *Ureaplasma urealyticum* and *Ureaplasma parvum*," *J Microbiol Methods*, 2005, 60(1):13-9.

McDonagh S, Maidji E, Ma W, et al, "Viral and Bacterial Pathogens at the Maternal-Fetal Interface," *J Infect Dis*, 2004, 190(4):826-34.

Simpson T and Oh MK, "Urethritis and Cervicitis in Adolescents," *Adolesc Med Clin*, 2004, 15(2):253-71.

Taylor-Robinson D, "*Ureaplasma urealyticum, Mycoplasma hominis,* and *Mycoplasma genitalium*" *Principles and Practice of Infectious Diseases*, 5th ed, Mandell GL, Bennett JE, and Dolin R, eds, New York, NY: Churchill Livingstone, 2000, 2027-32.

Waites KB, Bébéar C, Robertson JA, et al, "Laboratory Diagnosis of Mycoplasmal and Ureaplasmal Infections," *Clin Microbiol Newslett*, 1996, 18(14):105-11.

Waites KB, Crouse DT, and Cassell GH, "Antibiotic Susceptibilities and Therapeutic Options for *Ureaplasma urealyticum* Infections in Neonates," *Pediatr Infect Dis J*, 1992, 11(1):23-9.

Yoon BH, Romero R, Lim JH, et al, "The Clinical Significance of Detecting *Ureaplasma urealyticum* by the Polymerase Chain Reaction in the Amniotic Fluid of Patients With Preterm Labor," *Am J Obstet Gynecol*, 2003, 189(4):919-24.

Urethritis, Nongonococcal

Synonyms NGU; Nongonococcal Urethritis

Clinical Presentation Urethral discharge is more prominent in men than women and is less seen in NGU than gonococcal urethritis. The discharge may vary from a scant

clear mucopurulent to frank pus. Men typically complain of pain at the meatus or distal portion of the penis and may have dysuria. Rarely, men complain of discomfort during ejaculation. Women may complain of dysuria and usually have symptoms of cervicitis although they may be asymptomatic.

Differential Diagnosis Gonococcal urethritis; prostatitis; epididymitis; cervicitis; salpingitis; urinary tract infection, cystitis; noninfectious urethritis

Likely Pathogens

Chlamydia trachomatis on page 74
Trichomonas vaginalis on page 339
Herpes Simplex Virus *on page 172*
Ureaplasma urealyticum on page 342

Diagnostic Tests/Procedures

Chlamydia Culture *on page 413*
Chlamydia trachomatis by Molecular Probe *on page 415*
Genital Culture for *Ureaplasma urealyticum on page 471*
Herpes Simplex Virus Culture *on page 494*
Trichomonas Preparation *on page 600*

Empiric Drug Therapy

Recommended:

Doxycycline *on page 787*
Tetracycline *on page 1106*
Azithromycin *on page 674*

Alternate:

Erythromycin *on page 807*

Urinary Tract Infection, Catheter-Associated

Synonyms Catheter-Associated Urinary Tract Infection

Clinical Presentation Patient may have low-grade fever, chills, hematuria, pyuria, and peripheral leukocytosis.

Differential Diagnosis Colonization; trauma; infection - bacterial, fungal

Likely Pathogens

Escherichia coli on page 142
Enterococcus Species *on page 134*
Pseudomonas aeruginosa on page 282
Candida Species *on page 67*

Diagnostic Tests/Procedures

•Blood Culture, Aerobic and Anaerobic *on page 391*
•Gram Stain *on page 473*
•Urine Culture, Clean Catch *on page 609*
Complete Blood Count *on page 420*
Fungus Culture, Urine *on page 468*
Leukocyte Esterase, Urine *on page 520*
Nitrite, Urine *on page 549*

Drug Therapy Comment It is recommended that all catheter-related UTIs be confirmed by removing the catheter and obtaining a sterile straight catheter urine specimen to evaluate for leukocytes and organisms. Colonization should not be treated. Therapy should be pathogen directed. For *Candida albicans* and fluconazole susceptible isolates: Fluconazole renal adjusted for 10-14 days. For fluconazole-resistant fungal isolates: Voriconazole or caspofungin for 10-14 days.

Empiric Drug Therapy

Recommended:

Ampicillin *on page 657*
plus
Aminoglycosides *on page 641*

Alternate:

Vancomycin *on page 1144*
plus
Aminoglycosides *on page 641*

Selected Readings

Warren JW, "Catheter-Associated Urinary Tract Infections," *Infect Dis Clin North Am*, 1997, 11(3):609-22.

Urinary Tract Infection/Colonization, Asymptomatic *see* Asymptomatic Bacteriuria *on page 39*

Urinary Tract Infection, Perinephric Abscess

Synonyms Perinephric Abscess

Clinical Presentation Often a complication of untreated (or insufficiently treated) urinary tract infection or pyelonephritis. Patient may have fever, flank pain, leukocytosis. Pain may be severe or dull and chronic.
(Continued)

Urinary Tract Infection, Perinephric Abscess *(Continued)*

Differential Diagnosis Kidney stones; staghorn calculi; malignancy; infection - bacterial, fungal

Likely Pathogens

Escherichia coli on page 142

Staphylococcus aureus, Methicillin-Susceptible *on page 307*

Diagnostic Tests/Procedures

•Computed Transaxial Tomography, Abdomen Studies *on page 423*

•Ultrasound, Kidneys *on page 604*

•Urine Culture, Clean Catch *on page 609*

Cystometrogram, Simple *on page 434*

Empiric Drug Therapy

Recommended:

Cefazolin *on page 700*

Sulfamethoxazole and Trimethoprim *on page 1087*

Selected Readings

Dalla Palma L, Pozzi-Mucelli F, and Ene V, "Medical Treatment of Renal and Perirenal Abscesses: CT Evaluation," *Clin Radiol*, 1999, 54(12):792-7.

Dembry LM and Andriole VT, "Renal and Perirenal Abscesses," *Infect Dis Clin North Am*, 1997, 11(3):663-80.

Urinary Tract Infection, Pyelonephritis

Synonyms Pyelonephritis; Upper Urinary Tract Infection

Clinical Presentation Most commonly occurs in young females but may occur in any population. Patients may have fever, frequency, dysuria, urgency, hesitancy, plus flank pain. Leukocytosis, pyuria, and hematuria is common.

Differential Diagnosis Kidney stones; staghorn calculi, malignancy, infection - bacterial, fungal.

Likely Pathogens

Escherichia coli on page 142

Proteus Species *on page 278*

Diagnostic Tests/Procedures

•Blood Culture, Aerobic and Anaerobic *on page 391*

•Urine Culture, Clean Catch *on page 609*

Computed Transaxial Tomography, Abdomen Studies *on page 423*

Gram Stain *on page 473*

Drug Therapy Comment Most experts treat for 14 days with I.V. antibiotics unless there is an oral equivalent that can achieve adequate drug levels. Most would not switch to oral agent until fever and leukocytosis has resolved.

Empiric Drug Therapy

Recommended:

Monotherapy:

Sulfamethoxazole and Trimethoprim *on page 1087*

Fluoroquinolones *on page 824*

Combination therapy:

Ampicillin *on page 657*

plus

Gentamicin *on page 841*

Alternate:

Cephalosporins, 3rd Generation *on page 730*

Nitrofurantoin *on page 971*

Selected Readings

Barnett BJ and Stephens DS, "Urinary Tract Infection: An Overview," *Am J Med Sci*, 1997, 314(4):245-9.

Friedman AL, "Urinary Tract Infection," *Curr Opin Pediatr*, 1998, 10(2):197-200.

Hooton TM and Stamm WE, "Diagnosis and Treatment of Uncomplicated Urinary Tract Infection," *Infect Dis Clin North Am*, 1997, 11(3):551-81.

Talan DA, Stamm WE, Hooton TM, et al, "Comparison of Ciprofloxacin (7 days) and Trimethoprim-sulfamethoxazole (14 days) for Acute Uncomplicated Pyelonephritis in Women: A Randomized Trial," *JAMA*, 2000, 283(12):1583-90.

Warren JW, Abrutyn E, Hebel JR, et al, "Guidelines for Antimicrobial Treatment of Uncomplicated Acute Bacterial Cystitis and Acute Pyelonephritis in Women," *Clin Infect Dis*, 1999 29(4):745-58.

Urinary Tract Infection, Uncomplicated

Synonyms Cystitis; Uncomplicated Urinary Tract Infection; UTI, Uncomplicated

Clinical Presentation Patients with only lower tract disease (cystitis) present with dysuria, frequency, urgency, and suprapubic tenderness. Patients with both lower and upper tract disease present with cystitis, fever, and flank pain. Urinalysis reveals pyuria with or without hematuria. Elderly and diabetic patients may be asymptomatic.

Differential Diagnosis Urethritis; pyelonephritis; prostatitis; cervicitis

Likely Pathogens

Escherichia coli on page 142
Klebsiella Species *on page 200*
Proteus Species *on page 278*
Staphylococcus saprophyticus on page 312

Diagnostic Tests/Procedures

Urinalysis *on page 606*
Urine Culture, Clean Catch *on page 609*

Drug Therapy Comment Treatment duration may be from 3-7 days. An increasing proportion of *E. coli* isolates are resistant to sulfamethoxazole and trimethoprim. Local resistant patterns should influence empiric drug selection.

Empiric Drug Therapy

Recommended:

Sulfamethoxazole and Trimethoprim *on page 1087*

Alternate:

Amoxicillin and Clavulanate Potassium *on page 645*
Fluoroquinolones *on page 824*

Selected Readings

Barnett BJ and Stephens DS, "Urinary Tract Infection: An Overview." *Am J Med Sci*, 1997, 314(4):245-9.
Friedman AL, "Urinary Tract Infection," *Curr Opin Pediatr*, 1998, 10(2):197-200.
Hooton TM and Stamm WE, "Diagnosis and Treatment of Uncomplicated Urinary Tract Infection," *Infect Dis Clin North Am*, 1997, 11(3):551-81.

UTI, Uncomplicated *see* Urinary Tract Infection, Uncomplicated *on page 346*

Vaginosis, Bacterial

Related Information

Treatment of Sexually Transmitted Infections *on page 1311*

Synonyms Bacterial Vaginosis; Nonspecific Vaginosis

Clinical Presentation Patients complain of vaginal odor, and a majority note a mild to moderate clear, gray discharge. Patients rarely complain of dysuria or dyspareunia. Physical exam of vagina and cervix are unremarkable except for presence of thin, homogeneous, gray, bubbly discharge.

Differential Diagnosis Other vaginal infections; noninfectious vulvovaginitis

Likely Pathogens

Gardnerella vaginalis on page 153
Bacteroides and *Prevotella* Species *on page 46*
Streptococcus-Related Gram-Positive Cocci *on page 325*

Diagnostic Tests/Procedures The pH of the vaginal discharge should be tested.

Genital Culture *on page 470*
Trichomonas Preparation *on page 600*

Drug Therapy Comment Clindamycin as a vaginal cream; metronidazole as a vaginal gel or metronidazole orally.

Empiric Drug Therapy

Recommended:

Clindamycin *on page 752*
Metronidazole *on page 940*

Selected Readings

Joesoef MR, Schmid GP, and Hillier SL, "Bacterial Vaginosis: Review of Treatment Options and Potential Clinical Indications for Therapy," *Clin Infect Dis*, 1999, 28 (Suppl 1):S57-65.
Spiegel CA, "Bacterial Vaginosis: Changes in Laboratory Practice," *Clin Microbiol Newslett*, 1999, 21(5):33-7.

Valley Fever *see Coccidioides immitis on page 91*
VAP *see* Pneumonia, Ventilator-Associated *on page 273*

Varicella-Zoster Virus

Related Information

Prophylaxis for Patients Exposed to Common Communicable Diseases *on page 1309*
USPHS / IDSA Guidelines for the Prevention of Opportunistic Infections in Persons Infected With HIV *on page 1237*

Synonyms Herpes Zoster; VZV

Microbiology VZV is the cause of two different clinical entities, chickenpox (also called varicella) and shingles (also called zoster or herpes zoster).

Epidemiology Chickenpox (varicella): Approximately 3 million cases of primary chickenpox occur annually, leading to over 500,000 physician visits. Most cases occur in the late winter and spring. Humans are the only known reservoir for VZV. Transmission is probably via respiratory secretions, although this point has been difficult to substantiate. Intimate contact between a susceptible host (who is seronegative) and an individual actively shedding virus is necessary for transmission. Chickenpox still (Continued)

Varicella-Zoster Virus *(Continued)*

remains predominantly a pediatric disease, with >90% of all cases reported in children younger than 3 years of age. Household contacts of infected children are at high risk for varicella. The estimated secondary attack rate in susceptible family members is about 90%; the secondary attack rate in susceptible school mates approaches 40%. The incubation period between exposure and clinical disease is about 14 days, with a range of 10-20 days. Patients can be infectious and spread virus to others for about 2 days prior to the appearance of any skin rash. Patients remain infectious until all skin vesicles have crusted over (5 days or more).

Shingles (zoster): This is also a common disorder, with nearly 10% of the general population afflicted at some time. Almost 1.5 million physician office visits are for management of shingles. Shingles is predominantly a disease of the elderly, although immunocompromised patients are accounting for an increasing fraction. Cases appear sporadically in the population rather than in clusters, due to the pathogenesis of the disease. Herpes zoster results from reactivation of VZV which has remained latent in dorsal root ganglia of peripheral or cranial nerves since the original episode of chickenpox. The factors that govern both latency and reactivation are still under study, but clearly host immune competency is important. Shingles is not spread from one individual to another in the same manner as chickenpox, although the lesions of herpes zoster do contain active VZV and can potentially infect susceptible individuals.

Clinical Syndromes

- **Chickenpox in the normal child:** In the otherwise healthy child, chickenpox is generally a benign, self-limited infection. Typically, the child presents with fever, malaise, and a new generalized skin eruption. The skin rash is distinctive and consists of hundreds of discrete circular lesions. An individual lesion will pass through several stages over time: lesions first appear as vesicles with clear fluid ("dew drops"), then vesicles containing purulent fluid (pustules), then ruptured pustules, and then hard scabs. New vesicles continue to emerge for several days as older ones reach the scab stage. Thus, the rash of chickenpox characteristically has lesions in all stages of evolution at any single point in time. Patients complain of fatigue, pruritus, and anorexia. Lesions can be found in nearly all areas of the skin, and in some cases, the mucous membranes as well. The disease remains active for about 5 days. Complications are unusual in healthy children. Secondary bacterial infection of excoriated skin lesions is the most common complication in children. A variety of unusual neurologic syndromes has been reported in association with chickenpox including cerebellar ataxia (characterized by vertigo, abnormal gait, fever, and vomiting; usually resolves over weeks without treatment), encephalitis (characterized by confusion, personality changes, and seizures; a particularly worrisome complication, with up to 20% of cases resulting in death), cerebral angiitis, meningitis, and Reye's syndrome (particularly if aspirin is given). In clinical trials, acyclovir has demonstrated a statistically significant benefit in normal children (2-12 years of age) with chickenpox. This benefit, however, is small. New lesion formation was decreased from 2.5 days to 2 days, and the number of lesions was decreased from 350 to 300. Acyclovir did not alter the rate of serious complications or spread of infection within the family. The U.S. Food and Drug Administration has supported the use of acyclovir in this setting. The cost:benefit ratio of routine acyclovir use in normal children is likely to be low, since the disease is usually benign. Supportive care remains the mainstay of treatment.
- **Chickenpox in the healthy adult:** About 10% of adults do not acquire VZV infection in childhood and thus remain susceptible to primary infection later in life. Infection in the adult is more severe than in childhood, with varicella pneumonitis a significant concern. Data derived from studies of military recruits suggest that varicella pneumonia may be underdiagnosed. Pulmonary infiltrates were found on chest x-ray in 16% of all recruits with primary varicella, most of whom had no respiratory complaints.

  Perinatal varicella can occur when a pregnant woman develops chickenpox. This is unusual because most adult females are seropositive and immune. Maternal varicella can result in transmission to the fetus, especially if maternal infection occurs several days before delivery. The fetus may be born with visceral VZV dissemination, central nervous system abnormalities, skin scarring, and other defects collectively called the congenital varicella syndrome. Potentially infected neonates are candidates for varicella zoster immune globulin (with or without antiviral drugs).

  Clinical trials examining chickenpox in normal adolescents and adults have shown acyclovir to be effective when administered within 24 hours of symptoms. The treatment effect demonstrated in this older age group is greater than similar studies in children. The U.S. FDA has also approved the use of oral acyclovir for

chickenpox in healthy adults and teenagers. Pregnant women who contract varicella pneumonia are frequently given intravenous acyclovir because of the high mortality of this complication in pregnancy. Newborns with perinatal varicella probably benefit from acyclovir, although formal data to support this practice are limited.

- **Chickenpox in the immunocompromised host:** Morbidity and mortality are high in this population, with >50% of children suffering visceral complications. Mortality approaches 20% overall. Most reported cases of life-threatening varicella have been described in leukemic children. Other risk groups include patients with solid tumors, lymphoproliferative malignancies, and organ transplant recipients. The skin rash tends to be more severe, with delayed time to crusting of lesions. Pneumonitis, hepatitis, and encephalitis are common.

  HIV-infected children who develop chickenpox are also at risk for serious disease. In addition to the visceral complications as noted above, these children are at risk for an unusual, chronic form of the infection, where recurrent vesicular eruptions take place. Several clinical trials have been performed to examine the efficacy of antiviral agents in this setting. Acyclovir decreased the incidence of varicella pneumonia but did not alter the natural history of skin lesions. Intravenous acyclovir has been recommended for both adults and children who are immunosuppressed.

- **Shingles in the normal host:** Most cases of shingles occur in normal individuals 60-90 years of age, although cases have been reported in all age groups including children. Reactivation of VZV is heralded by localized pain along a dermatomal distribution, the phase of "acute neuritis". After 2-3 days of pain, the skin erupts with papules and vesicles along the same unilateral dermatomal distribution. As with primary varicella, the skin lesions evolve from fluid-filled vesicles into pustules and later scabs. The number of skin lesions is variable. Pain can be quite severe and may require narcotics. New lesions continue to form over 3-5 days. The disease stays active for about 1 week, but complete healing requires several additional weeks, particularly in the elderly.

  Selective involvement of the ophthalmic branch of the trigeminal nerve (cranial nerve V) is called herpes zoster ophthalmicus. Keratitis, uveitis, and other ocular complications may result in visual loss if untreated. Involvement of the geniculate ganglion results in the Ramsay Hunt syndrome - vesicles in the external auditory canal, facial palsy, and loss of taste in the anterior two-thirds of the tongue. Other serious complications of herpes zoster in the normal host include cutaneous dissemination and aseptic meningitis. Unlike chickenpox, visceral complications such as pneumonitis and hepatitis are rare. The most common complication of herpes zoster is postherpetic neuralgia, particularly problematic in the elderly. The incidence of this is unclear. Pain persists in the involved dermatome for months after the skin eruption has resolved. Narcotics are only partially helpful, and patients may be quite disabled from the pain; nerve blocks have been attempted with variable success.

  Several clinical trials have been conducted to evaluate the efficacy of acyclovir in herpes zoster in the normal adult. Acyclovir improved the healing time of skin lesions (only by 24 hours) but had a variable and often negligible effect on postherpetic neuralgia. This is an important limitation because postherpetic neuralgia is the most commonly encountered complication and a particularly frustrating problem for physicians. The U.S. FDA has recommended licensure of acyclovir in this setting, but other experts believe the benefit of acyclovir to be small and decisions regarding treatment should by made on a case-by-case basis. Certainly herpes zoster ophthalmicus and other complications warrant prompt treatment.

- **Shingles in the immunocompromised host:** Severe herpes zoster has been described in patients with lymphoma, leukemia, organ transplant recipients, solid malignancies, and those receiving chemotherapy or chronic corticosteroids. Skin lesions frequently extend beyond the original dermatomal distribution. The period of new lesion formation may continue for weeks, and healing is delayed. Generalized skin dissemination has been observed in nearly 25% of patients. Fifty percent of those patients with cutaneous dissemination will progress to visceral dissemination. In HIV-infected individuals, herpes zoster is also severe and potentially life-threatening. Often multiple dermatomes are involved, and recurrences are common. A chronic form of herpes zoster has been described in patients with advanced AIDS.

  Acyclovir has been shown to clearly benefit the immunocompromised host. It is generally given intravenously for 7 days or more. Chronic suppressive doses of oral acyclovir have been given to HIV-infected patients with recurrent herpes

(Continued)

Varicella-Zoster Virus *(Continued)*

zoster. Acyclovir-resistant VZV has been isolated from some individuals on chronic therapy, but this appears to still be uncommon.

Diagnostic Tests/Procedures

Herpes Cytology *on page 491*
Polymerase Chain Reaction *on page 567*
Skin Biopsy *on page 580*
Varicella-Zoster Virus Culture *on page 612*
Varicella-Zoster Virus Serology *on page 612*
Virus Detection by DFA *on page 619*

Treatment Immunization for varicella is recommended for all children to prevent chickenpox. For most immunocompetent children, chickenpox is a self-limiting disease and does not require treatment. In immunocompromised children, acyclovir I.V. should be started as soon as possible after diagnosis, especially in those who have not been passively immunized.

Varicella-zoster immune globulin should be administered in patients who are severely immunosuppressed within 4 days of exposure to varicella. Some authors believe that all patients with a negative VZV serology should receive VZIG.

Acyclovir, valacyclovir, and famciclovir are all effective in shortening the duration of viral shedding, stopping the formation of new lesions, and improving lesion healing rates. All three prevent postherpetic neuralgia better than placebo, with valacyclovir and famciclovir potentially decreasing the duration of pain. Acyclovir is effective in the treatment of herpes zoster in patients with HIV. Limited data is available for famciclovir or valacyclovir in these patients.

Drug Therapy

Recommended:

Treatment:

Acyclovir *on page 629*
Valacyclovir *on page 1140*
Famciclovir *on page 815*

Prophylaxis:

Varicella Virus Vaccine *on page 1148*

Selected Readings

Arvin AM, "Varicella-Zoster Virus," *Clin Microbiol Rev*, 1996, 9(3):361-81.
Brunell PA, "Varicella in Pregnancy, the Fetus, and the Newborn: Problems in Management," *J Infect Dis*, 1992, 166(Suppl 1):S42-7.
Hambleton S, "Chickenpox," *Curr Opin Infect Dis*, 2005, 18(3):235-40.
Liesegang TJ, "Herpes Zoster Virus Infection," *Curr Opin Ophthalmol*, 2004, 15(6):531-6.
Oxman MN, Levin MJ, Johnson GR, et al, "A Vaccine to Prevent Herpes Zoster and Postherpetic Neuralgia in Older Adults," *N Engl J Med*, 2005, 352(22):2271-84.
Wallace MR, Bowler WA, Murray NB, et al, "Treatment of Adult Varicella With Oral Acyclovir. A Randomized, Placebo-Controlled Trial," *Ann Intern Med*, 1992, 117(5):358-63.
Whitley RJ, "Varicella-Zoster Virus," *Principles and Practice of Infectious Diseases*, 5th ed, Mandell GL, Bennett JE, and Dolin R, eds, New York, NY: Churchill Livingstone, 2000, 1580-6.
Wu JJ, Pang KR, Huang DB, et al, "Advances in Antiviral Therapy," *Dermatol Clin*, 2005, 23(2):313-22.

Variola

Synonyms Smallpox

Microbiology A member of the family Poxviridae, subfamily Chordopoxvirinae, genus orthopoxvirus, variola is enveloped, and has a characteristic brick-shaped structure, measuring approximately 250-300 nm by 200 nm. The virus has a dumbell-shaped core, and its genetic material consists of linear, double-stranded DNA. One of the largest and structurally most complex of viruses, it is possible to image the refractile virion using a high-quality UV microscope. Variola has a complex interaction with the immune system, and replicates within the host cell cytoplasm. It is closely related to three other viruses which may infect humans (monkeypox, vaccinia, and cowpox); however, smallpox is the only disease from among this group which may be readily transmitted from human to human. Humans are the only known host, and the virus does not survive for more than a few days outside of the host. The virus is usually contracted via the respiratory route (aerosolization or fomites), but may also be spread through direct contact.

Epidemiology Smallpox has officially been eradicated. The last naturally-occurring case was reported in 1977 in Zaire, and the World Health Organization (WHO) declared formal eradication in 1980. However, variola virus has been discussed as a possible biological weapon which may be used in aerosol form or by inoculation onto fomites. Widespread smallpox vaccinations were discontinued in the 1980s; therefore, the use of this virus as a weapon constitutes a significant threat. In the United States, virtually no person under the age of 30 has been previously vaccinated. Exceptions may include military and primary healthcare workers.

Secondary transmission rates among unvaccinated contacts have been estimated to range from 37% to 88%. Patients are most infective from the onset of exanthema through the first 7-10 days of rash.

Clinical Syndromes Smallpox is an acute exanthematous disease caused by infection with the poxvirus variola. Following inhalation, mucous membranes and local lymph nodes are rapidly infected. The virus replicates within the reticuloendothelial system during the latent period. Overall, the incubation period for smallpox is between 7 and 17 days. A 2-4 day prodromal period, characterized by pharyngitis, high fever, malaise, rigors, headache, backache, and vomiting are followed by a generalized vesicular or pustular eruption. Enanthema of the oral mucosa normally precedes the development of rash by approximately 24 hours. The rash is generalized and centrifugal, following a rapid succession from papule to vesicle to pustules which crust over during a period of 7-14 days. Development of lesions is synchronous across multiple body sites. Smallpox eruption may be more prevalent on the face and distal extremities, with fewer lesions on the abdomen and back. The presence of lesions on the palms and soles of the patient are important diagnostic features. Fever may reappear 7 days after the onset of the rash. Mortality has been estimated between 20% to 50%.

The classic symptoms pattern is termed variola major, and accounts for approximately 90% of cases. However, less common presentations have also been described. Modified smallpox cases have been reported to occur in approximately 2% of unvaccinated contacts and up to 25% of vaccinated contacts. These cases are associated with milder symptomatology, superficial lesions, and a low mortality rate. Flat-type smallpox, which involves a slow evolution of flat, soft, focal skin lesions along with severe systemic toxicity, has been noted in 2% to 5% of patients. Mortality for flat-type smallpox was 66% in vaccinated patients and up to 97% in unvaccinated contacts. In addition, 3% of patients may have a hemorrhagic form of smallpox characterized by extensive petechiae, mucosal hemorrhage, and intense toxemia. Mortality associated with this presentation is extremely high, and death typically occurs prior to development of typical pox lesions. Finally, a fifth form of smallpox has been described in previously vaccinated patients (and in infants with maternal antibodies). Patients may be asymptomatic, or symptoms may be mild, including headache, fever and influenza-like symptoms, and mortality is <1%.

Diagnostic Tests/Procedures Possible cases of smallpox constitute a public health emergency. State health officials should be immediately contacted, who then should contact the CDC and WHO. Airborne and contact precautions should be used. Scrapings from papules, vesicular fluid, pus, or scabs may be collected for rapid identification by electron microscopy (EM). Skin samples may also be used for agar gel immunoprecipitation, immunofluorescence, or polymerase chain reaction (PCR) assay. PCR allows differentiation from other pox viruses. In the event of known exposures, early postexposure (0-24 hours) nasal swabs and induced respiratory secretions may be collected for viral culture, fluorescent antibody assay, and PCR assay. After 2 days, blood or serum may be collected for viral culture. Serological tests may be useful for confirmation or early presumptive diagnosis.

Immunofluorescent Studies, Biopsy *on page 507*
Polymerase Chain Reaction *on page 567*

Treatment Vaccination in the early phase of the disease may attenuate the course of the disease and may prevent manifestations. The United States currently has sufficient quantities of the vaccine to vaccinate every single person in the country in an emergency. Strict respiratory and contact isolation must be enforced, and patients should be placed in a negative-pressure room when possible. Several antiviral agents are under investigation. Cidofovir has proven effective *in vitro* and shown to be effective in animal models. Supportive treatment should be given. See Smallpox Vaccine *on page 1066.*

Selected Readings

Breman JG and Henderson DA, "Diagnosis and Management of Smallpox," *N Engl J Med*, 2002, 346(17):1300-8.

Frey SE, Newman FK, Yan L, et al, "Response to Smallpox Vaccine in Persons Immunized in the Distant Past," *JAMA*, 2003, 289(24):3295-9.

Henderson DA, Inglesby TV, Bartlett JG, et al, "Smallpox as a Biological Weapon: Medical and Public Health Management. Working Group on Civilian Biodefense," *JAMA*, 1999, 281(22):2127-37.

LeDuc JW and Jahrling PB, "Strengthening National Preparedness for Smallpox: An Update," *Emerg Infect Dis*, 2001, 7(1):155-7.

Ventilator-Associated Pneumonia *see* Pneumonia, Ventilator-Associated *on page 273*

Vibrio cholerae

Related Information

Clinical Syndromes Associated With Foodborne Diseases *on page 1276*
(Continued)

Vibrio cholerae (Continued)

Microbiology *Vibrio cholerae* is an oxidase-positive, fermentative, gram-negative rod that can have a comma-shaped appearance on initial isolation. *V. cholerae* can be subdivided by the production of endotoxin and agglutination in 0-1 antisera with the nomenclature of *V. cholerae* 0-1, atypical or nontoxigenic 0-1, or non-0-1. The serogroup 0-1 can further be subdivided into the El Tor and Classic cholera biotypes which can be further subdivided into a variety of serotypes. The major virulence factor of *V. cholerae* is the extracellular enterotoxin produced by the 0-1 strain, although nontoxin-producing organisms have been implicated in some outbreaks.

V. cholerae is a facultative anaerobe which grows best at a pH of 7.0 and at a wide temperature range (18°C to 37°C). *Vibrio* species can be differentiated from other gram-negative bacilli by their sensitivity to 0129 and may be speciated by a variety of biochemical tests.

Epidemiology Cholera is usually spread by contamination of water and food by infected feces, with fecal contamination of water being the principal vehicle of transmission. Person-to-person transmission is less common due to the large organism load necessary for infection. Asymptomatic carriers play a minor role in cholera outbreaks. Outbreaks may be seasonally dependent based on either temperature or rainfall. Transmission by food can be eliminated by thorough cooking. Adequate sanitation is the best means of cholera prevention.

There have been several pandemics of cholera reported since 1817, originating in Bengal and subsequently spreading to a variety of geographic locations, responsible for hundreds of thousands of deaths. The latest pandemic originated in Indonesia in 1961 and moved to the Western hemisphere. In 1991, a cholera outbreak in Peru and 20 other countries in the Western hemisphere accounted for over 600,000 cases with 5000 deaths caused by El Tor 0-1.

Clinical Syndromes After a 2- to 5-day incubation period, classic cholera is characterized by an abrupt onset of vomiting and profuse watery diarrhea with flecks of mucus (rice water stool). Fluid losses can be significant (up to 20 L/day). Hypovolemic shock and metabolic acidosis can cause death within a few hours of onset, especially in children. Mortality, in untreated cases, is as high as 60%. Milder forms of the disease also occur, especially with the non-0-1 cholera.

Diagnosis Organisms can be identified by darkfield microscopy showing large numbers of comma-shaped organisms with significant motility. However, this test is relatively insensitive and is nonspecific. Thiosulfate-citrate-bile salt-sucrose agar (TCBS) or alkaline peptone broth are used to facilitate growth and identification. Positive identification depends on serologic and biochemical testing.

Diagnostic Tests/Procedures

Fecal Leukocyte Stain *on page 455*

Stool Culture, Uncommon Organisms *on page 588*

Treatment Early and rapid replacement of fluid and electrolytes can decrease the mortality to <1%. Oral rehydration is usually successful, but in severe cases, intravenous replacement is required. When fluid and electrolyte imbalances are corrected, cholera is a short, self-limiting disease lasting a few days. According to the *MMWR*, doxycycline, tetracycline, sulfamethoxazole and trimethoprim, erythromycin, and furazolidone have all demonstrated effectiveness in decreasing the diarrhea and bacterial shedding in this disease. The usual recommendation is doxycycline 300 mg as a single dose for adults, and sulfamethoxazole and trimethoprim 5 mg/kg, twice daily for 3 days.

Pediatric Drug Therapy

Recommended:

<7 years:

Sulfamethoxazole and Trimethoprim *on page 1087*

>7 years:

Tetracycline *on page 1106*

Doxycycline *on page 787*

Alternate:

>7 years:

Sulfamethoxazole and Trimethoprim *on page 1087*

Adult Drug Therapy

Recommended:

Doxycycline *on page 787*

Tetracycline *on page 1106*

Alternate:

Sulfamethoxazole and Trimethoprim *on page 1087*

Selected Readings

Bhattacharya SK, "An Evaluation of Current Cholera Treatment," *Expert Opin Pharmacother*, 2003, 4(2):141-6.

Guerrant RL, Carneiro-Filho BA, and Dillingham RA, "Cholera, Diarrhea, and Oral Rehydration Therapy: Triumph and Indictment," *Clin Infect Dis*, 2003, 37(3):398-405.

Ryan ET and Calderwood SB, "Cholera Vaccines," *Clin Infect Dis*, 2000, 31(2):561-5.

Shears P, "Recent Developments in Cholera," *Curr Opin Infect Dis*, 2001, 14(5):553-8.

Viral Encephalitis *see* Encephalitis, Viral *on page 121*

Viral Gastroenteritis *see* Gastroenteritis, Viral *on page 155*

Viridans Streptococci *see Streptococcus*, Viridans Group *on page 326*

Vulvovaginitis, Mycotic *see Candida* Species *on page 67*

VZV *see* Varicella-Zoster Virus *on page 347*

Western Equine Encephalitis *see* Arboviruses *on page 35*

West Nile Encephalitis *see* Arboviruses *on page 35*

West Nile Virus

Microbiology A member of the Flaviridae virus family, West Nile virions are 40-60 nm in size, enveloped, with an icosahedral nucleocapsid. Genetic material consists of a positive-sense, single-stranded RNA approximately 10,000-11,000 bases.

Epidemiology First isolated from a febrile adult woman in the West Nile District of Uganda in 1937, West Nile virus is recognized as a cause of severe human meningoencephalitis. West Nile virus is maintained in a primary enzootic cycle between birds and mosquitoes. Domestic and wild birds are known to be infected, and mortality in these species is high. Human and equine infections are transmitted from infected mosquitoes. West Nile virus has emerged in recent years in temperate regions of Europe and North America, presenting a threat to public, equine, and animal health. The first appearance in North America occurred in 1999, and cases were reported in both humans and horses. Originally reported on the East Coast, viral activity and human infection spread to wider regions each ensuing year. In 2002, West Nile virus cases extended across the United States. In addition to typical transmission, a small number of cases have been attributed to blood transfusions from infected individuals.

Clinical Syndromes The incubation period of West Nile virus is between 3 and 14 days. Most people who are infected with West Nile virus either have no symptoms or experience mild illness such as fever, headache, and body aches before fully recovering. Some persons may also develop mild rash or lymphadenopathy. Encephalitis is the most serious manifestation of viral infection. Fewer than 1% of people infected with West Nile virus develop encephalitis, and among those hospitalized with West Nile encephalitis, the case fatality rate changes from 3% to 15%. Therefore, fewer than 1 in 1000 people infected with West Nile virus die. The elderly are at increased risk for the development of encephalitis, which may cause permanent neurologic sequelae, paralysis, or death. In addition, a polio-like syndrome has been reported. Genetic factors may influence the potential for severe encephalitis. Symptoms of encephalitis (inflammation of the brain) include the abrupt onset of severe headache, high fever, nuchal rigidity, muscle weakness, confusion, or coma.

There is no evidence for person-to-person transmission of West Nile virus.

Diagnostic Tests/Procedures

West Nile Virus Diagnostic Procedures *on page 620*

IgM antibody capture testing by ELISA on serum or cerebrospinal fluid specimens. Recommended clinical and laboratory case definitions are available at www.cdc.gov/ncidod/dvbid/westnile/resources/wnv-guidelines-apr-2001.pdf. Detection of West Nile virus is also possible by the use of polymerase chain reaction. Contact the laboratory to determine availability of the test.

Treatment There is no specific treatment for West Nile virus encephalitis. Treatment is supportive in nature. *In vitro* evidence suggests ribavirin and interferon alfa-2b may have activity against the virus.

Selected Readings

Charatan F, "Organ Transplants and Blood Transfusions May Transmit West Nile Virus," *BMJ*, 2002, 325(7364):566.

Glaser A, "West Nile Virus and North America: An Unfolding Story," *Rev Sci Tech*, 2004, 23(2):557-68.

Michaelson PG and Mair EA, "West Nile Virus: A Primer for the Otolaryngologist," *Otolaryngol Head Neck Surg*, 2005, 132(3):347-52.

Petersen LR and Hayes EB, "Westward Ho? The Spread of West Nile Virus," *N Engl J Med*, 2004, 351(22):2257-9.

Petersen LR and Marfin AA, "West Nile Virus: A Primer for the Clinician," *Ann Intern Med*, 2002, 137(3):173-9.

Yim R, Posfay-Barbe KM, Nolt D, et al, "Spectrum of Clinical Manifestations of West Nile Virus Infection in Children," *Pediatrics*, 2004, 114(6):1673-5.

Whooping Cough *see Bordetella pertussis on page 53*

Wool Sorter's Disease *see Bacillus anthracis on page 41*

Wound Infection, Surgical

Synonyms Surgical Wound Infection

Clinical Presentation The Centers for Disease Control case definition of an incisional surgical wound infection is one that occurs at the incision site within 30 days of surgery and involves skin or subcutaneous tissue above muscle fascia. Infection should not be diagnosed by only the isolation of organisms from the wound site alone as this may represent colonization. The site should show signs of infection as manifested by purulence and breakdown of tissue. A deep surgical wound is one that occurs within 30 days of surgery if no implant is left in place or one that occurs within 1 year of placement of nonhuman-derived implantable foreign device. Infection must be related to site and involve tissues at or beneath the muscle fascia. The wound may spontaneously dehisce or require surgical opening especially if the patient has fever, localized pain, or tenderness.

Likely Pathogens

Staphylococcus epidermidis, Methicillin-Susceptible *on page 310*
Staphylococcus aureus, Methicillin-Susceptible *on page 307*
Staphylococcus epidermidis, Methicillin-Resistant *on page 309*
Staphylococcus aureus, Methicillin-Resistant *on page 304*
Gram-Negative Bacilli *on page 157*

Diagnostic Tests/Procedures

Aerobic Culture, Appropriate Site *on page 365*
Anaerobic Culture *on page 371*
Gram Stain *on page 473*

Empiric Drug Therapy

Recommended:

Penicillins, Penicillinase-Resistant *on page 997*
Vancomycin *on page 1144*

If gram-negative bacilli seen on gram stain:
Penicillins, Extended-Spectrum *on page 997*
with or without
Aminoglycosides *on page 641*

Xanthomonas maltophilia *see Stenotrophomonas maltophilia on page 312*

Yellow Fever *see* Arboviruses *on page 35*

Yersinia enterocolitica

Related Information

Clinical Syndromes Associated With Foodborne Diseases *on page 1276*

Microbiology *Yersinia enterocolitica* is a gram-negative bacillus named in honor of the French bacteriologist Alexander Yersin, who discovered *Yersinia pestis* (the cause of plague) in 1894. *Y. enterocolitica* is an unusual cause of enterocolitis, terminal ileitis mimicking acute appendicitis, and septicemia. The organism is an aerobic gram-negative rod, nonlactose fermenting, which is motile at 25°C. It is unusual in that it grows better at somewhat cooler temperatures than do other pathogenic gram-negative rods (25°C to 32°C). It also is able to grow well at 4°C, which is the basis for CEM.

Epidemiology *Yersinia enterocolitica* is endemic in many animals which serve as reservoirs: cattle, pigs, dogs, cats, and others. The usual route of human infection is via ingestion of contaminated food, milk, and water. There have been three major food-borne epidemics in the United States: June 1982 - outbreak in several states linked to consumption of milk pasteurized at a plant in Memphis, Tennessee; 172 positive cultures from cases in Tennessee, Arkansas, and Mississippi, where patients presented with diarrhea, fever, abdominal pain. It also included 24 cases of extraintestinal infections including throat, blood, urinary tract, central nervous system, and wounds; 1976 - contaminated chocolate milk in New York State; 1982 - contaminated tofu in Washington state.

Clinical Syndromes

- **Enterocolitis:** *Yersinia enterocolitica* is a rare cause of enterocolitis. The severity of symptoms can be quite variable and can range from mild fever, diarrhea and abdominal pain, to fulminant colitis with spiking fevers and rectal bleeding.
- **Mesenteric adenopathy with or without terminal ileitis:** This form of *Yersinia* infection is known to mimic acute appendicitis. Patients present with right lower quadrant pain, fever, and leukocytosis. Upon laparotomy the appendix is normal but enlarged mesenteric lymph nodes are palpable and when cultured will yield the organism. This has been described primarily in adolescents, although cases have been reported in adults.
- **Polyarthritis:** This has been described as the sole manifestation of *Yersinia enterocolitica* infection or as a secondary manifestation of gastrointestinal infection. Well documented cases have been described in Scandinavia, where up to 30% of cases

develop erythema nodosum, and 10% to 30% develop polyarthritis (especially associated with HLA-B27 haplotype). *Yersinia* antigens have recently been found in synovial fluid cells from patients suffering from reactive arthritis following *Yersinia* infection.

- **Liver abscess:** *Yersinia* is a rare but reported cause of liver abscess in the absence of typical enterocolitis symptoms.
- **Ascending infection of an extremity:** Recently, cases of infections of the hand and upper extremity due to *Yersinia enterocolitica* have been described. These infections occurred in adults preparing contaminated chitterlings (pig intestines) with local inoculation into the hand via small cuts.
- **Septicemia:** *Yersinia* is an unusual cause of community-acquired septicemia but may occur following ingestion of heavily contaminated food. Risk factors for septicemia are cirrhosis, malignancy, diabetes mellitus, and patients with iron overload syndromes (such as hemachromatosis, frequent blood transfusions). Typically, there is fever, myalgias, confusion, and possibly hypotension. Symptoms of enterocolitis, such as diarrhea and abdominal pain, may be completely absent, adding to the diagnostic confusion. Elevated liver enzymes and muscle enzymes may occur. Blood cultures are often positive for the organism.
- **Miscellaneous:** Other manifestations of *Yersinia* infection include osteomyelitis, meningitis, pharyngitis (without enterocolitis), and intra-abdominal abscess.

Diagnosis In the absence of an outbreak, the diagnosis of enterocolitis due to *Yersinia* is difficult to make on clinical grounds alone. Thus, laboratory confirmation is important in most cases. Appropriate specimens for culture include stool, blood, lymph node, pharyngeal exudates, ascites fluid, and cerebrospinal fluid. Joint aspiration fluid may be sent for *Yersinia* culture in the appropriate clinical setting (ie, reactive polyarthritis following a diarrheal illness), but the yield is extremely low. The laboratory should be notified if a stool specimen is being examined for *Yersinia*. Serologic tests for specific antibody production to *Yersinia enterocolitica* are available in some laboratories.

Diagnostic Tests/Procedures

Aerobic Culture, Appropriate Site *on page 365*
Stool Culture, Uncommon Organisms *on page 588*

Treatment Many cases of enterocolitis and mesenteric adenitis secondary to *Yersinia* are self-resolving, and the role of antibiotics is unclear. Patients with *Yersinia* septicemia, however, definitely require antibiotic therapy since the mortality approaches 50%. The organism is susceptible *in vitro* to a number of agents, including third generation cephalosporins, piperacillin, sulfamethoxazole and trimethoprim, and aminoglycosides. Most isolates are resistant to penicillin, ampicillin, and first generation cephalosporins. The optimal drug regimen *in vivo* has not been defined in the literature. For serious infections, it seems reasonable to treat initially with a combination (eg, third generation cephalosporin and aminoglycoside) until the patient has stabilized.

Adult Drug Therapy

Recommended:

Severe infection:

Cephalosporins, 3rd Generation *on page 730*

plus

Aminoglycosides *on page 641*

Selected Readings

Bottone E and Sheehan DJ, "*Yersinia enterocolitica*: Guidelines for Serologic Diagnosis of Human Infections," *Rev Infect Dis*, 1983, 5(5):898-906.

Bottone EJ, "*Yersinia enterocolitica*: The Charisma Continues," *Clin Microbiol Rev*, 1997, 10(2):257-76.

Centers for Disease Control, "*Yersinia enterocolitica* Bacteremia and Endotoxin Shock Associated With Red Blood Cell Transfusions - United States, 1991," *JAMA*, 1991, 256(17):2174-5.

Cover TL and Aber RC, "*Yersinia enterocolitica*," *N Engl J Med*, 1989, 321(1):16-24.

Gayraud M, Mollaret HH, et al, "Antibiotic Treatment of *Yersinia enterocolitica* Septicemia: A Retrospective Review of 43 Cases," *Clin Infect Dis*, 1993, 17(3):405-10.

Naqvi SH, Swierkosz EM, and Gerard J, "Presentation of *Yersinia enterocolitica* Enteritis in Children," *Pediatr Infect Dis J*, 1993, 12(5):386-9.

Yersinia pestis

Related Information

Bioterrorism Agents *on page 390*

Microbiology *Yersinia pestis* is the etiological agent of plague. All of the 11 species of *Yersinia* are aerobic, gram-negative rods, are well established members of the family Enterobacteriaceae, and have been isolated from human clinical specimens. At least three species of *Yersinia* are unequivocal human pathogens: *Y. pestis*, *Y. enterocolitica*, and *Y. pseudotuberculosis*.

Epidemiology Yersinioses are zoonotic infections that usually affect rodents, small animals, and birds. Rats are the natural reservoir of *Y. pestis* in areas of urban ("city") plague; small animals such as ground squirrels, wood rats, rabbits, and cats are the

(Continued)

Yersinia pestis (Continued)

natural reservoirs of *Y. pestis* in areas of sylvatic ("country") plague. Humans are accidental hosts of *Yersinia* species. Humans become infected with the bacterium after being bitten by fleas of the aforementioned animals, or, much less commonly, by handling infected animals or inhaling aerosolized *Y. pestis* generated by a person with pulmonary plague. Human *Yersinia pestis* are rare in the United States. From 1970 to 1991, 295 cases were reported to the Center for Disease Control and Prevention. Plague occurs worldwide; most cases occur in Asia and Africa. In the United States, plague occurs (rarely) in New Mexico, Arizona, California, Utah, and Colorado.

Clinical Syndromes

- **Plague:** Human plague presents in many different and protean clinical forms: bubonic, septicemic, pneumonic, cutaneous, and meningitis. After an incubation period of 2-8 days, most patients with **bubonic plague**, the most common form, experience fever, chills, headache, aches, extreme exhaustion, and lymphadenitis. At the same time, extremely painful bubos develop in the groin, axilla, or neck. These patients have overwhelming numbers of bacteria in their blood. Patients with **septicemic plague** also have tremendous numbers of bacteria in their blood; however, these patients have a more septic presentation, and bubos usually are not present. **Pneumonic plague** is a complication of bubonic plague and is characterized by cough, chest pain, difficulty breathing, and hemoptysis; bubos might or might not be present. Pneumonic plague, if not treated immediately, has a very high mortality rate and can be rapidly fatal within 1 day. The natural progression of plague is from the bubonic, to the septicemic, to the pneumonic forms. The overall mortality rate for untreated cases of plague is 50% to 60%.

Diagnosis Diagnosis of plague is mainly a clinical diagnosis. Laboratories must be notified if *Y. pestis* is suspected as an etiological agent because many laboratories do not routinely suspect *Y. pestis* or culture clinical specimens for *Y. pestis* because special media and techniques easily can be used to enhance isolation of the bacterium and because the colonial morphology of *Y. pestis* is not typical of many other gram-negative rods. Culture is the most productive test for the laboratory diagnosis of plague. *Yersinia pestis* is not fastidious and grows well on blood agar media and many enteric media. Many commercial bacterial identification systems do not include *Y. pestis* in their databases. The most appropriate clinical specimens for culture include blood, biopsy or aspirate of bubo, sputum, cerebrospinal fluid, and cutaneous biopsy.

Diagnostic Tests/Procedures

Aerobic Culture, Appropriate Site *on page 365*

Blood Culture, Aerobic and Anaerobic *on page 391*

Treatment Supportive care is essential. The antibiotic of choice is streptomycin. Gentamicin, tetracyclines, and chloramphenicol are all effective alternatives. Timely treatment can potentially reduce mortality from plague to 10%.

Travelers to endemic areas are generally at low risk for developing infection. The CDC does, however, recommend the following precautions: avoid rat-infested areas; generous use of insect repellents and insecticides including body, clothing, and bedding application; avoid handling sick or dead animals. The CDC also recommends the use of prophylactic antibiotics if the risk of exposure is high. Tetracycline or doxycycline should be used in adults, and sulfonamides used for children younger than 8 years of age. Plague vaccine requires multiple dosing over several months for protection and is therefore not recommended for immediate protection during outbreaks.

Drug Therapy

Recommended:

Streptomycin *on page 1078*

Alternate:

Gentamicin *on page 841*
Tetracycline *on page 1106*
Doxycycline *on page 787*
Chloramphenicol *on page 733*

Selected Readings

Butler T, "*Yersinia* Infections: Centennial of the Discovery of the Plague Bacillus," *Clin Infect Dis*, 1994, 19(4):655-63.

Butler TB, "*Yersinia* Species (Including Plague)," *Principles and Practice of Infectious Diseases*, 5th ed, Mandell GL, Bennett JE, and Dolin R, eds, New York, NY: Churchill Livingstone, 2000, 2406-14.

Crook LD and Tempest B, "Plague. A Review of 27 Cases," *Arch Intern Med*, 1992, 152(6):1253-6.

Evans RG, Crutcher JM, Shadel B, et al, "Terrorism From a Public Health Perspective," *Am J Med Sci*, 2002, 323(6):291-8.

Frean J, Klugman KP, Arntzen L, et al, "Susceptibility of *Yersinia pestis* to Novel and Conventional Antimicrobial Agents," *J Antimicrob Chemother*, 2003, 52(2):294-6.

"Human Plague - United States, 1993-1994," *MMWR*, 1994, 43(13):242-6.

Krishna G and Chitkara RK, "Pneumonic plague," *Semin Respir Infect*, 2003, 18(3):159-67.

Rollins SE, Rollins SM, and Ryan ET, "*Yersinia pestis* and the Plague," *Am J Clin Pathol*, 2003, 119 Suppl:S78-85.

Zygomycosis *see Mucor* Species *on page 225*

DIAGNOSTIC TESTS/PROCEDURES

Abdomen, CT *see* Computed Transaxial Tomography, Abdomen Studies *on page 423*
Abdomen Ultrasound *see* Ultrasound, Abdomen *on page 604*
Abdominal Paracentesis *see* Paracentesis *on page 555*

Abscess Aerobic and Anaerobic Culture

Related Information

Antimicrobial Susceptibility Testing, Aerobic and Facultatively Anaerobic Organisms *on page 379*
Antimicrobial Susceptibility Testing, Anaerobic Bacteria *on page 381*
Genital Culture *on page 470*
Wound Culture *on page 620*

Applies to Aerobic Culture, Abscess; Anaerobic Culture, Abscess

Test Includes Culture for aerobic and facultative anaerobic organisms. Culture for anaerobic organisms usually must be specifically requested and may require a separate specimen.

Patient Preparation Aseptic preparation of the aspiration site. The overlying and adjacent areas must be carefully decontaminated to eliminate isolation of potentially contaminating anaerobes which colonize the skin surface.

Special Instructions The laboratory should be informed of the specific site of specimen, age of patient, current antibiotic therapy, clinical diagnosis, and time of collection.

Clinical Observations Suggestive of Anaerobic Infection

Foul-smelling discharge
Location of infection in proximity to a mucosal surface
Necrotic tissue, gangrene, pseudomembrane formation
Gas in tissues or discharges
Endocarditis with negative routine blood cultures
Infection associated with malignancy or other process producing tissue destruction
Infection related to the use of aminoglycosides (oral, parenteral, or topical)
Septic thrombophlebitis
Bacteremic picture with jaundice
Infection resulting from human or other bites
Black discoloration of blood-containing exudates (may fluoresce red under ultraviolet light in *B. melaninogenicus* infections)
Presence of "sulfur granules" in discharges (actinomycosis)
Classical clinical features of gas gangrene
Clinical setting suggestive for anaerobic infection (septic abortion, infection after gastrointestinal surgery, genitourinary surgery, etc)

From Bartlett JG, "Anaerobic Bacterial Infections of the Lung," *Chest*, 1987, 91:901-9, with permission.

Specimen Fluid, pus, abscess wall tissue, or other material properly obtained from an abscess for optimal yield. Specimens for anaerobic culture should be accompanied by a specimen for aerobic culture from the same site. Aspirated fluid is acceptable for anaerobic culture if it is submitted in a properly capped syringe or an approved anaerobic transport device. Specimens collected on swabs are vastly inferior specimens.

Container Anaerobic transport container swab with anaerobic transport medium and aerobic transport media or swab may be used if aspirated fluid is not available. However, swabs always provide inferior specimens.

Collection Specimens are to be collected from a prepared site using sterile technique. Contamination with normal flora from skin, rectum, vaginal tract, all mucus membranes, or other body surfaces must be avoided. Some anaerobes will be killed by contact with oxygen for only a few seconds. Ideally, pus obtained by needle aspiration through an intact surface, which has been aseptically prepared, is put directly into an anaerobic transport device or transported directly to the laboratory in the original syringe. **Note:** The needle **must** be removed from the syringe before the syringe is sent to the laboratory. Sampling of open lesions is enhanced by deep aspiration using a sterile needle and syringe. Curettings of the base of an open lesion may also provide a good yield. If irrigation is necessary, nonbacteriostatic sterile normal saline may be used. Pulmonary samples may be obtained by transtracheal percutaneous needle aspiration by physicians trained in this procedure or by use of a special sheathed catheter. If swabs must be used, two should be collected; one for culture and one for Gram stain. Specimens collected and transported in syringes should be transported to the laboratory within 30 minutes of collection.

Storage Instructions If syringe is used to transport specimen to the laboratory, all air should be expelled, and the needle removed.

Causes for Rejection Specimens which have been exposed to air, refrigerated, or delayed in transit have a less-than-optimal yield. Specimens from sites which have anaerobic bacteria as normal flora (eg, throat, feces, colostomy stoma, rectal swabs, bronchial washes, cervical-vaginal mucosal swabs, sputums, skin and superficial wounds, voided or catheterized urine) **are not** acceptable for anaerobic culture because of contamination by the normal flora.

Turnaround Time Cultures showing no bacterial growth can generally be reported after 2-3 days. However, initial growth may not appear for up to 7 days. Complete reports of cultures with anaerobic bacteria may take as long as 2 weeks after receipt of culture, depending upon the nature and number of the organisms isolated.

Reference Range No growth of anaerobic bacteria

Use Determine microbial etiology of the abscess and provide a guide for therapy

Limitations The only sources for specimens with established validity for meaningful anaerobic culture in patients with pleuropulmonary infections are blood, pleural fluid, transtracheal aspirates, transthoracic pulmonary aspirates, specimens obtained at thoracotomy, and fiberoptic bronchoscopic aspirates using the protected brush or sheathed catheter. Aspirated pleural fluid is preferred for patients with empyema. Blood cultures yield positive results in <5% of cases of anaerobic pulmonary infection.

Mycobacterium sp or *Nocardia* sp which may cause abscesses will **not** be recovered even if present, since extended incubation periods, aerobic incubation, and special media are necessary for their isolation. Cultures for these organisms should be specifically requested.

Contraindications Bronchoscopically obtained specimens are extremely poor specimens because the instrument becomes contaminated by organisms normally contaminating the oropharynx during insertion. Culture of specimens from sites harboring endogenous anaerobic organisms or contaminated by endogenous organisms (usually sites at or contiguous with any mucus membrane) usually will be misleading with regard to etiology and selection of appropriate therapy.

Additional Information In open wounds, anaerobic organisms may play an etiologic role, whereas aerobes may represent superficial contamination. Serious anaerobic infections are often due to mixed flora which are pathologic synergists. Anaerobes frequently recovered from closed postoperative wound infections include *Bacteroides fragilis*, approximately 50%; *Bacteroides* sp, approximately 25%; *Peptostreptococcus* sp, approximately 15%; and *Fusobacterium* sp, approximately 25%. Anaerobes are seldom recovered in pure culture (10% to 15% of cultures). Aerobes and facultative anaerobes when present are frequently found in lesser numbers than the anaerobes. Anaerobic infection is most commonly associated with operations involving opening or manipulating the bowel, mucus membranes, or a hollow viscus (eg, appendectomy, cholecystectomy, colectomy, gastrectomy, bile duct exploration, etc). The ratio of anaerobes to facultative anaerobes is normally about 10:1 in the mouth, vagina, and sebaceous glands and at least 1000:1 in the colon.

Selected Readings

Brook I, "A 12 Year Study of Aerobic and Anaerobic Bacteria in Intra-abdominal and Postsurgical Abdominal Wound Infections," *Surg Gynecol Obstet*, 1989, 169(5):387-92.

Donskey CJ and Rice LB, "The Influence of Antibiotics on Spread of Vancomycin-Resistant *Enterococci*: The Potential Role of Selective Use of Antibiotics as a Control Measure," *Clin Microbiol Newslett*, 1999, 21(8):57-65.

Finegold SM, Jousimies-Somer HR, and Wexler HM, "Current Perspectives on Anaerobic Infections: Diagnostic Approaches," *Infect Dis Clin North Am*, 1993, 7(2):257-75.

Styrt B and Gorbach SL, "Recent Developments in the Understanding of the Pathogenesis and Treatment of Anaerobic Infections," *N Engl J Med*, 1989, 321(4):240-6.

Swenson RM, "Rationale for the Identification and Susceptibility Testing of Anaerobic Bacteria," *Rev Infect Dis*, 1986, 8(5):809-13.

Acid-Fast Stain

Related Information

Mycobacteria Culture, Cerebrospinal Fluid *on page 541*
Mycobacteria Culture, Sputum *on page 542*

Synonyms AFB Smear; Atypical *Mycobacterium* Smear; Kinyoun Stain; *Mycobacterium* Smear; TB Smear; Ziehl-Neelsen Stain

Applies to Auramine-Rhodamine Stain; Fluorochrome Stain

Test Includes Acid-fast stain. For diagnosis, acid-fast stain and culture are usually ordered together. For monitoring therapy, stain alone may be sufficient.

Abstract Acid-fast bacilli are so called because they are surrounded by a waxy envelope that is resistant to destaining by acid-alcohol. Either heat (classic Ziehl-Neelsen) or a detergent (Tergitol Kinyoun method) is required to allow the stain to penetrate the cell wall. Once stained, acid-fast bacteria resist decolorization, whereas other bacteria are destained with acid-alcohol.

Patient Preparation Same as for mycobacteria culture of given site

Special Instructions The laboratory should be informed of the source of the specimen. Specimens may be divided for fungus culture and stain (KOH) preparation,

(Continued)

Acid-Fast Stain *(Continued)*

mycobacteria culture and acid-fast smear, and routine bacterial culture and Gram stain only if the specimen is accompanied by appropriate requests for these procedures and if the specimen is of adequate volume for all tests requested.

Specimen The appropriate specimen for an acid-fast smear is the same as for culture. See specific site mycobacteria culture listings for details.

Container Same as for culture of specific site

Collection See specific mycobacteria culture listings for specific site.

Causes for Rejection Insufficient specimen volume, specimen received on a swab

Turnaround Time Routine: 24-48 hours; stat (if available): 2 hours

Reference Range No mycobacteria identified. Positive smears usually are reported in a quantitative manner such as a number of bacilli per field or entire smear.

Use Determine the presence of mycobacteria, monitor the course of antimycobacterial therapy; establish the diagnosis of mycobacterial infection in undiagnosed granulomatous disease, fever of unknown origin (FUO), and in patients suspected of having a defect in cellular immunity (eg, AIDS, lymphoma, etc)

Limitations Cultures are more sensitive than smears; therefore, the smear may be negative when culture is positive. Fluorochrome stains (auramine-rhodamine) are more sensitive than carbol-fuchsin stains. Nonpathogenic acid-fast bacilli can be present as normal flora. Culture is necessary to determine the specific species of *Mycobacterium* present, however a presumptive determination of whether *Mycobacterium tuberculosis* or mycobacteria other than *M. tuberculosis* (formerly called "atypical mycobacteria") are present can be made. DNA probes, which are more sensitive and specific than smears for the diagnosis of mycobacterial infection are now in use in some laboratories.

Methodology Acid-fast stain of concentrated or unconcentrated specimen

Additional Information A stat acid-fast smear can be performed by some laboratories upon special request. However, concentration procedures are not usually performed on a stat basis. Very active infection is required to produce a positive without concentration. In extrapulmonary tuberculosis, the acid-fast stain can be useful in yielding a rapid diagnosis. Routine acid-fast staining and culturing of CSF for AFB is rarely, if ever, productive. However, positive smears have been reported from CSF in 67% of cases of culture-proven tuberculous meningitis, lymph nodes biopsy in 80% of miliary tuberculosis cases, 75% peritoneal biopsies in peritonitis, and urine in 80% of the cases of renal tuberculosis.

Acid-fast stains performed on gastric aspirates and urine when positive are reliable indicators of true mycobacterial disease. However, tap water can contain *M. gordonae* and can be responsible for false-positive results. Klotz and Penn have reported the sensitivity, compared to culture, as approximately 30% for gastric aspirates and approximately 50% for urine. False-positives were negligible, <1%.

The sensitivity and specificity of acid-fast staining for the diagnosis of pulmonary mycobacteria tuberculosis infection in a large prospective study was 53.1% and 99.8%, respectively, and 81.5% and 98.4%, respectively, for culture.

Selected Readings

Gordin F and Slutkin G, "The Validity of Acid-Fast Smears in the Diagnosis of Pulmonary Tuberculosis," *Arch Pathol Lab Med*, 1990, 114(10):1025-7.

Levy H, Feldman C, Sacho H, et al, "A Re-evaluation of Sputum Microscopy and Culture in the Diagnosis of Pulmonary Tuberculosis," *Chest*, 1989, 95(6):1193-7.

Morris A, Reller LB, Salfinger M, et al, "Mycobacteria in Stool Specimens: The Nonvalue of Smears for Predicting Culture Results," *J Clin Microbiol*, 1993, 31(5):1385-7.

Acid-Fast Stain, Modified, *Cryptosporidium* *see Cryptosporidium* Diagnostic Procedures, Stool *on page 432*

Acid-Fast Stain, Modified, *Nocardia* Species

Related Information

Actinomyces Culture, All Sites *on page 363*
Gram Stain *on page 473*
Methenamine Silver Stain *on page 534*
Nocardia Culture, All Sites *on page 550*
Periodic Acid-Schiff Stain *on page 563*

Synonyms Hank's Stain; *Nocardia* Species Modified Acid-Fast Stain

Test Includes Modified acid-fast stain. Culture generally must be ordered specifically as such. The recovery of *Nocardia* sp usually requires special culture techniques.

Abstract Infections with *Nocardia* sp may resemble many other more common diseases. Because therapy differs, it is important to establish a definitive diagnosis, preferably by culture. The diagnosis of nocardiosis should be considered in unexplained cavitary lung disease, granulomatous lung disease of established cause not

responsive to appropriate therapy, brain abscess particularly in the presence of cavitary lung disease, alveolar proteinosis, with mycetoma, and in any patient in whom a disseminated granulomatous disease is considered.

Specimen Appropriate preparation, specimen and container for smear is the same as for culture

Causes for Rejection Insufficient specimen volume, specimen received on a dry swab

Reference Range No acid-fast organisms seen

Use Determine the presence or absence of *Nocardia* sp which are usually, but not invariably, acid-fast when stained by the modified acid-fast stain. *Actinomyces* and *Streptomyces* sp which may be microscopically similar to *Nocardia* on Gram stain, are negative with the modified acid-fast stain. Establish the etiology of maduromycosis and of fever of unknown origin in patients with suspected defects of cellular immunity (eg, AIDS, Hodgkin's disease, lymphoma, and so forth).

Limitations *Nocardia* sp do not always stain acid-fast by this method; consequently, the presence of branching, gram-positive bacilli on Gram stain suggests that Gram stain might have greater sensitivity. *Nocardia* sp, however, cannot be distinguished from *Actinomyces* sp and other closely related organisms by Gram stain. Organisms from clinical material are more likely to be "modified acid-fast" than those from culture.

Methodology Kinyoun stain followed by relatively less severe decolorization with 3% acid alcohol (940 mL of 95% ethanol and 60 mL of concentrated HCl). If clumps or granules are observed, they should be crushed between two glass slides and examined microscopically.

Additional Information Nocardiosis has also been reported with lupus, rheumatoid arthritis, and liver disease. Aggressive diagnostic procedures are often necessary to obtain appropriate specimen for definitive diagnosis. Organisms consistent with *Nocardia* sp can be identified presumptively on Gram stain and modified acid-fast stain pending more definitive diagnosis by culture. Examination of sputum with *Nocardia* may show thin, crooked, weakly to strongly gram-positive, modified acid-fast positive, irregularly staining or beaded filaments. Opaque or pigmented sulfur granules may occasionally be present in direct smear of pus. Colonization without apparent infection may occur.

Selected Readings

Beaman BL and Beaman L, "*Nocardia* Species: Host-Parasite Relationships," *Clin Microbiol Rev*, 1994, 7(2):213-64.

Javaly K, Horowitz HW, and Wormser GP, "Nocardiosis in Patients With Human Immunodeficiency Virus Infection. Report of 2 Cases and Review of the Literature," *Medicine (Baltimore)*, 1992, 71(3):128-38.

McNeil MM and Brown JM, "The Medically Important Aerobic Actinomycetes: Epidemiology and Microbiology," *Clin Microbiol Rev*, 1994, 7(3):357-417.

Osoagbaka OU and Njoku-Obi AN, "Presumptive Diagnosis of Pulmonary Nocardiosis: Value of Sputum Microscopy," *J Appl Bacteriol*, 1987, 63(1):27-38.

Acromioclavicular Joint, Left or Right, X-ray *see* Bone Films *on page 396*

Actinomyces Culture, All Sites

Related Information

Acid-Fast Stain, Modified, *Nocardia* Species *on page 362*
Gram Stain *on page 473*
Nocardia Culture, All Sites *on page 550*

Applies to IUD Culture; Intrauterine Device Culture; Sulfur Granule, Culture

Test Includes Anaerobic culture for *Actinomyces* sp and direct microscopic examination of Gram stain for sulfur granules and gram-positive branching bacilli

Abstract Actinomycosis is a chronic progressive suppurative disease characterized by the formation of multiple abscesses, draining sinuses, and dense fibrosis. The classic presentations include cervicofacial, thoracic, abdominal, and pelvic infections.

Patient Preparation Cleanse the skin around the opening of a draining sinus with an alcohol swab, allow to dry, and obtain the specimen from as deep within the sinus as possible. Submit aspirated material or tissue. Do not submit a swab specimen.

Special Instructions In tissues, *Actinomyces* sp produce chronic suppuration with formation of multiple draining sinuses. Examination of material from such sinuses often reveals tangled masses of filamentous elements and granules called sulfur granules. The presence of sulfur granules is highly suggestive of *Actinomyces* infection. If actinomycosis is suspected clinically, the laboratory should be informed. The specific site of specimen, current antibiotic therapy, and clinical diagnosis should be provided.

Specimen Exudate, material from draining sinus

Container Anaerobic specimen transport medium

Collection *Actinomyces* sp are fastidious anaerobic organisms. It is, therefore, essential that the specimen be placed into the appropriate anaerobic transport tube and delivered to the laboratory as quickly as possible. If a syringe is used, expel all air before transferring into the tube. Swabs invariably collect poor specimens, but if used,

(Continued)

Actinomyces Culture, All Sites *(Continued)*

should be transported in anaerobic transport medium. With a draining sinus, obtain the specimen by aspirating as far into the sinus as possible.

Storage Instructions Specimens should be transported immediately to the laboratory and processed as soon as possible.

Causes for Rejection Specimens exposed to air, specimens which have been refrigerated or have an excessive delay in transit, have a less than optimal yield. Specimens from sites which have anaerobic bacteria as normal flora (eg, throat, feces, colostomy stoma, rectal swabs, bronchial washes, cervical-vaginal mucosal swabs, sputums, skin and superficial wounds, voided or catheterized urine), may **not** be acceptable for anaerobic culture because of contamination by the normal flora.

Turnaround Time Preliminary reports are usually available after 7 days. Cultures with no growth may be reported after 14 days.

Reference Range No *Actinomyces* isolated. *A. israelii* is a normal inhabitant of the mouth, oropharynx, and gastrointestinal tract.

Use Detect infections due to *Actinomyces* sp; establish the etiology of granulomatous disease, chronic draining sinus, and fever of unknown origin (FUO) particularly in immunocompromised patients

Limitations Inform the laboratory that actinomycosis is clinically suspected, to ensure that cultures will be incubated long enough to permit recovery of *Actinomyces* sp; *Actinomyces* sp are relatively slow growing and will often fail to grow in the period in which most laboratories incubate routine cultures. Additionally, even when incubated appropriately, recovery of *Actinomyces* sp may be hindered by overgrowth with obligate and facultative anaerobic bacteria.

Methodology Anaerobic culture including thioglycolate broth media

Additional Information If granules are detected on the gauze pad covering a draining sinus, submit the granules to the laboratory. A Gram stain and culture should be performed on such granules. On smear branching gram-positive rods may be found. They may be similar in appearance to other actinomycetes including species of *Nocardia*, *Streptomyces*, and also *Mycobacterium*. Actinomycetes are not stained by the modified acid-fast stain used for *Nocardia* sp. Several species of *Actinomyces* are responsible for human infection. *Actinomyces israelii* is the most significant. *A. naeslundii*, *A. odontolyticus*, *A. viscosus*, and *Arachnia propionica* also have been reported as human pathogens. Pelvic and perirectal infections have been associated with intrauterine devices (IUDs). A classic presentation of actinomycosis is as a painless lump in the jaw. *Actinomyces* may be found in rare instances of recurrent ventral hernia following appendectomy for appendicitis. The diagnosis of actinomycosis in many settings requires consideration of the possibility followed by persistence on the part of laboratory personnel.

Selected Readings

Bellingan GJ, "Disseminated Actinomycosis," *BMJ*, 1990, 301(6764):1323-4.

Feder HM Jr, "Actinomycosis Manifesting as an Acute Painless Lump of the Jaw," *Pediatrics*, 1990, 85(5):858-64.

Holtz HA, Lavery DP, and Kapila R, "Actinomycetales Infection in the Acquired Immunodeficiency Syndrome," *Ann Intern Med*, 1985, 102:203-5.

Persson E, "Genital Actinomycosis and *Actinomyces israelii* in the Female Genital Tract," *Adv Contracept*, 1987, 3:115-23 (review).

Acute Phase Reactant *see* C-Reactive Protein *on page 428*

Adenovirus Antibody Titer

Related Information

Adenovirus Culture *on page 365*

Special Instructions Acute and convalescent sera should be tested simultaneously.

Specimen Serum

Container Red top tube or serum separator tube

Sampling Time Acute and convalescent sera drawn 12-21 days apart

Reference Range A fourfold increase in titer of paired sera is indicative of a virus infection. Titers suggestive of no previous exposure are usually ≤1:16.

Use Establish the diagnosis of adenovirus infection; can be useful in differential diagnosis of respiratory ailments, hemorrhagic cystitis, and keratoconjunctivitis

Limitations The specific adenovirus serotype responsible for infection and the distinction between IgG and IgM titers cannot be determined by complement fixation test. Complement fixation tests are of low sensitivity, particularly in children.

Methodology Complement fixation (CF), hemagglutination inhibition (HAI), enzyme-linked immunosorbent assay (ELISA), serum neutralization, indirect immunofluorescent assay (IFA)

Additional Information There are 41 different types of adenovirus, and many infections are both asymptomatic and persistent. Thus, serologic evidence of adenovirus,

and even isolation of an adenovirus from a patient, may be coincidental rather than the cause of the patient's present complaints.

Selected Readings

Bryan JA, "The Serologic Diagnosis of Viral Infections," *Arch Pathol Lab Med*, 1987, 111(11):1015-23.
Edson RS and Terrell CL, "The Aminoglycosides," *Mayo Clin Proc*, 1999, 74:519-28.

Adenovirus Culture

Related Information

Adenovirus Antibody Titer *on page 364*
Viral Culture, Throat *on page 617*

Test Includes Culture for adenovirus only; adenovirus usually is detected in a routine/general virus culture

Specimen Midstream urine, stool, nasopharyngeal secretions, eye exudates, throat swab or tissue

Container Sterile container. Swabs should be placed into cold viral transport medium.

Storage Instructions Keep specimens cold and moist. Adenoviruses are more stabile than are most other viruses; however, specimens should not be stored or refrigerated for long periods of time. Specimens should be delivered immediately to the clinical laboratory.

Causes for Rejection Dry specimen, specimen not in proper viral transport medium, specimen not refrigerated during transport, specimen fixed in formalin

Turnaround Time Variable (1-14 days) and depends on culture method used and amount of virus in the specimen

Reference Range No virus isolated

Use Aid in the diagnosis of disease caused by adenovirus (eg, conjunctivitis, cystitis, pneumonia, and pharyngoconjunctivitis)

Limitations Rule out or identify adenovirus **only**

Methodology Inoculation of specimen into cell cultures, incubation of cell cultures, observation of characteristic cytopathic effect, and identification by fluorescent monoclonal antibody

Additional Information Adenoviruses can be the etiologic agent of respiratory infections in children up to 6 years of age and of ocular infections in both children and adults. Adenovirus respiratory infections can mimic pertussis.

Serology to detect adenovirus antibodies is often helpful in establishing a diagnosis.

Selected Readings

Hierholzer JC, "Adenoviruses - A Spectrum of Human Diseases," *Clin Microbiol Newslett*, 1992, 14(15):113-20.
Hierholzer JC, "Adenoviruses in the Immunocompromised Host," *Clin Microbiol Rev*, 1992, 5(3):262-74.
Wadell G, Allard A, and Hierholzer JC, "Adenoviruses," *Manual of Clinical Microbiology*, 7th ed, Murray PR, Baron EJ, Pfaller MA, et al, eds, Washington, DC: American Society for Microbiology, 1999, 970-82.

Adenovirus Culture, Stool *see* Viral Culture, Stool *on page 616*
ADNase-B *see* Antideoxyribonuclease-B Titer, Serum *on page 376*
Aerobic Blood Culture *see* Blood Culture, Aerobic and Anaerobic *on page 391*
Aerobic Bone Marrow Culture *see* Bone Marrow Culture, Routine *on page 400*
Aerobic Culture, Abscess *see* Abscess Aerobic and Anaerobic Culture *on page 360*

Aerobic Culture, Appropriate Site

Refer to

Aerobic Culture, Body Fluid *on page 365*
Aerobic Culture, Cerebrospinal Fluid *on page 366*
Aerobic Culture, Sputum *on page 367*

Aerobic Culture, Body Fluid

Related Information

Anaerobic Culture *on page 371*
Histopathology *on page 496*

Synonyms Body Fluid Culture, Routine

Applies to Ascitic Fluid Culture; Bone Marrow Culture; Culture, Biopsy; Joint Fluid Culture; Pericardial Fluid Culture; Peritoneal Fluid Culture; Pleural Fluid Culture; Surgical Specimen Culture; Synovial Fluid Culture

Test Includes Aerobic culture of biopsy or body fluid specimens

Patient Preparation Aseptic preparation of biopsy site

Special Instructions The laboratory should be informed of the specific source of the specimen, age of patient, current antibiotic therapy, and clinical diagnosis. Specimens may be divided for fungus culture and stain, mycobacteria culture and acid-fast stain, and routine bacterial culture and Gram stain only if the specimen is of adequate volume for all tests requested. Many body fluids (especially peritoneal fluid) are best

(Continued)

Aerobic Culture, Body Fluid *(Continued)*

cultured by inoculation of the fluid into blood culture broth (bottles). Consult the laboratory to determine if that procedure is appropriate for a particular fluid.

Specimen Surgical tissue, bone marrow, biopsy material from normally sterile site or aseptically aspirated body fluid

Container Sterile container with lid, no preservative. Bone marrow aspirates and body fluids may be directly inoculated into blood culture media. Contact the laboratory and obtain approval before inoculating fluids into blood culture media.

Collection Do **not** submit fluid collected with a swab. This type of specimen is rarely productive. The portion of the fluid specimen submitted for culture should be separated (utilizing sterile technique) from the portion submitted for histopathology.

Storage Instructions The specimen should be transported immediately to the laboratory.

Causes for Rejection Specimens in fixative, specimens collected on swabs, specimens having an excess transit time to the laboratory. Specimens which have been refrigerated have a less than optimal yield.

Turnaround Time Preliminary reports are available at 24 hours. Cultures with no growth are reported after 48 hours. Reports on specimens from which pathogens are isolated require a minimum of 48 hours for completion.

Reference Range No growth

Use Isolate and identify aerobic organisms causing infections in tissue

Limitations If anaerobes are suspected submit a properly collected specimen. See listings Anaerobic Culture *on page 371* and Abscess Aerobic and Anaerobic Culture *on page 360.* If mycobacteria or fungi are suspected see Mycobacteria Culture, Biopsy or Body Fluid *on page 539*, or Fungus Culture, Body Fluid *on page 462* for detailed instructions.

Methodology Aerobic culture

Additional Information The specimen should be obtained before empiric antimicrobial therapy is started.

Selected Readings

Donskey CJ and Rice LB, "The Influence of Antibiotics on Spread of Vancomycin-Resistant *Enterococci*: The Potential Role of Selective Use of Antibiotics as a Control Measure," *Clin Microbiol Newslett*, 1999, 21(8):57-65.

Aerobic Culture, Cerebrospinal Fluid

Related Information

Cerebrospinal Fluid Analysis *on page 408*

Synonyms Cerebrospinal Fluid Aerobic Culture

Applies to Ventricular Fluid Culture

Test Includes Aerobic culture and Gram stain (stat) if requested. Gram stain, cell count, differential, glucose, and protein levels are usually requested. Additional fluid if available may be used for additional cultures and other diagnostic tests such as those for bacterial or cryptococcal antigen and/or for acid-fast stain.

Abstract The major tests to be performed on the CSF for meningitis are the Gram stain and the bacteriologic culture. The "gold standard" for the diagnosis of bacterial meningitis is the isolation of a bacterium from the cerebrospinal fluid. Diagnosis of meningitis is made by blood culture and examination and culture of CSF.

Patient Preparation Aseptic preparation of the aspiration site

Special Instructions The laboratory should be informed of the specific source of specimen, age of patient, current antibiotic therapy, clinical diagnosis, and time of collection.

Specimen Cerebrospinal fluid

Container Sterile CSF tube

Collection Tubes should be numbered 1, 2, 3 with tube #1 representing the first portion of the sample collected. Contamination with normal flora from skin or other body surfaces must be avoided. The second or third tube collected during lumbar puncture is most suitable for culture, as skin contaminants from the puncture usually are washed out with fluid collected in the first two tubes. Since blood cultures are often positive in subjects with bacterial meningitis, blood cultures should be requested as well. Peripheral blood white cell count and differential are usually abnormal in patients with meningitis and represent an important part of the clinical investigation.

Storage Instructions The specimen should be transported immediately to the laboratory. If the specimen cannot be processed immediately, it should be kept at room temperature or placed in an incubator. Refrigeration inhibits viability of certain anaerobic organisms and may prevent the recovery of the common aerobic pathogens *Streptococcus pneumoniae*, *Neisseria meningitidis*, and *Haemophilus influenzae*.

Turnaround Time Preliminary reports are usually available at 24 hours. Cultures with no growth can be reported after 72 hours. Reports of cultures from which pathogens are isolated require a minimum of 48 hours for completion.

Reference Range No growth

Use Isolate and identify pathogenic organisms causing meningitis, shunt infection, brain abscess, subdural empyema, cerebral or spinal epidural abscess, bacterial endocarditis with embolism. The time honored Gram stain and aerobic CSF cultures in suspected bacterial meningitis are fundamental to appropriate diagnosis and treatment.

Limitations Cultures may be negative in partially treated cases of meningitis. Gram stain is the single most useful laboratory test to diagnose bacterial meningitis. However, Gram stains should be interpreted with care. Gram-positive organisms may decolorize (ie, stain gram-negative in partially treated cases). Acridine orange stain (AO) may have better sensitivity than Gram stain in detecting the presence of organisms in partially treated cases of meningitis but it is not at all widely used.

Methodology Aerobic culture

Additional Information See table in Cerebrospinal Fluid Analysis *on page 408* for laboratory values of components of CSF from healthy persons and from persons with meningitis. *Haemophilus influenzae*, *Neisseria meningitidis*, and *Streptococcus pneumoniae*, the most commonly isolated pathogens, can be serotyped if requested. Infections of cerebrospinal fluid shunts pose a difficult clinical problem. Organisms cultured include coagulase-negative staphylococci, *S. aureus*, *Streptococcus*, viridans group, enterococci, and *H. influenzae*. Culture of CSF or shunt fluid is diagnostic. Simultaneous blood cultures are rarely positive. Removal of the catheter and later replacement are frequently required to eradicate the infection. Susceptibility testing will be performed if indicated. If the CSF is collected through or is associated with a VP shunt, this information **must** be indicated to the laboratory so the laboratory personnel can look for *Propionibacterium* spp. which can be an etiological agent in CNS infections.

Selected Readings

Askari S and Cartwright CP, "The Changing Epidemiology of Bacterial Meningitis: Implications for the Clinical Laboratory," *Clin Microbiol Newslett*, 1998, 20(5):33-6.

Feigin RD, McCracken GH Jr, and Klein JO, "Diagnosis and Management of Meningitis," *Pediatr Infect Dis J*, 1992, 11(9):785-814.

Gray LD and Fedorko DP, "Laboratory Diagnosis of Bacterial Meningitis," *Clin Microbiol Rev*, 1992, 5(2):130-45.

McMillan DA, Lin CY, Aronin SI, et al, "Community-Acquired Bacterial Meningitis in Adults: Categorization of Causes and Timing of Death," *Clin Infect Dis*, 2001, 33(7):969-75.

Neumann MA and Thompson KD, "Acute Bacterial Meningitis: Prevention and Treatment," *Clin Microbiol Newslett*, 1998, 20(22):181-4.

van Deuren M, Brandtzaeg P, and van der Meer JWM, "Update on Meningococcal Disease With Emphasis on Pathogenesis and Clinical Management," *Clin Microbiol Rev*, 2000, 13(1):144-66.

Aerobic Culture, Sputum

Related Information

Anaerobic Culture *on page 371*
Legionella pneumophila Culture *on page 516*
Mycoplasma pneumoniae Diagnostic Procedures *on page 544*

Synonyms Sputum Culture, Aerobic

Applies to Bronchial Washings Culture; Bronchoscopy Culture; Percutaneous Transtracheal Culture Routine; Tracheal Aspirate Culture; Transtracheal Aspirate Culture

Test Includes Culture of aerobic organisms and usually Gram stain

Patient Preparation The patient should be instructed to remove dentures, rinse mouth, and gargle with water. The patient should then be instructed to cough deeply and expectorate sputum into proper container.

Special Instructions The laboratory should be informed of the specific site of specimen, the age of patient, current antibiotic therapy, clinical diagnosis, and time of collection.

Specimen Sputum, first morning specimen preferred; tracheal aspiration, bronchoscopy specimen, or transtracheal aspirate

Container Sputum container, sputum trap, sterile tracheal aspirate, or bronchoscopy aspirate tube

Collection Specimen collected, at time of bronchoscopy, by aspiration or by transtracheal aspiration by a physician skilled in the procedure. The specimen should be transported to laboratory within 1 hour of collection for processing.

Storage Instructions Refrigerate if the specimen cannot be promptly processed.

Causes for Rejection Specimens spilled or leaking onto the outside of the container pose excessive risk to laboratory personnel and may not be acceptable to the laboratory.

(Continued)

Aerobic Culture, Sputum *(Continued)*

Turnaround Time Preliminary reports are usually available at 24 hours. Cultures with no growth or normal flora are usually reported after 48 hours. Reports on specimens from which pathogens are isolated require at least 48 hours for completion.

Reference Range Normal upper respiratory flora. Tracheal aspirate and bronchoscopy specimens usually are contaminated with normal oral flora. Transtracheal aspiration: no growth.

Use Isolate and identify potentially pathogenic organisms present in the lower respiratory tract. Presence or absence of normal upper respiratory flora is often reported.

Limitations An adequate sputum specimen should contain many neutrophils and few to no squamous epithelial cells, which are indicative of contamination with saliva. Results obtained by culture without evaluation for contamination may be noncontributory or misleading. A carefully collected and Gram-stained specimen with neutrophils and gram-positive lancet-shaped diplococci can provide strong support for a clinical diagnosis of pneumococcal pneumonia.

In bronchoscopy and aspirated specimens reduction of contamination may be accomplished by a head-down position to reduce gravitational flow of saliva, when combined with quantitative culture techniques. Oral contamination may successfully be reduced by using a protected brush (PBC) catheter. The use of the PBC and bronchoalveolar lavage increases the overall diagnostic yield. Quantitation aids interpretation. Qualitatively, a bronchial washing is no better than sputum. If anaerobic bacteria are suspected in a transtracheal aspiration, a properly collected specimen for anaerobic culture should be submitted.

Methodology Aerobic culture following appropriate specimen selection. The most important step in the evaluation of a specimen is to be certain that the secretions that are examined are the product of the inflammatory process in the bronchi and not oropharyngeal material. All laboratories should perform this step.

Additional Information Potential pathogens recovered by usual sputum culture methods include: *Staphylococcus aureus*, *Haemophilus influenzae*, *Streptococcus pneumoniae*, *Neisseria meningitidis*, *Haemophilus parainfluenzae*, *Pseudomonas aeruginosa*, *Escherichia coli*, *Proteus* sp, *Moraxella catarrhalis*, *Bacteroides fragilis*, and rarely many other organisms. *Haemophilus* sp and *Neisseria* sp may not be isolated and identified by routine procedures. Thus, if their presence is clinically suspected, specific isolation procedures should be requested. See table.

Bacterial Species Recovered From Sputa in 103 Acute Bronchitic Exacerbations

	Number	Percent of All Types Cultured	Percent of Sputa Cultured
H. influenzae	41	24.0	39.8
H. parainfluenzae	29	17.0	28.2
S. pneumoniae	34	19.9	33.0
M. catarrhalis	19	11.1	18.4
N. meningitidis	5	2.9	4.9
K. pneumoniae	8	4.7	7.8
P. aeruginosa	4	2.3	3.9
Other possible pathogens	14	8.2	13.6
Unlikely pathogens	17	9.9	16.5

From Chodosh S, "Acute Bacterial Exacerbations in Bronchitis and Asthma," *Am J Med*, 1987, 82(Suppl 4A):154-63, with permission.

Organisms such as *Bordetella pertussis*, *Chlamydia pneumoniae Corynebacterium diphtheriae*, *Legionella pneumophila*, *Mycoplasma pneumoniae*, and *Mycobacterium tuberculosis* require special laboratory tests for isolation. Clinical suspicion of involvement by these agents should be communicated to the laboratory. See also listings for the specific agents.

The critical criteria for the diagnosis of acute bacterial infection of the bronchi are obtained from examination and culture of the sputum. The presence of bacteria in numbers greater than when the patient's condition is stable and a significant increase (ie, doubling) in the numbers of neutrophils present are essential laboratory criteria for the diagnosis of an acute bronchitic exacerbation. Gram stain results more closely reflect the clinical outcome and along with the criterion of the number of neutrophils in the sputum should be laboratory basis for determining success. Other commonly recognized agents causing pneumonia are listed in the tables on the next page.

Selected Readings

Bartlett JG, Dowell SF, Mandell LA, et al, "Practice Guidelines for the Management of Community-Acquired Pneumonia in Adults," *Clin Infect Dis*, 2000, 31(2):347-82.

Boerner DF and Zwadyk P, "The Value of the Sputum Gram's Stain in Community-Acquired Pneumonia," *JAMA*, 1982, 247(5):642-5.

Kaplan SL and Mason EO Jr, "Management of Infections Due to Antibiotic-Resistant *Streptococcus pneumoniae*," *Clin Microbiol Rev*, 1998, 11(4):628-44.

Lyczak JB, Cannon CL, and Pier GB, "Lung Infections Associated With Cystic Fibrosis," *Clin Microbiol Rev*, 2002, 15(2):194-222.

Stratton CW, "Bacterial Pneumonias - An Overview With Emphasis on Pathogenesis, Diagnosis, and Treatment," *Heart Lung*, 1986, 15(3):226-44.

Whittier S, "Update on the Microbiology of Cystic Fibrosis: Traditional and Emerging Pathogens," *Clinical Micobiology Newsletter*, 2001, 23(9):67-71.

Community-Acquired Bacterial Pneumonias: Frequency of Various Pathogens	**%**
Streptococcus pneumoniae	40-60
Haemophilus influenzae	2.5-20
Gram-negative bacilli	6-37
Staphylococcus aureus	2-10
Anaerobic infections	5-10
Legionella	0-22.5
Mycoplasma pneumoniae	5-15
Nosocomial Pneumonias: Frequency of Various Pathogens	
Klebsiella	13
Pseudomonas aeruginosa	10-12
Staphylococcus aureus	3-10.6
Escherichia coli	4-7.2
Enterobacter	6.2
Group D *Streptococcus*	1.3
Proteus and *Providencia*	6
Serratia	3.5
Pneumococcus	10-20
Aspiration pneumonia anaerobic pneumonia[1]	5-25
Legionella[1]	0-15

[1]The specific incidence of pneumonias caused by *Mycoplasma, Legionella*, and anaerobes is difficult to document because of the technical problems in isolating the organisms.

From Verghese A and Berk SL, "Bacterial Pneumonia in the Elderly Medicine," 1983, 62:271-85, with permission.

Spectrum of Frequent Etiologic Agents in Pneumonia

Aerobic Bacteria	**Anaerobes**	**Fungi**
Gram-positive aerobes	*Bacteroides melaninogenicus*	*Aspergillus*
Streptococcus pneumoniae	*Fusobacterium*	*Coccidioides immitis*
Staphylococcus aureus	*Peptostreptococcus*	*Histoplasma capsulatum*
Streptococcus pyogenes	*Bacteroides fragilis*	*Blastomyces dermatitidis*
Gram-negative aerobes	*Actinomyces israelii*	*Cryptococcus neoformans*
Haemophilus influenzae		Zygomycetes
Legionella pneumophila		
Escherichia coli		
Klebsiella pneumoniae		
Pseudomonas aeruginosa		
Viruses	**Parasites**	**Other**
Respiratory syncytial virus	*Pneumocystis carinii*	*Mycoplasma pneumoniae*
Parainfluenza virus	*Ascaris lumbricoides*	*Chlamydia trachomatis*
Influenza virus	*Toxocara canis* and *catis*	*Chlamydia psittaci*
Adenovirus	*Filaria*	*Mycobacterium tuberculosis*
Enterovirus	*Strongyloides stercoralis*	*Chlamydia* TWAR strains
Rhinovirus	Hookworms	*Nocardia*
Measles virus	*Paragonimus*	
Varicella-zoster virus	*Echinococcus*	
Rickettsia	Schistosomes	
Coxiella burnetii		
Cytomegalovirus		
Hantavirus		

From Cohen GJ, "Management of Infections of the Lower Respiratory Tract in Children," *Pediatr Infect Dis*, 1987, 6:317-23, with permission.

(Continued)

Aerobic Culture, Tissue *see* Biopsy Culture, Routine *on page 390*

***Aeromonas*, Stool Culture** *see* Stool Culture, Uncommon Organisms *on page 588*

AFB Culture, Biopsy *see* Mycobacteria Culture, Biopsy or Body Fluid *on page 539*

AFB Culture, Bronchial Aspirate *see* Mycobacteria Culture, Sputum *on page 542*

AFB Culture, Gastric Aspirate *see* Mycobacteria Culture, Sputum *on page 542*

AFB Culture, Sputum *see* Mycobacteria Culture, Sputum *on page 542*

AFB Smear *see* Acid-Fast Stain *on page 361*

Agents of Bioterrorism *see* Bioterrorism Agents *on page 390*

AIDS Antigen *see* p24 Antigen *on page 555*

AIDS Blood Culture *see* Blood Culture, Mycobacteria *on page 395*

AIDS Virus Culture *see* Human Immunodeficiency Virus Culture *on page 506*

Amebiasis Serological Test *see* *Entamoeba histolytica* Serology *on page 452*

Amikacin Level

Related Information

Antibiotic Level, Serum *on page 375*

Synonyms Amikin® Level, Blood

Applies to Kanamycin (Kantrex®) Level

Abstract Aminoglycoside antibiotics, including amikacin, are used primarily to treat infections caused by aerobic gram-negative bacilli. Amikacin has a narrow therapeutic window. Its use in life-threatening infections makes it mandatory that effective levels be achieved without overdosing.

Specimen Serum

Container Red top tube or serum separator tube

Collection Not more than 30 minutes before the next dose for trough level; for peak level draw 15-30 minutes after completion of infusion or 45-75 minutes following intramuscular injection. Specify dosage, time of dosage, and all other coadministered antimicrobials. For send outs, ship specimen frozen in plastic vial on dry ice.

Storage Instructions Separate serum within 1 hour of collection, refrigerate or freeze until assayed.

Reference Range Therapeutic: peak: 15-25 mcg/mL (SI: 26-43 μmol/L) (depends in part on the minimal inhibitory concentration of the drug against the organism being treated); trough: <10 mcg/mL (SI: <17 μmol/L).

Critical Values Toxic: peak: >35 mcg/mL (SI: >60 μmol/L); trough: >10 mcg/mL (SI: >17 μmol/L)

Use Peak levels are necessary to assure adequate therapeutic levels for organism being treated. Trough levels are necessary to reduce the likelihood of nephrotoxicity.

Limitations High peak levels may not have strong correlation with toxicity.

Methodology High performance liquid chromatography (HPLC), fluorescence polarization immunoassay (FPIA), enzyme immunoassay (EIA)

Additional Information Amikacin is cleared by the kidney and accumulates in renal tubular cells. **Nephrotoxicity** is most closely related to the length of time that trough levels exceed 10 mcg/mL (SI: >17 μmol/L). Creatinine levels should be monitored every 2-3 days as an indicator of impending renal toxicity. The initial toxic result is nonoliguric renal failure that is usually reversible if the drug is discontinued. Continued administration of amikacin may produce oliguric renal failure. Nephrotoxicity may occur in as many as 10% to 25% of patients receiving aminoglycosides; most of this toxicity can be avoided by monitoring levels and adjusting dosing schedules accordingly.

Aminoglycosides may also cause irreversible **ototoxicity** that manifests itself clinically as hearing loss. Aminoglycoside ototoxicity is relatively uncommon and clinical trials in which levels were carefully monitored and dosing adjusted failed to show a correlation between auditory toxicity and plasma aminoglycoside levels. In situations where dosing is not adjusted, however, sustained high levels may be associated with ototoxicity. This association is far from clear cut, and new once-daily dosing regimens (and associated high peak serum concentrations) that fail to enhance toxicity further complicate the understanding of this issue.

Selected Readings

Edson RS and Terrell CL, "The Aminoglycosides," *Mayo Clin Proc*, 1999, 74:519-28.

Hammett-Stabler CA and Johns T, "Laboratory Guidelines for Monitoring of Antimicrobial Drugs. National Academy of Clinical Biochemistry," *Clin Chem*, 1998, 44(5):1129-40.

Porter WH, "Therapeutic Drug Monitoring," *Clin Chem*, Taylor EH, ed, New York, NY: John Wiley and Sons, 1989, 217-48.

Amikin® Level, Blood *see* Amikacin Level *on page 370*

Amphotericin B Level

Synonyms Fungizone® Level, Blood

Abstract Amphotericin B is a clinically useful but highly toxic antifungal agent. Newer, less toxic agents are available. However, for many serious fungal infections, amphotericin B is still used despite its toxicity.

Specimen Serum

Container Red top tube or serum separator tube

Reference Range Therapeutic range: 1.0-2.0 mcg/mL (SI: 1.0-2.2 μmol/L)

Use Monitor serum levels for potential toxicity and correlation with *in vitro* susceptibility data

Limitations Assays for amphotericin B are performed only in a few reference laboratories. In routine clinical use it is probably more prudent to follow creatinine, potassium, bicarbonate, and magnesium concentrations and the CBC, than to perform amphotericin B assays.

Methodology High performance liquid chromatography (HPLC), bioassay

Additional Information Amphotericin B therapy frequently induces fever, chills, nausea, and reversible bone marrow suppression.

Additionally, approximately 80% of patients develop increased creatinine concentrations, and occasional patients show an acute deterioration in **renal function**; when creatinine levels exceed 3.0 mcg/mL it is advisable to withhold amphotericin B for several days and resume therapy at a lower dose.

Because the pharmacokinetics and biodistribution of the drug are not clearly defined, it may be useful to correlate serum levels with desired concentrations determined by *in vitro* susceptibility testing. Susceptibility testing, however, is not widely available, is not well standardized, and may not accurately predict clinical response. Amphotericin B can increase digitalis toxicity and decrease the anti-*Candida* effect of miconazole, and its toxicities are additive with those of aminoglycosides.

Selected Readings

Patel R, "Antifungal Agents. Part 1. Amphotericin B Preparations and Flucytosine," *Mayo Clin Proc*, 1998, 73:1205-25.

Terrell CL and Hughes CE, "Antifungal Agents Used for Deep-Seated Mycotic Infections," *Mayo Clin Proc*, 1992, 67(1):69-91.

Amplicor™ HCV Monitor *see* Hepatitis C Viral RNA, Quantitative PCR *on page 488*

Anaerobic Bacterial Susceptibility *see* Antimicrobial Susceptibility Testing, Anaerobic Bacteria *on page 381*

Anaerobic Blood Culture *see* Blood Culture, Aerobic and Anaerobic *on page 391*

Anaerobic Culture

Related Information

Aerobic Culture, Body Fluid *on page 365*
Aerobic Culture, Sputum *on page 367*
Biopsy Culture, Routine *on page 390*

Applies to Biopsy Culture, Anaerobic; Body Fluid Anaerobic Culture; Bronchial Aspirate Anaerobic Culture; Cerebrospinal Fluid Anaerobic Culture; Cyst Culture, Anaerobic; Surgical Specimen Anaerobic Culture; Tissue Anaerobic Culture; Transtracheal Aspirate Anaerobic Culture

Test Includes Isolation and identification of anaerobic organisms; susceptibility testing may be performed if clinically warranted.

Patient Preparation Sterile preparation of the site

Special Instructions The following information will assist the laboratory in the proper processing of the specimen: specific site of specimen, current antibiotic therapy, age and sex of patient, collection time and date, and clinical diagnosis.

Specimen Surgical tissue, biopsy material from normally sterile site, aspirated fluids, etc. Specimen for anaerobic culture should be accompanied by a specimen for aerobic culture from the same site. Specimens collected on swabs are vastly inferior specimens.

Container Fluids: anaerobic transport container or original syringe; tissue: sterile container, no preservative

Collection Specimens are to be collected from a prepared site using sterile technique. Contamination with normal flora from skin, rectum, vagina, or other body surfaces **must** be avoided. **Note:** The needle **must** be removed from the syringe before the syringe is sent to the laboratory.

Storage Instructions Transport specimen to the laboratory within 30 minutes. Do not refrigerate. Refrigeration inhibits viability of certain anaerobic organisms and also the common important aerobic pathogens *Neisseria meningitidis*, *Streptococcus pneumoniae*, and *Haemophilus influenzae*.

(Continued)

Anaerobic Culture *(Continued)*

Causes for Rejection Specimen not received in appropriate transport container or sterile container, specimen in fixative. Specimens delayed in transport to the laboratory and specimens which have been refrigerated have a less than optimal yield. Specimens from unacceptable sites (see above) may not be acceptable for anaerobic culture because of contamination by the normal flora.

Turnaround Time Cultures showing no bacterial growth will be reported after 2 days. Complete reports of cultures with anaerobic bacteria may take as long as 2 weeks after receipt of culture depending upon the nature and number of the organisms isolated.

Reference Range No growth of anaerobic bacteria

Use Anaerobic cultures are indicated particularly when suspected infections are related to mucus membranes, gastrointestinal tract, pelvic organs, associated with malignancy, related to use of aminoglycosides, or occur in a setting where the diagnosis of gas gangrene or actinomycosis is considered. Anaerobic culture is especially indicated when an exudate has a foul odor or if the exudate has a grayish discoloration and is hemorrhagic. Frequently, more than one organism is recovered from an anaerobic infection.

Limitations Specimens received in anaerobic transport containers are less-than-optimal for aerobic or fungal cultures.

Contraindications Specimens absolutely contraindicated for anaerobic culture include the following: oral, GI, skin, urogenital, throat, sputum, bronchial wash, bowel contents, void urine, vaginal, cervical, material adjacent to a mucus membrane, and surface material from a wound or decubitus.

Additional Information Biopsy culture is particularly useful in establishing the diagnosis of anaerobic osteomyelitis, clostridial myonecrosis, intracranial actinomycosis and pleuropulmonary infections. In cases of osteomyelitis, biopsy is mandatory. Anaerobic infections of soft tissue include the following: anaerobic cellulitis, necrotizing fasciitis, clostridial myonecrosis (gas gangrene), anaerobic streptococcal myositis or myonecrosis, synergistic nonclostridial anaerobic myonecrosis, and infected vascular gangrene. These infections, particularly clostridial myonecrosis, necrotizing fasciitis, and nonclostridial anaerobic myonecrosis, may be fulminant and are frequently characterized by the presence of gas and foul-smelling necrotic tissue. Empiric therapy based on likely pathogens should be instituted as soon as appropriate cultures are collected.

Oral contamination of bronchial aspirates can be minimized by using a telescoping double catheter with a plug to protect the brush. Even by this method, many anaerobes might not survive transit to the laboratory because of aeration of specimens and transport to the laboratory in an inappropriate transport device. Because of difficulty in interpretation, the usefulness of bronchial aspirate anaerobic cultures collected in the usual manner by routine bronchoscopy (ie, contaminated with oral flora), has been questioned. Pleuropulmonary infections caused by anaerobic organisms are most often secondary to aspiration of oropharyngeal contents. They may also be caused by septic emboli or from intra-abdominal infections (ie, subphrenic abscess, diverticulitis, appendicitis, etc). Community-acquired aspiration pneumonia, necrotizing pneumonia with multiple small abscesses, frank lung abscess, and pulmonary empyema yield significant anaerobes, 60% to 95% of cases, if appropriate culture technique is employed. The characteristic foul smelling odor of an anaerobic infection may not be present early in the course.

Selected Readings

Anuradha DE, Saraswathi K, and Gogate A, "Anaerobic Bacteraemia: A Review of 17 Cases," *J Postgrad Med*, 1998, 44(3):63-6.

Chaudhry R, Mishra B, Dhawan B, et al, "Clinical Spectrum of Bacteroidaceae in a Tertiary Care Hospital," *J Commun Dis*, 1999, 31(3):169-72.

Cinat ME and Wilson SE, "New Advances in the Use of Antimicrobial Agents in Surgery: Intra-Abdominal Infections," *J Chemother*, 1999, 11(6):453-63.

Finegold SM, "Anaerobic Bacteria: General Concepts," *Principles and Practice of Infectious Dieases*, 5th ed, Mandell GL, Bennett JE, and Dolin R, eds, New York, NY: Churchill Livingstone, 2000, 2519-37.

James PA and al-Shafi KM, "Clinical Value of Anaerobic Blood Culture: A Retrospective Analysis of Positive Patient Episodes," *J Clin Pathol*, 2000, 53(3):231-3.

Anaerobic Culture, Abscess *see* Abscess Aerobic and Anaerobic Culture *on page 360*

Ancobon® Level *see* Flucytosine Level *on page 456*

Anergy Control Panel *see* Anergy Skin Test Battery *on page 372*

Anergy Skin Test Battery

Related Information

Fungal Skin Testing *on page 459*

Tuberculin Skin Testing, Intracutaneous *on page 601*

Synonyms Anergy Control Panel; Anergy Skin Testing; Delayed Reaction Intracutaneous Tests; Skin Test Battery

Test Includes Injection of several common antigenic substances into the skin, such as *Candida*, *Trichophyton*, and mumps antigens. Anergy skin testing is an *in vivo* means of evaluating the cell-mediated immune system. Skin injection sites are examined at 24, 48, and 72 hours. The development of local erythema and induration indicates an adequate delayed hypersensitivity response, and implies competent T-cell function. Failure to respond to any skin test antigen is termed cutaneous anergy, and is seen in a variety of systemic disorders.

Patient Preparation Procedure and risks are explained to the patient. No specific skin preparation is necessary. However, those patients with generalized skin disease, such as psoriasis, should be examined beforehand to ensure that there are suitable areas of normal appearing skin. Although testing need not be performed by a physician, one should be immediately available in the event of a systemic reaction.

Aftercare If no adverse reaction has occurred within 30 minutes, patient may be discharged from the testing center. Test sites should be kept reasonably clean for 72 hours. No restrictions on bathing are necessary. Patient should contact physician if severe local reactions develop, extensive erythema beyond the test site occurs, or if fever, dyspnea, or lightheadedness develops.

Special Instructions Requisition should include a list of all current medications, with attention to corticosteroids or other immunosuppressive agents.

Complications Anergy skin testing is generally quite safe. However, as with other forms of skin testing, immediate local reactions to antigens are distinctly unusual but possible. These reactions are usually IgE-mediated and lead to an immediate wheal and flare reaction. Rarely, serious local reactions have been reported to various antigens commonly included in the test battery; these include vesiculation, skin necrosis, and extensive erythema. Systemic reactions have been reported only on an individual case basis.

Equipment Antigens used for anergy testing are commercially prepared liquid extracts of a variety of foreign substances. These antigens are chosen because ubiquitous exposure to these substances is expected in the general population. Thus, in any randomly selected subgroup, a high rate of delayed hypersensitivity skin reactions would be anticipated. Commonly used bacterial antigens include streptococcal antigen (derived from *Streptococcus* group CH 46A), *Proteus* antigen (often from *Proteus mirabilis* IM 2104 strain), and in some centers, tuberculin is also included. Fungal antigens frequently employed include *Candida* antigen (derived from *Candida albicans* strain 2111), *Trichophyton* antigen (from *Trichophyton mentagrophytes*), and frequently histoplasmin is used (from *Histoplasma capsulatum*). Toxoids are also included in the test battery, usually tetanus toxoid (from *Clostridium tetani*, Harvard strain 401) and diphtheria toxoid (from *Corynebacterium diphtheriae*). Mumps skin test antigen is a viral antigen derived from inactivated mumps virus cultured in chick embryo. The choice of antigens and total number employed has yet to be standardized. Most test centers use less than five antigens in their routine battery, but considerable variation exists, with the total number ranging from 1-11. In studies, 90% of 750 hospitalized patients reacted to one or more of the following: mumps, *Candida*, *Trichophyton*, and tuberculin. Increasing the total number of antigens improved the rate of skin reactions by only 1%. With respect to the individual selection of antigens, a representative battery might therefore include mumps, *Candida*, and *Trichophyton*; this combination is commonly seen in practice. However, in one literature review, more than thirty different antigens were found to be in routine use at major centers. Disposable plastic or glass tuberculin syringes, 0.5-1 mL are also required, along with 26- or 27-gauge short (¼" to ½") beveled needles, some alcohol pads, and gauze. An alternative anergy testing technique has been developed in recent years to address the aforementioned lack of standardization in antigen selection and number. Termed the Multitest® CMI system, seven standardized antigens and one control are simultaneously injected by means of a multiple puncture device. Antigens used in the system are tetanus toxoid, diphtheria toxoid, streptococcal antigen, *Proteus*, tuberculin, *Candida*, and *Trichophyton*. This device obviates the need for separate syringes, needles, and antigens.

Technique Traditional method: Antigens are injected separately. Antigens are individually drawn up into tuberculin syringes immediately prior to testing. The volar aspects of the arms or forearms are the preferred test sites. Only normal appearing skin should be used. Sites are prepared with alcohol swabs. Using a 26- or 27-gauge needle, each antigen is injected intradermally at a 45° angle, bevel down. A small bleb approximately 2-3 mm in diameter should be raised; usually an injected volume of 0.05 mL is sufficient. Care should be taken to avoid deeper subcutaneous injections. Each antigen is separately planted in this fashion with adequate spacing between injection sites (>2 cm).

(Continued)

Anergy Skin Test Battery *(Continued)*

Multipuncture method: Antigens are placed simultaneous by means of the Multitest® CMI device. Seven antigens and one glycerol control are standardized with respect to selection and concentration and are preloaded onto this disposable plastic device. A different antigen coats each of seven multiple puncture heads, which are spaced approximately 2 cm apart, in two parallel rows of four. The skin over the forearm is held taut. The device is then oriented per manufacturer's instructions ("T" bar towards the head) and applied to the skin with a rocking motion. Each head must sufficiently puncture the skin.

Regardless of technique, all tests sites should be examined immediately and at 24, 48, and 72 hours. Date and time of injection must be recorded. The precise location, identity, and concentration of each antigen should be recorded, most often in a pictorial format or standardized table. It may be helpful to circle and label each antigen with a waterproof pen directly onto the skin, but this must not replace formal notations in the medical chart.

Data Acquired The transverse diameter of induration at each test site should be carefully measured by both inspection and palpation. Results are recorded in millimeters at the appropriate 24-hour intervals. Areas of erythema are also measured but play a minor role in most grading schemes.

Reference Range Normal individuals should demonstrate a positive skin reaction to one or more test antigens.

Critical Values A positive skin test is usually defined as the presence of induration and accompanying erythema ≥5 mm in transverse diameter at an injection site at 24, 48, or 72 hours. Immediate skin reactions (ie, within minutes) are due to mechanisms other than cellular immunity and do not define a positive test. When the Multitest® CMI system is used, induration ≥2 mm in transverse diameter is considered significant. This disparity in definition between the intradermal and multiple puncture technique results from a variety of technical factors including volume of antigen introduced, depth of skin penetration, etc. A state of anergy is defined as an inability to mount an appropriate delayed hypersensitivity response. In clinical practice this is manifested as a complete absence of reactivity to a skin test battery of at least four to five antigens. Some authorities require repetition of the test battery at least once before labeling a patient "anergic". Normal individuals are expected to develop a positive skin test in response to at least one antigen, barring technical error. Anergy may be present as a generalized defect in T-cell function, as in sarcoidosis, AIDS, or tuberculosis, or as a specific defect in cellular immunity, as in mucocutaneous candidiasis where T-cell response to *Candida* is selectively deficient. There are numerous causes of anergy and may be categorized as follows:

- infections: bacterial, tuberculosis, disseminated fungal infections, viral (influenza, mumps, mononucleosis, hepatitis, and others), parasitic
- congenital: cell-mediated deficiency (DiGeorge syndrome), combined cellular and humoral deficiency (Nezelof's, Wiskott-Aldrich syndrome, etc)
- acquired/iatrogenic: neoplasms (solid tumors, lymphomas, leukemias), medications (corticosteroids, antineoplastic agents, methotrexate, and others), AIDS
- rheumatic diseases: rheumatoid arthritis, lupus, Behçet's disease
- miscellaneous: uremia, diabetes mellitus, inflammatory bowel disease, sarcoidosis, extremes of age, malnutrition

However, anergy skin testing by itself does not distinguish amongst these conditions from a diagnostic viewpoint. Clinically, anergy testing is most useful in evaluating the patient who presents with chronic or recurrent infections, or infection with unusual organisms. In such cases, formal evaluation of the immune system may be warranted. This may include assessment of all four major components of the immune system: cell-mediated (T-cell) immunity, antibody-mediated (B-cell) immunity, phagocytic system (polymorphonuclear leukocytes, macrophages), and complement. Often a careful history and physical, with attention to infectious diseases, will identify the particular component deficiency. Anergy testing is an appropriate and recommended screening procedure for suspected deficiencies in cell-mediated immunity, often characterized by fungal, mycobacterial, or disseminated viral infections (eg, varicella-zoster, cytomegalovirus, herpes simplex virus). Among the many laboratory tests available to evaluate host defense, anergy testing is rightfully obtained soon after the history and physical (along with a complete blood count with differential) but prior to more elaborate *in vitro* investigation of T-cell function. These latter tests include T-cell surface marker studies, T-cell subsets, and response to mitogens (such as pokeweed mitogen, phytohemagglutinin, concanavalin A). Some individuals demonstrate partial or inconclusive responses to skin testing. This is seen as a "borderline" skin induration diameter (ie, 1-4 mm) or as a poor reactivity rate when a large antigen battery is employed (ie, one positive reaction out of ten tested). These patients have sometimes been called "hypoergic," which implies a partially impaired

delayed hypersensitivity response. The clinical significance of this phenomenon is unclear at present.

Use

- Objectively demonstrate cutaneous anergy in cases of suspected cellular immune system deficiency (T-cell dysfunction); often this procedure is performed as part of an initial immune system assessment, but may also be repeated in a serial fashion in cases of protracted or chronic illness
- Serve as a "control" skin test accompanying the tuberculin skin test (or other specific antigen tests); this allows more accurate interpretation of a negative tuberculin test; patients with generalized cutaneous anergy predictably fail to react to injected tuberculin despite prior exposure to *M. tuberculosis*
- Establish the presence of cutaneous anergy prior to more extensive *in vitro* evaluation of lymphocyte and monocyte function
- Less commonly, to help predict postoperative morbidity and mortality, especially in the patient with sepsis
- Occasionally, to provide general prognostic information in patients with cancer

Limitations "Traditional" skin test battery limitations, mentioned previously, include variation in selection and total number of antigens used as well as a lack of standardization of antigen potency. However, some practitioners consider the inability to select and interchange antigens in the Multitest® CMI system a major drawback. False-positive reactions may occur:

- when an immediate wheal and flare is interpreted as delayed hypersensitivity
- when intradermal bleeding is interpreted as erythema
- when dermographism is present

False-negative reactions may be caused by:

- lack of antigen potency
- subcutaneous injection
- inadequate dose or concentration
- incomplete skin puncture by the Multitest® device
- attenuated skin response, as in atopic dermatitis

Contraindications

- Prior systemic reaction to any antigen included in the skin test battery; alternate antigens may be substituted in most cases
- Known hypersensitivity to a stabilizer or diluent used in commercial antigen preparations; for example, mumps skin test antigen is derived from virus incubated in chicken embryo and preserved in thimerosal. Patients should therefore be questioned regarding feather and egg allergy as well as sensitivity to thimerosal prior to administering mumps antigen. Depending on the particular antigens selected, published manufacturer's warnings should be reviewed and potential hypersensitivity reactions avoided.

Selected Readings

Gordin FM, Hartigan PM, Klimas NG, et al, "Delayed-Type Hypersensitivity Skin Tests Are an Independent Predictor of Human Immunodeficiency Virus Disease Progression," *J Infect Dis*, 1994, 169(4):893-7.

Kniker WT, Anderson CT, McBryde JL, et al, "Multitest CMI for Standardized Measurement of Delayed Cutaneous Hypersensitivity and Cell-Mediated Immunity. Normal Values and Proposed Scoring System for Healthy Adults in the U.S.A.," *Ann Allergy*, 1984, 52(2):75-82.

Anergy Skin Testing *see* Anergy Skin Test Battery *on page 372*

Ankle Arthrogram *see* Arthrogram *on page 387*

Ankle, Left or Right, X-ray *see* Bone Films *on page 396*

Anti-B19 Parvovirus IgG Antibodies *see* Parvovirus B19 Serology *on page 560*

Anti-B19 Parvovirus IgM Antibodies *see* Parvovirus B19 Serology *on page 560*

Antibacterial Activity, Serum *see* Serum Bactericidal Test *on page 578*

Antibiotic-Associated Colitis Toxin Test *see Clostridium difficile* Toxin Assay *on page 418*

Antibiotic Level, Serum

Related Information

Amikacin Level *on page 370*
Chloramphenicol Serum Level *on page 417*
Flucytosine Level *on page 456*
Gentamicin Level *on page 472*
Tobramycin Level *on page 596*
Vancomycin Level *on page 611*

Synonyms Antimicrobial Assay

Abstract Assays for antimicrobial agents in serum are performed for two primary reasons: (1) to ensure therapeutic levels, and (2) to monitor for potentially toxic levels. In most situations, it is not necessary to monitor antimicrobial levels because serum levels are relatively predictable based on dosing; *in vitro* susceptibility testing uses

(Continued)

Antibiotic Level, Serum *(Continued)*

those predictable levels to determine clinical efficacy. Similarly, toxicity is not always related to serum levels. It may be more appropriate to monitor for toxicity by following determinants of hematologic, renal, or hepatic function. In certain situations however (eg, aminoglycoside antibiotics which have a narrow therapeutic range and a high potential for toxicity), it is essential to follow serum levels.

Specimen Serum

Container Red top tube or serum separator tube

Sampling Time Peak: 30 minutes after 30 minute I.V. infusion; 1 hour after I.M. dose. Trough: immediately prior to next dose.

Collection Keep frozen if not assayed immediately.

Causes for Rejection Incomplete clinical information (eg, specific antimicrobial, dosage and schedule, other concurrent antimicrobials)

Reference Range Therapeutic range depends on agent being tested for, and minimal inhibitory concentration of drug against organism. Selected ranges in mcg/mL are presented as a guide only.

Antibiotic Level, Serum

Drug	Peak		Trough	
	mcg/mL	SI: µmol/L	mcg/mL	SI: µmol/L
Amikacin	15-25	26-43	<10	<17
Chloramphenicol	25	77		
Flucytosine	100	775		
Gentamicin	4-10	8-21	<2	<4
Netilmicin	4-8	8.0-17.0	1-2	0.7-1.4
Streptomycin	5-20	9-34	<5	<9
Tobramycin	4-10	8-21	<2	<4
Vancomycin	20-40	13.6-27.2	5-10	3.4-6.8

Selected ranges in mcg/mL are presented as a guide only.

Possible Panic Range See entries on aminoglycoside drugs (eg, Gentamicin and Tobramycin).

Use Evaluate adequacy of serum antibiotic level; detection of toxic levels

Limitations May not be technically possible in a patient taking more than one antibiotic

Methodology Bioassay: cephalosporins, clindamycin, erythromycin, metronidazole, penicillins, polymyxin, tetracycline, trimethoprim. High performance liquid chromatography: chloramphenicol, flucytosine, mezlocillin. Fluorescence polarization immunoassay (FPIA): amikacin, gentamicin, tobramycin, kanamycin, streptomycin, vancomycin, neomycin.

Additional Information With the increasing availability of *in vitro* sensitivity testing expressed as the minimal inhibitory or bactericidal concentration of an antibiotic, measurement of serum levels of these drugs has taken on practical clinical importance. This is especially true for agents with narrow therapeutic ranges and significant toxicity. It should be remembered, however, that in most patients, cure of infection depends on numerous host factors as well as on antibiotics. Therefore, antibiotic levels should not be relied on as the sole guide to therapy.

Selected Readings

Cockerill FR III, "Conventional and Genetic Laboratory Tests Used to Guide Antimicrobial Therapy," *Mayo Clin Proc*, 1998, 73:1007-21.

Donowitz GR and Mandell GL, "Drug Therapy. Beta-Lactam Antibiotics," *N Engl J Med*, 1988, 318(8):490-500.

Antideoxyribonuclease-B Titer, Serum

Related Information

Antistreptolysin O Titer, Serum *on page 383*
Streptozyme *on page 589*

Synonyms ADNase-B; Anti-DNase-B Titer; Antistreptococcal DNase-B Titer; Streptodornase

Specimen Serum

Container Red top tube or serum separator tube

Causes for Rejection Excessive hemolysis, chylous serum

Reference Range Preschool: ≤60 units; school: ≤170 units; adult: ≤85 units; A rise in titer of two or more dilution increments between acute and convalescent sera is significant.

Use Document recent streptococcal infection

Limitations Normal ranges may vary in different populations

Contraindications Not valid in patients with hemorrhagic pancreatitis

Methodology Colorimetry based on hydrolysis of DNA

Additional Information Presence of antibodies to streptococcal DNase is an indicator of recent infection, especially if a rise in titer can be documented. This test has both theoretical and technical advantages over the ASO test: it is more sensitive to streptococcal pyoderma, it is not so subject to false-positives due to liver disease, and one need not worry about test invalidation due to oxidation of reagents.

Anti-DNase-B Titer *see* Antideoxyribonuclease-B Titer, Serum *on page 376*

Antifungal Susceptibility Testing

Related Information

Periodic Acid-Schiff Stain *on page 563*

Synonyms Fungi, Susceptibility Testing; Susceptibility Testing, Fungi

Test Includes Broth dilution, agar dilution and disc diffusion testing of antifungal agents. Results may be quantitative or qualitative.

Special Instructions Consult the laboratory to determine availability and choice of methods.

Specimen Pure isolate of the organism

Causes for Rejection Organism disposed of prior to request for testing.

Reference Range See tables below and on next page.

General Antifungal *In Vitro* Susceptibility Patterns of Candida Species[1]

Candida Species	Amphotericin B	Fluconazole	Flucytosine	Itraconazole
C. albicans	S	S	S	S
C. glabrata	S to I[5]	S-DD to R[3]	S	S-DD to R[4]
C. krusei	S to I[5]	R	I to R	S-DD to R[6]
C. lusitaniae	S to R[2]	S	S	S
C. parapsilosis	S	S	S	S
C. tropicalis	S	S	S	S

Adapted from Galgiani JN, Ampel NM, Catanzaro A, et al; "Practice Guidelines for the Treatment of Coccidioidomycosis," *Clin Infect Dis*, 2000, 30(4):658-61.

[1]S = susceptible; I = intermediate; R = resistant; S-DD = susceptible but dose/delivery-dependent (ie, maxiumum dosage and bioavailability are critical to successful therapy).

[2]Resistance has been reported in some isolates.

[3]15% resistance.

[4]46% resistance.

[5]A "significant" percentage of isolates has reduced susceptibility.

[6]31% resistance.

Use Determine susceptibility of isolated fungi to available therapeutic agents, predict probable clinical response, explain observed or suspected therapeutic failures, determine if primary or secondary resistance is present

Limitations This test procedure is usually available only from specialized laboratories. An increasing number of university, hospital, and community clinical laboratories are offering yeast antifungal susceptibility testing. Methods for fungal susceptibility testing are not as yet as standardized as for bacteria. Stability and solubility of some of the agents cause technical difficulty.

Methodology Standardized methods are evolving for the susceptibility of yeasts. The availability of a choice of therapeutic agents will continue to cause laboratories to attempt to provide susceptibility data with a useful predictive value for clinicians.

Additional Information Interpretation of *in vitro* susceptibility data for antifungal drugs is hindered by limited standardized test criteria and a paucity of interpretive criteria. Thus, it is extremely difficult to identify a clear relation between minimal inhibitory concentrations and clinical outcome. The situation appears more readily resolvable for yeast-like fungi than for filamentous fungi since the former are more easily quantified by standardized microbiologic techniques.

See table on page 379 for guidelines for the interpretation of MIC values for *Candida* species.

Selected Readings

Clinical and Laboratory Standards Institute, "Reference Methods for Broth Dilution Antifungal Susceptibility Testing of Yeasts," Approved Standard, 2nd ed, 2002, Document M27-A2.

Espinel-Ingroff A, "Clinical Relevance of Fungal Susceptibility Testing and Antifungal Resistance," *Clin Microbiol Newslett*, 2000, 22(18):137.

Liao RS and Dunne WM, "Current Concepts in Antifungal Susceptibility Testing, Part I," *Clin Microbiol Newslett*, 2003, 25(23):177.

Liao RS and Dunne WM, "Current Concepts in Antifungal Susceptibility Testing, Part II," *Clin Microbiol Newslett*, 2003, 25(24):185.

Mukherjee PK, Sheehan DJ, Hitchcock CA, et al, "Combination Treatment of Invasive Fungal Infections," *Clin Microbiol Rev*, 2005, 18(1):163-94.

(Continued)

Antifungal Susceptibility Testing *(Continued)*

General Antifungal Susceptibility Patterns of *Candida* Species[1,2]

Species of *Candida*	Relative Frequency of Isolation	Antifungal Agent					
		Fluconazole	Itraconazole	Voriconazole	Flucytosine	Amphotericin B	Candins[3]
C. albicans	1	S	S	S	S	S	S
C. glabrata	2	S-DD to R[4]	S-DD to R[5]	S to I	S	S to I[6]	S
C. parasilosis	3	S	S	S	S	S	S (to I?)
C. tropicalis	4	S	S	S	S	S	S
C. krusei	5	R	S-DD to R[7]	S to I	I to R	S to I[6]	S
C. lusitaniae	6	S	S	S	S	S to R[8]	S
C. dubliniensis	7	S	S		S	S	
C. guilliermondii	8	S	S			S to R	

[1]Sources of data: Rows 1-6, Pappas PG, Rex JH, Sobel JD, et al, "Guidelines for Treatment of Candidiasis, *Clin Infect Dis*, 2004, 38(2):161-89; rows 7-8, Perea S and Patterson TF, "Antifungal Resistance in Pathogenic Fungi," *Clin Infect Dis*, 2002, 35(9):1073-80.

[2]S = susceptible, I - intermediate, R = resistant, S-DD = susceptible-dose/delivery-dependent.

[3]Caspofungin, micafungin, and anidulafungin (clinical responses to the use of caspofungin to treat invasive diseases caused by all *Candida* spp have been observed.

[4]10% to 15% of isolates are resistant.

[5]46% to 53% of isolates are resistant.

[6]Significant reduced susceptibility has been reported in many isolates.

[7]31% of isolates are resistant.

[8]Resistance is relatively common.

Pfaller MA and Diekema DJ, "Rare and Emerging Opportunistic Fungal Pathogens: Concern for Resistance Beyond *Candida albicans* and *Aspergillus fumigatus*," *J Clin Microbiol*, 2004, 42(10):4419-31.

Pfaller MA, Sheehan DJ, Rex JH, et al, "Determination of Fungicidal Activities Against Yeasts and Molds: Lessons Learned From Bactericidal Testing and the Need for Standardization," *Clin Microbiol Rev*, 2004, 17(2):268-80.

Randhawa GK and Sharma G, "Echinocandins: A Promising New Antifungal Group," *Indian J Pharmacol*, 2004, 36(2):65-71.

Interpretative Guidelines for *In Vitro* Susceptibility Testing of *Candida* Species[1]

Antifungal Agent	Susceptible	Susceptible Dose-Dependent[2]	Intermediate[3]	Resistant
Fluconazole[4]	≤8[5]	16-32	–	≥64
Itraconazole[6]	≤0.125	0.25-0.5	–	≥1
Flucytocine	≤4	–	8-16	≥32
Amphotericin B	MIC values for most isolates are 0.25-1[7]			
Ketoconazole	MIC values for most isolates are 0.03-16[7]			
Voriconazole Raviconazole Posiconazole	MIC values for most isolates are 0.03-16[7]			

[1]Information in this table (except indicated personal communications) is from *Reference Method for Broth Dilution Antifungal Susceptibility Testing of Yeasts; Approved Standard Document M27-A2*, 2nd ed, Wayne, PA: Clinical and Laboratory Standards Institute, 2002.

[2]Susceptibility is dependent on achieving maximal possible blood level of agent.

[3]Susceptibility of "intermediate" isolates is not certain and is not clearly "susceptible" or "resistant."

[4]Interpretations are based substantially on experience with mucosal infections, but are consistent with limited information on invasive *Candida* infections. *C. krusei* is considered intrinsically resistant to fluconazole, and their MIC values should not be interpreted by using this table.

[5]All MIC values are in μg/mL.

[6]Interpretations are based entirely on experience with mucosal infections; data supporting breakpoints of *Candida* invasive infections have not been established.

[7]Data are from personal communications with and the practical experiences of a reference laboratories. Interpretations have not been established.

Anti-HCV (IgM) *see* Hepatitis C Serology *on page 484*

Antihepatitis E Virus *see* Hepatitis E Serology *on page 490*

Anti-HEV *see* Hepatitis E Serology *on page 490*

Antimicrobial Assay *see* Antibiotic Level, Serum *on page 375*

Antimicrobial Removal Device (ARD) Blood Culture *see* Blood Culture, Aerobic and Anaerobic *on page 391*

Antimicrobial Susceptibility Testing, Aerobic and Facultatively Anaerobic Organisms

Related Information

Abscess Aerobic and Anaerobic Culture *on page 360*
Serum Bactericidal Test *on page 578*

Synonyms Kirby-Bauer Susceptibility Test; MIC; Minimum Inhibitory Concentration Susceptibility Test; Susceptibility Testing, Aerobic and Facultatively Anaerobic Organisms

Test Includes Qualitative or quantitative determination of antimicrobial susceptibility of an isolated organism

Abstract The purpose of antimicrobial susceptibility testing is to determine the degree of activity of antimicrobial agents against specific pathogens.

Specimen Viable pure culture of aerobic or facultatively anaerobic rapidly growing organism

Turnaround Time Usually 1 day after isolation of a pure culture

Use Determine the antimicrobial susceptibility of organisms involved in infectious processes when the susceptibility of the organism cannot be predicted from its identity

Methodology Manual methods: Disc diffusion and E-test; automated methods: MicroScan®, Vitek®, and others.

Additional Information Effective antimicrobial therapy is usually selected with the intent of achieving peak level 2-4 times the MIC at the site of infection. An antimicrobial level many times the MIC is usually sought in urinary tract infections. The "breakpoints" indicate clinically achievable levels and relate to MICs above which organisms are resistant and would not be expected to respond to readily achievable levels of antimicrobial therapy.
(Continued)

Antimicrobial Susceptibility Testing, Aerobic and Facultatively Anaerobic Organisms *(Continued)*

Susceptible: This category implies that an infection due to the strain may be appropriately treated with the dosage of antimicrobial agent recommended for that type of infection and infecting species, unless otherwise contraindicated.

Intermediate: This interpretation implies clinical applicability in body sites where the agent is physiologically concentrated (eg, in urine) or when a high dose of agent can be administered (eg, penicillins). In some cases "intermediate" applies to an MIC literally between a "susceptible" MIC and a "resistant" MIC. Such MICs are due to small uncontrollable technical errors/factors.

Resistant: Strains falling in this category are not inhibited by the usually achievable systemic concentrations of the agent with normal dosage schedules and/or fall in the range where specific microbial resistance mechanisms are likely (eg, beta-lactamases), and clinical efficacy has not been reliable in treatment studies. See table.

Major Mechanisms of Bacterial Antimicrobial Resistance

Enzymatic inactivation or modification of drug

- β-lactamase hydrolysis of β-lactam ring with subsequent inactivation of β-lactam antibiotics
- Modification of aminoglycosides by acetylating, adenylating, or phosphorylating enzymes
- Modification of chloramphenicol by chloramphenicol acetyltransferase

Decreased drug uptake or accumulation

- Intrinsic or acquired lack of outer membrane permeability
- Faulty or lacking antibiotic uptake and transport system
- Antibiotic efflux system (eg, tetracycline resistance)

Altered or lacking antimicrobial target

- Altered penicillin-binding proteins (β-lactam resistance)
- Altered ribosomal target (eg, aminoglycoside, macrolide, and lincomycin resistance)
- Altered enzymatic target (eg, sulfonamide, trimethoprim, rifampin, and quinolone resistance)

Circumvention of drug action consequences

- Hyperproduction of drug targets or competitive substrates (eg, sulfonamide and trimethoprim resistance)

Uncoupling of antibiotic attack and cell death

- Bacterial tolerance and survival in presence of usually bactericidal drugs (eg, β-lactams and vancomycin)

Note: The Clinical and Laboratory Standards Institute has issued disease-specific, organism-specific and antimicrobial agent-specific interpretations for MIC values: For *S. pneumoniae* meningitis and nonmeningitis diseases, the breakpoints for susceptibility to cefotaxime/ceftriaxone are 0.5 and 1.0 mcg/mL, respectively. These recommendations are due to the fact that these agents reach different achievable levels in the blood and CSF.

Selected Readings

Clinical and Laboratory Standards Institute, "Performance Standards for Antimicrobial Susceptibility Testing," 15th Informational Supplement, 2005, Document M100-S15.

Colodner R, "Extended-Spectrum Beta-Lactamases: A Challenge for Clinical Microbiologists and Infection Control Specialists," *Am J Infect Control*, 2005, 33(2):104-7.

Golan Y, McDermott LA, Jacobus NV, et al, "Emergence of Fluoroquinolone Resistance Among *Bacteroides* Species," *J Antimicrob Chemother*, 2003, 52(2):208-13.

Graffunder EM, Preston KE, Evans AM, et al, "Risk Factors Associated With Extended-Spectrum Beta-Lactamase-Producing Organisms at a Tertiary Care Hospital," *J Antimicrob Chemother*, 2005, 56(1):139-45.

Rice LB, Sahm D, and Bonomo RA, "Mechanisms of Resistance to Antimicrobial Agents," *Manual of Clinical Microbiology*, 8th ed, Murray PR, Baron EJ, Jorgensen JH, et al, eds, Washington, DC: ASM Press, 2003, 1074-101.

Schreckenberger PC, "Conundrums in the Laboratory Detection of Antimicrobial-Resistant Gram-Negative Bacteria," *Reviews in Medical Microbiology*, Philadelphia, PA: Lippincott Williams & Wilkins, 2004, 15(2):45-9.

Turner PJ, "Extended-Spectrum Beta-Lactamases," *Clin Infect Dis*, 2005, 41(Suppl 4):S273-5.

Yao DC and Moellering RC, "Antibacterial Agents," *Manual of Clinical Microbiology*, 8th ed, Murray PR, Baron EJ, Jorgensen JH, et al, eds, Washington, DC: ASM Press, 2003, 1039-73.

Antimicrobial Susceptibility Testing, Anaerobic Bacteria

Related Information

Abscess Aerobic and Anaerobic Culture *on page 360*

Synonyms Anaerobic Bacterial Susceptibility; MIC, Anaerobic Bacteria; Susceptibility Testing, Antimicrobial, Anaerobic Bacteria

Special Instructions The laboratory should be consulted regarding appropriateness and scope of anaerobic susceptibility testing in a particular clinical setting.

Specimen Viable pure culture of anaerobic organism

Turnaround Time 2-5 days from time organism is isolated and identified

Reference Range See table on next page.

Use Susceptibility testing of anaerobes is not performed automatically or routinely. Susceptibility test results are usually reported on anaerobic bacterial isolates only on special request to the laboratory. It may be indicated for individual patient isolates when the selection of therapeutic agents is critical. This situation may occur because of failure of empiric therapy or because of lack of response to empiric therapy. Difficulty in making empiric decisions due to lack of precedent, specific infections which may be appropriate for the determination of anaerobic susceptibility include brain abscess, endocarditis, osteomyelitis, joint infection, infection of prosthetic devices or vascular grafts.

Limitations Anaerobic infections are frequently mixed involving aerobic and anaerobic flora, thus, the predictive value of an anaerobic susceptibility test for a successful clinical outcome may be limited by the complexity of the clinical infection.

Contraindications Anaerobe isolate from patient is not available or fails to give adequate growth for susceptibility testing.

Methodology Broth microdilution and agar dilution methods; beta-lactamase testing

Additional Information At present, routine susceptibility testing of anaerobic isolates is not recommended. Infections involving anaerobes frequently contain mixed flora and appropriate drainage rather than antimicrobial therapy seems to be the most crucial factor in the successful treatment of these infections.

Indications for anaerobic susceptibility testing include:

- determination of susceptibility of anaerobes to new antimicrobial agents
- monitoring susceptibility patterns by geographic area
- monitoring susceptibility patterns in local hospitals
- assisting in the management of selected individual patients.

Many anaerobes grow so slowly that by the time isolation and susceptibility testing is completed (6-14 days), the results are of little clinical value. Most anaerobes have very predictable *in vitro* susceptibility patterns that appear to have changed little over the years. For these reasons, many laboratories perform anaerobic susceptibility testing only on anaerobic isolates from blood, pleural fluid, peritoneal fluid, and CSF. In cases of chronic anaerobic infections (septic arthritis, osteomyelitis, etc), susceptibility testing may be done by special request. The physician should contact the laboratory regarding the specific antibiotic(s) to be tested and the testing method (broth disk, MICs, etc) available.

Organisms that are recognized as virulent (ie, *Bacteroides fragilis* group, pigmented *Bacteroides* sp, *Bacteroides gracilis*, certain *Fusobacterium*, *Clostridium perfringens*, and *Clostridium ramosum*) may also be considered for testing.

Selected Readings

Baumgartner JC and Xia T, "Antibiotic Susceptibility of Bacteria Associated With Endodontic Abscesses," *J Endod*, 2003, 29(1):44-7.

Clinical and Laboratory Standards Institute, "Methods for Antimicrobial Susceptibility Testing of Anaerobic Bacteria," Approved Standard, 6th ed, 2004, Document M11-A6.

Golan Y, McDermott LA, Jacobus NV, et al, "Emergence of Fluoroquinolone Resistance Among *Bacteroides* Species," *J Antimicrob Chemother*, 2003, 52(2):208-13.

Hecht DW, "Evolution of Anaerobe Susceptibility Testing in the United States," *Clin Infect Dis*, 2002, 35(Suppl 1):S28-35.

Hecht DW, "Resistance Trends in Anaerobic Bacteria," *Clin Microbiol Newslett*, 2000, 22(6):41-4.

Levison ME, "Anaerobic Pleuropulmonary Infection," *Curr Opin Infect Dis*, 2001, 14(2):187-91.

Rosenblatt JE, "Susceptibility Testing of Anaerobic Bacteria," *Clin Lab Med*, 1989, 9(2):239-54, (review).

Styrt B and Gorbach SL, "Recent Developments in the Understanding of the Pathogenesis and Treatment of Anaerobic Infections," *N Engl J Med*, 1989, Part I, 321(4):240-6 and Part II, 321(5):298-302.

Percent of Anaerobes Susceptible to Antimicrobial Agents

Bacterium	Number of Isolates Tested	β-lactam/β-lactam inhibitor combinations	Penicillin G	Cefotetan	Cefoxitin	Chloramphenicol	Clindamycin	Imienem	Metronidazole
Bacteroides									
B. fragilis	227	97-99	97-98	83	91	100	87	99	100
Others	285	76-100	4-20	10-69	80-90	100	63-81	100	100
Prevotella									
P. melanogenica	17	82-100	82	94	100	100	100	100	94
Others	41	92-100	75	100	100	100	86	100	100
Fusobacterium									
F. necrophorum	10	100	100	100	100	100	100	100	100
F. nucleatum	29	94-100	93	100	100	100	100	100	100
Actinomyces spp	8	88-100	88	88	88	100	75	100	100
Eubacterium spp	45	92-100	96-100	58-85	92-89	100	92-100	100	95-85
Propionibacterium acnes	161	100	100	100	100	100	98	100	13
Lactobacillus spp	70	90-100	97	10	21	90	94	99	4
Clostridium									
C. perfringens	57	100	100	98	100	100	91	100	100
C. difficile	37	100	100	100	29	100	84	100	100
C. innocuum	50	100	100	8	32	100	92	100	100
Others	86	94-100	85-100	91-100	96-100	100	80-100	100	100
Peptostreptococcus									
P. anaerobius	30	74-100	78	68	97	100	100	100	97
Others	316	98-100	93-98	98-100	98-100	100	89-98	100	90-98

Adapted from Koneman EW, Allen SD, Janda WM, et al, Color Atlas and Textbook of Diagnostic Microbiology, 5th ed, Philadelphia, PA: Lippincott-Raven Publishers, 1997, 718-9. Adapted from data generated by the Indiana University Medical Center Anaerobe Laboratory, and are based on 1997 breakpoints established by the National Committee for Clinical Laboratory Standards.

Antimycobacterial Susceptibility Testing

Related Information Mycobacteria Culture, Biopsy or Body Fluid *on page 539*

Synonyms Mycobacteria, Susceptibility Testing; Susceptibility Testing, Mycobacteria

Test Includes Panel of antimycobacterial agents tested against isolates at appropriate concentrations

Specimen Pure isolate of an organism

Causes for Rejection Specimen not available for testing.

Turnaround Time 4-6 weeks after organism is isolated

Use Determine the susceptibility of the isolated organism to a panel of antimycobacterial agents

Limitations Susceptibilities cannot be reported if the organism fails to grow on test media.

Methodology Agar dilution. Some laboratories use commercial broth systems to determine susceptibility to some antimycobacterial agents. The CDC recommends this broth method. See table.

Antimicrobials Commonly Used for Mycobacterial Susceptibility Testing

Antituberculosis Drugs		
Primary	**Secondary**	**Alternatives**
Ethambutol	Capreomycin	Amikacin
Isoniazid	Cycloserine	Ciprofloxacin
Pyrazinamide	Ethionamide	Ofloxacin
Rifampin	Kanamycin	Rifabutin
	Para-aminosalicylate	Rifapentine
	Streptomycin	
Other Mycobacterial Isolates[1]		
Amikacin	Ethambutol	Rifabutin
Azithromycin	Ethionamide	Rifampin
Cefoxitin	Imipenem	Streptomycin
Clarithromycin	Isoniazid	Sulfonamides
Ciprofloxacin	Minocycline	Tobramycin
Doxycycline		

[1]Drug regimens will depend on the mycobacterial species identified.

Additional Information Susceptibilities are usually performed on the first organism isolated from a patient, and at 3- to 6-month intervals if that organism continues to be isolated while the patient is on therapy. Susceptibility tests should be performed in patients with recurrent tuberculosis as resistant strains are common in recurrent infection. Failure to take all drugs in a multidrug regimen can lead to a shift toward resistant organisms and treatment failure. Atypical or environmental mycobacteria, particularly stains of the *M. avium* complex, have variable susceptibility within species. Frequently, they are resistant to oral therapy.

Selected Readings

Clinical and Laboratory Standards Institute, "Susceptibility Testing of Mycobacteria, Nocardiae, and Other Aerobic Actinomycetes," Approved Standard, 2003, Document M24-A.

Grassi C, "New Drugs for Tuberculosis," *Expert Opin Investig Drugs*, 1997, 6(9):1211-26.

Van Scoy RE and Wilkowske CJ, "Antimycobacterial Therapy," *Mayo Clin Proc*, 1999, 74:1038-48.

Woods GL, "Mycobacterial Susceptibility Testing and Reporting: When, How, and What to Test," *Clin Microbiol Newslett*, 2005, 27(9):67.

Antistreptococcal DNase-B Titer *see* Antideoxyribonuclease-B Titer, Serum *on page 376*

Antistreptolysin O Titer, Serum

Related Information

Antideoxyribonuclease-B Titer, Serum *on page 376*

Streptozyme *on page 589*

Synonyms ASO

Specimen Serum

Container Red top tube or serum separator tube

Causes for Rejection Excessive hemolysis

Reference Range Less than 2 years of age: usually <50 Todd units; 2-5 years: <100 Todd units; 5-19 years: <166 Todd units; adults: <125 Todd units. A rise in titer of four or more dilution increments from acute to convalescent specimens is considered to be significant regardless of the magnitude of the titer. For a single specimen, ASO titers ≤166 Todd units are considered normal, but higher titers may be "normal" in demographic groups, or may be associated with chronic pharyngeal carriage.

(Continued)

Antistreptolysin O Titer, Serum *(Continued)*

Use Document streptococcal infection. A marked rise in titer or a persistently elevated titer indicates that a *Streptococcus* infection or poststreptococcal sequelae are present. Elevated titers are seen in 80% to 85% of patients with acute rheumatic fever and in 95% of patients with acute glomerulonephritis.

Limitations False-positive ASO titers can be caused by increased levels of serum betalipoprotein produced in liver disease and by contamination of the serum with *Bacillus cereus* and *Pseudomonas* sp. ASO is usually not formed as a result of streptococcal pyoderma. Test is subject to technical false-positives due to oxidation of reagents.

Methodology Hemolysis inhibition, latex agglutination (LA)

Additional Information Streptolysin is a cytolysin produced by group A streptococci. In an infected individual streptolysin O acts as a protein antigen, and the patient mounts an antibody response. A rise in titer begins about 1 week after infection and peaks 2-4 weeks later. In the absence of complications or reinfection, the ASO titer will usually fall to preinfection levels within 6-12 months. Both clinical and laboratory findings should be correlated in reaching a diagnosis.

Selected Readings

Ayoub EM and Harden E, "Immune Response to Streptococcal Antigens: Diagnostic Methods," *Manual of Clinical Laboratory Immunology*, 5th ed, Rose NR, Conway de Macario E, Folds JD, et al, eds, Washington, DC: American Society for Microbiology, 1997, 450-7.

Arbovirus Serology *see* Encephalitis Viral Serology *on page 452*
ARD, Blood Culture *see* Blood Culture, Aerobic and Anaerobic *on page 391*
Arterial Line Culture *see* Intravenous Line Culture *on page 511*
Arthritis Series, X-ray *see* Bone Films *on page 396*

Arthrocentesis

Synonyms Closed Joint Aspiration; Joint Tap

Test Includes Passing a needle into a joint space and aspirating synovial fluid for diagnostic analysis

Patient Preparation Procedure and risks are explained and consent is obtained. No intravenous pain medications or sedatives are required.

Aftercare Determined by results of procedure, as outlined by physician. May range from joint immobilization with passive range of motion, as in septic arthritis, to full weight bearing, as in effusions secondary to osteoarthritis. No specific joint positioning postprocedure has been demonstrated to reduce complications.

Complications Arthrocentesis is usually a safe procedure, especially when performed on an easily accessible joint such as the knee. Potential complications include:

- iatrogenic joint space infection (if properly performed, incidence has been estimated at 1 in 15,000 cases)
- hemorrhage or hematoma formation (usually when alternative approaches are used and blood vessels are ruptured on the flexor surface of the joint)
- local pain caused by needle trauma to the periosteum
- injury to cartilage, particularly problematic due to slow repair rate
- tendon rupture
- nerve palsies

Equipment Alcohol swabs, povidone-iodine prep solution, sterile gloves and towels, gauze, and forceps. Local anesthesia with ethyl chloride vinyl spray and/or lidocaine 1% with appropriate syringes and subcutaneous needles. If the joint to be aspirated is large, use 18- or 20-gauge 1.5" needle on a 20 mL syringe (additional syringes should be available). If joint is small or effusion minimal, use 20- or 22-gauge 1.5" needle on 3 mL syringe. In this latter case, additional tubes for fluid collection will not be needed. Otherwise, use three sterile tubes for collection, the first one with either EDTA additive or a small amount of heparin. If gonococcal arthritis is suspected, obtain chocolate (Thayer-Martin) media. Glass slides and polarized microscope are necessary if crystalline arthropathy is suspected.

Technique The following description details the technique of knee arthrocentesis, a joint commonly aspirated by the generalist. Patient is instructed to lie supine and remain relaxed. Physician selects the type of approach: suprapatellar, parapatellar, or infrapatellar. The parapatellar approach is popular and effective with tense effusions. Here, the knee is placed in 20° flexion to relax the quadriceps. The preferred entry site is the midportion of the patella (approximately 2 cm superior to the inferior portion of the patella), preferably the medial aspect. This site is marked by indenting the skin with the retracted end of a ballpoint pen. The skin is prepped with alcohol first then povidone-iodine. Some clinicians prefer strict aseptic technique (5-minute scrub, masks, gowns, and drapes) whereas others do not use even sterile gloves or drapes. We prefer a middle-ground approach, using sterile gloves and drapes but foregoing masks and gowns. The use of local anesthesia also varies amongst practitioners. If the joint is tense, and anatomical landmarks easily palpable, we prefer cutaneous anesthesia with only a spray of ethyl chloride solution. Alternatively, a subcutaneous

wheal of lidocaine may be raised in the usual fashion. Injection of lidocaine into deeper structures is not usually required (where it may potentially interfere with culture results because of bacteriostatic properties). Following this, the needle-on-syringe is passed through the marked skin site and advanced slowly while aspirating. A "pop" may be felt as the needle penetrates the capsule. The needle should be directed parallel to the plane of the synovial capsule if the parapatellar approach is used. Once fluid is returned, the needle should not be advanced further in order to avoid cartilage damage. Only mild suction should be used to aspirate so that trauma and hemorrhage do not occur. In general, joint effusions should be drained completely. A blind "search" with the needle (often with vigorous aspiration) is hazardous and should not be attempted. Forceps may be used to stabilize the needle if several syringe changes are required. Once completed, withdraw the needle, apply pressure, and place adhesive tape over puncture site. If persistent pain is encountered during the procedure, trauma to cartilage or periosteum is likely. Do not reflexly anesthetize these deeper tissues with lidocaine; instead, withdraw the needle and redirect it along a new plane. Correct placement of the needle in the joint space is normally painless. In the case of a "dry tap," folds of synovium may be acting as a valve obstructing the needle lumen. Reposition the needle slightly, or if there is fluid in the syringe, inject a small amount to clear the needle bevel. This problem can be avoided by using the infrapatellar approach. The technique for suprapatellar and infrapatellar aspiration has been detailed elsewhere. The suprapatellar approach is most useful in tense effusions where the suprapatellar bursa (usually in communication with the joint space) is visibly distended. While easily performed, there is a potential for sinus tract formation especially if the entry site is directly over the bursa, rather than several centimeters away. The infrapatellar approach has a low risk of cartilage damage compared with the parapatellar approach and is useful for patients with marked flexion contractures of the knee. However, clinicians may not be familiar with the technical details of this approach. Similar principles apply to aspiration of joints other than the knee.

Data Acquired A wide array of tests on synovial fluid is available. Routine tests on effusions of unknown etiology include: cell count, glucose, Gram stain and routine culture, and microscopic examination for crystals (urate, calcium, pyrophosphate dihydrate). Optional tests include: viscosity, mucin clot test, uric acid level, and culture for *Neisseria gonorrhoeae*, tuberculosis, fungi, *Mycoplasma pneumoniae*, nontuberculous, acid-fast bacteria, etc. Occasionally, ordered tests include: synovial fluid protein, LDH, cytology, rheumatoid factor, complement.

Specimen Synovial fluid

Container For small fluid volumes, send capped syringe without needle to laboratory; otherwise, fluid may be carefully transferred to sterile tubes.

Collection Tube 1: Gram stain and culture; tube 2: mucin clot, if ordered (no heparin); tube 3: (add heparin or EDTA) cell count, chemistries, crystals, additional studies. If gonococcal arthritis is suspected, chocolate (Thayer-Martin) agar should be available either at the bedside or during specimen processing in the microbiology laboratory.

Storage Instructions Specimen should be hand carried to the laboratory. Delay in processing may cause spuriously low synovial fluid glucose levels or false-negative results.

Normal Findings In the absence of disease, synovial fluid usually cannot be aspirated. Normal synovial fluid is clear and viscous. A drop placed between the thumb and forefinger (or two microscope slides) can form a string >2 cm long as the fingers are separated, indicating high viscosity. Similarly, the mucin clot test is performed by adding 1 mL of synovial fluid to a 5% solution of acetic acid. Normally, a firm clot forms. Both tests reflect high viscosity of synovial fluid caused by leukocyte hyaluronic acid. Cell count and differential normally reveal <200 WBCs/mm^3 with <25% neutrophils. Chemistries show protein <2 g/dL, uric acid <8 mg/dL, synovial glucose nearly equal to serum glucose, and synovial LDH less than serum LDH. Gram stain and cultures are negative (acellular).

Critical Values Abnormal synovial fluid can be divided into four diagnostic categories. Considerable overlap exists among these categories and correlation with the clinical presentation is required.

Group I synovial fluids are seen commonly in degenerative joint disease (osteoarthritis) and trauma. Fluid is clear or yellow tinged, viscous and mucin clot firm. WBC count is <200/mm^3 with <25% neutrophils (often mononuclears >50%). Chemistries including glucose are normal and microbiologic cultures are negative. This is considered a "noninflammatory" effusion. Some inflammatory conditions may at times cause a group I fluid, such as acute rheumatic fever and systemic lupus erythematosus.

Group II fluids are "inflammatory" in nature. Diseases leading to this category include: crystal-induced arthropathies (gout, CPPD or "pseudogout"), rheumatoid arthritis, connective tissue diseases (SLE, polymyositis, etc), ankylosing spondylitis and other seronegative spondyloarthropathies (Reiter's syndrome, psoriatic arthritis), and acute rheumatic fever. Synovial fluid appears opaque and turbid from cellular fragmentation. Viscosity is similar to water and the "string test" yields only short strings. Mucin

(Continued)

Arthrocentesis *(Continued)*

clot testing results in a friable gel rather than a tight, rope-like clot. WBC counts are elevated, 5000-75,000/mm^3 with >50% neutrophils. Synovial glucose tends to be lower than serum glucose, especially if synovial WBCs are elevated (neutrophils consume glucose). Gram stain and cultures are negative.

Group III effusions are characteristic of septic arthritis. Fluid appears grossly turbid and may be frankly purulent. WBC count as a rule is >50,000/mm^3 and may be >1,000,000/mm^3. Differential shows preponderance of neutrophils (>90%), with the exception of tuberculous arthritis where lymphocytes may comprise 50% of leukocytes. Synovial glucose is characteristically <50% of simultaneous serum glucose and this finding strongly suggests septic arthritis. Glucose values <10 mg/dL have been reported and support classification into group III (rather than group II) in cases where WBC count is moderately elevated. However, sensitivity of low glucose levels in the septic joint is approximately 50%. Gram stain yield in group III effusions varies with the bacteria isolated. In patients with staphylococcal septic arthritis, the Gram stain is diagnostic in 75% of cases in patients with gram-negative arthritis, 50% of Gram stains are diagnostic, but with gonococcal arthritis, only 25% of Gram stains are positive. In nongonococcal septic arthritis, the bacterial culture is more helpful than the Gram stain, the former being positive in 85% to 95% of cases (provided no recent antibiotic use). However, with gonococcal arthritis, the culture is less sensitive, with only a 25% positive yield.

Group IV synovial effusions are grossly hemorrhagic. Etiologies include: systemic abnormalities (eg, excessive heparin anticoagulation, severe thrombocytopenia) and local joint pathology (eg, femur fracture, neuropathic joint).

As mentioned earlier, diagnostic groups are not mutually exclusive. Certain disease entities may fall into more than one diagnostic category. For example, synovial fluid in acute rheumatic fever may appear as either a group I or a group II effusion; neuropathic arthropathy may appear as group I or IV, and lupus-associated effusions as group I or II. In addition, an individual patient may suffer from more than one pathologic process over the course of time. For example, a joint effusion from rheumatoid arthritis (group II effusion) maybe a predisposing factor to the later development of bacterial arthritis (group III) and both may be present in the same patient. Finally, some diseases may change from one diagnostic category to another over a short time period. For example, septic arthritis in an early stage may present with a low synovial WBC count and normal glucose (group I) and only later on progress to a typical septic arthritis (group III) picture on subsequent arthrocentesis.

Use Diagnostic indications include:

- joint effusions of unknown etiology
- arthritis of unclear etiology
- all cases of suspected infectious arthritis (bacterial, fungal, tuberculous)
- confirmation of a diagnosis strongly suspected on clinical grounds, such as suspected gout in patients with podagra
- monitoring synovial fluid response to antibiotic therapy in established cases of septic arthritis

Therapeutic indications include:

- decompression of a tense, painful joint effusion
- evacuation of pus in bacterial arthritis (repeated closed drainage)
- removal of inflammatory cells and crystals in selected cases of gout or pseudogout
- intra-articular injection of corticosteroids

Contraindications

- local infection along the proposed needle entrance tract (eg, overlying cellulitis, periarticular infection)
- uncooperative patient, especially if unable to keep the joint immobile throughout procedure
- difficulty identifying boney landmarks
- a poorly accessible joint space, as in hip aspiration in the obese patient
- inability to demonstrate a joint effusion on physical examination, except when septic arthritis is strongly suspected (and effusions may be barely detectable)

In addition, some authors consider bacteremia (documented or suspected) a contraindication to arthrocentesis based on the theoretical concern of seeding a sterile joint when the entering needle ruptures surrounding capillaries. No data is available to support or refute this and clinical judgment must be individualized in each case. If infectious arthritis is suspected, arthrocentesis should be promptly performed even with documented bacteremia. However, more elective indications for the procedure, such as corticosteroid injection, should be deferred, at physician's discretion.

Additional Information Arthrocentesis is indispensable for the accurate diagnosis (or exclusion) of septic arthritis and crystal-induced arthropathy and therein lies its greatest utility. Despite the difficulties with the classification scheme described above, synovial fluid findings in both these treatable conditions is often pathognomonic. Practically, the procedure carries a low risk of complications and can be performed in minutes when an accessible joint is involved. The general physician often handles aspirations of the knee, elbow, and first metatarsal phalangeal joint. When septic arthritis is suspected in a less accessible area, such as the sacroiliac joint, aspiration should not be delayed due to a lack of familiarity. Rheumatologic or orthopedic consultation should be obtained.

Selected Readings

Concoff AI and Kalunian KC, "What Is the Relation Between Crystals and Osteoarthritis?" *Curr Opin Rheumatol*, 1999, 11(5):436-40.

Dubost JJ, Fis I, Denis P, et al, "Polyarticular Septic Arthritis," *Medicine (Baltimore)*, 1993, 72(5):296-310.

Dubost JJ, Soubrier M, and Sauvezie B, "Pyogenic Arthritis in Adults," *Joint Bone Spine*, 2000, 67(1):11-21.

Gatter RA, "Arthrocentesis Technique and Intrasynovial Therapy," *Arthritis and Allied Conditions: A Textbook of Rheumatology*, 11th ed, Chapter 39, McCarty DJ, ed, Philadelphia, PA: Lea & Febiger, 1989.

Mader JT, Shirtliff ME, Bergquist S, et al, "Bone and Joint Infections in the Elderly: Practical Treatment Guidelines," *Drugs Aging*, 2000, 16(1):67-80.

Schumacher HR Jr, "Arthritis of Recent Onset. A Guide to Evaluation and Initial Therapy for Primary Care Physicians," *Postgrad Med*, 1995, 97(4):52-4, 57-9, 63.

Shetty AK and Gedalia A, "Septic Arthritis in Children," *Rheum Dis Clin North Am*, 1998, 24(2):287-304.

Arthrogram

Synonyms Joint Study

Applies to Ankle Arthrogram; Elbow Arthrogram; Hip Arthrogram; Knee Arthrogram; Shoulder Arthrogram; Temporomandibular Joint Arthrogram; Wrist Arthrogram

Patient Preparation Informed consent is obtained

Aftercare No strenuous activity involving the joint of interest for 24 hours.

Equipment 22-gauge needle, contrast medium, and fluoroscopic and x-ray equipment

Technique Local anesthesia is instilled at the appropriate site. A small gauge needle is inserted into the joint space. Any fluid within the joint space is aspirated and sent for appropriate chemical or bacteriologic analysis. Contrast medium and air are then inserted into the joint space under fluoroscopic guidance. Radiographs and occasionally tomograms are then obtained in multiple projections.

Data Acquired Visualization of the components of the joint space including the cartilage, ligaments, menisci, and connecting bursa

Normal Findings The joint space should not contain fluid. The cartilaginous surfaces and menisci should be smooth without evidence for erosions, tears, or disintegration.

Use Evaluate damage to the cartilage, ligaments, and bony structures composing the joint

Limitations Large joint effusions can be difficult to aspirate completely, thus resulting in dilution of the contrast material and poor visualization of the joint space structures.

Contraindications Bleeding abnormalities

Selected Readings

Goldman AB, "Arthrography for Rheumatic Disease. When Why, and for Whom," *Rheum Dis Clin North Am*, 1991, 17(3):505-42.

Mader JT, Shirtliff ME, Bergquist S, et al, "Bone and Joint Infections in the Elderly: Practical Treatment Guidelines," *Drugs Aging*, 2000, 16(1):67-80.

Resnick D, "Arthrography, Tenography and Bursography," *Diagnosis of Bone and Joint Disorders*, 2nd ed, Resnick D and Niwayama G, eds, Philadelphia, PA: WB Saunders Co, 1988, 302-444.

Arthropod Identification

Synonyms Ectoparasite Identification; Insect Identification

Applies to *Cimex* Identification; *Ixodes scapularis* Identification; *Pediculus humanus* Identification; *Phthirus pubis* Identification; *Sarcoptes scabiei* Skin Scrapings Identification; Bed Bugs Identification; Body Lice Identification; Crab Lice Identification; Deer Tick Identification; Flea Identification; Head Lice Identification; Lice Identification; Mite Identification; Nits Identification; Pubic Lice Identification; Skin Scrapings for *Sarcoptes scabiei* Identification; Tick Identification

Specimen Gross arthropod, skin scrapings

Container Screw cap tube or screw cap jar

Collection Arthropods (gross) are to be submitted in alcohol (70%) or formaldehyde in tube or container with secure closure. To establish the diagnosis of scabies, skin scrapings may be collected with a scalpel and a drop of mineral oil. The liquid may be examined directly or alternatively the organism may be teased away from its burrow or papule with a needle or scalpel.

Storage Instructions Room temperature, fill the container with preservative as completely as possible to avoid damage to the specimen by air bubbles in the container

(Continued)

Arthropod Identification *(Continued)*

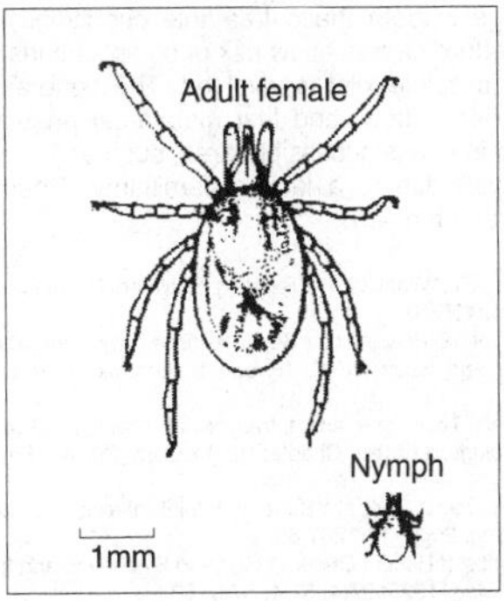

Black-legged (deer) tick (*Ixodes scapularis*)

Turnaround Time 1-2 hours; if referral to a state or federal laboratory is required, 2-4 weeks

Reference Range No arthropod identified

Use Identify arthropods affecting humans; establish the presence of ectoparasite infestation

Methodology Macroscopic evaluation

Selected Readings

Belman AL, "Tick-Borne Diseases," *Semin Pediatr Neurol*, 1999, 6(4):249-66.

Coon D and Versalovic J, "Tick-Borne Disease: A Review of the More Common Entities Found in the Northeastern United States," *Clin Microbiol Newslett*, 2002, 24(2):9-14.

Fritsche TR, "Arthropods of Medical Importance," *Manual of Clinical Microbiology*, 7th ed, Murray PR, Baron EJ, Pfaller MA, et al, eds, Washington, DC: American Society for Microbiology, 1999, 1449-66.

Hobbs GD and Harrell RE Jr, "Brown Recluse Spider Bites: A Common Cause of Necrotic Arachnidism," *Am J Emerg Med*, 1989, 7(3):309-12.

Nelson JA and Bouseman JK, "Human Tick-Borne Illnesses: United States," *Clin Microbiol Newslett*, 1992, 14(14):105-12.

Parola P and Raoult D, "Ticks and Tickborne Bacterial Diseases in Humans: An Emerging Infectious Threat," *Clin Infect Dis*, 2001, 32(6):897-928.

Ascites Fluid Tap *see* Paracentesis *on page 555*

Ascitic Fluid Culture *see* Aerobic Culture, Body Fluid *on page 365*

Ascitic Fluid Cytology *see* Cytology, Body Fluids *on page 438*

Ascitic Fluid Fungus Culture *see* Fungus Culture, Body Fluid *on page 462*

ASO *see* Antistreptolysin O Titer, Serum *on page 383*

***Aspergillus* Immunodiffusion** *see* Fungal Serology *on page 458*

Aspirates for Ova and Parasites *see* Ova and Parasites, Urine or Aspirates *on page 554*

Atypical *Mycobacterium* Smear *see* Acid-Fast Stain *on page 361*

Auramine-Rhodamine Stain *see* Acid-Fast Stain *on page 361*

B19 DNA *see* Parvovirus B19 DNA, Qualitative PCR *on page 559*

Bacterial Antigens, Rapid Detection Methods

Related Information

Group A *Streptococcus* Antigen Test *on page 475*

Group B *Streptococcus* Antigen Test *on page 476*

Synonyms Cerebrospinal Fluid Latex Agglutination for Bacterial Antigens; Latex Agglutination, Bacterial Antigens, Cerebrospinal Fluid

Test Includes Qualitative determination of the presence of antigens of *H. influenzae*, *S. pneumoniae*, *N. meningitidis*. Test may also identify subgroups of above organisms and may include testing for group B *Streptococcus* and *E. coli* K1 antigen in neonates. Gram stain and culture are preferable to bacterial antigen testing, and results of Gram stain must be coordinated with antigen testing by knowledgeable laboratory workers.

Abstract Rapid adjunctive tests include latex agglutination, which is more sensitive than coagglutination. False-negative results occur. *Clinical Microbiology Procedures Handbook* (Isenberg HD, ed) indicates that **these latex agglutination tests are not intended as a substitute for bacterial culture. Confirmatory diagnosis of bacterial meningitis infection is possible only with appropriate culture procedures.**

Similar observations are published by others as well. Concentration of antigen depends on variables including the number of bacteria, the duration of infection, and the presence or absence of specific antibodies which may prevent antigen detection. Several publications recognize these tests' shortcomings and describe the rapid diagnostic tests as not essential but note that they may be helpful in establishing an etiologic diagnosis rapidly.

Patient Preparation Usual aseptic aspiration

Specimen Cerebrospinal fluid, serum, urine

Container Sterile CSF tube, red top tube, sterile urine container

Storage Instructions Keep refrigerated

Reference Range Negative

Use Detect bacterial antigens in CSF for the rapid diagnosis of meningitis. The method may be applied to other body fluids, blood culture supernatants, and urine (depending on the body fluid tested and the test used).

Limitations May be negative in early meningitis. **Does not replace Gram stain and culture.** Group B *Streptococcus* and the *E. coli* K1 antigen are frequently not tested on infants over 6 months of age. The sensitivity of the tests vary from 55% to 100% depending on the specificity of the antibody and the concentration of antigen in the specimen. Nonspecific cross reactions occur. False-positive reactions and nonspecific agglutination occur. Antigenic crossover (cross reactions) are seen (eg, *E. coli* K1 and *N. meningitidis* group B). The sensitivity of commercial antigen detection kits remains imperfect, the sensitivity differing substantially with various organisms and in various clinical series. False-negative results occur, especially those taken early in the disease, with low antigen load. Pneumococcal and *Haemophilus* strains not possessing capsular antigens may not be detected by immunological techniques. Pneumococcal antigen is not detected in urine.

Many authors have stated that these tests are expensive and have, usually, no impact on patient care. Physicians are urged to order only Gram stain and culture. These tests can be used later if stain and culture results are negative. Counterimmunoelectrophoresis is no longer in common clinical use.

Methodology Latex agglutination and coagglutination

Additional Information Antigen detection methods should never be substituted for culture and Gram stain. Culture and Gram stain must always have priority when only very limited quantities of CSF are available.

The rapid diagnosis of group A and group B *Streptococcus* infection is discussed specifically in Group A *Streptococcus* Screen and Group B *Streptococcus* Screen test listings.

Selected Readings

Gray LD and Fedorko DP, "Laboratory Diagnosis of Bacterial Meningitis," *Clin Microbiol Rev*, 1992, 5(2):130-45.

Mein J and Lum G, "CSF Bacterial Antigen Detection Tests Offer No Advantage Over Gram's Stain in the Diagnosis of Bacterial Meningitis," *Pathology*, 1999, 31(1):67-9.

Negrini B, Kelleher KJ, and Wald ER, "Cerebrospinal Fluid Findings in Aseptic Versus Bacterial Meningitis," *Pediatrics*, 2000, 105(2):316-9.

Tarafdar K, Rao S, Recco RA, et al, "Lack of Sensitivity of the Latex Agglutination Test to Detect Bacterial Antigen in the Cerebrospinal Fluid of Patients With Culture-Negative Meningitis," *Clin Infect Dis*, 2001, 33(3):406-8.

Thomas JG, "Routine CSF Antigen Detection for Agents Associated With Bacterial Meningitis: Another Point of View," *Clin Microbiol Newslett*, 1994, 16(12):89-95.

Thomas JG, "Survey Results of Routine CSF Antigen Detection: Nothing to Be Proud Of," *Clin Microbiol Newslett*, 1994, 16(24):187-91.

Bacterial Inhibitory Level, Serum *see* Serum Bactericidal Test *on page 578*

Bacterial Smear *see* Gram Stain *on page 473*

Bacteria Screen, Urine *see* Leukocyte Esterase, Urine *on page 520*

Basement Membrane Antibodies *see* Skin Biopsy, Immunofluorescence *on page 583*

B Cells *see* Lymphocyte Subset Panels *on page 531*

bDNA Testing for HIV *see* HIV-1 RNA, Quantitative bDNA, 3rd Generation *on page 499*

Bed Bugs Identification *see* Arthropod Identification *on page 387*

Beta-Hemolytic Strep Culture, Throat *see* Throat Culture for Group A Beta-Hemolytic *Streptococcus on page 594*

Biopsy *see* Histopathology *on page 496*

Biopsy Culture, Aerobic *see* Biopsy Culture, Routine *on page 390*

Biopsy Culture, Anaerobic *see* Anaerobic Culture *on page 371*

Biopsy Culture, Fungus *see* Fungus Culture, Biopsy *on page 461*

Biopsy Culture, Routine

Related Information

Anaerobic Culture *on page 371*
Histopathology *on page 496*

Applies to *Brucella* Culture, Tissue; Aerobic Culture, Tissue; Biopsy Culture, Aerobic; Culture, Biopsy; Cyst Culture, Aerobic; Surgical Specimen Culture, Routine; Tissue Culture, *Brucella*; Tissue Culture, Routine

Patient Preparation Aseptic preparation of biopsy site

Special Instructions The following information must be provided to the laboratory and will assist the laboratory in the proper processing of the specimen; specific site of specimen, current antibiotic therapy, age and sex of patient, collection time and date, and clinical diagnosis.

Specimen Surgical tissue, bone marrow, biopsy material from normally sterile site or aseptically aspirated body fluid

Container Sterile container with lid, no preservative. Bone marrow aspirates and body fluids may be directly inoculated into blood culture media.

Collection The portion of the biopsy specimen submitted for culture should be separated from the portion submitted for histopathology by the surgeon or pathologist utilizing sterile technique.

Storage Instructions Transport specimen to the laboratory immediately.

Causes for Rejection Specimen not received in appropriate sterile container, specimen received in preservative, excessive delay in transport. If an unacceptable specimen is received the nursing station will be notified and another specimen will be requested before disposal of the original specimen.

Turnaround Time Preliminary reports are available at 24 hours. Cultures with no growth will be reported after 48 hours. Reports on specimens from which pathogens are isolated require a minimum of 48 hours for completion.

Reference Range No growth

Use Isolate and identify organisms causing infections in tissue

Limitations If anaerobes are suspected submit a properly collected specimen.

Additional Information The specimen should be obtained before empiric antimicrobial therapy is started.

Selected Readings

Bowler PG, Duerden BI, and Armstrong DG, "Wound Microbiology and Associated Approaches to Wound Management," *Clin Microbiol Rev*, 2001, 14(2):244-69.

Sharkawy A, Low DE, Saginur R, et al, "Severe Group a Streptococcal Soft-Tissue Infections in Ontario: 1992-1996," *Clin Infect Dis*, 2002, 34(4):454-60.

Biopsy *Legionella* Culture *see Legionella pneumophila* Culture *on page 516*

Biopsy of Lung (Transbronchial) for *Pneumocystis* *see Pneumocystis jiroveci* Test *on page 566*

Bioterrorism Agent *see* Blood Culture, *Brucella on page 394*

Bioterrorism Agents

Related Information

Bacillus anthracis on page 41
Brucella Species *on page 61*
Clostridium botulinum on page 83
Francisella tularensis on page 149
Variola *on page 350*
Yersinia pestis on page 355

Synonyms Agents of Bioterrorism

Special Instructions These agents are considered extremely dangerous to individual and public health and security. In cases of suspected bioterrorism, all aspects of specimen selection, collection, and testing vary with the suspected agent and should involve appropriate local, state, and national public health officials and law enforcement agencies. All diagnostic/clinical laboratories should be able to advise physicians in the aforementioned issues. It is imperative that physicians, laboratorians, and other healthcare workers:

- remain alert for the possibility and presentation of cases of disease caused by these and other agents of bioterrorism and
- be aware of necessary, mandatory, and immediate communication between local, state, and national public health officials and law enforcement agencies.

Additional Information Biological terrorism is the international use of bacteria, fungi, viruses, or toxins to (1) produce death or disease in humans, animals, or plants, and/or (2) intimidate governments or societies to promote an ideolistic cause or belief. Currently, the CDC has classified 31 agents which are more likely to be used as agents of bioterrorism and which can be classified into four biological groups (bacteria, viruses, protozoa, or toxins) and into three functional categories (A, B, and C). An agent is placed into category A, B, or C depending on its ease of transmission,

severity of morbidity/mortality it inflicts, and likelihood of use. Six of these agents have been placed into category A and have been given the highest priority:

- variola major (smallpox)
- *Yersinia pestis* (plague)
- *Bacillus anthracis* (anthrax)
- *Francisella tularensis* (tularensis)
- *Clostridium botulinum* toxin (botulism)
- hemorrhagic viruses (viral hemorrhagic fevers)

A member of category B also has been designated a status of highest priority:

- *Brucella* species

Selected Readings

Gilchrist MJR, McKinney WP, Miller JM, et al, "Laboratory Safety, Management, and Diagnosis of Biological Agents Associated With Bioterrorism," *Cumitech 33*, Synder JW, ed, Washington, D.C.: ASM Press, 2000.

Khardori N and Kanchanapoom T, "Overview of Biological Terrorism: Potential Agents and Preparedness," *Clin Microbiol Newslett*, 2005, 27(1):1.

Klietmann WF and Ruoff KL, "Bioterrorism: Implications for the Clinical Microbiologist," *Clin Microbiol Rev*, 2001, 14(2):364-81.

Miller JM, "Bioterrorism - A Perspective for the Community Hospital," *Clin Microbiol Newslett*, 2001, 23(23):179-86.

Perez-Castrillon JL, Bachiller-Luque P, Martin-Luquero M, et al, "Tularemia Epidemic in Northwestern Spain: Clinical Description and Therapeutic Response," *Clin Infect Dis*, 2001, 33(4):573-6.

Varkey P, Poland GA, Cockerill FR 3rd, et al, "Confronting Bioterrorism: Physicians on the Front Line," *Mayo Clin Proc*, 2002, 77(7):661-72.

Blastomycosis Immunodiffusion *see* Fungal Serology *on page 458*

Blind Liver Biopsy *see* Liver Biopsy *on page 521*

Blood Cell Profile *see* Complete Blood Count *on page 420*

Blood Count *see* Complete Blood Count *on page 420*

Blood Culture, Aerobic and Anaerobic

Related Information

Blood Culture, Fungus *on page 395*

Blood Culture, Mycobacteria *on page 395*

Synonyms Aerobic Blood Culture; Anaerobic Blood Culture; Culture, Blood

Applies to ARD, Blood Culture; Antimicrobial Removal Device (ARD) Blood Culture; Blood Culture With Antimicrobial Removal Device (ARD); Blood Culture, Lysis Centrifugation

Test Includes Isolation of both aerobic and anaerobic bacteria and susceptibility testing on all significant isolates

Patient Preparation The major difficulty in interpretation of blood cultures is contamination by skin flora. This difficulty can be markedly reduced by careful attention to the details of skin preparation and antisepsis prior to collection of the specimen.

After location of the vein by palpation, the venipuncture site should be vigorously scrubbed and cleansed with 70% alcohol (isopropyl or ethyl) and then swabbed in a circular motion concentrically from the center outward using tincture of iodine or a povidone iodine solution. **The iodine should be allowed to dry before the venipuncture is undertaken.** If palpation is required during the venipuncture, the glove covering the palpating finger tip should be disinfected.

In iodine sensitive patients, a double alcohol, green soap, or acetone alcohol preparation may be substituted.

Aftercare Iodine used in the skin preparation should be carefully removed from the skin after venipuncture.

Special Instructions The requisition should state current antibiotic therapy and clinical diagnosis.

Specimen Blood. The yield of positives is not increased by culturing arterial blood even in endocarditis.

Container Bottles of trypticase soy broth or other standard medium, one vented (for aerobes), one unvented (for anaerobes)

Collection A single blood culture is rarely indicated and to be discouraged unless medically necessary. More than three cultures in 24 hours is also not indicated (not necessary). Ideally, 2-3 cultures (1 hour apart) taken over 24 hours is adequate to recover bacteria causing septicemia.

Blood cultures should be drawn prior to initiation of antimicrobial therapy. If more than one culture is ordered at the same time (such should be ordered only in medically urgent situations), the specimens should be drawn from separately prepared sites. A syringe and needle, transfer set or pre-evacuated set of tubes containing culture media may be used to collect blood. Collection tubes should be held below the level

(Continued)

Blood Culture, Aerobic and Anaerobic *(Continued)*

of the venipuncture to avoid reflux. A sample volume of 10-20 mL (more is always better) in adults, 1-5 mL in pediatric patients is usually collected for each set.

If a syringe and needle or transfer set is used, the top of the blood culture bottles should also be aseptically prepared with alcohol only. See table.

Blood Culture Collection

Clinical Disease Suspected	Culture Recommendation	Rational
Sepsis, meningitis osteomyelitis, septic arthritis, bacterial pneumonia	Two cultures - one from each of two prepared sites, the second drawn after a brief time interval, then begin therapy.	Assure sufficient sampling in cases of intermittent or low level bacteremia. Minimize the confusion caused by a positive culture resulting from transient bacteremia or skin contamination.
Fever of unknown origin (eg, occult abscess, empyema, typhoid fever, etc)	Two cultures - one from each of two prepared sites, the second drawn after a brief time interval (30 minutes). If cultures are negative after 24-48 hours obtain two more cultures, preferably prior to an anticipated temperature rise.	The yield after four cultures is minimal. A maximum of three sets per patient per day for 3 consecutive days is recommended.
Endocarditis:		
Acute and subacute	Obtain at least four blood cultures.	The following will be positive for a typical microorganism consistent with infective endocarditis: • at least two positive blood cultures drawn more than 12 hours apart • all of three or a majority of four or more blood cultures (with the first and last drawn at least 1 hour apart)
Immunocompromised host (eg, AIDS):		
Septicemia, fungemia mycobacteremia	Obtain two cultures from each of two prepared sites; consider lysis concentration technique to enhance recovery for fungi and mycobacteria.	Low levels of fungemia and mycobacteremia frequently encountered.
Previous antimicrobial therapy:		
Septicemia, bacteremia; monitor effect of antimicrobial therapy	Obtain two cultures from each of two prepared sites; consider use of antimicrobial removal device (ARD) or increased volume >10 mL/culture.	Recovery of organisms is enhanced by dilution, increased sample volume, and removal of inhibiting antimicrobials.

Transient bacteremia caused by brushing teeth, bowel movements, etc or by local irritations caused by scratching of the skin, may cause positive blood cultures as can contamination by skin flora at the time of collection. Interpretation of results can be enhanced by collecting blood cultures separated by time intervals (1 hour is acceptable and useful). Cultures should be taken as early as possible in the course of a febrile episode.

Storage Instructions Specimens collected in tubes with SPS (sodium polyanetholesulfonate) should be processed without delay. The specimen should be transferred to appropriate blood culture media **immediately** to avoid any possible decrease in yield due to storage or prolonged contact with SPS.

Causes for Rejection Unlabeled bottles are not acceptable.

Interpretation of Positive Blood Cultures

Virtually **any** organism, including normal flora, **can** cause bacteremia.
A negative culture result does not necessarily rule out bacteremia; false-negative results occur when pathogens fail to grow.
A positive culture result does not necessarily indicate bacteremia; false-positive results occur when contaminants grow.
Gram-negative bacilli, anaerobes, and fungi should be considered pathogens until proven otherwise.
The most difficult interpretation problem is to determine whether an organism that is usually considered normal skin flora is a true pathogen.

From Flournoy DJ and Adkins L, "Understanding the Blood Culture Report," *Am J Infect Control*, 1986,14:41-6, with permission.

Turnaround Time Common laboratory procedure is to issue a final culture report after 5-7 days. A preliminary culture report based upon Gram stain and primary subculture is usually available at 24 hours. Positive blood cultures must be reported immediately by telephone and followed with a written report.

Reference Range Negative

Use Isolate and identify potentially pathogenic organisms causing bacteremia, septicemia, meningitis, and other microbiologic states

Limitations Three negative sets of blood cultures in the absence of antimicrobial therapy are usually sufficient to exclude the presence of bacteremia. One set is seldom, if ever, sufficient. Prior antibiotic therapy may cause negative blood cultures or delayed growth. Blood cultures from patients suspected of having *Brucella* or *Leptospira* must be requested as special cultures. Consultation with the laboratory for special culture procedures for the recovery of these organisms prior to collecting the specimen is recommended. See the listings *Leptospira* Culture *on page 518*, and Blood Culture, *Brucella on page 394* for the proper method of collection of these specimens. Yeast often are isolated from routine blood cultures. However, if yeast or other fungi are specifically suspected, a separate fungal blood culture should be drawn along with each of the routine blood culture specimens. See separate listing for proper collection of blood fungus culture. *Mycobacterium avium-intracellulare* (MAI) is frequently recovered from blood of immunocompromised patients particularly those with acquired immunodeficiency syndrome, AIDS. Special procedures are required for the recovery of these organisms (ie, lysis filtration concentration or use of a special mycobacteria blood culture medium). Radiometric methods facilitate the recovery of mycobacteria from blood.

Contraindications Use of a 2% iodine preparation is contraindicated in the preparation of patients sensitive to iodine. Green soap may be substituted for the iodine or alcohol acetone alone may be used.

Methodology Early subculture of aerobic bottle; visual, radiometric, or infrared monitoring. Aerobic and anaerobic culture in broth media usually with subculture to blood agar and chocolate agar. In the lysis centrifugation procedure, blood is lysed and centrifuged using a Du Pont Isolator™ tube or similar method. The sediment is divided to media appropriate for growing aerobic and anaerobic bacteria, fungi, and mycobacteria.

Additional Information Sequential blood cultures in nonendocarditis patients and using a 20 mL sample results in an 80% positive yield after the first set, a 90% yield after the second set, and a 99% yield after the third set. **Volume of blood** cultured seems to be more important than the specific culture technique being employed by the laboratory. The isolation of coagulase-negative *Staphylococcus* (CNS) poses a critical and difficult clinical dilemma. Although CNS is the most commonly isolated organism from blood cultures, only a few (6.3%) of the isolates represent "true" clinically significant bacteremia. Conversely, CNS is well recognized as a cause of infections involving prosthetic devices, cardiac valves, CSF shunts, dialysis catheters, and indwelling vascular catheters. Ultimately the physician is responsible for determining whether an organism is a contaminant or a pathogen. The decision is based on both laboratory and clinical data. Frequently this determination includes patient data (ie, patient history), physical examination, body temperatures, clinical course, and laboratory data (ie, culture results, white blood cell count, and differential). Clinical experience and judgment may play a significant role in resolving this clinical dilemma.

The use of a lysis centrifugation system or specific fungal blood culture media have been reported to increase the recovery rate and decrease the time of fungal recovery compared to traditional or biphasic blood culture systems. Recovery of mycobacteria and *Legionella* may also be enhanced by lysis filtration. In patients who have received antimicrobial drugs, four to six blood cultures may be necessary. Any organism isolated from the blood is usually tested for susceptibility. It is not recommended to culture blood while antimicrobials are present unless verification of an agent's efficacy is needed. This is confirmed with a single culture.

The use of antimicrobial removal devices (ARD) or resin bottles to attempt to increase the yield of blood cultures drawn from patients on antimicrobial therapy is controversial. Some microorganisms are occasionally not recovered with the use of ARD blood cultures. It is therefore advised that at least one culture in a series of three be requested without the use of the ARD bottles. ARD blood cultures are substantially more expensive than routine blood cultures. There is no consensus as to the effectiveness of the ARD cultures in enhancing recovery of organisms.

The diagnosis of bacterial meningitis is accomplished by blood culture, as well as culture and examination of the cerebrospinal fluid. Most children with bacterial meningitis are initially bacteremic.

(Continued)

Blood Culture, Aerobic and Anaerobic *(Continued)*

The following bacteria often are considered skin contaminants when they are isolated from only one blood culture of two or more blood cultures within a single 24-hour period.

- alpha-hemolytic *Streptococcus*
- *Micrococcus*
- *Bacillus* sp
- coagulase-negative *Staphylococcus*
- *Corynebacterium* sp (diphtheroids)
- *Propionibacterium* sp

Selected Readings

Aronson MD and Bor DH, "Blood Cultures," *Ann Intern Med*, 1987, 106(2):246-53.

Darouiche RO, "Anti-infective Efficacy of Silver-Coated Medical Prostheses," *Clin Infect Dis*, 1999, 29:1371-7.

Donskey CJ and Rice LB, "The Influence of Antibiotics on Spread of Vancomycin-Resistant Enterococci: The Potential Role of Selective Use of Antibiotics as a Control Measure," *Clin Microbiol Newslett*, 1999, 21(8):57-65.

Li JS, Sexton DJ, Mick N, et al, "Proposed Modifications to the Duke Criteria for the Diagnosis of Infective Endocarditis," *Clin Infect Dis*, 2000, 30(4):633-8.

Blood Culture, AIDS *see* Blood Culture, Mycobacteria *on page 395*

Blood Culture, *Brucella*

Synonyms *Brucella* Blood Culture; Undulant Fever, Culture

Applies to Bioterrorism Agent

Patient Preparation See preparation procedures under listing for Blood Culture, Aerobic and Anaerobic *on page 391.*

Special Instructions The laboratory must be informed of the request for *Brucella* blood culture. Collection time, date, age of patient, current antibiotic therapy, clinical diagnosis, and relevant history.

Specimen Blood

Container Castañeda bottle; *Brucella* broth and agar; conventional trypticase soy broth (TSB)

Collection Should be drawn prior to administration of antibiotics, and before an expected temperature rise. Follow collection procedure in Blood Culture, Aerobic and Anaerobic.

Causes for Rejection Specimens not received in appropriate bottles will have less than optimal yield.

Turnaround Time 6 weeks

Reference Range No growth

Use Establish the diagnosis of brucellosis

Limitations Blood cultures for *Brucella* are primarily useful in the early acute phase of the disease. Recovery of *Brucella* is limited by the relatively low level of bacteremia and the fastidious nature of the organism. Yield may be increased by culturing larger volumes of blood in a conventional trypticase soy broth or use of a lysis centrifugation concentration technique.

Methodology *Brucella* broth and agar culture. Most modern automated blood culture instruments can detect *Brucella* in the standard blood culture incubation time of 5 days. Trypticase soy broth (TSB) cultures yield acceptable results (93% of possible isolates). Blood clot cultures utilizing a variety of methods provide no advantage over more conventional TSB cultures for the isolation of *Brucella melitensis*. *Brucella* may be recovered using the Roche Septi-Chek® system with growth observed on the chocolate section of the paddle. The organism appears as a small slow-growing white colony. It is a gram-negative coccobacillus. **The handling of cultures and specimens as well as the inhalation of dust-containing *Brucella* organisms is dangerous to laboratory workers**. A biologic safety cabinet should be used for all suspected isolates.

Additional Information Bone marrow culture and serologic testing of acute and convalescent specimens for *Brucella* antibodies may be useful when cultures of peripheral blood are negative. In animals, brucellosis has a bacteremic phase followed by localization in the reproductive tract and reticuloendothelial system. The disease is common worldwide, particularly in the countries of the former Soviet Union, Mediterranean, Latin America, and Spain. One hundred and six cases were reported in the U.S. in 1986. Most brucellosis in the U.S. occurs in abattoir workers, farmers and rarely veterinarians. Symptoms may be subclinical, subacute, acute relapsing and chronic. Undulant fever is most typical of *B. melitensis*. Symptoms may include abdominal pain and may mimic appendicitis or cholecystitis. Unpasteurized milk may be a source of infection. Risk factors raising an index of suspicion include travel, food, and occupation. Serologic confirmation of the diagnosis may be helpful. **Note:** *Brucella* is a level B agent of bioterrorism.

Selected Readings

Pappas G, Akritidis N, Bosilkovski M, et al, "Brucellosis," *N Engl J Med*, 2005, 352(22):2325-36.
Shapiro DS and Wong JD, "*Brucella*," *Manual of Clinical Microbiology*, 7th ed, Murray PR, Baron EJ, Pfaller MA, et al, eds, Washington, DC: American Society for Microbiology, 1999, 625-31.
Young EJ, "*Brucella* Species," *Principles and Practice of Infectious Diseases*, 5th ed, Mandell GL, Bennett JE, and Dolin R, eds, New York, NY: Churchill Livingstone, 2000, 2386-93.

Blood Culture for CMV *see* Cytomegalovirus Culture, Blood *on page 439*

Blood Culture, Fungus

Related Information

Blood Culture, Aerobic and Anaerobic *on page 391*

Synonyms Fungus Blood Culture; Fungus Culture, Blood

Test Includes Routine blood culture and inoculation of specific fungal media at time of collection; identification of any fungi isolated

Patient Preparation See Blood Culture, Aerobic and Anaerobic *on page 391.*

Special Instructions Inform the laboratory of the specific request for fungus blood culture. The following information will assist the laboratory in the proper processing of the specimen: specific site of specimen, current antibiotic therapy, age and sex of patient, collection time and date, and clinical diagnosis.

Specimen Blood

Container Routine and special fungal blood culture media

Collection Standard blood culture collection procedures.

Storage Instructions Transport specimen to the laboratory immediately.

Turnaround Time Preliminary reports are usually available in one to two days. Negative cultures are commonly reported at 4-6 weeks.

Reference Range No fungi grown

Use Isolate and identify fungi; establish the diagnosis of fungemia, fungal endocarditis, and disseminated mycosis in immunocompromised patients, oncology patients, transplant patients, patients with leukemia and lymphoma, and patients with the acquired immunodeficiency syndrome (AIDS)

Limitations A single negative culture does not rule out the presence of fungal infection. Fungal blood cultures are most effective in isolating *Candida albicans* and *Candida glabrata* (*Torulopsis glabrata*). If other fungal species are suspected, a biopsy or bone marrow fungus culture should be considered. *Blastomyces dermatitidis* usually is not recovered from blood.

Additional Information Fungemia may complicate therapy with steroids, antineoplastic drugs, radiation therapy, broad-spectrum antibiotic therapy, venous or arterial catheterization, hyperalimentation, and the acquired immunodeficiency syndrome (AIDS). Intravenous drug abusers are prone to *Candida* endocarditis. Although many fungal species including *Histoplasma capsulatum*, *Coccidioides immitis*, *Cryptococcus neoformans*, and many other unusual isolates are recoverable from blood cultures, the most common cause of fungemia is *Candida albicans* followed by other *Candida* sp including *Candida glabrata* (*Torulopsis glabrata*). In most cases fungemia represents a failure of the host defense system. Fungemia may be caused by contamination of an indwelling catheter or, in the critically ill and immunocompromised patient, contamination of the gastrointestinal and less frequently the urinary tract.

Blood Culture, *Leptospira* *see Leptospira* Culture *on page 518*

Blood Culture, Lysis Centrifugation *see* Blood Culture, Aerobic and Anaerobic *on page 391*

Blood Culture, Mycobacteria

Related Information

Blood Culture, Aerobic and Anaerobic *on page 391*

Applies to AIDS Blood Culture; Blood Culture, AIDS

Patient Preparation Usual sterile preparation

Special Instructions Request test specifically. Not part of routine blood culture. Contact the laboratory prior to collecting blood.

Specimen Blood

Container Aerobic blood culture bottle

Storage Instructions Incubate if unable to deliver to the laboratory on the day of collection.

Causes for Rejection Other bacteria present

Use Isolate mycobacteria, especially *M. avium-intracellulare*

Additional Information Mycobacterial usually are identified to genus and species, and susceptibility tests will be done usually without special request. Contact the laboratory for details and special collection instructions.

Blood Culture With Antimicrobial Removal Device (ARD) *see* Blood Culture, Aerobic and Anaerobic *on page 391*

Blood Smear for Malarial Parasites *see* Peripheral Blood Smear, Thick and Thin *on page 563*

Blood Smear for Trypanosomal/Filarial Parasites *see* Microfilariae, Peripheral Blood Preparation *on page 535*

Body Cavity Fluid Cytology *see* Cytology, Body Fluids *on page 438*

Body Fluid Anaerobic Culture *see* Anaerobic Culture *on page 371*

Body Fluid Culture, Routine *see* Aerobic Culture, Body Fluid *on page 365*

Body Fluid Fungus Culture *see* Fungus Culture, Body Fluid *on page 462*

Body Lice Identification *see* Arthropod Identification *on page 387*

Bone Biopsy

Applies to Percutaneous Biopsy of Musculoskeletal Lesions and Synovial Membranes

Test Includes This procedure involves the passage of a needle, either under fluoroscopic or computed tomographic guidance, into an area of bony abnormality to facilitate precise histologic and/or bacteriologic diagnosis. In many clinical situations, this procedure can establish definitive diagnosis without the disadvantages of surgery making it a useful alternative to open biopsy. In selected cases of arthritis, examination of the synovium may provide precise diagnostic clues or useful information about the nature of the arthritic process. A biopsy of the synovium can be performed through an open arthrotomy, percutaneous biopsy, or as part of an arthroscopic procedure during which the synovium can be visualized.

Patient Preparation Biopsies are usually performed as a radiologic procedure. Skeletal biopsies are usually done under local anesthesia, with the exception of children and restless patients who are placed under general anesthesia or heavy sedation. Local anesthesia facilitates communication between the patient and the physician performing the procedure. Should the patient complain of radiating pain, the needle can be repositioned. Spinal biopsies may necessitate a 24-hour hospitalization. Other anatomic areas may be biopsied on an outpatient basis. The patient should not eat on the morning of the examination. An intravenous catheter is generally placed for I.V. access and the patient is usually administered both a sedative and a medication for pain.

Specimen There are a wide variety of commercially available needles for these procedures. A needle aspiration biopsy consists of aspiration of fluid for cytologic and/or bacteriologic analysis. A core biopsy, however, requires a larger needle and allows retrieval of a core of tissue for histopathologic interpretation.

Use When there is a need for a tissue or bacteriologic diagnosis in situations where it is desirable to forego open biopsy

Selected Readings

Anderson MW, Temple HT, Dussault RG, et al, "Compartmental Anatomy: Relevance to Staging and Biopsy of Musculoskeletal Tumors," *AJR Am J Roentgenol*, 1999, 173(6):1663-71.

Fraser-Hill MA, Renfrew DL, Hilsenrath PE, "Percutaneous Needle Biopsy of Musculoskeletal Lesions. 1. Effective Accuracy and Diagnostic Utility," *AJR Am J Roentgenol*, 1992, 158(4):809-12.

Fraser-Hill MA, Renfrew DL, Hilsenrath PE, "Percutaneous Needle Biopsy of Musculoskeletal Lesions. 2. Cost-Effectiveness," *AJR Am J Roentgenol*, 1992, 158(4):813-8.

Jelinek JS, Krasndorf MJ, Gray R, et al, "Percutaneous Transpedicular Biopsy of Vertebral Body Lesions," *Spine*, 1996, 21(17):2035-40.

Leffler SG and Chew FS, "CT-Guided Percutaneous Biopsy of Sclerotic Bone Lesions: Diagnostic Yield and Accuracy," *AJR Am J Roentgenol*, 1999, 172(5):1389-92.

Mader JT, Shirtliff ME, Bergquist S, et al, "Bone and Joint Infections in the Elderly: Practical Treatment Guidelines," *Drugs Aging*, 2000, 16(1):67-80.

Yao L, Nelson SD, Seeger LL, et al, "Primary Musculoskeletal Neoplasms: Effectiveness of Core-Needle Biopsy," *Radiology*, 1999, 212(3):682-6.

Bone Films

Applies to Acromioclavicular Joint, Left or Right, X-ray; Ankle, Left or Right, X-ray; Arthritis Series, X-ray; Calcaneus (heel), Left or Right, X-ray; Clavicle, Left or Right, X-ray; Elbow, Left or Right, X-ray; Femur, Left or Right, X-ray; Finger, Left or Right Hand, X-ray; Foot, Left or Right, X-ray; Forearm, Left or Right, X-ray; Hand, Left or Right, X-ray; Hands and Wrist Arthritis, X-ray; Hip, Left or Right, X-ray; Hip, Left or Right, and Pelvis, X-ray; Hips Arthritis, X-ray; Humerus, Left or Right, X-ray; Knee, Left or Right, X-ray; Knees Arthritis, X-ray; Patella of Knee, Left or Right, X-ray; Pelvis AP, X-ray; Pelvis Stereo, X-ray; Postreduction Films, X-ray; Scanogram, X-ray; Scapula, Left or Right, X-ray; Shoulder Stereo, Left or Right, X-ray; Shoulder to Include Axial View, Left or Right, X-ray; Shoulder, Left or Right, X-ray; Shoulders Arthritis, X-ray; Sternoclavicular Joint, Left or Right, X-ray; Thumb, Left or Right, X-ray; Tibia and Fibula, Left or Right, X-ray; Toes of Foot, Left or Right, X-ray; Wrist, Left or Right, X-ray

Test Includes Upper extremity and shoulder girdle: Fingers, thumb, hands, wrists, wrists for carpal tunnel, wrists for navicular views, PA hands and wrists for arthritis,

forearm, elbow, humerus, scapula, shoulder for trauma, shoulder for inflammatory process, shoulder to include axial view, clavicle, nonweight bearing and weight bearing views of acromioclavicular joints, bilateral comparison sternoclavicular joints, and postreduction films.

Lower extremity and pelvis: AP pelvis, stereo pelvis, pelvis and hips, hips for congenital deformity, hips for arthritis, femur, knee, weight bearing, knees for arthritis, knees with patellar views, knees with tunnel views, tibia-fibula, ankles, ankles with stress views, calcaneus, feet, toes.

Bony thorax: Ribs, unilateral or bilateral, sternum.

Patient Preparation If the area to be examined is covered by a dressing it should be the lightest possible dressing.

Special Instructions Requisition information should include: Whether it is safe for patient to sit, stand, and move extremities. If there is a question of fracture, how long ago injury occurred, and any previous fractures. In case of foreign bodies, state their nature since many are not visible on x-ray examination. If dressings, bivalved casts, and splints may be removed. If "wet reading" is desired. If a comparison with previous examinations is desired, it should be indicated.

Use Evaluate bones for the presence of metastatic and primary neoplasms, trauma, infectious disease, degenerative and reactive processes

Limitations Metal appliances, casts and dressings containing aluminum paste, lead water, or Epsom salts obscure or obliterate all detail.

Methodology The affected body part will be moved, if possible, into two or three different positions so films can be obtained.

Selected Readings

Mader JT, Shirtliff ME, Bergquist S, et al, "Bone and Joint Infections in the Elderly: Practical Treatment Guidelines," *Drugs Aging*, 2000, 16(1):67-80.

Bone Marrow *see* Bone Marrow Aspiration and Biopsy *on page 397*

Bone Marrow Aspiration and Biopsy

Applies to Bone Marrow Iron Stain; Bone Marrow Sampling; Bone Marrow Trephine Biopsy; Bone Marrow; Iron Stain

Test Includes Aspiration and/or biopsy of bone marrow (BM) for microscopic analysis. Both procedures are carried out under local anesthesia at the patient's bedside. For aspiration, a specialized hollow needle is advanced into the intramedullary cavity (usually iliac crest). Approximately 0.4 mL liquid marrow and bone fragments are aspirated into a syringe, then smeared onto a slide. Frequently, a bone marrow biopsy is performed as a complementary, but separate, procedure (different equipment and site). A specialized biopsy needle (eg, Jamshidi needle) is used to obtain a core of solid cortical bone. This technique preserves the normal marrow architecture of the biopsy sample and allows for formal for histologic analysis.

Patient Preparation Technique and risks of the procedure are explained to the patient and consent is obtained. Considerable patient apprehension often accompanies this procedure and requires thorough, step-by-step explanation beforehand. If coagulopathy is known or suspected, a recent CBC and PT/PTT should be drawn. Requisition must state in advance any special studies to be performed on specimen, such as AFB stain, Congo red stain for amyloid, cytogenetics studies, etc. Contact referring physician if any questions arise or contact appropriate laboratories directly. Patients are commonly premedicated with a short-acting benzodiazepine or analgesic such as meperidine.

Aftercare Needle puncture site(s) are covered with a dry sterile dressing. If the bone marrow biopsy is performed from the posterior iliac crest, patient must lie on back for a full 30 minutes before being discharged. In the presence of a low-grade coagulopathy or mild thrombocytopenia, direct pressure should be applied by operator (not patient) to puncture sites until local bleeding ceases. Instruct patient to keep dressings dry. Ideally, puncture sites should be examined approximately 24 hours later by nurse or physician, but this is not always feasible.

Special Instructions This procedure requires at least two operators. The first obtains the aspiration and/or biopsy specimen in a sterile fashion (usually a physician or specialized nurse clinician) and the second immediately examines and prepares the specimen (usually a nurse or technologist from the Hematology Laboratory).

Complications Bone marrow sampling is considered a relatively safe but invasive procedure. Minor complications include local bleeding, hematoma, and discomfort at the needle puncture site. Local infection is rarely seen if proper aftercare is followed. Major complications have been reported with sternal biopsy (Bahir 1963), including fatal puncture of mediastinal structures. Historical reports of fistula formation, osteomyelitis, and profuse bleeding were associated with biopsy of what are now considered nonstandard sites, such as the tibia. Minimal complications are associated with sampling of the iliac crest, the preferred site.

(Continued)

Bone Marrow Aspiration and Biopsy *(Continued)*

Equipment Commercially assembled trays for aspiration and biopsy are widely available. These prepackaged kits typically contain a bone marrow biopsy needle (usually Jamshidi needle), aspiration needle (usually Illinois needle), various syringes (5 mL, 10 mL, 20 mL), assorted needles (18-gauge, 25-gauge), and 1% lidocaine with epinephrine for local anesthesia. Also included are gauze, sterile gloves, drapes and towels, No 11 scalpel blade, and alcohol and iodine prep. The Jamshidi needle is a large-bore (usually 11-gauge), hollow needle with a tapered tip, thin metal stylet, and wide plastic grip to allow easy needle rotation. The Illinois needle is somewhat smaller, but likewise comes with a stylet and plastic sheath for improved grip. Smaller gauge needles are available for use in the pediatric population.

Technique The procedure is performed by experienced operators only. May be carried out at the bedside if adequate lighting is available, otherwise done in a procedure room.

Aspiration: Preferred site is the posterior superior iliac spine (PSIS), alternatively the sternum. Patient is placed on his side or lies prone. Landmarks are identified by palpation - the PSIS primarily, but the anterior superior iliac spine also. A wide circular area (approximately 5" in diameter) overlying the PSIS is prepped with povidone-iodine in the usual sterile fashion. Using the 25-gauge needle and lidocaine, the skin directly over the PSIS is anesthetized. Following this, deeper structures are liberally anesthetized with the 18-gauge needle, including a several centimeter area of the periosteum. A 4 mm long skin incision is made over the PSIS by means of the No 11 scalpel blade, then extended deeper through fatty tissues down to the anesthetized periosteum. The Illinois aspiration needle (with stylet in place) is advanced through this soft tissue incision and firmly into the cortex of the PSIS, using a constant rotary motion of the needle ("drilling"). Once the needle has penetrated approximately 1 cm into the marrow cavity, the stylet is removed and a 10 mL syringe is attached to the open (distal) end of the aspiration needle. At least 4-5 mL marrow is aspirated using firm suction. This volume is adequate for most routine hematologic studies, but larger volumes are usually needed for fungal or tuberculous cultures, cytogenetics, cell markers, etc. This step often causes the most patient discomfort. After aspiration, the syringe is detached and immediately handed over to the technologist in order to prevent the specimen from clotting (aspiration needle is still in the PSIS). The technologist examines the specimen grossly for marrow particles, which may be visible to the naked eye. If present, this signifies that an adequate marrow specimen has likely been obtained; if absent, the aspiration needle is redirected slightly and the previous listed steps repeated. After completion, the needle is removed and direct pressure applied.

Biopsy: May be carried out immediately following aspiration, while patient is still under local anesthesia. Preferred site is again the PSIS; however, unlike bone marrow aspiration, biopsy is never obtained from the sternum. A Jamshidi biopsy needle is passed through the same skin and soft tissue incision used for aspiration (alternatively, a completely new site may be used). However, a separate hole in the PSIS must be made. Once into the cortical bone, the needle is advanced using a pronounced clockwise/counterclockwise rotary motion. The needle is oriented along an imaginary line connecting the PSIS and the anterior superior iliac spine, forcing a slight angle of the needle with respect to the skin. The needle should **not** be advanced perpendicular to the skin; this results in poor quality biopsies (often with mostly cartilage). The stylet is then removed. The "drilling" is continued until the needle is at least 2 cm deep into the cortex. This may be estimated by periodically replacing the stylet into the needle and noting the distance the stylet protrudes. The biopsy core is subsequently "sheared off" by the following maneuvers:

- needle is rotated a full 10 turns clockwise then 10 turns counterclockwise
- needle is withdrawn slightly and redirected at a different angle
- needle is readvanced
- steps 1-3 are repeated (until the core is sheared off). The needle is withdrawn, again using rotary motions so as not to lose the core. The blunt obturator or "push wire" is passed through the sharp tip of the Jamshidi needle and the specimen pushed gently out of the needle base and onto a sterile gauze. The technologist immediately makes imprints of the core then places the specimen in fixative.

The techniques for aspiration and biopsy outlined are generally agreed upon in major textbooks. However, some clinicians strongly believe that bone marrow biopsy should always **precede** aspiration, despite the "textbook" recommendations. They argue that artifacts in the core biopsy may be induced by aspiration.

Specimen The bone marrow aspirate is immediately examined for visible bone spicules. The presence of these small spicules suggests an adequate specimen. Direct smears of the aspirate fluid are prepared by the technologist at the bedside. These smears consist of marrow particles and free marrow cells spread onto coverslips. This

technique helps to preserve the cytologic appearance of individual blood cells. Bone marrow biopsy samples are handled differently. In many institutions, touch preparations are made first, before specimen fixation. The marrow specimen is touched gently to a clean glass slide in several places, without smearing. These "touch preps" are allowed to air-dry and subsequently undergo routine staining. This technique also helps preserve cytologic detail. Once the touch preparations are completed, the remainder of the specimen is placed in a fixative such as formalin or Zenker's solution. The specimen is then processed according to individual laboratory protocol (eg, overnight fixation, decalcification, wash steps, dehydration, and serial sectioning). Routine stains are performed on processed specimens. These include hematoxylin and eosin (H & E), Wright-Giemsa stain, and iron stain. Optional studies may be obtained at physician request such as cytogenetic analysis, flow cytometry, electron microscopy, and amyloid stains. The Hematology Laboratory must be notified in advance for these studies. Bone marrow specimens may also be submitted for microbiological analysis. Cultures may be obtained for aerobic and anaerobic bacteria, fungi (eg, *Histoplasma capsulatum*), acid-fast bacilli (eg, *Mycobacterium tuberculosis* or *Mycobacterium avium-intracellulare*), and viruses (cytomegalovirus). Fixatives should **not** be added to specimens submitted for culture. Again, it is important to notify the Microbiology Laboratory in advance for these cultures.

Reference Range The bone marrow aspirate and biopsy are reviewed by a staff pathologist or hematologist. The preliminary report on the bone marrow aspirate may often be available several hours after the procedure, on request. Normal values for bone marrow cell lines in the adult are as follows:

Granulocytes
- blasts: 0% to 1%
- promyelocytes: 1% to 5%
- neutrophil myelocytes and metamyelocytes: 7% to 25%
- neutrophil bands and segs: 20% to 60%
- eosinophils: 0% to 3%
- basophils: 0% to 1%
- monocytes: 0% to 2%
- lymphocytes: 5% to 15%
- plasma cells: 0% to 2%

Erythrocytes
- proerythrocytes: 0% to 1%
- early erythrocytes: 1% to 4%
- late erythrocytes: 10% to 20%
- normoblasts: 5% to 10%

The above bone marrow differential cell counts are calculated from the bone marrow aspirate specimen. Other useful data provided by the bone marrow aspirate include:
- myeloid/erythroid ratio (normal ratio 3-4:1)
- total cells counted
- overall cellularity
- erythropoiesis
- granulopoiesis

The bone marrow biopsy provides additional information on marrow architecture (which cannot be obtained from the aspirate). When examining the biopsy specimen, the pathologist may comment on:
- gross description including size of sample
- overall cellularity
- presence of granulomas
- infiltrative marrow processes such as lymphoma, carcinoma, granulomas
- iron stores
- results of special stains

Use Bone marrow sampling is indicated in the evaluation of a wide variety of hematologic disorders, usually noted first on the CBC or peripheral smear. It is also useful in the diagnosis of systemic diseases which may potentially involve the marrow, such as infectious or granulomatous processes. Bone marrow aspiration and biopsy should be considered separate procedures, although indications often overlap. Indications for bone marrow **aspiration** include:
- evaluation of severe anemia, especially when etiology is in doubt and reticulocyte count is low
- evaluation of macrocytic anemia, to confirm the presence of megaloblastic anemia or to exclude sideroblastic anemia and normoblastic erythropoiesis
- leukopenia and/or thrombocytopenia, to differentiate excessive consumption from decreased production
- persistent leukocytosis of unknown etiology
- suspected myelodysplastic syndrome

(Continued)

Bone Marrow Aspiration and Biopsy *(Continued)*

- suspected leukemia, to confirm diagnosis and to classify subtype (FAB categorization)
- suspected immunoglobulin disorders, such as multiple myeloma, for diagnosis and staging
- evaluation of lipid storage diseases
- evaluation of suspected iron storage abnormalities
- acquisition of marrow for chromosomal analysis
- acquisition of tissue for microbiological culture (fungi, bacteria, mycobacteria, parasites)
- evaluation of response to therapy for hematologic malignancies

Bone marrow biopsy preserves the marrow architecture and is useful in evaluating systemic diseases secondarily involving the marrow. Bone marrow **biopsy** indications include:

- evaluation of pancytopenia
- evaluation of possible myelophthisic anemia (bone marrow infiltrated with leukemic cells, metastatic tumor, lymphoma, granulomas, etc)
- diagnosis and staging of solid tumors or lymphoma
- evaluation of selected cases of fever of unknown origin
- diagnosis of systemic amyloidosis when other methods have failed
- suspected cases of myelofibrosis
- evaluation of myeloproliferative syndromes (polycythemia vera, essential thrombocythemia, etc)
- failed bone marrow aspiration attempts (the so-called "dry tap")

Authorities differ on the exact indications for both bone marrow aspiration and biopsy. Some believe that most hematologic abnormalities are adequately evaluated by bone marrow aspiration alone (without biopsy). Bone marrow biopsy should not be routinely performed with aspiration, it is argued, due to the following reasons:

- diagnosis can often be made by aspiration
- significant patient discomfort accompanies biopsy
- there is needless expense and patient risk

Thus, bone marrow biopsy should only be performed if specific indications are present (as listed).

Other experts routinely include a biopsy whenever aspiration is performed. The following reasons are cited.

- Bone marrow biopsy may be diagnostic in cases where aspiration is negative or equivocal.
- It is nearly impossible to predict in advance which aspiration attempts will be technically difficult.
- Bone marrow biopsy actually causes less discomfort than aspiration in some cases.
- Cost-benefit analysis may favor the combined approach. The cost to physician, technologist, and patient may be doubled if patient is forced to undergo a separate bone marrow biopsy at a later date.

Contraindications

- uncooperative patient
- cellulitis, osteomyelitis, or radiation therapy involving the proposed site of needle entry
- severe, noncorrectable coagulopathy
- thoracic aortic aneurysm if a sternal approach is used
- Paget's disease involving the iliac bone represents a high risk situation, due to excessive bleeding at trephine biopsy site (but not necessarily a contraindication)

Selected Readings

Batjer JP, "Preparation of Optimal Bone Marrow Samples," *Laboratory Medicine*, 1979, 10:101-6.

Beckstead JH, "The Bone Marrow Biopsy: A Diagnostic Strategy," *Arch Pathol Lab Med*, 1986, 110(3):175-9.

Brynes RK, McKenna RW, and Sundberg RD, "Bone Marrow Aspiration and Trephine Biopsy: An Approach to a Thorough Study," *Am J Clin Pathol*, 1978, 70(5):753-9.

Williams WJ and Nelson DA, "Examination of the Marrow," *Hematology*, 4th ed, Chapter 3, WJ Williams, E Beutler, AJ Erslev, et al, eds, New York, NY: McGraw-Hill, 1990, 24-31.

Bone Marrow Culture *see* Aerobic Culture, Body Fluid *on page 365*

Bone Marrow Culture, Routine

Synonyms Aerobic Bone Marrow Culture; Routine Bone Marrow Culture

Test Includes Culture and Gram stain if requested. Properly collected specimens must also be cultured for anaerobes.

Patient Preparation Usual sterile preparation of aspiration site.

Special Instructions Add 0.1-0.2 mL heparin 10,000 units/mL to sterile tube or Anaport vial

Specimen Bone marrow

Container Sterile tube or Anaport vial containing 0.1-0.2 mL heparin 10,000 units/mL

Collection The specimen will be divided for aerobic, fungus, anaerobic, mycobacteria cultures and smears, volume permitting if accompanied by appropriate requisitions

Storage Instructions Transport specimen to the laboratory immediately. Do not refrigerate.

Causes for Rejection Clots, inadequate volume for studies requested. Specimen will not be discarded without consultation with the attending physician.

Turnaround Time Stat Gram stain: 1 hour. Physician will be notified of all positive smears or cultures. Preliminary results are reported at 24 hours with broth held for 5-7 days.

Reference Range No growth

Use Isolate and identify etiologic agent

Bone Marrow Iron Stain *see* Bone Marrow Aspiration and Biopsy *on page 397*

Bone Marrow Mycobacteria Culture *see* Mycobacteria Culture, Biopsy or Body Fluid *on page 539*

Bone Marrow Sampling *see* Bone Marrow Aspiration and Biopsy *on page 397*

Bone Marrow Trephine Biopsy *see* Bone Marrow Aspiration and Biopsy *on page 397*

Bone Scan

Synonyms Bone Scintigraphy; Radionuclide Bone Scan; Whole Body Bone Scan

Applies to Bone Scan With Flow; Three-Phase Bone Scan

Test Includes The patient receives an intravenous injection of a technetium-99m (^{99m}Tc) phosphonate radiopharmaceutical which localizes in bone with intensity proportional to the degree of metabolic activity present. Three hours after the injection, whole body and appropriate regional skeletal images are acquired. An initial dynamic flow study and/or early images may also be acquired if osteomyelitis, osteonecrosis, Legg-Calvé-Perthes disease, septic arthritis, or other inflammatory disease is suspected (three-phase technique).

Patient Preparation Patient should have all radioimmunoassay (RIA) blood work performed, or at least drawn, prior to injection of any radioactive material. The patient does not need to be fasting or NPO for this procedure. Patient should be encouraged to drink fluids during the waiting period before scanning and will be asked to void just before scanning begins.

Special Instructions The requisition should indicate the current patient diagnosis in order to select the most appropriate radiopharmaceutical and/or imaging technique. When ordering liver and bone scans for the same patient, schedule liver scan at least 1 day before the bone scan.

Duration of Procedure: 3-4.5 hours. This includes a 2-3 hour delay after tracer injection to allow adequate localization in bone.

Radiopharmaceutical: ^{99m}Tc phosphonate compound.

Technique The application of single-photon emission tomography (SPECT) techniques may contribute significantly to the diagnostic accuracy of this imaging study.

Causes for Rejection Other recent Nuclear Medicine procedures may interfere. If uncertain, call the consulting Nuclear Medicine Department.

Normal Findings Homogeneous and symmetric distribution of activity throughout all skeletal structures

Use Bone imaging is extremely sensitive for the detection of infection or malignancy involving any part of the skeleton. It is the most appropriate screening test for these conditions, since scan abnormalities are present long before structural defects develop radiographically. Bone scans are also accurate for localizing lesions for biopsy, excision, or debridement. Stress fractures can be diagnosed by bone scan when radiographs are completely normal.

Limitations In postoperative orthopedic patients and diabetics, additional imaging with gallium or indium-labeled white blood cells may help to confirm the presence of active infection and serve as a baseline for later comparison

Selected Readings

Datz FL, "Radionuclide Imaging of Joint Inflammation in the 90s," *J Nucl Med*, 1990, 31(5):684-7.

Duncan I, Dorai-Raj A, Khoo K, et al, "The Utility of Bone Scans in Rheumatology," *Clin Nucl Med*, 1999, 24(1):9-14.

Gupta NC and Prezio JA, "Radionuclide Imaging in Osteomyelitis," *Semin Nucl Med*, 1988, 18(4):287-99.

Jacobson AF, Cronin EB, Stomper PC, et al, "Bone Scans With One or Two Abnormalities in Cancer Patients With No Known Metastases: Frequency and Serial Scintigraphic Behavior of Benign and Malignant Lesions," *Radiology*, 1990, 175(1):229-32.

(Continued)

Bone Scan *(Continued)*

Lee BF, Chiu NT, Chang JK, et al, "Technetium-99m(V)-DMSA and Gallium-67 in the Assessment of Bone and Joint Infection," *J Nucl Med*, 1998, 39(12):2128-31.
Lusins JO, Danielski EF, and Goldsmith SJ, "Bone SPECT in Patients With Persistent Back Pain After Lumbar Spine Surgery," *J Nucl Med*, 1989, 30(4):490-6.
Matin P, "Basic Principles of Nuclear Medicine Techniques for Detection and Evaluation of Trauma and Sports Medicine Injuries," *Semin Nucl Med*, 1988, 18(2):90-112.
McDougall IR and Keeling CA, "Complications of Fractures and Their Healing," *Semin Nucl Med*, 1988, 18(2):113-25.
McNeil BJ, "Value of Bone Scanning in Neoplastic Disease," *Semin Nucl Med*, 1985, 14(4):277-86.
Palmer E, Henrikson B, McKusick K, et al, "Pain as an Indicator of Bone Metastasis," *Acta Radiol*, 1988, 29(4):445-9.
Schauwecker DS, "The Scintigraphic Diagnosis of Osteomyelitis," *AJR Am J Roentgenol*, 1992, 158(1):9-18.
Sutter CW and Shelton DK, "Three-Phase Bone Scan in Osteomyelitis and Other Musculoskeletal Disorders," *Am Fam Physician*, 1996, 54(5):1639-47.

Bone Scan With Flow *see* Bone Scan *on page 401*
Bone Scintigraphy *see* Bone Scan *on page 401*
***Bordetella pertussis* Antibodies** *see Bordetella pertussis* Serology *on page 404*

Bordetella pertussis Direct Fluorescent Antibody

Related Information

Bordetella pertussis Nasopharyngeal Culture *on page 403*
Bordetella pertussis Serology *on page 404*

Synonyms *Bordetella pertussis* Smear; Nasopharyngeal Smear for *Bordetella pertussis*

Test Includes Fluorescent antibody stain to detect *Bordetella pertussis* on smear

Patient Preparation Patient must not be on antimicrobial therapy.

Special Instructions Laboratory supervisor should be notified 24 hours before collection of specimen so that a special isolation medium can be prepared.

Specimen Nasopharyngeal swab

Container Nasopharyngeal swab, sterile saline

Collection Swab is passed through nose gently and into nasopharynx. Stay near septum and floor of nose. Rotate and remove. Specimen must be hand transported to the laboratory immediately following collection.

Storage Instructions Do not refrigerate. Transport to the laboratory immediately.

Causes for Rejection Specimen not received in appropriate sterile container or on appropriate isolation medium, specimen more than 2 hours old. Cough plates are unacceptable.

Reference Range No *B. pertussis* detected

Use Detect and identify *B. pertussis* and *B. parapertussis*; establish the diagnosis of whooping cough

Limitations Direct detection assays are always limited by the adequacy of the sample. Bacteria may be difficult to detect if there are few bacteria present in the specimen or too much mucoid material.

Contraindications Lack of clinical symptoms of pertussis; previous antibiotic therapy

Methodology Direct fluorescent antibody (DFA)

Additional Information Note: This DFA for *Bordetella pertussis* and culture for *B. pertussis* are **not** sensitive tests. The currently recommended test of choice is detection by molecular methods (eg, amplification by polymerase chain reaction (PCR) and subsequent detection by molecular probe). Molecular methods for *B. pertussis* are sensitive, specific, and rapid. The procedure enables early presumptive identification of *Bordetella pertussis*, the agent of whooping cough. Definitive cultural identification should be completed. There is also a test available for serum agglutinating antibodies, which, if present, may be titered over time to indicate exposure.

Bordetella pertussis, Molecular Methods

Related Information

Bordetella pertussis Direct Fluorescent Antibody *on page 402*
Bordetella pertussis Serology *on page 404*

Synonyms *Bordetella pertussis* PCR

Test Includes Amplification of specific *Bordetella pertussis*-specific nucleic acid sequences and use of molecular probes to detect the amplified product

Special Instructions Only experienced medical persons should collect specimens because collection of appropriate specimens can induce paroxysmal coughs. Contact testing laboratory prior to collection to determine if the laboratory has special requirements and will provide special collection kits and supplies. Specimens require special collection and transportation media.

Specimen Two pernasal nasopharyngeal specimens collected by using aluminum-shaft, minitip, Dacron swabs.

Container Contact testing laboratory for the required container.

Collection Gently rotate swab in place for several seconds. Repeat in the other naris. Pool the two specimens into the same container.

Turnaround Time One to three days from receipt by the testing laboratory. Depends on technical issues.

Use To detect *Bordetella pertussis* nucleic acid in clinical specimens

Limitations The test is relatively expensive, is available only in specialized laboratories, and cannot distinguish between live and dead organisms.

Methodology Most methods use (1) some form of nucleic acid amplification (most commonly PCR and *Bordetella pertussis*-specific primers) to amplify a *Bordetella pertussis*-specific region of the *Bordetella pertussis* genome and (2) sequence-specific molecular probes to detect the amplified product.

Additional Information A major advantage of this test is that detected organisms do not need to be viable. The test is extremely sensitive and specific, and is highly recommended over culture and DFA. Although very rare, false negative results can occur because (1) lower-than-detectable low numbers of organisms can be present in the nasopharynx or specimen, especially very early or late in the disease, (2) inhibitors in the specimen, and (3) technical issues. Likewise, false-positive results can occur because (1) cross reactions from other organisms and (2) carryover of amplified products from previous amplification in the same laboratory. "Real time" PCR has recently been described as a new molecular amplification method to detect *Bordetella pertussis* in clinical specimens in only a few hours.

Selected Readings

Farrell DJ, McKeon M, Daggard G, et al, "Rapid-Cycle PCR Method to Detect *Bordetella pertussis* That Fulfills All Consensus Recommendations for Use of PCR in Diagnosis of Pertussis," *J Clin Microbiol*, 2000, 38(12):4499-502.

Grimprel E, Begue P, Anjak I, et al, "Comparison of Polymerase Chain Reaction, Culture, and Western Immunoblot Serology for Diagnosis of *Bordetella pertussis* Infection," *J Clin Microbiol*, 1993, 31(10):2745-50.

Kosters K, Reischl U, Schmetz J, et al, "Real-Time LightCycler PCR for Detection and Discrimination of *Bordetella pertussis* and *Bordetella parapertussis*," *J Clin Microbiol*, 2002, 40(5):1719-22.

Lievano FA, Reynolds MA, Waring AL, et al, "Issues Associated With and Recommendations for Using PCR to Detect Outbreaks of Pertussis," *J Clin Microbiol*, 2002, 40(8):2801-5.

Reischl U, Lehn N, Sanden GN, et al, "Real-Time PCR Assay Targeting IS481 of *Bordetella pertussis* and Molecular Basis for Detecting *Bordetella holmesii*," *J Clin Microbiol*, 2001, 39(5):1963-6.

Bordetella pertussis Nasopharyngeal Culture

Related Information

Bordetella pertussis Direct Fluorescent Antibody *on page 402*
Bordetella pertussis, Molecular Methods *on page 402*
Bordetella pertussis Serology *on page 404*

Synonyms Nasopharyngeal Culture for *Bordetella pertussis*; Pertussis Culture; Whooping Cough Culture

Test Includes Specific culture and identification of *Bordetella pertussis* and *Bordetella parapertussis*

Patient Preparation Patient should not be on antimicrobial therapy prior to the collection of the specimen.

Special Instructions Consult the laboratory prior to collection of the specimen so that the special isolation medium can be obtained. The laboratory should be made aware of the specific request to screen for *Bordetella pertussis* with information relevant to current antibiotic therapy and current diagnosis. **Note: Culture for *B. pertussis* is not a sensitive test. The currently recommended test of choice is detection by molecular methods, eg, amplification by polymerase chain reaction (PCR) and subsequent detection by molecular probe. Molecular methods for *B. pertussis* are sensitive, specific, and rapid.**

Specimen Nasopharyngeal swab

Container Flexible calcium alginate swab (Calgiswab®) and Bordet-Gengou plate. Transport medium composed of half strength Oxoid charcoal agar CM19 supplemented with 40 mcg/mL cephalexin and 10% hemolyzed defibrinated horse blood may be used.

Collection Shape the flexible swab into the contour of the nares. Pass the swab gently through the nose. Leave swab in place near septum and floor of nose for 15-30 seconds. Rotate and remove. The recovery of the organism depends on collecting an adequate specimen. Inoculate the plate or transport medium directly at the bedside.

The following procedure optimizes the laboratory diagnosis of pertussis.

- Collect nasopharyngeal specimens in the early stage of illness. Providing specimen collection kits facilitates the appropriate specimen collection and transportation.

(Continued)

Bordetella pertussis Nasopharyngeal Culture *(Continued)*

- For swab collected specimens, use a transport medium consisting of half strength Oxoid charcoal agar supplemented with 10% hemolyzed, defibrinated horse blood, and 40 mcg/mL cephalexin.
- Inoculate a selective primary plating medium composed of Oxoid charcoal agar, 10% defibrinated horse blood, and 40 mcg/mL cephalexin. A nonselective medium without cephalexin may be used in addition to the selective medium.
- Perform direct fluorescent antibody (DFA) tests on appropriately collected nasopharyngeal secretions with *B. pertussis*- and *B. parapertussis*-conjugated antisera to facilitate an earlier diagnosis.
- After inoculating primary plating media, retain swabs in the original transport medium at room temperature. If cultures become overgrown with indigenous bacterial flora or fungi, use swabs to inoculate additional media.
- Identify suspicious isolates with appropriate cultural and biochemical tests. The DFA test performed on growth from isolated colonies is an excellent procedure for confirmatory or definitive identification.

Storage Instructions The specimen should not be refrigerated. It should be transported to the laboratory as soon as possible after collection.

Causes for Rejection Specimen not received on appropriate isolation medium. Excessive delay in transit to the laboratory results in less than optimal yield.

Turnaround Time Preliminary reports are generally available at 24 hours if pathogens other than *B. pertussis* are isolated. Growth of *Bordetella pertussis* takes at least 72 hours to be detected. Cultures with no growth are usually reported after 1 week. Reports on specimens from which *B. pertussis* has been isolated generally require at least 1 week for completion.

Reference Range No *B. pertussis* or *B. parapertussis* isolated

Use Isolate and identify *B. pertussis* and *B. parapertussis*; establish the diagnosis of whooping cough

Limitations Cough plates are less reliable than nasopharyngeal specimens.

Contraindications Lack of clinical symptoms of pertussis; previous antibiotic therapy; history of vaccination is a relative contraindication

Methodology Culture on selective medium (selective chocolate agar with 10% defibrinated horse blood and 40 mcg/mL cephalexin), presumptive confirmation by direct fluorescent antibody (DFA). Culture after enrichment in transport medium for 48 hours increases yield.

Additional Information Direct fluorescent antibody (DFA) procedures provide more rapid results and have been increasingly used in the diagnosis of *B. pertussis* infection. The DFA procedures are most useful in the first 2-3 weeks of the illness. DFA test detected 42 of 164 (26%) of patients who proved culture positive for *B. pertussis* and 8 of 38 (21%) of patients who proved culture positive for *B. parapertussis*. False-negatives may be caused by inadequate specimens having little cellular material (leukocytes and brush border epithelial cells).

Selected Readings

Heininger U, "Pertussis: An Old Disease That is Still With Us," *Curr Opin Infect Dis*, 2001, 14(3):329-35.

Heininger U, Schmidt-Schlapfer G, Cherry JD, et al, "Clinical Validation of a Polymerase Chain Reaction Assay for the Diagnosis of Pertussis by Comparison With Serology, Culture, and Symptoms During a Large Pertussis Vaccine Efficacy Trial," *Pediatrics*, 2000, 105(3):E31.

Lievano FA, Reynolds MA, Waring AL, et al, "Issues Associated With and Recommendations for Using PCR to Detect Outbreaks of Pertussis," *J Clin Microbiol*, 2002, 40(8):2801-5.

***Bordetella pertussis* PCR** *see* Bordetella pertussis, Molecular Methods *on page 402*

Bordetella pertussis Serology

Related Information

Bordetella pertussis Direct Fluorescent Antibody *on page 402*
Bordetella pertussis Nasopharyngeal Culture *on page 403*

Synonyms *Bordetella pertussis* Antibodies; *Bordetella pertussis* Titer; Pertussis Serology

Test Includes Enzyme-linked immunosorbent assay to detect antibodies to *Bordetella pertussis* and/or pertussis toxin

Specimen Serum

Container Red top tube

Storage Instructions Refrigerate serum at 4°C.

Reference Range Absent IgM antibody; less than fourfold rise in titer in paired sera

Use Evaluate acute infection with or immunity following vaccination for *Bordetella pertussis*

Methodology Microhemagglutination, enzyme-linked immunosorbent assay (ELISA)

Additional Information Note: Culture for *B. pertussis* is not a sensitive test. The currently recommended test of choice is detection by molecular methods, eg, amplification by polymerase chain reaction (PCR) and subsequent detection by

molecular probe. Molecular methods for *B. pertussis* are sensitive, specific, and rapid. Patients with acute infection develop IgG, IgM, and IgA antibodies to febrile agglutinogens; and IgM and IgA antibodies are probably diagnostic. Following vaccination, IgG and IgM antibodies can be demonstrated, except in infants. IgA antibodies do not develop.

Selected Readings

Hoppe JE, "*Bordetella*," *Manual of Clinical Laboratory Immunology*, 5th ed, Rose NR, Conway de Macario E, Folds JD, et al, eds, Washington, DC: American Society for Microbiology, 1997, 614-24.

Mertsola J, Ruuskanen O, Kuronen T, et al, "Serologic Diagnosis of Pertussis: Evaluation of Pertussis Toxin and Other Antigens in Enzyme-Linked Immunosorbent Assay," *J Infect Dis*, 1990, 161(5):966-71.

Tomoda T, Ogura H, and Kurashige T, "Immune Responses to *Bordetella pertussis* Infection and Vaccination," *J Infect Dis*, 1991, 163(3):559-63.

***Bordetella pertussis* Smear** *see Bordetella pertussis* Direct Fluorescent Antibody *on page 402*

***Bordetella pertussis* Titer** *see Bordetella pertussis* Serology *on page 404*

Borreliosis Serology *see* Lyme Disease Serology *on page 527*

Botulism, Diagnostic Procedure

Synonyms *Clostridium botulinum* Toxin Identification Procedure; Infant Botulism, Toxin Identification; Sudden Death Syndrome

Abstract A neurotoxin, botulin, may be produced by *C. botulinum* in foods which have been improperly preserved. Characteristics of this type of food poisoning include vomiting and abdominal pain, disturbances of vision, motor function and secretion, mydriasis, ptosis, dry mouth, and cough.

Special Instructions The laboratory must be notified prior to obtaining specimen in order to prepare for transport of the specimen to the State Health Laboratory or Center for Disease Control.

Specimen Vomitus, serum, stool, gastric washings, cerebrospinal fluid or autopsy tissue; food samples

Container Sterile wide-mouth, leakproof, screw-cap jar; red top tube

Storage Instructions Keep refrigerated at 4°C except for unopened food samples.

Turnaround Time 3-7 days

Reference Range No toxin identified, no *Clostridium botulinum* isolated

Use Diagnose infant botulism, sudden death syndrome, floppy baby syndrome, classic botulism in adults

Limitations The toxin from *C. botulinum* binds almost irreversibly to individual nerve terminals; thus, serum and cerebrospinal fluid specimens may yield false-negative results.

Contraindications Due to the difficulty in performance of the diagnostic test and because of the extensive epidemiological studies initiated upon receipt of the specimen, State Department of Health Laboratories require specific clinical symptomatology for infant botulism. Therefore, they should be consulted early to optimize handling of the suspect case.

Methodology Toxin neutralization test in mice, isolation of *Clostridium botulinum* from feces

Additional Information The classic presentation of **infant botulism** is hypotonia (floppy baby syndrome), constipation, difficulty in feeding, and a weak cry. Some cases of sudden death syndrome have been traced to ingesting honey containing *C. botulinum*. Both *C. botulinum* and *C. butyricum* have been identified as species capable of toxin production. Autointoxication may occur from toxin production during organism growth in tissue, the intestinal tract in both adults and infants, and in wounds. Botulism has been reported with cocaine-associated sinusitis. **Note:** Botulism toxin is a level A agent of bioterrorism.

Selected Readings

Fox CK, Keet CA, and Strober JB, "Recent Advances in Infant Botulism," *Pediatr Neurol*, 2005, 32(3):149-54.

Thompson JA, Filloux FM, Van Orman CB, et al, "Infant Botulism in the Age of Botulism Immune Globulin," *Neurology*, 2005, 64(12):2029-32.

Brain Biopsy

Related Information

Herpes Cytology *on page 491*
Herpes Simplex Antibody *on page 492*
Herpes Simplex Virus by Direct Immunofluorescence *on page 493*
Herpes Simplex Virus Culture *on page 494*
Herpes Simplex Virus Isolation, Rapid *on page 495*
Rabies Detection *on page 569*
Toxoplasma Serology *on page 596*
Toxoplasma Serology by ELISA *on page 597*
(Continued)

Brain Biopsy *(Continued)*

Test Includes Routine histopathologic diagnosis. Special tests are requested by physician.

Special Instructions Submit specimen in formalin for routine histology. Requisition must state operative diagnosis and source of specimen.

Specimen Brain tissue biopsy

Container Test tube

Collection For needle biopsies of brain, an open-end rather than side-opening needle should be used. All types of brain biopsies are best placed on saline-moistened Gelfoam®. Do not place on gauze or immerse in saline. Arrange for specimen to be in hands of neuropathologist in shortest possible time, otherwise store in refrigerator. Do not freeze.

Storage Instructions Any necessary storage should be done in formaldehyde in a closed container.

Causes for Rejection Unlabeled specimen container, insufficient material, improper fixative

Turnaround Time 24 hours to 3 weeks, depending on nature of clinical problem

Reference Range Results interpreted by neuropathologist

Use Morphologic evaluation of brain disease

Limitations The size of the tissue sample is often a limiting factor. Brain biopsy does not offer an answer in most obscure neurological diseases.

Additional Information The most commonly sought pathogens in brain biopsies are herpesvirus and *Toxoplasma*, especially in immunocompromised hosts. Special arrangements must be made for electron microscopy or immunoperoxidase studies.

Brain, CT *see* Computed Transaxial Tomography, Head Studies *on page 424*

Bronchial Aspirate Anaerobic Culture *see* Anaerobic Culture *on page 371*

Bronchial Aspirate Fungus Culture *see* Fungus Culture, Bronchial Aspirate *on page 463*

Bronchial Aspiration for *Pneumocystis* *see* *Pneumocystis jiroveci* Test *on page 566*

Bronchial Biopsy *see* Histopathology *on page 496*

Bronchial Washings Culture *see* Aerobic Culture, Sputum *on page 367*

Bronchoalveolar Lavage (BAL) *see* Fungus Culture, Bronchial Aspirate *on page 463*

Bronchopulmonary Lavage for *Pneumocystis* *see* *Pneumocystis jiroveci* Test *on page 566*

Bronchoscopic *Legionella* Culture *see* *Legionella pneumophila* Culture *on page 516*

Bronchoscopy Culture *see* Aerobic Culture, Sputum *on page 367*

Bronchoscopy, Fiberoptic

Synonyms Flexible Bronchoscopy

Test Includes Direct visual examination of upper airway, vocal cords, and tracheobronchial tree out to the fourth to sixth division bronchi. Other procedures such as washings, brush biopsy bronchoalveolar lavage, endobronchial and transbronchial biopsy are also included depending on the clinical indications.

Patient Preparation NPO after midnight for a morning bronchoscopy and NPO after light breakfast for afternoon procedures. Routine medications (especially antiasthmatic drugs) may be taken at any time with a small amount of water. Routine lab work including clotting times, BUN, CBC, and platelet count is essential to exclude a coagulopathy - especially if a biopsy is to be performed. Some measure of pulmonary function is useful (spirometry, blood gases) to assess pulmonary reserve and document bronchospasm. Premedication with a narcotic (meperidine 25-75 mg) or minor tranquilizer (diazepam 10 mg) is given parenterally 15-30 minutes before the procedure. Atropine 0.4 mg I.M. is given as a vagolytic agent at the same time unless contraindicated by the presence of arrhythmia, narrow angle glaucoma, or urinary retention.

Aftercare NPO for 2 hours or longer after the procedure until the gag reflex is fully recovered. Because of the premedication, outpatients should not drive until the following day. Transient fever and mild hemoptysis may be noted for the next 24 hours.

Equipment A fiberoptic bronchoscope and halogen or xenon light source are necessary for this examination. The bronchoscope is equipped with a thumb lever which allows angulation of the distal end of the instrument. A 2-2.6 mm hollow channel runs the length of the scope and allows injection of medication and aspiration of secretions for airway clearance and obtaining bronchial washings and lavage. It is also utilized for the passage of instruments, such as bronchial brushes and forceps.

Technique Procedure may be performed with the patient in supine or sitting position. Patient gargles with 2% lidocaine solution or alternatively tetracaine 2% aerosolized

spray (Cetacaine®) is used to anesthetize the pharynx. The bronchoscope tip is lubricated with Xylocaine® jelly and introduced transnasally or transorally with the use of a bite block. Lidocaine 2% solution is then injected through the bronchoscopic channel in 2 mL aliquots for anesthesia of the vocal cords and entire tracheobronchial tree. Lidocaine has definite toxicity (seizures and respiratory arrest) and the total dosage should generally not exceed 400 mg. The duration of action generally lasts 20-30 minutes. Once adequate anesthesia has been obtained, a detailed visual examination is performed. Subsequently other procedures such as biopsies, washings, and brushings can be carried out.

Data Acquired This examination provides information regarding the patency and normality of the central airways. It is used as a vehicle for sampling the airways and lung parenchyma itself via brushing and biopsy techniques.

Specimen Bronchial washings, brushings, biopsy, or lavage

Container Formalin jars, mucous specimen containers, slides in 95% alcohol

Turnaround Time Written report follows the procedure.

Normal Findings Normal endobronchial examination.

Use The major utility is in the assessment of malignant disease, early diagnosis of carcinoma, assessment of operability, transbronchial or endobronchial lung biopsy, hemoptysis (not massive), persistent chronic cough, removal of foreign bodies (minor role), and diagnosis of lung infections especially in immunocompromised hosts. Other uses include difficult endotracheal intubation.

Limitations Limited usefulness in retrieving foreign bodies and the management of massive hemoptysis.

Contraindications Asthma, severe hypoxemia, serious arrhythmia unstable angina pectoris, recent myocardial infarction, and poor patient cooperation. All of these are only relative contraindications and vary depending on the clinical situation and experience of the bronchoscopist. When bronchoscopy involves biopsy procedures, coagulopathies or bleeding tendencies are contraindications.

Additional Information The procedure is relatively low risk. Large reviews have shown that approximately 50% of the life-threatening complications are associated with premedication or topical anesthesia. The risk seems highest in patients with underlying cardiac disease and the elderly. Patients with underlying bronchospastic disease are particularly prone to bronchospasm and laryngospasm and thus should be under optimal treatment before undertaking bronchoscopy. A drop in pO_2 of approximately 20 mm Hg occurs, and therefore supplemental oxygen administration is indicated. Transient fever and pneumonia occur in a small number of patients. Bleeding can occur from the nose or tracheobronchial tree although this complication is mainly associated with transbronchial biopsy.

Selected Readings

Ahmad M and Dweik RA, "Future of Flexible Bronchoscopy," *Clin Chest Med*, 1999, 20(1):1-17.

Borchers SD and Beamis JF Jr, "Flexible Bronchoscopy," *Chest Surg Clin N Am*, 1996, 6(2):169-92.

Chung HS and Lee JH, "Bronchoscopic Assessment of the Evolution of Endobronchial Tuberculosis," *Chest*, 2000, 117(2):385-92.

"Medical Investigations. 4:Bronchoscopy," *Br J Nurs*, 1997, 6(10):592-3.

Shennib H and Baslaim G, "Bronchoscopy in the Intensive Care Unit," *Chest Surg Clin N Am*, 1996, 6(2):349-61.

Van Gundy K and Boylen CT, "Fiberoptic Bronchoscopy. Indications, Complications, Contraindications," *Postgrad Med*, 1988, 83(1):289-94.

Bronchoscopy Fungus Culture *see* Fungus Culture, Sputum *on page 466*

Bronchoscopy Mycobacteria Culture *see* Mycobacteria Culture, Sputum *on page 542*

***Brucella* Blood Culture** *see* Blood Culture, *Brucella on page 394*

***Brucella* Culture, Tissue** *see* Biopsy Culture, Routine *on page 390*

Buffy Coat Culture for CMV *see* Cytomegalovirus Culture, Blood *on page 439*

Buffy Coat Viral Culture *see* Cytomegalovirus Culture, Blood *on page 439*

Bullous Pemphigoid Antibodies *see* Skin Biopsy, Immunofluorescence *on page 583*

C6 Peptide EIA *see* Lyme (*Borrelia*) C6 Peptide Immunoassay *on page 527*

C 100-3 *see* Hepatitis C Serology *on page 484*

Calcaneus (heel), Left or Right, X-ray *see* Bone Films *on page 396*

***Campylobacter pylori*, Gastric Biopsy Culture** *see Helicobacter pylori* Culture, Gastric Biopsy *on page 480*

***Campylobacter pylori* Serology** *see Helicobacter pylori* Serology *on page 480*

***Campylobacter pylori* Urease Test and Culture** *see Helicobacter pylori* Culture and Urease Test *on page 479*

Casts, Urine *see* Urinalysis *on page 606*

Catheter Culture, Intravenous *see* Intravenous Line Culture *on page 511*

Catheter Tip Culture *see* Intravenous Line Culture *on page 511*

CBC *see* Complete Blood Count *on page 420*

Cell Sorting Fluorescence Activation *see* Lymph Node Biopsy *on page 529*

Cerebrospinal Fluid Aerobic Culture *see* Aerobic Culture, Cerebrospinal Fluid *on page 366*

Cerebrospinal Fluid Anaerobic Culture *see* Anaerobic Culture *on page 371*

Cerebrospinal Fluid Analysis

Related Information

Aerobic Culture, Cerebrospinal Fluid *on page 366*
Fungus Culture, Cerebrospinal Fluid *on page 464*
VDRL, Cerebrospinal Fluid *on page 613*
Viral Culture, Central Nervous System Symptoms *on page 614*

Synonyms CSF Analysis; Lumbar Puncture Analysis; Spinal Fluid Analysis; Spinal Tap

Test Includes Color of supernatant, turbidity, WBC/mm^3, polys/mm^3, lymphs/mm^3, RBC/mm^3, percent of crenated RBC, protein, sugar, and sometimes VDRL.

Abstract Examination of cerebrospinal fluid (CSF) contributes to diagnosis and sometimes management of infections of the central nervous system, meningitis, encephalitis, instances of vasculitis, demyelinating diseases, tumors, paraneoplastic entities, polyneuritis, instances of cerebrovascular disease, and cases of seizure disorders and confusional states.

Patient Preparation Aseptic preparation for aspiration

Special Instructions Specimen should be delivered to the laboratory **promptly**.

When a diagnosis of meningitis is considered, culture of blood, urine, and other sites, as well as culture of CSF may be helpful. Most children with bacterial meningitis are initially bacteremic, and blood cultures are of value. In neonates and small children, urine culture may be positive. Cultures and Gram stains of petechiae may provide immediate diagnosis.

Specimen Cerebrospinal fluid

Container Sterile test tubes from lumbar puncture tray

Collection Specimens of spinal fluid and blood, for culture, should be obtained prior to initiation of antibiotic treatment of meningitis. Tubes must be labeled with patient's name, date, and labeled with number indicating sequence in which tubes were obtained.

Storage Instructions Do **not** store; specimen should be processed as soon as possible.

Causes for Rejection Unlabeled tubes, insufficient specimen, clotted or refrigerated specimen, improper dispensation of specimen

Laboratory Values of Components of CSF From Healthy Persons and From Patients With Meningitis[1]

Source	CSF Laboratory Value			
	Protein (mg/dL)	Glucose (mg/dL)[2]	Leukocytes (/μL)	Predominant Cell Type (%)
Healthy persons				
newborns	15-170	34-119	0-30	
adults	15-50	40-80	0-10	Lymphocytes (63-99) Monocytes (3-37) PMN (0-15)
Adult patients with:				
bacterial meningitis	>100	<40	>1000	PMN (>50)
fungal meningitis	Increased	<30	Increased	Lymphocytes
viral or aseptic meningitis	<100	Normal[3]	<500	PMN (early) and lymphocytes (late)

[1]Data are commonly observed values. Notable exceptions to these values and overlap of values elicited by different etiological agents are not uncommon. PMN = polymorphonuclear leukocytes.

[2]CSF glucose/serum glucose ratio usually is 0.6 (adults) or 0.74-0.96 (neonates and preterm babies). In patients with bacterial meningitis, the ratios usually are <0.5 (adults) and <0.6 (neonates and preterm babies).

[3]Lower than normal glucose concentrations have been observed during some non-infectious disease processes and in some patients with viral meningoencephalitis due to herpesviruses, varicella-zoster virus, mumps virus, lymphocytic choriomeningitis virus, and enteroviruses.

From Gray LD and Fedorko DP, "Laboratory Diagnosis of Bacterial Meningitis," *Clin Microbiol Rev*, 1992, 5(2):133.

Reference Range Adults: 0-5 cells/mm^3, all lymphocytes and monocytes; 0 red blood cells; protein: lumbar 15-50 mg/dL, cisternal 15-25 mg/dL, ventricular 6-15 mg/dL; glucose 50-80 mg/dL. Younger than 1 month: <32 cells/mm^3, 1 month to 1 year: <10

cells/mm^3, 1-4 years: <8 cells/mm^3, 5 years to puberty: <5 cells/mm^3; in the premature neonate: <29 cells/mm^3

Possible Panic Range Increased number of cells

Use Evaluate bacterial or viral encephalitis, meningitis, meningoencephalitis, mycobacterial or fungal infection, parasitic infestations, primary or secondary malignancy, leukemia/malignant lymphoma of CNS, trauma, vascular occlusive disease, vasculitis, heredofamilial and/or degenerative processes. The tables outline findings, including those with subdural empyema, brain abscess, ventricular empyema, cerebral epidural, abscess, spinal epidural abscess, tuberculosis, syphilis, sarcoidosis, and other entities.

The nucleated blood cell count in the cerebrospinal fluid is described as superior to any combination of the other CSF tests for bacterial meningitis. In patients who have not received antimicrobial agents, the ultimate diagnosis of bacterial meningitis is based on results of culture. The cell count and differential count are mandatory, and a Gram stain must be examined promptly in work up of possible meningitis. The CSF must be cultured; glucose and protein are necessary, as well, in the work-up for possible meningitis. **Viral infection**, as well as **bacterial meningitis**, can elicit neutrophil leukocytosis in blood and CSF. Seasonal curves for viral and bacterial infection go in opposite directions; although viral meningitis is a disease of midsummer, bacterial meningitis is relatively more common in the winter.

Signals of possible meningeal infection in the newborn: leukocyte count >30 cells/mm^3 with >60% PMNs, CSF protein >100 mg/dL, and/or CSF glucose <40% than that in blood are found with bacterial meningitis. CSF WBC counts >10 cells/mm^3 in very young infants, and >5 cells/mm^3 in older infants, and children with >1 PMN/mm^3 are abnormal. See tables on following pages.

Limitations A traumatic (bloody) tap may make interpretation difficult. Normal CSF may be found early in meningitis.

Additional Information See table on following pages for laboratory values of components of CSF from healthy persons and from patients with meningitis.

More extensive testing: cytology, conventional cultures and cultures for mycobacteria, fungi, and viruses, additional chemistry and serologic determinations must usually be ordered separately.

Correction for traumatic tap: If cell counts and protein determinations are performed on CSF and blood obtained at the same time, correction for "bloody tap" can be calculated. All CSF measurements should be made from the same tube. The ratio of RBC count CSF to RBC count blood provides a factor which when multiplied by the blood WBC count or blood protein level indicates the expected level of contribution of these parameters from the blood to the spinal fluid. These contributed WBC or protein values can then be subtracted from the respective values measured in the spinal fluid. For example:

1. RBCs (CSF)/RBCs (blood) x WBCs (blood) or x protein (blood).
2. WBCs (CSF) or protein (CSF) - product calculated in 1 = true CSF WBC or true CSF protein.

If the peripheral blood is normal and traumatic tap had occurred, about 1 WBC is added to the CSF for each 700 RBCs that have been transferred into the CSF. RBC contamination from a traumatic tap does not adversely affect the laboratory diagnosis of bacterial meningitis.

Antigen detection methods cannot replace culture and Gram stain. Gram stain and culture must always have priority over antigen detection testing. A bacterial culture is the major test to be performed on cerebrospinal fluid for meningitis. It is the "gold standard" for diagnosis. A requirement for 50 or more leukocytes per μL of CSF has been proposed as justification for bacterial antigen testing. Another group found a CSF nucleated blood cell count <6/mm^3 provided a criterion for an abbreviated CSF evaluation. There is substantial mortality and morbidity in subjects with bacterial meningitis. Neurologic sequelae are found in as many as 33% of all survivors, especially newborns and children. Especially when bacterial meningitis follows an insidious pattern, diagnostic delay may be unavoidable. Eight of 21 survivors of neonatal meningitis were normal, 8 had mild and 5 had moderate to severe sequelae in a culture-proven series.

White cell pleocytosis is found in only 33% of patients with multiple sclerosis (MS). The white count rarely exceeds 20 cells/mm^3. Most patients with MS (66%) have normal total proteins. In contrast, patients with the demyelinating disease Guillain-Barré syndrome usually have no excess white cells but show elevated CSF protein of 100-500 mg/dL.

(Continued)

Initial Cerebrospinal Fluid Findings in SuppurativeDiseases of the Central Nervous System and Meninges

Condition	Pressure (mm H_2O)	Leukocytes/mm^3	Protein (mg/dL)	Glucose (mg/dL)	Specific Findings
Acute bacterial meningitis	Usually elevated; average, 300	Several hundred to >60,000; usually a few thousand; occasionally <100 (especially meningococcal or early in disease); PMNs[1] predominate	Usually 100-500, occasionally >1000	<40 in >50% of cases	Organism usually seen on smear or culture in >90% of cases
Subdural empyema	Usually elevated; average, 300	<100 to a few thousand; PMNs predominate	Usually 100-500	Normal	No organisms seen on smear or culture unless concurrent meningitis
Brain abscess	Usually elevated	Usually 10-200; fluid is rarely acellular; lymphocytes predominate	Usually 75-400	Normal	No organisms seen on smear or culture
Ventricular empyema (rupture of brain abscess)	Considerably elevated	Several thousand to 100,000; usually >90% PMNs	Usually several hundred	Usually <40	Organism may be seen on smear or culture
Cerebral epidural abscess	Slightly to modestly elevated	Few to several hundred or more cells; lymphocytes predominate	Usually 50-200	Normal	No organisms seen on smear or culture
Spinal epidural abscess	Usually reduced with spinal block	Usually 10-100; lymphocytes predominate	Usually several hundred	Normal	No organisms seen on smear or culture
Thrombophlebitis (often associated with subdural empyema)	Often elevated	Few to several hundred; PMNs and lymphocytes	Slightly to moderately elevated	Normal	No organisms seen on smear or culture

Initial Cerebrospinal Fluid Findings in Suppurative Diseases of the Central Nervous System and Meninges *(Continued)*

Condition	Pressure (mm H_2O)	Leukocytes/mm^3	Protein (mg/dL)	Glucose (mg/dL)	Specific Findings
Bacterial endocarditis (with embolism)	Normal or slightly elevated	Few to <100; lymphocytes and PMNs	Slightly elevated	Normal	No organisms seen on smear or culture
Acute hemorrhagic encephalitis	Usually elevated	Few to >1000; PMNs predominate	Moderately elevated	Normal	No organisms seen on smear or culture
Tuberculous infection	Usually elevated; may be low with dynamic block in advanced stages	Usually 25-100, rarely >500; lymphocytes predominate, except in early stages when PMNs may account for 80% of the cells	Nearly always elevated, usually 100-200; may be much higher if dynamic block	Usually reduced; <50 in 75% of cases	Acid-fast organisms may be seen on smear of protein coagulum (pellicle) or recovered from inoculated guinea pig or by culture
Cryptococcal infection	Usually elevated; average, 225	Average, 50 (0-800); lymphocytes predominate	Average, 100; usually 20-500	Reduced in >50% the cases; average 30; often higher in patients with concomitant diabetes mellitus	Organisms may be seen in India ink preparation and on culture (Sabouraud's medium); will usually grow on blood agar; may produce alcohol in cerebrospinal fluid from fermentation of glucose
Syphilis (acute)	Usually elevated	Average, 500; usually lymphocytes; rare PMNs	Average, 100; globulin often high, with abnormal colloidal gold curve	Normal (rarely reduced)	Positive results of reagin test for syphilis; spirochetes not demonstrable by usual techniques of smear or culture
Sarcoidosis	Normal to considerably elevated	0 to <100 mononuclear cells	Slight to moderate elevation	Normal	No specific findings

[1]Polymorphonuclear leukocytes.

From Feigin RD and Cherry JD, eds, *Textbook of Pediatric Infectious Diseases*, Vol 1, Philadelphia, PA: WB Saunders, 1992, 410, with permission.

Cerebrospinal Fluid Analysis *(Continued)*

Selected Readings

Attia J, Hatala R, Cook DJ, et al, "Does This Adult Patient Have Acute Meningitis?" *JAMA*, 1999, 282(2):175-81.

Bonadio WA, Smith DS, Goddard S, et al, "Distinguishing Cerebrospinal Fluid Abnormalities in Children With Bacterial Meningitis and Traumatic Lumbar Puncture," *J Infect Dis*, 1990, 162(1):251-4.

Feigin RD, McCracken GH Jr, and Klein JO, "Diagnosis and Management of Meningitis," *Pediatr Infect Dis J*, 1992, 11(9):785-814.

Gray LD and Fedorko DP, "Laboratory Diagnosis of Bacterial Meningitis," *Clin Microbiol Rev*, 1992, 5(2):130-45.

Mein J and Lum G, "CSF Bacterial Antigen Detection Tests Offer No Advantage Over Gram's Stain in the Diagnosis of Bacterial Meningitis," *Pathology*, 1999, 31(1):67-9.

Michelow IC, Nicol M, Tiemessen C, et al, "Value of Cerebrospinal Fluid Leukocyte Aggregation in Distinguishing the Causes of Meningitis in Children," *Pediatr Infect Dis J*, 2000, 19(1):66-72.

Moris G and Garcia-Monco JC, "The Challenge of Drug-Induced Aseptic Meningitis," *Arch Intern Med*, 1999, 159(11):1185-94.

Norris CM, Danis PG, and Gardner TD, "Aseptic Meningitis in the Newborn and Young Infant," *Am J Fam Phys*, 1999, 59(10):2761-70.

Schaumburg HH and Herskovitz S, "The Weak Child - A Cautionary Tale," *N Engl J Med*, 2000, 342(2):127-9.

Strampfer MJ, Domenico P, and Cunha BA, "Laboratory Aids in the Diagnosis of Bacterial Meningitis," *Heart Lung*, 1988, 17(6 Pt 1):605-7.

Cerebrospinal Fluid Cryptococcal Latex Agglutination *see* Cryptococcal Antigen Serology, Serum or Cerebrospinal Fluid *on page 431*

Cerebrospinal Fluid Fungus Culture *see* Fungus Culture, Cerebrospinal Fluid *on page 464*

Cerebrospinal Fluid India Ink Preparation *see* India Ink Preparation *on page 507*

Cerebrospinal Fluid Latex Agglutination for Bacterial Antigens *see* Bacterial Antigens, Rapid Detection Methods *on page 388*

Cerebrospinal Fluid Tap *see* Lumbar Puncture *on page 524*

Cerebrospinal Fluid VDRL *see* VDRL, Cerebrospinal Fluid *on page 613*

Cervical *Chlamydia* Culture *see Chlamydia* Culture *on page 413*

Cervical Culture *see* Genital Culture *on page 470*

Cervical Culture for T-Strain *Mycoplasma* *see* Genital Culture for *Ureaplasma urealyticum on page 471*

Cervical Culture for *Ureaplasma urealyticum* *see* Genital Culture for *Ureaplasma urealyticum on page 471*

Cervical *Trichomonas* Smear *see Trichomonas* Preparation *on page 600*

Cervix Culture *Neisseria gonorrhoeae* *see Neisseria gonorrhoeae* Culture *on page 547*

Cervix, *Mycoplasma* Culture *see Mycoplasma/Ureaplasma* Culture *on page 545*

Chest Films

Synonyms CXR; PA; PA and Lateral CXR

Test Includes PA and lateral exposures of the chest.

Patient Preparation Remove medals, lockets, and other jewelry from neck. Arrange hair, when long, high on head so that no locks hang over chest or shoulders.

Special Instructions The chest x-ray can be modified in various ways to answer specific questions. For example, while the standard PA view of the chest is obtained in full inspiration, a pneumothorax will be more readily appreciated when the film is exposed in expiration. Decubitus films are helpful in differentiating mobile fluid in the pleural space from fluid loculations or pleural thickening. A lordotic view of the chest may be helpful in evaluating the apices. Oblique views of the chest done with 45° angulation in the right anterior oblique projection and 60° angulation in the left anterior oblique projection with barium opacifying the esophagus at the time of exposure are helpful in evaluating the size of the various cardiac chambers. Modifications to the standard examination should be clearly communicated to the radiology consultant.

Use Evaluate lungs and thoracic bones for presence of metastatic and primary neoplasm, infectious disease, degenerative and reactive processes, trauma, and surgical change; evaluate the heart and great vessels

Additional Information Sagel and his colleagues published an article in 1974 questioning the efficacy of screening examinations of the chest and whether or not lateral views should be obtained. Both medical and economic factors were considered. The study was based on a review of PA and lateral views of the chest in 10,597 examinations and reached the following conclusions.

- Routine screening for hospital admission or for surgery was not warranted for patients younger than 20 years of age.
- Lateral projection could be eliminated in routine screening of patients 20-39 years of age.
- Lateral projection should be obtained at any age when disease of the chest is suspected.
- Lateral projection should be obtained in screening examinations of patients older than 40 years of age.

Selected Readings

Henschke CI, Yankelevitz DF, Wand A, et al, "Accuracy and Efficacy of Chest Radiography in the Intensive Care Unit," *Radiol Clin North Am*, 1996, 34(1):21-31.

Henschke CI, Yankelevitz DF, Wand A, et al, "Chest Radiography in the ICU," *Clin Imaging*, 1997, 21(2):90-103.

Sagel SS, Evens RG, Forrest JV, et al, "Efficacy of Routine Screening and Lateral Chest Radiographs in a Hospital-Based Population," *N Engl J Med*, 1974, 291(19):1001-4.

Tenholder MF, Greene LM, and Thomas AM, "The Role of Radiology in Pulmonary Infectious Disease," *Curr Opin Pulm Med*, 1998, 4(3):142-7

Chickenpox Culture *see* Varicella-Zoster Virus Culture *on page 612*

Chickenpox Titer *see* Varicella-Zoster Virus Serology *on page 612*

Chlamydia and *Chlamydophila* Species Serology

Related Information

Chlamydia Culture *on page 413*
Chlamydia trachomatis by Molecular Probe *on page 415*
Chlamydophila pneumoniae Serology *on page 416*
Chlamydophila psittaci Serology *on page 417*

Test Includes Detection of antibody titer to *Chlamydia* species

Specimen Serum

Container Red top tube

Collection Collect acute phase blood as soon as possible after onset (no later than 1 week). Convalescent blood should be drawn 1-2 weeks after acute (no less than 2 weeks after onset).

Reference Range Negative. A fourfold increase in titer in paired sera is usually indicative of chlamydial infection. Determination of IgM antibody may be helpful in differentiating acute infection from prior exposure.

Use Evaluate possible chlamydial infection

Limitations The antigen (lipopolysaccharide) used in the test is group specific and not species specific. In cases of conjunctivitis, nongonococcal urethritis, and pneumonia of the newborn, there is usually **not** an antibody response detectable by complement fixation. A very high "background" of immunity in the general population makes interpretation of results difficult.

Methodology Complement fixation (CF), indirect fluorescence antibody (IFA), enzyme immunoassay (EIA)

Additional Information Because of the high prevalence of antibodies to *Chlamydia*, especially in patients being evaluated for urethritis or possible venereal disease, results of serologic tests must be interpreted with caution. Very high titers, rising titers, or IgM specific antibody should be sought. In a patient being evaluated for chlamydial disease of the genitourinary tract, culture as well as serology should be obtained, as well as a serologic test for syphilis and a culture for *Neisseria gonorrhoeae*.

Selected Readings

Hammerschlag MR, "Current Status of Laboratory Diagnosis of *Chlamydia pneumoniae* and *Chlamydia psittaci*," *Clin Microbiol Newslett*, 2001, 23(14):107-11.

Mahony JB, Coombes BK, and Cherneseky MA, "*Chlamydia* and *Chlamydophila*," *Manual of Clinical Microbiology*, 8th ed, Murray PR, Baron EJ, Jorgensen JH, et al, eds, Washington, DC: American Society for Microbiology, 2003, 991-1004.

Miettinen A, Heinonen PK, Teisala K, et al, "Antigen-Specific Serum Antibody Response to *Chlamydia trachomatis* in Patients With Pelvic Inflammatory Disease," *J Clin Pathol*, 1990, 43(9):758-61.

Chlamydia Culture

Related Information

Chlamydia and *Chlamydophila* Species Serology *on page 413*
Chlamydia trachomatis by Molecular Probe *on page 415*
Chlamydophila pneumoniae Serology *on page 416*
Chlamydophila psittaci Serology *on page 417*
Genital Culture *on page 470*

Synonyms TRIC Agent Culture

Applies to Cervical *Chlamydia* Culture; Eye Swab *Chlamydia* Culture; Lymphogranuloma Venereum Culture; Urethral *Chlamydia* Culture

Test Includes Cell culture to detect *Chlamydia*

Special Instructions Availability and specific specimen collection requirements for *Chlamydia* cultures vary. Consult the laboratory for specific instructions, swabs, and transport materials prior to collection of the specimen.

Specimen *Chlamydia* is an intracellular organism; therefore, infected cells must be obtained by swabbing the urethra, cervix, rectum, conjunctiva, posterior nasopharynx, or throat.

Container Culturette® (Dacron) swabs should be used. Use specific *Chlamydia* transport medium.

(Continued)

Chlamydia Culture *(Continued)*

Collection

Urethra: Remove mucous/pus by using a separate swab; discard this swab. The swab should be inserted 2-4 cm into the urethra. Use firm pressure to scrape cells from the mucosal surface. If possible repeat with second swab. Patient should not urinate within 1 hour prior to specimen collection.

Cervix: Remove mucous/pus with a Culturette® and discard this swab. Use a new swab (Culturette®) and use firm and rotating pressure to obtain specimen. May be combined with a urethral swab into same transport medium. This two-swab method is highly recommended.

Rectum: Sample anal crypts with a Culturette®.

Conjunctiva: Remove mucous and exudate with a separate swab; discard this swab. Use a Culturette® and firm pressure to scrape away epithelial cells from upper and lower lids.

Posterior nasopharynx or throat: Collect epithelial cells by using a Culturette®.

Storage Instructions Deliver inoculated transport medium **immediately** to laboratory. **Specimens must be refrigerated** during storage and transportation or frozen at -70°C if stored more than 2 days.

Turnaround Time Cultures with no growth usually will be reported after 4-7 days. Rapid culture methods for detection of *Chlamydia* require a minimum of 48 hours.

Reference Range No *Chlamydia* isolated

Use Aid in the diagnosis of infections caused by *Chlamydia* (eg, cervicitis, trachoma, conjunctivitis, pelvic inflammatory disease, pneumonia, urethritis, nongonococcal urethritis, pneumonitis, and sexually transmitted diseases).

Limitations Culture may be negative in presence of *Chlamydia* infection. Culture is probably not the gold standard for the detection of *C. trachomatis*. The sensitivity of culture probably is only 70% to 90% because *C. trachomatis* does not always survive transit to the laboratory and because sampling is often inadequate even with (multiple) swabs.

Culture is likely to be negative if only mucus/discharge is submitted.

Methodology Inoculation of specimen onto McCoy cell culture and subsequent detection of *Chlamydia*-infected cells by immunofluorescence and monoclonal antibody

Additional Information This organism infects the endocervical columnar epithelial cells and will not be found in the inflammatory cells. In obtaining the specimen, clean the area of inflammatory cells and then attempt to scrape epithelial cells for culturing by using a new, separate swab. The results of cytological diagnosis of chlamydial infection of the female genital tract have been disappointing. Papanicolaou-stained cervical smears are not reliable enough to help establish or exclude the presence of *Chlamydia*. In patients with vaginal discharge or other genital tract symptomatology of unknown etiology, cervical cytology can be useful in identifying patients who should be cultured for *Chlamydia*. Direct immunofluorescence techniques and enzyme immunoassays are available to detect *Chlamydia* in clinical specimens. These methods usually provide reliable results in high-prevalence populations and detect both viable and nonviable organisms. Selection of the most efficient method for recovery of *Chlamydia* depends upon the incidence in the patient population and the local availability of the various methods. Urine culture for *Chlamydia* is not a sensitive procedure and generally should not be done. The incidence of cervical infection with *Chlamydia trachomatis* is two to three times that of gonorrhea: 4% to 9% in private office settings, 6% to 23% in family planning clinics, and 20% to 30% in sexually transmitted diseases clinics.

Culture should be the test-of-choice (i) in cases of child abuse, ascending pelvic infections, and rectal and throat infections, and (ii) when a test-for-cure is desired.

Chlamydia is a single genus and consists of the following:

- *C. trachomatis* (serotypes A-K): inclusion conjunctivitis, trachoma, and genital infections
- *C. trachomatis* (serotypes L1-L3): lymphogranuloma venereum

Two species closely related to *Chlamydia* are:

- *Chlamydophila psittaci* (psittacosis)
- *Chlamydophila pneumoniae* (respiratory infections)

Serology to detect antibodies to each of the three species of *Chlamydia* is available.

Laboratory diagnosis of *C. pneumoniae* infections is not widely available; commercial tests for *C. pneumoniae* are not available. *C. pneumoniae* is responsible for approximately 10% of community-acquired pneumonias. The cells (McCoy) usually used to culture *C. trachomatis* will not reliably support the growth of *C. pneumoniae*. Recent

studies have shown that other cell lines (H 292 and HEp-2) are more appropriate. However, culture using these cells is not generally available. An alternate, widely used method for the laboratory diagnosis of *C. pneumoniae* infection is serology by microimmunofluorescence. Currently, this serological test is the most sensitive and specific laboratory test for *C. pneumoniae.*

Selected Readings

Hammerschlag MR, "Current Status of Laboratory Diagnosis of *Chlamydia pneumoniae* and *Chlamydia psittaci*," *Clin Microbiol Newslett*, 2001, 23(14):107-11.

Hipp SS and Coles FB, "The Virtues of *Chlamydia* Culture," *Clin Microbiol Newslett*, 1994, 16(5):37-9.

Mahony JB, Coombes BK, and Cherneseky MA, "*Chlamydia* and *Chlamydophila*," *Manual of Clinical Microbiology*, 8th ed, Murray PR, Baron EJ, Jorgensen JH, et al, eds, Washington, DC: American Society for Microbiology, 2003, 991-1004.

Olshen E and Shrier LA, "Diagnostic Tests for Chlamydial and Gonorrheal Infections," *Semin Pediatr Infect Dis*, 2005, 16(3):192-8.

Taylor-Robinson D and Thomas BJ, "Sensitivity of Chlamydial Diagnostic Tests," *Int J STD AIDS*, 2000, 11(3):204-5.

***Chlamydia* Smear** *see* Ocular Cytology *on page 551*

Chlamydia trachomatis by Molecular Probe

Related Information

Chlamydia and *Chlamydophila* Species Serology *on page 413*
Chlamydia Culture *on page 413*
Chlamydophila pneumoniae Serology *on page 416*
Chlamydophila psittaci Serology *on page 417*

Synonyms *Chlamydia trachomatis* DNA Detection Test; DNA Hybridization Test for *Chlamydia trachomatis*; DNA Test for *Chlamydia trachomatis*

Test Includes Direct detection of *Chlamydia trachomatis* nucleic acid in swab specimens.

Patient Preparation When taking urethral specimens the patient should not have urinated for 1 hour prior to collection.

Specimen Swab specimen collected from the genitourinary tract of a male or female patient

Container Special transport medium is provided by the laboratory and should not be substituted. A commercially available kit containing a swab and a special transport medium is required for this test.

Collection Currently the molecular tests for *Chlamydia trachomatis* are FDA-approved only for urethral, cervical, and conjunctival specimens.

For a male the urethra is swabbed by rotating the swab 2-3 cm into the urethra. This should provide enough epithelial cells from the infected site to detect *C. trachomatis.* The swab is then placed in the transport tube for shipping to the laboratory.

For females, the cervix or endocervix should be swabbed and with one swab first to clean the area and the second swab is used to collect the specimen. The swab is inserted 2-3 cm into the endocervix and then rotated to collect the epithelial cells from the infected site. The swab is then put immediately into the transport tube and shipped to the laboratory.

For conjunctival specimens, use a "male" collection kit, clean away exudate with a separate swab and discard the swab, thoroughly swab the lower and upper conjunctiva each two to three times. Place the swab immediately into the transport tube with medium for transport to the laboratory.

Storage Instructions The specimens should be kept at room temperature or refrigerated. Do not freeze.

Causes for Rejection Contamination with urine; specimen frozen (which lyses the cells collected); gross blood in specimen

Turnaround Time Usually results are available within 24 hours of receipt of the specimen.

Reference Range The results of a normal test should be negative for *Chlamydia trachomatis* DNA. Sexually active, asymptomatic individuals may harbor *C. trachomatis* in rates ranging from 0% to 7%.

Use Rapid detection of *C. trachomatis* in clinical specimens

Limitations DNA detection test should not be done in child abuse cases. Although it is not as sensitive as molecular tests, cell culture is the only approved test in these cases. However, this test can be used to confirm positive culture results.

Methodology This test detects *C. trachomatis* ribosomal RNA directly from swab specimens. This requires denaturation of the RNA in the specimens by heating, hybridization with a specific DNA probe and detection of bound probe after several washing steps. Detection is done by using a probe labeled with an acridinium ester which releases a burst of light when in the presence of H_2O_2.

(Continued)

Chlamydia trachomatis by Molecular Probe *(Continued)*

An increasing number of clinical laboratories are offering molecular amplification of *Chlamydia* RNA in the specimen before detection. Such amplified methods are more sensitive than simple direct detection methods. Contact the testing laboratory for details before collecting specimens.

Additional Information Approximately 4 million cases of *C. trachomatis* occur annually in the United States, and it is considered a serious sexually transmitted disease problem. The detection of *C. trachomatis* RNA provides a diagnostic test that has several advantages over the traditional culture method. The turnaround time is shorter, it is less labor intensive, and it provides an objective result that makes interpretation easier. The RNA detection test for *C. trachomatis* has been proven to have an equivalent sensitivity to the antibody-based test (EIA and fluorescent antibody detection methods) and to have a greater specificity than these tests. However, at the present time this test cannot be done exclusively if a child abuse case is involved. These cases must be detected with a cell culture test.

Selected Readings

Barnes RC, "Laboratory Diagnosis of Human Chlamydial Infections," *Clin Microbiol Rev*, 1989, 2(2):119-36.

Black CM, "Current Methods of Laboratory Diagnosis of *Chlamydia trachomatis* Infections," *Clin Microbiol Rev*, 1997, 10(1):160-84.

Hammerschlag MR, "Current Status of Laboratory Diagnosis of *Chlamydia pneumoniae* and *Chlamydia psittaci*," *Clin Microbiol Newslett*, 2001, 23(14):107-11.

Mahony JB, Coombes BK, and Chernesky MA, "*Chlamydia* and *Chlamydophila*," *Manual of Clinical Microbiology*, 8th ed, Murray PR, Baron EJ, Jorgensen JH, et al, eds, Washington, DC: American Society for Microbiology, 2003, 991-1004.

Taylor-Robinson D and Thomas BJ, "Sensitivity of Chlamydial Diagnostic Tests," *Int J STD AIDS*, 2000, 11(3):204-5.

***Chlamydia trachomatis* DNA Detection Test** *see Chlamydia trachomatis* by Molecular Probe *on page 415*

Chlamydophila pneumoniae Serology

Related Information

Chlamydia and *Chlamydophila* Species Serology *on page 413*
Chlamydia Culture *on page 413*
Chlamydia trachomatis by Molecular Probe *on page 415*
Chlamydophila psittaci Serology *on page 417*
Community-Acquired Pneumonia in Adults *on page 1278*

Test Includes Pan-reactive for trachoma, psittacosis, LGV, and TWAR

Specimen Serum

Container Red top tube or serum separator tube

Storage Instructions Separate serum and refrigerate.

Causes for Rejection Excessive hemolysis, chylous serum, inadequate labeling

Reference Range Negative. Titers <1:64 suggest no current or previous infection. A fourfold or greater increase in antibody titer in paired specimens usually provides unequivocal evidence of recent infection. Contact the testing laboratory for specific reference ranges.

Use Evaluate possible chlamydial infection

Limitations The antigen (lipopolysaccharide) used in the test is group specific and not species specific. A very high "background" of immunity in the general population makes interpretation of results difficult.

Methodology Indirect fluorescent antibody (IFA)

Additional Information Recently, the genus *Chlamydia* was divided into the genera *Chlamydia* (*C. trachomatis*) and *Chlamydophila* (*C. psittaci* and *C. pneumoniae*). *C. pneumoniae* is a frequent cause of acute respiratory disease. *C. pneumoniae* antibody has been found in 25% to 60% of adults. The determination of species or type specific antibodies to *C. psittaci*, *C. trachomatis*, and *C. pneumoniae* strain is complicated by cross reactive antigens or nonspecific stimulation of antichlamydial antibodies. Thus, a panel of *Chlamydia* must be tested to determine specific titers and establish the strongest reactions. The panel to differentiate *C. pneumoniae, C. psittaci*, and *C. trachomatis* may be requested from a microbiology reference laboratory.

Selected Readings

Black CM, "Current Methods of Laboratory Diagnosis of *Chlamydia trachomatis* Infections," *Clin Microbiol Rev*, 1997, 10(1):160-84.

Hammerschlag MR, "Current Status of Laboratory Diagnosis of *Chlamydia pneumoniae* and *Chlamydia psittaci*," *Clin Microbiol Newslett*, 2001, 23(14):107-11.

Mahony JB, Coombes BK, and Chernesky MA, "*Chlamydia* and *Chlamydophila*," *Manual of Clinical Microbiology*, 8th ed, Murray PR, Baron EJ, Jorgensen JH, et al, eds, Washington, DC: American Society for Microbiology, 2003, 991-1004.

Starr JR and Jackson LA, "*Chlamydia pneumoniae* and Atherosclerotic Cardiovascular Disease," *Clin Microbiol Newslett*, 1999, 21(18):145-8.

***Chlamydophila psittaci* Antibody** *see Chlamydophila psittaci* Serology *on page 417*

Chlamydophila psittaci Serology

Related Information

Chlamydia and *Chlamydophila* Species Serology *on page 413*
Chlamydia Culture *on page 413*
Chlamydia trachomatis by Molecular Probe *on page 415*
Chlamydophila pneumoniae Serology *on page 416*
Community-Acquired Pneumonia in Adults *on page 1278*

Synonyms *Chlamydophila psittaci* Antibody

Special Instructions Acute and convalescent samples are recommended.

Specimen Serum

Container Red top tube or serum separator tube

Reference Range Less than a fourfold increase in titer in paired sera

Use Diagnose psittacosis

Limitations Antibody response may be suppressed if patient has been treated with antibiotics

Methodology Complement fixation (CF), microimmunofluorescence

Additional Information Most patients with psittacosis develop high titers of complement fixing antibody and in some with the proper clinical setting a single very high titer may be strongly supportive of the diagnosis. Specific IgM antibody can sometimes be demonstrated.

To detect psittacosis antibody, an antigen specific for *C. psittaci* must be included in the test system. There may be significant antibody titers in veterinarians and patients with Reiter's syndrome.

Selected Readings

Hammerschlag MR, "Current Status of Laboratory Diagnosis of *Chlamydia pneumoniae* and *Chlamydia psittaci*," *Clin Microbiol Newslett*, 2001, 23(14):107-11.

Mahony JB, Coombes BK, and Cherneseky MA, "*Chlamydia* and *Chlamydophila*," *Manual of Clinical Microbiology*, 8th ed, Murray PR, Baron EJ, Jorgensen JH, et al, eds, Washington, DC: American Society for Microbiology, 2003, 991-1004.

Chloramphenicol Serum Level

Related Information

Antibiotic Level, Serum *on page 375*

Synonyms Chloromycetin®; Mychel-S®

Abstract Chloramphenicol is an antimicrobial agent whose use has been greatly reduced in recent years because of the introduction of a wide variety of less toxic alternative agents. It is still appropriately used to treat certain rickettsial infections or penicillin-allergic patients with bacterial meningitis. Life-threatening bone marrow toxicity is not closely associated with high serum levels.

Specimen Serum

Container Red top tube or serum separator tube

Sampling Time Collect for trough level immediately before next dose; for peak level about 2 hours after oral dose, 30 minutes after I.V. dose (time to peak can be variable)

Storage Instructions Freeze processed specimen

Reference Range Therapeutic range: 10-25 mcg/mL (SI: 31-77 μmol/L), trough <5 mcg/mL (SI: <15 μmol/L)

Critical Values Toxic range: >25 mcg/mL (SI: >77 μmol/L)

Use Monitor drug therapy; monitor for potential toxicity

Limitations Reversible dose related bone marrow depression may occur when serum/plasma concentration >25 mcg/mL (SI: >77 μmol/L). Idiosyncratic bone marrow aplasia is a rare event that usually occurs weeks to months after completing therapy, but approximately 25% occur during the course of therapy. Hematologic studies should be performed before and during therapy.

Methodology High performance liquid chromatography (HPLC), gas-liquid chromatography (GLC), immunoassay

Additional Information Chloramphenicol is an extremely effective antibacterial agent which unfortunately has both idiosyncratic and dose-related toxicities. Half-life is 1.6-3.3 hours longer in infants and patients with hepatic and renal disease. The dose related toxicity is, in adults, bone marrow suppression. "Gray syndrome," a type of circulatory collapse, occurs primarily in infants whose livers are unable to metabolize chloramphenicol effectively. Idiosyncratic aplastic anemia occurs in between 1 in 20,000 and 1 in 40,000 exposures. There are a number of chloramphenicol drug interactions since chloramphenicol can inhibit hepatic microsomal metabolism, increasing the serum concentration of phenytoin, tolbutamide, and dicumarol. Phenobarbital may be elevated in the presence of chloramphenicol.

Selected Readings

Baselt RC, *Analytical Procedures for Therapeutic Drug Monitoring and Emergency Toxicology*, Davis, CA: Biomedical Publications, 1980, 71-5.

(Continued)

Chloramphenicol Serum Level *(Continued)*

de Louvois J, Mulhall A, and Hurley R, "Comparison of Methods Available for Assay of Chloramphenicol in Clinical Specimens," *J Clin Pathol*, 1980, 33(6):575-80.

Hammett-Stabler CA and Johns T, "Laboratory Guidelines for Monitoring of Antimicrobial Drugs. National Academy of Clinical Biochemistry," *Clin Chem*, 1998, 44(5):1129-40.

Smilack JD, Wilson WR, and Cockerill FR 3d, "Tetracyclines, Chloramphenicol, Erythromycin, Clindamycin, and Metronidazole," *Mayo Clin Proc*, 1991, 66(12):1270-80.

Chloromycetin® *see* Chloramphenicol Serum Level *on page 417*

***Cimex* Identification** *see* Arthropod Identification *on page 387*

Clavicle, Left or Right, X-ray *see* Bone Films *on page 396*

Closed Joint Aspiration *see* Arthrocentesis *on page 384*

***Clostridium botulinum* Toxin Identification Procedure** *see* Botulism, Diagnostic Procedure *on page 405*

Clostridium difficile Toxin Assay

Related Information

Fecal Leukocyte Stain *on page 455*

Synonyms Antibiotic-Associated Colitis Toxin Test; Pseudomembranous Colitis Toxin Assay; Toxin Assay, *Clostridium difficile*

Test Includes Toxin detection

Special Instructions When antibiotic-associated colitis is suspected a toxin assay rather than a *C. difficile* culture should be ordered on the stool.

Specimen Stool or proctoscopic specimen; one specimen per week is sufficient.

Container Stool container with lids (swabs are inadequate because of small volume)

Collection Keep specimen **cold** and transport immediately to prevent deterioration of toxin. Specimens can be frozen if transportation will be delayed.

Storage Instructions If the specimen cannot be processed immediately, it should be stored under refrigeration.

Turnaround Time 1-3 days depending on the availability and on the protocol of laboratory

Reference Range Presence of toxin is indicative of disease. Isolation of organism (*C. difficile*) may occur in a small percentage of normal adults (5% to 21%) and in normal newborns. Isolation of the organism without demonstration of toxin production is a nonspecific finding because only certain isolates are toxigenic.

Use Determine the presence or absence of antibiotic-related colitis caused by *C. difficile* toxin

Limitations Results given as titers are not significant as such because size/amounts of original specimens are usually not standardized. Results should be given as positive or negative, and any titer result should be interpreted as simply positive.

This test is **not** to be used as a "test of cure".

Methodology Toxin neutralization test in cell culture (to detect the toxin) probably is the standard. Enzyme immunoassay is a very sensitive test as an alternative to toxin neutralization, has a shorter turnaround time, and is being used increasingly more by many laboratories. Essentially all commercially available kits/products now detect both toxin A and toxin B.

Additional Information Antibiotic-associated pseudomembranous colitis has been shown to result from the action of toxins produced by the organism, *C. difficile*. The disease has been associated with clindamycin but now it is recognized that pseudomembranous colitis can follow administration of virtually any antibiotic. More than 70% of cases in a large study were associated with cephalosporin therapy. The clinical spectrum of antibiotic-induced syndromes caused by *C. difficile* includes patients with symptoms of acute abdomen with little or no diarrhea, as well as cases with fulminant life-threatening diarrhea. Nosocomial transmission and reinfection with different strains occurs as do spontaneous cases without prior antimicrobial therapy. In cases where cessation of antibiotic therapy does not produce a response, specific therapy with oral vancomycin, metronidazole or oral bacitracin may be effective. The detection of the toxin (rather than culture of the organism or detection of the organism by latex agglutination) is essential in determining the etiology of this potentially fatal disease. In a recent report of 40 patients with *C. difficile*-associated diarrhea, 70% were positive in the cytotoxin assay, 78% positive in the LA test, and 90% culture positive. Fifty-three control patients had a 2%, 8%, and 4% positive rate respectively (ie, a small percentage of false-positives). A reasonable strategy might be to screen with the LA test and perform the toxin assay in cases which are positive. The routine use of culture is not appropriate because of the costs and the high rate of recovery of strains which do not produce toxin. Cytotoxin results are slightly more predictive of *C. difficile* disease than latex-positive results. Neither method alone is able either to

predict or rule out all cases accurately. The organism is known to produce an enterotoxin, toxin A and a cytotoxin, toxin B. The exact role of each of these toxins, in clinical disease, remains unclear.

Selected Readings

Fekety R, and Shah AB, "Diagnosis and Treatment of *Clostridium difficile* Colitis," *JAMA*, 1993, 269(1):71-5.

Gorschluter M, Glasmacher A, Hahn C, et al, "*Clostridium difficile* Infection in Patients With Neutropenia," *Clin Infect Dis*, 2001, 33(6):786-91.

Knoop FC, Owens M, and Crocker IC, "*Clostridium difficile*: Clinical Disease and Diagnosis," *Clin Microbiol Rev*, 1993, 6(3):251-65.

McGowan KL and Kader HA, "*Clostridium difficile* Infection in Children," *Clin Microbiol Newslett*, 1999, 21(7):49-53.

CLO™ Test *see Helicobacter pylori* Culture and Urease Test *on page 479*

CMG *see* Cystometrogram, Simple *on page 434*

CMV Culture *see* Cytomegalovirus Culture, Blood *on page 439*

CMV DNA Hybrid Capture *see* Cytomegalovirus DNA Hybrid Capture *on page 440*

CMV Early Antigen FA Method *see* Cytomegalovirus Isolation, Rapid *on page 442*

CMV-IFA *see* Cytomegalovirus Serology *on page 442*

CMV-IFA, IgG *see* Cytomegalovirus Serology *on page 442*

CMV-IFA, IgM *see* Cytomegalovirus Serology *on page 442*

CMVS, Culture *see* Urine Culture, Clean Catch *on page 609*

CMV Shell Vial Method *see* Cytomegalovirus Isolation, Rapid *on page 442*

CMV Titer *see* Cytomegalovirus Serology *on page 442*

Coagglutination Test for Group A Streptococci *see* Group A *Streptococcus* Antigen Test *on page 475*

***Coccidioides* Immunodiffusion** *see* Fungal Serology *on page 458*

Cold Agglutinin Test

Test Includes Titer of patient's serum against type O blood cells at 2°C to 8°C

Special Instructions Transport blood immediately to laboratory.

Specimen Serum

Container Red top tube or serum separator tube

Storage Instructions After clotting at 37°C, separate serum from cells if specimen is to be stored overnight in refrigerator.

Causes for Rejection Refrigeration of the specimen before separating serum from cells; specimen not allowed to clot at 37°C

Reference Range Screen: negative; titer: <1:32

Use Because it is nonspecific, the test generally is not recommended. Occasionally, the cold agglutination titer is useful in supporting the diagnosis of primary atypical pneumonia (infection with *Mycoplasma pneumoniae*). Tests for specific antibodies to *Mycoplasma pneumoniae* are much more useful and specific than are tests for cold agglutinins.

Limitations False-negatives may occur if serum is refrigerated on the clot; only half of patients with *M. pneumoniae* infection will have positive test; many positive results are associated with a wide variety of nonspecific conditions

Additional Information The i and I RBC antigens appear to be ceramide heptasaccharides and decasaccharides. The fetal i RBCs change after birth so that by 18 months red cells carry largely I. The i substance has been found in saliva, milk, amniotic fluid, ovarian cyst fluid, and serum.

The most common cause of elevated cold agglutinin in high titers is an infection with *Mycoplasma pneumoniae. M. pneumoniae* has I-like antigen specificity. Fifty-five percent of patients with disease have rising titers. In primary atypical *Mycoplasma pneumoniae* pneumonia, cold agglutinins are demonstrated 1 week after onset; the titer increases in 8-10 days, peaks at 12-25 days, and rapidly falls after day 30. Antibiotic therapy may interfere with antibody formation. Ninety percent of those who are severely affected or have prolonged illness will have a positive cold agglutination titer.

Cold agglutinins are usually IgM autoantibodies directed against the Ii antigens of human RBCs. These antibodies may be found in patients with cold agglutinin disease or may occur transiently following a number of acute infectious illnesses. Cold agglutinins of cold agglutinin disease are usually monoclonal IgM kappa. Cold antibodies of IgG, IgA, or IgM type directed against Ii antigens may be found in infectious mononucleosis. Antibodies reacting near physiologic temperatures are more likely to be clinically important. Detection of cold agglutinins may be useful in patients where cold blood is to be used such as in a blood cardioplegia unit.

Complete Blood Count

Synonyms Blood Cell Profile; Blood Count; CBC; Hemogram

Test Includes WBC, Hct, Hgb, differential count, RBC, WBC and RBC morphology, RBC indices, platelet estimate, platelet count, RDW, and histograms. Although RBC, WBC, and platelet histograms are not available on patient charts, they are helpful to the technologist in detecting problems with patients and quality control. Even though the histograms are not on the chart, they can be viewed in the laboratory along with the blood smear. New analyzers also provide automated 5-part white cell differentials: granulocytes, monocytes, lymphocytes, eosinophils, and basophils.

Abstract The standard automated test for evaluation of RBC, WBC, and platelets

Specimen Whole blood

Container Lavender top (EDTA) tube

Collection Follow collection, mix the specimen 10 times by gentle inversion. If specimen is not immediately transported to the laboratory, refrigerate. If the anticipated delay in arrival is more than 4 hours, two blood smears should be prepared immediately after the venipuncture and submitted with the blood specimen.

Causes for Rejection Improper tube, clotted specimen, hemolyzed specimen, dilution of blood with I.V. fluid

Reference Range Accompanying tables summarize differences in red cell parameter normal ranges, note especially important age and sex variances. Refer to tables.

Critical Values Hematocrit: <18% or >54%; hemoglobin: <6.0 g/dL or >18.0 g/dL; WBC on admission: <2500/mm^3 or >30,000/mm^3

Use Evaluate anemia, leukemia, reaction to inflammation and infections, peripheral blood cellular characteristics, state of hydration and dehydration, polycythemia, hemolytic disease of the newborn; manage chemotherapy decisions

Limitations Hemoglobin may be falsely high if the plasma is lipemic or if the white count is >50,000 cells/mm^3. "Spun" (manual centrifuged) microhematocrits are approximately 3% higher (due to plasma trapping) compared to automated hematocrit levels. The increase is especially pronounced in cases of polycythemia (increased Hct levels) and when the cells are hypochromic and microcytic. The spun Hct level (as compared to Coulter S) may be 12% higher at Hct levels of 70% and MCV of 48 fL with decrease in change to 3% higher at Hct levels of 70% with MCV of 100 fL. Cold agglutinins (high titer) may cause spurious macrocytosis and low RBC count. This

Mean Hematologic Values for Low-Birth-Weight Infants[1]

Weight and Gestational Age at Birth	Age at Testing	Hemoglobin (g/dL)	Hematocrit (%)	Reticulocytes (%)
<1500 g, 28-32 wk	3 d	17.5±1.5	54±5	8.0±3.5
	1 wk	15.5±1.5	48±5	3.0±1.0
	2 wk	13.5±1.1	42±4	3.0±1.0
	3 wk	11.5±1.0	35±4	—
	4 wk	10.0±0.9	30±3	6.0±2.0
	6 wk	8.5±0.5	25±2	11.0±3.5
	8 wk	8.5±0.5	25±2	8.5±3.5
	10 wk	9.0±0.5	28±3	7.0±3.0
1500-2000 g, 32-36 wk	3 d	19.0±2.0	59±6	6.0±2.0
	1 wk	16.5±1.5	51±5	3.0±1.0
	2 wk	14.5±1.1	44±5	2.5±1.0
	3 wk	13.0±1.1	39±4	—
	4 wk	12.0±1.0	36±4	3.0±1.0
	6 wk	9.5±0.8	28±3	6.0±2.0
	8 wk	9.5±0.5	28±3	5.0±1.5
	10 wk	9.5±0.5	29±3	4.5±1.5
2000-2500 g, 36-40 wk	3 d	19.0±2.0	59±6	4.0±1.0
	1 wk	16.5±1.5	51±5	3.0±1.0
	2 wk	15.0±1.5	45±5	2.5±1.0
	3 wk	14.0±1.1	43±4	—
	4 wk	12.5±1.0	37±4	2.0±1.0
	6 wk	10.5±0.9	31±3	3.0±1.0
	8 wk	10.5±0.9	31±3	3.0±1.0
	10 wk	11.0±1.0	33±3	3.0±1.0

[1]Mean ±1 SD.

From Johnson TR, "How Growing Up Can Alter Lab Values in Pediatric Laboratory Medicine," *Diag Med* (special issue), 1982, 5:13-8, with permission.

results when RBC couplets are "seen" and processed as single cells by the detection circuitry. Keeping the blood warm and warming the diluent prior to and during counting can correct this problem.

Methodology Varies considerably between institutions. Most laboratories have high capacity multichannel instruments in place (available from multiple commercial sources). The majority measure RBC and WBC parameters on the basis of changes in electrical impedance as cells and platelets are pulled through a tiny aperture. These are highly automated devices with extensive computer processing of the electrical signals after analog/digital conversion. Accuracy (with proper standardization) and precision (usually in the 0.5% to 2% range) is significantly improved over older manual and semiautomated methods. Some instruments count light impulses that are generated as cells flow across a laser beam.

Red Cell Values on First Postnatal Day[1]

Gestational Age (wk)	24-25	26-27	28-29	30-31	32-33	34-35	36-37	Term
RBC ($\times 10^6/mm^3$)	4.65 ±0.43	4.73 ±0.45	4.62 ±0.75	4.79 ±0.74	5.0 ±0.76	5.09 ±0.5	5.27 ±0.68	5.14 ±0.7
Hgb (g/dL)	19.4 ±1.5	19.0 ±2.5	19.3 ±1.8	19.1 ±2.2	18.5 ±2.0	19.6 ±2.1	19.2 ±1.7	19.3 ±2.2
Hct (%)	63 ±4	62 ±8	60 ±7	60 ±8	60 ±8	61 ±7	64 ±7	61 ±7.4
MCV (fL)	135 ±0.2	132 ±14.4	131 ±13.5	127 ±12.7	123 ±15.7	122 ±10.0	121 ±12.5	119 ±9.4
Retic (%)	6.0 ±0.5	9.6 ±3.2	7.5 ±2.5	5.8 ±2.0	5.0 ±1.9	3.9 ±1.6	4.2 ±1.8	3.2 ±1.4

[1]Mean values ±1 SD.

From Zaizov R and Matoth Y, "Red Cell Values on the First Postnatal Day During the Last 16 Weeks of Gestation," *Amer J Hematol*, 1976, 1:2, 275-8, with permission.

Mean Hematologic Values for Full-Term Infants, Children, and Adults[1]

Age	Hgb (g/dL)	Hct (%)	RBC ($\times 10^6/mm^3$)	MCV (fL)	MCH (pg)	MCHC (g/dL)
Birth (cord blood)	17.1±1.8	52.0±5	4.64±0.5	113±6	37±2	33±1
1 d	19.4±2.1	58.0±7	5.30±0.5	110±6	37±2	33±1
2-6 d	19.8±2.4	66.0±8	5.40±0.7	122±14	37±4	30±3
14-23 d	15.7±1.5	52.0±5	4.92±0.6	106±11	32±3	30±2
24-37 d	14.1±1.9	45.0±7	4.35±0.6	104±11	32±3	31±3
40-50 d	12.8±1.9	42.0±6	4.10±0.5	103±11	31±3	30±2
2-2.5 mo	11.4±1.1	38.0±4	3.75±0.5	101±10	30±3	30±2
3-3.5 mo	11.2±0.8	37.0±3	3.88±0.4	95±9	29±3	30±2
5-7 mo	11.5±0.7	38.0±3	4.21±0.5	91±9	27±3	30±2
8-10 mo	11.7±0.6	39.0±2	4.35±0.4	90±8	27±3	30±1
11-13.5 mo	11.9±0.6	39.0±2	4.44±0.4	88±7	27±2	30±1
1.5-3 y	11.8±0.5	39.0±2	4.45±0.4	87±7	27±2	30±2
5 y	12.7±1.0	37.0±3	4.65±0.5	80±4	27±2	34±1
10 y	13.2±1.2	39.0±3	4.80±0.5	81±6	28±3	34±1
Male	15.5±1.1	46.0±3.1	5.11±0.38	90.1±4.8	30.2±1.8	33.7±1.1
Female	13.7±1.0	40.9±3	4.51±0.36	90.1±4.8	30.2±1.8	33.7±1.1

[1]Mean ±1 SD.

From Johnson TR, "How Growing Up Can Alter Lab Values in Pediatric Laboratory Medicine," *Diag Med* (special issue), 1982, 5:13-8, with permission.

Additional Information Presence of one or more of the following may be indications for further investigation: hemoglobin <10 g/dL, hemoglobin >18 g/dL, MCV >100 fL, MCV <80 fL, MCHC >37%, WBC >20,000/mm^3, WBC <2000/mm^3, presence of sickle cells, significant spherocytosis, basophilic stippling, stomatocytes,significant schistocytosis, oval macrocytes, tear drop red blood cells, eosinophilia (>10%) monocytosis (>15%), nucleated red blood cells in other than the newborn, malarial organisms or the possibility of malarial organisms, hypersegmented (five or more nuclear segments) PMNs, agranular PMNs, Pelger-Huët anomaly, Auer rods, Döhle bodies, marked toxic granulation, mononuclears in which apparent nucleoli are prominent (blast type cells), presence of metamyelocytes, myelocytes, promyelocytes, neutropenia, presence of plasma cells, peculiar atypical lymphocytes, significant increase or

(Continued)

Proposed Classification of Anemic Disorders Based on Red Cell Mean (MCV) and Heterogeneity (RDW)

MCV Low RDW Normal (microcytic homogeneous)	MCV Low RDW High (microcytic heterogeneous)	MCV Normal RDW Normal (normocytic homogeneous)	MCV Normal RDW High (normocytic heterogeneous)	MCV High RDW Normal (macrocytic homogeneous)	MCV High RDW High (macrocytic heterogeneous)
Heterozygous thalassemia[1]	Iron deficiency[1]	Normal	Mixed deficiency[1]	Aplastic anemia	Folate deficiency[1]
Chronic disease[1]	S/B-thalassemia	Chronic disease[1] chronic liver disease[1,2]	Early iron or folate deficiency[1]	Preleukemia[2]	Vitamin B_{12} deficiency
	Hemoglobin H	Nonanemic hemoglobinopathy (eg, AS, AC)	Anemic hemoglobinopathy (eg, SS, SC)[1]		Immune hemolytic anemia
	Red cell fragmentation	Transfusion[2]	Myelofibrosis		Cold agglutinins
		Chemotherapy	Sideroblastic[1]		Chronic lymphocytic leukemia, high count
		Chronic lymphocytic leukemia			
		Chronic myelocytic leukemia[2]			
		Hemorrhage			
		Hereditary spherocytosis			

[1]MCV alone <90% sensitive.

[2]RDW alone <90% sensitive.

From Bessman JD Jr, Gilmer PR, and Gardner FH, "Improved Classification of Anemias by MCV and RDW," *Am J Clin Pathol*, 1983, 80:324, with permission. The data for sensitivity of RDW and MCV in each disease category can be obtained from the authors.

decrease in platelets. Some quantitative elements of the CBC are related to each other, normally, such that examination of the results of any individual analysis allow for the application of a simple but effective case individualized quality control maneuver. The RBC count, hemoglobin, and hematocrit may be analyzed by applying a "rule of three." If red cells are normochromic/normocytic, the RBC count times 3 should approximately equal the hemoglobin and the hemoglobin multiplied by 3 should approximate the hematocrit. If there is significant deviation from this relation, one should check for supporting abnormalities in RBC indices and peripheral smear. The indices themselves offer a quick quality control check of the CBC. If patient transfusion can be excluded, then RBC indices should vary little consecutively from day to day. Anemias have been classified on the basis of their MCV and RDW (RBC heterogeneity). This classification has been especially helpful in the separation of iron deficiency from thalassemia. Heterozygous thalassemia has a normal RDW while RDW is high with iron deficiency.

In iron deficiency, the RDW is usually increased before the MCV decreases. Although this is somewhat controversial, it serves as an inexpensive screen for common iron deficiency anemia. See tables on previous pages.

Selected Readings

Fraser CG, Wilkinson SP, Neville RG, et al, "Biologic Variation of Common Hematologic Laboratory Quantities in the Elderly," *Am J Clin Pathol*, 1989, 92(4):465-70.

Fulwood R, Johnson CL, Bryner JD, et al, "Hematological and Nutritional Biochemistry Reference Data for Persons 6 Months - 74 Years of Age: United States 1976-1980," *Vital and Health Statistics*, Series 11, No. 232, DHHS Publication No (PHS) 83-1682, 1982.

Krantz SB, "Pathogenesis and Treatment of the Anemia of Chronic Disease," *Am J Med Sci*, 1994, 307(5):353-9.

Computed Transaxial Tomography, Abdomen Studies

Synonyms Abdomen, CT; CT, Lower Abdomen; CT, Total Abdomen; CT, Upper Abdomen

Test Includes CT scan of liver, spleen, kidneys, pancreas, aorta, retroperitoneum, gastrointestinal tract, pelvis. **Note:** In some departments, a request for a CT study of the abdomen will yield a study extending inferiorly to the pubic symphysis. In others, the study will extend only to the pelvic brim.

Patient Preparation Patient's oral intake restricted to fluid only for 4 hours prior to the examination. Medication schedule should not be interrupted. Should the patient have recently undergone a barium examination of the gastrointestinal tract, a digital radiograph obtained with the scanner prior to commencement of the procedure may be helpful in excluding the presence of barium within the bowel. The latter may produce significant artifact and thus render the study nondiagnostic. Where possible, all CT scan studies of the abdomen should be performed prior to normal GI barium studies. A recent serum creatinine is often requested on all patients 60 years of age and older, patients with known significant atherosclerotic disease, diabetes mellitus, or with pre-existing renal disease. Intravenous contrast material is routinely administered for this examination. Physician may opt to omit intravenous contrast. Patients undergoing a CT study of the abdomen are requested to drink approximately 450 mL of a dilute barium solution (approximately 1% barium) commencing 1 hour prior to the examination. Inclusion of the pelvis in the examination requires further patient preparation.

Special Instructions The abdominal area of interest should be specified along with pertinent clinical history. This will allow the diagnostic radiologist to tailor the examination for maximum diagnostic yield. For example, studies being performed for detection of renal calculi should be performed without contrast material, as the contrast, when excreted from the kidney, will mask the presence of small calculi within the collecting system. Adequate evaluation of small structures within the abdomen may require modification of technique such as thin slices or overlapping slices. A further example would be in the evaluation of the liver for primary or metastatic tumor. Maximum yield in the demonstration of such abnormalities requires examination both with and without contrast material.

Equipment This examination may be performed on any one of many commercially available computerized tomography scanners.

Technique Standard examination of the abdomen consists of 1 cm contiguous slices obtained from the dome of the diaphragm to the pelvic brim or pubic symphysis depending upon whether one groups the pelvis with the abdomen or treats it separately.

Causes for Rejection Patients with residual barium within the GI tract from a prior conventional barium study - this nondilute barium produces considerable artifact rendering the examination suboptimal and often nondiagnostic, uncooperative patients who are not candidates for sedation/anesthesia

Turnaround Time Written report usually provided within 24 hours.

(Continued)

Computed Transaxial Tomography, Abdomen Studies *(Continued)*

Use Diagnose and/or evaluate cysts, tumors, masses, aneurysm, metastases, abscesses, and trauma. The modality is also often used for staging of known tumors.

Contraindications Patient cooperation is of the utmost importance as the examination requires the patient to remain motionless for the duration of the study. The time of the study will vary from 20-40 minutes depending on the equipment being used. Children and uncooperative adults may require sedation.

Additional Information Patients should be informed that the examination may take 45 minutes to 1 hour and that oral contrast and intravenous contrast are commonly required. If the pelvis is included with the abdominal CT study, rectal contrast material and placement of a vaginal tampon in the case of females may also be required. The patient's medical record should accompany the patient. This will furnish the radiologist with sufficient information to tailor the examination as he/she deems appropriate. For example, patients suspected of an adrenal adenoma may require thin (2 mm) slices through the adrenal glands for the detection of such an abnormality.

Selected Readings

Fishman EK, "Spiral CT: Clinical Applications in the Gastrointestinal Tract," *Clin Imaging*, 1997, 21(2):111-21.

Halvorsen RA Jr and Thompson WM, "Computed Tomographic Staging of Gastrointestinal Tract Malignancies, Part I. Esophagus and Stomach," *Invest Radiol*, 1987, 22(1):2-16.

Thompson WM and Halvorsen RA Jr, "Computed Tomographic Staging of Gastrointestinal Tract Malignancies, Part II," *Invest Radiol*, 1987, 22(2):96-105.

Computed Transaxial Tomography, Appropriate Site

Refer to

Computed Transaxial Tomography, Abdomen Studies *on page 423*
Computed Transaxial Tomography, Head Studies *on page 424*
Computed Transaxial Tomography, Thorax *on page 426*

Computed Transaxial Tomography, Head Studies

Synonyms Brain, CT; Head Studies, CT

Test Includes CT scan of the brain

Patient Preparation The examination should be ordered and a requisition with information pertaining to the reason for the request and the clinical history should be completed by the referring physician. If there is the slightest possibility that intravenous contrast material will be administered, the patient's oral intake should be limited to liquids for at least 4 hours prior to the examination. Care must be taken to ensure the patient does not become dehydrated and medications should not be interrupted. A recent serum creatinine is requested on patients with pre-existing renal disease, diabetes mellitus, significant atherosclerotic disease, and advancing age (60 years and older). Agitated patients and children may require sedation prior to the examination. In these cases, an order for the appropriate sedative and dose should be recently recorded within the patient's chart. Sedatives should be administered by a physician within the Radiology Department.

Equipment Any commercially available computed tomographic scanner

Technique CT scans of the head are usually obtained at 15° angulation to the orbitomeatal line, a line connecting the lateral canthus of the eye with the external auditory canal. Contiguous slices 8 or 10 mm in thickness are obtained from the vertex of the skull to the foramen magnum. The orbital roof should be included. The patient is positioned supine for the examination. The head is placed securely in a head holder. The chin is flexed comfortably towards the chest. The appropriate 15° angulation can be obtained by angulation of the gantry if necessary.

Use Evaluate known or suspected primary or secondary neoplasm, cystic lesions, hydrocephalus, head trauma, seizure disorder, multiple sclerosis, atrophy, Alzheimer's disease, normal pressure hydrocephalus, Parkinson's disease, dementia, depression, organic brain syndrome, etc

Contraindications Assuming a cooperative or quiescent patient, there are no absolute contraindications to a CT scan of the head. A decision must be taken, however, as to whether the study is to be done with or without intravenous contrast material. While each case must be assessed individually, the following broad guidelines may be helpful. Those studies indicated by virtue of a recent infarct, cerebrovascular accident or stroke, or those being done for assessment of atrophy, Alzheimer's disease, normal pressure hydrocephalus, Parkinson's disease, hydrocephalus, evaluation of an intraventricular shunt, assessment of ventricular size, subdural hematoma, or suspected dementia are examined without contrast material. Patients for whom the indication is headache, psychiatric condition (such as anorexia or bulimia), tumor follow-up, rule out tumor, rule out metastasis, multiple sclerosis, seizure disorders,

depression, and organic brain syndrome are generally studied with contrast material. Patients in whom the indication is one of infection, abscess, meningitis, transient ischemic attack, arteriovenous malformation, remote subdural hematoma, or who have recently undergone a craniotomy and are being studied for postoperative evaluation are best studied with and without contrast material. Patients with a known diagnosis of plasmacytoma or multiple myeloma should not receive intravenous contrast material. Patients with compromised renal function may or may not benefit from intravenous contrast material. A recent serum creatinine and BUN will be helpful in deciding whether or not the latter group of patients receive contrast material.

Computed Transaxial Tomography, Paranasal Sinuses

Synonyms Paranasal Sinuses, CT; Sinuses, CT

Test Includes The examination is composed of contiguous 3-5 mm slices obtained from the inferior portion of the maxillary sinuses, cephalad to the superior extent of the frontal sinuses.

Patient Preparation Patients oral intake should be restricted to fluid for 4 hours prior to the examination. Medication schedule should not be interrupted. Administration of intravenous contrast material is at the discretion of the diagnostic radiologist. If a patient is being evaluated for trauma or inflammatory disease of the paranasal sinuses, no intravenous contrast material is usually administered. If a mass is identified in the course of the examination, or if a patient is known to have a tumor, then intravenous contrast material is usually given. Because of this, a recent serum creatinine is requested in all patients 60 years of age and older and those patients with known significant atherosclerotic disease, diabetes mellitus, or pre-existing renal disease. Children and uncooperative adults may require sedation.

Special Instructions If the nasopharynx is to be included in the examination, the study should be extended inferiorly to the hard palate or slightly below. The oral pharynx may be included by continuing to the base of the tongue. If there is a question of tumor invasion of the orbit from a sinus then coronal sections are very helpful.

Technique This examination may be performed in any one of many commercially available computerized tomographic scanners. Standard examination of the paranasal sinuses consist of 3-5 mm contiguous slices as previously described.

Turnaround Time Written report usually provided within 36 hours.

Use Diagnose and/or evaluate tumors, masses, metastases, inflammatory conditions, and traumatic involvement. The modality is commonly used for staging of tumors.

Contraindications Patients who are not candidates for sedation/anesthesia, uncooperative patient; patient cooperation is of the utmost importance as the examination requires the patient to remain motionless for the duration of the study.

Additional Information Some departments offer a limited CT study of the paranasal sinuses which is competitive with plain film radiographs of the sinus in terms of cost. This consists of 5 or 6 transaxial images through the sinus obtained parallel to Reid's baseline. The examination is achieved by obtaining a lateral digital image of the skull. From this the distance between the hard palate and the superior aspect of the frontal sinuses is measured. The distance is then divided by 5 or 6 to get the interslice distance. The slice thickness is 3-5 mm.

Kaliner MA, et al observed that sinusitis is one of the most commonly reported diseases in the United States, affecting an estimated 14% of the population. The prevalence of sinusitis is rising. Between 1990 and 1992, persons with sinusitis reported approximately 73 million restricted activity days (an increase from the 50 million restricted activity days reported between 1986 and 1988). Conrad DA and Jenson HB reported that acute bacterial rhinosinusitis, an infection of the nasal epithelium and paranasal sinus mucosa, is usually caused in children by *Streptococcus pneumoniae*, *Haemophilus influenzae*, *Moraxella catarrhalis*, and, less frequently, group A *Streptococcus* species. The clinical diagnosis is based on daytime cough that may be worse at night or purulent rhinorrhea, or both, lasting at least 10 days, often worsening after a period of initial improvement after initial symptoms of the common cold, and often associated with facial or dental pain, facial fullness, or swelling, headache, and fever. Sinusitis is diagnosed clinically; radiographic evaluation is not indicated for diagnosis. When the disease persists despite treatment, or is complicated by potential intracranial or orbital extension, CT is the preferred imaging modality.

Selected Readings

Conrad DA and Jenson HB, "Management of Acute Bacterial Rhinosinusitis," *Curr Opin Pediatr*, 2002, 14(1):86-90.

Harnsberger HR, Osborn AG, and Smoker RK, "CT in the Evaluation of the Normal and Diseased Paranasal Sinuses," *Seminars in the Ultrasound, CT and MR*, 1986, 7:68-90.

Kaliner MA, Osguthorpe JD, Fireman P, et al, "Sinusitis: Bench to Bedside. Current Findings, Future Directions," *J Allergy Clin Immunol*, 1997, 99(6 Pt 3):S829-48.

Computed Transaxial Tomography, Thorax

Test Includes CT study of the chest extending from the lung apices to the posterior costophrenic sulci. The study may extend inferiorly to image the adrenal glands because they are a relatively frequent site of metastasis from primary lung carcinoma.

Patient Preparation The patients should be limited to a liquid diet for at least 4 hours prior to the CT examination. Medication schedules should be maintained. The use of intravenous contrast material may be required at the discretion of the diagnostic radiologist. Because of this, a recent serum creatinine is requested in all patients 60 years of age and older, and those patients with known significant atherosclerotic disease, diabetes mellitus, or pre-existing renal disease. In the case of children who need sedation, a recent (within 30 days) recording of the child's weight and a written order by the child's physician must be in the patient's medical record. All children should be accompanied by a responsible adult. Opacification of the esophagus with thick barium paste may be of value in some cases and administration should be at the discretion of the diagnostic radiologist.

Special Instructions The exam may be requested by a practicing physician. The area of interest must be specified along with pertinent clinical history and reason for the CT scan. The test should be complete in 10-30 minutes. Intravenous contrast material may be administered.

Equipment The examination may be performed on any number of commercially available CT scanners.

Technique A routine CT study of the chest consists of sequential 1 cm slices obtained from the apices through the posterior costophrenic sulci. The study may be extended to include the adrenal glands if a diagnosis of primary bronchogenic carcinoma is known or suspected. The technique may vary depending upon the indications for the study. The examination may be tailored by the diagnostic radiologist to answer specific questions. For example, the questionably abnormal pulmonary hilum on conventional films may require 5 mm contiguous sections subsequent to the intravenous administration of contrast material. The latter will facilitate enhancement of major vascular structures thus highlighting normal and abnormal anatomy. Similarly, densitometric evaluation of a solitary pulmonary nodule will require contiguous 2 mm slices throughout the nodule without intravenous contrast material. This maneuver will facilitate evaluation of the nodule for the presence and distribution of calcium within it. All modifications of the conventional contiguous 1 cm slice protocol throughout the chest are made at the discretion of the radiologist. The patient's medical record should accompany the patient to the department in order to ensure that the radiologist is furnished with sufficient information to tailor the examination appropriately.

Causes for Rejection Inability of the patient to cooperate is the major problem. Should the uncooperative patient not be a candidate for sedation and/or anesthesia, the study cannot be performed.

Turnaround Time Written report usually available within 36 hours.

Use The examination facilitates evaluation of abnormalities of the lungs, mediastinum, pleura, and chest wall. Conventional PA and lateral views of the chest represent the basic screening tool in the identification of abnormalities involving the thorax. The axial anatomic display and superior density discrimination of computed tomography provides information pertaining to the extent of disease and more precise characterization of abnormalities initially noted on physical examination, chest films or on the barium swallow.

Contraindications Patient cooperation is of utmost importance as the examination requires the patient to remain motionless for the duration of the study. The time of the study will vary from 10-30 minutes depending on the equipment being used. Children and uncooperative adults may require sedation.

Selected Readings

Akira M, Hamada H, Sakatani M, et al, "CT Findings During Phase of Accelerated Deterioration in Patients With Idiopathic Pulmonary Fibrosis," *AJR Am J Roentgenol*, 1997, 168(1):79-83.

Miller WT Jr, Tino G, and Friedburg JS, "Thoracic CT in the Intensive Care Unit: Assessment of Clinical Usefulness," *Radiology*, 1998, 209(2):491-8.

Naidich DP, Zerhouni EA, Hutchins GM, et al, "Computed Tomography of the Pulmonary Parenchyma, Part 1: Distal Air-Space Disease," *J Thorac Imaging*, 1985, 1(1):39-53.

Zerhouni EA, Naidich DP, Stitik FP, et al, "Computed Tomography of the Pulmonary Parenchyma, Part 2: Interstitial Disease," *J Thorac Imaging*, 1985, 1(1):54-64.

Conjunctival Smear *see* Ocular Cytology *on page 551*

Corneal Culture, Bacterial and Fungal

Related Information

Gram Stain *on page 473*
Methenamine Silver Stain *on page 534*
Periodic Acid-Schiff Stain *on page 563*

Patient Preparation Most patients will benefit from topical corneal anesthetic. 0.5% proparacaine-HCl is the preferred anesthetic. This solution has a minimal effect on the viability of bacteria.

Special Instructions The minute amount of specimen obtained by scraping the cornea mandates physician inoculation of the specimens immediately and directly onto/into fresh, room temperature culture media used to culture both bacteria and fungi (the clinical appearance of fungal and bacterial keratitis can be similar). Solid media commonly used for bacterial culture of corneal specimens are 5% sheep blood, chocolate, and a nutritious broth such as tryptic soy or thioglycolate. Contact the laboratory for a supply of fresh media, any special instructions for the testing laboratory, and notification that a corneal culture is being sent to the laboratory.

Specimen Corneal scraping or biopsy

Container None. The specimen should be inoculated directly onto plated solid bacterial media as soon as it is collected and sent to the laboratory immediately.

Collection Use sterile technique and a sterile Kimura spatula, scalpel blade, or an L-bent needle to scrape tissue from the advancing edges of corneal ulcers or disrupted epithelium. A calcium alginate swab can be used. The swab should be moistened in culture broth (eg, trypticase soy broth) before obtaining the specimen. Collect as much specimen as reasonably possible.

Storage Instructions The specimen (inoculated media) should not be stored but, rather, sent to the laboratory immediately.

Causes for Rejection Dried media or specimen

Turnaround Time Most etiological agents of bacterial keratitis will grow in routine bacterial culture within 1-2 days. Most laboratories incubate eye cultures for 3-5 days before reporting "no growth." Most etiological agents of fungal keratitis will grow in routine fungal culture within 1-3 weeks. Most laboratories incubate eye cultures for 4-6 weeks before reporting "no growth."

Reference Range No bacteria or fungi isolated

Use Isolate and identify bacterial and fungal etiological agents and provide an isolate(s) for antimicrobial susceptibility testing

Limitations Normal conjunctival bacteria often grow in cultures of ulcerated cornea, in addition to the pathogens responsible for the keratitis. The clinical relevance of these isolates must be determined. Minimal specimens, such as corneal scrapings, often do not contain enough infected material to yield clinically relevant results. Therefore, negative or "no growth" results must be interpreted accordingly.

Additional Information Media should not be inoculated with the same specimen that was placed onto microscopic slides. However, if the instrument has come in contact with a microscope slide, resterilize the instrument and collect another specimen for culture.

Gram stain and/or a fungal stain should be ordered in addition to culture. The minute amount of specimen obtained by scraping the cornea mandates immediate physician preparation of a specimen for staining. Contact the testing laboratory for advice on which stain the laboratory offers and whether or not to fix the slide specimen before sending. Generally, most specimens should be air-dried and then fixed immediately in 95% methanol for 5 minutes. If the physician has microbiology experience in fixing extremely small pieces of air-dried tissue onto microscope slides, he/she should fix the specimen as above. Otherwise, the air-dried specimen should be sent to the microbiology laboratory immediately so it can be properly fixed by medical technologists. Specimens should be gently dabbed onto a microscope slide that has been thoroughly cleansed with 95% alcohol and allowed to air dry completely. At least two slides should be prepared for direct staining.

Selected Readings

Epley KD, Katz HR, Herling I, et al, "Platinum Spatula Versus Mini-Tip Culturette in Culturing Bacterial Keratitis," *Cornea*, 1998, 17(1):74-8.

Forster RK, "Conrad Berens Lecture. The Management of Infectious Keratitis as We Approach the 21st Century," *CLAO J*, 1998, 24(3):175-80.

Levey SB, Katz HR, Abrams DA, et al, "The Role of Cultures in the Management of Ulcerative Keratitis," *Cornea*, 1997, 16(4):383-6.

O'Brien TP, "Keratitis," *Principles and Practices of Infectious Diseases*, 5th ed, Mandell GL, et al, eds, New York, NY: Churchill Livingstone, 2000, 1257-67.

Corneal Smear *see* Ocular Cytology *on page 551*

***Corynebacterium diphtheriae* Culture, Throat** *see* Throat Culture for *Corynebacterium diphtheriae on page 593*

***Coxiella burnetii* Titer** *see* Q Fever Serology *on page 569*

Coxsackie A Virus Culture *see* Enterovirus Culture *on page 453*

Coxsackie A Virus Serology

Related Information

Enterovirus Culture *on page 453*

(Continued)

Coxsackie A Virus Serology *(Continued)*

Specimen Serum

Container Red top tube or serum separator tube

Sampling Time Acute and convalescent sera drawn at least 14 days apart are required

Reference Range Less than a fourfold increase in titer in paired sera. Most healthy people do not have titers >1:8. Titers ≥1:32 are especially diagnostic. Titers ≤1:8 could represent cross reactions with other enteroviruses. If serological testing is performed by enzyme immunoassay (EIA) on automated instrumentation, results are usually given in index units, not titers. In such cases, significant rises in antibody levels are determined by algorithms within the instrumentation, not by increases in titer.

Use Establish the diagnosis of Coxsackie A virus infection (eg, in viral myocarditis)

Limitations Neutralizing antibodies develop quickly and persist for many years after infection, making demonstration of a rise in titer difficult. There are at least 24 types/serotypes of Coxsackie A virus. Therefore, serotypes detected will depend on particular reagents used in a particular test. Consult the laboratory for serotypes detected.

Methodology Viral neutralization, complement fixation (CF), enzyme immunoassay (EIA)

Additional Information Coxsackie A virus produces a wide spectrum of disease including aseptic meningitis, myositis, encephalitis, respiratory illnesses, herpangina, hand-foot-and-mouth disease, rash, and generalized systemic infection. Documentation of infection by serology is difficult and diagnosis may depend on culture.

Selected Readings

Melnick JL, "Enteroviruses," *Manual of Clinical Laboratory Immunology*, 5th ed, Rose NR, Conway de Macario E, Folds JD, et al, eds, Washington, DC: American Society for Microbiology, 1997, 699-701.

Coxsackie B Virus Culture *see* Enterovirus Culture *on page 453*

Coxsackie B Virus Serology

Related Information

Enterovirus Culture *on page 453*

Test Includes Coxsackie B_1, B_2, B_3, B_4, B_5, B_6 virus titers

Specimen Serum

Container Red top tube or serum separator tube

Sampling Time Acute and convalescent sera drawn 10-14 days apart are required.

Reference Range Less than a fourfold increase in titer in paired sera. If serological testing is performed by enzyme immunoassay (EIA) on automated instrumentation, results are usually given in index units, not titers. In such cases, significant rises in antibody levels are determined by algorithms within the instrumentation, not by increases in titer.

Use Establish the diagnosis of Coxsackie B virus infection

Limitations Neutralizing antibodies arise quickly, last for years, and may make the demonstration of a rising titer difficult. Tests for complement fixing antibodies are insensitive and nonspecific. There are six types/serotypes of Coxsackie B virus. Consult the laboratory to determine if test detects some or all six types.

Methodology Complement fixation (CF), viral neutralization

Additional Information Coxsackie B virus causes a wide variety of clinical illness, including pleurodynia (Bornholm's disease), aseptic meningitis, carditis/myocarditis, rash, pulmonary infection, a generalized systemic infection, and several neonatal diseases and syndromes. Approximately 50% of clinical myocarditis and pericarditis is caused by Coxsackie B. Since culture is frequently unrewarding, diagnosis may depend on serologic studies.

Recently there has been interest in various viral assays for postviral fatigue syndrome. Antibody to Coxsackie B virus is not helpful in this assessment.

Selected Readings

Melnick JL, "Enteroviruses," *Manual of Clinical Laboratory Immunology*, 5th ed, Rose NR, Conway de Macario E, Folds JD, et al, eds, Washington, DC: American Society for Microbiology, 1997, 699-701.
Miller NA, Carmichael HA, Calder BD, et al, "Antibody to Coxsackie B Virus in Diagnosing Postviral Fatigue Syndrome," *BMJ*, 1991, 302(6769):140-3.

Coxsackie Virus Culture, Stool *see* Viral Culture, Stool *on page 616*
Crab Lice Identification *see* Arthropod Identification *on page 387*

C-Reactive Protein

Related Information

Sedimentation Rate, Erythrocyte *on page 576*
Serum Bactericidal Test *on page 578*

Synonyms Acute Phase Reactant; CRP

Specimen Serum

Container Red top tube or serum separator tube

Causes for Rejection Excessive hemolysis, chylous serum

Reference Range <8 mcg/mL

Use Used similarly to erythrocyte sedimentation rate. CRP is a nonspecific acute phase reactant protein used as an indicator of infectious disease and inflammatory states, including active rheumatic fever and rheumatoid arthritis. Progressive increases correlate with increases of inflammation/injury. CRP is a more sensitive, rapidly responding indicator than is ESR. CRP may be used to detect early postoperative wound infection and to follow therapeutic response to anti-inflammatory agents.

Limitations Frozen specimens may give false-positive results; oral contraceptives may affect results

Methodology Agglutination, nephelometry, radioimmunoassay (RIA)

Additional Information CRP is a pentameric globulin with mobility near the gamma zone. It is an acute phase reactant which rises rapidly, but nonspecifically, in response to tissue injury and inflammation. It is particularly useful in detecting occult infections, acute appendicitis, particularly in leukemia and in postoperative patients. In uncomplicated postoperative recovery, CRP peaks on the third postop day, and returns to preop levels by day 7. It may also be helpful in evaluating extension or reinfarction after myocardial infarction, and in following response to therapy in rheumatic disorders. It may help to differentiate Crohn's disease (high CRP) from ulcerative colitis (low CRP), and rheumatoid arthritis (high CRP) from uncomplicated lupus (low CRP). When used to evaluate patients with arthritis, serum is the preferred specimen. There is no advantage to examining synovial fluid for CRP.

Selected Readings

Babu ED, "Would Measurement of C-Reactive Protein Reduce the Rate of Negative Exploration for Acute Appendicitis?" *J R Coll Surg (Edinb)*, 2000, 45(3): 202-3.

Dowton SR and Colten HR, "Acute Phase Reactants in Inflammation and Infection," *Semin Hematol*, 1988, 25(2):84-90.

Hutchinson WL, Koenig W, Frohlich M, et al, "Immunoradiometric Assay of Circulating C-Reactive Protein: Age-Related Values in the Adult General Population," *Clin Chem*, 2000, 46(7):934-8.

Van Lente F, "The Diagnostic Utility of C-Reactive Protein," *Hum Pathol*, 1982, 13(12):1061-3.

Yilmaz Turay U, Yildirim Z, Turkoz Y, et al, "Use of Pleural Fluid C-Reactive Protein in Diagnosis of Pleural Effusions," *Respir Med*, 2000, 94(5):432-5.

Creatinine Clearance

Related Information

Body Surface Area of Adults and Children *on page 1173*

Creatinine Clearance Estimating Methods in Patients With Stable Renal Function *on page 1176*

Applies to GFR; Glomerular Filtration Rate

Test Includes Serum creatinine, urine creatinine

Patient Preparation Avoid cephalosporins. If possible, drugs should be stopped beforehand. Have patient drink water before the clearance is begun, and continue good hydration throughout the clearance.

Special Instructions Blood creatinine should be ordered at the same time. Requisition should state date and time collection started, date and time collection finished, patient's age, height, and weight.

Specimen 24-hour urine and serum; test can be done for shorter periods

Container Plastic urine container and red top tube

Collection Instruct the patient to void at 8 AM and discard the specimen. Then collect all urine including the final specimen voided at the end of the 24-hour collection period (ie, 8 AM the next morning). Keep specimen on ice during collection. Bottle must be labeled with patient's name, date and time for a 24-hour collection.

Especially for creatinine clearance, accuracy and precision of collection are important. Complete, carefully timed (usually 24-hour) collection is needed; 4-hour and 12-hour collections are acceptable.

Storage Instructions Refrigerate

Causes for Rejection No blood creatinine ordered, urine specimen not timed

Reference Range Clearance for:

- Children: 70-140 mL/minute/1.73 m^2 (SI: 1.17-2.33 mL/s/1.73 m^2)
- Adults: male: 85-125 mL/minute/1.73 m^2 (SI: 1.42-2.08 mL/s/1.73 m^2)
- Adults: female: 75-115 mL/minute/1.73 m^2 (SI: 1.25-1.92 mL/s/1.73 m^2).

For each age decade after 40, creatinine clearance decreases 6-7 mL/minute/1.73 m^2.

Critical Values Moderate renal impairment (adult): 30-40 mL/minute/1.73 m^2

Use Renal function test to estimate glomerular filtration rate (GFR); evaluate renal function in small or wasted subjects; follow possible progression of renal disease;

(Continued)

Creatinine Clearance *(Continued)*

adjust dosages of medications in which renal excretion is pivotal (eg, aminoglycosides, methotrexate, cisplatin)

Limitations Exercise may cause increased creatinine clearance. The glomerular filtration rate is substantially increased in pregnancy. Ascorbic acid, ketone bodies (acetoacetate), hydantoin, numerous cephalosporins and glucose may influence creatinine determinations. Trimethoprim, cimetidine, quinine, quinidine, procainamide reduce creatinine excretion. Icteric samples, lipemia, and hemolysis may interfere with determination of creatinine.

Since tubular secretion of creatinine is fractionally more important in progressing renal failure, the creatinine clearance overestimates GFR with high serum creatinine levels.

While ingestion of meats may cause some increase in creatinine excretion, in practice this seems to make little difference. Intraindividual variation in creatinine clearance is about 15%. Males excrete more creatinine and have slightly higher clearance than females.

Because of the exponential rise in serum creatinine concentration with decline of GFR, a 25% increase in serum creatinine actually represents a substantial diminution of GFR. When muscle mass and kidney function diminish in parallel with advancing age, an elderly woman with perceived normal creatinine concentration may have a GFR only 30% that of a young adult.

Methodology Jaffé reaction (alkaline picrate). The calculation for corrected creatinine clearance in mL/minute: = [(urine volume per minute x urine creatinine)/serum creatinine] x (1.73/surface area of body in square meters). Body surface area is obtained from nomograms which require age, height, and weight. See Appendix table Body Surface Area of Adults and Children *on page 1173*.

Additional Information Glomerular filtration rate declines about 10% per decade after age 50. Some patients with significant impairment of glomerular filtration rate have only slightly elevated serum creatinine.

Creatinine clearance is calculated on the basis of the surface area of the patient. The estimated error of determining creatinine clearance utilizing serum and 24-hour urine collection has been found to be in the range of 10% to 15%.

Any test requiring a 24-hour urine collection may also be run on the specimen (eg, protein, quantitative, 24-hour urine).

When **urine creatinine** is used to evaluate the completeness of a 24-hour urine collection in connection with the measurement of other analytes (eg, urine free cortisol, other steroids, albumin, total protein, phosphate, uric acid), the following reference intervals may be applied (Painter et al):

- Infants: 8-20 mg/kg/day (SI: 71-177 μmol/kg/day)
- Children: 8-22 mg/kg/day (SI: 71-194 μmol/kg/day)
- Adolescents: 8-30 mg/kg/day (SI: 71-265 μmol/kg/day)
- Adults: male: 14-26 mg/kg/day (SI: 124-230 μmol/kg/day)
- Adults: female: 11-20 mg/kg/day (SI: 97-177 μmol/kg/day)

For each decade after 40 years of age, the urine creatinine decreases approximately 10 mg/kg/day (SI: 0.0844 μg/kg/day).

- 90 years: male: 800-2000 mg/kg/day (SI: 7.1-17.7 μg/kg/day); female: 600-1800 mg/kg/day (SI: 5.2-15.9 μg/kg/day).

Selected Readings

Herget-Rosenthal S, Kribben A, Pietruck F, et al, "Two by Two-Hour Creatinine Clearance - Repeatable and Valid," *Clin Nephrol*, 1999, 51(6):348-54.

Levey AS, Bosch JP, Lewis JB, et al, "A More Accurate Method to Estimate Glomerular Filtration Rate From Serum Creatinine: A New Prediction Equation," Modification of Diet in Renal Disease Study Group, *Ann Intern Med*, 1999, 130(6):461-70.

Luke DR, Halstenson CE, Opsahl JA, et al, "Validity of Creatinine Clearance Estimates in the Assessment of Renal Function," *Clin Pharmacol Ther*, 1990, 48(5):503-8.

Painter PC, Cope JY, and Smith JL, "Reference Information for the Clinical Laboratory," *Tietz Textbook of Clinical Chemistry*, 3rd ed, Burtis CA and Ashwood ER, eds, Philadelphia, PA: WB Saunders Co, 1999, 1809.

Payne RB, "Biological Variation of Serum and Urine Creatinine and Creatinine Clearance," *Ann Clin Biochem*, 1989, 26(Pt 6):565-6.

Sokoll LJ, Russell RM, Sodowski JA, et al, "Establishment of Creatinine Clearance Reference Values for Older Women," *Clin Chem*, 1994, 40(12):2276-81.

Van Lente F and Suit P, "Assessment of Renal Function by Serum Creatinine and Creatinine Clearance: Glomerular Filtration Rate Estimated by Four Procedures," *Clin Chem*, 1989, 35(12):2326-30.

Young DS, *Effects of Drugs on Clinical Laboratory Tests*, 5th ed, Volume 1: Listing by Test, Washington, DC: AACC Press, American Association of Clinical Chemistry, 2000, Section 3, 258-61.

CRP *see* C-Reactive Protein *on page 428*

Cryptococcal Antigen Serology, Serum or Cerebrospinal Fluid

Related Information

Cryptococcus Serology *on page 431*
Fungus Culture, Cerebrospinal Fluid *on page 464*
India Ink Preparation *on page 507*
Methenamine Silver Stain *on page 534*
Periodic Acid-Schiff Stain *on page 563*

Synonyms Cerebrospinal Fluid Cryptococcal Latex Agglutination; *Cryptococcus* Antigen, Blood; *Cryptococcus* Latex Antigen Agglutination; Spinal Fluid Cryptococcal Latex Agglutination

Test Includes Testing patient's serum or CSF for the presence of cryptococcal antigen (with rheumatoid factor/nonspecific control)

Abstract Cryptococcal antigen testing is the single most useful diagnostic test for cryptococcal meningitis.

Specimen Serum or cerebrospinal fluid

Container Red top tube, sterile CSF tube

Reference Range Negative

Use Establish the diagnosis of *Cryptococcus neoformans* infection

Limitations False-positive results can occur in patients with rheumatoid arthritis, but test controls and procedures usually eliminate this possibility. The test is less frequently positive in serum than in CSF. Disseminated cryptococcal infections usually result in a positive serum test. False-negatives occur.

Methodology Latex agglutination with rheumatoid factor/nonspecific control and in some laboratories pronase pretreatment.

Additional Information Presence of cryptococcal capsular polysaccharide is indicative of cryptococcosis. Samples should either be treated to remove rheumatoid factor and other interfering factors or tested to distinguish between positivity due to cryptococcal antigen and that due to interfering factors. If this distinction cannot be made the test cannot be interpreted. Pretreatment of the specimen with pronase reduces false-positives and increases the likelihood of positivity of the method.

The cryptococcal antigen test is positive in about 85% to 90% of cases of cryptococcal meningitis, while the India ink test is positive in ≤50%. The cryptococcal antigen test has been reported to be able to detect antigen in 95% of AIDS patients with cryptococcal disease. Culture of cerebrospinal fluid for fungus should be performed in patients who are suspected of having cryptococcosis.

Selected Readings

Gray LD and Roberts GD, "Experience With the Use of Pronase to Eliminate Interference Factors in the Latex Agglutination Test for Cryptococcal Antigen," *J Clin Microbiol*, 1988, 26(11):2450-1.

Greenlee JE, "Approach to Diagnosis of Meningitis - Cerebrospinal Fluid Evaluation," *Infect Dis Clin North Am*, 1990, 4(4):583-98.

Kaufman L, Kovacs JA, and Reiss E, "Clinical Immunomycology," *Manual of Clinical Laboratory Immunology*, 5th ed, Rose NR, Conway de Macario E, Folds JD, et al, eds, Washington, DC: American Society for Microbiology, 1997, 585-604.

Saag MS, Graybill RJ, Larsen RA, et al, "Practice Guidelines for the Management of Cryptococcal Disease," *Clin Infect Dis*, 2000, 30(4):710-8.

Cryptococcosis, IFA *see Cryptococcus* Serology *on page 431*

Cryptococcosis, Indirect Fluorescent Antibody Titer *see Cryptococcus* Serology *on page 431*

***Cryptococcus* Antigen, Blood** *see* Cryptococcal Antigen Serology, Serum or Cerebrospinal Fluid *on page 431*

***Cryptococcus* Latex Antigen Agglutination** *see* Cryptococcal Antigen Serology, Serum or Cerebrospinal Fluid *on page 431*

***Cryptococcus* Preparation** *see* India Ink Preparation *on page 507*

Cryptococcus Serology

Related Information

Cryptococcal Antigen Serology, Serum or Cerebrospinal Fluid *on page 431*
Periodic Acid-Schiff Stain *on page 563*

Synonyms Cryptococcosis, IFA; Cryptococcosis, Indirect Fluorescent Antibody Titer

Special Instructions Sequential assays may be desirable

Specimen Serum

Container Red top tube or serum separator tube

Reference Range Negative

Use Diagnosis and prognosis of cryptococcal infections

Limitations A negative test result does not rule out infection because an antibody response may be reduced by circulating antigen bound to antibody. Cross reactions

(Continued)

Cryptococcus Serology *(Continued)*

of the IFA test have been reported with blastomycosis, histoplasmosis, and some other fungal infections.

Methodology Tube agglutination, indirect fluorescent antibody

Additional Information Antibody titers ≥1:2 are suggestive of infection with *Cryptococcus neoformans.* Antibody can be detected early in the course of the disease, but if the disease progresses, excess antigen may be produced and render antibodies undetectable. With effective chemotherapy, the antigen titer usually declines and antibody may once again be demonstrated. However, antibodies may persist for long periods even after cessation of chemotherapy.

Selected Readings

Heyworth MF, "Immunology of *Giardia* and *Cryptosporidium* Infections," *J Infect Dis*, 1992, 166(3):465-72.

Kaufman L, Kovacs JA, and Reiss E, "Clinical Immunomycology," *Manual of Clinical Laboratory Immunology*, 5th ed, Rose NR, Conway de Macario E, Folds JD, et al, eds, Washington, DC: American Society for Microbiology, 1997, 585-604.

Saag MS, Graybill RJ, Larsen RA, et al, "Practice Guidelines for the Management of Cryptococcal Disease," *Clin Infect Dis*, 2000, 30(4):710-8.

***Cryptococcus* Stain** *see* India Ink Preparation *on page 507*

Cryptosporidium Diagnostic Procedures, Stool

Related Information

Fecal Leukocyte Stain *on page 455*
Periodic Acid-Schiff Stain *on page 563*

Synonyms Acid-Fast Stain, Modified, *Cryptosporidium*

Test Includes Examination of stool for the presence of *Cryptosporidium*

Special Instructions Procedures for the detection of *Cryptosporidium* in humans have recently become available in most clinical laboratories. Consult the laboratory regarding availability of the procedure and specific specimen collection instructions before collecting the specimen.

Specimen Fresh stool; stool preserved with 10% formalin or sodium acetate-acetic acid formalin preservative

Container Stool container with lid

Collection Transport fresh specimen to laboratory promptly following collection. Specimen on outside of container poses excessive risk of contamination to laboratory personnel.

Reference Range Negative

Use A part of the differential work-up of diarrhea, particularly in immunocompromised hosts and suspected AIDS patients; establish the diagnosis of cryptosporidiosis by demonstration of the oocysts

Limitations The organisms are most readily demonstrated in diarrheal stools. Forms of *Blastocystis hominis* may cause confusion if Giemsa stain is used. Most recommended procedures cannot be performed on polyvinyl alcohol (PVA) preserved specimens.

Methodology Phase contrast microscopy after floatation concentration technique (Sheather's method) is not particularly sensitive; modified acid-fast stain on air-dried smears. Auramine and carbol-fuchsin stain is used by some laboratories for screening. An immunofluorescence test is also available.

Additional Information *Cryptosporidium* is a coccidian parasite of the intestines and respiratory tract of many animals including mice, sheep, snakes, turkeys, chickens, monkeys, and domestic cats. It is a cause of severe and chronic diarrhea in patients with hypogammaglobulinemia and the acquired immune deficiency syndrome. The organism is widely recognized as a disease of the immunocompromised patient, however it can also cause disease in immunocompetent patients. Animal contact, travel to an endemic area, living in a rural environment, and daycare attendance by toddlers have been recognized as risk factors for the development of cryptosporidiosis. Perinatal infection has been reported. Children are more prone to develop infection than are adults. In children, the disease is a self-limited gastroenteritis; in immunocompromised patients a profound enteropathy results. There is a seasonal variation in incidence with the highest frequency reported in summer and autumn. The organism can be demonstrated in biopsies of small bowel and colon, adherent to surface of the epithelial cells (Giemsa stain). Most therapeutic regimens for cryptosporidiosis are not successful unless immunosuppression is reversed.

Selected Readings

Baron EJ, Schenone C, and Tanenbaum B, "Comparison of Three Methods for Detection of *Cryptosporidium* Oocysts in a Low-Prevalence Population," *J Clin Microbiol*, 1989, 27(1):223-4.

Clark DP, "New Insights Into Human Cryptosporidiosis," *Clin Microbiol Rev*, 1999, 12(4):554-63.

Current WL, "The Biology of *Cryptosporidium*," *Am Soc Microbiol News*, 1988, 54:605-11 (review).

Current WL and Garcia LS, "Cryptosporidiosis," *Clin Microbiol Rev*, 1991, 4(3):325-58.

Gradus MS, "*Cryptosporidium* and Public Health: From Watershed to Water Glass," *Clin Microbiol Newslett*, 2000, 22(4):25-32.

Petersen C, "Cryptosporidiosis in Patients Infected With the Human Immunodeficiency Virus," *Clin Infect Dis*, 1992, 15(6):903-9.

Crystals, Urine *see* Urinalysis *on page 606*

CSF Analysis *see* Cerebrospinal Fluid Analysis *on page 408*

CSF Fungus Culture *see* Fungus Culture, Cerebrospinal Fluid *on page 464*

CSF Mycobacteria Culture *see* Mycobacteria Culture, Cerebrospinal Fluid *on page 541*

CSF VDRL *see* VDRL, Cerebrospinal Fluid *on page 613*

CT, Lower Abdomen *see* Computed Transaxial Tomography, Abdomen Studies *on page 423*

CT, Total Abdomen *see* Computed Transaxial Tomography, Abdomen Studies *on page 423*

CT, Upper Abdomen *see* Computed Transaxial Tomography, Abdomen Studies *on page 423*

Culdocentesis *see* Cytology, Body Fluids *on page 438*

Culture, Biopsy *see* Aerobic Culture, Body Fluid *on page 365*

Culture, Blood *see* Blood Culture, Aerobic and Anaerobic *on page 391*

Culture for *Leptospira* *see* *Leptospira* Culture *on page 518*

Culture, HSV Only *see* Herpes Simplex Virus Isolation, Rapid *on page 495*

Culture, *Legionella pneumophila* *see* *Legionella pneumophila* Culture *on page 516*

Culture, Protected Brush Catheter

Related Information

Aerobic Culture, Sputum *on page 367*
Bronchoscopy, Fiberoptic *on page 406*
Culture, Quantitative, Lower Respiratory Tract *on page 434*
Fungus Culture, Bronchial Aspirate *on page 463*
Mycobacteria Culture, Sputum *on page 542*
Pneumocystis jiroveci Test *on page 566*

Test Includes Culture of specimen collected by use of a protected brush catheter (PBC) and calculations to determine the number of organisms/mL in the specimen

Specimen Specimen collected by use of a protected brush catheter (PBC)

Container Sterile screw-cap container

Collection PBC specimens are collected by bronchoscopy performed by a specially trained physician

Storage Instructions PBC specimens should be kept cold.

Use Determine the major pathogens causing pneumonia and their absolute and relative quantity

Limitations The quantity of specimen collected by PBC is extremely small. Bronchoscopy to collect PBC specimens is not always available, is expensive, and involves risks to the patient. Not all clinical microbiology laboratories can perform quantitative cultures. Specimens can be contaminated with normal oropharyngeal flora. The reported sensitivity and specificity of this quantitative method vary widely (62% to 100% and 60% to 100%, respectively) and is influenced strongly by the threshold used during the studies. The clinical utility of quantitative culture of specimens by a PBC is controversial.

Methodology Routine methods are used to culture a known quantity of saline which has been used to wash the collected specimen from the brush of a PBC; calculations are used to determine the number of organisms/mL in the very dilute specimen

Additional Information An advantage of this quantitative method is several types of microscopic examinations can be performed on the specimen (Gram stain, fungal stain, cytology, etc.). Collection and culture of a PBC specimen along with culture of BAL fluid probably is more productive than is culture of either specimen alone. Thresholds for clinical relevance of isolated bacteria in this quantitative test have been as low as $\geq 10^2$ and as high as $\geq 10^6$, but commonly are $\geq 10^3$ or $\geq 10^4$ colony-forming units/mL of fluid. There is no well accepted value which provides both good sensitivity and good specificity. The disease for which this test has proven the most useful is hospital-acquired pneumonia.

Selected Readings

McFarlane JT and Baldwin DR, "Hospital-Acquired Pneumonia," *Infectious Diseases*, Armstrong D and Cohen J, eds, Philadelphia, PA: Mosby, 1999, 2.28.1-8.

Reimer LG and Carroll KC, "Role of the Microbiology Laboratory in the Diagnosis of Lower Respiratory Tract Infections," *Clin Infect Dis*, 1998, 26(3):742-8.

Strausbaugh LJ, "Nosocomial Respiratory Infections," *Principles and Practice of Infectious Diseases*, Mandell GL, Bennett JE, and Dolin R, eds, Philadelphia, PA: Churchill Livingstone, 2000, 3020-8.

Culture, Quantitative, Lower Respiratory Tract

Related Information

Aerobic Culture, Sputum *on page 367*
Bronchoscopy, Fiberoptic *on page 406*
Culture, Protected Brush Catheter *on page 433*
Fungus Culture, Bronchial Aspirate *on page 463*
Mycobacteria Culture, Sputum *on page 542*
Pneumocystis jiroveci Test *on page 566*

Test Includes Culture of known quantities of bronchoalveolar (BAL) fluid and calculations to determine the number of organisms/mL in the specimen

Specimen BAL fluid

Container Sterile screw-cap container

Collection BAL fluid is collected by bronchoscopy performed by a specially trained physician; large amounts (often separate 50 mL portions) of saline are used to lavage the distal alveoli of a large segment of the lung; the first portion of saline is essentially a bronchial wash and is more likely to be contaminated with normal oropharyngeal flora; subsequent withdrawn portions usually are pooled for culture or other tests

Storage Instructions BAL fluid for culture should be kept cold.

Use Determine the major pathogens causing pneumonia and their absolute and relative quantity

Limitations Most clinical laboratories do not offer this test. The clinical utility of quantitative culture of BAL fluid is controversial. Bronchoscopy to collect BAL fluid is not always available, is expensive, and involves risks to the patient. Not all clinical microbiology laboratories can perform quantitative cultures. Specimens can be contaminated with normal oropharyngeal flora. The reported sensitivity and specificity of this quantitative method vary widely (25% to 100% and 30% to 100%, respectively), and is influenced strongly by the threshold used during the studies.

Methodology Routine methods are used to culture a known quantity of BAL fluid, and calculations are used to determine the number of organisms/mL in the very dilute specimen.

Additional Information The advantage of this quantitative method is that an extremely large section of the lung can be sampled, and several types of microscopic examinations can be performed on the specimen (Gram stain, fungal stain, cytology, etc.). Collection and culture of a protected brush specimen along with culture of BAL fluid probably is more productive than culture of either specimen alone. Thresholds for clinical relevance of isolated bacteria in this quantitative test have been as low as $\geq 10^2$ and as high as $\geq 10^6$, but commonly are $\geq 10^3$ or $\geq 10^4$ colony-forming units/mL of fluid. There is no well accepted value which provides both good sensitivity and good specificity. The disease for which this test has proven the most useful is hospital-acquired pneumonia.

Selected Readings

McFarlane JT and Baldwin DR, "Hospital-Acquired Pneumonia," *Infectious Diseases*, Armstrong D and Cohen J, eds, Philadelphia, PA: Mosby, 1999, 2.28.1-8.

Reimer LG and Carroll KC, "Role of the Microbiology Laboratory in the Diagnosis of Lower Respiratory Tract Infections," *Clin Infect Dis*, 1998, 26(3):742-8.

Strausbaugh LJ, "Nosocomial Respiratory Infections," *Principles and Practice of Infectious Diseases*, Mandell GL, Bennett JE, and Dolin R, eds, Philadelphia, PA: Churchill Livingstone, 2000, 3020-8.

CXR *see* Chest Films *on page 412*

Cyst Culture, Aerobic *see* Biopsy Culture, Routine *on page 390*

Cyst Culture, Anaerobic *see* Anaerobic Culture *on page 371*

Cyst Culture, Fungus *see* Fungus Culture, Biopsy *on page 461*

Cystometrogram, Simple

Synonyms CMG; Cystometry; Filling Cystometrogram; Simple CMG; Urodynamic Testing of Bladder Function

Test Includes Bedside evaluation of urinary bladder function in selected patients with urinary incontinence or retention. The bladder is passively filled with sterile water through a transurethral Foley catheter. Intravesical pressures are measured with an open manometer as bladder volume increases. Information regarding bladder sensation, capacity, and contractility is obtained.

Patient Preparation Technique and risks of the procedure are explained to the patient and consent is obtained. Ideally, patient should be off sedatives, cholinergics, or anticholinergics prior to testing. Indwelling Foley catheters should be removed well in advance so that residual volume may be measured. No pain medications or anxiolytics are routinely necessary. Patient is asked to void, if possible, immediately prior to procedure.

Aftercare No specific postprocedure restrictions are required and previous activity level may be resumed. At physician discretion, a urinalysis (and possibly urine culture) may be ordered on follow-up, 48-72 hours later.

Special Instructions Simple cystometry may be easily performed by a trained nurse or physician assistant and in most cases does not require direct physician supervision. This is a considerable advantage over complex cystometry which is usually performed in the Urodynamics Laboratory.

Complications This procedure is considered relatively safe. The vast majority of patients tolerate simple cystometry with minimal problems. Reported complications are similar to those seen with straight catheterization, such as local urethral discomfort, hematuria, and urinary tract infection. The precise complication rate is not known, but in one study involving 171 incontinent geriatric patients, <8% developed new urinary symptoms consistent with infection and <2% required antibiotic therapy.

Equipment Standard Foley catheter or 14F red rubber catheter required. Alternatively, a 3-channel Foley catheter (often used for bladder irrigation) may be used. Also needed are a urinary catheterization tray (drapes, lubricant, iodine, gloves, syringes, etc), Y-connector, 50 mL syringe, sterile water in graduated container, sterile tubing, nonsterile measuring basin. An open manometer, such as a spinal manometer, is commonly used.

Technique Numerous minor variations in technique have been described with the choice depending on physician preference and patient logistics. In its simplest form, a manometer is not used. After voiding, patient is placed in supine position and a Foley catheter (or 14F red rubber straight catheter) is inserted transurethrally into the bladder. Residual urine volume is measured and the catheter is left in place. With the bladder empty, the patient is requested to relax completely and avoid all bladder or abdominal contractions for the remainder of the procedure. The inner piston of a 50 mL syringe is removed and the syringe tip inserted into the distal (open) end of the catheter. Using the syringe as a funnel, room temperature sterile water is infused through the syringe and catheter in 50 mL increments. The syringe is elevated so the highest level of the fluid column is always 15 cm above the symphysis pubis. Thus, fluid enters the bladder by gravity drainage and not forcibly by syringe pressure. After each 50 mL water, the height of the water column is observed. Patient subjectively reports first perceptible sensation of bladder fullness and first strong urge to void. When patient notes a strong voiding urge, additional volume is added in 25 mL increments until discomfort is reported or an involuntary bladder contraction occurs. A bladder contraction appears as a sharp and sustained rise in the water column despite attempted voluntary bladder relaxation (and may be seen at any time during the procedure). The procedure is terminated at this stage. This brief sequence of maneuvers has been described in several formal studies comparing simple and complex multichannel cystometry. A common and time-honored variation of this procedure requires the use of a spinal manometer. Initial steps are identical. After residual volume is measured, a Y-connector is attached to the distal end of the Foley. Through one arm of the Y-connector, sterile water in a calibrated reservoir is instilled by gravity drainage. The other arm is connected to an open spinal manometer via sterile connecting tubing. An anaeroid manometer (Lewis cystometer) may also be used. Pressure within the tubing system is "bled off" into the manometer port. As water incrementally fills the bladder, increasing intravesicular pressure is transmitted back through the tubing and is crudely estimated by the height of the water column in the manometer. A plot of bladder pressure versus volume may be constructed in this manner. Alternatively, a 3-channel Foley may be used. Again, fluid is introduced through 1-catheter channel, but in this technique the spinal manometer is connected to a physically separate channel. This allows more accurate intravesical pressure estimations. When bladder pressure is measured in the fluid in the flow channel (as in the Y-connector arrangement), several confounding variables are introduced, such as the internal resistance to fluid in the catheter. Some of these variables are eliminated by this simple maneuver.

Data Acquired

- residual volume (mL)
- threshold for sensation of bladder fullness (mL) - the volume at which patient reports first sensation of fullness
- maximum cystometric capacity (mL) - the volume at which patient describes a strong urge to void, or the volume just prior to an involuntary contraction
- bladder contractility (presence and number of involuntary bladder contractions, as defined)

If a manometer is used, additional data includes:

- pressure-volume characteristics of the bladder during filling, this is termed the cystometrogram - bladder pressure (ordinate) plotted against volume (abscissa)
- bladder compliance, defined as $\Delta V/\Delta P$ and is derived from the cystometrogram

(Continued)

Cystometrogram, Simple *(Continued)*

Normal Findings Approximated as follows:

- residual volume - usually minimal or no urine obtained
- threshold for sensation of bladder fullness, 100-200 mL
- maximum capacity, 400-500 mL
- bladder contractility, no involuntary contractions noted
- cystometrogram, normally divided into the following four phases: (see figure)
- compliance - normally very high in phase two of the cystometrogram (approaching infinity)

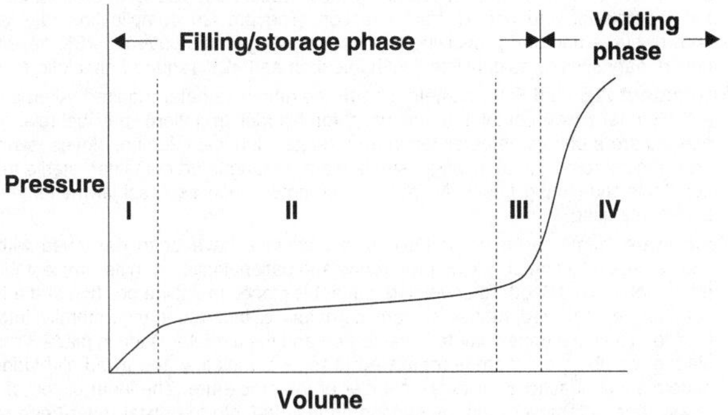

Phase 1: Initial pressure rise, stabilizes at the initial filling pressure or "resting pressure," normally approximately 10 cm H_2O.

Phase 2: The tonus limb, where compliance is high; pressure normally is low and remains constant as volume increases.

Phase 3: The limit of bladder elastic properties; increasing volume causes marked pressure increases. Patient normally can still voluntarily control micturition, even through maximum bladder capacity has almost been reached.

Phase 4: Voluntary voiding (not tested with simple cystometry).

Idealized cystometrogram. Note that the voiding phase is only assessed with complex cystometry. Reproduced with permission from Wein AJ, et al, *Urol Clin North Am*, 1988, 15(4):613.

Critical Values Residual volume: Significant postvoid residual may result from sensory neuropathy, lower motor neuron (LMN) disease, or bladder outlet resistance (functional or mechanical).

Threshold of sensation: Decreased sensation (ie, threshold >200 mL) is seen with sensory neuropathies such as diabetes mellitus, tabes dorsalis, cauda equina syndrome, or normal variant.

Maximum capacity: Decreased in a variety of disorders including upper motor neuron (UMN) disease, fibrotic bladder (eg, tuberculous interstitial cystitis), dysfunctionalized bladder, etc. Increased capacity (>500 mL) is seen with sensory neuropathy, LMN disease, chronic obstruction, bladder "training".

Contractility: Involuntary contractions at volumes less than capacity are abnormal. This condition has been called "detrusor hyper-reflexia" and "uninhibited" or "unstable" bladder. Increased contractility is found in various stroke syndromes, UMN lesions, hypertrophic bladder. Contractility is absent or weak in LMN lesions, sensory neuropathies, or voluntary inhibition.

Cystometrogram: Both the pattern of the tracing (pressure vs volume) and the absolute values should be compared against a standard normal curve. Some cystometrogram patterns may be diagnostic but tracings generated from simple cystometry are crude and may be difficult to interpret.

Compliance: A noncompliant bladder may result from a variety of disorders, including bladder wall fibrosis, bladder contraction, idiopathic male enuresis.

Use The exact indications for simple cystometry are controversial. Even amongst urologists, considerable debate exists in the medical/surgical literature considering

the optimal role of this procedure. Simple cystometry is useful in the patient with persistent urinary incontinence or retention felt to be secondary to impaired bladder filling or storage. Common clinical indications for this test include:

- suspected "neurogenic bladder"
- suspected detrusor motor instability, the hyper-reflexive bladder
- suspected abnormalities in bladder sensation, capacity, or contractility
- the geriatric patient with persistent urinary incontinence of unclear etiology (controversial)

Simple cystometry is less useful in evaluating the following conditions:

- suspected stress urinary incontinence in the female
- suspected psychogenic urinary incontinence in the male
- suspected urinary obstruction in the male

Limitations Procedure has questionable utility in the diagnosis of voiding disorders due to structural abnormalities, such as stress urinary incontinence or prostatic hypertrophy with retention, or complex voiding disorders. By nature, passive filling of the bladder is nonphysiologic and may potentially alter measured variables (eg, bladder capacity) in yet-to-be-understood ways. Only urologic function related to the bladder is assessed. Urine flow, force, urethral function, and myoneural coordination are not tested. Numerous technical factors may lead to false-positive or false-negative results. As previously mentioned, intravesical pressure is only crudely estimated by spinal manometry and is limited by confounding factors, such as inflow tubing resistance. Phase 4 of the standard cystometrogram is not evaluated (ie, the voiding phase of micturition). Complex cystometry is required for this. Increases in intra-abdominal pressure will alter pressure readings. This is not controlled for adequately in this procedure. Increases in manometric pressure readings may be due to increased intravesical pressure, increased abdominal wall pressure, or both. Thus, any abdominal muscle contraction may be misinterpreted as a bladder contraction. Although the examiner may simply observe the patient's abdomen for signs of muscle contraction, this is imprecise. With complex cystometry this is avoided by simultaneously recording intravesical and anorectal pressures (which estimate intra-abdominal pressure). The cystometrogram generated by manometer readings is discontinuous and crude. Provocative measures (position changes, medications, etc) are not routinely performed. These are usually reserved for complex cystometry.

Contraindications

- patient refusal
- the demented patient with severe cognitive impairment; this procedure requires the patient to accurately report sensations of bladder filling
- inability to pass transurethral Foley catheter
- active urinary tract infection

Additional Information The main advantage of simple cystometry is its convenience and low cost in comparison with more complex urodynamic testing. It may be performed by a trained nurse in less than minutes and need not be done in a hospital setting. Thus, it has been advocated for the evaluation of the nursing home patient or the elderly clinic patient. Several studies have compared simple and complex cystometry directly. Sutherst and Brown (1984) found that simple cystometry achieved a sensitivity of 100% for bladder instability with 89% specificity (when compared with complex cystometry as a gold standard). Ouslander (1988) also showed a high degree of correlation between the two tests in terms of bladder capacity and stability. However, the role of cystometry has not been clearly defined. Some authorities believe that only a small percentage of patients with voiding disorders need to undergo cystometry. This subpopulation may be identified using statistically derived algorithms based primarily on historical and physical examination findings. Others feel that the urologic history is misleading often enough (or inaccurate in the demented geriatric patient) to justify frequent use of simple cystometry. In many cases, it is argued, management of a voiding disorder will be influenced by the objective results from cystometry. In all cases, test results must be interpreted in conjunction with the clinical suspicion.

Selected Readings

Hilton P and Stanton SL, "Algorithmic Method for Assessing Urinary Incontinence in Elderly Women," *Br Med J [Clin Res]*, 1981, 282(6268):940-2.

Hinman F Jr, "Office Evaluation of Urodynamic Problems," *Urol Clin North Am*, 1979, 6(1):149-54.

Ouslander J, Leach G, Abelson S, et al, "Simple Versus Multichannel Cystometry in the Evaluation of Bladder Function in an Incontinent Geriatric Population," *J Urol*, 1988, 140(6):1482-6.

Sutherst JR and Brown MC, "Comparison of Single and Multichannel Cystometry in Diagnosing Bladder Instability," *Br Med J [Clin Res]*, 1984, 288(6432):1720-2.

Tanagho EA, "Urodynamic Studies," *Smith's General Urology*, Tanagho EA and McAninch JW, eds, 12th ed, Chapter 21, Norwalk, CT: Appleton and Lange, 1988, 452-72.

Wein AJ, English WS, and Whitmore KE, "Office Urodynamics," *Urol Clin North Am*, 1988, 15(4):609-23.

Cystometry *see* Cystometrogram, Simple *on page 434*

Cytology, Body Fluids

Synonyms Body Cavity Fluid Cytology; Effusion Cytology; Fluids Cytology

Applies to Ascitic Fluid Cytology; Culdocentesis; Paracentesis Fluid Cytology; Pericardial Fluid Cytology; Peritoneal Fluid Cytology; Pleural Fluid Cytology; Synovial Fluid Cytology; Thoracentesis Fluid Cytology

Test Includes Cytologic evaluation of smears, cytocentrifuge preparations, filters, and cell block when indicated

Patient Preparation Patient should sign informed consent prior to procedure. Puncture site should be carefully cleaned and prepped as for any tap.

Special Instructions Add 1 mL of heparin per 100 mL of fluid anticipated (each mL of heparin contains 1000 units). Include pertinent clinical information on requisition - previous malignancy, drugs, radiation therapy, history of alcohol abuse, or infection suspected.

Specimen Fresh body fluid

Container 150 mL vacuum heparinized bottle

Collection Gently agitate the flask as fluid is collected to mix the heparin with the fluid

Storage Instructions After hours place in the refrigerator

Causes for Rejection Fixation of any type, improper labeling or requisition, gross contamination due to spillage, prolonged period (over 24 hours) at room temperature

Use Establish the presence of primary or metastatic neoplasms; aid in the diagnosis of rheumatoid pleuritis, systemic lupus erythematosus, myeloproliferative and lymphoproliferative disorders, fungal and parasitic infestation of serous cavities, and fistulas involving serous cavities. Examination of synovial fluid from a joint effusion may aid in the diagnosis of metabolic arthritis (gout or pseudogout), rheumatoid arthritis, or traumatic arthritis. Examination of effusion is more sensitive and specific than blind pleural biopsy in the diagnosis of malignant pleural disease.

Limitations Allowing fluid to stand for prolonged period before processing may cause deterioration and artifact. Cells in fluids of long duration may be degenerated on first tap and a second tap may be required after reaccumulation for best cytologic detail. Clots may contain diagnostic cells which are unavailable for sampling. A cell block may enhance diagnostic yield.

Contraindications Documented bleeding diathesis is a relative contraindication

Additional Information Fluids should be submitted **fresh, unfixed**, and **heparinized** to provide well-preserved, representative, diagnostic material. Exfoliated cells deteriorate rapidly in the effusion, both in and out of the body. The amount of heparin recommended is minimal but adequate to prevent clotting of body cavity fluids and act as a preservative, though excess amounts will not alter cytologic detail. Cytologic evaluation may include the type of neoplasm and suggest its site of origin. The more clinical information provided, especially prior malignancy, prior radiation or chemotherapy, and relevant clinical findings, the better the diagnostic yield.

Venous blood drawn at the same time may be helpful; comparisons between serum and body fluid protein, LD, glucose, and other tests are often useful. When pleural fluid is sampled, a **pleural biopsy** may provide diagnosis, especially of granulomatous diseases as well as carcinoma.

Selected Readings

Dekker A and Bupp PA, "Cytology of Serous Effusions. An Investigation Into the Usefulness of Cell Blocks Versus Smears," *Am J Clin Pathol*, 1978, 70(6):855-60.

DeMay RM, "Fluids," *The Art and Science of Cytopathology*, Chapter 8, Chicago, IL: ASCP Press, American Society of Clinical Pathologists, 1996, 257-325.

Frist B, Kahan AV, and Koss LG, "Comparison of the Diagnostic Values of Biopsies of the Pleura and Cytologic Evaluation of Pleural Fluids," *Am J Clin Pathol*, 1979, 72(1):48-51.

Nathan NA, Narayan E, Smith MM, et al, "Cell Block Cytology. Improved Preparation and its Efficacy in Diagnostic Cytology," *Am J Clin Pathol*, 2000, 114(4):599-606.

Spieler P and Gloor F, "Identification of Types and Primary Sites of Malignant Tumors by Examination of Exfoliated Tumor Cells in Serous Fluids," *Acta Cytol*, 1985, 29(5):753-67.

Wahl RW, "Curschmann's Spirals in Pleural and Peritoneal Fluids," *Acta Cytol*, 1986, 30(2):147-51.

Cytomegalovirus Culture

Related Information

Cytomegalovirus Culture, Blood *on page 439*

Cytomegalovirus DNA Hybrid Capture *on page 440*

Cytomegalovirus Isolation, Rapid *on page 442*

Cytomegalovirus Serology *on page 442*

Synonyms CMV Culture; Viral Culture, Cytomegalovirus

Test Includes Culture for CMV only; CMV also is usually detected in a routine/general virus culture

Special Instructions Obtain viral transport medium from the laboratory prior to collecting the specimen.

Specimen Urine, throat, bronchoalveolar lavage, bronchial washings, lung biopsy

Container Sterile container; cold viral transport medium for swabs

Collection

Urine: A first morning clean catch urine should be submitted in a sterile screw cap container.

Throat: Rotate swab in both tonsillar crypts and against posterior oropharynx. Place swab in tube of viral transport medium, break off end of swab and tighten cap. This specimen is not particularly productive.

Storage Instructions Do not freeze specimens. Keep specimens cold and moist. Specimens should be delivered to the laboratory and handed to a technologist within 30 minutes of collection. If freezing is absolutely necessary, add an equal amount of 0.4 M sucrose-phosphate to the specimen before freezing.

Causes for Rejection Dry specimen, specimen not refrigerated during transport, specimen fixed in formalin, unlabeled specimen

Turnaround Time Variable (1-14 days) and depends on culture method used and amount of virus in the specimen

Reference Range No virus isolated

Use Aid in the diagnosis of disease caused by CMV (eg, viral infections, pneumonia, and organ transplant-related disease)

Methodology Inoculation of specimen into cell cultures, incubation of cultures, observation of characteristic cytopathic effect, and identification by fluorescent monoclonal antibody

Additional Information CMV infections are very common and are usually asymptomatic. CMV infections are frequently severe and life-threatening in immunocompromised patients including organ recipients and AIDS patients.

CMV is the most frequent cause of congenital viral infections in humans and occurs in about 1% of all newborns. Approximately 90% have no clinical symptoms at birth. Ten percent to 20% of these infants will develop complications before school age. Congenital infection may occur as a result of either primary or recurrent maternal infection.

Serology for the detection of cytomegalovirus is available, but the results are often of limited value unless a fourfold rise in titer can be documented.

Newer quantitative and qualitative molecular tests to detect cytomegalovirus DNA are considered to be more sensitive than in culture. Contact the testing laboratory for availability of molecular tests.

Selected Readings

Boeckh M and Boivin G, "Quantitation of Cytomegalovirus: Methodologic Aspects and Clinical Applications," *Clin Microbiol Rev*, 1998, 11(3):533-54.

Erice A, "Resistance of Human Cytomegalovirus to Antiviral Drugs," *Clin Microbiol Rev*, 1999, 12(2):286-97.

Griffiths PD and Grundy JE, "The Status of CMV as a Human Pathogen," *Epidemiol Infect*, 1988, 100(1):1-15.

Landini MP, "New Approaches and Perspectives in Cytomegalovirus Diagnosis," *Prog Med Virol*, 1993, 40:157-77.

Sia IG and Patel R, "New Strategies for Prevention and Therapy of Cytomegalovirus Infection and Disease in Solid-Organ Transplant Recipients," *Clin Microbiol Rev*, 2000, 13(1):83-121.

Yen-Lieberman B, "Diagnosis of Human Cytomegalovirus Disease," *Clin Microbiol Newslett*, 2000, 22(14):105-9.

Cytomegalovirus Culture, Blood

Related Information

Cytomegalovirus Culture *on page 438*
Cytomegalovirus DNA Hybrid Capture *on page 440*
Cytomegalovirus Isolation, Rapid *on page 442*
Cytomegalovirus Serology *on page 442*

Synonyms Blood Culture for CMV; Buffy Coat Culture for CMV; Buffy Coat Viral Culture; CMV Culture

Test Includes Culture of buffy coat for cytomegalovirus

Specimen Blood

Container Heparinized syringe or green top (heparin) tube

Collection Heparinize a 2 mL syringe with sterile preservative-free heparin. Invert the syringe several times after the blood is drawn to mix the blood thoroughly with the heparin. As an alternative, two 10 mL heparinized tubes may be used if transport of a syringe is difficult.

Storage Instructions Do not store specimen. Transport to the laboratory immediately in sealed plastic bag with request form.

Causes for Rejection Excessive hemolysis, delay in transport, leaking syringes

Turnaround Time Positive cultures will be reported when identification is made. Negative cultures will be reported after 28 days.

Reference Range No virus isolated

(Continued)

Cytomegalovirus Culture, Blood *(Continued)*

Use Detect cytomegaloviremia

Limitations Yield of CMV from this specimen may be high in patients with the acquired immunodeficiency syndrome (AIDS), but significantly lower in non-AIDS patients.

Methodology Cell culture for isolation and identification by indirect fluorescent antibody (IFA)

Selected Readings

Boeckh M and Boivin G, "Quantitation of Cytomegalovirus: Methodologic Aspects and Clinical Applications," *Clin Microbiol Rev*, 1998, 11(3):533-54.

Yen-Lieberman B, "Diagnosis of Human Cytomegalovirus Disease," *Clin Microbiol Newslett*, 2000, 22(14):105-9.

Cytomegalovirus DNA Hybrid Capture

Related Information

Cytomegalovirus Culture *on page 438*
Cytomegalovirus Culture, Blood *on page 439*
Cytomegalovirus Isolation, Rapid *on page 442*
Cytomegalovirus Serology *on page 442*

Synonyms CMV DNA Hybrid Capture; Digene CMV Hybrid Capture DNA; DNA Hybrid Capture, CMV; Murex CMV DNA Hybrid Capture Assay

Test Includes CMV hybrid capture (HC) is a molecular hybridization assay designed for the direct detection of CMV nucleic acid in white blood cells. This assay differs from polymerase chain reaction (PCR) assays since there are no viral amplification steps with HC. In the United States, the assay is commercially available as the Digene CMV Hybrid Capture System™ (Digene Corp, Silver Spring, MD).

HC is relatively simple to perform, rapid (6 hours), and does not require tissue culture techniques or molecular amplification steps. HC technology uses a CMV RNA probe which is capable of binding to a 40,000 base pair segment of the CMV genome. When the probe binds with the target CMV DNA, a "hybrid" of RNA-DNA is formed. The hybrids are then "captured" or immobilized within a special tube coated with antibodies specifically directed against the hybrids. A signal-amplified sandwich capture technique is used, and the hybrids are detected with chemiluminescent substrate. Light emitted is measured as relative light units. The intensity of light is proportional to the amount of target CMV DNA present in the specimen. The assay has been approved for qualitative determinations of CMV (virus absent or present) but can be set up for quantitative measurements (eg, copies/mL whole blood).

There are two versions of HC reported in the literature. Version 1 has a lower limit of detection of about 5000 copies of CMV per mL whole blood. Version 2 has a lower limit of about 700 copies per mL whole blood; only Version 2 is available commercially.

Specimen Whole blood

Container Lavender top (EDTA) tube

Storage Instructions Whole blood may be stored for up to 6 days at 4°C without a significant change in results. The ability to store the original specimen for several days is an important advantage for the HC assay and allows for flexible specimen collection on nights and weekends, and shipping specimens to reference laboratories is simplified. This is in contrast to the CMV antigenemia assay which requires prompt processing of fresh specimens within 6 hours.

For research purposes, a cell pellet can be extracted in several simple steps and frozen at -20°C for testing at a later date.

Turnaround Time Results available the same day or the following day, depending on the laboratory protocol.

Reference Range Laboratories may differ in how results are reported. Some laboratories may provide only a qualitative result for the detection of CMV (ie, yes/no); others will issue a quantitative result (eg, the number of CMV copies/mL whole blood).

Use

- Determine if the cause of a mononucleosis-like syndrome is from CMV (fever, myalgias, leukopenia, reactive lymphocytosis, pharyngitis, splenomegaly). CMV may cause a syndrome similar to infectious mononucleosis from Epstein-Barr virus in both immunocompetent and immunocompromised hosts.
- Determine if CMV infection is the cause of fever in an immunocompromised host who has no identifiable focus of infection (ie, the "CMV syndrome"). Laboratory testing in this setting must be interpreted cautiously since some patients may asymptomatically shed CMV in the blood during febrile episodes.
- Determine if CMV may be the cause of disease in a patient with an identified source of infection (ie, the transplant patient with a new pulmonary infiltrate of unknown etiology). Again, a positive DNA result must be interpreted carefully.

- Identify high-risk patients early in the course of CMV infection (ie, "pre-emptive therapy") (see Additional Information).

Limitations CMV hybrid capture is currently performed in a limited number of laboratories. In addition, some laboratories may require a specific request in advance for quantitative rather than qualitative HC results, since several control standards must be included in each test run to calculate a quantitative result.

Methodology A minimum of 3.5 mL whole blood is incubated for 15 minutes in a RBC-lysing solution. WBCs are spun down, washed, and resuspended. The sample is denatured with base which lyses the cells and separates the strands of DNA. A target-specific, single-stranded RNA probe to CMV DNA is added, creating an RNA:DNA hybrid. The RNA probe is large, containing approximately 38 kb of sequences. Hybridization takes place over 2 hours at 70°C. The captured hybrid is detected with a second set of RNA:DNA antibodies conjugated to alkaline phosphatase. Each 38 kb RNA:DNA hybrid binds approximately 1000 antibody conjugate molecules, and each is bound to three alkaline phosphatase molecules. Because each captured hybrid binds up to 3000 alkaline phosphatase molecules, the resulting signal is amplified at least 3000-fold. Substrate is then added. Upon cleavage by the alkaline phosphatase, the substrate produces light that is measured on a luminometer in relative light units. The intensity of the light emitted denotes the presence or absence of target DNA in the specimen.

Contact the testing laboratory for information on additional molecular tests for cytomegalovirus.

Additional Information CMV hybrid capture is one of several assays for CMV that have been used to identify patients at highest risk for serious CMV disease. Because HC is a relatively new assay, most of the studies have compared HC to CMV cell culture and to CMV pp65 antigenemia (see separate listings). It is hoped that the HC assay will prove to be equivalent to the pp65 antigenemia as part of a "pre-emptive approach" for management of CMV infection in many transplant centers. This therapeutic strategy is based on the identification of early subclinical disease by the use of a reliable laboratory test which can identify a subgroup of patients at the highest risk for clinical disease. CMV dissemination in the blood is now understood to be an important early step in the pathogenesis of CMV disease, and the early detection of CMV DNA ("DNA-emia") hopefully can identify infection before the development of disease. Pre-emptive therapy differs from prophylactic therapy in that pre-emptive therapy is based on a specific marker for disease (usually a positive laboratory test) which has sufficient predictive power to justify starting antimicrobial therapy. In contrast, prophylactic therapy is started before there is evidence of infection and involves treating larger numbers of people than the pre-emptive approach.

CMV antigenemia was one of the first assays used for pre-emptive therapy. HC and pp65 antigenemia appear to have comparable sensitivity and specificity based on the results of several comparison trials. How well the HC and pp65 antigenemia assays correlate in terms of quantitation of CMV is unknown. Larger studies are underway to study the quantitative aspects of HC. Several questions remain to be answered: (1) is there a "threshold" CMV DNA level as determined by HC that is associated with clinical disease, (2) what are the positive and negative predictive values of HC in predicting end-organ disease, (3) how does HC compare with other methods for CMV quantitation including pp65 antigenemia and quantitative PCR, and (4) how useful is HC in monitoring response to therapy?

HC has several advantages over existing assays for CMV. Because there are no target amplification steps, HC avoids the problem of contamination seen with PCR. In addition the problems with enzymatic inhibitors reported with PCR have not been noted with HC. HC also has several advantages over pp65 antigenemia, including the ease of specimen preparation, the stability of the original specimen for several days prior to laboratory processing, ability to batch specimens for large runs, and an objective, semiautomated means of viral quantification.

Selected Readings

Barrett-Muir WY, Aitken C, Templeton K, et al, "Evaluation of the Murex Hybrid Capture Cytomegalovirus DNA Assay Versus Plasma PCR and Shell Vial Assay for Diagnosis of Human Cytomegalovirus Viremia in Immunocompromised Patients," *J Clin Microbiol*, 1998, 36(9):2554-6.

Boeckh M and Boivin G, "Quantitation of Cytomegalovirus: Methodologic Aspects and Clinical Applications," *Clin Microbiol Rev*, 1998, 11(3):533-54.

Bossart W, Bienz K, and Wunderli W, "Surveillance of Cytomegalovirus After Solid-Organ Transplantation: Comparison of pp65 Antigenemia Assay With a Quantitative DNA Hybridization Assay," *J Clin Microbiol*, 1997, 35(12):3303-4.

Mazzulli T, Wood S, Chua R, et al, "Evaluation of the Digene Hybrid Capture System for Detection and Quantitation of Human Cytomegalovirus Viremia in Human Immunodeficiency Virus-Infected Patients," *J Clin Microbiol*, 1996, 34(12):2959-62.

Myers JB and Amsterdam D, "The Laboratory Diagnosis of Cytomegalovirus Infections," *Immunol Invest*, 1997, 26(3):383-94.

(Continued)

Cytomegalovirus DNA Hybrid Capture *(Continued)*

Nichols WG and Boeckh M, "Recent Advances in the Therapy and Prevention of CMV Infections," *J Clin Virol*, 2000, 16(1):25-40.
Veal N, Payan C, Fray D, et al, "Novel DNA Assay for Cytomegalovirus Detection: Comparison With Conventional Culture and pp65 Antigenemia Assay," *J Clin Microbiol*, 1996, 34(12):3097-100.
Yen-Lieberman B, "Diagnosis of Human Cytomegalovirus Disease," *Clin Microbiol Newslett*, 2000, 22(14):105-9.

Cytomegalovirus Isolation, Rapid

Related Information

Cytomegalovirus Culture *on page 438*
Cytomegalovirus Culture, Blood *on page 439*
Cytomegalovirus DNA Hybrid Capture *on page 440*
Cytomegalovirus Serology *on page 442*

Synonyms CMV Early Antigen FA Method; CMV Shell Vial Method

Test Includes Inoculation of cell cultures in shell vials, 16-hour incubation, and immunofluorescence staining of CMV early nuclear antigen with monoclonal antibodies; conventional cell culture inoculation

Specimen Urine, bronchoalveolar lavage, blood, tracheal aspirates, appropriate autopsy and biopsy specimens

Container Sterile container; cold viral transport medium for swabs

Collection

Urine: A first morning clean catch urine should be submitted in a sterile screw cap container.

Throat: Rotate swab in both tonsillar crypts and against posterior oropharynx. Place swab in tube of viral transport medium, break off end of swab and tighten cap. This specimen is not particularly productive.

Turnaround Time Overnight to 2 days depending on method and capability of laboratory

Reference Range No CMV detected

Use Aid in the diagnosis of disease caused by CMV (eg, viral infections, pneumonia, and organ transplant-related disease)

Limitations The rapid shell vial method for the detection of CMV has been reported to be more sensitive than conventional cell culture.

Methodology Specimens are centrifuged onto cell cultures grown on coverslips in the bottoms of 1-dram shell vials. Centrifugation greatly accelerates virus attachment and penetration. After incubation, fluorescein-labeled monoclonal antibodies are applied to the infected cells to detect viral antigens that are expressed in the membranes of the cells. Characteristic fluorescent foci indicate the presence of virus.

Some laboratories offer molecular testing for this organism. Contact the testing laboratory for the availability of amplified and nonamplified qualitative and quantitative molecular tests for this organism, and for information on selection and collection of appropriate specimens for specific molecular tests.

Selected Readings

Boeckh M and Boivin G, "Quantitation of Cytomegalovirus: Methodologic Aspects and Clinical Applications," *Clin Microbiol Rev*, 1998, 11(3):533-54.
Erice A, "Resistance of Human Cytomegalovirus to Antiviral Drugs," *Clin Microbiol Rev*, 1999, 12(2):286-97.
Yen-Lieberman B, "Diagnosis of Human Cytomegalovirus Disease," *Clin Microbiol Newslett*, 2000, 22(14):105-9.

Cytomegalovirus Serology

Related Information

Cytomegalovirus Culture *on page 438*
Cytomegalovirus Culture, Blood *on page 439*
Cytomegalovirus DNA Hybrid Capture *on page 440*
Cytomegalovirus Isolation, Rapid *on page 442*

Synonyms CMV-IFA; CMV Titer

Applies to CMV-IFA, IgG; CMV-IFA, IgM

Test Includes IgG and IgM testing of acute sera in neonates, patients suspected of post-transfusion CMV infection, immunosuppressed patients, and maternity cases; IgG testing of acute and convalescent sera

Specimen Serum

Container Red top tube or serum separator tube

Sampling Time Acute and convalescent sera drawn 10-14 days apart are required

Storage Instructions Store at 4°C or freeze.

Reference Range IgM <1:8 and IgG <1:16 is considered nondiagnostic. A fourfold increase in titer in paired sera drawn 10-14 days apart is usually indicative of acute infection.

Use Support the diagnosis of cytomegalovirus infection

Limitations Heterophil antibodies and presence of rheumatoid factor may cause false-positive IgM results. Fetal IgM antibody to maternal IgG may also cause false-positive results. Because of high levels of "background" antibody in adult populations, a single antibody determination is not useful. For rapid confirmation of new CMV infection, rapid shell vial culture for CMV is superior to serology.

Methodology Indirect fluorescent antibody (IFA), enzyme immunoassay (EIA).

If serological testing is performed by enzyme immunoassay (EIA) on automated instrumentation, results are usually given in index units, not titers. In such cases, significant rises in antibody levels are determined by algorithms within the instrumentation, not by increases in titers.

Additional Information A single titer is rarely significant if past history is unknown. A fourfold or greater rise in CMV titer between acute and convalescent specimens is evidence of infection. A single IgM specific titer >1:8 is also excellent evidence of acute infection. CMV causes an infectious mononucleosis syndrome clinically indistinguishable from heterophil positive mononucleosis, a very common disease. Significant CMV titers are found almost universally in patients with AIDS, and CMV genome has been demonstrated in the cells of Kaposi's sarcoma. CMV is a significant cause of postcardiotomy, post-transplant and postpump hepatitis syndromes.

Although serology is a useful method to detect CMV infections, the newer shell vial culture can more reliably identify symptomatic CMV infections in immunocompromised patients.

Several new EIA tests agree well with the IFA serology and provide a more objective measure of infection status than the subjective IFA test.

Selected Readings

Boeckh M and Boivin G, "Quantitation of Cytomegalovirus: Methodologic Aspects and Clinical Applications," *Clin Microbiol Rev*, 1998, 11(3):533-54.

Erice A, "Resistance of Human Cytomegalovirus to Antiviral Drugs," *Clin Microbiol Rev*, 1999, 12(2):286-97.

Sia IG and Patel R, "New Strategies for Prevention and Therapy of Cytomegalovirus Infection and Disease in Solid-Organ Transplant Recipients," *Clin Microbiol Rev*, 2000, 13(1):83-121.

Waner JL and Stewart JA, "Cytomegalovirus," *Manual of Clinical Laboratory Immunology*, 5th ed, Rose NR, Conway de Macario E, Folds JD, et al, eds, Washington, DC: American Society for Microbiology, 1997, 644-8.

Yen-Lieberman B, "Diagnosis of Human Cytomegalovirus Disease," *Clin Microbiol Newslett*, 2000, 22(14):105-9.

Darkfield Examination, Leptospirosis

Related Information

Leptospira Culture *on page 518*
Leptospira Serology *on page 519*
Mycoplasma pneumoniae Diagnostic Procedures *on page 544*

Synonyms Darkfield Microscopy, *Leptospira*; Leptospirosis, Darkfield Examination

Test Includes Examination of serum, urine, or CSF for organisms

Specimen Urine, serum, cerebrospinal fluid

Container Sterile plastic urine container, red top tube, or sterile CSF tube

Causes for Rejection Specimen dried out

Use Evaluate the presence of *Leptospira* to establish the diagnosis of leptospirosis. The failure to detect leptospires does not rule out their presence.

Limitations Most clinical laboratories do not perform this test. Culture for *Leptospira* is a more valuable and sensitive test. The concentration of leptospires in blood and CSF is low. Therefore, concentration by centrifugation with sodium oxalate or heparin can be useful. The incidence of false-positives is increased because fibrils and cellular extrusions can be mistaken for organisms. Extreme technical expertise is required.

Methodology A very small drop of fluid is distributed in a thin layer between a glass coverslip and slide. Positives should be confirmed by serologic or cultural methods. The typical morphology helicoidal, flexible organisms 6-20 μm long and 0.1 μm in diameter usually with semicircular hooked ends should be observed before a presumptive diagnosis is made. Artifacts are common.

Additional Information *Leptospira* are present in blood early in course of the disease (first week only). After 10-14 days they may be found in the urine. Urine must be neutral or alkaline. Culture has much greater value for diagnosis.

Darkfield microscopy is best used to demonstrate leptospires in specimens in which a high concentration of organisms is present, ie, tissue from animals (guinea pig or hamster), inoculation including blood, peritoneal fluid, or liver suspensions. Urine or kidney suspensions from swine, dogs, and domestic animals may also yield positive darkfield examination.

(Continued)

Darkfield Examination, Leptospirosis *(Continued)*

Selected Readings

Weyant RS, Bragg SL, and Kaufmann AF, "*Leptospira* and *Leptonema*," *Manual of Clinical Microbiology*, 7th ed, Murray PR, Baron EJ, Pfaller MA, et al, eds, Washington, DC: American Society for Microbiology, 1999, 739-45.

Darkfield Examination, Syphilis

Related Information

FTA-ABS, Serum *on page 457*
RPR *on page 574*
VDRL, Cerebrospinal Fluid *on page 613*

Synonyms Darkfield Microscopy, Syphilis; Syphilis, Darkfield Examination; *Treponema pallidum* Darkfield Examination

Test Includes Cleansing of chancre, procurement of specimen, and darkfield examination

Patient Preparation The test is usually performed by public health laboratories and public health facilities and clinics. The surface of the chancre is cleansed and roughened by the physician with a swab or gauze moistened with saline. This removes exudate and excess bacteria contamination. Serum is then collected from the surface of the chancre using a small pipette. The serum is placed on a slide or coverslip. Alternatively, the specimen can be collected by directly touching the slide to the lesion. The object is to obtain clear serum exudate from the subsurface of the lesion. It is then examined by darkfield microscopy.

Specimen Moist serum from the base of a cleansed unhealed chancre. The youngest lesion available is best. The chance of identification of treponemes decreases with the age of the lesion as it dries and heals.

Causes for Rejection Healed chancre, previous treatment, ointment, dried up specimen

Reference Range *Treponema pallidum* has a rapid and purposeful motion as it travels across the microscopic field. The organisms appear as a tight corkscrew. The organisms are 1.0 to 1.5 times the diameter of an RBC in length.

Use Determine the presence of characteristic spirochetes in lesions suspected of being syphilis

Limitations Most clinical laboratories do not perform this test. This test usually is performed in public health centers and clinics. Darkfield examination is of limited value in oral and rectal lesions because of the normal presence of other nonpathogenic spirochetes. Dry or bloody specimens render this examination worthless. The specimen should be examined within 15 minutes of collection because the organisms lose motility with decrease in temperature.

Contraindications Antibiotic therapy prior to the darkfield examination. The organisms are rapidly cleared following therapy.

Methodology Darkfield microscopy. Motile organisms are observed to rotate around their long axis and to bend, snap, and flex along their length. A smooth translational back and forth directed movement is also apparent.

Additional Information *Treponema* can be found in skin lesions and lymph nodes in secondary syphilis but are more plentiful in primary chancres. They cannot be grown in culture.

Selected Readings

Larsen SA, "Syphilis," *Clin Lab Med*, 1989, 9(3):545-57.
Larsen SA, Norris SJ, and Pope V, "*Treponema* and Other Host-Associated Spirochetes," *Manual of Clinical Microbiology*, 7th ed, Murray PR, Baron EJ, Pfaller MA, et al, eds, Washington, DC: American Society for Microbiology, 1999, 759-76.

Darkfield Microscopy, *Leptospira* *see* Darkfield Examination, Leptospirosis *on page 443*

Darkfield Microscopy, Syphilis *see* Darkfield Examination, Syphilis *on page 444*

Deer Tick Identification *see* Arthropod Identification *on page 387*

Delayed Hypersensitivity Fungal Skin Tests *see* Fungal Skin Testing *on page 459*

Delayed Reaction Intracutaneous Tests *see* Anergy Skin Test Battery *on page 372*

Delta Agent Serology *see* Hepatitis D Serology *on page 489*

Delta Hepatitis Serology *see* Hepatitis D Serology *on page 489*

Dermatitis Herpetiformis Antibodies *see* Skin Biopsy, Immunofluorescence *on page 583*

Dermatophyte Fungus Culture *see* Fungus Culture, Skin *on page 464*

Digene CMV Hybrid Capture DNA *see* Cytomegalovirus DNA Hybrid Capture *on page 440*

Diphtheria Culture *see* Throat Culture for *Corynebacterium diphtheriae on page 593*

Direct Detection of Virus *see* Virus Detection by DFA *on page 619*

Direct Fluorescent Antibody Smear for *Legionella pneumophila* *see* *Legionella pneumophila* Smear *on page 517*

Direct Fluorescent Antibody Test for Virus *see* Virus Detection by DFA *on page 619*

Direct Immunofluorescent Studies, Biopsy *see* Immunofluorescent Studies, Biopsy *on page 507*

DNA Hybrid Capture, CMV *see* Cytomegalovirus DNA Hybrid Capture *on page 440*

DNA Hybridization Test for *Chlamydia trachomatis* *see* *Chlamydia trachomatis* by Molecular Probe *on page 415*

DNA Hybridization Test for *Neisseria gonorrhoeae* *see* *Neisseria gonorrhoeae* by Nucleic Acid Probe *on page 546*

DNA Probe for *Legionella* *see* *Legionella* DNA Probe *on page 515*

DNA Probe for Mycobacteria *see* Mycobacteria Culture, Sputum *on page 542*

DNA Test for *Chlamydia trachomatis* *see* *Chlamydia trachomatis* by Molecular Probe *on page 415*

DNA Test for *Neisseria gonorrhoeae* *see* *Neisseria gonorrhoeae* by Nucleic Acid Probe *on page 546*

Eaton Agent Titer *see* *Mycoplasma* Serology *on page 545*

EB Nuclear Antigens *see* Epstein-Barr Virus Serology *on page 454*

EB Virus Titer *see* Epstein-Barr Virus Serology *on page 454*

EBV Titer *see* Epstein-Barr Virus Serology *on page 454*

Echocardiography, M-Mode

Synonyms M-Mode Echo; Unidimensional Echo

Test Includes M-mode echocardiography, the first form of cardiac ultrasound used in clinical practice, takes its name from the motion of the cardiac structures that was possible to visualize when this diagnostic method was introduced. M-mode echocardiography provides an "ice pick" view of the heart with a very high temporal and unidimensional space resolution, so that it provides an excellent method to measure chamber dimensions and to time cardiac events.

Patient Preparation No special patient preparation is required. Fasting is not necessary. The procedure can be done at any time. In scheduling patients that will have multiple cardiac diagnostic procedures it will be best to order the echocardiogram before Holter monitoring since the multiple electrodes placed on the chest for this procedure may interfere with the performance of the echocardiogram. Also, if a patient is to have a stress test on the same day, enough time (2-3 hours) should be allowed after the exercise test to perform the echocardiogram under basal conditions.

Special Instructions In most cases the M-mode echocardiogram is performed as part of a more complete cardiac ultrasound study that includes either 2-D echocardiography and/or Doppler echocardiography. The test that provides the most information should be requested, although sometimes this decision is left to the personnel in the Echo Laboratory. A complete cardiac ultrasound study takes anywhere from 60-90 minutes, the "M-mode" part of it takes approximately 30 minutes. To optimize the diagnostic yield of the echocardiogram a note relating the reason for the request should be made in the patient's chart or in a requisition form. Other useful information to be presented includes patient's age, weight, and height.

Normal M-Mode Echocardiographic Values

	Mean (cm)	Range (cm)
RVD	1.7	0.9-2.6
LVIDD	4.7	3.5-5.7
PLVWT	0.9	0.6-1.1
IVSWT	0.9	0.6-1.1
LA	2.9	1.9-4.0
AO	2.7	2.0-3.7
FS	36%	34%-44%

RVD = right ventricular dimension.

LVIDD = left ventricular internal dimension in diastole.

PLVWT = posterior left ventricular wall thickness.

IVSWT = interventricular wall thickness.

LA = left atrium.

AO = aorta.

FS = fractional shortening.

From Feigenbaum H, *Echocardiography*, 4th ed, Philadelphia, PA: Lea & Febiger, 1986, with permission.

(Continued)

Echocardiography, M-Mode *(Continued)*

Technique Three electrodes for EKG monitoring are placed on the chest and the patient is asked to lie in a left lateral decubitus position. Currently, most M-mode echocardiograms are obtained by using a 2-D echocardiographic probe and selecting M-mode information from it. Briefly, the transducer is placed at the left parasternal border, the long axis view is selected, and the M-mode line is moved from the left ventricle to the mitral valve and finally to the aorta and left atrium. Recordings at these levels are registered in a strip chart recorder, a video recorder, or a page printer. These recordings become part of the report and of the Echo Laboratory file.

Normal Findings Adequate interpretation of M-mode echocardiography requires knowledge of the normal values of the dimension of the cardiac chambers and great arteries (see table on previous page), and an understanding of the normal motion of the valves and different walls of the cardiac system. Distinct abnormalities can be characterized by M-mode echocardiography for many cardiovascular disorders.

Use The most common indications for this test include:

- wall thickness measurement of interventricular septum, posterior left ventricular wall and right ventricular free wall
- measurement of end-diastolic and end-systolic left ventricular internal dimensions
- percent of fractional shortening (difference between end-diastolic and end-systolic dimensions divided by end-diastolic dimension)
- measurement of right ventricular dimension; measurement of the anteroposterior diameter of the ascending aorta and left atrium.

M-mode echocardiography is **most useful** in:

- diagnosis of pericardial effusion
- left ventricular hypertrophy
- generalized left ventricular dysfunction
- hypertrophic obstructive cardiomyopathy
- mitral valve prolapse
- mitral stenosis
- left atrial myxoma

Contraindications There are no contraindications for M-mode echocardiography but patients with chronic obstructive lung disease or marked obesity will usually have tests of poor diagnostic quality.

Selected Readings

Sahn DJ, DeMaria A, Kisslo J, et al, "Recommendations Regarding Quantitation in M-Mode Echocardiography: Results of a Survey of Echocardiographic Measurements," *Circulation*, 1978, 58(6):1072-83.

Echovirus Culture *see* Enterovirus Culture *on page 453*

Echovirus Culture, Stool *see* Viral Culture, Stool *on page 616*

Ectoparasite Identification *see* Arthropod Identification *on page 387*

EEG *see* Electroencephalography *on page 447*

Effusion Cytology *see* Cytology, Body Fluids *on page 438*

Ehrlichia Serology

Related Information

Rocky Mountain Spotted Fever Serology *on page 573*

Test Includes Antibody to *Ehrlichia canis*

Specimen Serum

Container Red top tube or serum separator tube

Sampling Time Acute and convalescent serum 14-21 days apart are recommended.

Storage Instructions Separate serum and refrigerate.

Causes for Rejection Inadequate labeling, excessive hemolysis, chylous serum

Use Establish the diagnosis of ehrlichiosis

Methodology Indirect fluorescent antibody (IFA)

Additional Information Newly recognized human ehrlichiosis is a disease caused by a Rickettsiaceae (*Ehrlichia*) family member which is well known for causing disease in animals. Human infection with an *Ehrlichia canis*-like organism was first described in the United States in 1986. Preliminary data suggest that human ehrlichiosis is tick-borne, and that most human cases present with symptoms suggestive of RMSF without the rash or as "spotless" RMSF. *E. canis* is found in white blood cells, in particular, polymorphonuclear leukocytes and mononuclear cells. During acute illness, intracellular inclusions (in monocytes) of *E. canis* can be observed on peripheral blood smears. IgG titers of 1:16-1:32 are considered equivocal while IgG titers ≥1:64 are indicative of *E. canis* infection. Titers which show a fourfold or greater increase in IgG or the presence of IgM against *E. canis* is indicative of recent or current infection. Serological testing for *E. canis* is performed only in research and specialty reference laboratories.

Selected Readings

Bakken JS and Dumler JS, "Human Granulocytic Ehrlichiosis," *Clin Infect Dis*, 2000, 31(2):554-60.

Goldman DP, Artenstein AW, and Bolan CD, "Human Ehrlichiosis: A Newly Recognized Tick-Borne Disease," *Am Fam Physician*, 1992, 46(1):199-208.

McDade JE, "Ehrlichiosis - A Disease of Animals and Humans," *J Infect Dis*, 1990, 161(4):609-17.

Rikihisa Y, "The Tribe Ehrlichieae and Ehrlichial Diseases," *Clin Microbiol Rev*, 1991, 4(3):286-308.

Elbow Arthrogram *see* Arthrogram *on page 387*

Elbow, Left or Right, X-ray *see* Bone Films *on page 396*

Electrodiagnostic Study *see* Electromyography *on page 448*

Electroencephalogram *see* Electroencephalography *on page 447*

Electroencephalography

Synonyms EEG; Electroencephalogram

Applies to Somatosensory Evoked Potentials

Test Includes Analysis of the electrical activity of the brain using scalp electrodes. This procedure is based on the principle that neurons within the cerebral cortex will normally generate low-amplitude electrical potentials. Electrodes positioned over specific regions of the cortex are able to detect these signals. Brain rhythms are then amplified and transmitted to a multichannel polygraph which records waveforms with automatic ink pens on moving paper. This written document, often more than 100 pages, is called the electroencephalogram. It is a continuous plot of voltage (vertical axis) versus time (horizontal axis). Abnormalities in the EEG brain wave pattern may be diagnostic of specific neurologic diseases. EEG is an indispensable means of evaluating gray matter disease and it is the only electrophysiologic measure of ongoing cortical function.

Patient Preparation Details of the procedure are discussed with the patient. When possible, sedative medications should be discontinued well in advance. This includes benzodiazepines, barbiturates, ethanol, etc. Fasting prior to EEG is not necessary, in fact, relative hypoglycemia has been reported to alter the EEG. The patient should also be reasonably rested beforehand since sleep deprivation has been known to cause alpha-rhythm abnormalities. If the patient has already been receiving anticonvulsant agents (eg, phenytoin (Dilantin®), carbamazepine) the management is more complex. The decision to withdraw or continue anticonvulsants prior to EEG testing should be handled by the physician. When approaching the patient with a new-onset seizure disorder (witnessed or suspected), many clinicians will obtain the initial EEG while the patient is still on an anticonvulsant agent. If results are negative, the EEG may be repeated later after discontinuing anticonvulsants for 1-2 days. Although this approach is admittedly cautious, it reduces the chance of seizure "breakthrough". Patient should wash hair the night before the test. Hair cream, oils, spray, and lacquer should not be applied after washing.

Aftercare If an overnight sleep study has been performed, patient is not permitted to drive home afterwards. Otherwise, if a routine (wake) EEG is performed no specific postprocedure restrictions are necessary. If anticonvulsant medications were discontinued specifically for the EEG, the patient is instructed to restart medications until notified by physician.

Special Instructions Requisition for EEG from the ordering physician should state patient's age, brief clinical history, overall impression, and reason for EEG. Special requests can be made for overnight study, sleep study, nasopharyngeal leads, activation procedures, evoked response testing, etc.

Complications EEG is considered a safe procedure and is well tolerated. The following "activation" techniques may be successful in inducing a seizure, but this is a desired "complication".

Technique At the start of the procedure, surface electrodes are placed on the scalp over designated areas. From 8-20 electrodes may be used, each approximately 0.5 cm in diameter. The patient is asked to rest comfortably on the examining table, first with eyes open, then closed. The underlying electrical activity of the cerebral cortex is measured (deeper structures are more difficult to measure). The signals are amplified, filtered, and transmitted to a polygraph. The electrical signals detected at each electrode move a separate ink writing pen on the polygraph. Thus, activity within anatomically different areas of the brain (temporal lobe, occipital, frontal, etc) are recorded on separate "channels". A continuous graph is produced on moving paper plotting voltage (vertical axis) versus time (horizontal axis). The written record may be several hundred pages long. Testing requires approximately 1 hour. Several "activation" measures may be attempted in order to induce a seizure under controlled laboratory conditions. These include:

- hyperventilation (leads to acute respiratory alkalosis and cerebral vasoconstriction)
- stroboscopic stimulation
- sleep EEG (for suspected temporal lobe epilepsy)

(Continued)

Electroencephalography *(Continued)*

Use Common indications for EEG in general practice include:

- evaluation of the patient with a suspected seizure disorder; EEG is unique in its ability to objectively document the presence of seizure activity. In addition, EEG is crucial in localizing the site of a seizure focus and classifying the nature of epileptiform discharges. EEG is nearly always abnormal during an acute generalized seizure (eg, grand mal, petit mal), and frequently abnormal during an acute focal seizure (eg, Jacksonian). The EEG may also have diagnostic utility during the interictal period with abnormal discharges seen in 80% of patients with petit mal and 60% of patients with grand mal seizures.
- assessment of coma and other impairments in mental status; the EEG is abnormal in nearly every case of metabolic encephalopathy or ischemic encephalopathy, but is normal in most psychiatric conditions. In some instances, EEG may reveal important etiologic data not suspected clinically. For example, when coma is caused by hepatic encephalopathy, barbiturate overdose, or subclinical status epilepticus, distinctive and diagnostic EEG waveforms may be seen.
- diagnosis of certain infections of the central nervous system (CNS); characteristic EEG patterns may be seen in herpes simplex encephalitis, Creutzfeldt-Jakob disease, and subacute sclerosing panencephalitis.

Additional roles for EEG include:

- diagnosis of intracranial mass lesions; EEG is capable of diagnosing and localizing lesions such as brain tumors, abscesses, meningiomas, etc. However, this test cannot reliably distinguish between these entities. In recent years, the CT scan and MRI scan have supplanted the EEG in the evaluation of space occupying lesions.
- evaluation of cerebrovascular disease; in a patient who has suffered a recent cortical stroke, EEG can demonstrate regional electrical abnormalities in the distribution of the thrombosed vessel. In the patient who has suffered a subcortical stroke ("lacunar stroke"), the EEG is usually normal even though the patient is hemiplegic. Thus, EEG may play a role in distinguishing cortical from subcortical stroke syndromes. In addition, EEG has been used in the past to diagnose and localize subarachnoid hemorrhage. However, CT scan or MRI scan have become the diagnostic tests of choice for stroke and subarachnoid hemorrhage.
- assessment of head injury; following a cerebral concussion, EEG is usually normal, but after a cerebral contusion, EEG is usually abnormal (although nonspecific). EEG has also been used to predict the subset of patients with head trauma who will go on to develop a seizure disorder.
- evaluation of persistent sleep disorders; overnight EEG recording is included as part of the polysomnogram (along with other monitoring techniques).
- intraoperative monitoring of cerebral activity; EEG may be used during certain neurosurgical procedures, carotid endarterectomies, and some non-neurologic surgeries as well (eg, cardiothoracic surgery). It is also useful in assessing depth of anesthesia.
- evaluation of suspected pseudoseizures; the EEG is normal despite generalized clonic movements
- EEG is characteristically **normal** in the following: multiple sclerosis (in severe cases some nonspecific changes may be seen); delirium tremens; Wernicke-Korsakoff's syndrome; Alzheimer's disease; cryptococcal meningitis; cerebral concussion; psychiatric disturbances, including bipolar disorder; tension headache; pseudoseizures.

Contraindications No absolute contraindications exist for EEG.

Selected Readings

Adams RD and Victor M, *Principles of Neurology: Companion Handbook*, 6th ed, New York, NY: McGraw-Hill Book Co, 1997.

Aminoff MJ, *Electrodiagnosis in Clinical Neurology*, 4th ed, New York, NY: Churchill-Livingstone, 1999.

Aminoff MJ "Electrophysiologic Studies of the Central and Peripheral Nervous Systems," *Harrison's Principles of Internal Medicine*, 14th ed, Fauci AS, Braunwald E, Isselbacher KJ, et al, eds, New York, NY: McGraw-Hill Book Co, 1998, 2282-97.

Davis TL and Freemon FR, "Electroencephalography Should not Be Routine in the Evaluation of Syncope in Adults," *Arch Intern Med*, 1990, 150(10):2027-9.

Niedermeyer E and DaSilva FL, *Electroencephalography*, 4th ed, Baltimore, MD: Williams & Wilkins, 1999.

Spehlmann R, *EEG Primer*, Elsevier, North Holland: Biomedical Press, 1981.

Wee AS, "Is Electroencephalography Necessary in the Evaluation of Syncope?" *Arch Intern Med*, 1990, 150(10):2007-8.

Electromyography

Synonyms Electrodiagnostic Study; EMG

Test Includes Insertion of a needle electrode into skeletal muscle to measure electrical activity and assess physiologic function. In this procedure, percutaneous, extracellular needle electrodes are placed into a selected muscle group. Muscle action

potentials (AP) are detected by these electrodes, amplified, and displayed on a cathode ray oscilloscope. In addition, fluctuations in voltage are heard as "crackles" over a loudspeaker, permitting both auditory and visual analysis of the muscle APs. Testing is performed with the muscle at rest, with a mild voluntary contraction, and with maximal muscle contraction (where recruitment pattern and interference are noted). Unlike nerve conduction studies, EMG does not involve external electrical stimulation. Muscle APs (normal or abnormal) are physiologically generated. In various diseases of the motor system, typical electrical abnormalities may be present: increased insertional activity, abnormal motor unit potentials, fibrillations, fasciculations, positive sharp waves, decreased recruitment pattern, and others. EMG assesses the integrity of upper motor neurons, lower motor neurons, the neuromuscular junction, and the muscle itself. However, EMG is seldom diagnostic of a particular disease entity. Its major use lies in differentiating between the following disease classes: primary myopathy, peripheral motor neuron disease, and disease of the neuromuscular junction. As with nerve conduction velocity studies (with which EMG is usually paired), EMG should be considered an extension of the history and physical examination.

Patient Preparation Details of procedure are reviewed with the patient. Considerable patient apprehension often accompanies "needle tests" and calm reassurance from the medical team will go far in allaying such anxieties. Aspirin products should be discontinued 5-7 days beforehand. Nonsteroidal agents should also be stopped several days in advance. Routine medications may be taken on the morning of the examination. If coagulopathy is suspected, appropriate hematologic tests should be ordered (PT/PTT, CBC, bleeding time, etc). If a primary muscle disease is suspected, creatine phosphokinase (CPK) level should be drawn prior to needle examination. Routine EMG testing may cause minor elevations in CPK up to one and one-half times baseline. However, striking elevations in CPK, as seen with polymyositis or muscular dystrophy, are not associated with EMG testing.

Aftercare No specific activity restrictions are necessary. Patient may resume previous activity level.

Special Instructions Requisition from ordering physician should include brief clinical history, tentative neurologic diagnosis, and the specific limb(s) or muscle group(s) in question. Physician should also state whether nerve conduction studies are desired, although in some centers these may be added at the neurologist's discretion.

Complications Local discomfort at the site of needle insertion is common. This is often mild in severity and has no significant sequelae. Pneumothorax has been rarely documented in the literature. This was associated with needle examination of paraspinal muscles. Transient bacteremia has been reported, but routine antibiotic prophylaxis for patients with high-risk cardiac lesions is not generally recommended.

Equipment EMG is performed in a specially equipped procedure room, usually reserved for electrodiagnostic studies. Basic instrumentation includes:

- needle electrodes; these may be monopolar (sharpened, coated steel wires), coaxial, or bipolar (two wires within a needle). These needles record electrical activity from muscle fibers directly contacting the tip, as well as fibers within a several millimeter radius.
- amplifier with filters
- cathode ray oscilloscope with the vertical axis measuring voltage, the horizontal axis measuring time. This device usually has an audio amplifier and loudspeaker, which converts APs to sound energy.
- data storage apparatus (eg, magnetic tape recorder)

Technique A brief neurologic examination is performed prior to the start of the procedure. For EMG of the extremities, patient lies recumbent on the examination table. When paraspinal muscles are tested, the patient adopts a prone position. No intravenous sedatives or pain medications are used. Local anesthesia is also not required despite the generous number of needle insertions. The skin is cleansed thoroughly with alcohol pads, as necessary. Patient is instructed to relax as much as possible. The following steps are carried out.

- Recording needle electrode is inserted percutaneously into the muscle under consideration. The initial electrical activity of the muscle, as seen on the oscilloscope screen and heard over the loudspeaker, is termed the **insertional activity**.
- Next, the needle is held stationary and the muscle action potentials during voluntary relaxation are recorded.
- Patient performs a mild, submaximal contraction of the test muscle. The summed muscle action potentials - the motor unit potential - are observed on the oscilloscope.
- Finally, a maximal muscle contraction is carried out. The compound action potentials generated during this maneuver are studied for **interference** and **recruitment pattern**.

(Continued)

Electromyography *(Continued)*

Needle examination is, by nature, a slow and labor-intensive process. Numerous muscles must be tested individually including both symptomatic and clinically asymptomatic muscles. Within a specific muscle, several independent sites may need to be examined, particularly when the muscle has a large surface area. A number of myopathic processes are focal and sampling errors even within an individual muscle are possible (ie, disease process may effect proximal portion of a muscle, sparing distal fibers).

Normal Findings Results are interpreted by neurologist or physiatrist with preliminary impression written in chart immediately. A formal, typed report is completed several days later. The fundamental principles underlying test interpretation are as follows.

- Insertional activity: Immediately upon needle insertion, there is a brief burst of electrical activity lasting <300 msec. This "insertional activity" is heard over the loudspeaker and may be increased or decreased in various disease states.
- Electrical activity at rest: Muscle tissue is normally silent at rest. No action potentials are seen on the oscilloscope.
- Minimal muscle contraction: When a minimal contraction is performed, several motor unit potentials (MUPs) are activated. Several individual APs are normally visible on the oscilloscope at a rate of 4-5/second. The idealized configuration of a single MUP is depicted in the following figure (see normal column).
- Full voluntary contraction: As the strength of the muscle contraction increases, further muscle units are "recruited". On the oscilloscope the APs appear more disorganized and individual APs can no longer be recognized. At the peak of a contraction the "complete recruitment pattern" is seen, which represents a compilation of motor unit potentials firing asynchronously. The normal interference pattern is considered "full," that is, the amplitude of APs is high (≤5 mV) and firing rate is fast (40/second).

EMG FINDINGS

	EMG Steps \ LESION	NORMAL	NEUTOGENIC LESION: Lower Motor	NEUTOGENIC LESION: Upper Motor	MYOGENIC LESION: Myopathy	MYOGENIC LESION: Myotonia	MYOGENIC LESION: Polymyositis
1	Insertional Activity	Normal	Increased	Normal	Normal	Myotonic Discharge	Increased
2	Spontaneous Activity	—	Fibrillation; Positive Wave	—	—	—	Fibrillation; Positive Wave
3	Motor Unit Potential	0.5-1.0 mV; 5-10 ms	Large Unit Limited Recruitment	Normal	Small Unit Early Recruitment	Myotonic Discharge	Small Unit Early Recruitment
4	Interference Pattern	Full	Reduced Fast Firing Rate	Reduced Slow Firing Rate	Full Low Amplitude	Full Low Amplitude	Full Low Amplitude

Idealized EMG findings, normal, neurogenic lesions, and myogenic lesions. Reproduced with permission from Kimura J, Chapter 13, "Types of Abnormality," *Electrodiagnosis in Diseases of Nerve and Muscle: Principles and Practice*, 2nd ed, Philadelphia, PA: FA Davis, 1989, 263.

Critical Values Abnormalities in one or more of the previously stated parameters may be seen.

Insertional activity: Increased in both neurogenic disorders (eg, lower motor nerve disease) and myogenic disorders (eg, polymyositis), and thus is considered nonspecific. Decreased insertional activity is less common, but may be associated with far advanced denervation or myopathy, especially when muscle is replaced by fat or collagen. A distinctive insertional pattern is seen with myotonia, an unusual neurologic disorder, and is termed "myotonic discharge".

Abnormal activity at rest: Instead of the electrical silence which characterizes the muscle at rest, spontaneous action potentials in single muscle fibers ("fibrillation potentials") may be observed in several disease states.

Fibrillations are seen 1-3 weeks after destruction of a lower motor neuron. Denervated muscle fibers develop heightened chemosensitivity and individual muscle fibers contract spontaneously. The phenomenon of "positive sharp waves" may also be seen. Fibrillations may also occur with severe polymyositis when extensive areas of necrosis interrupt nerve innervation. The naked eye is unable to perceive fibrillations.

Fasciculations represent random contractions of a full motor unit, often visible through the skin. (A motor unit is comprised of an anterior horn cell, axon, neuromuscular junction, and the numerous muscle fibers supplied by the axon.) Fasciculations may be benign, with no other EMG abnormalities observed. They may also be associated with amyotrophic lateral sclerosis, other anterior horn cell diseases, nerve root compression, herniated nucleus pulposus syndrome, acute polyneuropathy, and others.

Abnormalities in the motor unit potential (MUP): Individual motor unit potentials are distinguishable during a submaximal muscle contraction. Abnormalities in amplitude, shape (number of phases, serrations, configuration), and duration are possible. Increased MUP amplitude is seen in lower motor neuron disease but is normal in upper motor neuron disease. Decreased MUP amplitude is characteristic of polymyositis and other myopathies and duration of the MUP is also decreased.

Abnormalities in interference pattern: The normal "full recruitment" pattern seen during maximal muscle contraction is often compromised in disease states. In myogenic lesions, such as polymyositis and myotonia, the amplitude of the MUPs is significantly decreased but the recruitment pattern is normal (ie, the number of activated motor units is normal but the number of muscle fibers per motor unit is diminished). In LMN lesions, the number of motor units recruited is decreased. In severe cases of neuropathy, the maximum interference pattern resembles that of a single MUP, with individual potentials visible. Amplitude of MUPs may be normal. These findings are summarized in the previous figure.

Use In the neurologic literature, EMG has been performed in a wide variety of clinical situations, many of which are experimental or highly specialized in nature. Common indications for EMG in general practice include the following.

Evaluation of the patient with clinical features of primary muscle disease (symmetric and proximal weakness, muscle atrophy, intact sensory system, etc). Examples include:

- muscular dystrophy
- glycogen storage disease
- myotonia
- inflammatory myopathies (systemic lupus, sarcoidosis, infectious myopathies)
- polydermatomyositis
- alcoholic myopathy
- endocrine myopathies, and others

Evaluation of the patient with lower motor neuron disease, including:

- suspected peripheral nerve lesions, such as diffuse peripheral neuropathies, spinal root lesions, and trauma
- suspected disease of the anterior horn cells (characterized by asymmetric weakness, muscle atrophy, fasciculations), as in amyotrophic lateral sclerosis or poliomyelitis

Assessment of the patient with suspected upper motor neuron disease, when prior imaging studies are inconclusive. This includes occult lesions of the corticospinal tract (syringomyelia, tumor) and, less commonly, lesions of the cerebral tract (tumor, CVA). Evaluation of the patient with suspected neuromuscular junction disease (NMJ). This includes myasthenia gravis and the paraneoplastic Eaton-Lambert syndrome. Conventional EMG, as described here, is not the diagnostic test of choice for myasthenia gravis. However, other forms of EMG such as single fiber EMG and repetitive stimulation tests are highly specific for NMJ disease. Assessment of the patient with severe and persistent muscle cramps. Serial documentation of response to therapy for known cases of myopathy or neuropathy. Identification of significantly diseased muscle groups to help guide muscle biopsy (if clinical examination is not inconclusive). EMG is less useful in:

- the restless legs syndrome
- transient, self-resolving muscle cramps
- uncomplicated cases of polymyalgia rheumatica unless the diagnosis is in doubt or underlying myositis is suspected
- routine cases of fibrositis/fibromyalgia (EMG abnormalities have recently been documented in the medical literature but needle examination is not routinely indicated)

Contraindications The following situations represent relative contraindications:

- severe coagulopathy, including hemophilia and marked thrombocytopenia. It should be noted that EMG has been performed safely with platelet counts as low as 20,000/mm^3, but this is not recommended.
- systemic anticoagulation (eg, intravenous heparin, oral Coumadin®)
- patients with an unusual susceptibility to systemic infections (EMG has been known to cause transient bacteremia)

(Continued)

Electromyography *(Continued)*

- patients undergoing a muscle biopsy after EMG require special consideration. It is well known that needle insertion and manipulation during EMG may cause local microscopic tissue damage on a traumatic basis. Histologically, this damage may be confused with a focal myopathy. Thus, some experts avoid detailed needle examinations of the specific muscle group which will be biopsied (although EMG testing of surrounding muscle groups is frequently performed).

Selected Readings

Adams RD and Victor M, *Principles of Neurology: Companion Handbook*, 6th ed, New York, NY: McGraw-Hill Book Co, 1997.

Aminoff MJ, *Electromyography in Clinical Practice*, 4th ed, New York, NY: Churchill-Livingstone, 1999.

Martin JB and Hauser SL, "Approach to the Patient With Neuromuscular Disease," *Harrison's Principles of Internal Medicine*, 14th ed, Fauci AS, Braunwald E, Isselbacher KJ, et al, eds, New York, NY: McGraw-Hill Book Co, 1998, 2277-93.

EMG *see* Electromyography *on page 448*

Encephalitis Viral Serology

Synonyms Arbovirus Serology

Abstract Encephalitogenic arboviruses commonly seen in North America (ie, West Nile Virus, California encephalitis (LaCrosse), Western equine encephalitis, Eastern equine encephalitis, and St Louis encephalitis viruses). Arboviruses (arthropod-borne viruses) are a taxonomically heterogeneous group of viruses grouped together because they are all transmitted to humans via arthropod vectors, usually mosquitoes.

Specimen Serum

Container Red top tube

Collection Acute and convalescent sera drawn 10-14 days apart

Reference Range Less than a fourfold titer increase in paired sera. CSF IgM: negative; hemagglutination inhibition: ≤1:80; complement fixation: ≤1:32; immunofluorescence: ≤1:128.

Use Support the diagnosis of infection with encephalitis viruses

Limitations Cross-reacting antibodies from previous infections or from immunization for yellow fever may produce false-positive results, particularly when assays are performed on unpaired sera.

Additional Information Central nervous system infection by California encephalitis (LaCrosse), Western equine encephalitis, Eastern equine encephalitis, or St Louis encephalitis viruses may manifest as aseptic meningitis, encephalitis, or meningoencephalitis. There is a seasonal distribution for these infections that reflects their mode of transmission to humans by mosquitoes. In the United States, the incidence of arboviral infection is low as is the prevalence of antibodies to these agents in the general population. Consequently, a positive result in an unpaired specimen is **presumptive** evidence for a recent infection. A fourfold increase in titer or a positive CSF IgM test is confirmatory. Antibody detection is the diagnostic test of choice as these viruses are essentially nonculturable in routine diagnostic virology laboratories.

Selected Readings

Asnis DS, Conetta R, Teixeira AA, et al, "The West Nile Virus Outbreak of 1999 in New York: The Flushing Hospital Experience," *Clin Infect Dis*, 2000, 30(3):413-8.

Bale JF Jr, "Viral Encephalitis," *Med Clin North Am*, 1993, 77(1):25-42.

Calisher CH, "Medically Important Arboviruses of the United States and Canada," *Clin Microbiol Rev*, 1994, 7(1):89-116.

Marfin AA and Gubler DJ, "West Nile Encephalitis: An Emerging Disease in the United States," *Clin Infect Dis*, 2001, 33(10):1713-9.

Tsai TF and Kuno G, "Arboviruses," *Manual of Clinical Laboratory Immunology*, 5th ed, Rose NR, Conway de Macario E, Folds JD, et al, eds, Washington, DC: American Society for Microbiology, 1997, 729-35.

Endocervical Culture *see* Genital Culture *on page 470*

Endoscopic Biopsy *see* Histopathology *on page 496*

Entamoeba histolytica Serology

Synonyms Amebiasis Serological Test

Patient Preparation Fasting blood sample required

Specimen Serum

Container Red top tube or serum separator tube

Reference Range IHA titer: <1:128; CF titer: <1:8; immunodiffusion test: negative

Use Diagnose systemic amebiasis

Limitations Sensitivity is highest in extraintestinal amebiasis, lower in amebic dysentery, and lowest in asymptomatic carriers. Some false-positives occur in patients with ulcerative colitis. Recently a serine-rich recombinant *Entamoeba histolytica* protein has proven to be a useful antigen to assist in the serodiagnosis of *Entamoeba* which has disseminated.

Methodology Complement fixation (CF), indirect hemagglutination (IHA), immunodiffusion (ID), indirect fluorescent antibody (IFA), enzyme immunoassay (EIA)

Additional Information Indirect hemagglutination is positive in 87% to 100% of patients with liver abscesses and >85% of patients with acute amebic dysentery. Fewer than 6% of uninfected individuals react in the test. Amebic serology when negative is strong evidence against amebic liver abscess. IHA titers ≥1:128 are considered to be clinically significant, and a fourfold rise in titer is diagnostic evidence. Although titers will decrease over time, serology may remain positive for as long as 2 years, even after curative therapy.

Selected Readings

Maddison SE, "Serodiagnosis of Parasitic Diseases," *Clin Microbiol Rev*, 1991, 4(4):457-69.

Petri WA Jr and Singh U, "Diagnosis and Management of Amebiasis," *Clin Infect Dis*, 1999, 29(5):1117-25.

Reed SL, "Amebiasis: An Update," *Clin Infect Dis*, 1992, 14(2):385-93.

Tanyuksel M and Petri WA Jr, "Laboratory Diagnosis of Amebiasis," *Clin Microbiol Rev*, 2003, 16(4):713-29.

Wilson M, Schantz PM, and Tsang VCW, "Clinical Immunoparasitology," *Manual of Clinical Laboratory Immunology*, 5th ed, Rose NR, Conway de Macario E, Folds JD, et al, eds, Washington, DC: American Society for Microbiology, 1997, 575-84.

Enteric Pathogens Culture, Routine *see* Stool Culture *on page 585*

Enterobiasis Test *see* Pinworm Preparation *on page 565*

***Enterobius vermicularis* Preparation** *see* Pinworm Preparation *on page 565*

Enterohemorrhagic *E. coli*, Stool Culture *see* Stool Culture, Diarrheagenic *E. coli on page 587*

Enteroinvasive *E. coli*, Stool Culture *see* Stool Culture, Diarrheagenic *E. coli on page 587*

Enteropathogenic *E. coli*, Stool Culture *see* Stool Culture, Diarrheagenic *E. coli on page 587*

Enterotoxigenic *E. coli*, Stool Culture *see* Stool Culture, Diarrheagenic *E. coli on page 587*

Enterovirus Culture

Related Information

Coxsackie A Virus Serology *on page 427*
Coxsackie B Virus Serology *on page 428*

Applies to Coxsackie A Virus Culture; Coxsackie B Virus Culture; Echovirus Culture; Poliovirus Culture

Test Includes Culture for Coxsackie A virus, Coxsackie B virus, echovirus, and poliovirus

Specimen Stool (best specimen), rectal swab, cerebrospinal fluid, upper and lower respiratory tract specimens, blood, throat swab (good specimen), various organs and tissues

Container Sterile container

Sampling Time It is important to obtain specimens very early in the disease; however, virus is shed in the stool for weeks.

Storage Instructions Enteroviruses are rather hardy; however, specimens should be refrigerated or placed into cold virus transport medium and delivered immediately to the clinical laboratory.

Causes for Rejection Dry specimen, specimen not in proper viral transport medium, specimen not refrigerated during transport, specimen fixed in formalin, unlabeled specimen

Turnaround Time Variable (1-4 days) and depends on culture method used and amount of virus in specimen

Reference Range No virus isolated

Use Aid in the diagnosis of disease caused by enteroviruses (eg, polio, congenital viral infections, and meningitis (aseptic))

Limitations Cell culture generally does not support the growth of Coxsackie A enteroviruses. Inoculation of suckling mice is the preferred method to isolate Coxsackie A virus.

Methodology Some laboratories offer molecular testing for this organism. Contact the testing laboratory for the availability of amplified and nonamplified qualitative and quantitative molecular tests for this organism, and for information on selection and collection of appropriate specimens for specific molecular tests.

Inoculation of specimens into cell culture, incubation, and observation of characteristic cytopathic effect. Specimens suspected of containing Coxsackie A virus are inoculated into suckling mice which are then observed for flaccid paralysis without encephalitis.

(Continued)

Enterovirus Culture *(Continued)*

Some (usually reference) laboratories can identify specific enteroviruses by using a battery of specific enterovirus-neutralizing antibodies. These antibodies are useful in identifying and typing Coxsackie A, Coxsackie B, echovirus, and poliovirus.

Additional Information Infrequently, aseptic meningitis is caused by Coxsackie A virus types which require animal inoculation for isolation.

Selected Readings

Dowsett EG, "Human Enteroviral Infections," *J Hosp Infect*, 1988, 11(2):103-15.
Modlin JF and Kinney JS, "Perinatal Enterovirus Infections," *Adv Pediatr Infect Dis*, 1987, 2:57-78.
Moore M and Morens DM, "Enteroviruses, Including Polioviruses," *Textbook of Human Virology*, Belshe RB, ed, Littleton, MA: PSG Publishing Co, 1984, 407-83.
Rotbart HA, "Enteroviruses," *Manual of Clinical Microbiology*, 7th ed, Murray PR, Baron EJ, Pfaller MA, et al, eds, Washington, DC: American Society for Microbiology, 1999, 990-1004.

Enterovirus Culture, Stool *see* Viral Culture, Stool *on page 616*

Enzyme Immunoassay for Group A *Streptococcus* Antigen *see* Group A *Streptococcus* Antigen Test *on page 475*

EPEC, Stool Culture *see* Stool Culture, Diarrheagenic *E. coli on page 587*

Epstein-Barr Early Antigens *see* Epstein-Barr Virus Serology *on page 454*

Epstein-Barr Viral Capsid Antigen *see* Epstein-Barr Virus Serology *on page 454*

Epstein-Barr Virus Serology

Related Information

Infectious Mononucleosis Serology *on page 509*

Synonyms EB Virus Titer; EBV Titer

Applies to EB Nuclear Antigens; Epstein-Barr Early Antigens; Epstein-Barr Viral Capsid Antigen

Test Includes Serology for several EBV antigens

Specimen Serum

Container Red top tube or serum separator tube

Reference Range

- Patients with no history of infectious mononucleosis: IgG anti-VCA: <1:10; IgM anti-VCA: <1:10; anti-EBNA: <1:5
- Patients with previous infectious mononucleosis by history: IgG anti-VCA: ≥1:10; IgM anti-VCA: ≤1:10; anti-EBNA: ≥1:50
- Patients with current or active infection: Many combinations of results are possible. Consult the laboratory for interpretation of specific results.

If serological testing is performed by enzyme immunoassay (EIA) on automated instrumentation, results are usually given in index units, not titers. In such cases, significant rises in antibody levels are determined by algorithms within the instrumentation, not by increases in titer.

Use Diagnose Epstein-Barr virus infection, heterophil-negative mononucleosis, hereditary sex-linked lymphadenopathy

Limitations Despite much publicity, these tests are neither sensitive nor specific for chronic fatigue syndrome

Contraindications The Epstein-Barr viral test need not be done on patients who have heterophil antibodies, symptoms, physical findings, and lymphocyte morphology consistent with infectious mononucleosis. Typically, this test is performed on the ~15% of patients who are heterophil-negative and are still suspected of having infectious mononucleosis.

Methodology Indirect fluorescent antibody (IFA), enzyme-linked immunosorbent assay (ELISA). Some laboratories offer molecular testing for this organism. Contact the testing laboratory for the availability of amplified and nonamplified qualitative and quantitative molecular tests for this organism, and for information on selection and collection of appropriate specimens for specific molecular tests.

Additional Information Epstein-Barr virus is a herpes group virus which is almost ubiquitous. It is the cause of classic infectious mononucleosis, and is causally implicated in the pathogenesis of Burkitt's lymphoma, some nasopharyngeal carcinomas, and rare hereditary lymphoproliferative disorders. The serologic response to EB virus includes antibody to early antigen, which is usually short lived, IgM and IgG antibodies to viral capsid antigen (VCA), and antibodies to nuclear antigen (EBNA). Antibody levels to early antigen are not particularly helpful in routine clinical practice.

Although most cases of infectious mononucleosis can be diagnosed on the basis of clinical findings, blood count and morphology, and a positive test for heterophil antibody, as many as 20% may be heterophil-negative, at least at presentation (heterophil may become positive when repeated in a few days). In some of these cases, a test for Epstein-Barr virus antibodies may be useful.

Of the numerous antibodies that may be assayed, viral capsid antibody is the most useful. A high presenting titer is good evidence for EB virus infection. Since titers are generally high by the time a patient is symptomatic, it may not be possible to demonstrate the fourfold rise in titer usually recommended. Even a very high titer may be due to past infection, so IgM titers should be measured to establish acute infection. Persistent absence of antibody to viral capsid is good evidence against EB virus infection.

Antibody to EB virus nuclear antigen (EBNA) usually develops 4-6 weeks after infection, so its presence early during an acute illness should lead one to consider diagnosis other than EB virus infectious mononucleosis.

Patients with nonkeratinizing squamous carcinoma of the nasopharynx may have elevated levels of IgG antibody to EB early antigen, but the rarity of this condition and the 10% to 20% false-positive rate vitiate its usefulness for screening. Such patients may also have IgA antibodies to VCA.

The most controversial use of EBV serology is in chronic fatigue syndrome, a complaint predominantly but not exclusively of young to middle-aged women, characterized by long persistent debilitating fatigue and a panoply of usually mild somatic complaints. In the initial reports of this illness, chronic infection with EBV was suggested as the cause, and EBV serology suggested as a diagnostic tool. In the past several years, although the legitimacy of a chronic fatigue syndrome seems to have been established, the inappropriateness of EBV serology for diagnosis has been realized. The high levels of EBV antibodies in the general population, their long persistence, and the poor correlation of antibody titers with symptoms combine to make EBV serology useless in diagnosing, following, or ruling out chronic fatigue syndrome.

IgG antibody to early antigen occurs in patients with Hodgkin's disease in higher titer than expected. This observation suggests the possibility that EB virus activation plays a pathogenetic role in Hodgkin's disease.

Selected Readings

Jenson HB, Ench Y, and Sumaya CV, "Epstein-Barr Virus," *Manual of Clinical Laboratory Immunology*, 5th ed, Rose NR, Conway de Macario E, Folds JD, et al, eds, Washington, DC: American Society for Microbiology, 1997, 634-43.

Merlin T, "Chronic Mononucleosis: Pitfalls in the Laboratory Diagnosis," *Hum Pathol*, 1986, 17(1):2-8.

Thiele GM and Okano M, "Diagnosis of Epstein-Barr Virus Infections in the Clinical Laboratory," *Clin Microbiol Newslett*, 1993, 15(6):41-8.

Esophageal Echo *see* Transesophageal Echocardiography *on page 598*

Esterase, Leukocyte, Urine *see* Leukocyte Esterase, Urine *on page 520*

Eye Smear for Cytology *see* Ocular Cytology *on page 551*

Eye Swab *Chlamydia* Culture *see Chlamydia* Culture *on page 413*

FA Smear for *Legionella pneumophila* *see Legionella pneumophila* Smear *on page 517*

5-FC Level *see* Flucytosine Level *on page 456*

Fecal Leukocyte Stain

Related Information

Clostridium difficile Toxin Assay *on page 418*

Cryptosporidium Diagnostic Procedures, Stool *on page 432*

Stool Culture *on page 585*

Stool Culture, Diarrheagenic *E. coli on page 587*

Test Includes Methylene blue, Gram, or Wright's stain of stool smear

Patient Preparation Collect specimen prior to barium procedures if possible.

Specimen Fresh random stool, rectal swab

Container Culturette®, sealed plastic stool container

Collection Transport specimen to laboratory as soon as possible after collection, significant deterioration of the specimen occurs with prolonged storage.

Storage Instructions Refrigerate

Causes for Rejection Insufficient specimen volume. Specimens which are delayed in transit are less than optimal.

Turnaround Time 1 hour

Reference Range Few, if any, leukocytes

Use Assist in the differential diagnosis of diarrheal disease

Limitations Ten percent to 15% of stools which yield an invasive bacterial pathogen have an absence of fecal leukocytes. Many bacterial intestinal pathogens do not elicit a leukocyte response in stool. Fecal leukocytes are present in idiopathic inflammatory bowel disease.

Methodology Smear of stool (preferably mucus) with one drop methylene blue (or other stain), coverslip, and observe the presence of leukocytes.

(Continued)

Fecal Leukocyte Stain *(Continued)*

Additional Information Conditions associated with varying degrees of fecal leukocytes, blood and/or mucus include diffuse antibiotic associated colitis, ulcerative colitis, shigellosis, *Campylobacter*, *Yersinia*, amebiasis, and some diarrheagenic *E. coli* infection. Conditions associated with an absence of fecal leukocytes include toxigenic bacterial infection, giardiasis, and viral infections. In a review the methylene blue stain for polymorpholeukocytes had a high sensitivity (85%) and specificity (88%) for bacterial diarrhea (*Shigella*, *Salmonella*, *Campylobacter*). Positive predictive value was poor (59%). Negative predicative value was 97%. In the presence of a history of abrupt onset, greater than four stools per day and no vomiting before the onset of diarrhea, the methylene blue stain for fecal polymorphonuclear leukocytes was a very effective presumptive diagnostic test for bacterial diarrhea. A positive occult blood test may also be suggestive of acute bacterial diarrhea. Neither method is sufficiently sensitive or specific to pre-empt the use of culture. Similar findings including a sensitivity of 81% and specificity 74% were observed when both tests were positive.

Selected Readings

Bishop WP and Ulshen MH, "Bacterial Gastroenteritis," *Pediatr Clin North Am*, 1988, 35(1):69-87.
DuBois D, Binder L, and Nelson B, "Usefulness of the Stool Wright's Stain in the Emergency Department," *J Emerg Med*, 1988, 6(6):483-6.
Harris JC, Dupont HL, and Hornick RB, "Fecal Leukocytes in Diarrheal Illness," *Ann Intern Med*, 1972, 76(5):697-703.
Siegel D, Cohen PT, Neighbor M, et al, "Predictive Value of Stool Examination in Acute Diarrhea," *Arch Pathol Lab Med*, 1987, 111(8):715-8.

Femur, Left or Right, X-ray *see* Bone Films *on page 396*
Filarial Infestation *see* Microfilariae, Peripheral Blood Preparation *on page 535*
Filariasis Peripheral Blood Preparation *see* Microfilariae, Peripheral Blood Preparation *on page 535*
Filling Cystometrogram *see* Cystometrogram, Simple *on page 434*
Finger, Left or Right Hand, X-ray *see* Bone Films *on page 396*
Flea Identification *see* Arthropod Identification *on page 387*
Flexible Bronchoscopy *see* Bronchoscopy, Fiberoptic *on page 406*

Flucytosine Level

Related Information

Antibiotic Level, Serum *on page 375*

Synonyms Ancobon® Level; 5-FC Level; 5-Fluorocytosine Level

Abstract Flucytosine is an antifungal agent often used in conjunction with amphotericin B for treatment of fungal meningitis and endocarditis. Bone marrow toxicity and hepatotoxicity are occasionally seen in patients being treated with flucytosine.

Specimen Serum

Container Red top tube

Sampling Time Peak serum levels are reached 4-6 hours after a single oral dose. During ongoing therapy, peak levels are reached 1-2 hours after successive doses.

Reference Range Therapeutic: 50-100 mcg/mL (SI: 390-775 μmol/L)

Possible Panic Range 100-125 mcg/mL (SI: 775-970 μmol/L)

Use Monitor for bone marrow toxicity; evaluate weekly if patient has normal renal function, more often if renal function is abnormal

Limitations Serum levels do not correlate well with clinical toxicity. The hypothesis of serum level associated adverse effects has been inferred from case reports but has not been definitively studied.

Methodology High performance liquid chromatography (HPLC), gas chromatography/mass spectrometry (GC/MS)

Additional Information Clinical use of flucytosine is associated with significant frequency of life-threatening bone marrow suppression which occurs most often when blood levels are >100 mcg/mL (SI: >775 μmol/L) for 2 or more weeks. The bone marrow suppression is usually reversible. It is most likely to occur in patients with underlying hematologic disorders or in patients undergoing myelosuppressive therapy.

Selected Readings

Bodey GP, "Topical and Systemic Antifungal Agents," *Med Clin North Am*, 1988, 72:637-59.
Edson RS and Terrell CL, "The Aminoglycosides," *Mayo Clin Proc*, 1999, 74(5):519-28.
Gerson B, "Flucytosine," *Clin Lab Med*, 1987, 7(3):541-4.

Fluids Cytology *see* Cytology, Body Fluids *on page 438*
Fluorescent Rabies Antibody Test *see* Rabies Detection *on page 569*
Fluorescent Treponemal Antibody Adsorption *see* FTA-ABS, Serum *on page 457*
Fluorochrome Stain *see* Acid-Fast Stain *on page 361*
5-Fluorocytosine Level *see* Flucytosine Level *on page 456*

Follow-up Ultrasound Abdomen *see* Ultrasound, Abdomen *on page 604*
Follow-up Ultrasound Retroperitoneal *see* Ultrasound, Abdomen *on page 604*
Foot, Left or Right, X-ray *see* Bone Films *on page 396*
Forearm, Left or Right, X-ray *see* Bone Films *on page 396*
***Francisella tularensis* Antibodies** *see* Tularemia Serology *on page 603*
FRA Test *see* Rabies Detection *on page 569*

FTA-ABS, Cerebrospinal Fluid

Related Information
VDRL, Cerebrospinal Fluid *on page 613*

Synonyms *Treponema pallidum* Antibodies, CSF

Test Includes CSF specimens are adsorbed (FTA - ABS) with nonpathogenic *Treponema* sp and tested.

Specimen Cerebrospinal fluid

Container Clean, sterile CSF tube

Causes for Rejection Bloody specimen

Reference Range Nonreactive

Use Test for the presence of *Treponema pallidum* antibodies; VDRL is preferred over the FTA when examining CSF.

Limitations The interpretation of FTA results when performed on CSF is not clearly defined. False-positive results may occur particularly if the specimen is not adsorbed prior to testing. VDRL on cerebrospinal fluid is recommended by the Center for Disease Control to help establish the diagnosis of neurosyphilis. However, while a positive CSF VDRL is strong evidence for active neurosyphilis, a negative does not rule it out. An FTA-ABS on CSF can be positive in cases of neurosyphilis when CSF VDRL is negative, but this combination of results is not common. Unfortunately, the CSF FTA-ABS test is less specific than CSF VDRL for distinguishing currently active neurosyphilis from past syphilis infection. Therefore, a correlation of the clinical facts with the serologic findings is essential for each case. One useful guide when screening for neurosyphilis is to first detect a serum FTA-ABS and/or a VDRL or RPR.

Methodology Indirect immunofluorescence of killed *Treponema* after serum adsorption of antibodies to nonpathogenic *Treponema* sp

Selected Readings

Pope V, Larsen SA, and Schriefer M, "Immunologic Methods for Diagnosis of Spirochetal Diseases," *Manual of Clinical Laboratory Immunology*, 5th ed, Rose NR, Conway de Macario E, Folds JD, et al, eds, Washington, DC: American Society for Microbiology, 1997, 510-25.

Singh AE and Romanowski B, "Syphilis: Review With Emphasis on Clinical Epidemiologic, and Some Biologic Features," *Clin Microbiol Rev*, 1999, 12(2):187-209.

Wicher V and Wicher K, "Pathogenesis of Maternal-Fetal Syphilis Revisited," *Clin Infect Dis*, 2001, 33(3):354-63.

FTA-ABS, Serum

Related Information
Darkfield Examination, Syphilis *on page 444*
RPR *on page 574*
VDRL, Cerebrospinal Fluid *on page 613*

Synonyms Fluorescent Treponemal Antibody Adsorption

Applies to Serologic Test for Syphilis

Patient Preparation Patient should be fasting if possible

Specimen Serum

Container Red top tube or serum separator tube

Reference Range Nonreactive

Use Confirm the presence of *Treponema pallidum* antibodies; establish the diagnosis of syphilis

Limitations FTA-ABS test for syphilis usually is positive in the treponemal diseases pinta, yaws and bejel, and falsely positive in patients with numerous diseases associated with increased or abnormal globulins, antinuclear antibodies, lupus erythematosus (beaded pattern), old age, pregnancy, and drug addiction (although drug addicts are likely to have true positives as well). As many as 2% of the general population may have a false-positive. Borderline results are inconclusive and cannot be interpreted; they may indicate a very low level of treponemal antibody or may be due to nonspecific factors. Further follow-up and serological confirmation with the treponemal immobilization test may be helpful.

Methodology Indirect immunofluorescence of killed *Treponema* after serum adsorption of antibodies to nonpathogenic *Treponema* sp

Additional Information FTA-ABS is the most sensitive test in all stages of syphilis, and is the best confirmatory test for a serum reactive to a screening test such as RPR. Occasionally, patients with ocular (uveitis) syphilis or otosyphilis will have a negative VDRL while their FTA-ABS is positive. FTA-ABS cannot be used to follow
(Continued)

FTA-ABS, Serum *(Continued)*

disease activity or response to treatment, because it will remain high for life. A modification of the test can detect IgM-specific antibodies, which may distinguish true congenital syphilis from placental transfer of maternal antibodies. However, tests for anti-*Treponema* IgM are not widely available. When a positive serum FTA-ABS is required before performing CSF VDRL examination, the specificity of the CSF test is markedly improved.

Although not officially recommended for testing cerebrospinal fluid, the FTA test, unabsorbed, can be performed on some spinal fluids with excellent specificity. At present this application of the test should be restricted to reference laboratories.

Selected Readings

Davis LE and Schmitt JW, "Clinical Significance of Cerebrospinal Fluid Tests for Neurosyphilis," *Ann Neurol*, 1989, 25(1):50-5.

Farnes SW and Setness PA, "Serologic Tests for Syphilis," *Postgrad Med*, 1990, 87(3):37-41, 45-6.

Pope V, Larsen SA, and Schriefer M, "Immunologic Methods for the Diagnosis of Spirochetal Diseases," *Manual of Clinical Laboratory Immunology*, 5th ed, Rose NR, Conway de Macario E, Folds JD, et al, eds, Washington, DC: American Society for Microbiology, 1997, 510-25.

Singh AE and Romanowski B, "Syphilis: Review With Emphasis on Clinical Epidemiologic, and Some Biologic Features," *Clin Microbiol Rev*, 1999, 12(2):187-209.

Wicher V and Wicher K, "Pathogenesis of Maternal-Fetal Syphilis Revisited," *Clin Infect Dis*, 2001, 33(3):354-63.

Fungal Immunodiffusion *see* Fungal Serology *on page 458*

Fungal Precipitin Test *see* Fungal Serology *on page 458*

Fungal Serology

Synonyms Fungal Immunodiffusion; Fungal Precipitin Test

Applies to *Aspergillus* Immunodiffusion; *Coccidioides* Immunodiffusion; Blastomycosis Immunodiffusion; Histoplasmosis Immunodiffusion

Specimen Serum

Container Red top tube or serum separator tube

Reference Range Negative or no bands identified

Use Confirm and aid in the differential diagnosis of aspergillosis, blastomycosis, histoplasmosis, and coccidioidomycosis

Limitations Results reported as positive or negative; no titer is given

Contraindications Prior skin test may give a single precipitin band ("M") with histoplasmin

Methodology Immunodiffusion (ID), enzyme-linked immunosorbent assay (ELISA)

Additional Information

Blastomycosis: A band of identity with the "A" reference antibody from an infected human indicates active infection or recent past infection. This detects about 80% of cases. A negative test has little value and in no way excludes the existence of blastomycosis. Cross-reacting antibodies producing lines of partial identity are seen in patients with histoplasmosis and coccidioidomycosis.

Aspergillosis: Sera can be tested against a polyvalent antigen mixture, or a series of species preparations. The greater the number of bands, the greater the likelihood of either a fungus ball or invasive aspergillosis. A negative test does not rule out aspergillosis. Nonidentity bands could be due to presence of CRP. Cross reactions occur in cases of histoplasmosis, coccidioidomycosis and blastomycosis, or may indicate antibody to an *Aspergillus* species other than *Aspergillus fumigatus*. Bands due to reaction with C-reactive protein can be removed by sodium citrate.

Coccidioidomycosis: A band of identity with coccidioidin indicates infection but may be negative early. Some individuals continue to produce detectable antibodies up to 1 year after clinical recovery from active disease. A negative test does not exclude coccidioidomycosis.

Histoplasmosis: "H" and "M" precipitin bands are of diagnostic significance and if both are present indicate active infection. "H" identity bands alone are rarely seen; they are always associated with active infection. "M" identity bands alone indicate active infection, recent past infection (within the past year), or recent positive histoplasmin skin test (within past 2 months). The absence of precipitin antibodies does not rule out histoplasmosis.

Unfortunately, because of poorly standardized reagents and inherent biologic cross-reactivity, and interference from complement, the general clinical utility of measuring or detecting fungal antibodies is low. Only the detection of CSF antibodies to *Coccidioides* is truly diagnostic. For this reason, much effort is now devoted to tests for detecting fungal antigens, of which the most useful presently is the latex agglutination test for cryptococcal antigen.

Selected Readings

Chapman SW, Bradsher RW Jr, Campbell GD Jr, et al, "Practice Guidelines for the Management of Patients With Blastomycosis," *Clin Infect Dis*, 2000, 30(4):679-83.

Drutz DJ, "Antigen Detection in Fungal Infections," *N Engl J Med*, 1986, 314(2):115-7.

Kaufman L, Kovacs JA, and Reiss E, "Clinical Immunomycology," *Manual of Clinical Laboratory Immunology*, 5th ed, Rose NR, Conway de Macario E, Folds JD, et al, eds, Washington, DC: American Society for Microbiology, 1997, 585-604.

Stevens DA, Kan VL, Judson MA, et al, "Practice Guidelines for Diseases Caused by *Aspergillus*," *Clin Infect Dis*, 2000, 30(4):696-709.

Wheat J, Sarosi G, McKinsey D, et al, "Practice Guidelines for the Management of Patients With Histoplasmosis. Infectious Diseases Society of America," *Clin Infect Dis*, 2000, 30(4):688-95.

Fungal Skin Testing

Related Information

Anergy Skin Test Battery *on page 372*

Tuberculin Skin Testing, Intracutaneous *on page 601*

Synonyms Delayed Hypersensitivity Fungal Skin Tests; Skin Tests for Histoplasmosis, Blastomycosis, Coccidioidomycosis

Test Includes Intradermal injection of fungal antigen(s) to determine if a delayed hypersensitivity reaction is present to a given fungus. Skin test sites are examined at 24, 48, and 72 hours for induration which, if present, implies prior infection with the tested fungus.

Patient Preparation Procedure and risks are explained to the patient. No specific skin preparation is necessary. However, those patients with generalized skin disorders such as extensive psoriasis should be examined beforehand for suitable areas of normal appearing skin. If immediate hypersensitivity to the fungal antigen is even remotely suspected, physician should be in attendance.

Aftercare Fifteen to 30 minutes after injections, sites should be examined for adverse reactions ranging from the IgE wheal and flare response to systemic reactions; otherwise, close observation postprocedure is generally not necessary and patients should be instructed to keep test sites clean for 72 hours. No restrictions on bathing or cleaning injection sites are necessary.

Special Instructions Requisition should state the specific fungal antigens to be planted, as well as whether a simultaneous skin anergy panel is desired. Current medications should also be included in the requisition, with attention to corticosteroids or other immunosuppressive agents.

Complications As with other forms of skin testing, immediate IgE-mediated local reactions are possible, although unusual. Erythema, vesiculation, and skin necrosis may be seen, at times involving large areas. Systemic reactions, including anaphylaxis, have rarely been reported. Patients with infection with *Coccidioides immitis* who manifest erythema nodosum may be at an increased risk of a major systemic reaction after skin testing. However, in the vast majority of cases, fungal skin testing is safe.

Equipment Skin test materials are derived from cultures of the appropriate fungi and most are available commercially in standardized concentrations. Common fungal antigens tested include *Histoplasma capsulatum*, *Coccidioides immitis*, *Blastomyces dermatitidis* (not available commercially), *Candida*, and *Trichophyton*. Disposable plastic or glass tuberculin syringes are required along with 26- or 27-gauge short ($^1/_4$" to $^1/_2$") beveled needles.

Technique The volar aspect of the forearm is prepped with alcohol swabs. Skin test material(s) are injected intradermally so that discrete wheals are raised. Generally, 0.1 mL skin test antigen is injected, but more dilute solutions may be used if a severe reaction is anticipated. Subcutaneous injections should be avoided. Multiple fungal antigens may be injected at separate sites using this method. Test sites should be examined at 24, 48, and 72 hours. Date and time of injection should be recorded along with the location of each fungal antigen.

Data Acquired The transverse diameter of induration should be carefully measured by inspection and palpation and results recorded (in millimeters) at 24-hour intervals. Areas of erythema, however, are not as important as induration and are excluded in most grading schemes unless extensive (>10 mm).

Normal Findings No induration or erythema

Critical Values A positive skin test is defined by many authorities as a diameter of induration ≥5 mm. Induration of 0-4 mm is considered negative. Alternatively, a standardized grading scale, which is popular with general delayed-type hypersensitivity skin testing, may be used:

- 0: no reaction
- 1+: erythema >10 mm and/or induration 1-5 mm
- 2+: induration 6-10 mm
- 3+: induration 11-20 mm
- 4+: induration >20 mm

The interpretation of a positive (or negative) skin test is so problematic that the clinical utility of fungal skin testing is significantly limited. A positive reaction indicates only

(Continued)

Fungal Skin Testing *(Continued)*

that exposure to the relevant fungus has occurred at some time in the past, whether recent or remote. In addition, fungal infections are endemic in many areas of the United States, where >90% of the local population may be skin test positive following asymptomatic or subclinical infections (eg, histoplasmosis in the Ohio River Valley). Thus, in the individual patient with suspected active fungal infection, a positive skin test adds little new diagnostic information and fails to establish the fungus as the infecting agent. This becomes especially relevant if the patient has ever lived in a known endemic area. In the patient with pulmonary nodules, the importance of a positive test is also unclear. Some authorities consider a positive histoplasmin test in an area of low prevalence as strong evidence for histoplasmosis. Others argue that lung nodules may still be due to bronchogenic carcinoma despite a positive histoplasmin test, and skin testing adds little to clinical decision making. Similarly, a negative skin test presents major problems in interpretation. Lack of reactivity may be seen in the following situations:

- no previous fungal infection
- previous fungal infection in an immunocompromised patient
- acute systemic fungal infection, where skin test positivity is often delayed for 2-4 weeks
- waning skin test reactivity to a given fungus, as occurs in the elderly
- technical errors in antigen placement

Even the documentation of skin test conversion (ie, negative test converting to positive or serial testing) is regarded as only indirect evidence of fungal exposure in the interim and does not necessarily imply active infection. Regarding the specific fungal antigens, the derivative of *Histoplasma capsulatum* is termed histoplasmin. An older preparation of histoplasmin cross reacted frequently with *Blastomyces* and *Coccidioides* and caused a rise in complement fixation titers to *Histoplasma*. A newer histoplasmin preparation ameliorates, but does not entirely eliminate, these problems. The histoplasmin skin test may cause a spurious increase in *Histoplasma* complement fixation titers. Since the CF serologic test is clinically more useful than the histoplasmin skin test, serologies should be drawn first in suspected cases. Coccidioidomycosis skin testing shares many of the same interpretive difficulties as histoplasmosis testing, such as waning reactivity over time, delay in test positivity during acute fungal infection, and areas of high prevalence. Two preparations of *Coccidioides* antigen are available, the older coccidioidin (derived from the mycelia phase) and Spherulin® (derived from lysed spherules). Spherulin® may have superior sensitivity and has been found to be positive in 30% more cases than coccidioidin. Although testing is not useful in the individual with suspected *Coccidioides* pneumonia, it may provide prognostic information in culture proven cases. In a classic study, patients with disseminated coccidioidomycosis had a higher survival rate if their skin test was positive (75%) compared with those who tested negative (15%). Patients with limited coccidioidomycosis almost always develop a positive test; failure to do so may predict impending disseminated disease. Use of the coccidioidin preparation may cause false-positive histoplasmosis serologic tests, but neither Spherulin® nor coccidioidin interferes with serologic tests for coccidioidomycosis. Coccidioidal skin tests are generally positive before coccidioidal serologic tests; some clinicians use this fact to justify skin testing in acute cases (despite its limited diagnostic utility). Skin tests for blastomycosis are presently of questionable value due to poor sensitivity and specificity, even in the study of epidemics. Fungal antigens derived from *Candida albicans* and *Trichophyton* are primarily used only for anergy testing because of high prevalence of positive skin tests in the general population.

Use Fungal skin testing has been applied for the following reasons:

- as an epidemiologic tool for defining geographic regions of endemic fungal infection
- as a diagnostic aid in individual cases of suspected primary fungal infection (limited usefulness)
- as a prognostic indicator in culture-proven cases of fungal infection (particularly coccidioidomycosis)
- as a component of a comprehensive cutaneous anergy panel, used to assess the integrity of a patient's cell-mediated immune system (T-cell function); this standardized panel is usually comprised of *Candida*, mumps, and *Trichophyton* antigens

Contraindications Prior systemic reaction to fungal skin testing; known immediate hypersensitivity (IgE-mediated) to the specific fungus to be tested; known immediate hypersensitivity to mercury, which is contained in some commercial preparations of *Coccidioides* antigen; the presence of erythema nodosum (high risk for adverse reaction - see following information).

Additional Information Fungal skin testing is a form of delayed hypersensitivity skin testing and as such is an assessment of cell-mediated immunity. Delayed hypersensitivity is a clinical phenomenon based on the reaction of the skin to intradermal injection of an antigen. It is a common form of immune protection against a wide range of infectious agents, including fungi. Following initial exposure to a fungus, a population of transformed T-lymphocytes is created, the so-called memory cells. When fungal antigen is introduced intradermally at a later date, these sensitized T cells are activated and initiate a cascade involving lymphokines, neutrophils, and macrophages. Clinically, this is manifested by the delayed formation of significant skin induration. Delayed hypersensitivity fungal skin testing should be differentiated from immediate hypersensitivity skin testing. The former is primarily T-cell mediated and the latter is mediated by IgE mechanisms. Skin testing for common allergies to molds or fungi is carried out using the percutaneous allergy testing method and is IgE-mediated. Similarly, skin tests for immediate hypersensitivity to *Aspergillus fumigatus* also use this method. This is commonly obtained in the evaluation of patients with suspected allergic bronchopulmonary aspergillosis.

Fungi, Susceptibility Testing *see* Antifungal Susceptibility Testing *on page 377*

Fungizone® Level, Blood *see* Amphotericin B Level *on page 371*

Fungus Blood Culture *see* Blood Culture, Fungus *on page 395*

Fungus Culture, Appropriate Site

Refer to

Fungus Culture, Biopsy *on page 461*
Fungus Culture, Body Fluid *on page 462*
Fungus Culture, Bronchial Aspirate *on page 463*
Fungus Culture, Cerebrospinal Fluid *on page 464*
Fungus Culture, Skin *on page 464*
Fungus Culture, Sputum *on page 466*
Fungus Culture, Urine *on page 468*

Fungus Culture, Biopsy

Related Information

Histopathology *on page 496*
Methenamine Silver Stain *on page 534*
Periodic Acid-Schiff Stain *on page 563*
Sporotrichosis Serology *on page 585*

Synonyms Biopsy Culture, Fungus; Fungus Culture, Tissue

Applies to Cyst Culture, Fungus; Fungus Culture, Surgical Specimen

Patient Preparation Usual sterile preparation of biopsy site

Special Instructions The following information will assist the laboratory in the proper processing of the specimen: specific site of specimen, current antibiotic therapy, age and sex of patient, collection time and date, and clinical diagnosis.

Specimen Surgical specimen. **Swab specimens are not acceptable. Tissue must be submitted.**

Container Sterile test tube or container

Collection The portion of the biopsy submitted for culture should be separated from the portion submitted for histopathology by the surgeon or pathologist utilizing sterile technique. The laboratory should be informed of the fungal species suspected. Every effort should be made to collect the specimen early in the day so that it may be processed promptly, assuring optimal yield.

Storage Instructions Transport specimen to the laboratory immediately. Do not store or refrigerate.

Causes for Rejection Specimen in fixative solution, specimen not received in a sterile container.

Turnaround Time Physician will be notified of positive cultures. Negatives are reported after 4 weeks.

Reference Range No growth

Use Isolate and identify fungi; establish the diagnosis of fungemia, fungal endocarditis, and disseminated mycosis in immunocompromised patients, oncology patients, transplant patients, patients with leukemia and lymphoma, and patients with the acquired immunodeficiency syndrome (AIDS)

Limitations A single negative culture does not rule out the presence of fungal infection

Additional Information Optimal isolation of fungi from tissue is accomplished by processing **as much tissue as possible. Swabs are not acceptable to collect specimens and to submit to the laboratory for this test because of the paucity of fungal organisms in many tissues.** Depending upon the geographic area *Histoplasma capsulatum, Blastomyces dermatitidis*, and *Coccidioides immitis*, among the deep pathogenic fungi, are most frequently isolated. Immunocompromised patients,

(Continued)

Fungus Culture, Biopsy *(Continued)*

transplant patients, and patients with acquired immunodeficiency syndrome (AIDS), are susceptible to opportunistic mycoses. The most frequently encountered are *Candida albicans*, *Cryptococcus neoformans*, and *Aspergillus* sp. The recovery of a recognized fungal pathogen from a wound culture or draining sinus is significant. Isolates such as *Candida* sp and *Aspergillus* sp are often environmental in origin and must be interpreted in the clinical context.

Selected Readings

Chapman SW, Bradsher RW Jr, Campbell GD Jr, et al, "Practice Guidelines for the Management of Patients With Blastomycosis. Infectious Diseases Society of America," *Clin Infect Dis*, 2000, 30(4):679-83.

Musial CE, Cockerill FR 3d, and Roberts GD, "Fungal Infections of the Immunocompromised Host: Clinical and Laboratory Aspects," *Clin Microbiol Rev*, 1988, 1(4):349-64.

Rex JH, Walsh TJ, Sobel JD, et al, "Practice Guidelines for the Treatment of Candidiasis. Infectious Diseases Society of America," *Clin Infect Dis*, 2000, 30(4):662-78.

Ribes JA, Vanover-Sams CL, and Baker DJ, "Zygomycetes in Human Disease," *Clin Microbiol Rev*, 2000, 13(2):236-301.

Stevens DA, Kan VL, Judson MA, et al, "Practice Guidelines for Diseases Caused by *Aspergillus*. Infectious Diseases Society of America," *Clin Infect Dis*, 2000, 30(4):696-709.

Wheat J, Sarosi G, McKinsey D, et al, "Practice Guidelines for the Management of Patients With Histoplasmosis. Infectious Diseases Society of America," *Clin Infect Dis*, 2000, 30(4):688-95.

Yeo SF and Wong B, "Current Status of Nonculture Methods for Diagnosis of Invasive Fungal Infections," *Clin Microbiol Rev*, 2002, 15(3):465-84.

Fungus Culture, Blood *see* Blood Culture, Fungus *on page 395*

Fungus Culture, Body Fluid

Related Information

Histopathology *on page 496*
Methenamine Silver Stain *on page 534*
Periodic Acid-Schiff Stain *on page 563*
Sporotrichosis Serology *on page 585*

Synonyms Body Fluid Fungus Culture

Applies to Ascitic Fluid Fungus Culture; Fungus Culture, Bone Marrow; Fungus Culture, Surgical Specimen; Fungus Culture, Tissue; Joint Fluid Fungus Culture; Pericardial Fluid Fungus Culture; Peritoneal Fluid Fungus Culture; Pleural Fluid Fungus Culture; Surgical Specimen Fungus Culture; Synovial Fluid Fungus Culture; Thoracentesis Fluid Fungus Culture Bone Marrow Fungus Culture; Tissue Fungus Culture; Wound Fungus Culture

Patient Preparation Aseptic preparation of biopsy site or site of body fluid aspiration

Special Instructions The laboratory should be informed of the specific source of specimen. Specimens may be divided for fungus culture, mycobacteria culture and acid-fast smear, and routine bacterial culture and Gram stain only if the specimen is of adequate volume for all tests requested.

Specimen Body fluid, blood, bone marrow

Container Sterile container with lid

Collection The portion of the fluid specimen submitted for culture should be separated from the portion submitted for cytology by the surgeon or pathologist utilizing sterile technique. The laboratory should be informed of the fungal species suspected. Every effort should be made to collect the specimen early in the day so as it may be processed promptly, assuring optimal yield. Multiple daily fungal blood cultures are not necessary. Single daily cultures for 2-3 days are sufficient.

Storage Instructions Specimens should not be stored or refrigerated. The specimen should be transported to the laboratory as soon as possible after collection.

Causes for Rejection Specimen in fixative

Turnaround Time Negatives are reported after 4 weeks

Reference Range No growth

Use Isolate and identify fungi; establish the diagnosis of fungemia, fungal endocarditis, and disseminated mycosis in immunocompromised patients, oncology patients, transplant patients, patients with leukemia and lymphoma, and patients with the acquired immunodeficiency syndrome (AIDS)

Methodology Culture under aerobic conditions on several media

Additional Information Optimal isolation of fungi from fluid is accomplished by processing as much tissue as possible. **Swab specimens of body fluids should not be submitted for fungal culture.** Specimen selection tables are provided in the listings for Fungus Culture, Sputum *on page 466* and Fungus Culture, Skin *on page 464*. Depending upon the geographic area *Histoplasma capsulatum*, *Blastomyces dermatitidis*, and *Coccidioides immitis*, among the deep pathogenic fungi, are most frequently isolated, but from tissue more commonly than from fluid. Immunocompromised patients, transplant patients, and patients with acquired immunodeficiency syndrome (AIDS), are susceptible to opportunistic mycoses. The recovery of a recognized fungal pathogen from a fluid or draining sinus is significant. Isolates such

as *Candida* sp and *Aspergillus* sp are often environmental in origin and must be interpreted in the clinical context.

Fungal peritonitis is clinically similar to bacterial peritonitis with pain, fever, and abdominal tenderness. Thirty-two fungal infections due to *Candida* sp (mostly *Candida albicans* and *Candida parapsilosis*), and rare single cases of *Aspergillus fumigatus* and the higher bacterium *Nocardia asteroides* have been reported in patients undergoing chronic dialysis. In a series of AIDS patients, bone marrow biopsy detected opportunistic fungal or mycobacterial infections in 20%. Eighty percent of the positive biopsies were associated with bone marrow granulomas. Fever, anemia, and neutropenia were often correlated with a positive biopsy. Neutrophil count <1000/mm^3 is associated with infection by *Candida*, *Aspergillus*, *Mucor*, *Rhizopus*, *Trichosporon*, and *Fusarium* sp. T-cell defects and/or impaired cell mediated immunity is associated with infection by *Candida*, *Cryptococcus neoformans*, *Histoplasma capsulatum*, *Coccidioides immitis*, and *Aspergillus* sp. Catheterization, arterial venous, or urinary and mechanical disruption of the skin is associated with *Candida* and *Rhodotorula* sp infections. Disruption of the natural barrier of the GI tract and respiratory tree by cytotoxic chemotherapy predispose to *Candida* sp infections.

Selected Readings

Fidel PL Jr, Vazquez JA, and Sobel JD, "*Candida glabrata*: Review of Epidemiology, Pathogenesis, and Clinical Disease With Comparison to *C. albicans*," *Clin Microbiol Rev*, 1999, 12(1):80-96.

Gray LD and Roberts GD, "Laboratory Diagnosis of Systemic Fungal Diseases," *Infect Dis Clin North Am*, 1988, 2(4):779-803.

Latgé JP, "*Aspergillus fumigatus* and Aspergillosis," *Clin Microbiol Rev*, 1999, 12(2):310-50.

Lyons RW and Andriole VT, "Fungal Infections of the CNS," *Neurol Clin*, 1986, 4(1):159-70.

Moser SA, "Laboratory Diagnosis of Histoplasmosis," *Clin Microbiol Newslett*, 1999, 21(12):95-101.

Musial CE, Cockerill FR 3d, and Roberts GD, "Fungal Infections of the Immunocompromised Host: Clinical and Laboratory Aspects," *Clin Microbiol Rev*, 1988, 1(4):349-64.

Ribes JA, Vanover-Sams CL, and Baker DJ, "Zygomycetes in Human Disease," *Clin Microbiol Rev*, 2000, 13(2):236-301.

Fungus Culture, Bone Marrow *see* Fungus Culture, Body Fluid *on page 462*

Fungus Culture, Bronchial Aspirate

Synonyms Bronchial Aspirate Fungus Culture; Lower Respiratory Fungus Culture

Applies to Bronchoalveolar Lavage (BAL); Fungus Culture, Tracheal Aspirate; Fungus Culture, Transtracheal Aspirate; Percutaneous Transtracheal Fungus Culture; Tracheal Aspirate Fungus Culture; Transtracheal Aspirate Fungus Culture

Test Includes Culture, Gram stain, KOH preparation

Special Instructions Requisition **must** state site of specimen

Specimen Bronchial aspirate, tracheal aspirate, transtracheal aspirate. These specimens are clinically equivalent to sputum (for microbiology purposes). **Do not submit specimen on a swab.**

Container Sterile tube, Lukens tube, or sputum container

Collection The specimen can be divided for fungus culture, mycobacteria culture and smear, and routine bacterial culture and Gram stain only if the specimen is accompanied by properly completed requisitions for these procedures and if the specimen is of adequate volume for all tests requested. Specify fungal species suspected.

Storage Instructions Specimen must be delivered to the laboratory as soon as possible. Refrigerate specimen until delivery is possible.

Causes for Rejection Specimen on outside of container, insufficient numbers of completed requisitions for the procedures requested

Turnaround Time Physicians will be notified of all positive cultures. Negative cultures are reported after 4 weeks.

Reference Range No fungi grown

Use Isolate and identify fungi

Limitations A single negative culture does not rule out presence of fungal infection

Additional Information Saprophytic fungi (especially yeast) isolated from respiratory aspirates are not uncommon. If mycobacteria are isolated, the isolate will be identified and referred for susceptibility testing on request.

Selected Readings

Chapman SW, Bradsher RW Jr, Campbell GD Jr, et al, "Practice Guidelines for the Management of Patients With Blastomycosis. Infectious Diseases Society of America," *Clin Infect Dis*, 2000, 30(4):679-83.

Galgiani JN, Ampel NM, Catanzaro A, et al, "Practice Guideline for the Treatment of Coccidioidomycosis. Infectious Diseases Society of America," *Clin Infect Dis*, 2000, 30(4):658-61.

Latgé JP, "*Aspergillus fumigatus* and Aspergillosis," *Clin Microbiol Rev*, 1999, 12(2):310-50.

Rex JH, Walsh TJ, Sobel JD, et al, "Practice Guidelines for the Treatment of Candidiasis. Infectious Diseases Society of America," *Clin Infect Dis*, 2000, 30(4):662-78.

Ribes JA, Vanover-Sams CL, and Baker DJ, "Zygomycetes in Human Disease," *Clin Microbiol Rev*, 2000, 13(2):236-301.

Stevens DA, Kan VL, Judson MA, et al, "Practice Guidelines for Diseases Caused by *Aspergillus*. Infectious Diseases Society of America," *Clin Infect Dis*, 2000, 30(4):696-709.

Wheat J, Sarosi G, McKinsey D, et al, "Practice Guidelines for the Management of Patients With Histoplasmosis. Infectious Diseases Society of America," *Clin Infect Dis*, 2000, 30(4):688-95.

Fungus Culture, Bronchoscopy *see* Fungus Culture, Sputum *on page 466*

Fungus Culture, Cerebrospinal Fluid

Related Information

Cerebrospinal Fluid Analysis *on page 408*
Cryptococcal Antigen Serology, Serum or Cerebrospinal Fluid *on page 431*
India Ink Preparation *on page 507*
Viral Culture, Central Nervous System Symptoms *on page 614*

Synonyms Cerebrospinal Fluid Fungus Culture; CSF Fungus Culture; Fungus Culture, CSF; Fungus Culture, Spinal Fluid; Spinal Fluid Fungus Culture

Test Includes Culture for fungi, India ink, fungus smear, and cryptococcal antigen test if requested (and depending on laboratory protocol)

Patient Preparation Aseptic preparation of aspiration site

Special Instructions The laboratory should be informed of the specific source of specimen.

Specimen Cerebrospinal fluid

Container Sterile CSF tube

Collection Tubes should be numbered 1, 2, 3 with tube #1 representing the first portion of the sample collected. Contamination with normal flora from skin or other body surfaces must be avoided. The third tube collected during lumbar puncture is most suitable for culture because skin contaminants from the puncture usually are washed out with fluid collected in the first two tubes.

Storage Instructions The specimen should be transported immediately to the laboratory. If it cannot be processed immediately, it should be kept at room temperature or placed in an incubator. Do not refrigerate.

Turnaround Time Negative cultures are usually reported after 4 weeks

Reference Range No growth

Use Isolate and identify fungi, particularly *Cryptococcus neoformans*. Diagnosis is established by detection of cryptococcal antigen.

Limitations Recovery of fungi from cerebrospinal fluid is directly related to the volume of cerebrospinal fluid cultured. ≥1 mL is recommended. Recovery is <100% on one specimen.

Methodology Aerobic culture of centrifuged sediment on several fungal media

Additional Information India ink preparations are not useful (sensitivity, <50%) in identifying the presence of *Cryptococcus neoformans*, the most common fungus isolated from cerebrospinal fluid. False positive results can occur with WBC appearing as *Cryptococcus* with a "capsule." Cryptococcal antigen titers of serum and cerebrospinal fluid provide rapid diagnosis and have greater sensitivity than India ink preparation. The diagnosis of central nervous system fungal infections is frequently complicated by the overlapping array of signs and symptoms which may accompany other clinical entities such as tuberculous meningitis, pyogenic abscess, brain tumor, hypersensitivity or allergic reactions, collagen vascular disease, leptomeningeal malignancy, chemical meningitis, meningeal inflammation secondary to contiguous suppuration, Behçet's disease, Mollaret's meningitis, and the uveomeningitic syndromes.

Especially in immunocompromised hosts, aspergillosis, mucormycosis, and candidiasis are observed. Infections with species which cause phaeohyphomycosis are described. Nocardiosis can infect the meninges. *Cryptococcus neoformans* has been isolated from up to 10% of patients with acquired immunodeficiency syndrome (AIDS).

Selected Readings

Greenlee JE, "Approach to Diagnosis of Meningitis - Cerebrospinal Fluid Evaluation," *Infect Dis Clin North Am*, 1990, 4(4):583-98.

Moser SA, "Laboratory Diagnosis of Histoplasmosis," *Clin Microbiol Newslett*, 1999, 21(12):95-101.

Ribes JA, Vanover-Sams CL, and Baker DJ, "Zygomycetes in Human Disease," *Clin Microbiol Rev*, 2000, 13(2):236-301.

Saag MS, Graybill RJ, Larsen RA, et al, "Practice Guidelines for the Management of Cryptococcal Disease. Infectious Diseases Society of America," *Clin Infect Dis*, 2000, 30(4):710-8.

Tunkel AR, Wispelwey B, and Scheld WM, "Pathogenesis and Pathophysiology of Meningitis," *Infect Dis Clin North Am*, 1990, 4(4):555-81.

Fungus Culture, CSF *see* Fungus Culture, Cerebrospinal Fluid *on page 464*
Fungus Culture, Dermatophytes *see* Fungus Culture, Skin *on page 464*
Fungus Culture, Gastric Aspirate *see* Fungus Culture, Sputum *on page 466*
Fungus Culture, Hair *see* Fungus Culture, Skin *on page 464*
Fungus Culture, Nail *see* Fungus Culture, Skin *on page 464*

Fungus Culture, Skin

Related Information

KOH Preparation *on page 513*

Methenamine Silver Stain *on page 534*
Periodic Acid-Schiff Stain *on page 563*
Skin Biopsy *on page 580*

Applies to Dermatophyte Fungus Culture; Fungus Culture, Dermatophytes; Fungus Culture, Hair; Fungus Culture, Nail; Hair Fungus Culture; Nail Fungus Culture

Patient Preparation Select fluorescent hairs or nonfluorescent hairs which are broken off and appear diseased and pluck them with sterile forceps. If diseased hair stubs are not apparent, scrape the edges of a skin lesion with a sterile scalpel. Cleanse skin lesions first with 70% alcohol to reduce bacteria and saprophytic fungi. Scrape from the outer edges of skin lesions. In infections of the nails, scrape out the friable material beneath the edge of the nails, or scrape or clip off portions of abnormal appearing nail and submit for examination and culture.

Special Instructions Careful choice of specimens for laboratory study is important. A Wood's lamp can occasionally be useful in the collection of specimens in tinea capitis infections because hairs infected by most members of the genus *Microsporum* frequently exhibit fluorescence under a Wood's lamp. However, in tinea capitis due to *Trichophyton* sp, infected hairs usually do not fluoresce. The laboratory should be informed of the specific site of the specimen. See table.

Selection of Specimens for the Diagnosis of Superficial Mycosis and Dermatomycosis

Diagnosis	Specimen of Choice
Superficial mycoses	
Piedra	Hair
Tinea nigra	Skin scraping
Tinea versicolor	Skin scraping
Dermatomycoses (cutaneous mycoses)	
Onychomycosis	Nail scraping
Tinea capitis	Hair (black dot)
Tinea corporis	Skin scraping
Tinea pedis	Skin scraping
Tinea cruris	Skin scraping
Candidiasis	
Thrush	Scraping of oral white patches
Diaper dermatitis	Scraping of pustules at margin
Paronychia	Scraping skin around nail
Cutaneous candidiasis	Scraping of pustules at margin
Erosio interdigitalis blastomycetia (coinfection with gram-negative rods)	Scrapings of interdigital space (routine culture also)
Congenital candidiasis	Scraping of scales, pustules and cutaneous debris, cultures of umbilical stump, mouth, urine and stool
Mucocutaneous candidiasis	Scraping of affected area

Specimen Skin scrapings, exudates, nail clippings, whole nail, debris under nail, hair. **Swab specimens are never adequate.**

Container Petri dish, urine container, envelope

Collection Enclose hair specimens, skin scrapings, or nail clippings or scrapings in clean clear container, test tube, urine container, or Petri dish. Label the specimen with the patient's name. Do not put specimens in cotton-plugged tubes, because the specimen may become trapped among the cotton fibers and lost. Do not put specimen into closed containers, such as rubber-stoppered tubes, because this keeps the specimen moist and allows overgrowth of bacteria and saprophytic fungi. The laboratory should be informed of the fungal species suspected.

Storage Instructions Keep specimen at room temperature until delivered to the laboratory

Turnaround Time Cultures positive for *Candida* sp are usually reported within 1 week. Cultures positive for dermatophytes are usually reported within 2-3 weeks. Negative cultures are usually reported after 1 month. Cultures in which suspicion of systemic fungal infection has been indicated are usually reported upon becoming positive, or negative after 4 weeks.

Reference Range No growth

Use Isolate and identify fungi

Limitations A single negative specimen does not rule out fungal infections. If infection with mycobacteria or aerobic organisms cannot be excluded clinically, a separate culture should be submitted as indicated.

Methodology Aerobic culture on selective media usually including nonselective Sabouraud's agar

(Continued)

Fungus Culture, Skin *(Continued)*

Additional Information *Candida* sp may colonize skin. Clinical diagnosis of *Candida* infection involves consideration of predisposing factors such as occlusion, maceration altered cutaneous barrier function. Signs of *Candida* infection include bright erythema, fragile papulopustules, and satellite lesions.

Selected Readings

Chapman SW, Bradsher RW Jr, Campbell GD Jr, et al, "Practice Guidelines for the Management of Patients With Blastomycosis. Infectious Diseases Society of America," *Clin Infect Dis*, 2000, 30(4):679-83.

Cohn MS, "Superficial Fungal Infections. Topical and Oral Treatment of Common Types," *Postgrad Med*, 1992, 91(2):239-44, 249-52.

McKay M, "Cutaneous Manifestations of Candidiasis," *Am J Obstet Gynecol*, 1988, 158(4):991-3.

Rex JH, Walsh TJ, Sobel JD, et al, "Practice Guidelines for the Treatment of Candidiasis. Infectious Diseases Society of America," *Clin Infect Dis*, 2000, 30(4):662-78.

Wheat J, Sarosi G, McKinsey D, et al, "Practice Guidelines for the Management of Patients With Histoplasmosis. Infectious Diseases Society of America," *Clin Infect Dis*, 2000, 30(4):688-95.

Fungus Culture, Spinal Fluid *see* Fungus Culture, Cerebrospinal Fluid *on page 464*

Fungus Culture, Sputum

Related Information

Methenamine Silver Stain *on page 534*
Periodic Acid-Schiff Stain *on page 563*

Selection of Specimens for the Diagnosis of Systemic and Subcutaneous Mycosis

Diagnosis	Specimen of Choice in Order of Usefulness
	Systemic Mycoses
Aspergillosis	Sputum Bronchial aspirate Biopsy (lung)
Blastomycosis	Skin scrapings Abscess drainage (pus) Urine Sputum Bronchial aspirate
Candidiasis	Sputum Bronchial aspirate Blood Cerebrospinal fluid Urine Stool
Coccidioidomycosis	Sputum Bronchial aspirate Cerebrospinal fluid Urine Skin scrapings Abscess drainage (pus)
Cryptococcosis	Cerebrospinal fluid Sputum Abscess drainage (pus) Skin scraping Urine
	Subcutaneous Mycoses
Chromoblastomycosis	Skin scrapings Biopsy (skin) Drainage (pus)
Maduromycosis (mycetoma)	Drainage (pus) Abscess drainage Biopsy (lesion)
Sporotrichosis	Drainage (pus) Abscess drainage Biopsy (skin, lymph node)

Synonyms Sputum Fungus Culture

Applies to Bronchoscopy Fungus Culture; Fungus Culture, Bronchoscopy; Fungus Culture, Gastric Aspirate; Fungus Culture, Tracheal Aspirate; Fungus Culture, Transtracheal Aspirate; Gastric Aspirate Fungus Culture; Percutaneous Transtracheal Fungus Culture; Tracheal Aspirate Fungus Culture; Transtracheal Aspirate Fungus Culture

Patient Preparation The patient should be instructed to remove dentures, rinse mouth with water and cough deeply expectorating sputum into the sputum collection cup.

Special Instructions The laboratory should be informed of the specific source of specimen and the suspected clinical diagnosis should be stated.

Specimen First morning sputum. Microbiologically, this specimen is equivalent to the following: gastric aspirate, induced sputum, aspirated sputum, bronchial aspirate, tracheal aspirate, transtracheal aspirate. **Swab specimens are never adequate.** See table on previous page.

Container Sterile sputum cup, sputum trap, sterile tracheal aspirate tube, or sterile bronchoscopy tube

Collection Every effort should be made to collect the specimen early in the day so that it may be processed by the laboratory for optimal recovery. A recommended screening procedure is three first morning specimens submitted on three successive days. The specimen can be divided for fungus culture, mycobacteria culture and smear, and routine bacterial culture and Gram stain only if the specimen is of adequate volume for all tests requested.

Storage Instructions Refrigerate the specimen if storage is in excess of 1 hour

Causes for Rejection Specimens contaminated on the outside of the container pose excessive risk to laboratory personnel and may not be acceptable to the laboratory.

Turnaround Time Negative cultures are reported after 4 weeks

Reference Range No growth; yeast from the oropharynx may be present.

Use Establish the presence of potentially pathogenic fungi

Limitations The yield may be reduced by bacterial overgrowth during storage or on standing; therefore, fresh sputum is preferred. A single negative culture does not rule out the presence of fungal infection. If two specimens are received simultaneously, many laboratories will pool them and process them as one specimen unless specific instructions are provided.

Methodology Culture on selective and nonselective media

Additional Information Deeply coughed sputum, transtracheal aspirate, bronchial washing or brushing, or deep tracheal aspirate are preferred specimens. Oncology patients, transplant patients, and patients with the acquired immunodeficiency syndrome (AIDS) are particularly prone to infection with fungi.

Primary fungal pulmonary infections frequently result in granulomatous disease. Classically, *Histoplasma capsulatum*, *Coccidioides immitis*, *Cryptococcus neoformans*, and *Blastomyces dermatitidis* have been implicated. The incidence was largely related to geographic exposure and many cases occurred in seemingly normal hosts. Recently increasing numbers of reports of opportunistic fungal pulmonary infections due to a wide variety of etiologic agents which are ubiquitous in the environment, are being published. Definitive diagnosis depends upon the following: presence of clinical signs of pulmonary infection including rales, rhonchi and fever, and a chest x-ray picture revealing consolidation of granuloma; laboratory isolation of a potentially significant organism from a suitable specimen; histologic documentation of tissue invasion by the isolated organism. Many lists of documented etiologic agents of pulmonary fungal disease have been reported (see table).

Pulmonary Fungal Infections

Endemic Fungi	Opportunistic Fungi
Histoplasma capsulatum	*Candida albicans*
Blastomyces dermatitidis	*Candida tropicalis*
Coccidioides immitis	*Aspergillus niger*
Paracoccidioides brasiliensis	*Aspergillus fumigatus*
	Mucor
	Rhizopus
	Absidia
	Cryptococcus neoformans

From Haque AK, "Pathology of Common Pulmonary Fungal Infections," *J Thorac Imaging*, 1992, 7:1-11, with permission.

(Continued)

Fungus Culture, Sputum *(Continued)*

In practice a diagnosis sufficient for therapy can frequently be established by observation of hyphae, pseudohyphae or yeast cells in tissue sections; recovery of the organism from a normally sterile site; repeated isolation of the same suspect organism from the same or different sites; seroconversion (ie, the development of an immune response to the suspected organism). *Candida* and *Aspergillus* sp are the most frequently isolated usually pathogenic organisms. However, they are frequently present as the result of contamination from the patient's normal flora or airborne sources. Their presence may represent colonization rather than invasion. Recovery of *Candida* from blood (see Blood Culture, Fungus *on page 395*) is a major adjunct to definitive diagnosis. Even without invasion *Aspergillus* may cause IgE-mediated asthma, allergic alveolitis cell mediated hypersensitivity, mucoid impaction, and bronchocentric granulomatosis. Fungal tracheobronchitis has recently been recognized to present as a pseudomembranous form involving the circumference of the bronchial wall or as multiple or discrete plaques. The plaques or pseudomembranes are composed of necrotic tissue exudate and fungal hyphae.

Selected Readings

Chapman SW, Bradsher RW Jr, Campbell GD Jr, et al, "Practice Guidelines for the Management of Patients With Blastomycosis. Infectious Diseases Society of America," *Clin Infect Dis*, 2000, 30(4):679-83.

Galgiani JN, Ampel NM, Catanzaro A, et al, "Practice Guideline for the Treatment of Coccidioidomycosis. Infectious Diseases Society of America," *Clin Infect Dis*, 2000, 30(4):658-61.

Latgé JP, "*Aspergillus fumigatus* and Aspergillosis," *Clin Microbiol Rev*, 1999, 12(2):310-50.

Rex JH, Walsh TJ, Sobel JD, et al, "Practice Guidelines for the Treatment of Candidiasis. Infectious Diseases Society of America," *Clin Infect Dis*, 2000, 30(4):662-78.

Saag MS, Graybill RJ, Larsen RA, et al, "Practice Guidelines for the Management of Cryptococcal Disease. Infectious Diseases Society of America," *Clin Infect Dis*, 2000, 30(4):710-8.

Stevens DA, Kan VL, Judson MA, et al, "Practice Guidelines for Diseases Caused by *Aspergillus*. Infectious Diseases Society of America," *Clin Infect Dis*, 2000, 30(4):696-709.

Wheat J, Sarosi G, McKinsey D, et al, "Practice Guidelines for the Management of Patients With Histoplasmosis. Infectious Diseases Society of America," *Clin Infect Dis*, 2000, 30(4):688-95.

Fungus Culture, Surgical Specimen *see* Fungus Culture, Body Fluid *on page 462*

Fungus Culture, Tissue *see* Fungus Culture, Body Fluid *on page 462*

Fungus Culture, Tracheal Aspirate *see* Fungus Culture, Sputum *on page 466*

Fungus Culture, Transtracheal Aspirate *see* Fungus Culture, Sputum *on page 466*

Fungus Culture, Urine

Related Information

Methenamine Silver Stain *on page 534*

Periodic Acid-Schiff Stain *on page 563*

Synonyms Urine Fungus Culture

Patient Preparation Usual preparation for clean catch midvoid urine specimen collection. See listing Urine Culture, Clean Catch *on page 609.*

Special Instructions The laboratory should be informed of the specific source of the specimen and the fungal species suspected.

Specimen Urine

Container Sterile plastic container or tube

Collection The specimen should be transported to laboratory within 2 hours of collection if not refrigerated. The patient must be instructed to thoroughly cleanse skin and collect midstream specimen.

Causes for Rejection Unrefrigerated specimen more than 2 hours old may be subject to overgrowth and may not yield valid results

Reference Range No growth

Use Isolate and identify fungi

Limitations A single negative culture does not rule out the presence of fungal infection.

Additional Information Patients with candiduria may or may not have candidemia; positive urine culture for fungi often may be followed by positive blood culture for fungi. Ascending infections occur in patients with diabetes, prolonged antimicrobial therapy, or following instrumentation. Urinary obstruction due to "fungus balls" may occur in diabetes and following renal transplantation. Candiduria associated with hematogenous infections is observed in patients with granulocytopenia, corticosteroid therapy, and with immunosuppression. The source is frequently the gastrointestinal tract or indwelling catheters particular with hyperalimentation. A blood fungus culture is useful in defining invasive disease. However, proof of invasive *Candida* infection requires direct cystoscopic or operative visualization of fungus balls, or pyelonephritis, or histological evidence of mucosa invasion. Urine is a useful specimen for culture in cryptococcosis, blastomycosis, and candidiasis. See table for fungus culture specimen selection in Fungus Culture, Sputum *on page 466.* The incidence of genitourinary fungal infections is increasing. They are usually associated with

broad-spectrum antibiotic therapy, corticosteroid therapy, underlying general debility, and AIDS. In addition to *Candida*, opportunistic pathogens in the genitourinary tract include *Aspergillus* and *Cryptococcus*. Endemic pathogens such as *Histoplasma*, *Blastomyces*, and *Coccidioides* are also encountered.

Selected Readings

Bryant K, Maxfield C, and Rabalais G, "Renal Candidiasis in Neonates With Candiduria," *Pediatr Infect Dis J*, 1999, 18(11):959-63.

Chapman SW, Bradsher RW Jr, Campbell GD Jr, et al, "Practice Guidelines for the Management of Patients With Blastomycosis. Infectious Diseases Society of America," *Clin Infect Dis*, 2000, 30(4):679-83.

Rex JH, Walsh TJ, Sobel JD, et al, "Practice Guidelines for the Treatment of Candidiasis. Infectious Diseases Society of America," *Clin Infect Dis*, 2000, 30(4):662-78.

Saag MS, Graybill RJ, Larsen RA, et al, "Practice Guidelines for the Management of Cryptococcal Disease. Infectious Diseases Society of America," *Clin Infect Dis*, 2000, 30(4):710-8.

Stevens DA, Kan VL, Judson MA, et al, "Practice Guidelines for Diseases Caused by *Aspergillus*. Infectious Diseases Society of America," *Clin Infect Dis*, 2000, 30(4):696-709.

Wheat J, Sarosi G, McKinsey D, et al, "Practice Guidelines for the Management of Patients With Histoplasmosis. Infectious Diseases Society of America," *Clin Infect Dis*, 2000, 30(4):688-95.

Gallium Abscess Scan *see* Gallium Scan *on page 469*

Gallium Scan

Applies to Gallium Abscess Scan; Gallium Tumor Scan; Soft Tissue Scan

Test Includes The patient receives an intravenous injection of gallium-67 citrate. Images are then acquired for some combination of 24, 48, and 72 hours after injection.

Patient Preparation Patient should have all RIA blood work performed, or at least drawn, prior to injection of any radioactive material. The patient does not need to be fasting or NPO for this procedure.

Special Instructions Requisition should indicate the current patient diagnosis in order to select the most appropriate radiopharmaceutical and/or imaging technique. Other Nuclear Medicine procedures (bone, liver, lung) should be completed prior to gallium injection. If abdominal abscess/infection is suspected, laxatives, and/or enemas may be ordered for the patient prior to delayed imaging at 48 or 72 hours. This will help clear normal intestinal gallium activity from the colon.

Duration of Procedure: 24-72 hours

Radiopharmaceutical: Gallium-67 citrate

Technique The application of single-photon emission tomography (SPECT) techniques may contribute significantly to the diagnostic accuracy of this imaging study.

Normal Findings Gallium will localize to some degree in liver and spleen, bone, nasopharynx, lacrimal glands, and breast tissue. There is normally some secretion of gallium into the bowel. This may require laxatives and/or enemas for the patient to evacuate this normal activity before additional imaging of possible abdominal infection or abscess. Abnormal accumulation of gallium will usually be asymmetric, increase in later images, and remain in the same location (normal bowel luminal gallium activity will transit).

Use Gallium localizes at sites of active inflammation or infection as well as in some neoplasms. Gallium imaging is very sensitive in detection of abscesses, pneumonia, pyelonephritis, active sarcoidosis, and active tuberculosis. Even in immunocompromised patients (eg, those with AIDS), gallium imaging can detect early complications such as *Pneumocystis jiroveci* pneumonitis. The nonspecificity of gallium activity, however, requires that correlation with other radiographic studies and clinical findings be given close attention. Gallium imaging is very useful in the differential diagnosis and staging of some neoplasms, notably Hodgkin's disease, lymphoma, hepatocellular carcinoma, bronchogenic carcinoma, melanoma, and leukemia. Recent evidence has shown a correlation of gallium localization in the lungs with the activity of disease in pulmonary fibrosis and asbestosis. Gallium is also used in addition to bone scintigraphy for detecting osteomyelitis, especially in its chronic stages. A common indication for gallium imaging is as a screening procedure for infection in fever of unknown origin (FUO).

Limitations There is variable normal excretion of gallium via the intestinal tract. This contributes to the nonspecificity of gallium imaging in suspected abdominal or pelvic infections. Previous treatment with antibiotics or high doses of steroids may decrease the inflammatory response and result in false-negative gallium imaging.

Additional Information Other isotope studies may need to be postponed up to 7 days after a gallium scan has been done due to its slow elimination from soft tissue.

Selected Readings

Bisson G, Lamoureux G, and Bégin R, "Quantitative Gallium-67 Lung Scan to Assess the Inflammatory Activity in the Pneumoconioses," *Semin Nucl Med*, 1987, 17(1):72-80.

Israel O, Front D, Epelbaum R, et al, "Residual Mass and Negative Gallium Scintigraphy in Treated Lymphoma," *J Nucl Med*, 1990, 31(3):365-8.

Lee BF, Chiu NT, Chang JK, et al, "Technetium-99m(V)-DMSA and Gallium-67 in the Assessment of Bone and Joint Infection," *J Nucl Med*, 1998, 39(12):2128-31.

(Continued)

Gallium Scan *(Continued)*

Maderazo EG, Hickingbotham NB, Woronick CL, et al, "The Influence of Various Factors on the Accuracy of Gallium-67 Imaging for Occult Infection," *J Nucl Med*, 1988, 29(5):608-15.

Rossleigh MA, Murray IP, Mackey DW, et al, "Pediatric Solid Tumors: Evaluation by Gallium-67 SPECT Studies," *J Nucl Med*, 1990, 31(2):168-72.

Turoglu HT, Akisik MF, Naddaf SY, et al, "Tumor and Infection Localization in AIDS Patients: Ga-67 and Tl-201 Findings," *Clin Nucl Med*, 1998, 23(7):446-59.

Yen TC, Tsai MF, and Tzen KY, "Biliary and Liver Abscesses Demonstrated With Tc-99m DISIDA and Ga-67 Imaging," *Clin Nucl Med*, 1998, 23(12):853-4.

Gallium Tumor Scan *see* Gallium Scan *on page 469*

Garamycin®, Blood *see* Gentamicin Level *on page 472*

Gastric Aspirate Fungus Culture *see* Fungus Culture, Sputum *on page 466*

Gastric Aspirate Mycobacteria Culture *see* Mycobacteria Culture, Sputum *on page 542*

Gastric Biopsy Culture for *Helicobacter pylori* *see Helicobacter pylori* Culture and Urease Test *on page 479*

GC Culture *see Neisseria gonorrhoeae* Culture *on page 547*

GC Culture, Throat *see Neisseria gonorrhoeae* Culture *on page 547*

Genital Culture

Related Information

Abscess Aerobic and Anaerobic Culture *on page 360*
Chlamydia Culture *on page 413*
Genital Culture for *Ureaplasma urealyticum on page 471*
Group B *Streptococcus* Antigen Test *on page 476*
Neisseria gonorrhoeae Culture *on page 547*
Trichomonas Preparation *on page 600*

Applies to Cervical Culture; Endocervical Culture; Prostatic Fluid Culture; Vaginal Culture

Test Includes Culture for aerobic organisms and *Candida* sp. *Neisseria gonorrhoeae*, *Gardnerella*, *Mobiluncus*, Gram stain, and fungal stain require separate requests. Each laboratory has a different protocol for processing and working up growth from genital cultures. Contact the laboratory to determine the particular laboratory's approach to genital cultures and which organisms are considered reportable.

Special Instructions The laboratory should be informed of the specific source of specimen, age of patient, current antibiotic therapy, clinical diagnosis, and time of collection.

Specimen Swab of vagina, cervix, discharge, aspirated endocervical, endometrial, prostatic fluid, or urethral discharge. Specimens to be cultured for *N. gonorrhoeae* **must** be cultured at bedside (onto special medium at room temperature) and be in the laboratory within 30 minutes.

Container Sterile Culturette® or sterile tube

Collection The specimen (except specimen for *N. gonorrhoeae*) should be transported to laboratory within 2 hours of collection. Refrigeration may reduce yield.

Turnaround Time Preliminary reports are usually available at 24 hours. Cultures with no growth are usually reported after 48 hours. Cultures from which pathogens are isolated usually require a minimum of 48 hours for completion.

Reference Range Normal flora; properly collected prostatic fluid and endocervical cultures are normally sterile.

Use Isolate and identify common and potentially pathogenic aerobic bacteria and yeast. Infectious causes of abnormal vaginal discharge or vulvovaginitis include *Candida albicans, Trichomonas vaginalis, Gardnerella vaginalis, Mobiluncus* sp, *Chlamydia trachomatis*, herpes simplex virus, human papillomavirus, *Enterobius vermicularis* (pinworms), *Giardia lamblia* and other microorganisms. Normal vaginal secretions have a pH ≤4.5, characteristic appearance, and consist of clear mucus, epithelial cells, and have no unusual odor. Many bacterial organisms and perhaps *Candida albicans* are present in a stable symbiotic relationship. Culture may allow documentation of a change in balance of normal organism populations or detection of a specific pathogen. Also used to document presence of *Staphylococcus aureus* in cases of suspected toxic shock syndrome.

Limitations *Chlamydia*, *Ureaplasma urealyticum*, viruses, and parasites are not recovered by this procedure. Generally, the clinical utility of genital cultures is limited because it is difficult to determine the clinical relevance of most growth from such cultures.

Methodology Aerobic culture with selective (Thayer-Martin) and nonselective media incubated at 35°C to 37°C with CO_2. Some laboratories offer molecular testing for *Candida, Gardnerella*, and *Trichomonas*. Contact the testing laboratory for the availability of amplified and nonamplified qualitative and quantitative molecular tests for

this organism, and for information on selection and collection of appropriate specimens for specific molecular tests.

Additional Information Rapid growing aerobic organisms which predominate are usually identified. Susceptibility testing can be performed if indicated. Routine culture often includes culture for *N. gonorrhoeae*, *Candida albicans*, *Staphylococcus aureus*, group B streptococci, and *Gardnerella vaginalis*. Presence or absence of normal flora will usually be reported. Normal flora of the vagina is dependent upon age, glycogen content, pH, exogenous hormone therapy, etc. Normal vaginal flora includes anaerobes, corynebacteria, enteric gram-negative rods, enterococci, lactobacilli, *Moraxella* sp, staphylococci, streptococci (alpha and nonhemolytic), *Mycobacterium smegmatis*. The laboratory should be consulted to arrange for special toxin identification procedures if toxic shock syndrome is suspected and *Staphylococcus aureus* is recovered.

Vaginitis is one of the most commonly encountered complaints of female patients. The majority of cases (approximately 90%) are caused by *Candida*, *Gardnerella*, or *Trichomonas*. Diagnosis and effective treatment depend upon accurate identification of the etiologic agent, effective specific therapy, and restoration of the normal ecosystem of the vagina. Proper hygiene, dietary control, and management of stress also are important factors in control of recurrent vaginal infections.

Candida sp are frequently present as normal flora in vagina. A saline wet mount may demonstrate yeast cells or pseudohyphae and may provide rapid diagnostic information. The most common clinical presentation is a characteristic clumpy white cottage cheese appearance with vaginal or vulvar itching. Vaginitis frequently complicates pregnancy and diabetes, and is seen with broad-spectrum antibiotic therapy as well as in conditions which lower host resistance.

Selected Readings

Knapp JS, "Antimicrobial Resistance in *Neisseria gonorrhoeae* in the United States," *Clin Microbiol Newslett*, 1999, 21(1):1-7.

Schuchat A, "Group B Streptococcal Disease: From Trials and Tribulations to Triumph and Trepidation," *Clin Infect Dis*, 2001, 33(6):751-6.

Sobel JD, "Vaginal Infections in Adult Women," *Med Clin North Am*, 1990, 74(6):1573-602.

Sobel JD, "Vulvovaginitis. When *Candida* Becomes a Problem," *Dermatol Clin*, 1998, 16(4):763-8.

Spiegel CA, "Bacterial Vaginosis," *Clin Microbiol Rev*, 1991, 4(4):485-502.

Zenilman JM, "Gonorrhea: Clinical and Public Health Issues," *Hosp Pract (Off Ed)*, 1993, 28(2A):29-35, 39-40, 43-50.

Genital Culture for *Mycoplasma* T-Strain *see* Genital Culture for *Ureaplasma urealyticum on page 471*

Genital Culture for *Ureaplasma urealyticum*

Related Information

Genital Culture *on page 470*
Mycoplasma/Ureaplasma Culture *on page 545*
Neisseria gonorrhoeae Culture *on page 547*

Synonyms Genital Culture for *Mycoplasma* T-Strain; *Mycoplasma* T-Strain Culture, Genital; *Ureaplasma urealyticum* Culture, Genital

Applies to Cervical Culture for *Ureaplasma urealyticum*; Cervical Culture for T-Strain *Mycoplasma*; Urethral Culture for T-Strain *Mycoplasma*

Special Instructions *Ureaplasma* and *Mycoplasma* are sensitive to delays in processing and storage. Consult the laboratory prior to collecting the specimen for optimal handling instructions and to determine (1) if the lab performs the test, and (2) how to obtain **special collection and transport fluid/medium**.

Specimen Culturette® swab of urethra or cervix

Container Culturette® swab

Storage Instructions Keep specimen refrigerated. **Organism is remarkably sensitive to drying**; swab must be placed promptly into Culturette® and hand delivered to the Microbiology Laboratory.

Turnaround Time 8 days if negative, up to 2 weeks if positive

Reference Range Frequently isolated from asymptomatic individuals

Use Establish the diagnosis of *Ureaplasma urealyticum* infection in suspected cases of nongonococcal urethritis and cervicitis

Limitations Culture may be negative in the presence of infection, and the presence of *Ureaplasma urealyticum* or *Mycoplasma hominis* does not always indicate infection, although there is a significant association with symptomatic disease. Most clinical laboratories do not offer this test. It is usually available at reference laboratories.

Methodology Culture on selective media

Additional Information *Ureaplasma* and *Mycoplasma* can be isolated from urethral and genital swabs and from urine of sexually active individuals. Sixty percent or more of all women asymptomatically carry *U. urealyticum* in their genital tract. Usual prevalence of these organisms in patients with urethral symptoms also is high; thus,

(Continued)

Genital Culture for *Ureaplasma urealyticum* (Continued)

conclusions regarding the etiologic role of an isolate in a given patient are difficult to make. *U. urealyticum* is usually associated with cases of nongonococcal urethritis.

Selected Readings

Aydin D, Kucukbasmaci O, Gonullu N, et al, "Susceptibilities of *Neisseria gonorrhoeae* and *Ureaplasma urealyticum* Isolates From male patients With Urethritis to Several Antibiotics Including Telithromycin," *Chemotherapy*, 2005, 51(2-3):89-92.

Cassell GH, Waites KB, Watson HL, et al, "*Ureaplasma urealyticum* Intrauterine Infection: Role in Prematurity and Disease in Newborns," *Clin Microbiol Rev*, 1993, 6(1):69-87.

Salari MH and Karimi A, "Prevalence of *Ureaplasma urealyticum* and *Mycoplasma genitalium* in Men With Nongonococcal Urethritis," *East Mediterr Health J*, 2003, 9(3):291-5.

Waites KB, Rikihisa Y, and Taylor-Robinson D, "*Mycoplasma* and *Ureaplasma*," *Manual of Clinical Microbiology*, 8th ed, Murray PR, Baron EJ, Jorgensen JH, et al, eds, Washington, DC: American Society for Microbiology, 2003, 972-90.

Genotyping, HCV *see* Hepatitis C Viral RNA Genotyping *on page 486*

Gentamicin Level

Related Information

Antibiotic Level, Serum *on page 375*

Synonyms Garamycin®, Blood

Abstract Aminoglycoside antibiotics, including gentamicin, are used primarily to treat infections caused by aerobic gram-negative bacilli. Additionally, when used in combination with penicillins, they may have synergistic bactericidal activity against gram-positive cocci such as *Staphylococcus aureus* and *Enterococcus*. Gentamicin has a narrow therapeutic window, and its use in life-threatening infections makes it mandatory that effective levels be achieved without overdosage.

Specimen Serum, urine

Container Red top tube, plastic urine container

Sampling Time Peak: 30-60 minutes after end of 30 minute I.V. infusion or 60 minutes post I.M. dose; trough: immediately prior to next dose. Specimens should be drawn at steady-state, usually after fifth dose, if drug given every 8 hours, or after third dose, if drug given every 12 hours.

Storage Instructions Separate within 1 hour of collection and refrigerate or freeze until assayed. Must be frozen if a β-lactam antibiotic is also present because of potential inactivation of aminoglycosides.

Reference Range Therapeutic: peak: 4-10 mcg/mL (SI: 8-21 μmol/L) (depends in part on the minimal inhibitory concentration of the drug against the organism being treated); trough: <2 mcg/mL (SI: <4 μmol/L)

Possible Panic Range Toxic: peak: >12 mcg/mL (SI: >25 μmol/L); trough: >2 mcg/mL (SI: >4 μmol/L)

Use Peak levels are necessary to assure adequate therapeutic levels for organism being treated. Trough levels are necessary to reduce the likelihood of nephrotoxicity.

Limitations High peak levels may not have strong correlation with toxicity.

Methodology Enzyme immunoassay (EIA), fluorescence polarization immunoassay (FPIA), high performance liquid chromatography (HPLC)

Additional Information Gentamicin is cleared by the kidney and accumulates in renal tubular cells. Nephrotoxicity is most closely related to the length of time that trough levels exceed 2 mcg/mL (SI: >4 μmol/L). Creatinine levels should be monitored every 2-3 days as an indicator of impending renal toxicity. The initial toxic result is nonoliguric renal failure that is usually reversible if the drug is discontinued. Continued administration of gentamicin may produce oliguric renal failure. Nephrotoxicity may occur in as many as 10% to 25% of patients receiving aminoglycosides; most of this toxicity can be avoided by monitoring levels and adjusting dosing schedules accordingly.

Aminoglycosides may also cause irreversible ototoxicity that manifests itself clinically as hearing loss. Aminoglycoside ototoxicity is relatively uncommon and clinical trials where levels were carefully monitored and dosing adjusted failed to show a correlation between auditory toxicity and plasma aminoglycoside levels. In situations where dosing is not monitored and adjusted, however, sustained high levels may be associated with ototoxicity. This association is far from clear cut, and new once-daily dosing regimens (and associated high peak serum concentrations) that fail to enhance toxicity further complicate this issue.

Selected Readings

Dipersio JR, "Gentamicin and Other Aminoglycosides," *Clinical Chemistry Theory, Analysis, and Correlation*, 2nd ed, Kaplan LA and Pesce AJ, eds, St Louis, MO: CV Mosby Co, 1989, 1102-8.

Edson RS and Terrell CL, "The Aminoglycosides," *Mayo Clin Proc*, 1999, 74(5):519-28.

Hammett-Stabler CA and Johns T, "Laboratory Guidelines for Monitoring of Antimicrobial Drugs. National Academy of Clinical Biochemistry," *Clin Chem*, 1998, 44(5):1129-40.

Pancoast SJ, "Aminoglycoside Antibiotics in Clinical Use," *Med Clin North Am*, 1987, 72(3):581-612.

German Measles Culture *see* Rubella Virus Culture *on page 575*

German Measles Serology *see* Rubella Serology *on page 575*
GFR *see* Creatinine Clearance *on page 429*
***Giardia* Antigen** *see Giardia* Specific Antigen (GSA65) *on page 473*
***Giardia* Immunoassay** *see Giardia* Specific Antigen (GSA65) *on page 473*
***Giardia* Screen** *see Giardia* Specific Antigen (GSA65) *on page 473*

Giardia Specific Antigen (GSA65)

Synonyms *Giardia* Antigen; *Giardia* Immunoassay; *Giardia* Screen

Test Includes A solid-phase immunoassay based on specific antibody to *Giardia* specific antigen (GSA65)

Specimen

- Fresh random stool, collected in a clean sealable plastic container - refrigerated or frozen until testing.
- Stool in 10% formalin - refrigerated or frozen.
- Stool in Cary-Blair medium - refrigerated or frozen.
- Rectal swabs, transported in Stewart's Culturette® or Ames Charcoal Culturette®. Swabs should not be allowed to dry out.
- Stool in PVA fixative **is not** acceptable.

Reference Range Negative

Use Diagnose giardiasis; monitor effectiveness of anti-*Giardia* therapy

Methodology Solid phase immunoassay

Additional Information A positive result indicates the presence of *Giardia* specific antigen (GGSA65). Secretion of GSA65 is present only when *Giardia* infection is present. GSA65 does not cross react with other enteric parasites, bacteria, or yeast. This test is more sensitive for the diagnosis of *Giardia* than the routine ova and parasite examination. It is not a substitute for the broad screen provided by the ova and parasite examination. An equivalent screening test (immunofluorescent antibody) is available in some laboratories.

Selected Readings

Gardner TB and Hill DR, "Treatment of Giardiasis," *Clin Microbiol Rev*, 2001, 14(1):114-28.
Maddison SE, "Serodiagnosis of Parasitic Diseases," *Clin Microbiol Rev*, 1991, 4(4):457-69.
Wolfe MS, "Giardiasis," *Clin Microbiol Rev*, 1992, 5(1):93-100.

Glomerular Filtration Rate *see* Creatinine Clearance *on page 429*
GMS Stain *see* Methenamine Silver Stain *on page 534*
Gomori-Methenamine Silver Stain *see* Methenamine Silver Stain *on page 534*
Gonorrhea Culture *see Neisseria gonorrhoeae* Culture *on page 547*
Gonorrhea Culture, Throat *see Neisseria gonorrhoeae* Culture *on page 547*

Gram Stain

Related Information

Acid-Fast Stain, Modified, *Nocardia* Species *on page 362*
Actinomyces Culture, All Sites *on page 363*
Interpretation of Gram Stain Results Guidelines *on page 1289*
Methenamine Silver Stain *on page 534*
Periodic Acid-Schiff Stain *on page 563*
Skin Biopsy *on page 580*

Synonyms Bacterial Smear; Smear, Gram Stain

Patient Preparation Same as for routine culture of specific site

Special Instructions The laboratory should be informed of the specific site of specimen, age of patient, current antibiotic therapy, and clinical diagnosis.

Specimen Duplicate of specimen appropriate for routine culture of the specific site

Container Sterile specimen container, or sterile tube or appropriate tube for swab

Collection Collection procedure same as for routine culture of the specific site. Specimen must be collected to avoid contamination with skin, adjacent structures, and nonsterile surfaces.

Storage Instructions Same as for a culture of the specimen

Causes for Rejection Insufficient specimen volume

Turnaround Time Usually same day

Reference Range Depends on site of specimen

Use Determine the presence or absence of bacteria, yeast, neutrophils, and epithelial cells; establish the presence of potentially pathogenic organisms. Also used by microbiology technologists to guide them in the evaluation and identification of growth from virtually all cultures. The Gram stain is essential in the evaluation of all suspected cases of bacterial meningitis.

Limitations Organism isolation and identification will usually be performed only if culture is requested. Request for Gram stain will not lead to stain for mycobacteria (TB). For detection of tubercle bacilli, an acid-fast stain must also be requested. Certain organisms do not stain or do not stain well with Gram stain, eg, *Legionella*
(Continued)

Gram Stain *(Continued)*

pneumophila and *Campylobacter* sp. As many as 30% of cases of bacterial meningitis have a negative Gram stain. Yield may be increased by use of the acridine orange stain (AO) particularly in cases of partially treated meningitis, but few laboratories elect to use this method. Gram stain is **not** reliable for diagnosis of cervical, rectal, pharyngeal, or asymptomatic urethral gonococcal infection, except for gonococcal urethritis in males.

Methodology Gram stain technique:

- Make a thin smear of the material for study and allow to air dry.
- Fix the material to the slide by passing the slide 3 or 4 times through the flame of a Bunsen burner so that the material does not wash off during the staining procedure. Some workers now recommend the use of alcohol for the fixation of material to be Gram stained (flood the smear with methanol or ethanol for a few minutes or warm for 10 minutes at 60°C on a slide warmer).
- Place the smear on a staining rack and overlay the surface with crystal violet solution.
- After 1 minute (less time may be used with some solutions) of exposure to the crystal violet stain, wash thoroughly with distilled water or buffer.
- Overlay the smear with Gram iodine solution for 1 minute. Wash again with water.
- Hold the smear between the thumb and forefinger and flood the surface with acetone-alcohol decolorizer until no violet color washes off. This usually takes 1-3 seconds.
- Wash with running water and again place the smear on the staining rack. Overlay the surface with safranin counterstain for 1 minute. Wash with running water.
- Use paper towels to blot the smear dry.
- Examine the stained smear under the 100x (oil) immersion objective of the microscope. Gram-positive bacteria stain dark blue; gram-negative bacteria appear pink-red.

Additional Information Grams' stain is the single most useful test in clinical microbiology. Gram stains are usually scanned for the presence or absence of white blood cells (indicative of infection) and squamous epithelial cells (indicative of mucosal contamination). A sputum specimen showing more than 25 squamous epithelial cells per low powered field, regardless of the number of white blood cells, is indicative that the specimen is grossly contaminated with saliva and the culture results cannot be properly interpreted. Additional sputum specimens should be submitted to the laboratory if evidence of contamination by saliva is revealed.

The Gram stain can be a reliable indicator to guide initial antibiotic therapy in community acquired pneumonia. It is imperative that a valid sputum specimen be obtained for Gram stain. In a well designed trial, valid expectorated sputum was obtained in 41% (59 of 144 patients). The Gram stain is reliable but not infallible.

Although mycobacteria have classically been considered to be gram-positive or faintly gram-positive, they are more correctly characterized as "gram-neutral" on routine stains. A careful search for mycobacteria should be undertaken when purulent sputum without stainable organisms is encountered.

Gram stains revealing 1 bacterium per high powered (100x) field in an uncentrifuged urine specimen (or any fluid) suggest a colony count of 10^5 bacteria/mL. Bacteria in the majority of fields suggests 10^6 bacteria/mL, a level associated with significant bacteriuria.

Gram stain is the most valuable immediately available diagnostic test in bacterial meningitis. Organisms are detectable in 60% to 80% of patients who have not been treated, and in 40% to 60% of those who have been given antibiotics. Its sensitivity relates to the number of organisms present. The sensitivity of the Gram stain is greater in gram-positive infections, and is only positive in half of the instances of gram-negative meningitis. It is positive even less frequently with listeriosis meningitis or with anaerobic infections.

Culture and Gram stain should always have priority over antigen detection methods.

Selected Readings

Gleckman R, DeVita J, Hibert D, et al, "Sputum Gram's Stain Assessment in Community-Acquired Bacteremic Pneumonia," *J Clin Microbiol*, 1988, 26(5):846-9.

Gray LD and Fedorko DP, "Laboratory Diagnosis of Bacterial Meningitis," *Clin Microbiol Rev*, 1992, 5(2):130-45.

Kobayashi N, Bauer TW, Togawa D, et al, "A Molecular Gram Stain Using Broad Range PCR and Pyrosequencing Technology: A Potentially Useful Tool for Diagnosing Orthopaedic Infections," *Diagn Mol Pathol*, 2005, 14(2):83-9.

Poppert S, Essig A, Stoehr B, et al, "Rapid Diagnosis of Bacterial Meningitis by Real-Time PCR and Fluorescence *in situ* Hybridization," *J Clin Microbiol*, 2005, 43(7):3390-7.

Provine H and Gardner P, "The Gram's Stained Smear and Its Interpretation," *Hosp Pract*, 1974, 9:85-91.

Shigemura K, Shirakawa T, Okada H, et al, "Rapid Detection and Differentiation of Gram-Negative and Gram-Positive Pathogenic Bacteria in Urine Using TaqMan® Probe," *Clin Exp Med*, 2005, 4(4):196-201.

Grocott's Modified Silver Stain *see* Methenamine Silver Stain *on page 534*

Gross and Microscopic Pathology *see* Histopathology *on page 496*

Group A Beta-Hemolytic *Streptococcus* Culture, Throat *see* Throat Culture for Group A Beta-Hemolytic *Streptococcus on page 594*

Group A *Streptococcus* Antigen Test

Related Information

Bacterial Antigens, Rapid Detection Methods *on page 388*
Throat Culture for Group A Beta-Hemolytic *Streptococcus on page 594*

Synonyms Coagglutination Test for Group A Streptococci; *Streptococcus* Group A Latex Screen; Throat Swab for Group A Streptococcal Antigen

Applies to Enzyme Immunoassay for Group A *Streptococcus* Antigen

Test Includes Latex agglutination test for group A *Streptococcus* (GAS) antigen

Special Instructions Some laboratories favor submission of dry swabs for antigen testing. Consult the laboratory for their specific recommendations.

Specimen Throat swab; many laboratories request two swabs, one for culture if the rapid screen is negative. Specimens negative by this test must be cultured to confirm the negative result.

Container Rayon or Dacron swabs rather than cotton swabs enhance the chance of detection.

Collection Rigorous swabbing of the tonsillar pilars and posterior throat increases the probability of detection of streptococcal antigen.

Use Detect the presence of group A streptococcal antigen in throat specimens

Limitations Many reviews have indicated a sensitivity of 75% to 80% and a specificity of 95% to 98% for the rapid methods. Sensitivity varies between manufacturers. Some kits are capable of detecting as few as 10 colony forming units (CFU) on culture while others require 100-1000 CFU on culture. Specimens which yield <10 colonies on culture usually are negative by rapid method. Adequate specimen collection on younger patients may be difficult, and thus, contribute to the false-negative rate. A positive result can be relied upon as a rational basis to begin therapy. **A negative result is only presumptive and a molecular probe test or culture should be performed to reasonably exclude the diagnosis of group A streptococcal infection.** Careful attention to the details of the method and the use of appropriate controls are required to assume adequate performance. Group A streptococcal antigen disappears rapidly following antibiotic therapy. Thus a history of prior therapy should be sought when assessing pharyngitis.

Contraindications The test may become negative 4 hours after therapy has been started.

Methodology The streptococcal group carbohydrate antigen is extracted from the swab used for collection by use of acid or enzyme reagents. The extraction mixture is added to particles coated with antistreptococcal antibody. If the streptococcal antigen is present visible agglutination occurs due to antigen cross links with antibody coated latex within 10 minutes. Enzyme immunoassay methods (EIA) are also used. Nucleic acid (molecular probe) tests are available in some laboratories.

Some laboratories offer molecular testing for this organism. Contact the testing laboratory for the availability of amplified and nonamplified qualitative and quantitative molecular tests for this organism, and for information on selection and collection of appropriate specimens for specific molecular tests.

Additional Information Rheumatic fever remains a concern in the United States and serious complications including sepsis, soft tissue invasion, and toxic shock-like syndrome have been reported to be increasing in frequency; therefore, timely diagnosis and early institution of appropriate therapy remains important. Timely therapy may reduce the acute symptoms and overall duration of streptococcal pharyngitis. The sequelae of poststreptococcal glomerulonephritis and rheumatic fever are diminished by early therapy.

The Infectious Diseases Society of America (IDSA) recently published updated practice guidelines based on a "laboratory algorithm" for the diagnosis and management of group A streptococcal pharyngitis. The IDSA recommendation emphasizes the importance of laboratory confirmation (ie, throat culture or antigen testing) in the diagnosis. The IDSA states, "The diagnosis of acute group A streptococcal pharyngitis should be suspected on clinical and epidemiological grounds and then supported by performance of a laboratory test."

(Continued)

Group A *Streptococcus* Antigen Test *(Continued)*

In contrast to these guidelines, the American College of Physicians - American Society of Internal Medicine in collaboration with the CDC has published an alternative "clinical algorithm" in which laboratory testing plays little, if any role in the diagnosis of group A streptococcal pharyngitis.

Selected Readings

Bisno AL, Gerber MA, Gwaltney JM Jr, et al, "Practice Guidelines for the Diagnosis and Management of Group A Streptococcal Pharyngitis. Infectious Diseases Society of America," *Clin Infect Dis*, 2002, 35(2):113-25.

Bisno AL, Peter GS, and Kaplan EL, "Diagnosis of Strep Throat in Adults: Are Clinical Criteria Really Good Enough?" *Clin Infect Dis*, 2002, 35(2):126-9.

Dagnelie CF, Bartelink ML, van der Graaf Y, et al, "Towards a Better Diagnosis of Throat Infections (With Group A Beta-Haemolytic *Streptococcus*) in General Practice," *Br J Gen Pract*, 1998, 48(427):959-62.

DiMatteo L, "Managing Streptococcal Pharyngitis: A Review of Clinical Decision-Managing Strategies, Diagnostic Evaluation, and Treatment," *J Am Acad Nurse Pract*, 1999, 11(2):57-62.

Gerber MA and Shulman ST, "Rapid Diagnosis of Pharyngitis Caused by Group A Streptococci," *Clin Microbiol Rev*, 2004, 17(3):571-80.

Snow V, Mottur-Pilson C, Cooper RJ, et al, "Principles of Appropriate Antibiotic Use for Acute Pharyngitis in Adults," *Ann Intern Med*, 2001, 134(6):506-8.

Group B *Streptococcus* Antigen Test

Related Information

Bacterial Antigens, Rapid Detection Methods *on page 388*

Genital Culture *on page 470*

Synonyms *Streptococcus agalactiae*, Latex Screen; *Streptococcus* Group B Latex Screen

Test Includes Latex screen for group B beta *Streptococcus*

Special Instructions The specimen should be tested as soon as possible after collection.

Specimen Cerebrospinal fluid, serum, urine, endocervical, vaginal, or amniotic fluid

Container Sterile container, red top tube

Storage Instructions If the specimen cannot be tested immediately it may be stored at 2°C to 8°C for 1 day or frozen at -20°C for longer storage.

Turnaround Time Routine: 24 hours; stat: 1 hour

Use Detect group B *Streptococcus* antigen in body fluids. Detection of group B *Streptococcus* antigen at the time of delivery is usually an indication for chemoprophylaxis.

Limitations Sensitivity is extremely low, 15% to 21%, for rapid group B streptococcal antigen tests, especially in women with low colonization counts. The low sensitivity of the test when used with vaginal and/or rectal specimens precludes its use to detect vaginal colonization prior to delivery. False-positives are rare. Concentrated urine is a good specimen. Testing CSF and serum, as well as culture for the organism, should be considered to establish the definitive diagnosis.

Methodology Latex agglutination (LA). Polystyrene latex particles coated with antibodies specific for the group B *Streptococcus* antigen agglutinate in the presence of the homologous antigen. Controls for nonspecific agglutination of latex particles are generally used. The specimen is heat inactivated and cooled to room temperature before testing. Urine may be concentrated. The infection can be diagnosed by detection of the group B specific carbohydrate antigen of the organism's cell wall which may be present in body fluids, serum and cerebrospinal fluid and which is excreted in urine. Enzyme immunoassay and nucleic acid (molecular probe) tests are available in some laboratories. Culture is the recommended test to detect even low levels of colonization prior to delivery.

Some laboratories offer molecular testing for this organism. Contact the testing laboratory for the availability of amplified and nonamplified qualitative and quantitative molecular tests for this organism, and for information on selection and collection of appropriate specimens for specific molecular tests.

Additional Information Group B *Streptococcus* is currently one of the most significant human pathogens in the neonatal period. The most common mode of acquisition by the neonate is exposure to the maternal genital flora *in utero* through ruptured membranes or by contamination during passage through the birth canal. Rapid identification of group B *Streptococcus* carriers is important in management of premature rupture of the membranes because the effectiveness of intrapartum prophylactic ampicillin may be compromised by awaiting the results of conventional cultures. Infection is manifested in two major forms, early onset septicemic infection manifest in the first few days of life and late onset meningitis which occurs during the first few months of life.

Isolates of group B *Streptococcus* resistant to erythromycin, intermediate to clindamycin, and resistant to cefoxitin, as well as strains with multiple antimicrobial resistance, have been reported. Susceptibility testing may be useful in selecting alternate antibiotic regimens.

Selected Readings

Bergeron MG, Ke D, Menard C, et al, "Rapid Detection of Group B Streptococci in Pregnant Women at Delivery," *N Engl J Med*, 2000, 343(3):175-9.

Centers for Diasease Control and Prevention, "Prevention of Perinatal Group B Streptococcal Disease. Revised Guidelines From CDC," *MMWR*, 2002, 51(RR-11):1-22.

Davies HD, Miller MA, Faro S, et al, "Multicenter Study of a Rapid Molecular-Based Assay for the Diagnosis of Group B *Streptococcus* Colonization in Pregnant Women," *Clin Infect Dis*, 2004, 39(8):1129-35.

Newton ER and Clark M, "Group B *Streptococcus* and Preterm Rupture of Membranes," *Obstet Gynecol*, 1988, 71(2):198-202.

Quinlan JD, Hill DA, Maxwell BD, et al, "The Necessity of Both Anorectal and Vaginal Cultures for Group B *Streptococcus* Screening During Pregnancy," *J Fam Pract*, 2000, 49(5):447-8.

Schuchat A, "Neonatal Group B Streptococcal Disease - Screening and Prevention," *N Engl J Med*, 2000, 343(3):209-10.

HAG *see Histoplasma capsulatum* Antigen Assay *on page 497*

Hair Fungus Culture *see* Fungus Culture, Skin *on page 464*

Hand, Left or Right, X-ray *see* Bone Films *on page 396*

Hands and Wrist Arthritis, X-ray *see* Bone Films *on page 396*

Hanging Drop Mount for *Trichomonas* *see Trichomonas* Preparation *on page 600*

Hank's Stain *see* Acid-Fast Stain, Modified, *Nocardia* Species *on page 362*

Hantavirus Pulmonary Syndrome *see* Hantavirus Serology *on page 477*

Hantavirus Serology

Synonyms Muerto Canyon Strain Virus

Applies to Hantavirus Pulmonary Syndrome

Test Includes Detection of IgM and IgG antibody specific for the Muerto Canyon strain of hantavirus.

Abstract An outbreak of severe respiratory illness associated with respiratory failure, shock, and high mortality was recognized in May, 1993 in the southwestern part of the United States. The cause of the illness was identified as a unique hantavirus now known as the Muerto Canyon strain, and the disease is now called hantavirus pulmonary syndrome (HPS). Since the recognition of this disease, other cases have been recognized in 17 states, with most of the cases occurring west of the Mississippi. HPS begins with nonspecific symptoms such as fever and myalgia, which is followed in 3-6 days by progressive cough and shortness of breath. Common findings during this later stage include tachypnea, tachycardia, fever, and hypotension. Bilateral abnormalities on the chest radiograph are detected, and pleural effusions are common. Hemoconcentration, thrombocytopenia, prolonged activated partial thromboplastin time, an increased proportion of immature granulocytes on the peripheral blood smear, leukocytosis, and elevated levels of serum lactate dehydrogenase and aspartate aminotransferase are found. Serum antibodies are detectable at the time of clinical presentation.

Special Instructions Specimens should be sent to the CDC through state health departments.

Specimen Serum from acute phase of illness

Container Red top tube

Storage Instructions Serum can be stored at 4°C up to 1 week; serum should be stored at -70°C after 1 week and during shipping

Reference Range No detectable hantavirus IgM or less than a fourfold increase in IgG specific for the N and G1 proteins of the Muerto Canyon virus.

Use Confirm the diagnosis of hantavirus pulmonary syndrome

Limitations Assays for the detection of antibody to hantavirus are experimental and none have been approved by the Food and Drug Administration for use in the United States. All requests for testing must be sent to the CDC.

Methodology Western blot; enzyme-linked immunosorbent assay (ELISA)

Additional Information Hantaviruses are single-stranded RNA viruses of the family Bunyaviridae. The Muerto Canyon strain of hantavirus has been found in a proportion of the deer mouse (*Peromyscus maniculatus*) population which is prevalent in the western United States. Thus, this rodent species is thought to be the reservoir for the etiologic agent of HPS. Recommendations for prevention include avoidance of contact with the deer mouse and excreta from deer mice. Currently, no evidence exists for person-to-person transmission of HPS.

HPS can also be diagnosed by detection of hantavirus antigen in tissue by immunohistochemistry with a monoclonal antibody reactive with conserved hantaviral nucleoproteins. In addition, hantaviral nucleotide sequences can be detected in tissue using a reverse transcriptase polymerase chain reaction.

Selected Readings

Butler JC and Peters CJ, "Hantaviruses and Hantavirus Pulmonary Syndrome," *Clin Infect Dis*, 1994, 19(3):387-95.

(Continued)

Hantavirus Serology *(Continued)*

Duchin JS, Koster FT, Peters CJ, et al, "Hantavirus Pulmonary Syndrome: A Clinical Description of 17 Patients With a Newly Recognized Disease. The Hantavirus Study Group," *N Engl J Med*, 1994, 330(14):949-55.

From the Centers for Disease Control and Prevention, "Progress in the Development of Hantavirus Diagnostic Assays - United States," *JAMA*, 1993, 270:1920-1.

Jenison S, Yamada T, Morris C, et al, "Characterization of Human Antibody Responses to Four Corners Hantavirus Infections Among Patients With Hantavirus Pulmonary Syndrome," *J Virol*, 1994, 68(5):3000-6.

HCV Branched DNA *see* Hepatitis C Viral RNA, Quantitative bDNA *on page 487*

HCV Genotyping *see* Hepatitis C Viral RNA Genotyping *on page 486*

HCV Monitor *see* Hepatitis C Viral RNA, Quantitative PCR *on page 488*

HCV PCR *see* Hepatitis C Viral RNA, Quantitative PCR *on page 488*

HCV RNA, bDNA *see* Hepatitis C Viral RNA, Quantitative bDNA *on page 487*

HCV Serology *see* Hepatitis C Serology *on page 484*

HCV Viral Load by bDNA *see* Hepatitis C Viral RNA, Quantitative bDNA *on page 487*

HCV Viral Load by PCR *see* Hepatitis C Viral RNA, Quantitative PCR *on page 488*

Head Lice Identification *see* Arthropod Identification *on page 387*

Head Studies, CT *see* Computed Transaxial Tomography, Head Studies *on page 424*

Helicobacter pylori Antigen, Direct

Related Information

Helicobacter pylori Culture and Urease Test *on page 479*
Helicobacter pylori Culture, Gastric Biopsy *on page 480*
Helicobacter pylori Serology *on page 480*
Helicobacter pylori Urea Breath Test (UBT) *on page 481*

Test Includes Extraction and direct assay for *Helicobacter pylori* antigen in stool

Specimen Fresh liquid, semiliquid, or formed stool; watery specimen is not appropriate for this test and should **not** be tested

Container Clean container, no preservative

Collection Do not place specimen in preservative, transport media, or collect on swab.

Storage Instructions Refrigerate specimen (up to 72 hours if necessary) at 4°C until testing. If testing will be delayed more than 72 hours, specimen should be frozen at -20°C or lower.

Reference Range Negative

Use Detect *Helicobacter pylori* antigens during active infection; monitor drug therapy

Limitations A positive result (antigen detected) is indicative of *H. pylori* presence (96% sensitivity); however some individuals may have *H. pylori* but no disease. A negative result (antigen not detected) indicates absence of *H. pylori* or an antigenic level below the assay limit of detection (184 ng *H. pylori* protein/mL of stool) (96% specificity). False-negative results may be obtained on specimens from patients who have ingested selected compounds (antimicrobial agents, proton pump inhibitors, and bismuth preparations) within 2 weeks prior to specimen collection. In such cases, another specimen should be collected more than 2 weeks after stopping the use of these agents. The test is not recommended for patients younger than 18 years of age.

Methodology Enzyme immunoassay (EIA) using a polyclonal antibody specific for *H. pylori* antigens

Additional Information *Helicobacter pylori* is associated with peptic ulcer disease (duodenal and gastric) and chronic active gastritis. *H. pylori* is also an independent risk factor for gastric cancer and primary malignant lymphoma of the stomach.

A positive result ≥7 days post therapy is indicative of treatment failure. A negative result ≥4 weeks post-therapy indicates eradication of the infection. Repeat testing may be desirable to document sustained eradication beyond 4 weeks post therapy.

In patients highly suspected of having a *H. pylori* infection, this test could be an alternative to endoscopy, urea breath test, and serology. Direct antigen testing is preferable to serology because the presence of IgG antibody indicates past exposure but not necessarily current infection. 50% of patients with positive serology results do not have active *H. pylori* infections.

Selected Readings

Chey W, "Diagnosis of *H. pylori*," *Practical Gastroenterology*, April 2001:28.

Dunn BE, Cohen H, and Blaser MJ, "*Helicobacter pylori*," *Clin Microbiol Rev*, 1997, 10(4):720-41.

Koletzko S, "Noninvasive Diagnostic Tests for *Helicobacter pylori* Infection in Children," *Can J Gastroenterol*, 2005, 19(7):433-9.

Makristhathis A, Pasching E, Schutze K, et al, "Detection of *Helicobacter pylori* in Stool Specimens by PCR and Antigen Enzyme Immunoassay," *J Clin Microbiol*, 1998, 36(9):2772-4.

Ni YH, Lin JT, Huang SF, et al, "Accurate Diagnosis of *Helicobacter pylori* Infection by Stool Antigen Test and 6 Other Currently Available Tests in Children," *J Pediatr*, 2000, 136(6):823-7.

Passaro DJ, Chosy EJ, and Parsonnet J, "*Helicobacter pylori*: Consensus and Controversy," *Clin Infect Dis*, 2002, 35(3):298-304.

Solnick JV and Schauer DB, "Emergence of Diverse *Helicobacter* Species in the Pathogenesis of Gastric and Enterohepatic Diseases," *Clin Microbiol Rev*, 2001, 14(1):59-97.

Vakil N and Fendrick AM, "How to Test for *Helicobacter pylori* in 2005," *Cleve Clin Med J*, 2005, 72(Suppl 2):S8-13.

Veijola L, Oksanen A, Lofgren T, et al, "Comparison of Three Stool Antigen Tests in Confirming *Helicobacter pylori* Eradication in Adults," *Scand J Gastroenterol*, 2005, 40(4):395-401.

Versalovic J, "Intestinal *Helicobacters*," *Clin Microbiol Newslett*, 2002, 24(13):97-101.

Helicobacter pylori Culture and Urease Test

Related Information

Helicobacter pylori Antigen, Direct *on page 478*
Helicobacter pylori Culture, Gastric Biopsy *on page 480*
Helicobacter pylori Serology *on page 480*
Helicobacter pylori Urea Breath Test (UBT) *on page 481*

Synonyms *Campylobacter pylori* Urease Test and Culture; CLO™ Test; Gastric Biopsy Culture for *Helicobacter pylori*; Urease Test and Culture, *Helicobacter pylori*

Test Includes Screening for the presence of urease activity indirectly indicating the presence of *Helicobacter pylori*, culture of the organism from gastric biopsy specimens

Specimen Gastric mucosal biopsy

Container Sterile container; **no fixative** for these microbiologic tests

Storage Instructions If specimen cannot be transported immediately to the laboratory, it should be placed in 0.5 mL transport medium (normal saline).

Turnaround Time 24 hours for urease final report; up to 7 days for culture

Reference Range Negative for urease activity, negative culture, biopsy negative for gastritis and negative for *H. pylori*

Use Establish the presence and possible etiologic role of *Helicobacter pylori* in cases of chronic gastric ulcer, chronic active gastritis, and a relationship with duodenal ulcers

Limitations Culture and urease testing alone, without biopsies, may allow occult neoplasms to go undetected.

Methodology **Urease test**: Gastric biopsies are incubated on slightly buffered medium. A change of phenol red to alkaline (pink color) persisting more than 5 minutes is considered positive and presumptively indicative of the presence of *Helicobacter pylori* even if the organism cannot be grown in culture. Specimens negative at 30 minutes should be re-examined periodically up to 24 hours. The sensitivity of urease testing leaves something to be desired and depends on the selected gold standard. It was only 62% at 24 hours in a 1991 report. This method is also is characterized by false-positive results.

Culture: Most laboratories do not offer this test. Contact the testing laboratory before ordering this test to determine if it is offered. Culture media may include enriched chocolate, Thayer-Martin with antibiotics, brain heart infusion (BHI) with 7% horse blood, and Mueller-Hinton with 5% sheep blood. The organism is microaerophilic and grows best in a reduced O_2 atmosphere or in a Campy-Pak™ system at 42°C. Cultures are usually observed for 7 days before being reported as negative.

Cytology: Touch cytology preparations (ie, imprints from biopsies) may provide a rapid diagnosis and preserve the biopsy specimen for histopathology or culture.

Smear: A direct smear can be Gram stained.

Approximate sensitivities of methods for detection of *H. pylori*:

- 24-hour urease: 62%
- direct Gram stain: 69%
- culture: 90%
- histology: 93%

Additional Information *Helicobacter pylori* is a major cause of chronic active gastritis. Its importance and etiologic relationship with duodenal ulcer requires further study. Seventy-eight percent to 100% of subjects who have duodenal ulcer have *H. pylori* infection, but 3% to 70% of patients without duodenal ulcer have *H. pylori* as well. The organism may be seen in biopsies stained with Gram stain, hematoxylin-eosin (H & E), Giemsa or Warthin-Starry silver stain. It is most often recognized in biopsies of the antrum but may also be seen in the fundic mucosa, metaplastic gastric mucosa of esophagus (Barrett's esophagus), or duodenum. Biopsy may also establish the diagnosis of carcinoma or lymphoma. *H. pylori* was not found in the gastric mucosa of Meckel's diverticula. Gram stains performed by a reuse imprint technique on biopsies from both the antrum and fundus yielded positives in 100% of 32 culture positive cases.

Most peptic ulcers related to *H. pylori* infection are reported as curable.
(Continued)

Helicobacter pylori Culture and Urease Test *(Continued)*

Breath isotope methods measuring bacterial urease by detection of labeled CO_2 and serologic tests for the detection of antibody are also useful but are rarely available. The breath test is preferred as a means of documenting presence of active infection and eradication of infection after therapy in the absence of endoscopy.

The serologic tests can be very helpful but are limited because they can remain positive for months following therapy. Use of specific IgA enhances the value of serology in monitoring therapy.

Past *H. pylori* infection increases risk of carcinoma of stomach. Chronic atrophic gastritis and intestinal metaplasia are related to *H. pylori* infection, which induces as well development of lymphoid tissue in the gastric mucosa. A possible role for *H. pylori* in the development of primary malignant lymphoma of stomach has been postulated.

Selected Readings

Blaser MJ, "*Helicobacter pylori*: Its Role in Disease," *Clin Infect Dis*, 1992, 15(3):386-91.

Hoek FJ, Noach LA, Rauws EJ, et al, "Evaluation of the Performance of Commercial Test Kits for Detection of *Helicobacter pylori* Antibodies in Serum," *J Clin Microbiol*, 1992, 30(6):1525-8.

Passaro DJ, Chosy EJ, and Parsonnet J, "*Helicobacter pylori*: Consensus and Controversy," *Clin Infect Dis*, 2002, 35(3):298-304.

Peterson WL, "*Helicobacter pylori* and Peptic Ulcer Disease," *N Engl J Med*, 1991, 324(15):1043-8.

Solnick JV and Schauer DB, "Emergence of Diverse *Helicobacter* Species in the Pathogenesis of Gastric and Enterohepatic Diseases," *Clin Microbiol Rev*, 2001, 14(1):59-97.

Versalovic J, "Intestinal *Helicobacters*," *Clin Microbiol Newslett*, 2002, 24(13):97-101.

Helicobacter pylori Culture, Gastric Biopsy

Related Information

Helicobacter pylori Antigen, Direct *on page 478*
Helicobacter pylori Culture and Urease Test *on page 479*
Helicobacter pylori Serology *on page 480*
Helicobacter pylori Urea Breath Test (UBT) *on page 481*

Synonyms *Campylobacter pylori*, Gastric Biopsy Culture

Special Instructions Notify laboratory before biopsy to obtain additional instructions and transport media.

Specimen Gastric mucosal biopsy

Container Sterile container, no fixative

Collection Special instructions from laboratory

Storage Instructions Transport specimen to the laboratory immediately. If specimen cannot be transported immediately to the laboratory it should be placed in 0.5 mL transport medium (normal saline).

Causes for Rejection Excessive delay in transport.

Reference Range No *Helicobacter pylori* detected

Use Establish the presence and possible etiologic role of *Helicobacter pylori* in cases of chronic gastric ulcer, gastritis, duodenal ulcer, dyspepsia, etc

Limitations *C. pylori* infections can be very focal. A negative culture does not rule out *C. pylori* or disease that may have been caused by *C. pylori*.

Additional Information *Helicobacter pylori* has been implicated as a factor associated with chronic gastritis. The clinical significance of the organism in regard to gastric or duodenal ulcers, dyspepsia, and gastric carcinoma remains unclear. Other factors such as pepsin, nonsteroidal anti-inflammatory agents (NSAIDs), aspirin, ischemia, stress, alcohol, and bile salts as well as *H. pylori* all may have a role in altering the material mucosal barrier. The relative etiologic role of *H. pylori* remains a subject of speculation. Large numbers of small bacteria, *Helicobacter pylori*, can be cultured from, or seen microscopically (especially with Dieterle stain) in gastric biopsies from most patients with chronic gastritis and/or peptic ulcers. They can also be found in significant numbers of asymptomatic patients who have histologic gastritis, and from some individuals with no abnormality.

Helicobacter pylori Serology

Related Information

Helicobacter pylori Antigen, Direct *on page 478*
Helicobacter pylori Culture and Urease Test *on page 479*
Helicobacter pylori Culture, Gastric Biopsy *on page 480*
Helicobacter pylori Urea Breath Test (UBT) *on page 481*

Synonyms *Campylobacter pylori* Serology

Abstract Persons with peptic ulcer disease either are users of nonsteroidal anti-inflammatory agents or have infection with *H. pylori*. Patients with peptic ulcer disease associated with *H. pylori* have elevated levels of serum antibody against this bacterium. *H. pylori* is very strongly associated with duodenal and gastric ulcer and

chronic active gastritis. It is an independent risk factor for gastric cancer. Antibodies persist as long as a year after treatment.

Specimen Serum or plasma

Container Red top tube; some laboratories use EDTA or heparin tubes

Collection Acute and convalescent samples may be helpful.

Reference Range Undetectable or lower than cutoff limits in commercial assays

Use Increased antibody levels are associated with *H. pylori* infection, chronic active gastritis, and peptic ulcer. Negative serological results provide evidence against these diagnoses.

Limitations Serologic findings provide evidence of past or present infection. A large number of people are infected with the organism but do not have apparent disease. Commercially available assays for diagnosis have sensitivities of 59% to 100% and specificities of 29% to 65%. (In contrast, the sensitivity and specificity of histopathologic examination of gastric mucosal biopsy are well above 90%.) If used to follow response to therapy, long-term follow-up is necessary.

Additional Information *Helicobacter pylori* causes chronic active gastritis. Strong evidence exists that it contributes to the pathogenesis of peptic ulcer diseases. It is linked to gastric carcinoma and lymphoma.

Large numbers of small, spiral-shaped bacteria, *H. pylori*, can be cultured from, or seen microscopically (especially with Dieterle or Giemsa stain) in gastric biopsies from most patients with chronic active gastritis and/or peptic ulcers. They can also be found in significant numbers of asymptomatic patients who have histologic gastritis, and from some individuals with no abnormality. Similarly, patients with chronic gastritis usually have elevated titers of IgG antibodies to *H. pylori*. The association of *H. pylori* infection in development of carcinoma and primary malignant lymphoma of stomach is recognized.

Strong correlation between carbon-13 labeled urea breath testing and serologic testing has been shown in symptom-free subjects.

Selected Readings

Blecker U, Lanciers S, Hauser B, et al, "Serology as a Valid Screening Test for *Helicobacter pylori* Infection in Asymptomatic Subjects," *Arch Pathol Lab Med*, 1995, 119(1):30-2.

Breslin NP and O'Morain CA, "Noninvasive Diagnosis of *Helicobacter pylori* Infection: A Review," *Helicobacter*, 1997, 2(3):111-7.

Harris A, Danesh J, and Forman D, "*Helicobacter pylori* Infection," *Lancet*, 1997, 349(9055):879-80.

Mendall MA, "Serology for Diagnosis of *Helicobacter pylori* Infection," *Helicobacter*, 1997, 2(1):54-5.

Passaro DJ, Chosy EJ, and Parsonnet J, "*Helicobacter pylori*: Consensus and Controversy," *Clin Infect Dis*, 2002, 35(3):298-304.

Solnick JV and Schauer DB, "Emergence of Diverse *Helicobacter* Species in the Pathogenesis of Gastric and Enterohepatic Diseases," *Clin Microbiol Rev*, 2001, 14(1):59-97.

Sung JJ, Chung SC, Ling TK, et al, "Antibacterial Treatment of Gastric Ulcers Associated With *Helicobacter pylori*," *N Engl J Med*, 1995, 332(3):139-42.

Bersalovic J, "Intestinal Helicobacters," *Clin Microbiol Newslett*, 2002, 24(13):97-101.

Helicobacter pylori Urea Breath Test (UBT)

Related Information

Helicobacter pylori Antigen, Direct *on page 478*
Helicobacter pylori Culture and Urease Test *on page 479*
Helicobacter pylori Culture, Gastric Biopsy *on page 480*
Helicobacter pylori Serology *on page 480*

Synonyms Meretek UBT®; UBT; Urea Breath Test

Specimen Two room temperature tubes of a baseline breath sample (1 tube minimum) and 2 tubes of a post ^{13}C-urea ingestion breath sample (1 tube minimum)

Follow patient preparation and sample collection instructions in the Meretek UBT® Collection Kit. When monitoring therapy, collect samples 4 or more weeks after the end of treatment.

Use Therapeutic monitoring in patients with *Helicobacter pylori* infection; differential diagnosis of patients with peptic ulcer disease and chronic active gastritis

Methodology Gas isotope ratio mass spectrometry (GIRMS) is used to detect a change in the ratio of $^{13}CO_2/^{12}CO_2$ in a patient's breath before and after ingestion of ^{13}C-urea (ie, urea labeled with a naturally-occurring, nonradioactive carbon isotope). When *H. pylori*-associated urease degrades urea, the resultant $^{13}CO_2$ is absorbed in blood and exhaled, raising the ratio of $^{13}CO_2/^{12}CO_2$ in the breath. Results are reported as the delta over baseline (DOB), the difference between the $^{13}CO_2/^{12}CO_2$ ratios of the baseline and post ^{13}C-urea ingestion breath samples.

Additional Information *Helicobacter pylori* is associated very strongly with peptic ulcer disease (duodenal and gastric) and chronic active gastritis. *H. pylori* is also an independent risk factor for gastric cancer and primary malignant lymphoma of the stomach. *H. pylori* infection can be treated successfully with a combination of drugs for 10-14 days.

(Continued)

Helicobacter pylori Urea Breath Test (UBT) *(Continued)*

Four methods can be used to diagnose *H. pylori*:

1. Upper GI tract biopsy, microscopic exam, rapid urease testing, culture
2. Urea breath test employing ^{14}C or ^{13}C-urea
3. Antibody detection
4. Antigen detection

This UBT method detects the action of *H. pylori*-associated urease by measuring a change in the $^{13}CO_2/^{12}CO_2$ ratio in the patient's breath.

A delta-over-baseline (DOB) <2.4 indicates the absence of *H. pylori*-associated urease; a negative result, however, does not rule out the possibility of *H. pylori* infection. False-negative results may be due to antimicrobials, proton pump inhibitors (PPIs), and bismuth preparations ingested by the patient within 2 weeks prior to testing or due to collection of a test sample before the recommended interval following ^{13}C-urea ingestion. When clinical signs warrant, a repeat test should be considered with this, or an alternative test method.

A DOB ≥2.4 is associated with the presence of *H. pylori* infection, other gastric spiral organisms such as *H. hellmannii*, and achlorhydria.

Helminths, Blood Preparation *see* Microfilariae, Peripheral Blood Preparation *on page 535*
Helper Cell/Suppressor Ratio *see* T4/T8 Ratio *on page 590*
Hemoflagellates *see* Microfilariae, Peripheral Blood Preparation *on page 535*
Hemogram *see* Complete Blood Count *on page 420*
Hemovac® Tip Culture *see* Intravenous Line Culture *on page 511*
Hepatitis C Gene Product *see* Hepatitis C Serology *on page 484*

Hepatitis A Profile

Related Information

Hepatitis Laboratory Diagnosis and Management *on page 1201*

Test Includes Determination of IgG and IgM antibody to hepatitis A virus and confirmation of all new IgM positives by repeat testing

Specimen Serum

Container Red top tube or serum separator tube

Storage Instructions Transport specimen to the laboratory immediately. Separate serum and freeze.

Reference Range IgG: negative; IgM: negative

Use Determine recent or past infection with hepatitis A virus

Methodology Radioimmunoassay (RIA) or enzyme immunoassay (EIA)

Additional Information Hepatitis A is transmitted by the fecal-oral route, usually food-borne. Its incubation period is 2-7 weeks. Hepatitis A virus is a picornavirus, and antibody is made to capsid proteins. Fecal excretion of HAV peaks before symptoms

HEPATITIS A PROFILE

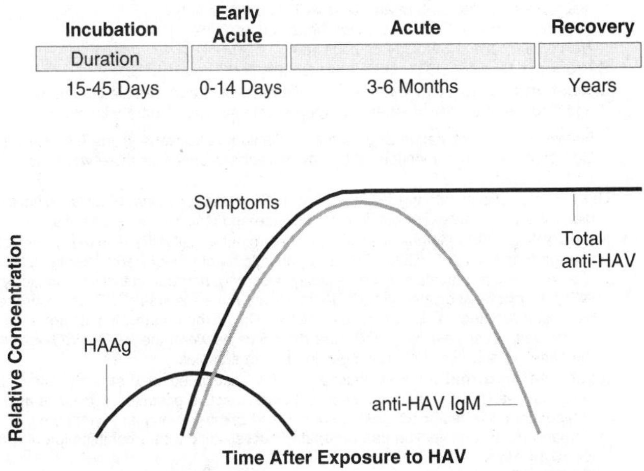

develop. If hepatitis A antibody is IgM, the hepatitis A infection is probably acute. IgM antibody develops within a week of symptom onset, peaks in 3 months, and is usually gone after 6 months. Hepatitis A antibody of IgG type is indicative of old infection, is found in almost half of adults, and is not usually clinically relevant. Many cases of hepatitis A are subclinical, particularly in children. Presence of IgG antibody to HAV does not exclude acute hepatitis B or non-A, non-B hepatitis.

Selected Readings

Cuthbert JA, "Hepatitis A: Old and New," *Clin Microbiol Rev*, 2001, 14(1):38-58.

Hollinger FB and Dreesman GR, "Hepatitis Viruses," *Manual of Clinical Laboratory Immunology*, 5th ed, Rose NR, Conway de Macario E, Folds JD, et al, eds, Washington, DC: American Society for Microbiology, 1997, 702-18.

Mbithi JN, Springthorpe VS, Boulet JR, et al, "Survival of Hepatitis A Virus on Human Hands and Its Transfer on Contact With Animate and Inanimate Surfaces," *J Clin Microbiol*, 1992, 30(4):757-63.

Mishu B, Hadler SC, Boaz VA, et al, "Food-Borne Hepatitis A: Evidence That Microwaving Reduces Risk?" *J Infect Dis*, 1990, 162(3):655-8.

Narbey A, "Update on Viral Hepatitis," *Nurs Times*, 2005, 101(20):55-7.

Summers PL, DuBois DR, Houston Cohen WH, et al, "Solid-Phase Antibody Capture Hemadsorption Assay for Detection of Hepatitis A Virus Immunoglobulin M Antibodies," *J Clin Microbiol*, 1993, 31(5):1299-302.

Wilson TR, "The ABCs of Hepatitis," *Nurse Pract*, 2005, 30(6):12-21.

Hepatitis B Profile

Related Information

Hepatitis Laboratory Diagnosis and Management *on page 1201*

Test Includes Detection of hepatitis B surface antigen (HB_sAg), antibody to hepatitis B surface antigen (anti-HB_s), hepatitis B core antibody (anti-HB_c), and confirmation of all new positives by repeat testing

Specimen Serum

Container Red top tube or serum separator tube

Storage Instructions Transport specimen to the laboratory immediately. Do not store blood.

Causes for Rejection Recently administered radioisotopes if assay performed by RIA, excessive hemolysis

Reference Range Negative

HEPATITIS B PROFILE

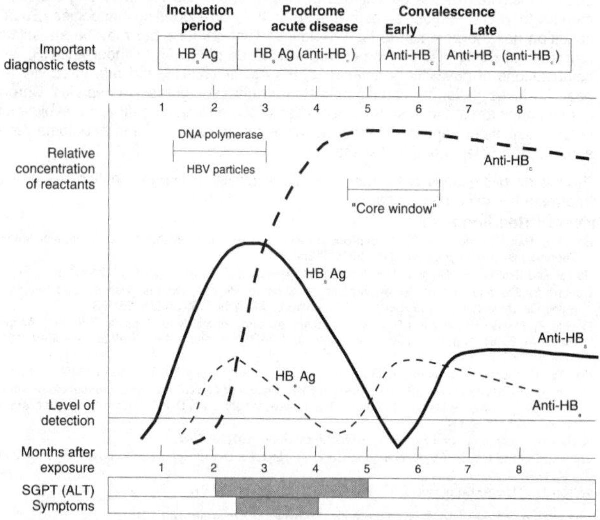

Serologic and clinical patterns observed during acute hepatitis B viral infection. From Hollinger FB and Dreesman GR, *Manual of Clinical Immunology*, 2nd ed, Rose NR and Friedman H, eds, Washington, DC: American Society for Microbiology, 1980, with permission.

Use Determine serological status to hepatitis B virus

Limitations Patients who are negative for HB_sAg may still have acute type B viral hepatitis. There is sometimes a "window" stage when HB_sAg has become negative

(Continued)

Hepatitis B Profile *(Continued)*

and the patient has not yet developed the antibody (anti-HB_sAg). On such occasions the anti-HB_cAg (IgM) is usually positive, and the patient should be treated as potentially infectious until anti-HB_sAg is detected, at which time immunity is probable. In cases with strong clinical suspicion of viral hepatitis, serologic testing should not be limited to detecting HB_sAg but should include a battery of tests to evaluate different stages of acute and convalescent hepatitis. These should include a test for hepatitis A antibody (IgM), and HB_sAg, HB_sAb, HB_cAb (IgM), and hepatitis C virus (HCV).

Presence of HB_sAb is not an absolute indicator of resolved hepatitis infection, nor of protection from future infection. Since there are different serologic subtypes of hepatitis B virus, it is possible (and has been reported) for a patient to have antibody to one surface antigen type and to be acutely infected with virus of a different subtype. Thus, a patient may have coexisting HB_sAg and HB_sAb. Transfused individuals or hemophiliacs receiving plasma components may give false-positive tests for antibody to hepatitis B surface antigen. Individuals vaccinated with HBV vaccine will have antibodies to the surface protein.

Contraindications Patients on heparin therapy may demonstrate weak positive results.

Methodology Radioimmunoassay (RIA); enzyme immunoassay (EIA). Some laboratories offer molecular testing for this organism. Contact the testing laboratory for the availability of amplified and nonamplified qualitative and quantitative molecular tests for this organism, and for information on selection and collection of appropriate specimens for specific molecular tests.

Additional Information Hepatitis B virus (HBV) is a DNA virus with a protein coat, surface antigen (HB_sAg), and a core consisting of nucleoprotein, (HB_cAg is the core antigen). There are eight different serotypes. Early in infection, HB_sAg, HBV DNA, and DNA polymerase can all be detected in serum.

Transmission is parenteral, sexual or perinatal. The incubation period of hepatitis B is 2-6 months. HB_sAg can be detected 1-7 weeks **before** liver enzyme elevation or the appearance of clinical symptoms. Three weeks after the onset of acute hepatitis about 50% of the patients will still be positive for HB_sAg, while at 17 weeks only 10% are positive. The best available markers for infectivity are HB_sAg and HB_eAg. The presence of HB_sAb and HB_eAb is associated with noninfectivity. The chronic carrier state is indicated by the persistence of HB_sAg and/or HB_eAg over long periods (6 months to years) without seroconversion to the corresponding antibodies. Such a condition has the potential to lead to serious liver damage but may be an isolated asymptomatic serologic phenomenon. Persistence of HB_sAg, without anti-HB_s, with combinations of positivity of anti-HB_{core}, HB_eAg, or anti-HB_e indicate infectivity and need for investigation for chronic persistent or chronic aggressive hepatitis. Chronic carrier states are found in up to 10% of cases. Some remain healthy, but evolution to chronic persistent hepatitis, chronic active hepatitis, cirrhosis, and hepatoma represent major problems of this disease.

Prevention of hepatitis B for those at risk is available via vaccination, as well as treatment for some chronic carriers.

Selected Readings

Boal WL, Hales T, and Ross CS, "Blood-Borne Pathogens Among Firefighters and Emergency Medical Technicians," *Prehosp Emerg Care*, 2005, 9(2):236-47.

Buti M and Esteban R, "Drugs in Development for Hepatitis B," *Drugs*, 2005, 65(11):1451-60.

Centers for Disease Control, "Screening Donors of Blood, Plasma, Organs, Tissues, and Semen for Evidence of Hepatitis B and Hepatitis C," *Laboratory Medicine*, 1991, 22(8):555-63.

Devine P, Taswell HF, Moore SB, et al, "Passively Acquired Antibody to Hepatitis B Surface Antigen. Pitfall in Evaluating Immunity to Hepatitis B Viral Infections," *Arch Pathol Lab Med*, 1989, 113(5):529-31.

Fry DE, "Occupational Blood-Borne Diseases in Surgery," *Am J Surg*, 2005, 190(2):249-54.

Hollinger FB and Dreesman GR, "Hepatitis Viruses," *Manual of Clinical Laboratory Immunology*, 5th ed, Rose NR, Conway de Macario E, Folds JD, et al, eds, Washington, DC: American Society for Microbiology, 1997, 702-18.

Narbey A, "Update on Viral Hepatitis," *Nurs Times*, 2005, 101(20):55-7.

Wieland SF and Chisari FV, "Stealth and Cunning: Hepatitis B and Hepatitis C Viruses," *J Virol*, 2005, 79(15):9369-80.

Wilson TR, "The ABCs of Hepatitis," *Nurse Pract*, 2005, 30(6):12-21.

Hepatitis E Antibody, IgG *see* Hepatitis E Serology *on page 490*

Hepatitis C Serology

Related Information

Hepatitis C Viral RNA Genotyping *on page 486*
Hepatitis C Viral RNA, Quantitative bDNA *on page 487*
Hepatitis C Viral RNA, Quantitative PCR *on page 488*
Hepatitis Laboratory Diagnosis and Management *on page 1201*

Synonyms HCV Serology

Applies to Anti-HCV (IgM); C 100-3; Hepatitis C Gene Product; Non-A, Non-B Hepatitis; Surrogate Tests for Non-A, Non-B Hepatitis

Test Includes Detection of antibody specific for hepatitis C in patient's serum

Abstract Most cases of post-transfusion non-A, non-B viral hepatitis are caused by HCV. Application of this test has caused a great decrease of post-transfusion hepatitis.

Patient Preparation Avoid recent administration of radioisotopes if assay is RIA

Specimen Serum

Container Red top tube

Causes for Rejection Recently administered radioisotopes if assay is RIA

Reference Range Negative

Use Differential diagnosis of acute hepatitis; screen blood units for transfusion safety

Limitations Since as many as 90% of commercial intravenous immunoglobulins test positive for hepatitis C antibody, a false-positive can result briefly after such transfusion.

Methodology Radioimmunoassay (RIA), enzyme-linked immunosorbent assay (ELISA). Some laboratories offer molecular testing for this organism. Contact the testing laboratory for the availability of amplified and nonamplified qualitative and quantitative molecular tests for this organism, and for information on selection and collection of appropriate specimens for specific molecular tests.

Additional Information Before initiation of hepatitis B surface antigen testing in the 1970's, most significant post-transfusion hepatitis was due to hepatitis B. Following the development of sensitive and specific testing for hepatitis B, greater than 90% of post-transfusion hepatitis became so called "non-A, non-B." Hepatitis C virus is the most common cause of non-A, non-B hepatitis in the United States. Chiron Corporation has isolated a gene product (c100-3) of hepatitis C virus (HCV) and developed an assay for antibodies to it. The assay detects antibody to the flavivirus which is the etiologic agent of hepatitis C. Non-A, non-B, and non-C hepatitis can still occur, probably due to CMV, hepatitis E, and to other viruses that have not been identified.

For blood donors, hepatitis C serology correlates with surrogate tests for non-A, non-B hepatitis (ALT and anti-HB_c). Since hepatitis C serology identifies a broader group of infected individuals than surrogate testing, it reduces risk of HCV during transfusion. Studies in hemophiliacs indicate that antibody to HCV is a reliable marker of HCV. Recently, IgM anti-HCV core has been shown to be a useful acute marker for HCV infection. Transmission is by intravenous drug abuse, dialysis, and other needlesticks. Sexual transmission also occurs. Before screening for hepatitis C antibody was in place, non-A, non-B hepatitis was said to occur in as many as 10% of transfusions. With the introduction of first generation hepatitis C screening tests, the number has fallen to 1 in 3300 units. With the introduction of a more sensitive second generation hepatitis C test in 1992, safety has increased even more. Chronic carrier states develop in more than half the patients, and chronic liver disease is a major problem. Substantial risk of chronic active hepatitis and cirrhosis exists in those who develop chronic non-A, non-B hepatitis, of whom, about 80% develop anti-HCV. A risk of hepatocellular carcinoma exists for these patients, as well as a risk of liver failure.

Selected Readings

Alter MJ, Margolis HS, Krawczynski K, et al, "The Natural History of Community-Acquired Hepatitis C in the United States," *N Engl J Med*, 1992, 327(27):1899-905.

Bhopale GM and Nanda RK, "Emerging Drugs for Chronic Hepatitis C," *Hepatol Res*, 2005, Jul 12; [Epub ahead of print].

Boal WL, Hales T, and Ross CS, "Blood-Borne Pathogens Among Firefighters and Emergency Medical Technicians," *Prehosp Emerg Care*, 2005, 9(2):236-47.

Braitstein P, Montessori V, Chan K, et al, "Quality of Life, Depression and Fatigue Among Persons Co-infected With HIV and Hepatitis C: Outcomes From a Population-Based Cohort," *AIDS Care*, 2005, 17(4):505-15.

Chandler L, "Diagnostic Tests for Hepatitis C Virus," *Clin Microbiol Newslett*, 2000, 22(19): 145-9.

Chevaliez S and Pawlotsky JM, "Use of Virologic Assays in the Diagnosis and Management of Hepatitis C Virus Infection," *Clin Liver Dis*, 2005, 9(3):371-82.

Cook L, "Hepatitis C Virus Diagnosis and Therapeutic Monitoring: Methods and Interpretation," *Clin Microbiol Newslett*, 1999, 21(9):67-73.

Curry MP and Afdhal NH, "Use of Growth Factors With Antiviral Therapy for Chronic Hepatitis C," *Clin Liver Dis*, 2005, 9(3):439-51.

Everson GT, Trotter J, Forman L, et al, "Treatment of Advanced Hepatitis C With a Low Accelerating Dosage Regimen of Antiviral Therapy," *Hepatology*, 2005, 42(2):255-62.

Fry DE, "Occupational Blood-Borne Diseases in Surgery," *Am J Surg*, 2005, 190(2):249-54.

Gretch DR, "Diagnostic Tests for Hepatitis C," *Hepatology*, 1997, 26(3 Suppl 1):43S-7S.

Jerome KR and Gretch DR, "Laboratory Approaches to the Diagnosis of Hepatitis C Virus Infection," *Minerva Gastroenterol Dietol*, 2004, 50(1):9-20.

Narbey A, "Update on Viral Hepatitis," *Nurs Times*, 2005, 101(20):55-7.

Sethi A and Shiffman ML, "Approach to the Management of Patients With Chronic Hepatitis C Who Failed to Achieve Sustained Virologic Response," *Clin Liver Dis*, 2005, 9(3):453-71.

Wieland SF and Chisari FV, "Stealth and Cunning: Hepatitis B and Hepatitis C Viruses," *J Virol*, 2005, 79(15):9369-80.

(Continued)

Hepatitis C Serology *(Continued)*

Wilson TR, "The ABCs of Hepatitis," *Nurse Pract*, 2005, 30(6):12-21.
Zein NN, "Clinical Significance of Hepatitis C Virus Genotypes," *Clin Microbiol Rev*, 2000, 13(2):223-35.

Hepatitis C Viral RNA Genotyping

Related Information

Hepatitis C Serology *on page 484*
Hepatitis C Viral RNA, Quantitative bDNA *on page 487*
Hepatitis C Viral RNA, Quantitative PCR *on page 488*
Hepatitis Laboratory Diagnosis and Management *on page 1201*

Synonyms Genotyping, HCV; HCV Genotyping

Abstract Hepatitis C virus (HCV) is the primary cause of non-A, non-B hepatitis (NANBH) in the United States. Acute HCV infection is usually without symptoms; however, 85% of infected individuals develop chronic liver infection and frequently progress to cirrhosis and hepatocellular carcinoma. Alpha interferon therapy has been the treatment of choice, although only 20% of patients demonstrate a sustained response. Low pretreatment HCV RNA levels and the absence of cirrhosis prior to treatment are independent, favorable predictors of therapeutic response.

HCV genotype is also an independent predictor of therapeutic response. Subpopulations having genotype 1 respond less favorably than subpopulations having a genotype other than 1 (ie, genotypes 2-6). For example, in two recent studies demonstrating increased response following interferon and ribavirin combination therapy, the subpopulations having genotypes other than 1 had response rates more than twice that of subpopulations with genotype 1, 73% vs 30% (Davis GL, et al) and 66% vs 28% (McHutchison JG, et al). By combining genotype and HCV RNA levels, risk was further stratified. The subpopulation with both a genotype other than 1 and a low pretreatment HCV RNA level ($\leq 2 \times 10^6$ copies/mL) had a response rate of 100%. Thus, HCV genotype, alone or in combination with viral load, can stratify patients according to their likelihood of response to drug therapy.

Special Instructions Use of HCV genotyping should be limited to patients with detectable hepatitis C viral RNA

Specimen Serum

Container Red top tube; yellow top (ACD) tube and lavender top (EDTA) tube are also acceptable

Storage Instructions Separate serum (plasma) from cells within 1 hour of collection and freeze.

Use Predict the likelihood of therapeutic response in patients with hepatitis C infection

Methodology The method used by Quest Diagnostics Inc Nichols Institute includes reverse transcription-polymerase chain reaction (RT-PCR) and DNA sequencing of the NS5B region of the HCV genome (nucleotide positions 7975-8196) and detects HCV genotypes 1-6 and subtypes 1a, 1b, 1cE, 1cO, 2a, 2b, 2c, 3a, 3b, 3c, 3(10a), 4a, 4c, 4d, 4e, 4f, 4g, 4h, 5a, 6a, 6e, 6g, 6i, and 6l, as well as novel subtypes.

Additional Information A HCV genotype 1 indicates a poor potential for response to alpha interferon therapy when used alone or in combination with ribavirin. Conversely, genotypes other than 1 (2-6 and associated subtypes) indicate a significantly higher likelihood for sustained response. HCV genotype should be interpreted in conjunction with pretreatment HCV viral load, pretreatment cirrhosis status, and other clinical and laboratory findings. Any decision to withhold drug therapy must be made very carefully since individual patients may not respond as predicted.

Multiple HCV subtypes indicate multiple infections.

Worldwide HCV Genotypic Subtype Distribution

HCV Genotype	Predominant Geographic Location
1	North America, Europe, East Asia
2	North America, Europe, East Asia
3	North America, Europe, East Asia
4	Middle East, Central Africa
5	South Africa, Southeast Asia
6	South Africa, Southeast Asia

Selected Readings

Boyer N and Marcellin P, "Pathogenesis, Diagnosis, and Management of Hepatitis C," *J Hepatol*, 2000, 32(1 Suppl):98-112.
Chandler L, "Diagnostic Tests for Hepatitis C Virus," *Clin Microbiol Newslett*, 2000, 22(19): 145-9.
Cook L, "Hepatitis C Virus Diagnosis and Therapeutic Monitoring: Methods and Interpretation," *Clin Microbiol Newslett*, 1999, 21(9):67-73.

Distribution of HCV Genotypic Subtypes in the United States

HCV Subtype	Frequency
1a	58%
1b	21%
2b	13%
3a	5%
Other	3%

Davis GL, Esteban-Mur R, Rustgi V, et al, "Interferon Alfa-2b Alone or in Combination With Ribavirin for the Treatment of Relapse of Chronic Hepatitis C. International Hepatitis Interventional Therapy Group," *N Engl J Med*, 1998, 339(21):1493-9.

Elsawy Em, Sobh MA, El-Chenawi FA, et al, "Serotyping of Hepatitis C Virus in Hemodialysis Patients: Comparison With a Standardized Genotyping Assay," *Diagn Microbiol Infect Dis*, 2005, 51(2):91-4.

Fried MW, "Clinical Application of Hepatitis C Virus Genotyping and Quantitation," *Clin Liver Dis*, 1997, 1(3):631-46.

Gerken G, Knolle P, Jakobs S, et al, "Quantification and Genotyping of Serum HCV-RNA in Patients With Chronic Hepatitis C Undergoing Interferon Treatment," *Arch Virol*, 1997, 142(3):459-64.

Gross JB Jr, "Clinician's Guide to Hepatitis C," *Mayo Clin Proc*, 1998, 73(4):355-60.

Hnatyszyn HJ, "Chronic Hepatitis C and Genotyping: The Clinical Significance of Determining HCV Genotypes," *Antivir Ther*, 2005, 10(1):1-11.

Knolle PA, Kremp S, Hohler T, et al, "Viral and Host Factors in the Prediction of Response to Interferon-Alpha Therapy in Chronic Hepatitis C After Long-Term Follow-up," *J Viral Hepat*, 1998, 5(6):399-406.

"Management of Hepatitis C," *NIH Consens Statement*, 1997, 15(3):1-41.

Martinot-Peignoux M, Boyer N, Pouteau M, et al, "Predictors of Sustained Response to Alpha Interferon Therapy in Chronic Hepatitis C," *J Hepatol*, 1998, 29(2):214-23.

McHutchison JG, Gordon SC, Schiff ER, et al, "Interferon Alfa-2b Alone or in Combination With Ribavirin as Initial Treatment for Chronic Hepatitis C. Hepatitis Interventional Therapy Group," *N Engl J Med*, 1998, 339(21):1485-92.

Rolfe KJ, Alexander GJ, Wreghitt TG, et al, "A Real-Time TaqMan® Method for Hepatitis C Virus Genotyping," *J Clin Virol*, 2005, May 11 [Epup ahead of print].

Zein NN, "Clinical Significance of Hepatitis C Virus Genotypes," *Clin Microbiol Rev*, 2000, 13(2):223-35.

Hepatitis C Viral RNA, Quantitative bDNA

Related Information

Hepatitis C Serology *on page 484*
Hepatitis C Viral RNA Genotyping *on page 486*
Hepatitis C Viral RNA, Quantitative PCR *on page 488*
Hepatitis Laboratory Diagnosis and Management *on page 1201*

Synonyms HCV Branched DNA; HCV RNA, bDNA; HCV Viral Load by bDNA

Abstract HCV RNA is a direct measurement of the level of hepatitis C virus. High levels of virus have been associated with lack of response to interferon treatment whereas low levels of virus have been associated with an increased rate of sustained response. Thus, quantitative HCV RNA testing can eliminate potentially ineffective and costly therapy by identifying nonresponders prior to initiation of therapy. Alanine aminotransferase (ALT), HCV RNA levels, or repeat liver biopsies can be used to assess response, or lack thereof, once therapy has been initiated. Patients who normalize ALT but do not have an appreciable change in HCV RNA within 3 months are less likely to benefit from further therapy. Quantitative HCV RNA levels need to be assessed in combination with all available clinical, biochemical, and liver biopsy information.

Specimen Serum

Container Red top tube

Storage Instructions Remove serum from clot within 1 hour of collection and freeze immediately.

Reference Range <0.2 million Eq/mL (lowest reportable value: 0.2 million Eq/mL); one equivalent (Eq) is approximately 1 copy of HCV RNA

Use Assess prognosis prior to initiation of antiviral therapy, predict response to alpha interferon therapy, monitor the effect of antiviral therapy, individualize antiviral therapy. HCV viral load is increased in active HCV infection, decreased likelihood of response to alpha interferon therapy (suggested by high initial viral load levels), insufficient therapeutic response (suggested by persistent elevation of viral load levels). HCV viral load is decreased in response to therapy and remission.

Limitations This test is for research use only. It is not to be used as a diagnostic procedure without confirmation of the diagnosis by another established product or procedure.

Methodology Branched DNA (bDNA) signal amplification in which viral RNA is captured on the surface of a microtiter well by synthetic oligonucleotides coating the

(Continued)

Hepatitis C Viral RNA, Quantitative bDNA *(Continued)*

well. The solid-phase bound viral RNA is hybridized to multiple-branched DNA molecules. Alkaline phosphatase-labeled probes are in turn hybridized to the branched DNA and reacted with a chemiluminescent substrate to produce a greatly amplified light signal. The amount of light emitted is directly proportional to the quantity of RNA in the specimen. This method demonstrates equal quantification of HCV genotypes 1-6.

Selected Readings

Alter HJ, "To C or Not to C: These Are the Questions," *Blood*, 1995, 85(7):1681-95.

Chandler L, "Diagnostic Tests for Hepatitis C Virus," *Clin Microbiol Newslett*, 2000, 22(19):145-9.

Cook L, "Hepatitis C Virus Diagnosis and Therapeutic Monitoring: Methods and Interpretation," *Clin Microbiol Newslett*, 1999, 21(9):67-73.

Davis GL, Lau JY, Urdea MS, et al, "Quantitative Detection of Hepatitis C Virus RNA With a Solid-Phase Signal Amplification Method: Definition of Optimal Conditions for Specimen Collection and Clinical Application in Interferon-Treated Patients," *Hepatology*, 1994, 19(6):1337-41.

Detmer J, Lagier R, Flynn J, et al, "Accurate Quantitation of Hepatitis C Virus (HCV) RNA From All HCV Genotypes by Using Branched-DNA Technology," *J Clin Microbiol*, 1996, 34(4):901-7.

Fried MW and Hoofnagle JH, "Therapy of Hepatitis C," *Semin Liver Dis*, 1995, 15(1):82-91.

Gretch DR, dela Rosa C, Carithers RL Jr, et al, "Assessment of Hepatitis C Viremia Using Molecular Amplification Technologies: Correlations and Clinical Implications," *Ann Intern Med*, 1995, 123(5):321-9.

Lau JY, Davis GL, Kniffen J, et al, "Significance of Serum Hepatitis C Virus RNA Levels in Chronic Hepatitis C," *Lancet*, 1993, 341(8859):1501-4.

Lau JY, Mizokami M, Ohno T, et al, "Discrepancy Between Biochemical and Virological Responses to Interferon-Alpha in Chronic Hepatitis C," *Lancet*, 1993, 342(8881):1208-9.

Martinot-Peignoux M, Marcellin P, Ponteau M, et al, "Pretreatment Serum Hepatitis C Virus RNA Levels and Hepatitis C Virus Genotype Are the Main and Independent Prognostic Factors of Sustained Response to Interferon Alfa Therapy in Chronic Hepatitis C, " *Hepatology*, 1995, 22(4 Pt 1):1050-6.

Nomura H, Kimura Y, Rikimaru N, et al, "Usefulness of HCV-RNA Assays in Efficacy Evaluation of Interferon Treatment for Chronic Hepatitis C: Amplicor HCV Assay and Branched DNA Probe Assay," *J Infect*, 1997, 34(3):249-55.

Shiratori Y, Kato N, Yokosuka O, et al, "Quantitative Assays for Hepatitis C Virus in Serum as Predictors of the Long-Term Response to Interferon," *J Hepatol*, 1997, 27(3):437-44.

Wada M, Kang KB, Nishigami T, et al, "Importance of Pretreatment Viral Load and Monitoring of Serum Hepatitis C Virus RNA in Predicting Response to Interferon-Alpha2a Treatment of Chronic Hepatitis C. Hanshin Chronic Hepatitis C Study Group," *J Interferon Cytokine Res*, 1997, 17(11):707-12.

Wilber JC and Polito A, "Serological and Virological Diagnostic Tests for Hepatitis C Virus Infection," *Semin Gastrointest Dis*, 1995, 6(1):13-9.

Zein NN, "Clinical Significance of Hepatitis C Virus Genotypes," *Clin Microbiol Rev*, 2000, 13(2):223-35.

Hepatitis C Viral RNA, Quantitative PCR

Related Information

Hepatitis C Serology *on page 484*
Hepatitis C Viral RNA Genotyping *on page 486*
Hepatitis C Viral RNA, Quantitative bDNA *on page 487*
Hepatitis Laboratory Diagnosis and Management *on page 1201*
Polymerase Chain Reaction *on page 567*

Synonyms Amplicor™ HCV Monitor; HCV Monitor; HCV PCR; HCV Viral Load by PCR

Abstract HCV RNA is a direct measurement of the level of hepatitis C virus. High levels of virus have been associated with lack of response to interferon treatment whereas low levels of virus have been associated with an increased rate of sustained response. Thus, quantitative HCV RNA testing can eliminate potentially ineffective and costly therapy by identifying nonresponders prior to initiation of therapy. Alanine aminotransferase (ALT), HCV RNA levels, or repeat liver biopsies can be used to assess response, or lack thereof, once therapy has been initiated. Patients who normalize ALT but do not have an appreciable change in HCV RNA within 3 months are less likely to benefit from further therapy. Quantitative HCV RNA levels need to be assessed in combination with all available clinical, biochemical, and liver biopsy information.

Specimen Serum

Container Red top tube

Storage Instructions Remove serum from clot within 1 hour of collection and freeze. Do not thaw.

Reference Range Not detected (lowest reportable value: 500 copies/mL)

Use Indicate infectivity, confirm HCV antibody test results, assess prognosis prior to initiation of antiviral therapy, predict response to alpha interferon therapy, monitor the effect of antiviral therapy, individualize antiviral therapy. HCV viral load is increased in active HCV infection, decreased likelihood of response to alpha interferon therapy (suggested by high initial viral load levels), insufficient therapeutic response (suggested by persistent elevation of viral load levels). HCV viral load is decreased in response to therapy and remission.

Limitations This test is for research only. It is not to be used as a diagnostic procedure without confirmation of the diagnosis by another established product or procedure.

Methodology Reverse transcription-polymerase chain reaction (RT-PCR) in which viral RNA is extracted from serum. RNA is then reverse-transcribed into DNA and amplified with biotin-labeled HCV-specific primers by the polymerase chain reaction (PCR). An internal quantitation standard (IQS) is also amplified. The amplification products are hybridized to capture probes and detected with an avidin-HRP conjugate in a colorimetric assay. Viral copy numbers are quantified as the ratio of viral and IQS products.

This method is more sensitive than the branched DNA (bDNA) method.

Selected Readings

Berger A, Braner J, Doerr HW, et al, "Quantification of Viral Load: Clinical Relevance for Human Immunodeficiency Virus, Hepatitis B Virus, and Hepatitis C Virus Infection," *Intervirology*, 1998, 41(1):24-34.

Bhopale GM and Nanda RK, "Emerging Drugs for Chronic Hepatitis C," *Hepatol Res*, 2005, Jul 12; [Epub ahead of print].

Braitstein P, Montessori V, Chan K, et al, "Quality of Life, Depression and Fatigue Among Persons Co-infected With HIV and Hepatitis C: Outcomes From a Population-Based Cohort," *AIDS Care*, 2005, 17(4):505-15.

Chandler L, "Diagnostic Tests for Hepatitis C Virus," *Clin Microbiol Newslett*, 2000, 22(19): 145-9.

Chevaliez S and Pawlotsky JM, "Use of Virologic Assays in the Diagnosis and Management of Hepatitis C Virus Infection," *Clin Liver Dis*, 2005, 9(3):371-82.

Cook L, "Hepatitis C Virus Diagnosis and Therapeutic Monitoring: Methods and Interpretation," *Clin Microbiol Newslett*, 1999, 21(9):67-73.

Curry MP and Afdhal NH, "Use of Growth Factors With Antiviral Therapy for Chronic Hepatitis C," *Clin Liver Dis*, 2005, 9(3):439-51.

Everson GT, Trotter J, Forman L, et al, "Treatment of Advanced Hepatitis C With a Low Accelerating Dosage Regimen of Antiviral Therapy," *Hepatology*, 2005, 42(2):255-62.

Fanning L, Kenny E, Sheehan M, et al, "Viral Load and Clinicopathological Features of Chronic Hepatitis C in a Homogeneous Patient Population," *Hepatology*, 1999, 29(3):904-7.

Fried MW and Hoofnagle JH, "Therapy of Hepatitis C," *Semin Liver Dis*, 1995, 15(1):82-91.

Fry DE, "Occupational Blood-Borne Diseases in Surgery," *Am J Surg*, 2005, 190(2):249-54.

Martinot-Peignoux M, Marcellin P, Ponteau M, et al, "Pretreatment Serum Hepatitis C Virus RNA Levels and Hepatitis C Virus Genotype Are the Main and Independent Prognostic Factors of Sustained Response to Interferon Alfa Therapy in Chronic Hepatitis C, " *Hepatology*, 1995, 22(4 Pt 1):1050-6.

Narbey A, "Update on Viral Hepatitis," *Nurs Times*, 2005, 101(20):55-7.

Sethi A and Shiffman ML, "Approach to the Management of Patients With Chronic Hepatitis C Who Failed to Achieve Sustained Virologic Response," *Clin Liver Dis*, 2005, 9(3):453-71.

Shiratori Y, Kato N, Yokosuka O, et al, "Quantitative Assays for Hepatitis C Virus in Serum As Predictors of the Long-Term Response to Interferon," *J Hepatol*, 1997, 27(3):437-44.

Wada M, Kang KB, Nishigami T, et al, "Importance of Pretreatment Viral Load and Monitoring of Serum Hepatitis C Virus RNA in Predicting Response to Interferon-Alpha2a Treatment of Chronic Hepatitis C. Hanshin Chronic Hepatitis C Study Group," *J Interferon Cytokine Res*, 1997, 17(11):707-12.

Wieland SF and Chisari FV, "Stealth and Cunning: Hepatitis B and Hepatitis C Viruses," *J Virol*, 2005, 79(15):9369-80.

Wilson TR, "The ABCs of Hepatitis," *Nurse Pract*, 2005, 30(6):12-21.

Zein NN, "Clinical Significance of Hepatitis C Virus Genotypes," *Clin Microbiol Rev*, 2000, 13(2):223-35.

Hepatitis D Serology

Related Information

Hepatitis Laboratory Diagnosis and Management *on page 1201*

Synonyms Delta Agent Serology; Delta Hepatitis Serology

Abstract Hepatitis D virus (HDV) was first recognized in 1977 by Rizzetto and colleagues. HDV always occurs as a simultaneous coinfection with hepatitis B (HBV). Patients coinfected with HDV and HBV have fulminant hepatitis more often than patients infected with HBV alone. Testing for serological markers of HDV should be considered when a patient shows clinical signs of acute or fulminant hepatitis.

Patient Preparation Avoid recent administration of radioisotopes

Specimen Serum

Container Red top tube

Causes for Rejection Recently administered radioisotopes

Reference Range Negative

Use Differential diagnosis of chronic, recurrent, and acute viral hepatitis

Methodology Radioimmunoassay (RIA), enzyme-linked immunosorbent assay (ELISA)

Additional Information Hepatitis D virus ("delta" agent) is an incomplete RNA virus, or viroid, that can only infect livers already infected by hepatitis B virus. It may occur, therefore, as coinfection with acute HBV hepatitis or super imposed on chronic HBV infection. It cannot occur in an HB_sAg-negative individual. IgG and IgM antibodies to HDV develop 5-7 weeks after infection. IgM antibody is most useful in distinguishing those patients with active liver disease. HDAg can be detected in serum or liver biopsies but is technically demanding and offers little to diagnosis. False-positive EIA results have been reported in patients with lipemia or high titer rheumatoid factor. Studies of liver transplants in patients with end-stage liver disease due to hepatitis B/D have shown, through serial biopsies post-transplant, that HDV viral reinfection occurs within 1 week but without damage. Not until HBV proliferation occurs several weeks to months later does one find histologic and clinical changes.

(Continued)

Hepatitis D Serology *(Continued)*

Hepatitis D Superinfection

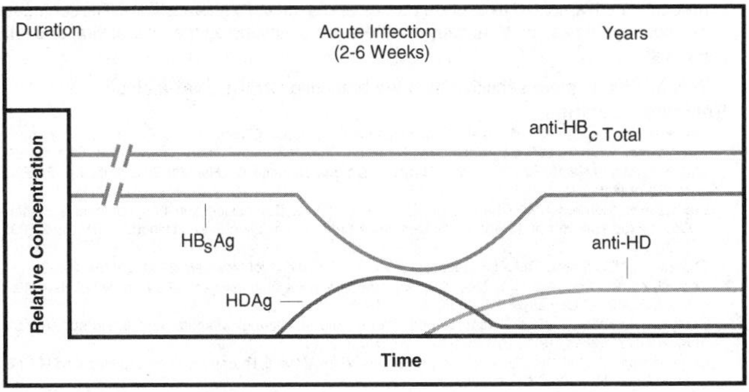

Reprinted from Abbott Diagnosis

Hepatitis D Coinfection

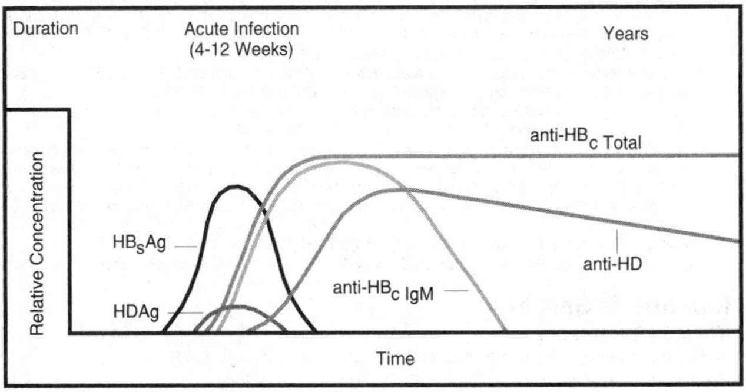

Reprinted from Abbott Diagnostics

Selected Readings

Craig JR, "Hepatitis Delta Virus - No Longer A Defective Virus," *Am J Clin Pathol*, 1992, 98(6):552-3, (editorial).

Davies SE, Lau JY, O'Grady JG, et al, "Evidence That Hepatitis D Virus Needs Hepatitis B Virus to Cause Hepatocellular Damage," *Am J Clin Pathol*, 1992, 98(6):554-8.

Ferenci P, Formann E, and Romeo R, "Successful Treatment of Chronic Hepatitis D With a Short Course of Peginterferon Alfa-2a," *Am J Gastroenterol*, 2005, 100(7):1626-7.

Narbey A, "Update on Viral Hepatitis," *Nurs Times*, 2005, 101(20):55-7.

Niro GA, Rosina F, and Rizzetto M, "Treatment of Hepatitis D," *J Viral Hepat*, 2005, 12(1):2-9.

Polish LB, Gallagher M, Fields HA, et al, "Delta Hepatitis: Molecular Biology and Clinical and Epidemiological Features," *Clin Microbiol Rev*, 1993, 6(3):211-29.

Wilson TR, "The ABCs of Hepatitis," *Nurse Pract*, 2005, 30(6):12-21.

Hepatitis E Serology

Related Information

Hepatitis Laboratory Diagnosis and Management *on page 1201*

Synonyms Antihepatitis E Virus; Anti-HEV; Hepatitis E Antibody, IgG; HEV Antibody, IgG

Specimen Serum

Collection Samples from individuals with suspected HEV infection should be collected as early in the course of illness as possible.

Storage Instructions Refrigerate serum.

Reference Range Nonreactive

Use Diagnose acute hepatitis E viral (HEV) infection; differential diagnosis of enteric hepatitis. HEV IgG increased in HEV infection; HEV decreased in the absence of HEV infection, early in HEV infection (prior to seroconversion), and in past, resolved HEV infection

Limitations A nonreactive test result does not rule out acute HEV infection (prior to seroconversion) or past HEV infection

Methodology Enzyme immunoassay (EIA); anti-HEV antibodies in the patient serum bind to two recombinant HEV antigens coating the polystyrene well. Following a wash to remove unbound material, HRP-conjugated goat antihuman IgG is added to bind to the antigen-antibody complexes. After a second wash, *o*-phenylenediamine (OPD) substrate is added, resulting in production of a yellow-orange color. The amount of color produced is directly proportional to the amount of antibody present in the patient specimen. Results are reported as nonreactive or repeatedly reactive.

Additional Information This test is for research use only. It is not to be used as a diagnostic procedure without confirmation of the diagnosis by another established product or procedure.

Hepatitis E virus (HEV) is the major etiologic agent of enterically transmitted non-A, non-B hepatitis in developing countries. In the United States, it is usually diagnosed in recent travelers to endemic areas (India, Asia, Africa, and Central America). Like hepatitis A, HEV occurs in both sporadic and epidemic forms and causes an acute, moderately severe, but not chronic, hepatitis that is frequently cholestatic. Unlike hepatitis A virus, HEV progresses to fatal fulminant hepatitis in at least 10% to 20% of pregnant patients, especially in the third trimester. The infection may also manifest without jaundice or be present subclinically.

Hepatitis E IgG antibodies have been detected in up to 93% of patients during the acute phase. In most patients, IgG antibodies are short lived, often being undetectable 6-12 months after onset; however, duration up to 4.5 years has been observed.

Selected Readings

Fields HA, Favorov MO, and Margolis II, "The Hepatitis E Virus: A Review," *J Clin Immunoassay*, 1993, 16:215-222.

Narbey A, "Update on Viral Hepatitis," *Nurs Times*, 2005, 101(20):55-7.

Purdy MA and Krawczynski K, "Hepatitis E," *Gastroenterol Clin North Am*, 1994, 23(3):537-46.

Schlauder GG and Dawson GJ, "Hepatitis E Virus," *Manual of Clinical Microbiology*, 8th ed, Murray PR, Baron EJ, Jorgensen JH, et al, eds, Washington, DC: American Society for Microbiology, 2003, 1495-511.

"Self-Learning Review, Hepatitis E," *Can Fam Physician*, 1998, 44:2648, 2652.

Wilson TR, "The ABCs of Hepatitis," *Nurse Pract*, 2005, 30(6):12-21.

Yang G and Vyas GN, "Immunodiagnosis of Viral Hepatitides A to E and Non-A to -E," *Clin Diagn Lab Immunol*, 1996, 3(3):247-56.

Herpes 1 and 2 *see* Herpes Simplex Antibody *on page 492*

Herpes Culture *see* Herpes Simplex Virus Culture *on page 494*

Herpes Cytology

Related Information

Herpes Simplex Antibody *on page 492*
Herpes Simplex Virus by Direct Immunofluorescence *on page 493*
Herpes Simplex Virus Culture *on page 494*
Herpes Simplex Virus Isolation, Rapid *on page 495*
Skin Biopsy *on page 580*

Synonyms Herpetic Inclusion Bodies, Cytology; Inclusion Body Stain; Tzanck Smear; Viral Study, Herpes

Test Includes Preparation of cytological smears, staining of smears, and microscopic evaluation for viral inclusions

Abstract Herpes simplex virus (HSV) infection may be asymptomatic or lead to ulcerated painful lesions of epithelial lined surfaces. Infected epithelial cells demonstrate characteristic nuclear changes including multinucleation, molding, and chromatin margination. In the Tzanck preparation, cells obtained from herpesvirus-induced vesicles are cytologically examined. This test may lead to a rapid diagnosis, but is only positive in ~50% of cases. Cytologic examination of gastrointestinal tract and genitourinary tract specimens can be used for diagnosis, but tissue biopsy is complimentary to these studies. Herpes simplex virus can also be detected in urine and CSF fluid. Genital herpes simplex virus infection can be associated with neonatal morbidity and mortality and therefore, its diagnosis in pregnant patients is important. Life-threatening herpesvirus infections include those in neonates and encephalitis.

Special Instructions A stat Pap stain can be requested at the time of delivery if active herpes is suspected.

Specimen Direct scrape of lesion

Collection Firmly scrape the edge of the lesion, preferably a bullous lesion after removal of the bulla. The edge of normal skin and ulcer is to be scraped. In sites other

(Continued)

Herpes Cytology *(Continued)*

than skin, a direct scrape is done. The scrape may be done with a wooden spatula, tongue blade, scalpel, or Culturette®.

Causes for Rejection Improper fixation, air drying artifact

Use Establish the presence of herpesvirus infection

Limitations Tzanck smears cannot provide distinction between HSV-1 and HSV-2. Neonatal herpes is most often due to type 2 infection. Herpes inclusions may not be seen in 50% of active lesions. Interpretation can be difficult. **Viral culture is the definitive diagnostic method.** Polymerase chain reaction has been utilized successfully in detection of HSV and VZV DNA sequences and has been reported as equivalent or superior to viral culture. Biopsy is also useful.

Methodology Pap stained smear, immunoperoxidase stain for herpes viral antigen

Additional Information Diagnostic yield is increased by immunoperoxidase or immunofluorescent procedures, which become positive before characteristic viral cytopathic changes develop. Smears with a heavy inflammatory exudate may be difficult to interpret because of nonspecific staining. Smears must be done with and without the primary antibody and positive and negative controls must be run concurrently.

Selected Readings

Arvin AM and Prober CG, "Herpes Simplex Viruses," *Manual of Clinical Microbiology*, 7th ed, Murray PR, Baron EJ, Pfaller MA, et al, eds, Washington, DC: American Society for Microbiology, 1999, 878-87.

Corey L and Holmes KK, "Genital Herpes Simplex Virus Infections: Current Concepts in Diagnosis, Therapy, and Prevention," *Ann Intern Med*, 1983, 98(6):973-83.

Corey L and Spear PG, "Infections With Herpes Simplex Viruses," *N Engl J Med*, 1986, 314(12):686-91 and 749-56.

Herpes Hominis 1 and 2 *see* Herpes Simplex Antibody *on page 492*

Herpes Simplex 1 and 2 Culture *see* Herpes Simplex Virus Culture *on page 494*

Herpes Simplex Antibody

Related Information

Herpes Cytology *on page 491*
Herpes Simplex Virus by Direct Immunofluorescence *on page 493*
Herpes Simplex Virus Culture *on page 494*
Herpes Simplex Virus Isolation, Rapid *on page 495*
Skin Biopsy *on page 580*

Synonyms Herpes 1 and 2; Herpes Hominis 1 and 2

Test Includes HSV 1 and 2

Specimen Serum

Container Red top tube or serum separator tube

Reference Range Interpretation depends on whether episode is initial or reinfection. IgG and IgM specific antibodies may give more useful information about an acute event.

Limitations Extensive background antibody in the population, and cross reaction of HSV 1 and HSV 2 responses make test useful only in epidemiology. The test is not generally useful except to determine rising titers.

Methodology Immunofluorescence, hemagglutination, complement fixation, enzyme immunoassay (EIA)

If serological testing is performed by enzyme immunoassay (EIA) on automated instrumentation, results are usually given in index units, not titers. In such cases, significant rises in antibody levels are determined by algorithms within the instrumentation, not by increases in titers.

Some laboratories offer molecular testing for this organism. Contact the testing laboratory for the availability of amplified and nonamplified qualitative and quantitative molecular tests for this organism, and for information on selection and collection of appropriate specimens for specific molecular tests.

Many reference laboratories now offer EIA which can discriminate between IgG antibodies to HSV-I and IgG antibodies to HSV-II. The test cannot discriminate between the two types of IgM antibodies. Contact the testing laboratory before ordering these tests.

Additional Information A primary HSV 1 or HSV 2 infection will produce a classical rising antibody titer. However, because exposure to herpesvirus is almost universal (50% to 90% of adults have antibodies) the background of antibody makes the serologic response in any particular episode of recurrence difficult to interpret. This is made especially true by the fact the antibody to one virus type may be stimulated by infection with the heterologous virus type. Both false-positive and false-negatives are common with currently licensed enzyme immunoassays. Collecting the requisite paired sera to delineate which titers are rising or stable generally adds nothing to clinical management, and thus herpes serology cannot be recommended in routine

clinical cases. However, in research settings or for epidemiologic studies serologic definition of the type of herpes infection have been worthwhile.

Herpes serology has not been proved clinically useful in determining whether cesarean delivery should be undertaken in pregnant patients with questionably active herpes. Pap smear or immunochemical demonstration of viral antigen is more useful for this. Nor is herpes serology usually helpful in the differential of a very sick infant with possible congenital herpes. Because of the fulminant course, even early IgM antibody may not be demonstrable in time to contribute to care.

Selected Readings

Ashley R, Cent A, Maggs V, et al, "Inability of Enzyme Immunoassays to Discriminate Between Infections With Herpes Simplex Virus Types 1 and 2," *Ann Intern Med*, 1991, 115(7):520-6.

Ashley RL and Wald A, "Genital Herpes: Review of the Epidemic and Potential Use of Type-Specific Serology," *Clin Microbiol Rev*, 1999, 12(1):1-8.

Corey L and Spear PG, "Infections With Herpes Simplex Viruses," *N Engl J Med*, 1986, 314(12):686-91 and 749-56.

Guerry SL, Bauer HM, Klausner JD, et al, "Recommendations for the Selective Use of Herpes Simplex Virus Type 2 Serological Tests," *Clin Infect Dis*, 2005, 40(1):38-45.

Stewart JA, "Herpes Simplex Virus," *Manual of Clinical Laboratory Immunology*, 5th ed, Rose NR, Conway de Macario E, Folds JD, et al, eds, Washington, DC: American Society for Microbiology, 1997, 625-30.

Wald A and Ashley-Morrow R, "Serological Testing for Herpes Simplex Virus (HSV)-1 and HSV-2 Infection," *Clin Infect Dis*, 2002, 35(Suppl 2):S173-82.

Herpes Simplex Virus Antigen Detection *see* Herpes Simplex Virus by Direct Immunofluorescence *on page 493*

Herpes Simplex Virus by Direct Immunofluorescence

Related Information

Herpes Cytology *on page 491*
Herpes Simplex Antibody *on page 492*
Herpes Simplex Virus Culture *on page 494*
Herpes Simplex Virus Isolation, Rapid *on page 495*
Skin Biopsy *on page 580*

Synonyms Herpes Simplex Virus Antigen Detection; HSV Antigen Detection, Direct

Test Includes Direct (nonculture) detection of HSV-infected cells

Special Instructions Make more than one slide preparation

Specimen Basal cells of a freshly unroofed lesion rolled onto a clean microscope slide

Sampling Time Preferably within 3 days of lesion eruption

Collection Make a preparation of cells taken from the suspected herpetic lesion onto a plain 1" x 3" glass slide. Cells from the bottom of an ulcer or vesicle should be scraped with a swab, scalpel or curette. Swabs should be **rolled** (**not** smeared) across a small area of the slide several times, and cells scraped with a scalpel should be gently dabbed onto the slide. The best specimen is a collection of the cells at the base of an intact vesicle. Cells from a diseased cornea can also be used. **The smear should be air dried at room temperature.**

Storage Instructions Do not store the specimen. Send it to the laboratory immediately.

Causes for Rejection Insufficient quantity of specimen on slide, poorly prepared or labeled slides

Turnaround Time Less than 1 day

Reference Range No herpes simplex virus-infected cells detected

Use Rapid detection of herpes simplex virus in oral or genital lesions

Limitations Some of the variables in this test include proper collection of specimens, stage and location of lesion, and community prevalence of the disease.

The efficiency of detection of HSV material depends in great part on the collection of a sufficiently large number of intact infected cells from the lesion. It is important to obtain cells from the base of an intact vesicle if at all possible. The presence of infected cells decreases as the lesion heals, and crusted lesions may have little or no herpes antigenic material remaining.

Methodology Immunoperoxidase or immunofluorescence staining of collected cells

Additional Information In certain situations, this direct antigen detection test can be more sensitive than cell culture; however, and in general, this test is only approximately 70% as sensitive as cell culture. In critical situations, clinicians should consider using both methods.

Air-dried preparations on slides can also be stained with Giemsa or Diff-Quik™ stains (Tzanck). Fixed preparations (usually 95% ethanol) can also be stained with the Papanicolaou or immunoperoxidase methods. Smears fixed with hairspray and subsequently stained with the Papanicolaou stain usually are excellent preparations.

HSV can also be detected by PCR and subsequent molecular probe testing.

(Continued)

Herpes Simplex Virus by Direct Immunofluorescence *(Continued)*

Selected Readings

Arvin AM and Prober CG, "Herpes Simplex Viruses," *Manual of Clinical Microbiology*, 7th ed, Murray PR, Baron EJ, Pfaller MA, et al, eds, Washington, DC: American Society for Microbiology, 1999, 878-87.

Coyle PV, Desai A, Wyatt D, et al, "A Comparison of Virus Isolation, Indirect Immunofluorescence and Nested Multiplex Polymerase Chain Reaction for the Diagnosis of Primary and Recurrent Herpes Simplex Type 1 and Type 2 Infections," *J Virol Methods*, 1999, 83(1-2):75-82.

Fredricks DN and Relman DA, "Application of Polymerase Chain Reaction to the Diagnosis of Infectious Diseases," *Clin Infect Dis*, 1999, 29:475-88.

Herpes Simplex Virus Culture

Related Information

Herpes Cytology *on page 491*
Herpes Simplex Antibody *on page 492*
Herpes Simplex Virus by Direct Immunofluorescence *on page 493*
Herpes Simplex Virus Isolation, Rapid *on page 495*

Synonyms Herpes Culture; Herpes Simplex 1 and 2 Culture; HSV 1 and 2 Culture; HSV Culture

Applies to Viral Culture, Eye; Viral Culture, Genital; Viral Culture, Skin

Test Includes Culture for HSV only; HSV also is usually detected in a routine/general virus culture

Special Instructions Special viral transport medium must be obtained from the laboratory prior to collection of specimen.

Specimen Specimen depends on type of infection:

- genital - vesicle fluid, lesion, endocervical
- conjunctivitis - conjunctival
- congenital - throat, vesicle, cerebrospinal fluid
- encephalitis - brain biopsy
- meningitis - cerebrospinal fluid
- respiratory/oral - throat, vesicle

Container Sterile container; cold viral transport medium for swabs

Collection All specimens should be kept cold and moist. As for most viral cultures, specimens should be collected in the acute stage of the disease, preferably within 3 days and no longer than 7 days after the onset of illness. Spinal fluid specimens should be submitted in the usual sterile tube; no special transport medium is necessary. All other specimens should be collected on a sterile swab as described and **the swab should be placed into cold viral transport medium immediately after collection**.

Endocervical: Swab cervix with enough force to obtain epithelial cells.

Vesicular lesion: Wash vesicles with sterile saline. Carefully open several vesicles and soak up vesicular fluid with swab. If vesicles are absent, vigorously swab base of lesion (specimen should be collected during first 3 days of eruption, because specimens collected later in the course of disease rarely yield virus).

Conjunctival: Using a moistened swab, firmly rub conjunctiva using sufficient force to obtain epithelial cells.

Throat, respiratory, oral: Rotate swab in both tonsillar crypts and against posterior oropharynx.

Storage Instructions Specimens should be delivered to the laboratory and handed to a technologist within 30 minutes of collection. Outpatient specimens: If transport is to be delayed more than 30 minutes after collection, specimen **must** be refrigerated (held at 4°C to 8°C) until it can be transported to the laboratory. Do not freeze specimen.

Causes for Rejection Dry specimen, specimen not refrigerated during transport, specimen fixed in formalin, unlabeled specimen

Turnaround Time Variable (1-14 days) and depends on culture method used and amount of virus in specimen

Reference Range No virus isolated

Use Aid in the diagnosis of HSV disease

Methodology Inoculation of specimen into cell cultures, incubation of cultures, observation of characteristic cytopathic effect, and identification by fluorescent monoclonal antibodies specific for type 1 or 2.

Some laboratories offer molecular testing for this organism. Contact the testing laboratory for the availability of amplified and nonamplified qualitative and quantitative molecular tests for this organism, and for information on selection and collection of appropriate specimens for specific molecular tests.

Additional Information HSV can only rarely be isolated from the CSF of patients with HSV 1 encephalitis. The virus is occasionally isolated from spinal fluid of patients with HSV 2 meningitis and of neonates with congenital herpes and from urine from patients with primary genital HSV infections concurrent with cystitis.

Serology for the detection of herpes simplex virus is available, but the results usually are of value only in the diagnosis of primary HSV infections. There is much cross-reaction between the antibodies to HSV 1 and HSV 2.

HSV can also be detected by PCR and subsequent molecular probe testing.

Selected Readings

Ashley RL and Wald A, "Genital Herpes: Review of the Epidemic and Potential Use of Type-Specific Serology," *Clin Microbiol Rev*, 1999, 12(1):1-8.

Brugha R, Brown D, Meheus A, et al, "Should We Be Screening for Asymptomatic HSV Infections?" *Sex Transm Infect*, 1999, 75(3):142-4.

Coyle PV, Desai A, Wyatt D, et al, "A Comparison of Virus Isolation, Indirect Immunofluorescence and Nested Multiplex Polymerase Chain Reaction for the Diagnosis of Primary and Recurrent Herpes Simplex Type 1 and Type 2 Infections," *J Virol Methods*, 1999, 83(1-2):75-82.

Fredricks DN and Relman DA, "Application of Polymerase Chain Reaction to the Diagnosis of Infectious Diseases," *Clin Infect Dis*, 1999, 29:475-88.

Jerome KR and Ashley RL, "Herpes Simplex Viruses and Herpes B Virus," *Manual of Clinical Microbiology*, 8th ed, Murray PR, et al, eds, Washington, DC: American Society for Microbiology, 2003, 1291-303.

LaRocco MT, "Evaluation of an Enzyme-Linked Viral Inducible System for the Rapid Detection of Herpes Simplex Virus," *Eur J Clin Microbiol Infect Dis*, 2000, 19(3):233-5.

Herpes Simplex Virus, Direct Detection *see* Virus Detection by DFA *on page 619*

Herpes Simplex Virus Isolation, Rapid

Related Information

Herpes Cytology *on page 491*
Herpes Simplex Antibody *on page 492*
Herpes Simplex Virus by Direct Immunofluorescence *on page 493*
Herpes Simplex Virus Culture *on page 494*

Synonyms HSV Shell Vial Method, Spin Amplification

Applies to Culture, HSV Only; HSV, Rapid Isolation; Skin Culture for HSV

Test Includes Inoculation of cell cultures in shell vials, 16-hour incubation, and immunofluorescence staining for HSV 1 and 2

Specimen Swab of genital, lip, or mucous membrane lesion; vesicular fluid; biopsy

Container Sterile container; cold viral transport medium for swabs

Collection All specimens should be kept cold and moist. As for most viral cultures, specimens should be collected in the acute stage of the disease, preferably within 3 days and no longer than 7 days after the onset of illness. Spinal fluid specimens should be submitted in the usual sterile tube; no special transport medium is necessary. All other specimens should be collected on a sterile swab as described and **the swab should be placed into cold viral transport medium immediately after collection**.

Endocervical: Swab cervix with enough force to obtain epithelial cells.

Vesicular lesion: Wash vesicles with sterile saline. Carefully open several vesicles and soak up vesicular fluid with swab. If vesicles are absent, vigorously swab base of lesion (specimen should be collected during first 3 days of eruption, because specimens collected later in the course of disease rarely yield virus).

Conjunctival: Using a moistened swab, firmly rub conjunctiva using sufficient force to obtain epithelial cells.

Throat, respiratory, oral: Rotate swab in both tonsillar crypts and against posterior oropharynx.

Turnaround Time Overnight to 2 days depending on method and capability of laboratory

Reference Range No HSV detected

Use Aid in the diagnosis of disease caused by HSV

Methodology Shell vial isolation technique with direct immunofluorescent staining for HSV 1 and HSV 2. Specimens are centrifuged onto cell cultures grown on coverslips in the bottoms of 1-dram shell vials. Centrifugation greatly accelerates virus attachment and penetration. After incubation, fluorescein-labeled monoclonal antibodies are applied to the infected cells to detect viral antigens that are expressed in the membranes of the cells. Characteristic fluorescent foci indicate the presence of virus.

Some laboratories offer molecular testing for this organism. Contact the testing laboratory for the availability of amplified and nonamplified qualitative and quantitative molecular tests for this organism, and for information on selection and collection of appropriate specimens for specific molecular tests.

(Continued)

Herpes Simplex Virus Isolation, Rapid *(Continued)*

Additional Information The rapid shell vial culture technique for the detection of HSV 1 and 2 has been reported to be as sensitive as conventional cell culture methods.

HSV can also be detected by PCR and subsequent molecular probe testing.

Selected Readings

Ashley RL and Wald A, "Genital Herpes: Review of the Epidemic and Potential Use of Type-Specific Serology," *Clin Microbiol Rev*, 1999, 12(1):1-8.

Fredricks DN and Relman DA, "Application of Polymerase Chain Reaction to the Diagnosis of Infectious Diseases," *Clin Infect Dis*, 1999, 29:475-88.

Jerome KR and Ashley RL, "Herpes Simplex Viruses and Herpes B Virus," *Manual of Clinical Microbiology*, 8th ed, Murray PR, et al, eds, Washington, DC: American Society for Microbiology, 2003, 1291-303.

Herpes Zoster Serology *see* Varicella-Zoster Virus Serology *on page 612*

Herpetic Inclusion Bodies, Cytology *see* Herpes Cytology *on page 491*

HEV Antibody, IgG *see* Hepatitis E Serology *on page 490*

HHV-6, IgM, IgG *see* Human Herpesvirus 6, IgG and IgM Antibodies, Quantitative *on page 506*

Hip Arthrogram *see* Arthrogram *on page 387*

Hip, Left or Right, X-ray *see* Bone Films *on page 396*

Hip, Left or Right, and Pelvis, X-ray *see* Bone Films *on page 396*

Hips Arthritis, X-ray *see* Bone Films *on page 396*

Histo Antigen *see* *Histoplasma capsulatum* Antigen Assay *on page 497*

Histopathology

Related Information

Aerobic Culture, Body Fluid *on page 365*
Biopsy Culture, Routine *on page 390*
Fungus Culture, Biopsy *on page 461*
Fungus Culture, Body Fluid *on page 462*
Liver Biopsy *on page 521*
Lymph Node Biopsy *on page 529*
Methenamine Silver Stain *on page 534*
Muscle Biopsy *on page 538*
Mycobacteria Culture, Biopsy or Body Fluid *on page 539*
Periodic Acid-Schiff Stain *on page 563*
Skin Biopsy *on page 580*
Virus Detection by DFA *on page 619*

Synonyms Biopsy; Gross and Microscopic Pathology; Pathologic Examination; Surgical Pathology; Tissue Examination

Applies to Bronchial Biopsy; Endoscopic Biopsy; Lung Biopsy; Medical Legal Specimens

Test Includes Gross and microscopic examination and diagnosis. Imprints may be made if the tissue is fresh and unfixed and if indications for imprints exist.

Abstract Surgical pathology has been defined as the discipline which deals with the anatomic pathology of tissues removed from living patients. Smears, aspirates, special stains, immunocytochemistry, flow cytometry, and molecular pathology may be included.

Patient Preparation It is essential that each specimen be accompanied by an adequate description of what it is thought to represent, as well as an appropriate clinical history.

Special Instructions Consult the laboratory prior to beginning the procedure for specific instructions. Requisition should state operative diagnosis and source of specimen, as well as patient's name, age, sex, room or location, name of surgeon, and names of other physicians who will need a copy of the pathology report.

Specimen Fresh tissue, tissue fixed in phosphate-buffered formalin or other appropriate fixative. Each specimen container must be labeled to include source as well as patient's name. Each specimen from a different anatomic site must be placed in a separate, correctly labeled container, designated "left," "right," "proximal," "distal," "ventral," "dorsal," and so forth.

Container Jars of assorted sizes, containing formalin or another appropriate fixative; the neck of the container should not be smaller than its diameter. Fresh specimens should be submitted on a sterile gauze pad moistened with sterile saline and should not be left on countertops; they must be placed in the hands of a responsible person.

Collection Small biopsy specimens are to be placed immediately in fixative, unless special needs such as frozen section exist. Use approximately 5-20 times as much

fixative solution as the bulk of the tissue. Small tissues such as those from bronchoscopic biopsy, bladder biopsy, and endometrium can be ruined in a very short time by drying out.

Storage Instructions Fixation in formalin solution or other appropriate fixative

Causes for Rejection Mislabeled specimen container, unlabeled specimen

Turnaround Time Biopsy reports commonly require a day or more. Delays are caused by need for clinical information, deeper sections, decalcification, or special stains.

Use Histopathologic diagnosis; evaluate extent of lesions and provision of classification and, when appropriate, grading in the case of tumors

Limitations Tissue fixed in formalin **cannot** be used for microbial culture, chemical estrogen or progesterone receptor assay, certain types of histochemistry, frozen sections, gene rearrangement, or optimal electron microscopy.

Additional Information A major advantage of conventional over frozen sections is that extensive sampling of the entire specimen can take place.

Cultures of tissue are best taken in the O.R., where a sterile field exists. A piece of tissue should be placed in an appropriate sterile container with requests for smear, culture, anaerobic culture, mycobacteria, and fungus culture if appropriate. It should be immediately taken to the Microbiology Laboratory. See test listings of suspected organism and specific site cultures.

Routine tissues are brought in fixative. Fixatives should be picked up prior to the biopsy. Commonly used fixatives include modified Zenker's fluid (for tiny specimens, eg, endometrial curettage, liver, and other needle biopsies, **not** skin), and formalin (for specimens thicker than 3 mm).

Bullets, shotgun pellets, and other metallic objects require special handling, but no fixative is needed. Of major importance in handling bullets and other specimens of possible forensic significance, including vaginal swabs obtained in rape cases, is the scrupulous maintenance of a chain-of-custody. Specimens must be accurately labeled, and transfer and receipt must be documented. Specimens must be kept under safeguards in the laboratory until turned over to law enforcement officials.

Bone biopsy for metabolic bone disease requires special handling.

Materials sometimes not sent for histopathologic examination, depending on the institution, include bullets, shotgun pellets, neonatal foreskins, grossly unremarkable placentas from uneventful deliveries, and orthopedic appliances. If a specimen is not sent to the Pathology Department, the surgeon should carefully describe the specimen in the operative report.

***Histoplasma capsulatum* Antibody and Antigen** *see* Histoplasmosis Serology *on page 498*

Histoplasma capsulatum Antigen Assay

Synonyms HAG; Histo Antigen; HPA

Test Includes Detection of *H. capsulatum* polysaccharide antigen

Special Instructions Call testing laboratory to determine availability of test.

Specimen Urine is the preferred specimen but can be done on blood, bronchoalveolar lavage, or other sterile body fluids

Container Sterile container for urine or body fluid, red top tube for blood

Storage Instructions Stable for 7 days at 4°C.

Reference Range Negative: <1.0 unit; indeterminate: 1.0-2.0 units; positive: >2.0 units

Use Assist in the diagnosis of disseminated histoplasmosis

Limitations Sensitivity of assay varies with the severity of infection: disseminated: 92%, acute pulmonary: 44%, chronic pulmonary: 21%, meningitis: 67%. Specificity of this assay is approximately 98%. False-positive results may occur with other systemic mycoses.

Methodology Enzyme immunoassay (EIA)

Some laboratories offer molecular testing for this organism. Contact the testing laboratory for the availability of amplified and nonamplified qualitative and quantitative molecular tests for this organism, and for information on selection and collection of appropriate specimens for specific molecular tests.

Additional Information The *Histoplasma* antigen is not only useful in the initial diagnosis but may be used to follow patients and for detection of relapse. Patients with suspected relapse experience a 2 unit rise in antigen, and patients with a definite relapse experience at least a 4 unit rise. Patients that are responding to therapy show a continual decline in antigen and approximately 70% of AIDS patients after 1 year of chronic suppressive therapy will have a urine HAG <4.0 units. Of note, there is

(Continued)

Histoplasma capsulatum Antigen Assay *(Continued)*

significant run variability, and one should not compare previous reported results with the most recent result. The last specimen has been stored and is run concurrently with the newly obtained specimen. Results of the repeated last specimen and the new specimen are available with an interpretation of these results by the Histoplasmosis Reference Laboratory.

Selected Readings

Bracca A, Tosello ME, Girardini JE, et al, "Molecular Detection of *Histoplasma capsulatum var. capsulatum* in Human Clinical Samples," *J Clin Microbiol*, 2003, 41(4):1753-5.

Durkin MM, Connolly PA, and Wheat LJ, "Comparison of Radioimmunoassay and Enzyme-Linked Immunoassay Methods for Detection of *Histoplasma capsulatum* var *capsulatum* Antigen," *J Clin Microbiol*, 1997, 35(9):2252-5.

Lee BL, Tauber MG, and Aberg JA, "Histoplasmosis" *The AIDS Knowledge Base*, 3rd ed, Chapter 59, Philadelphia, PA: Lippincott, Williams & Wilkins, 1999.

Moser SA, "Laboratory Diagnosis of Histoplasmosis," *Clin Microbiol Newslett*, 1999, 21(12):95-101.

Wheat JL, "Current Diagnosis of Histoplasmosis," *Trends Microbiol*, 2003, 11(10):488-94.

Wheat J, Sarosi G, McKinsey D, et al, "Practice Guidelines for the Management of Patients With Histoplasmosis," *Clin Infect Dis*, 2000, 30:688-95.

Wheat J, Wheat H, Connolly P, et al, "Cross-Reactivity in *Histoplasma capsulatum* Variety *capsulatum* Antigen Assays of Urine Samples From Patients With Endemic Mycoses," *Clin Infect Dis*, 1997, 24(6):1169-71.

Wheat LJ, Garringer T, Brizendine E, et al, "Diagnosis of Histoplasmosis by Antigen Detection Based Upon Experience at the Histoplasmosis Reference Laboratory," *Diagn Microbiol Infect Dis*, 2002, 43(1):29-37.

Histoplasmosis Immunodiffusion *see* Fungal Serology *on page 458*

Histoplasmosis Serology

Related Information

Periodic Acid-Schiff Stain *on page 563*

Applies to *Histoplasma capsulatum* Antibody and Antigen

Test Includes Reaction with yeast and mycelial antigens

Specimen Serum (antibody); urine (antigen)

Container Red top tube, plastic urine container

Collection Acute and convalescent sera are recommended, especially when acute titers are only presumptive

Reference Range Antibody: less than a fourfold change in titer between acute and convalescent samples; titers <1:4; negative CSF. Antigen: negative.

Use Diagnosis and prognosis of histoplasmosis

Limitations A negative result does not rule out histoplasmosis. Histoplasmin skin testing may interfere with results. Testing with both antigens must be performed. There are cross reactions with other fungi. Anticomplementary sera cannot be tested for complement fixing antibodies. The latex agglutination test gives some false-positives, and must be confirmed with another procedure.

Contraindications Previous skin testing

Methodology Complement fixation (CF), immunodiffusion (ID), latex agglutination (LA), radioimmunoassay (RIA) (antigen), enzyme immunoassay (EIA)

Additional Information CF titers of 1:8 or 1:16 are presumptive evidence of histoplasmosis. Titers ≥1:32 are highly suggestive of *H. capsulatum* infection but cannot be relied on as the sole means of diagnosis. Complement fixation and immunodiffusion each detect about 85% of disease. H and M bands on immunodiffusion indicate active disease. Complement fixation is less sensitive to disseminated or chronic disease. The latex agglutination test detects IgM antibodies and is positive early in disease, but not in late, chronic, or recurrent infection.

Tests for fungal antigen are now available and obviate some of the problems of ordinary serology - cross reactions, decreased immune response, need for paired specimens over time. The use of enzyme immunoassay and radioimmunoassay to detect *H. capsulatum* antigen has proven to be a useful approach in the diagnosis of histoplasmosis. Antigenuria or antigenemia is excellent evidence of disseminated disease.

In addition to histoplasmosis in immunologically intact individuals, this fungal infection is a serious opportunistic infection in patients with AIDS (occasionally as its first manifestation).

Selected Readings

Bracca A, Tosello ME, Girardini JE, et al, "Molecular Detection of *Histoplasma capsulatum var. capsulatum* in Human Clinical Samples," *J Clin Microbiol*, 2003, 41(4):1753-5.

Kaufman L, Kovacs JA, and Reiss E, "Clinical Immunomycology," *Manual of Clinical Laboratory Immunology*, 5th ed, Rose NR, Conway de Macario E, Folds JD, et al, eds, Washington, DC: American Society for Microbiology, 1997, 585-604.

Wheat JL, "Current Diagnosis of Histoplasmosis," *Trends Microbiol*, 2003, 11(10):488-94.

Wheat J, Sarosi G, McKinsey D, et al, "Practice Guidelines for the Management of Patients With Histoplasmosis," *Clin Infect Dis*, 2000, 30:688-95.

Wheat LJ, Garringer T, Brizendine E, et al, "Diagnosis of Histoplasmosis by Antigen Detection Based Upon Experience at the Histoplasmosis Reference Laboratory," *Diagn Microbiol Infect Dis*, 2002, 43(1):29-37.

HIV-1 Drug Resistance Testing *see* HIV Genotyping *on page 503*

HIV-1 Gene Sequencing *see* HIV Genotyping *on page 503*

HIV-1 Mutations Testing *see* HIV Genotyping *on page 503*

HIV-1 RNA, Expanded Range *see* HIV-1 RNA, Quantitative PCR, 2nd Generation *on page 500*

HIV-1 RNA, Qualitative PCR *see* HIV-1 RNA, Quantitative PCR, 2nd Generation *on page 500*

HIV-1 RNA, Quantitative bDNA, 3rd Generation

Related Information

HIV-1 RNA, Quantitative PCR, 2nd Generation *on page 500*
HIV-1 Serology *on page 501*
HIV Genotyping *on page 503*

Synonyms bDNA Testing for HIV; HIV bDNA; HIV Branched DNA; HIV Viral Load

Special Instructions This test is intended for use only in individuals with known HIV-1 infection. Qualitative tests may be used for diagnosis.

Specimen Plasma

Container Lavender top (EDTA) tube

Storage Instructions Remove plasma from cells within 6 hours of collection and freeze.

Reference Range 50 copies/mL

Use Monitor progression of HIV infection, assess prognosis, monitor the effect of antiretroviral drug therapy HIV viral load is increased in acute HIV infection, increased risk of progression to AIDS, disease progression, clinical AIDS, and drug resistance. HIV viral load is decreased in response to therapy and remission.

Methodology Branched DNA (bDNA) signal amplification in which viral RNA is extracted, captured by solid-phase bound synthetic oligonucleotides and hybridized to target probes and multiple-branched DNA molecules. Alkaline phosphatase-labeled probes are in turn hybridized to the branched DNA and reacted with a chemiluminescent substrate to produce a greatly amplified light signal. The amount of light emitted is directly proportional to the quantity of RNA in the specimen.

Additional Information The measurement of HIV-1 RNA provides the most direct and accurate assessment of HIV viral load, or viremia, by quantifying the amount of HIV-1 RNA in plasma. Levels of HIV RNA are elevated during primary HIV-1 infection preceding seroconversion. During the years of clinical latency, patients maintain a relatively constant, individually variable level of RNA. As infection progresses and the immune system weakens, HIV-1 RNA levels increase. The plasma viral RNA level has been shown to be a better independent predictor of progression to AIDS and death than the number of $CD4^+$ T-cells. Changes in RNA levels have been shown to be the most accurate indicator of the patient's response to therapy. Plasma HIV RNA levels must increase or decrease more than threefold (0.5 log) to be clinically significant in an individual patient.

Selected Readings

Cao Y, Ho DD, Todd J, et al, "Clinical Evaluation of Branched DNA Signal Amplification for Quantifying HIV Type 1 in Human Plasma," *AIDS Res Hum Retroviruses*, 1995, 11(3):353-61.

Carpenter CC, Fischl MA, Hammer SM, et al, "Antiretroviral Therapy for HIV Infection in 1998: Updated Recommendations of the International AIDS Society-USA Panel," *JAMA*, 1998, 280(1):78-86.

Christopherson C, Lu SD, and Kwok S, "Laboratory Markers of Antiviral Activity," *Antivir Ther*, 1998, 3(4):247-50.

Cu-Uvin S, "Women and HIV Infections," *Clin Microbiol Newslett*, 2000, 22(21):161-5.

Dewar RL, Highbarger HC, Sarmiento MD, et al, "Application of Branched DNA Signal Amplification to Monitor Human Immunodeficiency Virus Type 1 Burden in Human Plasma," *J Infect Dis*, 1994, 170(5):1172-9.

Ginocchio CC, "HIV Testing: The Next Step Beyond Viral Load," *Clin Microbiol Newslett*, 1999, 21(11):83-94.

Helbert M and Breuer J, "Monitoring Patients With HIV Disease," *J Clin Pathol*, 2000, 53(4):266-72.

Lange CG, "When to Start Antiretroviral Therapy in HIV-1 Infection," *Clin Microbiol Newslett*, 2001, 23(18):139-43.

Mellors JW, Kingsley LA, Rinaldo CR Jr, et al, "Quantitation of HIV-1 RNA in Plasma Predicts Outcome After Seroconversion," *Ann Intern Med*, 1995, 122(8):573-9.

Mellors JW, Rinaldo CR Jr, Gupta P, et al, "Prognosis in HIV-1 Infection Predicted by the Quantity of Virus in Plasma," *Science*, 1996, 272(5265):1167-70.

Pachl C, Todd JA, Kern DG, et al, "Rapid and Precise Quantification of HIV-1 RNA in Plasma Using a Branched DNA Signal Amplification Assay," *J Acquir Immune Defic Syndr Hum Retrovirol*, 1995, 8(5):446-54.

Perelson AS, Neumann AU, Markowitz M, et al, "HIV-1 Dynamics *in vivo*: Virion Clearance Rate, Infected Cell Life-Span, and Viral Generation Time," *Science*, 1996, 271(5255):1582-6.

Volberding PA, "HIV Quantification: Clinical Applications," *Lancet*, 1996, 347(8994):71-3.

HIV-1 RNA, Quantitative PCR, 1st Generation *see* HIV-1 RNA, Quantitative PCR, 2nd Generation *on page 500*

HIV-1 RNA, Quantitative PCR, 2nd Generation

Related Information

HIV-1 RNA, Quantitative bDNA, 3rd Generation *on page 499*
HIV-1 Serology *on page 501*
HIV Genotyping *on page 503*
Human Immunodeficiency Virus Culture *on page 506*
p24 Antigen *on page 555*
Polymerase Chain Reaction *on page 567*

Synonyms HIV-1 RNA, Quantitative PCR, Ultrasensitive; HIV Polymerase Chain Reaction; HIV Viral Load; Human Immunodeficiency Virus 1 RNA, 2nd Generation

Applies to HIV-1 RNA, Expanded Range; HIV-1 RNA, Qualitative PCR; HIV-1 RNA, Quantitative PCR, 1st Generation

Abstract The measurement of HIV-1 RNA provides the most direct and accurate assessment of HIV viral load, or viremia, by quantifying the amount of HIV-1 RNA in plasma. Levels of HIV RNA are elevated during primary HIV-1 infection preceding seroconversion. During the years of clinical latency, patients maintain a lower, and relatively constant, level of RNA. As the infection progresses and the immune system weakens, HIV-1 RNA levels increase. The HIV RNA level and the number of $CD4^+$ T-cells combined are a more accurate predictor of progression to AIDS and death than either marker alone. Change in the HIV RNA level is the most accurate individual marker of a patient's response to therapy. Levels must increase or decrease more than threefold (0.5 log) to be clinically significant in an individual patient.

Special Instructions This test is intended for use only in individuals with known HIV-1 infection. Qualitative tests may be used for diagnosis.

Specimen Plasma

Container Lavender top (EDTA) tube or yellow top (ACD) tube

Storage Instructions Remove plasma from cells within 6 hours of collection and freeze immediately.

Reference Range <40 copies/mL

HIV-1 Qualitative, Quantitative, and Genotyping Tests

Test Name	Sensitivity	Reference Range
HIV-1 DNA, Qualitative PCR	10 copies	Not detected
HIV-1 RNA, Qualitative PCR	10 copies	Not detected
HIV-1 RNA, Quantitative bDNA, 3rd Generation	50-500,000 copies/mL	<50 copies/mL; <1.60 log copies/mL
HIV-1 RNA, Quantitative PCR, 1st Generation	400-750,000 copies/mL	<400 copies/mL; <2.60 log copies/mL
HIV-1 RNA, Quantitative PCR, 2nd Generation	40-100,000 copies/mL	<40 copies/mL; <1.60 log copies/mL
HIV-1 RNA, Quantitative PCR, Expanded Range	40-7,500,000 copies/mL	<40 copies/mL; <1.60 log copies/mL
HIV-1 Genotyping for Drug Resistance to Protease Inhibitors (PrIs) and Reverse Transcriptase Inhibitors (RTs)	Do not genotype if viral load is <600 copies/mL; viral populations of >40% detected	No mutations detected None associated

Use Monitor the effect of antiretroviral drug therapy with maximum sensitivity, monitor progression of HIV infection, assess prognosis, individualize antiretroviral therapy

HIV viral load in increases in:

- acute HIV infection
- increased risk of progression to AIDS
- disease progression
- clinical AIDS
- drug resistance

HIV viral load is decreased in:

- response to therapy
- remission

Second generation assays can accurately quantify HIV RNA levels 10-fold lower than the first generation assay; thus, it is particularly useful for monitoring patients on combination antiretroviral therapy whom may routinely have HIV RNA levels <400 copies/mL. The first generation assay continues to be the method of choice for

patients with viral loads >100,000 copies/mL. Qualitative HIV-1 RNA assays can detect as few as 10 copies/mL.

Limitations Results obtained from different anticoagulants (EDTA, ACD) are not interchangeable; therefore, use of only one anticoagulant is recommended for patient monitoring

Methodology Enhanced reverse transcription-polymerase chain reaction (RT-PCR); increased sensitivity as a result of sample pretreatment methods

Additional Information Second generation assays can accurately quantify HIV RNA levels 10-fold lower than the first generation assay; thus, it is particularly useful for monitoring patients on combination antiretroviral therapy whom may routinely have HIV RNA levels <400 copies/mL. The first generation assay continues to be the method of choice for patients with viral loads >100,000 copies/mL. Qualitative HIV-1 RNA assays can detect as few as 10 copies/mL.

Selected Readings

Carpenter CC, Fischl MA, Hammer SM, et al, "Antiretroviral Therapy for HIV Infection in 1998: Updated Recommendations of the International AIDS Society-U.S.A. Panel," *JAMA*, 1998, 280(1):78-86.

Christopherson C, Lu SD, and Kwok S, "Laboratory Markers of Antiviral Activity," *Antivir Ther*, 1998, 3(4):247-50.

Cu-Uvin S, "Women and HIV Infections," *Clin Microbiol Newslett*, 2000, 22(21):161-5.

Detels R, Munoz A, McFarlane G, et al, "Effectiveness of Potent Antiretroviral Therapy on Time to AIDS and Death in Men With Known HIV Infection Duration. Multicenter AIDS Cohort Study Investigators," *JAMA*, 1998, 280(17):1497-503.

Ginocchio CC, "HIV Testing: The Next Step Beyond Viral Load," *Clin Microbiol Newslett*, 1999, 21(11):83-94.

Helbert M and Breuer J, "Monitoring Patients With HIV Disease," *J Clin Pathol*, 2000, 53(4):266-72.

Ho DD, Neumann AU, Perelson AS, et al, "Rapid Turnover of Plasma Virions and CD4 Lymphocytes in HIV-1 Infection," *Nature*, 1995, 373(6510):123-6.

Holodniy M, Mole L, Winters M, et al, "Diurnal and Short-Term Stability of HIV Virus Load as Measured by Gene Amplification," *J Acquir Immune Defic Syndr*, 1994, 7(4):363-8.

Hughes MD, Johnson VA, Hirsch MS, et al, "Monitoring Plasma HIV-1 RNA Levels in Addition to CD4$^+$ Lymphocyte Count Improves Assessment of Antiretroviral Therapeutic Response. ACTG 241 Protocol Virology Substudy Team," *Ann Intern Med*, 1997, 126(12):929-38.

Lange CG, "When to Start Antiretroviral Therapy in HIV-1 Infection," *Clin Microbiol Newslett*, 2001, 23(18):139-43.

Mellors JW, Kingsley LA, Rinaldo CR Jr, et al, "Quantitation of HIV-1 RNA in Plasma Predicts Outcome After Seroconversion," *Ann Intern Med*, 1995, 122(8):573-9.

Mellors JW, Rinaldo CR Jr, Gupta P, et al, "Prognosis in HIV-1 Infection Predicted by the Quantity of Virus in Plasma," *Science*, 1996, 272(5265):1167-70.

O'Brien WA, Hartigan PM, Daar ES, et al, "Changes in Plasma HIV RNA Levels and CD4$^+$ Lymphocyte Counts Predict Both Response to Antiretroviral Therapy and Therapeutic Failure. VA Cooperative Study Group on AIDS," *Ann Intern Med*, 1997, 126(12):939-45.

Paxton WB, Coombs RW, McElrath MJ, et al, "Longitudinal Analysis of Virologic Measures in Human Immunodeficiency Virus-Infected Subjects With ≥400 CD4 Lymphocytes: Implications for Applying Measurements to Individual Patients. National Institute of Allergy and Infectious Diseases AIDS Vaccine Evaluation Group," *J Infect Dis*, 1997, 175(2):247-54.

Saag MS, Holodniy M, Kuritzkes DR, et al, "HIV Viral Load Markers in Clinical Practice," *Nat Med*, 1996, 2(6):625-9.

Schockmel GA, Yerly S, and Perrin L, "Detection of Low HIV-1 RNA Levels in Plasma," *J Acquir Immune Defic Syndr Hum Retrovirol*, 1997, 14(2):179-83.

Volberding PA, "HIV Quantification: Clinical Applications," *Lancet*, 1996, 347(8994):71-3.

HIV-1 RNA, Quantitative PCR, Ultrasensitive *see* HIV-1 RNA, Quantitative PCR, 2nd Generation *on page 500*

HIV-1 Serology

Related Information

HIV-1 RNA, Quantitative bDNA, 3rd Generation *on page 499*
HIV-1 RNA, Quantitative PCR, 2nd Generation *on page 500*
HIV Genotyping *on page 503*
Human Immunodeficiency Virus Culture *on page 506*
p24 Antigen *on page 555*

Synonyms Human Immunodeficiency Virus Serology

Test Includes Screening test with confirmation of repeated positives

Patient Preparation In some states test may not be done or results revealed without express written or informed consent of the patient.

Special Instructions Blood and body fluid precautions must be observed

Specimen Serum

Reference Range Negative

Use Diagnose AIDS, exposure to HIV-1; screen blood and blood products for transfusion

Limitations There is a 2- to 12-week or longer interval after infection before antibody becomes detectable. Positive screening tests must be confirmed by more specific follow-up procedures (usually Western blot). Antibody is not protective against disease. There are some cross reactions in some test systems due to histocompatibility antigen mismatches (in particular, antibodies to HLA-DR4). Cross-reactions have been observed to other viral antigens as well. A recent influenza vaccine

(Continued)

HIV-1 Serology *(Continued)*

resulted in reactivity against p24 antigen and give false-positive enzyme-linked immunosorbent assays.

Methodology Enzyme-linked immunosorbent assay (ELISA), Western blot for confirmation

Additional Information Human immunodeficiency virus (HIV, formerly HTLV-III), a lentivirus, is the etiologic agent of AIDS. Acute infection, spread by blood or sexual contact, is usually followed within days by a flu-like illness, or no symptoms. During this time, HIV antigen, usually p24 core protein, may be detectable in serum. This becomes negative in 2 weeks to a month. There then follows a period of weeks to months during which an individual is infected with HIV, which may or may not be replicating at a low rate, but screening tests for antibody to HIV are **negative**.

Present screening tests for HIV antibodies are ELISA or EIA procedures which use disrupted virus or recombinant antigen products. Different antibodies are detected. Sensitivity and specificity of these tests are both extremely high, but positive results on a screen should be repeated; if positive a second time they should be confirmed with a Western blot procedure. Because of the grave implications of a positive result, confirmation of positive results by testing a second sample may be indicated.

Some individuals may have reactive screening tests, restricted to one test system, and completely negative Western blots. This may be due to HLA antibodies reacting with residual human cell surface proteins incorporated in the test kit. False-positives have been reported in individuals who have received intravenous gamma globulin. Since these proteins are due to antibodies in the transfused gamma globulin, repeat analysis in 3 months (half-life for IgG is about 3 weeks), will show a negative or much weaker EIA result.

Western blot analysis can identify the exact viral products with which patient antibody reacts. Criteria for a positive blot include two of the three bands for p24, gp41, and gp120/160 (Centers for Disease Control); or, one gag (p55, p24, p17), one pol (p64, p53, p31), and one env (gp41, gp120/160) (American Red Cross); or, p24, p31, and gp41 and/or gp120/160 (FDA license for Du Pont kit).

In donor screening programs, a low rate of false-positive (~0.00004%, 1 in 251,000) occurs. These cases usually lack Western blot reactivity to the p31 band.

HIV viral RNA testing is useful in the resolution of inconclusive Western blots.

HIV antibody can be detected in postmortem specimens of blood or vitreous humor.

Although **central nervous system involvement** is extremely common in AIDS, tests to detect HIV antigen or antibody in CSF lack both sensitivity and specificity. These tests do not help in differentiating neurologic symptoms secondary to HIV infection from those due to CNS neoplasm or opportunistic infection.

HIV-1 Infection Laboratory Tests

Test	Significance
HIV ELISA, EIA	Screening test for HIV infection. Sensitivity >99.9%. Reactive results must be confirmed by Western blot.
Western blot	Confirmatory test for HIV ELISA. Specificity when combined with ELISA >99.9%. Indeterminate results with early HIV infection, HIV-2 infection, autoimmune disease, pregnancy, and recent tetanus toxoid administration.
Absolute CD4 lymphocyte count	Most widely used predictor of HIV progression. Risk of progression is high with CD4 <200 cells/μL. Best short-term predictor for development of opportunistic infections.
CD4 lymphocyte percentage	Useful in conjunction with CD4 count. Risk of progression is high with percentage <20%.
B_2-Microglobulin	Cell surface protein indicative of macrophage-monocyte stimulation. Levels >3.5 mg/dL associated with rapid progression of disease. Limited usefulness.
p24 antigen	Indicates active HIV replication. Tends to be positive prior to seroconversion and with advanced disease. Relatively insensitive.
HIV DNA PCR	Most sensitive assay for diagnosing infection.
HIV RNA quantitative PCR or branched DNA	Most useful tests for determining prognosis and monitoring therapy.
HIV culture	Clinical research tool.

Chronology of Clinical and Laboratory Manifestations of HIV Infection

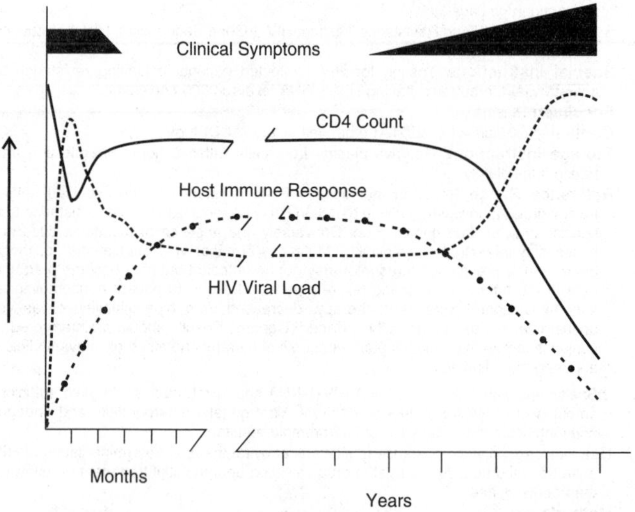

Primary infection may be asymptomatic or may be associated with transient flu-like symptoms which subside as the immune response develops. Rapid viral replication and high viral load levels are observed in the primary phase of infection. Prolonged "latent" period of dynamic host-virus quasi-equilibrium is associated with continuing viral replication and increased CD4 cell turnover. As the infection progresses, the host immune response wanes, viral replication increases, CD4 counts fall, and the clinical symptoms of AIDS manifest.

Selected Readings

Agbede OO, "HIV-1-Indeterminate Western Blot Results: Implications for Diagnosis and Subject Notification," *Clin Microbiol Newslett*, 1992, 14(16):121-5.

Brown AE, Jackson B, Fuller SA, et al, "Viral RNA in the Resolution of Human Immunodeficiency Virus Type 1 Diagnostic Serology," *Transfusion*, 1997, 37(9):926-9.

Burke DS, "Laboratory Diagnosis of Human Immunodeficiency Virus Infection," *Clin Lab Med*, 1989, 9(3):369-92.

Caliendo AM, "Methods, Interpretation, and Applications of HIV-1 Viral Load Measurements," *Clin Microbiol Newslett*, 1997, 19(1):1-7.

Cu-Uvin S, "Women and HIV Infections," *Clin Microbiol Newslett*, 2000, 22(21):161-5.

Ginocchio CC, "HIV Testing: The Next Step Beyond Viral Load," *Clin Microbiol Newslett*, 1999, 21(11):83-94.

"Interpretive Criteria Used to Report Western Blot Results in HIV-1 Antibody Testing - United States," *MMWR*, 1991, 40(40):692-5.

Kleinman S, Busch MP, Hall L, et al, "False-Positive HIV-1 Test Results in a Low-Risk Screening Setting of Voluntary Blood Donation," *JAMA*, 1998, 280(12):1080-5.

Krieger JN, "Acquired Immunodeficiency Syndrome Antibody Testing and Precautions," *J Urol*, 1992, 147(3):713-6.

O'Gorman MR, Weber D, Landis SE, et al, "Interpretive Criteria of the Western Blot Assay for Serodiagnosis of Human Immunodeficiency Virus Type 1 Infection," *Arch Pathol Lab Med*, 1991, 115(1):26-30.

Sloand EM, Pitt E, Chiarello RJ, et al, "HIV Testing - State of the Art," *JAMA*, 1991, 266(20):2861-6.

Yen-Lieberman B, "Rapid and Alternative Specimen Source Testing for HIV Antibody," *Clin Microbiol Newslett*, 1998, 20(16):133-6.

HIV bDNA *see* HIV-1 RNA, Quantitative bDNA, 3rd Generation *on page 499*

HIV Branched DNA *see* HIV-1 RNA, Quantitative bDNA, 3rd Generation *on page 499*

HIV Core Antigen *see* p24 Antigen *on page 555*

HIV Culture *see* Human Immunodeficiency Virus Culture *on page 506*

HIV Genotyping

Related Information

HIV-1 RNA, Quantitative bDNA, 3rd Generation *on page 499*

(Continued)

HIV Genotyping *(Continued)*

HIV-1 RNA, Quantitative PCR, 2nd Generation *on page 500*
HIV-1 Serology *on page 501*
Human Immunodeficiency Virus Culture *on page 506*
p24 Antigen *on page 555*

Synonyms HIV-1 Drug Resistance Testing; HIV-1 Gene Sequencing; HIV-1 Mutations Testing

Special Instructions Testing for HIV-1 infected patients exhibiting resistance to antiretroviral therapy and having HIV-1 RNA levels >2000 copies/mL.

Specimen Plasma

Container Lavender top (EDTA) tube, yellow top (ACD) tube

Storage Instructions Remove plasma from cells within 6 hours of collection and freeze immediately.

Reference Range Reported mutations indicate resistance to the specified antiretroviral drug(s); however, multiple mutations may be required to confer resistance to a specific drug or drug combination. Conversely, the absence of mutations does not necessarily infer drug susceptibility. Mutations in minor viral populations (ie, those below a 40% prevalence threshold) may not be detected but may become predominant in the future. Therapeutic failure may also be due to patient noncompliance, suboptimal antiretroviral drug therapy, decreased drug bioavailability, or as yet uncharacterized mutations in the Pr and RT genes. Results should be interpreted in conjunction with the patient's past antiretroviral therapy and all other relevant clinical and laboratory findings.

Specimens with fewer than 2000 HIV-1 RNA copies/mL may fail to yield sufficient amounts of cDNA for sequence analysis. Viral genetic heterogeneity and endogenous inhibitors may also yield uninterpretable results.

Use Detect genotypic resistance to HIV antiretroviral therapy; determine cause of HIV antiretroviral drug failure; assist in drug selection prior to initial treatment or following therapeutic failure

Methodology

- Reverse transcription and PCR amplification of plasma HIV-1 RNA followed by automated DNA sequencing
- Amplification of the entire sequence of the Pr gene and the amino-terminal 240 amino acids of the RT gene
- Sequencing in three overlapping reactions with d-Rhodamine-labeled terminators using an Applied Biosystems Model 377 automated sequencer
- Interpretation aided by a computer software program that compares the patient's HIV-1 sequence to the consensus clade B HIV-1 sequence
- Report includes detected mutations and associated drug resistance
- Clinical sensitivity: Viral populations >40% of the individual's HIV-1 population

Additional Information In HIV-1 infected patients, a large number of mutated virions are produced daily due to the high replication rate of HIV and the absence of replication error control mechanisms. Certain mutations are associated with resistance to specific therapeutic agents, thus resulting in the presence of resistant viral strains. Selective pressure favors replication of these resistant strains. As sensitive strains are eradicated by antiretroviral therapy, a resistant strain may become the dominant population in an individual patient, resulting in drug resistance and subsequent therapeutic failure. Mutations may occur in both the reverse transcriptase gene and the protease gene.

HIV-1 genotyping identifies mutations in individual patient viral populations, some of which are associated with therapeutic resistance. In this test, mutations currently known to be associated with resistance are reported.

Selected Readings

Angarano G and Monno L, "Genotype and Phenotype Resistance: An Overview," *J Biol Regul Homeost Agents*, 2000, 14(1):11-4.

Cohen J, "The Daunting Challenge of Keeping HIV Suppressed," *Science*, 1997, 277(5322):32-3.

Crandall KA, Vasco DA, Posada D, et al, "Advances in Understanding the Evolution of HIV," *AIDS*, 1999, 13 Suppl A:S39-47.

Deeks SG and Abrams DI, "Genotypic-Resistance Assays and Antiretroviral Therapy," *Lancet*, 1997, 349(9064):1489-90.

Deeks SG, Smith M, Holodniy M, et al, "HIV-1 Protease Inhibitors: A Review for Clinicians," *JAMA*, 1997, 277(2):145-53.

Ginocchio CC, "HIV Testing: The Next Step Beyond Viral Load," *Clin Microbiol Newslett*, 1999, 21(11):83-94.

Havlir DV and Richman DD, "Viral Dynamics of HIV: Implications for Drug Development and Therapeutic Strategies," *Ann Intern Med*, 1996, 124(11):984-94.

Hirsch MS, Conway B, D'Aquila RT, et al, "Antiretroviral Drug Resistance Testing in Adults With HIV Infection: Implications for Clinical Management. International AIDS Society-USA Panel," *JAMA*, 1998, 279(24):1984-91.

Katzenstein D, "Combination Therapies for HIV Infection and Genomic Drug Resistance," *Lancet*, 1997, 350(9083):970-1.

Larder BA, Kohli A, Kellam P, et al, "Quantitative Detection of HIV-1 Drug Resistance Mutations by Automated DNA Sequencing," *Nature*, 1993, 365(6447):671-3.
Mayers DL, "Drug-Resistant HIV-1: The Virus Strikes Back," *JAMA*, 1998, 279(24):2000-2.
Molla A, Korneyeva M, Gao Q, et al, "Ordered Accumulation of Mutations in HIV Protease Confers Resistance to Ritonavir," *Nat Med*, 1996, 2(7):260-6.
Romanelli F and Pomeroy C, "Human Immunodeficiency Virus Drug Resistance Testing: State of the Art in Genotypic and Phenotypic Testing of Antiretrovirals," *Pharmacotherapy*, 2000, 20(2):151-7.
Schinazi RF, Larder BA, and Mellors JW, "Mutations in Retroviral Genes Associated With Drug Resistance," *Intern Antivrial News*, 1996, 4:95-107.
Shafer RW, "Genotypic Testing for Human Immunodeficiency Virus Type 1 Drug Resistance," *Clin Microbiol Rev*, 2002, 15(2):247-77.
Tack PC, Bremer JW, Harris AA, et al, "Genotypic Analysis of HIV-1 Isolates to Identify Antiretroviral Resistance Mutations From Source Patients Involved in Health Care Worker Occupational Exposures," *JAMA*, 1999, 281(12):1085-6.
Wainberg MA and Friedland G, "Public Health Implications of Antiretroviral Therapy and HIV Drug Resistance," *JAMA*, 1998, 279(24):1977-83.

HIV Infection, Immune Status *see* Lymphocyte Subset Panels *on page 531*

HIV p24 Antigen *see* p24 Antigen *on page 555*

HIV Polymerase Chain Reaction *see* HIV-1 RNA, Quantitative PCR, 2nd Generation *on page 500*

HIV Viral Load *see* HIV-1 RNA, Quantitative PCR, 2nd Generation *on page 500*

HPA *see Histoplasma capsulatum* Antigen Assay *on page 497*

HSV 1 and 2 Culture *see* Herpes Simplex Virus Culture *on page 494*

HSV Antigen Detection, Direct *see* Herpes Simplex Virus by Direct Immunofluorescence *on page 493*

HSV Culture *see* Herpes Simplex Virus Culture *on page 494*

HSV, Rapid Isolation *see* Herpes Simplex Virus Isolation, Rapid *on page 495*

HSV Shell Vial Method, Spin Amplification *see* Herpes Simplex Virus Isolation, Rapid *on page 495*

HTLV-I/II Antibody

Synonyms Human T-Cell Leukemia Virus Type I and Type II; Human T-Lymphotropic Virus Type I Antibody

Specimen Serum

Container Red top tube

Reference Range Negative

Use Screen blood and blood products for transfusion; differential diagnosis of spastic myelopathy and adult T-cell acute lymphoblastic leukemia (ALL). HTLV-II has been associated with chronic neuromuscular diseases.

Limitations The combined assay for Anti HTLV-I/II is used mainly to screen blood donors. The assay detects 80% of patients with antibody to HTLV-II. The 20% of blood donors who are not detected by the assay for HTLV-II are not at sufficiently high risk to transmit the disease to warrant a separate assay.

Methodology Screen: enzyme immunoassay (EIA), confirmation: Western blot (WB) or radioimmunoprecipitation (RIPA)

Additional Information Human T-lymphotropic virus type I (HTLV-I) is a pathogenic retrovirus which is irregularly distributed in the world. Infection is generally uncommon in the U.S. and Europe. The virus is most commonly found in Japan and the Carribean. The virus can be asymptomatic for prolonged periods (20 years) but is strongly associated with myelopathies and adult T-cell leukemia. Less than 5% of those with antibody to HTLV-I develop myelopathies or leukemias even after 20 years. Adult T-cell leukemia is an aggressive malignancy of T lymphocytes often associated with skin infiltrates and hypercalcemia. The virus is tropic for T4 lymphocytes and is passed by sexual contact, blood products, from mother to fetus, and by breast milk. Pretransfusion testing for antibody to HTLV-I is now mandated by blood banks, in order to avoid transfusion transmitted HTLV-I infection from asymptomatic infected donors. The clinical course of HTLV-I infection, and the meaning of a positive serology are not yet well understood. Indeed, a recent study of hemophiliacs who were transfused regularly with plasma or its derivatives found no evidence of HTLV-I/II antibody in 179 patients.

Selected Readings

Blattner WA, "Human T-Lymphotropic Viruses and Diseases of Long Latency," *Ann Intern Med*, 1989, 111(1):4-6.
CDCP and USPHS Working Group, "Guidelines for Counseling Persons Infected With Human T-Lymphotropic Virus Type I (HTLV-I) and Type II (HTLV-II)," *Ann Intern Med*, 1993, 118(6):448-54.
Sullivan MT, Williams AE, Fang CT, et al, "Transmission of Human T-Lymphotropic Virus Types I and II by Blood Transfusion," *Arch Intern Med*, 1991, 151(10):2043-8.
Zaaijer HL, Cuypers HT, Dudok de Wit C, et al, "Results of 1-Year Screening of Donors in the Netherlands for Human T-Lymphotropic Virus (HTLV) Type I: Significance of Western Blot Patterns for Confirmation of HTLV Infection," *Transfusion*, 1994, 34(10):877-80.

HTLV-III Culture *see* Human Immunodeficiency Virus Culture *on page 506*

Human Herpesvirus 6, IgG and IgM Antibodies, Quantitative

Synonyms HHV-6, IgM, IgG

Specimen Serum

Container Red top tube or serum separator tube

Collection Specimens should be free from bacterial contamination and hemolysis

Storage Instructions Refrigerate serum

Causes for Rejection Gross lipemia

Use IgM HHV-6 may aid in the diagnosis of acute or recent infection with HHV-6. An increase in IgG HHV-6 (fourfold titer) between acute and convalescent samples is evidence for a recent HHV-6 infection.

Methodology Indirect fluorescent antibody (IFA)

Additional Information Human herpesvirus 6 (HHV-6) has recently been identified as the agent associated with both pediatric and adult infections. Most children have been infected by age 3 years. The acute infection in children is characterized clinically by an acute febrile illness, irritability, inflammation of tympanic membranes, and (uncommonly) a rash characteristic of roseola. When acute and convalescent (4-6 weeks later) serum samples are compared, a fourfold rise in HHV-6 IgG titer is typical. It has also been thought to be the etiological agent of exanthem subitum (roseola) in children.

In adults, HHV-6 has been associated with chronic fatigue and spontaneously resolving fever resembling a mononucleosis-like illness. During the acute episode an elevated IgM HHV-6 is useful. An increase in IgG HHV-6 between acute and convalescent serum sample is consistent with a recent HHV-6 infection. There is no antiviral agents directed toward this virus.

Selected Readings

De Bolle L, Naesens L, and De Clercq E, "Update on Human Herpesvirus 6 Biology, Clinical Features, and Therapy," *Clin Microbiol Rev*, 2005, 18(1):217-45.

Oren I and Sobel JD, "Human Herpesvirus Type 6: Review," *Clin Infect Dis*, 1992, 14(3):741-6.

Prober C, "Sixth Disease and the Ubiquity of Human Herpesviruses," *N Engl J Med*, 2005, 352(8):753-5.

Pruksananonda P, Hall CB, Insel RA, et al, "Primary Human Herpesvirus 6 Infection in Young Children," *N Engl J Med*, 1992, 326(22):1445-50.

Rathore MH, "Human Herpesvirus 6," *South Med J*, 1993, 86(11):1197-205.

Torre D, Mancuso R, and Ferrante P, "Pathogenic Mechanisms of Meningitis/Encephalitis Caused by Human Herpesvirus-6 in Immunocompetent Adult Patients," *Clin Infect Dis*, 2005, 41(3):422-3.

Whitley RJ and Lakeman FD, "Human Herpesvirus 6 Infection of the Central Nervous System: Is It Just a Case of Mistaken Association?" *Clin Infect Dis*, 2005, 40(6):894-5.

Human Immunodeficiency Virus 1 RNA, 2nd Generation *see* HIV-1 RNA, Quantitative PCR, 2nd Generation *on page 500*

Human Immunodeficiency Virus Culture

Related Information

HIV-1 RNA, Quantitative PCR, 2nd Generation *on page 500*
HIV-1 Serology *on page 501*
HIV Genotyping *on page 503*
p24 Antigen *on page 555*

Synonyms AIDS Virus Culture; HIV Culture; HTLV-III Culture

Specimen Blood (20-40 mL), cerebrospinal fluid (10 mL), other body fluids, biopsies. All specimens **must** be labeled with the patient's name or code and **must** be transported to the laboratory in a **sealed** plastic bag with the request form attached. Some laboratories will not accept patient names associated with HIV specimens.

Container Green top (heparin) tube for blood, sterile container for CSF and other fluids

Collection Routine venipuncture. Invert the tubes several times after drawing the blood to be sure the blood is thoroughly mixed with the heparin.

Storage Instructions Do not store the specimen. Send it to the laboratory immediately. Some laboratories require specimen to be received into the laboratory the same day the specimen is received.

Causes for Rejection Dry specimen, specimen not refrigerated during transport, specimen fixed in formalin, unlabeled specimen

Turnaround Time Positive cultures are usually reported after 2 consecutive positive reverse transcriptase assays. Blood cultures are usually incubated 4 weeks and some laboratories incubate CSF cultures 8 weeks before termination as negative.

Reference Range No virus isolated

Use Aid in the diagnosis of disease caused by HIV, research studies, recover virus for phenotyping

Limitations A negative culture cannot be assumed to rule out the presence of the virus.

Methodology Growth of virus in lymphocyte culture and subsequent (indirect) testing for presence of virus in culture fluids by EIA reverse transcriptase assay

Selected Readings

Cu-Uvin S, "Women and HIV Infections," *Clin Microbiol Newslett*, 2000, 22(21):161-5.

Erice A, Sannerud KJ, Leske VL, et al, "Sensitive Microculture Method for Isolation of Human Immunodeficiency Virus Type 1 From Blood Leukocytes," *J Clin Microbiol*, 1992, 30(2):444-8.

Garcia Rodriguez MC, Bates I, de Jose I, et al, "Prognostic Value of Immunological Data, *in vitro* Antibody Production, and Virus Culture in Vertical Infection With HIV-1," *Arch Dis Child*, 1995, 72(6):498-501.

Jackson JB, "Human Immunodeficiency Virus Type 1 Antigen and Culture Assays," *Arch Pathol Lab Med*, 1990, 114(3):249-53.

Jackson JB and Balfour HH Jr, "Practical Diagnostic Testing for Human Immunodeficiency Virus," *Clin Microbiol Rev*, 1988, 1(1):124-38.

Lange CG, "When to Start Antiretroviral Therapy in HIV-1 Infection," *Clin Microbiol Newslett*, 2001, 23(18):139-43.

MacGregor RR, Dubin G, Frank, I, et al, "Failure of Culture and Polymerase Chain Reaction to Detect Human Immunodeficiency Virus (HIV) in Seronegative Steady Sexual Partners of HIV-Infected Individuals," *Clin Infect Dis*, 1995, 21(1):122-7.

Markham PD and Salahuddin SZ, "*In Vitro* Cultivation of Human Leukocytes: Methods for the Expression and Isolation of Human Retroviruses," *BioTechniques*, 1987, 5:432-43.

Schleupner CJ, "Detection of HIV-1 Infection," *Principles and Practice of Infectious Diseases*, 4th ed, Mandell GL, Bennett JE, and Dolin R, eds, New York, NY: Churchill Livingstone, 1995, 1253-66.

Human Immunodeficiency Virus Serology *see* HIV-1 Serology *on page 501*

Human T-Cell Leukemia Virus Type I and Type II *see* HTLV-I/II Antibody *on page 505*

Human T-Lymphotropic Virus Type I Antibody *see* HTLV-I/II Antibody *on page 505*

Humerus, Left or Right, X-ray *see* Bone Films *on page 396*

Hyperalimentation Line Culture *see* Intravenous Line Culture *on page 511*

IgG Antibodies to Rubella *see* Rubella Serology *on page 575*

IgM Antibodies to Rubella *see* Rubella Serology *on page 575*

Iliac Arteries Ultrasound *see* Ultrasound, Peripheral Arteries and Veins *on page 605*

Immune Status HIV Infection *see* Lymphocyte Subset Panels *on page 531*

Immunofluorescent Studies, Biopsy

Related Information

Skin Biopsy *on page 580*

Synonyms Direct Immunofluorescent Studies, Biopsy

Test Includes Fluorescent stains for immunoglobulins, complement, fibrin, and routine histopathology

Special Instructions Consult the pathologist prior to biopsy procedure for specific instructions. Requisition **must** state operative diagnosis and source of specimen.

Specimen Biopsy of kidney, skin, muscle, and lung submitted fresh in saline-moistened gauze as soon as possible following removal

Container Jar with gauze pad moistened with sterile saline

Collection Container **must** be labeled with patient's full name, and date

Storage Instructions Transport specimen to the laboratory immediately.

Causes for Rejection Specimen allowed to dry

Reference Range Negative

Use Determine the presence of tissue deposits of IgG, IgM, IgA, C1q, C3, albumin, fibrinogen, and kappa and lambda light chains in immunological diseases of kidney (eg, immune complex glomerulonephritis and antiglomerular basement membrane glomerulonephritis), skin (pemphigus, bullous pemphigoid, dermatitis herpetiformis, lupus erythematosus), neoplasms (plasma cell myeloma, macroglobulinemia of Waldenström, malignant lymphoma), and lung (lupus erythematosus, Goodpasture's syndrome)

Additional Information Submit additional specimen in formalin for light microscopy. Electron microscopy is commonly needed in many of the same biopsies in which fluorescence is desired, but usually requires a different fixative than does light microscopy processing.

Inclusion Body Stain *see* Herpes Cytology *on page 491*

Inclusion Conjunctivitis *see* Ocular Cytology *on page 551*

India Ink Preparation

Related Information

Cryptococcal Antigen Serology, Serum or Cerebrospinal Fluid *on page 431*
Fungus Culture, Cerebrospinal Fluid *on page 464*
Methenamine Silver Stain *on page 534*
Periodic Acid-Schiff Stain *on page 563*

Synonyms Cerebrospinal Fluid India Ink Preparation; *Cryptococcus* Preparation; *Cryptococcus* Stain; Nigrosin Preparation

(Continued)

India Ink Preparation *(Continued)*

Patient Preparation Same as for culture of specific site

Specimen For all practical purposes, the only reasonably useful specimen is cerebrospinal fluid.

Container Sterile CSF tube

Collection The specimen may be divided for fungal culture, and mycobacteria culture and smear, and routine bacterial culture and Gram stain only if the specimen is of adequate volume for all tests requested.

Storage Instructions Do **not** refrigerate.

Causes for Rejection Insufficient specimen volume

Turnaround Time Routine: 24 hours; stat: 2 hours

Reference Range No encapsulated yeast identified

Use Establish the presence of *Cryptococcus* sp or other fungi

Limitations This technique is only 30% to 50% sensitive in cases of cryptococcal meningitis and is not highly recommended. WBC with an apparent "capsule" can easily be misinterpreted as *Cryptococcus* in this test (ie, a false positive result). Cultures and rapid latex agglutination (LA) methods are more sensitive than direct preparations; therefore, the India ink preparation may be negative when the culture or LA test is positive. Immunologic tests for *Cryptococcus* antigen have a sensitivity of 90% to 100%. Many laboratories have abandoned the use of the India ink preparation in favor of LA.

Methodology Wet mount with India ink (nigrosin) for contrast. Centrifugation may concentrate organisms and improve sensitivity.

Additional Information *Cryptococcus neoformans* is the most common central nervous system fungus in both normal hosts and patients with the acquired immunodeficiency syndrome (AIDS). Pigeon droppings act as a year round reservoir for dispersion of encapsulated yeast cells.

Selected Readings

Berlin L and Pincus JH, "Cryptococcal Meningitis. False-Negative Antigen Test Results and Cultures in Nonimmunosuppressed Patients," *Arch Neurol*, 1989, 46(12):1312-6.

Ellis DH and Pfeiffer TJ, "Ecology, Life Cycle, and Infectious Propagule of *Cryptococcus neoformans*," *Lancet*, 1990, 336(8720):923-5.

McGinnis MR, "Detection of Fungi in Cerebrospinal Fluid," *Am J Med*, 1983, 75(1B):129-38.

Indium-111 Labeled Leukocyte Scan *see* Indium Leukocyte Scan *on page 508*

Indium Leukocyte Scan

Synonyms Indium-111 Labeled Leukocyte Scan; Infection Scan; Infection Scintigraphy; Leukocyte Scintigraphy; WBC Scan; White Blood Cell Scan

Test Includes The patient receives an intravenous reinjection of radiolabeled leukocytes. The patient initially has a 60-80 mL sample of blood drawn for an *in vitro* process of labeling and separating the leukocyte component. Images are acquired at intervals between 2-24 hours after subsequent reinjection of radiolabeled cells.

Patient Preparation The patient does not need to be fasting or NPO for this procedure. Patient should have all RIA blood work performed, or at least drawn, prior to injection of any radioactive material.

Special Instructions Requisition must state the current patient diagnosis in order to select the most appropriate radiopharmaceutical and/or imaging technique.

Duration of Procedure: Two hours from blood draw to reinjection of labeled cells. 2-24 hours for imaging at intervals.

Radiopharmaceutical: Indium-111 labeled leukocytes

Causes for Rejection Other recent Nuclear Medicine procedures may interfere. If uncertain, call the consulting Nuclear Medicine Department.

Turnaround Time A written report will be sent to the patient's chart and/or to the referring physician.

Normal Findings Radiolabeled leukocytes will localize to some degree in the liver, spleen, and bone marrow. Focal accumulations in soft tissue or asymmetric uptake in bone will be seen in infected or inflamed sites. For osteomyelitis, a bone scan is usually performed first for comparison with the radiolabeled leukocyte scan findings.

Use Radiolabeled leukocyte imaging is useful either in determining the site of an occult infection or in confirming the presence or absence of infection at a suspected site. This technique has largely replaced gallium-67 imaging for acute infections because of the better image resolution and greater specificity. Some chronic infections, eg, chronic osteomyelitis, may be better imaged with gallium-67. Radiolabeled leukocyte imaging is especially helpful in detecting postoperative infection sites and in documenting lack of residual infection after a course of therapy.

Limitations Leukocyte radiolabeling is a complex process and is usually performed on-site only where there are dedicated radiopharmacy laboratories. Most commercial radiopharmacies will also provide this service locally.

Additional Information An alternative method of leukocyte radiolabeling with technetium-99m (^{99m}Tc) HMPAO is now available. Early reports show possible advantages with earlier imaging times and better sensitivity for infections in extremities with utilization of higher doses of ^{99m}Tc versus indium-111.

Selected Readings

Abreu SH, "Skeletal Uptake of Indium-111 Labeled White Blood Cells," *Semin Nucl Med*, 1989, 19(2):152-5.

Datz FL and Thorne DA, "Effect of Antibiotic Therapy on the Sensitivity of Indium-111 Labeled Leukocyte Scans," *J Nucl Med*, 1986, 27(12):1849-53.

Froelich JW and Field SA, "The Role of Indium-111 White Blood Cells in Inflammatory Bowel Disease," *Semin Nucl Med*, 1988, 18(4):300-7.

Ho Y and Hennessy O, "Indium-111 WBC Scan to Diagnose Mycotic Aneurysm," *Clin Nucl Med*, 1999, 24(11):903-4.

Kolindou A, Liu Y, Ozker K, et al, "In-111 WBC Imaging of Osteomyelitis in Patients With Underlying Bone Scan Abnormalities," *Clin Nucl Med*, 1996, 21(3):183-91.

Laitinen R, Tähtinen J, Lantto T, et al, "^{99m}Tc Labeled Leukocytes in Imaging of Patients With Suspected Acute Abdominal Inflammation," *Clin Nucl Med*, 1990, 15(9):597-602.

Larcos G, Brown ML, and Sutton RT, "Diagnosis of Osteomyelitis of the Foot in Diabetic Patients: Value of 111In-Leukocyte Scintigraphy," *AJR Am J Roentgenol*, 1991, 157(3):527-31.

Roddie ME, Peters AM, Danpure HJ, et al, "Inflammation: Imaging With ^{99m}Tc HMPAO-Labeled Leukocytes," *Radiology*, 1988, 166(3):767-72.

Induced Sputum Technique for *Pneumocystis* *see* Pneumocystis jiroveci Test *on page 566*

Infant Botulism, Toxin Identification *see* Botulism, Diagnostic Procedure *on page 405*

Infection Scan *see* Indium Leukocyte Scan *on page 508*

Infection Scintigraphy *see* Indium Leukocyte Scan *on page 508*

Infectious Mononucleosis Serology

Related Information

Epstein-Barr Virus Serology *on page 454*

Synonyms Monospot™ Test; Monosticon® Dri-Dot® Test; Mono Test

Test Includes Screening for the presence of heterophil antibodies

Specimen Serum

Container Red top tube or serum separator tube

Reference Range Negative

Use Diagnosis of infectious mononucleosis

Limitations Correlation with clinical findings is imperative since false-positive and negative results have been reported. About 15% of the adult population with infectious mononucleosis will not develop heterophil antibodies. Failure to develop heterophil antibodies occurs even more frequently in children. In these instances, patients usually are tested for specific Epstein-Barr virus antibodies. Less than 2% false-positives have been reported with Hodgkin's disease, lymphoma, acute lymphocytic leukemia, infectious hepatitis, pancreatic carcinoma, cytomegalovirus, Burkitt's lymphoma, rheumatoid arthritis, malaria, and rubella.

Overall, the Monospot™ test has 99% specificity and 86% sensitivity.

Methodology Latex agglutination (LA) and enzyme immunoassay (EIA)

If serological testing is performed by enzyme immunoassay (EIA) on automated instrumentation, results are usually given in index units, not titers. In such cases, significant rises in antibody levels are determined by algorithms within the instrumentation, not by increases in titers.

Additional Information The infectious mononucleosis heterophil antibody appears in the serum of patients by the sixth to tenth day of illness. Highest titers are usually found in the second to third week. Antibody levels may remain detectable for as little as 1 week or persist up to a year; usual persistence is 4-8 weeks. The level of antibody activity is not correlated with the severity of disease or the degree of lymphocytosis. A positive screening or differential test in the appropriate clinical and hematologic setting is sufficient to make the diagnosis of infectious mononucleosis.

If there is clinically a mononucleosis syndrome, but the screening test is negative, a differential absorption will add nothing. Instead, consider tests for EBV specific antibodies, CMV, and toxoplasmosis antibodies.

Selected Readings

Jenson HB, Ench Y, and Sumaya CV, "Epstein-Barr Virus," *Manual of Clinical Laboratory Immunology*, 5th ed, Rose NR, Conway de Macario E, Folds JD, et al, eds, Washington, DC: American Society for Microbiology, 1997, 634-43.

Influenza A and B Serology

Related Information

Influenza Virus Culture *on page 510*

Test Includes IgG and IgM antibody titers

Specimen Serum

(Continued)

Influenza A and B Serology *(Continued)*

Container Red top tube or serum separator tube

Collection Acute and convalescent sera drawn 10-14 days apart are required

Reference Range Less than a fourfold increase in titer in paired sera; IgG <1:10, IgM <1:10

Use Establish the diagnosis of influenza virus infection; epidemiologic surveillance and tracking; differentiate type A from B for treatment with amantadine

Methodology Complement fixation (CF), hemagglutination inhibition (HAI), single radial immunodiffusion (RID), enzyme immunoassay (EIA)

If serological testing is performed by enzyme immunoassay (EIA) on automated instrumentation, results are usually given in index units, not titers. In such cases, significant rises in antibody levels are determined by algorithms within the instrumentation, not by increases in titers.

Additional Information Influenza virus is typed by specifying a neuraminidase and hemagglutinin. Although serologic diagnosis is seldom practical (or necessary) during an influenza epidemic, serologic typing is valuable for epidemiology, and for planning therapy. Since type A influenza can be treated with amantadine, but type B cannot, this distinction may need to be made. Presence of specific IgM antibody indicates acute infection.

Many laboratories offer rapid (<1 hour) tests for influenza A and B. Although, these tests are rapid and have high specificity, they are not particularly sensitive. These tests have the greatest utility in settings where they are used within 48 hours of the onset of symptoms so anti-influenza therapy can be given within that timeframe.

Selected Readings

Rothbarth PH, Groen J, Bohnen AM, et al, "Influenza Virus Serology - A Comparative Study," *J Virol Methods*, 1999, 78(1-2):163-9.

Shaw MW, Arden NH, and Maassab HF, "New Aspects of Influenza Viruses," *Clin Microbiol Rev*, 1992, 5(1):74-92.

Wallace LA, McAulay KA, Douglas JD, et al, "Influenza Diagnosis: From Dark Isolation Into the Molecular Light. West Scotland Respiratory Virus Study Group," *J Infect*, 1999, 39(3):221-6.

Ziegler T, Katz JM, Cox NJ, et al, "Influenza Viruses," *Manual of Clinical Laboratory Immunology*, 5th ed, Rose NR, Conway de Macario E, Folds JD, et al, eds, Washington, DC: American Society for Microbiology, 1997, 673-8.

Influenza Virus Culture

Related Information

Influenza A and B Serology *on page 509*
Viral Culture, Throat *on page 617*

Test Includes Concurrent culture for other respiratory viruses (parainfluenza and respiratory syncytial virus)

Specimen Throat or nasopharyngeal swab, sputum, bronchial washings, bronchoalveolar lavage

Container Sterile container; cold virus transport medium for swabs

Sampling Time Specimens should be collected within 3 days of the onset of illness.

Storage Instructions Specimens should be placed into viral transport medium and kept cold at all times. Do not freeze specimens. Specimens should be delivered immediately to the laboratory.

Causes for Rejection Dry specimen, specimen not refrigerated during transport, specimen fixed in formalin, unlabeled specimen

Turnaround Time Variable (5-14 days) and depends on culture method used and the amount of virus in the specimen

Reference Range No virus isolated

Use Isolate and identify influenza virus as an etiologic agent in cases of influenza and viral pneumonia

Methodology Inoculation of specimens into cell cultures, incubation of cultures, observation of cultures for characteristic cytopathic effect, and identification/speciation by methods such as hemadsorption and fluorescent monoclonal antibodies specific for influenza virus A or B

Additional Information The shell vial technique to rapidly (within 24 hours) detect viruses has recently been adapted to detect influenza A and B viruses. Serology for the detection of influenza antibodies is available. A commercial and rapid (less than 15 minutes) enzyme immunoassay for the detection of influenza A virus in patient specimen is available.

Many laboratories offer rapid (<1 hour) tests for influenza A and B. Although, these tests are rapid and have high specificity, they are not particularly sensitive. These tests have the greatest utility in settings where they are used within 48 hours of the onset of symptoms so anti-influenza therapy can be given within that timeframe.

Selected Readings

Cox N and Ziegler T, "Influenza Viruses," *Manual of Clinical Microbiology*, 8th ed, Murray PR, et al, eds, Washington, DC: American Society for Microbiology, 2003, 1360-7.

Shaw MW, Arden NH, and Maassab HF, "New Aspects of Influenza Viruses," *Clin Microbiol Rev*, 1992, 5(1):74-92.

Subbarao K, "Influenza A Infections: From Chickens to Humans," *Clin Microbiol Newslett*, 2001, 23(2):9-13.

Influenza Virus, Direct Detection *see* Virus Detection by DFA *on page 619*

Infusion Pyelogram *see* Urography *on page 610*

Insect Identification *see* Arthropod Identification *on page 387*

Intercellular Antibody Basement Membrane Antibody *see* Skin Biopsy, Immunofluorescence *on page 583*

Intrauterine Device Culture *see Actinomyces* Culture, All Sites *on page 363*

Intravenous Devices Culture *see* Intravenous Line Culture *on page 511*

Intravenous Line Culture

Synonyms Arterial Line Culture; Catheter Culture, Intravenous; Catheter Tip Culture; Hemovac® Tip Culture; Hyperalimentation Line Culture; Intravenous Devices Culture; I.V. Catheter Culture; Shunt Culture; Swan-Ganz Tip Culture; Venous Catheter Culture

Test Includes Culture of foreign body organism identification, antibiotic susceptibilities of potential pathogens

Specimen Blood and **only** the distal 2" of I.V. catheter tip collected in a sterile manner (cut with sterile scissors and at a point just below the skin line)

Container Sterile container

Collection Aseptically prepare insertion site. Remove line without contact with adjacent skin and send only intra-arterial segment. Catheter tip aseptically removed and placed in sterile container. A procedure for quantitative comparative central and peripheral blood culture is as follows.

Separate blood samples (10 mL each) are obtained in a sterile manner from a peripheral blood vessel and from the central catheter. Aseptic technique at the catheter is as follows:

- The catheter is clamped and the needle adapter removed.
- The end of the catheter is swabbed once with 70% isopropyl alcohol and then with an iodine solution (allow to air dry).
- A sterile needle adapter is inserted into the end of the catheter.
- The clamp is removed and 2 mL of blood is drawn through a sterile syringe to clear the catheter.
- The blood for culture is then subsequently obtained in a separate sterile syringe.
- The catheter adapter is reattached to the intravenous tubing.

The paired blood specimens are placed in separate lysis centrifugation tubes after the stopper is swabbed three times with povidone-iodine. See also the listing Blood Culture, Aerobic and Anaerobic *on page 391*.

Storage Instructions Specimens should be transported to the laboratory within 1 hour of collection for optimal results. However, if specimens cannot be collected and delivered to the laboratory during regular hours specimen may be refrigerated overnight.

Reference Range No growth. For culture taken through a central catheter, a tenfold greater colony count than a simultaneous peripheral culture or >100 CFU/mL if only a central catheter culture is presumptive evidence of a colonized catheter. A culture of a catheter tip (rolled onto agar media) result of ≥15 CFU also is presumptive evidence which rules out contamination and, by interference, suggests a colonized catheter.

Use Identify a possible source of bacteremia or fungemia; particularly useful for the diagnosis of catheter-related sepsis (CRS) secondary to blood-borne seedling of catheters, and CRS associated with coagulase-negative staphylococci

Limitations Culture of blood obtained from intravenous lines is fraught with problems. Blood obtained from a line is easily and usually contaminated and interpretation of results usually is difficult.

Methodology Quantitative or semiquantitative culture with or without lysis centrifugation. A very simple and equally effective semiquantitative technique is to roll the culture tip on a blood or chocolate agar plate. Greater than 15 CFU rules out contamination and suggests infection; <15 CFU indicates a low probability of infection.

Additional Information Infections complicating therapy with indwelling central venous catheters pose a difficult problem. Catheter-related sepsis is defined when:

- Positive blood cultures collected through the central venous catheter can show a tenfold or greater colony count compared with peripheral quantitative blood culture or >100 CFU/mL if only central venous catheter blood culture is available
- A semiquantitative catheter tip culture result ≥15 CFU
- No obvious clinical or microbiologic source for the infection is apparent

(Continued)

Intravenous Line Culture *(Continued)*

Exit site infections are defined as purulent drainage or erythema at the catheter exit site. Tunnel infection is defined as spreading cellulitis with erythema, tenderness, and swelling of the skin surrounding the subcutaneous tunnel tract of the catheter. Successful therapy of catheter-related infection with antibiotics and local care has been reported. However, catheter removal almost always is required to achieve cure. *Staphylococcus aureus* and polymicrobial infections also are more difficult to eradicate. Intraluminal culture has been reported to correlate well with catheter tip cultures (87.5% identical) while skin puncture sites are usually less frequently identical (37.5%). See table.

Summary of Results of Prospective Studies Using Semiquantitative Techniques to Diagnose Vascular-Access Infections

Organism	No. With Same Organism in Semiquantitative Catheter Culture and Blood Culture
Coagulase-negative staphylococci	27
Staphylococcus aureus	26
Yeast	17
Enterobacter	7
Serratia	5
Enterococcus	5
Klebsiella	4
Streptococcus viridans group	3
Pseudomonas species	2
Proteus	2
Others: *Pseudomonas aeruginosa, Yersinia*	1 each

From Hampton A and Sheretz RJ, "Vascular-Access Infections in Hospitalized Patients," *Surg Clin North Am*, 1988, 68:57-72, with permission.

Selected Readings

Crnich CJ and Maki DG, "The Promise of Novel Technology for the Prevention of Intravascular Device-Related Bloodstream Infection. I. Pathogenesis and Short-Term Devices," *Clin Infect Dis*, 2002, 34(9):1232-42.

Garrison RN and Wilson MA, "Intravenous and Central Catheter Infections," *Surg Clin North Am*, 1994, 74(3):557-70.

Henderson DK, "Bacteremia Due to Percutaneous Intravascular Devices," *Principles and Practice of Infectious Diseases*, 4th ed, Mandell GL, Bennett JE and, eds, New York, NY: Churchill Livingstone, 1995, 2587-99.

Maki DG, Weise CE, and Sarafin HW, "A Semiquantitative Culture Method for Identifying Intravenous-Catheter-Related Infection," *N Engl J Med*, 1977, 296(23):1305-9.

Mermel LA, Farr BM, Sherertz RJ, et al, "Guidelines for the Management of Intravascular Catheter-Related Infections," *Clin Infect Dis*, 2001, 32(9):1249-72.

Nucci M and Anaissie E, "Should Vascular Catheters be Removed From All Patients With Candidemia? An Evidence-Based Review," *Clin Infect Dis*, 2002, 34(5):591-9.

Reimer LG, "Catheter-Related Infections and Blood Cultures," *Clin Lab Med*, 1994, 14(1):51-8.

Widmer AF, Nettleman M, Flint K, et al, "The Clinical Impact of Culturing Central Venous Catheters. A Prospective Study," *Arch Intern Med*, 1992, 152(6):1299-302.

Intravenous Pyelogram *see* Urography *on page 610*

Iron Stain *see* Bone Marrow Aspiration and Biopsy *on page 397*

Itraconazole Level

Synonyms Sporanox® Level, Blood

Abstract Itraconazole is an orally administered antifungal agent with a broad spectrum of activity.

Specimen Serum

Container Red top tube

Sampling Time 4 hours after oral dose and approximately 1-2 weeks after therapy has begun so that a steady-state is achieved

Reference Range Therapeutic: varies with methodology; see Additional Information.

Use May be useful to ensure therapeutic levels if poor absorption is suspected, or in cases of therapeutic failure or relapse

Limitations *In vitro* susceptibility testing of fungi against itraconazole is method dependent and may not accurately predict clinical success. Consequently, monitoring levels and adjusting dosage to attain therapeutic concentrations as determined by minimum inhibitory concentrations may not be helpful. Assays for itraconazole are performed only in a few reference laboratories.

Methodology Bioassay, high performance liquid chromatography (HPLC)

Additional Information Serum levels as determined by bioassay are approximately 10 times the levels determined by HPLC, presumably because bioassay also detects

an active metabolite. Consequently therapeutic levels vary with method. Concentrations >5 mcg/mL (bioassay) were predictive of therapeutic success in invasive aspergillosis, whereas serum concentrations <1 mcg/mL (bioassay) predicted therapeutic failure in cases of cryptococcal meningitis. Concentrations <0.25 mcg/mL (HPLC) predicted failure to prevent aspergillosis in granulocytopenic patients. Absorption is often depressed in bone marrow transplant and in AIDS patients.

Selected Readings

Bodey GP, "Topical and Systemic Antifungal Agents," *Med Clin North Am*, 1988, 72(3):637-59.
British Society for Antimicrobial Chemotherapy Working Party, "Laboratory Monitoring of Antifungal Chemotherapy," *Lancet*, 1991, 337(8757):1577-80.
Edson RS and Terrell CL, "The Aminoglycosides," *Mayo Clin Proc*, 1999, 74(5):519-28.

IUD Culture *see* *Actinomyces* Culture, All Sites *on page 363*
I.V. Catheter Culture *see* Intravenous Line Culture *on page 511*
IVP *see* Urography *on page 610*
***Ixodes scapularis* Identification** *see* Arthropod Identification *on page 387*
Joint Fluid Culture *see* Aerobic Culture, Body Fluid *on page 365*
Joint Fluid Fungus Culture *see* Fungus Culture, Body Fluid *on page 462*
Joint Study *see* Arthrogram *on page 387*
Joint Tap *see* Arthrocentesis *on page 384*
Kanamycin (Kantrex®) Level *see* Amikacin Level *on page 370*

Ketoconazole Level

Synonyms Nizoral

Abstract Ketoconazole is an orally administered antifungal agent that is appropriately used for a variety of nonlife-threatening fungal infections. Determining serum levels rarely contributes significantly to patient care.

Specimen Serum

Container Red top tube

Sampling Time 2 hours after administration

Reference Range Therapeutic: 5-20 mcg/mL, dependent on dose

Use Usually unnecessary. May be useful to ensure therapeutic levels if poor absorption is suspected, or in cases of therapeutic failure or relapse.

Limitations *In vitro* susceptibility testing of fungi against ketoconazole is method dependent and may not accurately predict clinical success. Consequently, monitoring levels and adjusting dosage to attain therapeutic concentrations as determined by minimum inhibitory concentrations may not be helpful. Assays for ketoconazole are performed only in a few reference laboratories.

Methodology Bioassay, high performance liquid chromatography (HPLC)

Additional Information Approximately 5% to 10% of patients receiving ketoconazole develop abnormally elevated serum transaminases, a transient and reversible state. Rarely, patients develop symptomatic hepatitis which is idiosyncratic and not dependent upon serum concentrations. Absorption is often depressed in bone marrow transplant and AIDS patients.

Selected Readings

Bodey GP, "Topical and Systemic Antifungal Agents," *Med Clin North Am*, 1988, 72(3):637-59.
British Society for Antimicrobial Chemotherapy Working Party, "Laboratory Monitoring of Antifungal Chemotherapy," *Lancet*, 1991, 337(8757):1577-80.
Edson RS and Terrell CL, "The Aminoglycosides," *Mayo Clin Proc*, 1999, 74(5):519-28.

Kidneys Ultrasound *see* Ultrasound, Kidneys *on page 604*
Kinyoun Stain *see* Acid-Fast Stain *on page 361*
Kirby-Bauer Susceptibility Test *see* Antimicrobial Susceptibility Testing, Aerobic and Facultatively Anaerobic Organisms *on page 379*
Knee Arthrogram *see* Arthrogram *on page 387*
Knee, Left or Right, X-ray *see* Bone Films *on page 396*
Knees Arthritis, X-ray *see* Bone Films *on page 396*

KOH Preparation

Related Information

Fungus Culture, Skin *on page 464*
Methenamine Silver Stain *on page 534*
Periodic Acid-Schiff Stain *on page 563*
Skin Biopsy *on page 580*

Synonyms Potassium Hydroxide Preparation

Test Includes Potassium hydroxide, (KOH) hydrolysis of proteinaceous debris, cells, etc. Microscopic examination under 10x and 40x.

Patient Preparation Same as for culture of specific site

Special Instructions The laboratory should be informed of the specific source of the specimen and the clinical diagnosis.

(Continued)

KOH Preparation *(Continued)*

Specimen Appropriate specimen for KOH preparation is a specimen composed mostly of keratin (hair, skin, nails). This test is not designed for the examination of body fluids.

Container Same as for culture of specific site

Collection The specimen may be divided for fungus culture and KOH preparation, mycobacteria culture and smear, and routine bacterial culture and Gram stain only if the specimen is of adequate volume for all tests requested.

Causes for Rejection Insufficient specimen volume

Reference Range No fungus elements identified

Use Determine presence of fungi in skin, nails, or hair

Limitations Cultures are more sensitive than smears; therefore, the KOH preparation may be negative when culture is positive. The test may require overnight incubation for complete disintegration of hair, nail, or skin debris.

Methodology 10% KOH with gentle heat, alternately 20% KOH or 10% KOH and 40% dimethyl sulfoxide (DMSO)

Additional Information See the specimen selection tables provided in the listings, Fungus Culture, Skin *on page 464* and Fungus Culture, Sputum *on page 466*. For the diagnosis of keratomycosis direct examination may have a higher yield than culture because of the presence of dead organisms in the corneal tissue.

Recent reports have emphasized the changing pattern of tinea capitis, particularly the fact that infection due to *Trichophyton tonsurans* has become increasingly common. When present it causes a less discrete, more diffuse pattern of alopecia. It is negative by Wood's light examination. The "black dot," a remnant of a broken infected hair shaft, is a good source for diagnostic material which should be sought with a magnifying glass and collected with forceps. Scale and pulled hairs are also useful specimens. Diagnostic specimens should be collected before antifungal therapy is instituted. Topic steroids should not be prescribed until fungal infection is excluded.

Selected Readings

Cohn MS, "Superficial Fungal Infections. Topical and Oral Treatment of Common Types," *Postgrad Med*, 1992, 91(2):239-44, 249-52.

Gray LD and Roberts GD, "Laboratory Diagnosis of Systemic Fungal Diseases," *Infect Dis Clin North Am*, 1988, 2(4):779-803.

Hebert AA and Burton-Esterly N, "Bacterial and Candidal Cutaneous Infections in the Neonate," *Dermatol Clin*, 1986, 4(1):3-21.

Ishibashi Y, Hommura S, and Matsumoto Y, "Direct Examination vs Culture of Biopsy Specimens for the Diagnosis of Keratomycosis," *Am J Ophthalmol*, 1987, 103(5):636-40.

Stein DH, "Superficial Fungal Infections," *Pediatr Clin North Am*, 1983, 30(3):545-61.

Latex Agglutination, Bacterial Antigens, Cerebrospinal Fluid *see* Bacterial Antigens, Rapid Detection Methods *on page 388*

LE Antibodies *see* Skin Biopsy, Immunofluorescence *on page 583*

Legionella Antigen, Urine

Related Information

Legionella pneumophila Culture *on page 516*

Synonyms Urine *Legionella* Antigen

Specimen Random urine

Container Sterile specimen container

Collection Early morning specimens yield highest bacterial counts from overnight incubation in the bladder, and are the best specimens. Forced fluids or random specimens dilute the urine and may cause reduced colony counts. Hair from perineum will contaminate the specimen. The stream from a male may be contaminated by bacteria from beneath the prepuce. Bacteria from vaginal secretions, vulva or distal urethra may contaminate. Organisms from hands or clothing might contaminate. Receptacle must be sterile.

Male: Wash your hands thoroughly with soap and water. Rinse them well and dry with a paper towel. Tear open the towelette packages so that the towels can be easily removed with one hand as they are needed. Open the urine container. Do not touch any of the inside surfaces of the container or the lid. Pull back the foreskin to completely expose the head of the penis. Wash the head of the penis thoroughly using first one towelette then the other. Discard the used towelettes into the toilet bowl. Pass a small amount of urine into the toilet bowl, then pass a sample into the container. Do not allow the container to touch the legs or the penis. Keep your fingers away from the rim and inner surface of the container. Fill the container half full. Replace the lid on the container. The urine specimen should be refrigerated within 10 minutes of collection or taken immediately to the laboratory.

Female: Wash your hands thoroughly with soap and water. Rinse them well and dry with a paper towel. Tear open the towelette packages so that the towels can be easily

removed with one hand as they are needed. Open the urine container. Do not touch any of the inside surfaces of the container or the lid. Remove your undergarments and sit on the toilet seat with your legs spread widely apart. With one hand, spread your labia apart to expose the vulva. Keep this hand in place during the washing and urinating procedure. Use one towelette to wash the vulva well passing the towelette only from front to back, not back and forth. Repeat this procedure using the second towelette. Discard the used towelettes into the toilet bowl. Begin urinating into the toilet bowl then without stopping the stream, insert the container to collect the specimen. Do not allow the container to touch the legs, vulva, or clothing. Keep your fingers away from the rim and inner surface of the container. Fill the container approximately half full. Replace the lid on the container. The urine specimen should be refrigerated within 10 minutes of collection or taken immediately to the laboratory. Apply the completed patient label to the specimen cup. Most patients, with instruction, do better with privacy than an attendant can.

Catheterized specimen: Do not collect urine from the drainage bag when an indwelling catheter is in place because growth of bacteria can occur in the bag itself. Rather, clean catheter with an alcohol sponge, puncture with sterile needle, collect in sterile syringe. Catheter tips are contaminated by the urethra as they are withdrawn; do not culture them.

Storage Instructions Specimen may be refrigerated if unable to transport immediately.

Causes for Rejection Specimen received in inappropriate or unlabeled container, specimen not received on ice, contaminated specimen. If an unacceptable specimen is received, the nursing unit will be notified and another specimen requested before disposal of the original specimen.

Reference Range Negative

Use Determine the presence of *Legionella* antigen in urine

Limitations This test detects antigen only to *L. pneumophilia* serotype 1. This test can remain positive for several weeks.

Methodology Radioimmunoassay (RIA)

Additional Information This test is sensitive, specific, and extremely clinically useful. However, this test should be confirmed by culture and serology for optimal chances of correct diagnosis.

Selected Readings

Breiman RF and Butler JC, "Legionnaires' Disease: Clinical, Epidemiological, and Public Health Perspectives," *Semin Respir Infect*, 1998, 13(2):84-9.

Cloud JL, Carroll KC, Pixton P, et al, "Detection of *Legionella* Species in Respiratory Specimens Using PCR With Sequencing Confirmation," *J Clin Microbiol*, 2000, 38(5):1709-12.

Pasculle W, "Update on *Legionella*," *Clin Microbiol Newslett*, 2000, 22(13):97-101.

Stout JE, "Laboratory Diagnosis of Legionnaires' Disease: The Expanding Role of the *Legionella* Urinary Antigen Test," *Clin Microbiol Newslett*, 2000, 22(8):62-4.

***Legionella* Assay** *see Legionella* DNA Probe *on page 515*

Legionella DNA Probe

Synonyms DNA Probe for *Legionella*; *Legionella* Assay

Applies to *Legionella* PCR

Specimen Respiratory secretions, sputum, bronchial washing, pleural fluid, lung biopsy

Container Sterile container

Storage Instructions Specimen should be received in the laboratory as soon as possible.

Reference Range Negative for *Legionella*

Use Determine the presence of *Legionella* species

Limitations Inconclusive results can be obtained.

Methodology DNA probe

Additional Information Culture for *Legionella* is the confirmatory test and should be done on all specimens received for *Legionella* DNA probe assay. The sensitivity and specificity of the DNA probe test is 60% to 75% and 98%, respectively. Recently, PCR methods have reported a sensitivity of 100% and a specificity of 93% compared to culture.

Selected Readings

Breiman RF and Butler JC, "Legionnaires' Disease: Clinical, Epidemiological, and Public Health Perspectives," *Semin Respir Infect*, 1998, 13(2):84-9.

Cloud JL, Carroll KC, Pixton P, et al, "Detection of *Legionella* Species in Respiratory Specimens Using PCR With Sequencing Confirmation," *J Clin Microbiol*, 2000, 38(5):1709-12.

Finkelstein R, Brown P, Palutke WA, et al, "Diagnostic Efficacy of a DNA Probe in Pneumonia Caused by *Legionella* Species," *J Med Microbiol*, 1993, 38(3):183-6.

Koide M and Saito A, "Diagnosis of *Legionella pneumophila* Infection by Polymerase Chain Reaction," *Clin Infect Dis*, 1995, 21(1):199-201.

Pasculle W, "Update on *Legionella*," *Clin Microbiol Newslett*, 2000, 22(13):97-101.

(Continued)

Legionella DNA Probe *(Continued)*

Stout JE, "Laboratory Diagnosis of Legionnaires' Disease: The Expanding Role of the *Legionella* Urinary Antigen Test," *Clin Microbiol Newslett*, 2000, 22(8):62-4.

***Legionella* PCR** *see Legionella* DNA Probe *on page 515*

***Legionella pneumophila* Antibodies** *see Legionella* Serology *on page 518*

Legionella pneumophila Culture

Related Information

Aerobic Culture, Sputum *on page 367*
Legionella Antigen, Urine *on page 514*
Legionella pneumophila Smear *on page 517*

Synonyms Culture, *Legionella pneumophila*

Applies to Biopsy *Legionella* Culture; Bronchoscopic *Legionella* Culture; Pleural Fluid *Legionella* Culture; Transtracheal Aspiration *Legionella* Culture

Test Includes Culture and, frequently, direct fluorescent antibody (DFA) smear for *Legionella pneumophila*

Specimen Lung tissue, other body tissue, pleural fluid, other body fluid, transtracheal aspiration, bronchoalveolar lavage, and bronchial brushing

Container Sterile container

Collection Contamination with normal flora from skin or other body surfaces should be avoided.

Turnaround Time Reports on specimens from which *Legionella* has been isolated require approximately 2-5 days.

Reference Range No growth

Use Isolate and identify *Legionella pneumophila*

Infections Caused by *Legionella*

Culture proven
Pneumonia
Empyema
Sinusitis
Prosthetic valve endocarditis
Wound infection
Associated with pneumonia
Bowel abscesses
Brain abscesses
Empyema
Lung abscesses
Myocarditis
Pericarditis
Peritonitis
Renal abscesses/pyelonephritis
Vascular graft infections
Strong seroepidemiological evidence
Pontiac fever
Weak seroepidemiological evidence
Encephalopathy without pneumonia
Myocarditis without pneumonia
Pericarditis without pneumonia

From Edelstein PH, "Laboratory Diagnosis of Infections Caused by *Legionella*," *Eur J Clin Microbiol*, 1987, 6:4-10, with permission.

Limitations Sputum (expectorated), bronchial aspirates, and other specimens having normal flora are subject to bacterial overgrowth and are not as desirable as transtracheal aspirates, pleural fluid, and biopsy material for culture. Sensitivity of cultures is relatively low (50% to 80%); however specificity is 100%. A direct fluorescent antibody smear without culture can be performed, but DFA alone is not recommended because cross reactions with *B. fragilis, Pseudomonas fluorescens*, and other species occur. Newer approaches utilizing monoclonal antibodies have enhanced the yield of fluorescent procedures.

Most clinical laboratories do not culture specifically for *Legionella* species. Contact testing laboratory for availability of the test.

Methodology Culture on selective and nonselective media (buffered charcoal yeast extract)

Some laboratories offer molecular testing for this organism. Contact the testing laboratory for the availability of amplified and nonamplified qualitative and quantitative molecular tests for this organism, and for information on selection and collection of appropriate specimens for specific molecular tests.

Additional Information Acute and convalescent sera for *Legionella* antibodies should also be considered to increase the chance of documenting the diagnosis. A fourfold rise to a titer of 1:128 is a diagnostic standard criterion. Seroconversion may be detected in many patients in the first weeks. Seroconversion 0-7 days after onset, 16%; 0-14 days, 52%; 0-21 days, 66%; 0-28 days, 71%. Twenty-five percent of patients may not have diagnostic titers. Methods to detect *Legionella* antigens in urine include radioimmunoassay, enzyme immunoassay, and latex agglutination. Sensitivity of these methods can be up to 80% under ideal conditions. Consult the laboratory regarding availability and selection of the most appropriate method. Nosocomial infections have been recognized with reservoirs, water distribution systems, cooling systems, and hot water systems of hospitals being reported. Twenty species in the Legionellaceae family of bacteria have been discovered since *Legionella pneumophila* was first recognized. Thirteen species have been implicated as causes of human pneumonia. See tables on previous page and below.

Clinical Clues to the Diagnosis of Legionnaires' Disease

- Gram's stain of respiratory secretions reveals numerous neutrophils, but few organisms
- Presence of hyponatremia (serum sodium ≤130 mmol/L)
- Failure to respond to B-lactam and aminoglycoside antibiotics
- Occurrence in hospital where potable water system is known to be contaminated with *Legionella*
- History of smoking and alcohol use
- Pleuritic chest pain
- Fever malaise, myalgia, headache

From Harrison TG and Taylor AG, "Timing of Seroconversion in Legionnaires' Disease," *Lancet*, Oct 1988, 795, with permission.

Selected Readings

Breiman RF and Butler JC, "Legionnaires' Disease: Clinical, Epidemiological, and Public Health Perspectives," *Semin Respir Infect*, 1998, 13(2):84-9.

Cloud JL, Carroll KC, Pixton P, et al, "Detection of *Legionella* Species in Respiratory Specimens Using PCR With Sequencing Confirmation," *J Clin Microbiol*, 2000, 38(5):1709-12.

Pasculle W, "Update on *Legionella*," *Clin Microbiol Newslett*, 2000, 22(13):97-101.

Rodgers FG, "New Perspectives on *Legionella* Infections," *Infect Med*, 1994, 11(2):137, 141-7.

Stout JE, "Laboratory Diagnosis of Legionnaires' Disease: The Expanding Role of the *Legionella* Urinary Antigen Test," *Clin Microbiol Newslett*, 2000, 22(8):62-4.

Legionella pneumophila Smear

Related Information

Legionella pneumophila Culture *on page 516*

Legionella Serology *on page 518*

Synonyms Direct Fluorescent Antibody Smear for *Legionella pneumophila*; FA Smear for *Legionella pneumophila*

Test Includes Direct fluorescent antibody (DFA) microscopic examination of specimen smear

Specimen Lung tissue, other body tissue, pleural fluid, other body fluid, transtracheal aspirate, sputum, bronchial washing

Container Sterile container

Collection Contamination with normal flora from skin or other body surfaces should be avoided

Causes for Rejection Saliva sent rather than sputum specimen

Reference Range No *Legionella pneumophila* seen in direct FA microscopic examination

Use Determine the presence of *Legionella pneumophila* organisms in direct FA smear of specimen, providing rapid diagnosis

Limitations Staining for several serogroups may be necessary. Most methods include antibodies only to *L. pneumophilia* and not to other *Legionella* species.

Methodology Direct fluorescent antibody (DFA)

Some laboratories offer molecular testing for this organism. Contact the testing laboratory for the availability of amplified and nonamplified qualitative and quantitative molecular tests for this organism, and for information on selection and collection of appropriate specimens for specific molecular tests.

Additional Information Community acquired and nosocomial infections caused by multiple serogroups of *Legionella* are increasingly recognized. Although culture is

(Continued)

Legionella pneumophila Smear *(Continued)*

now possible on buffered charcoal yeast extract agar, the demonstration of organisms in tissue or brushings is the fastest way to make the diagnosis. It also has the advantage of applicability to specimens contaminated with other bacteria. Development of monoclonal antibodies have increased sensitivity and specificity. False-positive reaction has been reported in a case of pleuropulmonary tularemia and in cases of *Campylobacter* infection. A combination of both culture and DFA is recommended.

Selected Readings

Andersen LP and Bangsborg J, "Cross-Reactions Between *Legionella* and *Campylobacter* Spp," *Lancet*, 1992, 340(8813):245.

Hart CA and Makin T, "*Legionella* in Hospitals: A Review," *J Hosp Infect*, 1991, 18(Suppl A):481-9.

Pasculle W, "Update on *Legionella*," *Clin Microbiol Newslett*, 2000, 22(13):97-101.

Roy TM, Fleming D, and Anderson WH, "Tularemic Pneumonia Mimicking Legionnaires' Disease With False-Positive Direct Fluorescent Antibody Stains for *Legionella*," *South Med J*, 1989, 82(11):1429-31.

Stout JE, "Laboratory Diagnosis of Legionnaires' Disease: The Expanding Role of the *Legionella* Urinary Antigen Test," *Clin Microbiol Newslett*, 2000, 22(8):62-4.

Legionella Serology

Related Information

Legionella pneumophila Smear *on page 517*

Synonyms *Legionella pneumophila* Antibodies; Legionnaires' Disease Antibodies

Specimen Serum

Container Red top tube

Collection A convalescent sample should be obtained 10-14 days after acute sample

Reference Range Negative. Less than a fourfold change in titer between acute and convalescent samples. Less than 1:256 in a single sample.

Use Detect antibody to *Legionella pneumophila*; support the clinical diagnosis of Legionnaires' disease

Limitations Testing for multiple serogroups may be necessary

Methodology Indirect fluorescent antibody assay using serogroup 1: Philadelphia, Knoxville, serogroup 2: Togus, serogroup 3: Los Angeles, serogroup 4: Bloomington. A polyvalent antigen which includes serogroup 1-6 may be utilized. IgG and IgM titers may be provided. Latex agglutination may be used in some laboratories.

Some laboratories offer molecular testing for this organism. Contact the testing laboratory for the availability of amplified and nonamplified qualitative and quantitative molecular tests for this organism, and for information on selection and collection of appropriate specimens for specific molecular tests.

Additional Information A fourfold rise in titer exceeding a titer of 1:128 from the acute to convalescent phase provides evidence of recent infection. A single titer ≥1:256 is evidence of infection at an undetermined time. However, due to the relatively high prevalence of antibodies to *Legionella pneumophila*, acute and convalescent titers are preferred to a single sample. Demonstration of a high titer in the proper clinical setting may allow timely institution of specific treatment, and may eliminate the need for an invasive procedure to obtain a specimen for culture or direct immunofluorescence. Demonstration of IgM antibody to serogroup I may allow rapid diagnosis. Recent availability of a latex agglutination test with 98.3% specificity and 97.6% sensitivity is well suited as a screening test. Serologic study is also valuable in evaluation of epidemic disease.

Selected Readings

Edelstein PH, "Detection of Antibodies to *Legionella* spp," *Manual of Clinical Laboratory Immunology*, 5th ed, Rose NR, Conway de Macario E, Folds JD, et al, eds, Washington, DC: American Society for Microbiology, 1997, 502-9

Holliday MG, "Use of Latex Agglutination Technique for Detecting *Legionella pneumophila* (Serogroup I) Antibodies," *J Clin Pathol*, 1990, 43(10):860-2.

Rodgers FG, "New Perspectives on *Legionella* Infections," *Infect Med*, 1994, 11(2):137, 141-7.

Legionnaires' Disease Antibodies *see Legionella* Serology *on page 518*

***Leptospira*, Blood Culture** *see Leptospira* Culture *on page 518*

Leptospira Culture

Related Information

Darkfield Examination, Leptospirosis *on page 443*

Leptospira Serology *on page 519*

Synonyms Culture for *Leptospira*

Applies to *Leptospira*, Blood Culture; Blood Culture, *Leptospira*

Patient Preparation Urine specimen: Thoroughly instruct patient in the proper collection technique for a midvoid urine specimen; avoid contamination with skin flora. See also Urine Culture, Clean Catch *on page 609* and Blood Culture, Aerobic and Anaerobic *on page 391* for detailed instructions.

Special Instructions The laboratory should be informed of the specific request for *Leptospira* culture, collection time, date, specific site of specimen, age of patient, current antibiotic therapy, date of onset of illness, and clinical diagnosis. Urine must be alkaline; *Leptospira* do not survive in acid urine. Repeated cultures may be required.

Specimen During the first week of illness: Blood and cerebrospinal fluid should be cultured. After the second week of illness: Urine should be cultured.

Container Sterile container or tube

Collection Specimen should be transported to laboratory within 1 hour of collection. For midvoid urine culture, patient should be instructed to clean skin thoroughly, do not collect first portion of stream, collect midportion of stream, and do not collect final portion of stream. Catheter or suprapubic puncture specimen may also be used.

Causes for Rejection Specimens delayed in transit to the laboratory have less than optimal yield.

Turnaround Time 4-8 weeks. Consult the laboratory prior to the collection of the specimen, so that appropriate processing of the specimen can be arranged.

Reference Range No *Leptospira* isolated

Use Confirm the clinical diagnosis of leptospirosis

Limitations Specimen will be cultured for *Leptospira*; other organisms may not be identified. The sensitivity of culture is very low. Usually the test is not particularly productive.

Contraindications Leptospiremia occurs during the septicemic acute phase of infection. This phase last 4-7 days after which organisms are not recoverable from blood. Cultures of blood should **not** be ordered after the first week of illness.

Methodology Urine or blood is inoculated onto specially prepared media containing rabbit serum or albumin and fatty acids. Incubation is for 4-6 weeks in the dark at 28°C to 29°C. Cultures are examined with darkfield or phase microscopy at weekly intervals; growth occurs 1-3 cm below the surface.

Additional Information Leptospirosis in humans is usually associated with occupational exposure. Veterinarians, dairymen, swineherds, abattoir workers, miners, fish and poultry processors, and those who work in a rat-infested environment are at increased risk. During the first week of disease, the most reliable means of detecting leptospires is by direct culturing of blood or spinal fluid on appropriate media. **Urine does not become positive for *Leptospira*** until the second week of disease and then can remain positive for several months. Concentration of *Leptospira* in human urine is low and shedding may be intermittent. Therefore, repeated isolation attempts should be made. Serology (acute and early convalescent) is recommended. Darkfield examination yields many false-positives.

Selected Readings

Levett PN, "Leptospirosis," *Clin Microbiol Rev*, 2001, 14(2):296-326.

Sperber SJ and Schleupner CJ, "Leptospirosis: A Forgotten Cause of Aseptic Meningitis and Multisystem Febrile Illness," *South Med J*, 1989, 82(10):1285-8.

Leptospira Serology

Related Information

Darkfield Examination, Leptospirosis *on page 443*
Leptospira Culture *on page 518*

Test Includes Testing of patient's serum for antibodies against *Leptospira biflexa* serovar *L. patoc*, and the following serovars of *Leptospira interrogans*: *L. copenhageni*, *L. canicola*, *L. pomona*, *L. autumnalis*, *L. grippotyphosa*, *L. wolffi*, and *L. djatzi*. Supplemental testing may be needed against serovars: *L. poi*, *L. castellonis*, *L. pyrogenes*, *L. borincana*, *L. szwajizak*, *L. bratislava*, *L. tarassovi*, *L. shermani*, *L. panama*, *L. celledoni*, *L. djasiman*, *L. cynopteri*, and *L. louisiana*.

Specimen Serum

Container Red top tube

Collection Acute and convalescent sera drawn 10-14 days apart are suggested

Causes for Rejection Inadequate labeling, excessive hemolysis, chylous serum, or gross contamination of the specimen

Reference Range Negative. A fourfold increase in titer is diagnostic of infection.

Use Support the diagnosis of leptospirosis

Limitations The antigens used in the test are the ones most commonly causing disease, but there are many other serovars which might not be detected. To optimize yield, a battery of antigens are used.

Methodology Microscopic agglutination test, macroagglutination, complement fixation, hemagglutination, enzyme-linked immunosorbent assay (ELISA)

Additional Information Leptospirosis is an acute febrile illness caused primarily by *Leptospira interrogans*, a large spirochete with over 180 serologic variants. Patients with extensive animal contact, either in the wild or with carcasses or excrement, are particularly at risk.

(Continued)

Leptospira Serology *(Continued)*

Although leptospires can be cultured from blood or urine during the first week of illness, this interval is often missed, and diagnosis must be based on the demonstration of rising antibody titers. Antibody appears at the end of the first week of illness and peaks at 3-4 weeks, after which it slowly disappears.

There has been an association between patients with leptospirosis and anticardiolipin antibodies which may induce vascular endothelial injury in severe cases.

Selected Readings

Levett PN, "Leptospirosis," *Clin Microbiol Rev*, 2001, 14(2):296-326.

Ribeiro MA, Sakata EE, Silva MV, et al, "Antigens Involved in the Human Antibody Response to Natural Infections With *Leptospira interrogans* serovar *copenhageni*," *J Trop Med Hyg*, 1992, 95(4):239-45.

Rugman FP, Pinn G, Palmer MF, et al, "Anticardiolipin Antibodies in Leptospirosis," *J Clin Pathol*, 1991, 44(6):517-9.

Leptospirosis, Darkfield Examination *see* Darkfield Examination, Leptospirosis *on page 443*

Lesion Culture *see* Wound Culture *on page 620*

Leukocyte Esterase, Urine

Related Information

Nitrite, Urine *on page 549*

Synonyms Bacteria Screen, Urine; Esterase, Leukocyte, Urine

Test Includes Screening of urine for leukocyte esterase activity by dipstick is usually a part of urinalysis

Abstract A rapid indirect test for detection of bacteriuria. A positive test reflects the presence of neutrophils. Evaluation of urinary tract infection includes nitrite (also on reagent strips) microscopy, Gram stain, urine culture with colony count, and other methods. **The best test for urinary tract infection is culture.**

Specimen Random clean catch urine; preferably midstream, clean catch collection, catheterized specimen, bladder aspiration

Container Plastic urine container

Storage Instructions If the specimen cannot be processed within 2 hours, it should be refrigerated for other portions of urine evaluation.

Reference Range Negative

Use The leukocyte esterase test is positive with intact or lysed white blood cells. The lysis of leukocytes that occurs when urine is allowed to stand intensifies the color reaction from release of esterase. The test performs best for specimens in which colony counts are $>10^5$ CFU/mL and when combined with nitrite: together the most enthusiastic reports find a specificity of 98.3%, sensitivity of 84%, positive predictive value of 84%, and negative predictive value of 98.3%. Sensitivity, however, was much worse in a Belgian study (Zaman, 1998).

Limitations Cephalexin; cephalothin; tetracycline; large amounts of oxalic acid (eg, iced tea drinkers); high glucose and high specific gravity may decrease or suppress positive results. Albumin and ascorbic acid inhibit the method. Tetracycline may cause decreased reactivity or false-negatives. Neutropenia can cause false-negative results.

There are numerous false positives and false negatives. **Leukocyte esterase** is unreliable as a screen. The urinalysis, including leukocyte esterase and nitrite, should not replace culture in symptomatic patients. For example, in women with symptomatic cystitis, both leukocyte esterase and nitrite miss approximately 1 in 5 patients who have positive cultures.

When laboratory testing is needed for a patient with symptoms of urinary sepsis, urine culture should be performed.

Methodology The substrate on the strip is indoxyl carbonic acid ester. Indoxyl is oxidized by atmospheric oxygen to indigo blue. The reaction time is 1 minute, but high sensitivity requires interpretation 5 minutes after immersion in the sample.

Selected Readings

Bachman JW, Heise RH, Naessens JM, et al, "A Study of Various Tests to Detect Asymptomatic Urinary Tract Infections in an Obstetric Population," *JAMA*, 1993, 270(16):1971-4.

Misdraji J and Nguyen PL, "Urinalysis. When - and When Not - To Order," *Postgrad Med*, 1996, 100(1):173-6, 181-2, 185-8 passim.

Semeniuk H and Church D, "Evaluation of the Leukocyte Esterase and Nitrite Urine Dipstick Screening Tests for Detection of Bacteriuria in Women With Suspected Uncomplicated Urinary Tract Infections," *J Clin Microbiol*, 1999, 37(9):3051-2.

Shaw ST Jr, Poon SY, and Wong ET, "Routine Urinalysis, Is the Dipstick Enough?" *JAMA*, 1985, 253(11):1596-600.

Van Nostrand JD, Junkins AD, and Bartholdi RK, "Poor Predictive Ability of Urinalysis and Microscopic Examination to Detect Urinary Tract Infection," *Am J Clin Pathol*, 2000, 113(5):709-13.

Zaman Z, Borremans A, Verhaegen J, et al, "Disappointing Dipstick Screening for Urinary Tract Infection in Hospital Inpatients," *J Clin Pathol*, 1998, 51(6):471-2.

Leukocyte Scintigraphy *see* Indium Leukocyte Scan *on page 508*

Lice Identification *see* Arthropod Identification *on page 387*

Liver Biopsy

Related Information

Histopathology *on page 496*

Synonyms Blind Liver Biopsy; Needle Biopsy of the Liver; Percutaneous Liver Biopsy

Applies to Percutaneous Needle Aspiration Biopsy Under Fluoroscopic, CT, or Ultrasound Guidance; Transjugular Needle Biopsy of the Liver

Test Includes Percutaneous biopsy of liver parenchyma in a "blind" fashion (ie, not under radiologic guidance). This is carried out at the bedside under local anesthesia. A specialized, thin-bore needle is advanced between the ribs overlying the region of hepatic dullness. Several 2 cm cores of deep liver tissue are excised. Fresh specimens may be sent for gross pathologic inspection, routine light microscopy, special stains for liver storage diseases, transmission and immune electron microscopy, immunohistochemistry (using monoclonal antibodies), DNA hybridization studies, and microbiologic culture. Liver biopsy is a valuable and time-honored means of diagnosing diffuse liver parenchymal disease as well as disseminated focal disease.

Patient Preparation Procedures and risks of the procedure are explained and consent is obtained. Procedure entails overnight hospitalization in most cases but some patients may be candidates for a "same day" outpatient biopsy. This latter group is in good general health, not jaundiced, and displays no signs of liver failure (ascites, encephalopathy). Postbiopsy, the patient should have access to hospital care if needed and should have supervision from family or friends. Scheduling arrangements for both in-hospital and outpatient liver biopsies are handled by gastroenterology team. All aspirin products and nonsteroidal agents must be discontinued at least 5 days prior to the procedure. If taking oral anticoagulants (Coumadin®), hospitalization is required to convert to heparin therapy before biopsy. Patient is NPO after midnight the evening prior. Daily medications may be taken on the day of procedure pending physician approval. In some hospitals, patient drinks 1-2 glasses of milk in the early AM on procedure day to empty the gallbladder. Screening laboratory studies ordered 24-48 hours in advance commonly include CBC, PT/PTT, BUN, bleeding time, and type and screen for possible transfusion. Electrolytes and liver function tests are optional. If pneumonia or pleural effusion suspected on examination, PA and lateral chest x-ray is obtained. Premedication with meperidine and/or diazepam may be administered at physician discretion. This is not routine in some centers due to possible toxicity.

Aftercare Protocols are individualized for each hospital. In general, patient is monitored in a recovery area with frequent vital signs postbiopsy. If no complications are apparent, patient is transferred back to hospital room by cart. Strict bedrest is enforced for 24 hours; for the first 2 hours patient is positioned on his right side. After 5 hours, patient may be allowed to sit up. Vitals (blood pressure, pulse) are checked every 15-30 minutes for 2 hours, every 30 minutes for the next 2 hours, and then every hour for 8 hours. Following this, vitals every 4 hours are permissible. Physician should be immediately notified if hypotension, tachycardia, fever, or uncontrolled pain occurs. Diet is restricted to clear liquids for several hours, then full liquids as tolerated. Acetaminophen is usually sufficient for pain control. Some physicians recheck hematocrit 24 hours after procedure before approving hospital discharge.

Special Instructions In the appropriate high-risk patient, antibiotic prophylaxis for infective endocarditis may be considered. Little data exists regarding the risk of bacteremia, however, much less endocarditis.

Complications Based on several large series, serious morbidity has been estimated at 0.1% to 0.2%. Fatality rates have ranged from 0% to 0.17%, both figures being derived from studies involving >20,000 biopsies each. The more commonly seen complications are:

- pain - the most common adverse event, noted in ≤50% of cases. Usually it is confined to the right shoulder, probably referred pain from diaphragmatic pleura. Analgesia is required in approximately 20% of patients with acetaminophen sufficient in most cases. Symptoms resolve in 1-2 days.
- hemorrhage - minor episodes are common. Self-limited oozing from the puncture site may persist for approximately 1 minute, but with loss of only 5-10 mL blood. Significant hemorrhage is less frequent but is the most common cause of death from liver biopsy. Several series have estimated an incidence of approximately 0.2%, but Sherlock (1984) reported 40 patients out of 6379 required transfusion for intraperitoneal bleeding. She felt these statistics may even underestimate the incidence since those with severe coagulopathies were excluded. Bleeding usually results from a tear of a distended portal or hepatic vein. Specific sites include the abdominal cavity (hemoperitoneum), liver capsule (capsular hematoma), liver parenchyma (intrahepatic hematoma), or biliary tree (hemobilia). Postulated risk factors are coagulopathy, amyloid liver, hepatocellular injury, hemangioma, and vascularized tumor. However, bleeding may be massive when

(Continued)

Liver Biopsy *(Continued)*

no risk factors are present. Not all episodes require surgery. In a study 4 of 7532 patients needed surgical intervention while 12 others with severe hemorrhage were transfused and observed.

- bile leakage with peritonitis - associated with severe obstruction of the larger bile ducts. This is felt to result from laceration of a small, distended duct or from puncture of the gallbladder. With the widespread use of noninvasive imaging, the size of the bile ducts is known prebiopsy and the complication rate has declined.
- laceration of internal organs and viscera - right kidney, gallbladder, colon, pancreas, and others
- others: right-sided pneumothorax, arteriovenous fistula - 5.4% of all biopsies, drug toxicity

Equipment Several biopsy needles are available.

- Menghini needle - 1.9 mm diameter steel shaft with sharpened beveled tip and syringe; specimen is obtained using suction/aspiration into a 10 mL syringe. Requires only 1 second within the liver ("1-second technique") and patient need not hold his breath. Disadvantages are small samples and fragmentation of biopsy specimens.
- "Trucut" needle - disposable 2.05 mm diameter needle designed to cut out cores of tissue. Specimens are less fragmented, even in the cirrhotic liver, and thus a high success rate. However, dwell time in liver is longer (5-10 seconds), patient must cooperate more, and several steps are necessary.
- Vim-Silverman needle - sheath with inner cutting blade (similar to a "punch" biopsy). Trucut needle is a modernized Vim-Silverman.

Technique Patient lies supine in bed with right hand behind his head. Liver margins are estimated by percussion. Two approaches are popular, transthoracic (intercostal) or subcostal (anterior). With the former, biopsy site is identified along the midaxillary line in the center of hepatic dullness, usually the eighth or ninth intercostal space. This approach avoids other abdominal organs but always penetrates the pleura. With the subcostal approach, the biopsy site lies below the bottom rib anteriorly, and is used when a liver mass is easily palpable below the right costal margin. The risk of visceral laceration is higher and this approach is infrequently used; fine needle aspiration under CT guidance has become more popular. A wide area is prepped and draped in sterile fashion with operators in gowns, gloves, and masks. The skin is anesthetized with 1% lidocaine, then deeper structures are infiltrated - subcutaneous tissue, intercostal muscles, and diaphragm. Some operators make a small superficial incision with a No 11 blade at the needle entry site to facilitate needle insertion. Techniques differ with the type of biopsy needle selected. In general, the biopsy needle is advanced as far as the diaphragm (depth estimated by a finder needle). If a Menghini needle is used, suction is applied to the syringe, the needle is pushed rapidly through the pleura and into the liver parenchyma. A 2.5 cm core of liver is aspirated and needle withdrawn, all within 1 second. If other needles are used, patient may need to hold his breath at end expiration to decrease the risk of pneumothorax. Several passes of the biopsy needle are performed to minimize sampling bias.

Specimen At least 2-3 liver cores, each >2 cm in length. A typical protocol would be as follows:

- tissue fixation - for light microscopy, specimen is routinely fixed in 10% buffered formalin within 1 minute. For transmission electron microscopy, 1 mm cubes of specimen are fixed immediately in glutaraldehyde with further processing in Pathology Laboratory.
- routine tissue stains including: H & E - general liver histology stain; reticulin stain - for connective tissue, especially cirrhosis, fibrosis, bridging necrosis; trichrome - fibrosis; iron stain - useful for hemosiderosis, hemochromatosis, bile pigments; diastase PAS stain - useful for $alpha_1$-antitrypsin globules, bile ducts, iron; orcein - for hepatitis B surface antigen (if present, fine granular brown material stains in hepatocytes). Also for copper-binding protein in Wilson's disease.
- cytologic preparation - fluid from aspirating syringe may be smeared on clean microscope slide, fixed, and sent to Cytology Laboratory
- microbiological culture - specimen sent without fixative in sterile container. Special stains (AFB, KOH, etc) and cultures (tuberculosis, viral, *Brucella*, parasites, fungi) as needed
- optional special stains (ie, congo red for amyloidosis, immunohistochemistry)

Use Candidates for liver biopsy must be carefully selected. This procedure, by nature, is invasive and histologic findings may often be reported as "consistent with" a particular disease (without being pathognomonic) or simply "nondiagnostic". In most cases, noninvasive imaging studies such as CT scan or ultrasound are now obtained first. With these considerations in mind, indications for liver biopsy include:

- suspected cases of liver cirrhosis, in order to confirm the diagnosis pathologically; establish etiology if possible (alcohol, alpha$_1$-antitrypsin deficiency, primary biliary cirrhosis, Wilson's disease, hemochromatosis, etc); assess and stage level of activity; assess complications
- chronic hepatitis, with or without cirrhosis, to identify cases of chronic activity hepatitis (liver biopsy mandatory for diagnosis) and differentiate this entity from chronic persistent hepatitis and lobular hepatitis
- suspected liver disease in the known alcoholic patient, to confirm alcoholic liver disease, exclude alternative causes of liver disease (which may be present in ≤20% of cases), stage and assess disease activity
- diagnosis of hepatoma or metastatic neoplasms
- suspected multisystem disease with liver involvement, where traditional diagnostic techniques have not been fruitful (eg, sarcoidosis, amyloidosis, tuberculosis, glycogen storage disease)
- staging of lymphoma
- unexplained hepatomegaly
- cholestasis of unknown etiology, where prior studies for biliary obstruction are negative
- persistently elevated liver enzyme tests
- selected cases of fever of unknown origin
- selected cases of hepatitis of unknown etiology, in order to differentiate viral from drug-induced etiologies (not always possible) or to assess complications, such as cholestasis
- evaluation of response to treatment

Liver biopsy is less useful in:

- acute hepatitis A or B infection, unless the diagnosis is in question
- extrahepatic biliary obstruction, where percutaneous transhepatic cholangiography and ERCP are considered first-line procedures
- fluid-filled liver cysts detected on ultrasound or CT scan, probably more amenable to guided thin needle aspiration first

Contraindications Mahal et al (1979) noted that failure to heed accepted contraindications led directly to 22 bleeding episodes in 3800 percutaneous liver biopsies. Contraindications include:

- impaired hemostasis, accepted as prothrombin time more than 3 seconds over control, PTT more than 20 seconds over control, thrombocytopenia, and markedly prolonged bleeding time
- severe anemia (Hgb <9.5 g/dL)
- local infection near needle entry site, such as right sided pleural effusion or empyema, right lower lobe pneumonia, local cellulitis, infected ascites or peritonitis
- tense ascites (low yield technically, risk of leakage)
- high-grade extrahepatic biliary obstruction with jaundice (increased risk of bile peritonitis)
- septic cholangitis
- possible hemangioma
- possible echinococcal (hydatid) cyst
- lack of compatible blood for transfusion
- uncooperative patient

Selected Readings

Lefkowitch JH, "Pathologic Diagnosis of Liver Disease," *Hepatology: A Textbook of Liver Disease*, 2nd ed, Chapter 29, Zakim D and Boyer TD, eds, Philadelphia, PA: WB Saunders Co, 1990, 711-32.

Mahal AS, Knauer CM, and Gregory PB, "Bleeding After Liver Biopsy," *West J Med*, 1981, 134(1):11-4.

Perrault J, McGill DB, Ott BJ, et al, "Liver Biopsy: Complications in 1000 Inpatients and Outpatients," *Gastroenterology*, 1978, 78(1):103-6.

Schaffner F and Thung SN, "Liver Biopsy," *Bockus Gastroenterology*, 5th ed, Chapter 97, Haubrich WS, Schaffner F, and Berk JE, eds, Philadelphia, PA: WB Saunders Co, 1995.

Sherlock S, Dick R, and van Leeuwen DJ, "Liver Biopsy Today. The Royal Free Hospital Experience," *J Hepatol*, 1984, 1(1):75-85.

Sherlock S and Dooley J, "Biopsy of the Liver," *Diseases of the Liver and Biliary System*, 10th ed, Chapter 3, Oxford, England: Blackwell Scientific Publications, 1997, 33-42.

Van Ness MM and Diehl AM, "Is Liver Biopsy Useful in the Evaluation of Patients With Chronically Elevated Liver Enzymes?" *Ann Intern Med*, 1989, 111(6):473-8.

Lower Respiratory Fungus Culture *see* Fungus Culture, Bronchial Aspirate *on page 463*

Lower Respiratory Mycobacteria Culture *see* Mycobacteria Culture, Sputum *on page 542*

LP *see* Lumbar Puncture *on page 524*

Lumbar Puncture

Synonyms Cerebrospinal Fluid Tap; LP; Spinal Tap

Test Includes Collection of cerebrospinal fluid (CSF) for chemical, cellular, and microbiological analysis. Performed as a bedside procedure under local anesthesia, a needle is passed into the L4-L5 vertebral interspace and subarachnoid fluid is withdrawn.

Patient Preparation Procedure and risks are explained and consent is obtained. If patient is confused or obtunded, obtain consent from guardians. If a coagulopathy is suspected, obtain platelet count and prothrombin/partial thromboplastin time if time permits. No intravenous pain medications such as meperidine are required routinely. Likewise, sedatives or anxiolytics may serve to confuse later assessments of mental status.

Aftercare Patient should be kept at strict bedrest for a minimum of 3 hours post-procedure to minimize post-LP headache. Regarding the optimal patient positioning, opinions vary. Some authors recommend the prone position post-LP based on a study involving >1000 subjects which demonstrated a 0.5% incidence of headache in patients kept prone versus 36.5% in the supine group. The frequency of obtaining vital signs and neurologic checks after the procedure should be based on the patient's overall status. Nursing staff should be familiar with potential LP complications, especially acute deteriorations in mental status (possible tonsillar herniation), sensory deficits, leg muscle weakness, and bladder and bowel incontinence (possible expanding spinal subdural hematoma). If no complications arise, activity may later be upgraded to *ad lib* as tolerated, with physician's approval.

Complications Although a wide range of complications has been reported, LP should generally be considered a safe procedure. The most common complication is "spinal headache" with an estimated incidence of 10% to 25%. This may be minimized by using a small gauge spinal needle and placing the patient in the prone position after the procedure. Another common complication is local bleeding, the "traumatic tap," which results from needle rupture of venous plexuses surrounding the spinal sack. Incidence may be as high as 20%. As long as no coagulation defect exists, the traumatic tap is clinically insignificant and rarely leads to spinal hematoma. Immediate painful paresthesias due to nerve root irritation is another common complication (≤13%), but usually resolves upon repositioning the spinal needle. Rare complications (<1%) include persistent pain or leg paresthesias; spinal epidural, subdural or subarachnoid hematomas; arachnoiditis from tracking in povidone-iodine on the needle; local infection (epidural or subdural empyema); transient cranial nerve palsies (especially CN VI when large volumes of CSF removed); rupture of nucleus pulposus; delayed formation of intraspinal epidermoid tumors (when stylet is not used); and vagal cardiac arrest. Note that the use of anticoagulants or presence of a coagulopathy significantly increases the risk of spinal hematoma formation (≤7%). Tonsillar herniation is an infrequent but potentially lethal complication of LP which occurs in patients with increased intracranial pressure. The exact incidence is not clear. In one series of patients with papilledema and increased intracranial pressure from a variety of causes, tonsillar herniation occurred after LP in <1.2% of cases. A particularly high risk group appears to be the patient with brain abscess or subdural empyema, with an estimated 10% to 20% incidence of LP-induced herniation and death. The herniation risk in patients with brain tumor is not known, although one study (which predated head CT scans) reported neurologic deterioration following LP in only 1 of 400 brain tumor cases. In general, due to incomplete data, a variety of clinical approaches have been adopted to avoid this fatal complication (see Additional Information).

Equipment Commercial LP trays are available. Common items include iodine, alcohol pads, sterile gloves and drapes, local anesthesia (usually 1% lidocaine) with appropriate needles and syringes, four sterile collecting tubes, 3-way stopcock with connecting tubing, manometer, and spinal needle with stylette. In general, a small bore spinal needle should be used, such as a 25-gauge, due to a lower incidence of spinal headache compared with a 20- or 22-gauge needle.

Technique In all cases, perform a careful fundoscopic and neurologic exam to rule out papilledema or a focal neurologic deficit. LP is then performed in one of two ways. In the standard method, patient is placed on a firm surface in the lateral recumbent position, curled with knees down in towards the chest and neck maximally flexed. The lumbar region should be close to the edge of the bed, with the plane of the back and shoulders as perpendicular to the bed as possible. Proper positioning is by far the most important step to ensure success and usually requires one or more assistants. The L4-L5 interspace is identified by drawing an imaginary line between the two posterior iliac crests. This area is cleaned, prepped, and draped. Skin and deeper subcutaneous tissues are infiltrated with lidocaine. The spinal needle with stylette is then passed into the L4-L5 interspace along the midline, bevel upwards. The needle is angled slightly cephalad along an imaginary line between the site of entry and the umbilicus. As the needle is advanced, the stylette should be frequently withdrawn and

replaced every 1-2 mm in order to identify the first drop of CSF (and avoid overpenetration). Once CSF fluid is seen in the needle hub, the manometer is immediately attached to the needle via connecting tubing. Opening pressure should be measured promptly (do not wait more than 1 minute) with the patient's legs and hips extended. If the opening pressure is elevated (>180 mm CSF), try to eliminate factors that may cause false elevations. Instruct patient to straighten his legs, breathe evenly, avoid Valsalva maneuvers, and relax his abdominal muscles. If the opening pressure remains markedly elevated, close the 3-way stopcock, collect only the CSF already in the manometer, disconnect all the tubing, reinsert stylette, and consider neurosurgical consultation. If opening pressure is normal, CSF is then collected in tubes 1-4 in sequence. Manometer is reconnected afterwards and a closing pressure recorded. Stylette is replaced and both needle and stylette removed together. Pressure is held over the puncture site. An alternate approach may be needed in the patient whose vertebral landmarks are difficult to palpate. Initially, patient is placed in a seated position with neck and spine maximally flexed, arms resting on a bedside table. The L4-L5 interspace is identified as before and the remainder of the procedure is identical. This may be used with the obese patient or the patient with ankylosing spondylitis or severe scoliosis. Variations of this procedure have been described including: a lateral approach through the paravertebral muscles, the "hanging drop" technique used by anesthesiologists for identifying entry into the subdural space, and suboccipital puncture of the cisterna magna. These techniques are not necessary in the majority of cases.

Data Acquired Estimation of spinal fluid pressure as described. CSF fluid analytic tests are ordered based on clinical suspicion. Routine tests include cell count and CSF glucose level. Optional tests (not all samples): protein, VDRL, bacterial antigen detection battery, fungal antigens (such as *Cryptococcus*), culture (bacterial, fungal, viral, tuberculous), India ink preparation for *Cryptococcus*, infectious antibody titers, Gram stain, acid-fast bacilli smear, and cytology. Specialized tests include oligoclonal bands and myelin basic protein (for multiple sclerosis). The interested reader should refer to the *Laboratory Test Handbook* for further details.

Specimen 10-12 mL maximum removed from the adult. Smaller volumes are sufficient for most routine tests (confirm with laboratory).

Container Sterile tubes, numbered 1 to 4

Collection Tube 1: CSF protein and glucose; tube 2: cell count and differential; tube 3: Gram stain and cultures; tube 4: save for optional studies

Storage Instructions Specimen should be sent to laboratory immediately, preferably hand carried by physician.

Normal Findings (Adults) opening pressure: 80-180 mm of CSF in lateral recumbent position, somewhat higher in sitting position. Respiratory variation of 5-10 mm normal. Clarity: normally very clear. CSF glucose: 60% to 70% of blood glucose. This estimation does not hold for blood glucose levels >300 mg/dL where CSF glucose empirically fails to rise. CSF protein: 15-55 mg/dL. CSF cell count and differential: 0-5 mononuclear white blood cells/mm^3 (lymphocytes and monocytes). The presence of even 1 or 2 polymorphonuclear cells (PMNs) is abnormal. Red blood cells: 0. Gram stain and culture: negative.

Critical Values Interpretation of CSF findings have been reviewed in detail elsewhere. As a rule, interpretation of abnormal CSF values must always be made in close conjunction with the individual patient's clinical presentation. Considerable overlap exists among the "classic" CSF patterns which are meant to characterize different disease entities. No constellation of CSF findings is entirely specific for a given disease. LP has its greatest value in the diagnosis of bacterial meningitis. A classic CSF "purulent profile" has been described for bacterial meningitis, characterized by elevated WBCs in CSF (often >500/mm^3), predominance of PMN cells on CSF differential (>5/mm^3, presumed high sensitivity, low specificity), depressed CSF glucose levels (<40 mg/dL, 58% sensitivity), low CSF glucose to blood glucose ratio (<0.3, sensitivity 70%). Gram stain of CSF is positive in most cases (60% to 90%) as is the culture (80%). However, even acute bacterial meningitis may present in an atypical fashion, with predominant CSF lymphocytosis (10%), negative Gram stain, or, rarely, normal CSF leukocyte counts. In addition, the "purulent profile" may also be seen in noninfectious conditions such as subarachnoid hemorrhage (≤20% of cases). In contrast, CSF findings in viral meningitis typically reveal <100 WBCs/mm^3, predominantly mononuclear cells on differential, normal glucose levels, normal or elevated protein levels, and negative Gram stain. However, some overlap exists with the profile for bacterial meningitis and 10% of patients with viral meningitis may have mostly PMNs, especially early in the course. Viral cultures are positive in <50% of the cases at best and may be as low as 5% for herpes simplex virus. Thus, viral cultures have a limited role and LP is most useful clinically in ruling out bacterial meningitis. Viral meningitis rarely presents with WBC counts in CSF >1000/mm^3, CSF protein levels >100 mg/dL, or glucose <40 mg/dL. Such patients should be treated as bacterial meningitis until proven otherwise. Fungal meningitis rarely presents a normal CSF

(Continued)

Lumbar Puncture *(Continued)*

picture but the abnormalities are very nonspecific (elevated protein, depressed glucose, and lymphocytic pleocytosis). For the diagnosis of cryptococcal meningitis, the cryptococcal antigen detection test is accurate very early on. Similar nonspecific CSF profiles are seen in tuberculous meningitis and sometimes may mimic bacterial meningitis. The acid-fast smear has notoriously low sensitivity (<25%) but acid-fast bacilli culture has a 90% sensitivity. Malignancy involving the meninges (primary or metastatic) often results in a CSF picture mimicking infectious meningitis. Typically, there is a CSF leukocytosis, elevated protein, and glucose may range from normal to markedly decreased. A completely normal CSF exam essentially rules out CNS malignancy. Sensitivity of CSF cytology varies considerably among studies and varies from 60% to 90%, independent of such factors as tumor type, metastases, or primary brain site. A significant 3% false-positive rate has been reported which has limited its role as a routine staging screen for patients with malignancy. LP may be useful in diagnosing selected cases of subarachnoid hemorrhage (SAH), especially those in which head CT scan is equivocal. Interpretation of LP results may be problematic since RBCs in CSF commonly arise from a traumatic tap. The presence of xanthochromia in CSF has traditionally been associated with SAH, but has also been found in nearly one-third of traumatic taps. Similarly, a decreased RBC count from tube 1-4 has usually meant a traumatic tap but studies have shown a specificity of only 56%. Because of these limitations and potential LP complications, head CT scan has supplanted LP as the major diagnostic test in cases of suspected SAH. The diagnosis of multiple sclerosis may be supported by special CSF studies including oligoclonal banding and myelin basic protein, but sensitivity and specificity are variable. Another demyelinating condition, Guillain-Barré syndrome, is characterized by an isolated CSF protein value >200 mg/dL, with the remainder of CSF parameters normal. The absence of an elevated protein level practically excludes Guillain-Barré. In general, LP is more useful in Guillain-Barré syndrome than multiple sclerosis.

Use Practitioners vary in their threshold for performing an LP. This procedure is clearly indicated in the following clinical settings:

- clinically suspected meningitis, either acute (where procedure is emergent), subacute, or chronic; also, suspected encephalitis or meningoencephalitis
- suspected central nervous system syphilis in clearly symptomatic patients (tertiary neurosyphilis)
- evaluation of potential CNS lymphoma, meningeal leukemia, and meningeal carcinomatosis
- staging of lymphoma, previously diagnosed from another site
- clinically suspected demyelinating disease such as multiple sclerosis or Guillain-Barré syndrome
- possible cases of subarachnoid hemorrhage

CSF findings in each of these indications is fairly distinctive and LP substantially aids in clinical diagnosis. In contrast, several diseases have abnormal, but nonspecific, CSF findings and LP has low sensitivity and specificity. These include brain abscess or subdural empyema, primary brain tumor, tumors metastatic to brain, subdural or epidural hematoma, connective tissue diseases with CNS involvement (such as CNS lupus or Sjögren's syndrome). Additional studies (such as head CT scan) are necessary to confirm each of these conditions. LP should usually be delayed in favor of other more accurate and less invasive tests. Controversial indications for LP include suspected spinal epidural abscess, evaluation of the acute stroke to identify those which are hemorrhagic, evaluation of dementia (arguably to exclude neurosyphilis or chronic meningitis), evaluation of the asymptomatic patient with a positive serologic test for syphilis (to exclude asymptomatic neurosyphilis).

Limitations When a "traumatic tap" occurs (iatrogenic trauma), white blood cells may be passively transferred to the CSF. In general, for every 700 RBCs found in the CSF, 1 WBC is also expected (applies to the traumatic tap **only**).

Contraindications Procedure is contraindicated if there is a local infection at the proposed site of needle entry due to the potential for infectious seeding of meninges (several literature case reports). The presence of a severe bleeding diathesis is a relative contraindication to LP and an increased risk of spinal subdural hematoma has been demonstrated. Elevated intracranial pressure is an absolute contraindication to LP because of the risk of uncal herniation (see Complications). The presence of septicemia is **not** considered a contraindication. Retrospective studies have failed to show an increased incidence of meningitis in septic patients undergoing LP compared with septic patients who do not undergo the procedure.

Additional Information Because of the risk of tonsillar herniation following LP, controversy exists concerning the routine use of head CT scan prior to LP. Data is incomplete and several clinical approaches are available. The conservative approach is to always perform a head CT prior to LP regardless of neurologic findings, so as never to overlook an intracranial mass lesion. Other clinicians follow a more flexible

approach and argue that tonsillar herniation only occurs with demonstrable papilledema or focal neurologic deficits; thus, when both of these physical signs are absent LP may be safely performed without prior head CT. A middle ground approach has been advocated where head CT scan is performed prior to LP in the following situations: papilledema, focal neurologic deficits, recent history of sinusitis or otitis media, severe and progressive headache, and deterioration of mental status.

Selected Readings

Brocker RJ, "Technique to Avoid Spinal Tap Headache," *JAMA*, 1958, 68:261-3.

Chun CH, Johnson JD, Hofstetter M, et al, "Brain Abscess: A Study of 45 Consecutive Cases," *Medicine (Baltimore)*, 1986, 65(6):415-31.

"Clinical Policy for the Initial Approach to Patients Presenting With Altered Mental Status," *Ann Emerg Med*, 1999, 33(2):251.

Dougherty JM and Roth RM, "Cerebral Spinal Fluid," *Emerg Med Clin North Am*, 1986, 4(2):281-97.

Eng RH and Seligman SJ, "Lumbar Puncture-Induced Meningitis," *JAMA*, 1981, 245(14):1456-9.

Fishman RA, *Cerebrospinal Fluid in Diseases of the Nervous System*, Philadelphia, PA: WB Saunders Co, 1980.

Keroack MA, "The Patient With Suspected Meningitis," *Emerg Med Clin North Am*, 1987, 5(4):807-26.

Korein J, Cravisto H, and Leicach M, "Re-evaluation of Lumbar Puncture: A Study of 129 Patients With Papilledema or Intracranial Hypertension," *Neurology*, 1959, 9:290-7.

Marton KI and Gean AD, "The Spinal Tap: A New Look at an Old Test," *Ann Intern Med*, 1986, 104(6):840-8.

Reik L, "Disorders That Mimic CNS Infections," *Neurol Clin*, 1986, 4(1):223-48.

Simon R and Brenner B, "Neurosurgical Procedures," *Emergency Medicine*, Chapter 149, Baltimore, MD: Williams & Wilkins, 1982, 156-67.

Lumbar Puncture Analysis *see* Cerebrospinal Fluid Analysis *on page 408*

Lung Biopsy *see* Histopathology *on page 496*

Lupus Band Test *see* Skin Biopsy, Immunofluorescence *on page 583*

Lyme Arthritis Serology *see* Lyme Disease Serology *on page 527*

Lyme (*Borrelia*) C6 Peptide Immunoassay

Synonyms C6 Peptide EIA

Test Includes Standard EIA for antibodies to a synthetic peptide specific for *Borrelia burgdorferi*, the etiological agent of Lyme disease (Lyme borreliosis).

Special Instructions This test is very clinically useful, but it is usually available only at reference laboratories. Therefore, the physician should contact the laboratory and (1) verbally inform the laboratory of the need for the test, and (2) inquire as to the availability of the test.

Specimen Serum (contact testing laboratory for confirmation)

Limitations This test does not differentiate between IgG and IgM, between early and chronic disease, and active and inactive infections.

Additional Information This test has several advantages over the standard EIA for antibodies to *Borrelia burgdorferi*.

- Can replace standard EIA and Western blot for antibodies to *Borrelia burgdorferi*
- Correlates well (better than the standard EIA and western blot) with clinical presentation
- Detects all strains of *Borrelia burgdorferi*
- Does not detect anti-*Borrelia burgdorferi* antibodies induced by previous *Borrelia burgdorferi* vaccination
- Very sensitive in the detection of early IgG and, therefore, early disease
- Extremely specific (no known cross reactivity, especially for chronic disease)

Selected Readings

Liang FT, Steere AC, Marques AR, et al, "Sensitive and Specific Serodiagnosis of Lyme Disease by Enzyme-Linked Immunosorbent Assay With a Peptide Based on an Immunodominant Conserved Region of *Borrelia burgdorferi* vlsE," *J Clin Microbiol*, 1999, 37(12):3990-6.

Marques AR, Martin DS, and Philipp MT, "Evaluation of the C6 Peptide Enzyme-Linked Immunosorbent Assay for Individuals Vaccinated With the Recombinant OspA Vaccine," *J Clin Microbiol*, 2002, 40(7):2591-3.

Lyme Borreliosis Antibody by Western Blot *see* Lyme Disease Serology by Western Blot *on page 528*

Lyme Disease Immunoblot *see* Lyme Disease Serology by Western Blot *on page 528*

Lyme Disease Serology

Related Information

Lyme Disease Serology by Western Blot *on page 528*

Synonyms Borreliosis Serology; Lyme Arthritis Serology

Specimen Serum or cerebrospinal fluid

Container Red top tube

Reference Range Values vary among laboratories

Use Laboratory confirmation of Lyme disease

Limitations Some cases are seronegative; there are cross reactions including those with antibodies to EB virus, *Rickettsia*, and syphilis. There is significant inter- and

(Continued)

Lyme Disease Serology *(Continued)*

intralaboratory variation in this assay which highlights limitations of currently available testing. Even the Western blot is not considered a definitive assay. Consequently, serologic evidence should not be the sole criterion for a diagnosis of Lyme disease. Serology is a confirmation test and should only **confirm** a clinical diagnosis.

Methodology Enzyme immunoassay (EIA), enzyme-linked immunosorbent assay (ELISA), indirect immunofluorescent antibody (IFA), Western blot

EIAs are often offered with a subsequent Western blot test to confirm positive results.

Some laboratories offer molecular testing for this organism. Contact the testing laboratory for the availability of amplified and nonamplified qualitative and quantitative molecular tests for this organism, and for information on selection and collection of appropriate specimens for specific molecular tests.

Some reference laboratories offer a newer test for Lyme borreliosis: C6 Lyme Peptide EIA. This test detects antibody to a synthetic peptide specific for *Borrelia burgdorferi.* The advantages of the test are the following.

- Does not cross-react with spirochetes
- Extremely specific, more so than standard EIA
- Detects both IgG and IgM
- Detects IgG earlier than can standard EIA
- Can replace standard EIA and subsequent Western blot tests
- Does not detect antibody elicited by vaccination

Use of the antibody to C6 peptide as an indicator of therapy outcome is controversial.

Additional Information Lyme disease is a multisystem disorder. A characteristic rash and arthritis are the hallmark symptoms. It is widespread in the US and is caused by *Borrelia burgdorferi*, a spirochete transmitted by the bite of the tick *Ixodes scapularis.* The disease has protean manifestations, can become chronic, and responds to antibiotics; prompt proper diagnosis is therefore important.

Assay is available for IgG and IgM antibody in both serum and CSF. In early disease a negative assay does not exclude the diagnosis because assay sensitivity is only 40% to 60%. Antibody response may be blunted by antibiotics. All patients with chronic disease will have positive assays.

Recent studies using recombinant outer surface protein A and B and flagellin hold out promise for better serologic testing in the near future.

Patients may harbor *B. burgdorferi* asymptomatically and have positive serology. Some individuals may have symptoms of other illnesses incorrectly attributed to Lyme disease and be given inappropriate and ineffective treatment.

Antibodies against Lyme disease antigens can interfere with the ANA test.

Selected Readings

Aguero-Rosenfeld ME, Wang G, Schwartz I, et al, "Diagnosis of Lyme Borreliosis," *Clin Microbiol Rev*, 2005, 18(3):484-509.

Fleming RV, Marques AR, Klempner MS, et al, "Pre-treatment and Post-treatment Assessment of the C(6) Test in Patients With Persistent Symptoms and a History of Lyme Borreliosis," *Eur J Clin Microbiol Infect Dis*, 2004, 23(8):615-8.

Heikkila T, Huppertz HI, Seppala I, et al, "Recombinant or Peptide Antigens in the Serology of Lyme Arthritis in Children," *J Infect Dis*, 2003, 187(12):1888-94.

Johnson RC and Johnson BJB, "Lyme Disease: Serodiagnosis of *Borrelia burgdorferi* Sensu Lato Infection," *Manual of Clinical Laboratory Immunology*, 5th ed, Rose NR, Conway de Macario E, Folds JD, et al, eds, Washington, DC: American Society for Microbiology, 1997, 526-33.

Khanna M, Fan J, Pehler-Harrington K, et al, "The Pneumoplex Assays, a Multiplex PCR-Enzyme Hybridization Assay That Allows Simultaneous Detection of Five Organisms, *Mycoplasma pneumoniae, Chlamydia (Chlamydophila) pneumoniae, Legionella pneumophila, Legionella micdadei,* and *Bordetella pertussis*, and Its Real-Time Counterpart," *J Clin Microbiol*, 2005, 43(2):565-71.

Koide M and Saito A, "Diagnosis of *Legionella pneumophila* Infection by Polymerase Chain Reaction," *Clin Infect Dis*, 1995, 21(1):199-201.

Philipp MT, Marques AR, Fawcett PT, et al, "C6 Test as an Indicator of Therapy Outcome for Patients With Localized or Disseminated Lyme Borreliosis," *J Clin Microbiol*, 2003, 41(11):4955-60.

Porwancher RB, "Cost-Effectiveness of Peptide-Antigen Immunoassays for Lyme Disease," *J Infect Dis*, 2004, 189(10):1962.

Rantakokko-Jalava K and Jalava J, "Development of Conventional and Real-Time PCR Assays for Detection of Legionella DNA in Respiratory Specimens," *J Clin Microbiol*, 2001, 39(8):2904-10.

Robertson J, Guy E, Andrews N, et al, "A European Multicenter Study of Immunoblotting in Serodiagnosis of Lyme Borreliosis," *J Clin Microbiol*, 2000, 38(6):2097-102.

Shapiro ED and Gerber MA, "Lyme disease," *Clin Infect Dis*, 2000, 31(2):533-42.

Strle F, "Principles of the Diagnosis and Antibiotic Treatment of *Lyme borreliosis*," *Wien Klin Wochenschr*, 1999, 111(22-23):911-5.

Lyme Disease Serology by Western Blot

Related Information

Lyme Disease Serology *on page 527*
Nitrite, Urine *on page 549*

Synonyms Borreliosis Serology; Lyme Disease Immunoblot

Applies to Lyme Borreliosis Antibody by Western Blot

Test Includes Confirmation Lyme disease antibody test

Specimen Serum

Container Red top tube

Storage Instructions Separate and freeze serum.

Causes for Rejection Inadequate labeling, excessive hemolysis, chylous serum

Reference Range Normal: number of bands is defined by individual laboratory

Use Confirm positive screening tests for Lyme disease

Limitations The Western blot assay is not sensitive for detecting early Lyme disease. Its utility is for confirming stage 2 and stage 3 Lyme disease and to identify false-positive results in patients suspected of late Lyme disease. This test is performed by reference laboratories. Each laboratory designates which bands are most significant. Significant interlaboratory variation exists.

Contraindications Negative screening test for Lyme disease

Methodology Western blot technique utilizing a mixture of proteins (antigens) that are extracted from *Borrelia burgdorferi* and separated by SDS-PAGE; subsequent reaction of serum with bands/proteins.

Selected Readings

Belman AL, "Tick-Borne Diseases," *Semin Pediatr Neurol*, 1999, 6(4):249-66.

Duffey PS and Salugsugan J, "Serodiagnosis of Lyme Borreliosis," *Clin Microbiol Newslett*, 1993, 15(11):81-5.

Johnson RC and Johnson BJB, "Lyme Disease: Serodiagnosis of *Borrelia burgdorferi* Sensu Lato Infection," *Manual of Clinical Laboratory Immunology*, 5th ed, Rose NR, Conway de Macario E, Folds JD, et al, eds, Washington, DC: American Society for Microbiology, 1997, 526-33.

Mitchell PD, "Lyme Borreliosis: A Persisting Diagnostic Dilemma," *Clin Microbiol Newslett*, 1993, 15(8):57-9.

Strle F, "Principles of the Diagnosis and Antibiotic Treatment of *Lyme borreliosis*," *Wien Klin Wochenschr*, 1999, 111(22-23):911-5.

Lymph Node Biopsy

Related Information

Histopathology *on page 496*

Skin Biopsy *on page 580*

Applies to Cell Sorting Fluorescence Activation

Test Includes Microscopic examination of frozen sections, paraffin and/or plastic sections, and often, touch preparations. Immunoperoxidase studies for immunoglobulin heavy and light chains are best done on snap frozen cryostat sections rather than paraffin sections.

Special Instructions The specimen should not be placed in fixative if it can be delivered immediately to the laboratory. Diagnostic difficulties in diseases of lymph nodes are compounded by poor fixation and improper handling. Lymph node biopsies should be immediately delivered to the Histology Laboratory uncut and in a small sterile jar or Petri dish. Requests for all examinations including Microbiology should accompany the specimen. All such specimens should be brought to the immediate attention of a pathologist. Bone marrow, blood studies, and other clinical information are commonly needed for appropriate work-up.

Specimen Lymph node or other tissues suspected of harboring lymphoma, ideally submitted fresh within minutes of the biopsy

Container Sterile saline moistened sponge or Petri dish

Collection Optimal selection of site of biopsy and the lymph nodes to be biopsied enhance ultimate correct diagnosis. Supraclavicular and cervical biopsies will most likely provide diagnostic specimens. The most accessible lymph nodes are not always the best choice. The whole, intact lymph node with its capsule, and adjacent fat or other tissue provides an optimal specimen.

The proper initial triage of the tissue is of utmost importance in establishing the correct diagnosis. Usually, sufficient tissue must be available for both permanent sections and for immunophenotypic analysis of frozen sections. Tissues allocated for immunotypic studies are also suitable for genotypic studies if necessary. Routine histopathologic study remains the gold standard in diagnostic hematopathology and optimal histology begins with proper fixation. Fine nuclear detail is best achieved using B5, zinc formalin, or a Zenker's-like fixative. These fixatives are also best for cell marker analysis in paraffin section. An ever expanding selection of antibodies is useful for establishing lineage of hematopoietic cells in paraffin section (see table). However, phenotypic indicators of clonal proliferation are most reliably established in frozen section. As morphologic detail in frozen sections is intrinsically limited, every precaution to minimize artifacts must be taken. Snap freezing small, thin slices of tissue using liquid nitrogen cooled isopentane yields tissues free of freezing artifacts. Special attention to fine details of cryostat sectioning is necessary to yield interpretable results. If a frozen section evaluation is necessary to initiate a "lymphoma

(Continued)

Lymph Node Biopsy *(Continued)*

Lymphocyte Markers Useful in Paraffin Section[1]

	LCA (CD45)	EMA	LN-2 (CD71w)	L26 (CD20)	UCHL-1 (CD45RO)	CD3	Leu-M1 (CD15)	Mono Ig's	Lysozyme	KP1 (CD68)	CAE
Non-Hodgkin's lymphoma											
B-cell lymphomas[2]	+	-	+	+	-	-	-	+	-	-	-
T-cell lymphomas[3]	+	-/+	-	-	+	+	-/+	-	-	-	-
Hodgkin's disease (NS, MC, LD)	-	-	+	-	-	-	+	-	-	-	-
Hodgkin's disease, LP	+	+/-	+	+	-	-	-	-	-	-	-
Myeloma/plasmacytoma	-/+	-/+	-	-	-	-	-	+	-	-	-
Granulocytic sarcoma[4]	+/-	-	-/+	-	-	-	+/-	-	+	+	+
True histiocytic lymphoma[4]	+/-	-/+	-/+	-	-	-	-	-	+	+	-

Abbreviations: LCA = leukocyte common antigen; EMA = epithelial membrane antigen; Mono Ig's = monoclonal immunoglobulins; CAE = chloroacetate esterase (an enzyme cytochemical stain rather than an immunostain); Hodgkin's disease (NS, MC, LD) = nodular sclerosing, mixed cellularity, and lymphocyte depleted subtypes, respectively; Hodgkin's disease, LP = lymphocyte predominate subtype. Designated reactions: + = characteristically positive; +/- = characteristically positive but may be negative; -/+ = characteristically negative but may be positive; - = characteristically negative.

Footnotes:

[1]Most lymphomas characteristically contain neoplastic and non-neoplastic lymphoid elements in variable proportions. Caution must be exercised in determining the phenotype of the neoplastic cells.

[2]Monoclonal immunoglobulins are best detected in frozen section. Large cell lymphomas and those with plasmacytic differentiation are more likely to display a convincing staining in paraffin section than other subtypes.

[3]T-cell clonal proliferation cannot be determined in paraffin section alone. The best phenotypic expression of clonal proliferation is aberrant expression of pan T-cell antigens which can be detected only by frozen section immunohistology, by flow cytometry using cell suspensions, or by gene rearrangement.

[4]Enzyme cytochemical profile using touch preparations is extremely useful in establishing these diagnoses.

protocol," the tissues used for this rapid diagnosis are often unsuitable for immunophenotypic analysis. If the size of biopsy is limiting, a routine frozen section evaluation should be discouraged as freezing distorts lymphoid tissue and may result in errors in final interpretation.

If tissues are to be sent to a reference laboratory for immunotyping, three basic options are available. First, the tissues may be snap frozen and stored at -70°C or colder until such time as immunotyping is considered necessary. If facilities for proper snap freezing and storage are not available, this option should be discouraged. Second, the tissues may be delivered in carrier media or saline soaked gauze immediately by courier to the reference laboratory, where experienced personnel will process the tissue. Third, tissues may be placed in a carrier media which may circumvent the need for immediate action for 24 hours without significantly compromising the immunologic studies.

Storage Instructions Snap frozen tissues should be maintained at -70°C or colder until immunophenotypic analysis can be performed. If the frozen tissues are to be transported to a reference laboratory, they should be shipped on dry ice, using an overnight courier if necessary. Tissues placed in carrier media should be maintained on wet ice or at room temperature and packaged in insulated containers to avoid large fluctuations in temperature during transit.

Causes for Rejection Desiccated specimen, formalin exposure, excessive freezing artifact

Use Diagnose various lymphadenopathies, including cat scratch disease, malignant lymphoma, and metastatic neoplasia

Limitations Formalin-fixed tissue cannot be used for culture or imprints and is suboptimal for electron microscopy.

Methodology Quality basic histology is of paramount importance in the evaluation of the lymph node biopsy. Interpretive errors are often due to deficient basic histology. Touch preparations should always be obtained and are often times invaluable for final diagnosis. Representative tissues should be allocated for immunotyping, taking the necessary precautions to minimize morphologic artifacts while maintaining maximal antigenicity. Immunoperoxidase stains on paraffin or frozen sections are accomplished according to the general procedures outlined in the test listing Immunoperoxidase Procedures. Immunologic markers on touch preparations and bone marrow smears are often best demonstrated by using an alkaline phosphatase enzyme detection system to minimize background staining. Cultures for infectious agents are sometimes indispensable.

Additional Information Correlation with peripheral blood, bone marrow, and other clinical laboratory studies is often desirable and sometimes mandatory. Flow cytometry on dissociated tissues or body fluids is often utilized instead of immunohistology for cell marker analysis. This methodology offers a more quantitative approach to cell markers but only at the critical expense of destroying the immunoarchitecture of tissues. In general, immunohistology provides the best approach for typing tissues while flow cytometry is best suited for blood, bone marrow, and other body fluids. Properly acquired and frozen tissue is suitable for gene probe analysis (gene rearrangement studies), which may be necessary to document B- or T-cell clonal proliferation in rare cases.

Selected Readings

Jaffe ES, "Surgical Pathology of the Lymph Nodes and Related Organs," *Major Problems in Pathology*, Vol 16, Philadelphia, PA: WB Saunders Co, 1985.

Knowles DM, *Neoplastic Hematopathology*, Baltimore, MD: Williams & Wilkins, 1992.

Wright DH and Isaacson PG, *Biopsy Pathology of the Lymphoreticular System*, Baltimore, MD: Williams & Wilkins, 1983.

Lymphocyte Subset Panels

Related Information

T4/T8 Ratio *on page 590*

Synonyms B Cells; HIV Infection, Immune Status; Immune Status HIV Infection; Natural Killer (NK) Cells; T Cells

Specimen Whole blood

Container 5 mL room temperature EDTA (lavender top) tube and 5 mL room temperature heparin (green top) or ACD solution B (yellow top) tube (1 mL minimum for each specimen)

Storage Instructions Samples must be assayed within 48 hours of collection.

Use Determine immune status of patients with HIV infection; monitor antiretroviral and immunosuppressive therapy; differential diagnosis of congenital and acquired immune deficiencies

Methodology In this four-color multiparametric flow cytometry method, whole blood is first incubated with fluorochrome-conjugated monoclonal antibodies targeted against the various cell surface antigens. Following red cell lysis, the sample is run through a flow cytometer. Using a CD45 vs side scatter gating technique, lymphocytes are

(Continued)

Lymphocyte Subset Panels *(Continued)*

selected and percentages of the various cell surface markers (CD3, CD4, CD8, CD19, and/or CD16/CD56) are determined. The absolute cell count of each marker is calculated using the absolute lymphocyte count (obtained from standard hematology instrumentation) and the marker percentage. Both the absolute cell count and the percentage are reported for each marker.

Additional Information The cellular and humoral immune systems are mediated by distinct lymphocyte classes or subsets, including T cells, B cells, and natural killer (NK) cells. T cells mediate the cellular immune system that combats intracellular infections, cancer cells, and foreign tissue. B cells mediate the humoral immune system that is targeted against bacterial and viral infections. Natural killer (NK) cells play a role in defense against viral infections and tumors. These lymphocyte subsets can be discerned by the antigenic properties of cell surface (membrane) markers. For example, T cells are CD3 positive, B cells are CD19 positive, and NK cells are CD3 negative, and CD16 and CD56 positive. T cells are further classified as helper cells (CD4 positive) or suppressor cells (CD8 positive).

Although there is a relatively fixed number and proportion of these lymphocyte subsets in normal individuals, the absolute number and proportions is altered in various diseases. For example, in individuals with human immunodeficiency virus (HIV), the number of CD4 cells and the proportion of CD4 cells relative to CD8 cells vary based on the stage of disease and therapeutic response. Thus, lymphocyte subset analysis can provide information regarding the immune status of the patient and assist in monitoring therapy as well as help characterize congenital and acquired immune deficiencies.

In patients with HIV infection, the CD4+ T cells and the CD4/CD8 ratio typically decline shortly after seroconversion. CD4+ levels >500 cells/mm^3 are usually associated with asymptomatic infection; whereas, levels <200 cells/mm^3 are consistent with a transition to AIDS. CD4 levels rise in response to effective antiretroviral therapy (opposite of the HIV viral load response). HIV-1 RNA has been shown to be a better independent predictor of progression to AIDS and death than the number of CD4+ T cells. The combined use of CD4 and HIV-1 RNA is recommended, however.

Selected Readings

Quest Diagnostics, "Nichols Institute Test Highlights," November 1999.

Lymphogranuloma Venereum Culture *see Chlamydia* Culture *on page 413*

Magnetic Resonance Scan, Brain

Applies to Magnetic Resonance Scan, Head

Patient Preparation Inpatient: Patient must be able to lie quietly while the scan is performed. The patient should be screened for metallic devices by nursing personnel. (See Contraindications.) This includes metal introduced into the patient either surgically or by trauma. All metallic objects must be removed from the patient including jewelry or any other metal objects which may be in the patient's bedding. Please remove dentures or other dental appliances. I.V.s which contain no metal are fine, but infusion pumps must be removed. Oxygen tanks and metallic backboards may come with the patient but will be removed prior to the patient entering the magnet room. Oxygen may be provided in the magnet room. Trauma, ICU, or CCU patients should be accompanied by a nurse. If the patient is restless, combative, or claustrophobic, proper sedation may be administered on the floor prior to the MRI, or at the MRI Center. Consult the MRI radiologists with questions on proper sedation. Outpatient: The patient should be screened for metallic devices. (See Contraindications.) If a question exists as to the patient's suitability for MRI, consult the radiologist. If the patient is claustrophobic, oral or parenteral sedation may be necessary. If so, the patient should be accompanied by another adult to provide transportation home after the examination.

Aftercare If the patient received an MRI contrast agent (Magnevist®) and develops a delayed hypersensitivity reaction (ie, hives or shortness of breath), the referring physician or MRI radiologist should be contacted immediately.

Data Acquired Digital information with film reproduction

Use Diagnose intracranial abnormalities including tumors, ischemia, infection, multiple sclerosis or any abnormalities relating to the brain or calvarium. MRI is an excellent modality for assessment of congenital brain abnormalities or relating to the status of brain maturation in the pediatric population.

Limitations Generally, the greatest limitation of magnetic resonance imaging results from the patient's fear of the procedure. The patient must remain quiet and still for several scans, each lasting from several minutes to 10 minutes in length. Total examination time is usually 30-45 minutes and occasionally up to 1 hour. If the patient is restless during the examination, motion artifacts will be present on the images limiting their diagnostic value. If the patient is claustrophobic, mild oral sedation or

occasionally parenteral sedation may be needed. Also the patient can be accompanied by a family member or friend during the examination which helps calm the patient's anxiety in many cases. Patients requiring life support equipment such as ventilators require special preparation. Please refer to Contraindications for further causes for rejection.

Contraindications Patients weighing more than 300 lb and patients unable to squeeze into the magnet cannot undergo MRI. An absolute contraindication for MRI is a cardiac pacemaker. Relative contraindications to magnetic resonance imaging include intracranial aneurysm clips, cochlear implants, insulin infusion and chemotherapy pumps, neurocutaneous stimulators and prosthetic heart valves, depending on date of manufacture and metallurgical composition, consult the radiologist. Patients who have metallic foreign bodies within the eye or who have undergone recent surgery within the last 6 weeks requiring placement of a vascular surgical clip, should also not undergo MRI. The safety of MRI in pregnant patients has not been determined. In such cases, prior consultation with the MRI physician is required. Generally, patients who have undergone recent surgery not requiring vascular clips or who have had coronary artery bypass surgery in the past may undergo MRI. Patients who have shrapnel wounds or orthopedic prostheses can generally safely undergo MRI unless the metallic device is in the anatomic region to be scanned which results in degradation of the images. Patients with surgically implanted intravascular vena cava filters to prevent pulmonary embolism can usually be scanned if the device has been in place for at least 6 weeks. Patients requiring life support equipment, including ventilators, require special preparation. Central venous lines, Swan-Ganz catheters, and nasogastric (NG) tubes usually present no problems.

Methodology Unlike most conventional radiologic procedures, magnetic resonance imaging does not utilize ionizing radiation, but relies upon radio frequency or radio signals induced within the patient by the magnetic field to obtain images. There are no known biologic effects secondary to the magnetic fields currently used in clinical MRI. Prior to the scan, the patient will be asked to remove all metallic objects from their person, including loose change, hair pins, earrings, belts, etc. This is for safety reasons as the strong magnetic field could result in these and any other metal objects becoming projectiles resulting in injury to the patient or MRI personnel. Also the patient should not carry a purse or wallet into the magnetic room, as the magnetic field can permanently erase bank cards or credit cards. The magnet is open on both ends and music can be played for the patient if desired. Fresh air is constantly circulated through the magnet room and the patient is continually monitored by the MRI technologist. An intercom system is provided for communication between the patient and the technologist. For MRI of the brain, a special coil surrounds, but does not touch the patient's head. The patient will be asked to remain very still while scans are being obtained. In certain cases, an MRI contrast agent, Gadopentetate Dimeglumine (Magnevist®) may be necessary to increase the diagnostic accuracy of the MRI examination. This is administered intravenously, via an antecubital vein in a small volume (<20 mL). This contrast agent may be used in patients who are allergic to conventional iodinated contrast agents such as is used in IVPs or CT examination without difficulty. There are very few contraindications to its use. (See Contraindications.)

Additional Information In some cases, an MRI contrast agent (Magnevist®) may be needed to increase the diagnostic accuracy of the MRI. This contrast agent can be administered to patients with a previous history of allergies to conventional iodinated x-ray agents as it contains no iodine. Contraindications to its use include previous allergy to the contrast agent itself, renal failure, certain types of anemia, and Wilson's disease. The contrast agent is generally very safe and increases the diagnostic efficacy of the MRI.

Selected Readings

Danielsen ER and Ross BD, "Neurospectroscopy," *Magn Reson Imaging*, 3rd ed, Stark DD and Bradley WG Jr, eds, St Louis, MO: CV Mosby Co, 1999, 1595-635.

Falcone S and Post MJ, "Encephalitis, Cerebritis, and Brain Abscess: Pathophysiology and Imaging Findings," *Neuroimaging Clin N Am*, 2000, 10(2):333-53.

Sorensen AG and Rosen BR, "Functional MRI of the Brain," *Magnetic Resonance Imaging of the Brain and Spine*, Philadelphia, PA: Lippincott Williams & Wilkins, 1996, 1501-45.

Magnetic Resonance Scan, Head *see* Magnetic Resonance Scan, Brain *on page 532*

Malarial Parasites *see* Peripheral Blood Smear, Thick and Thin *on page 563*

Malaria Smear *see* Peripheral Blood Smear, Thick and Thin *on page 563*

Mantoux Test *see* Tuberculin Skin Testing, Intracutaneous *on page 601*

Maximum Bactericidal Dilution *see* Serum Bactericidal Test *on page 578*

MBD *see* Serum Bactericidal Test *on page 578*

Measles Antibody

Test Includes IgG and IgM levels

Specimen Serum or cerebrospinal fluid

Container Red top tube

Reference Range Less than fourfold rise in titer; absent or stable IgM titer; HI >1:10, NT >1:20 indicates immunity. Consult laboratory for more specific (custom) information.

If serological testing is performed by enzyme immunoassay (EIA) on automated instrumentation, results are usually given in index units, not titers. In such cases, significant rises in antibody levels are determined by algorithms within the instrumentation, not by increases in titers.

Use Differential diagnosis of viral exanthemas, particularly in pregnant women; diagnosis of subacute sclerosing panencephalitis; document adequacy of measles immunization

Limitations Antibody sometimes present in multiple sclerosis

Methodology Hemagglutination inhibition, viral neutralization, enzyme-linked immunosorbent assay

Additional Information Measles (rubeola) is caused by a paramyxovirus. Despite vaccination programs, there have been several recent local epidemics. Revaccination appears to be of greater value at 11-12 years of age than at 4-6 years of age. Serologic study can be useful in establishing that an individual has effective immunity subsequent to vaccination. In many individuals **detectable** immunity does not persist.

In acute illness, hemagglutinating and neutralizing antibody peak two weeks after the rash appears. It is necessary to demonstrate rising titers over 2 weeks, or identify IgM antibody.

Very high serum titers in the absence of acute illness and/or high CSF titers are seen in subacute sclerosing panencephalitis.

Selected Readings

Markowitz LE, Albrecht P, Orenstein WA, et al, "Persistence of Measles Antibody After Revaccination," *J Infect Dis*, 1992, 166(1):205-8.

Wittler RR, Veit BC, McIntyre S, et al, "Measles Revaccination Response in a School-Age Population," *Pediatrics*, 1991, 88(5):1024-30.

Measles Culture, 3-Day *see* Rubella Virus Culture *on page 575*

Measles Virus, Direct Detection *see* Virus Detection by DFA *on page 619*

Medical Legal Specimens *see* Histopathology *on page 496*

Meretek UBT® *see Helicobacter pylori* Urea Breath Test (UBT) *on page 481*

Methenamine Silver Stain

Related Information

Acid-Fast Stain, Modified, *Nocardia* Species *on page 362*
Cryptococcal Antigen Serology, Serum or Cerebrospinal Fluid *on page 431*
Fungus Culture, Biopsy *on page 461*
Fungus Culture, Body Fluid *on page 462*
Fungus Culture, Skin *on page 464*
Fungus Culture, Sputum *on page 466*
Fungus Culture, Urine *on page 468*
Gram Stain *on page 473*
Histopathology *on page 496*
India Ink Preparation *on page 507*
KOH Preparation *on page 513*
Periodic Acid-Schiff Stain *on page 563*
Pneumocystis jiroveci Test *on page 566*
Skin Biopsy *on page 580*

Synonyms GMS Stain; Gomori-Methenamine Silver Stain; Grocott's Modified Silver Stain; Silver Stain

Test Includes Staining of organisms in a smear or histologic section with silver precipitate.

Patient Preparation If aspirate or biopsy, aseptic preparation of site is needed.

Specimen Bronchoalveolar lavage (BAL), lung biopsy, aspirated specimen, histopathology specimen

Container Sterile suction trap, sterile container for culture, jar with formalin for histopathology, clean glass slides air-dried or fixed in 95% alcohol for smears

Collection Touch preparation smears may be prepared by touching 8-10 glass slides to the cut surface of the fresh lung tissue. The slides should be fixed individually upon preparation in 95% alcohol. Each slide should be labeled with the patient's name on the frosted end.

Reference Range No organisms identified

Critical Values Fungi or *Pneumocystis jiroveci* detected

Use Rapid detection of *Pneumocystis* or fungi

Limitations Organisms may be present in low numbers making detection difficult. Cost and time may also be factors. The silver stain (GMS) requires approximately 1 hour, is technically demanding, and requires significant reagent preparation. Yeasts (*Candida* and *Histoplasma*) similar in size to *Pneumocystis jiroveci* may be confused with *Pneumocystis jiroveci* on silver-stained tissue sections. Culture for fungus is always recommended.

Methodology A black precipitate on the fungal or *Pneumocystis* cell walls is produced by the chromic acid oxidation of cell wall carbohydrate hydroxyl groups to aldehydes and the subsequent reaction of the aldehyde groups with the silver reagent. Fungi appear as yeast cells, pseudohyphae, or hyphae. *Pneumocystis* stains gray to black, has a characteristic cup shape appearance 5-8 μm in diameter, and may demonstrate intracystic bodies.

Additional Information Recent studies have suggested that a combination of Papanicolaou (PAP) stain and Diff-Quik stain (a modified Giemsa stain) may provide comparable results to the GMS stain more rapidly and at less cost. Neither method is as sensitive as immunofluorescence for the detection of *Pneumocystis*. Silver stains in conjunction with other stains and morphologic evaluation by a skilled observer can frequently speciate fungal organisms in tissue specimens.

Selected Readings

Delvenne P, Arrese JE, Thiry A, et al, "Detection of Cytomegalovirus, *Pneumocystis carinii*, and *Aspergillus* Species in Bronchoalveolar Lavage Fluid. A Comparison of Techniques," *Am J Clin Pathol*, 1993, 100(4):414-8.

Homer KS, Wiley EL, Smith AL, et al "Monoclonal Antibody to *Pneumocystis carinii*. Comparison With Silver Stain in Bronchial Lavage Specimens," *Am J Clin Pathol*, 1992, 97(5):619-24.

Naimey GL and Wuerker RB, "Comparison of Histologic Stains in the Diagnosis of *Pneumocystis carinii*," *Acta Cytol*, 1995, 39(6):1124-7.

Raab SS, Cheville JC, Bottles K, et al, "Utility of Gomori Methenamine Silver Stains in Bronchoalveolar Lavage Specimens," *Mod Pathol*, 1994, 7(5):599-604.

MHA-TP

Synonyms Microhemagglutination, *Treponema pallidum*; Serologic Test for Syphilis

Applies to Syphilis Serology

Patient Preparation Patient should be fasting, if possible.

Specimen Serum

Container Red top tube

Storage Instructions Refrigerate

Reference Range Less than 1:160

Use Confirmatory serologic test for syphilis

Limitations Moderate sensitivity in early (primary) stages of syphilis. False-positives may occur in systemic lupus, infectious mononucleosis, and lepromatous leprosy.

Methodology Hemagglutination

Additional Information This is a *Treponema*-specific test and should not be used as a screening test. It is as sensitive and specific as FTA-ABS in all stages of syphilis except primary, in which it is less sensitive (but more sensitive than the VDRL). It will be positive with treponemal infections other than syphilis (bejel, pinta, yaws). Like FTA-ABS, MHA-TP once positive remains so, and cannot be used to judge effect of treatment. The test is not applicable to CSF.

Selected Readings

Hart G, "Syphilis Tests in Diagnostic and Therapeutic Decision Making," *Ann Intern Med*, 1986, 104(3):368-76.

Romanowski B, Sutherland R, Fick GH, et al, "Serologic Response to Treatment of Infectious Syphilis," *Ann Intern Med*, 1991, 114(12):1005-9.

Wicher V and Wicher K, "Pathogenesis of Maternal-Fetal Syphilis Revisited," *Clin Infect Dis*, 2001, 33(3):354-63.

MIC *see* Antimicrobial Susceptibility Testing, Aerobic and Facultatively Anaerobic Organisms *on page 379*

MIC, Anaerobic Bacteria *see* Antimicrobial Susceptibility Testing, Anaerobic Bacteria *on page 381*

Microfilariae, Peripheral Blood Preparation

Related Information

Peripheral Blood Smear, Thick and Thin *on page 563*

Synonyms Blood Smear for Trypanosomal/Filarial Parasites; Filariasis Peripheral Blood Preparation; Helminths, Blood Preparation; Trypanosomiasis Peripheral Blood Preparation

Applies to Filarial Infestation; Hemoflagellates; Peripheral Blood Preparation

Test Includes Examination of both thick and thin smears, wet preparation

(Continued)

Microfilariae, Peripheral Blood Preparation *(Continued)*

Special Instructions If patient has traveled to an endemic area, the date of travel, the area, and the parasite suspected should be specified.

Specimen Fresh blood fingerstick

Container Slides

Collection Recommended procedure is for specimen to be obtained as follows: *Loa loa*, 10 AM - 2 PM; *Mansonella* and *Onchocerca*, anytime; *Wuchereria* and *Brugia*, 10 PM - 4 AM

Causes for Rejection Specimen clotted

Reference Range No parasites identified

Use Diagnose parasitic infestation of blood, including trypanosomiasis and microfilariasis

Limitations One negative result does not rule out the possibility of parasitic infestation. Since some species of blood parasites can be found during the day and others are nocturnal, both day and night specimens enhance identification. Most filariae generate microfilariae which can be found in peripheral blood, but *Onchocerca volvulus* and *Dipetalonema streptocerca* give rise to microfilariae which do not circulate.

Methodology Fresh wet blood film, with a coverslip, in which motile microfilariae cause agitation of adjacent red cells. Stained smears are used as well.

Additional Information Biopsy of skin and subcutaneous mass is used in diagnosis of *D. streptocerca* and *O. volvulus*. Differential diagnosis of species of circulating microfilariae requires distinction between the presence or absence of a sheath, the pattern of nuclei in the tail and the history of geographic exposure and time of sampling.

Selected Readings

Dacie JV and Lewis SM, "Blood Parasites in Preparation and Staining Methods for Blood and Bone-Marrow Films," *Practical Haematology*, 8th ed, Chapter 6, New York, NY: Churchill Livingstone, 1995, 93-6.

Freedman DO and Berry RS, "Rapid Diagnosis of Bancroftian Filariasis by Acridine Orange Staining of Centrifuged Parasites," *Am J Trop Med Hyg*, 1992, 47(6):787-93.

Maddocks S and O'Brien R, Images in Clinical Medicine, "African Trypanosomiasis in Australia," *N Engl J Med*, 2000, 342(17):1254.

Microhemagglutination, *Treponema pallidum* *see* MHA-TP *on page 535*

Microsporidia Diagnostic Procedures

Test Includes Examination of stool, fluid, wash, or biopsy for microsporidia (*Enterocytozoon*, *Encephalitozoon*, *Nosema*, *Septata*, *Pleistophora*, and others)

Special Instructions Even though the test is relatively simple to perform, very few laboratories offer this test at this time because demand for the test is relatively low. The laboratory must be notified that microsporidia are suspected. Consult laboratory before ordering test for advice on availability of test and instructions on specimen collection.

Specimen Many different types of specimens are appropriate. The specimen must be obtained from a mucosal surface or an epithelial-lined surface (the sites of microsporidia replication) that represents the probable site of infection. In general, there are two types of specimens: those for exfoliative cytology examination and those for histological examination. Both types of specimens often are very productive. The specimen that should be collected depends on the suspected type of infection.

- Intestinal infection: direct stool smear, biliary tract biopsy, small intestine wash, small intestine mucosal biopsy
- Ocular infection: corneal scraping or swab
- Respiratory infection: sputum, BAL, transbronchial biopsy, bronchial brushing, mucosal biopsy
- Sinonasal infection: scraping, smear, mucosal biopsy
- Urinary tract infection: concentrated urine, mucosal biopsy

Container Clean, screw-cap container appropriate for the particular specimen; contact testing laboratory for details before ordering test

Collection Appropriate for the site. Transport specimen to the laboratory as soon as possible. Biopsies should be fixed in formalin as soon as possible.

Many laboratories require stool be submitted fixed in 10% formalin if the stool is to be specially stained for *Microsporidium*.

Use A part of the differential diagnostic work-up of diarrhea and other microsporidia-associated diseases in immunocompromised patients, particularly AIDS patients; establish the diagnosis of microsporidiosis. Microsporidia have been demonstrated in immunocompetent persons.

Limitations Detection of microsporidia is entirely dependent on the adequacy of the specimen, staining and preparation of the specimen, and experience of the person who examines the specimen.

Methodology Microsporidia do not stain well with either hematoxylin, eosin, or the Papanicolaou stains. There are several good stains for microsporidia; however, not all of these stains stain the five major species of microsporidia. Microsporidia in paraffin-embedded tissues stain well with a tissue Gram stain (Brown and Hoop stain; Brown and Brenn stain). Microsporidia in plastic-embedded tissues stain well with toluidine blue and with methylene blue-azure II-basic fuchsin. Microsporidia in cytologic centrifugation, smears, and scrapings preparations usually stain well with Gram stain for specimens with little or no bacterial contamination. In these preparations, most microsporidia and bacteria are dark purple; some microsporidia are gram-negative or gram-variable. Weber's modified trichrome (chromotrope-based) stain works well with specimens with bacterial contamination; microsporidia are magenta-pink and the background (including bacteria) is blue-green. Some laboratories use Giemsa stain to stain stool smears and body fluids. Most stains cause microsporidia to appear as extremely fat bacteria which have a uniform oval shape, do not show budding, contain polar densities, and have a central clear band or area. The identification of microsporidia to species is very important in the selection of treatment. Speciation is accomplished most commonly by electron microscopy and, where available, molecular biology techniques. Cross reactions between the antibodies to the different types of microsporidia prevent serology from being clinically useful. Immunofluorescence staining techniques which include labeled antibody to specific microsporidia appear to work well in detecting microsporidia in clinical specimens and to be able to differentiate infections due to certain microsporidia. Some microsporidia have been cultured *in vitro*, but routine culture for microsporidia is not yet practical.

Selected Readings

Garcia LS, Shimuzu RY, and Brucker DA, "Detection of Microsporidial Spores in Fecal Specimens From Patients Diagnosed With Cryptosporidiosis," *J Clin Microbiol*, 1994, 32:1739-41.

Shadduck JA and Greely E, "Microsporidia and Human Infections," *Clin Microbiol Rev*, 1989, 2:158-65.

Sun T, "Microsporidiosis in the Acquired Immunodeficiency Syndrome," *Infect Dis Newslett*, 1993, 12:20-2.

Weber R and Bryan RT, "Microsporidial Infections in Immunodeficient and Immunocompetent Patients," *Clin Infect Dis*, 1994, 19:517-21.

Weber R, Bryan RT, Owen RL, et al, "Improved Light-Microscopical Detection of Microsporidia Spores in Stool and Duodenal Aspirates. The Enteric Opportunistic Infections Working Group," *N Engl J Med*, 1992, 326(3):161-6.

Midstream Urine Culture *see* Urine Culture, Clean Catch *on page 609*

Minimum Inhibitory Concentration Susceptibility Test *see* Antimicrobial Susceptibility Testing, Aerobic and Facultatively Anaerobic Organisms *on page 379*

Mite Identification *see* Arthropod Identification *on page 387*

M-Mode Echo *see* Echocardiography, M-Mode *on page 445*

Monospot™ Test *see* Infectious Mononucleosis Serology *on page 509*

Monosticon® Dri-Dot® Test *see* Infectious Mononucleosis Serology *on page 509*

Mono Test *see* Infectious Mononucleosis Serology *on page 509*

***M. pneumoniae* Titer** *see Mycoplasma* Serology *on page 545*

Mucicarmine Stain *see* Periodic Acid-Schiff Stain *on page 563*

Muerto Canyon Strain Virus *see* Hantavirus Serology *on page 477*

Mumps Serology

Related Information

Mumps Virus Culture *on page 538*

Specimen Serum

Container Red top tube

Collection Acute and convalescent sera drawn 10-14 days apart are required.

Reference Range A fourfold or greater increase in titer is indicative of recent mumps infection in the complement fixation test; a positive IgM immunofluorescent test is indicative of infection; an increasing hemagglutination inhibition titer indicates mumps **or parainfluenza virus** infection; a positive neutralization test indicates **immunity** to mumps.

Use Support the diagnosis of mumps virus infection; document previous exposure to mumps virus; document immunity

Limitations Several test systems are not specific for mumps

Methodology Complement fixation (CF), enzyme-linked immunosorbent assay (ELISA), immunofluorescence, hemagglutination inhibition (HAI), hemolysis-in-gel, virus neutralization

If serological testing is performed by enzyme immunoassay (EIA) on automated instrumentation, results are usually given in index units, not titers. In such cases, significant rises in antibody levels are determined by algorithms within the instrumentation, not by increases in titers.

(Continued)

Mumps Serology *(Continued)*

Additional Information Mumps is caused by a paramyxovirus. Serologic study may be undertaken to confirm a diagnosis in acute disease or to demonstrate established immunity. For diagnosis in an acute illness measuring the ratio of IgG to IgM antibody is simplest and fastest. Immunity depends on neutralizing antibody, which must be demonstrated in cell culture.

Selected Readings

Drew WL, "Diagnostic Virology," *Clin Lab Med*, 1987, 7(4):721-40.

Ukkonen P, Väisänen O, and Penttinen K, "Enzyme-Linked Immunosorbent Assay for Mumps and Parainfluenza Type 1 Immunoglobulin G and Immunoglobulin M Antibodies," *J Clin Microbiol*, 1980, 11(4):319-23.

Mumps Virus Culture

Related Information

Mumps Serology *on page 537*

Test Includes Concurrent culture for other viruses

Specimen Saliva, urine, cerebrospinal fluid

Container Sterile container for urine and CSF; tube with cold viral transport medium for swabs

Sampling Time At or within 5 days of the onset of illness

Collection It is desirable to collect specimens as early in the disease as possible. Saliva within 2 days of onset; spinal fluid of patients with meningoencephalitis within 6 days after onset. Virus is also excreted in urine for as long as 14 days.

In young patients, saliva is collected by a suitable suction device or by swabbing, especially the area around the orifices of Stensen's duct. The swabs must immediately be placed into cold viral transport medium. Spinal fluid is obtained in the usual manner and put into a sterile tube. For urine specimens, preferably the first voided morning urine is collected in a sterile container. All specimens must immediately be placed on ice and sent to the laboratory.

Storage Instructions Specimens should be delivered immediately on ice to the laboratory.

Causes for Rejection Dry specimen, specimen not refrigerated during transport, specimen fixed in formalin, unlabeled specimen

Turnaround Time Variable (5-14 days) and depends on methods used and amount of virus in the specimen

Reference Range No virus isolated

Use Aid in the diagnosis of disease caused by mumps virus

Methodology Inoculation of specimen into cell cultures, incubation, observation of characteristic cytopathic effect, and identification by methods such as hemadsorption and fluorescent monoclonal antibodies

Additional Information Although virus isolation is the most certain means for establishing the laboratory diagnosis, serologic methods are also useful and technically easier. Demonstration of IgM antibodies in acute serum is diagnostic of primary infection.

Selected Readings

Black FL, "Measles and Mumps," *Manual of Clinical Laboratory Immunology*, 5th ed, Rose NR, Conway de Macario E, Folds JD, et al, eds, Washington, DC: American Society for Microbiology, 1997, 688-92.

Swierkosz EM, "Mumps Virus," *Manual of Clinical Microbiology*, 7th ed, Murray PR, Baron EJ, Pfaller MA, et al, eds, Washington, DC: American Society for Microbiology, 1999, 959-63.

Tolpin MD and Schauf V, "Mumps Virus," *Textbook of Human Virology*, Belshe RB, ed, Littleton, MA: PSG Publishing Co, 1984, 311-31.

Mumps Virus, Direct Detection *see* Virus Detection by DFA *on page 619*

Murex CMV DNA Hybrid Capture Assay *see* Cytomegalovirus DNA Hybrid Capture *on page 440*

Muscle Biopsy

Related Information

Histopathology *on page 496*

Synonyms Skeletal Muscle Biopsy

Test Includes Examination of muscle biopsy by histopathology. The procedure frequently includes enzyme histochemistry and electron microscopy.

Abstract Diagnosis and classification of muscle disease.

Patient Preparation Clinical data is required and should include the patient's age and sex; the pattern, severity, and tempo of the muscle involvement; relevant laboratory results (ie, CPK, ESR); electromyographic (EMG) findings; and the presence of significant related conditions (ie, dermatitis, neoplasm, steroid/AZT therapy, AIDS).

Sampling Time The biopsy should be performed early in the day as the specimen will immediately require special handling and should arrive when histotechnical personnel

are available. The requisition should state a brief clinical history, pertinent laboratory findings, the biopsy site, and the name of the referring physician.

Collection Selection of muscle biopsy site: The muscle biopsies should be one that is familiar to the pathologist (ie, quadriceps, deltoid, biceps, gastrocnemius), unusual muscle groups such as oculomotor or pharyngeal muscles should be avoided as they have several unique and potentially confusing features. The biopsy should be from a muscle that is involved by the disease but has not reached "end-stage" atrophy. Injection sites, sites used for EMG, and sites near the myotendinous junction should be avoided as these biopsies will commonly exhibit artifactual changes.

Surgical technique: Except for children or exceptional adult cases, the procedure is done with local anesthesia. Ideally, the biopsied muscle should not be allowed to contract because this creates severe microscopic artifacts. To achieve an isometric specimen, it is best to use a surgical muscle clamp that prevents contraction.

If no clamp is available, pinning the muscle specimen to a tongue blade to prevent contraction may be used instead. A portion of the muscle, in continuity with that held in the clamp, should extend from the clamp so it can be cut off for freezing and histochemistry. A small piece should be placed in 1% glutaraldehyde for epon-embedding for electron microscopy, if necessary. Deliver on a saline-moistened gauze pad immediately to the Pathology Department. The moistened gauze pad is used to prevent drying. The specimen must not become saturated as this will cause severe ice crystal artifact, when the biopsy is subsequently snap frozen. The tissue should **not** be placed in fixative or frozen. It should ideally reach the Pathology Laboratory within 30 minutes to maintain enzyme activity.

Storage Instructions A small portion of the fresh material is usually stored deep frozen for possible later use as tissue for biochemical assays (eg, quantitation of glycogen, enzymes, or dystrophin levels).

Use Detect/diagnose trichinosis infection; evaluate muscle disease in terms of neurogenic atrophy, muscular dystrophies, myositis (infectious and "idiopathic," or autoimmune), endocrine myopathies, congenital myopathies, and enzyme deficiencies. Sometimes even with no observable clinical muscle disease, a muscle biopsy may shed light on a systemic condition such as systemic vasculitis.

Methodology A portion of the clamped muscle is oriented, frozen in isopentane/liquid nitrogen, and transverse sections are obtained for H & E, trichrome, and various histochemical preparations, some of which are listed below:

- Adenosine triphosphate (ATPase): At differing pH's, used to differentiates type I, IIa, and IIb myofibers and reveals abnormal fiber type distributions and diseases that selectively involve certain myofiber types.
- Succinate dehydrogenase (SDH): Stains mitochondria and shows abnormal aggregates or loss. Nicotinamide adenine dinucleotide-tetrazolium reductase (NADH-TR) may be used for the same purpose but is less sensitive.
- Oil red O: Stains lipids to detect abnormal accumulations.
- Periodic acid-Schiff (PAS): Used to detected glycogen in glycogenoses (ie, McArdle's disease, Pompe's disease, etc).

Extra frozen sections should be obtained and held in case additional, more specific, enzyme preparations are needed (ie, cytochrome C oxidase, phosphofructokinase, phosphorylase).

The remaining muscle tissue is formalin-fixed, paraffin-embedded, and stained for H & E and trichrome. These preparations are used to detect small foci of myositis or vasculitis which may be missed on the cryostat-cut sections, which are, of necessity, much smaller.

Selected Readings

Brooke MH, "Disorders of Skeletal Muscle," *Neurology in Clinical Practice*, Bradley WG, Daroff RB, Fenichel GM, et al, eds, Boston, MA: Butterworth-Heinemann, 1991, 1843-86.

DeGirolami U, Smith TW, Chad D, et al, "Skeletal Muscle," *Principles and Practice of Surgical Pathology*, Silverberg SG, ed, New York, NY: Churchill Livingstone, 1990, 545-92.

Heffner RR Jr, "Muscle Biopsy in Neuromuscular Disorders," *Diagnostic Surgical Pathology*, Sternberg SS, ed, New York, NY: Raven Press, 1989, 119-39.

Heffner RR Jr, "Skeletal Muscle," *Histology for Pathologists*, Sternberg SS, ed, New York, NY: Raven Press, 1992, 81-108.

Plotz PH, "Not Myositis: A Series of Chance Encounters," *JAMA*, 1992, 268(15):2074-7.

Mychel-S® *see* Chloramphenicol Serum Level *on page 417*

Mycobacteria Culture, Biopsy *see* Mycobacteria Culture, Biopsy or Body Fluid *on page 539*

Mycobacteria Culture, Biopsy or Body Fluid

Related Information

Antimycobacterial Susceptibility Testing *on page 383*
Histopathology *on page 496*
(Continued)

Mycobacteria Culture, Biopsy or Body Fluid *(Continued)*

Mycobacteria Culture, Sputum *on page 542*

Synonyms AFB Culture, Biopsy; Mycobacteria Culture, Biopsy; TB Culture, Biopsy

Applies to Bone Marrow Mycobacteria Culture; Mycobacteria Culture, Bone Marrow; Mycobacteria Culture, Surgical Specimen; Mycobacteria Culture, Tissue; Surgical Specimen Mycobacteria Culture; Tissue Mycobacteria Culture; Wound Mycobacteria Culture

Patient Preparation Aseptic preparation of biopsy site

Special Instructions The laboratory should be informed of the specific source of specimen, age of patient, current antibiotic therapy, clinical diagnosis, and time of collection. Specimens may be divided for fungus culture and KOH preparation, mycobacteria culture and acid-fast smear, and routine bacterial culture and Gram stain only if the specimen is of adequate volume for all tests requested.

Specimen Surgical tissue, bone marrow, biopsy material; **swab specimens are never adequate**

Container Sterile, screw cap container

Collection The portion of the surgical specimen submitted for culture should be separated from the portion submitted for histopathology by the surgeon or pathologist, utilizing sterile technique

Storage Instructions The specimen should be transported to laboratory as soon as possible after collection.

Causes for Rejection Specimen in fixative

Turnaround Time Negative cultures may be be reported after 8 weeks.

Reference Range No growth

Use Isolate and identify mycobacteria; establish the etiology of granulomatous disease, fever of unknown origin (FUO) particularly in immunocompromised patients and others with subtle defects of cellular immunity

Limitations Transbronchial biopsy cultures may be of assistance in documenting the diagnosis of tuberculosis in sputum smear negative cases; however, sputum culture and bronchial washing cultures have a higher percentage of positives.

If *Mycobacterium marinum* which may cause a localized cutaneous lesion that may be nodular, verrucous, ulcerative, or sporotrichoid and which may rarely involve deeper structure is suspected, the laboratory must be notified so that the culture may be incubated at an appropriate temperature (30°C). *Mycobacterium marinum* infection occurs in patients who have been exposed to the organism following an aquatic-related exposure involving a cutaneous abrasion or penetrating injury. Common histories include exposure while cleaning aquariums or clearing barnacles.

Methodology Culture on specialized selective media, usually including Löwenstein-Jensen (LJ) and frequently Middlebrook 7H11, incubated at 35°C with 5% to 10% CO_2 (30°C if *Mycobacterium marinum* or any mycobacterium suspected in causing a skin or soft tissue infection). Mycobacteria isolated are usually definitively identified and may be tested for antimicrobial susceptibility.

Some laboratories offer molecular testing for this organism. Contact the testing laboratory for the availability of amplified and nonamplified qualitative and quantitative molecular tests for this organism, and for information on selection and collection of appropriate specimens for specific molecular tests.

Susceptibility testing may be required because of the often unpredictable susceptibilities of the atypical mycobacteria. Susceptibility testing of mycobacteria is frequently referred to specialized laboratories and may only be offered by specific request.

Additional Information Occult infections with **atypical** mycobacteria (not *M. tuberculosis*), particularly *Mycobacterium avium* and *Mycobacterium intracellulare*, occur in patients with acquired immune deficiency syndrome (AIDS). In some institutions, the incidence of isolation of non-*Mycobacterium tuberculosis* species, specifically *M. avium-intracellulare* (*M. avium* complex), may exceed the rate of isolation of *M. tuberculosis*. Mycobacteria have been recovered from culture of Kaposi's sarcomas and bone marrow specimens, in which the characteristic granulomatous reaction has been absent. Optimal isolation of mycobacteria from tissue is accomplished by processing as much tissue as possible for culture. Swabs should be submitted only when adequate tissue is not available. Tuberculous spondylitis represents 50% to 60% of all cases of skeletal tuberculosis. It is seen in children in developing countries and adults older than 50 years of age in the United States and Europe. Frequently several vertebrae are involved and adjacent psoas muscle abscesses or paravertebral abscesses are not uncommon. Colony counts obtained from bone biopsies are low; however, >90% are culture positive. The diagnosis of vertebral tuberculosis should be considered in all cases of unexplained spondylitis.

Cases of sternal wound infection and of early onset prosthetic valve endocarditis have been recognized. *M. fortuitum* is the most commonly implicated mycobacterial species in these infections. Local environmental strains rather than contaminated commercial surgical materials or devices are considered to be the source of the organisms.

Pleural effusions frequently yield positive cultures in cases of pulmonary tuberculosis. The diagnosis of peritoneal tuberculosis is difficult and is usually made at laparotomy or after a considerable delay. Tuberculosis should be considered in any patient with ascitic fluid and chronic abdominal pain.

Notify laboratory if specimen is skin or soft tissue so laboratory can incubate culture at temperatures <37°C. Incubation at ~25°C enhances the recovery of Mycobacteria which causes such skin and soft tissue infections.

Selected Readings

Brown JW 3d and Sanders CV, "*Mycobacterium marinum* Infections: A Problem of Recognition, Not Therapy?" *Arch Intern Med*, 1987, 147(5):817-8.

Horsburgh CR Jr, Feldman S, and Ridzon R, "Practice Guidelines for the Treatment of Tuberculosis," *Clin Infect Dis*, 2000, 31(3):633-9.

Woods GI and Washington JA, "Mycobacteria Other Than *Mycobacterium tuberculosis*: Review of Microbiologic and Clinical Aspects," *Rev Infect Dis*, 1987, 9(2):275-94.

Mycobacteria Culture, Bone Marrow *see* Mycobacteria Culture, Biopsy or Body Fluid *on page 539*

Mycobacteria Culture, Bronchial Aspirate *see* Mycobacteria Culture, Sputum *on page 542*

Mycobacteria Culture, Cerebrospinal Fluid

Related Information

Acid-Fast Stain *on page 361*

Viral Culture, Central Nervous System Symptoms *on page 614*

Synonyms CSF Mycobacteria Culture; Mycobacteria Culture, CSF; Mycobacteria Culture, Spinal Fluid; Spinal Fluid Mycobacteria Culture

Test Includes Culture for mycobacteria and acid-fast stain if requested

Patient Preparation Usual sterile preparation

Specimen Cerebrospinal fluid

Container Sterile CSF tube

Collection The specimen may be divided for fungus culture and India ink preparation, cryptococcal antigen testing, fungus smear, mycobacteria culture and smear, and routine bacterial culture and Gram stain if the specimen is of adequate volume for all tests requested. Transport specimen to the laboratory as soon as possible.

Storage Instructions Do not refrigerate.

Turnaround Time Negative cultures are often reported after 6-8 weeks.

Reference Range No growth

Use Isolate and identify mycobacteria

Limitations Culture of cerebrospinal fluid for *M. tuberculosis* is usually nonproductive even in cases of tuberculosis meningitis. Culture of CSF for *M. tuberculosis* should be ordered only if such is truly suspected. Recovery of mycobacteria is directly related to the volume of specimen available to the laboratory for culture. 5-10 mL is recommended for optimal yield. Recovery of organisms can require as long as 6 weeks.

Methodology Culture on selective media usually including Löwenstein-Jensen (LJ) and Middlebrook 7H11 broth media may also be used with or without radiometric methodology

Additional Information A culture for mycobacteria is indicated if patient is immunocompromised and the Gram stain is negative and the white cell count is elevated. Tuberculous meningitis occurs in both children and adults. Early in the course neutrophils may predominate in the CSF. Lymphocytes, mononuclear cells, and granulocytes are found later. Rarely does the cell count exceed 1000 cells/mm^3. The CSF is clear and colorless early; later, a pellicle forms on standing. Low CSF glucose, <40 mg/dL, frequently is observed as is increased protein often >300 mg/dL. Other factors raising the index of suspicion include a positive tuberculin skin test (evidence of tuberculosis outside the CNS), previous active tuberculosis, significant recent exposure to tuberculosis, and suspicion of tuberculosis on imaging procedures. Acid-fast organisms can be identified on centrifuged sediments in 60% to 80% of cases.

Untreated tuberculous meningitis can be rapidly fatal. Blacks, Hispanics, and the elderly are most frequently affected. Alcohol abuse, drug abuse, steroid therapy, head trauma, pregnancy, and AIDS all may increase risk. Despite therapy, the mortality risk is high, approximately 30%. Evaluation of contacts is recommended.

(Continued)

Mycobacteria Culture, Cerebrospinal Fluid *(Continued)*

Selected Readings

Horsburgh CR Jr, Feldman S, and Ridzon R, "Practice Guidelines for the Treatment of Tuberculosis," *Clin Infect Dis*, 2000, 31(3):633-9.

Ogawa SK, Smith MA, Brennessel DJ, et al, "Tuberculous Meningitis in an Urban Medical Center," *Medicine (Baltimore)*, 1987, 66(4):317-26.

Mycobacteria Culture, CSF *see* Mycobacteria Culture, Cerebrospinal Fluid *on page 541*

Mycobacteria Culture, Gastric Aspirate *see* Mycobacteria Culture, Sputum *on page 542*

Mycobacteria Culture, Spinal Fluid *see* Mycobacteria Culture, Cerebrospinal Fluid *on page 541*

Mycobacteria Culture, Sputum

Related Information

Acid-Fast Stain *on page 361*
Mycobacteria Culture, Biopsy or Body Fluid *on page 539*

Synonyms AFB Culture, Sputum; Sputum; TB Culture, Sputum Culture, Mycobacteria

Applies to AFB Culture, Bronchial Aspirate; AFB Culture, Gastric Aspirate; Bronchoscopy Mycobacteria Culture; DNA Probe for Mycobacteria; Gastric Aspirate Mycobacteria Culture; Lower Respiratory Mycobacteria Culture; Mycobacteria Culture, Bronchial Aspirate; Mycobacteria Culture, Gastric Aspirate; Mycobacteria Culture, Tracheal Aspirate; Mycobacteria Culture, Transtracheal Aspirate; Mycobacteria, DNA Probe; Percutaneous Transtracheal Mycobacteria Culture; TB Culture, Bronchial Aspirate; TB Culture, Gastric Aspirate; Tracheal Aspirate Mycobacteria Culture; Transtracheal Aspirate Mycobacteria Culture

Test Includes Mycobacteria (AFB) culture and stain

Patient Preparation The patient should be instructed to remove dentures, rinse mouth with water, and then cough deeply expectorating sputum into the sputum collection cup.

Special Instructions Early morning specimen is preferred. Since at least 5 mL of sputum (**not saliva**) is required, the specimen may be collected over a 1- to 2-hour period in order to obtain sufficient quantity. However, 24-hour specimens are unacceptable because of bacterial overgrowth.

Specimen First morning sputum or induced sputum, fasting gastric aspirate, bronchial aspirate, tracheal aspirate, transtracheal aspirate, bronchial lavage

Container Sputum cup, sputum trap, sterile tracheal aspirate tube or sterile bronchoscopy tube

Sampling Time In children, the gastric aspirate should be done early in the morning as the child awakens before the stomach empties.

Collection A recommended screening procedure is three first morning specimens submitted on three successive days. The patient should be instructed to brush his/her teeth and/or rinse mouth well with water before attempting to collect the specimen to reduce the possibility of contaminating the specimen with food particles, oropharyngeal secretions, etc. After the specimen has been collected, the specimen should be examined to make sure it contains a sufficient quantity (at least 5 mL) of thick mucus (**not saliva**). If a two part collection system has been used, only the screw cap tube should be submitted to the laboratory. (The outer container is considered contaminated and its transport through the hospital constitutes a health hazard!) The specimen should be properly labeled and accompanied by a properly completed requisition. The specimen can be divided in the laboratory for fungal, mycobacterial, and routine cultures.

Storage Instructions The specimen should be refrigerated if it cannot be promptly processed. If a gastric aspirate cannot be processed immediately the pH should be neutralized for storage until it can be processed.

Causes for Rejection Specimens contaminated on the outside of the container pose excessive risk to laboratory personnel and may not be acceptable to the laboratory.

Turnaround Time Negative cultures are reported after 6-8 weeks.

Reference Range No growth

Use Isolate and identify mycobacteria

Limitations Bronchial washings are frequently diluted with topical anesthetics and irrigating fluids which may have an inhibitory effect on mycobacterial growth. Postbronchoscopy expectorated specimens may provide a better yield of organisms than those obtained during the procedure. Gastric aspirates yield organisms in <50% of cases of *M. tuberculosis* infection in children. Acid-fast stain of gastric aspirate has a sensitivity of 30%. Separate Cytology specimens must be submitted.

The relative yield of mycobacteria from clinical specimens is prebronchoscopy sputum > bronchial washings > postbronchoscopy sputum > bronchial biopsy.

Methodology Specimens to be cultured for Mycobacteria should be inoculated onto/into both solid and broth media. Selective solid media: Löwenstein-Jensen (LJ) and Middlebrook 7H11: Mycobacteria in clinical specimens can also be grown in broth media which are monitored by instruments. Detection times are more rapid than with conventional culture methods. Gas-liquid chromatography can be used to rapidly speciate mycobacteria. DNA probe technology using probes complementary to the ribosomal RNA of the *M. tuberculosis* complex (*M. tuberculosis, M. bovis*, BCG, *M. africanum*, and *M. microti*), as well as to *M. avium, M. intracellulare, M. kansasii*, and *M. gordonae* are available for culture confirmation. The probes can provide rapid confirmation of the species of mycobacteria isolated.

Some laboratories offer molecular testing for this organism. Contact the testing laboratory for the availability of amplified and nonamplified qualitative and quantitative molecular tests for this organism, and for information on selection and collection of appropriate specimens for specific molecular tests.

Additional Information Tuberculosis decreased in incidence in the United States in the 1970s and 1980s, however, high incidence populations exist in depressed inner city areas, some rural areas, amongst new immigrants, and in HIV-positive patients. The emergence of *M. tuberculosis* and *M. avium-intracellulare* infections complicating the acquired immunodeficiency syndrome has been striking. Primary pulmonary infections are common as case defining infections. Extrapulmonary mycobacterial infections are frequent in patients with an established diagnosis of AIDS.

See also listings Acid-Fast Stain *on page 361*, and Mycobacteria Culture, Biopsy or Body Fluid *on page 539* for additional discussion of mycobacterial disease in patients with the acquired immunodeficiency syndrome (AIDS).

Implication of *M. avium-intracellulare* as a pathogen usually requires at least one of the following criteria:

- Clinical evidence of a disease process that can be explained by atypical mycobacterial infection
- Repeated isolation of the same mycobacterial species from sputum over a period of weeks to months
- Exclusion of other possible etiologies
- Biopsy demonstrating acid-fast bacilli or diagnostic histopathologic changes

Endobronchial tuberculosis has been increasingly recognized because of its incidence in association with the acquired immunodeficiency syndrome and because it may mimic carcinoma.

Nosocomial transmission of multidrug-resistant *Mycobacterium tuberculosis* has been noted to occur from patient to patient and from patient to healthcare worker. Acid-fast bacilli isolation precautions and adherence to appropriate infection control procedures is recommended.

Selected Readings

Chaisson RE and Slutkin G, "Tuberculosis and Human Immunodeficiency Virus Infection," *J Infect Dis*, 1989, 159(1):96-100.

Inderlied CB, Kemper CA, and Bermudez LE, "The *Mycobacterium avium* Complex," *Clin Microbiol Rev*, 1993, 6(3):266-310.

Marmion BP, Williamson J, Worswick DA, et al, "Experience With Newer Techniques for the Laboratory Detection of *Mycoplasma pneumoniae* Infection: Adelaide, 1978-1992," *Clin Infect Dis*, 1993, 17(Suppl 1):S90-9.

Mehta JB and Morris F, "Impact of HIV Infection on Mycobacterial Disease," *Am Fam Physician*, 1992, 45(5):2203-11.

Pearson ML, Jereb JA, Frieden TR, et al, "Nosocomial Transmission of Multidrug-Resistant *Mycobacterium tuberculosis*. A Risk to Patients and Health Care Workers," *Ann Intern Med*, 1992, 117(3):191-6.

Stratton CW, "Mycobacterial Infections Other Than Tuberculosis in the AIDS Era," *Infect Dis Newslett*, 1992, 11(12):89-96.

Wellstood SA, "Diagnostic Mycobacteriology: Current Challenges and Technologies," *Laboratory Medicine*, 1993, 24(6):357-61.

Witebsky FG and Conville PS, "The Laboratory Diagnosis of Mycobacterial Diseases," *Infect Dis Clin North Am*, 1993, 7(2):359-76.

Mycobacteria Culture, Surgical Specimen *see* Mycobacteria Culture, Biopsy or Body Fluid *on page 539*

Mycobacteria Culture, Tissue *see* Mycobacteria Culture, Biopsy or Body Fluid *on page 539*

Mycobacteria Culture, Tracheal Aspirate *see* Mycobacteria Culture, Sputum *on page 542*

Mycobacteria Culture, Transtracheal Aspirate *see* Mycobacteria Culture, Sputum *on page 542*

Mycobacteria, DNA Probe *see* Mycobacteria Culture, Sputum *on page 542*

Mycobacteria, Susceptibility Testing *see* Antimycobacterial Susceptibility Testing *on page 383*

***Mycobacterium* Smear** *see* Acid-Fast Stain *on page 361*

***Mycoplasma genitalium* Culture** *see* *Mycoplasma/Ureaplasma* Culture *on page 545*

***Mycoplasma hominis* Culture** *see* *Mycoplasma/Ureaplasma* Culture *on page 545*

***Mycoplasma pneumoniae* Culture** *see* *Mycoplasma pneumoniae* Diagnostic Procedures *on page 544*

Mycoplasma pneumoniae Diagnostic Procedures

Related Information

Aerobic Culture, Sputum *on page 367*
Darkfield Examination, Leptospirosis *on page 443*
Mycoplasma Serology *on page 545*
Mycoplasma/Ureaplasma Culture *on page 545*

Synonyms *Mycoplasma pneumoniae* Culture

Test Includes Culture and identification of *Mycoplasma pneumoniae*

Abstract *Mycoplasma pneumoniae* commonly causes respiratory infections. Most involve the upper respiratory tract, but pneumonia and other manifestations can occur as well.

Specimen Throat or nasopharyngeal swabs

Collection Throat or nasopharyngeal swabs should be placed **immediately** in transport medium and sent immediately to the laboratory.

Turnaround Time 2-3 weeks

Reference Range No *Mycoplasma pneumoniae* identified

Use Aid in the diagnosis of pneumonia caused by *Mycoplasma pneumoniae*

Limitations The culture procedure is not often used because it is slow and insensitive; 2-3 weeks or more are often required for isolation and definitive identification of positive cultures.

Mycoplasma pneumoniae Clinical Manifestations of Infection

Respiratory	Pneumonia Pharyngitis Otitis media Bullous myringitis Sinusitis Laryngotracheobronchitis Bronchiolitis Nonspecific upper respiratory symptoms
Neurologic	Meningoencephalitis Encephalitis Transverse myelitis Cranial neuropathy Poliomyelitis-like syndrome Psychosis Cerebral infarction Guillain-Barré syndrome
Cardiac	Pericarditis Myocarditis Complete heart block Congestive heart failure Myocardial infarction
Gastrointestinal	Pancreatitis Hepatic dysfunction
Hematologic	Autoimmune hemolytic anemia Bone marrow suppression Thrombocytopenia Disseminated intravascular coagulation
Musculoskeletal	Myalgias Arthralgias Arthritis
Genitourinary	Glomerulonephritis Tubulointerstitial nephritis Tubo-ovarian abscess
Immunologic	Depressed cellular immunity and neutrophil chemotaxis

From Broughton RA, "Infections Due to *Mycoplasma pneumoniae* in Childhood," *Pediatr Infect Dis J*, 1986, 71-85, with permission.

Methodology Isolates are cultured in special broth and on special agar media and are identified by biochemical tests and ability to hemolyze erythrocytes. However, the most commonly used and currently recommended method of diagnosis is serology to measure acute and convalescent antibody levels to *M. pneumoniae.*

Some laboratories offer molecular testing for this organism. Contact the testing laboratory for the availability of amplified and nonamplified qualitative and quantitative molecular tests for this organism, and for information on selection and collection of appropriate specimens for specific molecular tests.

Additional Information *Mycoplasma pneumoniae* infection is acquired via the respiratory route from small-particle aerosols or large droplets of secretions. The organism can penetrate the mucociliary barrier of respiratory epithelium and produce cellular injury and ciliostasis which may account for the prolonged cough observed clinically. Most infections are observed in older children and young adults. Early infection in infancy or childhood may increase the severity of subsequent infections. Cold agglutinins and *Mycoplasma pneumoniae* complement fixation serology have been the mainstays of diagnosis because of the limitations and long turnaround time for cultures. However, immunofluorescence techniques and immunoassays to detect antibodies to *M. pneumoniae* are available and are the recommended diagnostic methods. DNA probes for *Mycoplasma* are not yet available for routine testing. Consult the laboratory for availability of specific tests and specific instructions for specimen collection. See table on previous page.

Selected Readings

Dorigo-Zetsma JW, Zaat SA, Wertheim-van Dillen PM, "Comparison of PCR, Culture, and Serological Tests for Diagnosis of *Mycoplasma pneumoniae* Respiratory Tract Infection in Children," *J Clin Microbiol*, 1999, 37(1):14-7.

Foy HM, "*Mycoplasma pneumoniae* Pneumonia: Current Perspectives," *Clin Infect Dis*, 1999, 28:237.

O'Handley JG and Gray LD, "The Incidence of *Mycoplasma pneumoniae* Pneumonia," *J Am Board Fam Pract*, 1997, 10(6):425-9.

"The Changing Role of *Mycoplasma* in Respiratory Disease and AIDS," *Clin Infect Dis*, 1993, 17(Suppl 1):S1-315.

***Mycoplasma pneumoniae* Titer** *see Mycoplasma* Serology *on page 545*

Mycoplasma Serology

Related Information

Mycoplasma pneumoniae Diagnostic Procedures *on page 544*

Synonyms Eaton Agent Titer; *M. pneumoniae* Titer; *Mycoplasma pneumoniae* Titer; PPLO Titer

Specimen Serum

Container Red top tube

Collection Acute and convalescent sera drawn 10-14 days apart are required

Reference Range Negative: IgG <1:10, IgM <1:10. A fourfold increase in titer in paired sera or a single complement fixation titer >1:256 suggests infection. Contact laboratory for specific cutoff values and significant titers.

Use Support the diagnosis of *Mycoplasma pneumoniae* infection

Limitations False-positives occur in pancreatitis.

Methodology Complement fixation, immunofluorescence, enzyme immunoassay

Additional Information *Mycoplasma pneumoniae* is the cause of the relatively common "primary atypical pneumonia." *Mycoplasma* is more difficult to culture than are bacteria; thus, serologic confirmation of the diagnosis is often desirable. The complement fixation test to detect antibody to a lipid antigen is more specific and more sensitive than is the cold agglutinin test. However, complement fixation requires paired sera, and is thus of limited clinical utility. Demonstration of specific IgG and IgM antibody by immunofluorescence is rapid, sensitive, and specific. IgM antibody indicates acute infection.

Selected Readings

Baum SG, "*Mycoplasma* Infection: Immunologic and Molecular Biologic Diagnostic Techniques," *Manual of Clinical Laboratory Immunology*, 5th ed, Rose NR, Conway de Macario E, Folds JD, et al, eds, Washington, DC: American Society for Microbiology, 1997, 547-51.

Foy HM, "*Mycoplasma pneumoniae* Pneumonia: Current Perspectives," *Clin Infect Dis*, 1999, 28:237.

Waites KB, Bébéar C, Robertson JA, et al, "Laboratory Diagnosis of Mycoplasmal and Ureaplasmal Infections," *Clin Microbiol Newslett*, 1996, 18(14):105-11.

***Mycoplasma* T-Strain Culture, Genital** *see* Genital Culture for *Ureaplasma urealyticum on page 471*

Mycoplasma/Ureaplasma Culture

Related Information

Genital Culture for *Ureaplasma urealyticum on page 471*

Mycoplasma pneumoniae on page 238

Mycoplasma pneumoniae Diagnostic Procedures *on page 544*

(Continued)

Mycoplasma/Ureaplasma Culture *(Continued)*

Synonyms PPLO Culture

Applies to *Mycoplasma genitalium* Culture; *Mycoplasma hominis* Culture; *Ureaplasma urealyticum* Culture; Cervix, *Mycoplasma* Culture; Urethra, *Mycoplasma* Culture; Urine, *Mycoplasma* Culture

Specimen The following specimens are appropriate: throat swabs (send two swabs), sputum, bronchial washings, tracheal aspiration, cerebrospinal fluid, heparinized blood, urethral swab, vaginal swab, cervical swab, placenta, and urine. Urine should **not** be clean catch midstream. Initial urine flow is best specimen.

Collection The laboratory **must** be contacted prior to collection for advice and for appropriate transport medium. Transport specimen to the laboratory within 1 hour. Do **not** use cotton swabs or swabs with wooden sticks.

Turnaround Time 1-6 weeks

Reference Range No *Mycoplasma* isolated

Use Isolate and identify *Mycoplasma*

Limitations Culture is frequently negative in presence of *Mycoplasma* infection.

Methodology Isolates are cultured in special broth and on special agar media and are identified by biochemical tests and ability to hemolyze erythrocytes. However, the most commonly used and currently recommended method of diagnosis is serology to measure acute and convalescent antibody levels to *M. pneumoniae.*

Some laboratories offer molecular testing for this organism. Contact the testing laboratory for the availability of amplified and nonamplified qualitative and quantitative molecular tests for this organism, and for information on selection and collection of appropriate specimens for specific molecular tests.

Additional Information *Mycoplasma pneumoniae* is the causative agent of mycoplasmal pneumonia or atypical pneumonia. This condition is generally mild, but may develop into severe illness. Other members of the *Mycoplasma* family are *M. hominis* and *Ureaplasma urealyticum*, which cause infection of the urogenital tract, namely pelvic inflammatory disease and 10% of the cases of nongonococcal urethritis. Both organisms can be isolated for identification and both respond to erythromycin and tetracycline.

Selected Readings

Waites KB and Thacker WL, "The Value of Culture and Serology for Detection of *Mycoplasma pneumoniae* Infections in the Clinical Laboratory in the Age of Molecular Diagnostics," *Clin Microbiol Newslett*, 2002, 23(16):123-9.

Neisseria gonorrhoeae by Nucleic Acid Probe

Related Information

Neisseria gonorrhoeae Culture *on page 547*

Synonyms DNA Hybridization Test for *Neisseria gonorrhoeae*; DNA Test for *Neisseria gonorrhoeae*; *Neisseria gonorrhoeae* DNA Detection Test

Test Includes Direct detection of *Neisseria gonorrhoeae* nucleic acid in clinical specimens from the urogenital site. This test cannot be used in legal cases or child protection cases.

Patient Preparation When taking urethral specimens, the patient should not have urinated for 1 hour prior to collection.

Specimen Swab specimen collected from the genitourinary site of a male or female patient

Container Special transport medium is provided by the laboratory and should not be substituted. A kit containing a swab and special transport medium is made by the manufacturer of the molecular tests and is **required** for this test.

Collection Currently the probe test for *Neisseria gonorrhoeae* is FDA approved only for genitourinary specimens. It has not yet been approved for testing of nongenital specimens (ie, ocular).

For a male, the urethra is swabbed by rotating the swab 2-3 cm into the urethra. This should provide enough specimen from the infected site to detect *N. gonorrhoeae* nucleic acid. The swab is then placed in the transport tube for shipment to the laboratory.

For females, most kits provide two swabs. The cervix or endocervix should be swabbed with one swab **first** to clean the area and then the **second** swab is used to collect the specimen. The swab is then put immediately into the transport tube and shipped to the laboratory. This is the same collection kit used for the *Chlamydia trachomatis* probe assay. A single swab specimen from each patient is sufficient to test for both *N. gonorrhoeae* and *C. trachomatis*.

Storage Instructions The specimens should be kept at room temperature or refrigerated. Do not freeze.

Causes for Rejection Contamination of specimen with urine

Turnaround Time Results are available within 24 hours of receipt of the specimen. However, most laboratories batch test every 2 or 3 days.

Reference Range Normal: Negative for *Neisseria gonorrhoeae* nucleic acid. A sexually active, asymptomatic female may harbor *N. gonorrhoeae* without overt clinical symptoms.

Use Rapid detection of *N. gonorrhoeae* in clinical urogenital specimens

Limitations Nucleic acid detection tests should not be done in child abuse cases. In these cases many laboratories perform more than one confirmatory test after culture of the isolate. The probe assay can be used to confirm the identification of organisms recovered by culture.

Methodology This test detects *N. gonorrhoeae* nucleic acid directly from swab specimens. This requires denaturation of the nucleic acid in the specimens by heating, hybridization with a specific nucleic acid probe, and detection of bound probe after several washing steps.

Additional Information Gonorrhea is a commonly reported sexually transmitted disease in the United States. The disease is manifest as acute urethritis in males and as cervicitis in females. *N. gonorrhoeae* can be isolated from asymptomatic females. Treatment of these individuals is critical because gonorrhea can result in more serious complications such as pelvic inflammatory disease, sterility, and ectopic pregnancy.

It is very important to control the spread of this disease between sexual partners, thus the use of a quick, reliable test system is essential. The DNA detection assay has a sensitivity and a specificity equal to traditional methods of organism isolation and identification. The current definitive method of detection for *N. gonorrhoeae* is the culture of the microorganism. However, this organism is fastidious and can be difficult to grow in culture when an established laboratory is not available. Loss of viability and overgrowth of contaminating microorganisms may limit recovery of *N. gonorrhoeae* by culture from clinical specimens that must be transported to a referral laboratory.

The major disadvantage of the probe method at the present time is that this test cannot be done in child abuse cases. These cases must be documented with the recovery of *N. gonorrhoeae* organism from the clinical specimen.

Selected Readings

Knapp JS, "Antimicrobial Resistance in *Neisseria gonorrhoeae* in the United States," *Clin Microbiol Newslett*, 1999, 21(1):1-7.

Koumans EH, Johnson RE, Knapp JS, et al, "Laboratory Testing for *Neisseria gonorrhoeae* by Recently Introduced Nonculture Tests: A Performance Review With Clinical and Public Health Considerations," *Clin Infect Dis*, 1998, 27(5):1171-80.

Panke ES, Yang LI, Leist PA, et al, "Comparison of Gen-Probe DNA Probe Test and Culture for the Detection of *Neisseria gonorrhoeae* in Endocervical Specimens," *J Clin Microbiol*, 1991, 29(5):883-8.

Neisseria gonorrhoeae Culture

Related Information

Genital Culture *on page 470*
Genital Culture for *Ureaplasma urealyticum* *on page 471*
Neisseria gonorrhoeae by Nucleic Acid Probe *on page 546*

Synonyms GC Culture; Gonorrhea Culture

Applies to Cervix Culture *Neisseria gonorrhoeae*; GC Culture, Throat; Gonorrhea Culture, Throat; Prostatic Fluid Culture *Neisseria gonorrhoeae*; Synovial Fluid Culture for *Neisseria gonorrhoeae*, Only; Throat Culture for *Neisseria gonorrhoeae*; Urethral Culture for *Neisseria gonorrhoeae*; Urine Culture, First Voided, for *Neisseria gonorrhoeae*; Vaginal Culture *Neisseria gonorrhoeae*

Patient Preparation Preparation same as for clean catch urine. See listing Urine Culture, Clean Catch *on page 609* for detailed information. *Neisseria gonorrhoeae* is very sensitive to lubricants and disinfectants. If possible avoid collecting urethral specimens until at least 1 hour after urinating.

(Continued)

Neisseria gonorrhoeae Culture *(Continued)*

Special Instructions The laboratory should be informed of the specific request for culture of *Neisseria gonorrhoeae* only, and the collection time, date, specific site of specimen, age of patient, current antibiotic therapy, and clinical diagnosis.

Specimen Body fluid, discharge, pus, swab of genital lesions, urethral discharge (best when available for men); endocervix (best when available for female); sediment of first 10 mL of centrifuged urine collected at least 2 hours after last micturition or first few drops of urine voided into a sterile cup for "first voided urine specimen" for asymptomatic males, or first void overnight urine, centrifuged.

Container Swab with transport medium or sterile container if transported to laboratory within a few minutes; otherwise, direct planting on **room temperature** transgrow medium, Jembec™, NYC, or Thayer-Martin medium

Collection

Urethral discharge: Collect male urethral discharge by endourethral swab after stripping toward the orifice to express exudate.

Rectal swab: Collect anorectal specimens from the crypts just inside the anal ring. Direct visualization with anoscopy is useful. Insert the swab past the anal sphincter. Move the swab circumferentially around the anal crypts. Allow 15-30 seconds for organisms to adsorb onto the swab. Replace the swab and crush the media compartment. Prostatic fluid yields fewer positives than does culture of urethral discharge. Cultures from the urethra or vagina are indicated from females when endocervical culture is not possible.

Endocervical/cervical: Gently compress cervix between speculum blades to express any endocervical exudate. Swab in a circular pattern.

Bartholin gland: Express exudate from duct. Abscesses should be aspirated with needle and syringe.

Urethra in women: Massage the urethra against the pubic symphysis to express discharge or use endourethral swab.

Vagina: Obtain the specimen from the vaginal vault. Allow 15-30 seconds for organisms to adsorb onto the swab.

The specimen should be transported to laboratory within 1 hour of collection.

Storage Instructions Specimen **must not** be refrigerated or exposed to a cold environment. If the specimen is directly inoculated on Thayer-Martin medium it should be transported to the laboratory as soon as possible and placed directly in CO_2 incubator or candle jar.

Selection of Culture Sites for the Isolation of *Neisseria gonorrhoeae*

Culture Site	Diagnostic Sensitivity (%)
Female (nonhysterectomized)	
Primary site	
Endocervical canal	86-96
Secondary sites	
Vagina	55-90
Urethra	60-86
Anal canal	70-85
Oropharynx	50-70
Female (hysterectomized)	
Primary site	
Urethra	88.9
Secondary sites	
Vagina	55.7
Anal canal	40.7
Male (heterosexuals)	
Primary site	
Urethra	94-98 (symptomatic) 84 (asymptomatic)
Male (homosexuals)	
Primary sites	
Urethra	60-98
Anal canal	40-85
Oropharynx	50-70

From Ehret JM and Knapp JS, "Gonorrhea," *Clin Lab Med*, 1989, 9:445-80, with permission.

Causes for Rejection Specimen not received in appropriate container, refrigerated specimens

Turnaround Time Preliminary reports are usually available at 24 hours. Cultures with no growth are commonly reported after 48 hours. Cultures from which *N. gonorrhoeae* is isolated require a minimum of 48 hours for completion.

Reference Range No *Neisseria gonorrhoeae* isolated

Use Isolate and identify *Neisseria gonorrhoeae*, establish the diagnosis of gonorrhea

Limitations See table on previous page. Cultures are usually screened only for *Neisseria gonorrhoeae*. No other organisms are usually identified. Overgrowth by *Proteus* and yeast may make it impossible to rule out presence of *N. gonorrhoeae*. The vancomycin in Thayer-Martin media may inhibit some stains of *N. gonorrhoeae*. Nongonococcal urethritis may be caused by *Ureaplasma urealyticum*, *Corynebacterium genitalium* type 1, *Trichomonas vaginalis*, *Chlamydia trachomatis*, herpes simplex virus, and rarely, *Candida albicans*.

Methodology Culture on selective medium, Thayer-Martin or NYC. Nucleic acid probes, monoclonal antibodies and enzyme-linked immunoassays are used as alternatives to culture in some laboratories. Advantages of the newer methods over traditional culture and smear techniques are not universally recognized.

Additional Information Thirty percent to 50% of patients infected with *N. gonorrhoeae* are also infected with *Chlamydia trachomatis*. In high prevalence populations, the recovery of *N. gonorrhoeae* is as follows: endocervix > urine sediment > anal canal > pharynx. A serologic test for syphilis (VDRL, RPR, or ART), HIV, and cervical/vaginal cytology should be considered in patients suspected of having gonorrhea.

Selected Readings

Judson FN, "Gonorrhea," *Med Clin North Am*, 1990, 74(6):1353-66.

Knapp JS, "Antimicrobial Resistance in *Neisseria gonorrhoeae* in the United States," *Clin Microbiol Newslett*, 1999, 21(1):1-7.

Neisseria gonorrhoeae **DNA Detection Test** *see Neisseria gonorrhoeae* by Nucleic Acid Probe *on page 546*

Nigrosin Preparation *see* India Ink Preparation *on page 507*

Nitrite, Urine

Related Information

Leukocyte Esterase, Urine *on page 520*

Lyme Disease Serology by Western Blot *on page 528*

Synonyms Bacteria Screen, Urine

Test Includes This test is usually part of a routine urinalysis

Abstract A rapid method for detection of bacteriuria. A positive test indicates the presence of bacteria which reduce urinary nitrate to nitrite.

Specimen Urine, first morning specimen is preferred; random urine is acceptable; preferably midstream, clean catch collection

Container Plastic urine container

Storage Instructions If the specimen cannot be processed within 2 hours it should be refrigerated.

Reference Range Negative

Use Detect the presence of potentially significant bacteriuria; aid to the diagnosis of cystitis, pyelonephritis, urinary tract infection

Limitations This test is not specific. The sensitivity of the nitrite test is decreased with high urine specific gravity and with high urine ascorbic acid content. False-negatives are relatively common and relate to varying retention times of urine in the bladder, varying urinary nitrate concentrations (diet dependent) and the presence and quantity of nitrate reducing organisms present. Storage of sample at room temperature for excessive periods (more than 2 hours) may lead to reduction of nitrite to nitrogen.

Some urinary tract infections are caused by organisms which do not contain reductase to convert nitrate to nitrite. These include infections caused by *Enterococcus faecalis* and other gram-positive cocci, *N. gonorrhoeae*, *M. tuberculosis*. Negative results are found when infecting organisms do not convert nitrate to nitrite. In addition, urine may not have been retained in the bladder for 4 hours or more to allow adequate reduction of nitrate to occur.

Methodology This reaction depends upon the conversion of nitrate to nitrite by the action of certain species of urinary bacteria. Nitrite from the urine reacts with p-arsanilic acid forming a diazonium compound. The diazonium compound couples with 1,2,3,4-tetrahydrobenzo(h)quinolin-3-ol.

Additional Information A positive nitrite test is strongly suggestive of urinary tract infection (ie, $\geq 10^5$ organisms/mL). Therefore, when positive, a urine culture is recommended, but urine culture is indicated in any case if the patient is symptomatic. The use of nitrate and leukocyte esterase together is more extensively discussed in the listing Leukocyte Esterase, Urine *on page 520.*

(Continued)

Nitrite, Urine *(Continued)*

Selected Readings

Damato JJ, Garis J, Hawley RJ, et al, "Comparative Leukocyte Esterase-Nitrite and BAC-T-SCREEN Studies Using Single and Multiple Urine Volumes," *Arch Pathol Lab Med*, 1988, 112(5):533-5.

Misdraji J and Nguyen PL, "Urinalysis. When - and When Not - To Order," *Postgrad Med*, 1996, 100(1):173-6, 181-2, 185-8 passim.

Semeniuk H and Church D, "Evaluation of the Leukocyte Esterase and Nitrite Dipstick Screening Tests for Detection of Bacteriuria in Women With Suspected Uncomplicated Urinary Tract Infections," *J Clin Microbiol*, 1999, 37(9):3051-2.

Zaman Z, Borremans A, Verhaegen J, et al, "Disappointing Dipstick Screening for Urinary Tract Infection in Hospital Inpatients," *J Clin Pathol*, 1998, 51(6):471-2.

Nits Identification *see* Arthropod Identification *on page 387*

Nizoral *see* Ketoconazole Level *on page 513*

Nocardia Culture, All Sites

Related Information

Acid-Fast Stain, Modified, *Nocardia* Species *on page 362*
Actinomyces Culture, All Sites *on page 363*

Test Includes Culture for *Nocardia* sp and direct microscopic examination of Gram stain for branching gram-positive bacilli, modified acid-fast stain

Abstract *Nocardia asteroides*, *N. brasiliensis*, and *N. caviae* cause two disease entities, nocardiosis and mycetoma. The latter relates to trauma.

Special Instructions Consultation with laboratory prior to collection of the specimen is recommended when nocardiosis is suspected clinically. Culture should be specifically ordered as Culture for *Nocardia*.

Specimen Pus, tissue, cerebrospinal fluid or other body fluid, aspirate, sputum. The usual portal of entry is the lung. Swabs are vastly inferior to aspirates and/or tissue specimens.

Collection Refer to listing for culture of specific site for complete collection and storage instructions (eg, Biopsy or Body Fluid Culture, Sputum Culture, or Wound Culture).

Turnaround Time Negative cultures are reported after 2-4 weeks.

Reference Range No *Nocardia* sp isolated

Critical Values *Nocardia* sp recovered from a central nervous system specimen

Use Establish the diagnosis of nocardiosis

Limitations *Nocardia* sp will not be recovered by routine culture techniques because of its relatively slow growth. Growth of *Nocardia* may be obscured by overgrowth of other organisms in mixed culture (ie, sputum). The diagnosis may not be made unless the laboratory is advised of the clinical suspicion of nocardiosis. *Nocardia* sp are not strongly gram-positive, but their branching pattern when visible is helpful. A modified acid-fast stain (see Acid-Fast Stain, Modified, *Nocardia* Species *on page 362*) is needed, since *Nocardia* are weakly acid-fast and may not be found with conventional acid-fast staining. Staining may be positive when cultures fail. Repeated sputum cultures may not yield a diagnosis of pulmonary nocardiosis. Bronchoscopic biopsy, transtracheal aspiration, or fine needle biopsy is often required.

Methodology Aerobic culture on blood agar and Löwenstein-Jensen (LJ) media with no antibiotics. Recent data supports the use of *Legionella* culture media (selective and nonselective buffered charcoal yeast agar) for recovery of *Nocardia*. *Nocardia* sp can also be cultured on noninhibitory fungal media. Cultures are usually held for 10-30 days. Cultures for *Nocardia* often need to be decontaminated similar to the decontamination process for *Mycobacterium*.

Additional Information *Nocardia* sp are aerobic, gram-positive bacteria which are filamentous, relatively slow growing, and variably acid fast. Human infection is seen most frequently in patients whose immune systems are suppressed by HIV infection, lymphoreticular malignancy, or chemotherapy. Nocardiosis frequently affects debilitated hosts and has been implicated in cases of infections in renal transplant patients, osteomyelitis, in patients on long-term steroid therapy and with peritonsillar abscess, and in cutaneous infections. The clinical picture may be similar to that observed with systemic mycobacterial or fungal infections. Infections may be acute, subacute, or chronic; and they may be disseminated or localized to cutaneous sites or the respiratory tract. Hematogenous dissemination occurs. Metastatic infection in brain, bone, skin, or subcutaneous infection in the presence of pulmonary involvement is suggestive of nocardiosis. *Nocardia asteroides* is the species most commonly recovered from clinical specimens and is usually associated with the respiratory tract; this species is phenotypically heterogeneous, and it has been proposed that the species be considered a complex which is subdivided. *Nocardia brasiliensis* and *Nocardia caviae* also produce human infections; of the two, *Nocardia brasiliensis* is far more common. The species found in mycetoma is usually *N. brasiliensis*.

Nocardia sp are variably acid-fast and may be frequently confused with *Actinomyces* sp or saprophytic fungi in Gram stains of clinical specimens. Prognosis is dependent on early diagnosis, treatment with appropriate antimicrobials, and the course of the underlying disease. In management of high-risk patients, a strong index of suspicion for the diagnosis of nocardiosis must be maintained.

Selected Readings

Bennett JE, "Actinomycosis and Nocardiosis," *Harrison's Principles of Internal Medicine*, 12th ed, Chapter 152, Wilson JD, Braunwald E, Isselbacher KJ, et al, eds, New York, NY: McGraw-Hill Inc, 1991, 752-3.

Filice GA, "Nocardiosis in Persons With Human Immunodeficiency Virus Infection, Transplant Recipients, and Large, Geographically Defined Populations," *J Lab Clin Med*, 2005, 145(3):156-62.

Javaly K, Horowitz HW, and Wormser GP, "Nocardiosis in Patients With Human Immunodeficiency Virus Infection. Report of 2 Cases and Review of the Literature," *Medicine (Baltimore)*, 1992, 71(3):128-38.

Kerr E, Snell H, Black BL, et al, "Isolation of *Nocardia asteroides* From Respiratory Specimens by Using Selective Buffered Charcoal-Yeast Extract Agar," *J Clin Microbiol*, 1992, 30(5):1320-2.

McNeil MM and Brown JM, "The Medically Important Aerobic Actinomycetes: Epidemiology and Microbiology," *Clin Microbiol Rev*, 1994, 7(3):357-417.

McNeil MM, Brown JM, Jarvis WR, et al, "Comparison of Species Distribution and Antimicrobial Susceptibility of Aerobic Actinomycetes From Clinical Specimens," *Rev Infect Dis*, 1990, 12(5):778-83.

Smeets LC, van Agtmael MA, and van der Vorm ER, "Successful Treatment of a Disseminated *Nocardia brasiliensis* Infection," *Eur J Clin Microbiol Infect Dis*, 2005, 24(5):350-1.

Schwartz JG and Tio FO, "Nocardial Osteomyelitis: A Case Report and Review of the Literature," *Diagn Microbiol Infect Dis*, 1987, 8:37-46, (review).

Wallace RJ Jr, Brown BA, Tsukamura M, et al, "Clinical and Laboratory Features of *Nocardia nova*," *J Clin Microbiol*, 1991, 29(11):2407-11.

***Nocardia* Species Modified Acid-Fast Stain** *see* Acid-Fast Stain, Modified, *Nocardia* Species *on page 362*

Non-A, Non-B Hepatitis *see* Hepatitis C Serology *on page 484*

Nucleic Acid Amplification *see* Polymerase Chain Reaction *on page 567*

Occult Blood, Semiquantitative, Urine *see* Urinalysis *on page 606*

Ocular Cytology

Synonyms *Chlamydia* Smear; Conjunctival Smear; Corneal Smear; Eye Smear for Cytology

Applies to Inclusion Conjunctivitis

Test Includes Papanicolaou stain and/or Giemsa stain

Specimen Direct smear of ocular lesion

Collection Swab lesion with cotton-tipped applicator or scrape with sterile ophthalmic spatula and smear on clean glass slides (2), **immediately** spray fix one slide, let other air dry. Label frosted end of slide with patient's name and date.

Causes for Rejection Inadequate fixation

Use Diagnose trachoma-inclusion conjunctivitis, adenovirus infection, vaccinia infection or herpetic conjunctivitis; evaluate possible dysplastic or malignant conjunctival lesions

Limitations The sensitivity of this test is very low. Positive results are only suggestive and should prompt subsequent culture.

Additional Information Diagnosis of viral and chlamydial infections is considerably improved by immunofluorescent and immunoperoxidase stains for organisms.

Selected Readings

Leibowitz HM, "The Red Eye," *N Engl J Med*, 2000, 343(5):345-51.

Sanderson TL, Pustai W, Shelley L, et al, "Cytologic Evaluation of Ocular Lesions," *Acta Cytol*, 1980, 24(5):391-400.

Schumann GB, O'Dowd GJ, and Spinnler PA, "Eye Cytology," *Laboratory Medicine*, 1980, 11:533-40.

Ova and Parasite, Pinworm Preparation *see* Pinworm Preparation *on page 565*

Ova and Parasites, Stool

Related Information

Pinworm Preparation *on page 565*
Stool Culture *on page 585*

Synonyms Parasites, Stool; Parasitology Examination, Stool; Stool for Ova and Parasites

Test Includes Gross appearance, direct wet mounts, saline and iodine, concentration procedure, hematoxylin smear or trichrome smear

Patient Preparation Specimens obtained with a warm saline enema or Fleet® Phospho®-Soda are acceptable. Specimens obtained with mineral oil, bismuth, or magnesium compounds are unsatisfactory. Wait 1 week or more after barium procedures before collecting stools for examination.

Aftercare Warning: Any stool collected by or from the patient may harbor pathogens which are **immediately infective.**

Specimen Fresh or preserved random stool. If pinworm is suspected, a Scotch® Tape preparation should be submitted to the laboratory instead of stool. See also test listing Pinworm Preparation *on page 565.*

(Continued)

Ova and Parasites, Stool *(Continued)*

Container Plastic stool container. The collection procedure of choice is to provide patients with containers with polyvinyl alcohol (PVA) and formalin into which they can place stool. This procedure assures that the specimen will be well preserved. Degradation of parasites during transportation to the laboratory will be markedly reduced.

Sampling Time Single specimens from a single day should be obtained and tested. The older rule of "three specimens collected over three days" is no longer recommended. Test a specimen, obtain the results, and retest if still clinically indicated.

Collection The specimen should be delivered within 1 hour of collection to laboratory. Direct wet preparation exams for motile trophozoite observation can be performed on stools which arrive in the laboratory not longer than 1 hour after collection. The old recommended screening procedure is the automatic ordering of three random stool specimens; one collected every other day. The current, and much more clinically relevant, recommendation is a single specimen and obtaining its result; then the ordering of additional specimens if indicated. Specimens may be preserved in polyvinyl alcohol (PVA) fixative which is suitable for the preparation of permanent stains and formalin or merthiolate-iodine-formalin (MIF), which is suitable for concentration preparations and direct examination.

Storage Instructions Liquid specimens should be brought directly to laboratory. Wet mounts can be performed immediately and the specimen placed in PVA and/or MIF preservatives to maintain ova and trophozoite states when applicable.

Causes for Rejection Because of risk to laboratory personnel, specimens sent on diaper or tissue paper, specimen contaminating outside of transport container may not be acceptable to the laboratory. Specimen containing interfering substances, eg, castor oil, bismuth, Metamucil®, barium specimens delayed in transit and those contaminated with urine will not have optimal yield.

Turnaround Time Variable, depending on method

Reference Range No parasites seen

Use Establish the diagnosis of parasitic infestation

Limitations Note: One negative result does not rule out the possibility of parasitic infestation. Stool examination for *Giardia* may be negative in early stages of infection, in patients who shed organisms cyclically, and in chronic infections. The sensitivity of microscopic methods for the detection of *Giardia* vary. Tests for *Giardia* antigen and immunofluorescence tests have a higher yield.

Contraindications Administration of barium, bismuth, Metamucil®, castor oil, mineral oil, tetracycline therapy, administration of antiamebic drugs within 1 week prior to test. Purgation contraindicated for pregnancy, ulcerative colitis, cardiovascular disease, child younger than 5 years of age, appendicitis or possible appendicitis.

Methodology Wet mount and trichrome stain after concentration, immunofluorescence (IF), counterimmunoelectrophoresis (CIE), or enzyme-linked immunosorbent assay (ELISA) for the detection of *Giardia* antigens. The use of pooled preserved specimens to contain costs is acceptable.

Additional Information Parasite exams on stool from patients hospitalized ≥3 days are rarely, if ever, productive and should not be ordered unless special circumstances exist.

Amebas and certain other parasites cannot be seen in stools containing barium. Optimal diagnostic yield is obtained by the examination of fresh, warm stool by an experienced technologist, during usual laboratory hours. Amebic cysts, *Giardia* cysts, and helminth eggs are often recovered from formed stools. Mushy or liquid stools (either normally passed or obtained by purgation) often yield trophozoites. Purgation does not enhance the yield of *Giardia*. Stools which can be processed by the laboratory in less than 1 hour need not be preserved. Mushy, loose, or watery stools which cannot reach the laboratory within 1 hour should be preserved in formalin or merthiolate-iodine-formalin (MIF) and/or polyvinyl alcohol (PVA). Formalin will preserve protozoan cysts and larvae and the eggs of helminths. It is used for concentration procedures. PVA will preserve the trophozoite stage of protozoa. A trichrome stained smear may be prepared from PVA fixed material. PVA cannot be concentrated; therefore, they should always be accompanied by a portion of the specimen in formalin. Formed stools may be preserved in formalin, or refrigerated in a secure container until they can be transported to the laboratory. The collection/preservation kits will preserve protozoan cysts, helminth eggs and larvae. It is meant to be sent home with the patient and mailed back to the laboratory.

Parasites commonly identified in the stool of AIDS patients include *Cryptosporidium*, *Entamoeba histolytica*, *Giardia lamblia*, and Microsporidia.

Blastocystis hominis which is commonly observed in stool of healthy and symptomatic patients is not currently deemed to be pathogenic. The current consensus is that there is no convincing proof of a causal relationship between *B. hominis* and

symptoms, that there is no correlation between resolution of symptoms with therapy or with the disappearance of the organism from stool, and that treatment directed at the indication of *B. hominis* is not indicated.

In a large children's hospital study of nosocomial diarrhea rotavirus, *C. difficile* and enteric adenovirus were recovered. Stool for ova and parasites and bacterial stool cultures yielded no pathogens.

OVA AND PARASITES, AMEBAE

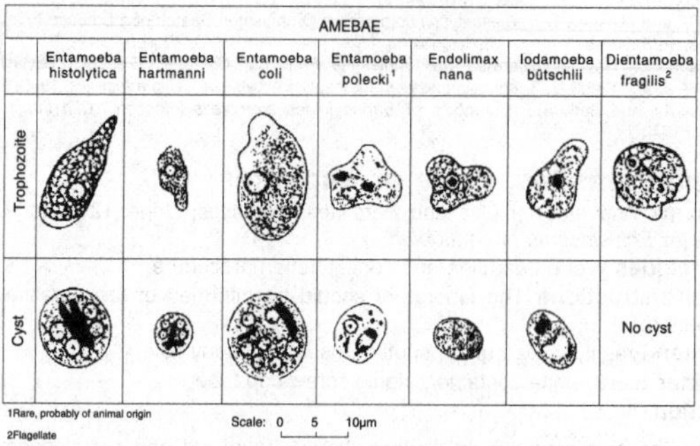

Amebae found in human stool specimens.

OVA AND PARASITES, COCCIDIA

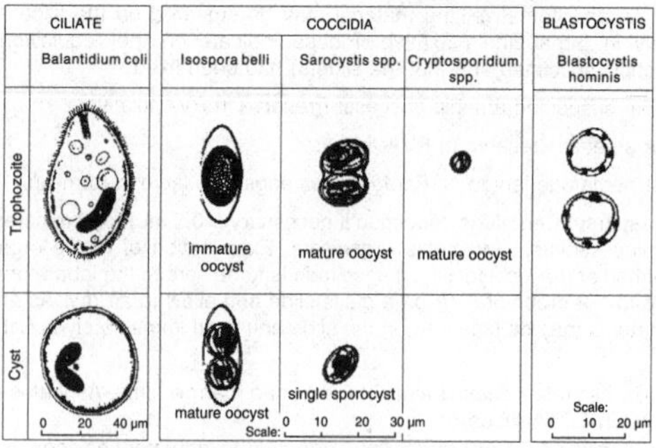

Ciliate, coccidia, and *B. hominis found in human stool specimens.*

OVA AND PARASITES, FLAGELLATES

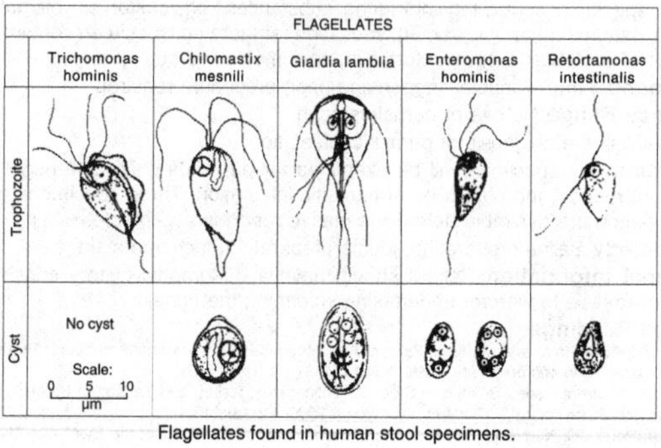

Flagellates found in human stool specimens.

(Continued)

Ova and Parasites, Stool *(Continued)*

Selected Readings

Clark DP, "New Insights Into Human Cryptosporidiosis," *Clin Microbiol Rev*, 1999, 12(4):554-63.
Espinosa-Cantellano M and Martinez-Palomo A, "Pathogenesis of Intestinal Amebiasis: From Molecules to Disease," *Clin Microbiol Rev*, 2000, 13(2):318-31.
Garcia LS, "Laboratory Identification of the Microsporidia," *J Clin Microbiol*, 2002, 40(6):1892-901.
Gardner TB and Hill DR, "Treatment of giardiasis," *Clin Microbiol Rev*, 2001, 14(1):114-28.
Herwaldt BL, "*Cyclospora cayetanensis*: A Review, Focusing on the Outbreaks of Cyclosporiasis in the 1990s," *Clin Infect Dis*, 2000, 31(4):1040-57.
Miller RA and Minshew BH, "*Blastocystis hominis*: An Organism in Search of a Disease," *Rev Infect Dis*, 1988, 10(5):930-8.
Okhuysen PC, "Traveler's Diarrhea Due to Intestinal Protozoa," *Clin Infect Dis*, 2001, 33(1):110-4.
Petri WA Jr and Singh U, "Diagnosis and Management of Amebiasis," *Clin Infect Dis*, 1999, 29:1117-25.
Siddiqui AA and Berk SL, "Diagnosis of *Strongyloides stercoralis* Infection," *Clin Infect Dis*, 2001, 33(7):1040-7.

Ova and Parasites, Urine or Aspirates

Synonyms Aspirates for Ova and Parasites; Parasites, Urine; Urine for Parasites; Urine for *Schistosoma haematobium*

Test Includes Wet preparation and concentration procedure

Special Instructions The laboratory should be informed of the parasite clinically suspected.

Specimen Freshly voided urine, sputum, aspirates, body fluid

Container Sterile urine container, sterile screw cap tube

Collection

Urine: The specimen should be less than 4 hours old and not refrigerated. The recommended screening procedure is to submit three first morning urines on successive days.

Sigmoidoscopic specimens: Mix material with 2-3 drops of PVA on a slide and allow to air dry. As an alternative, the material may be smeared on the slide and fixed immediately in Schaudinn's fixative. Please indicate on the requisition slip as sigmoidoscopic specimen and that the slide(s) has been fixed.

Material from suspected amebic abscess: Preserve in PVA fixative.

Sputum for ameba: Preserve in PVA fixative.

Sputum for nematode larvae or *Paragonimus* eggs: Preserve in formalin.

Duodenal aspirate: Centrifuge specimen if necessary (>0.5 mL) for 2 minutes at 1500 rpm. Examine sediment for motile organisms. Examination of motile organisms is best performed at the local facility. If specimen is to be sent to the laboratory, mix the sediment with 1-2 drops of PVA on a glass slide and allow to air dry. As an alternative, the material may be smeared on the slide and fixed immediately in Schaudinn's fixative.

Bone marrow aspirates: Submit alcohol fixed bone marrow films. Aspirates may also be submitted in EDTA tubes.

Storage Instructions Do **not** refrigerate. Transport to laboratory as soon as possible after collection.

Causes for Rejection Specimen more than 4 hours old, specimen sent on swab, specimen consisting entirely of saliva, specimen contaminated with urine and/or water, specimen containing interfering substances, eg, castor oil, bismuth, Metamucil®, barium (upper or lower GI); specimen refrigerated, specimen contaminated on outside of container, biopsy in formalin, specimen dried out

Turnaround Time Variable - depending upon procedure required

Reference Range No ova or parasites seen

Use Establish the diagnosis of parasitic infestation

Limitations The specimen will be examined for parasites only. One negative result does not rule out the possibility of parasitic infestation. Three specimens over 5- to 7-day period are desirable before a negative report is acceptable.

Methodology Saline preparation, iodine preparation, trichome stain

Additional Information Patient should have a geographic history consistent with schistosomiasis to warrant undertaking screening the urine.

Selected Readings

Espinosa-Cantellano M and Martinez-Palomo A, "Pathogenesis of Intestinal Amebiasis: From Molecules to Disease," *Clin Microbiol Rev*, 2000, 13(2):318-31.
Garcia LS, "Current Issues Related to Stool Collection, Processing, and Testing of Stool Specimens for Diagnostic Parasitology," *Clin Microbiol News*, 2000, 22(18):140-4.
Klotz SA, Penn CC, Negvesky GJ, et al, "Fungal and Parasitic Infections of the Eye," *Clin Microbiol Rev*, 2000, 13(4):662-85.
Petri WA Jr and Singh U, "Diagnosis and Management of Amebiasis," *Clin Infect Dis*, 1999, 29:1117-25.
Tsang VC and Wilkins PP, "Immunodiagnosis of Schistosomiasis. Screen With FAST-ELISA and Confirm With Immunoblot," *Clin Lab Med*, 1991, 11(4):1029-39.

p24 Antigen

Related Information

HIV-1 RNA, Quantitative PCR, 2nd Generation *on page 500*
HIV-1 Serology *on page 501*
HIV Genotyping *on page 503*
Human Immunodeficiency Virus Culture *on page 506*

Synonyms HIV Core Antigen; HIV p24 Antigen

Applies to AIDS Antigen

Special Instructions Observe strict blood and body fluid precautions. In some states written or informed patient consent is a prerequisite for the test. Results may need to be kept confidential.

Specimen Serum or cerebrospinal fluid

Container Red top tube

Reference Range Negative

Use Diagnose recent acute infection with HIV; may also be of prognostic significance in AIDS, if antigen becomes positive during infection, after having been negative. (Can also be used to test viral culture supernatants.)

Limitations Test is not as sensitive as culture for detecting HIV infection.

Methodology Enzyme immunoassay (EIA)

Additional Information p24 antigen is a 24 kD protein product of the **gag** gene of HIV. As a viral, rather than host, product, it appears concomitant with initial infection, and then generally becomes undetectable during periods of viral latency. It reappears with renewed viral replication; the reappearance of p24 antigen in serum generally heralds progression of clinical disease in AIDS. Measuring antigen may also be useful in assessing therapy. It has not been recommended as a further screening test for blood products for transfusion. However, recent studies indicate that an acid dissociation procedure that disrupts the p24 antigen-antibody complexes can increase the sensitivity of the procedure up to fivefold. This may improve its diagnostic utility.

Selected Readings

Bollinger RC Jr, Kline RL, Francis HL, et al, "Acid Dissociation Increases the Sensitivity of p24 Antigen Detection for the Evaluation of Antiviral Therapy and Disease Progression in Asymptomatic HIV-Infected Persons," *J Infect Dis*, 1992, 165(5):913-6.

Ledergerber B, Flepp M, Boni J, et al, "Human Immunodeficiency Virus Type 1 p24 Concentration Measured by Boosted ELISA of Heat-Denatured Plasma Correlates With Decline in CD4 Cells, Progression to AIDS, and Survival: Comparison With Viral RNA Measurement," *J Infect Dis*, 2000, 181(4):1280-8.

PA *see* Chest Films *on page 412*
PA and Lateral CXR *see* Chest Films *on page 412*

Paracentesis

Synonyms Abdominal Paracentesis; Ascites Fluid Tap

Test Includes At the bedside, physician introduces a needle into the peritoneal space of a patient with free ascites, and samples the fluid for diagnostic and/or therapeutic purposes.

Patient Preparation Technique and risks of the procedure are explained. Premedications (eg, sedatives or narcotics) are not routinely required. Laboratory requisitions are completed in advance to avoid delay in fluid processing later. Prothrombin and partial thromboplastin times prior to paracentesis are ordered at physician discretion (some elect to transfuse fresh frozen plasma immediately prior to procedure if PT/PTT are prolonged).

Aftercare No special limitations exist for the patient postprocedure. If large amounts of ascites are removed (several liters), frequent blood pressure measurements are needed to monitor possible hypotension. Patients may ambulate postprocedure if vital signs remain stable. Occasionally, ascites fluid may leak persistently from the puncture site; in this instance, the patient should remain supine with the site angled directly upwards, until the leak stops spontaneously.

Special Instructions In clinical practice, paracentesis is at times performed on patients with significant hepatic encephalopathy. Assistance may be required to properly position the patient.

Complications The medical literature is divided on the incidence of complications from paracentesis. Earlier literature was more negative and tended to emphasize the possible complications, based on retrospective analysis. Some authors suggested that paracentesis itself was the cause of many cases of ascites fluid infection. A recent prospective study concluded that paracentesis is a safe procedure, carrying <1% risk of major complications and <1% risk of minor complications. No deaths or bowel perforations were seen in 229 consecutive attempts. The most feared complication is needle perforation of an abdominal viscus or solid organ such as liver or spleen. Others include: intraperitoneal hemorrhage from laceration of an umbilical (Continued)

Paracentesis *(Continued)*

vein, scrotal or penile edema, abdominal wall hematoma, contamination of ascites by nonsterile technique. Hypotension can be seen when large amounts of ascites (>1500 mL) are removed rapidly.

Equipment Sterile gloves, drapes (optional), and adequate local anesthesia (26-gauge subcutaneous needle, 2% lidocaine). In clinical practice, various needles and angiocatheters are used. A 22-gauge, 1.5" metal needle with a plastic catheter is recommended. If a thick panniculus is encountered, a 3" to 5" 22-gauge needle may be substituted. Also required are a sterile 50 mL syringe and, if large volumes of ascites are to be removed, a sterile 1 L vacuum bottles with connecting tubing.

Technique Patient empties bladder prior to procedure. Physician confirms presence of ascites by physical examination with patient in a semirecumbent position. Preferred site of entry is in the midline, inferior to the umbilicus. If a midline scar is present from prior surgery or if percussion is not reliable, an area near the flank is selected. At times, physician may request patient to assume the hand-knees position if small amounts of ascites are present. The entry site is then caudad to the umbilicus. The site is prepped with iodine solution and skin and deeper tissues are infiltrated with lidocaine. The skin is retracted caudally and the 22-gauge needle (attached to syringe) is inserted into the anesthetized area and advanced while aspirating. When ascites fluid returns freely, the needle is held in position and not advanced further (avoiding bowel trauma). Multiple aliquots (50 mL) may be obtained in this manner. For larger volumes, the syringe is removed and connecting tubing is directly attached to the 22-gauge needle to allow drainage into vacuum bottles. Once the desired amount is collected, the needle is withdrawn quickly and the caudal skin retraction is released, allowing the skin to return to its normal position. This causes the entrance and exit needle sites to form a "Z-tract" which minimizes ascites leakage.

Data Acquired Ascites fluid is routinely analyzed for cell count and differential, chemistries including LD, albumin and protein, Gram stain, bacterial culture, and cytology. Additional tests include special cultures for tuberculosis or fungi, ascites fluid pH, amylase, lipase, glucose, triglycerides, lactate, CEA, and hyaluronic acid.

Specimen When the procedure is performed therapeutically, the maximum volume of ascites that can be removed safely depends on the presence or absence of peripheral edema. It is recommended that in patients without edema, the upper limit should be 1500 mL. Patients with peripheral edema may tolerate larger volumes without hypotension (in one study, ≤5 L). When performed for diagnostic purposes, smaller volumes (50-100 mL) are adequate for routine studies. If malignancy or fastidious infection is suspected, larger volumes (>100 mL) will improve laboratory yield.

Container Lavender top tube for cell count; red top tube for routine chemistries; aerobic and anaerobic culture media bottles for bacteriology. For cytology, send sterile vacuum bottles with 5000 units of heparin added. If ascites fluid pH desired, send specimen to laboratory in an anaerobic syringe (gas bubbles removed) on ice.

Collection Some authorities recommend inoculating the bacterial culture media with ascites fluid immediately at bedside. The average concentration of bacteria in ascites fluid is very low in most cases of spontaneous peritonitis. In addition, a significant number of organisms may not survive in the time needed for specimen transport and plating in the Microbiology Laboratory. Bedside inoculation of appropriate media (standard blood culture bottles) may improve the chances of obtaining a positive bacterial culture several fold.

Normal Findings Ascites fluid is traditionally categorized as either "exudative" or "transudative" based on laboratory analysis. Transudative ascites is caused for the most part by cirrhosis physiology; that is, increased portal venous pressure or decreased portal venous colloid osmotic pressure. Examples of transudates include hepatic cirrhosis, congestive heart failure, constrictive pericarditis, Budd-Chiari syndrome, inferior vena caval obstruction, and nephrotic syndrome. Exudative ascites is generally noncirrhotic in its pathophysiology and may be due to peritoneal membrane permeability defects. Examples of exudates include malignancy, spontaneous bacterial peritonitis (SBP), or other ascites infections (such as tuberculosis), vasculitis, pancreatitis, myxedema.

Critical Values Transudates are characteristically "low-protein" ascites and have been defined by ascites protein <3 g/dL; exudates >3 g/dL. Exceptions are common and other laboratory tests are often used in conjunction with the protein concentration. These include (for transudates): LD <200 units/L, protein ascites/serum ratio <0.5, LD ascites/serum ratio <0.6. Values outside these ranges support the diagnosis of an exudate. The "albumin gradient," defined as serum albumin minus ascites albumin, has recently been shown to accurately identify ascites caused by portal hypertension physiology (eg, cirrhosis). An albumin gradient >1.1 is considered transudative and is due to an oncotic (albumin) pressure gradient between the systemic arterial pressure and ascites fluid, as seen with elevated portal pressures. Exudates tend to have gradients <1.1. The early diagnosis of spontaneous bacterial peritonitis (SBP) prior to

bacterial culture results can frequently be made on routine analysis of ascites fluid. Patients with SBP, or other ascites fluid infections, have ascites WBC count >500/mm^3 along with many polymorphonuclear (PMN) cells on the differential (>250/mm^3). In addition, two other laboratory indices suggestive of SBP are ascites pH <7.35 and ascites lactate <25 ng/dL. The clinical utility of these last two criteria has not been as well established as the standard PMN count. Many physicians will begin empiric antibiotics on the basis of PMN >250/mm^3 alone. Gram stain of ascites fluid has low sensitivity for detecting SBP due to the low bacterial concentration, even on a centrifuged sample. Malignant ascites can be expected to have abnormal cytology in >50% of the cases. Indirect evidence of neoplasm include: grossly hemorrhagic fluid (may also be traumatic); ascites CEA >10 ng/mL with adenocarcinoma; ascites hyaluronic acid >0.25 mg/mL with mesothelioma; high ascites triglyceride levels with chronic chylous ascites (>80% of cases are lymphoma); ascites WBC count >500/mm^3 with peritoneal carcinomatosis (but PMN count low, <250/mm^3), pH <7.35, lactate <25 mg/dL. None of these values are considered diagnostic of malignancy and should be used only as supportive evidence.

Use Diagnostic indications include:

- patients with new onset of ascites
- ascites fluid of unknown etiology
- patients with clinically suspected ascites fluid infections (abdominal pain, unexplained fever, leukocytosis, declining mental status)

Therapeutic paracentesis is indicated when ascites fluid has accumulated enough to cause respiratory compromise, abdominal pain, or worsening of existing inguinal or umbilical hernias. Paracentesis should not be performed to diagnose the presence of ascites fluid. This should be known prior to the procedure (by physical examination or radiological imaging).

Limitations As described previously, the strict use of the ascites protein concentration alone in differentiating exudate from transudate has considerable potential for error. Multiple criteria should be considered, including the albumin gradient and relevant clinical findings.

Contraindications Severe coagulopathy not correctable by vitamin K, fresh frozen plasma, etc; inability of physician to demonstrate ascites fluid on physical examination; lack of patient cooperation. Recent literature suggests the following factors are **not** contraindications for paracentesis: morbid obesity, low grade coagulopathy, multiple abdominal surgical scars, and bacteremia.

Additional Information Paracentesis is a safe procedure when ascites is easily demonstrable on physical examination. When small amounts of ascites are present, a fluid wave may be difficult to demonstrate even when ≤1.5 L ascites are present. CT scan or abdominal ultrasound guided needle aspiration is particularly useful in these cases. Patients with ascites from cirrhosis may develop SBP and yet have minimal evidence of infection; some patients may be completely asymptomatic. A low threshold for performing paracentesis is recommended in this setting, despite the low-grade coagulopathy that frequently is seen.

Selected Readings

Aslam N and Marino CR, "Malignant Ascites: New Concepts in Pathophysiology, Diagnosis, and Management," *Arch Intern Med*, 2001, 161(22):2733-7.

Bender MD and Ockner RK, "Ascites," *Gastrointestinal Disease*, 4th ed, Sleisenger MH and Fordtran JS, eds, Philadelphia, PA: WB Saunders Co, 1988.

Conn HO, "Bacterial Peritonitis: Spontaneous or Paracentric?" *Gastroenterology*, 1979, 77(5):1145-6.

Hoefs JC and Runyon BA, "Spontaneous Bacterial Peritonitis," *Dis Mon*, 1985, 31(9):1-48.

Kao HW, Rakov NE, Savage E, et al, "The Effect of Large Volume Paracentesis on Plasma Volume - A Cause of Hypovolemia?" *Hepatology*, 1985, 5(3):403-7.

Liebowitz HR, "Hazards of Abdominal Paracentesis in the Cirrhotic Patient," *N Y State J Med*, 1962, 62:1822-6, 1997-2004, 2223-9.

Mallory A and Schaefer JW, "Complications of Diagnostic Paracentesis in Patients With Liver Disease," *JAMA*, 1978, 239(7):628-30.

Pare P, Talbot J, and Hoefs JC, "Serum Ascites Albumin Concentration Gradient: A Physiologic Approach to the Differential Diagnosis of Ascites," *Gastroenterology*, 1983, 85(2):240-4.

Pinzello G, Simonetti RG, and Craxi A, "Spontaneous Bacterial Peritonitis: A Prospective Investigation in Predominantly Nonalcoholic Cirrhotic Patients," *Hepatology*, 1983, 3(4):545-9.

Rocco VK and Ware AJ, "Cirrhotic Ascites: Pathophysiology, Diagnosis, and Management," *Ann Intern Med*, 1986, 105(4):573-85.

Runyon BA, Umland ET, and Merlin T, "Inoculation of Blood Culture Bottles With Ascitic Fluid; Improved Detection of Spontaneous Bacterial Peritonitis," *Arch Intern Med*, 1987, 147(1):73-5.

Yang CY, Liaw YF, Chu CM, et al, "White Count, pH, and Lactate in Ascites in the Diagnosis of Spontaneous Bacterial Peritonitis," *Hepatology*, 1985, 5(1):85-90.

Paracentesis Fluid Cytology *see* Cytology, Body Fluids *on page 438*

Parainfluenza 1, 2, and 3 Virus Culture *see* Parainfluenza Virus Culture *on page 558*

Parainfluenza Virus Antigen by Direct Fluorescent Antibody

Related Information

Parainfluenza Virus Culture *on page 558*
Parainfluenza Virus Serology *on page 559*

Test Includes Testing of appropriate clinical materials for presence of parainfluenza virus antigen

Special Instructions Before ordering, contact laboratory to determine if this test is available. DFA test should be performed as soon as possible.

Specimen Appropriate specimens include nasopharyngeal wash (specimen of choice), respiratory secretions (next most useful), nasopharyngeal swabs (less useful), tracheal aspirates, sputum, appropriate autopsy and biopsy specimens

Collection Specimen should be received fresh, not in fixative

Reference Range Negative

Use Identify parainfluenza antigen in clinical specimens

Methodology Direct fluorescent antibody (DFA)

Additional Information This procedure does not depend on a changing antibody titer over time, and is diagnostic for the presence of virus (although the virus may not be the cause of the clinical illness in question). There is also a nonimmunologic cytologic change, ciliocytophthoria, which may be seen in sputum cytology and suggests parainfluenza infection.

Selected Readings

Waner JL, "Parainfluenza Viruses," *Manual of Clinical Microbiology*, 7th ed, Murray PR, Baron EJ, Pfaller MA, et al, eds, Washington, DC: American Society for Microbiology, 1999, 936-41.

Parainfluenza Virus Culture

Related Information

Parainfluenza Virus Antigen by Direct Fluorescent Antibody *on page 558*
Parainfluenza Virus Serology *on page 559*
Viral Culture, Throat *on page 617*

Synonyms Parainfluenza 1, 2, and 3 Virus Culture

Test Includes Concurrent culture for other respiratory viruses (influenza, adenovirus, and respiratory syncytial viruses)

Specimen Throat or nasopharyngeal swab, nasopharyngeal washes and secretions

Container Sterile container; cold viral transport medium for swabs

Collection Place swabs into cold viral transport medium and keep cold. Infants and small children: soft catheters and suction devices (syringes and suction bulbs) can be used to collect nasal secretions (best specimens) as the catheter is withdrawn from far back in the nose. Another excellent method is to introduce 3-7 mL of sterile saline into the child's posterior nasal cavity and immediately aspirate the fluid.

Storage Instructions Keep specimens ice cold but **do not freeze specimens**.

Causes for Rejection Dry specimen, specimen not refrigerated during transport, specimen fixed in formalin, unlabeled specimen

Turnaround Time Variable (5-14 days) and depends on culture method and amount of virus in specimen

Reference Range No virus isolated

Use Aid in the diagnosis of disease caused by parainfluenza virus

Methodology Inoculation of specimens into cell cultures, incubation of cultures, observation of cultures for hemadsorption or characteristic cytopathic effect, and identification/speciation by fluorescent monoclonal antibodies specific for types 1, 2, or 3 or by virus neutralization

Additional Information Most virology laboratories hemadsorb all viral (especially respiratory) cultures at 14 days (prior to discarding the culture) to detect hemadsorbing viruses that have not produced cytopathic effect by that time. Positive hemadsorption tests are often reported preliminarily as "hemadsorbing virus present." This result suggests the presence of influenza, parainfluenza, measles, and/or mumps virus.

Serology for the detection of parainfluenza antibodies is available, but the results are often difficult to interpret.

Selected Readings

Waner JL, "Parainfluenza Viruses," *Manual of Clinical Microbiology*, 7th ed, Murray PR, Baron EJ, Pfaller MA, et al, eds, Washington, DC: American Society for Microbiology, 1999, 936-41.

Wright PF, "Parainfluenza Viruses," *Textbook of Human Virology*, Belshe RB, ed, Littleton, MA: PSG Publishing Co, 1984, 299-309.

Parainfluenza Virus, Direct Detection *see* Virus Detection by DFA *on page 619*

Parainfluenza Virus Serology

Related Information

Parainfluenza Virus Antigen by Direct Fluorescent Antibody *on page 558*
Parainfluenza Virus Culture *on page 558*

Test Includes Antibody titers to parainfluenza virus types 1, 2, and 3

Specimen Serum

Container Red top tube or serum separator tube

Sampling Time Acute and convalescent sera drawn 10-14 days apart are recommended.

Causes for Rejection Inadequate labeling, gross contamination of specimen

Reference Range A single low titer or less than a fourfold change in titer in paired sera

Use Support the diagnosis of parainfluenza virus infection

Limitations Need for convalescent specimen delays diagnosis. Heterotypic rises in parainfluenza titers may occur in infections with other viruses. Infant antibody response may be undetectable.

Methodology Complement fixation (CF), hemagglutination inhibition (HAI), enzyme-linked immunosorbent assay (ELISA)

Additional Information Since the demonstration of a fourfold rise in antibody titer requires testing a convalescent specimen, serologic diagnosis is seldom useful in clinical management of an acute illness. This is especially so since the rise may occur even in an infection caused by some other virus. Serologic studies are of value in epidemiology. Rapid diagnosis during acute illness may be accomplished by demonstrating viral antigen in smears or tissue by immunofluorescence. Since parainfluenza virus may respond to ribavirin, prompt accurate diagnosis could become important, particularly in the immunocompromised host.

If serological testing is performed by enzyme immunoassay (EIA) on automated instrumentation, results are usually given in index units, not titers. In such cases, significant rises in antibody levels are determined by algorithms within the instrumentation, not by increases in titers.

Selected Readings

Sperber SJ and Hayden FG, "Antiviral Chemotherapy and Prophylaxis of Viral Respiratory Disease," *Clin Lab Med*, 1987, 7(4):869-96.

Tristram DA and Welliver RC, "Respiratory Syncytial Virus," *Manual of Clinical Microbiology*, 7th ed, Murray PR, Baron EJ, Pfaller MA, et al, eds, Washington, DC: American Society for Microbiology, 1999, 942-50.

Paranasal Sinuses, CT *see* Computed Transaxial Tomography, Paranasal Sinuses *on page 425*

Parasites, Stool *see* Ova and Parasites, Stool *on page 551*

Parasites, Urine *see* Ova and Parasites, Urine or Aspirates *on page 554*

Parasitology Examination, Stool *see* Ova and Parasites, Stool *on page 551*

Parvovirus B19 DNA, Qualitative PCR

Related Information

Parvovirus B19 Serology *on page 560*
Polymerase Chain Reaction *on page 567*

Synonyms B19 DNA

Specimen Plasma, amniotic fluid, synovial fluid

Container Lavender top (EDTA) tube, yellow top (ACD) tube

Storage Instructions Separate plasma from cells and freeze.

Reference Range Not detected

Use Determine etiology of acute and chronic anemias, erythema infectiosum, and polyarthropathy; diagnose parvovirus infection as the causative agent for fetal hydrops; diagnose parvovirus infection in immunosuppressed individuals (HIV-infected individuals, transplant patients); diagnose parvovirus infection prior to seroconversion

Limitations Diagnosis of parvovirus infection should not rely solely on the result of a PCR test. A negative test result does not exclude the diagnosis of parvovirus infection. Sensitivity of test is 400 copies/mL.

Methodology Polymerase chain reaction (PCR) and enzyme immunoassay (EIA) in which DNA is extracted from the patient specimen and a viral DNA segment is then amplified by polymerase chain reaction (PCR). The amplified DNA is used as sample in an enzyme immunoassay utilizing a digoxigenin (DIG)-labeled probe specific for parvovirus B19. Results are reported as parvovirus B19 DNA detected, not detected, or indeterminate.

Additional Information Parvovirus B19 is an unenveloped single-stranded DNA virus which infects, replicates in and lyses red cell progenitors. Clinical symptoms of infection result from subsequent erythroid aplasia or from the host immune response.
(Continued)

Parvovirus B19 DNA, Qualitative PCR *(Continued)*

In children, the infection manifests as a nonspecific illness or with erythema infectiosum with a characteristic "slapped-cheek" malar rash. Parvovirus occasionally causes polyarthritis in adults and transient aplastic crisis may occur in patients with chronic hemolytic anemia (sickle cell, hereditary spherocytosis, beta thalassemia, etc). Although usually self-limiting, parvovirus infection may cause acute or chronic anemia in the immunocompromised host and is the leading cause of red cell aplasia in AIDS patients. In pregnant women, the infection may be transmitted to the fetus. Fetal anemia, hydrops fetalis, or fetal demise may occur in a small percentage of intrauterine infections.

In intense infection, viremia develops 7-14 days after parvovirus infection. Clinical symptoms occur with the onset of specific IgM production, followed shortly by IgG production. Detection of parvovirus DNA is an earlier and more sensitive marker of viral infection than antiviral antibodies and should be used in conjunction with antiparvovirus IgM detection for optimal diagnostic sensitivity. Parvovirus DNA is especially useful for immunosuppressed patients in whom antibody levels may be undetectable.

Selected Readings

Brown KE, "Parvovirus B19," *Principles and Practices of Infectious Dieases*, 5th ed, Mandell GL, et al, eds, New York, NY: Churchill Livingstone, 2000, 1685-93.

Clewley JP, "PCR Detection of Parvovirus B19," *Diagnostic Molecular Microbiology: Principles and Applications*, Persing DH, Smith TF, Tevover FC, et al, eds, Washington, DC: American Society for Microbiology, 1993, 367-73.

Heegaard ED and Brown KE, "Human Parvovirus B19," *Clin Microbiol Rev*, 2002, 15(3):485-505.

Heegaard ED, Myhre J, Hornsleth A, et al, "Parvovirus B19 Infections in Patients With Chronic Anemia," *Haematologica*, 1997, 82(4):402-5.

Lefrere JJ, Servant-Delmas A, Candotti D, et al, "Persistent B19 Infection in Immunocompetent Individuals: Implications for Transfusion Safety," *Blood*, 2005, Jun 23; [Epub ahead of print].

Petersson K, Norbeck O, Westgren M, et al, "Detection of Parvovirus B19, Cytomegalovirus, and Enterovirus Infections in Cases of Intrauterine Fetal Death," *Obstet Gynecol Surv*, 2005, 60(5):284-6.

Torok TJ, Wang Q, Gray GW Jr, et al, "Prenatal Diagnosis of Intrauterine Infection With Parvovirus B19 by the Polymerase Chain Reaction Technique," *Clin Infect Dis*, 1992, 14(1):149-55.

Weir E, "Parvovirus B19 Infection: Fifth Disease and More," *CMAJ*, 2005, 172(6):743.

Parvovirus B19 Serology

Related Information

Parvovirus B19 DNA, Qualitative PCR *on page 559*

Synonyms Anti-B19 Parvovirus IgG Antibodies; Anti-B19 Parvovirus IgM Antibodies

Test Includes Assays for parvovirus B19 IgM and IgG antibodies

Specimen Blood

Container Red top tube

Storage Instructions Separate serum and freeze.

Use Diagnose parvovirus B19 infection

Methodology Radioimmunoassay (RIA) or immunoblot assay (Western blot) for the detection of IgM and IgG antibodies to parvovirus B19

Additional Information Parvovirus B19 is a DNA virus and can cause a wide spectrum of disease ranging from outbreaks of self-limiting erythema infectiosum (Fifth disease) to persistent bone marrow failure and fetal death. Intrauterine transfusion has been suggested when there is evidence of B19 parvovirus-associated hydrops and anemia. In most people the low-titer parvovirus B19 viremia, which begins approximately 1 week after exposure and lasts 7-10 days, is associated with mild symptoms and a subclinical red cell aplasia. Because the virus destroys erythroid precursor cells, which leads to a reduction in normal red blood cell production, infection with parvovirus B19 can cause a transient aplastic crisis in patients already at maximum red cell production and in those with increased red cell destruction (sickle cell disease, β-thalassemia, and spherocytosis). In immunocompromised patients, parvovirus B19 infection can cause life-threatening anemia. IgM antibodies are detectable 2 weeks after exposure. IgG antibody production usually occurs 18-24 days after exposure and is probably immune-complex mediated. The presence of IgM antibodies to parvovirus B19 provide definite evidence of recent infection.

Selected Readings

Brown KE, "Parvovirus B19," *Principles and Practices of Infectious Dieases*, 5th ed, Mandell GL, et al, eds, New York, NY: Churchill Livingstone, 2000, 1685-93.

Cohen BJ, "Detection of Parvovirus B19-Specific IgM by Antibody Capture Radioimmunoassay," *J Virol Methods*, 1997, 66(1):1-4.

Heegaard ED and Brown KE, "Human Parvovirus B19," *Clin Microbiol Rev*, 2002, 15(3):485-505. Study," *Am J Obstet Gynecol*, 1991, 164(4 Pt 1):1363-4.

Lefrere JJ, Servant-Delmas A, Candotti D, et al, "Persistent B19 Infection in Immunocompetent Individuals: Implications for Transfusion Safety," *Blood*, 2005, Jun 23; [Epub ahead of print].

Petersson K, Norbeck O, Westgren M, et al, "Detection of Parvovirus B19, Cytomegalovirus, and Enterovirus Infections in Cases of Intrauterine Fetal Death," *Obstet Gynecol Surv*, 2005, 60(5):284-6.

Weir E, "Parvovirus B19 Infection: Fifth Disease and More," *CMAJ*, 2005, 172(6):743.

PAS Stain *see* Periodic Acid-Schiff Stain *on page 563*

Patella of Knee, Left or Right, X-ray *see* Bone Films *on page 396*
Pathologic Examination *see* Histopathology *on page 496*
PCR *see* Polymerase Chain Reaction *on page 567*
***Pediculus humanus* Identification** *see* Arthropod Identification *on page 387*
Pelvis AP, X-ray *see* Bone Films *on page 396*
Pelvis Stereo, X-ray *see* Bone Films *on page 396*
Pemphigus Antibodies *see* Skin Biopsy, Immunofluorescence *on page 583*

Penicillin Allergy Skin Testing

Synonyms Penicillin Skin Tests; Skin Tests for Penicillin Allergy

Test Includes Skin testing patients with suspected IgE-mediated penicillin allergy. The reagents used in this procedure are derivatives of the basic benzylpenicillin molecule. They are introduced into the epidermis by a skin prick or into the dermis by an intracutaneous (intradermal) injection. An immediate wheal-and-flare reaction confirms immediate hypersensitivity (Gell and Coombs' type I reaction). This is an important procedure in clinical practice and accurately identifies those individuals at high risk for a severe allergic reaction to penicillin.

Patient Preparation In some medical centers, penicillin skin testing is permitted only after formal consultation with the allergist performing the procedure. If the procedure appears necessary, the technique, risks, and benefits should be explained to the patient. As a preliminary screening measure, the physician should perform a brief dermatologic exam to ensure adequate areas of normal-appearing skin and to identify the rare patient with dermographism. Patient should be instructed to discontinue the following medications several days prior to testing: antihistamines, tricyclic antidepressants, hydroxyzine, phenothiazines. Newer antihistamines with extended half-lives may interfere with testing for over 1 week. All medication changes should be approved by the primary physician.

Aftercare If no complications have occurred, the patient may be discharged from the testing center following completion of the test. Skin sites should be kept clean but remain uncovered. Physician should be contacted immediately if symptoms of wheezing, lightheadedness, or shortness of breath develop several hours later (the unusual case of the "late phase response").

Special Instructions If skin testing is performed by a nurse or physician-assistant, a physician should be immediately available for the rare case of anaphylactic shock. Emergency equipment must be in the testing area, including defibrillation equipment, intubation blades, lidocaine (and other cardiac medications), aqueous epinephrine for injection needles, syringes, and tourniquets.

Complications When properly performed, serious adverse reactions are unusual. The incidence of systemic reactions has been estimated at <1%, with the majority of these being mild or self-limited. Local complications are more common, but generally resolve within hours. These include subcutaneous hemorrhage, localized pruritus, and nonspecific irritant reactions. The risk of hepatitis B, local infection, or human immunodeficiency virus (HIV) transmission is diminishingly small since needles are not reused between patients. The "late response" is a rare but reported complication of allergy skin testing.

Equipment The reagents used for skin testing include:

- The "major determinant," a derivative of the benzylpenicillin molecule called benzylpenicillin-polylysine. It is standardized, commercially available, and routinely used.
- The "minor determinant mixture (MDM)," either benzylpenicillin itself or another derivative (such as penicilloate or penicilloyl-amine). The MDM has not yet been standardized and is not commercially available. Nonetheless, the MDM is widely employed by many allergists and is clinically relevant.

Both the major and minor determinants are administered in most cases. If the major determinant is used alone, 10% to 25% of allergic individuals could be missed. If the minor determinant is used alone, perhaps 5% to 10% of cases could remain undetected, including potential cases of anaphylaxis. In addition to these two reagents, positive (histamine) and negative (diluent) controls are often given. Standard tuberculin syringes, 27-gauge needles, and prick test equipment are also needed.

Technique Ideally, skin test reagents are applied first by the prick test, followed by an intradermal test if the prick test is negative. The prick test is carried out by placing a drop of the reagent in a predetermined location on the skin, usually the forearm. A small needle is passed through the drop and into the epidermis, then removed. For intracutaneous testing, each reagent is individually drawn up into a tuberculin syringe. Again, the volar aspect of the forearm is the preferred site for testing. The reagent (or control) is injected into the dermis, using a 27-gauge needle. A small bleb is raised, usually 0.01-0.02 mL.

(Continued)

Penicillin Allergy Skin Testing *(Continued)*

Data Acquired Test sites are examined at 15-20 minutes for a local wheal-and-flare reaction. The largest diameter of the wheal and/or erythema is measured and recorded in millimeters.

Normal Findings No wheal or erythema after the major determinant, minor determinant, and diluent control. Administration of histamine control should result in a positive skin reaction, with induration >5 mm diameter.

Critical Values For both the prick test and the intracutaneous test, a wheal >5 mm in diameter (with erythema) is considered a positive test. For proper interpretation, the patient should be questioned regarding a history of penicillin allergy. If a reasonable history of penicillin allergy is obtained, a negative skin test essentially rules out a life-threatening allergic response to therapeutic doses of penicillin. No cases of anaphylaxis have been reported in patients who are skin test negative. However, ≤3% of patients who are skin test negative may develop minor reactions while on therapy, such as rash and pruritus. In the patient who has a positive skin test and a positive history of penicillin allergy, the odds of a serious allergic reaction to penicillin therapy are quite high, perhaps 50% to 70%. If skin tests are administered to patients who provide no history of penicillin allergy, the chances of a positive test are low (about 2%). Unfortunately, anaphylaxis during penicillin therapy has been reported in this patient population, although rare. Skin testing all patients prior to beta-lactam therapy, with or without a history of penicillin allergy, is not practical or cost-effective.

Use Theoretically, all patients about to receive a beta-lactam antibiotic should be skin tested. However, it has been demonstrated that such a comprehensive testing policy has a low yield and is not cost-effective. Most authorities recommend skin testing in the following situations:

- patients with a history of penicillin allergy who require penicillin as the drug of choice (eg, treatment of central nervous system syphilis)
- patients with a history of penicillin allergy who require a beta-lactam antibiotic (eg, semisynthetic penicillin, cephalosporin)
- patients with a history of multiple "antibiotic allergies;" skin testing can determine if a beta-lactam drug is a safe treatment option.

Limitations

- This procedure detects only IgE-mediated allergic reactions. Thus, a variety of adverse drug reactions may still occur in skin test negative patients, including serum sickness, drug fever, antibiotic associated colitis, interstitial nephritis, contact dermatitis, bone marrow suppression, and others.
- A number of factors can cause false-positive and false-negative results, as seen in other forms of skin testing.
- Test results apply to penicillin-type antibiotics (natural penicillins, semisynthetic penicillins), but not to cephalosporins, aztreonam, or imipenem.

Contraindications

- Documented history of penicillin-induced anaphylaxis, Stevens-Johnson syndrome, exfoliative dermatitis, or status asthmaticus. These conditions are life-threatening and contraindicate the use of penicillins in general; thus, there is little need to skin test.
- Recent use of medications known to inhibit the IgE-mediated skin response (wheal and flare); this includes antihistamines, hydroxyzine, tricyclic antidepressants, and phenothiazines

Selected Readings

Miles AM and Bain B, "Penicillin Anaphylaxis: A Review of Sensitization, Treatment, and Prevention," *J Assoc Acad Minor Phys*, 1992, 3(2):50-6.

Sarti W, "Routine Use of Skin Testing for Immediate Penicillin Allergy to 6764 Patients in an Outpatient Clinic," *Ann Allergy*, 1985, 55(2):157-61.

VanArsdel PP Jr, Martonick GJ, Johnson LE, et al, "The Value of Skin Testing for Penicillin Allergy Diagnosis," *West J Med*, 1986, 144(3):311-4.

Volz MA and Nelson HS, "Drug Allergy. Best Diagnostic and Treatment Approaches," *Postgrad Med*, 1990, 87(5):137-42, 149.

Weiss ME and Adkinson NF Jr, "β-Lactam Allergy," *Principles and Practice of Infectious Diseases*, 4th ed, Mandell GL, Bennett JE, and Dolin R, eds, New York, NY: Churchill Livingstone, 1995, 272-8.

Weiss ME and Adkinson NF, "Immediate Hypersensitivity Reactions to Penicillin and Related Antibiotics," *Clin Allergy*, 1988, 18(6):515-40.

Penicillin Skin Tests *see* Penicillin Allergy Skin Testing *on page 561*

Percutaneous Biopsy of Musculoskeletal Lesions and Synovial Membranes *see* Bone Biopsy *on page 396*

Percutaneous Liver Biopsy *see* Liver Biopsy *on page 521*

Percutaneous Needle Aspiration Biopsy Under Fluoroscopic, CT, or Ultrasound Guidance *see* Liver Biopsy *on page 521*

Percutaneous Transtracheal Culture Routine *see* Aerobic Culture, Sputum *on page 367*

Percutaneous Transtracheal Fungus Culture *see* Fungus Culture, Sputum *on page 466*

Percutaneous Transtracheal Mycobacteria Culture *see* Mycobacteria Culture, Sputum *on page 542*

Pericardial Fluid Culture *see* Aerobic Culture, Body Fluid *on page 365*

Pericardial Fluid Cytology *see* Cytology, Body Fluids *on page 438*

Pericardial Fluid Fungus Culture *see* Fungus Culture, Body Fluid *on page 462*

Periodic Acid-Schiff Stain

Related Information

Acid-Fast Stain, Modified, *Nocardia* Species *on page 362*
Antifungal Susceptibility Testing *on page 377*
Cryptococcal Antigen Serology, Serum or Cerebrospinal Fluid *on page 431*
Cryptococcus Serology *on page 431*
Cryptosporidium Diagnostic Procedures, Stool *on page 432*
Fungus Culture, Biopsy *on page 461*
Fungus Culture, Body Fluid *on page 462*
Fungus Culture, Skin *on page 464*
Fungus Culture, Sputum *on page 466*
Fungus Culture, Urine *on page 468*
Gram Stain *on page 473*
Histopathology *on page 496*
Histoplasmosis Serology *on page 498*
India Ink Preparation *on page 507*
KOH Preparation *on page 513*
Methenamine Silver Stain *on page 534*
Skin Biopsy *on page 580*
Sporotrichosis Serology *on page 585*

Synonyms PAS Stain

Applies to Mucicarmine Stain

Test Includes Staining of organisms in smear or histologic section with periodic acid-Schiff stain (PAS)

Specimen Bronchoalveolar lavage (BAL), lung biopsy, aspirated specimen, histopathology specimen

Container Sterile suction trap, sterile container for culture, jar with formalin for histopathology, clean glass slides air-dried or fixed in 95% alcohol for smears

Collection Touch preparation smears may be prepared by touching 8-10 glass slides to the cut surface of the fresh lung tissue. The slides should be fixed individually upon preparation in 95% alcohol. Each slide should be labeled with the patient's name on the frosted end.

Reference Range No organisms identified

Critical Values Fungal elements identified

Use Detect fungal elements in clinical specimens, primarily tissue and sputum. Stains fungal elements well; hyphae and yeast can be distinguished relatively easily.

Limitations Takes 1 hour to prepare stain. *Nocardia* species do not stain reliably. *Blastomyces dermatitidis* may vary in appearance. Interpretation requires recognition of PAS-positive artifacts which may appear as yeast cells.

Methodology Periodic acid oxidation of the hydroxyl group in fungal cell wall carbohydrate and reaction with Schiff's reagent to stain the hyphae pink-red

Additional Information In addition to the PAS stain, the methenamine silver stain and the mucicarmine stain are useful for the identification of fungi in tissue. The mucicarmine stain stains the polysaccharide capsular material of *Cryptococcus neoformans* bright pink. See also the listings Skin Biopsy *on page 580* and Methenamine Silver Stain *on page 534*.

Peripheral Arteries and Veins Ultrasound *see* Ultrasound, Peripheral Arteries and Veins *on page 605*

Peripheral Blood Preparation *see* Microfilariae, Peripheral Blood Preparation *on page 535*

Peripheral Blood Smear, *Bartonella* *see* Peripheral Blood Smear, Thick and Thin *on page 563*

Peripheral Blood Smear, Thick and Thin

Related Information

Microfilariae, Peripheral Blood Preparation *on page 535*

Synonyms Blood Smear for Malarial Parasites; Malarial Parasites; Malaria Smear; Thin and Thick Smears, Blood

Applies to Peripheral Blood Smear, *Bartonella*

(Continued)

Peripheral Blood Smear, Thick and Thin *(Continued)*

Test Includes Examination of thick and thin smears

Abstract Malaria is still one of the most common infectious disease in the world. Its rapid diagnosis in the laboratory is extremely important. With increased world travel, the number of cases diagnosed in the United States is increasing.

Special Instructions If the patient has traveled to a malaria-endemic area the date and area traveled should be communicated to the laboratory. Most cases of malaria seen in the U.S. are found in foreign nationals traveling in the United States.

Specimen Fresh blood - fresh fingerstick smears (two or three of each thick and thin film type) made at bedside preferred, EDTA anticoagulated blood for saponin lysis. Contact laboratory for preparation of thick and thin smears.

Container Slides and lavender top (EDTA) tube

Collection Several samples should be taken during a 24-hour period until diagnosis is established or excluded.

Causes for Rejection Specimen clotted

Reference Range No organisms identified

Use Diagnose malaria, parasitic infestation of blood; evaluate febrile disease of unknown origin

Limitations One negative result does not rule out the possibility of parasitic infestation. If protozoal, filarial, or trypanosomal infection is strongly suspected, test should be performed at least three times with samples obtained at different times in the fever cycle.

Malaria Species Infecting Human Red Cells

Plasmodium Species	Malaria	Length of Cycle (hours)
P. vivax	Tertian	45
P. falciparum	Malignant tertian	48
P. ovale	Ovale	48
P. malariae	Quartan	72

Methodology Microscopic examination of thick and thin Giemsa-stained smears. Thick films are more difficult to read and require considerable experience to interpret. Use of thick smears increases the number of cells examined in a given time period by a factor of about 12 because infected cells and organisms are concentrated. Screening by fluorescent microscopy using acridine orange and with gene probes have been described. Thin smears, although not as sensitive, are far superior for determining the species of *Plasmodium* on morphological grounds.

Additional Information Proper therapy depends upon identification of the specific variety of malaria parasite. Release of trophozoites and RBC debris results in a febrile response. Periodicity of fever correlates with type of malaria (see table). Organisms are most likely to be detected just before onset of fever which is predictable in many cases. Sampling immediately upon onset of fever is the most desirable time to obtain blood. Cases with a strong clinical history, which prove negative on initial laboratory screening, may require multiple sampling at different times in the fever cycle to document the diagnosis. Malarial parasites are destroyed in hemoglobin AS and SS patients. The cause of parasite death in AS cells is potassium loss, in SS cells Hb S aggregates destroy the parasites by physical penetration.

Changes in Infected RBCs Useful in Identification of Malaria Species

Plasmodium Species	Infected RBC Enlarged	Presence of Schüffner Dots	Presence of Maurer Dots	Multiple Parasites per RBC	Parasite With Double Chromatin Dots	Parasite With Sausage-Shaped Gametocytes
P. vivax	+	+	—	Rare	Rare	—
P. falciparum	—	—	+	+	+	+
P. ovale	±	+	—	—	—	—
P. malariae	—	—	+	—	—	—

Selected Readings

Orihel TC and Ash LR, "Tissue Helminths," *Manual of Clinical Microbiology*, 7th ed, Murray PR, Baron EJ, Pfaller MA, et al, eds, Washington, DC: American Society for Microbiology, 1999, 1436-48.

Pammenter MD, "Techniques for the Diagnosis of Malaria," *S Afr Med J*, 1988, 74(2):55-7.

Rogers WO, "*Plasmodium* and *Babesia*," *Manual of Clinical Microbiology*, 7th ed, Murray PR, Baron EJ, Pfaller MA, et al, eds, Washington, DC: American Society for Microbiology, 1999, 1355-64.

Peritoneal Fluid Culture *see* Aerobic Culture, Body Fluid *on page 365*

Peritoneal Fluid Cytology *see* Cytology, Body Fluids *on page 438*

Peritoneal Fluid Fungus Culture *see* Fungus Culture, Body Fluid *on page 462*
Pertussis Culture *see Bordetella pertussis* Nasopharyngeal Culture *on page 403*
Pertussis Serology *see Bordetella pertussis* Serology *on page 404*
***Phthirus pubis* Identification** *see* Arthropod Identification *on page 387*

Pinworm Preparation

Related Information
Ova and Parasites, Stool *on page 551*

Synonyms Enterobiasis Test; *Enterobius vermicularis* Preparation; Ova and Parasite, Pinworm Preparation; Scotch® Tape Test

Specimen Scotch® Tape slide preparation of perianal region

Container Scotch® Tape slide must be submitted in a covered container. Commercial kit products are also available for collection of pinworm specimens and are convenient, inexpensive, and highly recommended. **Caution**: Pinworm eggs are very infectious.

Collection The specimen is best obtained a few hours after the patient has retired (ie, 10 or 11 PM), or early in the morning before a bowel movement or bath. This collection procedure is essential if valid results are expected. Clear Scotch® Tape should be used. The nontransparent type is unsatisfactory. An 8 cm (3 in) piece of cellophane tape is placed over the end of a glass slide sticky side out. The anal folds are spread apart and the mucocutaneous junction is firmly pressed in all four quadrants. The tape is then pressed over the slide and the specimen is transported to the laboratory in a carefully sealed container. Refer to diagram.

PINWORM PREPARATION

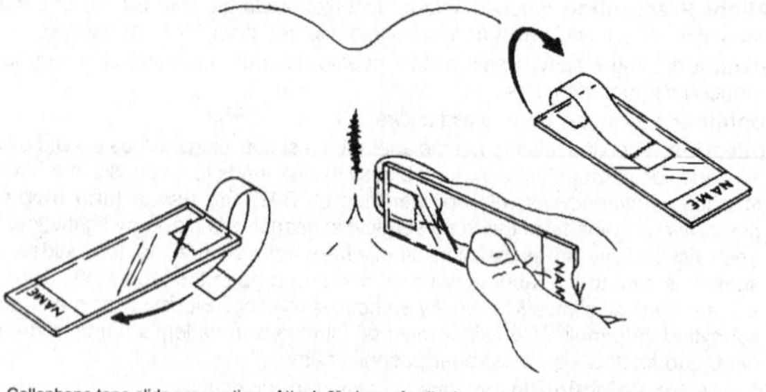

Cellophane tape slide preparation. Attach 3" piece of cellophane tape to undersurface of clear end of microscope slide, which has previously been identified (ground-glass end). Press sticky surface of tape against perianal skin. Then roll back tape onto slide, sticky surface down. Wash hands and nails well. From Bauer JD, *Clinical Laboratory Methods*, 9th ed, Mosby-Year Book Inc, St. Louis, MO: 1982, 989, with permission.

Causes for Rejection Use of nontransparent Scotch® Tape, Scotch® Tape on both sides of the slide, specimen which is not inside a covered container, use of frosted slide, tape sent sticky side up. Specimens which are not properly contained pose excessive risk to laboratory personnel and may not be acceptable to the laboratory.

Reference Range No pinworm eggs (*Enterobius vermicularis*) identified. Positives reported as few, moderate, or many eggs identified.

Use Detect cases of pinworm infestation (enterobiasis), *Enterobius vermicularis* parasitic infestation

Limitations Examination for pinworm only. One negative result does not rule out possibility of parasitic infestation. Stool specimens are not satisfactory for pinworm studies.

Contraindications Specimen collection at improper time

Additional Information The most satisfactory means of diagnosing pinworm infection is by the recovery of eggs or female worms from the perianal region. Only 5% to 10% of infected persons have demonstrable eggs in their stools. If feces is submitted for examination, only the surface should be sampled. Enterobiasis often is present in multiple family members. Therefore, it is recommended that all members of the family be tested. The responsible parent should be instructed how to collect samples using one kit per individual. Female worms or parts of them may be demonstrated on the tape by microscopic examination. Eggs, if present, may be immature, embryonated (with viable or dead larvae), or empty egg shells if the specimen is several days or more old. *Enterobius vermicularis* has been reported as a rare cause of appendicitis, salpingitis, epididymitis, and hepatic granuloma. Diagnosis at colonoscopy has also been reported.

(Continued)

Pinworm Preparation *(Continued)*

Selected Readings

Bauer JD, "Parasitology," *Clinical Laboratory Methods*, 9th ed, St Louis, MO: CV Mosby Co, 1982, 987-9.

***Plesiomonas*, Stool Culture** *see* Stool Culture, Uncommon Organisms *on page 588*

Pleural Fluid Culture *see* Aerobic Culture, Body Fluid *on page 365*

Pleural Fluid Cytology *see* Cytology, Body Fluids *on page 438*

Pleural Fluid Fungus Culture *see* Fungus Culture, Body Fluid *on page 462*

Pleural Fluid *Legionella* Culture *see Legionella pneumophila* Culture *on page 516*

Pleural Fluid Tap *see* Thoracentesis *on page 590*

Pneumocystis jiroveci Test

Related Information

Methenamine Silver Stain *on page 534*

Applies to Biopsy of Lung (Transbronchial) for *Pneumocystis*; Bronchial Aspiration for *Pneumocystis*; Bronchopulmonary Lavage for *Pneumocystis*; Induced Sputum Technique for *Pneumocystis*; Transthoracic Needle Aspiration for *Pneumocystis*

Test Includes Methenamine silver stain; toluidine blue stain and/or Giemsa and/or Wright's stain, or immunofluorescent stain with monoclonal antibodies to *Pneumocystis*

Abstract *Pneumocystis jiroveci* pneumonia is essentially an alveolar disease. The cornerstone of diagnosis is bronchoalveolar lavage (BAL). Of value in the diagnosis of *P.* pneumonia in any immunocompromised subject, including individuals with AIDS, postorgan transplant patients, those with hematologic malignant diseases, inflammatory disorders, and those receiving chemotherapeutic regimens.

Patient Preparation Induced sputum technique: Gargle with 30 mL 3% NaCl, then inhalation of 3% NaCl mist from an ultrasonic nebulizer for 5-15 minutes.

Specimen Lung biopsy, transthoracic needle aspirate, bronchopulmonary lavage or induced sputum technique

Container Sterile jar, clean glass slides

Collection When inoculating needle aspirate on slides, single drops should be applied. The addition of bronchoscopic lung biopsy to BAL leads to diagnosis in a few subjects in whom *Pneumocystis* was not identified by BAL. For **tissue lung biopsy**, touch preparations made from the fresh surgical specimen are made by lightly touching the fresh tissue in rapid succession along the length of three to four slides. Induced sputum is sent to the laboratory fresh, and prepared in the laboratory. They may be alcohol-fixed or allowed to air dry without spreading. Biopsy specimens should be submitted in formalin. Container must be labeled with patient's name, room number, date, and time. Slides must bear patient's name.

Causes for Rejection Inadequate specimen for diagnosis

Use Diagnose *Pneumocystis jiroveci* pneumonia (eg, in acquired immunodeficiency syndrome (AIDS) and other immunocompromised conditions)

Limitations *Pneumocystis* preparations applied to spontaneously expectorated sputum have an extremely low yield. However, in about 40% of individuals with AIDS and symptomatic pneumonia caused by other agents one may anticipate *P. jiroveci* in bronchoalveolar lavage fluid.

Methodology Methenamine silver stain (GMS), immunofluorescence, toluidine blue stain

Additional Information This organism is found in patients with clinical diffuse interstitial pneumonitis. Immunocompromised patients have a high incidence of *Pneumocystis jiroveci* infection (as high as 44% in some series). *Pneumocystis jiroveci* pneumonia may be, but is not always, rapidly progressive. It may be life-threatening, so that rapid diagnosis is important to allow prompt institution of therapy. *Pneumocystis jiroveci* is the most frequent cause of death in children with ALL in remission, such that some institutions routinely give prophylactic trimethoprim-sulfamethoxazole to their leukemic children undergoing antineoplastic therapy. It is also the most common infection and the most common cause of death in patients with AIDS.

P. jiroveci occasionally causes extrapulmonary infections in patients with or without AIDS, usually in patients with advanced HIV infection.

Selected Readings

Cameron RB, Watts JC, and Kasten BL, "*Pneumocystis carinii* Pneumonia. An Approach to Rapid Laboratory Diagnosis," *Am J Clin Pathol*, 1979, 72(1):90-3.

Goodell B, Jacobs JB, Powell RD, et al, "*Pneumocystis carinii*: The Spectrum of Diffuse Interstitial Pneumonia in Patients With Neoplastic Diseases," *Ann Intern Med*, 1970, 72(3):337-40.

Kim HK and Hughes WT, "Comparison of Methods for Identification of *Pneumocystis carinii* in Pulmonary Aspirates," *Am J Clin Pathol*, 1973, 60(4):462-6.

Smith JW and Bartlett MS, "Diagnosis of *Pneumocystis* Pneumonia," *Laboratory Medicine*, 1979, 10:429.

Zimmerman RL, "Testing for *Pneumocystis carinii* Pneumonia," *Laboratory Medicine*, 2000, 31(9):477-8.

Poliovirus Antibody *see* Poliovirus Serology *on page 567*

Poliovirus Culture *see* Enterovirus Culture *on page 453*
Poliovirus Culture, Stool *see* Viral Culture, Stool *on page 616*

Poliovirus Serology

Synonyms Poliovirus Antibody

Specimen Serum

Container Red top tube

Collection Acute and convalescent sera drawn 10-14 days apart are required

Reference Range A fourfold increase in titer in paired sera is diagnostic; presence of neutralizing antibody indicates adequate immunization; normal <1:8

Use Support the diagnosis of poliovirus infection; document previous exposure to poliovirus (complement fixing antibodies); document immunization (neutralizing antibodies)

Methodology Viral neutralization, complement fixation (CF)

Additional Information Poliovirus may also be cultured, producing a characteristic cytopathic effect in cell culture. Culture is more suitable than serology for diagnosis of acute infection.

Selected Readings

Melnick JL, "Enteroviruses," *Manual of Clinical Laboratory Immunology*, 5th ed, Rose NR, Conway de Macario E, Folds JD, et al, eds, Washington, DC: American Society for Microbiology, 1997, 699-701.

Polymerase Chain Reaction

Synonyms Nucleic Acid Amplification; PCR

Abstract The polymerase chain reaction is **not** a test; it is a method to amplify small quantities of the nucleic acid of a microorganism so the microorganism can be detected by other molecular biology means. The polymerase chain reaction is a molecular biology target amplification technique developed with much current and potential use in the medical laboratory. The technique was developed at the Cetus Corporation in Emeryville, California, and was first described for use in the prenatal diagnosis of sickle cell anemia. It may become as important as gene cloning itself. The PCR technique permits a numerous log-fold amplification of segments of DNA in several hours. The amplification is performed by multiple cycles of DNA polymerizing enzyme activity at the sites of known nucleotide sequences. (See figure.) Thus, the nucleotide sequence of the gene to be amplified must be known so oligonucleotide primers flanking the region to be amplified can be synthesized. The method has continually expanding applications not only in prenatal diagnosis, but also for cancer and infectious disease detection and diagnosis.

Specimen The specimen for the PCR assay depends on the type of analysis. For example, prenatal diagnosis will require amniotic fluid or chorionic villus biopsy whole blood will be required for human immunodeficiency virus (HIV) detection, other specimens such as cerebrospinal fluid, sputum, serum, biopsies, or discharge from wounds for other infectious agents, or solid tissue by biopsy for cancer diagnosis.

Collection Varies with type of specimen. Methods of collecting, storing, and transporting vary greatly and depend on the microorganism sought and the laboratory performing the test. Consult the laboratory before ordering the test and collecting the specimen.

Use Uses in the laboratory include prenatal diagnosis of sickle cell anemia, hemophilia, cystic fibrosis, and muscular dystrophy, as well as oncogene activation in the case of lymphoma and chronic myelogenous leukemia. Numerous infectious agents such as *Mycobacterium* species, the agent of Lyme disease, and viruses, have been detected using this amplification technique.

Limitations The tests must be carefully monitored with appropriate controls (especially negative controls) due to the great sensitivity of the amplification technique which may lead to false-positive results.

Methodology PCR is not a test. Actually, PCR is a technique for amplifying a segment of nucleic acid of an organism (pathogens) in a specimen, so that the nucleic acid (and therefore, the organism) will be more likely to be detected in the molecular probe test, which follows PCR. The PCR technique requires knowledge of the base sequence of the target gene. From the sequence data, oligonucleotide primers, 25 nucleotides in length, can be constructed using oligonucleotide synthesizers. These primers flank a 100-2000 base sequence in the nucleic acid segment of interest. The primers are constructed so that the primers bind to opposite strands of the target double helix. A special thermostable DNA polymerase is used because it can withstand the many denaturing, reannealing, and polymerizing cycles without the need for replenishment. The reaction requires the target DNA, the primers, polymerase, and the four deoxynucleotide triphosphates. The mixture is heated several minutes to 95°C to separate the target DNA double strands. The primers are then allowed to bind to the target DNA at 50°C to 60°C and the polymerase reaction allowed to

(Continued)

Polymerase Chain Reaction *(Continued)*

Polymerase Chain Reaction Cycles

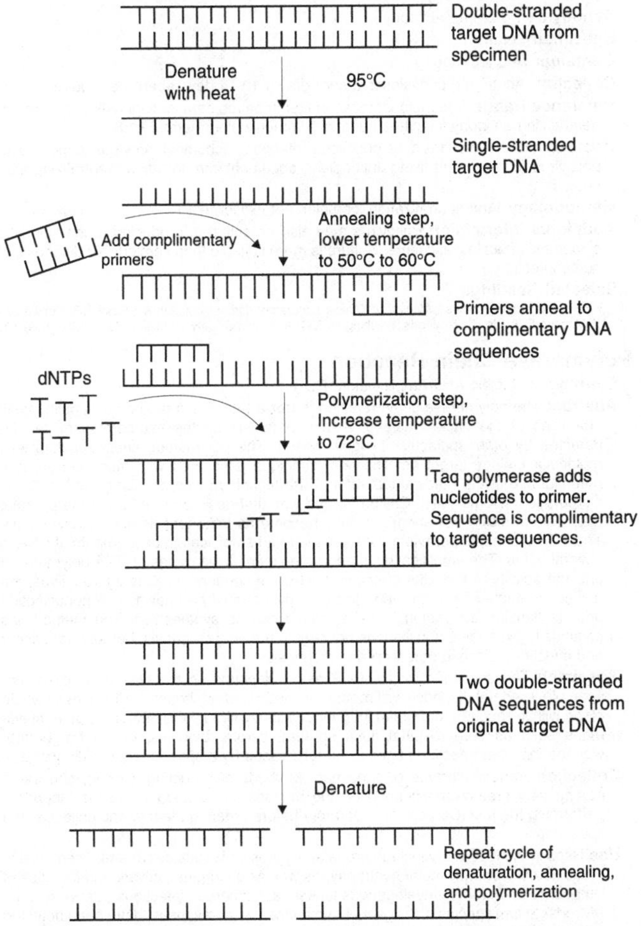

proceed for several minutes at 72°C. This cycle of denaturation, annealing, polymerization is repeated over and over as many as 25-35 times amplifying the sequence between the primers hundreds of thousands to millions of times (see figure). The amplified DNA can then be detected by agarose electrophoresis followed by ethidium bromide staining. The amplified bands can be seen with a UV light and photographed for analysis.

DNA can be extracted from paraffin-embedded tissue for PCR analysis. Such tissue is best fixed in 10% formalin. Genotype can be ascertained by selective ultraviolet radiation fractionation.

Note: Real-time PCR tests are becoming increasingly more available in clinical microbiology laboratories. In real-time PCR, amplification and internal detection of the product (rather than the usual detection that is done only after complete amplification) occur at the same time. Therefore, the product is detected in minutes or only an hour or so, as soon as there is enough product to detect. The result is an extremely short turnaround time.

Additional Information PCR is being expanded and refined. The procedure is automated with programmable heating blocks to cycle the reaction automatically. The technique has unprecedented amplification capability and is able to amplify nanogram quantities of target DNA and can, theoretically, be used to amplify the DNA from a single cell. Amplification reactions other than PCR are also being developed for use in the diagnostic laboratory.

Selected Readings

Bustin SA, "Quantification of mRNA Using Real-Time Reverse Transcription PCR (RT-PCR): Trends and Problems," *J Mol Endocrinol*, 2002, 29(1):23-39.

Crotty PL, Staggs RA, Porter PT, et al, "Quantitative Analysis in Molecular Diagnostics," *Hum Pathol*, 1994, 25(6):572-9.

Fredricks DN and Relman DA, "Application of Polymerase Chain Reaction to the Diagnosis of Infectious Diseases," *Clin Infect Dis*, 1999, 29(3):475-88.

Lee LG, Connell CR, and Bloch W, "Allelic Discrimination by Nick-Translation PCR With Fluorogenic Probes," *Nucleic Acids Res*, 1993, 21(16):3761-6.

Livak KJ, Flood SJ, Marmaro J, et al, "Oligonucleotides With Fluorescent Dyes at Opposite Ends Provide a Quenched Probe System Useful for Detecting PCR Product and Nucleic Acid Hybridization," *PCR Methods Appl*, 1995, 4(6):357-62.

Loda M, "Polymerase Chain Reaction-Based Methods for the Detection of Mutations in Oncogenes and Tumor Suppressor Genes," *Hum Pathol*, 1994, 25(6):564-71.

Mackay IM, Arden KE, and Nitsche A, "Real-time PCR in Virology," *Nucleic Acids Res*, 2002, 30(6):1292-305.

Popliteal Ultrasound *see* Ultrasound, Peripheral Arteries and Veins *on page 605*

Postreduction Films, X-ray *see* Bone Films *on page 396*

Potassium Hydroxide Preparation *see* KOH Preparation *on page 513*

PPD Test *see* Tuberculin Skin Testing, Intracutaneous *on page 601*

PPLO Culture *see Mycoplasma/Ureaplasma* Culture *on page 545*

PPLO Titer *see Mycoplasma* Serology *on page 545*

Prostatic Fluid Culture *see* Genital Culture *on page 470*

Prostatic Fluid Culture *Neisseria gonorrhoeae* *see Neisseria gonorrhoeae* Culture *on page 547*

Pseudomembranous Colitis Toxin Assay *see Clostridium difficile* Toxin Assay *on page 418*

Pubic Lice Identification *see* Arthropod Identification *on page 387*

Purified Protein Derivative (PPD) Test *see* Tuberculin Skin Testing, Intracutaneous *on page 601*

Q Fever Serology

Synonyms *Coxiella burnetii* Titer

Special Instructions Acute and convalescent samples are recommended.

Specimen Serum

Container Red top tube

Reference Range Titer of less than 1:2; comparison of acute and convalescent titers is of greatest diagnostic value

Use Support the diagnosis of Q fever due to *Coxiella burnetii*

Limitations Reagents prepared from fresh isolates (phase I organisms) react differently from those from multiply-passaged organism (phase II)

Methodology Complement fixation (CF), indirect fluorescent antibody (IFA)

Additional Information Q fever shows no reaction in the Weil-Felix test with *Proteus* antigen, so serologic diagnosis must be based on specific rickettsial antigen. Convalescent sera react best with phase II organism (see above), but sera from chronic persistent infection react best with phase I organisms. Cross reactions with *Legionella* have been described.

New Duke criteria for infective endocarditis includes a positive Q fever anti-phase I IgG antibody result of >1:800.

Selected Readings

Eisemann CS and Osterman JV, "*Rickettsia*," *Manual of Clinical Laboratory Immunology*, 3rd ed, Rose NR, Friedman H, and Fahey JL, eds, Washington, DC: American Society for Microbiology, 1986, 847-58.

Hechemy KE, "The Immunoserology of Rickettsiae," *Manual of Clinical Laboratory Immunology*, 5th ed, Rose NR, Conway de Macario E, Folds JD, et al, eds, Washington, DC: American Society for Microbiology, 1997, 558-69.

Reimer LG, "Q Fever," *Clin Microbiol Rev*, 1993, 6(3):193-8.

Rabbit Fever Antibodies *see* Tularemia Serology *on page 603*

Rabid Animals *see* Rabies Detection *on page 569*

Rabies Detection

Related Information

Animal and Human Bites *on page 1270*

Brain Biopsy *on page 405*

(Continued)

Rabies Detection *(Continued)*

Synonyms Rabid Animals

Applies to FRA Test; Fluorescent Rabies Antibody Test; Negri Bodies

Test Includes Examination of animal brain for Negri bodies or inoculation of mice with suspension of brain tissue

Abstract Rabies has been a recognized disease in humans and animals for more than 25 centuries. Zinke is credited with first demonstrating the virus in 1804. Unlike many other viruses, the rabies virus is capable of infecting a number of different animal species, allowing it to propagate and survive in nature. Individuals with a high risk of contact with rabid animals (veterinarians, animal control officers, etc) should consider vaccination against rabies.

Specimen Head of large animal or entire small animal suspected of rabies. Use gloves and mask when handling an animal carcass suspected of rabies.

Container Sealed container

Storage Instructions Ideally, animal brain should be examined in the fresh state. Transport using wet ice or place in absorbent material, then in two plastic bags, or, place half the brain in 50% glycerol, half in 10% formalin, depending on instructions from state laboratory. Local state laboratory must be consulted. Rabies virus may also be demonstrated by immunofluorescence in skin biopsies of patients suspected of having rabies (*vide infra*).

Causes for Rejection Unlabeled or improperly packaged specimen

Use Diagnose rabies; evaluate animal bites

Limitations Negri bodies are found in about 90% of rabid animals.

Contraindications Formalin fixation precludes fluorescent antibody application

Methodology Fluorescent antibody examination (but Negri bodies can be seen in H & E)

Representative Mortality Rates in Nonvaccinated Individuals Following Exposure to Rabid Canines

Location of Exposure	Extent of Exposure	Mortality (%)
Face	Bites (multiple and severe)	60
Other part of head	Bites (multiple and severe)	50
Face	Bite (single)	30
Fingers/hand	Bite (severe)	15
Face	Bites (multiple and superficial)	10
Hand	Bites (multiple and superficial)	5
Trunk/legs	Scratch	3
Hands/exposed skin	Bleeding and superficial wound	2
Skin covered by clothes	Superficial wound	0.5
Recent wound	Saliva	0.1
Wounds >24 h old	Saliva	0.0

From Whitley RJ and Middlebrooks M, "Rabies," *Infections of the Central Nervous System*, Chapter 7, Scheld WM, Whitley RJ, and Durack DT, eds, New York, NY: Raven Press, 1991, 134, with permission.

Additional Information Animals at risk for rabies include skunks, raccoons, dogs, cats, bats, cattle, foxes, and to a lesser extent, jackals, wolves, coyotes, mongooses, weasels, squirrels, and any escaped wild animal. Bites of rabbits, squirrels, hamsters, guinea pigs, gerbils, chipmunks, rats, mice, and other rodents have seldom if ever resulted in human rabies in the United States and are regarded as low risk. High risk species include bats, raccoons, skunks, and foxes among wild carnivorous animals.

Domestic animals should be kept alive if possible, to be quarantined. Animal bites, when unprovoked, are more likely to transmit rabies. Survival of animal for 10 days makes rabies unlikely. Signs of rabies among wild carnivorous animals cannot be reliably interpreted and any such animal that bites or scratches a person should be killed at once and the head submitted for rabies testing.

Rabies is a zoonosis caused by a neurotropic RNA virus which occurs in saliva, central nervous system, urine, and feces. Rabies virus produces Negri bodies (viral inclusions) in neurons.

The geographic area is important. Although a dog bite along the U.S.-Mexican border is considered a rabies exposure until proven otherwise, such bites in New York or Philadelphia are reported not to require prophylaxis. Most Americans dying of rabies were exposed in foreign countries. One patient, bitten by a rabid dog in Kenya, had even had pre-exposure prophylaxis with human diploid cell vaccine. This emphasizes the **necessity for postexposure therapy in appropriate cases.** Almost all rabies

follows bite exposure. However, rabies virus can (rarely) enter through nonbite exposure, such as an open wound, or by inhalation of aerosolized bat urine (eg, cave explorers) or by corneal transplantation. The following table lists location of exposure to rabid canine bites and extent of exposure as it relates to mortality rates. The proportion of cases for which the source of exposure is not known has been increasing since 1960.

Antemortem rabies virus has been isolated from human saliva, brain tissues, CSF, urine sediment, and tracheal secretions. Rabies virus may also be demonstrated by immunofluorescent rabies antibody staining of skin biopsy tissue. The most reliable and reproducible of the immunofluorescent studies that can aid in patient diagnosis is biopsy of the neck skin. A 6-8 mm full thickness wedge or punch biopsy specimen from the neck containing as many hair follicles as possible should be sampled, snap frozen, and shipped frozen at -70°C to a reference laboratory. Consult with reference laboratory for shipping instructions. False-negative results do occur especially after the development of neutralizing antibodies.

Selected Readings

Center for Disease Control, "Compendium of Animal Rabies Control, 1990," *MMWR*, 1990, 39(RR-4):1-8.
Center for Disease Control, "Human Rabies - Oregon," *MMWR*, 1989, 38(19):335-7.
Center for Disease Control, "Rabies Prevention - United States, 1991 - Recommendations of the Immunization Practices Advisory Committee (ACIP)," *MMWR*, 1991, 40(RR-3):1-19.
Fishbein DB and Baer GM, "Animal Rabies: Implications for Diagnosis and Human Treatment," *Ann Intern Med*, 1988, 109(12):935-7.
Fishbein DB and Bernard KW , "Rabies Virus," *Principles and Practice of Infectious Diseases*, Mandell GL, Bennett JE, and Dolin R, eds, New York, NY: Churchill Livingstone, 1995, 1527-43.
Mishu B, "A Rabies Primer for Clinicians," *Infect Dis Newslett*, 1993, 12(1):1-4
Mrak, RE and Young L, "Rabies Encephalitis in a Patient With No History of Exposure," *Hum Pathol*, 1992, 24(1):109-10.
Plotkin SA, "Rabies," *Clin Infect Dis*, 2000, 30:4-12.
Smith JS, "Rabies," *Clin Microbiol Newslett*, 1999, 21(3):17-23.
Smith JS, Fishbein DB, Rupprecht CE, et al, "Unexplained Rabies in Three Immigrants in the United States. A Virologic Investigation," *N Engl J Med*, 1991, 324(4):205-11.
Whitley RJ and Middlebrooks M, "Rabies," *Infections of the Central Nervous System*, Scheld WM, Whitley RJ, and Durack DT, eds, New York, NY: Raven Press, 1991, 134.

Rabies Virus, Direct Detection *see* Virus Detection by DFA *on page 619*
Radionuclide Bone Scan *see* Bone Scan *on page 401*
Rapid Plasma Reagin Test *see* RPR *on page 574*
Rectal Swab Culture *see* Stool Culture *on page 585*
Rectal Swab Culture for Diarrheagenic, *E. coli* *see* Stool Culture, Diarrheagenic *E. coli* *on page 587*
Rectal Swab, Unusual Organism *see* Stool Culture, Uncommon Organisms *on page 588*
Renal Ultrasound *see* Ultrasound, Kidneys *on page 604*

Respiratory Syncytial Virus Antigen by EIA

Related Information

Respiratory Syncytial Virus Culture *on page 572*
Respiratory Syncytial Virus Serology *on page 572*

Synonyms RSV Testing

Test Includes Enzyme immunoassay for respiratory syncytial virus infection

Specimen Nasopharyngeal washes or aspirates, sputum, appropriate autopsy or biopsy specimens

Container Capped syringe

Collection Send specimen fresh, not in fixative. Tissues may be snap frozen.

Causes for Rejection Inadequate specimen

Reference Range No virus detected.

Use Identify respiratory syncytial virus, particularly in infants and young children

Limitations Inadequate specimen collection, improper sample handling/transport or low levels of virus shedding may yield false-negative result. Accordingly, a negative result does not totally eliminate the possibility of RSV infection.

Methodology Enzyme immunoassay (EIA)

Additional Information This test allows rapid diagnosis of the presence of respiratory syncytial virus. It avoids the necessity of obtaining acute and convalescent specimens over a 2-week period. It may be particularly useful in children younger than 6 months of age, whose antibody response to infection may not be diagnostic. However, it must be remembered that showing the virus is present is not equivalent to showing that it is causing a particular disease.

Selected Readings

Domachowske JB and Rosenberg HF, "Respiratory Syncytial Virus Infection: Immune Response, Immunopathogenesis, and Treatment," *Clin Microbiol Rev*, 1999, 12(2):298-309.
Falsey AR and Walsh EE, "Respiratory Syncytial Virus Infection in Elderly Adults," *Drugs Aging*, 2005, 22(7):577-87.

(Continued)

Respiratory Syncytial Virus Antigen by EIA *(Continued)*

Falsey AR and Walsh EE, "Respiratory Syncytial Virus Infection in Adults," *Clin Microbiol Rev*, 2000, 13(3):371-84.
Ismail N and Reisner B, "Update on Human Respiratory Syncytial Virus," *Clin Microbiol Newslett*, 2001, 23(12):91-7.
Welliver RC, "Detection, Pathogenesis, and Therapy of Respiratory Syncytial Virus Infections," *Clin Microbiol Rev*, 1988, 1(1):27-39.

Respiratory Syncytial Virus Culture

Related Information

Respiratory Syncytial Virus Antigen by EIA *on page 571*
Respiratory Syncytial Virus Serology *on page 572*
Viral Culture, Throat *on page 617*

Synonyms RSV Culture

Test Includes Concurrent culture for other respiratory viruses (influenza and parainfluenza viruses)

Specimen Throat or nasopharyngeal swab, nasopharyngeal washes and secretions

Container Sterile container; cold viral transport medium for swabs

Collection Place swabs into cold viral transport medium and keep cold. Infants and small children: soft catheters and suction devices (syringes and suction bulbs) can be used to collect nasal secretions (best specimens) as the catheter is withdrawn from far back in the nose. Another excellent method is to introduce 3-7 mL of sterile saline into the child's posterior nasal cavity and immediately aspirate the fluid.

Storage Instructions Respiratory syncytial virus is extremely labile. **Do not freeze** specimens and send specimens to the laboratory **as soon as possible.**

Causes for Rejection Dry specimen, specimen not refrigerated during transport, specimen fixed in formalin, unlabeled specimen

Turnaround Time Variable (1-14 days) depending on culture method and amount of virus in specimen

Reference Range No virus isolated

Use Aid in the diagnosis of respiratory disease caused by respiratory syncytial virus

Methodology Inoculation of specimen into cell cultures, incubation of cultures, observation of cultures for characteristic cytopathic effect in 2-7 days, and identification by fluorescent monoclonal antibodies specific for respiratory syncytial virus. The use of a rapid shell viral culture technique may yield positive culture results overnight.

Additional Information Serology is available to detect antibodies to respiratory syncytial virus. Many laboratories offer enzyme immunoassay (EIA) tests for the direct detection of RSV in patient specimens. In general, these tests are very rapid, sensitive, and specific.

Selected Readings

Domachowske JB and Rosenberg HF, "Respiratory Syncytial Virus Infection: Immune Response, Immunopathogenesis, and Treatment," *Clin Microbiol Rev*, 1999, 12(2):298-309.
Falsey AR and Walsh EE, "Respiratory Syncytial Virus Infection in Adults," *Clin Microbiol Rev*, 2000, 13(3):371-84.
Hughes JH, Mann DR, and Hamparian VV, "Detection of Respiratory Syncytial Virus in Clinical Specimens by Viral Culture, Direct and Indirect Immunofluorescence, and Enzyme Immunoassay," *J Clin Microbiol*, 1988, 26(3):588-91.
Ismail N and Reisner B, "Update on Human Respiratory Syncytial Virus," *Clin Microbiol Newslett*, 2001, 23(12):91-7.
Welliver RC, "Detection, Pathogenesis, and Therapy of Respiratory Syncytial Virus Infections," *Clin Microbiol Rev*, 1988, 1(1):27-39.

Respiratory Syncytial Virus, Direct Detection *see* Virus Detection by DFA *on page 619*

Respiratory Syncytial Virus Serology

Related Information

Respiratory Syncytial Virus Antigen by EIA *on page 571*
Respiratory Syncytial Virus Culture *on page 572*

Synonyms RSV Titer

Specimen Serum

Container Red top tube

Reference Range IgG <1:5, IgM <1:5; less than fourfold rise in titer by CF

Use Establish the diagnosis of respiratory syncytial virus infection

Limitations Children younger than 6 months of age may not mount a diagnostic serologic response to infection

Methodology Complement fixation, enzyme linked immunosorbent assay

Additional Information Diagnosis by CF depends on demonstrating a rise in antibody titer over a 2- to 3-week period. As such, the test is seldom useful in planning clinical care in an acute illness. For rapid diagnosis the demonstration of viral antigen in nasopharyngeal washings or of IgM antibody is more useful.

Selected Readings

Domachowske JB and Rosenberg HF, "Respiratory Syncytial Virus Infection: Immune Response, Immunopathogenesis, and Treatment," *Clin Microbiol Rev*, 1999, 12(2):298-309.

Falsey AR and Walsh EE, "Respiratory Syncytial Virus Infection in Elderly Adults," *Drugs Aging*, 2005, 22(7):577-87.

Falsey AR and Walsh EE, "Respiratory Syncytial Virus Infection in Adults," *Clin Microbiol Rev*, 2000, 13(3):371-84.

Ismail N and Reisner B, "Update on Human Respiratory Syncytial Virus," *Clin Microbiol Newslett*, 2001, 23(12):91-7.

Rhinovirus Culture *see* Viral Culture, Throat *on page 617*

***Rickettsia rickettsii* Serology** *see* Rocky Mountain Spotted Fever Serology *on page 573*

Rocky Mountain Spotted Fever Serology

Related Information

Ehrlichia Serology *on page 446*

Synonyms *Rickettsia rickettsii* Serology

Special Instructions Acute and convalescent specimens are recommended.

Specimen Serum

Container Red top tube

Reference Range Less than a fourfold increase in titer in paired sera; IgG <1:64, IgM <1:8

Use Establish the diagnosis of Rocky Mountain spotted fever

Limitations Cross reactions with other organism in the spotted fever group. False-positive reactions may occur during pregnancy, especially in the last two trimesters.

Methodology Complement fixation, immunofluorescence, hemagglutination, enzyme linked immunosorbent assay

Additional Information Rocky Mountain spotted fever occurs primarily in the southeastern and western United States from April through October, but is also endemic on Long Island. It is a disease of variable clinical manifestation (some cases present with few or no "spots"), and since there is good specific therapy, and serious outcome if untreated, all aids to diagnosis are important. Serologic diagnosis may be made promptly enough to direct therapy.

Hemagglutination and immunofluorescent tests are least subject to cross reactions with other *Rickettsia*. The complement fixation test can be used with different concentration of antigen to minimize cross reactions. Tests for IgM specific antibody are helpful in early disease, since they appear in 3-8 days. Patients treated with antibiotics early in illness may not develop serologic responses. A direct fluorescent test is also available to demonstrate the *Rickettsia* in tissue.

As many as 71% of patients with Rocky Mountain spotted fever also develop antibodies against cardiolipin and endothelial cells.

Selected Readings

Amsden JR, Warmack S, and Gubbins PO, "Tick-Borne Bacterial, Rickettsial, Spirochetal, and Protozoal Infectious Diseases in the United States: A Comprehensive Review," *Pharmacotherapy*, 2005, 25(2):191-210.

Benson P, "Rocky Mountain Spotted Fever, Another Important Cause of Fever and Rash," *J Emerg Med*, 2004, 27(4):415-6.

Bratton RL and Corey R, "Tick-Borne Disease," *Am Fam Physician*, 2005, 71(12):2323-30.

Buckingham SC, "Tick-Borne Infections in Children: Epidemiology, Clinical Manifestations, and Optimal Management Strategies," *Paediatr Drugs*, 2005, 7(3):163-76.

Sexton DJ and Corey GR, "Rocky Mountain "Spotless" and "Almost Spotless" Fever: A Wolf in Sheep's Clothing," *Clin Infect Dis*, 1992, 15(3):439-48.

Rose Handlers Disease *see* Sporotrichosis Serology *on page 585*

Rotavirus, Direct Detection

Synonyms Rotavirus Rapid Detection

Applies to Viral Antigen Detection, Direct, Stool

Test Includes Direct (nonculture) detection of rotavirus in stool specimens

Specimen Stool from the acute, diarrheal phase of disease

Container Sterile container

Sampling Time As soon as possible after onset of disease, preferably 3-5 days after onset

Collection Several specimens during the course of illness should be submitted in an attempt to eliminate false-negative results.

Causes for Rejection Excessive transit time to laboratory, unlabeled specimen

Turnaround Time 1 day

Reference Range No virus detected

Use Detect rotavirus in stools of patients suspected of having viral gastroenteritis

(Continued)

Rotavirus, Direct Detection *(Continued)*

Limitations Quality of specimens cannot be evaluated, and specimens are collected randomly.

Methodology Commercially available (and often automated) enzyme immunoassays (EIA) are the preferred diagnostic methods. Commercial kits have not been standardized.

Additional Information Rotavirus is an extremely common cause of pediatric gastroenteritis. The illness is most common in winter, is highly contagious, involves 5-8 days of diarrhea, and is rarely fatal. Patients should also be evaluated for possible bacterial gastroenteritis.

Selected Readings

Christensen ML, "Human Viral Gastroenteritis," *Clin Microbiol Rev*, 1989, 2(1):51-89.

Christensen ML, "Rotaviruses," *Manual of Clinical Microbiology*, 7th ed, Murray PR, Baron EJ, Pfaller MA, et al, eds, Washington, DC: American Society for Microbiology, 1999, 999-1004.

Cunney RJ, Costigan P, McNamara EB, et al, "Investigation of an Outbreak of Gastroenteritis Caused by Norwalk-Like Virus, Using Solid Phase Immune Electron Microscopy," *J Hosp Infect*, 2000, 44(2):113-8.

Gray LD, "Novel Viruses Associated With Gastroenteritis," *Clin Microbiol Newslett*, 1991, 13(18):137-44.

Kapikian AZ, "The Discovery of the 27-nm Norwalk Virus: An Historic Perspective," *J Infect Dis*, 2000, 181 Suppl 2:S295-302.

Rotavirus Rapid Detection *see* Rotavirus, Direct Detection *on page 573*

Routine Bone Marrow Culture *see* Bone Marrow Culture, Routine *on page 400*

Routine Culture, Rectal Swab *see* Stool Culture *on page 585*

RPR

Related Information

Darkfield Examination, Syphilis *on page 444*
FTA-ABS, Serum *on page 457*
VDRL, Cerebrospinal Fluid *on page 613*

Synonyms Rapid Plasma Reagin Test; Serologic Test for Syphilis; STS; Syphilis Screening Test

Applies to Syphilis Serology

Test Includes Reactive specimens may be titered and/or an FTA-ABS test performed

Specimen Serum

Container Red top tube

Reference Range Negative

Use Screening test for syphilis

Limitations This is a nontreponemal test and is associated with false-positive reactions due to intercurrent infections, pregnancy, drug addiction, collagen-vascular diseases, and Gaucher's disease.

Methodology Cord agglutination test with reagin antibody

Additional Information This is a very sensitive (but nonspecific) screening test for syphilis and detects antibodies to reagin. These antibodies usually develop within 4-6 weeks of initial infection, peak during the secondary phase of disease, and then decrease. They also decrease with treatment. Greater than 90% of patients with primary syphilis will have positive tests. RPR titers are usually higher in HIV-infected patients than in those who do not have HIV infection.

Because of the many causes of false-positive tests any reactive serum should be tested by a treponemal-specific test (HAI or FTA-ABS). The RPR should not be done on cerebrospinal fluid.

False-negative tests may occur at birth in some infants with recently acquired congenital syphilis. Therefore, especially in areas where the disease is prevalent, a serologic test for syphilis should be included in evaluating febrile infants even if they had a negative screen at birth. False-negatives have also been due to the prozone effect. Therefore, pregnant women in areas with high syphilis prevalence should have dilution performed on negative screening tests.

Selected Readings

Dorfman DH and Glaser JH, "Congenital Syphilis Presenting in Infants After the Newborn Period," *N Engl J Med*, 1990, 323(19):1299-302.

Hart G, "Syphilis Tests in Diagnostic and Therapeutic Decision Making," *Ann Intern Med*, 1986, 104(3):368-76.

Singh AE and Romanowski B, "Syphilis: Review With Emphasis on Clinical Epidemiologic, and Some Biologic Features," *Clin Microbiol Rev*, 1999, 12(2):187-209.

van Voorst and Vader PC, "Syphilis Management and Treatment," *Dermatol Clin*, 1998, 16(4):699-711, xi.

Wicher V and Wicher K, "Pathogenesis of Maternal-Fetal Syphilis Revisited," *Clin Infect Dis*, 2001, 33(3):354-63.

Young H, "Syphilis. Serology," *Dermatol Clin*, 1998, 16(4):691-8.

RSV Culture *see* Respiratory Syncytial Virus Culture *on page 572*

RSV Testing *see* Respiratory Syncytial Virus Antigen by EIA *on page 571*

RSV Titer *see* Respiratory Syncytial Virus Serology *on page 572*

Rubella Antibodies *see* Rubella Serology *on page 575*

Rubella Serology

Synonyms German Measles Serology; Rubella Antibodies

Applies to IgG Antibodies to Rubella; IgM Antibodies to Rubella

Test Includes Detection of serologic response to rubella infection or vaccination

Abstract German measles is a viral infection usually characterized by a macular exanthem, an incubation period of 14-21 days and lymphadenopathy, pharyngitis, and conjunctivitis. Severe transplacental infections occur in the first trimester.

Specimen Serum

Container Red top tube

Reference Range Absence of antibody indicates susceptibility to rubella. Presence of IgM antibody indicates acute infection or vaccination. Presence of IgG antibody requires interpretation.

Possible Panic Range Evidence of susceptibility in a pregnant woman recently exposed to rubella

Use Aid in the diagnosis of congenital rubella infections; evaluate susceptibility to infections

Limitations Requires clinical correlation and judgment. Low levels of antibody are poorly detected by enzyme immunoassays.

Methodology Indirect fluorescent antibody (IFA), hemagglutination, enzyme-linked immunosorbent assay (ELISA), radioimmunoassay (RIA), complement fixation (CF), latex agglutination (LA), enzyme immunoassay (EIA)

If serological testing is performed by enzyme immunoassay (EIA) on automated instrumentation, results are usually given in index units, not titers. In such cases, significant rises in antibody levels are determined by algorithms within the instrumentation, not by increases in titers.

Additional Information Rubella virus is the cause of German measles, usually a mild exanthem, often subclinical. However, when acquired *in utero*, rubella virus can cause the congenital rubella syndrome, and lead to fetal demise, cataracts, malformation, deafness, and mental retardation. For this reason the federal government and many states support programs to immunize women against rubella before they have children. There has been a resurgence of congenital rubella in the early 1990s and more widespread screening for rubella serology is recommended.

The role of serologic testing for antibodies to rubella is different in different clinical settings. The simplest and most straight forward application is in premarital assessment of immunity. If a woman has antibodies against rubella, even of low titer, demonstrated by any of multiple methods, she need not worry about infection during subsequent pregnancy. If she is not immune, and is not pregnant, she can receive rubella vaccine.

A second, more complex, role is in the management of a pregnant woman who has been exposed to rubella. Here the questions include susceptibility, present acute infection, and risk to the fetus. Several flowcharts are available to assess these possibilities, utilizing antibody titers, class of antibody, and changes in titer over time. Management of such a case requires individualized expert consultation. Of particular concern is that some enzyme-linked immunoassays are not as sensitive and specific as hemagglutination inhibition.

Still a third role is in the evaluation of an infant born with an illness which may be congenital rubella. Problems here include evaluating whether antibody is present, and whether it represents antibody passively acquired by transplacental passage or is indicative of true neonatal infection. In this setting determining the immunoglobulin class is particularly important; IgM antibody strongly supports congenital infection.

Selected Readings

Amanna I and Slifka MK, "Public Fear of Vaccination: Separating Fact From Fiction," *Viral Immunol*, 2005, 18(2):307-15.

Edlich RF, Winters KL, Long WB 3rd, et al, "Rubella and Congenital Rubella (German Measles)," *J Long Term Eff Med Implants*, 2005, 15(3):319-28.

Lee SH, Ewert DF, Frederick PD, et al, "Resurgence of Congenital Rubella Syndrome in the 1990s. Report on Missed Opportunities and Failed Prevention Policies Among Women of Childbearing Age," *JAMA*, 1992, 267(19):2616-20.

Weir E and Sider D, "A Refresher on Rubella," *CMAJ*, 2005, 172(13):1680-1.

Zhang T, Mauracher CA, Mitchell LA, et al, "Detection of Rubella Virus-Specific Immunoglobulin G (IgG), IgM, and IgA Antibodies by Immunoblot Assays," *J Clin Microbiol*, 1992, 30(4):824-30.

Rubella Virus Culture

Synonyms German Measles Culture; Measles Culture, 3-Day

Test Includes Isolation and identification of rubella virus in cell culture

Specimen Two throat swabs, 10 mL urine, cerebrospinal fluid, tissues, amniotic fluid

Container Sterile urine container

(Continued)

Rubella Virus Culture *(Continued)*

Sampling Time Virus is more likely to be isolated if specimen is collected within 5 days after onset of illness.

Storage Instructions Specimens should not be stored. Specimens should be delivered immediately to the laboratory. If unavoidable delays occur the specimen can be stored at 4°C for up to 3 days, but there is a loss of infectivity when culture is delayed.

Causes for Rejection Dry specimen, specimen not refrigerated during transport, specimen fixed in formalin, unlabeled specimen

Turnaround Time Positive cultures are detected in 3-7 days. Negative cultures are usually reported after 3 weeks.

Reference Range No virus isolated

Use Aid in the diagnosis of disease caused by rubella virus (eg, congenital viral infection)

Limitations Isolation of rubella virus is usually of little help in the diagnosis of rubella except in cases of severe rubella complications, epidemiological purposes, and fatality. Serological diagnosis is much more useful.

Methodology Cell culture, isolation, and confirmation/identification by antibody-specific neutralization

Additional Information The incidence of rubella has been reduced dramatically by the wide use of immunization in children. However, rubella can still occur in older people who were not vaccinated or people who have immigrated to the United States from countries where vaccination for rubella is not common. Pregnant women, who become infected with rubella, have a very high chance of the virus crossing the placenta and infecting the fetus. Congenital rubella infections have disastrous effects, causing fetal death, premature delivery, and severe congenital defects including deafness and congenital heart disease. Neonates with congenital rubella excrete rubella virus in nasopharyngeal secretions and urine for many months after birth. These children pose a risk to susceptible pregnant women. Serology is available for diagnostic purposes. Usually immune status can be determined by examining a single serum sample.

Selected Readings

Centers for Disease Control, "Increase in Rubella and Congenital Rubella Syndrome - United States, 1988-1990," *MMWR*, 1991, 40(6):93-9.

Herrmann KL, "Rubella Virus," *Laboratory Diagnosis of Viral Infections*, Lennette EH, ed, New York, NY: Marcel Dekker Inc, 1992, 731-47.

Wadell G, Allard A, and Hierholzer JC, "Rubella Virus," *Manual of Clinical Microbiology*, 7th ed, Murray PR, Baron EJ, Pfaller MA, et al, eds, Washington, DC: American Society for Microbiology, 1999, 970-82.

***Sarcoptes scabiei* Skin Scrapings Identification** *see* Arthropod Identification *on page 387*

Scanogram, X-ray *see* Bone Films *on page 396*

Scapula, Left or Right, X-ray *see* Bone Films *on page 396*

Schlichter Test *see* Serum Bactericidal Test *on page 578*

Scotch® Tape Test *see* Pinworm Preparation *on page 565*

Screening Culture for Group A Beta-Hemolytic *Streptococcus* *see* Throat Culture for Group A Beta-Hemolytic *Streptococcus on page 594*

Sedimentation Rate, Erythrocyte

Related Information

C-Reactive Protein *on page 428*

Synonyms Westergren Sed Rate

Abstract The erythrocyte sedimentation rate (ESR) is a nonspecific measure of inflammation which is applied to the detection/evaluation of infectious and immune based (in particular rheumatic type) inflammatory disease. It is commonly used to follow management of rheumatology patients. The test is a measure of the acute phase inflammatory response. Test result is derived from the sedimentation of patient's red blood cells through his/her plasma. As such, ESR is accelerated by increase in the plasma level of acute phase proteins of large molecular size, (fibrinogen in particular) and by anemia. Thus, the ESR may reflect both the hyperproteinemia and anemia of inflammatory disease. ESR methodology has undergone modification in order to increase precision and decrease biohazard exposure.

Special Instructions If EDTA anticoagulated blood is used for the standard Westergren method, 1 volume of 109 mmol/L of trisodium citrate is added to 4 volumes of blood just before performing the test.

Specimen Whole blood

Container Lavender top (EDTA) tube or citrated plasma in 4:1 dilution (4 volumes of blood to 1 volume of 109 mmol/L of trisodium citrate)

Collection Specimen must be received and test carried out within 4-6 hours of collection.

Storage Instructions Keep specimen at 4°C prior to testing

Causes for Rejection Insufficient blood, clotted, hemolyzed specimen

Turnaround Time 1-2 hours, some recent automated methods can determine an ESR endpoint in as little as 20 minutes

Reference Range Male: younger than 50 years of age: 0-15 mm/hour, older than 50 years of age: 0-20 mm/hour; female: younger than 50 years of age: 0-25 mm/hour, older than 50 years of age: 0-30 mm/hour by Westergren method. See reference by Wolfe and Michaud for their extensive study of and application of the ESR in a number of different settings. Their study indicates that in a rheumatology clinic women younger than 60 years of age who have noninflammatory disorders have upper limit of normal for ESR of 38 mm/hour.

Use Evaluate the activity of infections, inflammatory states, autoimmune disorders, and plasma cell dyscrasias; in particular to screen for, to assess severity of and follow clinical activity of rheumatic diseases, especially rheumatoid arthritis; important in clinical evaluation of temporal arteritis and polymyalgia rheumatica

Limitations Anemia and paraproteinemia invalidate results; High-thermal-amplitude cold agglutinins cause less rapid sedimentation (lower ESR) as the temperature rises towards 37°C. The ESR is usually reduced in stored blood. Some procedural methods may be associated with hazardous exposure of medical technologists to fresh whole blood.

Methodology Westergren: A 30 cm long glass tube, 2.55 mm in diameter, is filled with mixed sample of blood up to the 200 mm mark of a Westergren tube. After 1 hour the column of clear plasma above the upper limit of sedimenting red cells is measured. The result is given as number of mm in 1 hour.

Additional Information Elevations in fibrinogen, alpha- and beta-globulins (acute phase reactants), and immunoglobulins increase the sedimentation rate of red cells through plasma. The test is important in the diagnosis and management of temporal arthritis and of polymyalgia rheumatica (PMR), which are nearly always but not uniformly, characterized by a significantly elevated ESR. Presence of a normal ESR in a PMR-like clinical setting could lead to delay in diagnosis and therapy.

The ESR, while lacking in specificity, is elevated in a very broad-spectrum of conditions characterized by inflammation. For decades the ESR has played a prominent role in the evaluation and monitoring of rheumatoid inflammatory processes, notably rheumatoid arthritis and its variants including ankylosing spondylitis. ESR continues to be actively utilized in this manner being further defined and itself further defining rheumatoid inflammatory conditions and their therapy.

In a study by Wolfe comparing IgM rheumatoid factor (RF) methods, serial measures of RF did correlate with changes in clinical activity but repeat testing to determine clinical status was found to be only a "fair predictor" and to have little utility in clinical

Table 1. Factors That May Affect Erythrocyte Sedimentation Rate

Factor	Effect on rate
Red blood cell aggregation (plasma proteins raised in infection, inflammation, and malignant conditions)	Increased[1]
Pregnancy	Increased[1]
Anemia (decreased hematocrit)	Increased[1]
Obesity	Possibly increased[1]
Drug therapy (eg, steroids, anti-inflammatories)	Decreased[1]
Female sex	Slightly increased[1]
Old age	Increased,[1] possibly due to higher prevalence of disease
Red blood cell abnormalities	
Macrocytosis	Increased[1]
Microcytosis	Decreased
Sickle cell disease	Decreased
Polycythemia	Decreased
Protein abnormalities (hypofibrinogenemia, hypogammaglobulinemia, dysproteinemia with hyperviscosity state)	Decreased

[1]Upper limit of normal: Age ≤50 years: men: 15 mm/hour; women: 25 mm/hour. Age >50 years: men: 20 mm/hour; women: 30 mm/hour.

Adapted from Sox and Liang, *Postgrad Med*, 1998, 103(5):258.

(Continued)

Sedimentation Rate, Erythrocyte *(Continued)*

practice. ESR and C-reactive protein (CRP) were found to be more effective in following clinical activity.

In a study comparing the value of ESR vs CRP in measuring disease activity in ankylosing spondylitis (AS) the positive predictive values of both CRP and ESR were low, neither CRP nor ESR was considered superior in assessment of disease activity. On the basis of literature review (Ruof and Stucki, 1967 through April 1998), it was concluded that neither ESR or CRP is superior in terms of validity and it was considered that acute phase reactants "do not comprehensively represent the disease process" in AS.

Lurie et al found that an ESR >100 mm/hour, in a patient with back pain, has a likelihood ratio of 55 for presence of a serious underlying cause. See tables on previous page and below.

Table 2. Comparison of Erythrocyte Sedimentation Rate, Plasma Viscosity, and C-Reactive Protein Tests

Test	Advantages	Disadvantages
Erythrocyte sedimentation rate (ESR)	Inexpensive, quick, simple to perform	Affected by anemia and red blood cell size, not sensitive enough for screening
Plasma viscosity	Not affected by anemia or red blood cell size	Cumbersome apparatus, expensive, not widely available
C-reactive protein	Rapid response to inflammation, complementary to ESR	Wide reference range necessitates sequential recording of values, expensive, batch processing may delay individual results

Selected Readings

Lurie JD, Gerber PD, and Sox HC, "A Pain in the Back," *N Engl J Med*, 2000, 343(10):723-6.

Paulus HE, Ramos B, Wong WK, et al, "Equivalence of the Acute Phase Reactants C-Reactive Protein, Plasma Viscosity, and Westergren Erythrocyte Sedimentation Rate When Used to Calculate American College of Rheumatology 20% Improvement Criteria or the Disease Activity Score in Patients With Early Rheumatoid Arthritis," *J Rheumatol*, 1999, 26(11):2324-31.

Ruof J and Stucki G, "Validity Aspects of Erythrocyte Sedimentation Rate and C-reactive Protein in Ankylosing Spondylitis: A Literature Review," *J Rheumatol*, 1999, 26(4):966-70.

Wolfe F, "A Comparison of IgM Rheumatoid Factor by Nephelometry and Latex Methods: Clinical and Laboratory Significance," *Arthritis Care Res*, 1998, 11(2):89-93.

Serologic Test for Syphilis *see* FTA-ABS, Serum *on page 457*

Serologic Test for Syphilis, CSF *see* VDRL, Cerebrospinal Fluid *on page 613*

Serum Antibacterial Titer *see* Serum Bactericidal Test *on page 578*

Serum Bactericidal Level *see* Serum Bactericidal Test *on page 578*

Serum Bactericidal Test

Related Information

Antimicrobial Susceptibility Testing, Aerobic and Facultatively Anaerobic Organisms *on page 379*

C-Reactive Protein *on page 428*

Synonyms Antibacterial Activity, Serum; Bacterial Inhibitory Level, Serum; Maximum Bactericidal Dilution; MBD; Schlichter Test; Serum Antibacterial Titer; Serum Bactericidal Level; Serum Inhibitory Titer; Susceptibility Testing, Schlichter Test; Susceptibility Testing, Serum Bactericidal Dilution Method

Special Instructions If a serum bactericidal test is desired, the physician **must** request that the laboratory save the patient's isolate within 48 hours of submission of the specimen for initial culture. **If the isolate has not been saved, the test cannot be performed.** The laboratory **must** be informed of current antibiotic therapy including date and time of last dosage, route of administration on all antimicrobial agents patient is receiving and clinical diagnosis. Time of specimen collection should be indicated on requisition.

Specimen Serum or body fluid. Bacterial isolate causing infection prepared by laboratory.

Container Red top tube; sterile tube for body fluid

Sampling Time The peak level for intravenously (I.V.) administered drugs is obtained 30-60 minutes after the drug is absorbed and distributed. The trough level is obtained within 30 minutes or less of the next dose. For intramuscularly (I.M.) administered drugs and oral drugs, the peak should be drawn later at 2-4 hours. Vancomycin peak is drawn 2 hours post dose.

Collection Specimen should be transported to laboratory within 1 hour of collection.

Storage Instructions Separate serum using aseptic technique and freeze.

Causes for Rejection Isolate discarded before request for testing.

Turnaround Time 2-3 days

Reference Range Peak bactericidal activity should be observed at ≥1:8 dilution, trough at ≥1:2

Use Determine the maximum bactericidal dilution of the serum or body fluid, MBD, which is bactericidal for the patient's infecting organism; monitor total therapeutic effect. Frequently used to evaluate therapy in endocarditis, osteomyelitis, and suppurative arthritis. Serum bactericidal titers ≥1:8 are often recommended for the optimal treatment of infective endocarditis, osteomyelitis and suppurative arthritis.

Limitations There is no universal agreement on the clinical utility and prognostic value of this test. New infective endocarditis guidelines recommend against using this test. The serum bactericidal assay has many ill-defined variables, ie, no widely accepted standard procedure, no consensus as to whether dilutions should be performed with serum or broth, the unknown inhibitory effect of serum if used as a diluent, etc. The use of pooled serum diluent may not accurately predict actual bactericidal titers in patients with abnormal protein binding.

Results will reflect the combined *in vitro* effect of all antimicrobial agents present in the patient's serum or body fluid on his/her infecting organism(s). Results are accurate to plus or minus 1 dilution, and are not necessarily equivalent to a serum assay. Maximum inhibitory concentration (MIC) may also be reported. An apparently adequate ratio may represent a highly susceptible organism responding to a relatively low blood level, or a moderately resistant organism responding to an unexpectedly high blood level. A serum inhibitory titer might suggest an adequate therapeutic level, but would give no clue to potential toxicity, when an extremely narrow margin exists between a therapeutically adequate dose and a possibly toxic one (eg, aminoglycosides).

Contraindications The bacterium isolated from patient is not available or fails to grow for the serum bactericidal test.

Methodology Serial dilution of patient's serum; each dilution is incubated with an inoculum of the patient's isolate. Subsequent steps are complicated and vary from laboratory to laboratory.

Additional Information It is preferable to perform this test with paired specimens, one obtained approximately 15 minutes before an antibiotic dose (predose trough), and one obtained 30-60 minutes after an antibiotic dose (postdose peak).

In patients with chronic osteomyelitis, the observation of peak levels <1:16 and trough levels <1:2 accurately predicted treatment failure. In acute osteomyelitis, peak levels >1:16 and trough levels >1:2 accurately predicted medical cure. The serum bactericidal test alone is not sufficient to predict outcome in endocarditis. The therapeutic outcome of endocarditis depends on many clinical factors including cardiac status, underlying medical disease, embolic complications, and clinical management of patient. In granulocytopenic patient, titers 1:8-1:16 or greater in patients on combination therapy was associated with a more favorable outcome.

The serum bactericidal test has been applied to detect antimicrobial activity in cerebrospinal fluid and joint fluid. It is also useful in determining whether serum antimicrobial activity remains adequate after a shift from parenteral to oral therapy.

Selected Readings

MacLowry JD, "Perspective: The Serum Dilution Test," *J Infect Dis*, 1989, 160(4):624-6.

Stratton CW, "Serum Bactericidal Test," *Clin Microbiol Rev*, 1988, 1(1):19-26.

Serum Inhibitory Titer *see* Serum Bactericidal Test *on page 578*

Shiga Toxin Test, Direct

Test Includes Direct assay for *E. coli* Shiga toxin in stool

Specimen Fresh stool

Container Clean container, no preservative

Storage Instructions Refrigerate specimen (up to 7 days if necessary) at 4°C until testing.

Reference Range Negative

Use Detect Shiga-like cytotoxin in the stool of persons with diarrhea suspected of being caused by EHEC

Limitations The test detects Shiga toxin produced by *Shigella dysenteriae*; this Shiga toxin is almost identical to that produced by EHEC

Methodology Enzyme immunoassay (EIA) using a monoclonal antibody specific for the Shiga-like toxin

Additional Information Most culture techniques for EHEC are able to detect only the O157:H7 serotype of *E. coli*, by far the most common serotype of EHEC. However, many serotypes other than O157:H7 produce Shiga-like toxin. Therefore, an obvious advantage of this enzyme immunoassay test over culture is the fact that this test can

(Continued)

Shiga Toxin Test, Direct *(Continued)*

detect the presence of EHEC other than serotype O157:H7 and can detect O157:H- strains which are sorbitol fermenting and are not detectable by culture on sorbitol MacConkey's agar. The level of the detected toxin has not been shown to correlate with the severity of EHEC-induced diarrhea. A positive test in the presence of clinical symptoms is highly significant. All positives may not be associated with clinical symptoms. Therefore, the results of the test should be interpreted in relation to the clinical presentation and patient history. The Shiga toxin test is widely available from national reference laboratories. Most state Department of Health laboratories use the test in investigation of outbreaks.

Selected Readings

Acheson DWK and Jaeger JL, "Shiga Toxin-Producing *Escherichia coli*," *Clin Microbiol Newslett*, 1999, 21(23):183-8.

Acheson DWK and Keusch GT, "Which Shiga Toxin-Producing Types of *E. coli* Are Important," *ASM News*, 1996, 62(6):302-6.

Nataro JP and Kaper JB, "Diarrheagenic *Escherichia coli*," *Clin Microbiol Rev*, 1998, 11(1):142-201.

Osek J, "Rapid and Specific Identification of Shiga Toxin-Producing *Escherichia coli* in Faeces by Multiplex PCR," *Lett Appl Microbiol*, 2002, 34(4):304-10.

Park CH, Kim HJ, Hixon DL, et al, "Evaluation of the Duopath Verotoxin Test for Detection of Shiga Toxins in Cultures of Human Stools," *J Clin Microbiol*, 2003, 41(6):2650-3.

Perelle S, Dilasser F, Grout J, et al, "Detection of *Escherichia coli* Serogroup O103 by Real-Time Polymerase Chain Reaction," *J Appl Microbiol*, 2005, 98(5):1162-8.

Shingles Culture *see* Varicella-Zoster Virus Culture *on page 612*
Shoulder Arthrogram *see* Arthrogram *on page 387*
Shoulder, Left or Right, X-ray *see* Bone Films *on page 396*
Shoulders Arthritis, X-ray *see* Bone Films *on page 396*
Shoulder Stereo, Left or Right, X-ray *see* Bone Films *on page 396*
Shoulder to Include Axial View, Left or Right, X-ray *see* Bone Films *on page 396*
Shunt Culture *see* Intravenous Line Culture *on page 511*
Silver Stain *see* Methenamine Silver Stain *on page 534*
Simple CMG *see* Cystometrogram, Simple *on page 434*
Sinuses, CT *see* Computed Transaxial Tomography, Paranasal Sinuses *on page 425*
Skeletal Muscle Biopsy *see* Muscle Biopsy *on page 538*

Skin Biopsy

Related Information

Fungus Culture, Skin *on page 464*
Gram Stain *on page 473*
Herpes Cytology *on page 491*
Herpes Simplex Virus by Direct Immunofluorescence *on page 493*
Histopathology *on page 496*
Immunofluorescent Studies, Biopsy *on page 507*
KOH Preparation *on page 513*
Lymph Node Biopsy *on page 529*
Methenamine Silver Stain *on page 534*
Periodic Acid-Schiff Stain *on page 563*
Varicella-Zoster Virus Culture *on page 612*
Varicella-Zoster Virus Serology *on page 612*

Applies to Skin Lesions

Abstract This section deals with sampling and procurement techniques and with a selected group of diagnostic skin problems.

Container 10% neutral formalin is satisfactory for submission of most specimens, but there are special requirements for culture, immunofluorescence, and electron microscopy.

Collection Techniques for procuring skin specimens:

Shave biopsy: A technique for obtaining superficial samples of predominantly epidermal or projecting lesions by cutting them flush with the adjacent skin as illustrated in Figure 1. This technique is usually used for nonmalignant lesions but may be useful for the patch phase of mycosis fungoides. **Since shave biopsy provides the most limited specimen, a serious potential for histopathologic misdiagnosis exists, especially in regard to melanocytic lesions.**

Punch biopsy: Very popular with dermatologists because it can be done easily, quickly, and repetitively at low cost in office practice. Biopsy punches, illustrated in Figure 2, range from 3-6 mm in size. The punch is pressed into the skin and rotated. It yields a plug or core of tissue which is cut from its base by scissors as the punch is withdrawn. It may be difficult to adequately sample subcutanea by punch. Punch

Figure 1. Shave Biopsy

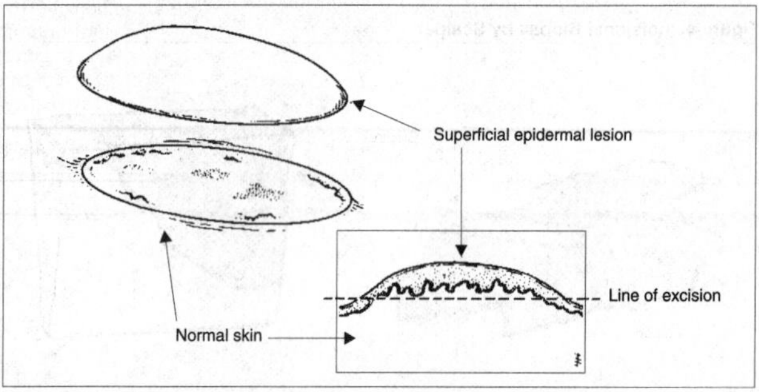

biopsies may be submitted for culture. They may be particularly useful in the diagnosis of cutaneous myosis and mycobacterial disease. Pathologists prefer the largest possible sample.

Figure 2. Punch Biopsy

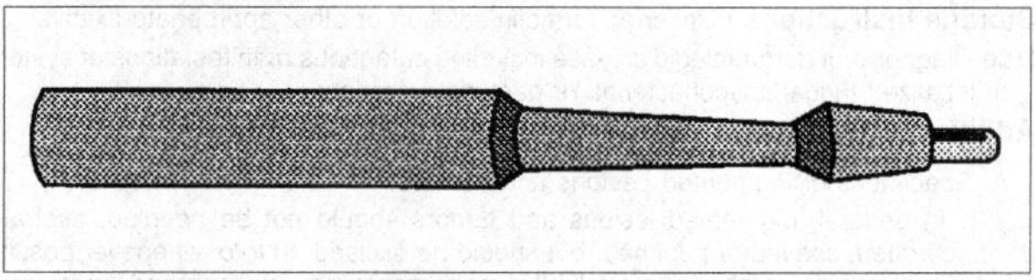

Excisional biopsy: This usually implies total removal of a skin lesion, most commonly a tumor, with a scalpel as illustrated in Figure 3. It is a preferred technique for removal of pigmented lesions and tumors.

Figure 3. Excisional Biopsy by Scalpel

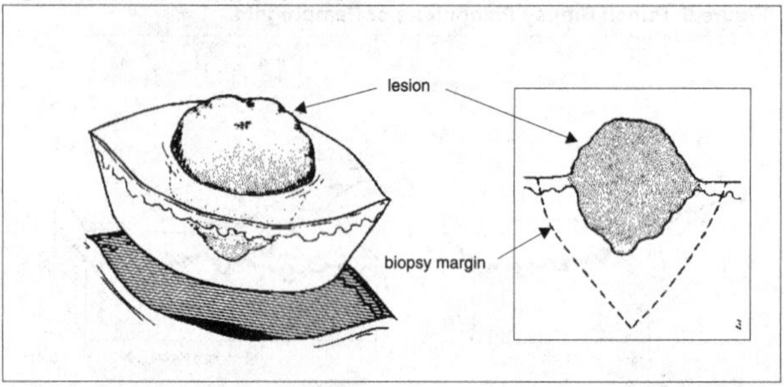

Incisional biopsy: The removal of a portion of a lesion by scalpel as illustrated in Figure 4. It is performed when a non-neoplastic lesion (ie, necrobiosis lipoidica) is too large to be totally excised but definitive diagnosis mandates a large sample to evaluate overall architectural detail or, in the case of tumors, for which complete excision would require extensive surgery and/or would produce cosmetic deformity which would not be warranted until accurate histologic diagnosis is established.

Smears and/or aspirates: Stained with Wright or Giemsa type stains may suffice to demonstrate polys or eosinophils (as in toxic erythema or pustular melanosis of newborns). Gram, acid-fast, PAS and GMS stains, and cultures are used to establish the presence of bacterial or fungal organisms. Finding multinucleated giant cells in smears in a proper clinical context suggests herpes or related viral infection. Aspirates may be adequate for cultures for bacteria, fungi, and viruses. Scrapings are often utilized in the diagnosis of dermatomycoses. Cytologic techniques (Tzanck smears) are rarely used in practice to evaluate acantholytic processes or tumors.
(Continued)

Skin Biopsy *(Continued)*

Figure 4. Incisional Biopsy by Scalpel

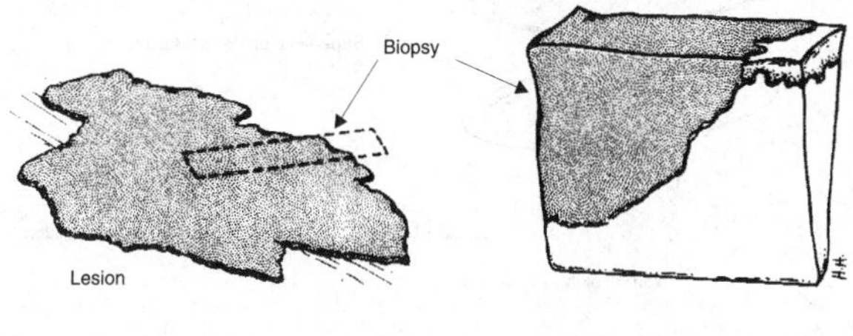

Curettings: Most frequently used when nodular basal cell carcinoma is suspected, and used as well for actinic and seborrheic keratoses. **Contraindicated for suspicious melanotic lesions.**

Storage Instructions Fixation in formalin solution or other appropriate fixative

Use Diagnosis of dermatologic disease including cutaneous manifestations of systemic or localized fungal, mycobacterial, or bacterial infections.

Additional Information Selected Problems in Dermatopathology:

A. Specimens of Pigmented Lesions and Tumors
   1. In general, pigmented lesions and tumors should not be needled, aspirated, curetted, shaved or punched, but should be excised, *in toto*, whenever possible, to permit comprehensive evaluation and measurements appropriate for melanoma.

B. Specimens of Vesiculobullous Lesions
   1. If the diagnostic impression is pemphigus or pemphigoid, fresh lesions are preferred. Figure 5 illustrates appropriate biopsy technique.

Figure 5. Punch Biopsy Pemphigus or Pemphigoid

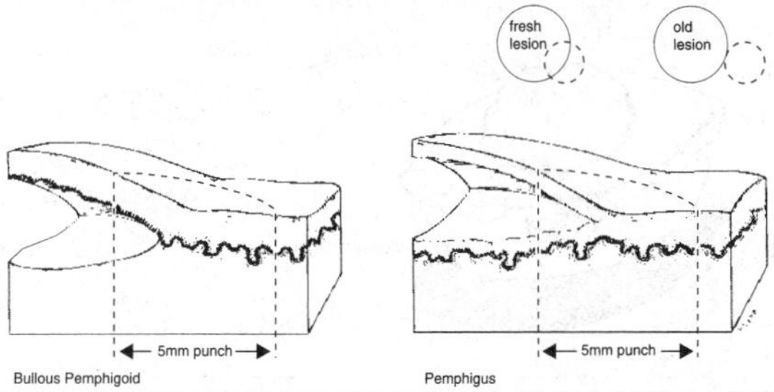

   2. If the diagnostic impression is dermatitis herpetiformis, take the biopsy at the edge of the lesion (to study the change in the dermal papillae) as shown in Figure 6, rather than the lesion itself.
   3. If the diagnostic impression is epidermolysis bullosa, the clinician should be aware of the availability of four special regional reference centers in the U.S. for special studies of mechanobullous lesion.
   4. Immunofluorescent studies of vesiculobullous lesions: Vesiculobullous lesions which require biopsy should be considered for immunofluorescent studies (IF). In many laboratories, skin samples for immunofluorescent studies are separately submitted in vials of isopentane prior to snap freezing in liquid nitrogen by the laboratory. Some reference laboratories provide special solutions in which to store specimens for their analysis.

C. Specimens for Lupus Erythematosus (LE)

Figure 6. Punch Biopsy: Dermatitis Herpetiformis

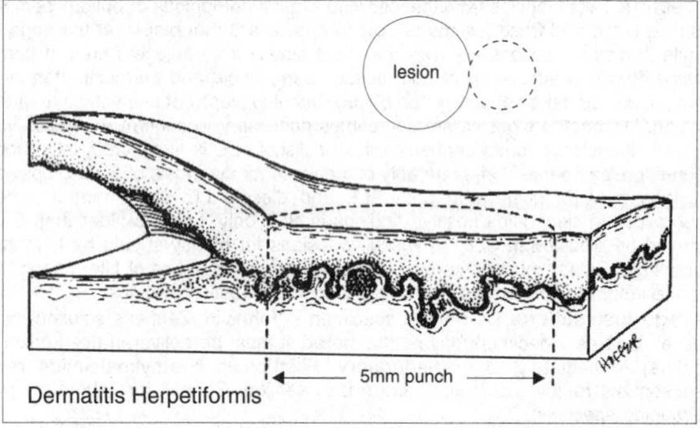

1. Direct immunofluorescence was first utilized on cutaneous biopsies in LE. The procedure (the lupus band test) was widely utilized to study SLE, DLE, and MCTD. Recent data suggests the band test is much less specific and sensitive than previously thought, that it is not clinically useful in discriminating SLE from other CT disorders or in predicting which patients with undifferentiated CT disease would develop SLE. Serologic evaluation is more sensitive, more efficient , and more cost effective in discriminating DLE and SLE.

Biopsy Site	SLE	DLE
Lesional Tissue	+	+
Uninvolved, Sun-exposed	+	-

D. Specimens of Epidermolysis Bullosa Acquisita (EBA)
   1. Recent studies suggest that from 5% to 10% of patients regarded as bullous pemphigoid by routine direct immunofluorescence can be shown to be EBA based on indirect immunofluorescence on salt-split skin.

E. Special Studies for Hematopoietic Disorders
   1. Special studies for T and B cells and markers for lymphocytes are considered elsewhere.

Pitfalls and artifacts to avoid: The biopsy technique should provide adequate and representative lesional tissue. Specimens should be handled gently without crushing by forceps. Cautery of lesions may burn or coagulate tissue making pathologic diagnosis impossible. If specimens are mailed to a reference laboratory in freezing weather, they may freeze after fixation. Formation of ice crystals may render interpretation hazardous if not impossible. Send in Lillie's "winter fixative" (acetic acid alcohol and formaldehyde).

Selected Readings

Dimino-Emme L and Gurevitch AW, "Cutaneous Manifestations of Disseminated Cryptococcosis," *J Am Acad Dermatol*, 1995, 32(5 Pt 2):844-50.

Skin Biopsy Antibodies *see* Skin Biopsy, Immunofluorescence *on page 583*

Skin Biopsy for Bullous or Collagen Disease *see* Skin Biopsy, Immunofluorescence *on page 583*

Skin Biopsy for Pemphigus *see* Skin Biopsy, Immunofluorescence *on page 583*

Skin Biopsy, Immunofluorescence

Synonyms Basement Membrane Antibodies; Bullous Pemphigoid Antibodies; Dermatitis Herpetiformis Antibodies; Intercellular Antibody Basement Membrane Antibody; LE Antibodies; Lupus Band Test; Pemphigus Antibodies; Skin Biopsy Antibodies; Skin Biopsy for Bullous or Collagen Disease; Skin Biopsy for Pemphigus

Test Includes Anti-IgG, anti-IgA, anti-IgM, anti-C3, anti-C1q, antialbumin, antifibrinogen, antikappa and lambda light chains immunofluorescence

Specimen 3 mm skin punch biopsy and serum

Container Covered Petri dish or screw cap glass vial, red top tube for blood

(Continued)

Skin Biopsy, Immunofluorescence *(Continued)*

Collection Take biopsies from the following sites: If pemphigus or bullous pemphigoid is suspected and fresh lesions are present, take a 3 mm biopsy at the edge of the bulla. If only old lesions are available, take biopsy from adjacent area. If dermatitis herpetiformis is suspected or both bullous pemphigoid and dermatitis herpetiformis are suspected, take not only lesion biopsy, but also biopsy of uninvolved area around lesions. Repeated biopsies are sometimes necessary to confirm dermatitis herpetiformis. If systemic lupus erythematosus or discoid LE is suspected, take biopsy of sun-exposed normal skin, preferably of the wrist, for diagnosis of SLE. Biopsies from lesions may be positive in both SLE and discoid LE while normal appearing sun-exposed skin yields positive findings in SLE only. Lesions older than 6 weeks should be biopsied in SLE. In vasculitis lesions for biopsy should be less than 24 hours old. Biopsy must be kept moist on saline soaked gauze or filter paper. Deliver to the laboratory on wet ice immediately upon completion of biopsy.

Storage Instructions Do not put specimen in formalin, Zenker's solution, or other usual fixatives. Specimen may not be stored, it must be delivered (iced or on moist saline) immediately to the laboratory. Fixation in N-ethylmaleimide requires subsequent removal of fixative and frozen section. Consult the laboratory prior to obtaining specimen.

Causes for Rejection Specimen in formalin, drying out of specimen

Reference Range No deposition of immunoglobulins, complement, or fibrinogen

Use Detect immune complexes, complement, and immunoglobulin deposition in SLE, DLE, pemphigus, bullous pemphigoid, and dermatitis herpetiformis; differential diagnosis of bullous skin diseases

Limitations Many skin lesions which may clinically resemble SLE and DLE also have deposits of Ig at the basement membrane. These include psoriasis, polymorphous light eruption, and drug eruptions.

Contraindications Specimen should not be taken from heavily keratinized body areas if possible. Failure to demonstrate IgG in some biopsies may be due to a secondary change in the tissue due to infection and inflammatory reaction.

Methodology Direct fluorescent antibody (DFA), indirect fluorescent antibody (IFA)

Additional Information Distinctive patterns of IgG, IgA, IgM, and complement components in epidermis, basement membrane, and dermal vessels may contribute to the differential diagnosis of bullous skin diseases, and discoid and systemic lupus erythematosus.

- Pemphigus: Fixation of IgG or other immunoglobulin along intercellular bridges of squamous cells; C3 can be fixed.
- Bullous pemphigoid: Fixation of IgG and C3 along epidermal basement membrane.
- Dermatitis herpetiformis: Fixation of IgA immunoglobulin deposits near the epidermal-dermal junction of skin adjacent to bulla.
- Lupus erythematosus: Fixation of IgG or other immunoglobulin deposits and complement along the epidermal-dermal junction. IgG, IgM, and C3 are the most common.

Serum antibodies to the same skin components can also be demonstrated, using a tissue substrate (usually monkey or guinea pig esophagus), and these may correlate with disease activity. Steroid therapy can convert findings to negative in previously positive patients. In bullous disease antibody levels often reflect disease activity and rising titers may foretell clinical relapse.

Skin Culture for HSV *see* Herpes Simplex Virus Isolation, Rapid *on page 495*

Skin Lesions *see* Skin Biopsy *on page 580*

Skin Scrapings for *Sarcoptes scabiei* Identification *see* Arthropod Identification *on page 387*

Skin Test Battery *see* Anergy Skin Test Battery *on page 372*

Skin Tests for Histoplasmosis, Blastomycosis, Coccidioidomycosis *see* Fungal Skin Testing *on page 459*

Skin Tests for Penicillin Allergy *see* Penicillin Allergy Skin Testing *on page 561*

Smear, Gram Stain *see* Gram Stain *on page 473*

Soft Tissue Scan *see* Gallium Scan *on page 469*

Somatosensory Evoked Potentials *see* Electroencephalography *on page 447*

Spinal Fluid Analysis *see* Cerebrospinal Fluid Analysis *on page 408*

Spinal Fluid Cryptococcal Latex Agglutination *see* Cryptococcal Antigen Serology, Serum or Cerebrospinal Fluid *on page 431*

Spinal Fluid Fungus Culture *see* Fungus Culture, Cerebrospinal Fluid *on page 464*

Spinal Fluid Mycobacteria Culture *see* Mycobacteria Culture, Cerebrospinal Fluid *on page 541*

Spinal Fluid VDRL *see* VDRL, Cerebrospinal Fluid *on page 613*

Spinal Tap *see* Cerebrospinal Fluid Analysis *on page 408*
Sporanox® Level, Blood *see* Itraconazole Level *on page 512*
***Sporothrix* Antibodies** *see* Sporotrichosis Serology *on page 585*

Sporotrichosis Serology

Related Information

Fungus Culture, Biopsy *on page 461*
Fungus Culture, Body Fluid *on page 462*
Periodic Acid-Schiff Stain *on page 563*
Sporothrix schenckii on page 302

Synonyms *Sporothrix* Antibodies

Applies to Rose Handlers Disease

Test Includes Detection of serological response to *Sporothrix schenckii*

Abstract Sporotrichosis is a fungal disease classically beginning in a distal extremity, often at a site of inoculation, spreading proximally involving lymphatics. The organisms in tissue and in 37°C culture exist as yeast, which are often difficult or impossible to see in tissue sections. Extracutaneous disease includes monarticular arthritis. Pulmonary sporotrichosis is much less frequently found than osteoarticular infection.

Specimen Serum or cerebrospinal fluid

Container Red top tube; sterile CSF tube

Reference Range Latex agglutinating titer: <1:4; ELISA: <1:16 in serum, <1:8 in CSF

Use Diagnose sporotrichosis, especially extracutaneous disease

Limitations A negative test result does not rule out infection. Serial titers are not prognostically useful. There are occasional low titer false-positives from nonfungal disease. This test is not widely available.

Methodology Tube agglutination, latex agglutination (LA), enzyme-linked immunosorbent assay (ELISA)

Additional Information Titer ≥1:4 is presumptive evidence for sporotrichosis. Titers >1:128, rising titers, and persistent elevation are common with pulmonary or systemic disease. Positive reaction in CSF is diagnostic, and is particularly useful in chronic meningitis caused by this organism, which is difficult to culture.

Selected Readings

Bhumbra NA and McCullough SG, "Skin and Subcutaneous Infections," *Prim Care*, 2003, 30(1):1-24.
Gonzalez GM, Fothergill AW, Sutton DA, et al, "*In vitro* Activities of New and Established Triazoles Against Opportunistic Filamentous and Dimorphic Fungi," *Med Mycol*, 2005, 43(3):281-4.
Guimaraes AJ, Pizzini CV, De Matos Guedes HL, et al, "ELISA for Early Diagnosis of Histoplasmosis," *J Med Microbiol*, 2004, 53(Pt 6):509-14.
Kauffman CA, "Sporotrichosis," *Clin Infect Dis*, 1999, 29:231-7.
Kauffman CA, Hajjeh R, and Chapman SW, "Practice Guidelines for the Management of Patients With Sporotrichosis," *Clin Infect Dis*, 2000, 30:684-7.
Pang KR, Wu JJ, Huang DB, et al, "Subcutaneous Fungal Infections," *Dermatol Ther*, 2004, 17(6):523-31.
Rex JH and Okhuysen PC, "*Sporothrix schenckii*," *Principles and Practice of Infectious Diseases*, Mandell GL, Bennett JE, and Dolin R, eds, New York, NY: Churchill Livingstone, 2000, 2695-99.

Sputum *see* Mycobacteria Culture, Sputum *on page 542*
Sputum Culture, Aerobic *see* Aerobic Culture, Sputum *on page 367*
Sputum Fungus Culture *see* Fungus Culture, Sputum *on page 466*
Sternoclavicular Joint, Left or Right, X-ray *see* Bone Films *on page 396*

Stool Culture

Related Information

Fecal Leukocyte Stain *on page 455*
Ova and Parasites, Stool *on page 551*

Synonyms Enteric Pathogens Culture, Routine; Stool for Culture

Applies to Rectal Swab Culture; Routine Culture, Rectal Swab

Test Includes Screening culture for *Salmonella*, *Shigella*, *Helicobacter*, and, if requested, *Staphylococcus.*

Special Instructions The laboratory should be informed of the specific pathogen suspected if not *Salmonella*, *Shigella*, or *Campylobacter.*

Specimen Fresh random stool, rectal swab

Container Plastic stool container, Culturette®

Sampling Time If present, most bacterial stool pathogens are detected by culture of only a single specimen, collected on a single day.

Collection If stool is collected in a clean bedpan, it must not be contaminated with urine, residual soap, or disinfectants. Swabs of lesions of the rectal wall during proctoscopy or sigmoidoscopy are preferred.

Rectal swab: Insert the swab past the anal sphincter, move the swab circumferentially around the rectum. Allow 15-30 seconds for organisms to adsorb onto the swab. Withdraw swab, place in Culturette® tube, and crush media compartment.

Storage Instructions Refrigerate if the specimen cannot be processed promptly.
(Continued)

Stool Culture *(Continued)*

Causes for Rejection Because of risk to laboratory personnel, specimens sent on diaper or tissue paper, specimen contaminating outside of transport container may not be acceptable to the laboratory. Specimen containing interfering substances (eg, castor oil, bismuth, Metamucil®, barium), specimens delayed in transit and those contaminated with urine may not have optimal yield.

Turnaround Time Minimum 48 hours if negative

Reference Range Negative for *Salmonella*, *Shigella*, *Campylobacter*, and/or *E. coli* O157:H7. In endemic areas the isolation of a pathogen may not indicate the cause or only cause of diarrhea. Some clinical laboratories also look for and report *Aeromonas* spp and *Pleisiomonas* spp.

Use Screen for common bacterial pathogenic organisms in the stool; diagnose typhoid fever, enteric fever, bacillary dysentery, *Salmonella* infection

Indications for stool culture include:

- bloody diarrhea
- fever
- tenesmus
- severe or persistent symptoms
- recent travel to a third world country
- known exposure to a bacterial agent
- presence of fecal leukocytes

Limitations *Yersinia* species and *Vibrio* species usually are not isolated or sought by the laboratory unless specifically requested.

Contraindications A rectal swab culture is not as effective as a stool culture for detection of the carrier state.

Methodology Aerobic culture on selective media

Additional Information Stool cultures on patients hospitalized ≥3 days are not productive and should not be ordered unless special circumstances exist.

In enteric fever caused by *Salmonella typhi*, *S. choleraesuis*, or *S. enteritidis*, blood culture may be positive before stool cultures, and blood cultures are indicated early. Diarrhea is common in patients with the acquired immunodeficiency syndrome (AIDS). Diarrhea in AIDS is frequently caused by the classic bacterial pathogens; however, parasitic infestation is also common with *Giardia* and *Cryptosporidium*. Rectal swabs are useful for the diagnosis of *Neisseria gonorrhoeae* and *Chlamydia* infections.

In acute or subacute diarrhea, three common syndromes are recognized: gastroenteritis, enteritis, and colitis (dysenteric syndrome). With colitis, patients have fecal urgency and tenesmus. Stool are frequently small in volume and contain blood, mucus, and leukocytes. External hemorrhoids are common and painful. Diarrhea of small bowel origin is indicated by the passage of few large volume stools. This is due to accumulation of fluid in the large bowel before passage. Leukocytes indicate colonic inflammation rather than a specific pathogen. Bacterial diarrhea may be

Diarrhea Syndromes Classified by Predominant Features

Syndrome (anatomic site)	Features	Characteristic Etiologies
Gastroenteritis (stomach)	Vomiting	Rotavirus Norwalk virus Staphylococcal food poisoning *Bacillus cereus* food poisoning
Enteritis (small bowel)	Watery diarrhea Large-volume stools, few in number	Enterotoxigenic *Escherichia coli* *Vibrio cholerae* Any enteric microbe Inflammatory bowel disease
Dysentery, colitis (colon)	Small-volume stools containing blood and/or mucus and many leukocytes	*Shigella* *Campylobacter* *Salmonella* Invasive *E. coli* *Plesiomonas shigelloides* *Aeromonas hydrophila* *Vibrio parahaemolyticus* *Clostridium difficile* *Entamoeba histolytica* Inflammatory bowel disease

present in the absence of fecal leukocytes and fecal leukocytes may be present in the absence of bacterial or parasitic agents (ie, idiopathic inflammatory bowel disease). See table. Although most bacterial diarrhea is transient (1-30 days) cases of persistent symptoms (10 months) have been reported. The etiologic agent in the reported case was *Shigella flexneri* diagnosed by culture of rectal swab. In infants younger than 1 year of age, a history of blood in the stool, more than 10 stools in 24 hours, and temperature >39°C have a high probability of having bacterial diarrhea.

Selected Readings

Acheson DWK and Jaeger JL, "Shiga Toxin-Producing *Escherichia coli*," *Clin Microbiol Newslett*, 1999, 21(23):183-8.

Allos BM, "*Campylobacter jejuni* Infections: Update on Emerging Issues and Trends," *Clin Infect Dis*, 2001, 32(8):1201-6.

Guerrant RL and Lima AAM, "Inflammatory Enteritides," *Principles and Practices of Infectious Diseases*, 5th ed, Mandell GL, et al, eds, New York, NY: Churchill Livingstone, 2000, 1126-36.

Guerrant RL, Wanke CA, Barrett LJ, et al, "A Cost Effective and Effective Approach to the Diagnosis and Management of Acute Infectious Diarrhea," *Bull N Y Acad Med*, 1987, 63(6):484-99.

Pickering LK, "Therapy for Acute Infectious Diarrhea in Children," *J Pediatr*, 1991, 118(4 Pt 2):S118-28.

Stool Culture, Diarrheagenic *E. coli*

Related Information

Fecal Leukocyte Stain *on page 455*

Applies to EPEC, Stool Culture; Enterohemorrhagic *E. coli*, Stool Culture; Enteroinvasive *E. coli*, Stool Culture; Enteropathogenic *E. coli*, Stool Culture; Enterotoxigenic *E. coli*, Stool Culture; Rectal Swab Culture for Diarrheagenic, *E. coli*; Stool Culture, EPEC; Verocytotoxin Producing *E. coli*, Stool Culture

Special Instructions Routine stool culture is usually performed on all requests for enteropathogenic *E. coli*, but usually detects only enterohemorrhagic *E. coli* O157:H7. The laboratory **must** be notified if other *E. coli* are suspected.

Specimen Rectal swab, fresh stool

Container Plastic stool container, Culturette®

Collection If stool is collected in sterile bedpan, must not be contaminated with urine or residual soap or disinfectants. Swabs of lesions of the rectal wall during proctoscopy or sigmoidoscopy preferred.

Rectal swab: Insert the swab past the anal sphincter, move the swab circumferentially around the anus. Allow 15-30 seconds for organisms to adsorb onto the swab. Withdraw swab, place in Culturette® tube, and crush media compartment.

Storage Instructions Do not refrigerate

Causes for Rejection Because of risk to laboratory personnel, specimen sent on diaper or tissue paper, specimen contaminating outside of transport container may not be acceptable to the laboratory. Specimen containing interfering substances (eg, castor oil, bismuth, Metamucil®, barium), specimens delayed in transit, and those contaminated with urine may not have optimal yield.

Turnaround Time Preliminary report available at 24 hours; minimum 72 hours for final reports

Reference Range Normal colonic flora

Use Establish diarrheagenic *E. coli* as the cause of clinical illness

Limitations Many laboratories are not equipped to perform elaborate diagnostic procedures needed to definitively characterize diarrheagenic *E. coli*. Clinical diagnosis and exclusion of other more readily characterized pathogens form the practical basis of presumptive diagnosis of diarrheagenic *E. coli* illness.

Methodology Cultures may be screened for sorbitol-negative (colorless) colonies on sorbitol-MacConkey agar; EHEC is confirmed by serotyping. Culture filtrate can be incubated with Vero cells. Changes observed in the presence of toxin include rounding up at 36 hours and destruction of the monolayer with detachment at 72 hours. Shiga-like toxin is most frequently associated with the O157:H7 serotype.

Additional Information Factors common to diarrheagenic *E. coli* include the presence of critical virulence factors encoded in plasmids, characteristic interaction with intestinal mucosa, production of enterotoxin or cytotoxin, and the observation that within each category the strains fall into certain O:H serotypes. See table.

Four Major Categories of Diarrheagenic *E. coli*

Category	Abbreviation	Clinical Manifestation
Enterotoxigenic	ETEC	Travelers diarrhea and infant diarrhea in less developed countries
Enteropathogenic	EPEC	Infant diarrhea
Enterohemorrhagic	EHEC	Hemorrhagic colitis Hemolytic uremic syndrome Thrombotic thrombocytopenia purpura
Enteroinvasive	EIEC	Dysentery

(Continued)

Stool Culture, Diarrheagenic *E. coli* (Continued)

Hemorrhagic colitis can be differentiated from other causes of diarrhea by its progression from watery to bloody diarrhea over a few days time. The fecal leukocytes are markedly increased. Fever is usually absent. The disease is mediated by the production of a Shiga-like toxin which interferes with colonic brush border cells, protein synthesis, and ultimately causes cell death. Enterohemorrhagic *E. coli* (EHEC), differ from other strains of bacteria in the large amount of toxin they produce. Virtually all O157:H7 organisms produce this toxin.

Enterotoxigenic *E. coli* (ETEC) infection is acquired by ingesting contaminated food or water. The organisms colonize the proximal small intestine and there they elaborate enterotoxins. Clinical features of ETEC infection include watery diarrhea, nausea, abdominal cramps, and low grade fever. Enterotoxigenic *E. coli* is the most common agent of travelers diarrhea. Symptoms start early in the visit, typically on day 3. The illness may typically last 3-4 days.

Enteropathogenic *E. coli* (EPEC) produce a cytotoxin similar or identical to that produced by *Shigella dysenteriae* type 1. The clinical symptoms of EPEC illness include fever, malaise, vomiting, and diarrhea with large amounts of mucus but not grossly bloody. EPEC diarrhea in infants may persist for longer than 14 days and is frequently severe.

Enteroinvasive *E. coli* (EIEC) invade and proliferate within epithelial cells and cause eventual cell death, like *Shigella*. Clinical illness is characterized by fever, severe abdominal cramps, malaise, toxemia, and watery diarrhea. The illness progresses to gross dysentery with scant stools consisting of blood and mucus. The methylene blue stain of stool reveals sheets of leukocytes.

Selected Readings

Acheson DWK and Jaeger JL, "Shiga Toxin-Producing *Escherichia coli*," *Clin Microbiol Newslett*, 1999, 21(23):183-8.

Bopp CA, Brenner FW, Wells JG, et al, "*Escherichia*, *Shigella*, and *Salmonella*," *Manual of Clinical Microbiology*, 7th ed, Murray PR, Baron EJ, Pfaller MA, et al, eds, Washington, DC: American Society for Microbiology, 1999, 459-74.

Doyle MP, "Pathogenic *Escherichia coli*, *Yersinia enterocolitica*, and *Vibrio parahaemolyticus*," *Lancet*, 1990, 336(8723):1111-5.

Fedorko DP, Engler HD, O'Shaughnessy EM, et al, "Evaluation of Two Rapid Assays for Detection of *Clostridium difficile* Toxin A in Stool Specimens," *J Clin Microbiolo*, 1999, 37(9):3044-7.

Guerrant RL and Lima AAM, "Inflammatory Enteritides," *Principles and Practices of Infectious Diseases*, 5th ed, Mandell GL, et al, eds, New York, NY: Churchill Livingstone, 2000, 1126-36.

Kehl SC, "Role of the Laboratory in the Diagnosis of Enterohemorrhagic *Escherichia coli* Infections," *J Clin Microbiol*, 2002, 40(8):2711-5.

Nataro JP and Kaper JB, "Diarrheagenic *Escherichia coli*," *Clin Microbiol Rev*, 1998, 11(1):142-201

Wanke CA, "To Know *Escherichia coli* Is to Know Bacterial Diarrheal Disease," *Clin Infect Dis*, 2001, 32(12):1710-2.

Stool Culture, EPEC *see* Stool Culture, Diarrheagenic *E. coli on page 587*

Stool Culture, Uncommon Organisms

Applies to *Aeromonas*, Stool Culture; *Plesiomonas*, Stool Culture; *Vibrio cholerae*, Stool Culture; *Vibrio parahaemolyticus*, Stool Culture; *Yersinia enterocolitica*, Stool Culture; Rectal Swab, Unusual Organism

Special Instructions Laboratory must be contacted prior to collecting specimen

Specimen Rectal swab or fresh stool

Container Culturette® or plastic stool container

Collection If collected in sterile bedpan, must not be contaminated with urine or residual soap or disinfectants. Specimen must be less than 3 hours old.

Storage Instructions Do not refrigerate.

Causes for Rejection Specimen more than 3 hours old, rectal swabs in which the medium compartment is not broken, insufficient specimen volume, specimen contaminated with urine and/or water, specimen containing interfering substances (eg, castor oil, bismuth, Metamucil®, barium); specimen refrigerated; more than two specimens submitted to the laboratory per day; specimen not submitted as sealed swab or in a sealed plastic stool container. **Diapers are not acceptable.**

Reference Range No organisms detected.

Use Identify an etiologic agent in cases of diarrhea

Limitations Special media necessary for the isolation of these specific pathogens may have to be prepared **prior** to collection of specimen. Most clinical laboratories do not routinely culture for *Yersinia*, *Vibrio*, *Aeromonas*, and *Plesiomonas*.

Selected Readings

Acheson DWK and Jaeger JL, "Shiga Toxin-Producing *Escherichia coli*," *Clin Microbiol Newslett*, 1999, 21(23):183-8.

Kehl SC, "Role of the Laboratory in the Diagnosis of Enterohemorrhagic *Escherichia coli* Infections," *J Clin Microbiol*, 2002, 40(8):2711-5.

Wanke CA, "To Know *Escherichia coli* Is to Know Bacterial Diarrheal Disease," *Clin Infect Dis*, 2001, 32(12):1710-2.

Stool for Culture *see* Stool Culture *on page 585*
Stool for Ova and Parasites *see* Ova and Parasites, Stool *on page 551*
Stool Viral Culture *see* Viral Culture, Stool *on page 616*
Strep Throat Screening Culture *see* Throat Culture for Group A Beta-Hemolytic *Streptococcus on page 594*
***Streptococcus agalactiae*, Latex Screen** *see* Group B *Streptococcus* Antigen Test *on page 476*
***Streptococcus* Group A Latex Screen** *see* Group A *Streptococcus* Antigen Test *on page 475*
***Streptococcus* Group B Latex Screen** *see* Group B *Streptococcus* Antigen Test *on page 476*
***Streptococcus pyogenes* Culture** *see* Throat Culture for Group A Beta-Hemolytic *Streptococcus on page 594*
Streptodornase *see* Antideoxyribonuclease-B Titer, Serum *on page 376*

Streptozyme

Related Information

Antideoxyribonuclease-B Titer, Serum *on page 376*
Antistreptolysin O Titer, Serum *on page 383*

Test Includes Screening for anti-NADase, anti-DNase B, antistreptokinase, antistreptolysin O (ASO), antihyaluronidase. Sheep red blood cells are sensitized with these the five streptococcal exoenzymes.

Specimen Serum

Container Red top tube

Reference Range <100 streptozyme units

Use Screen for antibodies to streptococcal antigens: NADase, DNase B, streptokinase, streptolysin O, and hyaluronidase

Limitations A single determination is less useful than a series. May not be as sensitive in children as in adults.

Methodology Hemagglutination

Additional Information Streptozyme is a screening test for antibodies to several streptococcal antigens. It has the advantages of detecting several antibodies in a single assay (although which one has been detected cannot be ascertained), of being technically quick and easy, and of being unaffected by several factors producing false-positives in the ASO test. A serially rising titer is more significant than a single determination.

A disadvantage of the test is that borderline antibody elevations, which could be clinically significant particularly in children, may not be detected.

Selected Readings

Ayoub EM and Harden E, "Immune Response to Streptococcal Antigens: Diagnostic Methods," *Manual of Clinical Laboratory Immunology*, 5th ed, Rose NR, Conway de Macario E, Folds JD, et al, eds, Washington, DC: American Society for Microbiology, 1997, 450-7.

Ayoub EM, "Immune Response to Group A Streptococcal Infections," *Pediatr Infect Dis J*, 1991, 10(10 Suppl):S15-9.

el-Kholy A, Hafez K, and Krause RM, "Specificity and Sensitivity of the Streptozyme Test for the Detection of Streptococcal Antibodies," *Appl Microbiol*, 1974, 27(4):748-52.

STS *see* RPR *on page 574*
Sudden Death Syndrome *see* Botulism, Diagnostic Procedure *on page 405*
Sulfur Granule, Culture *see Actinomyces* Culture, All Sites *on page 363*
Surgical Pathology *see* Histopathology *on page 496*
Surgical Specimen Anaerobic Culture *see* Anaerobic Culture *on page 371*
Surgical Specimen Culture *see* Aerobic Culture, Body Fluid *on page 365*
Surgical Specimen Culture, Routine *see* Biopsy Culture, Routine *on page 390*
Surgical Specimen Fungus Culture *see* Fungus Culture, Body Fluid *on page 462*
Surgical Specimen Mycobacteria Culture *see* Mycobacteria Culture, Biopsy or Body Fluid *on page 539*
Surrogate Tests for Non-A, Non-B Hepatitis *see* Hepatitis C Serology *on page 484*
Susceptibility Testing, Aerobic and Facultatively Anaerobic Organisms *see* Antimicrobial Susceptibility Testing, Aerobic and Facultatively Anaerobic Organisms *on page 379*
Susceptibility Testing, Antimicrobial, Anaerobic Bacteria *see* Antimicrobial Susceptibility Testing, Anaerobic Bacteria *on page 381*
Susceptibility Testing, Fungi *see* Antifungal Susceptibility Testing *on page 377*
Susceptibility Testing, Mycobacteria *see* Antimycobacterial Susceptibility Testing *on page 383*
Susceptibility Testing, Schlichter Test *see* Serum Bactericidal Test *on page 578*
Susceptibility Testing, Serum Bactericidal Dilution Method *see* Serum Bactericidal Test *on page 578*

Swan-Ganz Tip Culture *see* Intravenous Line Culture *on page 511*

Synovial Fluid Culture *see* Aerobic Culture, Body Fluid *on page 365*

Synovial Fluid Culture for *Neisseria gonorrhoeae*, Only *see* *Neisseria gonorrhoeae* Culture *on page 547*

Synovial Fluid Cytology *see* Cytology, Body Fluids *on page 438*

Synovial Fluid Fungus Culture *see* Fungus Culture, Body Fluid *on page 462*

Syphilis, Darkfield Examination *see* Darkfield Examination, Syphilis *on page 444*

Syphilis Screening Test *see* RPR *on page 574*

Syphilis Serology *see* MHA-TP *on page 535*

T4/T8 Ratio

Synonyms Helper Cell/Suppressor Ratio

Test Includes Quantitation of T4 and T8 cells

Specimen Blood

Container Yellow top (ACD) tube or green top (heparin) tube

Collection Routine venipuncture

Storage Instructions Maintain specimen at room temperature.

Causes for Rejection Excessive hemolysis, lipemia

Use Evaluate patients with suspected AIDS

Limitations Not diagnostic for AIDS

Methodology Flow cytometry

Additional Information Normal immunity requires a balance between thymus-derived helper cells (T4) and suppressor cells (T8). The quantitation of the T4 (helper) and T8 (suppressor) is helpful in the evaluation of a patient with suspected AIDS. In AIDS, the T4 cells are severely reduced, and the T4/T8 ratio is <1.

TB Culture, Biopsy *see* Mycobacteria Culture, Biopsy or Body Fluid *on page 539*

TB Culture, Bronchial Aspirate *see* Mycobacteria Culture, Sputum *on page 542*

TB Culture, Gastric Aspirate *see* Mycobacteria Culture, Sputum *on page 542*

TB Culture, Sputum Culture, Mycobacteria *see* Mycobacteria Culture, Sputum *on page 542*

TB Smear *see* Acid-Fast Stain *on page 361*

T Cells *see* Lymphocyte Subset Panels *on page 531*

TEE *see* Transesophageal Echocardiography *on page 598*

Teichoic Acid Antibody

Specimen Serum

Container Red top tube

Reference Range Titer ≤1:2. Less than a fourfold rise between acute and convalescent serum. (Reference ranges vary among laboratories.)

Use Assess therapy in chronic infections caused by *Staphylococcus aureus*

Limitations Clinical utility is not well established and is equivocal. Technical variability.

Methodology Gel diffusion assay, enzyme-linked immunosorbent assay (ELISA)

Additional Information Teichoic acid is a component of the cell wall of gram-positive bacteria. Antibodies to teichoic acid can be demonstrated in some patients with infections due to such organisms, particularly staphylococcal endocarditis and osteomyelitis. Serial determinations of teichoic acid antibodies have been used by some to assess the adequacy of therapy for these conditions, but this or other clinical applications are not yet established.

Selected Readings

Herzog C, Wood HC, Noel I, et al, "Comparison of a New Enzyme-Linked Immunosorbent Assay Method With Counterimmunoelectrophoresis for Detection of Teichoic Acid Antibodies in Sera From Patients With *Staphylococcus aureus* Infections," *J Clin Microbiol*, 1984, 19(4):511-15.

Jacob E, Durham LC, Falk MC, et al, "Antibody Response to Teichoic Acid and Peptidoglycan in *Staphylococcus aureus* Osteomyelitis," *J Clin Microbiol*, 1987, 25(1):122-7.

Temporomandibular Joint Arthrogram *see* Arthrogram *on page 387*

Thin and Thick Smears, Blood *see* Peripheral Blood Smear, Thick and Thin *on page 563*

Thoracentesis

Synonyms Pleural Fluid Tap

Test Includes At the bedside, a physician utilizes a needle and catheter system to withdraw fluid from a patient with radiographically demonstrable pleural effusion for diagnostic or therapeutic purposes.

Patient Preparation Technique and risks of procedure are explained and consent is obtained. Chest x-ray is routinely performed prior to procedure, including a PA, lateral, and lateral decubitus view, and should be available for physician review. Recent prothrombin, partial thromboplastin time, and platelet count on the chart.

Laboratory requisitions completed in advance. Premedication for pain (such as parenteral meperidine) is rarely required and local anesthesia during the procedure is usually sufficient.

Aftercare Immediately postprocedure, a "stat" chest x-ray is performed, usually at end-expiration. Vital signs must be monitored closely, especially if >1 L fluid is removed. Hypoxemia is a known complication of thoracentesis and some patients may require temporary supplemented oxygen. If dyspnea or hypotension develops, physician must be contacted promptly. Otherwise, if vital signs and postprocedure chest x-ray are satisfactory, patient activity may be ad lib.

Complications Although numerous complications have been reported, diagnostic thoracentesis is generally at low risk. Complications may be classified as traumatic or nontraumatic. Nontraumatic complications are related to predictable physiologic responses and include:

- syncope
- cough
- hypotension, either immediate (vasovagal reaction) or delayed (fluid shifts)
- noncardiogenic pulmonary edema (following rapid expansion of a collapsed lung, especially on removal of large volumes of a chronic effusion)
- hypoxemia; PaO_2 may drop by 10 mm Hg within minutes and not return to baseline until the following day. Some authorities recommend supplemental oxygen routinely.

Traumatic complications are iatrogenic and include:

- pneumothorax, simple or tension (requiring chest tube); lateral decubitus radiograph demonstrating a pleural effusion <10 mm thick substantially increases the risk of pneumothorax
- hemothorax
- laceration of intercostal artery, potentially lethal
- puncture of liver or spleen
- miscellaneous, subcutaneous emphysema, air embolism, infection

Of note, the recovery of a grossly bloody pleural effusion (RBC >100,000/mm^3) does not automatically imply needle trauma since blood may be seen in several pleural diseases as well. To differentiate this, traumatic effusions tend to clot rapidly and become more clear as serial samples are withdrawn; bloody effusions from pleural disease generally are slow to clot due to defibrination over time. In doubtful cases, a hematocrit should be obtained on the bloody effusion and compared with plasma hematocrit.

Equipment Several complete thoracentesis kits are available commercially. Alternatively, individual components commonly found in most clinics and hospitals may be assembled separately. Common items include sterile drapes, iodine, alcohol pads, gauze, local anesthesia (1% lidocaine), at least four sterile tubes, syringes, and anaerobic culture media. Two red top tubes and two lavender top (EDTA containing) tubes may be used in place of the four sterile tubes. If cytologic studies are planned, heparin (1:1000) is needed as an additive. If pleural fluid pH is planned, a heparinized syringe and ice bag are needed. Several needle and catheter assemblies are available. For diagnostic thoracentesis (only 50-100 mL fluid removed), a 2" angiocatheter is convenient (18- or 20-gauge needle within catheter). For therapeutic thoracentesis with >1 L removed, a catheter within needle arrangement is effective. A 12" long plastic catheter (16-gauge) within a 14-gauge needle allows more complete pleural space drainage. Also required are liter-sized vacuum bottles and connecting tubing for collection of large volumes of fluid. Commercial thoracentesis kits represent variations of the above and are most useful when >1 L fluid is to be removed.

Technique Ideally, patient is positioned so that he/she is seated and leaning forward slightly, arms crossed in front and resting comfortably on a bedside table. The highest level of pleural effusion is determined on physical examination and a mark is placed one intercostal space below. The area is prepped and draped, and the skin and subcutaneous tissues are infiltrated with local anesthetic. Generally, the site is located 5-10 cm lateral to the spine, near the posterior axillary line. At this point technique varies with equipment used. If a catheter within needle is used, the needle (14-gauge) is passed bevel down over the superior aspect of the rib in the anesthetized intercostal space (avoiding the neurovascular bundle). Once the needle has penetrated the parietal pleura and fluid easily aspirated, the smaller plastic catheter (16-gauge) can be advanced its entire length into the pleural space. The needle is then completely withdrawn through the skin. Pleural fluid can be aspirated through the plastic catheter into a 50 mL syringe. Multiple samples of 50 mL may be obtained in this fashion. Alternatively, the catheter may be attached to sterile connecting tubing and fluid collected with liter-sized vacuum bottles. Once the desired amount is obtained, the catheter is pulled out completely and pressure held over the puncture site. If an angiocatheter is used (needle within catheter), the technique is similar. (Continued)

Thoracentesis *(Continued)*

Immediately after collection, serum is drawn for LDH, protein, and further additional studies depending on the clinical situation (see Additional Information).

Specimen For diagnostic thoracentesis, 50-100 mL is adequate for routine studies. If cytology desired, larger volumes have been recommended (100-250 mL), although occasionally as little as 5 mL have been sufficient. For therapeutic thoracentesis, removal of 1000-1500 mL is generally well tolerated.

Container Lavender top tube for cell count, red top tube for chemistries, sterile syringe adequate for transport to Microbiology Laboratory. For cytology samples add 5000-10,000 units of heparin into syringe or vacuum bottle and label. For pleural fluid pH send specimen in anaerobic syringe (air bubbles removed) on ice immediately to blood gas laboratory.

Collection Samples should be hand carried to respective laboratories immediately.

Causes for Rejection Lack of heparin additive to cytology (or cell count, if plain glass tube used in place of lavender top tube), improper collection technique for pH (not on ice)

Normal Findings Pleural effusions are traditionally classified as either "transudates" or "exudates" based on the underlying mechanism of pleural fluid formation. This is the first and most crucial step in pleural fluid analysis. Transudates are ultrafiltrates of plasma which result from alterations in the osmotic or hydrostatic forces across pleural membranes. The pleural surface itself is usually disease-free. Examples include congestive heart failure (elevated hydrostatic pressure), nephrotic syndrome, and other hypoproteinemic states (decreased oncotic pressure), cirrhosis, myxedema, sarcoidosis, and Meig's syndrome. Exudates occur when the pleural membrane is involved in a disease process which increases pleural capillary permeability or obstructs lymphatics. Causes of exudates include pulmonary infections (pneumonia, empyema, abscess), malignancy (mesothelioma or metastases), collagen vascular diseases, pulmonary embolism, gastrointestinal diseases (pancreatitis, esophageal rupture), hemothorax, chylothorax, and miscellaneous causes such as postmyocardial infarction syndrome, uremia, and postradiation. In general, discovering a transudate allows therapy to be focused on the underlying systemic disease causing the effusion (eg, cirrhosis). Further studies of the pleural space are not necessary. Discovering an exudate, however, is more ominous and mandates additional, thorough diagnostic testing to rule out entities such as occult malignancy and pleural space infection.

Critical Values The following biochemical criteria were found by Light to accurately predict an exudate:

- pleural fluid protein to serum protein ratio >0.5
- pleural fluid LDH to serum LDH ratio >0.6
- pleural fluid LDH >200 units/L (or >two-thirds the upper limit of normal serum LDH)

Exudates satisfy one or more of these three criteria. Effusions are classified as transudates only if none of the these criteria are met. Misclassification rate is <1%, based on several prospective studies. In the past, specific gravity (SG) was used as the sole criteria for separating transudates (SG <1.016) from exudates (SG >1.016). Despite its appeal as a simple and inexpensive test, it is no longer recommended due to its high misclassification rate (≤30%). Similarly, older criteria using pleural fluid protein alone to differentiate transudates (protein <3.0 mg/dL) from exudates (>3 mg/dL) carries a misclassification rate near 15% and should no longer be used.

Use The major diagnostic indication is the presence of pleural fluid of unclear etiology. In those instances where the etiology of a pleural effusion is clinically apparent, thoracentesis may be deferred at physician's discretion. For example, the patient with recurrent congestive heart failure who presents with typical left ventricular failure and pleural effusion may appropriately undergo a trial of diuresis prior to thoracentesis. The major therapeutic indication for thoracentesis is respiratory compromise secondary to a large pleural effusion. Less commonly, the procedure may be used to evacuate trapped air in the pleural space (rather than fluid) as with a tension pneumothorax.

Contraindications Platelet count <50,000/mm^3; severe, uncorrectable coagulopathy; effusions <10 mm thick on decubitus radiograph (or effusions not freely movable on decubitus radiograph); inability to define rib landmarks (necessary for proper needle placement); an uncooperative patient, unable to sit immobile. Other high-risk situations, not necessarily representing contraindications, include: mechanical ventilation with positive end expiratory pressure (PEEP); severe emphysema with blebs; patients who have undergone pneumonectomy with pleural effusion located on the side of the remaining lung. In these instances, ultrasound or CT guided aspiration of pleural fluid may be more prudent; a common complication such as pneumothorax could have profound consequences.

Additional Information Supplemental tests are available for more specific evaluation of the exudate. To minimize expense, test selection should be based on the differential diagnosis of an individual case. Malignant effusions are often grossly bloody with RBCs from 5000-100,000/mm^3. Cytologic exam is initially positive for malignancy in approximately 60% of cases of later documented pleural malignancy; if three separate samples are sent, yield improves to 90%. Pleural fluid pH is often <7.3 and glucose is low (<60 mg/dL) in 15% of cases. In patients with empyema, enormous numbers of polymorphonuclear cells are present in pleural fluid. Parapneumonic effusions are sterile effusions secondary to pneumonia and require pleural pH measurement for optimal management. A pH <7.2, in the absence of systemic acidosis, indicates that the effusion will behave clinically like an empyema and will require chest tube drainage for resolution. Note that pleural fluid pH <7.2 may occur in other conditions (malignancy, TB, rheumatoid arthritis) which do not necessarily require tube thoracotomy. Tuberculosis effusions are characterized by WBC count >10,000/mm^3 with >50% small lymphocytes. This latter finding is highly suggestive of either TB or malignancy and may warrant pleural biopsy. Mesothelial cells are absent in tuberculous effusions; some authors feel that the presence >1% mesothelial cells effectively rules out TB. AFB stains alone are initially positive in only 25% of proven cases. Rheumatoid effusions characteristically have low glucose levels and a value >30 mg/dL makes the diagnosis doubtful. Pleural pH levels are quite low (often <7). Rheumatoid factor testing on pleural fluid is nonspecific and not clinically useful. In suspected lupus effusions, the finding of lupus erythematosus (LE) cells in pleural fluid is pathognomonic for systemic lupus erythematosus. Effusions associated with both pancreatitis and esophageal rupture have similar laboratory profiles. Amylase levels are elevated >160 units/L with both esophageal rupture (salivary amylase) and pancreatitis (pancreatic amylase). Pleural fluid pH is low in both cases, and may be <7 with esophageal rupture.

Selected Readings

Bartter T, Santarelli R, Akers SM, et al, "The Evaluation of Pleural Effusion," *Chest*, 1994, 106(4):1209-14.

Grogan DR, Irwin RS, Channick R, et al, "Complications Associated With Thoracentesis. A Prospective, Randomized Study Comparing Three Different Methods," *Arch Intern Med*, 1990, 150(4):873-7.

Health and Public Policy Committee, American College of Physicians, "Diagnostic Thoracentesis and Pleural Biopsy in Pleural Effusions," *Ann Intern Med*, 1985, 103(5):799-802.

Jay SJ, "Pleural Effusions: Preliminary Evaluation - Recognition of the Transudate," *Postgrad Med*, 1986, 80(5):164-7, 170-7.

Light RW, Macgregor MI, Luchsinger PC, et al, "Pleural Effusions: The Diagnostic Separation of Transudates and Exudates," *Ann Intern Med*, 1972, 77(4):507-13.

McVay PA and Toy PT, "Lack of Increased Bleeding After Paracentesis and Thoracentesis in Patients With Mild Coagulation Abnormalities," *Transfusion*, 1991, 31(2):164-71.

Norris AM and Burke CM, "Diagnostic Thoracentesis," *Chest*, 1990, 98(5):1251-2.

Ogirala RG and Azrieli FM, "Thoracentesis and Closed Pleural Biopsy," *Interventional Pulmonology*, Beamis JF Jr and Mathur PN, eds, New York, NY: McGraw-Hill Book Co, 1999, 223-40.

Prakash UB, "Malignant Pleural Effusions," *Postgrad Med*, 1986, 80(5):201-9.

Qureshi N, Momin ZA, and Brandstetter RD, "Thoracentesis in Clinical Practice," *Heart Lung*, 1994, 23(5):376-83.

Stogner SW and Campbell GD, "Pleural Effusion. What You Can Learn From the Results of a Tap," *Postgrad Med*, 1992, 91(5):439-42, 445-54. Thoracentesis. A Prospective, Randomized Study Comparing Three Different Methods," *Arch Intern Med*, 1990, 150(4):873-7.

Norris AM and Burke CM, "Diagnostic Thoracentesis," *Chest*, 1990, 98(5):1251-2.

Ogirala RG and Azrieli FM, "Thoracentesis and Closed Pleural Biopsy," *Interventional Pulmonology*, Beamis JF Jr and Mathur PN, eds, New York, NY: McGraw-Hill Book Co, 1999, 223-40.

Qureshi N, Momin ZA, and Brandstetter RD, "Thoracentesis in Clinical Practice," *Heart Lung*, 1994, 23(5):376-83.

Stogner SW and Campbell GD, "Pleural Effusion. What You Can Learn From the Results of a "Tap"," *Postgrad Med*, 1992, 91(5):439-42, 445-54.

Thoracentesis Fluid Cytology *see* Cytology, Body Fluids *on page 438*

Thoracentesis Fluid Fungus Culture Bone Marrow Fungus Culture *see* Fungus Culture, Body Fluid *on page 462*

Three-Phase Bone Scan *see* Bone Scan *on page 401*

Throat Culture for *Corynebacterium diphtheriae*

Synonyms *Corynebacterium diphtheriae* Culture, Throat; Diphtheria Culture

Applies to Nasopharyngeal Culture for *Corynebacterium diphtheriae*

Abstract Diphtheria causes pseudomembranes. It may be found in the anterior nasal mucosa, but classically it is a disease of the oropharynx. It may spread to or begin in the larynx and can involve the tracheobronchial tree. The major effects of the exotoxin are on the heart and nervous system.

Aftercare Observe for laryngospasm following collection of specimen.

Special Instructions The laboratory should be notified before collection of specimens so that special isolation media can be made available. The laboratory should be informed of the specific site of specimen, age of patient, current antibiotic therapy, and clinical diagnosis.

Specimen Throat swab, nasopharyngeal swab

(Continued)

Throat Culture for *Corynebacterium diphtheriae* (Continued)

Container Sterile Mini-Tip Culturette® or flexible calcium alginate swab, Calgiswab®, is recommended for obtaining nasopharyngeal culture.

Collection The tongue should be depressed while both the tonsillar crypts and nasopharynx and throat lesions are swabbed. If a pseudomembrane is present, the swab should be taken from the membrane and beneath its edge if possible. Separate swabs for throat and nasopharynx are desirable. Avoid swabbing the tongue and uvula. Specimen must be transported to the laboratory immediately following collection.

Storage Instructions Refrigerate the specimen if it cannot be promptly processed.

Turnaround Time Preliminary reports are usually available at 24 hours. Cultures with no growth are usually reported after 72 hours. Final reports on specimens from which *C. diphtheriae* has been isolated usually take at least 4 days.

Reference Range No *C. diphtheriae* isolated

Use Isolate *C. diphtheriae* from patients suspected of having diphtheria. The organisms remain superficial in the respiratory tract and skin, but the potent exotoxin is responsible for the virulence of the disease.

Limitations Cultures should be taken from nasopharynx, as well as, the throat; culture of both sites increases the chance of recovery of the organism. Stain results are presumptive and are commonly reported out as "gram-positive pleomorphic bacilli suggestive of *C. diphtheriae*". Definitive diagnosis depends on isolation of the organism because of the similar appearance of other organisms commonly found in the oropharynx.

Contraindications Lack of clinical symptoms or signs of diphtheria, valid history of immunization

Methodology Culture on selective medium (Löeffler's), cystine tellurite agar, and blood agar smear stained with Löeffler's methylene blue stain and/or Gram stain. *C. diphtheriae* may appear as V, Y, or L figures. Metachromatic granules which stain deep blue may also be seen.

Additional Information Routine throat culture should be ordered in addition. *C. diphtheriae* may occasionally cause skin infections, wound infections, pulmonary infections, and endocarditis and may be recovered from the oropharynx of healthy carriers. *C. diphtheriae* is spread through respiratory secretions by convalescent and healthy carriers. The clinical presentation includes a grayish pseudomembrane, overlying superficial ulcers in the oropharynx. The organism is noninvasive, however, the exotoxin elaborated in the throat affects primarily the heart and nervous system. Mortality is 10% to 30%. Only strains of *C. diphtheriae* infected by B-phage are capable of producing toxin. Nontoxigenic strains are commonly recovered and are capable of producing pharyngitis. Confirmation of exotoxin production requires animal testing and is rarely done for clinical testing. *C. ulcerans* may also produce a diphtheria-like disease.

Selected Readings

Farizo KM, Strebel PM, Chen RT, et al, "Fatal Respiratory Disease Due to *Corynebacterium diphtheriae*: Case Report and Review of Guidelines for Management, Investigation, and Control," *Clin Infect Dis*, 1993, 16(1):59-68.

Larsson P, Brinkhoff B, and Larsson L, "*Corynebacterium diphtheriae* in the Environment of Carriers and Patients," *J Hosp Infect*, 1987, 10:282-6.

MacGregor RR, "*Corynebacterium diphtheriae*," *Principles and Practice of Infectious Diseases*, 5th ed, Mandell GL, Bennett JE, and Dolin R, eds, New York, NY: Churchill Livingstone, 2000, 2190-8.

Rappuoli R, Perugini M, and Falsen E, "Molecular Epidemiology of the 1984-1986 Outbreak of Diphtheria in Sweden," *N Engl J Med*, 1988, 318:12-4.

Walters RF, "Diphtheria Presenting in the Accident and Emergency Department," *Arch Emerg Med*, 1987, 4:47-51.

Throat Culture for Group A Beta-Hemolytic *Streptococcus*

Related Information

Group A *Streptococcus* Antigen Test *on page 475*

Synonyms Beta-Hemolytic Strep Culture, Throat; Group A Beta-Hemolytic *Streptococcus* Culture, Throat; Screening Culture for Group A Beta-Hemolytic *Streptococcus*; Strep Throat Screening Culture; *Streptococcus pyogenes* Culture

Patient Preparation Do not swab throat in cases of acute epiglottitis unless provisions to establish an alternate airway are readily available.

Special Instructions The laboratory should be informed of the specific site of specimen, age of patient, current antibiotic therapy, and clinical diagnosis.

Specimen Throat swab

Container Sterile Culturette®; Dacron or rayon swabs are acceptable.

Collection The tongue should be depressed while both tonsillar pillars and the oropharynx are swabbed. Exudates should be swabbed and the tongue and uvula should be avoided.

Turnaround Time Reports are usually available within 24 hours. Cultures with no beta-hemolytic streptococci are usually reported after 24 or 48 hours. Reports on specimens from which beta-hemolytic streptococci group A have been isolated require a minimum of 24-48 hours for completion.

Reference Range No beta-hemolytic *Streptococcus pyogenes* isolated

Use Isolate and identify group A beta-hemolytic streptococci; establish the diagnosis of strep throat

Limitations Cultures are usually screened for beta-hemolytic strep group A only. No other organisms are usually reported. Interpretation of throat cultures requires a significant level of experience and technical proficiency in order to avoid false-positives and false-negatives.

Methodology Culture on blood agar plate, serological latex agglutination identification as group A.

Some laboratories offer molecular testing for this organism. Contact the testing laboratory for the availability of amplified and nonamplified qualitative and quantitative molecular tests for this organism, and for information on selection and collection of appropriate specimens for specific molecular tests.

Additional Information *Streptococcus pyogenes* (group A beta-hemolytic strep) is susceptible to penicillin and other beta-lactam antimicrobial agents; therefore, susceptibility need not be routinely determined. The principal reason for considering an alternative drug for individual patients is allergy to penicillin. Erythromycin or a cephalosporin might be substituted in these cases. Patients allergic to penicillins may also be allergic to cephalosporins.

Use of rapid tests providing confirmation of the presence of group A streptococci is common. The sensitivity of the rapid methods is 80% to 95% in overt clinical pharyngitis. The screening method is far less sensitive in cases where concomitant cultures yield <10 colonies.

The Infectious Diseases Society of America (IDSA) recently published updated practice guidelines based on a "laboratory algorithm" for the diagnosis and management of group A streptococcal pharyngitis. The IDSA recommendation emphasizes the importance of laboratory confirmation (ie, throat culture or antigen testing) in the diagnosis. The IDSA states, "The diagnosis of acute group A streptococcal pharyngitis should be suspected on clinical and epidemiological grounds and then supported by performance of a laboratory test."

In contrast to these guidelines, the American College of Physicians - American Society of Internal Medicine in collaboration with the CDC has published an alternative "clinical algorithm" in which laboratory testing plasys little, if any role in the diagnosis of group A streptococcal pharyngitis.

In the late 1980s, a resurgence of serious *Streptococcus pyogenes* infection was observed. Complications including rheumatic fever, sepsis, severe soft tissue invasion, and toxic shock-like syndrome (TSLS) are reported to be most common with the M1 serotype and that a unique invasive clone has become the predominant cause of severe streptococcal infections.

Selected Readings

Bisno AL, Gerber MA, Gwaltney JM Jr, et al, "Practice Guidelines for the Diagnosis and Management of Group A Streptococcal Pharyngitis. Infectious Diseases Society of America," *Clin Infect Dis*, 2002, 35(2):113-25.

Bisno AL, Peter GS, and Kaplan EL, "Diagnosis of Strep Throat in Adults: Are Clinical Criteria Really Good Enough?" *Clin Infect Dis*, 2002, 35(2):126-9.

Hahn RG, Knox LM, and Forman TA, "Evaluation of Poststreptococcal Illness," *Am Fam Physician*, 2005, 71(10):1949-54.

Lindbaek M, Hoiby EA, Lermark G, et al, "Which is the Best Method to Trace Group A Streptococci in Sore Throat Patients: Culture or GAS Antigen Test?" *Scand J Prim Health Care*, 2004, 22(4):233-8.

Nimishikavi S and Stead L, "Images in Clinical Medicine. Streptococcal pharyngitis," *N Engl J Med*, 2005, 352(11):e10.

Singh S and Dolan J, "Diagnosis and Treatment of Group A Pharyngitis Strep," *Am Fam Physician*, 2005, 71(6):1064, 1066.

Snow V, Mottur-Pilson C, Cooper RJ, et al, "Principles of Appropriate Antibiotic Use for Acute Pharyngitis in Adults," *Ann Intern Med*, 2001, 134(6):506-8.

Stollerman GH, "Rheumatic Fever in the 21st Century," *Clin Infect Dis*, 2001, 33(6):806-14.

Throat Culture for *Neisseria gonorrhoeae* *see* Neisseria gonorrhoeae Culture *on page 547*

Throat Swab for Group A Streptococcal Antigen *see* Group A *Streptococcus* Antigen Test *on page 475*

Throat Viral Culture *see* Viral Culture, Throat *on page 617*

Thumb, Left or Right, X-ray *see* Bone Films *on page 396*

Tibia and Fibula, Left or Right, X-ray *see* Bone Films *on page 396*
Tick Identification *see* Arthropod Identification *on page 387*
Tissue Anaerobic Culture *see* Anaerobic Culture *on page 371*
Tissue Culture, *Brucella* *see* Biopsy Culture, Routine *on page 390*
Tissue Culture, Routine *see* Biopsy Culture, Routine *on page 390*
Tissue Examination *see* Histopathology *on page 496*
Tissue Fungus Culture *see* Fungus Culture, Body Fluid *on page 462*
Tissue Mycobacteria Culture *see* Mycobacteria Culture, Biopsy or Body Fluid *on page 539*

Tobramycin Level

Related Information

Antibiotic Level, Serum *on page 375*

Synonyms Nebcin®, Blood

Abstract Aminoglycoside antibiotics, including tobramycin, are used primarily to treat infections caused by aerobic gram-negative bacilli. Tobramycin has a narrow therapeutic window, and its use in life-threatening infections makes it mandatory that effective levels be achieved without overdosing.

Specimen Serum

Container Red top tube

Sampling Time Peak: 30 minutes after I.V. infusion; trough: immediately before next dose. Levels should be drawn at steady-state, usually 24-36 hours after starting treatment, depending on dosing schedule.

Storage Instructions Separate serum and refrigerate; must be frozen if a β-lactam is also present

Reference Range Therapeutic: peak: 4-10 mcg/mL (SI: 8-21 μmol/L) (depends in part on the minimal inhibitory concentration of the drug against the organism being treated); trough: <2 mcg/mL (SI: <4 μmol/L)

Possible Panic Range Toxic: peak: >12 mcg/mL (SI: >25 μmol/L); trough: >2 mcg/mL (SI: >4 μmol/L)

Use Peak levels are necessary to assure adequate therapeutic levels for organism being treated. Trough levels are necessary to reduce the likelihood of nephrotoxicity.

Limitations High peak levels may not have strong correlation with toxicity.

Methodology Immunoassay, fluorescence polarization immunoassay (FPIA)

Additional Information Tobramycin is cleared by the kidney, and accumulates in renal tubular cells. Nephrotoxicity is most closely related to the length of time that trough levels exceed 2 mcg/mL (SI: >4 μmol/L). Creatinine levels should be monitored every 2-3 days as this serves as a useful indicator of impending renal toxicity. The initial toxic result is nonoliguric renal failure that is usually reversible if the drug is discontinued. Continued administration of tobramycin may produce oliguric renal failure. Nephrotoxicity may occur in as many as 10% to 25% of patients receiving aminoglycosides; most of this toxicity can be eliminated by monitoring levels and adjusting dosing schedules accordingly.

Aminoglycosides may also cause irreversible ototoxicity that manifests itself clinically as hearing loss. Aminoglycoside ototoxicity is relatively uncommon and clinical trials where levels were carefully monitored and dosing adjusted failed to show a correlation between auditory toxicity and plasma aminoglycoside levels. In situations where dosing is not adjusted, however, sustained high levels may be associated with ototoxicity. This association is far from clear cut, and new once-daily dosing regimens (and associated high peak serum concentrations) that fail to enhance toxicity further complicates the understanding of this issue.

Selected Readings

Edson RS and Terrell CL, "The Aminoglycosides," *Mayo Clin Proc*, 1999, 74(5):519-28.
Gilbert DN, "Once-Daily Aminoglycoside Therapy," *Antimicrob Agents Chemother*, 1991, 35(3):399-405.
Hammett-Stabler CA and Johns T, "Laboratory Guidelines for Monitoring of Antimicrobial Drugs. National Academy of Clinical Biochemistry," *Clin Chem*, 1998, 44(5):1129-40.
Pancoast SJ, "Aminoglycoside Antibiotics in Clinical Use," *Med Clin North Am*, 1987, 72(3):581-612.
Townsend PL, Fink MP, Stein KL, et al, "Aminoglycoside Pharmacokinetics: Dosage Requirements and Nephrotoxicity in Trauma Patients," *Crit Care Med*, 1989, 17(2):154-7.

Toes of Foot, Left or Right, X-ray *see* Bone Films *on page 396*
Toxin Assay, *Clostridium difficile* *see* *Clostridium difficile* Toxin Assay *on page 418*

Toxoplasma Serology

Related Information

Toxoplasma Serology by ELISA *on page 597*

Synonyms Toxoplasmosis Titer

Test Includes IgG and IgM antibodies to *Toxoplasma*. IgA anti-*Toxoplasma* may also be available.

Special Instructions Acute and convalescent specimens are recommended.

Specimen Serum

Container Red top tube

Reference Range Titer: <1:64 by immunofluorescence; <1:256 by indirect hemagglutination; significance of titers varies by laboratory and methodology.

Use Support the diagnosis of toxoplasmosis; document past exposure and/or immunity to *Toxoplasma gondii*

Limitations Diagnosis of neonatal infection may be difficult because the clinical course of infection outstrips demonstrable antibody response

Methodology Indirect fluorescent antibody (IFA), indirect hemagglutination (IHA), enzyme-linked immunosorbent assay (ELISA)

If serological testing is performed by enzyme immunoassay (EIA) on automated instrumentation, results are usually given in index units, not titers. In such cases, significant rises in antibody levels are determined by algorithms within the instrumentation, not by increases in titers.

Some laboratories offer molecular testing for this organism. Contact the testing laboratory for the availability of amplified and nonamplified qualitative and quantitative molecular tests for this organism, and for information on selection and collection of appropriate specimens for specific molecular tests.

Additional Information *Toxoplasma gondii* is endemic in cats and is excreted by them. Humans are easily exposed to cyst forms, either in caring for pets or in casual environmental contact. The majority of individuals develop antibody without any clinical disease. A self-limited lymphadenitis is the most common clinical presentation in symptomatic infection.

Congenital toxoplasmosis and infection in an immunocompromised host (AIDS) are more serious, and can produce a fatal cerebritis or disseminated illness. Congenital toxoplasmosis can now be diagnosed *in utero* by detection of IgM antibody in fetal blood.

The diagnosis of toxoplasmosis is supported by high or rising IgG antibody titer, or the demonstration of IgM antibody. The recent availability of IgA anti-*Toxoplasma* may be useful in detection of congenital toxoplasmosis. However, IgM is still the established technique.

A few special reference laboratories offer a newer serological test for anti-*Toxoplasma* antibody: The *Toxoplasma* IgA acidity test. The test is designed to detect IgG and to determine the acidity (ie, the degree of attachment of the antibody to its specific antigen) of the IgG for the *Toxoplasma* antigen. The degree of acidity can indicate approximately when during pregnancy a pregnant woman was infected with *Toxoplasma*.

Selected Readings

Bessieres MH, Roques C, Berrebi A, et al, "IgA Antibody Response During Acquired and Congenital Toxoplasmosis," *J Clin Pathol*, 1992, 45(7):605-8.

Daffos F, Forestier F, Capella-Pavlovsky M, et al, "Prenatal Management of 746 Pregnancies at Risk for Congenital Toxoplasmosis," *N Engl J Med*, 1988, 318(5):271-5.

Wilson M and McAuley JB, "Laboratory Diagnosis of Toxoplasmosis," *Clin Lab Med*, 1991, 11(4):923-39.

Toxoplasma Serology by ELISA

Related Information

Toxoplasma Serology *on page 596*

Synonyms Toxoplasmosis Antibodies; Toxoplasmosis Titer

Test Includes Detection of *Toxoplasma* antigen by ELISA. IgG and IgM antibodies to *Toxoplasma gondii* may also be included. This test may also be available as a component of the TORCH serology battery.

Special Instructions Collection of convalescent specimen 10-14 days after acute specimen is collected facilitates interpretation of the results.

Specimen Serum

Container Red top tube

Storage Instructions Separate serum and refrigerate if the specimen cannot be delivered to the laboratory within 2 hours of collection.

Causes for Rejection Excessive hemolysis, chylous serum, gross contamination of the specimen.

Reference Range Results are given in EIA units and, generally, are interpreted as negative (or antibody not detected), equivocal (or indeterminate), and positive (or antibody detected).

Use Support the diagnosis of toxoplasmosis; document past exposure

Limitations Very limited availability

Methodology Enzyme-linked immunosorbent assay (ELISA)

(Continued)

Toxoplasma Serology by ELISA *(Continued)*

If serological testing is performed by enzyme immunoassay (EIA) on automated instrumentation, results are usually given in index units, not titers. In such cases, significant rises in antibody levels are determined by algorithms within the instrumentation, not by increases in titers.

Additional Information Toxoplasmosis infection in an immunocompromised patient is serious and can produce fatal cerebritis or disseminated illness. The majority of exposed individuals who are immunocompetent develop antibody without clinical disease. A few special reference laboratories offer a newer serological test for anti-*Toxoplasma* antibody: The *Toxoplasma* IgG acidity test. The test is designed to detect IgG and to determine the acidity (ie, the degree of attachment of the antibody to its specific antigen) of the IgG for the *Toxoplasma* antigen. The degree of acidity can indicate approximately when during pregnancy a pregnant woman was infected with *Toxoplasma.*

Toxoplasmosis Antibodies *see Toxoplasma* Serology by ELISA *on page 597*

Toxoplasmosis Titer *see Toxoplasma* Serology *on page 596*

Tracheal Aspirate Culture *see* Aerobic Culture, Sputum *on page 367*

Tracheal Aspirate Fungus Culture *see* Fungus Culture, Sputum *on page 466*

Tracheal Aspirate Mycobacteria Culture *see* Mycobacteria Culture, Sputum *on page 542*

Transesophageal Echocardiography

Synonyms Esophageal Echo; TEE

Test Includes Transesophageal echocardiography (TEE) has been developed to solve one of the limitations of echocardiography, that is, the poor imaging quality seen in some patients in whom the bony structures as well as increased lung interface degrade the quality of the images obtained with conventional echocardiography. By placing an echo transducer at the tip of a gastroscope and advancing it into the esophagus, the heart can be imaged from behind without any lung or chest cage interference. Additionally, the closer proximity to the heart allows for utilization of higher frequency transducers which provide higher resolution images. Transesophageal echocardiography has provided a new window through which the heart can be examined with far greater detail than was once thought possible. The mild inconvenience of having to pass a transesophageal probe has been by far outweighed by the enhanced images obtained with it. Presently, transesophageal echocardiography includes 2-D echocardiography, pulsed Doppler, and color flow imagings. Continuous wave Doppler may also be available.

Special Instructions To minimize the risk of aspiration, a period of 6-8 hours fasting is recommended. An intravenous line to keep a vein open for administration of I.V. antibiotics is needed, and sedation as required is advised. Patients with prosthetic valves, native valve stenosis or insufficiency, and congenital heart disease should receive I.V. antibiotic prophylaxis as recommended by the American Heart Association. After the antibiotics have been given the patient should be expected to be in the laboratory for approximately 1 hour to allow for the performance of the procedure and recovery from sedation and analgesic when used. There is no need for repeated antibiotic prophylaxis after initial dose is completed. Most patients will be able to resume full activity after the procedure. Outpatients are advised to have a companion drive them back home to minimize risks from sedation and analgesics.

Technique A fasting period of 6-8 hours is confirmed, the reasons indicated for the test are reviewed, vital signs are obtained, symptomatic status is determined, history of allergies is determined, and a detailed explanation of the procedure is made. SBE antibiotic prophylaxis is completed as recommended by the AHA. Electrocardiographic and blood pressure monitoring will be performed throughout the procedure. A local anesthetic is given to the back of the throat through a spray, and a fast-acting hypnotic and analgesic is given I.V. (currently we use Versed 0.5-2 mg I.V. and Demend® 25-100 mg I.V.). The patient is then placed on left lateral decubitus and the esophageal probe is passed. A dental suction set minimizes flow of saliva out of the mouth. Patient stays awake and comfortable throughout the procedure in most cases. A systematic and complete study should be performed on each patient. Additionally, the area of specific concern should be evaluated with further detail. A complete study will include 2-D imaging and color flow Doppler study of all cardiac chambers, valves, and great vessels. The study is initiated with the probe placed most distally, which provides a short axis view of the left ventricle as the probe is removed a view equivalent to an apical 4-chamber is obtained. This allows for the best view of the mitral and tricuspid valves. Further removal of the probe allows for visualization of the outflow tract of the left ventricle and aortic valve, after this the left atrium atrial appendage, interatrial septum, and pulmonary veins can be studied. Finally, with further removal of the probe, the aortic arch is visualized. The color Doppler is turned

on during the study to evaluate normal and abnormal flow patterns. A continuous video recording is obtained throughout the study for later study and analysis. After completion of the study, the transesophageal probe is removed and the patient is kept under observation until regaining a prestudy status.

Normal Findings Transesophageal echocardiography has provided a new window to the heart. However, the interpreter must recognize and become familiar with the different orientation of the cardiac structures and tomographic planes as seen from a different perspective. There is a limitation in the number of tomographic planes than can be obtained through TEE since the motion of the probe is somewhat limited in the esophagus. With these limitations in mind, the interpretation of images through TEE is similar to that of color Doppler echocardiography.

Use Transesophageal echocardiography currently is being used intraoperatively to follow cardiac function during cardiac and noncardiac surgery, in the intensive care units to follow and evaluate critically ill patients, and in the study of ambulatory patients to better evaluate a variety of cardiovascular disorders. Transesophageal echocardiography has been found most useful in the evaluation of prosthetic valve dysfunction, particularly mitral valve prosthesis, in the quantitation and diagnostic characterization of native mitral valve insufficiency, in the evaluation of left atrial thrombosis and masses, in the evaluation of bacterial endocarditis and its complications, and in the evaluation of intracardiac shunts.

Contraindications TEE is contraindicated in patients with esophageal obstructions or with respiratory failure if not intubated.

Selected Readings

Seward JB, Khandheria BK, Oh JK, et al, "Transesophageal Echocardiography: Technique, Anatomic Correlations, Implementation, and Clinical Applications," *Mayo Clin Proc*, 1988, 63(7):649-80.

Transjugular Needle Biopsy of the Liver *see* Liver Biopsy *on page 521*

Transthoracic Needle Aspiration for *Pneumocystis* *see Pneumocystis jiroveci* Test *on page 566*

Transtracheal Aspirate Anaerobic Culture *see* Anaerobic Culture *on page 371*

Transtracheal Aspirate Culture *see* Aerobic Culture, Sputum *on page 367*

Transtracheal Aspirate Fungus Culture *see* Fungus Culture, Sputum *on page 466*

Transtracheal Aspirate Mycobacteria Culture *see* Mycobacteria Culture, Sputum *on page 542*

Transtracheal Aspiration *Legionella* Culture *see Legionella pneumophila* Culture *on page 516*

***Treponema pallidum* Antibodies, CSF** *see* FTA-ABS, Cerebrospinal Fluid *on page 457*

***Treponema pallidum* Darkfield Examination** *see* Darkfield Examination, Syphilis *on page 444*

TRIC Agent Culture *see Chlamydia* Culture *on page 413*

***Trichinella* Antibody** *see Trichinella* Serology *on page 599*

Trichinella Serology

Related Information

Trichinella spiralis on page 338

Synonyms *Trichinella* Antibody; Trichinosis Serology

Specimen Serum

Container Red top tube

Reference Range Negative; Interpretation of positive results vary by method and by laboratory. Consult laboratory for specific interpretations.

Use Screen for antibodies to *Trichinella spiralis* to establish the diagnosis of trichinosis

Limitations Low titers may represent antibody from previous rather than current infection. The bentonite flocculation test cannot be used for testing lightly infected pigs. The test may have a high false-negative rate of 15% to 22% during the first period of the infection.

Methodology Bentonite flocculation test (BFT), indirect fluorescent antibody (IFA), complement fixation (CF), latex agglutination (LA), enzyme-linked immunosorbent assay (ELISA)

Additional Information The bentonite flocculation test is sensitive and specific. Antibody becomes detectable 3 weeks after infection, rises for several weeks, and then declines slowly so that most individuals will test negative in 2-3 years. Immunofluorescence is more sensitive for light infection in pigs. In humans, diagnosis can also be made by finding cysts in a muscle biopsy.

Selected Readings

Bruschi F, Tassi C, and Pozio E, "Parasite-Specific Antibody Response in *Trichinella* sp. 3 Human Infection: A One Year Follow-up," *Am J Trop Med Hyg*, 1990, 43(2):186-93.

Wilson M, Schantz PM, and Tsang VCW, "Clinical Immunoparasitology," *Manual of Clinical Laboratory Immunology*, 5th ed, Rose NR, Conway de Macario E, Folds JD, et al, eds, Washington, DC: American Society for Microbiology, 1997, 575-84.

Trichinosis Serology *see Trichinella* Serology *on page 599*
***Trichomonas* Culture** *see Trichomonas* Preparation *on page 600*
***Trichomonas* Pap Smear** *see Trichomonas* Preparation *on page 600*

Trichomonas Preparation

Related Information
Genital Culture *on page 470*

Synonyms Hanging Drop Mount for *Trichomonas*; *Trichomonas vaginalis* Wet Preparation; Trich Prep; Wet Prep; Wet Preparation for *Trichomonas vaginalis*

Applies to *Trichomonas* Culture; *Trichomonas* Pap Smear; *Trichomonas* Wet Preparation, Urine; Cervical *Trichomonas* Smear; Urethral *Trichomonas* Smear; Urine *Trichomonas* Wet Mount; Vaginal *Trichomonas* Smear

Test Includes Wet mount and microscopic examination. Pap smear and/or culture may also be performed.

Special Instructions The laboratory should be informed of the specific source of the specimen.

Specimen Vaginal, cervical, or urethral swabs, prostatic fluid, urine sediment

Container Sterile tube containing 1 mL of sterile nonbacteriostatic saline

Collection The specimen should be collected using a speculum without lubricant. The mucosa of the posterior vagina may be swabbed or the secretions may be collected with a pipette. The swab **must** be expressed into the saline for transport to the laboratory. The specimen should be examined as soon as possible.

Storage Instructions Transport the specimen to the laboratory as soon as possible after collection. Do not refrigerate.

Causes for Rejection Specimen dried out

Turnaround Time Same day; culture in Kupferberg's medium is examined for 5 days

Reference Range Negative: no trichomonads identified; positive: demonstration of actively motile flagellates or positive culture

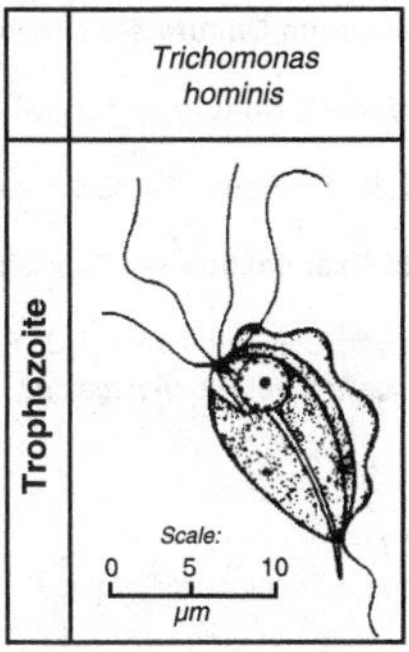

From Brooks MM and Melvin DM, *Morphology of Diagnostic Stages of Intestinal Parasites of Humans,* 2nd ed, Atlanta, GA: U.S. Department of Health and Human Services, Publication No. 84-8116, Centers for Disease Control, 1984, with permission.

Use Establish the presence of *Trichomonas vaginalis*

Limitations The specimen will be examined for *Trichomonas vaginalis* only. A separate swab (Culturette®) must be collected for culture of bacteria or fungus cultures, if required. One negative result does not rule out the possibility of *Trichomonas vaginalis* infection. The sensitivity of the wet mount procedure is low (50% to 70%); therefore, the wet mount is negative in 30% to 50% of women with trichomoniasis.

Contraindications Douching within 3 days prior to specimen collection

Methodology Wet mount microscopic examination, Pap smear, direct immunofluorescent technique with monoclonal antibody. Culture may be performed using Kupferberg's liquid medium or Hirsch charcoal agar.

Some laboratories offer molecular testing for this organism. Contact the testing laboratory for the availability of amplified and nonamplified qualitative and quantitative

molecular tests for this organism, and for information on selection and collection of appropriate specimens for specific molecular tests.

Additional Information The absence of the classical yellow, frothy discharge does not exclude trichomoniasis. Culture usually yield positive results when wet preparations are negative. Cultures are the gold standard and are sensitive; however, they are expensive and have limited availability. The high rate of false-negatives, 48.4%, and false-positives observed with stained preparations (Pap smears) requires that confirmation by wet mount or culture be considered when the reported results are inconsistent with the clinical findings. Immunofluorescence tests are being adopted which have increased sensitivity. The false-positives observed when immunofluorescent methods are compared to culture may represent failure of culture in patients with few organisms. Culture is not available in many laboratories.

In a series of 600 "high risk" women, 88 *Trichomonas* infected patients were observed. Coinfection was noted as follows: *Ureaplasma urealyticum* 96%, *Gardnerella vaginalis* 91%, *Mycoplasma hominis* 89%, bacterial vaginosis 57%, *Neisseria gonorrhoeae* 29%, and *Chlamydia trachomatis* 15%. *Candida albicans* and other *Candida* sp are frequently implicated in vulvovaginitis. A vaginal pH above 5 is suggestive of *Trichomonas*.

In males a milky white fluid discharge and urethral irritation present for more than 4 weeks is frequently associated with urethritis caused by *T. vaginalis*.

Selected Readings

Bennett JR, "The Emergency Department Diagnosis of *Trichomonas vaginalis*," *Ann Emerg Med*, 1989, 18(5):564-6.

Clay JC, Veeravahu M, and Smyth RW, "Practical Problems of Diagnosing Trichomoniasis in Women," *Genitourin Med*, 1988, 64(2):115-7.

Krieger JN, Tam MR, Stevens CE, et al, "Diagnosis of Trichomoniasis, Comparison of Conventional Wet-Mount Examination With Cytologic Studies, Cultures, and Monoclonal Antibody Staining of Direct Specimens," *JAMA*, 1988, 259(8):1223-7.

Pastorek JG 2d, "Common Types of Vaginitis," *Hosp Med*, 1992, 73-88.

Petrin D, Delgaty K, Bhatt R, et al, "Clinical and Microbiological Aspects of *Trichomonas vaginalis*," *Clin Microbiol Rev*, 1998, 11(2):300-17.

Sobel JD, "Vaginal Infections in Adult Women," *Med Clin North Am*, 1990, 74(6):1573-602.

Spiegel CA, "Bacterial Vaginosis: Changes in Laboratory Practice," *Clin Microbiol Newslett*, 1999, 21(5):33-7.

***Trichomonas vaginalis* Wet Preparation** *see Trichomonas* Preparation *on page 600*

***Trichomonas* Wet Preparation, Urine** *see Trichomonas* Preparation *on page 600*

Trich Prep *see Trichomonas* Preparation *on page 600*

Trypanosomiasis Peripheral Blood Preparation *see* Microfilariae, Peripheral Blood Preparation *on page 535*

Tuberculin Skin Testing *see* Tuberculin Skin Testing, Intracutaneous *on page 601*

Tuberculin Skin Testing, Intracutaneous

Related Information

Anergy Skin Test Battery *on page 372*
Fungal Skin Testing *on page 459*
Tuberculosis *on page 1315*

Synonyms Mantoux Test; PPD Test; Purified Protein Derivative (PPD) Test; Tuberculin Skin Testing

Test Includes Intradermal injection of culture extracts of *Mycobacterium tuberculosis* (MTB). This is an *in vivo* means of evaluating delayed hypersensitivity to MTB. Skin test sites are examined at 24, 48, and 72 hours for signs of induration and erythema. A positive skin test indicates prior exposure to MTB (either recent or remote), with an adequate cell-mediated immune response.

Patient Preparation The procedure is explained to the patient. Inquiries should be made regarding past PPD reactions. No specific skin preparation is necessary; however, patients with severe skin disease, such as psoriasis, should be examined beforehand to ensure that there are suitable areas of normal appearing skin. Although testing need not be performed by a physician, one should be immediately available for systemic reactions.

Aftercare If no adverse reaction has occurred within several minutes, the patient may be discharged from the testing center. In some centers, patients are given written instructions on measurement and recording of a positive skin reaction at home. Other centers prefer patients to return to the test center at 48 and 72 hours for formal skin test reading by a nurse or physician. Test sites should be kept clean for 72 hours. No bathing restrictions are necessary. Patient should contact physician if a severe local reaction develops or if fever and dyspnea occurs.

Special Instructions If skin testing is performed in a separate department, requisition should state:

- the strength of tuberculin test (1 TU, 5 TU, 250 TU)

(Continued)

Tuberculin Skin Testing, Intracutaneous *(Continued)*

- whether an anergy skin battery is also desired (see Anergy Skin Test Battery *on page 372*)

Complications In general, adverse reactions are uncommon. Rare complications include fever, lymphangitis, adenopathy, and local ulcers or vesicles. If local lesions develop, these should be treated with dry sterile dressings. The use of topical ointments is optional.

Equipment Culture extracts of MTB (tuberculins) are available for injection in preparations termed "purified protein derivatives" or PPD. Commercial preparations of PPD are available in different doses, standard test dose being 5 tuberculin unit dose (5 TU). Also required are a disposable glass or plastic tuberculin syringe, a short 1/4" to 1/2" 26- or 27-gauge needle.

Technique The standard 5 TU tuberculin test is performed as follows. A skin site on the volar surface of the forearm is cleaned. 0.1 mL 5 TU PPD is drawn up into a tuberculin syringe and the needle is inserted bevel upwards intradermally and a discrete wheel (5-10 mL) is produced. If the test is improperly performed, a second dose can be given at an alternate location. Test sites are examined at 24, 48, and 72 hours for the presence of induration, by palpation and inspection. The largest transverse diameter of induration is measured along the long axis of the forearm. Areas of erythema are disregarded. The following should be **carefully** recorded in the chart: Strength of PPD used, date of testing, date of reading, and size of induration. The applied method described also applies to testing with nonstandard tuberculin doses (1 TU or 250 TU).

Normal Findings No reaction to the 5 TU PPD test, but a normal skin reaction to anergy skin testing.

Critical Values Interpretation of the tuberculin skin test is highly dependent on the background diseases of the person being tested. There is no single cutoff point for interpreting a positive or negative test. In 1990, the Centers for Disease Control recommended the following scheme for interpreting results of the 5 TU PPD test.

1. A skin reaction ≥5 mm is positive in those persons with:
   - HIV infection
   - chest x-ray with fibrotic lesions likely to be old healed TB
   - recent close contact with a patient with known infectious TB
2. A skin reaction of ≥10 mm is positive in the following groups.
   - Persons with medical risk factors known to increase the risk of active TB once infection has occurred (silicosis, diabetes mellitus, corticosteroids and other immunosuppressive therapies, hematologic disease, lymphoproliferate diseases, end-stage renal disease, intestinal bypass, postgastrectomy, carcinomas of head and neck, being 10% below ideal body weight)
   - Foreign born from areas (such as Asia, Africa, Latin America) where the prevalence of TB is high
   - Low income, high-risk minorities (African-American, Hispanics, American Indians)
   - I.V. drug users
   - Residents of long-term care facilities (jails, nursing homes)
3. A skin reaction ≥15 mm is positive in all other persons, including otherwise healthy persons.

Use In general, the tuberculin skin test is used to evaluate individuals with suspected MTB infection. Testing is routinely indicated in the following situations:

- patient with clinical signs and symptoms of active tuberculosis, either pulmonary or extrapulmonary
- patient with a chest radiograph compatible with past tuberculosis
- individuals who have been recently exposed to a proven (index) case of active tuberculosis; this includes close household contacts and healthcare workers with significant exposure
- individuals who have a history of tuberculosis in the remote past, never treated
- selected patients who are to start a prolonged course of steroids (or other immunosuppressives), particularly if there has been past exposure to MTB; this includes most solid organ transplantation candidates
- patients at increased risk for developing tuberculosis on the basis of their underlying disease (eg, silicosis, gastrectomy)
- routine surveillance of persons with ongoing exposure to MTB, such as nursing personnel, respiratory therapists, etc
- immigrants from areas where MTB is endemic
- epidemiologic and public health surveys (eg, nursing homes, innercity residents, etc)

Some clinicians will skin test any patient with a serious underlying illness, such as hepatitis, cirrhosis, AIDS, peptic ulcer disease, cardiomyopathy, severe pulmonary

disease, end-stage renal failure, carcinoma, leukemia, and others. A positive tuberculin skin test in patients with these conditions is usually an indication for prolonged isoniazid prophylaxis.

Limitations For best results, trained personnel are necessary for administering and reading the test.

Contraindications Testing is contraindicated in the rare patient with known sensitivity to tuberculin. This includes severe local reactions (extensive erythema, vesiculations, ulcers) and anaphylaxis. Note that the development of local skin erythema (only) on a prior tuberculin skin test does not usually constitute a true hypersensitivity reaction. Some clinicians feel that the Mantoux test is contraindicated in the patient who has had a clearly documented positive PPD test in the past. The incidence and significance of this complication has not been studied formally; some physicians fear a hyperimmune local response when the patient is rechallenged with tuberculin.

Additional Information The tuberculin test is a measure of delayed (cellular) immunity to MTB. As such, a positive test indicates only exposure to MTB and does not distinguish current from past infections. False-positive tests may be seen with exposure to nontuberculous (atypical) *Mycobacterium* or previous inoculation with BCG vaccine. False-negative tests are common and can be difficult to interrupt. Causes for false-negative tests relate not only to the technique of administration, but also the age and immune status of the person being tested. Insignificant reactions are commonly seen secondary to anergy from immunosuppressive therapy, neoplastic disease, various bacterial or viral infections, and vaccinations. Thus, the tuberculin test is often performed along with skin tests for common antigens, such as *Candida* and mumps, to assess possible anergic states. In addition, hypersensitivity to tuberculin may diminish gradually with age. A "booster phenomenon" has been described in the elderly whereby waning tuberculin sensitivity is augmented by repeating 5 TU skin testing at 1 week intervals. Although controversy exists concerning the interpretation of both the booster phenomenon and of the standard tuberculin test itself, this test remains an invaluable aid in diagnosing tuberculous infection.

Selected Readings

Huebner RE, Schein MF, and Bass JB Jr, "The Tuberculin Skin Test," *Clin Infect Dis*, 1993, 17(6):968-75.

Reichman LB, "Tuberculin Skin Testing, The State of the Art," *Chest*, 1979, 76(6 Suppl):764-70.

Snider DE Jr, "Bacille Calmette-Guérin Vaccinations and Tuberculin Skin Tests," *JAMA*, 1985, 253(23):3438-9.

Stead WW and To T, "The Significance of the Tuberculin Skin Test in Elderly Persons," *Ann Intern Med*, 1987, 107(6):837-42.

The American Thoracic Society, "The Tuberculin Skin Test," *Am Rev Respir Dis*, 1981, 124:356-63.

Thompson NJ, Glassroth JL, Snider DE Jr, "The Booster Phenomenon in Serial Tuberculin Testing," *Am Rev Respir Dis*, 1979, 119(4):587-97.

Tularemia Serology

Synonyms *Francisella tularensis* Antibodies; Rabbit Fever Antibodies

Abstract *Francisella tularensis*, found in wild rabbits and in a number of other animals, may be transmitted to man by direct contact and by ticks and deer flies.

Specimen Serum

Container Red top tube

Collection Paired sera collected 2-3 weeks apart is recommended.

Reference Range Less than a fourfold increase in titer or single agglutination titer ≤1:40.

Critical Values Presumptive evidence for tularemia is provided by a single agglutination titer ≥1:160; a fourfold increase in titer is more convincing.

Use Investigation of illness characterized by an ulcerative lesion at a site of inoculation, with regional lymphadenopathy, fever, and pneumonia. Liver and spleen are affected. Conjunctivitis may occur. **Agglutinins represent the key laboratory evaluation in many cases.**

Limitations There is serologic cross reactivity with *Brucella* sp, *Proteus* OX-19, and *Yersinia* sp. IgM and IgG titers may remain elevated for over a decade after infection, limiting the value of unpaired specimens.

Methodology Agglutination, hemagglutination, enzyme-linked immunosorbent assay (ELISA)

Additional Information Although laboratory diagnosis of tularemia is often established by serologic methods, *F. tularensis* may be recovered in culture from a variety of clinical specimens. Blood cultures are often negative. *F. tularensis* is an extremely hazardous infectious agent responsible for several laboratory acquired infections. **If tularemia is clinically suspected, contact the laboratory so that appropriate precautions can be taken.**

Antibodies to *F. tularensis* develop 2-3 weeks after infection and peak at 4-5 weeks. Although *F. tularensis* antibodies may develop as a result of infection with cross-reacting organisms, titers are usually highest to the homologous agent.

(Continued)

Tularemia Serology *(Continued)*

Selected Readings

Fortier AH, Green SJ, Polsinelli T, et al, "Life and Death of an Intracellular Pathogen: *Francisella tularensis* and the Macrophage," *Immunol Ser*, 1994, 60:349-61.

Chu MC and Weyant RS, "*Francisella*," *Manual of Clinical Microbiology*, 8th ed, Murray PR, Baron EJ, Pfaller MA, et al, eds, Washington, DC: American Society for Microbiology, 2003, 789-808.

Tzanck Smear *see* Herpes Cytology *on page 491*

UA *see* Urinalysis *on page 606*

UBT *see Helicobacter pylori* Urea Breath Test (UBT) *on page 481*

Ultrasound, Abdomen

Synonyms Abdomen Ultrasound

Applies to Follow-up Ultrasound Abdomen; Follow-up Ultrasound Retroperitoneal; Ultrasound Retroperitoneal

Test Includes Liver, spleen, gallbladder, pancreas, and biliary tree

Patient Preparation The patient should not have had a barium study within the 3 days prior to study. The examinations may require up to 1 hour. **Note**: Ultrasound examination is usually scheduled before endoscopy, endoscopic retrograde cholangiopancreatography, colonoscopy, or a barium study. If barium study was done, bowel preparation is needed before doing ultrasound examination. **No** barium studies should have been done for **at least** 2 days preceding exam. NPO after midnight before day of examination.

Special Instructions Patients will generally be asked to remain in the radiology facility after the examination until films are reviewed by the radiologist. Ultrasound uses sound waves to image the different organs. There is **no** radiation involved, therefore, it is not harmful to the patient.

Equipment Standard B-mode real time ultrasonic imager with 2-5 MHz transducer

Technique A gel is applied to the skin and a handheld transducer is swept across the abdomen to image the appropriate organs. Sound waves are used for the imaging and no radiation exposure is present. Images are recorded on x-ray film.

Data Acquired Transverse, sagittal, and oblique images of upper abdominal organs

Causes for Rejection Bowel gas, barium, eating or drinking, unresponsive or poorly responsive patient, open wound(s) overlying area of study

Turnaround Time A written report is usually provided within 36 hours.

Normal Findings Absence of abnormal masses, fluid collections, enlarged structures, or calcifications

Use Determine the presence of neoplasms, cystic lesions, enlarged lymph nodes, bile ducts, abdominal abscesses, pancreatic mass or pseudocysts, gallbladder calculi, or any malignancies

Contraindications Open wound or incision overlying examination area, recent barium study

Additional Information Request for this study will result in imaging of liver, gallbladder, pancreas, and spleen. Individual study of any of these organs may be requested as a specific examination (eg, gallbladder, ultrasound). Solid and cystic abnormalities of each of these organs may be detected as well as adenopathy or retroperitoneal masses. It is not uncommon to be unable to visualize the pancreas and/or retroperitoneum in its entirety due to overlying bowel gas. Common abnormalities detected by this modality include cholelithiasis, biliary tree dilatation, primary carcinomas of liver, gallbladder, and pancreas as well as metastatic disease to any organ studied. Ascites as well as inflammatory masses or collections of fluid are also readily detected.

Selected Readings

Bernardino ME, "The Liver: Anatomy and Examination Techniques," *Radiology*, Taveras JT and Ferrucci JT, eds, Philadelphia, PA: JB Lippincott, 1988.

Cooperberg PL and Rowley VA, "Abdominal Sonographic Examination Technique," *Radiology*, Taveras JT and Ferrucci JT, eds, Philadelphia, PA: JB Lippincott, 1988.

Fisher AJ, Paulson EK, Sheafor DH, et al, "Small Lymph Nodes of the Abdomen, Pelvis, and Retroperitoneum: Usefulness of Sonographically Guided Biopsy," *Radiology*, 1997, 205(1):185-90.

Goldberg BB, *Abdominal Ultrasonography*, New York, NY: John Wiley and Sons Inc, 1984.

Memel DS, Dodd GD 3rd, and Esola CC, "Efficacy of Sonography as a Guidance Technique for Biopsy of Abdominal, Pelvic, and Retroperitoneal Lymph Nodes," *AJR Am J Roentgenol*, 1996, 167(4):957-62.

Netzer P, Binek J, Hammer B, et al, "Utility of Abdominal Sonography in Patients With Idiopathic Deep Vein Thrombosis," *J Clin Ultrasound*, 1999, 27(4):177-81.

Tous F and Busto M, "Assessment of Abdominal Sonography in the Diagnosis of Tumors of the Gastroduodenal Tract," *J Clin Ultrasound*, 1997, 25(5):243-7.

Ultrasound, Kidneys

Synonyms Kidneys Ultrasound; Renal Ultrasound

Test Includes Kidneys

Patient Preparation The examination may require up to 1 hour including waiting time. **Note**: Ultrasound exam to be scheduled before a barium study. If barium study was done, bowel preparation is needed before doing ultrasound examination.

Special Instructions All outpatient examinations are by appointment only. All inpatients are placed on the daily schedule as time permits and are performed as scheduled. Nonemergent examinations are given secondary priority and therefore may not be able to be performed the same day scheduled. Patients will generally be asked to remain in the radiology facility after the examination until films are reviewed by the radiologist.

Equipment Standard B-mode real time ultrasonic imager with 2-5 MHz transducer.

Technique A gel is applied to the skin and a handheld transducer is swept across the area of interest to image the appropriate organs. Sound waves are used for the imaging and no radiation exposure is present. Images are recorded on x-ray film.

Data Acquired Longitudinal and transverse images of each kidney

Causes for Rejection Patient unable to cooperate with positioning and respiratory maneuvers; bowel gas, barium, obesity

Turnaround Time A written report usually provided within 36 hours.

Use Evaluate cysts and neoplasms, calcifications, abscess, and hydronephrosis and hydroureter

Additional Information Rapid, sensitive evaluation for the presence of hydronephrosis. Useful in confirming the cystic nature of lesions. Detection of hydroureter is often problematic.

Selected Readings

Goldberg BB, *Abdominal Ultrasonography*, New York, NY: John Wiley and Sons Inc, 1984.

Grant DC, "Ultrasound of the Genitourinary Tract," *Radiology*, Taveras JT and Ferrucci JT, eds, Philadelphia, PA: JB Lippincott, 1988.

Nass K and O'Neill WC, "Bedside Renal Biopsy: Ultrasound Guidance by the Nephrologist," *Am J Kidney Dis*, 1999, 34(5):955-9.

Platt JF, Rubin JM, and Ellis JH, "Lupus Nephritis: Predictive Value of Conventional and Doppler US and Comparison With Serologic and Biopsy Parameters," *Radiology*, 1997, 203(1):82-6.

Richter F, Kasabian NG, Irwin RJ Jr, et al, "Accuracy of Diagnosis by Guided Biopsy of Renal Mass Lesions Classified Indeterminate by Imaging Studies," *Urology*, 2000, 55(3):348-52.

Ultrasound, Peripheral Arteries and Veins

Synonyms Iliac Arteries Ultrasound; Peripheral Arteries and Veins Ultrasound; Popliteal Ultrasound

Test Includes Peripheral arteries and/or veins

Patient Preparation The examination may require up to 1 hour.

Special Instructions Specific vessels of interest to be studied as well as location must be specified. Patients will generally be asked to remain in the radiology facility after the examination until films are reviewed by the radiologist.

Equipment Standard B-mode real time ultrasonic imager with Doppler capability with 5-10 MHz transducer.

Technique A gel is applied to the skin and a handheld transducer is swept across the area of interest to image the appropriate organs. Sound waves are used for the imaging and no radiation exposure is present. Images are recorded on x-ray film.

Turnaround Time A written report is usually provided within 36 hours.

Normal Findings Presence of appropriate flow, compressibility of venous structures

Use Determine aneurysm, cysts, pseudoaneurysm, deep vein thrombosis (DVT), arterial insufficiency

Additional Information Examination is valuable in the detection of pseudoaneurysms, aneurysms, arterial insufficiency, and deep venous thrombosis (DVT)

Selected Readings

Bimbaum Y, Fishbein MC, Luo H, et al, "Regional Remodeling of Atherosclerotic Arteries: A Major Determinant of Clinical Manifestations of Disease," *J Am Coll Cardiol*, 1997, 30(5):1149-64.

Keyes LE, Frazee BW, Snoey ER, et al, "Ultrasound-Guided Brachial and Basilic Vein Cannulation in Emergency Department Patients With Difficult Intravenous Access," *Ann Emerg Med*, 1999, 34(6):711-4.

Libertiny G and Hands L, "Lower Limb Deep Vein Flow in Patients With Peripheral Vascular Disease," *J Vasc Surg*, 1999, 29(6):1065-70.

Sofocleous CT, Schur I, Cooper SG, et al, "Sonographically Guided Placement of Peripherally Inserted Central Venous Catheters: Review of 355 Procedures," *AJR Am J Roentgenol*, 1998, 170(6):1613-6.

Ultrasound Retroperitoneal *see* Ultrasound, Abdomen *on page 604*

Undulant Fever, Culture *see* Blood Culture, *Brucella on page 394*

Unidimensional Echo *see* Echocardiography, M-Mode *on page 445*

Urea Breath Test *see Helicobacter pylori* Urea Breath Test (UBT) *on page 481*

***Ureaplasma urealyticum* Culture** *see Mycoplasma/Ureaplasma* Culture *on page 545*

***Ureaplasma urealyticum* Culture, Genital** *see* Genital Culture for *Ureaplasma urealyticum on page 471*

Urease Test and Culture, *Helicobacter pylori* *see* *Helicobacter pylori* Culture and Urease Test *on page 479*

Urethral *Chlamydia* Culture *see* *Chlamydia* Culture *on page 413*

Urethral Culture for *Neisseria gonorrhoeae* *see* *Neisseria gonorrhoeae* Culture *on page 547*

Urethral Culture for T-Strain *Mycoplasma* *see* Genital Culture for *Ureaplasma urealyticum on page 471*

Urethral *Trichomonas* Smear *see* *Trichomonas* Preparation *on page 600*

Urethra, *Mycoplasma* Culture *see* *Mycoplasma/Ureaplasma* Culture *on page 545*

Urinalysis

Synonyms UA

Applies to Casts, Urine; Crystals, Urine; Occult Blood, Semiquantitative, Urine; Urine Crystals

Test Includes Opacity, color, appearance, specific gravity, pH, protein, glucose, occult blood, ketones, bilirubin, and in some laboratories, urobilinogen and microscopic examination of urine sediment. Some laboratories include screening for leukocyte esterase and nitrite and do not perform a microscopic examination unless one of the chemical screening (macroscopic) tests is abnormal or unless a specific request for microscopic examination is made.

Abstract The examination of urine is one of the oldest practices in medicine. A carefully performed urinalysis still provides a wealth of information about the patient, both in terms of differential diagnosis, and by exclusion of many conditions when the urinalysis is "normal."

Patient Preparation Instructions should be given in method of collection. Both males and females need instruction in cleansing the urethral meatus. "Midstream collections" are performed by initiating urination into the toilet, then bringing the collection device into the urine stream to catch the midportion of the void.

Specimen Urine

Container Plastic urine container

Urinalysis

Test	Reference Range
Specific gravity	1.003-1.029
pH	4.5-7.8
Protein	Negative
Glucose	Negative
Ketones	Negative
Bilirubin	Negative
Occult blood	Negative
Leukocyte esterase	Negative
Nitrite	Negative
Urobilinogen	0.1-1.0 EU/dL
WBCs	0-4/hpf
RBCs	male: 0-3/hpf female: 0-5/hpf
Casts	0-4/lpf hyaline
Bacteria	Negative

hpf = high power field.
lpf = low power field.
EU = Ehrlich units.

Collection A voided specimen is usually suitable. If the specimen is likely to be contaminated by vaginal discharge or hemorrhage, a clean catch specimen is desirable. If the specimen is collected by catheter, it should be so labeled. The timing of urine collection will vary with the purpose of the test. To check for casts or renal concentration ability, a first voided morning specimen may be preferred. For screening purposes, this is also the best time, as a later and more dilute specimen may make small increases in protein, RBC, or WBC excretion harder to detect. The upright position increases protein excretion by hemodynamic factors. Midmorning urine is likely to give the highest albumin excretion, but early morning urine is best when attempting to detect Bence Jones protein.

Storage Instructions Transport specimen to the laboratory as soon as possible after collection. If the specimen cannot be processed immediately by the laboratory it

should be refrigerated. Refrigeration preserves formed elements in the urine, but may precipitate crystals not originally present.

Causes for Rejection Specimen delayed in transport, fecal contamination, decomposition, or bacterial overgrowth

Reference Range See table. **Crystals** are interpreted by the physician. Warm, freshly voided urine sediment from normal subjects almost never contains crystals, despite maximal concentration. Xanthine, cystine, and uric acid crystal (and stone) formation is favored by a consistently acid urine (pH <5.5-6). Calcium oxalate and apatite stones are associated with no particular disturbance of urine pH. Calcium carbonate, calcium phosphate, and especially magnesium ammonium phosphate stones are associated with pH >7. Urine pH >7.5 may briefly follow meals (alkaline tide) but more commonly indicate systemic alkali intake ($NaHCO_3$, etc) or urine infected by bacteria which split urea to ammonia.

Possible Panic Range The presence of massive amounts of oxalate crystals in fresh urine should be reported promptly to the physician, as this finding may represent ethylene glycol intoxication.

Use Screen for abnormalities of urine; diagnose and manage renal diseases, urinary tract infection, urinary tract neoplasms, systemic diseases, and inflammatory or neoplastic diseases adjacent to the urinary tract

Limitations Insufficient volume, less than 2 mL, may limit the extent of procedures performed. Metabolites of Pyridium® may interfere with the dipstick reactions by producing color interference. High vitamin C intake may cause an underestimate of glucosuria, or a false-negative nitrate test. Survival of WBCs is decreased by low osmolality, alkalinity, and lack of refrigeration. Formed elements in the urine including casts disintegrate rapidly, therefore the specimen should be analyzed as soon as possible after collection. Specific gravity is affected by glucosuria, mannitol infusion, or prior administration of iodinated contrast material for radiologic studies (IVP dye). Some brands of test strips give a "trace positive" protein indication if not stored in dry atmosphere (cap of test strip bottle not on tight). Ambient humidity exposure of the test strips over time also causes some reduction of sensitivity for occult blood and nitrate and increased sensitivity for glucose (false-positive). This can be detected by using tap water as a negative control. False-positive tests for protein can also be due to contamination of the urine by an ammonium-containing cleansing solution. Problems relevant to the sensitivity of protein detection have led to development of methods described in the listing Microalbuminuria.

Methodology The chemical portion of the urinalysis is done by test strip, with confirming chemical method for protein (sulfosalicylic acid precipitation).

Additional Information

MICROSCOPY:

Crystalluria is frequently observed in urine specimens stored at room temperature or refrigerated. Such crystals are diagnostically useful when observed in warm, fresh urine by a physician evaluating microhematuria, nephrolithiasis, or toxin ingestion.

In abundance, **calcium oxalate** and/or **hippurate crystals** may suggest ethylene glycol ingestion (especially if known to be accompanied by neurological abnormalities, appearance of drunkenness, hypertension, and a high anion gap acidosis.) Urine is usually supersaturated in calcium oxalate, often in calcium phosphate, and acid urine is often saturated in uric acid. Yet crystalluria is uncommon (in warm, fresh urine) because of the normal presence of crystal inhibitors, the lack of available nidus, and the time factor. When properly observed in fresh urine, crystals may provide a clue to the composition of renal stones even not yet passed, the nidus for such stones, or, as such, have been associated with microhematuria.

Uric acid crystals are reddish brown, rectangular, rhomboidal, or flower-like structures of narrow rectangular petals. **Ammonium urates,** in alkaline urine, are irregular blobs and crescents, sometimes resembling fragmented red cell shapes.

Calcium oxalate crystals are fairly uniform small double pyramids, base to base, which under the microscope look like little crosses on a square.

Calcium phosphate crystallizes in urine as flowers of narrow rectangular needles.

Cystine crystals, uniquely in urine, form large irregular hexagonal plates, which may dissolve if alkalinized. They occur only in the urine of subjects with cystinuria.

Calcium magnesium ammonium phosphate, or "triple phosphate," forms unique "coffin lid" angularly domed rectangles which may be present in massive quantities in alkaline urine. They usually are associated with urine infected by urea splitting bacteria which cause "infection," or "triple phosphate" stones.

Leukocyturia may indicate inflammatory disease in the genitourinary tract, including bacterial infection, glomerulonephritis, chemical injury, autoimmune diseases, or

(Continued)

Urinalysis *(Continued)*

inflammatory disease adjacent to the urinary tract such as appendicitis or diverticulitis.

White cell casts indicate the renal origin of leukocytes, and are most frequently found in acute pyelonephritis. White cell casts are also found in glomerulonephritis such as lupus nephritis, and in acute and chronic interstitial nephritis. When nuclei degenerate, such leukocyte casts resemble renal tubular casts.

Red cell casts indicate renal origin of hematuria and suggest glomerulonephritis, including lupus nephritis. Red cell casts may also be found in subacute bacterial endocarditis, renal infarct, vasculitis, Goodpasture's syndrome, sickle cell disease, and in malignant hypertension. Degenerated red cell casts may be called **"hemoglobin casts"**. Orange to red casts may be found with myoglobinuria as well.

Dysmorphic red cells are observed in glomerulonephritis. "Dysmorphic" red cells refer to heterogeneous sizes, hypochromia, distorted irregular outlines and frequently small blobs extruding from the cell membrane. Phase contrast microscopy best demonstrates RBC and WBC morphology. Nonglomerular urinary red blood cells resemble peripheral circulating red blood cells. Schramek et al have used the presence or absence of dysmorphic red cells to direct the degree of work-up for hematuria and for follow-up.

Crenated RBCs provide no implication regarding RBC source.

Dark brown or smoky urine suggests a renal source of hematuria.

A **pink or red urine** suggests an extrarenal source.

Hyaline casts occur in physiologic states (eg, after exercise) and many types of renal diseases. They are best seen in phase contrast microscopy or with reduced illumination.

Renal tubular (epithelial) casts are most suggestive of tubular injury, as in acute tubular necrosis. They are also found in other disorders, including eclampsia, heavy metal poisoning, ethylene glycol intoxication, and acute allograft rejection.

Granular casts: Very finely granulated casts may be found after exercise and in a variety of glomerular and tubulointerstitial diseases; coarse granular casts are abnormal and are present in a wide variety of renal diseases.

"Dirty brown" granular casts are typical of acute tubular necrosis.

Waxy casts are found especially in chronic renal diseases, and are associated with chronic renal failure; they occur in diabetic nephropathy, malignant hypertension, and glomerulonephritis, among other conditions. They are named for their waxy or glossy appearance. They often appear brittle and cracked.

Fatty casts are generally found in the nephrotic syndromes, diabetic nephropathy, other forms of chronic renal diseases, and glomerulonephritis. The fat droplets originate in renal tubular cells when they exceed their capacity to reabsorb protein of glomerular origin. Their inclusions have the features and significance of oval fat bodies.

Broad casts originate from dilated, chronically damaged tubules or the collecting ducts. They can be granular or waxy. **Broad waxy casts** are called "renal failure casts."

Spermatozoa may be seen in male urine related to recent or retrograde ejaculation. In female urine, the presence of spermatozoa may provide evidence of vaginal contamination following recent intercourse.

Automation of the urinalysis is routine in many laboratories. Some authors wish to abandon microscopic evaluation of the urine, which is not easily automated, on urine samples testing "normal" by dipstick screening. A urine sample that is normal to inspection and dipstick will be normal to microscopic exam 95% of the time.

One instrument for automating the entire urinalysis, the Yellow IRIS®, includes a module that automates the microscopic sediment exam. This has been found to be more consistent than the manual method for routine urinalysis and has increased the number of abnormal urines detected.

Selected Readings

Carlson D and Statland BE, "Automated Urinalysis," *Clin Lab Med*, 1988, 8(3):449-61.

Cohen HT and Spiegel DM, "Air-Exposed Urine Dipsticks Give False-Positive Results for Glucose and False-Negative Results for Blood," *Am J Clin Pathol*, 1991, 96(3):398-400.

Haber MH, "Quality Assurance in Urinalysis," *Clin Lab Med*, 1988, 8(3):431-47.

Haber MH, *Urinary Sediment: A Textbook Atlas*, American Society of Clinical Pathologists, 1981.

Kiel DP and Moskowitz MA, "The Urinalysis: A Critical Appraisal," *Med Clin North Am*, 1987, 71(4):607-24.

Mariani AJ, Luangphinith S, Loo S, et al, "Dipstick Chemical Urinalysis: An Accurate Cost-Effective Screening Test," *J Urol*, 1984, 132(1):64-6.

Rizzoni G, Braggion F, and Zacchello G, "Evaluation of Glomerular and Nonglomerular Hematuria by Phase Contrast Microscopy," *J Pediatr*, 1983, 103:370-4.

Roe CE, Carlson DA, Daigneault RW, et al, "Evaluation of the Yellow IRIS®. An Automated Method for Urinalysis," *Am J Clin Pathol*, 1986, 86(5):661-5.

Schramek P, Schuster FX, Georgopoulos M, et al, "Value of Urinary Erythrocyte Morphology in Assessment of Symptomless Microhaematuria," *Lancet*, 1989, 2(8675):1316-9.

Schumann GB, "Cytodiagnostic Urinalysis for the Nephrology Practice," *Semin Nephrol*, 1986, 6(4):308-45.

Scott JH, "Abnormal Urinalysis in Appendicitis," *J Urol*, 1983, 129:1015.

Segasothy M, Lau TM, Birch DF, et al, "Immunocytologic Dissection of the Urine Sediment Using Monoclonal Antibodies," *Am J Clin Pathol*, 1988, 90(6):691-6.

Sheets C and Lyman JL, "Urinalysis," *Emerg Med Clin North Am*, 1986, 4(2):263-80.

Shenoy UA, "Current Assessment of Microhematuria and Leukocyturia," *Clin Lab Med*, 1985, 5:317-29, (review).

Threatti GA and Henry JB, "Urine and Other Body Fluids," *Clinical Diagnosis and Management by Laboratory Methods*, Henry JB, ed, Philadelphia, PA: WB Saunders Co, 2001, 367-401.

Wargotz ES, Hyde JE, Karcher DS, et al, "Urine Sediment Analysis by the Yellow IRIS® Automated Urinalysis Workstation," *Am J Clin Pathol*, 1987, 88(6):746-8.

Wenz B and Lampasso JA, "Eliminating Unnecessary Urine Microscopy - Results and Performance Characteristics of an Algorithm Based on Chemical Reagent Strip Testing," *Am J Clin Pathol*, 1989, 92(1):78-81.

Yager HM and Harrington JT, "Urinalysis and Urinary Electrolytes," *The Principles and Practice of Nephrology*, Chapter 28, Jacobson HR, Striker GE, and Klahr S, eds, Philadelphia, PA: BC Decker Inc, 1991, 167-77.

Urine Crystals *see* Urinalysis *on page 606*

Urine Culture *see* Urine Culture, Clean Catch *on page 609*

Urine Culture, Clean Catch

Synonyms CMVS, Culture; Midstream Urine Culture; Urine Culture; Urine Culture, Midvoid Specimen

Applies to Urine Culture, Foley Catheter

Patient Preparation Thoroughly instruct patient for proper collection of "clean catch" specimen. Wash hands thoroughly. Wash penis or vulva using downward strokes four times with four soapy sponges, then once with sponge wet with warm water. Urethral meatus and perineum must be washed. Each sponge must be discarded after one use. Urinate about 30 mL (1 ounce) of urine directly into toilet or bedpan and take middle portion of urine sample. Screw cap securely on container without touching the inside rim. Apply the completed patient label to the specimen cup. Most patients, with instruction, do better with privacy than with an attendant.

Specimen Random urine

Container Plastic urine container or sterile tube

Collection Early morning specimens yield highest bacterial counts from overnight incubation in the bladder. Forced fluids dilute the urine and may cause reduced colony counts. Hair from perineum will contaminate the specimen. The stream from a male may be contaminated by bacteria from beneath the prepuce. Bacteria from vaginal secretions, vulva or distal urethra may also contaminate the specimen as may organisms from hands or clothing. Receptacle must be sterile.

Storage Instructions The specimen should be refrigerated if it cannot be promptly transported to the laboratory. A transport stabilizer may be used to preserve the specimen if refrigeration is not available.

Causes for Rejection Unrefrigerated specimen more than 2 hours old may be subject to overgrowth, may not yield valid results, and will be rejected.

Turnaround Time Preliminary reports are usually available at 24 hours. Cultures with no growth are usually reported after 24 hours. Reports on specimens from which an organism or organisms have been isolated require a minimum of 48 hours for completion.

Reference Range No growth. Significant bacteriuria is usually considered to be $\geq 10^4$ CFU/mL (colony forming units). A break point of 10^2 maximizes diagnostic sensitivity. Urethral contamination particularly in women may cause colony counts of 10^3 or 10^4; thus, a breakpoint of 10^2 CFU/mL causes inclusion of a large number of normal women without significant bacteriuria.

Use Isolate and identify potentially pathogenic organisms causing urinary tract infection

Limitations Bacteria present in numbers $\geq 10^4$ CFU/mL may not be detected by routine methods used by most clinical microbiology labs.

Methodology Quantitative aerobic culture

Additional Information A single culture is about 80% accurate in the female; two containing the same organism with count of 10^5 or more represents 95% chance of true bacteriuria; three such specimens mean virtual certainty of true bacteriuria. Urinary tract infection is significantly higher in women who use diaphragm-spermicide contraception, perhaps secondary to increased vaginal pH and a higher frequency of vaginal colonization with *E. coli.* A single clean voided specimen from an adult male
(Continued)

Urine Culture, Clean Catch *(Continued)*

may be considered diagnostic with proper preparation and care in specimen collection. If the patient is receiving antimicrobial therapy at the time the specimen is collected, any level of bacteriuria may be significant. When more than two organisms are recovered, the likelihood of contamination is high; thus, the significance of definitive identification of the organisms and susceptibility testing in this situation is severely limited. A repeat culture with proper specimen collection patient preparation is often indicated. Periodic screening of diabetics and pregnant women for asymptomatic bacteriuria has been recommended. Cultures of specimens from Foley catheters yielding multiple organisms with high colony counts may represent colonization of the catheter and not true significant bacteriuria. Most laboratories limit the number of organisms which will be identified when recovered from urine to two and similarly do not routinely perform susceptibility tests on isolates from presumably contaminated specimens.

Failure to recover aerobic organisms from patients with pyuria or positive Gram stains of urinary sediment may indicate the presence of mycobacteria or anaerobes.

Selected Readings

Aughey DR and Aschbacher C, "Evaluating Dysuria in Adolescent Females," *Minn Med*, 2005, 88(5):50-1.

Bitsori M, Maraki S, Raissaki M, et al, "Community-Acquired Enterococcal Urinary Tract Infections," *Pediatr Nephrol*, 2005, Jun 22; [Epub ahead of print].

Stamm WE, Counts GW, Running KR, et al, "Diagnosis of Coliform Infection in Acutely Dysuric Women," *N Engl J Med*, 1982, 307(8):462-8.

Stamm WE, Hooton TM, Johnson JR, et al, "Urinary Tract Infections: From Pathogenesis to Treatment," *J Infect Dis*, 1989, 159(3):400-6.

Urine Culture, First Voided, for *Neisseria gonorrhoeae* *see Neisseria gonorrhoeae* Culture *on page 547*

Urine Culture, Foley Catheter *see* Urine Culture, Clean Catch *on page 609*

Urine Culture, Midvoid Specimen *see* Urine Culture, Clean Catch *on page 609*

Urine for Parasites *see* Ova and Parasites, Urine or Aspirates *on page 554*

Urine for *Schistosoma haematobium* *see* Ova and Parasites, Urine or Aspirates *on page 554*

Urine Fungus Culture *see* Fungus Culture, Urine *on page 468*

Urine *Legionella* Antigen *see Legionella* Antigen, Urine *on page 514*

Urine, *Mycoplasma* Culture *see Mycoplasma/Ureaplasma* Culture *on page 545*

Urine *Trichomonas* Wet Mount *see Trichomonas* Preparation *on page 600*

Urodynamic Testing of Bladder Function *see* Cystometrogram, Simple *on page 434*

Urography

Synonyms Infusion Pyelogram; Intravenous Pyelogram; IVP

Test Includes Intravenous administration of a contrast material. The contrast material is concentrated and excreted by the kidneys. Appropriate radiographs are exposed during the concentration and excretion of the contrast material for evaluation of the morphology and function of the urinary tract.

Patient Preparation Patients are encouraged to take nothing by mouth after midnight the night before the examination. This degree of fluid restriction will not produce significant dehydration but will improve the overall quality of the examination. If the urography examination is to be performed in the afternoon, a light liquid breakfast may be consumed. Views on the necessity and the usefulness of cathartics in the preparation of patients for urography vary. Some physicians advocate the routine use of 10 oz of magnesium citrate the evening before the examination. Alternatives would include a mild laxative such as $1^1/_4$ oz of a standard extract of senna fruit the evening before the examination.

Aftercare Encourage hydration by fluid ingestion.

Special Instructions All patients undergoing this examination should be questioned specifically with regard to drug allergies, particularly iodine. A recent serum creatinine is requested on patients 60 years of age or older, those with significant atherosclerotic disease, those with a known diagnosis of diabetes mellitus or with known pre-existing renal disease.

Complications Reactions to contrast material and specific treatment for such reactions are beyond the scope of this handbook. An appropriately equipped emergency cart should be immediately available should resuscitation be necessary.

Equipment Overhead radiography tube with float top table. Tomographic capabilities are desirable.

Use This examination accurately demonstrates normal anatomy and a wide range of abnormalities involving the urinary tract.

Limitations Urography should be performed prior to barium studies of the gastrointestinal tract. The presence of barium within the abdomen will compromise the urographic examination.

Contraindications Allergy to iodine or a previous serious adverse reaction, advanced renal failure. A known diagnosis of multiple myeloma constitutes a relative contraindication. Every attempt should be made to hydrate patients with multiple myeloma or diabetes mellitus prior to performance of a urogram as these patients run an increased risk of acute renal failure. Helical CT may be considered as an alternative for these patients.

Selected Readings

Hattery RR, Williamson B Jr, Hartman GW, et al, "Intravenous Urographic Technique," *Radiology*, 1988, 167(3):593-9.

Katzberg RW, "Urography into the 21st Century: New Contrast Media, Renal Handling, Imaging Characteristics, and Nephrotoxicity," *Radiology*, 1997, 204(2):297-312.

Miller DL, Chang R, Wells WT, et al, "Intravascular Contrast Media: Effect of Dose on Renal Function," *Radiology*, 1988, 167(3):607-11.

Sourtzis S, Thibeau JF, Damry N, et al, "Radiologic Investigation of Renal Colic: Unenhanced Helical CT Compared With Excretory Urography," *AJR Am J Roentgenol*, 1999, 172(6):1491-4.

Vaginal Culture *see* Genital Culture *on page 470*

Vaginal Culture *Neisseria gonorrhoeae* *see Neisseria gonorrhoeae* Culture *on page 547*

Vaginal *Trichomonas* Smear *see Trichomonas* Preparation *on page 600*

Vancocin®, Blood *see* Vancomycin Level *on page 611*

Vancoled®, Blood *see* Vancomycin Level *on page 611*

Vancomycin Level

Related Information

Antibiotic Level, Serum *on page 375*

Synonyms Vancocin®, Blood; Vancoled®, Blood

Abstract Vancomycin is an antimicrobial agent with potent activity against most gram-positive bacteria. Its use has occasionally been associated with nephrotoxicity and/or ototoxicity, though the frequency of these toxicities has decreased as vancomycin preparations have become more purified.

Specimen Serum, body fluid

Container Red top tube, sterile fluid container

Sampling Time Peak: 30 minutes following dose; trough: immediately prior to next dose

Storage Instructions Separate serum using aseptic technique and place in freezer

Causes for Rejection Specimen more than 4 hours old

Reference Range Therapeutic concentration: peak: 20-40 mcg/mL (SI: 14-27 μmol/L) (depends in part on minimum inhibitory concentration of organism being treated); trough: 5-10 mcg/mL (SI: 3.4-6.8 μmol/L)

Possible Panic Range Toxic: >80 mcg/mL (>54 μmol/L)

Use Monitor therapeutic levels and potential toxicities, particularly in patients with impaired renal function and in patients also being treated with aminoglycoside antibiotics

Methodology High performance liquid chromatography (HPLC), gas-liquid chromatography (GLC), immunoassay

Additional Information Vancomycin is currently being used in its intravenous form to treat a variety of gram-positive bacterial infections, particularly those due to methicillin-resistant staphylococci. Additionally, vancomycin is often used in its oral form to treat pseudomembranous colitis due to *Clostridium difficile*. When administered orally, serum vancomycin levels are undetectable due to poor absorption from the gastrointestinal tract. When administered intravenously, vancomycin may be ototoxic and nephrotoxic, though nephrotoxicity is rare with newer preparations. Ototoxicity is seen primarily in patients with extremely high serum concentrations (80-100 mcg/mL; SI: 54-68 μmol/L) and rarely occurs when serum concentrations are maintained at ≤30 mcg/mL (SI: 20 μmol/L). Both oto- and nephrotoxicity are enhanced by concurrent administration of aminoglycosides.

Selected Readings

Fogarty KA and McClain WJ, "Vancomycin: Current Perspectives and Guidelines for Use in the NICU," *Neonatal Netw*, 1989, 7(5):31-5.

Hammett-Stabler CA and Johns T, "Laboratory Guidelines for Monitoring of Antimicrobial Drugs. National Academy of Clinical Biochemistry," *Clin Chem*, 1998, 44(5):1129-40.

Ingerman MJ and Santoro J, "Vancomycin. A New Old Agent," *Infect Dis Clin North Am*, 1989, 3(3):641-51.

Levine JF, "Vancomycin: A Review," *Med Clin North Am*, 1987, 71(6):1135-45.

Wilhelm MP and Estes L, "Symposium on Antimicrobial Agents - Part XII. Vancomycin," *Mayo Clin Proc*, 1999, 74(9):928-35.

Varicella-Zoster Serology *see* Varicella-Zoster Virus Serology *on page 612*

Varicella-Zoster Virus Culture

Related Information

Skin Biopsy *on page 580*
Varicella-Zoster Virus Serology *on page 612*

Synonyms Chickenpox Culture; Shingles Culture

Applies to Viral Culture, Rash; Viral Culture, Skin

Test Includes Culture for VZV only; VZV also is usually detected in a routine/general virus culture

Specimen Swab specimens of the base of fresh, unroofed lesions, vesicle fluid, vesicle scrapings. In addition, acute and convalescent sera should be collected at appropriate times to document a clinically significant rise in antibody titer.

Container Cold viral transport medium

Sampling Time Specimens should be collected during the acute phase of the disease (within 3 days of lesion eruption).

Collection Unroofed lesions should be cleaned before specimens are taken. Vesicle fluid from several vesicles can be pooled and added to viral transport medium. Alternatively, the bases of several freshly unroofed lesions can be vigorously sampled with a sterile swab which subsequently should be placed into cold viral transport medium and sent to the laboratory as soon as possible.

Storage Instructions Keep specimens cold and moist. **Do not freeze specimens.**

Causes for Rejection Dry specimen, specimen not refrigerated during transport, specimen fixed in formalin, unlabeled specimen

Turnaround Time Variable (1-14 days) and depends on cell culture method used and amount of virus in the specimen

Reference Range No virus isolated

Use Aid in the diagnosis of disease caused by varicella-zoster virus (ie, chickenpox and shingles)

Methodology Inoculation of specimens into cell cultures, incubation of cultures, observation of characteristic cytopathic effect, and identification by fluorescent monoclonal antibody

Some laboratories offer molecular testing for this organism. Contact the testing laboratory for the availability of amplified and nonamplified qualitative and quantitative molecular tests for this organism, and for information on selection and collection of appropriate specimens for specific molecular tests.

Additional Information Varicella-zoster virus is a single virus which causes two diseases: **chickenpox** (varicella) in children and, after reactivation from latency, **shingles** (zoster) in adults.

Disease caused by VZV is usually self-limited. However, the disease can be life-threatening in pregnant persons, immunocompromised persons, and children who receive cancer therapy. In addition, congenital chickenpox can result in neonatal systemic disease and/or congenital malformations.

Serology for the detection of VZV antibodies is available. Rapid turnaround time of serological tests can be especially important in detecting the presence of antibody (prior exposure) in pregnant persons who have been exposed to persons with chickenpox because VZIG (varicella immune globulin) should be given within 3 days (maximum) of exposure.

Cell culture of VZV is considered less sensitive than direct antigen detection of VZV by immunofluorescence.

Selected Readings

Arvin A, "Aging, Immunity, and the Varicella-Zoster Virus," *N Engl J Med*, 2005, 352(22):2266-7.
Hambleton S, "Chickenpox," *Curr Opin Infect Dis*, 2005, 18(3):235-40.
Leung TF, Chik KW, Li CK, et al, "Incidence, Risk Factors and Outcome of Varicella-Zoster Virus Infection in Children After Haematopoietic Stem Cell Transplantation," *Bone Marrow Transplant*, 2000, 25(2):167-72.
Sauerbrei A, Eichhorn U, Schacke M, et al, "Laboratory Diagnosis of Herpes Zoster," *J Clin Virol*, 1999, 14(1):31-6.
Schmader K, "Herpes Zoster in Older Adults," *Clin Infect Dis*, 2001, 32(10):1481-6.
Strommen GL, Pucino F, Tight RR, et al, "Human Infection With Herpes Zoster: Etiology, Pathophysiology, Diagnosis, Clinical Course, and Treatment," *Pharmacotherapy*, 1988, 8(1):52-68.
Whitley RJ, "Changing Dynamics of Varicella-Zoster Virus Infections in the 21st Century: The Impact of Vaccination," *J Infect Dis*, 2005, 191(12):1999-2001.

Varicella-Zoster Virus, Direct Detection *see* Virus Detection by DFA *on page 619*

Varicella-Zoster Virus Serology

Related Information

Skin Biopsy *on page 580*
Varicella-Zoster Virus Culture *on page 612*

Synonyms Chickenpox Titer; Zoster Titer

Applies to Herpes Zoster Serology; Varicella-Zoster Serology

Special Instructions Acute and convalescent sera drawn 10-14 days apart are recommended.

Specimen Serum

Container Red top tube

Reference Range A single low titer or less than a fourfold increase in titer in paired sera by complement fixation; undetectable antibody by FAMA test

Use Establish the diagnosis of varicella-zoster infection; determine adult susceptibility to infection

Limitations Complement fixation test is insensitive and has heterologous reactions with herpesvirus

Methodology Fluorescent antibody to membrane antigen (FAMA), hemagglutination (HA), complement fixation (CF), enzyme-linked immunosorbent assay (ELISA)

If serological testing is performed by enzyme immunoassay (EIA) on automated instrumentation, results are usually given in index units, not titers. In such cases, significant rises in antibody levels are determined by algorithms within the instrumentation, not by increases in titers.

Additional Information Although most cases of varicella or zoster are clinically unambiguous, serology may be occasionally useful in the differential diagnosis of other blistering illnesses or when infection shows an unusual complication, such as hepatitis. It may also be important to establish whether an individual is susceptible when clinical history is unclear, or when VZIG (varicella immune globulin) may be needed, as in the immunocompromised host or cancer patient on toxic chemotherapy.

Zoster is more common with aging and may occur in the face of significant antibody titers, demonstrating that cell-mediated immunity is also significant.

Selected Readings

Leung TF, Chik KW, Li CK, et al, "Incidence, Risk Factors and Outcome of Varicella-Zoster Virus Infection in Children After Haematopoietic Stem Cell Transplantation," *Bone Marrow Transplant*, 2000, 25(2):167-72.

Schmader K, "Herpes Zoster in Older Adults," *Clin Infect Dis*, 2001, 32(10):1481-6.

Straus SE, Ostrove JM, Inchauspe G, et al, "Varicella-Zoster Virus Infections: Biology, Natural History, Treatment, and Prevention," *Ann Intern Med*, 1988, 108(2):221-36.

VDRL, Cerebrospinal Fluid

Related Information

Cerebrospinal Fluid Analysis *on page 408*
Darkfield Examination, Syphilis *on page 444*
FTA-ABS, Cerebrospinal Fluid *on page 457*
FTA-ABS, Serum *on page 457*
RPR *on page 574*

Synonyms Cerebrospinal Fluid VDRL; CSF VDRL; Serologic Test for Syphilis, CSF; Spinal Fluid VDRL; VDRL, CSF

Test Includes Titer of reactive specimens

Specimen Cerebrospinal fluid

Container Clean, sterile container or glass tube

Reference Range Nonreactive

Use Test for syphilis, neurosyphilis

Limitations VDRL, CSF is the only laboratory test for neurosyphilis approved by the Center for Disease Control. It is quite specific and has acceptable sensitivity.

Methodology Flocculation test detects reagin, antibody to nontreponemal antigen

Additional Information A positive VDRL in a spinal fluid uncontaminated by serum is essentially diagnostic of neurosyphilis. However, a negative test may occur in 30% of patients with tabes dorsalis. The CSF VDRL may take years to become nonreactive after adequate therapy. In AIDS patients, serial CSF VDRL determinations may be needed when neurosyphilis is suspected. By requiring either a positive serum RPR or FTA-ABS, seropositivity of CSF VDRL could increase to 90%.

Selected Readings

Albright RE Jr, Christenson RH, Emlet JL, et al, "Issues in Cerebrospinal Fluid Management. CSF Venereal Disease Research Laboratory Testing," *Am J Clin Pathol*, 1991, 95(3):397-401.

Davis LE and Schmitt JW, "Clinical Significance of Cerebrospinal Fluid Tests for Neurosyphilis," *Ann Neurol*, 1989, 25(1):50-5.

Hart G, "Syphilis Tests in Diagnostic and Therapeutic Decision Making," *Ann Intern Med*, 1986, 104(3):368-76.

Singh AE and Romanowski B, "Syphilis: Review With Emphasis on Clinical Epidemiologic, and Some Biologic Features," *Clin Microbiol Rev*, 1999, 12(2):187-209.

Wicher V and Wicher K, "Pathogenesis of Maternal-Fetal Syphilis Revisited," *Clin Infect Dis*, 2001, 33(3):354-63.

VDRL, CSF *see* VDRL, Cerebrospinal Fluid *on page 613*

Venous Catheter Culture *see* Intravenous Line Culture *on page 511*

Ventricular Fluid Culture *see* Aerobic Culture, Cerebrospinal Fluid *on page 366*

Verocytotoxin Producing *E. coli*, Stool Culture *see* Stool Culture, Diarrheagenic *E. coli on page 587*

***Vibrio cholerae*, Stool Culture** *see* Stool Culture, Uncommon Organisms *on page 588*

***Vibrio parahaemolyticus*, Stool Culture** *see* Stool Culture, Uncommon Organisms *on page 588*

Viral Antigen Detection, Direct, Stool *see* Rotavirus, Direct Detection *on page 573*

Viral Culture, Brain *see* Viral Culture, Central Nervous System Symptoms *on page 614*

Viral Culture, Bronchial Wash *see* Viral Culture, Throat *on page 617*

Viral Culture, Central Nervous System Symptoms

Related Information

Cerebrospinal Fluid Analysis *on page 408*
Fungus Culture, Cerebrospinal Fluid *on page 464*
Mycobacteria Culture, Cerebrospinal Fluid *on page 541*

Applies to Viral Culture, Brain; Viral Culture, CSF

Test Includes Isolation and identification of virus

Abstract Viral meningitis is by far the most important cause of aseptic meningitis. The latter includes multiple entities, both infectious and noninfectious. Most instances of aseptic meningitis are caused by viruses, especially enteroviruses, most often in the late summer. Subjects are usually children and young adults. Enteroviruses include polioviruses, Coxsackie viruses, and echoviruses. Aseptic meningitis syndrome is characterized by an acute disease with signs and symptoms of meningeal inflammation associated with pleocytosis (usually mononuclear), variable increase in protein content, normal glucose level, and no demonstrable organism by smear and routine culture of the cerebrospinal fluid (CSF).

By definition, the cerebrospinal fluid in aseptic meningitis will show a pleocytosis of white blood cells but no growth on bacterial culture.

Specimen Cerebrospinal fluid (do not put into virus transport medium), brain biopsy, lesions, throat or throat washings, stool, urine

Container Sterile tube for CSF; sterile screw cap container for biopsy, tissue, urine, or throat washing; sterile viral transport medium for swab specimens

Sampling Time As soon as possible after the onset of illness

Collection Always consult the laboratory for specific details prior to collecting specimen. Specimen should be collected during the acute phase of the disease, as follows:

Cerebrospinal fluid: Collect 1 mL CSF aseptically in a sterile dry screw cap vial. **Keep cold and bring to laboratory immediately.**

The following may be relevant to CNS viral infection: Specimens useful for diagnosis of CNS viral infections:

Eye swab or scraping: Use a Virocult® or Culturette® swab to collect conjunctival material or take conjunctival scrapings with a fine sterile spatula and transfer the scraping to a viral transport medium. **Keep cold and bring to laboratory immediately.**

Skin lesions: Open the vesicle and absorb exudate into a dry swab, and/or vigorously scrape base of freshly exposed lesion with a swab to obtain cells which contain viruses. If enough vesicle fluid is available, aspirate the fluid with a fine gauge needle and tuberculin syringe, and place the fluid into cold viral transport medium. Use Virocult® or Culturette® swabs for specimen collection. **Keep cold and bring to laboratory immediately.** The clinical appearance of herpes zoster or the vesicles of herpes simplex may suggest the diagnosis.

Throat swab: Carefully rub the posterior wall of the nasopharynx with a dry, sterile swab. Avoid touching the tongue or buccal mucosa. Use Virocult® or Culturette® swabs for specimen collection. **Keep cold and bring to laboratory immediately.** Coxsackie, mumps, adenovirus, herpes type 1, Epstein-Barr virus may be recovered from throat washings.

Feces: Collect 4-8 g of feces (about the size of a thumbnail), and place in a clean, leakproof container. Do **not** dilute the specimen (into virus transport medium) or use preservatives. **Keep cold and bring to laboratory immediately.** Enteroviruses, adenovirus.

Urine: Collect clean-catch, midstream urine in a leakproof, sterile, plastic container. **Keep cold and bring to laboratory immediately.** Mumps virus, cytomegalovirus.

Genital swab: See skin. **Keep cold and bring to laboratory immediately.**

Storage Instructions Keep all specimens cold and moist. Transport to laboratory immediately. Enteroviruses are relatively stable from -70°C to 4°C but are labile if allowed to dry or to be at room temperature for several hours.

Causes for Rejection Dry specimen, specimen not refrigerated during transport, specimen fixed in formalin, unlabeled specimen

Turnaround Time Variable (1-14 days) and depends on culture method used and amount of virus in specimen

Reference Range No virus isolated

Use Determine etiological agent of viral CNS diseases (eg, meningitis (aseptic), meningoencephalitis, polio, and encephalitis)

Limitations The CSF findings in tuberculous meningitis may simulate those of viral meningitis, especially herpes simplex and mumps.

Methodology Inoculation of specimen into cell cultures, incubation of cultures, observation of characteristic cytopathic effect, and identification/speciation by methods such as hemadsorption and fluorescent monoclonal antibodies. If specific viruses such as HSV, CMV, VZV, or adenovirus are suspected, the laboratory might be able to use rapid (1-2 days) culture (shell vial) methods to detect these viruses. Suckling mice are usually inoculated with the specimen if group A Coxsackie virus is suspected. The mice are observed for the development of flaccid paralysis. Bacterial culture, Gram stain, cell count, glucose, and protein are needed to rule out bacterial meningitis, with antigen agglutination when indicated.

Some laboratories offer molecular testing for this organism. Contact the testing laboratory for the availability of amplified and nonamplified qualitative and quantitative molecular tests for this organism, and for information on selection and collection of appropriate specimens for specific molecular tests.

Additional Information Arthropod-borne (arbo) viruses and reoviruses are not considered culturable and may be detected indirectly by viral serology.

The seasonal peak of viral meningitis in late summer is widely recognized and clinically significant in differential diagnosis. Meningitis caused by HIV, Epstein-Barr virus, CMV, or herpes simplex lacks seasonal variation. The significance of seasonal curves for viral meningitis (more frequent in summer) versus bacterial meningitis is greater than most physicians recognize.

Mumps meningitis is usually self limited and benign. As with lymphocytic choriomeningitis and herpes simplex meningoencephalitis, hypoglycorrhachia may be found.

In the differential diagnosis between viral and bacterial meningitis, much higher WBC count (>1180 x 10^6/L) and protein (>220 mg/dL) may be found in many cases of bacterial meningitis. In Spanos' series, no patient with acute viral meningitis had glucose <30.6 mg/dL but 43% with acute bacterial meningitis did. Although aseptic meningitis is usually characterized by mononuclear cells, PMNs may predominate early.

Five patients with mixed viral-bacterial meningitis among 276 patients with viral and/or bacterial culture proven meningitis are described.

A high frequency of negative lumbar punctures in babies presenting with fever but without other specific findings is recognized. In a series of children with high fever, 57% of patients with bacterial meningitis and 37% of those with aseptic meningitis had vomiting. In a study of 171 children with febrile convulsions, only one had bacterial meningitis and four had aseptic meningitis.

Complications of lumbar puncture (LP) are between 0.19% and 0.43%, reaching up to 35.5% when minor complications are included. Instances of meningitis and local infection are described following LP in subjects with bacteremia, who may be at risk for meningeal seeding during the puncture.

Nonviral aseptic causes of aseptic meningitis include meningeal carcinomatosis, collagen diseases, sarcoidosis, drugs including antineoplastic agents, immunosuppressants, materials used in radiology units, Mollaret's meningitis, and many other entities.

Selected Readings

Boeckh M and Boivin G, "Quantitation of Cytomegalovirus: Methodologic Aspects and Clinical Applications," *Clin Microbiol Rev*, 1998, 11(3):533-54.

Chonmaitree T, Baldwin CD, and Lucia HL, "Role of the Virology Laboratory in Diagnosis and Management of Patients With Central Nervous System Disease," *Clin Microbiol Rev*, 1989, 2(1):1-14.

Connolly KJ and Hammer SM, "The Acute Aseptic Meningitis Syndrome," *Infect Dis Clin North Am*, 1990, 4(4):599-622.

(Continued)

Viral Culture, Central Nervous System Symptoms *(Continued)*

Erice A, "Resistance of Human Cytomegalovirus to Antiviral Drugs," *Clin Microbiol Rev*, 1999, 12(2):286-97.
Falsey AR and Walsh EE, "Respiratory Syncytial Virus Infection in Adults," *Clin Microbiol Rev*, 2000, 13(3):371-84.
Greenlee JE, "Approach to Diagnosis of Meningitis - Cerebrospinal Fluid Evaluation," *Infect Dis Clin North Am*, 1990, 4(4):583-98.
Hammer SM and Connolly KJ, "Viral Aseptic Meningitis in the United States: Clinical Features, Viral Etiologies, and Differential Diagnosis," *Curr Clin Top Infect Dis*, 1992, 12:1-25.
Mishu B, "A Rabies Primer for Clinicians," *Infect Dis Newslett*, 1993, 12(1):1-4.
Yen-Lieberman B, "Diagnosis of Human Cytomegalovirus Disease," *Clin Microbiol Newslett*, 2000, 22(14):105-9.

Viral Culture, CSF *see* Viral Culture, Central Nervous System Symptoms *on page 614*
Viral Culture, Cytomegalovirus *see* Cytomegalovirus Culture *on page 438*
Viral Culture, Eye *see* Herpes Simplex Virus Culture *on page 494*
Viral Culture, Genital *see* Herpes Simplex Virus Culture *on page 494*
Viral Culture, Nasopharyngeal *see* Viral Culture, Throat *on page 617*
Viral Culture, Pulmonary Biopsy *see* Viral Culture, Throat *on page 617*
Viral Culture, Rash *see* Varicella-Zoster Virus Culture *on page 612*
Viral Culture, Skin *see* Herpes Simplex Virus Culture *on page 494*

Viral Culture, Stool

Synonyms Stool Viral Culture

Applies to Adenovirus Culture, Stool; Coxsackie Virus Culture, Stool; Echovirus Culture, Stool; Enterovirus Culture, Stool; Poliovirus Culture, Stool

Test Includes Isolation and identification of viruses

Specimen Stool or rectal swab. Freshly passed stool is much more preferable than a rectal swab.

Container Stool: screw cap container. Do not use cardboard or waxed containers. Swab: cold viral transport medium

Collection Collect stools into a clean and dry container. Insert swab gently into rectum and hold there for 10-15 seconds, moisten with contents of Culturette® bulb, and send to laboratory.

Storage Instructions Keep specimens cold

Causes for Rejection Dry specimen, specimen not refrigerated during transport, specimen fixed in formalin, unlabeled specimen

Turnaround Time Variable (usually 1-14 days) and depends on cell culture methods and amount of virus in the specimen

Viruses Typically Isolated From Clinical Specimens

Specimen	Virus[1]
Blood	CMV, enteroviruses,[2,3] HSV,[3] VZV[3]
CSF and CNS tissues	Enteroviruses, mumps virus, HSV, CMV
Dermal lesions	HSV, VZV, adenovirus, enteroviruses
Eye	HSV, VZV, adenovirus, enteroviruses, CMV, *Chlamydia*
Genital	HSV, CMV, *Chlamydia*
Mucosal	HSV, VZV
Oral	HSV, VZV
Rectal	HSV, VZV, enterovirus
Respiratory tract	
upper	Adenovirus, rhinovirus, influenza, parainfluenza, enteroviruses, RSV, reovirus, HSV
lower	Adenovirus, influenza, parainfluenza, RSV, CMV[4]
Stool	Enteroviruses, adenoviruses
Tissues	CMV, HSV, enteroviruses
Urine	CMV, adenovirus, enteroviruses, mumps

[1]Abbreviations:
HSV = herpes simplex virus.
CMV = cytomegalovirus.
VZV = varicella-zoster virus.
RSV = respiratory syncytial virus.
[2]Enteroviruses: coxsackie virus, poliovirus, echovirus, and enterovirus.
[3]Rarely isolated.
[4]Usually in immunocompromised hosts.

Reference Range No virus isolated

Use Identify carriage or excretion of a virus in stool; isolate and identify an enterovirus which could be the cause of meningitis

Limitations Children convalescing from upper respiratory illness or aseptic meningitis can shed virus in the stool for weeks; children recently vaccinated against polio can shed poliovirus in the stool for months after vaccination; sampling errors; presence of nonculturable, disease-causing virus (eg, encephalitis, hepatitis, and gastroenteritis viruses)

Methodology Inoculation of specimen into cell cultures, incubation of cultures, observation of characteristic cytopathic effect, and identification/speciation by methods such as hemadsorption and fluorescent monoclonal antibodies. If specific viruses such as HSV, CMV, VZV, or adenovirus are suspected, the laboratory might be able to use rapid (1-2 days) culture (shell vial) methods to detect these viruses.

Additional Information See table for viruses most likely to be isolated from stool specimens. The viruses most likely to be isolated from stool specimen are those which are extremely hardy and which do not have a lipid membrane envelope (ie, adenovirus and enterovirus (polio, Coxsackie, and echoviruses)).

Selected Readings

Miller JM, Holmes HT, and Krisher K, "General Principles of Specimen Collection and Handling," *Manual of Clinical Microbiology*, 8th ed, Murray PR, et al, eds, Washington, DC: American Society for Microbiology, 2003, 55-66.

Viral Culture, Throat

Related Information

Adenovirus Culture *on page 365*
Influenza Virus Culture *on page 510*
Parainfluenza Virus Culture *on page 558*
Respiratory Syncytial Virus Culture *on page 572*

Synonyms Throat Viral Culture; Viral Culture, Bronchial Wash; Viral Culture, Nasopharyngeal; Viral Culture, Pulmonary Biopsy; Viral Culture, Throat Swab

Applies to Rhinovirus Culture

Test Includes Isolation and identification of virus most likely to cause respiratory disease

Patient Preparation Local anesthesia might be necessary

Specimen Throat swab; throat washing; nasopharyngeal washing, aspirates, or secretions; sputum; bronchial washings or lavage; lung biopsy

Container Cold and sterile viral transport medium for swabs; sterile cup for feces, washings, aspirates, and sputum

Sampling Time As soon as possible after onset of illness

Collection Methods are the same as those used for collecting most respiratory specimens (see Specimen). If respiratory syncytial virus or parainfluenza virus is suspected, see collection techniques in Parainfluenza Virus Culture *on page 558*.

Storage Instructions Keep specimen cold and moist. Transport to laboratory immediately.

Causes for Rejection Dry specimen, specimen not refrigerated during transport, specimen fixed in formalin, unlabeled specimen

Turnaround Time Variable (1-14 days) and depends on culture method and amount of virus in specimen

Reference Range No virus isolated

Use Determine etiological agent of viral respiratory infections (eg, pneumonia, pneumonitis, croup, and influenza)

Limitations Sampling errors; presence of nonculturable, disease-causing virus (eg, encephalitis, hepatitis, and gastroenteritis viruses); invasive procedures. Many persons carry and shed viruses which might not be related to the patient's illness.

Methodology Inoculation of specimen into cell cultures, incubation of cultures, observation of characteristic cytopathic effect, and identification/speciation by methods such as hemadsorption and the use of fluorescent monoclonal antibodies. If specific viruses such as HSV, CMV, VZV, or adenovirus are suspected, the laboratory might be able to use rapid (1-2 days) culture (shell vial) methods to detect these viruses. Most laboratories use hemadsorption to help determine the presence of a respiratory virus in cell culture and usually will report "hemadsorbing virus present." Some laboratories are capable of using specific virus-neutralizing antibodies to determine the particular type of virus which caused the observed hemadsorption. This final identification can require as many as several days and often is done only by reference laboratories.

Some laboratories offer molecular testing for this organism. Contact the testing laboratory for the availability of amplified and nonamplified qualitative and quantitative molecular tests for this organism, and for information on selection and collection of appropriate specimens for specific molecular tests.

(Continued)

Viral Culture, Throat *(Continued)*

Additional Information Viruses to be considered as causes of viral respiratory illness include the following: influenza virus, parainfluenza virus, rhinovirus, RSV, adenovirus, CMV, and reovirus. Contact the Virology Laboratory and inform the staff if influenza or parainfluenza is suspected.

Selected Readings

Falsey AR and Walsh EE, "Respiratory Syncytial Virus Infection in Adults," *Clin Microbiol Rev*, 2000, 13(3):371-84.

Miller JM, Holmes HT, and Krisher K, "General Principles of Specimen Collection and Handling," *Manual of Clinical Microbiology*, 8th ed, Murray PR, et al, eds, Washington, DC: American Society for Microbiology, 2003, 55-66.

Ruben FL and Cate TR, "Influenza Pneumonia," *Semin Respir Infect*, 1987, 2(2):122-9.

Welliver RC, "Detection, Pathogenesis, and Therapy of Respiratory Syncytial Virus Infections," *Clin Microbiol Rev*, 1988, 1(1):27-39.

Viral Culture, Throat Swab *see* Viral Culture, Throat *on page 617*

Viral Direct Detection by Fluorescent Antibody *see* Virus Detection by DFA *on page 619*

Viral Serology

Test Includes Detection of IgG and/or IgM formed in response to infection by a specific virus

Special Instructions For the determination of immune status, a single specimen is sufficient. For the determination of acute disease, both acute and convalescent specimens must be tested.

Specimen Serum

Container Red top tube

Collection Two specimens should be collected, an acute specimen obtained as soon as possible after the onset of symptoms and a convalescent specimen obtained 10-14 days later. Both specimens should be tested when the convalescent specimen is obtained.

Reference Range Varies greatly and depends on the antibody being tested

Use Determine the immune status of a patient; help in the diagnosis of a viral infection when culture for the virus or methods for the detection of viral antigen(s) are not available or do not exist

Limitations Serological tests for antibodies to viruses can provide valuable diagnostic information. The detection of virus-specific IgM or more than a fourfold rise (from acute disease to convalescence) in virus-specific IgG titer can confirm acute infection, and viral serology is the only laboratory method for the laboratory diagnosis of many viral diseases. On the other hand, such tests can be fraught with many problems: The results obtained by testing a single specimen are rarely (only if the titer is obviously and extremely high), if ever, useful; for the results of viral serological test to be clinically relevant, both acute and convalescent serum must be tested at the same time; and false-positive results can result if interfering rheumatoid factor is in the specimen or when virus-specific antibody is attracted to Fc receptors in cell substrates used in viral serology assays.

Methodology Several methods are used to detect and semiquantitate antibodies to viruses: indirect fluorescent antibody (IFA), enzyme immunoassay (EIA), complement fixation (CF), and Western blot (WB)

Additional Information IMPORTANT: "Viral serology" can mean many things to medical technologists and other personnel of testing laboratories. Physicians **must** specify the specific viruses for which they want "viral serology."

For viral serology studies to be effective, specific serological tests for specific viruses must be ordered. Orders for "TORCH titers", "TORCH serology", "viral studies", "virus serology", "encephalitis titers", etc are useless, confusing, and wasteful orders which usually lead to results of equally useless value. Laboratories usually issue reports of antibody levels in terms of titers (usually determined by dilution and immunofluorescence) or index values (usually determined by enzyme immunoassay), each of which when interpreted alone usually is not of much clinical value. A fourfold rise in titer or an appropriately higher index value after testing of acute and convalescent specimens is considered clinically relevant and significant. IgM antibody levels are not always observed/detected immediately following a primary viral infection. With the herpes viruses (HSV, CMV, VZV, and EBV), IgM can appear more than once and suggest a reinfection or reactivation. Complement fixation tests detect both IgG and IgM at the same time, but the test is not able to differentiate between the two classes of antibodies.

See table for a list of viruses for which serological testing methods exist. The table also shows infectious diseases and medical conditions in which testing for specific antibodies to multiple viruses (panels/batteries) might be indicated. Some laboratories offer these or similar serology panels.

Viral Serology Tests Available

Infectious Disease or Medical Condition	Viruses and/or Serology Panels to Be Considered
AIDS	Human immunodeficiency virus
CNS infections	Western, eastern, California, St Louis equine encephalitis, lymphocytic choriomeningitis, measles, mumps, Epstein-Barr, rabies
Exanthems	Measles, rubella, parvovirus
Vesicles	Herpes simplex, varicella-zoster
Hepatitis A/B/C/E	Hepatitis A/B/C/E
Heterophil-negative syndrome	Cytomegalovirus, Epstein-Barr
Myocarditis-pericarditis	Coxsackie, influenza, cytomegalovirus
Respiratory	Influenza, parainfluenza, respiratory syncytial virus, adenovirus
Determination of immune status (single specimen)	Measles, mumps, rubella, varicella-zoster, cytomegalovirus, hepatitis B

Selected Readings

Asnis DS, Conetta R, Teixeira AA, et al, "The West Nile Virus Outbreak of 1999 in New York: The Flushing Hospital Experience," *Clin Infect Dis*, 2000, 30(3):413-8.

Ashley RL and Wald A, "Genital Herpes: Review of the Epidemic and Potential Use of Type-Specific Serology," *Clin Microbiol Rev*, 1999, 12(1):1-8.

Marfin AA and Gubler DJ, "West Nile Encephalitis: An Emerging Disease in the United States," *Clin Infect Dis*, 2001, 33(10):1713-9.

Specter S, "Viral Diseases," *Manual of Clinical Laboratory Immunology*, 5th ed, Rose, NR, Conway de Macario E, Folds JD, et al, eds, Washington, DC: American Society for Microbiology, 1997, 605-754.

Subbarao K, "Influenza A Infections: From Chickens to Humans," *Clin Microbiol Newslett*, 2001, 23(2):9-13.

Thompson RB, "Laboratory Methods in Basic Virology," *Bailey and Scott's Diagnostic Microbiology*, 9th ed, Baron EJ, Peterson LP, and Finegold SM, eds, St. Louis, MO: Mosby-Year Book Inc, 1994, 634-88.

Viral Study, Herpes *see* Herpes Cytology *on page 491*

Virus Detection by DFA

Related Information

Histopathology *on page 496*

Synonyms Direct Detection of Virus; Direct Fluorescent Antibody Test for Virus; Viral Direct Detection by Fluorescent Antibody; Virus Fluorescent Antibody Test

Applies to Herpes Simplex Virus, Direct Detection; Influenza Virus, Direct Detection; Measles Virus, Direct Detection; Mumps Virus, Direct Detection; Parainfluenza Virus, Direct Detection; Rabies Virus, Direct Detection; Respiratory Syncytial Virus, Direct Detection; Varicella-Zoster Virus, Direct Detection

Test Includes Direct (nonculture) detection of virus-infected cells

Special Instructions Make at least four impression smears or place four frozen sections on four separate slides. Cell suspensions should be centrifuged, resuspended to slight turbidity, and applied to prewelled slides.

Specimen Impression smears of tissues, lesion scrapings and swabs, frozen sections, cell suspensions, upper respiratory tract swabs

Causes for Rejection Insufficient material, slides broken or badly scratched, fixative used on slide preparation (generally, the laboratory is responsible for fixing specimens)

Turnaround Time Less than 1 day

Reference Range No virus detected

Use Rapid diagnosis of HSV, VZV, RSV, parainfluenza, influenza, and rabies infections

Limitations Physicians must specify the particular viruses they suspect or desire to be tested. Only a few viruses (HSV, VZV, RSV, influenza, parainfluenza, measles, mumps, and rabies virus) can be detected in this manner. It is possible for the test to be negative in the presence of viral infection. Expertly trained and experienced personnel, excellent quality reagents and adequate numbers of cells are required. **Contact laboratory prior to requesting test to determine if laboratory offers this/these tests.**

Methodology Monoclonal antibody reagents and immunofluorescence microscopy are used to detect viruses/viral antigens in specimen cells.

Additional Information Generally, this test is not as sensitive as cell culture.

Selected Readings

Drew WL, "Controversies in Viral Diagnosis," *Rev Infect Dis*, 1986, 8(5):814-24.

Drew WL, "Diagnostic Virology," *Clin Lab Med*, 1987, 7(4):721-40.

Smith TF, "Rapid Methods for the Diagnosis of Viral Infections," *Laboratory Medicine*, 1987, 18:16-20.

Virus Fluorescent Antibody Test *see* Virus Detection by DFA *on page 619*

WBC Scan *see* Indium Leukocyte Scan *on page 508*

Westergren Sed Rate *see* Sedimentation Rate, Erythrocyte *on page 576*

West Nile Virus Diagnostic Procedures

Related Information

Encephalitis Viral Serology *on page 452*

Abstract West Nile virus infections usually cause a febrile illness characterized by rash, lymphadenopathy, and polyarthropathy. Severe neurologic disease develops in 1 of 150 infections. Advanced age is a pivotal risk factor. Encephalitis is more common than meningitis/meningoencephalitis. The agent is an arbovirus spread by *Culex* mosquito vectors and by more than 110 species of birds, especially crows and jays.

Specimen Serum, cerebrospinal fluid, brain tissue (humans), mosquitoes, avian samples

Turnaround Time Specimens may be sent to state or provincial (in Canada) departments of health.

Use Evidence of encephalitis, myelitis, or meningoencephalitis, profound muscle weakness, fever, and flaccid paralysis may indicate West Nile virus (WNV) infection. Other clinical observations include rash, lymphadenopathy, and polyarthropathy.

Limitations Cross-reactions may occur in subjects who have recently been vaccinated against related flaviviruses or recently infected with one of these agents; but cross-reactivity was not reported to represent a problem in acute-phase samples tested for IgM antibody.

Methodology IgM antibody testing, TaqMan reverse transcriptase-PCR testing.

If serological testing is performed by enzyme immunoassay (EIA) on automated instrumentation, results are usually given in index units, not titers. In such cases, significant rises in antibody levels are determined by algorithms within the instrumentation, not by increases in titers.

Some laboratories offer molecular testing for this organism. Contact the testing laboratory for the availability of amplified and nonamplified qualitative and quantitative molecular tests for this organism, and for information on selection and collection of appropriate specimens for specific molecular tests.

IgM capture and IgG enzyme-linked immunosorbent assays (ELISA). IgM antibody may be found without IgG virus-specific IgG in the first week of illness. Switch to IgG antibody is reported following 4-5 days of illness and is found earlier in CSF.

TaqMan reverse transcriptase-PCR testing is reported as specific. It is described as providing greater sensitivity than traditional RT-PCR methods.

WNV may be identified by immunocytochemistry, immunofluorescent assays.

Additional Information Monitoring for West Nile virus activity includes mosquitoes, chickens, wild birds, and susceptible mammals, including horses as well as humans.

The virus appears to survive in donated blood, but a low risk of transmission by blood transfusion is postulated for the Queens epidemic.

Selected Readings

"All You Need to Know About West Nile Virus," *Nurs Times*, 2005, 101(26):28.

Centers for Disease Control and Prevention (CDC), "West Nile Virus Activity - United States, 2005," *MMWR*, 2005, 54(27):678-9.

Gottfried K, Quinn R, and Jones T, "Clinical Description and Follow-up Investigation of Human West Nile Virus Cases," *South Med J*, 2005, 98(6):603-6.

Mazurek JM, Winpisinger K, Mattson BJ, et al, "The Epidemiology and Early Clinical Features of West Nile Virus Infection," *Am J Emerg Med*, 2005, 23(4):536-43.

Tilley PA, Zachary GA, Walle R, et al, "West Nile Virus Detection and Commercial Assays," *Emerg Infect Dis*, 2005, 11(7):1154-5.

Wet Prep *see Trichomonas* Preparation *on page 600*

Wet Preparation for *Trichomonas vaginalis* *see Trichomonas* Preparation *on page 600*

White Blood Cell Scan *see* Indium Leukocyte Scan *on page 508*

Whole Body Bone Scan *see* Bone Scan *on page 401*

Whooping Cough Culture *see Bordetella pertussis* Nasopharyngeal Culture *on page 403*

Wound Culture

Related Information

Abscess Aerobic and Anaerobic Culture *on page 360*

Synonyms Lesion Culture

Test Includes Culture for aerobic organisms and usually Gram stain

Patient Preparation Sterile preparation of the aspiration site

Special Instructions The laboratory should be informed of the specific site of specimen, the age of patient, current antibiotic therapy, clinical diagnosis, and time of collection. The submission of biopsy specimens or specimens from normally sterile sites should be clearly indicated to the laboratory. Procedures for laboratory work-up of wound cultures which may contain contamination from the skin surface are different than those from sites which are expected to be sterile. Drainage cultured by aspiration away from a sinus tract may provide more useful information.

Specimen Tissue or aspirated pus/fluid properly obtained from a wound site or abscess

Container Sterile tube or screw-cap container. **Do not submit lesion specimens collected with swabs. Swab specimens are extremely inadequate for almost all specimens except for throat, cervix, and other small openings.**

Collection The specimen should be transported to laboratory as soon as possible after collection. Contamination with normal flora from skin, rectum, vaginal tract, or other body surfaces must be avoided.

Storage Instructions Refrigerate the specimen if it cannot be promptly processed.

Causes for Rejection Specimens delayed in transit to the laboratory may have less than optimal yields.

Turnaround Time Preliminary reports are usually available at 24 hours. Cultures with no growth are usually reported after 72 hours. Reports on specimens from which pathogens are isolated require a minimum of 48 hours for completion.

Reference Range No growth. A simultaneous Gram stain should always be performed to facilitate interpretation. Gram-negative organisms, frequently colonize wounds and mixed culture results are common.

Use Isolate and identify potentially pathogenic organisms

Limitations Only rapid-growing, nonfastidious aerobic organisms will be screened for and identified by routine methods. Often only organisms which predominate will be completely identified. Unless specifically requested by the physician or mandated by the specimen source (ie, genital specimen) fastidious organisms such as *N. gonorrhoeae* may not be isolated. Fungal and mycobacterial pathogens should be considered and appropriate cultures requested if indicated.

Contraindications Culture of contaminated open wounds which have not been cleansed or debrided

Additional Information Susceptibility testing is performed if laboratory personnel determine such is appropriate; such testing is not always performed automatically when "culture and sensitivity" is ordered by a physician. If anaerobes are suspected a properly collected specimen for anaerobic culture should also be submitted. See table.

Classification of Soft-Tissue Infections

Tissue Level	Common Surgical Pathogens				
				Mixed Bacteria	
	S. pyogenes	*S. aureus*	*C. perfringens*	Staph & Strep	Enteric
Epidermis	Ecthyma contagiosum	Scalded-skin syndrome		Possibly impetigo	
Dermis and subdermis	Erysipelas/ cellulitis	Folliculitis / abscess	Abscess / cellulitis	Meleny's ulcer (synergistic gangrene)	Tropical ulcer
Fascial planes	Strep gangrene	Carbuncle	Fasciitis	Necrotizing fasciitis	
Muscle tissue	Strep myositis	Muscular abscess / pyomyositis	Myonecrosis	Nonclostridial myonecrosis	

From Ahrenholz DH, "Necrotizing Soft Tissue Infections," *Surg Clin North Am*, 1988, 68:198-214, with permission.

Effective treatment of wound infection usually includes drainage, removal of foreign bodies, infected prosthetic devices, and retained foreign objects such as suture material. Suction irrigation may be helpful in resolving wound infections. Species commonly recovered from wounds include *Escherichia coli*, *Proteus* sp, *Klebsiella* sp, *Pseudomonas* sp, *Enterobacter* sp, enterococci, streptococci, staphylococci, *Bacteroides* sp, and *Clostridium* sp.

Selected Readings

Erlich KS and Rumack JS, "Evaluation and Management of Nonhealing Infected Wounds in Diabetics," *Infect Med*, 1993, 10(8):21-7.

Gerding DN, Piziak VK, and Rowbotham JL, "Saving the Diabetic Foot," *Patient Care*, 1991.

Goldstein EJ, "Management of Human and Animal Bite Wounds," *J Am Acad Dermatol*, 1989, 21(6):1275-9.

(Continued)

Wound Culture *(Continued)*

Pollock AV and Evans M, "Microbiologic Prediction of Abdominal Surgical Wound Infection," *Arch Surg*, 1987, 122(1):33-7.

Wound Fungus Culture *see* Fungus Culture, Body Fluid *on page 462*

Wound Mycobacteria Culture *see* Mycobacteria Culture, Biopsy or Body Fluid *on page 539*

Wrist Arthrogram *see* Arthrogram *on page 387*

Wrist, Left or Right, X-ray *see* Bone Films *on page 396*

***Yersinia enterocolitica*, Stool Culture** *see* Stool Culture, Uncommon Organisms *on page 588*

Ziehl-Neelsen Stain *see* Acid-Fast Stain *on page 361*

Zoster Titer *see* Varicella-Zoster Virus Serology *on page 612*

ANTIMICROBIAL THERAPY

A200® Lice [OTC] *see* Permethrin *on page 1001*

A-200® Maximum Strength [OTC] *see* Pyrethrins and Piperonyl Butoxide *on page 1023*

Abacavir (a BAK a veer)

Related Information

Antiretroviral Agents *on page 1206*

Antiretroviral Therapy for HIV Infection *on page 1219*

Management of Healthcare Worker Exposures to HBV, HCV, and HIV *on page 1227*

U.S. Brand Names Ziagen®

Canadian Brand Names Ziagen®

Synonyms Abacavir Sulfate; ABC

Generic Available No

Use Treatment of HIV infections in combination with other antiretroviral agents

Drug of Choice or Alternative for

Organism(s):

Human Immunodeficiency Virus *on page 181*

Restrictions An FDA-approved medication guide is available at www.fda.gov/cder/Offices/ODS/labeling.htm; distribute to each patient to whom this medication is dispensed.

Pregnancy Risk Factor C

Pregnancy Implications It is not known if abacavir crosses the human placenta. Cases of lactic acidosis/hepatic steatosis syndrome have been reported in pregnant women receiving nucleoside analogues. It is not known if pregnancy itself potentiates this known side effect; however, pregnant women may be at increased risk of lactic acidosis and liver damage. Hepatic enzymes and electrolytes should be monitored frequently during the 3rd trimester of pregnancy in women receiving nucleoside analogues. The pharmacokinetics of abacavir during pregnancy are currently under study. The Perinatal HIV Guidelines Working Group considers abacavir to be an alternative NRTI in dual nucleoside combination regimens. Health professionals are encouraged to contact the antiretroviral pregnancy registry to monitor outcomes of pregnant women exposed to antiretroviral medications (1-800-258-4263 or www.APRegistry.com).

Contraindications Hypersensitivity to abacavir (or carbovir) or any component of the formulation (do not rechallenge patients who have experienced hypersensitivity to abacavir); moderate-to-severe hepatic impairment

Warnings/Precautions Should always be used as a component of a multidrug regimen. Serious and sometimes fatal hypersensitivity reactions have occurred. **Patients exhibiting symptoms from two or more of the following: Fever, skin rash, constitutional symptoms (malaise, fatigue, aches), respiratory symptoms (eg, pharyngitis, dyspnea, cough) and GI symptoms (eg, abdominal pain, diarrhea, nausea, vomiting) should discontinue therapy immediately and call for medical attention. Abacavir should be permanently discontinued if hypersensitivity cannot be ruled out, even when other diagnoses are possible. Abacavir SHOULD NOT be restarted because more severe symptoms may occur within hours, including LIFE-THREATENING HYPOTENSION AND DEATH. Fatal hypersensitivity reactions have occurred following the reintroduction of abacavir in patients whose therapy was interrupted (interruption in drug supply, temporary discontinuation while treating other conditions). Reactions occurred within hours. In some cases, signs of hypersensitivity may have been previously present, but attributed to other medical conditions (acute onset respiratory diseases, gastroenteritis, reactions to other medications). If abacavir is restarted following an interruption in therapy, evaluate the patient for previously unsuspected symptoms of hypersensitivity. Do not restart if hypersensitivity is suspected or if hypersensitivity cannot be ruled out. To report these events on abacavir hypersensitivity, a registry has been established (1-800-270-0425).** Use with caution in patients with mild hepatic dysfunction (contraindicated in moderate-to-severe dysfunction). Lactic acidosis and severe hepatomegaly with steatosis (sometimes fatal) have occurred with antiretroviral nucleoside analogues; female gender, obesity, and prolonged treatment may increase the risk of hepatotoxicity.

Adverse Reactions Hypersensitivity reactions (which may be fatal) occur in ~5% of patients (see Warnings/Precautions). Symptoms may include anaphylaxis, fever, rash (including erythema multiforme), fatigue, diarrhea, abdominal pain; respiratory symptoms (eg, pharyngitis, dyspnea, cough, adult respiratory distress syndrome, or respiratory failure); headache, malaise, lethargy, myalgia, myolysis, arthralgia, edema, paresthesia, nausea and vomiting, mouth ulcerations, conjunctivitis, lymphadenopathy, hepatic failure, and renal failure.

Note: Rates of adverse reactions were defined during combination therapy with other antiretrovirals (lamivudine and efavirenz **or** lamivudine and zidovudine). Only reactions which occurred at a higher frequency than in the comparator group are noted. Adverse reaction rates attributable to abacavir alone are not available.

>10%:

Central nervous system: Headache (7% to 13%), fatigue and malaise (7% to 12%)

Gastrointestinal: Nausea (7% to 19%, children 9%)

1% to 10%:

Central nervous system: Depression (6%), dizziness (6%), fever (6%, children 9%), anxiety (5%), abnormal dreams (10%)

Dermatologic: Rash (5% to 6%, children 7%)

Gastrointestinal: Diarrhea (7%), vomiting (2% to 10%, children 9%), abdominal pain (6%)

Hematologic: Thrombocytopenia (1%)

Hepatic: AST increased (6%)

Neuromuscular and skeletal: Musculoskeletal pain (5% to 6%)

Respiratory: Bronchitis (4%), respiratory viral infection (5%)

Miscellaneous: Hypersensitivity reactions (9%; may include reactions to other components of antiretroviral regimen), infection (EENT 5%)

<1% (Limited to important or life-threatening): Erythema multiforme, hepatotoxicity, lactic acidosis, pancreatitis, Stevens-Johnson syndrome, toxic epidermal necrolysis

Drug Interactions

Increased Effect/Toxicity: Abacavir increases the blood levels of amprenavir. Abacavir may decrease the serum concentration of methadone in some patients. Concomitant use of ribavirin and nucleoside analogues may increase the risk of developing lactic acidosis (includes adefovir, didanosine, lamivudine, stavudine, zalcitabine, zidovudine).

Ethanol/Nutrition/Herb Interactions Ethanol: Ethanol may increase the risk of toxicity.

Stability Store oral solution and tablets at controlled room temperature of 20°C to 25°C (68°F to 77°F). Oral solution may be refrigerated; do not freeze.

Mechanism of Action Nucleoside reverse transcriptase inhibitor. Abacavir is a guanosine analogue which is phosphorylated to carbovir triphosphate which interferes with HIV viral RNA dependent DNA polymerase resulting in inhibition of viral replication.

Pharmacodynamics/Kinetics

Absorption: Rapid and extensive absorption

Distribution: V_d: 0.86 L/kg

Protein binding: 50%

Metabolism: Hepatic via alcohol dehydrogenase and glucuronyl transferase to inactive carboxylate and glucuronide metabolites

Bioavailability: 83%

Half-life elimination: 1.5 hours

Time to peak: 0.7-1.7 hours

Excretion: Primarily urine (as metabolites, 1.2% as unchanged drug); feces (16% total dose)

Dosage Oral:

Children: 3 months to 16 years: 8 mg/kg body weight twice daily (maximum 300 mg twice daily) in combination with other antiretroviral agents

Adults: 300 mg twice daily or 600 mg once daily in combination with other antiretroviral agents

Dosage adjustment in hepatic impairment:

Mild dysfunction (Child-Pugh score 5-6): 200 mg twice daily (oral solution is recommended)

Moderate-to-severe dysfunction: Use is contraindicated by the manufacturer

Dietary Considerations May be taken with or without food.

Administration May be administered with or without food.

Patient Information If you experience any of the following: Fever, skin rash, fatigue, nausea, vomiting, diarrhea, abdominal pain, contact your prescriber **immediately**. This is not a cure for HIV infection, nor will it reduce the risk of transmission to others. You will need frequent blood tests to adjust dosage for maximum therapeutic effect. Take as directed; do not discontinue (even if feeling better). You may experience headache or muscle pain or weakness. If you are instructed to stop the medication, **do not take this medication in the future.** Do not restart without specific instructions by your prescriber.

Additional Information A medication guide is available and should be dispensed with each prescription or refill for abacavir. A warning card is also available and patients should be instructed to carry this card with them.

(Continued)

Abacavir *(Continued)*

A high rate of early virologic nonresponse was observed when abacavir, lamivudine, and tenofovir were used as the initial regimen in treatment-naive patients. Use of this combination is not recommended; patients currently on this regimen should be closely monitored for modification of therapy.

Dosage Forms

Solution, oral: 20 mg/mL (240 mL) [strawberry-banana flavor]

Tablet: 300 mg

Selected Readings

Havlir DV and Lange JM, "New Antiretrovirals and New Combinations," *AIDS*, 1998, 12(Suppl A):S165-74.

Hervey PS and Perry CM, "Abacavir: A Review of Its Clinical Potential in Patients With HIV Infection," *Drugs*, 2000, 60(2):447-79.

Schmit JC and Weber B, "Recent Advances in Antiretroviral Therapy and HIV Infection Monitoring," *Intervirology*, 1997, 40(5-6)304-21.

"Three New Drugs for HIV Infection," *Med Lett Drugs Ther*, 1998, 40(1041):114-6.

Weverling GJ, Lange JM, Jurriaans S, et al, "Alternative Multidrug Regimen Provides Improved Suppression of HIV-1 Replication Over Triple Therapy," *AIDS*, 1998, 12(11):F117-22.

Abacavir and Lamivudine (a BAK a veer & la MI vyoo deen)

Related Information

Antiretroviral Agents *on page 1206*

Antiretroviral Therapy for HIV Infection *on page 1219*

U.S. Brand Names Epzicom™

Synonyms Abacavir Sulfate and Lamivudine; Lamivudine and Abacavir

Generic Available No

Use Treatment of HIV infections in combination with other antiretroviral agents

Restrictions An FDA-approved medication guide is available at www.fda.gov/cder/Offices/ODS/labeling.htm; distribute to each patient to whom this medication is dispensed.

Pregnancy Risk Factor C

Pregnancy Implications See individual agents.

Contraindications Hypersensitivity to abacavir, lamivudine, or any component of the formulation; hepatic impairment. Do not rechallenge patients who have experienced hypersensitivity to abacavir.

Warnings/Precautions Should always be used as a component of a multidrug regimen. Serious and sometimes fatal hypersensitivity reactions have occurred in patients taking abacavir. **Patients exhibiting symptoms from two or more of the following: Fever, skin rash, constitutional symptoms (eg, malaise, fatigue, aches), respiratory symptoms (eg, pharyngitis, dyspnea, cough) and GI symptoms (eg, abdominal pain, nausea, vomiting) should discontinue therapy immediately and seek medical attention. Abacavir should be permanently discontinued if hypersensitivity cannot be ruled out, even when other diagnoses are possible. Abacavir SHOULD NOT be restarted because more severe symptoms may occur within hours, including LIFE-THREATENING HYPOTENSION AND DEATH. Fatal hypersensitivity reactions have occurred following the reintroduction of abacavir in patients whose therapy was interrupted (interruption in drug supply, temporary discontinuation while treating other conditions). Reactions occurred within hours. In some cases, signs of hypersensitivity may have been previously present, but attributed to other medical conditions (acute onset respiratory diseases, gastroenteritis, reactions to other medications). If abacavir is restarted following an interruption in therapy, evaluate the patient for previously unsuspected symptoms of hypersensitivity. Do not restart if hypersensitivity is suspected or if hypersensitivity cannot be ruled out. To report these events on abacavir hypersensitivity, a registry has been established (1-800-270-0425).**

Following discontinuation of lamivudine, severe acute exacerbations of hepatitis B in patients coinfected with HBV and HIV have been reported. Monitor patients closely for several months following discontinuation of therapy for chronic hepatitis B; clinical exacerbations may occur.

Lactic acidosis and severe hepatomegaly with steatosis (sometimes fatal) have occurred with antiretroviral nucleoside analogues; female gender, obesity, and prolonged treatment may increase the risk of hepatotoxicity. Due to fixed dose of combination product, use is not recommended with renal or hepatic impairment or in pediatric patients.

Adverse Reactions Percentages reported with once daily abacavir, lamivudine, and efavirenz administration. Also see individual agents.

1% to 10%:

Central nervous system: Fatigue/malaise (7%), headache/migraine (7%), insomnia (7%), dizziness/vertigo (6%), pyrexia (5%), abnormal dreams (4%), anxiety (3%)

Dermatologic: Rash (5%)

Gastrointestinal: Nausea (6%), diarrhea (5%), abdominal pain/gastritis (4%)

Miscellaneous: Hypersensitivity (9%)

Overdosage/Toxicology See individual agents.

Drug Interactions

Increased Effect/Toxicity: See individual agents.

Decreased Effect: See individual agents.

Stability Store at controlled room temperature of 25°C (77°F).

Mechanism of Action Nucleoside reverse transcriptase inhibitor combination.

Abacavir is a guanosine analogue which is phosphorylated to carbovir triphosphate which interferes with HIV viral RNA-dependent DNA polymerase resulting in inhibition of viral replication.

Lamivudine is a cytosine analog. After lamivudine is triphosphorylated, the principle mode of action is inhibition of HIV reverse transcription via viral DNA chain termination; inhibits RNA-dependent DNA polymerase activities of reverse transcriptase.

Pharmacodynamics/Kinetics See individual agents.

Dosage Oral: Adults: HIV: One tablet (abacavir 600 mg and lamivudine 300 mg) once daily

Dosage adjustment in renal impairment: Cl_{cr} <50 mL/minute: Use not recommended

Dosage adjustment in hepatic impairment: Use not recommended.

Dietary Considerations May be taken with or without food.

Administration May be administered with or without food.

Monitoring Parameters Amylase, bilirubin, liver enzymes, hematologic parameters, viral load, and CD4 count

Additional Information A medication guide is available and should be dispensed with each new prescription or refill. A warning card is also available and patients should be instructed to carry this card with them.

A high rate of early virologic nonresponse was observed when abacavir, lamivudine, and tenofovir were used as the initial regimen in treatment-naive patients. Use of this combination is not recommended; patients currently on this regimen should be closely monitored for modification of therapy.

Dosage Forms Tablet, film-coated: Abacavir 600 mg and lamivudine 300 mg

Abacavir, Lamivudine, and Zidovudine

(a BAK a veer, la MI vyoo deen, & zye DOE vyoo deen)

Related Information

Abacavir *on page 624*
Antiretroviral Agents *on page 1206*
Antiretroviral Therapy for HIV Infection *on page 1219*
Lamivudine *on page 905*
Zidovudine *on page 1159*

U.S. Brand Names Trizivir®

Synonyms Azidothymidine, Abacavir, and Lamivudine; AZT, Abacavir, and Lamivudine; Compound S, Abacavir, and Lamivudine; Lamivudine, Abacavir, and Zidovudine; 3TC, Abacavir, and Zidovudine; ZDV, Abacavir, and Lamivudine; Zidovudine, Abacavir, and Lamivudine

Generic Available No

Use Treatment of HIV infection (either alone or in combination with other antiretroviral agents) in patients whose regimen would otherwise contain the components of Trizivir®

Drug of Choice or Alternative for Organism(s):

Human Immunodeficiency Virus *on page 181*

Restrictions An FDA-approved medication guide is available at www.fda.gov/cder/Offices/ODS/labeling.htm; distribute to each patient to whom this medication is dispensed.

Pregnancy Risk Factor C

Pregnancy Implications See individual agents.

Contraindications Hypersensitivity to abacavir, lamivudine, zidovudine, or any component of the formulation. Do not rechallenge patients who have experienced hypersensitivity to abacavir (as Trizivir® or Ziagen®); life-threatening and fatal reactions have been reported.

(Continued)

Abacavir, Lamivudine, and Zidovudine *(Continued)*

Warnings/Precautions Fatal hypersensitivity reactions have occurred in patients taking abacavir (in Trizivir®). **Patients exhibiting symptoms of fever, skin rash, fatigue, respiratory symptoms (eg, pharyngitis, dyspnea, cough) and/or GI symptoms (eg, abdominal pain, nausea, vomiting, diarrhea) should discontinue therapy immediately and call for medical attention. Trizivir® should be permanently discontinued if hypersensitivity cannot be ruled out, even when other diagnoses are possible. Trizivir® SHOULD NOT be restarted because more severe symptoms may occur within hours, including LIFE-THREATENING HYPOTENSION AND DEATH. Fatal hypersensitivity reactions have occurred following the reintroduction of abacavir in patients whose therapy was interrupted (interruption in drug supply, temporary discontinuation while treating other conditions). Reactions occurred within hours. In some cases, signs of hypersensitivity may have been previously present, but attributed to other medical conditions (acute onset respiratory diseases, gastroenteritis, reactions to other medications). If Trizivir® is to be restarted following an interruption in therapy, first evaluate the patient for previously unsuspected symptoms of hypersensitivity. Do not restart if hypersensitivity is suspected or if hypersensitivity cannot be ruled out. To report these events on Trizivir® hypersensitivity, a registry has been established (1-800-270-0425).** Trizivir®, as a fixed-dose combination tablet, should not be used in patients <40 kg or those requiring dosage adjustment; should not be used in patients with Cl_{cr} ≤50 mL/minute; not intended for use in pediatric patients; should not be administered concomitantly with abacavir, lamivudine, or zidovudine. Prior liver disease, prolonged use, and obesity may be risk factors for development of lactic acidosis and severe hepatomegaly with steatosis. Dose reductions may be required for zidovudine in patients with hepatic impairment. Trizivir® is a fixed-dose combination; it is not recommended (per manufacturer) in hepatic impairment. Use with caution in patients with bone marrow compromise; myopathy and myositis have been associated with prolonged use of zidovudine (in Trizivir®).

Adverse Reactions Fatal hypersensitivity reactions have occurred in patients taking abacavir (in Trizivir®). If Trizivir® is to be restarted following an interruption in therapy, first evaluate the patient for previously unsuspected symptoms of hypersensitivity. Do not restart if hypersensitivity is suspected or if hypersensitivity cannot be ruled out.

The following information is based on CNAAB3003 study data concerning effects noted in patients receiving abacavir, lamivudine, and zidovudine. See individual agent monographs for additional information.

>10%:

- Endocrine & metabolic: Triglycerides increased (25%)
- Gastrointestinal: Nausea (47%), nausea and vomiting (16%), diarrhea (12%), loss of appetite/anorexia (11%)

1% to 10%:

- Central nervous system: Insomnia (7%)
- Miscellaneous: Hypersensitivity (5% based on abacavir component)

Other (frequency unknown): Pancreatitis, GGT increased

Postmarketing and/or case reports (limited to important or life-threatening): Redistribution/accumulation of body fat, anaphylaxis, cardiomyopathy, hepatic steatosis, lactic acidosis, Stevens-Johnson syndrome

Overdosage/Toxicology Symptoms of overdose with zidovudine include nausea, vomiting, headache, dizziness, drowsiness, lethargy, confusion, and hematologic changes. Myocardial degeneration has been documented in animals during long-term high-dose toxicology studies; clinical relevance is unknown. Peritoneal dialysis and hemodialysis have little to no effect on the removal of the components of Trizivir®.

Drug Interactions

Increased Effect/Toxicity: See individual agents.

Decreased Effect: See individual agents.

Stability Store at room temperature 25°C (77°F)

Mechanism of Action The combination of abacavir, lamivudine, and zidovudine is believed to act synergistically to inhibit reverse transcriptase via DNA chain termination after incorporation of the nucleoside analogue as well as to delay the emergence of mutations conferring resistance

Pharmacodynamics/Kinetics Bioavailability studies of Trizivir® show no difference in AUC or C_{max} when compared to abacavir, lamivudine, and zidovudine given together as individual agents. See individual agents.

Dosage Oral: Adolescents and Adults: 1 tablet twice daily; **Note:** Not recommended for patients <40 kg

Elderly: Use with caution

Dosage adjustment in renal impairment: Because lamivudine and zidovudine require dosage adjustment in renal impairment, Trizivir® should not be used in patients with Cl_{cr} ≤50 mL/minute

Dosage adjustment in hepatic impairment: Use not recommended.

Dietary Considerations May be taken without regard to food or water.

Administration Administer without regard to food or water.

Dosage Forms Tablet [film coated]: Abacavir 300 mg, lamivudine 150 mg, and zidovudine 300 mg

Abacavir Sulfate *see* Abacavir *on page 624*

Abacavir Sulfate and Lamivudine *see* Abacavir and Lamivudine *on page 626*

ABC *see* Abacavir *on page 624*

ABCD *see* Amphotericin B Cholesteryl Sulfate Complex *on page 649*

Abelcet® *see* Amphotericin B (Lipid Complex) *on page 653*

ABLC *see* Amphotericin B (Lipid Complex) *on page 653*

Abreva® [OTC] *see* Docosanol *on page 787*

Absorbine Jr.® Antifungal [OTC] *see* Tolnaftate *on page 1127*

Acetasol® HC *see* Acetic Acid, Propylene Glycol Diacetate, and Hydrocortisone *on page 629*

Acetic Acid, Hydrocortisone, and Propylene Glycol Diacetate *see* Acetic Acid, Propylene Glycol Diacetate, and Hydrocortisone *on page 629*

Acetic Acid, Propylene Glycol Diacetate, and Hydrocortisone

(a SEE tik AS id, PRO pa leen GLY kole dye AS e tate, & hye droe KOR ti sone)

U.S. Brand Names Acetasol® HC; VoSol® HC

Canadian Brand Names VoSoL® HC

Synonyms Acetic Acid, Hydrocortisone, and Propylene Glycol Diacetate; Hydrocortisone, Acetic Acid, and Propylene Glycol Diacetate; Hydrocortisone, Propylene Glycol Diacetate, and Acetic Acid; Propylene Glycol Diacetate, Acetic Acid, and Hydrocortisone; Propylene Glycol Diacetate, Hydrocortisone, and Acetic Acid

Generic Available Yes

Use Treatment of superficial infections of the external auditory canal caused by organisms susceptible to the action of the antimicrobial, complicated by swelling

Adverse Reactions Frequency not defined: Otic: Transient burning or stinging may be noticed occasionally when the solution is first instilled into the acutely inflamed ear

Drug Interactions

Cytochrome P450 Effect: Hydrocortisone: **Substrate** of CYP3A4 (minor); **Induces** CYP3A4 (weak)

Dosage Adults: Otic: Instill 4 drops in ear(s) 3-4 times/day

Dosage Forms Solution, otic drops: Acetic acid 2%, propylene glycol diacetate 3%, and hydrocortisone 1% (10 mL)

Achromycin *see* Tetracycline *on page 1106*

Aciclovir *see* Acyclovir *on page 629*

ActHIB® *see Haemophilus* b Conjugate Vaccine *on page 848*

Acticin® *see* Permethrin *on page 1001*

Activated Protein C, Human, Recombinant *see* Drotrecogin Alfa *on page 793*

ACU-dyne® [OTC] *see* Povidone-Iodine *on page 1016*

ACV *see* Acyclovir *on page 629*

Acycloguanosine *see* Acyclovir *on page 629*

Acyclovir (ay SYE kloe veer)

U.S. Brand Names Zovirax®

Canadian Brand Names Alti-Acyclovir; Apo-Acyclovir®; Gen-Acyclovir; Nu-Acyclovir; ratio-Acyclovir; Zovirax®

Synonyms Aciclovir; ACV; Acycloguanosine

Generic Available Yes: Excludes cream, ointment

Use Treatment of genital herpes simplex virus (HSV), herpes labialis (cold sores), herpes zoster (shingles), HSV encephalitis, neonatal HSV, mucocutaneous HSV, varicella-zoster (chickenpox)

Unlabeled/Investigational Use Prevention of HSV reactivation in HIV positive patients; prevention of HSV reactivation in hematopoietic stem cell transplant (HSCT); prevention of CMV infection after bone marrow transplants in HSV and CMV seropositive individuals

(Continued)

Acyclovir *(Continued)*

Drug of Choice or Alternative for Disease/Syndrome(s):

Encephalitis, Viral *on page 121*
Esophagitis *on page 147*

Organism(s):

Herpes Simplex Virus *on page 172*
Varicella-Zoster Virus *on page 347*

Pregnancy Risk Factor B

Pregnancy Implications Teratogenic effects were not observed in animal studies. Acyclovir has been shown to cross the human placenta. Results from a pregnancy registry, established in 1984 and closed in 1999, did not find an increase in the number of birth defects with exposure to acyclovir when compared to those expected in the general population. However, due to the small size of the registry and lack of long-term data, the manufacturer recommends using during pregnancy with caution and only when clearly needed. Data from the pregnancy registry may be obtained from GlaxoSmithKline.

Contraindications Hypersensitivity to acyclovir, valacyclovir, or any component of the formulation

Warnings/Precautions Use with caution in immunocompromised patients; thrombocytopenic purpura/hemolytic uremic syndrome (TTP/HUS) has been reported. Use caution in the elderly, pre-existing renal disease or in those receiving other nephrotoxic drugs. Maintain adequate hydration during I.V. therapy. Use I.V. preparation with caution in patients with underlying neurologic abnormalities, serious hepatic or electrolyte abnormalities, or substantial hypoxia.

Chickenpox: Treatment should begin within 24 hours of appearance of rash; oral route not recommended for routine use in otherwise healthy children with varicella, but may be effective in patients at increased risk of moderate to severe infection (>12 years of age, chronic cutaneous or pulmonary disorders, long-term salicylate therapy, corticosteroid therapy).

Genital herpes: Physical contact should be avoided when lesions are present; transmission may also occur in the absence of symptoms. Treatment should begin with the first signs or symptoms.

Herpes labialis: For external use only to the lips and face; do not apply to eye or inside the mouth or nose. Treatment should begin with the first signs or symptoms.

Herpes zoster: Acyclovir should be started within 72 hours of appearance of rash to be effective.

Adverse Reactions

Systemic: Oral:

1% to 10%:
- Central nervous system: Lightheadedness, headache
- Gastrointestinal: Diarrhea, nausea, vomiting, abdominal pain

Systemic: Parenteral:

>10%:
- Central nervous system: Lightheadedness
- Gastrointestinal: Anorexia

1% to 10%:
- Dermatologic: Hives, itching, rash
- Gastrointestinal: Nausea, vomiting
- Hepatic: Liver function tests increased
- Local: Inflammation at injection site or phlebitis
- Renal: Acute renal failure, BUN increased, creatinine increased

Topical:

>10%: Mild pain, burning, or stinging
1% to 10%: Itching

All forms: <1%, postmarketing, and/or case reports: Abdominal pain, aggression, agitation, alopecia, anaphylaxis, anemia, angioedema, anorexia, ataxia, coma, confusion, consciousness decreased, delirium, diarrhea, dizziness, dysarthria, encephalopathy, erythema multiforme, fatigue, fever, gastrointestinal distress, hallucinations, hematuria, hepatitis, hyperbilirubinemia, insomnia, jaundice, leukocytoclastic vasculitis, leukopenia, local tissue necrosis (following extravasation), mental depression, myalgia, paresthesia, peripheral edema, photosensitization, pruritus, psychosis, renal failure, seizure, somnolence, sore throat, Stevens-Johnson syndrome, thrombocytopenia, thrombocytopenic purpura/hemolytic uremic syndrome (TTP/HUS), toxic epidermal necrolysis, tremor, urticaria, visual disturbances

Overdosage/Toxicology Symptoms include seizures, somnolence, confusion, elevated serum creatinine, and renal failure. In the event of an overdose, sufficient urine flow must be maintained to avoid drug precipitation within the renal tubules. Hemodialysis has resulted in up to 60% reductions in serum acyclovir levels.

Drug Interactions

Increased Effect/Toxicity: Increased CNS side effects when taken with zidovudine or probenecid.

Ethanol/Nutrition/Herb Interactions Food: Does not appear to affect absorption of acyclovir.

Stability

Capsule, tablet: Store at controlled room temperature of 15°C to 25°C (59°F to 77°F); protect from moisture.

Cream, suspension: Store at controlled room temperature of 15°C to 25°C (59°F to 77°F).

Ointment: Store at controlled room temperature of 15°C to 25°C (59°F to 77°F) in a dry place.

Injection: Store powder at controlled room temperature of 15°C to 25°C (59°F to 77°F). Reconstitute acyclovir 500 mg with SWFI 10 mL; do not use bacteriostatic water containing benzyl alcohol or parabens. For intravenous infusion, dilute to a final concentration of ≤7 mg/mL. Concentrations >10 mg/mL increase the risk of phlebitis. Reconstituted solutions remain stable for 12 hours at room temperature. Do not refrigerate reconstituted solutions as they may precipitate. Once diluted for infusion, use within 24 hours.

Mechanism of Action Acyclovir is converted to acyclovir monophosphate by virus-specific thymidine kinase then further converted to acyclovir triphosphate by other cellular enzymes. Acyclovir triphosphate inhibits DNA synthesis and viral replication by competing with deoxyguanosine triphosphate for viral DNA polymerase and being incorporated into viral DNA.

Pharmacodynamics/Kinetics

Absorption: Oral: 15% to 30%

Distribution: Widely (ie, brain, kidney, lungs, liver, spleen, muscle, uterus, vagina, CSF)

Protein binding: 9% to 33%

Metabolism: Converted by viral enzymes to acyclovir monophosphate, and further converted to diphosphate then triphosphate (active form) by cellular enzymes

Bioavailability: Oral: 10% to 20% with normal renal function (bioavailability decreases with increased dose)

Half-life elimination: Terminal: Neonates: 4 hours; Children 1-12 years: 2-3 hours; Adults: 3 hours

Time to peak, serum: Oral: Within 1.5-2 hours

Excretion: Urine (62% to 90% as unchanged drug and metabolite)

Dosage Note: Obese patients should be dosed using ideal body weight

Genital HSV:

I.V.: Children ≥12 years and Adults (immunocompetent): Initial episode, severe: 5 mg/kg every 8 hours for 5-7 days

Oral:

Children:

Initial episode (unlabeled use): 40-80 mg/kg/day divided into 3-4 doses for 5-10 days (maximum: 1 g/day)

Chronic suppression (unlabeled use; limited data): 80 mg/kg/day in 3 divided doses (maximum: 1 g/day), re-evaluate after 12 months of treatment

Adults:

Initial episode: 200 mg every 4 hours while awake (5 times/day) for 10 days (per manufacturer's labeling); 400 mg 3 times/day for 5-10 days has also been reported

Recurrence: 200 mg every 4 hours while awake (5 times/day) for 5 days (per manufacturer's labeling; begin at earliest signs of disease); 400 mg 3 times/day for 5 days has also been reported

Chronic suppression: 400 mg twice daily or 200 mg 3-5 times/day, for up to 12 months followed by re-evaluation (per manufacturer's labeling); 400-1200 mg/day in 2-3 divided doses has also been reported

Topical: Adults (immunocompromised): Ointment: Initial episode: 1/2" ribbon of ointment for a 4" square surface area every 3 hours (6 times/day) for 7 days

Herpes labialis (cold sores): Topical: Children ≥12 years and Adults: Cream: Apply 5 times/day for 4 days

Herpes zoster (shingles):

Oral: Adults (immunocompetent): 800 mg every 4 hours (5 times/day) for 7-10 days

(Continued)

Acyclovir *(Continued)*

I.V.:
- Children <12 years (immunocompromised): 20 mg/kg/dose every 8 hours for 7 days
- Children ≥12 years and Adults (immunocompromised): 10 mg/kg/dose or 500 mg/ m^2/dose every 8 hours for 7 days

HSV encephalitis: I.V.:
- Children 3 months to 12 years: 20 mg/kg/dose every 8 hours for 10 days (per manufacturer's labeling); dosing for 14-21 days also reported
- Children ≥12 years and Adults: 10 mg/kg/dose every 8 hours for 10 days (per manufacturer's labeling); 10-15 mg/kg/dose every 8 hours for 14-21 days also reported

Mucocutaneous HSV:

I.V.:
- Children <12 years (immunocompromised): 10 mg/kg/dose every 8 hours for 7 days
- Children ≥12 years and Adults (immunocompromised): 5 mg/kg/dose every 8 hours for 7 days (per manufacturer's labeling); dosing for up to 14 days also reported

Oral: Adults (immunocompromised, unlabeled use): 400 mg 5 times a day for 7-14 days

Topical: Ointment: Adults (nonlife-threatening, immunocompromised): ½" ribbon of ointment for a 4" square surface area every 3 hours (6 times/day) for 7 days

Neonatal HSV: I.V.: Neonate: Birth to 3 months: 10 mg/kg/dose every 8 hours for 10 days (manufacturer's labeling); 15 mg/kg/dose or 20 mg/kg/dose every 8 hours for 14-21 days has also been reported

Varicella-zoster (chickenpox): Begin treatment within the first 24 hours of rash onset:

Oral:
- Children ≥2 years and ≤40 kg (immunocompetent): 20 mg/kg/dose (up to 800 mg/ dose) 4 times/day for 5 days
- Children >40 kg and Adults (immunocompetent): 800 mg/dose 4 times a day for 5 days

I.V.:
- Children <1 year (immunocompromised, unlabeled use): 10 mg/kg/dose every 8 hours for 7-10 days
- Children ≥1 year and Adults (immunocompromised, unlabeled use): 1500 mg/m^2/ day divided every 8 hours or 10 mg/kg/dose every 8 hours for 7-10 days

Prevention of HSV reactivation in HIV-positive patients, for use only when recurrences are frequent or severe (unlabeled use): Oral:
- Children: 80 mg/kg/day in 3-4 divided doses
- Adults: 200 mg 3 times/day or 400 mg 2 times/day

Prevention of HSV reactivation in HSCT (unlabeled use): Note: Start at the beginning of conditioning therapy and continue until engraftment or until mucositis resolves (~30 days)

Oral: Adults: 200 mg 3 times/day

I.V.:
- Children: 250 mg/m^2/dose every 8 hours or 125 mg/m^2/dose every 6 hours
- Adults: 250 mg/m^2/dose every 12 hours

Bone marrow transplant recipients (unlabeled use): I.V.: Children and Adults: Allogeneic patients who are HSV and CMV seropositive: 500 mg/m^2/dose (10 mg/ kg) every 8 hours; for clinically-symptomatic CMV infection, consider replacing acyclovir with ganciclovir

Dosing adjustment in renal impairment:

Oral:
- Cl_{cr} 10-25 mL/minute: Normal dosing regimen 800 mg every 4 hours: Administer 800 mg every 8 hours
- Cl_{cr} <10 mL/minute:
  - Normal dosing regimen 200 mg every 4 hours, 200 mg every 8 hours, or 400 mg every 12 hours: Administer 200 mg every 12 hours
  - Normal dosing regimen 800 mg every 4 hours: Administer 800 mg every 12 hours

I.V.:
- Cl_{cr} 25-50 mL/minute: Administer recommended dose every 12 hours
- Cl_{cr} 10-25 mL/minute: Administer recommended dose every 24 hours
- Cl_{cr} <10 mL/minute: Administer 50% of recommended dose every 24 hours

Hemodialysis: Administer dose after dialysis

Peritoneal dialysis: No supplemental dose needed
CAVH: 3.5 mg/kg/day
CVVHD/CVVH: Adjust dose based upon Cl_{cr} 30 mL/minute

Dietary Considerations May be taken with or without food. Acyclovir 500 mg injection contains sodium ~50 mg (~2 mEq).

Administration

Oral: May be administered with or without food.
I.V.: Avoid rapid infusion; infuse over 1 hour to prevent renal damage; maintain adequate hydration of patient; check for phlebitis and rotate infusion sites
Topical: Not for use in the eye. Apply using a finger cot or rubber glove to avoid transmission to other parts of the body or to other persons.

Monitoring Parameters Urinalysis, BUN, serum creatinine, liver enzymes, CBC

Patient Information This is not a cure for herpes (recurrences tend to continually reappear every 3-6 months after original infection), nor will this medication reduce the risk of transmission to others when lesions are present; avoid sexual intercourse when visible lesions are present. Take as directed for full course of therapy; do not discontinue even if feeling better. Oral doses may be taken with food.

Dosage Forms

Capsule: 200 mg
Cream, topical: 5% (2 g)
Injection, powder for reconstitution, as sodium: 500 mg, 1000 mg
  Zovirax®: 500 mg
Injection, solution, as sodium [preservative free]: 25 mg/mL (20 mL, 40 mL); 50 mg/mL (10 mL, 20 mL)
Ointment, topical: 5% (15 g)
Suspension, oral: 200 mg/5 mL (480 mL) [banana flavor]
Tablet: 400 mg, 800 mg

Selected Readings

"Drugs for Non-HIV Viral Infections," *Med Lett Drugs Ther*, 1994, 36(919):27.
Dunkle LM, Arvin AM, Whitley RJ, et al, "A Controlled Trial of Acyclovir for Chickenpox in Normal Children," *N Engl J Med*, 1991, 325(22):1539-44.
Keating MR, "Antiviral Agents," *Mayo Clin Proc*, 1992, 67(2):160-78.
Wallace MR, Bowler WA, Murray NB, et al, "Treatment of Adult Varicella With Oral Acyclovir," *Ann Intern Med*, 1992, 117(5):358-63.
Whitley RJ and Gnann JW Jr, "Acyclovir: A Decade Later," *N Engl J Med*, 1992, 327(11):782-3.

Aczone™ *see* Dapsone *on page 766*

Adacel™ *see* Diphtheria, Tetanus Toxoids, and Acellular Pertussis Vaccine *on page 782*

Adamantanamine Hydrochloride *see* Amantadine *on page 636*

Adefovir (a DEF o veer)

U.S. Brand Names Hepsera™

Synonyms Adefovir Dipivoxil

Generic Available No

Use Treatment of chronic hepatitis B with evidence of active viral replication (based on persistent elevation of ALT/AST or histologic evidence), including patients with lamivudine-resistant hepatitis B

Pregnancy Risk Factor C

Pregnancy Implications There are no adequate and well-controlled studies in pregnant women. Use in pregnancy only when clearly needed.

Contraindications Hypersensitivity to adefovir or any component of the formulation

Warnings/Precautions Use with caution in patients with renal dysfunction or in patients at risk of renal toxicity (including concurrent nephrotoxic agents or NSAIDs). Chronic administration may result in nephrotoxicity. Dosage adjustment is required in patients with renal dysfunction or in patients who develop renal dysfunction during therapy. May cause the development of resistance in patients with unrecognized or untreated HIV infection. Lactic acidosis and severe hepatomegaly with steatosis (sometimes fatal) have occurred with antiretroviral nucleoside analogues; female gender, obesity, and prolonged treatment may increase the risk of hepatotoxicity. Treatment should be discontinued in patients with lactic acidosis or signs/symptoms of hepatotoxicity (which may occur without marked transaminase elevations). Acute exacerbations of hepatitis may occur (in up to 25% of patients) when antihepatitis therapy is discontinued. Exacerbations typically occur within 12 weeks; monitor patients following discontinuation of therapy. Safety and efficacy in pediatric patients have not been established.

Adverse Reactions

>10%: Renal: Hematuria (11% vs. 10% in placebo-treated)
1% to 10%:
  Central nervous system: Fever, headache
  Dermatologic: Rash, pruritus
(Continued)

Adefovir *(Continued)*

Gastrointestinal: Dyspepsia (3%), nausea, vomiting, flatulence, diarrhea, abdominal pain
Hepatic: AST/ALT increased, abnormal liver function, hepatic failure
Neuromuscular & skeletal: Weakness
Renal: Serum creatinine increased (4%), renal failure, renal insufficiency
Note: In patients with baseline renal dysfunction, frequency of increased serum creatinine has been observed to be as high as 26% to 37%; the role of adefovir in these changes could not be established.
Respiratory: Cough increased, sinusitis, pharyngitis

Overdosage/Toxicology Limited experience in acute overdose. Chronic overdose may be associated with renal toxicity and gastrointestinal adverse effects. Hemodialysis may be effective in the removal of adefovir (35% of a 10 mg dose removed in 4 hours).

Drug Interactions

Increased Effect/Toxicity: Ibuprofen increases the bioavailability of adefovir. Concurrent use of nephrotoxic agents (including aminoglycosides, cyclosporine, NSAIDs, tacrolimus, vancomycin) may increase the risk of nephrotoxicity.

Ethanol/Nutrition/Herb Interactions

Ethanol: Should be avoided in hepatitis B infection due to potential hepatic toxicity.
Food: Does not have a significant effect on adefovir absorption.

Stability Store at 25°C (77 °F); excursions permitted to 15°C to 30°C (59°F to 86°F).

Mechanism of Action Acyclic nucleotide reverse transcriptase inhibitor (adenosine analog) which interferes with HBV viral RNA dependent DNA polymerase resulting in inhibition of viral replication.

Pharmacodynamics/Kinetics

Distribution: 0.35-0.39 L/kg
Protein binding: ≤4%
Metabolism: Prodrug; rapidly converted to adefovir (active metabolite) in intestine
Bioavailability: 59%
Half-life elimination: 7.5 hours; prolonged in renal impairment
Time to peak: 1.75 hours
Excretion: Urine (45% as active metabolite within 24 hours)

Dosage Oral: Adults: 10 mg once daily

Dosage adjustment in renal impairment:

Cl_{cr} 20-49 mL/minute: 10 mg every 48 hours
Cl_{cr} 10-19 mL/minute: 10 mg every 72 hours

Hemodialysis: 10 mg every 7 days (following dialysis)

Dietary Considerations May be taken without regard to food.

Administration May be administered without regard to food.

Monitoring Parameters HIV status (prior to initiation of therapy); serum creatinine (prior to initiation and during therapy)

Patient Information Not a cure for hepatitis B, nor will it reduce the risk of transmission. Report persistent lethargy, acute headache, severe nausea or vomiting, difficulty breathing, loss of sensation, or rash. Do not discontinue unless instructed by prescriber; additional monitoring is required after discontinuation to ensure the disease does not recur.

Additional Information Adefovir dipivoxil is a prodrug, rapidly converted to the active component (adefovir). It was previously investigated as a treatment for HIV infections (at dosages substantially higher than the approved dose for hepatitis B). The NDA was withdrawn, and no further studies in the treatment of HIV are anticipated (per manufacturer).

Dosage Forms Tablet, as dipivoxil: 10 mg

Adefovir Dipivoxil *see* Adefovir *on page 633*

Adoxa™ *see* Doxycycline *on page 787*

Aftate® Antifungal [OTC] *see* Tolnaftate *on page 1127*

Agenerase® *see* Amprenavir *on page 662*

$AgNO_3$ *see* Silver Nitrate *on page 1064*

Akne-Mycin® *see* Erythromycin *on page 807*

AK-Poly-Bac® *see* Bacitracin and Polymyxin B *on page 681*

AK-Spore® H.C. [DSC] *see* Bacitracin, Neomycin, Polymyxin B, and Hydrocortisone *on page 682*

AKTob® *see* Tobramycin *on page 1122*

AK-Tracin® [DSC] *see* Bacitracin *on page 679*

AK-Trol® *see* Neomycin, Polymyxin B, and Dexamethasone *on page 965*

Alatrofloxacin Mesylate *see* Trovafloxacin *on page 1134*

Albendazole (al BEN da zole)

U.S. Brand Names Albenza®

Generic Available No

Use Treatment of parenchymal neurocysticercosis caused by *Taenia solium* and cystic hydatid disease of the liver, lung, and peritoneum caused by *Echinococcus granulosus*

Unlabeled/Investigational Use Albendazole has activity against *Ascaris lumbricoides* (roundworm); *Ancylostoma caninum*; *Ancylostoma duodenale* and *Necator americanus* (hookworms); cutaneous larva migrans; *Enterobius vermicularis* (pinworm); *Gnathostoma spinigerum*; *Gongylonema* sp; *Hymenolepis nana* sp (tapeworms); *Mansonella perstans* (filariasis); *Opisthorchis sinensis* and *Opisthorchis viverrini* (liver flukes); *Strongyloides stercoralis* and *Trichuris trichiura* (whipworm); visceral larva migrans (toxocariasis); activity has also been shown against the liver fluke *Clonorchis sinensis*, *Giardia lamblia*, *Cysticercus cellulosae*, and *Echinococcus multilocularis*. Albendazole has also been used for the treatment of intestinal microsporidiosis (*Encephalitozoon intestinalis*), disseminated microsporidiosis (*E. hellem, E. cuniculi, E. intestinalis, Pleistophora* sp, *Trachipleistophora* sp, *Brachiola vesicularum*), and ocular microsporidiosis (*E. hellem, E. cuniculi, Vittaforma corneae*).

Drug of Choice or Alternative for Organism(s):

Cestodes *on page 72*

Giardia lamblia *on page 155*

Microsporidia *on page 220*

Pregnancy Risk Factor C

Pregnancy Implications Albendazole has been shown to be teratogenic in laboratory animals and should not be used during pregnancy, if at all possible. Women should be advised to avoid pregnancy for at least 1 month following therapy. Discontinue if pregnancy occurs during treatment.

Contraindications Hypersensitivity to albendazole or any component of the formulation

Warnings/Precautions Discontinue therapy if LFT elevations are significant; may restart treatment when decreased to pretreatment values. Becoming pregnant within 1 month following therapy is not advised.

Neurocysticercosis: Corticosteroids should be administered 1-2 days before albendazole therapy to minimize inflammatory reactions. Steroid and anticonvulsant therapy should be used concurrently during the first week of therapy to prevent cerebral hypertension. If retinal lesions exist, weigh risk of further retinal damage due to albendazole-induced changes to the retinal lesion vs benefit of disease treatment.

Adverse Reactions

N = Neurocysticercosis; H = Hydatid disease

>10%:
- Central nervous system: Headache (11% - N; 1% - H)
- Hepatic: LFTs Increased (~15% - H; <1% - N)

1% to 10%:
- Central nervous system: Dizziness, vertigo, fever (≤1%); intracranial pressure increased (1% - N), meningeal signs (1% - N)
- Dermatologic: Alopecia (2% - H; <1% - N)
- Gastrointestinal: Abdominal pain (6% - H; 0% - N); nausea/vomiting (3% to 6%)
- Hematologic: Leukopenia (reversible) (<1%)
- Miscellaneous: Allergic reactions (<1%)

<1%: Acute renal failure, agranulocytopenia, allergic reaction, granulocytopenia, pancytopenia, rash, thrombocytopenia, urticaria

Drug Interactions

Cytochrome P450 Effect: Substrate (minor) of CYP1A2, 3A4; **Inhibits** CYP1A2 (weak)

Ethanol/Nutrition/Herb Interactions Food: Albendazole serum levels may be increased if taken with a fatty meal (increases the oral bioavailability by 4-5 times).

Mechanism of Action Active metabolite, albendazole, causes selective degeneration of cytoplasmic microtubules in intestinal and tegmental cells of intestinal helminths and larvae; glycogen is depleted, glucose uptake and cholinesterase secretion are impaired, and desecratory substances accumulate intracellulary. ATP production decreases causing energy depletion, immobilization, and worm death.

Pharmacodynamics/Kinetics

Absorption: <5%; may increase up to 4-5 times when administered with a fatty meal

Distribution: Well inside hydatid cysts and CSF

Protein binding: 70%

Metabolism: Hepatic; extensive first-pass effect; pathways include rapid sulfoxidation (major), hydrolysis, and oxidation

(Continued)

Albendazole *(Continued)*

Half-life elimination: 8-12 hours
Time to peak, serum: 2-2.4 hours
Excretion: Urine (<1% as active metabolite); feces

Dosage Oral:

Children:

Cysticercus cellulosae (unlabeled use): 15 mg/kg/day (maximum: 800 mg/day) in 2 divided doses for 8-30 days; may be repeated as necessary

Echinococcus granulosus (tapeworm) (unlabeled use): 15 mg/kg/day (maximum: 800 mg) divided twice daily for 1-6 months

Children and Adults:

Neurocysticercosis:

<60 kg: 15 mg/kg/day in 2 divided doses (maximum: 800 mg/day) for 8-30 days
≥60 kg: 400 mg twice daily for 8-30 days

Note: Give concurrent anticonvulsant and steroid therapy during first week.

Hydatid:

<60 kg: 15 mg/kg/day in 2 divided doses (maximum: 800 mg/day)
≥60 kg: 400 mg twice daily

Note: Administer dose for three 28-day cycles with a 14-day drug-free interval in between.

Ancylostoma caninum, *Ascaris lumbricoides* (roundworm), *Ancylostoma duodenale*, and *Necator americanus* (hookworms) (unlabeled use): 400 mg as a single dose

Clonorchis sinensis (Chinese liver fluke) (unlabeled use): 10 mg/kg for 7 days

Cutaneous larva migrans (unlabeled use): 400 mg once daily for 3 days

Enterobius vermicularis (pinworm) (unlabeled use): 400 mg as a single dose; may repeat in 2 weeks

Gnathostoma spinigerum (unlabeled use): 400 mg twice daily for 21 days

Gongylonemiasis (unlabeled use): 10 mg/kg/day for 3 days

Mansonella perstans (unlabeled use): 400 mg twice daily for 10 days

Visceral larva migrans (toxocariasis) (unlabeled use): 400 mg twice daily for 5 days

Adults:

Cysticercus cellulosae (unlabeled use): 400 mg twice daily for 8-30 days; may be repeated as necessary

Disseminated microsporidiosis (unlabeled use): 400 mg twice daily

Echinococcus granulosus (tapeworm) (unlabeled use): 400 mg twice daily for 1-6 months

Intestinal microsporidiosis (unlabeled use): 400 mg twice daily for 21 days

Ocular microsporidiosis (unlabeled use): 400 mg twice daily, in combination with fumagillin

Dietary Considerations Should be taken with a high-fat meal.

Administration Administer with meals; administer anticonvulsant and steroid therapy during first week of neurocysticercosis therapy

Monitoring Parameters Monitor fecal specimens for ova and parasites for 3 weeks after treatment; if positive, retreat; monitor LFTs, and clinical signs of hepatotoxicity; CBC at start of each 28-day cycle and every 2 weeks during therapy

Dosage Forms Tablet: 200 mg

Selected Readings

de Silva N, Guyatt H, and Bundy D, "Anthelmintics. A Comparative Review of Their Clinical Pharmacology," *Drugs*, 1997, 53(5):769-88.
Liu LX and Weller PF, "Antiparasitic Drugs," *N Engl J Med*, 1996, 334(18):1178-84.

Albenza® *see* Albendazole *on page 635*
Alcomicin® (Can) *see* Gentamicin *on page 841*
Aldara™ *see* Imiquimod *on page 864*
Alinia® *see* Nitazoxanide *on page 970*
Aloe Vesta® 2-n-1 Antifungal [OTC] *see* Miconazole *on page 945*
Alti-Acyclovir (Can) *see* Acyclovir *on page 629*
Alti-Amoxi-Clav (Can) *see* Amoxicillin and Clavulanate Potassium *on page 645*
Alti-Clindamycin (Can) *see* Clindamycin *on page 752*
Alti-Minocycline (Can) *see* Minocycline *on page 947*

Amantadine (a MAN ta deen)

Related Information

USPHS / IDSA Guidelines for the Prevention of Opportunistic Infections in Persons Infected With HIV *on page 1237*

U.S. Brand Names Symmetrel®

Canadian Brand Names Endantadine®; PMS-Amantadine; Symmetrel®

Synonyms Adamantanamine Hydrochloride; Amantadine Hydrochloride

Generic Available Yes

Use Prophylaxis and treatment of influenza A viral infection; treatment of parkinsonism; treatment of drug-induced extrapyramidal symptoms

Drug of Choice or Alternative for Organism(s):

Influenza Virus *on page 193*

Pregnancy Risk Factor C

Pregnancy Implications Teratogenic effects were observed in animal studies; limited data in humans. Impaired fertility has also been reported during animal studies and during human *in vitro* fertilization.

Contraindications Hypersensitivity to amantadine, rimantadine, or any component of the formulation

Warnings/Precautions Use with caution in patients with liver disease, history of recurrent and eczematoid dermatitis, uncontrolled psychosis or severe psychoneurosis, seizures, and in those receiving CNS stimulant drugs; reduce dose in renal disease. When treating Parkinson's disease, do not discontinue abruptly. In many patients, the therapeutic benefits of amantadine are limited to a few months. Elderly patients may be more susceptible to CNS effects (using 2 divided daily doses may minimize this effect). Has been associated with neuroleptic malignant syndrome (associated with dose reduction or abrupt discontinuation). Has not been shown to prevent bacterial infection or complications when used as prophylaxis or treatment of influenza A. Use with caution in patients with CHF, peripheral edema, or orthostatic hypotension. Avoid in angle closure glaucoma.

Adverse Reactions

1% to 10%:

Cardiovascular: Orthostatic hypotension, peripheral edema

Central nervous system: Insomnia, depression, anxiety, irritability, dizziness, hallucinations, ataxia, headache, somnolence, nervousness, dream abnormality, agitation, fatigue, confusion

Dermatologic: Livedo reticularis

Gastrointestinal: Nausea, anorexia, constipation, diarrhea, xerostomia

Respiratory: Dry nose

<1%: Amnesia, CHF, decreased libido, dyspnea, eczematoid dermatitis, euphoria, hyperkinesis, hypertension, instances of convulsions, leukopenia, neutropenia, oculogyric episodes, photosensitivity, psychosis, rash, slurred speech, urinary retention, visual disturbances, vomiting, weakness; withdrawal reactions may include delirium, hallucinations and psychosis

Overdosage/Toxicology Symptoms include nausea, vomiting, slurred speech, blurred vision, lethargy, hallucinations, seizures, and myoclonic jerking. Acute toxicity may be primarily due to anticholinergic effects. The minimum lethal dose may be as low as 1 g. Following GI decontamination, treatment should be directed at reducing CNS stimulation and at maintaining cardiovascular function. Seizures can be treated with diazepam, while lidocaine infusion may be required for cardiac dysrhythmias.

Drug Interactions

Increased Effect/Toxicity: Anticholinergics (benztropine and trihexyphenidyl) may potentiate CNS side effects of amantadine. Hydrochlorothiazide, triamterene, and/or trimethoprim may increase toxicity of amantadine; monitor for altered response.

Ethanol/Nutrition/Herb Interactions Ethanol: Avoid ethanol (may increase CNS adverse effects).

Stability Store at 15°C to 30°C (59°F to 86°F); protect from freezing

Mechanism of Action As an antiviral, blocks the uncoating of influenza A virus preventing penetration of virus into host; antiparkinsonian activity may be due to its blocking the reuptake of dopamine into presynaptic neurons or by increasing dopamine release from presynaptic fibers

Pharmacodynamics/Kinetics

Onset of action: Antidyskinetic: Within 48 hours

Absorption: Well absorbed

Distribution: V_d: Normal: 1.5-6.1 L/kg; Renal failure: 5.1 ± 0.2 L/kg; in saliva, tear film, and nasal secretions; in animals, tissue (especially lung) concentrations higher than serum concentrations; crosses blood-brain barrier

Protein binding: Normal renal function: ~67%; Hemodialysis: ~59%

Metabolism: Not appreciable; small amounts of an acetyl metabolite identified

Bioavailability: 86% to 90%

Half-life elimination: Normal renal function: 16 ± 6 hours (9-31 hours); End-stage renal disease: 7-10 days

(Continued)

Amantadine *(Continued)*

Excretion: Urine (80% to 90% unchanged) by glomerular filtration and tubular secretion

Total clearance: 2.5-10.5 L/hour

Dosage Oral:

Children:

Influenza A treatment:

1-9 years: 5 mg/kg/day in 2 divided doses (manufacturers range: 4.4-8.8 mg/kg/day); maximum dose: 150 mg/day

≥10 years and <40 kg: 5 mg/kg/day; maximum dose: 150 mg/day

≥10 years and ≥40 kg: 100 mg twice daily

Note: Initiate within 24-48 hours after onset of symptoms; discontinue as soon as possible based on clinical response (generally within 3-5 days or within 24-48 hours after symptoms disappear)

Influenza A prophylaxis: Refer to "Influenza A treatment" dosing

Note: Continue treatment throughout the peak influenza activity in the community or throughout the entire influenza season in patients who cannot be vaccinated. Development of immunity following vaccination takes ~2 weeks; amantadine therapy should be considered for high-risk patients from the time of vaccination until immunity has developed. For children <9 years receiving influenza vaccine for the first time, amantadine prophylaxis should continue for 6 weeks (4 weeks after the first dose and 2 weeks after the second dose)

Adults:

Drug-induced extrapyramidal symptoms: 100 mg twice daily; may increase to 300-400 mg/day, if needed

Parkinson's disease or Creutzfeldt-Jakob disease (unlabeled use): 100 mg twice daily as sole therapy; may increase to 400 mg/day if needed with close monitoring; initial dose: 100 mg/day if with other serious illness or with high doses of other anti-Parkinson drugs

Influenza A viral infection: 100 mg twice daily; initiate within 24-48 hours after onset of symptoms; discontinue as soon as possible based on clinical response (generally within 3-5 days or within 24-48 hours after symptoms disappear)

Influenza A prophylaxis: 100 mg twice daily

Note: Continue treatment throughout the peak influenza activity in the community or throughout the entire influenza season in patients who cannot be vaccinated. Development of immunity following vaccination takes ~2 weeks; amantadine therapy should be considered for high-risk patients from the time of vaccination until immunity has developed

Elderly: Adjust dose based on renal function; some patients tolerate the drug better when it is given in 2 divided daily doses (to avoid adverse neurologic reactions). Influenza A prophylaxis or treatment: ≤100 mg/day in patients ≥65 years

Dosing interval in renal impairment:

Cl_{cr} 30-50 mL/minute: Administer 200 mg on day 1, then 100 mg/day

Cl_{cr} 15-29 mL/minute: Administer 200 mg on day 1, then 100 mg on alternate days

Cl_{cr} <15 mL/minute: Administer 200 mg every 7 days

Hemodialysis: Administer 200 mg every 7 days

Peritoneal dialysis: No supplemental dose is needed

Continuous arteriovenous or venous-venous hemofiltration: No supplemental dose is needed

Monitoring Parameters Renal function, Parkinson's symptoms, mental status, influenza symptoms, blood pressure

Patient Information Do not abruptly discontinue therapy, it may precipitate a parkinsonian crisis; may impair ability to perform activities requiring mental alertness or coordination; must take throughout flu season or for at least 10 days following vaccination for effective prophylaxis; take second dose of the day in early afternoon to decrease incidence of insomnia

Additional Information Patients with intolerable CNS side effects often do better with rimantadine.

Dosage Forms [DSC] = Discontinued product

Capsule, as hydrochloride: 100 mg

Syrup, as hydrochloride: 50 mg/5 mL (480 mL)

Symmetrel®: 50 mg/5 mL (480 mL) [raspberry flavor] [DSC]

Tablet, as hydrochloride (Symmetrel®): 100 mg

Selected Readings

Arden NH, Patriarca PA, Fasano MB, et al, "The Roles of Vaccination and Amantadine Prophylaxis in Controlling an Outbreak of Influenza A (H3N2) in a Nursing Home," *Arch Intern Med*, 1988, 148(4):865-8.

Douglas RG Jr, "Prophylaxis and Treatment of Influenza," *N Engl J Med*, 1990, 322(7):443-50.

"Drugs for Non-HIV Viral Infections," *Med Lett Drugs Ther*, 1994, 36(919):27.

Keating MR, "Antiviral Agents," *Mayo Clin Proc*, 1992, 67(2):160-78.

Somani SK, Degelau J, Cooper SL, et al, "Comparison of Pharmacokinetic and Safety Profiles of Amantadine 50- and 100-mg Daily Doses in Elderly Nursing Home Residents," *Pharmacotherapy*, 1991, 11(6):460-6.

Amantadine Hydrochloride *see* Amantadine *on page 636*

AmBisome® *see* Amphotericin B (Liposomal) *on page 655*

Amikacin (am i KAY sin)

Related Information

Aminoglycoside Dosing and Monitoring *on page 1267*
Antimicrobial Activity Against Selected Organisms *on page 1165*
Tuberculosis *on page 1315*

U.S. Brand Names Amikin®

Canadian Brand Names Amikin®

Synonyms Amikacin Sulfate

Generic Available Yes

Use Treatment of serious infections due to organisms resistant to gentamicin and tobramycin including *Pseudomonas*, *Proteus*, *Serratia*, and other gram-negative bacilli (bone infections, respiratory tract infections, endocarditis, and septicemia); documented infection of mycobacterial organisms susceptible to amikacin

Drug of Choice or Alternative for

Disease/Syndrome(s):

Endophthalmitis, Bacterial and Fungal *on page 128*
Pneumonia, Hospital-Acquired *on page 272*
Pneumonia, Ventilator-Associated *on page 273*

Organism(s):

Mycobacterium avium-intracellulare (Complex) *on page 228*

Pregnancy Risk Factor D

Contraindications Hypersensitivity to amikacin sulfate or any component of the formulation; cross-sensitivity may exist with other aminoglycosides

Warnings/Precautions Dose and/or frequency of administration must be monitored and modified in patients with renal impairment; drug should be discontinued if signs of ototoxicity, nephrotoxicity, or hypersensitivity occur; ototoxicity is proportional to the amount of drug given and the duration of treatment; tinnitus or vertigo may be indications of vestibular injury and impending bilateral irreversible damage; renal damage is usually reversible

Adverse Reactions

1% to 10%:

Central nervous system: Neurotoxicity
Otic: Ototoxicity (auditory), ototoxicity (vestibular)
Renal: Nephrotoxicity

<1%: Hypotension, headache, drowsiness, drug fever, rash, nausea, vomiting, eosinophilia, paresthesia, tremor, arthralgia, weakness, dyspnea, allergic reaction

Overdosage/Toxicology Symptoms include ototoxicity, nephrotoxicity, and neuromuscular toxicity. Treatment of choice, following a single acute overdose, appears to be the maintenance of good urine output of at least 3 mL/kg/hour. Dialysis is of questionable value in the enhancement of aminoglycoside elimination. If required, hemodialysis is preferred over peritoneal dialysis in patients with normal renal function.

Drug Interactions

Increased Effect/Toxicity: Amikacin may increase or prolong the effect of neuromuscular blocking agents. Concurrent use of amphotericin (or other nephrotoxic drugs) may increase the risk of amikacin-induced nephrotoxicity. The risk of ototoxicity from amikacin may be increased with other ototoxic drugs.

Stability Stable for 24 hours at room temperature and 2 days at refrigeration when mixed in D_5W, $D_5{}^1\!/_4NS$, $D_5{}^1\!/_2NS$, NS, LR

Mechanism of Action Inhibits protein synthesis in susceptible bacteria by binding to 30S ribosomal subunits

Pharmacodynamics/Kinetics

Absorption: I.M.: May be delayed in the bedridden patient

Distribution: Primarily into extracellular fluid (highly hydrophilic); penetrates blood-brain barrier when meninges inflamed; crosses placenta

Relative diffusion of antimicrobial agents from blood into CSF: Good only with inflammation (exceeds usual MICs)

CSF:blood level ratio: Normal meninges: 10% to 20%; Inflamed meninges: 15% to 24%

Half-life elimination (renal function and age dependent):

Infants: Low birth weight (1-3 days): 7-9 hours; Full-term >7 days: 4-5 hours
Children: 1.6-2.5 hours

(Continued)

Amikacin *(Continued)*

Adults: Normal renal function: 1.4-2.3 hours; Anuria/end-stage renal disease: 28-86 hours

Time to peak, serum: I.M.: 45-120 minutes

Excretion: Urine (94% to 98%)

Dosage Individualization is critical because of the low therapeutic index

Use of ideal body weight (IBW) for determining the mg/kg/dose appears to be more accurate than dosing on the basis of total body weight (TBW)

In morbid obesity, dosage requirement may best be estimated using a dosing weight of IBW + 0.4 (TBW - IBW)

Initial and periodic peak and trough plasma drug levels should be determined, particularly in critically-ill patients with serious infections or in disease states known to significantly alter aminoglycoside pharmacokinetics (eg, cystic fibrosis, burns, or major surgery)

Infants, Children, and Adults: I.M., I.V.: 5-7.5 mg/kg/dose every 8 hours

Some clinicians suggest a daily dose of 15-20 mg/kg for all patients with normal renal function. This dose is at least as efficacious with similar, if not less, toxicity than conventional dosing.

Dosing interval in renal impairment: Some patients may require larger or more frequent doses if serum levels document the need (ie, cystic fibrosis or febrile granulocytopenic patients)

Cl_{cr} ≥60 mL/minute: Administer every 8 hours

Cl_{cr} 40-60 mL/minute: Administer every 12 hours

Cl_{cr} 20-40 mL/minute: Administer every 24 hours

Cl_{cr} <20 mL/minute: Loading dose, then monitor levels

Hemodialysis: Dialyzable (50% to 100%); administer dose postdialysis or administer $^2/_3$ normal dose as a supplemental dose postdialysis and follow levels

Peritoneal dialysis: Dose as Cl_{cr} <20 mL/minute: Follow levels

Continuous arteriovenous or venovenous hemodiafiltration effects: Dose as for Cl_{cr} 10-40 mL/minute and follow levels

Dietary Considerations Sodium content of 1 g: 29.9 mg (1.3 mEq)

Administration Administer I.M. injection in large muscle mass

Monitoring Parameters Urinalysis, BUN, serum creatinine, appropriately timed peak and trough concentrations, vital signs, temperature, weight, I & O, hearing parameters

Reference Range

Sample size: 0.5-2 mL blood (red top tube) or 0.1-1 mL serum (separated)

Therapeutic levels:

Peak:

Life-threatening infections: 25-30 mcg/mL

Serious infections: 20-25 mcg/mL

Urinary tract infections: 15-20 mcg/mL

Trough:

Serious infections: 1-4 mcg/mL

Life-threatening infections: 4-8 mcg/mL

Toxic concentration: Peak: >35 mcg/mL; Trough: >10 mcg/mL

Timing of serum samples: Draw peak 30 minutes after completion of 30-minute infusion or at 1 hour following initiation of infusion or I.M. injection; draw trough within 30 minutes prior to next dose

Test Interactions Penicillin may decrease aminoglycoside serum concentrations *in vitro*

Patient Information Report loss of hearing, ringing or roaring in the ears, or feeling of fullness in head

Additional Information Aminoglycoside levels measured from blood taken from Silastic® central catheters can sometimes give falsely high readings (draw levels from alternate lumen or peripheral stick, if possible)

Dosage Forms Injection, solution, as sulfate: 50 mg/mL (2 mL, 4 mL); 62.5 mg/mL (8 mL); 250 mg/mL (2 mL, 4 mL) [contains metabisulfite]

Selected Readings

Begg EJ and Barclay ML, "Aminoglycosides - 50 Years On," *Br J Clin Pharmacol*, 1995, 39(6):597-603.

Cunha BA, "Aminoglycosides: Current Role in Antimicrobial Therapy," *Pharmacotherapy*, 1988, 8(6):334-50.

Edson RS and Terrell CL, "The Aminoglycosides," *Mayo Clin Proc*, 1999, 74(5):519-28.

Gilbert DN, "Once-Daily Aminoglycoside Therapy," *Antimicrob Agents Chemother*, 1991, 35(3):399-405.

Iseman MD, "Treatment of Multidrug-Resistant Tuberculosis," *N Engl J Med*, 1993, 329(11):784-91.

Lortholary O, Tod M, Cohen Y, et al, "Aminoglycosides," *Med Clin North Am*, 1995, 79(4):761-87.

McCormack JP and Jewesson PJ, "A Critical Re-evaluation of the "Therapeutic Range" of Aminoglycosides," *Clin Infect Dis*, 1992, 14(1):320-39

Van der Auwera P, "Pharmacokinetic Evaluation of Single Daily Dose Amikacin," *J Antimicrob Chemother*, 1991, 27(Suppl C):63-71.

Amikacin Sulfate *see* Amikacin *on page 639*
Amikin® *see* Amikacin *on page 639*
Aminobenzylpenicillin *see* Ampicillin *on page 657*

Aminoglycosides

Refer to

Amikacin *on page 639*
Gentamicin *on page 841*
Kanamycin *on page 901*
Neomycin *on page 962*
Streptomycin *on page 1078*
Tobramycin *on page 1122*

Drug of Choice or Alternative for Disease/Syndrome(s):

Cholangitis, Acute *on page 79*
Diverticulitis *on page 116*
Fever, Neutropenic *on page 148*
Keratitis, Bacterial and Fungal *on page 199*
Otitis Externa, Severe (Malignant) *on page 252*
Peritonitis, CAPD-Associated *on page 262*
Pneumonia, Community-Acquired *on page 270*
Sepsis *on page 295*
Urinary Tract Infection, Catheter-Associated *on page 345*
Wound Infection, Surgical *on page 354*

Organism(s):

Alcaligenes Species *on page 31*
Bordetella bronchiseptica on page 52
Pseudomonas aeruginosa on page 282
Yersinia enterocolitica on page 354

Aminosalicylate Sodium *see* Aminosalicylic Acid *on page 641*

Aminosalicylic Acid (a mee noe sal i SIL ik AS id)

U.S. Brand Names Paser®

Canadian Brand Names Nemasol® Sodium

Synonyms Aminosalicylate Sodium; 4-Aminosalicylic Acid; Para-Aminosalicylate Sodium; PAS; Sodium PAS

Generic Available No

Use Adjunctive treatment of tuberculosis used in combination with other antitubercular agents

Unlabeled/Investigational Use Crohn's disease

Pregnancy Risk Factor C

Pregnancy Implications Teratogenic effects have been reported in animals, however, adequate studies have not been done in humans. Use during pregnancy only if clearly needed.

Contraindications Hypersensitivity to aminosalicylic acid or any component of the formulation

Warnings/Precautions Use with caution in patients with hepatic or renal dysfunction and patients with gastric ulcer.

Adverse Reactions Frequency not defined.

Cardiovascular: Pericarditis, vasculitis
Central nervous system: Encephalopathy, fever
Dermatologic: Skin eruptions
Endocrine & metabolic: Goiter (with or without myxedema), hypoglycemia
Gastrointestinal: Abdominal pain, diarrhea, nausea, vomiting
Hematologic: Agranulocytosis, anemia (hemolytic), leukopenia, thrombocytopenia
Hepatic: Hepatitis, jaundice
Ocular: Optic neuritis
Respiratory: Eosinophilic pneumonia

Overdosage/Toxicology Acute overdose results in crystalluria and renal failure, nausea, and vomiting. Alkalinization of the urine with sodium bicarbonate and forced diuresis can prevent crystalluria and nephrotoxicity.

Drug Interactions

Decreased Effect: Aminosalicylic acid may decrease serum levels of digoxin and vitamin B_{12}.

Stability Prior to dispensing, store granules below 15°C (59°F). Once dispensed, packets may be stored at room temperature for short periods of time. Do not use if packet is swollen or if granules are dark brown or purple.

(Continued)

Aminosalicylic Acid *(Continued)*

Mechanism of Action Aminosalicylic acid (PAS) is a highly specific bacteriostatic agent active against *M. tuberculosis*. Structurally related to para-aminobenzoic acid (PABA) and its mechanism of action is thought to be similar to the sulfonamides, a competitive antagonism with PABA; disrupts plate biosynthesis in sensitive organisms.

Pharmacodynamics/Kinetics

Absorption: Readily, >90%
Protein binding: 50% to 60%
Metabolism: Hepatic (>50%) via acetylation
Half-life elimination: Reduced with renal impairment
Time to peak, serum: 6 hours
Excretion: Urine (>80% as unchanged drug and metabolites)

Dosage Oral:

Children: Tuberculosis: 200-300 mg/kg/day in 3-4 equally divided doses
Adults:
Tuberculosis: 150 mg/kg/day in 2-3 equally divided doses
Crohn's disease (unlabeled use): 1.5 g/day

Dosing adjustment in renal impairment:

Cl_{cr} 10-50 mL/minute: Administer 50% to 75% of dose
Cl_{cr} <10 mL/minute: Administer 50% of dose
Administer after hemodialysis: Administer 50% of dose
Continuous arteriovenous hemofiltration: Dose for Cl_{cr} <10 mL/minute

Dietary Considerations May be taken with food.

Administration Do not use granules if packet is swollen or if granules are discolored (ie, brown or purple). Granules may be sprinkled on applesauce or yogurt (do not chew) or suspended in tomato or orange juice.

Patient Information Notify prescriber if persistent sore throat, fever, unusual bleeding or bruising, persistent nausea, vomiting, or abdominal pain occurs; do not stop taking before consulting your prescriber; take with food or meals; do not use products that are brown or purple; store in a cool, dry place away from sunlight

Dosage Forms Granules: 4 g/packet (30s) [contains talc]

Selected Readings

Davidson PT and Le HQ, "Drug Treatment of Tuberculosis - 1992," *Drugs*, 1992, 43(5):651-73.
"Drugs for Tuberculosis," *Med Lett Drugs Ther*, 1993, 35(908):99-101.
Iseman MD, "Treatment of Multidrug-Resistant Tuberculosis," *N Engl J Med*, 1993, 329(11):784-91.

4-Aminosalicylic Acid *see* Aminosalicylic Acid *on page 641*

Amoxicillin (a moks i SIL in)

Related Information

Animal and Human Bites *on page 1270*
Antimicrobial Activity Against Selected Organisms *on page 1165*
Community-Acquired Pneumonia in Adults *on page 1278*
Helicobacter pylori Treatment *on page 1288*

U.S. Brand Names Amoxil®; DisperMox™; Moxilin®; Trimox®

Canadian Brand Names Amoxil®; Apo-Amoxi®; Gen-Amoxicillin; Lin-Amox; Novamoxin®; Nu-Amoxi; pms-Amoxicillin

Synonyms Amoxicillin Trihydrate; Amoxycillin; *p*-Hydroxyampicillin

Generic Available Yes: Excludes tablet for oral suspension

Use Treatment of otitis media, sinusitis, and infections caused by susceptible organisms involving the respiratory tract, skin, and urinary tract; prophylaxis of bacterial endocarditis in patients undergoing surgical or dental procedures; as part of a multidrug regimen for *H. pylori* eradication

Unlabeled/Investigational Use Postexposure prophylaxis for anthrax exposure with documented susceptible organisms

Drug of Choice or Alternative for Disease/Syndrome(s):

Bronchitis *on page 60*
Cervicitis *on page 71*
Otitis Media, Acute *on page 253*
Pharyngitis *on page 264*
Pneumonia, Community-Acquired *on page 270*
Sinusitis, Community-Acquired, Acute *on page 299*

Organism(s):

Borrelia burgdorferi on page 56
Haemophilus influenzae on page 159
Helicobacter pylori on page 162
Streptococcus agalactiae on page 313
Streptococcus pneumoniae, Drug-Susceptible *on page 319*

Pregnancy Risk Factor B

Contraindications Hypersensitivity to amoxicillin, penicillin, or any component of the formulation

Warnings/Precautions In patients with renal impairment, doses and/or frequency of administration should be modified in response to the degree of renal impairment; a high percentage of patients with infectious mononucleosis have developed rash during therapy with amoxicillin; a low incidence of cross-allergy with other beta-lactams and cephalosporins exists

Adverse Reactions Frequency not defined.

Central nervous system: Hyperactivity, agitation, anxiety, insomnia, confusion, convulsions, behavioral changes, dizziness

Dermatologic: Acute exanthematous pustulosis, erythematous maculopapular rash, erythema multiforme, Stevens-Johnson syndrome, exfoliative dermatitis, toxic epidermal necrolysis, hypersensitivity vasculitis, urticaria

Gastrointestinal: Nausea, vomiting, diarrhea, hemorrhagic colitis, pseudomembranous colitis, tooth discoloration (brown, yellow, or gray; rare)

Hematologic: Anemia, hemolytic anemia, thrombocytopenia, thrombocytopenia purpura, eosinophilia, leukopenia, agranulocytosis

Hepatic: Elevated AST (SGOT) and ALT (SGPT), cholestatic jaundice, hepatic cholestasis, acute cytolytic hepatitis

Renal: Crystalluria

Overdosage/Toxicology Symptoms of penicillin overdose include neuromuscular hypersensitivity (eg, agitation, hallucinations, asterixis, encephalopathy, confusion, and seizures). Interstitial nephritis and/or crystalluria, possibly resulting in renal failure, may occur; hydration and diuresis may be beneficial. Electrolyte imbalance may occur if the preparation contains potassium or sodium salts, especially in renal failure. A study of 51 pediatric overdose victims suggests that ingestion of doses ≤250 mg/kg does not manifest significant clinical symptoms, and thus does not require gastric lavage. Hemodialysis may be helpful to aid in removal of the drug from blood; otherwise, treatment is symptom-directed and supportive.

Drug Interactions

Increased Effect/Toxicity: Disulfiram and probenecid may increase amoxicillin levels. Amoxicillin may increase the effects of oral anticoagulants (warfarin). Theoretically, allopurinol taken with amoxicillin has an additive potential for amoxicillin rash. Penicillins may increase the exposure to methotrexate during concurrent therapy; monitor.

Decreased Effect: Decreased effectiveness with tetracyclines and chloramphenicol. Although anecdotal reports suggest oral contraceptive efficacy could be reduced by penicillins, this has been refuted by more rigorous scientific and clinical data.

Stability

Amoxil®: Oral suspension remains stable for 14 days at room temperature or if refrigerated (refrigeration preferred); unit-dose antibiotic oral syringes are stable for 48 hours.

DisperMox™: Dissolve 1 tablet in ~10 mL water immediately before use.

Mechanism of Action Inhibits bacterial cell wall synthesis by binding to one or more of the penicillin binding proteins (PBPs); which in turn inhibits the final transpeptidation step of peptidoglycan synthesis in bacterial cell walls, thus inhibiting cell wall biosynthesis. Bacteria eventually lyse due to ongoing activity of cell wall autolytic enzymes (autolysins and murein hydrolases) while cell wall assembly is arrested.

Pharmacodynamics/Kinetics

Absorption: Oral: Rapid and nearly complete; food does not interfere

Distribution: Widely to most body fluids and bone; poor penetration into cells, eyes, and across normal meninges

Pleural fluids, lungs, and peritoneal fluid; high urine concentrations are attained; also into synovial fluid, liver, prostate, muscle, and gallbladder; penetrates into middle ear effusions, maxillary sinus secretions, tonsils, sputum, and bronchial secretions; crosses placenta; low concentrations enter breast milk

CSF:blood level ratio: Normal meninges: <1%; Inflamed meninges: 8% to 90%

Protein binding: 17% to 20%

Metabolism: Partially hepatic

Half-life elimination:

Neonates, full-term: 3.7 hours

Infants and Children: 1-2 hours

Adults: Normal renal function: 0.7-1.4 hours

Cl_{cr} <10 mL/minute: 7-21 hours

Time to peak: Capsule: 2 hours; Suspension: 1 hour

Excretion: Urine (80% as unchanged drug); lower in neonates

(Continued)

Amoxicillin *(Continued)*

Dosage Oral:

Children ≤3 months: 20-30 mg/kg/day divided every 12 hours

Children: >3 months and <40 kg: Dosing range: 20-50 mg/kg/day in divided doses every 8-12 hours

Ear, nose, throat, genitourinary tract, or skin/skin structure infections:

Mild to moderate: 25 mg/kg/day in divided doses every 12 hours **or** 20 mg/kg/day in divided doses every 8 hours

Severe: 45 mg/kg/day in divided doses every 12 hours **or** 40 mg/kg/day in divided doses every 8 hours

Acute otitis media: 80-90 mg/kg/day divided every 12 hours

Lower respiratory tract infections: 45 mg/kg/day in divided doses every 12 hours **or** 40 mg/kg/day in divided doses every 8 hours

Subacute bacterial endocarditis prophylaxis: 50 mg/kg 1 hour before procedure

Anthrax exposure (unlabeled use): **Note:** Postexposure prophylaxis only with documented susceptible organisms:

<40 kg: 15 mg/kg every 8 hours

≥40 kg: 500 mg every 8 hours

Adults: Dosing range: 250-500 mg every 8 hours or 500-875 mg twice daily

Ear, nose, throat, genitourinary tract or skin/skin structure infections:

Mild to moderate: 500 mg every 12 hours **or** 250 mg every 8 hours

Severe: 875 mg every 12 hours **or** 500 mg every 8 hours

Lower respiratory tract infections: 875 mg every 12 hours **or** 500 mg every 8 hours

Endocarditis prophylaxis: 2 g 1 hour before procedure

Helicobacter pylori eradication: 1000 mg twice daily; requires combination therapy with at least one other antibiotic and an acid-suppressing agent (proton pump inhibitor or H_2 blocker)

Anthrax exposure (unlabeled use): **Note:** Postexposure prophylaxis only with documented susceptible organisms: 500 mg every 8 hours

Dosing interval in renal impairment: The 875 mg tablet should not be used in patients with Cl_{cr} <30 mL/minute.

Cl_{cr} 10-30 mL/minute: 250-500 mg every 12 hours

Cl_{cr} <10 mL/minute: 250-500 mg every 24 hours

Dialysis: Moderately dialyzable (20% to 50%) by hemo- or peritoneal dialysis; approximately 50 mg of amoxicillin per liter of filtrate is removed by continuous arteriovenous or venovenous hemofiltration; dose as per Cl_{cr} <10 mL/minute guidelines

Dietary Considerations May be taken with food. Amoxil® chewable contains phenylalanine 1.82 mg per 200 mg tablet, phenylalanine 3.64 mg per 400 mg tablet. DisperMox™ contains phenylalanine 5.6 mg in each 200 mg and 400 mg tablet.

Administration Administer around-the-clock to promote less variation in peak and trough serum levels. The appropriate amount of suspension may be mixed with formula, milk, fruit juice, water, ginger ale or cold drinks; administer dose immediately after mixing.

DisperMox™: Dissolve 1 tablet in ~10 mL of water immediately before administration. Rinse container with additional water and drink entire contents to ensure that complete dose is taken. Do not chew or swallow tablet whole.

Monitoring Parameters With prolonged therapy, monitor renal, hepatic, and hematologic function periodically; assess patient at beginning and throughout therapy for infection; monitor for signs of anaphylaxis during first dose

Test Interactions May interfere with urinary glucose tests using cupric sulfate (Benedict's solution, Clinitest®); may inactivate aminoglycosides *in vitro*

Patient Information Report diarrhea promptly; take entire course of medication; females should report symptoms of vaginitis; pediatric drops may be placed on child's tongue or added to formula, milk, etc

Dosage Forms [DSC] = Discontinued product

Capsule, as trihydrate: 250 mg, 500 mg

Amoxil®: 250 mg [DSC], 500 mg

Moxilin®, Trimox®: 250 mg, 500 mg

Powder for oral suspension, as trihydrate: 125 mg/5 mL (80 mL, 100 mL, 150 mL); 200 mg/5 mL (50 mL, 75 mL, 100 mL); 250 mg/5 mL (80 mL, 100 mL, 150 mL); 400 mg/5 mL (50 mL, 75 mL, 100 mL)

Amoxil®: 125 mg/5 mL (150 mL) [contains sodium benzoate; strawberry flavor] [DSC]; 200 mg/5 mL (5 mL, 50 mL, 75 mL, 100 mL) [contains sodium benzoate; bubble gum flavor]; 250 mg/5 mL (100 mL, 150 mL) [contains sodium benzoate; bubble gum flavor]; 400 mg/5 mL (5 mL, 50 mL, 75 mL, 100 mL) [contains sodium benzoate; bubble gum flavor]

Moxilin®: 250 mg/5 mL (100 mL, 150 mL)

Trimox®: 125 mg/5 mL (80 mL, 100 mL, 150 mL); 250 mg/5 mL (80 mL, 100 mL, 150 mL) [contains sodium benzoate; raspberry-strawberry flavor]

Powder for oral suspension, as trihydrate [drops] (Amoxil®): 50 mg/mL (15 mL [DSC], 30 mL) [bubble gum flavor]

Tablet, as trihydrate [film coated] (Amoxil®): 500 mg, 875 mg

Tablet, chewable, as trihydrate: 125 mg, 200 mg, 250 mg, 400 mg

Amoxil®: 200 mg [contains phenylalanine 1.82 mg/tablet; cherry banana peppermint flavor]; 400 mg [contains phenylalanine 3.64 mg/tablet; cherry banana peppermint flavor]

Tablet, for oral suspension, as trihydrate (DisperMox™): 200 mg [contains phenylalanine 5.6 mg; strawberry flavor]; 400 mg [contains phenylalanine 5.6 mg; strawberry flavor]; 600 mg [contains phenylalanine 11.23 mg; strawberry flavor]

Selected Readings

Donowitz GR and Mandell GL, "Beta-Lactam Antibiotics," *N Engl J Med*, 1988, 318(7):419-26 and 318(8):490-500.

Wright AJ, "The Penicillins," *Mayo Clin Proc*, 1999, 74(3):290-307.

Amoxicillin and Clavulanate Potassium

(a moks i SIL in & klav yoo LAN ate poe TASS ee um)

Related Information

Animal and Human Bites *on page 1270*
Antimicrobial Activity Against Selected Organisms *on page 1165*
Community-Acquired Pneumonia in Adults *on page 1278*
Neutropenic Fever Guidelines *on page 1295*

U.S. Brand Names Augmentin®; Augmentin ES-600®; Augmentin XR™

Canadian Brand Names Alti-Amoxi-Clav; Apo-Amoxi-Clav®; Augmentin®; Clavulin®; Novo-Clavamoxin; ratio-Aclavulanate

Synonyms Amoxicillin and Clavulanic Acid

Generic Available Yes: Excludes extended release

Use Treatment of otitis media, sinusitis, and infections caused by susceptible organisms involving the lower respiratory tract, skin and skin structure, and urinary tract; spectrum same as amoxicillin with additional coverage of beta-lactamase producing *B. catarrhalis*, *H. influenzae*, *N. gonorrhoeae*, and *S. aureus* (not MRSA). The expanded coverage of this combination makes it a useful alternative when amoxicillin resistance is present and patients cannot tolerate alternative treatments.

Drug of Choice or Alternative for

Disease/Syndrome(s):

Bronchitis *on page 60*
Erysipelas *on page 141*
Fever, Neutropenic *on page 148*
Mastitis *on page 214*
Osteomyelitis, Diabetic Foot *on page 249*
Pneumonia, Aspiration, Community-Acquired *on page 269*
Pneumonia, Community-Acquired *on page 270*
Sinusitis, Community-Acquired, Acute *on page 299*
Urinary Tract Infection, Uncomplicated *on page 346*

Organism(s):

Capnocytophaga Species *on page 69*
Haemophilus influenzae *on page 159*
Moraxella catarrhalis *on page 223*
Pasteurella multocida *on page 258*
Streptococcus-Related Gram-Positive Cocci *on page 325*

Pregnancy Risk Factor B

Pregnancy Implications Both amoxicillin and clavulanate potassium cross the human placenta. Teratogenic effects have not been reported. Use in women with premature rupture of fetal membranes may increase risk of necrotizing enterocolitis in neonates.

Contraindications Hypersensitivity to amoxicillin, clavulanic acid, penicillin, or any component of the formulation; history of cholestatic jaundice or hepatic dysfunction with amoxicillin/clavulanate potassium therapy; Augmentin XR™: severe renal impairment (Cl_{cr} <30 mL/minute) and hemodialysis patients

Warnings/Precautions Hypersensitivity reactions, including anaphylaxis (some fatal), have been reported. Prolonged use may result in superinfection, including *Pseudomembranous colitis.* In patients with renal impairment, doses and/or frequency of administration should be modified in response to the degree of renal impairment. High percentage of patients with infectious mononucleosis have developed rash during therapy. Incidence of diarrhea is higher than with amoxicillin alone. Use caution in patients with hepatic dysfunction. Hepatic dysfunction, although rare, is more common in elderly and/or males, and occurs more frequently with prolonged treatment, and may occur after therapy is complete. Due to differing content of

(Continued)

Amoxicillin and Clavulanate Potassium *(Continued)*

clavulanic acid, not all formulations are interchangeable. Low incidence of cross-allergy with cephalosporins exists. Some products contain phenylalanine.

Adverse Reactions

>10%: Gastrointestinal: Diarrhea (3% to 34% incidence varies upon dose and regimen used)

1% to 10%:

Dermatologic: Diaper rash, skin rash, urticaria

Gastrointestinal: Abdominal discomfort, loose stools, nausea, vomiting

Genitourinary: Vaginitis, vaginal mycosis

Miscellaneous: Moniliasis

<1%: Cholestatic jaundice, flatulence, headache, hepatic dysfunction, prothrombin time increased, thrombocytosis

Additional adverse reactions seen with **ampicillin-class antibiotics:** Agitation, agranulocytosis, alkaline phosphatase increased, anaphylaxis, anemia, angioedema, anxiety, behavioral changes, bilirubin increased, black "hairy" tongue, confusion, convulsions, crystalluria, dizziness, enterocolitis, eosinophilia, erythema multiforme, exanthematous pustulosis, exfoliative dermatitis, gastritis, glossitis, hematuria, hemolytic anemia, hemorrhagic colitis, indigestion, insomnia, hyperactivity, interstitial nephritis, leukopenia, mucocutaneous candidiasis, pruritus, pseudomembranous colitis, serum sickness-like reaction, Stevens-Johnson syndrome, stomatitis, transaminases increased, thrombocytopenia, thrombocytopenic purpura, tooth discoloration, toxic epidermal necrolysis

Overdosage/Toxicology Symptoms of overdose may include abdominal pain, diarrhea, drowsiness, rash, hyperactivity, stomach pain, and vomiting. Interstitial nephritis and/or crystalluria, possibly resulting in renal failure, may occur; hydration and diuresis may be beneficial. Electrolyte imbalance may occur, especially in renal failure. A study of 51 pediatric overdose victims suggests that ingestion of amoxicillin at doses ≤250 mg/kg do not manifest significant clinical symptoms, and thus do not require gastric lavage. Hemodialysis may be helpful to aid in removal of the drug from blood; otherwise, treatment is supportive or symptom-directed.

Drug Interactions

Increased Effect/Toxicity: Probenecid may increase amoxicillin levels (concomitant use is not recommended). Increased effect of anticoagulants with amoxicillin. Allopurinol taken with Augmentin® has an additive potential for rash. Penicillins may increase the exposure to methotrexate during concurrent therapy; monitor.

Decreased Effect: Although anecdotal reports suggest oral contraceptive efficacy could be reduced by penicillins, this has been refuted by more rigorous scientific and clinical data.

Stability

Powder for oral suspension: Store dry powder at room temperature of 25°C (77°F). Reconstitute powder for oral suspension with appropriate amount of water as specified on the bottle. Shake vigorously until suspended. Reconstituted oral suspension should be kept in refrigerator. Discard unused suspension after 10 days. Unit-dose antibiotic oral syringes are stable for 48 hours.

Tablet: Store at room temperature of 25°C (77°F).

Mechanism of Action Clavulanic acid binds and inhibits beta-lactamases that inactivate amoxicillin resulting in amoxicillin having an expanded spectrum of activity. Amoxicillin inhibits bacterial cell wall synthesis by binding to one or more of the penicillin binding proteins (PBPs); which in turn inhibits the final transpeptidation step of peptidoglycan synthesis in bacterial cell walls, thus inhibiting cell wall biosynthesis. Bacteria eventually lyse due to ongoing activity of cell wall autolytic enzymes (autolysins and murein hydrolases) while cell wall assembly is arrested.

Pharmacodynamics/Kinetics Amoxicillin pharmacokinetics are not affected by clavulanic acid.

Amoxicillin: See Amoxicillin monograph.

Clavulanic acid:

Metabolism: Hepatic

Excretion: Urine (30% to 40% as unchanged drug)

Dosage Note: Dose is based on the amoxicillin component; see "Augmentin® Product-Specific Considerations" table on next page.

Infants <3 months: 30 mg/kg/day divided every 12 hours using the 125 mg/5 mL suspension

Children ≥3 months and <40 kg:

Otitis media (Augmentin® ES-600): 90 mg/kg/day divided every 12 hours for 10 days in children with severe illness and when coverage for β-lactamase postitive *H. influenzae* and *M. catarrhalis* is needed.

Lower respiratory tract infections, severe infections, sinusitis: 45 mg/kg/day divided every 12 hours **or** 40 mg/kg/day divided every 8 hours

Less severe infections: 25 mg/kg/day divided every 12 hours or 20 mg/kg/day divided every 8 hours

Children >40 kg and Adults: 250-500 mg every 8 hours or 875 mg every 12 hours

Children ≥16 years and Adults:

Acute bacterial sinusitis: Extended release tablet: Two 1000 mg tablets every 12 hours for 10 days

Community-acquired pneumonia: Extended release tablet: Two 1000 mg tablets every 12 hours for 7-10 days

Dosing interval in renal impairment:

Cl_{cr} <30 mL/minute: Do not use 875 mg tablet or extended release tablets

Cl_{cr} 10-30 mL/minute: 250-500 mg every 12 hours

Cl_{cr} <10 mL/minute: 250-500 every 24 hours

Hemodialysis: Moderately dialyzable (20% to 50%)

250-500 mg every 24 hours; administer dose during and after dialysis. Do not use extended release tablets.

Peritoneal dialysis: Moderately dialyzable (20% to 50%)

Amoxicillin: Administer 250 mg every 12 hours

Clavulanic acid: Dose for Cl_{cr} <10 mL/minute

Continuous arteriovenous or venovenous hemofiltration effects:

Amoxicillin: ~50 mg of amoxicillin/L of filtrate is removed

Clavulanic acid: Dose for Cl_{cr} <10 mL/minute

Augmentin® Product-Specific Considerations

Strength	Form	Consideration
125 mg	CT, S	q8h dosing
	S	For adults having difficulty swallowing tablets, 125 mg/5 mL suspension may be substituted for 500 mg tablet.
200 mg	CT, S	q12h dosing
	CT	Contains phenylalanine
	S	For adults having difficulty swallowing tablets, 200 mg/5 mL suspension may be substituted for 875 mg tablet.
250 mg	CT, S, T	q8h dosing
	CT	Contains phenylalanine
	T	Not for use in patients <40 kg
	CT, T	Tablet and chewable tablet are not interchangeable due to differences in clavulanic acid.
	S	For adults having difficulty swallowing tablets, 250 mg/5 mL suspension may be substituted for 500 mg tablet.
400 mg	CT, S	q12h dosing
	CT	Contains phenylalanine
	S	For adults having difficulty swallowing tablets, 400 mg/5 mL suspension may be substituted for 875 mg tablet.
500 mg	T	q8h or q12h dosing
600 mg	S	q12h dosing
		Contains phenylalanine
		Not for use in adults or children ≥40 kg
		600 mg/5 mL suspension is not equivalent to or interchangeable with 200 mg/5 mL or 400 mg/5 mL due to differences in clavulanic acid.
875 mg	T	q12h dosing; not for use in Cl_{cr} <30 mL/minute
1000 mg	XR	q12h dosing
		Not for use in children <16 years of age
		Not interchangeable with two 500 mg tablets
		Not for use if Cl_{cr} <30 mL/minute or hemodialysis

Legend: CT = chewable tablet, S = suspension, T = tablet, XR = extended release.

Dietary Considerations May be taken with meals or on an empty stomach; take with meals to increase absorption and decrease GI intolerance; may mix with milk, formula, or juice. Extended release tablets should be taken with food. Some products contain phenylalanine; avoid use in phenylketonurics. All dosage forms contain potassium.

Administration Administer around-the-clock to promote less variation in peak and trough serum levels. Administer with food to decrease stomach upset; shake suspension well before use. Extended release tablets should be administered with food.

(Continued)

Amoxicillin and Clavulanate Potassium *(Continued)*

Monitoring Parameters Assess patient at beginning and throughout therapy for infection; with prolonged therapy, monitor renal, hepatic, and hematologic function periodically; monitor for signs of anaphylaxis during first dose

Test Interactions May interfere with urinary glucose tests using cupric sulfate (Benedict's solution, Clinitest®, Fehling's solution); may inactivate aminoglycosides *in vitro*

Patient Information Take extended release tablets with food. Report diarrhea promptly; take entire course of medication; females should report onset of symptoms of candidal vaginitis

Additional Information Two 250 mg tablets are not equivalent to a 500 mg tablet (both tablet sizes contain equivalent clavulanate). Two 500 mg tablets are not equivalent to a single 1000 mg extended release tablet.

Dosage Forms

Powder for oral suspension: 200: Amoxicillin 200 mg and clavulanate potassium 28.5 mg per 5 mL (100 mL) [contains phenylalanine]; 400: Amoxicillin 400 mg and clavulanate potassium 57 mg per 5 mL (100 mL) [contains phenylalanine]

Augmentin®:

125: Amoxicillin 125 mg and clavulanate potassium 31.25 mg per 5 mL (75 mL, 100 mL, 150 mL) [banana flavor]

200: Amoxicillin 200 mg and clavulanate potassium 28.5 mg per 5 mL (50 mL, 75 mL, 100 mL) [contains phenylalanine 7 mg/5 mL; orange-raspberry flavor]

250: Amoxicillin 250 mg and clavulanate potassium 62.5 mg per 5 mL (75 mL, 100 mL, 150 mL) [orange flavor]

400: Amoxicillin 400 mg and clavulanate potassium 57 mg per 5 mL (50 mL, 75 mL, 100 mL) [contains phenylalanine 7 mg/5 mL; orange-raspberry flavor]

Augmentin ES-600®: Amoxicillin 600 mg and clavulanic potassium 42.9 mg per 5 mL (75 mL, 125 mL, 200 mL) [contains phenylalanine 7 mg/5 mL; orange flavor]

Tablet: 500: Amoxicillin trihydrate 500 mg and clavulanate potassium 125 mg; 875: Amoxicillin trihydrate 875 mg and clavulanate potassium 125 mg

Augmentin®:

250: Amoxicillin trihydrate 250 mg and clavulanate potassium 125 mg

500: Amoxicillin trihydrate 500 mg and clavulanate potassium 125 mg

875: Amoxicillin trihydrate 875 mg and clavulanate potassium 125 mg

Tablet, chewable: 200: Amoxicillin trihydrate 200 mg and clavulanate potassium 28.5 mg [contains phenylalanine]; 400: Amoxicillin trihydrate 400 mg and clavulanate potassium 57 mg [contains phenylalanine]

Augmentin®:

125: Amoxicillin trihydrate 125 mg and clavulanate potassium 31.25 mg [lemon-lime flavor]

200: Amoxicillin trihydrate 200 mg and clavulanate potassium 28.5 mg [contains phenylalanine 2.1 mg/tablet; cherry-banana flavor]

250: Amoxicillin trihydrate 250 mg and clavulanate potassium 62.5 mg [lemon-lime flavor]

400: Amoxicillin trihydrate 400 mg and clavulanate potassium 57 mg [contains phenylalanine 4.2 mg/tablet; cherry-banana flavor]

Tablet, extended release (Augmentin XR™): Amoxicillin 1000 mg and clavulanic acid 62.5 mg [contains potassium 29.3 mg (1.27 mEq) and sodium 12.6 mg (0.32 mEq)

Selected Readings

Donowitz GR and Mandell GL, "Beta-Lactam Antibiotics," *N Engl J Med*, 1988, 318(7):419-26 and 318(8):490-500.

Todd PA and Benfield P, "Amoxicillin/Clavulanic Acid. An Update of Its Antibacterial Activity, Pharmacokinetic Properties and Therapeutic Use," *Drugs*, 1990, 39(2):264-307.

Wright AJ, "The Penicillins," *Mayo Clin Proc*, 1999, 74(3):290-307.

Amoxicillin and Clavulanic Acid *see* Amoxicillin and Clavulanate Potassium *on page 645*

Amoxicillin, Lansoprazole, and Clarithromycin *see* Lansoprazole, Amoxicillin, and Clarithromycin *on page 908*

Amoxicillin Trihydrate *see* Amoxicillin *on page 642*

Amoxil® *see* Amoxicillin *on page 642*

Amoxycillin *see* Amoxicillin *on page 642*

Amphocin® *see* Amphotericin B (Conventional) *on page 650*

Amphotec® *see* Amphotericin B Cholesteryl Sulfate Complex *on page 649*

Amphotericin B Cholesteryl Sulfate Complex

(am foe TER i sin bee kole LES te ril SUL fate KOM plecks)

U.S. Brand Names Amphotec®

Canadian Brand Names Amphotec®

Synonyms ABCD; Amphotericin B Colloidal Dispersion

Generic Available No

Use Treatment of invasive aspergillosis in patients who have failed amphotericin B deoxycholate treatment, or who have renal impairment or experience unacceptable toxicity which precludes treatment with amphotericin B deoxycholate in effective doses.

Unlabeled/Investigational Use Effective in patients with serious *Candida* species infections

Drug of Choice or Alternative for Organism(s):

Aspergillus Species *on page 38*

Fusarium Species *on page 151*

Pregnancy Risk Factor B

Contraindications Hypersensitivity to amphotericin B or any component of the formulation

Warnings/Precautions Anaphylaxis has been reported with other amphotericin B-containing drugs. Facilities for cardiopulmonary resuscitation should be available during administration due to the possibility of anaphylactic reaction. If severe respiratory distress occurs, the infusion should be immediately discontinued. During the initial dosing, the drug should be administered under close clinical observation. Infusion reactions, sometimes, severe, usually subside with continued therapy - manage with decreased rate of infusion and pretreatment with antihistamines/corticosteroids; pulmonary reactions may occur in neutropenic patients receiving leukocyte transfusions; separation of the infusions as much as possible is advised.

Adverse Reactions

>10%: Central nervous system: Chills, fever

1% to 10%:

- Cardiovascular: Hypotension, tachycardia
- Central nervous system: Headache
- Dermatologic: Rash
- Endocrine & metabolic: Hypokalemia, hypomagnesemia
- Gastrointestinal: Nausea, diarrhea, abdominal pain
- Hematologic: Thrombocytopenia
- Hepatic: LFT change
- Neuromuscular & skeletal: Rigors
- Renal: Elevated creatinine
- Respiratory: Dyspnea

Note: Amphotericin B colloidal dispersion has an improved therapeutic index compared to conventional amphotericin B, and has been used safely in patients with amphotericin B-related nephrotoxicity; however, continued decline of renal function has occurred in some patients.

Overdosage/Toxicology Symptoms include renal dysfunction, anemia, thrombocytopenia, granulocytopenia, fever, nausea, and vomiting. Treatment is supportive.

Drug Interactions

Increased Effect/Toxicity: Toxic effect with other nephrotoxic drugs (eg, cyclosporine and aminoglycosides) may be additive. Corticosteroids may increase potassium depletion caused by amphotericin. Amphotericin B may predispose patients receiving digitalis glycosides or neuromuscular blocking agents to toxicity secondary to hypokalemia.

Decreased Effect: Pharmacologic antagonism may occur with azole antifungals (eg, ketoconazole, miconazole).

Stability

Store intact vials under refrigeration.

Reconstitute 50 mg and 100 mg vials with 10 mL and 20 mL of SWI, respectively. The reconstituted vials contain 5 mg/mL of amphotericin B. Shake the vial gently by hand until all solid particles have dissolved. After reconstitution, the solution should be refrigerated at 2°C to 8°C/36°F to 46°F and used within 24 hours.

Further dilute amphotericin B colloidal dispersion with dextrose 5% in water. Concentrations of 0.1-2 mg/mL in dextrose 5% in water are stable for 14 days at 4°C and 23°C if protected from light, however, due to the occasional formation of subvisual particles, solutions should be used within 48 hours.

Incompatible with sodium chloride solutions

(Continued)

Amphotericin B Cholesteryl Sulfate Complex *(Continued)*

Mechanism of Action Binds to ergosterol altering cell membrane permeability in susceptible fungi and causing leakage of cell components with subsequent cell death. Proposed mechanism suggests that amphotericin causes an oxidation-dependent stimulation of macrophages (Lyman, 1992).

Pharmacodynamics/Kinetics

Distribution: V_d: Total volume increases with higher doses, reflects increasing uptake by tissues (with 4 mg/kg/day = 4 L/kg); predominantly distributed in the liver; concentrations in kidneys and other tissues are lower than observed with conventional amphotericin B

Half-life elimination: 28-29 hours; prolonged with higher doses

Dosage Children and Adults: I.V.:

Premedication: For patients who experience chills, fever, hypotension, nausea, or other nonanaphylactic infusion-related immediate reactions, premedicate with the following drugs, 30-60 minutes prior to drug administration: a nonsteroidal (eg, ibuprofen, choline magnesium trisalicylate) with or without diphenhydramine; or acetaminophen with diphenhydramine; or hydrocortisone 50-100 mg. If the patient experiences rigors during the infusion, meperidine may be administered.

Range: 3-4 mg/kg/day (infusion of 1 mg/kg/hour); maximum: 7.5 mg/kg/day

Administration Avoid injection faster than 1 mg/kg/hour. For a patient who experiences chills, fever, hypotension, nausea, or other nonanaphylactic infusion-related reactions, premedication with the following drugs, 30-60 minutes prior to drug administration: A nonsteroidal (eg, ibuprofen, choline magnesium trisalicylate) with or without diphenhydramine; or acetaminophen with diphenhydramine, or hydrocortisone 50-100 mg. If the patient experiences rigors during the infusion, meperidine may be administered. If severe respiratory distress occurs, the infusion should be immediately discontinued.

Monitoring Parameters Liver function tests, electrolytes, BUN, Cr, temperature, CBC, I/O, signs of hypokalemia (muscle weakness, cramping, drowsiness, ECG changes)

Additional Information Controlled trials which compare the original formulation of amphotericin B to the newer liposomal formulations (ie, Amphotec®) are lacking. Thus, comparative data discussing differences among the formulations should be interpreted cautiously. Although the risk of nephrotoxicity and infusion-related adverse effects may be less with Amphotec®, the efficacy profiles of Amphotec® and the original amphotericin formulation are comparable. Consequently, Amphotec® should be restricted to those patients who cannot tolerate or fail a standard amphotericin B formulation.

Dosage Forms Injection, powder for reconstitution: 50 mg, 100 mg

Selected Readings

Hiemenz JW and Walsh TJ, "Lipid Formulations of Amphotericin B: Recent Progress and Future Directions," *Clin Infect Dis*, 1996, 22 Suppl 2:S133-44.

Patel R, "Antifungal Agents. Part I. Amphotericin B Preparations and Flucytosine," *Mayo Clin Proc*, 1998, 73(12):1205-25.

Slain D, "Lipid-Based Amphotericin B for the Treatment of Fungal Infections," *Pharmacotherapy*, 1999, 19(3):306-23.

Amphotericin B Colloidal Dispersion *see* Amphotericin B Cholesteryl Sulfate Complex *on page 649*

Amphotericin B (Conventional)

(am foe TER i sin bee con VEN sha nal)

U.S. Brand Names Amphocin®

Canadian Brand Names Fungizone®

Synonyms Amphotericin B Desoxycholate

Generic Available Yes

Use Treatment of severe systemic and central nervous system infections caused by susceptible fungi such as *Candida* species, *Histoplasma capsulatum*, *Cryptococcus neoformans*, *Aspergillus* species, *Blastomyces dermatitidis*, *Torulopsis glabrata*, and *Coccidioides immitis*; fungal peritonitis; irrigant for bladder fungal infections; used in fungal infection in patients with bone marrow transplantation, amebic meningoencephalitis, ocular aspergillosis (intraocular injection), candidal cystitis (bladder irrigation), chemoprophylaxis (low-dose I.V.), immunocompromised patients at risk of aspergillosis (intranasal/nebulized), refractory meningitis (intrathecal), coccidioidal arthritis (intra-articular/I.M.).

Low-dose amphotericin B has been administered after bone marrow transplantation to reduce the risk of invasive fungal disease.

Drug of Choice or Alternative for Disease/Syndrome(s):

Endocarditis, Prosthetic Valve, Early *on page 124*

Endocarditis, Prosthetic Valve, Late *on page 125*
Endophthalmitis, Bacterial and Fungal *on page 128*
Esophagitis *on page 147*
Keratitis, Bacterial and Fungal *on page 199*
Peritonitis, CAPD-Associated *on page 262*
Thrombophlebitis, Suppurative *on page 330*

Organism(s):
Aspergillus Species *on page 38*
Blastomyces dermatitidis on page 50
Candida Species *on page 67*
Coccidioides immitis on page 91
Cryptococcus neoformans on page 102
Dematiaceous Fungi *on page 112*
Dermatophytes *on page 114*
Fusarium Species *on page 151*
Histoplasma capsulatum on page 177
Malassezia furfur on page 213
Mucor Species *on page 225*
Penicillium marneffei on page 260
Prototheca Species *on page 280*
Sporothrix schenckii on page 302

Pregnancy Risk Factor B

Contraindications Hypersensitivity to amphotericin or any component of the formulation

Warnings/Precautions Anaphylaxis has been reported with other amphotericin B-containing drugs. During the initial dosing, the drug should be administered under close clinical observation. Avoid use with other nephrotoxic drugs; drug-induced renal toxicity usually improves with interrupting therapy, decreasing dosage, or increasing dosing interval. Infusion reactions are most common 1-3 hours after starting the infusion and diminish with continued therapy. Use amphotericin B with caution in patients with decreased renal function. Pulmonary reactions may occur in neutropenic patients receiving leukocyte transfusions; separation of the infusions as much as possible is advised.

Adverse Reactions

>10%:
- Central nervous system: Fever, chills, headache, malaise, generalized pain
- Endocrine & metabolic: Hypokalemia, hypomagnesemia
- Gastrointestinal: Anorexia
- Hematologic: Anemia
- Renal: Nephrotoxicity

1% to 10%:
- Cardiovascular: Hypotension, hypertension, flushing
- Central nervous system: Delirium, arachnoiditis, pain along lumbar nerves
- Gastrointestinal: Nausea, vomiting
- Genitourinary: Urinary retention
- Hematologic: Leukocytosis
- Local: Thrombophlebitis
- Neuromuscular & skeletal: Paresthesia (especially with I.T. therapy)
- Renal: Renal tubular acidosis, renal failure

<1%: Cardiac arrest, bone marrow suppression, convulsions, maculopapular rash, coagulation defects, thrombocytopenia, agranulocytosis, leukopenia, acute liver failure, vision changes, hearing loss, anuria, dyspnea

Overdosage/Toxicology Symptoms include cardiac arrest, renal dysfunction, anemia, thrombocytopenia, granulocytopenia, fever, nausea, and vomiting. Treatment is supportive.

Drug Interactions

Increased Effect/Toxicity: Use of amphotericin with other nephrotoxic drugs (eg, cyclosporine and aminoglycosides) may result in additive toxicity. Amphotericin may increase the toxicity of flucytosine. Antineoplastic agents may increase the risk of amphotericin-induced nephrotoxicity, bronchospasms, and hypotension. Corticosteroids may increase potassium depletion caused by amphotericin. Amphotericin B may predispose patients receiving digitalis glycosides or neuromuscular-blocking agents to toxicity secondary to hypokalemia.

Decreased Effect: Pharmacologic antagonism may occur with azole antifungal agents (ketoconazole, miconazole).

Stability Store intact vials under refrigeration; protect from light. Add 10 mL of SWFI (without a bacteriostatic agent) to each vial of amphotericin B. Further dilute with 250-500 mL D_5W; final concentration should not exceed 0.1 mg/mL (peripheral infusion) or 0.25 mg/mL (central infusion).

(Continued)

Amphotericin B (Conventional) *(Continued)*

Reconstituted vials are stable, protected from light, for 24 hours at room temperature and 1 week when refrigerated. Parenteral admixtures are stable, protected from light, for 24 hours at room temperature and 2 days under refrigeration. Short-term exposure (<24 hours) to light during I.V. infusion does**not** appreciably affect potency.

Mechanism of Action Binds to ergosterol altering cell membrane permeability in susceptible fungi and causing leakage of cell components with subsequent cell death. Proposed mechanism suggests that amphotericin causes an oxidation-dependent stimulation of macrophages (Lyman, 1992).

Pharmacodynamics/Kinetics

Distribution: Minimal amounts enter the aqueous humor, bile, CSF (inflamed or noninflamed meninges), amniotic fluid, pericardial fluid, pleural fluid, and synovial fluid

Protein binding, plasma: 90%

Half-life elimination: Biphasic: Initial: 15-48 hours; Terminal: 15 days

Time to peak: Within 1 hour following a 4- to 6-hour dose

Excretion: Urine (2% to 5% as biologically active form); ~40% eliminated over a 7-day period and may be detected in urine for at least 7 weeks after discontinued use

Dosage

I.V.: Premedication: For patients who experience infusion-related immediate reactions, premedicate with the following drugs, 30-60 minutes prior to drug administration: NSAID (with or without diphenhydramine) **or** acetaminophen with diphenhydramine **or** hydrocortisone 50-100 mg. If the patient experiences rigors during the infusion, meperidine may be administered.

Infants and Children:

Test dose: I.V.: 0.1 mg/kg/dose to a maximum of 1 mg; infuse over 30-60 minutes. Many clinicians believe a test dose is unnecessary.

Maintenance dose: 0.25-1 mg/kg/day given once daily; infuse over 2-6 hours. Once therapy has been established, amphotericin B can be administered on an every-other-day basis at 1-1.5 mg/kg/dose; cumulative dose: 1.5-2 g over 6-10 week.

Adults:

Test dose: 1 mg infused over 20-30 minutes. Many clinicians believe a test dose is unnecessary.

Maintenance dose: Usual: 0.25-1.5 mg/kg/day; 1-1.5 mg/kg over 4-6 hours every other day may be given once therapy is established; aspergillosis, mucormycosis, rhinocerebral phycomycosis often require 1-1.5 mg/kg/day; do not exceed 1.5 mg/kg/day

Duration of therapy varies with nature of infection: Usual duration is 4-12 weeks or cumulative dose of 1-4 g

I.T.: Meningitis, coccidioidal or cryptococcal:

Children.: 25-100 mcg every 48-72 hours; increase to 500 mcg as tolerated

Adults: Initial: 25-300 mcg every 48-72 hours; increase to 500 mcg to 1 mg as tolerated; maximum total dose: 15 mg has been suggested

Bladder irrigation: Candidal cystitis: Irrigate with 50 mcg/mL solution instilled periodically or continuously for 5-10 days or until cultures are clear

Dosing adjustment in renal impairment: If renal dysfunction is due to the drug, the daily total can be decreased by 50% or the dose can be given every other day; I.V. therapy may take several months

Dialysis: Poorly dialyzed; no supplemental dosage necessary when using hemo- or peritoneal dialysis or continuous arteriovenous or venovenous hemodiafiltration effects

Administration in dialysate: Children and Adults: 1-2 mg/L of peritoneal dialysis fluid either with or without low-dose I.V. amphotericin B (a total dose of 2-10 mg/kg given over 7-14 days). Precipitate may form in ionic dialysate solutions.

Administration May be infused over 4-6 hours. For a patient who experiences chills, fever, hypotension, nausea or other nonanaphylactic infusion-related reactions, premedication with the following drugs, 30-60 minutes prior to drug administration: A nonsteroidal (eg, ibuprofen, choline magnesium trisalicylate) with or without diphenhydramine; or acetaminophen with diphenhydramine, or hydrocortisone 50-100 mg. If the patient experiences rigors during the infusion, meperidine may be administered. Bolus infusion of normal saline immediately preceding, or immediately preceding and following amphotericin B may reduce drug-induced nephrotoxicity. Risk of nephrotoxicity increases with amphotericin B doses >1 mg/kg/day. Infusion of admixtures more concentrated than 0.25 mg/mL should be limited to patients absolutely requiring volume contraction.

Monitoring Parameters Renal function (monitor frequently during therapy), electrolytes (especially potassium and magnesium), liver function tests, temperature, PT/

PTT, CBC; monitor input and output; monitor for signs of hypokalemia (muscle weakness, cramping, drowsiness, ECG changes, etc)

Reference Range Therapeutic: 1-2 mcg/mL (SI: 1-2.2 µmol/L)

Additional Information Premedication with diphenhydramine and acetaminophen may reduce the severity of acute infusion-related reactions. Meperidine reduces the duration of amphotericin B-induced rigors and chilling. Hydrocortisone may be used in patients with severe or refractory infusion-related reactions. Bolus infusion of normal saline immediately preceding, or immediately preceding and following amphotericin B may reduce drug-induced nephrotoxicity. Risk of nephrotoxicity increases with amphotericin B doses >1 mg/kg/day. Infusion of admixtures more concentrated than 0.25 mg/mL should be limited to patients absolutely requiring volume restriction. Amphotericin B does not have a bacteriostatic constituent, subsequently admixture expiration is determined by sterility more than chemical stability.

Dosage Forms

Injection, powder for reconstitution, as desoxycholate (Amphocin®): 50 mg

Selected Readings

Bianco JA, Almgren J, Kern DL, et al, "Evidence That Oral Pentoxifylline Reverses Acute Renal Dysfunction in Bone Marrow Transplant Recipients Receiving Amphotericin B and Cyclosporine," *Transplantation*, 1991, 51(4):925-7.

Branch RA, "Prevention of Amphotericin B-Induced Renal Impairment. A Review on the Use of Sodium Supplementation," *Arch Intern Med*, 1988, 148(11):2389-94.

Cruz JM, Peacock JE Jr, Loomer L, et al, "Rapid Intravenous Infusion of Amphotericin B: A Pilot Study," *Am J Med*, 1992, 93:123-30.

Gallis HA, Drew RH, and Pickard WW, "Amphotericin B: 30 Years of Clinical Experience," *Rev Infect Dis*, 1990, 12(2):308-29.

Kauffman CA and Carver PL, "Antifungal Agents in the 1990s. Current Status and Future Developments," *Drugs*, 1997, 53(4):539-49.

Lyman CA and Walsh TJ, "Systemically Administered Antifungal Agents. A Review of Their Clinical Pharmacology and Therapeutic Applications," *Drugs*, 1992, 44(1):9-35.

Patel R, "Antifungal Agents. Part I. Amphotericin B Preparations and Flucytosine," *Mayo Clin Proc*, 1998, 73(12):1205-25.

Slain D, "Lipid-Based Amphotericin B for the Treatment of Fungal Infections," *Pharmacotherapy*, 1999, 19(3):306-23.

Amphotericin B Desoxycholate *see* Amphotericin B (Conventional) *on page 650*

Amphotericin B (Lipid Complex)

(am foe TER i sin bee LIP id KOM pleks)

U.S. Brand Names Abelcet®

Canadian Brand Names Abelcet®

Synonyms ABLC

Generic Available No

Use Treatment of aspergillosis or any type of progressive fungal infection in patients who are refractory to or intolerant of conventional amphotericin B therapy

Unlabeled/Investigational Use Effective in patients with serious *Candida* species infections

Drug of Choice or Alternative for Organism(s):

Aspergillus Species *on page 38*
Candida Species *on page 67*
Cryptococcus neoformans on page 102
Fusarium Species *on page 151*
Mucor Species *on page 225*

Pregnancy Risk Factor B

Contraindications Hypersensitivity to amphotericin or any component of the formulation

Warnings/Precautions Anaphylaxis has been reported with other amphotericin B-containing drugs. Facilities for cardiopulmonary resuscitation should be available during administration due to the possibility of anaphylactic reaction. If severe respiratory distress occurs, the infusion should be immediately discontinued. During the initial dosing, the drug should be administered under close clinical observation. Acute reactions (including fever and chills) may occur 1-2 hours after starting an intravenous infusion. These reactions are usually more common with the first few doses and generally diminish with subsequent doses. Pulmonary reactions may occur in neutropenic patients receiving leukocyte transfusions; separation of the infusions as much as possible is advised.

Adverse Reactions Nephrotoxicity and infusion-related hyperpyrexia, rigor, and chilling are reduced relative to amphotericin deoxycholate.

>10%:

Central nervous system: Chills, fever
Renal: Increased serum creatinine

1% to 10%:

Cardiovascular: Hypotension, cardiac arrest

(Continued)

Amphotericin B (Lipid Complex) *(Continued)*

Central nervous system: Headache, pain

Dermatologic: Rash

Endocrine & metabolic: Bilirubinemia, hypokalemia, acidosis

Gastrointestinal: Nausea, vomiting, diarrhea, gastrointestinal hemorrhage, abdominal pain

Renal: Renal failure

Respiratory: Respiratory failure, dyspnea, pneumonia

Drug Interactions

Increased Effect/Toxicity: See Drug Interactions - Increased Effect/Toxicity in Amphotericin B (Conventional) *on page 650.*

Decreased Effect: See Drug Interactions - Decreased Effect in Amphotericin B (Conventional) *on page 650.*

Stability Intact vials should be stored at 2°C to 8°C (35°F to 46°F) and protected from exposure to light; do not freeze intact vials. Solutions for infusion are stable for 48 hours under refrigeration and for 6 hours at room temperature. Shake the vial gently until there is no evidence of any yellow sediment at the bottom. Dilute with D_5W to 1-2 mg/mL. Protect from light.

Do not dilute with saline solutions or mix with other drugs or electrolytes - compatibility has not been established

Do not use an in-line filter during administration.

Mechanism of Action Binds to ergosterol altering cell membrane permeability in susceptible fungi and causing leakage of cell components with subsequent cell death. Proposed mechanism suggests that amphotericin causes an oxidation-dependent stimulation of macrophages.

Pharmacodynamics/Kinetics

Distribution: V_d: Increases with higher doses; reflects increased uptake by tissues (131 L/kg with 5 mg/kg/day)

Half-life elimination: ~24 hours

Excretion: Clearance: Increases with higher doses (5 mg/kg/day): 400 mL/hour/kg

Dosage Children and Adults: I.V.:

Premedication: For patients who experience infusion-related immediate reactions, premedicate with the following drugs, 30-60 minutes prior to drug administration: a nonsteroidal anti-inflammatory agent ± diphenhydramine; or acetaminophen with diphenhydramine; or hydrocortisone 50-100 mg. If the patient experiences rigors during the infusion, meperidine may be administered.

Range: 2.5-5 mg/kg/day as a single infusion

Dosing adjustment in renal impairment: None necessary; effects of renal impairment are not currently known

Hemodialysis: No supplemental dosage necessary

Peritoneal dialysis: No supplemental dosage necessary

Continuous arteriovenous or venovenous hemofiltration: No supplemental dosage necessary

Administration Patients who experience nonanaphylactic infusion-related reactions, premedication 30-60 minutes prior to drug administration with a nonsteroidal anti-inflammatory agent ± diphenhydramine; acetaminophen with diphenhydramine or hydrocortisone 50-100 mg. If the patient experiences rigors during the infusion, meperidine may be administered.

Invert infusion container several times prior to administration and every 2 hours during infusion.

Monitoring Parameters Renal function (monitor frequently during therapy), electrolytes (especially potassium and magnesium), liver function tests, temperature, PT/PTT, CBC; monitor input and output; monitor for signs of hypokalemia (muscle weakness, cramping, drowsiness, ECG changes, etc)

Additional Information As a modification of dimyristoyl phosphatidylcholine:dimyristoyl phosphatidylglycerol 7:3 (DMPC:DMPG) liposome, amphotericin B lipid-complex has a higher drug to lipid ratio and the concentration of amphotericin B is 33 M. ABLC is a ribbon-like structure, not a liposome.

Controlled trials which compare the original formulation of amphotericin B to the newer liposomal formulations (ie, Abelcet®) are lacking. Thus, comparative data discussing differences among the formulations should be interpreted cautiously. Although the risk of nephrotoxicity and infusion-related adverse effects may be less with Abelcet®, the efficacy profiles of Abelcet® and the original amphotericin formulation are comparable. Consequently, Abelcet® should be restricted to those patients who cannot tolerate or fail a standard amphotericin B formulation.

Dosage Forms Injection, suspension [preservative free]: 5 mg/mL (20 mL)

Selected Readings

De Marie S, "Clinical Use of Liposomal and Lipid-Complexed Amphotericin B," *J Antimicrob Chemother*, 1994, 33(5):907-16.

Hiemenz JW and Walsh TJ, "Lipid Formulations of Amphotericin B: Recent Progress and Future Directions," *Clin Infect Dis*, 1996, 22 Suppl 2:S133-44.

Kline S, Larsen TA, Fieber L, et al, "Limited Toxicity of Prolonged Therapy With High Doses of Amphotericin B Lipid Complex," *Clin Infect Dis*, 1995, 21(5):1154-8.

Patel R, "Antifungal Agents. Part I. Amphotericin B Preparations and Flucytosine," *Mayo Clin Proc*, 1998, 73(12):1205-25.

Rapp RP, Gubbins PO, and Evans ME, "Amphotericin B Lipid Complex," *Ann Pharmacother*, 1997, 31(10):1174-86.

Slain D, "Lipid-Based Amphotericin B for the Treatment of Fungal Infections," *Pharmacotherapy*, 1999, 19(3):306-23.

Amphotericin B (Liposomal) (am foe TER i sin bee lye po SO mal)

U.S. Brand Names AmBisome®

Canadian Brand Names AmBisome®

Synonyms L-AmB

Generic Available No

Use Empirical therapy for presumed fungal infection in febrile, neutropenic patients. Treatment of patients with *Aspergillus* species, *Candida* species and/or *Cryptococcus* species infections refractory to amphotericin B desoxycholate, or in patients where renal impairment or unacceptable toxicity precludes the use of amphotericin B desoxycholate. Treatment of cryptococcal meningitis in HIV-infected patients. Treatment of visceral leishmaniasis.

Unlabeled/Investigational Use Effective in patients with serious *Candida* species infections

Drug of Choice or Alternative for Organism(s):

Aspergillus Species *on page 38*
Candida Species *on page 67*
Fusarium Species *on page 151*
Mucor Species *on page 225*

Pregnancy Risk Factor B

Contraindications Hypersensitivity to amphotericin B or any component of the formulation unless, in the opinion of the treating physician, the benefit of therapy outweighs the risk

Warnings/Precautions Although amphotericin B (liposomal) has been shown to be significantly less toxic than amphotericin B desoxycholate, adverse events may still occur. Patients should be under close clinical observation during initial dosing. As with other amphotericin B-containing products, anaphylaxis has been reported. Facilities for cardiopulmonary resuscitation should be available during administration, and the drug should be administered by medically-trained personnel. Acute reactions (including fever and chills) may occur 1-2 hours after starting infusions; reactions are more common with the first few doses and generally diminish with subsequent doses. Immediately discontinue infusion if severe respiratory distress occurs; the patient should not receive further infusions. Safety and efficacy have not been established in patients <1 year of age.

Adverse Reactions Percentage of adverse reactions is dependent upon population studied and may vary with respect to premedications and underlying illness. Incidence of decreased renal function and infusion-related events are lower than rates observed with amphotericin B deoxycholate.

>10%:

Cardiovascular: Peripheral edema (15%), edema (12% to 14%), tachycardia (9% to 18%), hypotension (7% to 14%), hypertension (8% to 20%), chest pain (8% to 12%), hypervolemia (8% to 12%)

Central nervous system: Chills (29% to 48%), insomnia (17% to 22%), headache (9% to 20%), anxiety (7% to 14%), pain (14%), confusion (9% to 13%)

Dermatologic: Rash (5% to 25%), pruritus (11%)

Endocrine & metabolic: Hypokalemia (31% to 51%), hypomagnesemia (15% to 50%), hyperglycemia (8% to 23%), hypocalcemia (5% to 18%), hyponatremia (8% to 12%)

Gastrointestinal: Nausea (16% to 40%), vomiting (10% to 32%), diarrhea (11% to 30%), abdominal pain (7% to 20%), constipation (15%), anorexia (10% to 14%)

Hematologic: Anemia (27% to 48%), blood transfusion reaction (9% to 18%), leukopenia (15% to 17%), thrombocytopenia (6% to 13%)

Hepatic: Increased alkaline phosphatase (7% to 22%), increased BUN (7% to 21%), bilirubinemia (9% to 18%), increased ALT (15%), increased AST (13%), abnormal liver function tests (not specified) (4% to 13%)

Local: Phlebitis (9% to 11%)

Neuromuscular & skeletal: Weakness (6% to 13%), back pain (12%)

(Continued)

Amphotericin B (Liposomal) *(Continued)*

Renal: Increased creatinine (18% to 40%), hematuria (14%)

Respiratory: Dyspnea (18% to 23%), lung disorder (14% to 18%), increased cough (2% to 18%), epistaxis (8% to 15%), pleural effusion (12%), rhinitis (11%)

Miscellaneous: Sepsis (7% to 14%), infection (11% to 12%)

2% to 10%:

Cardiovascular: Arrhythmia, atrial fibrillation, bradycardia, cardiac arrest, cardiomegaly, facial swelling, flushing, postural hypotension, valvular heart disease, vascular disorder

Central nervous system: Agitation, abnormal thinking, coma, convulsion, depression, dysesthesia, dizziness (7% to 8%), hallucinations, malaise, nervousness, somnolence

Dermatologic: Alopecia, bruising, cellulitis, dry skin, maculopapular rash, petechia, purpura, skin discoloration, skin disorder, skin ulcer, urticaria, vesiculobullous rash

Endocrine & metabolic: Acidosis, increased amylase, fluid overload, hypernatremia (4%), hyperchloremia, hyperkalemia, hypermagnesemia, hyperphosphatemia, hypophosphatemia, hypoproteinemia, increased lactate dehydrogenase, increased nonprotein nitrogen

Gastrointestinal: Constipation, dry mouth, dyspepsia, enlarged abdomen, eructation, fecal incontinence, flatulence, gastrointestinal hemorrhage (10%), hematemesis, hemorrhoids, gum/oral hemorrhage, ileus, mucositis, rectal disorder, stomatitis, ulcerative stomatitis

Genitourinary: Vaginal hemorrhage

Hematologic: Coagulation disorder, hemorrhage, decreased prothrombin, thrombocytopenia

Hepatic: Hepatocellular damage, hepatomegaly, veno-occlusive liver disease

Local: Injection site inflammation

Neuromuscular & skeletal: Arthralgia, bone pain, dystonia, myalgia, neck pain, paresthesia, rigors, tremor

Ocular: Conjunctivitis, dry eyes, eye hemorrhage

Renal: Abnormal renal function, acute kidney failure, dysuria, kidney failure, toxic nephropathy, urinary incontinence

Respiratory: Asthma, atelectasis, cough, dry nose, hemoptysis, hyperventilation, lung edema, pharyngitis, pneumonia, respiratory alkalosis, respiratory insufficiency, respiratory failure, sinusitis, hypoxia (6% to 8%)

Miscellaneous: Allergic reaction, cell-mediated immunological reaction, flu-like syndrome, graft versus host disease, herpes simplex, hiccup, procedural complication (8% to 10%), diaphoresis (7%)

Postmarketing and/or case reports: Angioedema, erythema, urticaria, cyanosis/hypoventilation, pulmonary edema, agranulocytosis, hemorrhagic cystitis

Overdosage/Toxicology Toxicity due to overdose has not been defined. Repeated daily doses up to 7.5 mg/kg have been administered in clinical trials with no reported dose-related toxicity. If overdosage should occur, cease administration immediately. Symptomatic supportive measures should be instituted. Particular attention should be given to monitoring renal function.

Drug Interactions

Increased Effect/Toxicity: Drug interactions have not been studied in a controlled manner; however, drugs that interact with conventional amphotericin B may also interact with amphotericin B liposome for injection. See Drug Interactions - Increased Effect/Toxicity in Amphotericin B (Conventional) monograph.

Stability Unopened vials should be stored at temperatures ≤25°C (77°F). Must be reconstituted using sterile water for injection, USP (without a bacteriostatic agent). Follow package insert instructions carefully for preparation. Do not reconstitute with saline or add saline to the reconstituted concentration, or mix with other drugs. The use of any solution other than those recommended, or the presence of a bacteriostatic agent in the solution, may cause precipitation.

Must be diluted with 5% dextrose injection to a final concentration of 1-2 mg/mL prior to administration. Lower concentrations (0.2-0.5 mg/mL) may be appropriate for infants and small children to provide sufficient volume for infusion.

Injection should commence within 6 hours of dilution with 5% dextrose injection.

An in-line membrane filter may be used for the intravenous infusion; provided, THE MEAN PORE DIAMETER OF THE FILTER SHOULD NOT BE LESS THAN 1 (one) MICRON.

Mechanism of Action Binds to ergosterol altering cell membrane permeability in susceptible fungi and causing leakage of cell components with subsequent cell death. Proposed mechanism suggests that amphotericin causes an oxidation-dependent stimulation of macrophages.

Pharmacodynamics/Kinetics

Distribution: V_d: 131 L/kg

Half-life elimination: Terminal: 174 hours

Dosage Children and Adults: I.V.:

Note: Premedication: For patients who experience chills, fever, hypotension, nausea, or other nonanaphylactic infusion-related immediate reactions, premedicate with the following drugs, 30-60 minutes prior to drug administration: a nonsteroidal (eg, ibuprofen, choline magnesium trisalicylate) with or without diphenhydramine; or acetaminophen with diphenhydramine; or hydrocortisone 50-100 mg. If the patient experiences rigors during the infusion, meperidine may be administered.

Empiric therapy: Recommended initial dose: 3 mg/kg/day

Systemic fungal infections (*Aspergillus*, *Candida*, *Cryptococcus*): Recommended initial dose of 3-5 mg/kg/day

Cryptococcal meningitis in HIV-infected patients: 6 mg/kg/day

Treatment of visceral leishmaniasis:

Immunocompetent patients: 3 mg/kg/day on days 1-5, and 3 mg/kg/day on days 14 and 21; a repeat course may be given in patients who do not achieve parasitic clearance

Immunocompromised patients: 4 mg/kg/day on days 1-5, and 4 mg/kg/day on days 10, 17, 24, 31, and 38

Dosing adjustment in renal impairment: None necessary; effects of renal impairment are not currently known

Hemodialysis: No supplemental dosage necessary

Peritoneal dialysis effects: No supplemental dosage necessary

Continuous arteriovenous or venovenous hemofiltration: No supplemental dosage necessary

Administration Should be administered by intravenous infusion, using a controlled infusion device, over a period of approximately 2 hours. Infusion time may be reduced to approximately 1 hour in patients in whom the treatment is well-tolerated. If the patient experiences discomfort during infusion, the duration of infusion may be increased. Administer at a rate of 2.5 mg/kg/hour. Existing intravenous line should be flushed with D_5W prior to infusion (if not feasible, administer through a separate line). An in-line membrane filter (not less than 1 micron) may be used.

Monitoring Parameters Renal function (monitor frequently during therapy), electrolytes (especially potassium and magnesium), liver function tests, temperature, PT/PTT, CBC; monitor input and output; monitor for signs of hypokalemia (muscle weakness, cramping, drowsiness, ECG changes, etc)

Additional Information Amphotericin B (liposomal) is a true single bilayer liposomal drug delivery system. Liposomes are closed, spherical vesicles created by mixing specific proportions of amphophilic substances such as phospholipids and cholesterol so that they arrange themselves into multiple concentric bilayer membranes when hydrated in aqueous solutions. Single bilayer liposomes are then formed by microemulsification of multilamellar vesicles using a homogenizer. Amphotericin B (liposomal) consists of these unilamellar bilayer liposomes with amphotericin B intercalated within the membrane. Due to the nature and quantity of amphophilic substances used, and the lipophilic moiety in the amphotericin B molecule, the drug is an integral part of the overall structure of the amphotericin B liposomal liposomes. Amphotericin B (liposomal) contains true liposomes that are <100 nm in diameter.

Dosage Forms Injection, powder for reconstitution: 50 mg

Selected Readings

Hiemenz JW and Walsh TJ, "Lipid Formulations of Amphotericin B: Recent Progress and Future Directions," *Clin Infect Dis*, 1996, 22 Suppl 2:S133-44.

Patel R, "Antifungal Agents. Part I. Amphotericin B Preparations and Flucytosine," *Mayo Clin Proc*, 1998, 73(12):1205-25.

Slain D, "Lipid-Based Amphotericin B for the Treatment of Fungal Infections," *Pharmacotherapy*, 1999, 19(3):306-23.

Ampicillin (am pi SIL in)

Related Information

Animal and Human Bites *on page 1270*

Antibiotic Treatment of Adults With Infective Endocarditis *on page 1271*

Antimicrobial Activity Against Selected Organisms *on page 1165*

U.S. Brand Names Principen®

Canadian Brand Names Apo-Ampi®; Novo-Ampicillin; Nu-Ampi

Synonyms Aminobenzylpenicillin; Ampicillin Sodium; Ampicillin Trihydrate

Generic Available Yes

Use Treatment of susceptible bacterial infections (nonbeta-lactamase-producing organisms); susceptible bacterial infections caused by streptococci, pneumococci, nonpenicillinase-producing staphylococci, *Listeria*, meningococci; some strains of *H. influenzae*, *Salmonella*, *Shigella*, *E. coli*, *Enterobacter*, and *Klebsiella*

(Continued)

Ampicillin *(Continued)*

Drug of Choice or Alternative for Disease/Syndrome(s):

Brain Abscess *on page 58*
Diverticulitis *on page 116*
Meningitis, Community-Acquired, Adult *on page 216*
Meningitis, Neonatal (<1 month of age) *on page 217*
Urinary Tract Infection, Catheter-Associated *on page 345*
Urinary Tract Infection, Pyelonephritis *on page 346*

Organism(s):

Actinomyces Species *on page 27*
Borrelia burgdorferi on page 56
Enterococcus Species *on page 134*
Escherichia coli on page 142
Gardnerella vaginalis on page 153
Haemophilus influenzae on page 159
Leptospira interrogans on page 205
Listeria monocytogenes on page 208
Salmonella Species *on page 291*
Shigella Species *on page 297*
Staphylococcus saprophyticus on page 312
Streptococcus agalactiae on page 313

Pregnancy Risk Factor B

Pregnancy Implications Teratogenic effects were not observed in animal studies. Ampicillin crosses the human placenta.

Contraindications Hypersensitivity to ampicillin, any component of the formulation, or other penicillins

Warnings/Precautions Dosage adjustment may be necessary in patients with renal impairment; a low incidence of cross-allergy with other beta-lactams exists; high percentage of patients with infectious mononucleosis have developed rash during therapy with ampicillin. Appearance of a rash should be carefully evaluated to differentiate a nonallergic ampicillin rash from a hypersensitivity reaction. Ampicillin rash occurs in 5% to 10% of children receiving ampicillin and is a generalized dull red, maculopapular rash, generally appearing 3-14 days after the start of therapy. It normally begins on the trunk and spreads over most of the body. It may be most intense at pressure areas, elbows, and knees.

Adverse Reactions Frequency not defined.

Central nervous system: Fever, penicillin encephalopathy, seizure

Dermatologic: Erythema multiforme, exfoliative dermatitis, rash, urticaria

Note: Appearance of a rash should be carefully evaluated to differentiate (if possible) nonallergic ampicillin rash from hypersensitivity reaction. Incidence is higher in patients with viral infection, *Salmonella* infection, lymphocytic leukemia, or patients that have hyperuricemia.

Gastrointestinal: Black hairy tongue, diarrhea, enterocolitis, glossitis, nausea, pseudomembranous colitis, sore mouth or tongue, stomatitis, vomiting

Hematologic: Agranulocytosis, anemia, hemolytic anemia, eosinophilia, leukopenia, thrombocytopenia purpura

Hepatic: AST increased

Renal: Interstitial nephritis (rare)

Respiratory: Laryngeal stridor

Miscellaneous: Anaphylaxis, serum sickness-like reaction

Overdosage/Toxicology Symptoms of penicillin overdose include neuromuscular hypersensitivity (agitation, hallucinations, asterixis, encephalopathy, confusion, and seizures) and electrolyte imbalance (with potassium or sodium salts), especially in renal failure. Hemodialysis may be helpful to aid in the removal of the drug from the blood, otherwise most treatment is supportive or symptom-directed.

Drug Interactions

Increased Effect/Toxicity: Ampicillin increases the effect of disulfiram and anticoagulants. Probenecid may increase penicillin levels. Theoretically, allopurinol taken with ampicillin has an additive potential for rash. Penicillins may increase the exposure to methotrexate during concurrent therapy; monitor.

Decreased Effect: Although anecdotal reports suggest oral contraceptive efficacy could be reduced by penicillins, this has been refuted by more rigorous scientific and clinical data.

Ethanol/Nutrition/Herb Interactions Food: Food decreases ampicillin absorption rate; may decrease ampicillin serum concentration.

Stability

Oral: Oral suspension is stable for 7 days at room temperature or for 14 days under refrigeration.

I.V.:

Minimum volume: Concentration should not exceed 30 mg/mL due to concentration-dependent stability restrictions.

Solutions for I.M. or direct I.V. should be used within 1 hour. Solutions for I.V. infusion will be inactivated by dextrose at room temperature. If dextrose-containing solutions are to be used, the resultant solution will only be stable for 2 hours versus 8 hours in the 0.9% sodium chloride injection. D_5W has limited stability.

Stability of parenteral admixture in NS at room temperature (25°C) is 8 hours.

Stability of parenteral admixture in NS at refrigeration temperature (4°C) is 2 days.

Standard diluent: 500 mg/50 mL NS; 1 g/50 mL NS; 2 g/100 mL NS

Mechanism of Action Inhibits bacterial cell wall synthesis by binding to one or more of the penicillin binding proteins (PBPs); which in turn inhibits the final transpeptidation step of peptidoglycan synthesis in bacterial cell walls, thus inhibiting cell wall biosynthesis. Bacteria eventually lyse due to ongoing activity of cell wall autolytic enzymes (autolysins and murein hydrolases) while cell wall assembly is arrested.

Pharmacodynamics/Kinetics

Absorption: Oral: 50%

Distribution: Bile, blister, and tissue fluids; penetration into CSF occurs with inflamed meninges only, good only with inflammation (exceeds usual MICs)

Normal meninges: Nil; Inflamed meninges: 5% to 10%

Protein binding: 15% to 25%

Half-life elimination:

Children and Adults: 1-1.8 hours

Anuria/end-stage renal disease: 7-20 hours

Time to peak: Oral: Within 1-2 hours

Excretion: Urine (~90% as unchanged drug) within 24 hours

Dosage

Infants and Children:

Mild-to-moderate infections:

I.M., I.V.: 100-150 mg/kg/day in divided doses every 6 hours (maximum: 2-4 g/day)

Oral: 50-100 mg/kg/day in doses divided every 6 hours (maximum: 2-4 g/day)

Severe infections/meningitis: I.M., I.V.: 200-400 mg/kg/day in divided doses every 6 hours (maximum: 6-12 g/day)

Endocarditis prophylaxis: I.M., I.V.:

Dental, oral, respiratory tract, or esophageal procedures: 50 mg/kg within 30 minutes prior to procedure in patients unable to take oral amoxicillin

Genitourinary and gastrointestinal tract (except esophageal) procedures:

High-risk patients: 50 mg/kg (maximum: 2 g) within 30 minutes prior to procedure, followed by ampicillin 25 mg/kg (or amoxicillin 25 mg/kg orally) 6 hours later; must be used in combination with gentamicin.

Moderate-risk patients: 50 mg/kg within 30 minutes prior to procedure

Adults:

Susceptible infections:

Oral: 250-500 mg every 6 hours

I.M., I.V.: 250-500 mg every 6 hours

Sepsis/meningitis: I.M., I.V.: 150-250 mg/kg/24 hours divided every 3-4 hours (range: 6-12 g/day)

Endocarditis prophylaxis: I.M., I.V.:

Dental, oral, respiratory tract, or esophageal procedures: 2 g within 30 minutes prior to procedure in patients unable to take oral amoxicillin

Genitourinary and gastrointestinal tract (except esophageal) procedures:

High-risk patients: 2 g within 30 minutes prior to procedure, followed by ampicillin 1 g (or amoxicillin 1 g orally) 6 hours later; must be used in combination with gentamicin

Moderate-risk patients: 2 g within 30 minutes prior to procedure

Dosing interval in renal impairment:

Cl_{cr} >50 mL/minute: Administer every 6 hours

Cl_{cr} 10-50 mL/minute: Administer every 6-12 hours

Cl_{cr} <10 mL/minute: Administer every 12-24 hours

Hemodialysis: Moderately dialyzable (20% to 50%); administer dose after dialysis

Peritoneal dialysis: Moderately dialyzable (20% to 50%)

Administer 250 mg every 12 hours

Continuous arteriovenous or venovenous hemofiltration effects: Dose as for Cl_{cr} 10-50 mL/minute; ~50 mg of ampicillin per liter of filtrate is removed

Dietary Considerations Take on an empty stomach 1 hour before or 2 hours after meals.

Sodium content of 5 mL suspension (250 mg/5 mL): 10 mg (0.4 mEq)

Sodium content of 1 g: 66.7 mg (3 mEq)

(Continued)

Ampicillin *(Continued)*

Administration Administer around-the-clock to promote less variation in peak and trough serum levels.

Oral: Administer on an empty stomach (ie, 1 hour prior to, or 2 hours after meals) to increase total absorption.

I.V.: Administer over 3-5 minutes (125-500 mg) or over 10-15 minutes (1-2 g). More rapid infusion may cause seizures. Ampicillin and gentamicin should not be mixed in the same I.V. tubing or administered concurrently.

Monitoring Parameters With prolonged therapy monitor renal, hepatic, and hematologic function periodically; observe signs and symptoms of anaphylaxis during first dose

Test Interactions May interfere with urinary glucose tests using cupric sulfate (Benedict's solution, Clinitest®); may inactivate aminoglycosides *in vitro*

Patient Information Report diarrhea promptly; take entire course of medication; females should report onset of symptoms of candidal vaginitis

Dosage Forms

Capsule (Principen®): 250 mg, 500 mg

Injection, powder for reconstitution, as sodium: 125 mg, 250 mg, 500 mg, 1 g, 2 g, 10 g

Powder for oral suspension (Principen®): 125 mg/5 mL (100 mL, 200 mL); 250 mg/5 mL (100 mL, 200 mL)

Selected Readings

Donowitz GR and Mandell GL, "Beta-Lactam Antibiotics," *N Engl J Med*, 1988, 318(7):419-26 and 318(8):490-500.

Wright AJ, "The Penicillins," *Mayo Clin Proc*, 1999, 74(3):290-307.

Ampicillin and Sulbactam (am pi SIL in & SUL bak tam)

Related Information

Antimicrobial Activity Against Selected Organisms *on page 1165*

U.S. Brand Names Unasyn®

Canadian Brand Names Unasyn®

Synonyms Sulbactam and Ampicillin

Generic Available Yes

Use Treatment of susceptible bacterial infections involved with skin and skin structure, intra-abdominal infections, gynecological infections; spectrum is that of ampicillin plus organisms producing beta-lactamases such as *S. aureus*, *H. influenzae*, *E. coli*, *Klebsiella*, *Acinetobacter*, *Enterobacter*, and anaerobes

Drug of Choice or Alternative for Disease/Syndrome(s):

Amnionitis *on page 33*
Cholangitis, Acute *on page 79*
Diverticulitis *on page 116*
Endocarditis, Acute Native Valve *on page 124*
Endocarditis, Subacute Native Valve *on page 126*
Endometritis *on page 127*
Epididymitis/Orchitis *on page 138*
Intra-abdominal Abscess *on page 194*
Liver Abscess *on page 211*
Lung Abscess *on page 212*
Mastitis *on page 214*
Osteomyelitis, Diabetic Foot *on page 249*
Pancreatitis/Pancreatic Abscess *on page 253*
Pelvic Inflammatory Disease *on page 260*
Peritonitis, Secondary *on page 263*
Peritonitis, Spontaneous Bacterial *on page 264*
Pneumonia, Aspiration, Community-Acquired *on page 269*
Pneumonia, Community-Acquired *on page 270*
Pneumonia, Hospital-Acquired *on page 272*
Pneumonia, Ventilator-Associated *on page 273*

Organism(s):

Acinetobacter Species *on page 24*
Bacteroides and *Prevotella* Species *on page 46*
Pasteurella multocida on page 258
Streptococcus-Related Gram-Positive Cocci *on page 325*

Pregnancy Risk Factor B

Contraindications Hypersensitivity to ampicillin, sulbactam, penicillins, or any component of the formulations

Warnings/Precautions Dosage adjustment may be necessary in patients with renal impairment; a low incidence of cross-allergy with other beta-lactams exists; high

percentage of patients with infectious mononucleosis have developed rash during therapy with ampicillin. Appearance of a rash should be carefully evaluated to differentiate a nonallergic ampicillin rash from a hypersensitivity reaction. Ampicillin rash occurs in 5% to 10% of children receiving ampicillin and is a generalized dull red, maculopapular rash, generally appearing 3-14 days after the start of therapy. It normally begins on the trunk and spreads over most of the body. It may be most intense at pressure areas, elbows, and knees.

Adverse Reactions Also see Ampicillin monograph

>10%: Local: Pain at injection site (I.M.)

1% to 10%:

- Dermatologic: Rash
- Gastrointestinal: Diarrhea
- Local: Pain at injection site (I.V.), thrombophlebitis
- Miscellaneous: Allergic reaction (may include serum sickness, urticaria, bronchospasm, hypotension, etc)

<1%: Abdominal distension, candidiasis, chest pain, chills, dysuria, edema, epistaxis, erythema, facial swelling, fatigue, flatulence, glossitis, hairy tongue, headache, interstitial nephritis, itching, liver enzymes increased, malaise, mucosal bleeding, nausea, pseudomembranous colitis, seizure, substernal pain, throat tightness, thrombocytopenia, urine retention, vomiting

Overdosage/Toxicology Symptoms of penicillin overdose include neuromuscular hypersensitivity (agitation, hallucinations, asterixis, encephalopathy, confusion, and seizures) and electrolyte imbalance (with potassium or sodium salts), especially in renal failure. Hemodialysis may be helpful to aid in the removal of the drug from the blood, otherwise most treatment is supportive or symptom-directed.

Drug Interactions

Increased Effect/Toxicity: Disulfiram or probenecid can increase ampicillin levels. Theoretically, allopurinol taken with ampicillin has an additive potential for rash. Penicillins may increase the exposure to methotrexate during concurrent therapy; monitor.

Decreased Effect: Although anecdotal reports suggest oral contraceptive efficacy could be reduced by penicillins, this has been refuted by more rigorous scientific and clinical data.

Stability Prior to reconstitution, store at ≤30°C (86°F).

I.M. and direct I.V. administration: Use within 1 hour after preparation; reconstitute with sterile water for injection or 0.5% or 2% lidocaine hydrochloride injection (I.M.); sodium chloride 0.9% (NS) is the diluent of choice for I.V. piggyback use, solutions made in NS are stable up to 72 hours when refrigerated whereas dextrose solutions (same concentration) are stable for only 4 hours

Mechanism of Action The addition of sulbactam, a beta-lactamase inhibitor, to ampicillin extends the spectrum of ampicillin to include some beta-lactamase producing organisms; inhibits bacterial cell wall synthesis by binding to one or more of the penicillin binding proteins (PBPs); which in turn inhibits the final transpeptidation step of peptidoglycan synthesis in bacterial cell walls, thus inhibiting cell wall biosynthesis. Bacteria eventually lyse due to ongoing activity of cell wall autolytic enzymes (autolysins and murein hydrolases) while cell wall assembly is arrested.

Pharmacodynamics/Kinetics

Ampicillin: See Ampicillin monograph.

Sulbactam:

- Distribution: Bile, blister, and tissue fluids
- Protein binding: 38%
- Half-life elimination: Normal renal function: 1-1.3 hours
- Excretion: Urine (~75% to 85% as unchanged drug) within 8 hours

Dosage Unasyn® (ampicillin/sulbactam) is a combination product. Dosage recommendations for Unasyn® are based on the ampicillin component.

Children ≥1 year: I.V.:

- Mild-to-moderate infections: 100-150 mg ampicillin/kg/day (150-300 mg Unasyn®) divided every 6 hours; maximum: 8 g ampicillin/day (12 g Unasyn®)
- Severe infections: 200-400 mg ampicillin/kg/day divided every 6 hours; maximum: 8 g ampicillin/day (12 g Unasyn®)

Adults: I.M., I.V.: 1-2 g ampicillin (1.5-3 g Unasyn®) every 6 hours; maximum: 8 g ampicillin/day (12 g Unasyn®)

Dosing interval in renal impairment:

- Cl_{cr} 15-29 mL/minute: Administer every 12 hours
- Cl_{cr} 5-14 mL/minute: Administer every 24 hours

Dietary Considerations Sodium content of 1.5 g injection: 115 mg (5 mEq)

Administration Administer around-the-clock to promote less variation in peak and trough serum levels. Administer by slow injection over 10-15 minutes or I.V. over

(Continued)

Ampicillin and Sulbactam *(Continued)*

15-30 minutes. Ampicillin and gentamicin should not be mixed in the same I.V. tubing or administered concurrently.

Monitoring Parameters With prolonged therapy, monitor hematologic, renal, and hepatic function; monitor for signs of anaphylaxis during first dose

Test Interactions May interfere with urinary glucose tests using cupric sulfate (Benedict's solution, Clinitest®); may inactivate aminoglycosides *in vitro*

Dosage Forms Injection, powder for reconstitution: 3 g [ampicillin sodium 2 g and sulbactam sodium 1 g]; 15 g [ampicillin sodium 10 g and sulbactam sodium 5 g] [bulk package]

Unasyn®: 1.5 g [ampicillin sodium 1 g and sulbactam sodium 0.5 g]; 3 g [ampicillin sodium 2 g and sulbactam sodium 1 g]; 15 g [ampicillin sodium 10 g and sulbactam sodium 5 g] [bulk package]

Selected Readings

Donowitz GR and Mandell GL, "Beta-Lactam Antibiotics," *N Engl J Med*, 1988, 318(7):419-26 and 318(8):490-500.

Itokazu GS and Danziger LH, "Ampicillin-Sulbactam and Ticarcillin-Clavulanic Acid: A Comparison of Their *In Vitro* Activity and Review of Their Clinical Efficacy," *Pharmacotherapy*, 1991, 11(5):382-414.

Wright AJ, "The Penicillins," *Mayo Clin Proc*, 1999, 74(3):290-307.

Ampicillin Sodium *see* Ampicillin *on page 657*

Ampicillin Trihydrate *see* Ampicillin *on page 657*

Amprenavir (am PREN a veer)

Related Information

Antiretroviral Agents *on page 1206*

Antiretroviral Therapy for HIV Infection *on page 1219*

Management of Healthcare Worker Exposures to HBV, HCV, and HIV *on page 1227*

U.S. Brand Names Agenerase®

Canadian Brand Names Agenerase®

Generic Available No

Use Treatment of HIV infections in combination with at least two other antiretroviral agents; oral solution should only be used when capsules or other protease inhibitors are not therapeutic options

Drug of Choice or Alternative for Organism(s):

Human Immunodeficiency Virus *on page 181*

Pregnancy Risk Factor C

Pregnancy Implications It is not known if amprenavir crosses the human placenta and there are no clinical studies currently underway to evaluate its use in pregnant women. Use of oral solution is contraindicated during pregnancy. Pregnancy and protease inhibitors are both associated with an increased risk of hyperglycemia. Glucose levels should be closely monitored. Health professionals are encouraged to contact the antiretroviral pregnancy registry to monitor outcomes of pregnant women exposed to antiretroviral medications (1-800-258-4263 or www.APRegistry.com).

Contraindications Hypersensitivity to amprenavir or any component of the formulation; concurrent therapy with cisapride, ergot derivatives, midazolam, pimozide, and triazolam; severe previous allergic reaction to sulfonamides; oral solution is contraindicated in infants or children <4 years of age, pregnant women, patients with renal or hepatic failure, and patients receiving concurrent metronidazole or disulfiram

Warnings/Precautions Because of hepatic metabolism and effect on cytochrome P450 enzymes, amprenavir should be used with caution in combination with other agents metabolized by this system (see Contraindications and Drug Interactions). Avoid use of lovastatin or simvastatin (risk of rhabdomyolysis may be increased). Avoid concurrent use of hormonal contraceptives, rifampin, and/or St John's wort (may lead to loss of virologic response and/or resistance). Use with caution in patients with diabetes mellitus, sulfonamide allergy, hepatic impairment, or hemophilia. Redistribution of fat may occur (eg, buffalo hump, peripheral wasting, cushingoid appearance). Additional vitamin E supplements should be avoided. Certain ethnic populations (Asians, Eskimos, Native Americans) may be at increased risk of propylene glycol-associated adverse effects; use of the oral solution of amprenavir should be avoided. Use oral solution only when capsules or other protease inhibitors are not options. Dosage adjustment is required for combination therapy with amprenavir and ritonavir; in addition, the risk of hyperlipidemia may be increased during concurrent therapy.

Adverse Reactions Protease inhibitors cause dyslipidemia which includes elevated cholesterol and triglycerides and a redistribution of body fat centrally to cause increased abdominal girth, buffalo hump, facial atrophy, and breast enlargement. These agents also cause hyperglycemia.

>10%:
- Central nervous system: Paresthesia (peripheral 10% to 14%)
- Dermatologic: Rash (22%)
- Endocrine & metabolic: Hyperglycemia (>160 mg/dL: 37% to 41%), hypertriglyceridemia (>399 mg/dL: 36% to 47%; >750 mg/dL: 8% to 13%)
- Gastrointestinal: Nausea (43% to 74%), vomiting (24% to 34%), diarrhea (39% to 60%), abdominal symptoms
- Miscellaneous: Perioral tingling/numbness (26% to 31%)

1% to 10%:
- Central nervous system: Depression (4% to 15%), headache, fatigue, depression, mood disorder
- Dermatologic: Stevens-Johnson syndrome (1% of total, 4% of patients who develop a rash)
- Endocrine & metabolic: Hyperglycemia (>251 mg/dL: 2% to 3%)
- Gastrointestinal: Taste disorders (2% to 10%)
- Hepatic: AST increased (3% to 5%), ALT increased (4%), amylase increased (3% to 4%)

Overdosage/Toxicology Monitor for signs and symptoms of propylene glycol toxicity (seizures, stupor, tachycardia, hyperosmolality, lactic acidosis, renal toxicity, hemolysis) if the oral solution is administered.

Drug Interactions

Cytochrome P450 Effect: Substrate of CYP2C8/9 (minor), 3A4 (major); **Inhibits** CYP2C19 (weak), 3A4 (strong)

Increased Effect/Toxicity: Concurrent use of cisapride, midazolam, pimozide, quinidine, or triazolam is contraindicated. Concurrent use of ergot alkaloids (dihydroergotamine, ergotamine, ergonovine, methylergonovine) with amprenavir is also contraindicated (may cause vasospasm and peripheral ischemia). Concurrent use of oral solution with disulfiram or metronidazole is contraindicated, due to the risk of propylene glycol toxicity.

Serum concentrations of amiodarone, bepridil, lidocaine, quinidine and other antiarrhythmics may be increased, potentially leading to toxicity; when amprenavir is coadministered with ritonavir, flecainide and propafenone are contraindicated. HMG-CoA reductase inhibitors serum concentrations may be increased by amprenavir, increasing the risk of myopathy/rhabdomyolysis; lovastatin and simvastatin are not recommended; fluvastatin and pravastatin may be safer alternatives.

Amprenavir may increase the levels/effects of selected benzodiazepines (midazolam and triazolam are contraindicated), calcium channel blockers, cyclosporine, mirtazapine, nateglinide, nefazodone, quinidine, sildenafil (and other PDE-5 inhibitors), tacrolimus, venlafaxine, and other CYP3A4 substrates. When used with strong CYP3A4 inhibitors, dosage adjustment/limits are recommended for sildenafil and other PDE-5 inhibitors; refer to individual monographs.

Concurrent therapy with ritonavir may result in increased serum concentrations: dosage adjustment is recommended; avoid concurrent use of amprenavir and ritonavir oral solutions due to metabolic competition between formulation components. Clarithromycin, indinavir, nelfinavir may increase serum concentrations of amprenavir.

Decreased Effect: Serum concentrations of estrogen (oral contraceptives) may be decreased, use alternative (nonhormonal) forms of contraception. Dexamethasone may decrease the therapeutic effect of amprenavir. Serum concentrations of delavirdine may be decreased; may lead to loss of virologic response and possible resistance to delavirdine; concomitant use is not recommended. Efavirenz and nevirapine may decrease serum concentrations of amprenavir (dosing for combinations not established). Avoid St John's wort (may lead to subtherapeutic concentrations of amprenavir). Effect of amprenavir may be diminished when administered with methadone (consider alternative antiretroviral); in addition, effect of methadone may be reduced (dosage increase may be required). The levels/effects of amprenavir may be decreased by include aminoglutethimide, carbamazepine, nafcillin, nevirapine, phenobarbital, phenytoin, rifamycins, and other CYP3A4 inducers. The administration of didanosine (buffered formulation) should be separated from amprenavir by 1 hour to limit interaction between formulations.

Ethanol/Nutrition/Herb Interactions

Ethanol: Avoid ethanol with amprenavir oral solution.

Food: Levels increased sixfold with high-fat meals.

Herb/Nutraceutical: Amprenavir serum concentration may be decreased by St John's wort; avoid concurrent use. Formulations contain vitamin E; avoid additional supplements.

Mechanism of Action Binds to the protease activity site and inhibits the activity of the enzyme. HIV protease is required for the cleavage of viral polyprotein precursors into

(Continued)

Amprenavir *(Continued)*

individual functional proteins found in infectious HIV. Inhibition prevents cleavage of these polyproteins, resulting in the formation of immature, noninfectious viral particles.

Pharmacodynamics/Kinetics

Absorption: 63%
Distribution: 430 L
Protein binding: 90%
Metabolism: Hepatic via CYP (primarily CYP3A4)
Bioavailability: Not established; increased sixfold with high-fat meal
Half-life elimination: 7.1-10.6 hours
Time to peak: 1-2 hours
Excretion: Feces (75%); urine (14% as metabolites)

Dosage Oral: **Note:** Capsule and oral solution are **not** interchangeable on a mg-per-mg basis.

Capsule:

Children 4-12 years **or** 13-16 years (<50 kg): 20 mg/kg twice daily or 15 mg/kg 3 times daily; maximum: 2400 mg/day

Children >13 years (≥50 kg) and Adults: 1200 mg twice daily

Note: Dosage adjustments for amprenavir when administered in combination therapy:

Efavirenz: Adjustments necessary for both agents:
Amprenavir 1200 mg 3 times/day (single protease inhibitor) **or**
Amprenavir 1200 mg twice daily plus ritonavir 200 mg twice daily

Ritonavir: Adjustments necessary for both agents:
Amprenavir 1200 mg plus ritonavir 200 mg once daily **or**
Amprenavir 600 mg plus ritonavir 100 mg twice daily
Note: Oral solution of ritonavir and amprenavir should not be coadministered.

Solution:

Children 4-12 years **or** 13-16 years (<50 kg): 22.5 mg/kg twice daily or 17 mg/kg 3 times daily; maximum: 2800 mg/day

Children >13 years (≥50 kg) and Adults: 1400 mg twice daily

Dosage adjustment in renal impairment: Oral solution is contraindicated in renal failure.

Dosage adjustment in hepatic impairment:

Child-Pugh score between 5-8:
Capsule: 450 mg twice daily
Solution: 513 mg twice daily; contraindicated in hepatic failure

Child-Pugh score between 9-12:
Capsule: 300 mg twice daily
Solution: 342 mg twice daily; contraindicated in hepatic failure

Dietary Considerations May be taken with or without food; do not take with high-fat meal.

Patient Information Advise prescriber of any previous reactions to sulfonamides. Do not take this medication with antacids or high-fat meals. Do not take additional vitamin E supplements. Do not take any prescription medications, over-the-counter products, or herbal products without consulting prescriber.

Additional Information The 150 mg capsules contain 109 int. units of vitamin E per capsule; oral solution contains 46 int. units of vitamin E per mL. Propylene glycol is included in the oral solution; a dose of 22.5 mg/kg twice daily corresponds to an intake of 1650 mg/kg of propylene glycol. Capsule and oral solution are not interchangeable on a mg-per-mg basis.

Dosage Forms [DSC] = Discontinued product

Capsule: 50 mg, 150 mg [DSC]

Solution, oral [use only when there are no other options]: 15 mg/mL (240 mL) [contains propylene glycol 550 mg/mL and vitamin E 46 int. units/mL; grape-bubble gum-peppermint flavor]

Selected Readings

Kaul DR, Cinti SK, Carver PL, et al, "HIV Protease Inhibitors: Advances in Therapy and Adverse Reactions, Including Metabolic Complications," *Pharmacotherapy*, 1999, 19(3):281-98.

Noble S and Goa KL, "Amprenavir: A Review of Its Clinical Potential in Patients With HIV Infection," *Drugs*, 2000, 60(6):1383-410.

Anadrol® *see* Oxymetholone *on page 986*
Ancef® *see* Cefazolin *on page 700*
Ancobon® *see* Flucytosine *on page 822*
Andriol® (Can) *see* Testosterone *on page 1100*
Androderm® *see* Testosterone *on page 1100*
AndroGel® *see* Testosterone *on page 1100*

Andropository (Can) *see* Testosterone *on page 1100*

Ansamycin *see* Rifabutin *on page 1045*

Anthrax Vaccine Adsorbed (AN thraks vak SEEN ad SORBED)

U.S. Brand Names BioThrax™

Synonyms AVA

Generic Available No

Use Immunization against *Bacillus anthracis*. Recommended for individuals who may come in contact with animal products which come from anthrax endemic areas and may be contaminated with *Bacillus anthracis* spores; recommended for high-risk persons such as veterinarians and other handling potentially infected animals. Routine immunization for the general population is not recommended.

The Department of Defense is implementing an anthrax vaccination program against the biological warfare agent anthrax, which will be administered to all active duty and reserve personnel.

Unlabeled/Investigational Use Postexposure prophylaxis in combination with antibiotics

Restrictions Not commercially available in the U.S.; presently, all anthrax vaccine lots are owned by the U.S. Department of Defense. The Centers for Disease Control (CDC) does not currently recommend routine vaccination of the general public.

Pregnancy Risk Factor D

Pregnancy Implications Reproduction studies have not been conducted. Use during pregnancy only if clearly needed. Unpublished data from the Department of Defense suggest the vaccine may be linked with an increased number of birth defects when given during pregnancy.

Contraindications Hypersensitivity to anthrax vaccine or any component of the formulation; severe anaphylactic reaction to a previous dose of anthrax vaccine; history of anthrax; history of Guillain-Barré syndrome; pregnancy

Warnings/Precautions Immediate treatment for anaphylactic/anaphylactoid reaction should be available during vaccine use. Patients with a history of Guillain-Barré syndrome should not be given the vaccine unless there is a clear benefit that outweighs the potential risk of recurrence. Defer dosing during acute respiratory disease or other active infection; defer dosing during short-term corticosteroid therapy, chemotherapy or radiation; additional dose required in patients on long-term corticosteroid therapy; discontinue immunization in patients with chills or fever associated with administration; use caution with latex allergy; immune response may be decreased with immunodeficiency. Safety and efficacy in children <18 years of age or adults >65 years of age have not been established.

Adverse Reactions (Includes pre- and postlicensure data; systemic reactions reported more often in women than in men)

>10%:

- Central nervous system: Malaise (4% to 11%)
- Local: Tenderness (58% to 71%), erythema (12% to 43%), subcutaneous nodule (4% to 39%), induration (8% to 21%), warmth (11% to 19%), local pruritus (7% to 19%)
- Neuromuscular & skeletal: Arm motion limitation (7% to 12%)

1% to 10%:

- Central nervous system: Headache (4% to 7%), fever (<1% to 7%)
- Gastrointestinal: Anorexia (4%), vomiting (4%), nausea (<1% to 4%)
- Local: Mild local reactions (edema/induration <30mm) (9%), edema (8%)
- Neuromuscular & skeletal: Myalgia (4% to 7%)
- Respiratory: Respiratory difficulty (4%)

<1%: Chills, body aches, delayed hypersensitivity reaction (started approximately day 17), moderate local reactions (edema/induration >30 mm and <120 mm), severe local reactions (edema/induration >120 mm in diameter or accompanied by marked limitation of arm motion or marked axillary node tenderness)

Postmarketing and/or case reports: Anaphylaxis, angioedema, aplastic anemia, arthralgia, aseptic meningitis, asthma, atrial fibrillation, cardiomyopathy, cellulitis, cerebrovascular accident, CNS lymphoma, cysts, collagen vascular disease, dizziness, encephalitis, endocarditis, facial palsy, fatigue, glomerulonephritis, Guillain-Barré syndrome, hearing disorder, idiopathic thrombocytopenia purpura, immune deficiency, inflammatory arthritis, injection site pain/tenderness, leukemia, liver abscess, lymphoma, mental status change, multiple sclerosis, myocarditis, neutropenia, pemphigus vulgaris, peripheral swelling, polyarteritis nodosa, psychiatric disorders, renal failure, seizure, sepsis, spontaneous abortion, sudden cardiac arrest, suicide, syncope, transverse myelitis, tremor, systemic lupus erythematosus, visual disorder

(Continued)

Anthrax Vaccine Adsorbed *(Continued)*

Drug Interactions

Decreased Effect: Effect of vaccine may be decreased with chemotherapy, corticosteroids (high doses, ≥14 days), immunosuppressant agents and radiation therapy; consider waiting at least 3 months between discontinuing therapy and administering vaccine.

Stability Store under refrigeration at 2°C to 8°C (36°F to 46°F); do not freeze

Mechanism of Action Active immunization against *Bacillus anthracis*. The vaccine is prepared from a cell-free filtrate of *B. anthracis*, but no dead or live bacteria.

Pharmacodynamics/Kinetics Duration: Unknown; may be 1-2 years following two inoculations based on animal data

Dosage SubQ:

Children <18 years: Safety and efficacy have not been established

Children ≥18 years and Adults:

Primary immunization: Three injections of 0.5 mL each given 2 weeks apart, followed by three additional injections given at 6-, 12-, and 18 months; it is not necessary to restart the series if a dose is not given on time; resume as soon as practical

Subsequent booster injections: 0.5 mL at 1-year intervals are recommended for immunity to be maintained

Elderly: Safety and efficacy have not been established for patients >65 years of age

Administration Administer SubQ; shake well before use. Do not use if discolored or contains particulate matter. Do not use the same site for more than one injection. Do not mix with other injections. After administration, massage injection site to disperse the vaccine. Federal law requires that the date of administration, the vaccine manufacturer, lot number of vaccine, and the administering person's name, title and address be entered into the patient's permanent medical record.

Monitoring Parameters Monitor for local reactions, chills, fever, anaphylaxis

Patient Information Immunization using the vaccine consists of a series of 6 injections. The vaccine should be used by people who may be exposed to the anthrax bacteria, such as laboratory workers, veterinarians, and military personnel. You should not use the vaccine if you have already had anthrax disease. Most people receiving the vaccine will experience soreness, redness, or itching at the injection site, which should clear up within 48 hours. Contact your prescriber immediately if you experience a fever, difficulty breathing, hoarseness, wheezing, fast heart beat, hives, dizziness, paleness, or swelling of the throat.

Additional Information Not commercially available in the U.S.

Local reactions increase in severity by the fifth dose. Moderate local reactions (>5 cm) may be pruritic and may occur if given to a patient with a previous history of anthrax infection. Federal law requires that the date of administration, the vaccine manufacturer, lot number of vaccine, and the administering person's name, title and address be entered into the patient's permanent medical record.

Dosage Forms Injection, suspension: 5 mL [vial stopper contains dry natural rubber]

AntibiOtic® Ear *see* Neomycin, Polymyxin B, and Hydrocortisone *on page 966*

Antifungal, Topical

Refer to

Betamethasone and Clotrimazole *on page 685*
Butenafine *on page 691*
Butoconazole *on page 691*
Ciclopirox *on page 739*
Clotrimazole *on page 758*
Econazole *on page 795*
Gentian Violet *on page 845*
Iodoquinol and Hydrocortisone *on page 891*
Ketoconazole *on page 903*
Miconazole *on page 945*
Naftifine *on page 956*
Nystatin and Triamcinolone *on page 977*
Nystatin *on page 976*
Oxiconazole *on page 985*
Sertaconazole *on page 1064*
Sulconazole *on page 1080*
Terbinafine *on page 1097*
Tolnaftate *on page 1127*
Triacetin *on page 1129*
Undecylenic Acid and Derivatives *on page 1139*

Drug of Choice or Alternative for Organism(s):
Candida Species *on page 67*
Dermatophytes *on page 114*

Antituberculars

Refer to
Capreomycin *on page 692*
CycloSERINE *on page 763*
Ethambutol *on page 812*
Ethionamide *on page 814*
Isoniazid *on page 893*
Pyrazinamide *on page 1022*
Rifabutin *on page 1045*
Rifampin and Isoniazid *on page 1050*
Rifampin, Isoniazid, and Pyrazinamide *on page 1050*
Rifampin *on page 1046*
Rifapentine *on page 1051*
Streptomycin *on page 1078*

Drug of Choice or Alternative for Organism(s):
Mycobacterium bovis on page 229
Mycobacterium tuberculosis on page 234

Aplisol® *see* Tuberculin Tests *on page 1136*
Apo-Acyclovir® (Can) *see* Acyclovir *on page 629*
Apo-Amoxi® (Can) *see* Amoxicillin *on page 642*
Apo-Amoxi-Clav® (Can) *see* Amoxicillin and Clavulanate Potassium *on page 645*
Apo-Ampi® (Can) *see* Ampicillin *on page 657*
Apo-Cefaclor® (Can) *see* Cefaclor *on page 697*
Apo-Cefadroxil® (Can) *see* Cefadroxil *on page 698*
Apo-Cefuroxime® (Can) *see* Cefuroxime *on page 725*
Apo-Cephalex® (Can) *see* Cephalexin *on page 727*
Apo-Chlorhexadine® (Can) *see* Chlorhexidine Gluconate *on page 735*
Apo-Ciproflox® (Can) *see* Ciprofloxacin *on page 742*
Apo-Clindamycin® (Can) *see* Clindamycin *on page 752*
Apo-Cloxi® (Can) *see* Cloxacillin *on page 760*
Apo-Doxy® (Can) *see* Doxycycline *on page 787*
Apo-Doxy Tabs® (Can) *see* Doxycycline *on page 787*
Apo-Erythro Base® (Can) *see* Erythromycin *on page 807*
Apo-Erythro E-C® (Can) *see* Erythromycin *on page 807*
Apo-Erythro-ES® (Can) *see* Erythromycin *on page 807*
Apo-Erythro-S® (Can) *see* Erythromycin *on page 807*
Apo-Fluconazole® (Can) *see* Fluconazole *on page 819*
Apo-Hydroxyquine® (Can) *see* Hydroxychloroquine *on page 859*
Apo-Ketoconazole® (Can) *see* Ketoconazole *on page 903*
Apo-Mefloquine® (Can) *see* Mefloquine *on page 929*
Apo-Megestrol® (Can) *see* Megestrol *on page 932*
Apo-Metronidazole® (Can) *see* Metronidazole *on page 940*
Apo-Minocycline® (Can) *see* Minocycline *on page 947*
Apo-Nitrofurantoin® (Can) *see* Nitrofurantoin *on page 971*
Apo-Norflox® (Can) *see* Norfloxacin *on page 973*
Apo-Oflox® (Can) *see* Ofloxacin *on page 977*
Apo-Ofloxacin® (Can) *see* Ofloxacin *on page 977*
Apo-Pen VK® (Can) *see* Penicillin V Potassium *on page 998*
Apo-Quin-G® (Can) *see* Quinidine *on page 1027*
Apo-Quinidine® (Can) *see* Quinidine *on page 1027*
Apo-Quinine® (Can) *see* Quinine *on page 1030*
Apo-Sulfatrim® (Can) *see* Sulfamethoxazole and Trimethoprim *on page 1087*
Apo-Terbinafine® (Can) *see* Terbinafine *on page 1097*
Apo-Tetra® (Can) *see* Tetracycline *on page 1106*
Apo-Tobramycin® (Can) *see* Tobramycin *on page 1122*
Apo-Trimethoprim® (Can) *see* Trimethoprim *on page 1130*
Apo-Zidovudine® (Can) *see* Zidovudine *on page 1159*
APPG *see* Penicillin G Procaine *on page 995*

Aptivus® *see* Tipranavir *on page 1120*
Aqueous Procaine Penicillin G *see* Penicillin G Procaine *on page 995*
Aralen® *see* Chloroquine *on page 737*

Atazanavir (at a za NA veer)

Related Information

Antiretroviral Agents *on page 1206*
Antiretroviral Therapy for HIV Infection *on page 1219*

U.S. Brand Names Reyataz®

Canadian Brand Names Reyataz®

Synonyms Atazanavir Sulfate; BMS-232632

Generic Available No

Use Treatment of HIV-1 infections in combination with at least two other antiretroviral agents

Note: In patients with prior virologic failure, coadministration with ritonavir is recommended.

Drug of Choice or Alternative for Organism(s):

Human Immunodeficiency Virus *on page 181*

Pregnancy Risk Factor B

Pregnancy Implications Teratogenic effects not observed in animal studies. It is not known if atazanavir crosses the human placenta. Pregnancy and protease inhibitors are both associated with an increased risk of hyperglycemia. Glucose levels should be closely monitored. It is not known if atazanavir will exacerbate hyperbilirubinemia in neonates. Health professionals are encouraged to contact the antiretroviral pregnancy registry to monitor outcomes of pregnant women exposed to antiretroviral medications (1-800-258-4263 or www.APRegistry.com).

Contraindications Hypersensitivity to atazanavir or any component of the formulation. Concurrent therapy with: Bepridil; cisapride; ergot derivatives (dihydroergotamine, ergonovine, ergotamine, methylergonovine); indinavir; irinotecan; lovastatin; midazolam; pimozide; proton pump inhibitors (esomeprazole, lansoprazole, omeprazole); rifampin; simvastatin; St John's wort; or triazolam.

Warnings/Precautions Atazanavir is hepatically metabolized and has multiple drug interactions. A listing of medications that should not be used is available with each bottle and patients should be provided with this information. Use caution with medications metabolized by CYP3A4 and/or UGT1A1 (many are contraindicated). Additional CYP3A4 substrates include calcium channel blockers, immunosuppressants, and sildenafil.

Atazanavir may prolong PR interval, use with caution in patients with pre-existing conduction abnormalities or with medications which prolong AV conduction (dosage adjustment required with some agents); rare cases of AV block have been reported. May exacerbate pre-existing hepatic dysfunction; use caution in patients with hepatitis B or C or in patients with cirrhosis. Asymptomatic elevations in bilirubin (unconjugated) occur commonly during therapy with atazanavir; consider alternative therapy if bilirubin is >5 times ULN. Evaluate alternative etiologies if transaminase elevations also occur.

Use with caution in patients with hemophilia A or B; increased bleeding during protease inhibitor therapy has been reported. Changes in glucose tolerance, hyperglycemia, exacerbation of diabetes, DKA, and new-onset diabetes mellitus have been reported in patients receiving protease inhibitors. May be associated with fat redistribution (buffalo hump, increased abdominal girth, breast engorgement, facial atrophy). Atazanavir has been associated with development of rash (median onset 8 weeks); if mild-moderate, treatment may be continued (rash may resolve); discontinue therapy in cases of severe rash. Optimal dosing in pediatric patients has not been established; do not use in children <3 months of age due to potential for kernicterus.

Adverse Reactions Protease inhibitors cause dyslipidemia which includes elevated cholesterol and triglycerides and a redistribution of body fat centrally to cause increased abdominal girth, buffalo hump, facial atrophy, and breast enlargement. These agents also cause hyperglycemia.

>10%:

Dermatologic: Rash (21%; median onset 8 weeks)
Gastrointestinal: Nausea (6% to 14%)
Hepatic: Bilirubin increased (>2.6 times ULN: 35% to 47%), amylase increased (14%)

3% to 10%:

Central nervous system: Depression (4% to 8%), dizziness (1% to 2%), fatigue (2% to 5%), fever (4% to 5%), headache (1% to 6%), insomnia (1% to 3%), pain (1% to 3%), peripheral neuropathy (1% to 4%)

Endocrine & metabolic: Lipodystrophy (1% to 8%)
Gastrointestinal: Abdominal pain (4%), vomiting (3% to 4%), diarrhea (1% to 11%)
Hepatic: Jaundice (7% to 8%), transaminases increased (2% to 9%)
Neuromuscular & skeletal: Myalgia (4%)
Respiratory: Cough increased (3% to 5%)

<3%: Abnormal dreams, acholia, agitation, allergic reaction, alopecia, amenorrhea, amnesia, angioedema, anorexia, anxiety, aphthous stomatitis, bone pain, buffalo hump, cardiac arrest, chest pain, colitis, confusion, constipation, crystalluria, dehydration, diabetes mellitus, diaphoresis increased, dyslipidemia, dyspepsia, dyspnea, ecchymosis, eczema, edema, emotional lability, esophageal ulcer, esophagitis, facial atrophy, fertility (male) decreased, gastritis, gout, gynecomastia, hallucination, heart block, hematuria, hepatitis, hepatomegaly, hiccup, hyperkinesias, hypertension, impotence, infection, lactic acidosis, libido decreased, malaise, menstrual disorder, myasthenia, myocarditis, myopathy, nail disorder, nervousness, otitis, palpitation, pancreatitis, peptic ulcer, photosensitivity, polyuria, pruritus, psychosis, purpura, reflexes decreased, renal calculus, renal failure, seborrhea, seizure, sleep disorder, suicide attempt, syncope, taste perversion, tinnitus, urinary frequency, urticaria, vasodilation, vesiculobullous rash, weakness, weight gain/loss

Postmarketing and/or case reports: Erythema multiforme, PR interval prolongation (first-degree AV block; rarely second-degree AV block), Stevens-Johnson syndrome

Overdosage/Toxicology Limited experience in overdose. Treatment is symptomatic and supportive. Dialysis is not likely to remove significant amounts of drug.

Drug Interactions

Cytochrome P450 Effect: Substrate of CYP3A4 (major); **Inhibits** CYP1A2 (weak), 2C9 (weak), 3A4 (strong)

Increased Effect/Toxicity: Serum concentrations of medications significantly metabolized by CYP3A4 or UGT1A1 may be elevated by atazanavir. Concurrent therapy with bepridil, cisapride, ergot derivatives (dihydroergotamine, ergonovine, ergotamine, methylergonovine), indinavir, irinotecan, lovastatin, midazolam, pimozide, simvastatin or triazolam is contraindicated (or not recommended, per manufacturer).

Atazanavir may increase the levels/effects of selected benzodiazepines, calcium channel blockers, cyclosporine, mirtazapine, nateglinide, nefazodone, quinidine, sildenafil (and other PDE-5 inhibitors), tacrolimus, tenofovir, venlafaxine, and other CYP3A4 substrates. When used with strong CYP3A4 inhibitors, dosage adjustment/limits are recommended for sildenafil and other PDE-5 inhibitors; consult individual monographs. Serum concentrations of antiarrhythmics (amiodarone, lidocaine, and quinidine) may be increased; monitor serum concentrations of these agents. Serum concentrations/effects of trazodone may be increased; use caution and reduce trazodone dose.

The levels/effects of atazanavir may be increased by azole antifungals, ciprofloxacin, clarithromycin, diclofenac, doxycycline, erythromycin, imatinib, isoniazid, nefazodone, nicardipine, propofol, protease inhibitors, quinidine, telithromycin, verapamil, and other CYP3A4 inhibitors. When used with strong Serum concentrations of atazanavir are increased by ritonavir. Specific dosing adjustment of atazanavir in combination with ritonavir and efavirenz has been established. Serum concentrations of saquinavir may be increased by atazanavir. Dosing recommendations for the combination have not been established. Tenofovir concentrations are increased by atazanavir. Concurrent use of indinavir may increase the risk of hyperbilirubinemia. Concurrent administration is not recommended. Serum concentrations of orally inhaled corticosteroids (fluticasone, budesonide) may be increased by atazanavir (with or without ritonavir) resulting in decreased serum cortisol, HPA axis suppression; concurrent use with atazanavir plus ritonavir not recommended.

Atazanavir may increase warfarin's hypoprothrombinemic effect; monitor INR closely. Serum levels of the hormones in oral contraceptives may increase significantly with administration of atazanavir; use with caution at lowest effective dose. Atazanavir may increase serum concentrations of clarithromycin, potentially increasing the risk of QT_c prolongation. A 50% reduction in clarithromycin dose or an alternative agent (except in *M. avium* complex infections) should be considered. An increase in rifabutin plasma AUC (>200%) has been observed when coadministered with atazanavir (decrease rifabutin's dose by up to 75%).

Decreased Effect: Concurrent use of proton pump inhibitors may reduce atazanavir absorption; avoid concurrent use. Antacids and buffered formulations (ie, didanosine buffered tablets) may reduce the serum concentrations of atazanavir. Administer atazanavir 2 hours before or 1 hour after these medications. H_2 antagonists may reduce the absorption of atazanavir; avoid concurrent use or administer at least 12 hours apart.

(Continued)

Atazanavir *(Continued)*

The levels/effects of atazanavir may be decreased by aminoglutethimide, carbamazepine, nafcillin, nevirapine, phenobarbital, phenytoin, rifamycins, and other CYP3A4 inducers. Rifampin decreases bioavailability of protease inhibitors by ~90%; loss of virologic response and resistance may occur; the two drugs should not be administered together. St John's wort (*Hypericum perforatum*) decreases serum concentrations of protease inhibitors and may lead to treatment failures; concurrent use is contraindicated. Tenofovir may decrease serum concentrations of atazanavir, resulting in a loss of virologic response (specific atazanavir dosing recommendations provided by manufacturer).

Ethanol/Nutrition/Herb Interactions

Food: Atazanavir taken with food increases bioavailability.

Herb/Nutraceutical: St John's wort (*Hypericum perforatum*) decreases serum concentrations of protease inhibitors and may lead to treatment failures; concurrent use is contraindicated.

Stability Store at 25°C (77°F); excursions permitted to 15°C to 30°C (59°F to 86°F).

Mechanism of Action Inhibits the HIV-1 protease; inhibition of the viral protease prevents cleavage of the gag-pol polyprotein resulting in the production of immature, noninfectious virus

Pharmacodynamics/Kinetics

Protein binding: 86%

Metabolism: Hepatic, via multiple pathways including CYP3A4; forms 2 metabolites (inactive)

Half-life elimination: ~7 hours

Time to peak, plasma: 2.5 hours

Excretion: Feces (79% as metabolites, 20% as unchanged drug); urine (13% as metabolites, 7% as unchanged drug)

Dosage Oral: Adolescents ≥16 years and Adults:

Antiretroviral-naive patients: 400 mg once daily; administer with food

Antiretroviral-experienced patients: 300 mg once daily **plus** ritonavir 100 mg once daily; administer with food

Coadministration with efavirenz: Adults:

Antiretroviral-naive patients: It is recommended that atazanavir 300 mg plus ritonavir 100 mg be given with efavirenz 600 mg (all as a single daily dose); administer with food

Antiretroviral-experienced patients: Recommendations have not been established.

Coadministration with didanosine buffered formulations: Administer atazanavir 2 hours before or 1 hour after didanosine buffered formulations

Coadministration with tenofovir: Adults: The manufacturer recommends that atazanavir 300 mg plus ritonavir 100 mg be given with tenofovir 300 mg (all as a single daily dose); administer with food

Dosage adjustment in renal impairment: No recommendation

Dosage adjustment in hepatic impairment:

Moderate hepatic insufficiency (Child-Pugh Class B): Reduce dose to 300 mg once daily

Severe hepatic insufficiency (Child-Pugh Class C): Avoid use

Note: Data unavailable for patients with underlying hepatitis B or C.

Dietary Considerations Should be taken with food to enhance absorption.

Administration Administer with food.

Monitoring Parameters Viral load, CD4, serum glucose; liver function tests, bilirubin

Patient Information This drug may interact with many medications. Check with prescriber before taking any medication, including OTC and herbal medicines. This drug is not a cure for HIV and has not been shown to reduce the risk of transmitting HIV to others. Do not miss doses. If you miss a dose, take as soon as possible and return to your regular schedule (never take a double dose). Frequent blood tests may be required with prolonged therapy. May cause nausea or vomiting (small, frequent meals, frequent mouth care, chewing gum, or sucking lozenges may help). Report rash; difficulty breathing; CNS changes (migraine, confusion, suicidal ideation); muscular or skeletal pain, weakness, or tremors; or other adverse reactions.

Additional Information A listing of medications that should not be used is available with each bottle and patients should be provided with this information.

Dosage Forms Capsules, as sulfate: 100 mg, 150 mg, 200 mg

Atazanavir Sulfate *see* Atazanavir *on page 668*

Atovaquone (a TOE va kwone)

Related Information

USPHS / IDSA Guidelines for the Prevention of Opportunistic Infections in Persons Infected With HIV *on page 1237*

U.S. Brand Names Mepron®

Canadian Brand Names Mepron®

Generic Available No

Use Acute oral treatment of mild to moderate *Pneumocystis carinii* pneumonia (PCP) in patients who are intolerant to co-trimoxazole; prophylaxis of PCP in patients intolerant to co-trimoxazole; treatment/suppression of *Toxoplasma gondii* encephalitis, primary prophylaxis of HIV-infected persons at high risk for developing *Toxoplasma gondii* encephalitis

Drug of Choice or Alternative for Organism(s):

Babesia microti on page 40

Pneumocystis jiroveci on page 266

Pregnancy Risk Factor C

Contraindications Life-threatening allergic reaction to the drug or formulation

Warnings/Precautions Has only been indicated in mild to moderate PCP; use with caution in elderly patients due to potentially impaired renal, hepatic, and cardiac function

Adverse Reactions Note: Adverse reaction statistics have been compiled from studies including patients with advanced HIV disease; consequently, it is difficult to distinguish reactions attributed to atovaquone from those caused by the underlying disease or a combination, thereof.

>10%:

- Central nervous system: Headache, fever, insomnia, anxiety
- Dermatologic: Rash
- Gastrointestinal: Nausea, diarrhea, vomiting
- Respiratory: Cough

1% to 10%:

- Central nervous system: Dizziness
- Dermatologic: Pruritus
- Endocrine & metabolic: Hypoglycemia, hyponatremia
- Gastrointestinal: Abdominal pain, constipation, anorexia, dyspepsia, increased amylase
- Hematologic: Anemia, neutropenia, leukopenia
- Hepatic: Elevated liver enzymes
- Neuromuscular & skeletal: Weakness
- Renal: Elevated BUN/creatinine
- Miscellaneous: Oral moniliasis

Drug Interactions

Increased Effect/Toxicity: Possible increased toxicity with other highly protein-bound drugs.

Decreased Effect: Rifamycins (rifampin) used concurrently decrease the steady-state plasma concentrations of atovaquone.

Ethanol/Nutrition/Herb Interactions Food: Ingestion with a fatty meal increases absorption.

Stability Do not freeze

Mechanism of Action Has not been fully elucidated; may inhibit electron transport in mitochondria inhibiting metabolic enzymes

Pharmacodynamics/Kinetics

Absorption: Significantly increased with a high-fat meal
Distribution: 3.5 L/kg
Protein binding: >99%
Metabolism: Undergoes enterohepatic recirculation
Bioavailability: Tablet: 23%; Suspension: 47%
Half-life elimination: 2-3 days
Excretion: Feces (94% as unchanged drug)

Dosage Oral: Adolescents 13-16 years and Adults:

Prevention of PCP: 1500 mg once daily with food
Treatment of mild to moderate PCP: 750 mg twice daily with food for 21 days

Patient Information Take as directed. Take with high-fat meals.

Dosage Forms Suspension, oral: 750 mg/5 mL (5 mL, 210 mL) [contains benzyl alcohol; citrus flavor]

Selected Readings

Artymowicz RJ and James VE, "Atovaquone: A New Antipneumocystis Agent," *Clin Pharm*, 1993, 12(8):563-70.

El-Sadr WM, Murphy RL, Yurik TM, et al, "Atovaquone Compared With Dapsone for the Prevention of *Pneumocystis carinii* in Patients With HIV Infection Who Cannot Tolerate Trimethoprim, Sulfonamides, or Both," *N Engl J Med*, 1998, 339(26):1889-95.

Haile LG and Flaherty JF, "Atovaquone: A Review," *Ann Pharmacother*, 1993, 27(12):1488-94.

(Continued)

Atovaquone *(Continued)*

Hughes W, Leoung G, Kramer F, et al, "Comparison of Atovaquone (566C80) With Trimethoprim-Sulfamethoxazole to Treat *Pneumocystis carinii* Pneumonia in Patients With AIDS," *N Engl J Med*, 1993, 328(21):1521-7.

Spencer CM and Goa KL, "Atovaquone. A Review of Its Pharmacological Properties and Therapeutic Efficacy in Opportunistic Infections," *Drugs*, 1995, 50(1):176-96.

Atovaquone and Proguanil (a TOE va kwone & pro GWA nil)

Related Information

Malaria Treatment *on page 1292*

U.S. Brand Names Malarone®

Canadian Brand Names Malarone®

Synonyms Proguanil and Atovaquone

Generic Available No

Use Prevention or treatment of acute, uncomplicated *P. falciparum* malaria

Drug of Choice or Alternative for Organism(s):

Plasmodium Species *on page 265*

Pregnancy Risk Factor C

Pregnancy Implications Use in pregnant women only if the potential benefit outweighs the possible risk to the fetus. Because falciparum malaria can cause maternal death and fetal loss, pregnant women traveling to malaria-endemic areas must use personal protection against mosquito bites.

Contraindications Hypersensitivity to atovaquone, proguanil, or any component of the formulation; prophylactic use in severe renal impairment

Warnings/Precautions Not indicated for severe or complicated malaria. Absorption of atovaquone may be decreased in patients who have diarrhea or vomiting; monitor closely and consider use of an antiemetic. If severe, consider use of an alternative antimalarial. Do not use with other medications containing proguanil. Administer with caution to patients with pre-existing renal disease. Not for use in patients <5 kg (treatment) or <11 kg (prophylaxis). Delayed cases of *P. falciparum* malaria may occur after stopping prophylaxis; travelers returning from endemic areas who develop febrile illnesses should be evaluated for malaria. Recrudescent infections or infections following prophylaxis with this agent should be treated with alternative agent(s).

Adverse Reactions The following adverse reactions were reported in patients being treated for malaria. When used for prophylaxis, reactions are similar to those seen with placebo.

>10%: Gastrointestinal: Abdominal pain (17%), nausea (12%), vomiting (children 10% to 13%, adults 12%)

1% to 10%:

- Central nervous system: Headache (10%), dizziness (5%)
- Dermatologic: Pruritus (children 6%)
- Gastrointestinal: Diarrhea (children 6%, adults 8%), anorexia (5%)
- Neuromuscular & skeletal: Weakness (8%)

Postmarketing and/or case reports: Anaphylaxis, angioedema, erythema multiforme, hallucinations, photosensitivity, psychotic episodes, rash, seizure, Stevens-Johnson syndrome, urticaria

Overdosage/Toxicology

Atovaquone: Overdoses of up to 31,500 mg have been reported. Rash has been reported as well as methemoglobinemia in one patient also taking dapsone. There is no known antidote and it is unknown if it is dialyzable.

Proguanil: Single doses of 1500 mg and 700 mg twice daily for two weeks have been reported without toxicity. Reversible hair loss, scaling of skin, reversible aphthous ulceration, and hematologic side effects have occurred. Epigastric discomfort and vomiting would also be expected.

There have been no reported overdoses with the atovaquone/proguanil combination.

Drug Interactions

Cytochrome P450 Effect: Proguanil: **Substrate** (minor) of 1A2, 2C19, 3A4

Decreased Effect: Metoclopramide decreases bioavailability of atovaquone. Rifabutin decreases atovaquone levels by 34%. Rifampin decreases atovaquone levels by 50%. Tetracycline decreases plasma concentrations of atovaquone by 40%.

Ethanol/Nutrition/Herb Interactions Food: Atovaquone taken with dietary fat increases the rate and extent of absorption.

Stability Store tablets at 25°C (77°F)

Mechanism of Action

Atovaquone: Selectively inhibits parasite mitochondrial electron transport.

Proguanil: The metabolite cycloguanil inhibits dihydrofolate reductase, disrupting deoxythymidylate synthesis. Together, atovaquone/cycloguanil affect the erythrocytic and exoerythrocytic stages of development.

Pharmacodynamics/Kinetics

Atovaquone: See Atovaquone monograph.

Proguanil:

Absorption: Extensive

Distribution: 42 L/kg

Protein binding: 75%

Metabolism: Hepatic to active metabolites, cycloguanil (via CYP2C19) and 4-chlorophenylbiguanide

Half-life elimination: 12-21 hours

Excretion: Urine (40% to 60%)

Dosage Oral:

Children (dosage based on body weight):

Prevention of malaria: Start 1-2 days prior to entering a malaria-endemic area, continue throughout the stay and for 7 days after returning. Take as a single dose, once daily.

11-20 kg: Atovaquone/proguanil 62.5 mg/25 mg
21-30 kg: Atovaquone/proguanil 125 mg/50 mg
31-40 kg: Atovaquone/proguanil 187.5 mg/75 mg
>40 kg: Atovaquone/proguanil 250 mg/100 mg

Treatment of acute malaria: Take as a single dose, once daily for 3 consecutive days.

5-8 kg: Atovaquone/proguanil 125 mg/50 mg
9-10 kg: Atovaquone/proguanil 187.5 mg/75 mg
11-20 kg: Atovaquone/proguanil 250 mg/100 mg
21-30 kg: Atovaquone/proguanil 500 mg/200 mg
31-40 kg: Atovaquone/proguanil 750 mg/300 mg
>40 kg: Atovaquone/proguanil 1 g/400 mg

Adults:

Prevention of malaria: Atovaquone/proguanil 250 mg/100 mg once daily; start 1-2 days prior to entering a malaria-endemic area, continue throughout the stay and for 7 days after returning

Treatment of acute malaria: Atovaquone/proguanil 1 g/400 mg as a single dose, once daily for 3 consecutive days

Elderly: Use with caution due to possible decrease in renal and hepatic function, as well as possible decreases in cardiac function, concomitant diseases, or other drug therapy.

Dosage adjustment in renal impairment: Should not be used as prophylaxis in severe renal impairment (Cl_{cr} <30 mL/minute). Alternative treatment regimens should be used in patients with Cl_{cr} <30 mL/minute. No dosage adjustment required in mild to moderate renal impairment.

Dosage adjustment in hepatic impairment: No dosage adjustment required in mild to moderate hepatic impairment. No data available for use in severe hepatic impairment.

Dietary Considerations Must be taken with food or a milky drink.

Administration Administer with food or milk at the same time each day. If vomiting occurs within 1 hour of administration, repeat the dose. For children who have difficulty swallowing tablets, tablets may be crushed and mixed with condensed milk just prior to administration.

Patient Information Take at the same time each day with food or a milky drink. If vomiting occurs within 1 hour of taking your dose, you may repeat the dose. Notify your prescriber if you develop a fever after returning from or while visiting a malaria-endemic area.

Dosage Forms

Tablet: Atovaquone 250 mg and proguanil hydrochloride 100 mg

Tablet, pediatric: Atovaquone 62.5 mg and proguanil hydrochloride 25 mg

A/T/S® *see* Erythromycin *on page 807*
Attenuvax® *see* Measles Virus Vaccine (Live) *on page 927*
Augmentin® *see* Amoxicillin and Clavulanate Potassium *on page 645*
Augmentin ES-600® *see* Amoxicillin and Clavulanate Potassium *on page 645*
Augmentin XR™ *see* Amoxicillin and Clavulanate Potassium *on page 645*
AVA *see* Anthrax Vaccine Adsorbed *on page 665*
Avagard™ [OTC] *see* Chlorhexidine Gluconate *on page 735*
Avaxim® (Can) *see* Hepatitis A Vaccine *on page 853*
Avaxim®-Pediatric (Can) *see* Hepatitis A Vaccine *on page 853*
Avelox® *see* Moxifloxacin *on page 949*

Avelox® I.V. *see* Moxifloxacin *on page 949*

Avita® *see* Tretinoin (Topical) *on page 1127*

Azactam® *see* Aztreonam *on page 677*

Azidothymidine *see* Zidovudine *on page 1159*

Azidothymidine, Abacavir, and Lamivudine *see* Abacavir, Lamivudine, and Zidovudine *on page 627*

Azithromycin (az ith roe MYE sin)

Related Information

Antimicrobial Activity Against Selected Organisms *on page 1165*
Community-Acquired Pneumonia in Adults *on page 1278*
USPHS / IDSA Guidelines for the Prevention of Opportunistic Infections in Persons Infected With HIV *on page 1237*

U.S. Brand Names Zithromax®; Zmax™

Canadian Brand Names Zithromax®

Synonyms Azithromycin Dihydrate; Zithromax® TRI-PAK™; Zithromax® Z-PAK®

Generic Available No

Use Treatment of acute otitis media due to *H. influenzae*, *M. catarrhalis*, or *S. pneumoniae*; pharyngitis/tonsillitis due to *S. pyogenes*; treatment of mild-to-moderate upper and lower respiratory tract infections, infections of the skin and skin structure, community-acquired pneumonia, pelvic inflammatory disease (PID), sexually-transmitted diseases (urethritis/cervicitis), pharyngitis/tonsillitis (alternative to first-line therapy), and genital ulcer disease (chancroid) due to susceptible strains of *C. trachomatis*, *M. catarrhalis*, *H. influenzae*, *S. aureus*, *S. pneumoniae*, *Mycoplasma pneumoniae*, and *C. psittaci*; acute bacterial exacerbations of chronic obstructive pulmonary disease (COPD) due to *H. influenzae*, *M. catarrhalis*, or *S. pneumoniae*; acute bacterial sinusitis

Unlabeled/Investigational Use Prevention of (or to delay onset of) or treatment of MAC in patients with advanced HIV infection; prophylaxis of bacterial endocarditis in patients who are allergic to penicillin and undergoing surgical or dental procedures

Drug of Choice or Alternative for Disease/Syndrome(s):

Bronchitis *on page 60*
Cervicitis *on page 71*
Erysipelas *on page 141*
Traveler's Diarrhea *on page 333*
Urethritis, Nongonococcal *on page 344*

Organism(s):

Babesia microti on page 40
Bordetella pertussis on page 53
Chlamydophila pneumoniae on page 78
Haemophilus ducreyi on page 158
Legionella pneumophila on page 202
Moraxella catarrhalis on page 223
Mycobacterium avium-intracellulare (Complex) *on page 228*
Mycoplasma pneumoniae on page 238
Ureaplasma urealyticum on page 342

Pregnancy Risk Factor B

Pregnancy Implications Azithromycin has been shown to cross the placenta. It has been used as an alternative treatment of *Chlamydia* in late-term pregnancy. There are no adequate and well-controlled studies in pregnant women; use during pregnancy only if clearly needed.

Contraindications Hypersensitivity to azithromycin, other macrolide antibiotics, or any component of the formulation

Warnings/Precautions Use with caution in patients with hepatic dysfunction; hepatic impairment with or without jaundice has occurred chiefly in older children and adults; it may be accompanied by malaise, nausea, vomiting, abdominal colic, and fever; discontinue use if these occur. May mask or delay symptoms of incubating gonorrhea or syphilis, so appropriate culture and susceptibility tests should be performed prior to initiating azithromycin. Pseudomembranous colitis has been reported with use of macrolide antibiotics; use caution with renal dysfunction. Prolongation of the QT_c interval has been reported with macrolide antibiotics; use caution in patients at risk of prolonged cardiac repolarization. Safety and efficacy have not been established in children <6 months of age with acute otitis media, acute bacterial sinusitis, or community-acquired pneumonia, or in children <2 years of age with pharyngitis/tonsillitis. Suspensions (immediate release and extended release) are not interchangeable.

Adverse Reactions

>10%: Gastrointestinal: Diarrhea (4% to 11%)

1% to 10%:

Central nervous system: Headache

Gastrointestinal: Nausea, abdominal pain, cramping, vomiting (especially with high single-dose regimens)

<1%: Agitation, allergic reaction, anemia, anorexia, candidiasis, chest pain, conjunctivitis, constipation, dermatitis (fungal), dizziness, dyspepsia, eczema, enteritis, facial edema, fatigue, gastritis, hyperkinesia, increased cough, insomnia, jaundice, leukopenia, malaise, oral moniliasis, pain, palpitations, pharyngitis, pleural effusion, pruritus, rash, rhinitis, taste perversion, urticaria, vaginitis, vertigo, weakness

Postmarketing and/or case reports: Acute renal failure, aggressive behavior, anaphylaxis, angioedema, anxiety, arrhythmia (including ventricular tachycardia), arthralgia, cholestatic jaundice, convulsion, deafness, dehydration, edema, erythema multiforme (rare), hearing loss, hepatic necrosis (rare), hepatitis, hypertrophic pyloric stenosis, hypotension, interstitial nephritis, LFTs increased, neutropenia (mild), oral candidiasis, pancreatitis, paresthesia, pseudomembranous colitis, QT_c prolongation (rare), seizure, somnolence, Stevens-Johnson syndrome (rare), syncope, thrombocytopenia, tinnitus, tongue discoloration (rare), torsade de pointes (rare)

Overdosage/Toxicology Symptoms include nausea, vomiting, diarrhea, and prostration. Treatment is supportive and symptomatic.

Drug Interactions

Cytochrome P450 Effect: Substrate of CYP3A4 (minor); **Inhibits** CYP3A4 (weak)

Increased Effect/Toxicity: Concurrent use of pimozide is contraindicated due to potential cardiotoxicity. The manufacturer warns that azithromycin potentially may increase levels of tacrolimus, phenytoin, ergot alkaloids, alfentanil, bromocriptine, carbamazepine, cyclosporine, digoxin, disopyramide, and triazolam. However, azithromycin did not affect the response/levels of carbamazepine, theophylline, or warfarin in specific interaction studies; caution is advised when administered together. Nelfinavir may increase azithromycin serum levels (monitor for adverse effects).

Decreased Effect: Decreased azithromycin peak serum concentrations with aluminum- and magnesium-containing antacids (by 24%), however, total absorption is unaffected.

Ethanol/Nutrition/Herb Interactions Food: Rate and extent of GI absorption may be altered depending upon the formulation. Azithromycin suspension, not tablet form, has significantly increased absorption (46%) with food.

Stability

Injection: Store intact vials of injection at room temperature. Reconstitute the 500 mg vial with 4.8 mL of sterile water for injection and shake until all of the drug is dissolved. Each mL contains 100 mg azithromycin. Reconstituted solution is stable for 24 hours when stored below 30°C/86°F.

The initial solution should be further diluted to a concentration of 1 mg/mL (500 mL) to 2 mg/mL (250 mL) in 0.9% sodium chloride, 5% dextrose in water, or lactated Ringer's. The diluted solution is stable for 24 hours at or below room temperature (30°C or 86°F) and for 7 days if stored under refrigeration (5°C or 41°F).

Other medications should not be infused simultaneously through the same I.V. line.

Suspension, immediate release: Store dry powder below 30°C (86°F); following reconstitution, store at 5°C to 30°C (41°F to 86°F).

Suspension, extended release: Store dry powder below 30°C (86°F); following reconstitution, store at 15°C to 30°C (59°F to 86°F); do not freeze; should be consumed within 12 hours following reconstitution

Tablets: Store between 15°C to 30°C (59°F to 86°F).

Mechanism of Action Inhibits RNA-dependent protein synthesis at the chain elongation step; binds to the 50S ribosomal subunit resulting in blockage of transpeptidation

Pharmacodynamics/Kinetics

Absorption: Rapid

Distribution: Extensive tissue; distributes well into skin, lungs, sputum, tonsils, and cervix; penetration into CSF is poor; I.V.: 33.3 L/kg; Oral: 31.1 L/kg

Protein binding (concentration dependent): 7% to 51%

Metabolism: Hepatic

Bioavailability: 38%, decreased by 17% with extended release suspension; variable effect with food (increased with immediate or delayed release oral suspension, unchanged with tablet)

Half-life elimination: Terminal: Immediate release: 68-72 hours; Extended release: 59 hours

Time to peak, serum: Immediate release: 2-3 hours; Extended release: 5 hours

Excretion: Biliary (major route); urine (6%)

(Continued)

Azithromycin *(Continued)*

Dosage

Note: Extended release suspension (Zmax™) is not interchangeable with immediate release formulations. Use should be limited to approved indications. All doses are expressed as immediate release azithromycin unless otherwise specified.

Oral:

Children ≥6 months:

Community-acquired pneumonia: 10 mg/kg on day 1 (maximum: 500 mg/day) followed by 5 mg/kg/day once daily on days 2-5 (maximum: 250 mg/day)

Bacterial sinusitis: 10 mg/kg once daily for 3 days (maximum: 500 mg/day)

Otitis media:

1-day regimen: 30 mg/kg as a single dose (maximum dose: 1500 mg)

3-day regimen: 10 mg/kg once daily for 3 days (maximum: 500 mg/day)

5-day regimen: 10 mg/kg on day 1 (maximum: 500 mg/day) followed by 5 mg/kg/day once daily on days 2-5 (maximum: 250 mg/day)

Children ≥2 years: Pharyngitis, tonsillitis: 12 mg/kg/day once daily for 5 days (maximum: 500 mg/day)

Children:

M. avium-infected patients with acquired immunodeficiency syndrome (unlabeled use): 5 mg/kg/day once daily (maximum dose: 250 mg/day) or 20 mg/kg (maximum dose: 1200 mg) once weekly given alone or in combination with rifabutin

Treatment and secondary prevention of disseminated MAC (unlabeled use): 5 mg/kg/day once daily (maximum dose: 250 mg/day) in combination with ethambutol, with or without rifabutin

Prophylaxis for bacterial endocarditis (unlabeled use): 15 mg/kg 1 hour before procedure

Uncomplicated chlamydial urethritis or cervicitis (unlabeled use): Children ≥45 kg: 1 g as a single dose

Adolescents ≥16 years and Adults:

Community-acquired pneumonia: Extended release suspension (Zmax™): 2 g as a single dose

Respiratory tract, skin and soft tissue infections: 500 mg on day 1 followed by 250 mg/day on days 2-5 (maximum: 500 mg/day)

Alternative regimen: Bacterial exacerbation of COPD: 500 mg/day for a total of 3 days

Bacterial sinusitis: 500 mg/day for a total of 3 days

Extended release suspension (Zmax™): 2 g as a single dose

Urethritis/cervicitis:

Due to *C. trachomatis*: 1 g as a single dose

Due to *N. gonorrhoeae*: 2 g as a single dose

Chancroid due to *H. ducreyi*: 1 g as a single dose

Prophylaxis of disseminated *M. avium* complex disease in patient with advanced HIV infection (unlabeled use): 1200 mg once weekly (may be combined with rifabutin)

Treatment of disseminated *M. avium* complex disease in patient with advanced HIV infection (unlabeled use): 600 mg daily (in combination with ethambutol 15 mg/kg)

Prophylaxis for bacterial endocarditis (unlabeled use): 500 mg 1 hour prior to the procedure

I.V.: Adults:

Community-acquired pneumonia: 500 mg as a single dose for at least 2 days, follow I.V. therapy by the oral route with a single daily dose of 500 mg to complete a 7-10 day course of therapy

Pelvic inflammatory disease (PID): 500 mg as a single dose for 1-2 days, follow I.V. therapy by the oral route with a single daily dose of 250 mg to complete a 7-day course of therapy

Dosage adjustment in renal impairment: Use caution in patients with Cl_{cr} <10 mL/minute

Dosage adjustment in hepatic impairment: Use with caution due to potential for hepatotoxicity (rare). Specific guidelines for dosing in hepatic impairment have not been established.

Dietary Considerations

Oral suspension, immediate release, may be administered with or without food.

Oral suspension, extended release, should be taken on an empty stomach (at least 1 hour before or 2 hours following a meal).

Tablet may be administered with food to decrease GI effects.

Sodium content:

Injection: 114 mg (4.96 mEq) per vial

Oral suspension, immediate release: 3.7 mg per 100 mg/5 mL of constituted suspension; 7.4 mg per 200 mg/5 mL of constituted suspension; 37 mg per 1 g single-dose packet

Oral suspension, extended release: 148 mg per 2 g constituted suspension

Tablet: 0.9 mg/250 mg tablet; 1.8 mg/500 mg tablet; 2.1 mg/600 mg tablet

Administration

I.V.: Infusate concentration and rate of infusion for azithromycin for injection should be either 1 mg/mL over 3 hours or 2 mg/mL over 1 hour. Other medications should not be infused simultaneously through the same I.V. line.

Oral: Immediate release suspension and tablet may be taken without regard to food; extended release suspension should be taken on an empty stomach (at least 1 hour before or 2 hours following a meal), within 12 hours of reconstitution.

Monitoring Parameters Liver function tests, CBC with differential

Patient Information Take entire course of medication. Do not discontinue until prescription is completed. Take extended release oral suspension 1 hour before or 2 hours after meals; immediate release suspension may be taken with or without food; tablet form may be taken with meals to decrease GI effects. Do not take with aluminum- or magnesium-containing antacids.

Additional Information

Capsules are no longer being produced in the United States.

Zithromax® tablets and immediate release suspension may be interchanged (eg, two 250 Zithromax® tablets may be substituted for a 500 mg Zithromax® tablet or the tablets may be substituted with the immediate release suspension); however, the extended release suspension (Zmax™) is not bioequivalent with Zithromax® and therefore should not be interchanged.

Dosage Forms

Injection, powder for reconstitution, as dihydrate: 500 mg [contains sodium 114 mg (4.96 mEq) per vial]

Microspheres for oral suspension, extended release, as dihydrate (Zmax™): 2 g [single-dose bottle; contains sodium 148 mg per bottle; cherry and banana flavor]

Powder for oral suspension, immediate release, as dihydrate: 100 mg/5 mL (15 mL) [contains sodium 3.7 mg/ 5 mL; cherry creme de vanilla and banana flavor]; 200 mg/5 mL (15 mL, 22.5 mL, 30 mL) [contains sodium 7.4 mg/5 mL; cherry creme de vanilla and banana flavor]; 1 g [single-dose packet; contains sodium 37 mg per packet; cherry creme de vanilla and banana flavor]

Tablet, as dihydrate: 250 mg, 500 mg, 600 mg [contains sodium 0.9 mg per 250 mg tablet, 1.8 mg per 500 mg tablet, 2.1 mg per 600 mg tablet]

Zithromax® TRI-PAK™ [unit-dose pack]: 500 mg (3s)

Zithromax® Z-PAK® [unit-dose pack]: 250 mg (6s)

Selected Readings

Amsden GW, "Erythromycin, Clarithromycin, and Azithromycin: Are the Differences Real?" *Clin Ther*, 1996, 18(1):56-72.

Drew RH and Gallis HA, "Azithromycin-Spectrum of Activity, Pharmacokinetics, and Clinical Applications," *Pharmacotherapy*, 1992, 12(3):161-73.

Goldman MP and Longworth DL, "The Role of Azithromycin and Clarithromycin in Clinical Practice," *Cleve Clin J Med*, 1993, 60(5):359-64.

Tartaglione TA, "Therapeutic Options for the Management and Prevention of *Mycobacterium avium* Complex Infection in Patients With the Acquired Immunodeficiency Syndrome," *Pharmacotherapy*, 1996, 16(2):171-82.

Zuckerman JM and Kaye KM, "The Newer Macrolides. Azithromycin and Clarithromycin," *Infect Dis Clin North Am*, 1995, 9(3):731-45.

Azithromycin Dihydrate *see* Azithromycin *on page 674*

AZT™ (Can) *see* Zidovudine *on page 1159*

AZT + 3TC (error-prone abbreviation) *see* Zidovudine and Lamivudine *on page 1162*

AZT, Abacavir, and Lamivudine *see* Abacavir, Lamivudine, and Zidovudine *on page 627*

AZT (error-prone abbreviation) *see* Zidovudine *on page 1159*

Azthreonam *see* Aztreonam *on page 677*

Aztreonam (AZ tree oh nam)

Related Information

Antimicrobial Activity Against Selected Organisms *on page 1165*

U.S. Brand Names Azactam®

Canadian Brand Names Azactam®

Synonyms Azthreonam

Generic Available No

(Continued)

Aztreonam *(Continued)*

Use Treatment of patients with urinary tract infections, lower respiratory tract infections, septicemia, skin/skin structure infections, intra-abdominal infections, and gynecological infections caused by susceptible gram-negative bacilli

Drug of Choice or Alternative for Disease/Syndrome(s):

Intra-abdominal Abscess *on page 194*
Osteomyelitis, Diabetic Foot *on page 249*
Pneumonia, Community-Acquired *on page 270*

Organism(s):

Acinetobacter Species *on page 24*
Alcaligenes Species *on page 31*
Klebsiella Species *on page 200*
Serratia Species *on page 296*

Pregnancy Risk Factor B

Pregnancy Implications Teratogenic effects were not observed in animal studies. Aztreonam crosses the human placenta and enters fetal circulation.

Contraindications Hypersensitivity to aztreonam or any component of the formulation

Warnings/Precautions Rare cross-allergenicity to penicillins and cephalosporins has been reported. Use caution in renal impairment; dosing adjustment required.

Adverse Reactions As reported in adults:

1% to 10%:
- Dermatologic: Rash
- Gastrointestinal: Diarrhea, nausea, vomiting
- Local: Thrombophlebitis, pain at injection site

<1%: Abdominal cramps, abnormal taste, anaphylaxis, anemia, angioedema, aphthous ulcer, breast tenderness, bronchospasm, *C. difficile*-associated diarrhea, chest pain, confusion, diaphoresis, diplopia, dizziness, dyspnea, eosinophilia, erythema multiforme, exfoliative dermatitis, fever, flushing, halitosis, headache, hepatitis, hypotension, insomnia, jaundice, leukopenia, liver enzymes increased, muscular aches myalgia, neutropenia, numb tongue, pancytopenia, paresthesia, petechiae, pruritus, pseudomembranous colitis, purpura, seizure, sneezing, thrombocytopenia, tinnitus, toxic epidermal necrolysis, urticaria, vaginitis, vertigo, weakness, wheezing

Overdosage/Toxicology Symptoms include seizures. If necessary, dialysis can reduce the drug concentration in the blood.

Drug Interactions

Decreased Effect: Avoid antibiotics that induce beta-lactamase production (cefoxitin, imipenem).

Stability Prior to reconstitution, store at room temperature; avoid excessive heat. Reconstituted solutions are colorless to light yellow straw and may turn pink upon standing without affecting potency. Use reconstituted solutions and I.V. solutions (in NS and D_5W) within 48 hours if kept at room temperature (25°C) or 7 days under refrigeration (4°C).

I.M.: Reconstitute with at least 3 mL SWFI, sterile bacteriostatic water for injection, NS, or bacteriostatic sodium chloride.

I.V.:
- Bolus injection: Reconstitute with 6-10 mL SWFI.
- Infusion: Reconstitute to a final concentration ≤2%. Solution for infusion may be frozen at less than -2°C (less than -4°F) for up to 3 months. Thawed solution should be used within 24 hours if thawed at room temperature or within 72 hours if thawed under refrigeration. **Do not refreeze.**

Mechanism of Action Inhibits bacterial cell wall synthesis by binding to one or more of the penicillin binding proteins (PBPs); which in turn inhibits the final transpeptidation step of peptidoglycan synthesis in bacterial cell walls, thus inhibiting cell wall biosynthesis. Bacteria eventually lyse due to ongoing activity of cell wall autolytic enzymes (autolysins and murein hydrolases) while cell wall assembly is arrested. Monobactam structure makes cross-allergenicity with beta-lactams unlikely.

Pharmacodynamics/Kinetics

Absorption: I.M.: Well absorbed; I.M. and I.V. doses produce comparable serum concentrations

Distribution: Widely to most body fluids and tissues; crosses placenta; enters breast milk
- V_d: Children: 0.2-0.29 L/kg; Adults: 0.2 L/kg
- Relative diffusion of antimicrobial agents from blood into CSF: Good only with inflammation (exceeds usual MICs)
- CSF:blood level ratio: Meninges: Inflamed: 8% to 40%; Normal: ~1%

Protein binding: 56%
Metabolism: Hepatic (minor %)
Half-life elimination:
Children 2 months to 12 years: 1.7 hours
Adults: Normal renal function: 1.7-2.9 hours
End-stage renal disease: 6-8 hours
Time to peak: I.M., I.V. push: Within 60 minutes; I.V. infusion: 1.5 hours
Excretion: Urine (60% to 70% as unchanged drug); feces (~13% to 15%)

Dosage

Children >1 month: I.M., I.V.:
Mild-to-moderate infections: 30 mg/kg every 8 hours
Moderate-to-severe infections: 30 mg/kg every 6-8 hours; maximum: 120 mg/kg/day (8 g/day)
Cystic fibrosis: 50 mg/kg/dose every 6-8 hours (ie, up to 200 mg/kg/day); maximum: 8 g/day

Adults:
Urinary tract infection: I.M., I.V.: 500 mg to 1 g every 8-12 hours
Moderately-severe systemic infections: 1 g I.V. or I.M. or 2 g I.V. every 8-12 hours
Severe systemic or life-threatening infections (especially caused by *Pseudomonas aeruginosa*): I.V.: 2 g every 6-8 hours; maximum: 8 g/day

Dosing adjustment in renal impairment: Adults: Following initial dose, maintenance doses should be given as follows:
Cl_{cr} 10-30 mL/minute: 50% of usual dose at the usual interval
Cl_{cr} <10 mL/minute: 25% of usual dosage at the usual interval

Hemodialysis: Moderately dialyzable (20% to 50%); 1/8 of initial dose after each hemodialysis session (given in addition to the maintenance doses)
Peritoneal dialysis: Administer as for Cl_{cr} <10 mL/minute
Continuous arteriovenous or venovenous hemofiltration: Dose as for Cl_{cr} 10-30 mL/minute

Administration Doses >1 g should be administered I.V.

I.M.: Administer by deep injection into large muscle mass, such as upper outer quadrant of gluteus maximus or the lateral part of the thigh
I.V.: Administer by IVP over 3-5 minutes or by intermittent infusion over 20-60 minutes at a final concentration not to exceed 20 mg/mL

Monitoring Parameters Periodic liver function test; monitor for signs of anaphylaxis during first dose

Test Interactions May interfere with urine glucose tests containing cupric sulfate (Benedict's solution, Clinitest®); positive Coombs' test

Additional Information Although marketed as an agent similar to aminoglycosides, aztreonam is a monobactam antimicrobial with almost pure gram-negative aerobic activity. It cannot be used for gram-positive infections. Aminoglycosides are often used for synergy in gram-positive infections.

Dosage Forms

Infusion [premixed]: 1 g (50 mL); 2 g (50 mL)
Injection, powder for reconstitution: 500 mg, 1 g, 2 g

Selected Readings

Brogden RN and Heel RC, "Aztreonam. A Review of Its Antibacterial Activity, Pharmacokinetic Properties and Therapeutic Use," *Drugs*, 1986, 31(2):96-130.

Donowitz GR and Mandell GL, "Beta-Lactam Antibiotics," *N Engl J Med*, 1988, 318(7):419-26 and 318(8):490-500.

Hellinger WC and Brewer NS, "Carbapenems and Monobactams: Imipenem, Meropenem, and Aztreonam," *Mayo Clin Proc*, 1999, 74(4):420-34.

Johnson DH and Cunha BA, "Aztreonam," *Med Clin North Am*, 1995, 79(4):733-43.

BabyBIG® *see* Botulism Immune Globulin (Intravenous-Human) *on page 690*

Baciguent® [OTC] *see* Bacitracin *on page 679*

BaciiM® *see* Bacitracin *on page 679*

Baciject® (Can) *see* Bacitracin *on page 679*

Bacillus Calmette-Guérin (BCG) Live *see* BCG Vaccine *on page 683*

Bacitracin (bas i TRAY sin)

U.S. Brand Names AK-Tracin® [DSC]; Baciguent® [OTC]; BaciiM®

Canadian Brand Names Baciguent®; Baciject®

Generic Available Yes

Use Treatment of susceptible bacterial infections mainly; has activity against gram-positive bacilli; due to toxicity risks, systemic and irrigant uses of bacitracin should be limited to situations where less toxic alternatives would not be effective

Unlabeled/Investigational Use Oral administration: Successful in antibiotic-associated colitis; has been used for enteric eradication of vancomycin-resistant enterococci (VRE)

(Continued)

Bacitracin *(Continued)*

Drug of Choice or Alternative for Disease/Syndrome(s):

Blepharitis *on page 52*

Pregnancy Risk Factor C

Contraindications Hypersensitivity to bacitracin or any component of the formulation; I.M. use is contraindicated in patients with renal impairment

Warnings/Precautions Prolonged use may result in overgrowth of nonsusceptible organisms; I.M. use may cause renal failure due to tubular and glomerular necrosis; **do not administer intravenously** because severe thrombophlebitis occurs

Adverse Reactions 1% to 10%:

Cardiovascular: Hypotension, edema of the face/lips, tightness of chest
Central nervous system: Pain
Dermatologic: Rash, itching
Gastrointestinal: Anorexia, nausea, vomiting, diarrhea, rectal itching
Hematologic: Blood dyscrasias
Miscellaneous: Diaphoresis

Overdosage/Toxicology Symptoms include nephrotoxicity (parenteral), nausea, and vomiting (oral).

Drug Interactions

Increased Effect/Toxicity: Nephrotoxic drugs, neuromuscular blocking agents, and anesthetics (increased neuromuscular blockade).

Stability For I.M. use; bacitracin sterile powder should be dissolved in 0.9% sodium chloride injection containing 2% procaine hydrochloride; once reconstituted, bacitracin is stable for 1 week under refrigeration (2°C to 8°C); sterile powder should be stored in the refrigerator; do not use diluents containing parabens

Mechanism of Action Inhibits bacterial cell wall synthesis by preventing transfer of mucopeptides into the growing cell wall

Pharmacodynamics/Kinetics

Duration: 6-8 hours
Absorption: Poor from mucous membranes and intact or denuded skin; rapidly following I.M. administration; not absorbed by bladder irrigation, but absorption can occur from peritoneal or mediastinal lavage
Distribution: CSF: Nil even with inflammation
Protein binding, plasma: Minimal
Time to peak, serum: I.M.: 1-2 hours
Excretion: Urine (10% to 40%) within 24 hours

Dosage Do not administer I.V.:

Infants: I.M.:
- ≤2.5 kg: 900 units/kg/day in 2-3 divided doses
- >2.5 kg: 1000 units/kg/day in 2-3 divided doses

Children: I.M.: 800-1200 units/kg/day divided every 8 hours

Adults: Oral:
- Antibiotic-associated colitis: 25,000 units 4 times/day for 7-10 days
- VRE eradication (unlabeled use): 25,000 units 4 times/day for 7-10 days

Children and Adults:
- Topical: Apply 1-5 times/day
- Ophthalmic, ointment: Instill 1/4" to 1/2" ribbon every 3-4 hours into conjunctival sac for acute infections, or 2-3 times/day for mild to moderate infections for 7-10 days
- Irrigation, solution: 50-100 units/mL in normal saline, lactated Ringer's, or sterile water for irrigation; soak sponges in solution for topical compresses 1-5 times/day or as needed during surgical procedures

Administration For I.M. administration only, **do not administer I.V.**; confirm any orders for parenteral use; pH of urine should be kept >6 by using sodium bicarbonate; bacitracin sterile powder should be dissolved in 0.9% sodium chloride injection containing 2% procaine hydrochloride; do not use diluents containing parabens

Monitoring Parameters I.M.: Urinalysis, renal function tests

Patient Information

Ophthalmic: Tilt head back, place medication in conjunctival sac and close eyes; apply light finger pressure on lacrimal sac for 1 minute following instillation. Ophthalmic ointment may cause blurred vision; do not share eye medications with others.

Topical: Do not be use for longer than 1 week unless directed by prescriber.

Additional Information 1 unit is equivalent to 0.026 mg

Dosage Forms [DSC] = Discontinued product

Injection, powder for reconstitution (BaciiM®): 50,000 units
Ointment, ophthalmic (AK-Tracin® [DSC]): 500 units/g (3.5 g)

Ointment, topical: 500 units/g (0.9 g, 15 g, 30 g, 120 g, 454 g)
Baciguent®: 500 units/g (15 g, 30 g)

Extemporaneous Preparations In some institutions, oral formulations have been prepared either by preparation of capsules from powder or oral administration of I.V. solution.

Selected Readings

Kelly CP, Pothoulakis C, and LaMont JT, "*Clostridium difficile* colitis," *N Engl J Med*, 1994, 330(4):257-62.

Bacitracin and Polymyxin B (bas i TRAY sin & pol i MIKS in bee)

Related Information

Bacitracin *on page 679*
Polymyxin B *on page 1012*

U.S. Brand Names AK-Poly-Bac®; Betadine® First Aid Antibiotics + Moisturizer [OTC]; Polysporin® Ophthalmic; Polysporin® Topical [OTC]

Canadian Brand Names LID-Pack®; Optimyxin®; Polycidin® Ophthalmic Ointment

Synonyms Polymyxin B and Bacitracin

Generic Available Yes

Use Treatment of superficial infections caused by susceptible organisms

Pregnancy Risk Factor C

Adverse Reactions 1% to 10%: Local: Rash, itching, burning, anaphylactoid reactions, swelling, conjunctival erythema

Mechanism of Action See individual monographs for Bacitracin and Polymyxin B

Pharmacodynamics/Kinetics See individual agents.

Dosage Children and Adults:

Ophthalmic ointment: Instill 1/2" ribbon in the affected eye(s) every 3-4 hours for acute infections or 2-3 times/day for mild to moderate infections for 7-10 days

Topical ointment/powder: Apply to affected area 1-4 times/day; may cover with sterile bandage if needed

Additional Information Complete prescribing information for this medication should be consulted for additional detail.

Dosage Forms

Ointment, ophthalmic (AK-Poly-Bac®, Polysporin®): Bacitracin 500 units and polymyxin B sulfate 10,000 units per g (3.5 g)

Ointment, topical [OTC]: Bacitracin 500 units and polymyxin B sulfate 10,000 units per g in white petrolatum (15 g, 30 g)

Betadine® First Aid Antibiotics + Moisturizer: Bacitracin 500 units and polymyxin B sulfate 10,000 units per g (14 g)

Polysporin®: Bacitracin 500 units and polymyxin B sulfate 10,000 units per g (15 g, 30 g)

Powder, topical (Polysporin®): Bacitracin 500 units and polymyxin B sulfate 10,000 units per g (10 g)

Bacitracin, Neomycin, and Polymyxin B

(bas i TRAY sin, nee oh MYE sin, & pol i MIKS in bee)

Related Information

Bacitracin *on page 679*
Neomycin *on page 962*
Polymyxin B *on page 1012*

U.S. Brand Names Neosporin® Neo To Go® [OTC]; Neosporin® Ophthalmic Ointment; Neosporin® Topical [OTC]

Canadian Brand Names Neosporin® Ophthalmic Ointment; Neotopic®

Synonyms Neomycin, Bacitracin, and Polymyxin B; Polymyxin B, Bacitracin, and Neomycin; Triple Antibiotic

Generic Available Yes

Use Helps prevent infection in minor cuts, scrapes and burns; short-term treatment of superficial external ocular infections caused by susceptible organisms

Pregnancy Risk Factor C

Contraindications Hypersensitivity to neomycin, polymyxin B, zinc bacitracin, or any component of the formulation; epithelial herpes simplex keratitis; mycobacterial or fungal infections; topical ointments for external use only

Warnings/Precautions

Ophthalmic ointment: Bacterial keratitis has been reported with the use of topical ophthalmic products in multiple-dose containers. Care should be taken to not contaminate the container.

Topical ointment: When used for self-medication (OTC use), patients should notify healthcare provider if needed for >1 week. Should not be used for self-medication on deep or puncture wounds, animal bites, or serious burns. Not for application to large areas of the body.

(Continued)

Bacitracin, Neomycin, and Polymyxin B *(Continued)*

Adverse Reactions Frequency not defined.

Dermatologic: Reddening, allergic contact dermatitis

Local: Itching, failure to heal, swelling, irritation

Ophthalmic: Conjunctival edema

Miscellaneous: Anaphylaxis

Mechanism of Action Refer to individual monographs for Bacitracin; Neomycin Sulfate; and Polymyxin B Sulfate

Pharmacodynamics/Kinetics See individual agents.

Dosage Children and Adults:

Ophthalmic: Ointment: Instill 1/2" into the conjunctival sac every 3-4 hours for 7-10 days for acute infections

Topical: Apply 1-3 times/day to infected area; may cover with sterile bandage as needed

Dosage Forms

Ointment, ophthalmic (Neosporin®): Bacitracin 400 units, neomycin 3.5 mg, and polymyxin B 10,000 units per g (3.5 g)

Ointment, topical: Bacitracin 400 units, neomycin 3.5 mg, and polymyxin B 5000 units per g (0.9 g, 15 g, 30 g, 454 g)

Neosporin®: Bacitracin 400 units, neomycin 3.5 mg, and polymyxin B 5000 units per g (15 g, 30 g)

Neosporin® Neo To Go®: Bacitracin 400 units, neomycin 3.5 mg, and polymyxin B 5000 units per g (0.9 g)

Bacitracin, Neomycin, Polymyxin B, and Hydrocortisone

(bas i TRAY sin, nee oh MYE sin, pol i MIKS in bee, & hye droe KOR ti sone)

Related Information

Bacitracin *on page 679*

Neomycin *on page 962*

Polymyxin B *on page 1012*

U.S. Brand Names AK-Spore® H.C. [DSC]; Cortisporin® Ointment

Canadian Brand Names Cortisporin® Topical Ointment

Synonyms Hydrocortisone, Bacitracin, Neomycin, and Polymyxin B; Neomycin, Bacitracin, Polymyxin B, and Hydrocortisone; Polymyxin B, Bacitracin, Neomycin, and Hydrocortisone

Generic Available Yes: Ophthalmic ointment

Use Prevention and treatment of susceptible inflammatory conditions where bacterial infection (or risk of infection) is present

Pregnancy Risk Factor C

Contraindications Hypersensitivity to any component of the formulation; not for use in viral infections, fungal diseases, mycobacterial infections

Warnings/Precautions Prolonged use of corticosteroids may result in systemic effects. May suppress immune response, predisposing to secondary infections. May mask or enhance purulent infections; may increase severity of viral infections.

Ophthalmic ointment: Should never be directly introduced into the anterior chamber. May retard corneal healing. Prolonged use may result in ocular hypertension/glaucoma, corneal and scleral thinning, potentially resulting in perforation. Use with caution in glaucoma. Avoid use following ocular cataract surgery.

Adverse Reactions Frequency not defined.

Dermatologic: Rash, generalized itching

Ocular: Irritation

Respiratory: Apnea

Miscellaneous: Secondary infection

Drug Interactions

Cytochrome P450 Effect: Hydrocortisone: **Substrate** of CYP3A4 (minor); **Induces** CYP3A4 (weak)

Stability Store at controlled room temperature of 15°C to 25°C (59°F to 77°F).

Mechanism of Action Refer to individual monographs for Bacitracin, Neomycin, Polymyxin B, and Hydrocortisone

Pharmacodynamics/Kinetics See individual agents.

Dosage Children and Adults:

Ophthalmic: Ointment: Instill 1/2" ribbon to inside of lower lid every 3-4 hours until improvement occurs

Topical: Apply sparingly 2-4 times/day. Therapy should be discontinued when control is achieved; if no improvement is seen, reassessment of diagnosis may be necessary.

Monitoring Parameters If ophthalmic ointment is used >10 days or in patients with glaucoma, monitor intraocular pressure (IOP).

Dosage Forms [DSC] = Discontinued product

Ointment, ophthalmic (AK-Spore® H.C. [DSC], Cortisporin®): Bacitracin 400 units, neomycin sulfate 3.5 mg, polymyxin B 10,000 units, and hydrocortisone 10 mg per g (3.5 g)

Ointment, topical (Cortisporin®): Bacitracin 400 units, neomycin 3.5 mg, polymyxin B 5000 units, and hydrocortisone 10 mg per g (15 g)

Bacitracin, Neomycin, Polymyxin B, and Pramoxine

(bas i TRAY sin, nee oh MYE sin, pol i MIKS in bee, & pra MOKS een)

Related Information

Bacitracin *on page 679*
Neomycin *on page 962*
Polymyxin B *on page 1012*

U.S. Brand Names Neosporin® + Pain Ointment [OTC]; Spectrocin Plus™ [OTC]

Synonyms Neomycin, Bacitracin, Polymyxin B, and Pramoxine; Polymyxin B, Neomycin, Bacitracin, and Pramoxine; Pramoxine, Neomycin, Bacitracin, and Polymyxin B

Generic Available Yes

Use Prevention and treatment of susceptible superficial topical infections and provide temporary relief of pain or discomfort

Contraindications Hypersensitivity to bacitracin, neomycin, polymyxin B, pramoxine, or any component of the formulation

Warnings/Precautions For external use only; not for use over large areas of the body or for longer than 1 week.

Dosage Children ≥2 years and Adults: Apply 1-3 times/day to infected areas; cover with sterile bandage if needed

Dosage Forms Ointment, topical: Bacitracin 500 units, neomycin base 3.5 mg, polymyxin B sulfate 10,000 units, and pramoxine hydrochloride 10 mg (15 g, 30 g)

Spectrocin Plus™: Bacitracin 500 units, neomycin base 3.5 mg, polymyxin B sulfate 10,000 units, and pramoxine hydrochloride 10 mg (30 g)

Neosporin® + Pain Ointment: Bacitracin 500 units, neomycin base 3.5 mg, polymyxin B sulfate 10,000 units, and pramoxine hydrochloride 10 mg (15 g, 30 g)

BactoShield® CHG [OTC] *see* Chlorhexidine Gluconate *on page 735*
Bactrim™ *see* Sulfamethoxazole and Trimethoprim *on page 1087*
Bactrim™ DS *see* Sulfamethoxazole and Trimethoprim *on page 1087*
Bactroban® *see* Mupirocin *on page 953*
Bactroban® Nasal *see* Mupirocin *on page 953*
Baraclude™ *see* Entecavir *on page 803*
BayGam® *see* Immune Globulin (Intramuscular) *on page 866*
BayHep B® *see* Hepatitis B Immune Globulin *on page 855*
BayRab® *see* Rabies Immune Globulin (Human) *on page 1034*
BayRho-D® Full-Dose *see* Rh_o(D) Immune Globulin *on page 1038*
BayRho-D® Mini-Dose *see* Rh_o(D) Immune Globulin *on page 1038*
BayTet™ *see* Tetanus Immune Globulin (Human) *on page 1103*
Baza® Antifungal [OTC] *see* Miconazole *on page 945*
BCG, Live *see* BCG Vaccine *on page 683*

BCG Vaccine (bee see jee vak SEEN)

U.S. Brand Names TheraCys®; TICE® BCG

Canadian Brand Names ImmuCyst®; Oncotice™; Pacis™

Synonyms Bacillus Calmette-Guérin (BCG) Live; BCG, Live

Generic Available No

Use Immunization against tuberculosis and immunotherapy for cancer; treatment of bladder cancer

BCG vaccine is not routinely recommended for use in the U.S. for prevention of tuberculosis

BCG vaccine is strongly recommended for infants and children with negative tuberculin skin tests who:

- are at high risk of intimate and prolonged exposure to persistently untreated or ineffectively treated patients with infectious pulmonary tuberculosis, and
- cannot be removed from the source of exposure, and
- cannot be placed on long-term preventive therapy
- are continuously exposed with tuberculosis who have bacilli resistant to isoniazid and rifampin

(Continued)

BCG Vaccine *(Continued)*

BCG is also recommended for tuberculin-negative infants and children in groups in which the rate of new infections exceeds 1% per year and for whom the usual surveillance and treatment programs have been attempted but are not operationally feasible

Pregnancy Risk Factor C

Contraindications Hypersensitivity to BCG vaccine or any component of the formulation; immunocompromized, AIDS, and burn patients; tuberculin-positive individual

Warnings/Precautions Protection against tuberculosis is only relative, not permanent, nor entirely predictable; for live bacteria vaccine, proper aseptic technique and disposal of all equipment in contact with BCG vaccine as a biohazardous material is recommended; systemic reactions have been reported in patients treated as immunotherapy for bladder cancer

BCG should be administered with caution to persons in groups at high risk for HIV infection or persons known to be severely immunocompromised. Although limited data suggest that the vaccine may be safe for use in asymptomatic children infected with HIV, BCG vaccination is not recommended for HIV-infected adults or for persons with symptomatic disease. Until further research can clearly define the risks and benefits of BCG vaccination for this population, vaccination should be restricted to persons at exceptionally high risk for tuberculosis infection. HIV infected persons thought to be infected with *Mycobacterium tuberculosis* should be strongly recommended for tuberculosis preventive therapy.

Adverse Reactions All serious adverse reactions must be reported to the U.S. Department of Health and Human Services (DHHS) Vaccine Adverse Event Reporting System (VAERS) 1-800-822-7967.

>10%:
- Gastrointestinal: Nausea and vomiting (3% to 16%)
- Genitourinary: Dysuria (62%), polyuria (42%), hematuria (26% to 40%), cystitis (6% to 30%), urinary urgency (6% to 18%)
- Miscellaneous: Flu-like syndrome including fever, chills (42%)

1% to 10%:
- Central nervous system: Fatigue, headache, dizziness
- Gastrointestinal: Anorexia, diarrhea
- Genitourinary: Urinary incontinence (2% to 6%)

<1%: Abscesses, anemia, bladder irritation, coagulation abnormalities, hepatitis, hepatic granuloma, leukopenia, prostatitis, rash, skin ulceration, thrombocytopenia

Stability Refrigerate, protect from light

TheraCys®: Reconstitute with 3 mL of diluent provided and shake gently. Add contents to 50 mL of 0.9% NaCl (preservative free) provided.

TICE® BCG: Reconstitute with 1 mL 0.9% NaCl (preservative free) using a 3 mL syringe. Mix by drawing and expelling solution into ampul 3 times. Add to a catheter tip syringe containing 49 mL of 0.9% NaCl (preservative free). Use within 2 hours of mixing

Mechanism of Action BCG live is an attenuated strain of bacillus Calmette-Guérin used as a biological response modifier; BCG live, when used intravesicular for treatment of bladder carcinoma *in situ*, is thought to cause a local, chronic inflammatory response involving macrophage and leukocyte infiltration of the bladder. By a mechanism not fully understood, this local inflammatory response leads to destruction of superficial tumor cells of the urothelium. Evidence of systemic immune response is also commonly seen, manifested by a positive PPD tuberculin skin test reaction, however, its relationship to clinical efficacy is not well-established. BCG is active immunotherapy which stimulates the host's immune mechanism to reject the tumor.

Dosage Children >1 month and Adults:

Immunization against tuberculosis (TICE® BCG): 0.2-0.3 mL percutaneous; initial lesion usually appears after 10-14 days consisting of small red papule at injection site and reaches maximum diameter of 3 mm in 4-6 weeks; conduct postvaccinal tuberculin test (ie, 5 TU of PPD) in 2-3 months; if test is negative, repeat vaccination

Immunotherapy for bladder cancer:
- Intravesical treatment: Instill into bladder for 2 hours
- TheraCys®: One dose instilled into bladder once weekly for 6 weeks followed by one treatment at 3, 6, 12, 18, and 24 months after initial treatment
- TICE® BCG: One dose instilled into the bladder once weekly for 6 weeks followed by once monthly for 6-12 months

Administration Should only be given intravesicularly or percutaneously; **do not administer I.V., SubQ, or intradermally;** can be used for bladder irrigation

Test Interactions PPD intradermal test

Additional Information When used for immunization against tuberculosis, Federal law requires that the date of administration, the vaccine manufacturer, lot number of vaccine, and the administering person's name, title and address be entered into the patient's permanent medical record.

Dosage Forms Injection, powder for reconstitution, intravesical:
TheraCys®: 81 mg [with diluent]
TICE® BCG: 50 mg

Behenyl Alcohol *see* Docosanol *on page 787*
BenzaClin® *see* Clindamycin and Benzoyl Peroxide *on page 756*
Benzamycin® *see* Erythromycin and Benzoyl Peroxide *on page 811*
Benzamycin® Pak *see* Erythromycin and Benzoyl Peroxide *on page 811*
Benzathine Benzylpenicillin *see* Penicillin G Benzathine *on page 991*
Benzathine Penicillin G *see* Penicillin G Benzathine *on page 991*
Benzene Hexachloride *see* Lindane *on page 913*
Benzoyl Peroxide and Clindamycin *see* Clindamycin and Benzoyl Peroxide *on page 756*
Benzoyl Peroxide and Erythromycin *see* Erythromycin and Benzoyl Peroxide *on page 811*
Benzylpenicillin Benzathine *see* Penicillin G Benzathine *on page 991*
Benzylpenicillin Potassium *see* Penicillin G (Parenteral/Aqueous) *on page 993*
Benzylpenicillin Sodium *see* Penicillin G (Parenteral/Aqueous) *on page 993*
Betadine® [OTC] *see* Povidone-Iodine *on page 1016*
Betadine® First Aid Antibiotics + Moisturizer [OTC] *see* Bacitracin and Polymyxin B *on page 681*
Betadine® Ophthalmic *see* Povidone-Iodine *on page 1016*

Betamethasone and Clotrimazole

(bay ta METH a sone & kloe TRIM a zole)

U.S. Brand Names Lotrisone®

Canadian Brand Names Lotriderm®

Synonyms Clotrimazole and Betamethasone

Generic Available Yes

Use Topical treatment of various dermal fungal infections (including tinea pedis, cruris, and corpora in patients ≥17 years of age)

Pregnancy Risk Factor C

Pregnancy Implications There are no adequate and well-controlled studies using topical betamethasone during pregnancy. However, intrauterine growth retardation has been reported with another topical steroid. Avoid use in large amounts for long periods of time during pregnancy. Clotrimazole is poorly absorbed when used topically.

Contraindications Hypersensitivity to betamethasone dipropionate, clotrimazole, other corticosteroids or imidazoles, or any component of the formulation

Warnings/Precautions Systemic absorption of topical corticosteroids may cause hypothalamic-pituitary-adrenal (HPA) axis suppression (reversible); may lead to manifestations of Cushing's syndrome, hyperglycemia, and glucosuria; risk is increased when used over large surface areas, for prolonged periods of time, or with occlusive dressings; not for use in patients <17 years of age (striae and growth retardation have been reported with use in infants and children); do not use for diaper dermatitis.

Adverse Reactions Also see individual agents.

1% to 10%:
- Dermatologic: Dry skin (2%)
- Local: Burning (2%)
- Neuromuscular & skeletal: Paresthesia (2%)

<1%: Cushing's syndrome, edema, glycosuria, HPA axis suppression (higher in children), hyperglycemia, rash, secondary infection, stinging. Growth suppression, intracranial hypertension, and striae have also been reported with use in children.

Postmarketing/case reports: Skin atrophy, skin ulceration (rare)

Drug Interactions

Cytochrome P450 Effect:
- Betamethasone: **Inhibits** CYP3A4 (weak)
- Clotrimazole: **Inhibits** CYP1A2 (weak), 2A6 (weak), 2B6 (weak), 2C8/9 (weak), 2C19 (weak), 2D6 (weak), 2E1 (weak), 3A4 (moderate)

Stability
Cream: Store between 2°C to 30°C (36°F to 86°F)
Lotion: Store upright between 15°C to 30°C (59°F to 86°F)
(Continued)

Betamethasone and Clotrimazole *(Continued)*

Mechanism of Action Betamethasone dipropionate is a corticosteroid. Clotrimazole is an antifungal agent.

Pharmacodynamics/Kinetics See individual agents.

Dosage

Children <17 years: Do not use

Children ≥17 years and Adults:

Allergic or inflammatory diseases: Topical: Apply to affected area twice daily, morning and evening

Tinea corporis, tinea cruris: Topical: Massage into affected area twice daily, morning and evening; do not use for longer than 2 weeks; re-evaluate after 1 week if no clinical improvement; do not exceed 45 g cream/week or 45 mL lotion/week

Tinea pedis: Topical: Massage into affected area twice daily, morning and evening; do not use for longer than 4 weeks; re-evaluate after 2 weeks if no clinical improvement; do not exceed 45 g cream/week or 45 mL lotion/week

Elderly: Use with caution; skin atrophy and skin ulceration (rare) have been reported in patients with thinning skin; do not use for diaper dermatitis or under occlusive dressings

Administration For external use only; do not use on open wounds; do not cover with occlusive dressings; shake lotion well prior to use

Monitoring Parameters Urinary free cortisol test, morning plasma cortisol test, and ACTH stimulation test may be used to evaluate HPA axis suppression; signs of infection

Dosage Forms

Cream: Betamethasone dipropionate 0.05% and clotrimazole 1% (15 g, 45 g) [contains benzyl alcohol]

Lotion: Betamethasone dipropionate 0.05% and clotrimazole 1% (30 mL) [contains benzyl alcohol]

Selected Readings

Reed, BD, "Dermatologic Drugs, Pregnancy, and Lactation. A Conservative Guide," *Arch Dermatol*, 1997, 133: 894-8.

Betasept® [OTC] *see* Chlorhexidine Gluconate *on page 735*

Biaxin® *see* Clarithromycin *on page 749*

Biaxin® XL *see* Clarithromycin *on page 749*

Bicillin® L-A *see* Penicillin G Benzathine *on page 991*

Bicillin® C-R *see* Penicillin G Benzathine and Penicillin G Procaine *on page 992*

Bicillin® C-R 900/300 *see* Penicillin G Benzathine and Penicillin G Procaine *on page 992*

BIG-IV *see* Botulism Immune Globulin (Intravenous-Human) *on page 690*

Biltricide® *see* Praziquantel *on page 1017*

Biocef® *see* Cephalexin *on page 727*

BioQuin® Durules™ (Can) *see* Quinidine *on page 1027*

Bio-Statin® *see* Nystatin *on page 976*

BioThrax™ *see* Anthrax Vaccine Adsorbed *on page 665*

Bismatrol *see* Bismuth *on page 686*

Bismuth (BIZ muth)

Related Information

Helicobacter pylori Treatment *on page 1288*

U.S. Brand Names Children's Kaopectate® *(reformulation)* [OTC] [DSC]; Diotame® [OTC]; Kaopectate® [OTC]; Kaopectate® Extra Strength [OTC]; Kaopectolin *(new formulation)* [OTC]; Pepto-Bismol® [OTC]; Pepto-Bismol® Maximum Strength [OTC]

Synonyms Bismatrol; Bismuth Subgallate; Bismuth Subsalicylate; Pink Bismuth

Generic Available Yes

Use

Subsalicylate formulation: Symptomatic treatment of mild, nonspecific diarrhea; control of traveler's diarrhea (enterotoxigenic *Escherichia coli*); as part of a multidrug regimen for *H. pylori* eradication to reduce the risk of duodenal ulcer recurrence

Subgallate formulation: An aid to reduce fecal odors from a colostomy or ileostomy

Drug of Choice or Alternative for Organism(s):

Helicobacter pylori on page 162

Pregnancy Risk Factor C/D (3rd trimester)

Contraindications Hypersensitivity to bismuth or any component of the formulation

Subsalicylate formulation: Do not use subsalicylate in patients with influenza or chickenpox because of risk of Reye's syndrome; hypersensitivity to salicylates or any component of the formulation; history of severe GI bleeding; history of coagulopathy; pregnancy (3rd trimester)

Warnings/Precautions Subsalicylate should be used with caution if patient is taking aspirin; use with caution in children, especially those <3 years of age and those with viral illness; may be neurotoxic with very large doses.

When used for self-medication (OTC labeling): Children and teenagers who have or are recovering from chickenpox or flu-like symptoms should not use subsalicylate. Changes in behavior (along with nausea and vomiting) may be an early sign of Reye's syndrome; patients should be instructed to contact their healthcare provider if these occur. Patients should be instructed to contact healthcare provider for diarrhea lasting >2 days, hearing loss, or ringing in the ears. Not labeled for OTC use in children <12 years of age.

Adverse Reactions Frequency not defined; subsalicylate formulation:

Central nervous system: Anxiety, confusion, headache, mental depression, slurred speech

Gastrointestinal: Discoloration of the tongue (darkening), grayish black stools, impaction may occur in infants and debilitated patients

Neuromuscular & skeletal: Muscle spasms, weakness

Ocular: Hearing loss, tinnitus

Overdosage/Toxicology

Symptoms of toxicity: **Subsalicylate**: Hyperpnea, nausea, vomiting, tinnitus, hyperpyrexia, metabolic acidoses/respiratory alkalosis, tachycardia, and confusion; seizures in severe overdose, pulmonary or cerebral edema, respiratory failure, cardiovascular collapse, coma, and death. **Note:** Each 262.4 mg tablet of bismuth subsalicylate contains an equivalent of 130 mg aspirin; 150 mg/kg of aspirin is considered to be toxic. Serious life-threatening toxicity occurs with >300 mg/kg.

Treatment: Gastrointestinal decontamination (activated charcoal for immediate release formulations (10 x dose of ASA in g), whole bowel irrigation for enteric coated tablets or when serially increasing ASA plasma levels indicate the presence of an intestinal bezoar), supportive and symptomatic treatment with emphasis on correcting fluid, electrolyte, blood glucose and acid-base disturbances; elimination is enhanced with urinary alkalinization (sodium bicarbonate infusion with potassium), multiple-dose activated charcoal, and hemodialysis.

Symptoms of toxicity: **Bismuth**: Rare with short-term administrations of bismuth salts; encephalopathy, methemoglobinemia, seizures

Treatment: Gastrointestinal decontamination; chelation with dimercaprol in doses of 3 mg/kg or penicillamine 100 mg/kg/day for 5 days can hasten recovery from bismuth-induced encephalopathy; methylene blue 1-2 mg/kg in a 1% sterile aqueous solution I.V. push over 4-6 minutes for methemoglobinemia. This may be repeated within 60 minutes if necessary, up to a total dose of 7 mg/kg. Seizures usually respond to I.V. diazepam.

Drug Interactions

Increased Effect/Toxicity: Toxicity of aspirin, warfarin, and/or hypoglycemics may be increased.

Decreased Effect: The effects of tetracyclines and uricosurics may be decreased.

Mechanism of Action Bismuth subsalicylate exhibits both antisecretory and antimicrobial action. This agent may provide some anti-inflammatory action as well. The salicylate moiety provides antisecretory effect and the bismuth exhibits antimicrobial directly against bacterial and viral gastrointestinal pathogens.

Pharmacodynamics/Kinetics

Absorption: Bismuth: <1%; Subsalicylate: >90%

Metabolism: Bismuth subsalicylate is converted to salicylic acid and insoluble bismuth salts in the GI tract.

Half-life elimination: Terminal: Bismuth: Highly variable

Excretion: Bismuth: Urine and feces; Salicylate: Urine

Dosage Oral:

Treatment of nonspecific diarrhea, control/relieve traveler's diarrhea: Subsalicylate (doses based on 262 mg/15 mL liquid or 262 mg tablets):

Children: Up to 8 doses/24 hours:

3-6 years: 1/3 tablet or 5 mL every 30 minutes to 1 hour as needed

6-9 years: 2/3 tablet or 10 mL every 30 minutes to 1 hour as needed

9-12 years: 1 tablet or 15 mL every 30 minutes to 1 hour as needed

Children >12 years and Adults: 2 tablets or 30 mL every 30 minutes to 1 hour as needed up to 8 doses/24 hours

Helicobacter pylori eradication: Adults: 524 mg 4 times/day with meals and at bedtime; requires combination therapy

(Continued)

Bismuth *(Continued)*

Control of fecal odor in ileostomy or colostomy: Children ≥12 years and Adults: Subgallate: 200-400 mg up to 4 times/day

Dosing adjustment in renal impairment: Should probably be avoided in patients with renal failure

Dietary Considerations Drink plenty of fluids to help prevent dehydration caused by diarrhea. Different dosage forms contain variable amounts of sodium; consult individual product labeling.

Administration Subsalicylate tablets should be taken at least 3 hours apart from other medications.

Test Interactions Increased uric acid, increased AST; bismuth absorbs x-rays and may interfere with diagnostic procedures of GI tract

Patient Information Chew tablet well or shake suspension well before using; may darken stools; if diarrhea persists for more than 2 days, consult prescriber; can turn tongue black; tinnitus may indicate toxicity and use should be discontinued

Dosage Forms [DSC] = Discontinued product

Caplet, as subsalicylate (Pepto-Bismol®): 262 mg [sugar free; contains sodium 2 mg]

Liquid, as subsalicylate: 262 mg/15 mL (240 mL, 360 mL, 480 mL); 525 mg/15 mL (240 mL, 360 mL)

Children's Kaopectate®: 87 mg/5 mL (180 mL) [contains sodium 3.3 mg/5 mL; cherry flavor] [DSC]

Diotame®: 262 mg/15 mL (30 mL)

Kaopectate®: 262 mg/15 mL (180 mL, 240 mL, 360 mL) [contains sodium 10 mg/15 mL; regular and peppermint flavor]

Kaopectate® Extra Strength: 525 mg/15 mL (240 mL) [contains sodium 11 mg/15 mL; peppermint flavor]

Pepto-Bismol®: 262 mg/15 mL (120 mL, 240 mL, 360 mL, 480 mL) [sugar free; contains sodium 6 mg/15 mL and benzoic acid; wintergreen flavor]

Pepto-Bismol® Maximum Strength: 525 mg/15 mL (120 mL, 240 mL, 360 mL) [sugar free; contains sodium 6 mg/15 mL and benzoic acid; wintergreen flavor]

Suspension (Kaopectolin): 262 mg/15 mL (480 mL)

Tablet, as subgallate: 200 mg

Tablet, chewable, as subsalicylate: 262 mg

Diotame®: 262 mg

Pepto-Bismol®: 262 mg [sugar free; contains sodium <1 mg; cherry flavor]

Selected Readings

Graham DY, Lew GM, Evans DG, et al, "Effect of Triple Therapy (Antibiotics Plus Bismuth) on Duodenal Ulcer Healing," *Ann Intern Med*, 1991, 115(4):266-9.

Graham DY, Lew GM, Klein PD, et al, "Effect of Treatment of *Helicobacter pylori* Infection on the Long-Term Recurrence of Gastric or Duodenal Ulcer," *Ann Intern Med*, 1992, 116(9):705-8.

Ormand JE and Talley NJ, "*Helicobacter pylori*: Controversies and an Approach to Management," *Mayo Clin Proc*, 1990, 65(3):414-26.

Bismuth Subgallate *see* Bismuth *on page 686*

Bismuth Subsalicylate *see* Bismuth *on page 686*

Bismuth Subsalicylate, Metronidazole, and Tetracycline

(BIZ muth sub sa LIS i late, me troe NI da zole, & tet ra SYE kleen)

Related Information

Bismuth *on page 686*

Metronidazole *on page 940*

Tetracycline *on page 1106*

U.S. Brand Names Helidac®

Synonyms Bismuth Subsalicylate, Tetracycline, and Metronidazole; Metronidazole, Bismuth Subsalicylate, and Tetracycline; Metronidazole, Tetracycline, and Bismuth Subsalicylate; Tetracycline, Bismuth Subsalicylate, and Metronidazole; Tetracycline, Metronidazole, and Bismuth Subsalicylate

Generic Available No

Use In combination with an H_2 antagonist, as part of a multidrug regimen for *H. pylori* eradication to reduce the risk of duodenal ulcer recurrence

Pregnancy Risk Factor D (tetracycline); B (metronidazole)

Contraindications Hypersensitivity to salicylates, bismuth, metronidazole, tetracycline, or any component of the formulation; children; significant renal/hepatic impairment; pregnancy (tetracycline)

Warnings/Precautions See individual agents.

Adverse Reactions See individual agents.

>1%:

Central nervous system: Dizziness

Gastrointestinal: Nausea, diarrhea, abdominal pain, vomiting, anal discomfort, anorexia

Neuromuscular & skeletal: Paresthesia

Drug Interactions

Cytochrome P450 Effect:

Metronidazole: **Inhibits** CYP2C8/9 (weak), 3A4 (moderate)

Tetracycline: **Substrate** of CYP3A4 (major); **Inhibits** CYP3A4 (moderate)

Increased Effect/Toxicity: See individual agents.

Decreased Effect: See individual agents.

Mechanism of Action Bismuth subsalicylate, metronidazole, and tetracycline individually have demonstrated *in vitro* activity against most susceptible strains of *H. pylori* isolated from patients with duodenal ulcers. Resistance to metronidazole is increasing in the U.S.; an alternative regimen, not containing metronidazole, if *H. pylori* is not eradicated follow therapy.

Pharmacodynamics/Kinetics See individual agents.

Dosage Adults: Chew 2 bismuth subsalicylate 262.4 mg tablets, swallow 1 metronidazole 250 mg tablet, and swallow 1 tetracycline 500 mg capsule 4 times/day at meals and bedtime, plus an H_2 antagonist (at the appropriate dose) for 14 days; follow with 8 oz of water; the H_2 antagonist should be continued for a total of 28 days

Monitoring Parameters See individual agents.

Dosage Forms Combination package [each package contains 14 blister cards (2-week supply); each card contains the following]:

Capsule: Tetracycline hydrochloride: 500 mg (4)

Tablet: Bismuth subsalicylate [chewable]: 262.4 mg (8)

Tablet: Metronidazole: 250 mg (4)

Bismuth Subsalicylate, Tetracycline, and Metronidazole *see* Bismuth Subsalicylate, Metronidazole, and Tetracycline *on page 688*

Bleph®-10 *see* Sulfacetamide *on page 1081*

Blephamide® *see* Sulfacetamide and Prednisolone *on page 1082*

Blis-To-Sol® [OTC] *see* Tolnaftate *on page 1127*

BMS-232632 *see* Atazanavir *on page 668*

Boostrix® *see* Diphtheria, Tetanus Toxoids, and Acellular Pertussis Vaccine *on page 782*

Botulinum Pentavalent (ABCDE) Toxoid

(BOT yoo lin num pen ta VAY lent TOKS oyd)

Synonyms Botulinum Toxoid, Pentavalent Vaccine (Against Types A / B / C / D / E Strains of *C. botulinum*)

Unlabeled/Investigational Use Investigational: Prophylaxis for *C. botulinum* exposure (high-risk research laboratory personnel actively working with, or expect to work with, known cultures and purified botulinum toxin)

Drug of Choice or Alternative for Organism(s):

Clostridium botulinum on page 83

Adverse Reactions Moderate-to-severe effects (initial series 5.6%, booster 12.3%, systemic 4.5% initial & booster)

Central nervous system: Fever, headache

Dermatologic: Rash

Local: Pain/soreness at injection site

Neuromuscular & skeletal: Muscle pain

Dosage Do not inject intracutaneously or into superficial structures.

Initial vaccination series: 0.5 mL deep SubQ at 0-, 2-, and 12 weeks

First booster: 0.5 mL deep SubQ 12 months after first injection of the initial series

Subsequent boosters: 0.5 mL deep SubQ at 2-year intervals based on antitoxin titers as checked by CDC

Additional Information Each vial contains 0.022% formaldehyde and 1:10,000 thimerosal as a preservative; manufactured by Michigan Biologic Products Institute, Lansing, Michigan, 48909.

For advice on vaccine administration and contraindications, contact the Division of Immunization, CDC, Atlanta, GA 30333 (404-639-3670, FAX 404-639-3717).

Botulinum Toxoid, Pentavalent Vaccine (Against Types A / B / C / D / E Strains of *C. botulinum*) *see* Botulinum Pentavalent (ABCDE) Toxoid *on page 689*

Botulism Immune Globulin (Intravenous-Human)

(BOT yoo lism i MYUN GLOB you lin, in tra VEE nus, YU man)

U.S. Brand Names BabyBIG®

Synonyms BIG-IV

Generic Available No

Use Treatment of infant botulism caused by toxin type A or B

Drug of Choice or Alternative for Organism(s):

Clostridium botulinum on page 83

Restrictions Available from the California Department of Health

Pregnancy Implications Reproduction studies have not been conducted.

Contraindications Hypersensitivity to human immune globulin preparations or any component of the formulation; selective immunoglobulin A deficiency

Warnings/Precautions Use caution with renal dysfunction or those at increased risk for renal disease, including concomitant nephrotoxic drugs, diabetes mellitus, paraproteinemia, sepsis, or volume depletion. Patients should not be volume depleted prior to therapy. For I.V. infusion only; do not exceed recommended rate of administration. Not indicated for use in adults or children; safety and efficacy established for infants <1 year of age.

Adverse Reactions Percentages reported in open-label study except where otherwise noted; may reflect pathophysiology of infant botulism.

>10%:

- Cardiovascular: Blood pressure increased (transient, 75%); pallor (28%); edema (18%); blood pressure decreased (transient, 16%); cardiac murmur (15%)
- Central nervous system: Irritability (41%), pyrexia (17%), body temperature decreased (16%)
- Dermatologic: Contact dermatitis (24%); erythematous rash (22%, reported as 14% vs 8% in placebo-controlled study)
- Gastrointestinal: Dysphagia (65%), loose stools (25%), vomiting (20%), abdominal distension (11%)
- Otic: Otitis media (11%, reported in placebo-controlled study)
- Respiratory: Atelectasis (39%), rhonchi (34%), nasal congestion (18%), oxygen saturation decreased (17%), cough (13%), rales (13%)

1% to 10%:

- Cardiovascular: Tachycardia (7%), peripheral coldness (7%)
- Central nervous system: Agitation (10%)
- Endocrine & metabolic: Dehydration (10%), hyponatremia (6%), metabolic acidosis (5%)
- Hematologic: Hemoglobin decreased (9%), anemia (5%)
- Local: Injection site reaction (7%), injection site erythema (5%)
- Renal: Neurogenic bladder
- Respiratory: Breath sounds decreased (10%), stridor (9%), lower respiratory tract infection (8%), dyspnea (6%), tachypnea (5%)
- Miscellaneous: Oral candidiasis (8%); intubation (5%); infusion rate reactions (<5%, includes chills, back pain, fever, muscle cramps, nausea, vomiting, wheezing)

Overdosage/Toxicology Limited data; adverse reactions related to volume overload may be expected

Drug Interactions

Decreased Effect: Immune globulins may interfere with live virus vaccines, defer vaccination for ~5 months following therapy; revaccinations may be needed if given shortly before or after BIG-IV administration.

Stability Prior to reconstitution, store between 2°C to 8°C (35.6°F to 46.4°F). Infusion should begin within 2 hours of reconstitution and be completed within 4 hours of reconstitution. Reconstitute with SWFI 2 mL; swirl gently to wet powder, do not shake. Powder should dissolve in ~30 minutes.

Mechanism of Action BIG-IV is purified immunoglobulin derived from the plasma of adults immunized with botulinum toxoid types A and B. BIG-IV provides antibodies to neutralize circulating toxins.

Pharmacodynamics/Kinetics

Duration: Protective neutralizing antibody levels: 6 months

Half-life elimination: 28 days

Dosage I.V.: Children <1 year: Infant botulism: 1 mL/kg (50 mg/kg) as a single dose; infuse at 0.5 mL/kg/hour (25 mg/kg/hour) for the first 15 minutes; if well tolerated, may increase to 1 mL/kg/hour (50 mg/kg/hour)

Administration For I.V. infusion only. Do not administer if solution is turbid. Epinephrine should be available for the treatment of acute allergic reaction. Administer using low volume tubing and infusion pump with an in-line or syringe tip 18 μm filter. Infuse

at 0.5 mL/kg/hour (25 mg/kg/hour) for the first 15 minutes; if well tolerated, may increase to 1 mL/kg/hour (50 mg/kg/hour). Infusion should take ~67.5 minutes. Infusion should be slowed or temporarily interrupted for minor side effects; discontinue in case of hypotension or anaphylaxis.

Monitoring Parameters Renal function (BUN, serum creatinine, urinary output); vital signs (continuously during infusion); aseptic meningitis syndrome (may occur hours to days following IGIV therapy); signs of relapse (may occur up to 1 month following recovery)

Patient Information Defer vaccination for ~5 months following therapy.

Dosage Forms Injection, powder for reconstitution [preservative free]: ~100 mg [contains albumin 1% and sucrose 5%; packaged with SWFI]

Butenafine (byoo TEN a feen)

U.S. Brand Names Lotrimin® Ultra™ [OTC]; Mentax®

Synonyms Butenafine Hydrochloride

Generic Available No

Use Topical treatment of tinea pedis (athlete's foot), tinea cruris (jock itch), tinea corporis (ringworm), and tinea versicolor

Pregnancy Risk Factor B

Contraindications Hypersensitivity to butenafine or any component of the formulation

Warnings/Precautions Only for topical use (not ophthalmic, vaginal, or internal routes); patients sensitive to other allylamine antifungals may cross-react with butenafine; has not been studied in immunocompromised patients

Adverse Reactions

>1%: Dermatologic: Burning, stinging, irritation, erythema, pruritus (2%)

<1%: Contact dermatitis

Stability Store at 5°C to 30°C (41°F to 86°F).

Mechanism of Action Butenafine exerts antifungal activity by blocking squalene epoxidation, resulting in inhibition of ergosterol synthesis (antidermatophyte and *Sporothrix schenckii* activity). In higher concentrations, the drug disrupts fungal cell membranes (anticandidal activity).

Pharmacodynamics/Kinetics

Absorption: Minimal systemic

Metabolism: Hepatic via hydroxylation

Half-life elimination: 35 hours

Time to peak, serum: 6 hours

Dosage Children >12 years and Adults: Topical:

Tinea corporis, tinea cruris, or tinea versicolor: Apply once daily for 2 weeks to affected area and surrounding skin

Tinea pedis: Apply once daily for 4 weeks or twice daily for 7 days to affected area and surrounding skin (7-day regimen may have lower efficacy)

Monitoring Parameters Culture and KOH exam, clinical signs of tinea pedis

Patient Information Report any signs of rash or allergy to your prescriber immediately; do not apply other topical medications on the same area as butenafine unless directed by your prescriber

Dosage Forms Cream, as hydrochloride:

Lotrimin® Ultra™: 1% (12 g, 24 g) [contains benzyl alcohol and sodium benzoate]

Mentax®: 1% (15 g, 30 g) [contains benzyl alcohol and sodium benzoate]

Selected Readings

McNeely W and Spencer CM, "Butenafine," *Drugs*, 1998, 55(3):405-12.

"Topical Butenafine for Tinea Pedis," *Med Lett Drugs Ther*, 1997, 39(1004):63-4.

Butenafine Hydrochloride *see* Butenafine *on page 691*

Butoconazole (byoo toe KOE na zole)

U.S. Brand Names Gynazole-1®; Mycelex®-3 [OTC]

Canadian Brand Names Femstat® One; Gynazole-1®

Synonyms Butoconazole Nitrate

Generic Available No

Use Local treatment of vulvovaginal candidiasis

Pregnancy Risk Factor C (use only in 2nd or 3rd trimester)

Pregnancy Implications There are no adequate and well-controlled studies have been conducted in pregnant women. However, butoconazole has been used during pregnancy. Use should be limited to the 2nd or 3rd trimesters only.

Contraindications Hypersensitivity to butoconazole or any component of the formulation

(Continued)

Butoconazole *(Continued)*

Warnings/Precautions If irritation or sensitization occurs, discontinue use. Contains mineral oil which may weaken latex or rubber products (condoms, vaginal contraceptive diaphragms); do not use these products within 72 hours of treatment. HIV infection should be considered in sexually-active women with difficult to eradicate recurrent vaginal yeast infections. OTC product is not for use in women with a first-time vaginal yeast infection. Safety and efficacy in females <12 years have not been established.

Adverse Reactions Frequency not defined.

Gastrointestinal: Abdominal pain or cramping

Genitourinary: Pelvic pain; vulvar/vaginal burning, itching, soreness, and swelling

Stability Store at 15°C to 30°C (59°F to 86°F)

Mechanism of Action Increases cell membrane permeability in susceptible fungi (*Candida*)

Pharmacodynamics/Kinetics

Absorption: 2%

Metabolism: Not reported

Time to peak: 12-24 hours

Dosage Adults: Female:

Femstat®-3 [OTC]: Insert 1 applicatorful (~5 g) intravaginally at bedtime for 3 consecutive days

Gynazole-1®: Insert 1 applicatorful (~5 g) intravaginally as a single dose; treatment may need to be extended for up to 6 days in pregnant women (use in pregnancy during 2nd or 3rd trimester only)

Patient Information May cause burning or stinging on application; dispose of applicator after use. If symptoms of vaginitis persist, contact prescriber. Do not use OTC product if you have abdominal pain, fever, or foul-smelling discharge. Contact prescriber if infection does not clear within 3 days. Do not use tampons while using this medication. This medication contains mineral oil, which may cause damage to condoms or diaphragms; use another method of birth control during treatment.

Additional Information Gynazole-1®: This product is delivered in a base allowing the active ingredient to remain vaginally for 4 days. It is associated with less leakage and can therefore be applied at anytime during the day or night (per product information, Gynazole-1®).

Dosage Forms

Cream, vaginal, as nitrate:

Mycelex®-3: 2% (5 g) [prefilled applicator], (20 g) [with disposable applicator]

Gynazole-1®: 2% (5 g) [prefilled applicator]

Butoconazole Nitrate *see* Butoconazole *on page 691*

BW524W91 *see* Emtricitabine *on page 799*

Cancidas® *see* Caspofungin *on page 695*

Candistatin® (Can) *see* Nystatin *on page 976*

Canesten® Topical (Can) *see* Clotrimazole *on page 758*

Canesten® Vaginal (Can) *see* Clotrimazole *on page 758*

Capastat® Sulfate *see* Capreomycin *on page 692*

Capreomycin (kap ree oh MYE sin)

Related Information

Tuberculosis *on page 1315*

U.S. Brand Names Capastat® Sulfate

Synonyms Capreomycin Sulfate

Generic Available No

Use Treatment of tuberculosis in conjunction with at least one other antituberculosis agent

Pregnancy Risk Factor C

Pregnancy Implications Capreomycin has been shown to be teratogenic in animal studies. There are no adequate and well-controlled studies in pregnant women; use during pregnancy only if the potential benefit to the mother outweighs the possible risk to the fetus.

Contraindications Hypersensitivity to capreomycin sulfate or any component of the formulation

Warnings/Precautions Use in patients with renal insufficiency or pre-existing auditory impairment must be undertaken with great caution, and the risk of additional eighth nerve impairment or renal injury should be weighed against the benefits to be derived from therapy. Since other parenteral antituberculous agents (eg, streptomycin) also have similar and sometimes irreversible toxic effects, particularly on eighth cranial nerve and renal function, simultaneous administration of these agents

with capreomycin is not recommended. Use with nonantituberculous drugs (ie, aminoglycoside antibiotics) having ototoxic or nephrotoxic potential should be undertaken only with great caution. Use caution with renal dysfunction and in the elderly.

Adverse Reactions

>10%:

Otic: Ototoxicity [subclinical hearing loss (11%), clinical loss (3%)], tinnitus

Renal: Nephrotoxicity (36%, increased BUN)

1% to 10%: Hematologic: Eosinophilia (dose related, mild)

<1%: Vertigo, hypokalemia, leukocytosis, thrombocytopenia (rare); pain, induration, and bleeding at injection site; hypersensitivity (urticaria, rash, fever)

Postmarketing and/or case reports: Acute tubular necrosis, Bartter's syndrome

Overdosage/Toxicology Symptoms include renal failure, ototoxicity, and thrombocytopenia. Treatment is supportive.

Drug Interactions

Increased Effect/Toxicity: May increase effect/duration of nondepolarizing neuromuscular blocking agents. Additive toxicity (nephrotoxicity and ototoxicity), respiratory paralysis may occur with aminoglycosides (eg, streptomycin).

Stability Powder for injection should be stored at room temperature of 15°C to 30°C (59°F to 86°F). Dissolve powder in 2 mL of NS or SWFI; allow 2-3 minutes for dissolution. For I.V. administration, further dilute in NS 100 mL. For I.M. administration, dose <1 g may be further diluted to concentrations of 200-350 mg/mL. Following reconstitution, may store under refrigeration for up to 24 hours.

Mechanism of Action Capreomycin is a cyclic polypeptide antimicrobial. It is administered as a mixture of capreomycin IA and capreomycin IB. The mechanism of action of capreomycin is not well understood. Mycobacterial species that have become resistant to other agents are usually still sensitive to the action of capreomycin. However, significant cross-resistance with viomycin, kanamycin, and neomycin occurs.

Pharmacodynamics/Kinetics

Half-life elimination: Normal renal function: 4-6 hours

Time to peak, serum: I.M.: ~1 hour

Excretion: Urine (as unchanged drug)

Dosage I.M., I.V.:

Infants and Children: 15-30 mg/kg/day, up to 1 g/day maximum

Adults: 1 g/day (not to exceed 20 mg/kg/day) for 60-120 days, followed by 1 g 2-3 times/week

Elderly: Refer to Adults dosing; use with caution due to the increased potential for pre-existing renal dysfunction or impaired hearing

Dosing interval in renal impairment: Adults:

Cl_{cr} >100 mL/minute: Administer 13-15 mg/kg every 24 hours

Cl_{cr} 80-100 mL/minute: Administer 10-13 mg/kg every 24 hours

Cl_{cr} 60-80 mL/minute: Administer 7-10 mg/kg every 24 hours

Cl_{cr} 40-60 mL/minute: Administer 11-14 mg/kg every 48 hours

Cl_{cr} 20-40 mL/minute: Administer 10-14 mg/kg every 72 hours

Cl_{cr} <20 mL/minute: Administer 4-7 mg/kg every 72 hours

Administration

I.M.: Administer by deep I.M. injection into a large muscle mass.

I.V.: Administer over 60 minutes.

Monitoring Parameters Audiometric measurements and vestibular function at baseline and during therapy; renal function at baseline and weekly during therapy; serum potassium; liver function tests

Reference Range 10 mcg/mL

Patient Information Report any hearing loss immediately. Do not discontinue without notifying prescriber.

Dosage Forms Injection, powder for reconstitution, as sulfate: 1 g

Selected Readings

Davidson PT and Le HQ, "Drug Treatment of Tuberculosis - 1992," *Drugs*, 1992, 43(5):651-73.

"Drugs for Tuberculosis," *Med Lett Drugs Ther*, 1993, 35(908):99-101.

Iseman MD, "Treatment of Multidrug-Resistant Tuberculosis," *N Engl J Med*, 1993, 329(11):784-91.

Capreomycin Sulfate *see* Capreomycin *on page 692*

Carbapenems

Refer to

Ertapenem *on page 805*

Imipenem and Cilastatin *on page 861*

Meropenem *on page 936*

Drug of Choice or Alternative for Disease/Syndrome(s):

Osteomyelitis, Diabetic Foot *on page 249*

(Continued)

Carbapenems *(Continued)*

Organism(s):

Bacteroides and *Prevotella* Species *on page 46*
Burkholderia cepacia on page 62
Clostridium perfringens on page 88
Escherichia coli on page 142
Proteus Species *on page 278*
Providencia Species *on page 281*

Carbenicillin (kar ben i SIL in)

Related Information

Antimicrobial Activity Against Selected Organisms *on page 1165*

U.S. Brand Names Geocillin®

Synonyms Carbenicillin Indanyl Sodium; Carindacillin

Generic Available No

Use Treatment of serious urinary tract infections and prostatitis caused by susceptible gram-negative aerobic bacilli

Pregnancy Risk Factor B

Contraindications Hypersensitivity to carbenicillin, penicillins, or any component of the formulation

Warnings/Precautions Do not use in patients with severe renal impairment (Cl_{cr} <10 mL/minute); dosage modification required in patients with impaired renal and/or hepatic function; oral carbenicillin should be limited to treatment of urinary tract infections. Use with caution in patients with history of hypersensitivity to cephalosporins.

Adverse Reactions

>10%: Gastrointestinal: Diarrhea

1% to 10%: Gastrointestinal: Nausea, bad taste, vomiting, flatulence, glossitis

<1%: Headache, skin rash, urticaria, anemia, thrombocytopenia, leukopenia, neutropenia, eosinophilia, hyperthermia, itchy eyes, vaginitis, hypokalemia, hematuria, thrombophlebitis

Overdosage/Toxicology Symptoms include neuromuscular hypersensitivity and convulsions. Many beta-lactam containing antibiotics have the potential to cause neuromuscular hyperirritability or convulsive seizures. Hemodialysis may be helpful to aid in the removal of the drug from the blood, otherwise, most treatment is supportive or symptom-directed.

Drug Interactions

Increased Effect/Toxicity: Increased bleeding effects if taken with high doses of heparin or oral anticoagulants. Aminoglycosides may be synergistic against selected organisms. Penicillins may increase the exposure to methotrexate during concurrent therapy; monitor. Probenecid and disulfiram may increase levels of penicillins (carbenicillin).

Decreased Effect: Decreased effectiveness with tetracyclines. Although anecdotal reports suggest oral contraceptive efficacy could be reduced by penicillins, this has been refuted by more rigorous scientific and clinical data.

Mechanism of Action Inhibits bacterial cell wall synthesis by binding to one or more of the penicillin binding proteins (PBPs); which in turn inhibits the final transpeptidation step of peptidoglycan synthesis in bacterial cell walls, thus inhibiting cell wall biosynthesis. Bacteria eventually lyse due to ongoing activity of cell wall autolytic enzymes (autolysins and murein hydrolases) while cell wall assembly is arrested.

Pharmacodynamics/Kinetics

Absorption: 30% to 40%

Distribution: Crosses placenta; small amounts enter breast milk; distributes into bile; low concentrations attained in CSF

Protein binding: ~50%

Half-life elimination: Children: 0.8-1.8 hours; Adults: 1-1.5 hours, prolonged to 10-20 hours with renal insufficiency

Time to peak, serum: Normal renal function: 0.5-2 hours; concentrations are inadequate for treatment of systemic infections

Excretion: Urine (~80% to 99% as unchanged drug)

Dosage Oral:

Children: 30-50 mg/kg/day divided every 6 hours; maximum dose: 2-3 g/day

Adults: 1-2 tablets every 6 hours for urinary tract infections or 2 tablets every 6 hours for prostatitis

Dosing interval in renal impairment: Adults:

Cl_{cr} 10-50 mL/minute: Administer 382-764 mg every 12-24 hours

Cl_{cr} <10 mL/minute: Administer 382-764 mg every 24-48 hours

Moderately dialyzable (20% to 50%)

Dietary Considerations Should be taken with water on empty stomach. Sodium content of 382 mg tablet: 23 mg (1 mEq).

Administration Administer around-the-clock to promote less variation in peak and trough serum levels. Give at least 1 hour before aminoglycosides.

Monitoring Parameters Renal, hepatic, and hematologic function tests

Reference Range Therapeutic: Not established; Toxic: >250 mcg/mL (SI: >660 μmol/L)

Test Interactions May interfere with urinary glucose tests using cupric sulfate (Benedict's solution, Clinitest®); may inactivate aminoglycosides *in vitro*; false-positive urine or serum proteins

Patient Information Tablets have a bitter taste; take with a full glass of water, preferably on an empty stomach; take entire course of medication

Dosage Forms Tablet [film coated]: 382 mg [contains sodium 23 mg/tablet]

Selected Readings

Donowitz GR and Mandell GL, "Beta-Lactam Antibiotics," *N Engl J Med*, 1988, 318(7):419-26 and 318(8):490-500.

Wright AJ, "The Penicillins," *Mayo Clin Proc*, 1999, 74(3):290-307.

Carbenicillin Indanyl Sodium *see* Carbenicillin *on page 694*

Carimune™ [DSC] *see* Immune Globulin (Intravenous) *on page 867*

Carimune™ NF *see* Immune Globulin (Intravenous) *on page 867*

Carindacillin *see* Carbenicillin *on page 694*

Carmol® Scalp *see* Sulfacetamide *on page 1081*

Carrington Antifungal [OTC] *see* Miconazole *on page 945*

Caspofungin (kas poe FUN jin)

U.S. Brand Names Cancidas®

Canadian Brand Names Cancidas®

Synonyms Caspofungin Acetate

Generic Available No

Use Treatment of invasive *Aspergillus* infections in patients who are refractory or intolerant of other therapy; treatment of candidemia and other *Candida* infections (intra-abdominal abscesses, esophageal, peritonitis, pleural space); empirical treatment for presumed fungal infections in febrile neutropenic patient

Drug of Choice or Alternative for Disease/Syndrome(s):

Endophthalmitis, Bacterial and Fungal *on page 128*
Esophagitis *on page 147*

Organism(s):

Aspergillus Species *on page 38*
Candida Species *on page 67*

Pregnancy Risk Factor C

Pregnancy Implications There are no adequate and well-controlled studies in pregnant women. Should be used during pregnancy only if potential benefit justifies the potential risk to the fetus. Embryotoxicity has been demonstrated in animal studies.

Contraindications Hypersensitivity to caspofungin or any component of the formulation

Warnings/Precautions Has not been studied as initial therapy for invasive *Aspergillus*. Concurrent use of cyclosporine should be limited to patients for whom benefit outweighs risk, due to a high frequency of hepatic transaminase elevations observed during concurrent use. Limited data are available concerning treatment durations longer than 4 weeks; however, treatment appears to be well tolerated. Use caution in hepatic impairment; dosage reduction required in moderate impairment. Safety and efficacy in pediatric patients have not been established.

Adverse Reactions

>10%:

Central nervous system: Headache (up to 11%), fever (3% to 26%), chills (up to 14%)
Endocrine & metabolic: Hypokalemia (4% to 11%)
Hematologic: Hemoglobin decreased (1% to 12%)
Hepatic: Serum alkaline phosphatase (3% to 11%) increased, transaminases increased (up to 13%)
Local: Infusion site reactions (2% to 12%), phlebitis/thrombophlebitis (up to 16%)

1% to 10%:

Cardiovascular: Flushing (2% to 3%), facial edema (up to 3%), hypertension (1% to 2%), tachycardia (1% to 2%), hypotension (1%)
Central nervous system: Dizziness (2%), pain (1% to 5%), insomnia (1%)
Dermatologic: Rash (<1% to 6%), pruritus (1% to 3%), erythema (1% to 2%)

(Continued)

Caspofungin *(Continued)*

Gastrointestinal: Nausea (2% to 6%), vomiting (1% to 4%), abdominal pain (1% to 4%), diarrhea (1% to 4%), anorexia (1%)

Hematologic: Eosinophils increased (3%), neutrophils decreased (2% to 3%), WBC decreased (5% to 6%), anemia (up to 4%), platelet count decreased (2% to 3%)

Hepatic: Bilirubin increased (3%)

Local: Induration (up to 3%)

Neuromuscular & skeletal: Myalgia (up to 3%), paresthesia (1% to 3%), tremor (≤2%)

Renal: Nephrotoxicity (8%)*, proteinuria (5%), hematuria (2%), serum creatinine increased (<1% to 4%), urinary WBCs increased (up to 8%), urinary RBCs increased (1% to 4%), blood urea nitrogen increased (1%)

*Nephrotoxicity defined as serum creatinine ≥2X baseline value or ≥1 mg/dL in patients with serum creatinine above ULN range (patients with Cl_{cr} <30 mL/minute were excluded)

Miscellaneous: Flu-like syndrome (3%), diaphoresis (up to 3%)

<1%: Adult respiratory distress syndrome (ARDS), jaundice, pulmonary edema, renal insufficiency, serum bicarbonate decreased, tachypnea; histamine-mediated reactions (including facial swelling, bronchospasm, sensation of warmth) have been reported

Postmarketing and/or case reports: Anaphylaxis, dyspnea, dystonia, hepatic dysfunction, hypercalcemia, peripheral edema, swelling, stridor

Overdosage/Toxicology No experience with overdosage has been reported. Caspofungin is not dialyzable. Treatment is symptomatic and supportive.

Drug Interactions

Increased Effect/Toxicity: Concurrent administration of cyclosporine may increase caspofungin concentrations; hepatic serum transaminases may be observed.

Decreased Effect: Caspofungin may decrease blood concentrations of tacrolimus. Dosage adjustment of caspofungin to 70 mg is required for patients on rifampin.

Stability Store vials at 2°C to 8°C (36°F to 46°F). Reconstituted solution may be stored at less than 25°C (77°F) for 1 hour prior to preparation of infusion solution. Infusion solutions may be stored at less than 25°C (77°F) and should be used within 24 hours; up to 48 hours if stored at 2°C to 8°C (36°F to 46°F).

Bring refrigerated vial to room temperature. Reconstitute vials using 0.9% sodium chloride for injection, SWFI, or bacteriostatic water for injection. Mix gently until clear solution is formed; do not use if cloudy or contains particles. Solution should be further diluted with 0.9%, 0.45%, or 0.225% sodium chloride or LR. Do not mix with dextrose-containing solutions. Do not coadminister with other medications.

Mechanism of Action Inhibits synthesis of β(1,3)-D-glucan, an essential component of the cell wall of susceptible fungi. Highest activity in regions of active cell growth. Mammalian cells do not require β(1,3)-D-glucan, limiting potential toxicity.

Pharmacodynamics/Kinetics

Protein binding: 97% to albumin

Metabolism: Slowly, via hydrolysis and *N*-acetylation as well as by spontaneous degradation, with subsequent metabolism to component amino acids. Overall metabolism is extensive.

Half-life elimination: Beta (distribution): 9-11 hours; Terminal: 40-50 hours

Excretion: Urine (41% as metabolites, 1% to 9% unchanged) and feces (35% as metabolites)

Dosage I.V.:

Children: Safety and efficacy in pediatric patients have not been established

Adults: **Note:** Duration of caspofungin treatment should be determined by patient status and clinical response. Empiric therapy should be given until neutropenia resolves. In patients with positive cultures, treatment should continue until 14 days after last positive culture. In neutropenic patients, treatment should be given at least 7 days after both signs and symptoms of infection **and** neutropenia resolve.

Empiric therapy: Initial dose: 70 mg on day 1; subsequent dosing: 50 mg/day; may increase up to 70 mg/day if tolerated, but clinical response is inadequate

Invasive *Aspergillus*, candidiasis: Initial dose: 70 mg on day 1; subsequent dosing: 50 mg/day

Esophageal candidiasis: 50 mg/day; **Note:** The majority of patients studied for this indication also had oropharyngeal involvement.

Concomitant use of an enzyme inducer:

Patients receiving rifampin: 70 mg caspofungin daily

Patients receiving carbamazepine, dexamethasone, efavirenz, nevirapine, **or** phenytoin (and possibly other enzyme inducers) may require an increased daily dose of caspofungin (70 mg/day).

Elderly: The number of patients >65 years of age in clinical studies was not sufficient to establish whether a difference in response may be anticipated.

Dosage adjustment in renal impairment: No specific dosage adjustment is required; supplemental dose is not required following dialysis

Dosage adjustment in hepatic impairment:

Mild hepatic insufficiency (Child-Pugh score 5-6): No adjustment necessary

Moderate hepatic insufficiency (Child-Pugh score 7-9): 35 mg/day; initial 70 mg loading dose should still be administered in treatment of invasive infections

Severe hepatic insufficiency (Child-Pugh score >9): No clinical experience

Administration Infuse slowly, over 1 hour; monitor during infusion; isolated cases of possible histamine-related reactions have occurred during clinical trials (rash, flushing, pruritus, facial edema); do not coadminister with other medications

Patient Information Report immediately any pain, burning, or swelling at infusion site, or any signs of allergic reaction (eg, difficulty breathing or swallowing, back pain, chest tightness, rash, hives, or swelling of lips or mouth). Report nausea, vomiting, abdominal pain, or diarrhea.

Dosage Forms Injection, powder for reconstitution, as acetate: 50 mg [contains sucrose 39 mg], 70 mg [contains sucrose 54 mg]

Caspofungin Acetate *see* Caspofungin *on page 695*

Ceclor® (Can) *see* Cefaclor *on page 697*

Cedax® *see* Ceftibuten *on page 719*

Cefaclor (SEF a klor)

Related Information

Antimicrobial Activity Against Selected Organisms *on page 1165*

U.S. Brand Names Raniclor™

Canadian Brand Names Apo-Cefaclor®; Ceclor®; Novo-Cefaclor; Nu-Cefaclor; PMS-Cefaclor

Generic Available Yes: Excludes chewable tablet

Use Treatment of susceptible bacterial infections including otitis media, lower respiratory tract infections, acute exacerbations of chronic bronchitis, pharyngitis and tonsillitis, urinary tract infections, skin and skin structure infections

Drug of Choice or Alternative for Organism(s):

Haemophilus influenzae on page 159

Pregnancy Risk Factor B

Contraindications Hypersensitivity to cefaclor, any component of the formulation, or other cephalosporins

Warnings/Precautions Modify dosage in patients with severe renal impairment. Prolonged use may result in superinfection. Use with caution in patients with a history of penicillin allergy especially IgE-mediated reactions (eg, anaphylaxis, urticaria). Beta-lactamase-negative, ampicillin-resistant (BLNAR) strains of *H. influenzae* should be considered resistant to cefaclor. Extended release tablets are not approved for use in children <16 years of age.

Adverse Reactions

1% to 10%:

Dermatologic: Rash (maculopapular, erythematous, or morbilliform) (1% to 2%)

Gastrointestinal: Diarrhea (3%)

Genitourinary: Vaginitis (2%)

Hematologic: Eosinophilia (2%)

Hepatic: Transaminases increased (3%)

Miscellaneous: Moniliasis (2%)

<1%: Agitation, agranulocytosis, anaphylaxis, angioedema, aplastic anemia, arthralgia, cholestatic jaundice, CNS irritability, confusion, dizziness, hallucinations, hemolytic anemia, hepatitis, hyperactivity, insomnia, interstitial nephritis, nausea, nervousness, neutropenia, paresthesia, pruritus, pseudomembranous colitis, PT prolonged, seizure, serum-sickness, somnolence, Stevens-Johnson syndrome, urticaria, thrombocytopenia, toxic epidermal necrolysis, vomiting

Reactions reported with other cephalosporins include fever, abdominal pain, superinfection, renal dysfunction, toxic nephropathy, hemorrhage, cholestasis

Overdosage/Toxicology Symptoms of overdose include diarrhea, epigastric distress, nausea, and vomiting. Many beta-lactam antibiotics have the potential to cause neuromuscular hyperirritability or seizures. Hemodialysis may be helpful to aid in removal of the drug from the blood, but is not usually indicated; otherwise, most treatment is supportive and symptom-directed.

(Continued)

Cefaclor *(Continued)*

Drug Interactions

Increased Effect/Toxicity: Probenecid may decrease cephalosporin elimination. Furosemide, aminoglycosides when taken with cefaclor may result in additive nephrotoxicity.

Ethanol/Nutrition/Herb Interactions

Food: Cefaclor serum levels may be decreased slightly if taken with food. The bioavailability of cefaclor extended release tablets is decreased 23% and the maximum concentration is decreased 67% when taken on an empty stomach.

Stability Store at controlled room temperature. Refrigerate suspension after reconstitution. Discard after 14 days. Do not freeze.

Mechanism of Action Inhibits bacterial cell wall synthesis by binding to one or more of the penicillin-binding proteins (PBPs) which in turn inhibits the final transpeptidation step of peptidoglycan synthesis in bacterial cell walls, thus inhibiting cell wall biosynthesis. Bacteria eventually lyse due to ongoing activity of cell wall autolytic enzymes (autolysins and murein hydrolases) while cell wall assembly is arrested.

Pharmacodynamics/Kinetics

Absorption: Well absorbed, acid stable

Distribution: Widely throughout the body and reaches therapeutic concentration in most tissues and body fluids, including synovial, pericardial, pleural, peritoneal fluids; bile, sputum, and urine; bone, myocardium, gallbladder, skin and soft tissue; crosses placenta; enters breast milk

Protein binding: 25%

Metabolism: Partially hepatic

Half-life elimination: 0.5-1 hour; prolonged with renal impairment

Time to peak: Capsule: 60 minutes; Suspension: 45 minutes

Excretion: Urine (80% as unchanged drug)

Dosage Oral:

Children >1 month: Dosing range: 20-40 mg/kg/day divided every 8-12 hours; maximum dose: 1 g/day

Otitis media: 40 mg/kg/day divided every 12 hours

Pharyngitis: 20 mg/kg/day divided every 12 hours

Adults: Dosing range: 250-500 mg every 8 hours

Dosing adjustment in renal impairment:

Cl_{cr} 10-50 mL/minute: Administer 50% to 100% of dose

Cl_{cr} <10 mL/minute: Administer 50% of dose

Hemodialysis: Moderately dialyzable (20% to 50%)

Dietary Considerations Capsule, chewable tablet, and suspension may be taken with or without food. Raniclor™ contains phenylalanine 2.8 mg/cefaclor 125 mg.

Administration Administer around-the-clock to promote less variation in peak and trough serum levels.

Chewable tablet: Should be chewed before swallowing; should not be swallowed whole

Oral suspension: Shake well before using.

Monitoring Parameters Assess patient at beginning and throughout therapy for infection; monitor for signs of anaphylaxis during first dose

Test Interactions Positive direct Coombs', false-positive urinary glucose test using cupric sulfate (Benedict's solution, Clinitest®, Fehling's solution), false-positive serum or urine creatinine with Jaffé reaction

Patient Information Chilling of the oral suspension improves flavor (do not freeze); report persistent diarrhea; take entire course of medication; may interfere with oral contraceptives; females should report symptoms of vaginitis

Dosage Forms

Capsule: 250 mg, 500 mg

Powder for oral suspension: 125 mg/5 mL (75 mL, 150 mL); 187 mg/5 mL (50 mL, 100 mL); 250 mg/5 mL (75 mL, 150 mL); 375 mg/5 mL (50 mL, 100 mL)

Tablet, chewable (Raniclor™): 125 mg [contains phenylalanine 2.8 mg; fruity flavor], 187 mg [contains phenylalanine 4.2 mg; fruity flavor], 250 mg [contains phenylalanine 5.6 mg; fruity flavor], 375 mg [contains phenylalanine 8.4 mg; fruity flavor]

Selected Readings

Donowitz GR and Mandell GL, "Beta-Lactam Antibiotics," *N Engl J Med*, 1988, 318(7):419-26 and 318(8):490-500.

Marshall WF and Blair JE, "The Cephalosporins," *Mayo Clin Proc*, 1999, 74(2):187-95.

Smith GH, "Oral Cephalosporins in Perspective," *DICP*, 1990, 24(1):45-51.

Cefadroxil (sef a DROKS il)

Related Information

Antimicrobial Activity Against Selected Organisms *on page 1165*

U.S. Brand Names Duricef®

Canadian Brand Names Apo-Cefadroxil®; Duricef®; Novo-Cefadroxil

Synonyms Cefadroxil Monohydrate

Generic Available Yes: Capsule, tablet

Use Treatment of susceptible bacterial infections, including those caused by group A beta-hemolytic *Streptococcus*; prophylaxis against bacterial endocarditis in patients who are allergic to penicillin and undergoing surgical or dental procedures

Pregnancy Risk Factor B

Contraindications Hypersensitivity to cefadroxil, other cephalosporins, or any component of the formulation

Warnings/Precautions Modify dosage in patients with severe renal impairment; prolonged use may result in superinfection; use with caution in patients with a history of penicillin allergy especially IgE-mediated reactions (eg, anaphylaxis, angioedema, urticaria). May cause antibiotic-associated colitis or colitis secondary to *C. difficile.*

Adverse Reactions

1% to 10%: Gastrointestinal: Diarrhea

<1%: Anaphylaxis, rash (maculopapular and erythematous), erythema multiforme, Stevens-Johnson syndrome, serum sickness, arthralgia, urticaria, pruritus, angioedema, pseudomembranous colitis, abdominal pain, dyspepsia, nausea, vomiting, cholestasis, vaginitis, neutropenia, agranulocytosis, thrombocytopenia, transaminases increased, fever

Reactions reported with other cephalosporins include toxic epidermal necrolysis, abdominal pain, superinfection. renal dysfunction, toxic nephropathy, aplastic anemia, hemolytic anemia, hemorrhage, prolonged prothrombin time, increased BUN, increased creatinine, eosinophilia, pancytopenia, seizure

Overdosage/Toxicology After acute overdose, most agents cause only nausea, vomiting, and diarrhea, although neuromuscular hypersensitivity and seizures are possible, especially in patients with renal insufficiency. Many beta-lactam antibiotics have the potential to cause neuromuscular hyperirritability or seizures. Hemodialysis may be helpful to aid in removal of the drug from the blood, but is not usually indicated; otherwise, most treatment is supportive or symptom-directed, following GI decontamination.

Drug Interactions

Increased Effect/Toxicity: Bleeding may occur when administered with anticoagulants. Probenecid may decrease cephalosporin elimination.

Ethanol/Nutrition/Herb Interactions Food: Concomitant administration with food, infant formula, or cow's milk does **not** significantly affect absorption.

Stability Refrigerate suspension after reconstitution; discard after 14 days

Mechanism of Action Inhibits bacterial cell wall synthesis by binding to one or more of the penicillin-binding proteins (PBPs) which in turn inhibits the final transpeptidation step of peptidoglycan synthesis in bacterial cell walls, thus inhibiting cell wall biosynthesis. Bacteria eventually lyse due to ongoing activity of cell wall autolytic enzymes (autolysins and murein hydrolases) while cell wall assembly is arrested.

Pharmacodynamics/Kinetics

Absorption: Rapid and well absorbed

Distribution: Widely throughout the body and reaches therapeutic concentrations in most tissues and body fluids, including synovial, pericardial, pleural, and peritoneal fluids; bile, sputum, and urine; bone, myocardium, gallbladder, skin and soft tissue; crosses placenta; enters breast milk

Protein binding: 20%

Half-life elimination: 1-2 hours; Renal failure: 20-24 hours

Time to peak, serum: 70-90 minutes

Excretion: Urine (>90% as unchanged drug)

Dosage Oral:

Children: 30 mg/kg/day divided twice daily up to a maximum of 2 g/day

Adults: 1-2 g/day in 2 divided doses

Prophylaxis against bacterial endocarditis:

- Children: 50 mg/kg 1 hour prior to the procedure
- Adults: 2 g 1 hour prior to the procedure

Dosing interval in renal impairment:

- Cl_{cr} 10-25 mL/minute: Administer every 24 hours
- Cl_{cr} <10 mL/minute: Administer every 36 hours

Administration Administer around-the-clock to promote less variation in peak and trough serum levels.

Monitoring Parameters Observe for signs and symptoms of anaphylaxis during first dose

Test Interactions Positive direct Coombs', false-positive urinary glucose test using cupric sulfate (Benedict's solution, Clinitest®, Fehling's solution), false-positive serum or urine creatinine with Jaffé reaction

(Continued)

Cefadroxil *(Continued)*

Patient Information Report persistent diarrhea; take entire course of medication; may interfere with oral contraceptives; females should report symptoms of vaginitis

Dosage Forms

Capsule, as monohydrate: 500 mg

Powder for oral suspension, as monohydrate: 250 mg/5 mL (50 mL, 100 mL); 500 mg/5 mL (75 mL, 100 mL) [contains sodium benzoate; orange-pineapple flavor]

Tablet, as monohydrate: 1 g

Selected Readings

Donowitz GR and Mandell GL, "Beta-Lactam Antibiotics," *N Engl J Med*, 1988, 318(7):419-26 and 318(8):490-500.

Marshall WF and Blair JE, "The Cephalosporins," *Mayo Clin Proc*, 1999, 74(2):187-95.

Smith GH, "Oral Cephalosporins in Perspective," *DICP*, 1990, 24(1):45-51.

Cefadroxil Monohydrate *see* Cefadroxil *on page 698*

Cefazolin (sef A zoe lin)

Related Information

Animal and Human Bites *on page 1270*

Antibiotic Treatment of Adults With Infective Endocarditis *on page 1271*

Antimicrobial Activity Against Selected Organisms *on page 1165*

U.S. Brand Names Ancef®

Synonyms Cefazolin Sodium

Generic Available Yes

Use Treatment of respiratory tract, skin and skin structure, genital, urinary tract, biliary tract, bone and joint infections, and septicemia due to susceptible gram-positive cocci (except enterococcus); some gram-negative bacilli including *E. coli*, *Proteus*, and *Klebsiella* may be susceptible; perioperative prophylaxis

Unlabeled/Investigational Use Prophylaxis against bacterial endocarditis

Drug of Choice or Alternative for Disease/Syndrome(s):

Catheter Infection, Intravascular *on page 70*

Intra-abdominal Abscess *on page 194*

Joint Replacement, Late Infection *on page 198*

Mastitis *on page 214*

Peritonitis, CAPD-Associated *on page 262*

Urinary Tract Infection, Perinephric Abscess *on page 345*

Pregnancy Risk Factor B

Contraindications Hypersensitivity to cefazolin sodium, any component of the formulation, or other cephalosporins

Warnings/Precautions Modify dosage in patients with severe renal impairment; prolonged use may result in superinfection; use with caution in patients with a history of penicillin allergy especially IgE-mediated reactions (eg, anaphylaxis, angioedema, urticaria). May cause antibiotic-associated colitis or colitis secondary to *C. difficile*.

Adverse Reactions Frequency not defined.

Central nervous system: Fever, seizure

Dermatologic: Rash, pruritus, Stevens-Johnson syndrome

Gastrointestinal: Diarrhea. nausea, vomiting, abdominal cramps, anorexia, pseudomembranous colitis, oral candidiasis

Genitourinary: Vaginitis

Hepatic: Transaminases increased, hepatitis

Hematologic: Eosinophilia, neutropenia, leukopenia, thrombocytopenia, thrombocytosis

Local: Pain at injection site, phlebitis

Renal: BUN increased, serum creatinine increased, renal failure

Miscellaneous: Anaphylaxis

Reactions reported with other cephalosporins include toxic epidermal necrolysis, abdominal pain, cholestasis, superinfection, toxic nephropathy, aplastic anemia, hemolytic anemia, hemorrhage, prolonged prothrombin time, pancytopenia

Overdosage/Toxicology Symptoms include neuromuscular hypersensitivity and convulsions especially with renal insufficiency. Many beta-lactam antibiotics have the potential to cause neuromuscular hyperirritability or seizures. Hemodialysis may be helpful to aid in removal of the drug from the blood; otherwise, most treatment is supportive or symptom-directed.

Drug Interactions

Increased Effect/Toxicity: High-dose probenecid decreases clearance and increases effect of cefazolin. Aminoglycosides increase nephrotoxic potential when taken with cefazolin. Cefazolin may increase the hypothrombinemic response to warfarin (due to alteration of GI microbial flora).

Stability Store intact vials at room temperature and protect from temperatures exceeding 40°C. Dilute large vial with 2.5 mL SWFI; 10 g vial may be diluted with 45 mL to yield 1 g/5 mL or 96 mL to yield 1 g/10 mL. May be injected or further dilution for I.V. administration in 50-100 mL compatible solution. Standard diluent is 1 g/50 mL D_5W or 2 g/50 mL D_5W.

Reconstituted solutions of cefazolin are light yellow to yellow. Protection from light is recommended for the powder and for the reconstituted solutions. Reconstituted solutions are stable for 24 hours at room temperature and for 10 days under refrigeration. Stability of parenteral admixture at room temperature (25°C) is 48 hours. Stability of parenteral admixture at refrigeration temperature (4°C) is 14 days.

DUPLEX™: Store at 20°C to 25°C (68°F to 77°F); excursions permitted to 15°C to 30°C (59°F to 86°F) prior to activation. Following activation, stable for 24 hours at room temperature and for 7 days under refrigeration.

Mechanism of Action Inhibits bacterial cell wall synthesis by binding to one or more of the penicillin-binding proteins (PBPs) which in turn inhibits the final transpeptidation step of peptidoglycan synthesis in bacterial cell walls, thus inhibiting cell wall biosynthesis. Bacteria eventually lyse due to ongoing activity of cell wall autolytic enzymes (autolysins and murein hydrolases) while cell wall assembly is arrested.

Pharmacodynamics/Kinetics

Distribution: Widely into most body tissues and fluids including gallbladder, liver, kidneys, bone, sputum, bile, pleural, and synovial; CSF penetration is poor; crosses placenta; enters breast milk

Protein binding: 74% to 86%

Metabolism: Minimally hepatic

Half-life elimination: 90-150 minutes; prolonged with renal impairment

Time to peak, serum: I.M.: 0.5-2 hours

Excretion: Urine (80% to 100% as unchanged drug)

Dosage I.M., I.V.:

Children >1 month: 25-100 mg/kg/day divided every 6-8 hours; maximum: 6 g/day

Adults: 250 mg to 2 g every 6-12 (usually 8) hours, depending on severity of infection; maximum dose: 12 g/day

Prophylaxis against bacterial endocarditis (unlabeled use):

Infants and Children: 25 mg/kg 30 minutes before procedure; maximum dose: 1 g

Adults: 1 g 30 minutes before procedure

Dosing adjustment in renal impairment:

Cl_{cr} 10-30 mL/minute: Administer every 12 hours

Cl_{cr} <10 mL/minute: Administer every 24 hours

Hemodialysis: Moderately dialyzable (20% to 50%); administer dose postdialysis or administer supplemental dose of 0.5-1 g after dialysis

Peritoneal dialysis: Administer 0.5 g every 12 hours

Continuous arteriovenous or venovenous hemofiltration: Dose as for Cl_{cr} 10-30 mL/minute; removes 30 mg of cefazolin per liter of filtrate per day

Dietary Considerations Sodium content of 1 g: 48 mg (2 mEq)

Administration

I.M.: Inject deep I.M. into large muscle mass

I.V.: Inject direct I.V. over 5 minutes. Infuse intermittent infusion over 30-60 minutes.

Monitoring Parameters Renal function periodically when used in combination with other nephrotoxic drugs, hepatic function tests, CBC; monitor for signs of anaphylaxis during first dose

Test Interactions Positive direct Coombs', false-positive urinary glucose test using cupric sulfate (Benedict's solution, Clinitest®, Fehling's solution), false-positive serum or urine creatinine with Jaffé reaction

Dosage Forms

[DSC] = Discontinued product

Infusion [premixed in D_5W]: 500 mg (50 mL); 1 g (50 mL)

Injection, powder for reconstitution: 500 mg, 1 g, 10 g, 20 g

Ancef®: 1 g; 10 g [DSC]

Selected Readings

Donowitz GR and Mandell GL, "Beta-Lactam Antibiotics," *N Engl J Med*, 1988, 318(7):419-26 and 318(8):490-500.

Gentry LO, Zeluff BJ, and Cooley DA, "Antibiotic Prophylaxis in Open-Heart Surgery: A Comparison of Cefamandole, Cefuroxime, and Cefazolin," *Ann Thorac Surg*, 1988, 46(2):167-71.

Marshall WF and Blair JE, "The Cephalosporins," *Mayo Clin Proc*, 1999, 74(2):187-95.

Peterson CD, Lake KD, Arom KV, et al, "Antibiotic Prophylaxis in Open-Heart Surgery Patients: Comparison of Cefamandole and Cefuroxime," *Drug Intell Clin Pharm*, 1987, 21(9):728-32.

Cefazolin Sodium *see* Cefazolin *on page 700*

Cefdinir (SEF di ner)

U.S. Brand Names Omnicef®

Canadian Brand Names Omnicef®

Synonyms CFDN

Generic Available No

Use Treatment of community-acquired pneumonia, acute exacerbations of chronic bronchitis, acute bacterial otitis media, acute maxillary sinusitis, pharyngitis/tonsillitis, and uncomplicated skin and skin structure infections.

Pregnancy Risk Factor B

Pregnancy Implications Teratogenic effects were not observed in animal studies. There are no adequate and well-controlled studies in pregnant women.

Contraindications Hypersensitivity to cefdinir, other cephalosporins, related antibiotics, or any component of the formulation

Warnings/Precautions Administer cautiously to penicillin-sensitive patients, especially IgE-mediated reactions (eg, anaphylaxis, urticaria). There is evidence of partial cross-allergenicity and cephalosporins cannot be assumed to be an absolutely safe alternative to penicillin in the penicillin-allergic patient. Serum sickness-like reactions have been reported. Signs and symptoms occur after a few days of therapy and resolve a few days after drug discontinuation with no serious sequelae. Pseudomembranous colitis occurs; consider its diagnosis in patients who develop diarrhea with antibiotic use. Use caution with renal dysfunction; dose adjustment may be required.

Adverse Reactions

>10%: Gastrointestinal: Diarrhea (8% to 15%)

1% to 10%:

- Central nervous system: Headache (2%)
- Dermatologic: Rash (≤3%)
- Gastrointestinal: Nausea (≤3%), abdominal pain (≤1%), vomiting (≤1%)
- Genitourinary: Vaginal moniliasis (≤4%), urine leukocytes increased (2%), urine protein increased (1% to 2%), vaginitis (≤1%)
- Hematologic: Eosinophils increased (1%)
- Hepatic: Alkaline phosphatase increased (≤1%), platelets increased (1%)
- Renal: Microhematuria (1%)
- Miscellaneous: Lymphocytes increased (≤2%), GGT increased (1%), lactate dehydrogenase increased (≤1%), bicarbonate decreased (≤1%), lymphocytes decreased (≤1%), PMN changes (≤1%)

<1% (Limited to importantor life-threatening): Anorexia, constipation, cutaneous moniliasis, dizziness, dyspepsia, flatulence, hyperkinesia, insomnia, leukopenia, leukorrhea, maculopapular rash, moniliasis, pruritus, somnolence, stools abnormal, weakness, xerostomia

Postmarketing and/or case reports: Allergic vasculitis, amylase increased, anaphylaxis, bleeding tendency, bloody diarrhea, cardiac failure, chest pain, cholestasis, coagulation disorder, conjunctivitis, disseminated intravascular coagulation, enterocolitis (acute), eosinophilic pneumonia, erythema multiforme, erythema nodosum, exfoliative dermatitis, facial edema, fever, fulminant hepatitis, granulocytopenia, hemolytic anemia, hemorrhagic colitis, hepatic failure, hepatitis (acute), hypertension, idiopathic thrombocytopenia purpura, ileus, interstitial pneumonia (idiopathic), involuntary movement, jaundice, laryngeal edema, loss of consciousness, melena, myocardial infarction, nephropathy, pancytopenia, peptic ulcer, pneumonia (drug-induced), pseudomembranous colitis, renal failure (acute), respiratory failure (acute), rhabdomyolysis, serum sickness, shock, Stevens-Johnson syndrome, stomatitis, thrombocytopenia, toxic epidermal necrolysis, upper GI bleed

Reactions reported with other cephalosporins include dizziness, fever, encephalopathy, asterixis, neuromuscular excitability, seizure, aplastic anemia, interstitial nephritis, toxic nephropathy, angioedema, hemorrhage, prolonged PT, and superinfection

Overdosage/Toxicology After acute overdose, most agents cause only nausea, vomiting, and diarrhea, although neuromuscular hypersensitivity and seizures are possible, especially in patients with renal insufficiency. Hemodialysis may be helpful to aid in the removal of the drug from the blood but not usually indicated, otherwise, most treatment is supportive or symptom-directed following GI decontamination.

Drug Interactions

Increased Effect/Toxicity: Probenecid may increase the effects of cefdinir by decreasing renal elimination (peak plasma levels of cefdinir are increased by 54% and half-life is prolonged by 50%).

Decreased Effect: Coadministration with iron or antacids reduces the rate and extent of cefdinir absorption.

Stability Capsules and unmixed powder should be stored at room temperature of 25°C (77°F). Oral suspension should be mixed with 38 mL water for the 60 mL bottle and

63 mL of water for the 120 mL bottle. After mixing, the suspension can be stored at room temperature of 25°C (77°F) for 10 days.

Mechanism of Action Inhibits bacterial cell wall synthesis by binding to one or more of the penicillin-binding proteins (PBPs) which in turn inhibits the final transpeptidation step of peptidoglycan synthesis in bacterial cell walls, thus inhibiting cell wall biosynthesis. Bacteria eventually lyse due to ongoing activity of cell wall autolytic enzymes (autolysins and murein hydrolases) while cell wall assembly is arrested.

Pharmacodynamics/Kinetics

Distribution: V_d:

Children 6 months to 12 years: 0.29-1.05 L/kg

Adults: 0.06-0.64 L/kg

Protein binding: 60% to 70%

Metabolism: Minimally hepatic

Bioavailability: Capsule: 16% to 21%; suspension 25%

Half-life elimination: 100 minutes

Excretion: Primarily urine

Dosage Oral:

Children 6 months to 12 years:

Acute bacterial otitis media, pharyngitis/tonsillitis: 7 mg/kg/dose twice daily for 5-10 days **or** 14 mg/kg/dose once daily for 10 days (maximum: 600 mg/day)

Acute maxillary sinusitis: 7 mg/kg/dose twice daily **or** 14 mg/kg/dose once daily for 10 days (maximum: 600 mg/day)

Uncomplicated skin and skin structure infections: 7 mg/kg/dose twice daily for 10 days (maximum: 600 mg/day)

Adolescents and Adults:

Community-acquired pneumonia, uncomplicated skin and skin structure infections: 300 mg twice daily for 10 days

Acute exacerbations of chronic bronchitis, pharyngitis/tonsillitis: 300 mg twice daily for 5-10 days **or** 600 mg once daily for 10 days

Acute maxillary sinusitis: 300 mg twice daily **or** 600 mg once daily for 10 days

Dosing adjustment in renal impairment: Cl_{cr} <30 mL/minute:

Children: 7 mg/kg once daily (maximum: 300 mg/day)

Adults: 300 mg once daily

Hemodialysis removes cefdinir; recommended initial dose: 300 mg (or 7 mg/kg/dose) every other day. At the conclusion of each hemodialysis session, 300 mg (or 7 mg/kg/dose) should be given. Subsequent doses (300 mg or 7 mg/kg/dose) should be administered every other day.

Dietary Considerations Suspension contains sucrose 2.86 g/5 mL

Administration Twice daily doses should be given every 12 hours. May be taken with or without food. The suspension should be shaken well before each administration.

Monitoring Parameters Observe for signs and symptoms of anaphylaxis during first dose

Dosage Forms

Capsule: 300 mg

Powder for oral suspension: 125 mg/5 mL (60 mL, 100 mL) [contains sodium benzoate and sucrose 2.86 g/5 mL; strawberry flavor]; 250 mg/5 mL (60 mL, 100 mL) [contains sodium benzoate and sucrose 2.86 g/5 mL; strawberry flavor]

Selected Readings

Guay DR, "Cefdinir: An Expanded-Spectrum Oral Cephalosporin," *Ann Pharmacother*, 2000, 34(12):1469-77.

Marshall WF and Blair JE, "The Cephalosporins," *Mayo Clin Proc*, 1999, 74(2):187-95.

Cefditoren (sef de TOR en)

U.S. Brand Names Spectracef™

Synonyms Cefditoren Pivoxil

Generic Available No

Use Treatment of acute bacterial exacerbation of chronic bronchitis or community-acquired pneumonia (due to susceptible organisms including *Haemophilus influenzae*, *Haemophilus parainfluenzae*, *Streptococcus pneumoniae*-penicillin susceptible only, *Moraxella catarrhalis*); pharyngitis or tonsillitis (*Streptococcus pyogenes*); and uncomplicated skin and skin-structure infections (*Staphylococcus aureus* - not MRSA, *Streptococcus pyogenes*)

Pregnancy Risk Factor B

Pregnancy Implications There are no adequate and well-controlled studies in pregnant women; use only if clearly needed.

Contraindications Hypersensitivity to cefditoren, other cephalosporins, milk protein, or any component of the formulation; carnitine deficiency

(Continued)

Cefditoren *(Continued)*

Warnings/Precautions Use with caution in patients with a history of penicillin allergy, especially IgE-mediated reactions (eg, anaphylaxis, urticaria). May cause antibiotic-associated colitis or colitis secondary to *C. difficile*. Modify dosage in patients with severe renal impairment. Caution in individuals with seizure disorders. Prolonged use may result in superinfection. Use caution in patients with renal or hepatic impairment. Cefditoren causes renal excretion of carnitine, do not use in patients with carnitine deficiency; not for long-term therapy due to the possible development of carnitine deficiency over time. Cefditoren tablets contain sodium caseinate, which may cause hypersensitivity reactions in patients with milk protein hypersensitivity; this does not affect patients with lactose intolerance. Safety and efficacy have not been established in children <12 years of age.

Adverse Reactions

>10%: Gastrointestinal: Diarrhea (11% to 15%)

1% to 10%:

Central nervous system: Headache (2% to 3%)

Endocrine & metabolic: Glucose increased (1%)

Gastrointestinal: Nausea (4% to 6%), abdominal pain (2%), dyspepsia (1% to 2%), vomiting (1%)

Genitourinary: Vaginal moniliasis (3% to 6%)

Hematologic: Hematocrit decreased (2%)

Renal: Hematuria (3%), urinary white blood cells increased (2%)

<1%: Abnormal dreams, acute renal failure, serum albumin decreased, allergic reaction, anorexia, appetite increased, arthralgia, BUN increased, serum calcium, decreased serum chloride, increased serum cholesterol, coagulation time increased, constipation, diaphoresis, dizziness, dry mouth, eosinophilic pneumonia, eosinophils increased, eructation, fever, flatulence, fungal infection, gastritis, gastrointestinal disorder, hemoglobin decreased, hyperglycemia, inorganic phosphorus decreased, insomnia, interstitial pneumonia, leukopenia, lymphocytes increased, mouth ulceration, myalgia, nervousness, neutrophils decreased, oral moniliasis, pain, peripheral edema, pharyngitis, platelet count increased, positive direct Coombs' test, potassium increased, pseudomembranous colitis, proteinuria, pruritus, rash, rhinitis, SGOT increased, SGPT increased, sinusitis, somnolence, stomatitis, taste perversion, thrombocytopenia, urinary frequency, urticaria, vaginitis, weakness, weight loss, white blood cell increase/decrease

Additional adverse effects seen with cephalosporin antibiotics: Anaphylaxis, aplastic anemia, cholestasis, erythema multiforme, hemorrhage, hemolytic anemia, renal dysfunction, reversible hyperactivity, serum sickness-like reaction, Stevens-Johnson syndrome, toxic epidermal necrolysis, toxic nephropathy

Drug Interactions

Increased Effect/Toxicity: Increased levels of cefditoren with probenecid.

Decreased Effect: Antacids and H_2 receptor antagonists decrease cefditoren levels.

Ethanol/Nutrition/Herb Interactions Food: Moderate- to high-fat meals increase bioavailability and maximum plasma concentration.

Stability Store at controlled room temperature of 25°C (77°F). Protect from light and moisture.

Mechanism of Action Inhibits bacterial cell wall synthesis by binding to one or more of the penicillin binding proteins (PBPs); which in turn inhibits the final transpeptidation step of peptidoglycan synthesis in bacterial cell walls, thus inhibiting cell wall biosynthesis. Bacteria eventually lyse due to ongoing activity of cell wall autolytic enzymes (autolysins and murein hydrolases) while cell wall assembly is arrested.

Pharmacodynamics/Kinetics

Distribution: 9.3 ± 1.6 L

Protein binding: 88% (*in vitro*), primarily to albumin

Metabolism: Cefditoren pivoxil is hydrolyzed to cefditoren (active) and pivalate

Bioavailability: ~14% to 16%, increased by moderate to high-fat meal

Half-life elimination: 1.6 ± 0.4 hours

Time to peak: 1.5-3 hours

Excretion: Urine (as cefditoren and pivaloylcarnitine)

Dosage Oral: Children ≥12 years and Adults:

Acute bacterial exacerbation of chronic bronchitis: 400 mg twice daily for 10 days

Community-acquired pneumonia: 400 mg twice daily for 14 days

Pharyngitis, tonsillitis, uncomplicated skin and skin structure infections: 200 mg twice daily for 10 days

Treatment of dental infections (unlabeled use): 400 mg twice daily for 10 days

Elderly: Refer to adult dosing

Dosage adjustment in renal impairment:

Cl_{cr} 30-49 mL/minute: Maximum dose: 200 mg twice daily

Cl_{cr} <30 mL/minute: Maximum dose: 200 mg once daily
End-stage renal disease: Appropriate dosing not established

Dosage adjustment in hepatic impairment:
Mild or moderate impairment: Adjustment not required
Severe impairment (Child-Pugh Class C): Specific guidelines not available

Dietary Considerations Cefditoren should be taken with meals. Plasma carnitine levels are decreased during therapy (39% with 200 mg dosing, 63% with 400 mg dosing); normal concentrations return within 7-10 days after treatment is discontinued.

Administration Should be administered with meals.

Monitoring Parameters Assess patient at beginning and throughout therapy for infection; monitor for signs of anaphylaxis during first dose.

Test Interactions May cause a false-negative ferricyanide test; false-positive urine glucose test when using Clinitest®

Patient Information Take entire course of medication. Report persistent diarrhea. Females should report symptoms of vaginitis.

Dosage Forms Tablet, as pivoxil: 200 mg [equivalent to cefditoren; contains sodium caseinate]

Selected Readings

Darkes MJ and Plosker GL, "Cefditoren Pivoxil," *Drugs*, 2002, 62(2):319-36.

Cefditoren Pivoxil *see* Cefditoren *on page 703*

Cefepime (SEF e pim)

Related Information

Antimicrobial Activity Against Selected Organisms *on page 1165*
Neutropenic Fever Guidelines *on page 1295*

U.S. Brand Names Maxipime®

Canadian Brand Names Maxipime®

Synonyms Cefepime Hydrochloride

Generic Available No

Use Treatment of uncomplicated and complicated urinary tract infections, including pyelonephritis caused by typical urinary tract pathogens; monotherapy for febrile neutropenia; uncomplicated skin and skin structure infections caused by *Streptococcus pyogenes*; moderate to severe pneumonia caused by pneumococcus, *Pseudomonas aeruginosa*, and other gram-negative organisms; complicated intra-abdominal infections (in combination with metronidazole). Also active against methicillin-susceptible staphylococci, *Enterobacter* sp, and many other gram-negative bacilli.

Children 2 months to 16 years: Empiric therapy of febrile neutropenia patients, uncomplicated skin/soft tissue infections, pneumonia, and uncomplicated/complicated urinary tract infections.

Drug of Choice or Alternative for Disease/Syndrome(s):

Endocarditis, Acute, I.V. Drug Abuse *on page 123*
Endocarditis, Prosthetic Valve, Early *on page 124*
Endocarditis, Prosthetic Valve, Late *on page 125*
Fever, Neutropenic *on page 148*
Intra-abdominal Abscess *on page 194*
Meningitis, Postsurgical *on page 218*
Peritonitis, Spontaneous Bacterial *on page 264*
Pneumonia, Community-Acquired *on page 270*
Pneumonia, Hospital-Acquired *on page 272*
Pneumonia, Ventilator-Associated *on page 273*

Organism(s):

Enterobacter Species *on page 132*
Pseudomonas aeruginosa on page 282

Pregnancy Risk Factor B

Contraindications Hypersensitivity to cefepime, any component of the formulation, or other cephalosporins

Warnings/Precautions Modify dosage in patients with severe renal impairment; prolonged use may result in superinfection; use with caution in patients with a history of penicillin or cephalosporin allergy, especially IgE-mediated reactions (eg, anaphylaxis, urticaria). May cause antibiotic-associated colitis or colitis secondary to *C. difficile*.

Adverse Reactions

>10%: Hematologic: Positive Coombs' test without hemolysis

1% to 10%:

Central nervous system: Fever (1%), headache (1%)

(Continued)

Cefepime *(Continued)*

Dermatologic: Rash, pruritus
Gastrointestinal: Diarrhea, nausea, vomiting
Local: Pain, erythema at injection site

<1%: Anaphylactic shock, anaphylaxis, agranulocytosis, coma, encephalopathy, hallucinations, leukopenia, myoclonus, neuromuscular excitability, neutropenia, seizure, thrombocytopenia

Reactions reported with other cephalosporins include aplastic anemia, erythema multiforme, hemolytic anemia, hemorrhage, pancytopenia, prolonged PT, renal dysfunction, Stevens-Johnson syndrome, superinfection, toxic epidermal necrolysis, toxic nephropathy, vaginitis

Overdosage/Toxicology Symptoms include neuromuscular hypersensitivity and CNS toxicity (including hallucinations, confusion, seizures, and coma). Many beta-lactam antibiotics have the potential to cause neuromuscular hyperirritability or seizures. Hemodialysis may be helpful to aid in the removal of the drug from the blood, however, most often treatment is supportive and symptom-directed.

Drug Interactions

Increased Effect/Toxicity: High-dose probenecid decreases clearance and increases effect of cefepime. Aminoglycosides increase nephrotoxic potential when taken with cefepime.

Stability Cefepime is **compatible** and stable with normal saline, D_5W, and a variety of other solutions for 24 hours at room temperature and 7 days refrigerated

Mechanism of Action Inhibits bacterial cell wall synthesis by binding to one or more of the penicillin-binding proteins (PBPs) which in turn inhibits the final transpeptidation step of peptidoglycan synthesis in bacterial cell walls, thus inhibiting cell wall biosynthesis. Bacteria eventually lyse due to ongoing activity of cell wall autolytic enzymes (autolysis and murein hydrolases) while cell wall assembly is arrested.

Pharmacodynamics/Kinetics

Absorption: I.M.: Rapid and complete
Distribution: V_d: Adults: 14-20 L; penetrates into inflammatory fluid at concentrations ~80% of serum levels and into bronchial mucosa at levels ~60% of those reached in the plasma; crosses blood-brain barrier
Protein binding, plasma: 16% to 19%
Metabolism: Minimally hepatic
Half-life elimination: 2 hours
Time to peak: 0.5-1.5 hours
Excretion: Urine (85% as unchanged drug)

Dosage

Children:
Febrile neutropenia: I.V.: 50 mg/kg every 8 hours for 7-10 days
Uncomplicated skin/soft tissue infections, pneumonia, and complicated/uncomplicated UTI: I.V.: 50 mg/kg twice daily

Adults:
Most infections: I.V.: 1-2 g every 12 hours for 7-10 days; higher doses or more frequent administration may be required in pseudomonal infections
Urinary tract infections, mild to moderate: I.M., I.V.: 500-1000 mg every 12 hours
Monotherapy for febrile neutropenic patients: I.V.: 2 g every 8 hours for 7 days or until the neutropenia resolves

Dosing adjustment in renal impairment: Adults: Recommended maintenance schedule based on creatinine clearance (mL/minute), compared to normal dosing schedule: See table.

Cefepime Hydrochloride

Creatinine Clearance (mL/minute)	Recommended Maintenance Schedule			
>60 Normal recommended dosing schedule	500 mg every 12 hours	1 g every 12 hours	2 g every 12 hours	2 g every 8 hours
30-60	500 mg every 24 hours	1 g every 24 hours	2 g every 24 hours	2 g every 12 hours
11-29	500 mg every 24 hours	500 mg every 24 hours	1 g every 24 hours	2 g every 24 hours
<11	250 mg every 24 hours	250 mg every 24 hours	500 mg every 24 hours	1 g every 24 hours

Hemodialysis: Initial: 1 g (single dose) on day 1. Maintenance: 500 mg once daily (1 g once daily in febrile neutropenic patients). Dosage should be administered after dialysis on dialysis days.

Peritoneal dialysis: Removed to a lesser extent than hemodialysis; administer 250 mg every 48 hours

Continuous arteriovenous or venovenous hemofiltration: Dose as normal Cl_{cr} (eg, >30 mL/minute)

Administration May be administered either I.M. or I.V.

Monitoring Parameters Obtain specimen for culture and sensitivity prior to the first dose; monitor for signs of anaphylaxis during first dose

Test Interactions Positive direct Coombs', false-positive urinary glucose test using cupric sulfate (Benedict's solution, Clinitest®, Fehling's solution), false-positive serum or urine creatinine with Jaffé reaction, false-positive urinary proteins and steroids

Patient Information Report side effects such as diarrhea, dyspepsia, headache, blurred vision, and lightheadedness.

Dosage Forms Injection, powder for reconstitution, as hydrochloride: 500 mg, 1 g, 2 g

Selected Readings

Barradell LB and Bryson HM, "Cefepime. A Review of Its Antibacterial Activity, Pharmacokinetic Properties, and Therapeutic Use," *Drugs*, 1994, 47(3):471-505.

Cunha BA and Gill MV, "Cefepime," *Med Clin North Am*, 1995, 79(4):721-32.

Marshall WF and Blair JE, "The Cephalosporins," *Mayo Clin Proc*, 1999, 74(2):187-95.

Okamoto MP, Nakahiro RK, Chin A, et al, "Cefepime: A New Fourth-Generation Cephalosporin," *Am J Hosp Pharm*, 1994, 51(4):463-77.

Sanders CC, "Cefepime: The Next Generation?" *Clin Infect Dis*, 1993, 17(3):369-79.

Wynd MA and Paladino JA, "Cefepime: A Fourth-Generation Parenteral Cephalosporin," *Ann Pharmacother*, 1996, 30(12):1414-24.

Cefepime Hydrochloride *see* Cefepime *on page 705*

Cefixime (sef IKS eem)

Related Information

Antimicrobial Activity Against Selected Organisms *on page 1165*

U.S. Brand Names Suprax®

Canadian Brand Names Suprax®

Generic Available No

Use Treatment of urinary tract infections, otitis media, respiratory infections due to susceptible organisms including *S. pneumoniae* and *S. pyogenes*, *H. influenzae* and many Enterobacteriaceae; uncomplicated cervical/urethral gonorrhea due to *N. gonorrhoeae*

Drug of Choice or Alternative for

Disease/Syndrome(s):

Cervicitis *on page 71*

Organism(s):

Neisseria gonorrhoeae on page 244

Pregnancy Risk Factor B

Contraindications Hypersensitivity to cefixime, any component of the formulation, or other cephalosporins

Warnings/Precautions Prolonged use may result in superinfection; modify dosage in patients with renal impairment; use with caution in patients with a history of penicillin allergy especially IgE-mediated reactions (eg, anaphylaxis, urticaria). May cause antibiotic-associated colitis or colitis secondary to *C. difficile*.

Adverse Reactions

>10%: Gastrointestinal: Diarrhea (16%)

2% to 10%: Gastrointestinal: Abdominal pain, nausea, dyspepsia, flatulence, loose stools

<2%: Acute renal failure, anaphylactic/anaphylactoid reactions, angioedema, BUN increased, candidiasis, creatinine increased, dizziness, drug fever, eosinophilia, erythema multiforme, facial edema, fever, headache, hepatitis, hyperbilirubinemia, jaundice, leukopenia, neutropenia, prolonged PT, pruritus, pseudomembranous colitis, rash, seizure, serum sickness-like reaction, Stevens-Johnson syndrome, thrombocytopenia, toxic epidermal necrolysis, transaminases increased, urticaria, vaginitis, vomiting

Reactions reported with other cephalosporins include interstitial nephritis, aplastic anemia, hemolytic anemia, hemorrhage, pancytopenia, agranulocytosis, colitis, superinfection

Overdosage/Toxicology After acute overdose, most agents cause only nausea, vomiting, and diarrhea, although neuromuscular hypersensitivity and seizures are possible, especially in patients with renal insufficiency. Many beta-lactam antibiotics have the potential to cause neuromuscular hyperirritability or seizures. Hemodialysis may be helpful to aid in removal of the drug from the blood but is not usually indicated; otherwise, most treatment is supportive or symptom-directed, following GI decontamination.

(Continued)

Cefixime *(Continued)*

Drug Interactions

Increased Effect/Toxicity: Aminoglycosides and furosemide may be possible additives to nephrotoxicity. Probenecid increases cefixime concentration. Cefixime may increase carbamazepine. Cefixime may increase prothrombin time when administered with warfarin.

Ethanol/Nutrition/Herb Interactions Food: Delays cefixime absorption.

Stability After reconstitution, suspension may be stored for 14 days at room temperature or under refrigeration.

Mechanism of Action Inhibits bacterial cell wall synthesis by binding to one or more of the penicillin binding proteins (PBPs); which in turn inhibits the final transpeptidation step of peptidoglycan synthesis in bacterial cell walls, thus inhibiting cell wall biosynthesis. Bacteria eventually lyse due to ongoing activity of cell wall autolytic enzymes (autolysins and murein hydrolases) while cell wall assembly is arrested.

Pharmacodynamics/Kinetics

Absorption: 40% to 50%

Distribution: Widely throughout the body and reaches therapeutic concentration in most tissues and body fluids, including synovial, pericardial, pleural, peritoneal; bile, sputum, and urine; bone, myocardium, gallbladder, and skin and soft tissue

Protein binding: 65%

Half-life elimination: Normal renal function: 3-4 hours; Renal failure: Up to 11.5 hours

Time to peak, serum: 2-6 hours; delayed with food

Excretion: Urine (50% of absorbed dose as active drug); feces (10%)

Dosage Oral:

Children ≥6 months: 8 mg/kg/day divided every 12-24 hours

Children >50 kg or >12 years and Adults: 400 mg/day divided every 12-24 hours

Uncomplicated cervical/urethral gonorrhea due to *N. gonorrhoeae*: 400 mg as a single dose

For *S. pyogenes* infections, treat for 10 days

Dosing adjustment in renal impairment:

Cl_{cr} 21-60 mL/minute or with renal hemodialysis: Administer 75% of the standard dose

Cl_{cr} <20 mL/minute or with CAPD: Administer 50% of the standard dose

Moderately dialyzable (10%)

Dietary Considerations May be taken with food.

Administration May be administered with or without food; administer with food to decrease GI distress

Monitoring Parameters With prolonged therapy, monitor renal and hepatic function periodically; observe for signs and symptoms of anaphylaxis during first dose

Test Interactions Positive direct Coombs', false-positive urinary glucose test using cupric sulfate (Benedict's solution, Clinitest®, Fehling's solution), false-positive serum or urine creatinine with Jaffé reaction

Patient Information Report diarrhea promptly; take entire course of medication; may interfere with oral contraceptives, females should report symptoms of vaginitis

Additional Information Otitis media should be treated with the suspension since it results in higher peak blood levels than the tablet.

Dosage Forms

Powder for oral suspension: 100 mg/5 mL (50 mL, 75 mL, 100 mL) [contains sodium benzoate; strawberry flavor]

Selected Readings

Donowitz GR and Mandell GL, "Beta-Lactam Antibiotics," *N Engl J Med*, 1988, 318(7):419-26 and 318(8):490-500.

Markham A and Brogden RN, "Cefixime. A Review of Its Therapeutic Efficacy in Lower Respiratory Tract Infections," *Drugs*, 1995, 49(6):1007-22.

Marshall WF and Blair JE, "The Cephalosporins," *Mayo Clin Proc*, 1999, 74(2):187-95.

Schatz BS, Karavokiros KT, Taeubel MA, et al, "Comparison of Cefprozil, Cefpodoxime Proxetil, Loracarbef, Cefixime, and Ceftibuten," *Ann Pharmacother*, 1996, 30(3):258-68.

Smith GH, "Oral Cephalosporins in Perspective," *DICP*, 1990, 24(1):45-51.

Cefizox® *see* Ceftizoxime *on page 720*

Cefotan® *see* Cefotetan *on page 710*

Cefotaxime (sef oh TAKS eem)

Related Information

Antimicrobial Activity Against Selected Organisms *on page 1165*

Community-Acquired Pneumonia in Adults *on page 1278*

U.S. Brand Names Claforan®

Canadian Brand Names Claforan®

Synonyms Cefotaxime Sodium

Generic Available Yes: Powder

Use Treatment of susceptible infection in respiratory tract, skin and skin structure, bone and joint, urinary tract, gynecologic as well as septicemia, and documented or suspected meningitis. Active against most gram-negative bacilli (not *Pseudomonas*) and gram-positive cocci (not enterococcus). Active against many penicillin-resistant pneumococci.

Drug of Choice or Alternative for Disease/Syndrome(s):

Intra-abdominal Abscess *on page 194*
Liver Abscess *on page 211*
Meningitis, Community-Acquired, Adult *on page 216*
Meningitis, Neonatal (<1 month of age) *on page 217*
Meningitis, Pediatric (>1 month of age) *on page 218*
Meningitis, Post-traumatic *on page 219*
Peritonitis, Spontaneous Bacterial *on page 264*
Pneumonia, Community-Acquired *on page 270*

Organism(s):

Borrelia burgdorferi on page 56
Neisseria gonorrhoeae on page 244
Neisseria meningitidis on page 245
Streptococcus pneumoniae, Drug-Resistant *on page 316*

Pregnancy Risk Factor B

Contraindications Hypersensitivity to cefotaxime, any component of the formulation, or other cephalosporins

Warnings/Precautions Modify dosage in patients with severe renal impairment; prolonged use may result in superinfection; a potentially life-threatening arrhythmia has been reported in patients who received a rapid bolus injection via central line. Use caution in patients with colitis; minimize tissue inflammation by changing infusion sites when needed. Use with caution in patients with a history of penicillin allergy especially IgE-mediated reactions (eg, anaphylaxis, urticaria). May cause antibiotic-associated colitis or colitis secondary to *C. difficile*.

Adverse Reactions

1% to 10%:

Dermatologic: Rash, pruritus
Gastrointestinal: Diarrhea, nausea, vomiting, colitis
Local: Pain at injection site

<1%: Anaphylaxis, arrhythmia (after rapid IV injection via candidiasis, central catheter), BUN increased, creatinine increased, eosinophilia, erythema multiforme, fever, headache, interstitial nephritis, neutropenia, phlebitis, pseudomembranous colitis, Stevens-Johnson syndrome, thrombocytopenia, toxic epidermal necrolysis, transaminases increased, urticaria, vaginitis

Reactions reported with other cephalosporins include agranulocytosis, aplastic anemia, cholestasis, hemolytic anemia, hemorrhage, pancytopenia, renal dysfunction, seizure, superinfection, toxic nephropathy.

Overdosage/Toxicology Usually well tolerated even in overdose; convulsions are possible. Many beta-lactam antibiotics have the potential to cause neuromuscular hyperirritability or seizures. Hemodialysis may be helpful to aid in removal of the drug from the blood; otherwise, most treatment is supportive or symptom-directed.

Drug Interactions

Increased Effect/Toxicity: Probenecid may decrease cephalosporin elimination resulting in increased levels. Furosemide, aminoglycosides in combination with cefotaxime may result in additive nephrotoxicity.

Stability Reconstituted solution is stable for 12-24 hours at room temperature and 7-10 days when refrigerated and for 13 weeks when frozen; for I.V. infusion in NS or D_5W, solution is stable for 24 hours at room temperature, 5 days when refrigerated, or 13 weeks when frozen in Viaflex® plastic containers; thawed solutions previously of frozen premixed bags are stable for 24 hours at room temperature or 10 days when refrigerated

Mechanism of Action Inhibits bacterial cell wall synthesis by binding to one or more of the penicillin-binding proteins (PBPs) which in turn inhibits the final transpeptidation step of peptidoglycan synthesis in bacterial cell walls, thus inhibiting cell wall biosynthesis. Bacteria eventually lyse due to ongoing activity of cell wall autolytic enzymes (autolysins and murein hydrolases) while cell wall assembly is arrested.

Pharmacodynamics/Kinetics

Distribution: Widely to body tissues and fluids including aqueous humor, ascitic and prostatic fluids, bone; penetrates CSF best when meninges are inflamed; crosses placenta; enters breast milk

Metabolism: Partially hepatic to active metabolite, desacetylcefotaxime

(Continued)

Cefotaxime *(Continued)*

Half-life elimination:

Cefotaxime: Premature neonates <1 week: 5-6 hours; Full-term neonates <1 week: 2-3.4 hours; Adults: 1-1.5 hours; prolonged with renal and/or hepatic impairment

Desacetylcefotaxime: 1.5-1.9 hours; prolonged with renal impairment

Time to peak, serum: I.M.: Within 30 minutes

Excretion: Urine (as unchanged drug and metabolites)

Dosage

Infants and Children 1 month to 12 years: I.M., I.V.: <50 kg: 50-180 mg/kg/day in divided doses every 4-6 hours

Meningitis: 200 mg/kg/day in divided doses every 6 hours

Children >12 years and Adults:

Uncomplicated infections: I.M., I.V.: 1 g every 12 hours

Moderate/severe infections: I.M., I.V.: 1-2 g every 8 hours

Infections commonly needing higher doses (eg, septicemia): I.V.: 2 g every 6-8 hours

Life-threatening infections: I.V.: 2 g every 4 hours

Preop: I.M., I.V.: 1 g 30-90 minutes before surgery

C-section: 1 g as soon as the umbilical cord is clamped, then 1 g I.M., I.V. at 6- and 12-hour intervals

Dosing interval in renal impairment:

Cl_{cr} 10-50 mL/minute: Administer every 8-12 hours

Cl_{cr} <10 mL/minute: Administer every 24 hours

Hemodialysis: Moderately dialyzable

Dosing adjustment in hepatic impairment: Moderate dosage reduction is recommended in severe liver disease

Continuous arteriovenous or venovenous hemodiafiltration effects: Administer 1 g every 12 hour

Dietary Considerations Sodium content of 1 g: 50.5 mg (2.2 mEq)

Administration Can be administered IVP over 3-5 minutes or I.V. intermittent infusion over 15-30 minutes

Monitoring Parameters Observe for signs and symptoms of anaphylaxis during first dose; CBC with differential (especially with long courses)

Test Interactions Positive direct Coombs', false-positive urinary glucose test using cupric sulfate (Benedict's solution, Clinitest®, Fehling's solution), false-positive serum or urine creatinine with Jaffé reaction

Dosage Forms

Infusion, as sodium [premixed in D_5W] (Claforan®): 1 g (50 mL); 2 g (50 mL)

Injection, powder for reconstitution, as sodium: 500 mg, 1 g, 2 g, 10 g, 20 g

Claforan®: 500 mg, 1 g, 2 g, 10 g [contains sodium 50.5 mg (2.2 mEq) per cefotaxime 1 g]

Selected Readings

Brogden RN and Spencer CM, "Cefotaxime. A Reappraisal of Its Antibacterial Activity and Pharmacokinetic Properties, and a Review of Its Therapeutic Efficacy When Administered Twice Daily for the Treatment of Mild to Moderate Infections," *Drugs*, 1997, 53(3):483-510.

Donowitz GR and Mandell GL, "Beta-Lactam Antibiotics," *N Engl J Med*, 1988, 318(7):419-26 and 318(8):490-500.

Klein NC and Cunha BA, "Third-Generation Cephalosporins," *Med Clin North Am*, 1995, 79(4):705-19.

Marshall WF and Blair JE, "The Cephalosporins," *Mayo Clin Proc*, 1999, 74(2):187-95.

Cefotaxime Sodium *see* Cefotaxime *on page 708*

Cefotetan (SEF oh tee tan)

Related Information

Animal and Human Bites *on page 1270*

Antimicrobial Activity Against Selected Organisms *on page 1165*

U.S. Brand Names Cefotan®

Canadian Brand Names Cefotan®

Synonyms Cefotetan Disodium

Generic Available No

Use Surgical prophylaxis; intra-abdominal infections and other mixed infections; respiratory tract, skin and skin structure, bone and joint, urinary tract and gynecologic as well as septicemia; active against gram-negative enteric bacilli including *E. coli*, *Klebsiella*, and *Proteus*; less active against staphylococci and streptococci than first generation cephalosporins, but active against anaerobes including *Bacteroides fragilis*

Drug of Choice or Alternative for Disease/Syndrome(s):

Endometritis *on page 127*

Liver Abscess *on page 211*

Pancreatitis/Pancreatic Abscess *on page 253*
Pelvic Inflammatory Disease *on page 260*
Peritonitis, Spontaneous Bacterial *on page 264*

Organism(s):

Bacteroides and *Prevotella* Species *on page 46*

Pregnancy Risk Factor B

Contraindications Hypersensitivity to cefotetan, any component of the formulation, or other cephalosporins; previous cephalosporin-associated hemolytic anemia

Warnings/Precautions Modify dosage in patients with severe renal impairment; prolonged use may result in superinfection; although cefotetan contains the methyltetrazolethiol side chain, bleeding has not been a significant problem; use with caution in patients with a history of penicillin allergy especially IgE-mediated reactions (eg, anaphylaxis, urticaria). Cefotetan has been associated with a higher risk of hemolytic anemia relative to other cephalosporins (approximately threefold); monitor carefully during use and consider cephalosporin-associated immune anemia in patients who have received cefotetan within 2-3 weeks (either as treatment or prophylaxis). May cause antibiotic-associated colitis or colitis secondary to *C. difficile.*

Adverse Reactions

1% to 10%:

- Gastrointestinal: Diarrhea (1%)
- Hepatic: Transaminases increased (1%)
- Miscellaneous: Hypersensitivity reactions (1%)

<1%: Anaphylaxis, urticaria, rash, pruritus, pseudomembranous colitis, nausea, vomiting, eosinophilia, thrombocytosis, agranulocytosis, hemolytic anemia, leukopenia, thrombocytopenia, prolonged PT, bleeding, elevated BUN, elevated creatinine, nephrotoxicity, phlebitis, fever

Reactions reported with other cephalosporins include seizure, Stevens-Johnson syndrome, toxic epidermal necrolysis, renal dysfunction, toxic nephropathy, cholestasis, aplastic anemia, hemolytic anemia, hemorrhage, pancytopenia, agranulocytosis, colitis, superinfection

Overdosage/Toxicology Symptoms include neuromuscular hypersensitivity and convulsions especially with renal insufficiency. Many beta-lactam antibiotics have the potential to cause neuromuscular hyperirritability or seizures. Hemodialysis may be helpful to aid in removal of the drug from the blood; otherwise, most treatment is supportive or symptom-directed.

Drug Interactions

Increased Effect/Toxicity: Disulfiram-like reaction may occur if ethanol is consumed by a patient taking cefotetan. Probenecid may increase cefotetan plasma levels. Cefotetan may increase risk of bleeding in patients receiving warfarin.

Ethanol/Nutrition/Herb Interactions Ethanol: Avoid ethanol (may cause a disulfiram-like reaction).

Stability Reconstituted solution is stable for 24 hours at room temperature and 96 hours when refrigerated; for I.V. infusion in NS or D_5W solution and after freezing, thawed solution is stable for 24 hours at room temperature or 96 hours when refrigerated; frozen solution is stable for 12 weeks

Mechanism of Action Inhibits bacterial cell wall synthesis by binding to one or more of the penicillin-binding proteins (PBPs) which in turn inhibits the final transpeptidation step of peptidoglycan synthesis in bacterial cell walls, thus inhibiting cell wall biosynthesis. Bacteria eventually lyse due to ongoing activity of cell wall autolytic enzymes (autolysins and murein hydrolases) while cell wall assembly is arrested.

Pharmacodynamics/Kinetics

Distribution: Widely to body tissues and fluids including bile, sputum, prostatic, peritoneal; low concentrations enter CSF; crosses placenta; enters breast milk

Protein binding: 76% to 90%

Half-life elimination: 3-5 hours

Time to peak, serum: I.M.: 1.5-3 hours

Excretion: Primarily urine (as unchanged drug); feces (20%)

Dosage

Children (unlabeled use): I.M., I.V.:

- Severe infections: 20-40 mg/kg/dose every 12 hours; maximum: 6 g/day
- Preoperative prophylaxis: I.M., I.V.: 40 mg/kg 30-60 minutes prior to surgery

Adolescents and Adults: I.V.: Pelvic inflammatory disease: 2 g every 12 hours; used in combination with doxycycline

Adults: I.M., I.V.: 1-6 g/day in divided doses every 12 hours; usual dose: 1-2 g every 12 hours for 5-10 days; 1-2 g may be given every 24 hours for urinary tract infection

- Preoperative prophylaxis: I.M., I.V.: 1-2 g 30-60 minutes prior to surgery; when used for cesarean section, dose should be given as soon as umbilical cord is clamped

(Continued)

Cefotetan *(Continued)*

Dosing interval in renal impairment:

Cl_{cr} 10-30 mL/minute: Administer every 24 hours

Cl_{cr} <10 mL/minute: Administer every 48 hours

Hemodialysis: Dialyzable (5% to 20%); administer 1/4 the usual dose every 24 hours on days between dialysis; administer 1/2 the usual dose on the day of dialysis.

Continuous arteriovenous or venovenous hemodiafiltration effects: Administer 750 mg every 12 hours

Dietary Considerations Contains sodium of 80 mg (3.5 mEq) per cefotetan 1 g

Administration

I.M.: Inject deep I.M. into large muscle mass.

I.V.: Inject direct I.V. over 3-5 minutes. Infuse intermittent infusion over 30 minutes

Monitoring Parameters Observe for signs and symptoms of anaphylaxis during first dose; monitor for signs and symptoms of hemolytic anemia, including hematologic parameters where appropriate.

Test Interactions Positive direct Coombs', false-positive urinary glucose test using cupric sulfate (Benedict's solution, Clinitest®, Fehling's solution), false-positive serum or urine creatinine with Jaffé reaction

Dosage Forms [DSC] = Discontinued product

Infusion [premixed iso-osmotic solution]: 1 g (50 mL); 2 g (50 mL) [contains sodium 80 mg/g (3.5 mEq/g)]

Injection, powder for reconstitution: 1 g, 2 g [contains sodium 80 mg/g (3.5 mEq/g)] [DSC]

Selected Readings

"Antimicrobial Prophylaxis in Surgery," *Med Lett Drugs Ther*, 1993, 35(906):91-4.

Donowitz GR and Mandell GL, "Beta-Lactam Antibiotics," *N Engl J Med*, 1988, 318(7):419-26 and 318(8):490-500.

Marshall WF and Blair JE, "The Cephalosporins," *Mayo Clin Proc*, 1999, 74(2):187-95.

Cefotetan Disodium *see* Cefotetan *on page 710*

Cefoxitin (se FOKS i tin)

Related Information

Antimicrobial Activity Against Selected Organisms *on page 1165*

U.S. Brand Names Mefoxin®

Canadian Brand Names Mefoxin®

Synonyms Cefoxitin Sodium

Generic Available Yes: Powder for injection

Use Less active against staphylococci and streptococci than first generation cephalosporins, but active against anaerobes including *Bacteroides fragilis*; active against gram-negative enteric bacilli including *E. coli*, *Klebsiella*, and *Proteus*; used predominantly for respiratory tract, skin and skin structure, bone and joint, urinary tract and gynecologic as well as septicemia; surgical prophylaxis; intra-abdominal infections and other mixed infections; indicated for bacterial *Eikenella corrodens* infections

Drug of Choice or Alternative for

Disease/Syndrome(s):

Amnionitis *on page 33*
Endometritis *on page 127*
Liver Abscess *on page 211*
Osteomyelitis, Diabetic Foot *on page 249*
Pancreatitis/Pancreatic Abscess *on page 253*
Pelvic Inflammatory Disease *on page 260*
Peritonitis, Spontaneous Bacterial *on page 264*

Organism(s):

Bacteroides and *Prevotella* Species *on page 46*

Pregnancy Risk Factor B

Contraindications Hypersensitivity to cefoxitin, any component of the formulation, or other cephalosporins

Warnings/Precautions Use with caution in patients with history of colitis; cefoxitin may increase resistance of organisms by inducing beta-lactamase; modify dosage in patients with severe renal impairment; prolonged use may result in superinfection; use with caution in patients with a history of penicillin allergy especially IgE-mediated reactions (eg, anaphylaxis, urticaria). May cause antibiotic-associated colitis or colitis secondary to *C. difficile*.

Adverse Reactions

1% to 10%: Gastrointestinal: Diarrhea

<1%: Anaphylaxis, angioedema, bone marrow suppression, BUN increased, creatinine increased, dyspnea, eosinophilia, exacerbation of myasthenia gravis, exfoliative dermatitis, fever, hemolytic anemia, hypotension, interstitial nephritis, jaundice, leukopenia, nausea, nephrotoxicity increased (with aminoglycosides), phlebitis, prolonged PT, pruritus, pseudomembranous colitis, rash, thrombocytopenia, thrombophlebitis, toxic epidermal necrolysis, transaminases increased, urticaria, vomiting

Reactions reported with other cephalosporins include Agranulocytosis, aplastic anemia, cholestasis, colitis, erythema multiforme, hemolytic anemia, hemorrhage, pancytopenia, renal dysfunction, serum-sickness reactions, seizure, Stevens-Johnson syndrome, superinfection, toxic nephropathy, vaginitis

Overdosage/Toxicology Symptoms include neuromuscular hypersensitivity and convulsions especially with renal insufficiency. Many beta-lactam antibiotics have the potential to cause neuromuscular hyperirritability or seizures. Hemodialysis may be helpful to aid in removal of the drug from the blood; otherwise, most treatment is supportive or symptom-directed.

Drug Interactions

Increased Effect/Toxicity: Probenecid may decrease cephalosporin elimination. Furosemide, aminoglycosides in combination with cefoxitin may result in additive nephrotoxicity.

Stability Reconstitute vials with SWFI, bacteriostatic water for injection, NS, or D_5W. For I.V. infusion, solutions may be further diluted in NS, D_5¼NS, D_5½NS, D_5NS, D_5W, $D_{10}W$, LR, D_5LR, mannitol 10%, or sodium bicarbonate 5%. Reconstituted solution is stable for 6 hours at room temperature or 7 days when refrigerated; I.V. infusion in NS or D_5W solution is stable for 18 hours at room temperature or 48 hours when refrigerated. Premixed frozen solution, when thawed, is stable for 24 hours at room temperature or 21 days when refrigerated.

Mechanism of Action Inhibits bacterial cell wall synthesis by binding to one or more of the penicillin-binding proteins (PBPs) which in turn inhibits the final transpeptidation step of peptidoglycan synthesis in bacterial cell walls, thus inhibiting cell wall biosynthesis. Bacteria eventually lyse due to ongoing activity of cell wall autolytic enzymes (autolysins and murein hydrolases) while cell wall assembly is arrested.

Pharmacodynamics/Kinetics

Distribution: Widely to body tissues and fluids including pleural, synovial, ascitic, bile; poorly penetrates into CSF even with inflammation of the meninges; crosses placenta; small amounts enter breast milk

Protein binding: 65% to 79%

Half-life elimination: 45-60 minutes; significantly prolonged with renal impairment

Time to peak, serum: I.M.: 20-30 minutes

Excretion: Urine (85% as unchanged drug)

Dosage

Infants >3 months and Children: I.M., I.V.:

Mild to moderate infection: 80-100 mg/kg/day in divided doses every 4-6 hours

Severe infection: 100-160 mg/kg/day in divided doses every 4-6 hours; maximum dose: 12 g/day

Perioperative prophylaxis: 30-40 mg/kg 30-60 minutes prior to surgery followed by 30-40 mg/kg/dose every 6 hours for no more than 24 hours after surgery depending on the procedure

Adolescents and Adults: I.M., I.V.: Perioperative prophylaxis: 1-2 g 30-60 minutes prior to surgery followed by 1-2 g every 6-8 hours for no more than 24 hours after surgery depending on the procedure

Adults: I.M., I.V.: 1-2 g every 6-8 hours (I.M. injection is painful); up to 12 g/day

Pelvic inflammatory disease:

Inpatients: I.V.: 2 g every 6 hours **plus** doxycycline 100 mg I.V. or 100 mg orally every 12 hours until improved, followed by doxycycline 100 mg orally twice daily to complete 14 days

Outpatients: I.M.: 2 g **plus** probenecid 1 g orally as a single dose, followed by doxycycline 100 mg orally twice daily for 14 days

Dosing interval in renal impairment:

Cl_{cr} 30-50 mL/minute: Administer 1-2 g every 8-12 hours

Cl_{cr} 10-29 mL/minute: Administer 1-2 g every 12-24 hours

Cl_{cr} 5-9 mL/minute: Administer 0.5-1 g every 12-24 hours

Cl_{cr} <5 mL/minute: Administer 0.5-1 g every 24-48 hours

Hemodialysis: Moderately dialyzable (20% to 50%); administer a loading dose of 1-2 g after each hemodialysis; maintenance dose as noted above based on Cl_{cr}

Continuous arteriovenous or venovenous hemodiafiltration effects: Dose as for Cl_{cr} 10-50 mL/minute

Dietary Considerations Sodium content of 1 g: 53 mg (2.3 mEq)

Administration

I.M.: Inject deep I.M. into large muscle mass.

(Continued)

Cefoxitin *(Continued)*

I.V.: Can be administered IVP over 3-5 minutes at a maximum concentration of 100 mg/mL or I.V. intermittent infusion over 10-60 minutes at a final concentration for I.V. administration not to exceed 40 mg/mL

Monitoring Parameters Monitor renal function periodically when used in combination with other nephrotoxic drugs; observe for signs and symptoms of anaphylaxis during first dose

Test Interactions Positive direct Coombs', false-positive urinary glucose test using cupric sulfate (Benedict's solution, Clinitest®, Fehling's solution), false-positive serum or urine creatinine with Jaffé reaction

Dosage Forms

Infusion, as sodium [premixed iso-osmotic solution]: 1 g (50 mL); 2 g (50 mL) [contains sodium 53.8 mg/g (2.3 mEq/g)]

Injection, powder for reconstitution, as sodium: 1 g, 2 g, 10 g [contains sodium 53.8 mg/g (2.3 mEq/g)]

Selected Readings

"Antimicrobial Prophylaxis in Surgery," *Med Lett Drugs Ther*, 1993, 35(906):91-4.

Donowitz GR and Mandell GL, "Beta-Lactam Antibiotics," *N Engl J Med*, 1988, 318(7):419-26 and 318(8):490-500.

Marshall WF and Blair JE, "The Cephalosporins," *Mayo Clin Proc*, 1999, 74(2):187-95.

Cefoxitin Sodium *see* Cefoxitin *on page 712*

Cefpodoxime (sef pode OKS eem)

Related Information

Antimicrobial Activity Against Selected Organisms *on page 1165*

Community-Acquired Pneumonia in Adults *on page 1278*

U.S. Brand Names Vantin®

Canadian Brand Names Vantin®

Synonyms Cefpodoxime Proxetil

Generic Available Yes: Tablet

Use Treatment of susceptible acute, community-acquired pneumonia caused by *S. pneumoniae* or nonbeta-lactamase producing *H. influenzae*; acute uncomplicated gonorrhea caused by *N. gonorrhoeae*; uncomplicated skin and skin structure infections caused by *S. aureus* or *S. pyogenes*; acute otitis media caused by *S. pneumoniae*, *H. influenzae*, or *M. catarrhalis*; pharyngitis or tonsillitis; and uncomplicated urinary tract infections caused by *E. coli*, *Klebsiella*, and *Proteus*

Drug of Choice or Alternative for Disease/Syndrome(s):

Pneumonia, Community-Acquired *on page 270*

Pregnancy Risk Factor B

Contraindications Hypersensitivity to cefpodoxime, any component of the formulation, or other cephalosporins

Warnings/Precautions Modify dosage in patients with severe renal impairment; prolonged use may result in superinfection. Use with caution in patients with a history of penicillin allergy especially IgE-mediated reactions (eg, anaphylaxis, urticaria).

Adverse Reactions

>10%:

Dermatologic: Diaper rash (12%)

Gastrointestinal: Diarrhea in infants and toddlers (15%)

1% to 10%:

Central nervous system: Headache (1%)

Dermatologic: Rash (1%)

Gastrointestinal: Diarrhea (7%), nausea (4%), abdominal pain (2%), vomiting (1% to 2%)

Genitourinary: Vaginal infection (3%)

<1%: Anaphylaxis, chest pain, hypotension, fungal skin infection, pseudomembranous colitis, vaginal candidiasis, pruritus, flatulence, decreased salivation, malaise, fever, decreased appetite, cough, epistaxis, dizziness, fatigue, anxiety, insomnia, flushing, weakness, nightmares, taste alteration, eye itching, tinnitus, purpuric nephritis

Reactions reported with other cephalosporins include seizure, Stevens-Johnson syndrome, toxic epidermal necrolysis, erythema multiforme, urticaria, serum-sickness reactions, renal dysfunction, interstitial nephritis toxic nephropathy, cholestasis, aplastic anemia, hemolytic anemia, hemorrhage, pancytopenia, agranulocytosis, colitis, vaginitis, superinfection

Overdosage/Toxicology After acute overdose, most agents cause only nausea, vomiting, and diarrhea, although neuromuscular hypersensitivity and seizures are possible, especially in patients with renal insufficiency. Many beta-lactam antibiotics have the potential to cause neuromuscular hyperirritability or seizures. Hemodialysis

may be helpful to aid in removal of the drug from the blood but not usually indicated; otherwise, most treatment is supportive or symptom-directed, following GI decontamination.

Drug Interactions

Increased Effect/Toxicity: Probenecid may decrease cephalosporin elimination. Furosemide, aminoglycosides in combination with cefpodoxime may result in additive nephrotoxicity.

Decreased Effect: Antacids and H_2-receptor antagonists reduce absorption and serum concentration of cefpodoxime.

Ethanol/Nutrition/Herb Interactions Food: Food delays absorption; cefpodoxime serum levels may be increased if taken with food.

Stability After mixing, keep suspension in refrigerator, shake well before using; discard unused portion after 14 days

Mechanism of Action Inhibits bacterial cell wall synthesis by binding to one or more of the penicillin-binding proteins (PBPs) which in turn inhibits the final transpeptidation step of peptidoglycan synthesis in bacterial cell walls, thus inhibiting cell wall biosynthesis. Bacteria eventually lyse due to ongoing activity of cell wall autolytic enzymes (autolysins and murein hydrolases) while cell wall assembly is arrested.

Pharmacodynamics/Kinetics

Absorption: Rapid and well absorbed (50%), acid stable; enhanced in the presence of food or low gastric pH

Distribution: Good tissue penetration, including lung and tonsils; penetrates into pleural fluid

Protein binding: 18% to 23%

Metabolism: De-esterified in GI tract to active metabolite, cefpodoxime

Half-life elimination: 2.2 hours; prolonged with renal impairment

Time to peak: Within 1 hour

Excretion: Urine (80% as unchanged drug) in 24 hours

Dosage Oral:

Children 2 months to 12 years:

Acute otitis media: 10 mg/kg/day divided every 12 hours (400 mg/day) for 5 days (maximum: 200 mg/dose)

Acute maxillary sinusitis: 10 mg/kg/day divided every 12 hours for 10 days (maximum: 200 mg/dose)

Pharyngitis/tonsillitis: 10 mg/kg/day in 2 divided doses for 5-10 days (maximum: 100 mg/dose)

Children ≥12 years and Adults:

Acute community-acquired pneumonia and bacterial exacerbations of chronic bronchitis: 200 mg every 12 hours for 14 days and 10 days, respectively

Acute maxillary sinusitis: 200 mg every 12 hours for 10 days

Skin and skin structure: 400 mg every 12 hours for 7-14 days

Uncomplicated gonorrhea (male and female) and rectal gonococcal infections (female): 200 mg as a single dose

Pharyngitis/tonsillitis: 100 mg every 12 hours for 5-10 days

Uncomplicated urinary tract infection: 100 mg every 12 hours for 7 days

Dosing adjustment in renal impairment: Cl_{cr} <30 mL/minute: Administer every 24 hours

Hemodialysis: Administer dose 3 times/week following hemodialysis

Dietary Considerations May be taken with food.

Administration Administer around-the-clock to promote less variation in peak and trough serum levels.

Monitoring Parameters Observe for signs and symptoms of anaphylaxis during first dose

Test Interactions Positive direct Coombs', false-positive urinary glucose test using cupric sulfate (Benedict's solution, Clinitest®, Fehling's solution), false-positive serum or urine creatinine with Jaffé reaction

Patient Information Take with food; chilling improves flavor (do not freeze); report persistent diarrhea; take entire course of medication; may interfere with oral contraceptives; females should report symptoms of vaginitis

Dosage Forms

Granules for oral suspension: 50 mg/5 mL (50 mL, 75 mL, 100 mL); 100 mg/5 mL (50 mL, 75 mL, 100 mL) [contains sodium benzoate; lemon creme flavor]

Tablet [film coated]: 100 mg, 200 mg

Selected Readings

Adam D, Bergogne-Berezin E, and Jones RN, "Symposium on Cefpodoxime Proxetil: A New Third Generation Oral Cephalosporin," *Drugs*, 1991, 42(Suppl 3):1-66.

Cohen R, "Clinical Experience With Cefpodoxime Proxetil in Acute Otitis Media," *Pediatr Infect Dis J*, 1995, 14(Suppl 4):S12-8.

Marshall WF and Blair JE, "The Cephalosporins," *Mayo Clin Proc*, 1999, 74(2):187-95.

(Continued)

Cefpodoxime *(Continued)*

Schatz BS, Karavokiros KT, Taeubel MA, et al, "Comparison of Cefprozil, Cefpodoxime Proxetil, Loracarbef, Cefixime, and Ceftibuten," *Ann Pharmacother*, 1996, 30(3):258-68.

Cefpodoxime Proxetil *see* Cefpodoxime *on page 714*

Cefprozil (sef PROE zil)

Related Information

Community-Acquired Pneumonia in Adults *on page 1278*

U.S. Brand Names Cefzil®

Canadian Brand Names Cefzil®

Generic Available No

Use Treatment of otitis media and infections involving the respiratory tract and skin and skin structure; active against methicillin-sensitive staphylococci, many streptococci, and various gram-negative bacilli including *E. coli*, some *Klebsiella*, *P. mirabilis*, *H. influenzae*, and *Moraxella*.

Drug of Choice or Alternative for Disease/Syndrome(s):

Pneumonia, Community-Acquired *on page 270*

Pregnancy Risk Factor B

Contraindications Hypersensitivity to cefprozil, any component of the formulation, or other cephalosporins

Warnings/Precautions Modify dosage in patients with severe renal impairment; prolonged use may result in superinfection; use with caution in patients with a history of penicillin allergy especially IgE-mediated reactions (eg, anaphylaxis, urticaria). May cause antibiotic-associated colitis or colitis secondary to *C. difficile*.

Adverse Reactions

1% to 10%:

- Central nervous system: Dizziness (1%)
- Dermatologic: Diaper rash (2%)
- Gastrointestinal: Diarrhea (3%), nausea (4%), vomiting (1%), abdominal pain (1%)
- Genitourinary: Vaginitis, genital pruritus (2%)
- Hepatic: Transaminases increased (2%)
- Miscellaneous: Superinfection

<1%: Anaphylaxis, angioedema, pseudomembranous colitis, rash, urticaria, erythema multiforme, serum sickness, Stevens-Johnson syndrome, hyperactivity, headache, insomnia, confusion, somnolence, leukopenia, eosinophilia, thrombocytopenia, elevated BUN, elevated creatinine, arthralgia, cholestatic jaundice, fever

Reactions reported with other cephalosporins include seizure, toxic epidermal necrolysis, renal dysfunction, interstitial nephritis, toxic nephropathy, aplastic anemia, hemolytic anemia, hemorrhage, pancytopenia, agranulocytosis, colitis, vaginitis, superinfection

Overdosage/Toxicology After acute overdose, most agents cause only nausea, vomiting, and diarrhea, although neuromuscular hypersensitivity and seizures are possible, especially in patients with renal insufficiency. Many beta-lactam antibiotics have the potential to cause neuromuscular hyperirritability or seizures. Hemodialysis may be helpful to aid in removal of the drug from the blood but not usually indicated; otherwise, most treatment is supportive or symptom-directed, following GI decontamination.

Drug Interactions

Increased Effect/Toxicity: Probenecid may decrease cephalosporin elimination. Furosemide, aminoglycosides in combination with cefprozil may result in additive nephrotoxicity.

Ethanol/Nutrition/Herb Interactions Food: Food delays cefprozil absorption.

Mechanism of Action Inhibits bacterial cell wall synthesis by binding to one or more of the penicillin-binding proteins (PBPs) which in turn inhibits the final transpeptidation step of peptidoglycan synthesis in bacterial cell walls, thus inhibiting cell wall biosynthesis. Bacteria eventually lyse due to ongoing activity of cell wall autolytic enzymes (autolysins and murein hydrolases) while cell wall assembly is arrested.

Pharmacodynamics/Kinetics

- Absorption: Well absorbed (94%)
- Distribution: Low amounts enter breast milk
- Protein binding: 35% to 45%
- Half-life elimination: Normal renal function: 1.3 hours
- Time to peak, serum: Fasting: 1.5 hours
- Excretion: Urine (61% as unchanged drug)

Dosage Oral:

Infants and Children >6 months to 12 years: Otitis media: 15 mg/kg every 12 hours for 10 days

Pharyngitis/tonsillitis:
Children 2-12 years: 7.5 -15 mg/kg/day divided every 12 hours for 10 days (administer for >10 days if due to *S. pyogenes*); maximum: 1 g/day
Children >13 years and Adults: 500 mg every 24 hours for 10 days
Uncomplicated skin and skin structure infections:
Children 2-12 years: 20 mg/kg every 24 hours for 10 days; maximum: 1 g/day
Children >13 years and Adults: 250 mg every 12 hours, or 500 mg every 12-24 hours for 10 days
Secondary bacterial infection of acute bronchitis or acute bacterial exacerbation of chronic bronchitis: 500 mg every 12 hours for 10 days

Dosing adjustment in renal impairment: Cl_{cr} <30 mL/minute: Reduce dose by 50%
Hemodialysis: Reduced by hemodialysis; administer dose after the completion of hemodialysis

Dietary Considerations May be taken with food. Oral suspension contains phenylalanine 28 mg/5 mL.

Administration Administer around-the-clock to promote less variation in peak and trough serum levels. Chilling the reconstituted oral suspension improves flavor (do not freeze).

Monitoring Parameters Assess patient at beginning and throughout therapy for infection; monitor for signs of anaphylaxis during first dose

Test Interactions Positive direct Coombs', false-positive urinary glucose test using cupric sulfate (Benedict's solution, Clinitest®, Fehling's solution), false-positive serum or urine creatinine with Jaffé reaction

Patient Information Chilling improves flavor; report persistent diarrhea; take entire course of medication; may interfere with oral contraceptives; females should report symptoms of vaginitis

Dosage Forms

Powder for oral suspension, as anhydrous: 125 mg/5 mL (50 mL, 75 mL, 100 mL); 250 mg/5 mL (50 mL, 75 mL, 100 mL) [contains phenylalanine 28 mg/5 mL and sodium benzoate; bubble gum flavor]
Tablet, as anhydrous: 250 mg, 500 mg

Selected Readings

Gainer RB 2nd, "Cefprozil: A New Cephalosporin; Its Use in Various Clinical Trials," *South Med J*, 1995, 88(3):338-46.
Marshall WF and Blair JE, "The Cephalosporins," *Mayo Clin Proc*, 1999, 74(2):187-95.
Schatz BS, Karavokiros KT, Taeubel MA, et al, "Comparison of Cefprozil, Cefpodoxime Proxetil, Loracarbef, Cefixime, and Ceftibuten," *Ann Pharmacother*, 1996, 30(3):258-68.

Ceftazidime (SEF tay zi deem)

Related Information

Antimicrobial Activity Against Selected Organisms *on page 1165*
Neutropenic Fever Guidelines *on page 1295*

U.S. Brand Names Ceptaz® [DSC]; Fortaz®; Tazicef®

Canadian Brand Names Fortaz®

Generic Available No

Use Treatment of documented susceptible *Pseudomonas aeruginosa* infection and infections due to other susceptible aerobic gram-negative organisms; empiric therapy of a febrile, granulocytopenic patient

Drug of Choice or Alternative for Disease/Syndrome(s):

Endocarditis, Acute, I.V. Drug Abuse *on page 123*
Endophthalmitis, Bacterial and Fungal *on page 128*
Fever, Neutropenic *on page 148*
Intra-abdominal Abscess *on page 194*
Joint Replacement, Early Infection *on page 197*
Meningitis, Postsurgical *on page 218*
Osteomyelitis, Diabetic Foot *on page 249*
Otitis Externa, Severe (Malignant) *on page 252*
Peritonitis, CAPD-Associated *on page 262*
Pneumonia, Hospital-Acquired *on page 272*
Pneumonia, Ventilator-Associated *on page 273*
Sepsis *on page 295*
Sinusitis, Hospital-Acquired *on page 300*

Organism(s):

Burkholderia cepacia on page 62
Pseudomonas aeruginosa on page 282
Stenotrophomonas maltophilia on page 312

Pregnancy Risk Factor B

Contraindications Hypersensitivity to ceftazidime, any component of the formulation, or other cephalosporins

(Continued)

Ceftazidime *(Continued)*

Warnings/Precautions Modify dosage in patients with severe renal impairment; prolonged use may result in superinfection; use with caution in patients with a history of penicillin allergy especially IgE-mediated reactions (eg, anaphylaxis, urticaria). May cause antibiotic-associated colitis or colitis secondary to *C. difficile*.

Adverse Reactions

1% to 10%:

Gastrointestinal: Diarrhea (1%)

Local: Pain at injection site (1%)

Miscellaneous: Hypersensitivity reactions (2%)

<1%: Anaphylaxis, angioedema, asterixis, BUN increased, candidiasis, creatinine increased, dizziness, encephalopathy, eosinophilia, erythema multiforme, fever, headache, hemolytic anemia, hyperbilirubinemia, jaundice, leukopenia, myoclonus, nausea, neuromuscular excitability, paresthesia, phlebitis, pruritus, pseudomembranous colitis, rash, Stevens-Johnson syndrome, thrombocytosis, toxic epidermal necrolysis, transaminases increased, vaginitis, vomiting

Reactions reported with other cephalosporins include seizure, urticaria, serum-sickness reactions, renal dysfunction, interstitial nephritis, toxic nephropathy, elevated BUN, elevated creatinine, cholestasis, aplastic anemia, hemolytic anemia, pancytopenia, agranulocytosis, colitis, prolonged PT, hemorrhage, superinfection

Overdosage/Toxicology Symptoms include neuromuscular hypersensitivity and convulsions, especially with renal insufficiency. Many beta-lactam antibiotics have the potential to cause neuromuscular hyperirritability or seizures. Hemodialysis may be helpful to aid in removal of the drug from the blood, otherwise, most treatment is supportive or symptom-directed.

Drug Interactions

Increased Effect/Toxicity: Probenecid may decrease cephalosporin elimination. Aminoglycosides: *in vitro* studies indicate additive or synergistic effect against some strains of Enterobacteriaceae and *Pseudomonas aeruginosa*. Furosemide, aminoglycosides in combination with ceftazidime may result in additive nephrotoxicity.

Stability Reconstituted solution and I.V. infusion in NS or D_5W solution are stable for 24 hours at room temperature, 10 days when refrigerated, or 12 weeks when frozen; after freezing, thawed solution is stable for 24 hours at room temperature or 4 days when refrigerated; 96 hours under refrigeration, after mixing

Mechanism of Action Inhibits bacterial cell wall synthesis by binding to one or more of the penicillin-binding proteins (PBPs) which in turn inhibits the final transpeptidation step of peptidoglycan synthesis in bacterial cell walls, thus inhibiting cell wall biosynthesis. Bacteria eventually lyse due to ongoing activity of cell wall autolytic enzymes (autolysins and murein hydrolases) while cell wall assembly is arrested.

Pharmacodynamics/Kinetics

Distribution: Widely throughout the body including bone, bile, skin, CSF (higher concentrations achieved when meninges are inflamed), endometrium, heart, pleural and lymphatic fluids

Protein binding: 17%

Half-life elimination: 1-2 hours, prolonged with renal impairment; Neonates <23 days: 2.2-4.7 hours

Time to peak, serum: I.M.: ~1 hour

Excretion: Urine (80% to 90% as unchanged drug)

Dosage

Infants and Children 1 month to 12 years: I.V.: 30-50 mg/kg/dose every 8 hours; maximum dose: 6 g/day

Adults: I.M., I.V.: 500 mg to 2 g every 8-12 hours

Urinary tract infections: 250-500 mg every 12 hours

Dosing interval in renal impairment:

Cl_{cr} 30-50 mL/minute: Administer every 12 hours

Cl_{cr} 10-30 mL/minute: Administer every 24 hours

Cl_{cr} <10 mL/minute: Administer every 48-72 hours

Hemodialysis: Dialyzable (50% to 100%)

Continuous arteriovenous or venovenous hemodiafiltration effects: Dose as for Cl_{cr} 30-50 mL/minute

Dietary Considerations Sodium content of 1 g: 2.3 mEq

Administration Any carbon dioxide bubbles that may be present in the withdrawn solution should be expelled prior to injection; administer around-the-clock to promote less variation in peak and trough serum levels; ceftazidime can be administered deep I.M. into large mass muscle, IVP over 3-5 minutes, or I.V. intermittent infusion over 15-30 minutes; do not admix with aminoglycosides in same bottle/bag; final concentration for I.V. administration should not exceed 100 mg/mL

Monitoring Parameters Observe for signs and symptoms of anaphylaxis during first dose

Test Interactions Positive direct Coombs', false-positive urinary glucose test using cupric sulfate (Benedict's solution, Clinitest®, Fehling's solution), false-positive serum or urine creatinine with Jaffé reaction

Additional Information With some organisms, resistance may develop during treatment (including *Enterobacter* spp and *Serratia* spp); consider combination therapy or periodic susceptibility testing for organisms with inducible resistance

Dosage Forms [DSC] = Discontinued product

Infusion, as sodium [premixed iso-osmotic solution] (Fortaz®): 1 g (50 mL); 2 g (50 mL)

Injection, powder for reconstitution:

Ceptaz® [DSC]: 10 g [L-arginine formulation]

Fortaz®: 500 mg, 1 g, 2 g, 6 g [contains sodium carbonate]

Tazicef®: 1 g, 2 g, 6 g [contains sodium carbonate]

Selected Readings

Donowitz GR and Mandell GL, "Beta-Lactam Antibiotics," *N Engl J Med*, 1988, 318(7):419-26 and 318(8):490-500.

Klein NC and Cunha BA, "Third-Generation Cephalosporins," *Med Clin North Am*, 1995, 79(4):705-19.

Marshall WF and Blair JE, "The Cephalosporins," *Mayo Clin Proc*, 1999, 74(2):187-95.

Rains CP, Bryson HM, and Peters DH, "Ceftazidime. An Update of Its Antibacterial Activity, Pharmacokinetic Properties and Therapeutic Efficacy," *Drugs*, 1995, 49(4):577-617.

Vlasses PH, Bastion WA, Behal R, et al, "Ceftazidime Dosing in the Elderly: Economic Implications," *Ann Pharmacother*, 1993, 27(7-8):967-71.

Ceftibuten (sef TYE byoo ten)

U.S. Brand Names Cedax®

Generic Available No

Use Oral cephalosporin for treatment of bronchitis, otitis media, and pharyngitis/tonsillitis due to *H. influenzae* and *M. catarrhalis*, both beta-lactamase-producing and nonproducing strains, as well as *S. pneumoniae* (weak) and *S. pyogenes*

Pregnancy Risk Factor B

Contraindications Hypersensitivity to ceftibuten, any component of the formulation, or other cephalosporins

Warnings/Precautions Modify dosage in patients with severe renal impairment, prolonged use may result in superinfection; use with caution in patients with a history of penicillin allergy, especially IgE-mediated reactions (eg, anaphylaxis, urticaria). May cause antibiotic-associated colitis or colitis secondary to *C. difficile*.

Adverse Reactions

1% to 10%:

Central nervous system: Headache (3%), dizziness (1%)

Gastrointestinal: Nausea (4%), diarrhea (3%), dyspepsia (2%), vomiting (1%), abdominal pain (1%)

Hematologic: Increased eosinophils (3%), decreased hemoglobin (2%), thrombocytosis

Hepatic: Increased ALT (1%), increased bilirubin (1%)

Renal: Increased BUN (4%)

<1%: Anorexia, agitation, constipation, creatinine increased, diaper rash, dry mouth, dyspnea, dysuria, fatigue, candidiasis, rash, urticaria, irritability, paresthesia, nasal congestion, insomnia, rigors, transaminases increased, leukopenia

Reactions reported with other cephalosporins include anaphylaxis, fever, paresthesia, pruritus, Stevens-Johnson syndrome, toxic epidermal necrolysis, erythema multiforme, angioedema, pseudomembranous colitis, hemolytic anemia, candidiasis, vaginitis, encephalopathy, asterixis, neuromuscular excitability, seizure, serum-sickness reactions, renal dysfunction, interstitial nephritis, toxic nephropathy, cholestasis, aplastic anemia, hemolytic anemia, pancytopenia, agranulocytosis, colitis, prolonged PT, hemorrhage, superinfection

Overdosage/Toxicology After acute overdose, most agents cause only nausea, vomiting, and diarrhea, although neuromuscular hypersensitivity and seizures are possible, especially in patients with renal insufficiency. Many beta-lactam antibiotics have the potential to cause neuromuscular hyperirritability or seizures. Hemodialysis may be helpful to aid in removal of the drug from the blood but not usually indicated; otherwise, most treatment is supportive or symptom-directed, following GI decontamination.

Drug Interactions

Increased Effect/Toxicity: High-dose probenecid decreases clearance. Aminoglycosides in combination with ceftibuten may increase nephrotoxic potential.

Stability Reconstituted suspension is stable for 14 days in the refrigerator

Mechanism of Action Inhibits bacterial cell wall synthesis by binding to one or more of the penicillin-binding proteins (PBPs) which in turn inhibits the final transpeptidation

(Continued)

Ceftibuten *(Continued)*

step of peptidoglycan synthesis in bacterial cell walls, thus inhibiting cell wall biosynthesis. Bacteria eventually lyse due to ongoing activity of cell wall autolytic enzymes (autolysins and murein hydrolases) while cell wall assembly is arrested.

Pharmacodynamics/Kinetics

Absorption: Rapid; food decreases peak concentrations, delays T_{max}, and lowers AUC

Distribution: V_d: Children: 0.5 L/kg; Adults: 0.21 L/kg

Half-life elimination: 2 hours

Time to peak: 2-3 hours

Excretion: Urine

Dosage Oral:

Children <12 years: 9 mg/kg/day for 10 days; maximum daily dose: 400 mg

Children ≥12 years and Adults: 400 mg once daily for 10 days; maximum: 400 mg

Dosage adjustment in renal impairment:

Cl_{cr} 30-49 mL//minute: Administer 4.5 mg/kg or 200 mg every 24 hours

Cl_{cr} <29 mL/minute: Administer 2.25 mg/kg or 100 mg every 24 hours

Dietary Considerations

Capsule: Take without regard to food.

Suspension: Take 2 hours before or 1 hour after meals; contains 1 g of sucrose per 5 mL

Administration Shake suspension well before use.

Monitoring Parameters Observe for signs and symptoms of anaphylaxis during first dose; with prolonged therapy, monitor renal, hepatic, and hematologic function periodically

Test Interactions Positive direct Coombs', false-positive urinary glucose test using cupric sulfate (Benedict's solution, Clinitest®, Fehling's solution), false-positive serum or urine creatinine with Jaffé reaction

Patient Information Must be administered at least 2 hours before meals or 1 hour after a meal; discard any unused portion after 14 days; report prolonged diarrhea; take entire course of medication; may interfere with oral contraceptive; females should report symptoms of vaginitis

Dosage Forms

Capsule: 400 mg

Powder for oral suspension: 90 mg/5 mL (30 mL, 60 mL, 120 mL) [contains sodium benzoate; cherry flavor]

Selected Readings

Guay DR, "Ceftibuten: A New Expanded-Spectrum Oral Cephalosporin," *Ann Pharmacother*, 1997, 31(9):1022-33.

Owens RC Jr, Nightingale CH, and Nicolau DP, "Ceftibuten: An Overview," *Pharmacotherapy*, 1997, 17(4):707-20.

Schatz BS, Karavokiros KT, Taeubel MA, et al, "Comparison of Cefprozil, Cefpodoxime Proxetil, Loracarbef, Cefixime, and Ceftibuten," *Ann Pharmacother*, 1996, 30(3):258-68.

Wiseman LR and Balfour JA, "Ceftibuten: A Review of Its Antibacterial Activity Pharmacokinetic Properties and Clinical Efficacy," *Drugs*, 1994, 47(5):784-808.

Ceftin® *see* Cefuroxime *on page 725*

Ceftizoxime (sef ti ZOKS eem)

Related Information

Antimicrobial Activity Against Selected Organisms *on page 1165*

U.S. Brand Names Cefizox®

Canadian Brand Names Cefizox®

Synonyms Ceftizoxime Sodium

Generic Available No

Use Treatment of susceptible bacterial infection, mainly respiratory tract, skin and skin structure, bone and joint, urinary tract and gynecologic, as well as septicemia; active against many gram-negative bacilli (not *Pseudomonas*), some gram-positive cocci (not *Enterococcus*), and some anaerobes

Drug of Choice or Alternative for

Disease/Syndrome(s):

Intra-abdominal Abscess *on page 194*

Peritonitis, Spontaneous Bacterial *on page 264*

Organism(s):

Neisseria gonorrhoeae on page 244

Pregnancy Risk Factor B

Contraindications Hypersensitivity to ceftizoxime, any component of the formulation, or other cephalosporins

Warnings/Precautions Modify dosage in patients with severe renal impairment, prolonged use may result in superinfection; use with caution in patients with a history

of penicillin allergy, especially IgE-mediated reactions (eg, anaphylaxis, urticaria). May cause antibiotic-associated colitis or colitis secondary to *C. difficile*.

Adverse Reactions

1% to 10%:

Central nervous system: Fever

Dermatologic: Rash, pruritus

Hematologic: Eosinophilia, thrombocytosis

Hepatic: Alkaline phosphatase increased, transaminases increased

Local: Pain, burning at injection site

<1%: Anaphylaxis, diarrhea, nausea, vomiting, injection site reactions, phlebitis, paresthesia, numbness, increased bilirubin, increased BUN, increased creatinine, anemia, leukopenia, neutropenia, thrombocytopenia, vaginitis

Other reactions reported with cephalosporins include Stevens-Johnson syndrome, toxic epidermal necrolysis, erythema multiforme, pseudomembranous colitis, angioedema, hemolytic anemia, candidiasis, encephalopathy, asterixis, neuromuscular excitability, seizure, serum-sickness reactions, renal dysfunction, interstitial nephritis, toxic nephropathy, cholestasis, aplastic anemia, hemolytic anemia, pancytopenia, agranulocytosis, colitis, prolonged PT, hemorrhage, superinfection

Overdosage/Toxicology Symptoms include neuromuscular hypersensitivity and convulsions especially with renal insufficiency. Many beta-lactam antibiotics have the potential to cause neuromuscular hyperirritability or seizures. Hemodialysis may be helpful to aid in removal of the drug from the blood; otherwise, most treatment is supportive or symptom-directed.

Drug Interactions

Increased Effect/Toxicity: Probenecid may decrease cephalosporin elimination. Furosemide, aminoglycosides in combination with ceftizoxime may result in additive nephrotoxicity.

Stability Reconstituted solution is stable for 24 hours at room temperature and 96 hours when refrigerated; for I.V. infusion in NS or D_5W solution is stable for 24 hours at room temperature, 96 hours when refrigerated or 12 weeks when frozen; after freezing, thawed solution is stable for 24 hours at room temperature or 10 days when refrigerated

Mechanism of Action Inhibits bacterial cell wall synthesis by binding to one or more of the penicillin-binding proteins (PBPs) which in turn inhibits the final transpeptidation step of peptidoglycan synthesis in bacterial cell walls, thus inhibiting cell wall biosynthesis. Bacteria eventually lyse due to ongoing activity of cell wall autolytic enzymes (autolysins and murein hydrolases) while cell wall assembly is arrested.

Pharmacodynamics/Kinetics

Distribution: V_d: 0.35-0.5 L/kg; widely into most body tissues and fluids including gallbladder, liver, kidneys, bone, sputum, bile, pleural and synovial fluids; has good CSF penetration; crosses placenta; small amounts enter breast milk

Protein binding: 30%

Half-life elimination: 1.6 hours; Cl_{cr} <10 mL/minute: 25 hours

Time to peak, serum: I.M.: 0.5-1 hour

Excretion: Urine (as unchanged drug)

Dosage I.M., I.V.:

Children ≥6 months: 150-200 mg/kg/day divided every 6-8 hours (maximum of 12 g/24 hours)

Adults: 1-2 g every 8-12 hours, up to 2 g every 4 hours or 4 g every 8 hours for life-threatening infections

Dosing adjustment in renal impairment: Adults:

Cl_{cr} 10-30 mL/minute: Administer 1 g every 12 hours

Cl_{cr} <10 mL/minute: Administer 1 g every 24 hours

Moderately dialyzable (20% to 50%)

Continuous arteriovenous or venovenous hemodiafiltration effects: Dose as for Cl_{cr} 10-50 mL/minute

Dietary Considerations Sodium content of 1 g: 60 mg (2.6 mEq)

Administration

I.M.: Inject deep I.M. into large muscle mass.

I.V.: Inject direct I.V. over 3-5 minutes. Infuse intermittent infusion over 30 minutes.

Monitoring Parameters Observe for signs and symptoms of anaphylaxis during first dose

Test Interactions Positive direct Coombs', false-positive urinary glucose test using cupric sulfate (Benedict's solution, Clinitest®, Fehling's solution), false-positive serum or urine creatinine with Jaffé reaction

Dosage Forms

Infusion [premixed iso-osmotic solution]: 1 g (50 mL); 2 g (50 mL)

Injection, powder for reconstitution: 1 g, 2 g, 10 g

(Continued)

Ceftizoxime *(Continued)*

Selected Readings

Donowitz GR and Mandell GL, "Beta-Lactam Antibiotics," *N Engl J Med*, 1988, 318(7):419-26 and 318(8):490-500.

Klein NC and Cunha BA, "Third-Generation Cephalosporins," *Med Clin North Am*, 1995, 79(4):705-19.

Marshall WF and Blair JE, "The Cephalosporins," *Mayo Clin Proc*, 1999, 74(2):187-95.

Ceftizoxime Sodium *see* Ceftizoxime *on page 720*

Ceftriaxone (sef trye AKS one)

Related Information

Animal and Human Bites *on page 1270*

Antibiotic Treatment of Adults With Infective Endocarditis *on page 1271*

Antimicrobial Activity Against Selected Organisms *on page 1165*

Community-Acquired Pneumonia in Adults *on page 1278*

U.S. Brand Names Rocephin®

Canadian Brand Names Rocephin®

Synonyms Ceftriaxone Sodium

Generic Available Yes

Use Treatment of lower respiratory tract infections, acute bacterial otitis media, skin and skin structure infections, bone and joint infections, intra-abdominal and urinary tract infections, pelvic inflammatory disease (PID), uncomplicated gonorrhea, bacterial septicemia, and meningitis; used in surgical prophylaxis

Unlabeled/Investigational Use Treatment of chancroid, epididymitis, complicated gonococcal infections; sexually-transmitted diseases (STD); periorbital or buccal cellulitis; salmonellosis or shigellosis; atypical community-acquired pneumonia; Lyme disease; used in chemoprophylaxis for high-risk contacts and persons with invasive meningococcal disease; sexual assault

Drug of Choice or Alternative for

Disease/Syndrome(s):

Arthritis, Septic *on page 36*

Cervicitis *on page 71*

Epididymitis/Orchitis *on page 138*

Intra-abdominal Abscess *on page 194*

Joint Replacement, Late Infection *on page 198*

Liver Abscess *on page 211*

Meningitis, Community-Acquired, Adult *on page 216*

Meningitis, Pediatric (>1 month of age) *on page 218*

Meningitis, Post-traumatic *on page 219*

Necrotizing Fasciitis *on page 243*

Osteomyelitis, Diabetic Foot *on page 249*

Peritonitis, Spontaneous Bacterial *on page 264*

Pneumonia, Community-Acquired *on page 270*

Pneumonia, Hospital-Acquired *on page 272*

Pneumonia, Ventilator-Associated *on page 273*

Prostatitis *on page 277*

Organism(s):

Borrelia burgdorferi on page 56

Haemophilus ducreyi on page 158

Neisseria gonorrhoeae on page 244

Neisseria meningitidis on page 245

Streptococcus pneumoniae, Drug-Resistant *on page 316*

Streptococcus, Viridans Group *on page 326*

Treponema pallidum on page 334

Pregnancy Risk Factor B

Contraindications Hypersensitivity to ceftriaxone sodium, any component of the formulation, or other cephalosporins; **do not use in hyperbilirubinemic neonates**, particularly those who are premature since ceftriaxone is reported to displace bilirubin from albumin binding sites

Warnings/Precautions Modify dosage in patients with severe renal impairment, prolonged use may result in superinfection. Use with caution in patients with a history of penicillin allergy, especially IgE-mediated reactions (eg, anaphylaxis, urticaria). May cause antibiotic-associated colitis or colitis secondary to *C. difficile*. Discontinue in patients with signs and symptoms of gallbladder disease.

Adverse Reactions

1% to 10%:

Dermatologic: Rash (2%)

Gastrointestinal: Diarrhea (3%)

Hematologic: Eosinophilia (6%), thrombocytosis (5%), leukopenia (2%)

Hepatic: Transaminases increased (3.1% to 3.3%)

Local: Pain, induration at injection site (I.V. 1%); warmth, tightness, induration (5% to 17%) following I.M. injection

Renal: BUN increased (1%)

<1%: Agranulocytosis, allergic pneumonitis, anaphylaxis, anemia, basophilia, bronchospasm, candidiasis, chills, colitis, diaphoresis, dizziness, dysgeusia, flushing, gallstones, glycosuria, headache, hematuria, hemolytic anemia, jaundice, leukocytosis, lymphocytosis, lymphopenia, monocytosis, nausea, neutropenia, phlebitis, prolonged or decreased PT, pruritus, pseudomembranous colitis, renal stones, seizure, serum sickness, thrombocytopenia, urinary casts, vaginitis, vomiting; increased alkaline phosphatase, bilirubin, and creatinine

Postmarketing and/or case reports: Nephrolithiasis, renal precipitations

Reactions reported with other cephalosporins include angioedema, aplastic anemia, asterixis, cholestasis, encephalopathy, erythema multiforme, hemorrhage, interstitial nephritis, neuromuscular excitability, pancytopenia, paresthesia, renal dysfunction, Stevens-Johnson syndrome, superinfection, toxic epidermal necrolysis, toxic nephropathy

Overdosage/Toxicology Symptoms include neuromuscular hypersensitivity and convulsions especially with renal insufficiency. Many beta-lactam antibiotics have the potential to cause neuromuscular hyperirritability or seizures. Hemodialysis may be helpful to aid in removal of the drug from the blood; otherwise, most treatment is supportive or symptom-directed.

Drug Interactions

Increased Effect/Toxicity: Cephalosporins may increase the anticoagulant effect of coumarin derivatives (eg, dicumarol, warfarin).

Decreased Effect: Uricosuric agents (eg, probenecid, sulfinpyrazone) may decrease the excretion of cephalosporin; monitor for toxic effects.

Stability

Powder for injection: Prior to reconstitution, store at room temperature of 25°C (77°F); protect from light.

Premixed solution (manufacturer premixed): Store at -20°C; once thawed, solutions are stable for 3 days at room temperature of 25°C (77°F) or for 21 days refrigerated at 5°C (41°F). Do not refreeze.

Stability of reconstituted solutions:

10-40 mg/mL: Reconstituted in D_5W or NS: Stable for 2 days at room temperature of 25°C (77°F) or for 10 days when refrigerated at 5°C (41°F).

100 mg/mL:

Reconstituted in D_5W or NS: Stable for 2 days at room temperature of 25°C (77°F) or for 10 days when refrigerated at 5°C (41°F). Stable for 26 weeks when frozen at -20°C. Once thawed, solutions are stable for 2 days at room temperature of 25°C (77°F) or for 10 days when refrigerated at 5°C (41°F); does not apply to manufacturer's premixed bags. Do not refreeze.

Reconstituted in lidocaine 1% solution: Stable for 24 hours at room temperature of 25°C (77°F) or for 10 days when refrigerated at 5°C (41°F).

250-350 mg/mL: Reconstituted in D_5W, NS, lidocaine 1% solution, or SWFI: Stable for 24 hours at room temperature of 25°C (77°F) or for 3 days when refrigerated at 5°C (41°F).

Reconstitution:

I.M. injection: Vials should be reconstituted with appropriate volume of diluent (including D_5W, NS, or 1% lidocaine) to make a final concentration of 250 mg/mL or 350 mg/mL.

Volume to add to create a **250 mg/mL** solution:

250 mg vial: 0.9 mL
500 mg vial: 1.8 mL
1 g vial: 3.6 mL
2 g vial: 7.2 mL

Volume to add to create a **350 mg/mL** solution:

500 mg vial: 1.0 mL
1 g vial: 2.1 mL
2 g vial: 4.2 mL

I.V. infusion: Infusion is prepared in two stages: Initial reconstitution of powder, followed by dilution to final infusion solution.

Vials: Reconstitute powder with appropriate I.V. diluent (including SWFI, D_5W, NS) to create an initial solution of ~100 mg/mL. Recommended volume to add:

250 mg vial: 2.4 mL
500 mg vial: 4.8 mL
1 g vial: 9.6 mL
2 g vial: 19.2 mL

Note: After reconstitution of powder, further dilution into a volume of compatible solution (eg, 50-100 mL of D_5W or NS) is recommended.

(Continued)

Ceftriaxone *(Continued)*

Piggyback bottle: Reconstitute powder with appropriate I.V. diluent (D_5W or NS) to create a resulting solution of ~100 mg/mL. Recommended initial volume to add:

1 g bottle:10 mL

2 g bottle: 20 mL

Note: After reconstitution, to prepare the final infusion solution, further dilution to 50 mL or 100 mL volumes with the appropriate I.V. diluent (including D_5W or NS) is recommended.

Mechanism of Action Inhibits bacterial cell wall synthesis by binding to one or more of the penicillin-binding proteins (PBPs) which in turn inhibits the final transpeptidation step of peptidoglycan synthesis in bacterial cell walls, thus inhibiting cell wall biosynthesis. Bacteria eventually lyse due to ongoing activity of cell wall autolytic enzymes (autolysins and murein hydrolases) while cell wall assembly is arrested.

Pharmacodynamics/Kinetics

Absorption: I.M.: Well absorbed

Distribution: Widely throughout the body including gallbladder, lungs, bone, bile, CSF (higher concentrations achieved when meninges are inflamed); crosses placenta; enters amniotic fluid and breast milk

Protein binding: 85% to 95%

Half-life elimination: Normal renal and hepatic function: 5-9 hours

Time to peak, serum: I.M.: 1-2 hours

Excretion: Urine (33% to 65% as unchanged drug); feces

Dosage

Infants and Children:

Usual dose: I.M., I.V.:

Mild-to-moderate infections: 50-75 mg/kg/day in 1-2 divided doses every 12-24 hours (maximum: 2 g/day); continue until at least 2 days after signs and symptoms of infection have resolved

Serious infections: 80-100 mg/kg/day in 1-2 divided doses (maximum: 4 g/day)

Gonococcal infection, uncomplicated: I.M.: 125 mg in a single dose

Gonococcal conjunctivitis, complicated (unlabeled use): I.M.:

<45 kg: 50 mg/kg in a single dose (maximum: 1 g)

>45 kg: 1 g in a single dose

Gonococcal endocarditis (unlabeled use):

<45 kg: I.M., I.V.: 50 mg/kg/day every 12 hours (maximum: 2 g/day) for at least 28 days

>45 kg: I.V.: 1-2 g every 12 hours, for at least 28 days

Gonococcal infection, disseminated (unlabeled use): I.M., I.V.:

<45 kg: 25-50 mg/kg once daily (maximum: 1 g)

>45 kg: 1 g once daily for 7 days

Meningitis: I.M., I.V.:

Uncomplicated: Loading dose of 100 mg/kg (maximum: 4 g), followed by 100 mg/kg/day divided every 12-24 hours (maximum: 4 g/day); usual duration of treatment is 7-14 days

Gonococcal, complicated:

<45 kg: 50 mg/kg/day given every 12 hours (maximum: 2 g/day); usual duration of treatment is 10-14 days

>45 kg: I.V.: 1-2 g every 12 hours; usual duration of treatment is 10-14 days

Otitis media: I.M., I.V.:

Acute: 50 mg/kg in a single dose (maximum: 1 g)

Persistent or relapsing (unlabeled use): 50 mg/kg once daily for 3 days

STD, sexual assault (unlabeled uses): 125 mg in a single dose

Children >8 years (≥45 kg) and Adolescents (unlabeled use): Epididymitis, acute: I.M.: 125 mg in a single dose

Children ≤15 years: Chemoprophylaxis for high-risk contacts and persons with invasive meningococcal disease (unlabeled use): I.M.: 125 mg in a single dose. Children >15 years: Refer to Adults dosing.

Adults: Usual dose: I.M., I.V.: 1-2 g every 12-24 hours, depending on the type and severity of infection

Gonococcal conjunctivitis, complicated (unlabeled use): I.M.: 1 g in a single dose

Gonococcal endocarditis (unlabeled use): I.M., I.V.: 1-2 g every 12 hours for at least 28 days

Gonococcal infection, disseminated (unlabeled use): I.M., I.V.: 1 g once daily for 7 days

Gonococcal infection, uncomplicated: I.M.: 125-250 mg in a single dose

PID: I.M.: 250 mg in a single dose

Surgical prophylaxis: I.V.: 1 g 30 minutes to 2 hours before surgery

Epididymitis, acute (unlabeled use): I.M.: 250 mg in a single dose

Chemoprophylaxis for high-risk contacts and persons with invasive meningococcal disease (unlabeled use): I.M.: 250 mg in a single dose

Dosage adjustment in renal/hepatic impairment: No adjustment necessary

Hemodialysis: Not dialyzable (0% to 5%); administer dose postdialysis

Peritoneal dialysis effects: Administer 750 mg every 12 hours

Continuous arteriovenous or venovenous hemofiltration: Removes 10 mg of ceftriaxone of liter of filtrate per day

Dietary Considerations Sodium contents: 83 mg (3.6 mEq) per ceftriaxone 1 g

Administration Do not admix with aminoglycosides in same bottle/bag.

I.M.: Inject deep I.M. into large muscle mass; a concentration of 250 mg/mL or 350 mg/mL is recommended for all vial sizes except the 250 mg size (250 mg/mL is suggested); can be diluted with 1:1 water and 1% lidocaine for I.M. administration

I.V.: Infuse intermittent infusion over 30 minutes

Monitoring Parameters Observe for signs and symptoms of anaphylaxis

Test Interactions Positive direct Coombs', false-positive urinary glucose test using cupric sulfate (Benedict's solution, Clinitest®, Fehling's solution), false-positive serum or urine creatinine with Jaffé reaction

Dosage Forms Note: Contains sodium 83 mg (3.6 mEq) per ceftriaxone 1 g

Infusion [premixed in dextrose]: 1 g (50 mL); 2 g (50 mL)

Injection, powder for reconstitution: 250 mg, 500 mg, 1 g, 2 g, 10 g

Selected Readings

Donowitz GR and Mandell GL, "Beta-Lactam Antibiotics," *N Engl J Med*, 1988, 318(7):419-26 and 318(8):490-500.

Klein NC and Cunha BA, "Third-Generation Cephalosporins," *Med Clin North Am*, 1995, 79(4):705-19.

Lamb HM, Ormrod D, Scott LJ, et al, "Ceftriaxone: An Update of Its Use in the Management of Community-Acquired and Nosocomial Infections," *Drugs*, 2002, 62(7):1041-89.

Marshall WF and Blair JE, "The Cephalosporins," *Mayo Clin Proc*, 1999, 74(2):187-95.

Schaad UB, Suter S, Gianella-Borradori A, et al, "A Comparison of Ceftriaxone and Cefuroxime for the Treatment of Bacterial Meningitis in Children," *N Engl J Med*, 1990, 322(3):141-7.

Ceftriaxone Sodium *see* Ceftriaxone *on page 722*

Cefuroxime (se fyoor OKS eem)

Related Information

Antimicrobial Activity Against Selected Organisms *on page 1165*

Community-Acquired Pneumonia in Adults *on page 1278*

U.S. Brand Names Ceftin®; Zinacef®

Canadian Brand Names Apo-Cefuroxime®; Ceftin®; Kefurox®; ratio-Cefuroxime; Zinacef®

Synonyms Cefuroxime Axetil; Cefuroxime Sodium

Generic Available Yes

Use Treatment of infections caused by staphylococci, group B streptococci, *H. influenzae* (type A and B), *E. coli*, *Enterobacter*, *Salmonella*, and *Klebsiella*; treatment of susceptible infections of the lower respiratory tract, otitis media, urinary tract, skin and soft tissue, bone and joint, sepsis and gonorrhea

Drug of Choice or Alternative for Disease/Syndrome(s):

Intra-abdominal Abscess *on page 194*

Osteomyelitis, Diabetic Foot *on page 249*

Pneumonia, Community-Acquired *on page 270*

Organism(s):

Borrelia burgdorferi on page 56

Pregnancy Risk Factor B

Contraindications Hypersensitivity to cefuroxime, any component of the formulation, or other cephalosporins

Warnings/Precautions Modify dosage in patients with severe renal impairment, prolonged use may result in superinfection; use with caution in patients with a history of penicillin allergy, especially IgE-mediated reactions (eg, anaphylaxis, urticaria). May cause antibiotic-associated colitis or colitis secondary to *C. difficile*. May be associated with increased INR, especially in nutritionally-deficient patients, prolonged treatment, hepatic or renal disease. Tablets and oral suspension are not bioequivalent (do not substitute on a mg-per-mg basis).

Adverse Reactions

1% to 10%:

Endocrine & metabolic: Alkaline phosphatase increased (2%)

Hematologic: Eosinophilia (7%), decreased hemoglobin and hematocrit (10%)

Hepatic: Transaminases increased (4%)

Local: Thrombophlebitis (2%)

<1%: Anaphylaxis, angioedema, cholestasis, colitis, diarrhea, dizziness, erythema multiforme, fever, GI bleeding, headache, hemolytic anemia, increased BUN,

(Continued)

Cefuroxime *(Continued)*

increased creatinine, interstitial nephritis, leukopenia, nausea, neutropenia, pain at injection site, pancytopenia, prolonged PT/INR, pseudomembranous colitis, rash, seizure, stomach cramps, thrombocytopenia, toxic epidermal necrolysis, vaginitis, vomiting

Reactions reported with other cephalosporins include agranulocytosis, aplastic anemia, asterixis, encephalopathy, hemorrhage, neuromuscular excitability, serum-sickness reactions, superinfection, toxic nephropathy

Overdosage/Toxicology After acute overdose, most agents cause only nausea, vomiting, and diarrhea, although neuromuscular hypersensitivity and seizures are possible, especially in patients with renal insufficiency. Many beta-lactam antibiotics have the potential to cause neuromuscular hyperirritability or seizures. Hemodialysis may be helpful to aid in removal of the drug from the blood but not usually indicated; otherwise, most treatment is supportive or symptom-directed, following GI decontamination.

Drug Interactions

Increased Effect/Toxicity: High-dose probenecid decreases clearance. Aminoglycosides in combination with cefuroxime may result in additive nephrotoxicity.

Ethanol/Nutrition/Herb Interactions Food: Bioavailability is increased with food; cefuroxime serum levels may be increased if taken with food or dairy products.

Stability Reconstituted solution is stable for 24 hours at room temperature and 48 hours when refrigerated; I.V. infusion in NS or D_5W solution is stable for 24 hours at room temperature, 7 days when refrigerated, or 26 weeks when frozen; after freezing, thawed solution is stable for 24 hours at room temperature or 21 days when refrigerated

Mechanism of Action Inhibits bacterial cell wall synthesis by binding to one or more of the penicillin-binding proteins (PBPs) which in turn inhibits the final transpeptidation step of peptidoglycan synthesis in bacterial cell walls, thus inhibiting cell wall biosynthesis. Bacteria eventually lyse due to ongoing activity of cell wall autolytic enzymes (autolysins and murein hydrolases) while cell wall assembly is arrested.

Pharmacodynamics/Kinetics

Absorption: Oral (cefuroxime axetil): Increases with food

Distribution: Widely to body tissues and fluids; crosses blood-brain barrier; therapeutic concentrations achieved in CSF even when meninges are not inflamed; crosses placenta; enters breast milk

Protein binding: 33% to 50%

Bioavailability: Tablet: Fasting: 37%; Following food: 52%

Half-life elimination: Adults: 1-2 hours; prolonged with renal impairment

Time to peak, serum: I.M.: ~15-60 minutes; I.V.: 2-3 minutes

Excretion: Urine (66% to 100% as unchanged drug)

Dosage Note: Cefuroxime axetil film-coated tablets and oral suspension are not bioequivalent and are not substitutable on a mg/mg basis

Children ≥3 months to 12 years:

- Pharyngitis, tonsillitis: Oral:
  - Suspension: 20 mg/kg/day (maximum: 500 mg/day) in 2 divided doses for 10 days
  - Tablet: 125 mg every 12 hours for 10 days
- Acute otitis media, impetigo: Oral:
  - Suspension: 30 mg/kg/day (maximum: 1 g/day) in 2 divided doses for 10 days
  - Tablet: 250 mg twice daily for 10 days
  - I.M., I.V.: 75-150 mg/kg/day divided every 8 hours; maximum dose: 6 g/day
- Meningitis: Not recommended (doses of 200-240 mg/kg/day divided every 6-8 hours have been used); maximum dose: 9 g/day
- Acute bacterial maxillary sinusitis:
  - Suspension: 30 mg/kg/day in 2 divided doses for 10 days; maximum dose: 1 g/day
  - Tablet: 250 mg twice daily for 10 days

Children ≥13 years and Adults:

- Oral: 250-500 mg twice daily for 10 days (5 days in selected patients with acute bronchitis)
  - Uncomplicated urinary tract infection: 125-250 mg every 12 hours for 7-10 days
  - Uncomplicated gonorrhea: 1 g as a single dose
  - Early Lyme disease: 500 mg twice daily for 20 days
- I.M., I.V.: 750 mg to 1.5 g/dose every 8 hours or 100-150 mg/kg/day in divided doses every 6-8 hours; maximum: 6 g/24 hours

Dosing adjustment in renal impairment:

- Cl_{cr} 10-20 mL/minute: Administer every 12 hours
- Cl_{cr} <10 mL/minute: Administer every 24 hours

Hemodialysis: Dialyzable (25%)

Continuous arteriovenous or venovenous hemodiafiltration effects: Dose as for Cl_{cr} 10-20 mL/minute

Dietary Considerations May be taken with food.

Zinacef®: Sodium content: 4.8 mEq (111 mg) per 750 mg

Ceftin®: Powder for oral suspension 125 mg/5 mL contains phenylalanine 11.8 mg/5 mL; 250 mg/5 mL contains phenylalanine 25.2 mg/5 mL.

Administration

Oral: Administer around-the-clock to promote less variation in peak and trough serum levels.

Oral suspension: Administer with food. Shake well before use.

I.M.: Inject deep I.M. into large muscle mass.

I.V.: Inject direct I.V. over 3-5 minutes. Infuse intermittent infusion over 15-30 minutes.

Monitoring Parameters Observe for signs and symptoms of anaphylaxis during first dose; with prolonged therapy, monitor renal, hepatic, and hematologic function periodically; monitor prothrombin time in patients at risk of prolongation during cephalosporin therapy (nutritionally-deficient, prolonged treatment, renal or hepatic disease)

Test Interactions Positive direct Coombs', false-positive urinary glucose test using cupric sulfate (Benedict's solution, Clinitest®, Fehling's solution), false-positive serum or urine creatinine with Jaffé reaction

Patient Information Report prolonged diarrhea; take entire course of medication; may interfere with oral contraceptives; females should report symptoms of vaginitis

Dosage Forms [DSC] = Discontinued product

Infusion, as sodium [premixed] (Zinacef®): 750 mg (50 mL); 1.5 g (50 mL) [contains sodium 4.8 mEq (111 mg) per 750 mg]

Injection, powder for reconstitution, as sodium (Zinacef®): 750 mg, 1.5 g, 7.5 g [contains sodium 4.8 mEq (111 mg) per 750 mg]

Powder for oral suspension, as axetil (Ceftin®): 125 mg/5 mL (100 mL) [contains phenylalanine 11.8 mg/5 mL; tutti-frutti flavor]; 250 mg/5 mL (50 mL, 100 mL) [contains phenylalanine 25.2 mg/5 mL; tutti-frutti flavor]

Tablet, as axetil: 250 mg, 500 mg

Ceftin®: 250 mg, 500 mg

Selected Readings

"Antimicrobial Prophylaxis in Surgery," *Med Lett Drugs Ther*, 1993, 35(906):91-4.

Donowitz GR and Mandell GL, "Beta-Lactam Antibiotics," *N Engl J Med*, 1988, 318(7):419-26 and 318(8):490-500.

Gentry LO, Zeluff BJ, and Cooley DA, "Antibiotic Prophylaxis in Open-Heart Surgery: A Comparison of Cefamandole, Cefuroxime, and Cefazolin," *Ann Thorac Surg*, 1988, 46(2):167-71.

Marshall WF and Blair JE, "The Cephalosporins," *Mayo Clin Proc*, 1999, 74(2):187-95.

Perry CM and Brogden RN, "Cefuroxime Axetil. A Review of Its Antibacterial Activity, Pharmacokinetic Properties and Therapeutic Efficacy," *Drugs*, 1996, 52(1):125-58.

Peterson CD, Lake KD, Arom KV, et al, "Antibiotic Prophylaxis in Open-Heart Surgery Patients: Comparison of Cefamandole and Cefuroxime," *Drug Intell Clin Pharm*, 1987, 21(9):728-32.

Scott LJ, Ormrod D, and Goa KL, "Cefuroxime Axetil: An Updated Review of Its Use in the Management of Bacterial Infections," *Drugs*, 2001, 61(10):1455-500.

Cefuroxime Axetil *see* Cefuroxime *on page 725*

Cefuroxime Sodium *see* Cefuroxime *on page 725*

Cefzil® *see* Cefprozil *on page 716*

Centany™ *see* Mupirocin *on page 953*

Cephalexin (sef a LEKS in)

Related Information

Animal and Human Bites *on page 1270*

Antimicrobial Activity Against Selected Organisms *on page 1165*

U.S. Brand Names Biocef®; Keflex®; Panixine DisperDose™

Canadian Brand Names Apo-Cephalex®; Keftab®; Novo-Lexin; Nu-Cephalex

Synonyms Cephalexin Monohydrate

Generic Available Yes: Excludes tablet for oral suspension

Use Treatment of susceptible bacterial infections including respiratory tract infections, otitis media, skin and skin structure infections, bone infections and genitourinary tract infections, including acute prostatitis; alternative therapy for acute bacterial endocarditis prophylaxis

Drug of Choice or Alternative for Disease/Syndrome(s):

Osteomyelitis, Diabetic Foot *on page 249*

Pregnancy Risk Factor B

Contraindications Hypersensitivity to cephalexin, any component of the formulation, or other cephalosporins

Warnings/Precautions Modify dosage in patients with severe renal impairment, prolonged use may result in superinfection; use with caution in patients with a history (Continued)

Cephalexin *(Continued)*

of penicillin allergy, especially IgE-mediated reactions (eg, anaphylaxis, urticaria). May cause antibiotic-associated colitis or colitis secondary to *C. difficile.*

Adverse Reactions Frequency not defined.

Central nervous system: Agitation, confusion, dizziness, fatigue, hallucinations, headache

Dermatologic: Angioedema, erythema multiforme (rare), rash, Stevens-Johnson syndrome (rare), toxic epidermal necrolysis (rare), urticaria

Gastrointestinal: Abdominal pain, diarrhea, dyspepsia, gastritis, nausea (rare), pseudomembranous colitis, vomiting (rare)

Genitourinary: Genital pruritus, genital moniliasis, vaginitis, vaginal discharge

Hematologic: Eosinophilia, neutropenia, thrombocytopenia

Hepatic: AST/ALT increased, cholestatic jaundice (rare), transient hepatitis (rare)

Neuromuscular & skeletal: Arthralgia, arthritis, joint disorder

Renal: Interstitial nephritis (rare)

Miscellaneous: Allergic reactions

Overdosage/Toxicology Symptoms of overdose include epigastric distress, diarrhea, hematuria, nausea, and vomiting. Many beta-lactam containing antibiotics have the potential to cause neuromuscular hyperirritability or seizures. Hemodialysis may be helpful to aid in removal of the drug from blood; otherwise, treatment is supportive and symptom-directed.

Drug Interactions

Increased Effect/Toxicity: High-dose probenecid may decrease clearance of cephalexin. Aminoglycosides in combination with cephalexin may result in additive nephrotoxicity.

Ethanol/Nutrition/Herb Interactions Food: Peak antibiotic serum concentration is lowered and delayed, but total drug absorbed is not affected. Cephalexin serum levels may be decreased if taken with food.

Stability Refrigerate suspension after reconstitution; discard after 14 days.

Tablet for oral suspension (Panixine DisperDose™): Tablets must be dissolved in ~10 mL water prior to administration, and should be used immediately after dissolving.

Mechanism of Action Inhibits bacterial cell wall synthesis by binding to one or more of the penicillin-binding proteins (PBPs) which in turn inhibits the final transpeptidation step of peptidoglycan synthesis in bacterial cell walls, thus inhibiting cell wall biosynthesis. Bacteria eventually lyse due to ongoing activity of cell wall autolytic enzymes (autolysins and murein hydrolases) while cell wall assembly is arrested.

Pharmacodynamics/Kinetics

Absorption: Delayed in young children

Distribution: Widely into most body tissues and fluids, including gallbladder, liver, kidneys, bone, sputum, bile, and pleural and synovial fluids; CSF penetration is poor; crosses placenta; enters breast milk

Protein binding: 6% to 15%

Half-life elimination: Adults: 0.5-1.2 hours; prolonged with renal impairment

Time to peak, serum: ~1 hour

Excretion: Urine (80% to 100% as unchanged drug) within 8 hours

Dosage Oral:

Children >1 year: Dosing range: 25-50 mg/kg/day every 6-8 hours; more severe infections: 50-100 mg/kg/day in divided doses every 6-8 hours; maximum: 4 g/24 hours

Otitis media: 75-100 mg/kg/day in 4 divided doses

Streptococcal pharyngitis, skin and skin structure infections: 25-50 mg/kg/day divided every 12 hours

Uncomplicated cystitis: Children >15 years: Refer to Adults dosing

Prophylaxis of bacterial endocarditis (dental, oral, respiratory tract, or esophageal procedures): 50 mg/kg 1 hour prior to procedure (maximum: 2 g)

Adults: Dosing range: 250-1000 mg every 6 hours; maximum: 4 g/day

Streptococcal pharyngitis, skin and skin structure infections: 500 mg every 12 hours

Uncomplicated cystitis: 500 mg every 12 hours for 7-14 days

Prophylaxis of bacterial endocarditis (dental, oral, respiratory tract, or esophageal procedures): 2 g 1 hour prior to procedure

Dosing adjustment in renal impairment: Adults: Cl_{cr} <10 mL/minute: 250-500 mg every 12 hours

Hemodialysis: Moderately dialyzable (20% to 50%)

Dietary Considerations Take without regard to food. If GI distress, take with food. Panixine DisperDose™ contains phenylalanine 2.8 mg/cephalexin 125 mg.

Administration Take without regard to food. If GI distress, take with food. Give around-the-clock to promote less variation in peak and trough serum levels.

Panixine DisperDose™: Tablets should be mixed in ~10 mL of water immediately prior to administration. Drink entire solution, then rinse glass with additional water and drink contents to ensure entire dose has been taken. Tablets should not be chewed or swallowed whole.

Monitoring Parameters With prolonged therapy monitor renal, hepatic, and hematologic function periodically; monitor for signs of anaphylaxis during first dose

Test Interactions Positive direct Coombs', false-positive urinary glucose test using cupric sulfate (Benedict's solution, Clinitest®, Fehling's solution), false-positive serum or urine creatinine with Jaffé reaction, false-positive urinary proteins and steroids

Patient Information Report prolonged diarrhea; take entire course of medication; may interfere with oral contraceptives; females should report symptoms of vaginitis

Dosage Forms

Capsule: 250 mg, 500 mg

Biocef®: 500 mg

Keflex®: 250 mg, 500 mg

Powder for oral suspension: 125 mg/5 mL (100 mL, 200 mL); 250 mg/5 mL (100 mL, 200 mL)

Biocef®: 125 mg/5 mL (100 mL); 250 mg/5 mL (100 mL)

Keflex®: 125 mg/5 mL (100 mL, 200 mL); 250 mg/5 mL (100 mL, 200 mL)

Tablet, for oral suspension (Panixine DisperDose™): 125 mg [contains phenylalanine 2.8 mg; peppermint flavor], 250 mg [contains phenylalanine 5.6 mg; peppermint flavor]

Selected Readings

Donowitz GR and Mandell GL, "Beta-Lactam Antibiotics," *N Engl J Med*, 1988, 318(7):419-26 and 318(8):490-500.

Marshall WF and Blair JE, "The Cephalosporins," *Mayo Clin Proc*, 1999, 74(2):187-95.

Smith GH, "Oral Cephalosporins in Perspective," *DICP*, 1990, 24(1):45-51.

Cephalexin Monohydrate *see* Cephalexin *on page 727*

Cephalosporins, 1st Generation

Refer to

Cefadroxil *on page 698*
Cefazolin *on page 700*
Cephalexin *on page 727*
Cephalothin *on page 730*
Cephradine *on page 731*

Drug of Choice or Alternative for Disease/Syndrome(s):

Asymptomatic Bacteriuria *on page 39*
Erysipelas *on page 141*
Furunculosis *on page 151*
Impetigo *on page 193*
Keratitis, Bacterial and Fungal *on page 199*
Osteomyelitis, Healthy Adult *on page 250*
Osteomyelitis, Pediatric *on page 251*
Pharyngitis *on page 264*
Skin and Soft Tissue *on page 300*

Organism(s):

Erysipelothrix rhusiopathiae on page 141
Escherichia coli on page 142
Klebsiella Species *on page 200*
Proteus Species *on page 278*
Staphylococcus aureus, Methicillin-Susceptible *on page 307*
Staphylococcus epidermidis, Methicillin-Susceptible *on page 310*
Staphylococcus saprophyticus on page 312
Streptococcus agalactiae on page 313
Streptococcus pneumoniae, Drug-Susceptible *on page 319*
Streptococcus pyogenes on page 321
Streptococcus-Related Gram-Positive Cocci *on page 325*
Streptococcus, Viridans Group *on page 326*

Cephalosporins, 2nd Generation

Refer to

Cefaclor *on page 697*
Cefotetan *on page 710*
Cefoxitin *on page 712*
Cefprozil *on page 716*
Cefuroxime *on page 725*
(Continued)

Cephalosporins, 2nd Generation *(Continued)*

Drug of Choice or Alternative for Disease/Syndrome(s):

Bronchitis *on page 60*
Cholangitis, Acute *on page 79*
Diverticulitis *on page 116*
Epiglottitis *on page 139*
Otitis Media, Acute *on page 253*
Sinusitis, Community-Acquired, Acute *on page 299*

Organism(s):

Escherichia coli on page 142
Haemophilus influenzae on page 159
Klebsiella Species *on page 200*
Moraxella catarrhalis on page 223
Proteus Species *on page 278*
Providencia Species *on page 281*

Cephalosporins, 3rd Generation

Refer to

Cefdinir *on page 702*
Cefixime *on page 707*
Cefotaxime *on page 708*
Cefpodoxime *on page 714*
Ceftazidime *on page 717*
Ceftibuten *on page 719*
Ceftizoxime *on page 720*
Ceftriaxone *on page 722*

Drug of Choice or Alternative for Disease/Syndrome(s):

Amnionitis *on page 33*
Brain Abscess *on page 58*
Catheter Infection, Intravascular *on page 70*
Cholangitis, Acute *on page 79*
Diverticulitis *on page 116*
Epiglottitis *on page 139*
Osteomyelitis, Diabetic Foot *on page 249*
Urinary Tract Infection, Pyelonephritis *on page 346*

Organism(s):

Acinetobacter Species *on page 24*
Aeromonas Species *on page 30*
Alcaligenes Species *on page 31*
Bordetella bronchiseptica on page 52
Burkholderia mallei on page 64
Citrobacter Species *on page 81*
Enterobacter Species *on page 132*
Escherichia coli on page 142
HACEK Group *on page 158*
Haemophilus influenzae on page 159
Klebsiella Species *on page 200*
Moraxella catarrhalis on page 223
Proteus Species *on page 278*
Providencia Species *on page 281*
Salmonella Species *on page 291*
Serratia Species *on page 296*
Shigella Species *on page 297*
Yersinia enterocolitica on page 354

Cephalothin (sef A loe thin)

Related Information

Antimicrobial Activity Against Selected Organisms *on page 1165*

Synonyms Cephalothin Sodium

Generic Available Yes

Use Treatment of infections when caused by susceptible strains in respiratory, genitourinary, gastrointestinal, skin and soft tissue, bone and joint infections; septicemia; treatment of susceptible gram-positive bacilli and cocci (never enterococcus); some gram-negative bacilli including *E. coli*, *Proteus*, and *Klebsiella* may be susceptible

Pregnancy Risk Factor B

Contraindications Hypersensitivity to cephalothin, any component of the formulation, or other cephalosporins

Warnings/Precautions Modify dosage in patients with severe renal impairment, prolonged use may result in superinfection; use with caution in patients with a history of penicillin allergy, especially IgE-mediated reactions (eg, anaphylaxis, urticaria). May cause antibiotic-associated colitis or colitis secondary to *C. difficile.*

Adverse Reactions Frequency not defined.

Dermatologic: Maculopapular and erythematous rash

Gastrointestinal: Diarrhea, nausea, vomiting, dyspepsia, pseudomembranous colitis

Local: Bleeding, pain and induration at injection site

Reactions reported with other cephalosporins include anaphylaxis, erythema multiforme, toxic epidermal necrolysis, Stevens-Johnson syndrome, dizziness, fever, headache, CNS irritability, seizure, decreased hemoglobin, neutropenia, leukopenia, agranulocytosis, pancytopenia, aplastic anemia, hemolytic anemia, interstitial nephritis, toxic nephropathy, vaginitis, angioedema, cholestasis, hemorrhage, prolonged PT, serum-sickness reactions, superinfection

Stability After freezing, thawed solution is stable for 12 hours at room temperature.

Mechanism of Action Inhibits bacterial cell wall synthesis by binding to one or more of the penicillin-binding proteins (PBPs) which in turn inhibits the final transpeptidation step of peptidoglycan synthesis in bacterial cell walls, thus inhibiting cell wall biosynthesis. Bacteria eventually lyse due to ongoing activity of cell wall autolytic enzymes (autolysins and murein hydrolases) while cell wall assembly is arrested.

Pharmacodynamics/Kinetics

Distribution: Does not penetrate CSF unless meninges are inflamed; crosses placenta; small amounts enter breast milk

Protein binding: 65% to 80%

Metabolism: Partially hepatic and renal via deacetylation

Half-life elimination: 30-60 minutes

Excretion: Urine (50% to 75% as unchanged drug)

Dosage I.V.:

Neonates:

- Postnatal age <7 days:
  - <2000 g: 20 mg every 12 hours
  - >2000 g: 20 mg every 8 hours
- Postnatal age >7 days:
  - <2000 g: 20 mg every 8 hours
  - >2000 g: 20 mg every 6 hours

Children: 75-125 mg/kg/day divided every 4-6 hours; maximum dose: 10 g in a 24-hour period

Adults: 500 mg to 2 g every 4-6 hours

Dosing interval in renal impairment:

- Cl_{cr} 10-50 mL/minute: Administer every 6-8 hours
- Cl_{cr} <10 mL/minute: Administer every 12 hours

Continuous arteriovenous or venovenous hemodiafiltration effects: Administer 1 g every 8 hours

Monitoring Parameters Observe for signs and symptoms of anaphylaxis during first dose

Test Interactions Positive direct Coombs', false-positive urinary glucose test using cupric sulfate (Benedict's solution, Clinitest®, Fehling's solution), false-positive serum or urine creatinine with Jaffé reaction, false-positive urinary proteins and steroids

Dosage Forms [DSC] = Discontinued product

Infusion, as sodium [frozen]: 1 g (50 mL); 2 g (50 mL) [DSC]

Selected Readings

Donowitz GR and Mandell GL, "Beta-Lactam Antibiotics," *N Engl J Med*, 1988, 318(7):419-26 and 318(8):490-500.

Marshall WF and Blair JE, "The Cephalosporins," *Mayo Clin Proc*, 1999, 74(2):187-95

Cephalothin Sodium *see* Cephalothin *on page 730*

Cephradine (SEF ra deen)

Related Information

Antimicrobial Activity Against Selected Organisms *on page 1165*

U.S. Brand Names Velosef®

Generic Available No

Use Treatment of infections when caused by susceptible strains in respiratory, genitourinary, gastrointestinal, skin and soft tissue, bone and joint infections; treatment of susceptible gram-positive bacilli and cocci (never enterococcus); some gram-negative bacilli including *E. coli*, *Proteus*, and *Klebsiella* may be susceptible

Pregnancy Risk Factor B

Contraindications Hypersensitivity to cephradine, any component of the formulation, or cephalosporins

(Continued)

Cephradine *(Continued)*

Warnings/Precautions Use caution with renal impairment; dose adjustment required. Prolonged use may result in superinfection; use with caution in patients with a history of penicillin allergy, especially IgE-mediated reactions (eg, anaphylaxis, urticaria). May cause antibiotic-associated colitis or colitis secondary to *C. difficile*.

Adverse Reactions Frequency not defined.

Central nervous system: Dizziness
Dermatologic: Rash, pruritus
Gastrointestinal: Diarrhea, nausea, vomiting, pseudomembranous colitis
Hematologic: Leukopenia, neutropenia, eosinophilia
Neuromuscular & skeletal: Joint pain
Renal: BUN increased, creatinine increased

Reactions reported with other cephalosporins include anaphylaxis, erythema multiforme, toxic epidermal necrolysis, Stevens-Johnson syndrome, fever, headache, encephalopathy, asterixis, neuromuscular excitability, seizure, agranulocytosis, pancytopenia, aplastic anemia, hemolytic anemia, interstitial nephritis, toxic nephropathy, vaginitis, angioedema, cholestasis, hemorrhage, prolonged PT, serum-sickness reactions, superinfection

Overdosage/Toxicology Symptoms include neuromuscular hypersensitivity and convulsions especially with renal insufficiency. Many beta-lactam antibiotics have the potential to cause neuromuscular hyperirritability or seizures. Hemodialysis may be helpful to aid in removal of the drug from the blood; otherwise, most treatment is supportive or symptom-directed.

Drug Interactions

Increased Effect/Toxicity: High-dose probenecid decreases clearance of cephradine. Aminoglycosides in combination with cephradine may result in additive nephrotoxicity.

Ethanol/Nutrition/Herb Interactions Food: Food delays cephradine absorption but does not decrease extent.

Stability

Capsule: Store at controlled room temperature.

Powder for oral suspension: Store at controlled room temperature. Following reconstitution, refrigerated storage of oral suspension maintains potency for 14 days. Room temperature storage maintains potency for 7 days.

Mechanism of Action Inhibits bacterial cell wall synthesis by binding to one or more of the penicillin-binding proteins (PBPs) which in turn inhibits the final transpeptidation step of peptidoglycan synthesis in bacterial cell walls, thus inhibiting cell wall biosynthesis. Bacteria eventually lyse due to ongoing activity of cell wall autolytic enzymes (autolysins and murein hydrolases) while cell wall assembly is arrested.

Pharmacodynamics/Kinetics

Absorption: Well absorbed

Distribution: Widely into most body tissues and fluids including gallbladder, liver, kidneys, bone, sputum, bile, and pleural and synovial fluids; CSF penetration is poor; crosses placenta; enters breast milk

Protein binding: 18% to 20%

Half-life elimination: 1-2 hours; prolonged with renal impairment

Time to peak, serum: 1-2 hours

Excretion: Urine (~80% to 90% as unchanged drug) within 6 hours

Dosage Oral:

Children ≥9 months: Usual dose: 25-50 mg/kg/day in divided doses every 6 hours

Otitis media: 75-100 mg/kg/day in divided doses every 6 or 12 hours (maximum: 4 g/day)

Adults: 250-500 mg every 6-12 hours

Dosing adjustment in renal impairment: Adults:

Cl_{cr} 10-50 mL/minute: 250 mg every 6 hours

Cl_{cr} <10 mL/minute: 125 mg every 6 hours

Dietary Considerations May administer with food to decrease GI distress.

Administration Administer around-the-clock to promote less variation in peak and trough serum levels. Shake oral suspension well.

Monitoring Parameters Observe for signs and symptoms of anaphylaxis during first dose

Test Interactions Positive direct Coombs', false-positive urinary glucose test using cupric sulfate (Benedict's solution, Clinitest®, Fehling's solution), false-positive serum or urine creatinine with Jaffé reaction, false-positive urinary proteins and steroids

Patient Information Take until gone, do not miss doses; report diarrhea promptly; take entire course of medication; may interfere with oral contraceptives; females should report symptoms of vaginitis

Dosage Forms [DSC] = Discontinued product

Capsule: 250 mg, 500 mg [DSC]
Powder for oral suspension: 250 mg/5 mL (100 mL) [fruit flavor]

Selected Readings

Donowitz GR and Mandell GL, "Beta-Lactam Antibiotics," *N Engl J Med*, 1988, 318(7):419-26 and 318(8):490-500.
Marshall WF and Blair JE, "The Cephalosporins," *Mayo Clin Proc*, 1999, 74(2):187-95.
Smith GH, "Oral Cephalosporins in Perspective," *DICP*, 1990, 24(1):45-51.

Ceptaz® [DSC] *see* Ceftazidime *on page 717*
Cetamide™ (Can) *see* Sulfacetamide *on page 1081*
CFDN *see* Cefdinir *on page 702*
CHG *see* Chlorhexidine Gluconate *on page 735*
Chicken Pox Vaccine *see* Varicella Virus Vaccine *on page 1148*
Children's Kaopectate® *(reformulation)* [OTC] [DSC] *see* Bismuth *on page 686*

Chloramphenicol (klor am FEN i kole)

Related Information

Antimicrobial Activity Against Selected Organisms *on page 1165*

U.S. Brand Names Chloromycetin® Sodium Succinate

Canadian Brand Names Chloromycetin®; Diochloram®; Pentamycetin®

Generic Available Yes

Use Treatment of serious infections due to organisms resistant to other less toxic antibiotics or when its penetrability into the site of infection is clinically superior to other antibiotics to which the organism is sensitive; useful in infections caused by *Bacteroides*, *H. influenzae*, *Neisseria meningitidis*, *Salmonella*, and *Rickettsia*; active against many vancomycin-resistant enterococci

Drug of Choice or Alternative for Disease/Syndrome(s):

Meningitis, Community-Acquired, Adult *on page 216*
Meningitis, Neonatal (<1 month of age) *on page 217*
Meningitis, Pediatric (>1 month of age) *on page 218*

Organism(s):

Bordetella pertussis on page 53
Burkholderia cepacia on page 62
Burkholderia mallei on page 64
Coxiella burnetii on page 100
Ehrlichia Species *on page 119*
Enterococcus Species *on page 134*
Francisella tularensis on page 149
Haemophilus influenzae on page 159
Neisseria meningitidis on page 245
Rickettsia rickettsii on page 289
Salmonella Species *on page 291*
Streptococcus pneumoniae, Drug-Susceptible *on page 319*
Yersinia pestis on page 355

Pregnancy Risk Factor C

Pregnancy Implications Embryotoxic and teratogenic in animals, but there are no adequate and well-controlled studies in pregnant women. Has been shown to cross placental barrier. "Gray syndrome" has been reported in a neonate following administration to the mother during labor.

Contraindications Hypersensitivity to chloramphenicol or any component of the formulation

Warnings/Precautions Serious and fatal blood dyscrasias have occurred after both short-term and prolonged therapy including reports associated with topical treatment. Should not be used when less potentially toxic agents are effective; prolonged use may result in superinfection. Use with caution in patients with impaired renal or hepatic function and in neonates; reduce dose with impaired liver function; use with care in patients with glucose 6-phosphate dehydrogenase deficiency.

Adverse Reactions

Three (3) major toxicities associated with chloramphenicol include:

Aplastic anemia, an idiosyncratic reaction which can occur with any route of administration; usually occurs 3 weeks to 12 months after initial exposure to chloramphenicol

Bone marrow suppression is thought to be dose related with serum concentrations >25 mcg/mL and reversible once chloramphenicol is discontinued; anemia and neutropenia may occur during the first week of therapy

Gray syndrome is characterized by circulatory collapse, cyanosis, acidosis, abdominal distention, myocardial depression, coma, and death; reaction appears to be associated with serum levels ≥50 mcg/mL; may result from drug accumulation in patients with impaired hepatic or renal function

(Continued)

Chloramphenicol *(Continued)*

Additional adverse reactions, frequency not defined:

Central nervous system: Confusion, delirium, depression, fever, headache

Dermatologic: Angioedema, rash, urticaria

Gastrointestinal: Diarrhea, enterocolitis, glossitis, nausea, stomatitis, vomiting

Hematologic: Granulocytopenia, hypoplastic anemia, pancytopenia, thrombocytopenia

Ocular: Optic neuritis

Miscellaneous: Anaphylaxis, hypersensitivity reactions

Overdosage/Toxicology Symptoms include anemia, metabolic acidosis, hypotension, and hypothermia. Treatment is supportive following GI decontamination.

Drug Interactions

Cytochrome P450 Effect: Inhibits CYP2C8/9 (weak), 3A4 (weak)

Increased Effect/Toxicity: Chloramphenicol increases serum concentrations of chlorpropamide, phenytoin, and oral anticoagulants.

Decreased Effect: Phenobarbital and rifampin may decrease serum concentrations of chloramphenicol.

Ethanol/Nutrition/Herb Interactions Food: May decrease intestinal absorption of vitamin B_{12} may have increased dietary need for riboflavin, pyridoxine, and vitamin B_{12}.

Stability Store at room temperature prior to reconstitution; reconstituted solutions remain stable for 30 days; use only clear solutions; frozen solutions remain stable for 6 months

Mechanism of Action Reversibly binds to 50S ribosomal subunits of susceptible organisms preventing amino acids from being transferred to growing peptide chains thus inhibiting protein synthesis

Pharmacodynamics/Kinetics

Distribution: To most tissues and body fluids; readily crosses placenta; enters breast milk

CSF:blood level ratio: Normal meninges: 66%; Inflamed meninges: >66%

Protein binding: 60%

Metabolism: Extensively hepatic (90%) to inactive metabolites, principally by glucuronidation; chloramphenicol sodium succinate is hydrolyzed by esterases to active base

Half-life elimination

Normal renal function: 1.6-3.3 hours

End-stage renal disease: 3-7 hours

Cirrhosis: 10-12 hours

Excretion: Urine (5% to 15%)

Dosage

Meningitis: I.V.: Infants >30 days and Children: 50-100 mg/kg/day divided every 6 hours

Other infections: I.V.:

Infants >30 days and Children: 50-75 mg/kg/day divided every 6 hours; maximum daily dose: 4 g/day

Adults: 50-100 mg/kg/day in divided doses every 6 hours; maximum daily dose: 4 g/day

Dosing adjustment/comments in hepatic impairment: Avoid use in severe liver impairment as increased toxicity may occur

Hemodialysis: Slightly dialyzable (5% to 20%) via hemo- and peritoneal dialysis; no supplemental doses needed in dialysis or continuous arteriovenous or veno-venous hemofiltration

Dietary Considerations May have increased dietary need for riboflavin, pyridoxine, and vitamin B_{12}. Sodium content of 1 g injection: ~52 mg (2.25 mEq).

Administration Do not administer I.M.; can be administered IVP over at least 1 minute at a concentration of 100 mg/mL, or I.V. intermittent infusion over 15-30 minutes at a final concentration for administration of ≤20 mg/mL

Monitoring Parameters CBC with reticulocyte and platelet counts, periodic liver and renal function tests, serum drug concentration

Reference Range

Therapeutic levels:

Meningitis:

Peak: 15-25 mcg/mL; toxic concentration: >40 mcg/mL

Trough: 5-15 mcg/mL

Other infections:

Peak: 10-20 mcg/mL

Trough: 5-10 mcg/mL

Timing of serum samples: Draw levels 0.5-1.5 hours after completion of I.V. dose

Dosage Forms Injection, powder for reconstitution (Chloromycetin® Sodium Succinate): 1 g [contains sodium ~52 mg/g (2.25 mEq/g)]

Selected Readings

Smilack JD, Wilson WR, and Cockerill FR 3d, "Tetracyclines, Chloramphenicol, Erythromycin, Clindamycin, and Metronidazole," *Mayo Clin Proc*, 1991, 66(12):1270-80.

Tunkel AR, Wispelwey B, and Scheld M, "Bacterial Meningitis: Recent Advances in Pathophysiology and Treatment," *Ann Intern Med*, 1990, 112(8):610-23.

ChloraPrep® [OTC] *see* Chlorhexidine Gluconate *on page 735*

Chlorhexidine Gluconate (klor HEKS i deen GLOO koe nate)

U.S. Brand Names Avagard™ [OTC]; BactoShield® CHG [OTC]; Betasept® [OTC]; ChloraPrep® [OTC]; Dyna-Hex® [OTC]; Hibiclens® [OTC]; Hibistat® [OTC]; Operand® Chlorhexidine Gluconate [OTC]; Peridex®; PerioChip®; PerioGard®

Canadian Brand Names Apo-Chlorhexadine®; Hibidil® 1:2000; ORO-Clense; SpectroGram 2™

Synonyms CHG; 3M™ Avagard™ [OTC]

Generic Available Yes: Oral liquid

Use Skin cleanser for surgical scrub, cleanser for skin wounds, preoperative skin preparation, germicidal hand rinse, and as antibacterial dental rinse. Chlorhexidine is active against gram-positive and gram-negative organisms, facultative anaerobes, aerobes, and yeast.

Orphan drug: Peridex®: Oral mucositis with cytoreductive therapy when used for patients undergoing bone marrow transplant

Pregnancy Risk Factor B

Contraindications Hypersensitivity to chlorhexidine gluconate or any component of the formulation

Warnings/Precautions

Oral: Staining of oral surfaces (mucosa, teeth, tooth restorations, dorsum of tongue) may occur; may be visible as soon as 1 week after therapy begins and is more pronounced when there is a heavy accumulation of unremoved plaque and when teeth fillings have rough surfaces. Stain does not have a clinically adverse effect, but because removal may not be possible, patient with frontal restoration should be advised of the potential permanency of the stain.

Topical: For topical use only. Keep out of eyes and ears. May stain fabric. There have been case reports of anaphylaxis following chlorhexidine disinfection. Not for preoperative preparation of face or head; avoid contact with meninges.

Adverse Reactions

Oral:

- >10%: Increase of tartar on teeth, changes in taste. Staining of oral surfaces (mucosa, teeth, dorsum of tongue) may be visible as soon as 1 week after therapy begins and is more pronounced when there is a heavy accumulation of unremoved plaque and when teeth fillings have rough surfaces. Stain does not have a clinically adverse effect but because removal may not be possible, patient with frontal restoration should be advised of the potential permanency of the stain.
- 1% to 10%: Gastrointestinal: Tongue irritation, oral irritation
- <1%: Facial edema, nasal congestion, dyspnea

Topical: Skin erythema and roughness, dryness, sensitization, allergic reactions

Overdosage/Toxicology Symptoms of oral overdose include gastric distress, nausea, or signs of ethanol intoxication

Stability Store at room temperature

Avagard™: Avoid excessive heat. Ethanol-containing products are flammable; keep away from flames or fire. Hand lotions and gel hand sanitizers are incompatible. The thickeners used in these products (eg, carbomer) react to form an insoluble salt and cause loss of antibacterial action.

Mechanism of Action The bactericidal effect of chlorhexidine is a result of the binding of this cationic molecule to negatively charged bacterial cell walls and extramicrobial complexes. At low concentrations, this causes an alteration of bacterial cell osmotic equilibrium and leakage of potassium and phosphorous resulting in a bacteriostatic effect. At high concentrations of chlorhexidine, the cytoplasmic contents of the bacterial cell precipitate and result in cell death.

Pharmacodynamics/Kinetics

Topical hand sanitizer (Avagard™): Duration of antimicrobial protection: 6 hours

Oral rinse (Peridex®, PerioGard®):

- Absorption: ~30% retained in the oral cavity following rinsing and slowly released into oral fluids; poorly absorbed
- Time to peak, plasma: Oral rinse: Detectable levels not present after 12 hours
- Excretion: Feces (~90%); urine (<1%)

(Continued)

Chlorhexidine Gluconate *(Continued)*

Dosage Adults:

Oral rinse (Peridex®, PerioGard®):

Floss and brush teeth, completely rinse toothpaste from mouth and swish 15 mL (one capful) undiluted oral rinse around in mouth for 30 seconds, then expectorate. Caution patient not to swallow the medicine and instruct not to eat for 2-3 hours after treatment. (Cap on bottle measures 15 mL.)

Treatment of gingivitis: Oral prophylaxis: Swish for 30 seconds with 15 mL chlorhexidine, then expectorate; repeat twice daily (morning and evening). Patient should have a re-evaluation followed by a dental prophylaxis every 6 months.

Periodontal chip: One chip is inserted into a periodontal pocket with a probing pocket depth ≥5 mm. Up to 8 chips may be inserted in a single visit. Treatment is recommended every 3 months in pockets with a remaining depth ≥5 mm. If dislodgment occurs 7 days or more after placement, the subject is considered to have had the full course of treatment. If dislodgment occurs within 48 hours, a new chip should be inserted. The chip biodegrades completely and does not need to be removed. Patients should avoid dental floss at the site of PerioChip® insertion for 10 days after placement because flossing might dislodge the chip.

Insertion of periodontal chip: Pocket should be isolated and surrounding area dried prior to chip insertion. The chip should be grasped using forceps with the rounded edges away from the forceps. The chip should be inserted into the periodontal pocket to its maximum depth. It may be maneuvered into position using the tips of the forceps or a flat instrument.

Cleanser:

Surgical scrub: Scrub 3 minutes and rinse thoroughly, wash for an additional 3 minutes

Hand sanitizer (Avagard™): Dispense 1 pumpful in palm of one hand; dip fingertips of opposite hand into solution and work it under nails. Spread remainder evenly over hand and just above elbow, covering all surfaces. Repeat on other hand. Dispense another pumpful in each hand and reapply to each hand up to the wrist. Allow to dry before gloving.

Hand wash: Wash for 15 seconds and rinse

Hand rinse: Rub 15 seconds and rinse

Administration

Hand sanitizer (Avagard™): To facilitate drying, continue rubbing hand prep into hands until dry.

Periodontal chip insertion: Pocket should be isolated and surrounding area dried prior to chip insertion. The chip should be grasped using forceps with the rounded edges away from the forceps. The chip should be inserted into the periodontal pocket to its maximum depth. It may be maneuvered into position using the tips of the forceps or a flat instrument. The chip biodegrades completely and does not need to be removed. Patients should avoid dental floss at the site of PerioChip® insertion for 10 days after placement because flossing might dislodge the chip.

Topical: Keep out of eyes, ears, and mouth. Do not routinely apply to wounds which involve more than superficial layers of skin.

Patient Information

Oral rinse: Do not swallow, do not rinse after use; may cause reduced taste perception which is reversible; may cause discoloration of teeth

Topical administration is for external use only

Dosage Forms

Chip, for periodontal pocket insertion (PerioChip®): 2.5 mg

Liquid, topical [surgical scrub]:

Avagard™: 1% (500 mL) [contains ethyl alcohol and moisturizers]

BactoShield® CHG: 2% (120 mL, 480 mL, 750 mL, 1000 mL, 3800 mL); 4% (120 mL, 480 mL, 750 mL, 1000 mL, 3800 mL) [contains isopropyl alcohol]

Betasept®: 4% (120 mL, 240 mL, 480 mL, 960 mL, 3840 mL) [contains isopropyl alcohol]

ChloraPrep®: 2% (0.67 mL, 1.5 mL, 3 mL, 10.5 mL) [contains isopropyl alcohol 70%; prefilled applicator]

Dyna-Hex®: 2% (120 mL, 960 mL, 3840 mL); 4% (120 mL, 960 mL, 3840 mL)

Hibiclens®: 4% (15 mL, 120 mL, 240 mL, 480 mL, 960 mL, 3840 mL) [contains isopropyl alcohol]

Operand® Chlorhexidine Gluconate: 2% (120 mL); 4% (120 mL, 240 mL, 480 mL, 960 mL, 3840 mL) [contains isopropyl alcohol]

Liquid, oral rinse: 0.12% (480 mL)

Peridex®: 0.12% (480 mL) [contains alcohol 11.6%]

PerioGard®: 0.12% (480 mL) [contains alcohol 11.6%; mint flavor]

Pad [prep pad]: Hibistat®: 0.5% (50s) [contains isopropyl alcohol]

Sponge/Brush (BactoShield® CHG): 4% per sponge/brush [contains isopropyl alcohol]

Selected Readings

Emerson D and Pierce C, "A Case of a Single Ingestion of 4% Hibiclens®," *Vet Hum Toxicol*, 1988, 30(6):583.

Massano G, Ciocatto E, Rosabianca C, et al, "Striking Aminotransferase Rise After Chlorhexidine Self-Poisoning," *Lancet*, 1982, 1(8266):289.

Quinn MW and Bini RM, "Bradycardia Associated With Chlorhexidine Spray," *Arch Dis Child*, 1989, 64(6):892-3.

Yong D, Parker FC, and Foran SM, "Severe Allergic Reactions and Intraurethral Chlorhexidine Gluconate," *Med J Aust*, 1995, 162(5):257-8.

Chloromycetin® (Can) *see* Chloramphenicol *on page 733*

Chloromycetin® Sodium Succinate *see* Chloramphenicol *on page 733*

Chloroquine (KLOR oh kwin)

Related Information

Malaria Treatment *on page 1292*

U.S. Brand Names Aralen®

Canadian Brand Names Aralen®; Novo-Chloroquine

Synonyms Chloroquine Phosphate

Generic Available Yes

Use Suppression or chemoprophylaxis of malaria; treatment of uncomplicated or mild to moderate malaria; extraintestinal amebiasis

Unlabeled/Investigational Use Rheumatoid arthritis; discoid lupus erythematosus

Drug of Choice or Alternative for

Organism(s):

Plasmodium Species *on page 265*

Pregnancy Risk Factor C

Pregnancy Implications There are no adequate and well-controlled studies using chloroquine during pregnancy. However, based on clinical experience and because malaria infection in pregnant women may be more severe than in nonpregnant women, chloroquine prophylaxis may be considered in areas of chloroquine-sensitive *P. falciparum* malaria. Pregnant women should be advised not to travel to areas of *P. falciparum* resistance to chloroquine.

Contraindications Hypersensitivity to chloroquine or any component of the formulation; retinal or visual field changes

Warnings/Precautions Use with caution in patients with liver disease, G6PD deficiency, alcoholism or in conjunction with hepatotoxic drugs. May exacerbate psoriasis or porphyria. Retinopathy (irreversible) has occurred with long or high-dose therapy; discontinue drug if any abnormality in the visual field or if muscular weakness develops during treatment. Use caution in patients with pre-existing auditory damage; discontinue immediately if hearing defects are noted. Use caution in patients with seizure disorders.

Adverse Reactions Frequency not defined.

Cardiovascular: Hypotension (rare), ECG changes (rare; including T-wave inversion), cardiomyopathy

Central nervous system: Fatigue, personality changes, headache, psychosis, seizure, delirium, depression

Dermatologic: Pruritus, hair bleaching, pleomorphic skin eruptions, alopecia, lichen planus eruptions, alopecia, mucosal pigmentary changes (blue-black), photosensitivity

Gastrointestinal: Nausea, diarrhea, vomiting, anorexia, stomatitis, abdominal cramps

Hematologic: Aplastic anemia, agranulocytosis (reversible), neutropenia, thrombocytopenia

Neuromuscular & skeletal: Rare cases of myopathy, neuromyopathy, proximal muscle atrophy, and depression of deep tendon reflexes have been reported

Ocular: Retinopathy (including irreversible changes in some patients long-term or high-dose therapy), blurred vision

Otic: Nerve deafness, tinnitus, reduced hearing (risk increased in patients with pre-existing auditory damage)

Overdosage/Toxicology Symptoms of overdose include headache, visual changes, cardiovascular collapse, shock, seizures, abdominal cramps, vomiting, cyanosis, methemoglobinemia, leukopenia, and respiratory and cardiac arrest. Following initial measures (immediate GI decontamination), treatment is supportive and symptomatic.

Drug Interactions

Cytochrome P450 Effect: Substrate (major) of CYP2D6, 3A4; **Inhibits** CYP2D6 (moderate)

Increased Effect/Toxicity: Chloroquine may increase the levels/effects of dextromethorphan, fluoxetine, lidocaine, mirtazapine, nefazodone, paroxetine, risperidone, ritonavir, thioridazine, tricyclic antidepressants, venlafaxine, and other

(Continued)

Chloroquine *(Continued)*

CYP2D6 substrates. Chloroquine may increase the levels/effects of cyclosporine. The levels/effects of chloroquine may be increased by azole antifungals, chlorpromazine, cimetidine, ciprofloxacin, clarithromycin, delavirdine, diclofenac, doxycycline, erythromycin, fluoxetine, imatinib, isoniazid, miconazole, nefazodone, nicardipine, paroxetine, pergolide, propofol, protease inhibitors, quinidine, quinine, ritonavir, ropinirole, telithromycin, verapamil, and other CYP2D6 or 3A4 inhibitors.

Decreased Effect: Chloroquine levels may be decreased by antacids or kaolin. Chloroquine may decrease ampicillin and/or praziquantel levels. Chloroquine may decrease the levels/effects of CYP2D6 prodrug substrates; example prodrug substrates include codeine, hydrocodone, oxycodone, and tramadol. The levels/effects of chloroquine may be decreased by aminoglutethimide, carbamazepine, nafcillin, nevirapine, phenobarbital, phenytoin, rifamycins, and other CYP3A4 inducers.

Ethanol/Nutrition/Herb Interactions Ethanol: Avoid ethanol (may increase GI irritation).

Stability Store tablets at 25°C (77°F); excursions permitted at 15°C to 30°C (59°F to 86°F).

Mechanism of Action Binds to and inhibits DNA and RNA polymerase; interferes with metabolism and hemoglobin utilization by parasites; inhibits prostaglandin effects; chloroquine concentrates within parasite acid vesicles and raises internal pH resulting in inhibition of parasite growth; may involve aggregates of ferriprotoporphyrin IX acting as chloroquine receptors causing membrane damage; may also interfere with nucleoprotein synthesis

Pharmacodynamics/Kinetics

Duration: Small amounts may be present in urine months following discontinuation of therapy

Absorption: Oral: Rapid (~89%)

Distribution: Widely in body tissues (eg, eyes, heart, kidneys, liver, lungs) where retention prolonged; crosses placenta; enters breast milk

Metabolism: Partially hepatic

Half-life elimination: 3-5 days

Time to peak, serum: 1-2 hours

Excretion: Urine (~70% as unchanged drug); acidification of urine increases elimination

Dosage Oral:

Suppression or prophylaxis of malaria:

Children: Administer 5 mg base/kg/week on the same day each week (not to exceed 300 mg base/dose); begin 1-2 weeks prior to exposure; continue for 4-6 weeks after leaving endemic area; if suppressive therapy is not begun prior to exposure, double the initial loading dose to 10 mg base/kg and administer in 2 divided doses 6 hours apart, followed by the usual dosage regimen

Adults: 500 mg/week (300 mg base) on the same day each week; begin 1-2 weeks prior to exposure; continue for 4-6 weeks after leaving endemic area; if suppressive therapy is not begun prior to exposure, double the initial loading dose to 1 g (600 mg base) and administer in 2 divided doses 6 hours apart, followed by the usual dosage regimen

Acute attack:

Children: 10 mg/kg (base) on day 1, followed by 5 mg/kg (base) 6 hours later and 5 mg/kg (base) on days 2 and 3

Adults: 1 g (600 mg base) on day 1, followed by 500 mg (300 mg base) 6 hours later, followed by 500 mg (300 mg base) on days 2 and 3

Extraintestinal amebiasis:

Children: 10 mg/kg (base) once daily for 2-3 weeks (up to 300 mg base/day)

Adults: 1 g/day (600 mg base) for 2 days followed by 500 mg/day (300 mg base) for at least 2-3 weeks

Rheumatoid arthritis, lupus erythematosus (unlabeled uses): Adults: 250 mg (150 mg base) once daily; reduce dosage following maximal response (taper to discontinue after response in lupus); generally requires 3-6 weeks

Note: Not considered first-line agent.

Dosing adjustment in renal impairment: Cl_{cr} <10 mL/minute: Administer 50% of dose

Hemodialysis: Minimally removed by hemodialysis

Dietary Considerations May be taken with meals to decrease GI upset.

Administration Chloroquine phosphate tablets have also been mixed with chocolate syrup or enclosed in gelatin capsules to mask the bitter taste.

Monitoring Parameters Periodic CBC, examination for muscular weakness, and ophthalmologic examination in patients receiving prolonged therapy

Patient Information Take with meals; report any visual disturbances or difficulty in hearing or ringing in the ears; tablets are bitter tasting; may cause diarrhea, loss of appetite, nausea, stomach pain; notify prescriber if these become severe

Dosage Forms

Tablet, as phosphate: 250 mg [equivalent to 150 mg base]; 500 mg [equivalent to 300 mg base]

Aralen®: 500 mg [equivalent to 300 mg base]

Extemporaneous Preparations A 10 mg chloroquine base/mL suspension is made by pulverizing two Aralen® 500 mg phosphate = 300 mg base/tablet, levigating with sterile water, and adding by geometric proportion, a significant amount of the cherry syrup and levigating until a uniform mixture is obtained; qs ad to 60 mL with cherry syrup, stable for up to 4 weeks when stored in the refrigerator or at a temperature of 29°C

Mirochnick M, Barnett E, Clarke DF, et al, "Stability of Chloroquine in an Extemporaneously Prepared Suspension Stored at Three Temperatures," *Pediatr Infect Dis J*, 1994, 13(9):827-8.

Selected Readings

Panisko DM and Keystone JS, "Treatment of Malaria - 1990," *Drugs*, 1990, 39(2):160-89.
White NJ, "The Treatment of Malaria," *N Engl J Med*, 1996, 335(11):800-6.
Wyler DJ, "Malaria Chemoprophylaxis for the Traveler," *N Engl J Med*, 1993, 329(1):31-7.
Wyler DJ, "Malaria: Overview and Update," *Clin Infect Dis*, 1993, 16(4):449-56.

Chloroquine Phosphate *see* Chloroquine *on page 737*

Ciclopirox (sye kloe PEER oks)

U.S. Brand Names Loprox®; Penlac®

Canadian Brand Names Loprox®; Penlac®

Synonyms Ciclopirox Olamine

Generic Available Yes: Cream, topical suspension

Use

Cream/suspension: Treatment of tinea pedis (athlete's foot), tinea cruris (jock itch), tinea corporis (ringworm), cutaneous candidiasis, and tinea versicolor (pityriasis)

Gel: Treatment of tinea pedis (athlete's foot), tinea corporis (ringworm); seborrheic dermatitis of the scalp

Lacquer (solution): Topical treatment of mild-to-moderate onychomycosis of the fingernails and toenails due to *Trichophyton rubrum* (not involving the lunula) and the immediately-adjacent skin

Shampoo: Treatment of seborrheic dermatitis of the scalp

Pregnancy Risk Factor B

Pregnancy Implications Teratogenic effects were not observed in animal studies, however, there are no adequate and well-controlled studies in pregnant women. Use during pregnancy only if clearly needed.

Contraindications Hypersensitivity to ciclopirox or any component of the formulation; avoid occlusive wrappings or dressings

Warnings/Precautions For external use only; avoid contact with eyes; nail lacquer is for topical use only and has not been studied in conjunction with systemic therapy or in patients with type 1 diabetes mellitus (insulin dependent, IDDM).

Adverse Reactions

>10%: Local: Burning sensation (gel: 34%; ≤1% with other forms)

1% to 10%:

Central nervous system: Headache

Dermatologic: Erythema, nail disorder, pruritus, rash

Local: Irritation, redness, or pain

<1%: Alopecia, dry skin, facial edema

Stability

Cream, suspension: Store between 5°C to 25°C (41°F to 77°F)

Lacquer (solution): Store at room temperature of 15°C to 30°C (59°F to 86°F); protect from light. Flammable; keep away from heat and flame.

Gel, shampoo: Store at room temperature of 15°C to 30°C (59°F to 86°F)

Mechanism of Action Inhibiting transport of essential elements in the fungal cell disrupting the synthesis of DNA, RNA, and protein

Pharmacodynamics/Kinetics

Absorption: Cream, solution: <2% through intact skin; increased with gel; <5% with lacquer

Distribution: Scalp application: To epidermis, corium (dermis), including hair, hair follicles, and sebaceous glands

Protein binding: 94% to 98%

Half-life elimination: Biologic: 1.7 hours (solution); elimination: 5.5 hours (gel)

Excretion: Urine (gel: 3% to 10%); feces (small amounts)

(Continued)

Ciclopirox *(Continued)*

Dosage Topical:

Children >10 years and Adults: Tinea pedis, tinea cruris, tinea corporis, cutaneous candidiasis, and tinea versicolor: Cream/suspension: Apply twice daily, gently massage into affected areas; if no improvement after 4 weeks of treatment, re-evaluate the diagnosis

Children >16 years and Adults:

Tinea pedis, tinea corporis, seborrheic dermatitis of the scalp: Gel: Apply twice daily, gently massage into affected areas and surrounding skin; if no improvement after 4 weeks of treatment, re-evaluate diagnosis

Seborrheic dermatitis of the scalp: Shampoo: Apply to wet hair, lather, and leave in place ~3 minute; rinse. Repeat twice weekly for 4 weeks; allow a minimum of 3 days between applications.

Onychomycosis of the fingernails and toenails: Children ≥12 years and Adults: Lacquer (solution): Apply to adjacent skin and affected nails daily (as a part of a comprehensive management program for onychomycosis). Remove with alcohol every 7 days

Administration Topical:

Cream, suspension: Gently massage into affected areas.

Gel: Gently massage into affected areas and adjacent skin.

Lacquer (solution): Apply evenly over nail and surrounding skin at bedtime (or allow 8 hours before washing); apply daily over previous coat for 7 days; after 7 days, may remove with alcohol and continue cycle.

Shampoo: Apply to wet hair; lather and leave in place for ~3 minutes; rinse.

Patient Information Avoid contact with eyes; if sensitivity or irritation occurs, discontinue use

Dosage Forms

Cream, as olamine (Loprox®): 0.77% (15 g, 30 g, 90 g)
Gel (Loprox®): 0.77% (30 g, 45 g, 100 g)
Shampoo (Loprox®): 1% (120 mL)
Solution, topical [nail lacquer] (Penlac®): 8% (6.6 mL)
Suspension, topical, as olamine (Loprox®): 0.77% (30 mL, 60 mL)

Ciclopirox Olamine *see* Ciclopirox *on page 739*
Cidecin *see* Daptomycin *on page 768*

Cidofovir (si DOF o veer)

Related Information

USPHS / IDSA Guidelines for the Prevention of Opportunistic Infections in Persons Infected With HIV *on page 1237*

U.S. Brand Names Vistide®

Generic Available No

Use Treatment of cytomegalovirus (CMV) retinitis in patients with acquired immunodeficiency syndrome (AIDS). **Note:** Should be administered with probenecid.

Drug of Choice or Alternative for

Disease/Syndrome(s):

Esophagitis *on page 147*

Organism(s):

Cytomegalovirus *on page 107*
Herpes Simplex Virus *on page 172*

Pregnancy Risk Factor C

Pregnancy Implications Cidofovir was shown to be teratogenic and embryotoxic in animal studies, some at doses which also produced maternal toxicity. Reduced testes weight and hypospermia were also noted in animal studies. There are no adequate and well-controlled studies in pregnant women; use during pregnancy only if the potential benefit to the mother outweighs the possible risk to the fetus. Women of childbearing potential should use effective contraception during therapy and for 1 month following treatment. Males should use a barrier contraceptive during therapy and for 3 months following treatment.

Contraindications Hypersensitivity to cidofovir; history of clinically-severe hypersensitivity to probenecid or other sulfa-containing medications; serum creatinine >1.5 mg/dL; Cl_{cr} <55 mL/minute; urine protein ≥100 mg/dL (≥2+ proteinuria); use with or within 7 days of nephrotoxic agents; direct intraocular injection

Warnings/Precautions Dose-dependent nephrotoxicity requires dose adjustment or discontinuation if changes in renal function occur during therapy (eg, proteinuria, glycosuria, decreased serum phosphate, uric acid or bicarbonate, and elevated creatinine); neutropenia and ocular hypotony have also occurred; safety and efficacy have not been established in children or the elderly; administration must be accompanied

by oral probenecid and intravenous saline prehydration; prepare admixtures in a class two laminar flow hood, wearing protective gear; dispose of cidofovir as directed

Adverse Reactions

>10%:

Central nervous system: Chills, fever, headache, pain
Dermatologic: Alopecia, rash
Gastrointestinal: Nausea, vomiting, diarrhea, anorexia
Hematologic: Anemia, neutropenia
Neuromuscular & skeletal: Weakness
Ocular: Intraocular pressure decreased, iritis, ocular hypotony, uveitis
Renal: Creatinine increased, proteinuria, renal toxicity
Respiratory: Cough, dyspnea
Miscellaneous: Infection, oral moniliasis, serum bicarbonate decreased

1% to 10%:

Renal: Fanconi syndrome
Respiratory: Pneumonia

<1%: Hepatic failure, metabolic acidosis, pancreatitis

Frequency not defined (limited to important or life-threatening reactions):

Cardiovascular: Cardiomyopathy, cardiovascular disorder, CHF, edema, postural hypotension, shock, syncope, tachycardia
Central nervous system: Agitation, amnesia, anxiety, confusion, convulsion, dizziness, hallucinations, insomnia, malaise, vertigo
Dermatologic: Photosensitivity reaction, skin discoloration, urticaria
Endocrine & metabolic: Adrenal cortex insufficiency
Gastrointestinal: Abdominal pain, aphthous stomatitis, colitis, constipation, dysphagia, fecal incontinence, gastritis, GI hemorrhage, gingivitis, melena, proctitis, splenomegaly, stomatitis, tongue discoloration
Genitourinary: Urinary incontinence
Hematologic: Hypochromic anemia, leukocytosis, leukopenia, lymphadenopathy, lymphoma-like reaction, pancytopenia, thrombocytopenia, thrombocytopenic purpura
Hepatic: Hepatomegaly, hepatosplenomegaly, jaundice, liver function tests abnormal, liver damage, liver necrosis
Local: Injection site reaction
Neuromuscular & skeletal: Tremor
Ocular: Amblyopia, blindness, cataract, conjunctivitis, corneal lesion, diplopia, vision abnormal
Otic: Hearing loss
Miscellaneous: Allergic reaction, sepsis

Overdosage/Toxicology Hemodialysis and hydration may reduce drug plasma concentrations. Probenecid may assist in decreasing active tubular secretion.

Drug Interactions

Increased Effect/Toxicity: Drugs with nephrotoxic potential (eg, amphotericin B, aminoglycosides, foscarnet, and I.V. pentamidine) should not be used with or within 7 days of cidofovir therapy. Due to concomitant probenecid administration, temporarily discontinue or decrease zidovudine dose by 50% on the day of cidofovir administration only.

Stability Store at controlled room temperature 20°C to 25°C (68°F to 77°F). Dilute dose in NS 100 mL prior to infusion. Store admixtures under refrigeration for ≤24 hours. Cidofovir infusion admixture should be administered within 24 hours of preparation at room temperature or refrigerated. Admixtures should be allowed to equilibrate to room temperature prior to use.

Mechanism of Action Cidofovir is converted to cidofovir diphosphate which is the active intracellular metabolite; cidofovir diphosphate suppresses CMV replication by selective inhibition of viral DNA synthesis. Incorporation of cidofovir into growing viral DNA chain results in reductions in the rate of viral DNA synthesis.

Pharmacodynamics/Kinetics The following pharmacokinetic data is based on a combination of cidofovir administered with probenecid:

Distribution: V_d: 0.54 L/kg; does not cross significantly into CSF
Protein binding: <6%
Metabolism: Minimal; phosphorylation occurs intracellularly
Half-life elimination, plasma: ~2.6 hours
Excretion: Urine

Dosage Adults:

Induction: 5 mg/kg I.V. over 1 hour once weekly for 2 consecutive weeks
Maintenance: 5 mg/kg over 1 hour once every other week

Note: Administer with probenecid 2 g orally 3 hours prior to each cidofovir dose and 1 g at 2 hours and 8 hours after completion of the infusion (total: 4 g)

(Continued)

Cidofovir *(Continued)*

Hydrate with 1 L of 0.9% NS I.V. prior to cidofovir infusion; a second liter may be administered over a 1- to 3-hour period immediately following infusion, if tolerated

Dosing adjustment in renal impairment:

Changes in renal function during therapy: If the creatinine increases by 0.3-0.4 mg/dL, reduce the cidofovir dose to 3 mg/kg; discontinue therapy for increases ≥0.5 mg/dL or development of ≥3+ proteinuria

Pre-existing renal impairment: Use is contraindicated with serum creatinine >1.5 mg/dL, Cl_{cr} <55 mL/minute, or urine protein ≥100 mg/dL (≥2+ proteinuria)

Administration For I.V. infusion only. Infuse over 1 hour. Hydrate with 1 L of 0.9% NS I.V. prior to cidofovir infusion; a second liter may be administered over a 1- to 3-hour period immediately following infusion, if tolerated

Monitoring Parameters Renal function (Cr, BUN, UAs) within 48 hours of each dose, LFTs, WBCs; intraocular pressure and visual acuity, signs and symptoms of uveitis/iritis

Patient Information Cidofovir is not a cure for CMV retinitis; regular follow-up ophthalmologic exams and careful monitoring of renal function are necessary; probenecid must be administered concurrently with cidofovir; report rash immediately; avoid use during pregnancy; use contraception during and for 3 months following treatment

Dosage Forms Injection, solution [preservative free]: 75 mg/mL (5 mL)

Selected Readings

Akler ME, Johnson DW, Burman WJ, et al, "Anterior Uveitis and Hypotony After Intravenous Cidofovir for the Treatment of Cytomegalovirus Retinitis," *Ophthalmology*, 1998, 105(4):651-7.

Alrabiah FA and Sacks SL, "New Antiherpesvirus Agents. Their Targets and Therapeutic Potential," *Drugs*, 1996, 52(1):17-32.

Garcia CR, Torriani FJ, and Freeman WR, "Cidofovir in the Treatment of Cytomegalovirus (CMV) Retinitis," *Ocul Immunol Inflamm*, 1998, 6(3):195-203.

Hitchcock MJ, Jaffe HS, Martin JC, et al, "Cidofovir, a New Agent With Potent Anti-Herpes Virus Activity," *Antivir Chem Chemother*, 1996, 7:115-27.

Lalezari JP, Holland GN, Kramer F, et al, "Randomized, Controlled Study of the Safety and Efficacy of Intravenous Cidofovir for the Treatment of Relapsing Cytomegalovirus Retinitis in Patients With AIDS," *J Acquir Immune Defic Syndr Hum Retrovirol*, 1998, 17(4):339-44.

Lea AP and Bryson HM, "Cidofovir," *Drugs*, 1996, 52(2):225-30.

Taskintuna I, Rahhal FM, Capparelli EV, et al, "Intravitreal and Plasma Cidofovir Concentrations After Intravitreal and Intravenous Administration in AIDS Patients With Cytomegalovirus Retinitis," *J Ocul Pharmacol Ther*, 1998, 14(2):147-51.

Whitley RJ, Jacobson MA, Friedberg DN, et al, "Guidelines for the Treatment of Cytomegalovirus Diseases in Patients With AIDS in the Era of Potent Antiretroviral Therapy: Recommendations of an International Panel. International AIDS Society-USA," *Arch Intern Med*, 1998, 158(9):957-69.

Ciloxan® *see* Ciprofloxacin *on page 742*

Cipro® *see* Ciprofloxacin *on page 742*

Cipro® XL (Can) *see* Ciprofloxacin *on page 742*

Ciprodex® *see* Ciprofloxacin and Dexamethasone *on page 748*

Ciprofloxacin (sip roe FLOKS a sin)

Related Information

Antimicrobial Activity Against Selected Organisms *on page 1165*

Neutropenic Fever Guidelines *on page 1295*

Tuberculosis *on page 1315*

USPHS / IDSA Guidelines for the Prevention of Opportunistic Infections in Persons Infected With HIV *on page 1237*

U.S. Brand Names Ciloxan®; Cipro®; Cipro® XR; Proquin® XR

Canadian Brand Names Apo-Ciproflox®; Ciloxan®; Cipro®; Cipro® XL; CO Ciprofloxacin; Gen-Ciprofloxacin; Novo-Ciprofloxacin; pms-Ciprofloxacin; ratio-Ciprofloxacin; Rhoxal-ciprofloxacin

Synonyms Ciprofloxacin Hydrochloride

Generic Available Yes: Suspension, tablet

Use

Children: Complicated urinary tract infections and pyelonephritis due to *E. coli.* **Note:** Although effective, ciprofloxacin is not the drug of first choice in children.

Children and adults: To reduce incidence or progression of disease following exposure to aerolized *Bacillus anthracis.* Ophthalmologically, for superficial ocular infections (corneal ulcers, conjunctivitis) due to susceptible strains

Adults: Treatment of the following infections when caused by susceptible bacteria: Urinary tract infections; acute uncomplicated cystitis in females; chronic bacterial prostatitis; lower respiratory tract infections (including acute exacerbations of chronic bronchitis); acute sinusitis; skin and skin structure infections; bone and joint infections; complicated intra-abdominal infections (in combination with metronidazole); infectious diarrhea; typhoid fever due to *Salmonella typhi* (eradication of chronic typhoid carrier state has not been proven); uncomplicated cervical and

urethra gonorrhea (due to *N. gonorrhoeae*); nosocomial pneumonia; empirical therapy for febrile neutropenic patients (in combination with piperacillin)

Unlabeled/Investigational Use Acute pulmonary exacerbations in cystic fibrosis (children); cutaneous/gastrointestinal/oropharyngeal anthrax (treatment, children and adults); disseminated gonococcal infection (adults); chancroid (adults); prophylaxis to *Neisseria meningitidis* following close contact with an infected person

Drug of Choice or Alternative for Disease/Syndrome(s):

Cervicitis *on page 71*
Cholangitis, Acute *on page 79*
Endocarditis, Acute Native Valve *on page 124*
Endocarditis, Subacute Native Valve *on page 126*
Endometritis *on page 127*
Fever, Neutropenic *on page 148*
Gastroenteritis, Bacterial *on page 154*
Intra-abdominal Abscess *on page 194*
Joint Replacement, Early Infection *on page 197*
Liver Abscess *on page 211*
Osteomyelitis, Diabetic Foot *on page 249*
Otitis Externa, Mild *on page 252*
Otitis Externa, Severe (Malignant) *on page 252*
Pelvic Inflammatory Disease *on page 260*
Peritonitis, Spontaneous Bacterial *on page 264*
Pneumonia, Community-Acquired *on page 270*
Pneumonia, Hospital-Acquired *on page 272*
Pneumonia, Ventilator-Associated *on page 273*
Prostatitis *on page 277*
Traveler's Diarrhea *on page 333*

Organism(s):

Burkholderia cepacia on page 62
Burkholderia mallei on page 64
Calymmatobacterium granulomatis on page 65
Francisella tularensis on page 149
Haemophilus ducreyi on page 158
Isospora belli on page 196
Mycobacterium avium-intracellulare (Complex) *on page 228*
Neisseria gonorrhoeae on page 244
Pseudomonas aeruginosa on page 282
Rickettsia rickettsii on page 289
Salmonella Species *on page 291*
Shigella Species *on page 297*

Pregnancy Risk Factor C

Pregnancy Implications Ciprofloxacin crosses the placenta and concentrates in amniotic fluid; maternal serum levels may be decreased during pregnancy. Reports of arthropathy (observed in immature animals and reported rarely in humans) have limited the use of fluoroquinolones in pregnancy. According to the FDA, the Teratogen Information System concluded that therapeutic doses during pregnancy are unlikely to produce substantial teratogenic risk, but data are insufficient to say that there is no risk. In general, reports of exposure have been limited to short durations of therapy in the first trimester. When considering treatment for life-threatening infection and/or prolonged duration of therapy (such as in anthrax), the potential risk to the fetus must be balanced against the severity of the potential illness.

Contraindications Hypersensitivity to ciprofloxacin, any component of the formulation, or other quinolones

Warnings/Precautions CNS stimulation may occur (tremor, restlessness, confusion, and very rarely hallucinations or seizures). Use with caution in patients with known or suspected CNS disorder. Prolonged use may result in superinfection. Tendon inflammation and/or rupture have been reported with ciprofloxacin and other quinolone antibiotics. Risk may be increased with concurrent corticosteroids, particularly in the elderly. Discontinue at first sign of tendon inflammation or pain. Adverse effects, including those related to joints and/or surrounding tissues, are increased in pediatric patients. Rare cases of peripheral neuropathy may occur.

Severe hypersensitivity reactions, including anaphylaxis, have occurred with quinolone therapy. Quinolones may exacerbate myasthenia gravis, use with caution (rare, potentially life-threatening weakness of respiratory muscles may occur). Use caution in renal impairment. Avoid excessive sunlight; may cause moderate-to-severe phototoxicity reactions.

(Continued)

Ciprofloxacin *(Continued)*

Adverse Reactions

1% to 10%:

Central nervous system: Neurologic events (children 2%, includes dizziness, insomnia, nervousness, somnolence); fever (children 2%); headache (I.V. administration); restlessness (I.V. administration)

Dermatologic: Rash (children 2%, adults 1%)

Gastrointestinal: Nausea (children/adults 3%); diarrhea (children 5%, adults 2%); vomiting (children 5%, adults 1%); abdominal pain (children 3%, adults <1%); dyspepsia (children 3%)

Hepatic: ALT/AST increased (adults 1%)

Local: Injection site reactions (I.V. administration)

Respiratory: Rhinitis (children 3%)

<1%: Abnormal gait, acute renal failure, agitation, allergic reactions, anaphylaxis, anemia, angina pectoris, angioedema, anorexia, arthralgia, ataxia, atrial flutter, breast pain, bronchospasm, candidiasis, cardiopulmonary arrest, cerebral thrombosis, chills, cholestatic jaundice, confusion, chromatopsia, crystalluria (particularly in alkaline urine), cylindruria, depersonalization, depression, dizziness, drowsiness, dyspnea, edema, eosinophilia, erythema nodosum, fever (adults), gastrointestinal bleeding, hallucinations, headache (oral), hematuria, hyperpigmentation, hyper-/hypotension, insomnia, interstitial nephritis, intestinal perforation, irritability, joint pain, laryngeal edema, lightheadedness, lymphadenopathy, malaise, manic reaction, migraine, MI, nephritis, nightmares, palpitation, paranoia, paresthesia, peripheral neuropathy, petechia, photosensitivity, pulmonary edema, seizure, syncope, tachycardia, thrombophlebitis, tinnitus, tremor, urethral bleeding, vaginitis, ventricular ectopy, visual disturbance, weakness

Postmarketing and/or case reports: Agranulocytosis, albuminuria, anaphylactic shock, anosmia, bone marrow depression (life-threatening), candiduria, constipation, delirium, dyspepsia (adults), dysphagia, erythema multiforme, exfoliative dermatitis, fixed eruption, flatulence, hemolytic anemia, hepatic failure, hepatic necrosis, hyperesthesia, hyperglycemia, hypertonia, jaundice, methemoglobinemia, moniliasis, myalgia, myasthenia gravis, myoclonus, nystagmus, orthostatic hypotension, pancreatitis, pancytopenia (life-threatening or fatal), prolongation of PT/INR, pseudomembranous colitis, psychosis, renal calculi, serum cholesterol increased, serum glucose increased, serum sickness-like reactions, serum triglycerides increased, Stevens-Johnson syndrome, taste loss, tendon rupture, tendonitis, toxic epidermal necrolysis (Lyell's syndrome), torsade de pointes, twitching, vaginal candidiasis, vasculitis

Overdosage/Toxicology Symptoms of overdose include acute renal failure and seizures. Treatment is supportive and should include adequate hydration and renal function monitoring. Magnesium or calcium containing antacids may be given to decrease absorption of oral ciprofloxacin. Only a small amount of ciprofloxacin (<10%) is removed from the body after hemodialysis or peritoneal dialysis.

Drug Interactions

Cytochrome P450 Effect: Inhibits CYP1A2 (strong), 3A4 (weak)

Increased Effect/Toxicity: Ciprofloxacin may increase the effects/toxicity of caffeine, CYP1A2 substrates (eg, aminophylline, fluvoxamine, mexiletine, mirtazapine, ropinirole, and trifluoperazine), glyburide, methotrexate, ropivacaine, theophylline, and warfarin. Concomitant use with corticosteroids may increase the risk of tendon rupture. Concomitant use with foscarnet may increase the risk of seizures. Probenecid may increase ciprofloxacin levels.

Decreased Effect: Concurrent administration of metal cations, including most antacids, oral electrolyte supplements, quinapril, sucralfate, some didanosine formulations (chewable/buffered tablets and pediatric powder for oral suspension), and other highly-buffered oral drugs, may decrease quinolone levels; separate doses. Ciprofloxacin may decrease phenytoin levels.

Ethanol/Nutrition/Herb Interactions

Food: Food decreases rate, but not extent, of absorption. Ciprofloxacin serum levels may be decreased if taken with dairy products or calcium-fortified juices. Ciprofloxacin may increase serum caffeine levels if taken with caffeine.

Enteral feedings may decrease plasma concentrations of ciprofloxacin probably by >30% inhibition of absorption. Ciprofloxacin should not be administered with enteral feedings. The feeding would need to be discontinued for 1-2 hours prior to and after ciprofloxacin administration. Nasogastric administration produces a greater loss of ciprofloxacin bioavailability than does nasoduodenal administration.

Herb/Nutraceutical: Avoid dong quai, St John's wort (may also cause photosensitization).

Stability

Injection:

Premixed infusion: Store between 5°C to 25°C (41°F to 77°F); protect from light; avoid freezing.

Vial: Store between 5°C to 30°C (41°F to 86°F); protect from light; avoid freezing. May be diluted with NS, D_5W, SWFI, $D_{10}W$, $D_5{}^1/_4NS$, $D_5{}^1/_2NS$, LR. Diluted solutions of 0.5-2 mg/mL are stable for up to 14 days refrigerated or at room temperature.

Ophthalmic solution/ointment: Store at 36°F to 77°F (2°C to 25°C); protect from light.

Microcapsules for oral suspension: Prior to reconstitution, store below 25°C (77°F); protect from freezing. Following reconstitution, store below 30°C (86°F) for up to 14 days; protect from freezing.

Tablet:

Immediate release: Store below 30°C (86°F).

Extended release: Store at room temperature of 15°C to 30°C (59°F to 86°F).

Mechanism of Action Inhibits DNA-gyrase in susceptible organisms; inhibits relaxation of supercoiled DNA and promotes breakage of double-stranded DNA

Pharmacodynamics/Kinetics

Absorption: Oral: Immediate release tablet: Rapid (~50% to 85%)

Distribution: V_d: 2.1-2.7 L/kg; tissue concentrations often exceed serum concentrations especially in kidneys, gallbladder, liver, lungs, gynecological tissue, and prostatic tissue; CSF concentrations: 10% of serum concentrations (noninflamed meninges), 14% to 37% (inflamed meninges); crosses placenta; enters breast milk

Protein binding: 20% to 40%

Metabolism: Partially hepatic; forms 4 metabolites (limited activity)

Half-life elimination: Children: 2.5 hours; Adults: Normal renal function: 3-5 hours

Time to peak: Oral:

Immediate release tablet: 0.5-2 hours

Extended release tablet: Cipro® XR: 1-2.5 hours, Proquin® XR: 3.5-8.7 hours

Excretion: Urine (30% to 50% as unchanged drug); feces (15% to 43%)

Dosage Note: Extended release tablets and immediate release formulations are not interchangeable. Unless otherwise specified, oral dosing reflects the use of immediate release formulations.

Children (see Warnings/Precautions):

Oral:

Complicated urinary tract infection or pyelonephritis: Children 1-17 years: 20-30 mg/kg/day in 2 divided doses (every 12 hours) for 10-21 days; maximum: 1.5 g/day

Cystic fibrosis (unlabeled use): Children 5-17 years: 40 mg/kg/day divided every 12 hours administered following 1 week of I.V. therapy has been reported in a clinical trial; total duration of therapy: 10-21 days

Anthrax:

Inhalational (postexposure prophylaxis): 15 mg/kg/dose every 12 hours for 60 days; maximum: 500 mg/dose

Cutaneous (treatment, CDC guidelines): 10-15 mg/kg every 12 hours for 60 days (maximum: 1 g/day); amoxicillin 80 mg/kg/day divided every 8 hours is an option for completion of treatment after clinical improvement. **Note:** In the presence of systemic involvement, extensive edema, lesions on head/neck, refer to I.V. dosing for treatment of inhalational/gastrointestinal/oropharyngeal anthrax

I.V.:

Complicated urinary tract infection or pyelonephritis: Children 1-17 years: 6-10 mg/kg every 8 hours for 10-21 days (maximum: 400 mg/dose)

Cystic fibrosis (unlabeled use): Children 5-17 years: 30 mg/kg/day divided every 8 hours for 1 week, followed by oral therapy, has been reported in a clinical trial

Anthrax:

Inhalational (postexposure prophylaxis): 10 mg/kg/dose every 12 hours for 60 days; do **not** exceed 400 mg/dose (800 mg/day)

Inhalational/gastrointestinal/oropharyngeal (treatment, CDC guidelines): Initial: 10-15 mg/kg every 12 hours for 60 days (maximum: 500 mg/dose); switch to oral therapy when clinically appropriate; refer to Adults dosing for notes on combined therapy and duration

Adults: Oral:

Urinary tract infection:

Acute uncomplicated: Immediate release formulation: 250 mg every 12 hours for 3 days

Acute uncomplicated pyelonephritis: Extended release formulation (Cipro® XR): 1000 mg every 24 hours for 7-14 days

Uncomplicated/acute cystitis: Extended release formulation (Cipro® XR, Proquin® XR): 500 mg every 24 hours for 3 days

(Continued)

Ciprofloxacin *(Continued)*

Mild/moderate: Immediate release formulation: 250 mg every 12 hours for 7-14 days
Severe/complicated:
Immediate release formulation: 500 mg every 12 hours for 7-14 days
Extended release formulation (Cipro® XR): 1000 mg every 24 hours for 7-14 days
Lower respiratory tract, skin/skin structure infections: 500-750 mg twice daily for 7-14 days depending on severity and susceptibility
Bone/joint infections: 500-750 mg twice daily for 4-6 weeks, depending on severity and susceptibility
Infectious diarrhea: 500 mg every 12 hours for 5-7 days
Intra-abdominal (in combination with metronidazole): 500 mg every 12 hours for 7-14 days
Typhoid fever: 500 mg every 12 hours for 10 days
Urethral/cervical gonococcal infections: 250-500 mg as a single dose (CDC recommends concomitant doxycycline or azithromycin due to developing resistance; avoid use in Asian or Western Pacific travelers)
Disseminated gonococcal infection (CDC guidelines): 500 mg twice daily to complete 7 days of therapy (initial treatment with ceftriaxone 1 g I.M./I.V. daily for 24-48 hours after improvement begins)
Chancroid (CDC guidelines): 500 mg twice daily for 3 days
Sinusitis (acute): 500 mg every 12 hours for 10 days
Chronic bacterial prostatitis: 500 mg every 12 hours for 28 days
Anthrax:
Inhalational (postexposure prophylaxis): 500 mg every 12 hours for 60 days
Cutaneous (treatment, CDC guidelines): Immediate release formulation: 500 mg every 12 hours for 60 days. **Note:** In the presence of systemic involvement, extensive edema, lesions on head/neck, refer to I.V. dosing for treatment of inhalational/gastrointestinal/oropharyngeal anthrax

Adults: I.V.:
Bone/joint infections:
Mild to moderate: 400 mg every 12 hours for 4-6 weeks
Severe or complicated: 400 mg every 8 hours for 4-6 weeks
Lower respiratory tract, skin/skin structure infections:
Mild to moderate: 400 mg every 12 hours for 7-14 days
Severe or complicated: 400 mg every 8 hours for 7-14 days
Nosocomial pneumonia (mild to moderate to severe): 400 mg every 8 hours for 10-14 days
Prostatitis (chronic, bacterial): 400 mg every 12 hours for 28 days
Sinusitis (acute): 400 mg every 12 hours for 10 days
Urinary tract infection:
Mild to moderate: 200 mg every 12 hours for 7-14 days
Severe or complicated: 400 mg every 12 hours for 7-14 days
Febrile neutropenia (with piperacillin): 400 mg every 8 hours for 7-14 days
Intra-abdominal infection (with metronidazole): 400 mg every 12 hours for 7-14 days
Anthrax:
Inhalational (postexposure prophylaxis): 400 mg every 12 hours for 60 days
Inhalational/gastrointestinal/oropharyngeal (treatment, CDC guidelines): 400 mg every 12 hours. **Note:** Initial treatment should include two or more agents predicted to be effective (per CDC recommendations). Agents suggested for use in conjunction with ciprofloxacin or doxycycline include rifampin, vancomycin, imipenem, penicillin, ampicillin, chloramphenicol, clindamycin, and clarithromycin. May switch to oral antimicrobial therapy when clinically appropriate. Continue combined therapy for 60 days.

Elderly: No adjustment needed in patients with normal renal function

Ophthalmic:
Solution: Children >1 year and Adults:
Bacterial conjunctivitis: Instill 1-2 drops in eye(s) every 2 hours while awake for 2 days and 1-2 drops every 4 hours while awake for the next 5 days
Corneal ulcer: Instill 2 drops into affected eye every 15 minutes for the first 6 hours, then 2 drops into the affected eye every 30 minutes for the remainder of the first day. On day 2, instill 2 drops into the affected eye hourly. On days 3-14, instill 2 drops into affected eye every 4 hours. Treatment may continue after day 14 if re-epithelialization has not occurred.
Ointment: Children >2 years and Adults: Bacterial conjunctivitis: Apply a ½" ribbon into the conjunctival sac 3 times/day for the first 2 days, followed by a ½" ribbon applied twice daily for the next 5 days

Dosing adjustment in renal impairment: Adults:

Cl_{cr} 30-50 mL/minute: Oral: 250-500 mg every 12 hours

Cl_{cr} <30 mL/minute: Acute uncomplicated pyelonephritis or complicated UTI: Oral: Extended release formulation: 500 mg every 24 hours

Cl_{cr} 5-29 mL/minute:

Oral: 250-500 mg every 18 hours

I.V.: 200-400 mg every 18-24 hours

Dialysis: Only small amounts of ciprofloxacin are removed by hemo- or peritoneal dialysis (<10%); usual dose: Oral: 250-500 mg every 24 hours following dialysis

Continuous arteriovenous or venovenous hemodiafiltration effects: Administer 200-400 mg I.V. every 12 hours

Dietary Considerations

Food: Drug may cause GI upset; take without regard to meals (manufacturer prefers that immediate release tablet is taken 2 hours after meals). Extended release tablet may be taken with meals that contain dairy products (calcium content <800 mg), but not with dairy products alone.

Dairy products, calcium-fortified juices, oral multivitamins, and mineral supplements: Absorption of ciprofloxacin is decreased by divalent and trivalent cations. The manufacturer states that the usual dietary intake of calcium (including meals which include dairy products) has not been shown to interfere with ciprofloxacin absorption. Immediate release ciprofloxacin and Cipro® XR may be taken 2 hours before or 6 hours after, and Proquin® XR may be taken 4 hours before or 6 hours after, any of these products.

Caffeine: Patients consuming regular large quantities of caffeinated beverages may need to restrict caffeine intake if excessive cardiac or CNS stimulation occurs.

Administration

Oral: May administer with food to minimize GI upset; avoid antacid use; maintain proper hydration and urine output. Administer immediate release ciprofloxacin and Cipro® XR at least 2 hours before or 6 hours after, and Proquin® XR at least 4 hours before or 6 hours after antacids or other products containing calcium, iron, or zinc (including dairy products or calcium-fortified juices). Separate oral administration from drugs which may impair absorption (see Drug Interactions).

Oral suspension: Should not be administered through feeding tubes (suspension is oil-based and adheres to the feeding tube). Patients should avoid chewing on the microcapsules.

Nasogastric/orogastric tube: Crush immediate-release tablet and mix with water. Flush feeding tube before and after administration. Hold tube feedings at least 1 hour before and 2 hours after administration.

Tablet, extended release: Do not crush, split, or chew. May be administered with meals containing dairy products (calcium content <800 mg), but not with dairy products alone. Proquin® XR should be administered with a main meal of the day; evening meal is preferred.

Parenteral: Administer by slow I.V. infusion over 60 minutes to reduce the risk of venous irritation (burning, pain, erythema, and swelling); final concentration for administration should not exceed 2 mg/mL

Monitoring Parameters Patients receiving concurrent ciprofloxacin, theophylline, or cyclosporine should have serum levels monitored; CBC, renal and hepatic function during prolonged therapy

Reference Range Therapeutic: 2.6-3 mcg/mL; Toxic: >5 mcg/mL

Patient Information Take as directed, preferably on an empty stomach, 2 hours after meals. Extended release tablet may be taken with meals containing dairy products, but not with dairy products alone; do not crush, split, or chew extended release tablet. Swallow oral suspension, do not chew microcapsules. Take entire prescription even if feeling better. Maintain adequate hydration (2-3 L/day of fluids unless instructed to restrict fluid intake) to avoid concentrated urine and crystal formation. You may experience nausea, vomiting, or anorexia (small frequent meals, frequent mouth care, sucking lozenges, or chewing gum may help). You may experience increased sensitivity to sunlight; use sunblock, wear protective clothing and dark glasses, or avoid direct exposure to sunlight. Report immediately any signs of skin rash, joint or back pain, or difficulty breathing. Report unusual fever or chills; vaginal itching or foul-smelling vaginal discharge; easy bruising or bleeding. Report immediately any pain, inflammation, or rupture of tendon.

Dosage Forms

Infusion, [premixed in D_5W] (Cipro®): 200 mg (100 mL); 400 mg (200 mL) [latex free]

Injection, solution (Cipro®): 10 mg/mL (20 mL, 40 mL, 120 mL)

Microcapsules for oral suspension (Cipro®): 250 mg/5 mL (100 mL); 500 mg/5 mL (100 mL) [strawberry flavor]

Ointment, ophthalmic, as hydrochloride (Ciloxan®): 3.33 mg/g [0.3% base] (3.5 g)

Solution, ophthalmic, as hydrochloride (Ciloxan®): 3.5 mg/mL [0.3% base] (2.5 mL, 5 mL, 10 mL) [contains benzalkonium chloride]

(Continued)

Ciprofloxacin *(Continued)*

Tablet: 250 mg, 500 mg, 750 mg
  Cipro®: 100 mg, 250 mg, 500 mg, 750 mg
Tablet, extended release
  Cipro® XR: 500 mg [equivalent to ciprofloxacin hydrochloride 287.5 mg and ciprofloxacin base 212.6 mg]; 1000 mg [equivalent to ciprofloxacin hydrochloride 574.9 mg and ciprofloxacin base 425.2 mg]
  Proquin® XR: 500 mg

Selected Readings

Davis R, Markham A, and Balfour JA, "Ciprofloxacin. An Updated Review of Its Pharmacology, Therapeutic Efficacy and Tolerability," *Drugs*, 1996, 51(6):1019-74.
Hooper DC and Wolfson JS, "Fluoroquinolone Antimicrobial Agents," *N Engl J Med*, 1991, 324(6):384-94.
Lomaestro BM and Bailie GR, "Quinolone-Cation Interactions: A Review," *DICP*, 1991, 25(11):1249-58.
Sanders CC, "Ciprofloxacin: *In Vitro* Activity, Mechanism of Action, and Resistance," *Rev Infect Dis*, 1988, 10(3):516-27.
Stein GE, "The 4-Quinolone Antibiotics: Past, Present, and Future," *Pharmacotherapy*, 1988, 8(6):301-14.
Walker RC and Wright AJ, "The Fluoroquinolones," *Mayo Clin Proc*, 1991, 66(12):1249-59.

Ciprofloxacin and Dexamethasone

(sip roe FLOKS a sin & deks a METH a sone)

U.S. Brand Names Ciprodex®

Canadian Brand Names Ciprodex®

Synonyms Ciprofloxacin Hydrochloride and Dexamethasone; Dexamethasone and Ciprofloxacin

Generic Available No

Use Treatment of acute otitis media in pediatric patients with tympanostomy tubes or acute otitis externa in children and adults

Pregnancy Risk Factor C

Pregnancy Implications Refer to individual agents. Reproduction studies have not been conducted with the otic preparation. Ciprofloxacin is detectable in the serum following otic administration.

Contraindications Hypersensitivity to ciprofloxacin, other quinolones, dexamethasone, or any component of the formulation; not for use in viral infection of the external canal

Warnings/Precautions For otic use only; not intended for injection or ophthalmic use. Safety and efficacy have been established in pediatric patients ≥6 months of age, however, the manufacturer states that there are no safety concerns which would preclude the use of this product in younger children. Prior to instillation, suspension should be warmed in hands to prevent dizziness which may occur following use of a cold solution.

Adverse Reactions

1% to 10%: Otic: Discomfort (3%), pain (<1% to 2%), pruritus (1%)
<1%: Hearing decreased, ear congestion, ear erythema, ear residue, ear tingling, irritability, taste perversion

Drug Interactions

Cytochrome P450 Effect:

Ciprofloxacin: **Inhibits** CYP1A2 (strong), 3A4 (weak)
Dexamethasone: **Substrate** of CYP3A4 (minor); **Induces** CYP2A6 (weak), 2B6 (weak), 2C8/9 (weak), 3A4 (weak)

Stability Store at controlled room temperature of 15°C to 30°C (59°F to 86°F); protect from light; do not freeze

Mechanism of Action Ciprofloxacin is a quinolone antibiotic; dexamethasone is a corticosteroid used to decrease inflammation accompanying bacterial infections

Pharmacodynamics/Kinetics

Absorption: Otic: Ciprofloxacin: Minor systemic absorption
Time to peak, plasma: Otic: Ciprofloxacin: 15 minutes to 2 hours

Dosage Otic:

Children: Acute otitis media in patients with tympanostomy tubes or acute otitis externa: Instill 4 drops into affected ear(s) twice daily for 7 days
Adults: Acute otitis externa: Instill 4 drops into affected ear(s) twice daily for 7 days

Administration Otic: Prior to instillation, bottle should be warmed in hands for 1-2 minutes. Shake suspension well immediately before using. Patient should lie with affected ear upward and remain in this position for 60 seconds following application. Drops should be instilled directly into tympanostomy tube (if present) and tragus should be pumped 5 times to facilitate penetration into the middle ear.

Patient Information For use only in the ear. Before use, bottle should be warmed in hands for 1-2 minutes. Shake suspension well immediately before using. Patient should lie with affected ear upward and remain in this position for 60 seconds after application. Drops should be instilled directly into tympanostomy tube (if present). Discard unused portion of suspension after therapy is complete.

Dosage Forms Suspension, otic: Ciprofloxacin 0.3% and dexamethasone 0.1% (7.5 mL) [contains benzalkonium chloride]

Ciprofloxacin and Hydrocortisone

(sip roe FLOKS a sin & hye droe KOR ti sone)

Related Information

Ciprofloxacin *on page 742*

U.S. Brand Names Cipro® HC

Canadian Brand Names Cipro® HC

Synonyms Hydrocortisone and Ciprofloxacin

Generic Available No

Use Treatment of acute otitis externa, sometimes known as "swimmer's ear"

Drug Interactions

Cytochrome P450 Effect:

Ciprofloxacin: **Inhibits** CYP1A2 (strong), 3A4 (weak)

Hydrocortisone: **Substrate** of CYP3A4 (minor); **Induces** CYP3A4 (weak)

Pharmacodynamics/Kinetics See individual agents.

Dosage Children >1 year of age and Adults: Otic: The recommended dosage for all patients is three drops of the suspension in the affected ear twice daily for seven day; twice-daily dosing schedule is more convenient for patients than that of existing treatments with hydrocortisone, which are typically administered three or four times a day; a twice-daily dosage schedule may be especially helpful for parents and caregivers of young children

Dosage Forms Suspension, otic: Ciprofloxacin hydrochloride 0.2% and hydrocortisone 1% (10 mL) [contains benzyl alcohol]

Ciprofloxacin Hydrochloride *see* Ciprofloxacin *on page 742*

Ciprofloxacin Hydrochloride and Dexamethasone *see* Ciprofloxacin and Dexamethasone *on page 748*

Cipro® HC *see* Ciprofloxacin and Hydrocortisone *on page 749*

Cipro® XR *see* Ciprofloxacin *on page 742*

Claforan® *see* Cefotaxime *on page 708*

Clarithromycin

(kla RITH roe mye sin)

Related Information

Antimicrobial Activity Against Selected Organisms *on page 1165*

Community-Acquired Pneumonia in Adults *on page 1278*

Helicobacter pylori Treatment *on page 1288*

USPHS / IDSA Guidelines for the Prevention of Opportunistic Infections in Persons Infected With HIV *on page 1237*

U.S. Brand Names Biaxin®; Biaxin® XL

Canadian Brand Names Biaxin®; Biaxin® XL; ratio-Clarithromycin

Generic Available Yes: Tablet

Use

Children:

- Pharyngitis/tonsillitis, acute maxillary sinusitis, uncomplicated skin/skin structure infections, and mycobacterial infections due to the above organisms
- Acute otitis media (*H. influenzae, M. catarrhalis*, or *S. pneumoniae*)
- Prevention of disseminated mycobacterial infections due to MAC disease in patients with advanced HIV infection

Adults:

- Pharyngitis/tonsillitis due to susceptible *S. pyogenes*
- Acute maxillary sinusitis and acute exacerbation of chronic bronchitis due to susceptible *H. influenzae, M. catarrhalis*, or *S. pneumoniae*
- Pneumonia due to susceptible *H. influenzae, Mycoplasma pneumoniae, S. pneumoniae*, or *Chlamydia pneumoniae* (TWAR)
- Uncomplicated skin/skin structure infections due to susceptible *S. aureus, S. pyogenes*
- Disseminated mycobacterial infections due to *M. avium* or *M. intracellulare*
- Prevention of disseminated mycobacterial infections due to *M. avium* complex (MAC) disease (eg, patients with advanced HIV infection)
- Duodenal ulcer disease due to *H. pylori* in regimens with other drugs including amoxicillin and lansoprazole or omeprazole, ranitidine bismuth citrate, bismuth subsalicylate, tetracycline, and/or an H_2 antagonist
- Alternate antibiotic for prophylaxis of bacterial endocarditis in patients who are allergic to penicillin and undergoing surgical or dental procedures

Drug of Choice or Alternative for Disease/Syndrome(s):

Bronchitis *on page 60*

(Continued)

Clarithromycin *(Continued)*

Erysipelas *on page 141*

Organism(s):

Bordetella pertussis on page 53
Chlamydophila pneumoniae on page 78
Legionella pneumophila on page 202
Moraxella catarrhalis on page 223
Mycobacterium avium-intracellulare (Complex) *on page 228*
Mycobacterium kansasii on page 231
Mycoplasma pneumoniae on page 238
Ureaplasma urealyticum on page 342

Pregnancy Risk Factor C

Pregnancy Implications There are no adequate and well-controlled studies in pregnant women. Due to adverse fetal effects reported in animal studies, the manufacturer recommends that clarithromycin not be used in a pregnant woman unless there are no alternatives to therapy.

Contraindications Hypersensitivity to clarithromycin, erythromycin, or any macrolide antibiotic; use with ergot derivatives, pimozide, cisapride; combination with ranitidine bismuth citrate should not be used in patients with history of acute porphyria or Cl_{cr} <25 mL/minute

Warnings/Precautions Dosage adjustment required with severe renal impairment, decreased dosage or prolonged dosing interval may be appropriate; antibiotic-associated colitis has been reported with use of clarithromycin. Macrolides (including clarithromycin) have been associated with rare QT prolongation and ventricular arrhythmias, including torsade de pointes. The extended release formulation consists of drug within a nondeformable matrix; following drug release/absorption, the matrix/shell is expelled in the stool. The use of nondeformable products in patients with known stricture/narrowing of the GI tract has been associated with symptoms of obstruction. Safety and efficacy in children <6 months of age have not been established.

Adverse Reactions

1% to 10%:

Central nervous system: Headache (adults and children 2%)
Dermatologic: Rash (children 3%)
Gastrointestinal: Diarrhea (adults 6%, children 6%); vomiting (children 6%); nausea (adults 3%); abnormal taste (adults 7%); heartburn (adults 2%); abdominal pain (adults 2%, children 3%)
Hepatic: Prothrombin time increased (1%)
Renal: BUN increased (4%)

<1%, postmarketing, and/or case reports (limited to important or life-threatening); *Clostridium difficile* colitis, alkaline phosphatase increased, anaphylaxis, anorexia, anxiety, AST increased, bilirubin increased, dizziness, dyspnea, glossitis, hallucinations, hearing loss (reversible), hepatic failure, hepatitis, hypoglycemia, jaundice, leukopenia, manic behavior, neuromuscular blockade (case reports), neutropenia, pancreatitis, psychosis, QT prolongation, seizure, serum creatinine increased, Stevens-Johnson syndrome, thrombocytopenia, tongue discoloration, tooth discoloration, torsade de pointes, toxic epidermal necrolysis, tremor, ventricular tachycardia, vertigo, vomiting

Overdosage/Toxicology Symptoms include nausea, vomiting, diarrhea, prostration, reversible pancreatitis, hearing loss with or without tinnitus, or vertigo. Treatment includes symptomatic and supportive care.

Drug Interactions

Cytochrome P450 Effect: Substrate of CYP3A4 (major); **Inhibits** CYP1A2 (weak), 3A4 (strong)

Increased Effect/Toxicity: Avoid concomitant use of the following with clarithromycin due to increased risk of malignant arrhythmias: Cisapride, gatifloxacin, moxifloxacin, pimozide, sparfloxacin, thioridazine. Other agents that prolong the QT_c interval, including type Ia (eg, quinidine) and type III antiarrhythmic agents, and selected antipsychotic agents (eg, mesoridazine, thioridazine) should be used with extreme caution.

Clarithromycin is a strong CYP3A4 inhibitor, and may increase the levels/effects of selected benzodiazepines, calcium channel blockers, cyclosporine, mirtazapine, nateglinide, nefazodone, quinidine, sildenafil (and other PDE-5 inhibitors), tacrolimus, venlafaxine, and other CYP3A4 substrates. Selected benzodiazepines (midazolam, triazolam), cisapride, ergot alkaloids, selected HMG-CoA reductase inhibitors (lovastatin and simvastatin), and pimozide are generally contraindicated with strong CYP3A4 inhibitors. When used with strong CYP3A4 inhibitors, dosage

adjustment/limits are recommended for sildenafil and other PDE-5 inhibitors; refer to individual monographs.

The effects of neuromuscular-blocking agents and warfarin have been potentiated by clarithromycin. Clarithromycin serum concentrations may be increased by amprenavir (and possibly other protease inhibitors). Digoxin serum levels may be increased by clarithromycin; digoxin toxicity and potentially fatal arrhythmias have been reported; monitor digoxin levels. Fluconazole increases clarithromycin levels and AUC by ~25%. Peak levels (but not AUC) of zidovudine may be increased; other studies suggest levels may be decreased.

The levels/effects of clarithromycin may be increased by azole antifungals, ciprofloxacin, diclofenac, doxycycline, erythromycin, imatinib, isoniazid, nefazodone, nicardipine, propofol, protease inhibitors, quinidine, telithromycin, verapamil, and other CYP3A4 inhibitors.

Decreased Effect: Clarithromycin may decrease the serum concentrations of zafirlukast. Clarithromycin may antagonize the therapeutic effects of clindamycin and lincomycin. Peak levels (but not AUC) of zidovudine may be increased; other studies suggest levels may be decreased. The levels/effects of clarithromycin may be decreased by aminoglutethimide, carbamazepine, nafcillin, nevirapine, phenobarbital, phenytoin, rifamycins, and other CYP3A4 inducers.

Ethanol/Nutrition/Herb Interactions

Food: Delays absorption; total absorption remains unchanged.

Herb/Nutraceutical: St John's wort may decrease clarithromycin levels.

Stability Store tablets and granules for oral suspension at controlled room temperature. Reconstituted oral suspension should not be refrigerated because it might gel; microencapsulated particles of clarithromycin in suspension is stable for 14 days when stored at room temperature

Mechanism of Action Exerts its antibacterial action by binding to 50S ribosomal subunit resulting in inhibition of protein synthesis. The 14-OH metabolite of clarithromycin is twice as active as the parent compound against certain organisms.

Pharmacodynamics/Kinetics

Absorption: Highly stable in presence of gastric acid (unlike erythromycin); food delays but does not affect extent of absorption

Distribution: Widely into most body tissues except CNS

Metabolism: Partially hepatic; converted to 14-OH clarithromycin (active metabolite)

Bioavailability: 50%

Half-life elimination: 5-7 hours

Time to peak: 2-4 hours

Excretion: Primarily urine

Clearance: Approximates normal GFR

Dosage Oral:

Children ≥6 months: 15 mg/kg/day divided every 12 hours for 10 days

- Mycobacterial infection (prevention and treatment): 7.5 mg/kg twice daily, up to 500 mg twice daily
- Prophylaxis of bacterial endocarditis: 15 mg/kg 1 hour before procedure (maximum dose: 500 mg)

Adults:

- Usual dose: 250-500 mg every 12 hours **or** 1000 mg (two 500 mg extended release tablets) once daily for 7-14 days
- Upper respiratory tract: 250-500 mg every 12 hours for 10-14 days
  - Pharyngitis/tonsillitis: 250 mg every 12 hours for 10 days
  - Acute maxillary sinusitis: 500 mg every 12 hours **or** 1000 mg (two 500 mg extended release tablets) once daily for 14 days
- Lower respiratory tract: 250-500 mg every 12 hours for 7-14 days
  - Acute exacerbation of chronic bronchitis due to:
    - *M. catarrhalis* and *S. pneumoniae*: 250 mg every 12 hours **or** 1000 mg (two 500 mg extended release tablets) once daily for 7-14 days
    - *H. influenzae*: 500 mg every 12 hours for 7-14 days
  - Pneumonia due to:
    - *C. pneumoniae, M. pneumoniae*, and *S. pneumoniae*: 250 mg every 12 hours for 7-14 days **or** 1000 mg (two 500 mg extended release tablets) once daily for 7 days
    - *H. influenzae*: 250 mg every 12 hours for 7 days **or** 1000 mg (two 500 mg extended release tablets) once daily for 7 days
  - Mycobacterial infection (prevention and treatment): 500 mg twice daily (use with other antimycobacterial drugs, eg, ethambutol, clofazimine, or rifampin)
- Prophylaxis of bacterial endocarditis: 500 mg 1 hour prior to procedure
- Uncomplicated skin and skin structure: 250 mg every 12 hours for 7-14 days

(Continued)

Clarithromycin *(Continued)*

Helicobacter pylori: Combination regimen with bismuth subsalicylate, tetracycline, clarithromycin, and an H_2-receptor antagonist; or combination of omeprazole and clarithromycin; 250 mg twice daily to 500 mg 3 times/day

Dosing adjustment in renal impairment:

Cl_{cr} <30 mL/minute: Half the normal dose or double the dosing interval

In combination with ritonavir:

Cl_{cr} 30-60 mL/minute: Decrease clarithromycin dose by 50%

Cl_{cr} <30 mL/minute: Decrease clarithromycin dose by 75%

Dosing adjustment in hepatic impairment: No dosing adjustment is needed as long as renal function is normal

Elderly: Pharmacokinetics are similar to those in younger adults; may have age-related reductions in renal function; monitor and adjust dose if necessary

Dietary Considerations May be taken with or without meals; may be taken with milk. Biaxin® XL should be taken with food.

Administration Clarithromycin may be given with or without meals. Give every 12 hours rather than twice daily to avoid peak and trough variation.

Biaxin® XL: Should be given with food. Do not crush or chew extended release tablet.

Patient Information May be taken with meals; finish all medication; do not skip doses; do not refrigerate oral suspension, more palatable when taken at room temperature; do not crush or chew extended-release tablets

Dosage Forms

Granules for oral suspension (Biaxin®): 125 mg/5 mL (50 mL, 100 mL); 250 mg/5 mL (50 mL, 100 mL) [fruit punch flavor]

Tablet [film coated] (Biaxin®): 250 mg, 500 mg

Tablet, extended release [film coated] (Biaxin® XL): 500 mg

Selected Readings

Amsden GW, "Erythromycin, Clarithromycin, and Azithromycin: Are the Differences Real?" *Clin Ther*, 1996, 18(1):56-72.

Barradell LB, Plosker GL, and McTavish D, "Clarithromycin. A Review of Its Pharmacological Properties and Therapeutic Use in *Mycobacterium avium-intracellulare* Complex Infection in Patients With Acquired Immune Deficiency Syndrome," *Drugs*, 1993, 46(2):289-312.

Goldman MP and Longworth DL, "The Role of Azithromycin and Clarithromycin in Clinical Practice," *Cleve Clin J Med*, 1993, 60(5):359-64.

Langtry HD and Brogden RN, "Clarithromycin. A Review of Its Efficacy in the Treatment of Respiratory Tract Infections in Immunocompetent Patients," *Drugs*, 1997, 53(6):973-1004.

Tartaglione TA, "Therapeutic Options for the Management and Prevention of *Mycobacterium avium* Complex Infection in Patients With the Acquired Immunodeficiency Syndrome," *Pharmacotherapy*, 1996, 16(2):171-82.

Zuckerman JM and Kaye KM, "The Newer Macrolides. Azithromycin and Clarithromycin," *Infect Dis Clin North Am*, 1995, 9(3):731-45.

Clarithromycin, Lansoprazole, and Amoxicillin *see* Lansoprazole, Amoxicillin, and Clarithromycin *on page 908*

Clavulin® (Can) *see* Amoxicillin and Clavulanate Potassium *on page 645*

Cleocin® *see* Clindamycin *on page 752*

Cleocin HCl® *see* Clindamycin *on page 752*

Cleocin Pediatric® *see* Clindamycin *on page 752*

Cleocin Phosphate® *see* Clindamycin *on page 752*

Cleocin T® *see* Clindamycin *on page 752*

Clindagel® *see* Clindamycin *on page 752*

ClindaMax™ *see* Clindamycin *on page 752*

Clindamycin (klin da MYE sin)

Related Information

Animal and Human Bites *on page 1270*

Antimicrobial Activity Against Selected Organisms *on page 1165*

Community-Acquired Pneumonia in Adults *on page 1278*

Malaria Treatment *on page 1292*

U.S. Brand Names Cleocin®; Cleocin HCl®; Cleocin Pediatric®; Cleocin Phosphate®; Cleocin T®; Clindagel®; ClindaMax™; Clindesse™; Clindets®; Evoclin™

Canadian Brand Names Alti-Clindamycin; Apo-Clindamycin®; Clindoxyl®; Dalacin® C; Dalacin® T; Dalacin® Vaginal; Novo-Clindamycin

Synonyms Clindamycin Hydrochloride; Clindamycin Palmitate; Clindamycin Phosphate

Generic Available Yes: Excludes foam, vaginal suppositories, vaginal cream

Use Treatment against aerobic and anaerobic streptococci (except enterococci), most staphylococci, *Bacteroides* sp and *Actinomyces*; bacterial vaginosis (vaginal cream, vaginal suppository); pelvic inflammatory disease (I.V.); topically in treatment of severe acne; vaginally for *Gardnerella vaginalis*

Unlabeled/Investigational Use May be useful in PCP; alternate treatment for toxoplasmosis

Drug of Choice or Alternative for Disease/Syndrome(s):

Acne Vulgaris *on page 27*
Amnionitis *on page 33*
Brain Abscess *on page 58*
Endometritis *on page 127*
Furunculosis *on page 151*
Impetigo *on page 193*
Joint Replacement, Late Infection *on page 198*
Lung Abscess *on page 212*
Mastitis *on page 214*
Myositis *on page 242*
Necrotizing Fasciitis *on page 243*
Osteomyelitis, Diabetic Foot *on page 249*
Osteomyelitis, Healthy Adult *on page 250*
Osteomyelitis, Pediatric *on page 251*
Pelvic Inflammatory Disease *on page 260*
Pneumonia, Aspiration, Community-Acquired *on page 269*
Pneumonia, Community-Acquired *on page 270*
Sinusitis, Community-Acquired, Chronic *on page 299*
Skin and Soft Tissue *on page 300*
Vaginosis, Bacterial *on page 347*

Organism(s):

Babesia microti on page 40
Bacteroides and *Prevotella* Species *on page 46*
Clostridium perfringens on page 88
Gardnerella vaginalis on page 153
Mycoplasma hominis and *Mycoplasma genitalium on page 237*
Staphylococcus aureus, Methicillin-Susceptible *on page 307*
Staphylococcus epidermidis, Methicillin-Susceptible *on page 310*
Streptococcus-Related Gram-Positive Cocci *on page 325*
Toxoplasma gondii on page 331

Pregnancy Risk Factor B

Contraindications Hypersensitivity to clindamycin or any component of the formulation; previous pseudomembranous colitis; regional enteritis, ulcerative colitis

Warnings/Precautions Dosage adjustment may be necessary in patients with severe hepatic dysfunction; can cause severe and possibly fatal colitis; discontinue drug if significant diarrhea, abdominal cramps, or passage of blood and mucus occurs. Vaginal products may weaken latex or rubber condoms, or contraceptive diaphragms. Barrier contraceptives are not recommended concurrently or for 3-5 days (depending on the product) following treatment. Some dosage forms contain benzyl alcohol or tartrazine. Use caution in atopic patients.

Adverse Reactions

Systemic:

>10%: Gastrointestinal: Diarrhea, abdominal pain

1% to 10%:
- Cardiovascular: Hypotension
- Dermatologic: Urticaria, rash, Stevens-Johnson syndrome
- Gastrointestinal: Pseudomembranous colitis, nausea, vomiting
- Local: Thrombophlebitis, sterile abscess at I.M. injection site
- Miscellaneous: Fungal overgrowth, hypersensitivity

<1% (Limited to important or life-threatening): Renal dysfunction (rare), neutropenia, granulocytopenia, thrombocytopenia, polyarthritis

Topical:

>10%: Dermatologic: Dryness, burning, itching, scaliness, erythema, or peeling of skin (lotion, solution); oiliness (gel, lotion)

1% to 10%: Central nervous system: Headache

<1% (Limited to important or life-threatening): Pseudomembranous colitis, nausea, vomiting, diarrhea (severe), abdominal pain, folliculitis, hypersensitivity reactions

Vaginal:

>10%: Genitourinary: Fungal vaginosis, vaginitis or vulvovaginal pruritus (from *Candida albicans*)

1% to 10%:
- Central nervous system: Back pain, headache
- Gastrointestinal: Constipation, diarrhea
- Genitourinary: Urinary tract infection
- Respiratory: Nasopharyngitis
- Miscellaneous: Fungal infection

(Continued)

Clindamycin *(Continued)*

<1% (Limited to important or life-threatening): Atrophic vaginitis, bladder infection, bladder spasm, cervical dysplasia, diarrhea, dizziness, epistaxis, erythema, fever, hypersensitivity, hyperthyroidism, local edema, menstrual disorder, nausea, pain, palpable lymph node, pruritus, pyelonephritis, pyrexia, rash, sciatica, stomach cramps, upper respiratory urticaria, uterine cervical disorder, uterine spasm, vaginal burning, vertigo, vomiting, vulvar erythema, vulvar laceration, wheezing

Overdosage/Toxicology Following GI decontamination, symptoms of overdose include diarrhea, nausea, and vomiting. Treatment is supportive.

Drug Interactions

Increased Effect/Toxicity: Increased duration of neuromuscular blockade when given in conjunction with tubocurarine and pancuronium.

Ethanol/Nutrition/Herb Interactions

Food: Peak concentrations may be delayed with food.

Herb/Nutraceutical: St John's wort may decrease clindamycin levels.

Stability

Capsule: Store at room temperature of 20°C to 25°C (68°F to 77°F)

Cream: Store at room temperature

Foam: Store at room temperature of 20°C to 25°C (68°F to 77°F); avoid fire, flame, or smoking during or following application

Gel: Store at room temperature

Clindagel®: Do not store in direct sunlight

I.V.: Infusion solution in NS or D_5W solution is stable for 16 days at room temperature

Lotion: Store at room temperature of 20°C to 25°C (68°F to 77°F)

Oral solution: Do not refrigerate reconstituted oral solution (it will thicken); following reconstitution, oral solution is stable for 2 weeks at room temperature of 20°C to 25°C (68°F to 77°F)

Ovule: Store at room temperature of 15°C to 30°C (68°F to 77°F)

Pledget: Store at room temperature

Topical solution: Store at room temperature of 20°C to 25°C (68°F to 77°F)

Mechanism of Action Reversibly binds to 50S ribosomal subunits preventing peptide bond formation thus inhibiting bacterial protein synthesis; bacteriostatic or bactericidal depending on drug concentration, infection site, and organism

Pharmacodynamics/Kinetics

Absorption: Topical: ~10%; Oral: Rapid (90%)

Distribution: High concentrations in bone and urine; no significant levels in CSF, even with inflamed meninges; crosses placenta; enters breast milk

Metabolism: Hepatic

Bioavailability: Topical: <1%

Half-life elimination: Neonates: Premature: 8.7 hours; Full-term: 3.6 hours; Adults: 1.6-5.3 hours (average: 2-3 hours)

Time to peak, serum: Oral: Within 60 minutes; I.M.: 1-3 hours

Excretion: Urine (10%) and feces (~4%) as active drug and metabolites

Dosage

Infants and Children:

Oral: 8-20 mg/kg/day as hydrochloride; 8-25 mg/kg/day as palmitate in 3-4 divided doses; minimum dose of palmitate: 37.5 mg 3 times/day

I.M., I.V.:

<1 month: 15-20 mg/kg/day

>1 month: 20-40 mg/kg/day in 3-4 divided doses

Children: Prevention of bacterial endocarditis (unlabeled use): Oral: 20 mg/kg 1 hour before procedure with no follow-up dose needed; for patients allergic to penicillin and unable to take oral medications: 20 mg/kg I.V. within 30 minutes before procedure

Children ≥12 years and Adults: Topical:

Gel, pledget, lotion, solution: Apply a thin film twice daily

Foam (Evoclin™): Apply once daily

Adults:

Oral: 150-450 mg/dose every 6-8 hours; maximum dose: 1.8 g/day

Prevention of bacterial endocarditis in patients unable to take amoxicillin (unlabeled use): Oral: 600 mg 1 hour before procedure with no follow-up dose needed; for patients allergic to penicillin and unable to take oral medications: 600 mg I.V. within 30 minutes before procedure

I.M., I.V.: 1.2-1.8 g/day in 2-4 divided doses; maximum dose: 4.8 g/day

Pelvic inflammatory disease: I.V.: 900 mg every 8 hours with gentamicin 2 mg/kg, then 1.5 mg/kg every 8 hours; continue after discharge with doxycycline 100 mg twice daily to complete 14 days of total therapy

Pneumocystis carinii pneumonia (unlabeled use):

Oral: 300-450 mg 4 times/day with primaquine

I.M., I.V.: 1200-2400 mg/day with pyrimethamine

I.V.: 600 mg 4 times/day with primaquine

Bacterial vaginosis: Intravaginal:

Suppositories: Insert one ovule (100 mg clindamycin) daily into vagina at bedtime for 3 days

Cream:

Cleocin®: One full applicator inserted intravaginally once daily before bedtime for 3 or 7 consecutive days in nonpregnant patients or for 7 consecutive days in pregnant patients

Clindesse™: One full applicator inserted intravaginally as a single dose at anytime during the day in nonpregnant patients

Dosing adjustment in hepatic impairment: Adjustment recommended in patients with severe hepatic disease

Dietary Considerations May be taken with food.

Administration

I.M.: Deep I.M. sites, rotate sites; do not exceed 600 mg in a single injection

Intravaginal:

Cream: Insertion should be as far as possible into the vagina without causing discomfort

Ovule: The foil should be removed; if the applicator is used for insertion, it should be washed for additional use

I.V.: **Never administer as bolus**; administer by I.V. intermittent infusion over at least 10-60 minutes, at a rate **not** to exceed 30 mg/minute (not exceed 1200 mg/hour); final concentration for administration should not exceed 18 mg/mL

Oral: Administer with a full glass of water to minimize esophageal ulceration; give around-the-clock to promote less variation in peak and trough serum levels

Topical foam: Dispense directly into cap or onto a cool surface; do not dispense directly into hands

Monitoring Parameters Observe for changes in bowel frequency, monitor for colitis and resolution of symptoms; during prolonged therapy monitor CBC, liver and renal function tests periodically

Patient Information Report any severe diarrhea immediately and do not take antidiarrheal medication; take each oral dose with a full glass of water; finish all medication; do not skip doses; should not engage in sexual intercourse during treatment with vaginal product; avoid contact of topical gel/solution with eyes, abraded skin, or mucous membranes

Dosage Forms Note: Strength is expressed as base

Capsule, as hydrochloride: 150 mg, 300 mg

Cleocin HCl®: 75 mg [contains tartrazine], 150 mg [contains tartrazine], 300 mg

Cream, vaginal, as phosphate:

Cleocin®: 2% (40 g) [contains benzyl alcohol and mineral oil; packaged with 7 disposable applicators]

Clindesse™: 2% (5 g) [contains mineral oil; prefilled single disposable applicator]

Foam, topical, as phosphate (Evoclin™): 1% (50 g, 100 g) [contains ethanol 58%]

Gel, topical, as phosphate: 1% [10 mg/g] (30 g, 60 g)

Cleocin T®: 1% [10 mg/g] (30 g, 60 g)

Clindagel®: 1% [10 mg/g] (40 mL, 75 mL)

ClindaMax™: 1% (30 g, 60 g)

Granules for oral solution, as palmitate (Cleocin Pediatric®): 75 mg/5 mL (100 mL) [cherry flavor]

Infusion, as phosphate [premixed in D_5W] (Cleocin Phosphate®): 300 mg (50 mL); 600 mg (50 mL); 900 mg (50 mL)

Injection, solution, as phosphate (Cleocin Phosphate®): 150 mg/mL (2 mL, 4 mL, 6 mL, 60 mL) [contains benzyl alcohol and disodium edetate 0.5 mg]

Lotion, as phosphate (Cleocin T®, ClindaMax™): 1% [10 mg/mL] (60 mL)

Pledgets, topical: 1% (60s) [contains alcohol]

Clindets®: 1% (69s) [contains isopropyl alcohol 52%]

Cleocin T®: 1% (60s) [contains isopropyl alcohol 50%]

Solution, topical, as phosphate (Cleocin T®): 1% [10 mg/mL] (30 mL, 60 mL) [contains isopropyl alcohol 50%]

Suppository (ovule), vaginal, as phosphate (Cleocin®): 100 mg (3s) [contains oleaginous base; single reusable applicator]

Selected Readings

Falagas ME and Gorbach SL, "Clindamycin and Metronidazole," *Med Clin North Am*, 1995, 79(4):845-67.

Smilack JD, Wilson WR, and Cockerill FR 3d, "Tetracyclines, Chloramphenicol, Erythromycin, Clindamycin, and Metronidazole," *Mayo Clin Proc*, 1991, 66(12):1270-80.

Clindamycin and Benzoyl Peroxide

(klin da MYE sin & BEN zoe il peer OKS ide)

U.S. Brand Names BenzaClin®; Duac™

Canadian Brand Names BenzaClin®

Synonyms Benzoyl Peroxide and Clindamycin; Clindamycin Phosphate and Benzoyl Peroxide

Generic Available No

Use Topical treatment of acne vulgaris

Drug of Choice or Alternative for Disease/Syndrome(s):

Acne Vulgaris *on page 27*

Pregnancy Risk Factor C

Pregnancy Implications Reproduction studies have not been conducted; use during pregnancy only if clearly needed.

Contraindications Hypersensitivity to benzoyl peroxide, lincomycin, clindamycin, or any component of the formulation; history of regional enteritis, ulcerative colitis, or antibiotic-associated colitis; concurrent use of erythromycin and clindamycin

Warnings/Precautions Diarrhea, bloody diarrhea, and colitis (including pseudomembranous colitis) have been reported with topical clindamycin. Stop the drug if significant diarrhea occurs. Use concomitant topical acne therapy with caution; cumulative irritancy may occur. Bacterial overgrowth of nonsusceptible organisms may occur. Avoid contact with eyes and mucous membranes; not for ophthalmic use. May bleach hair or colored fabric. Safety and efficacy in children <12 years of age have not been established.

Adverse Reactions >10%: Dermatologic: Peeling (2% to 17%), dry skin (1% to 15%)

1% to 10%: Dermatologic: Pruritus (2%), erythema (1% to 5%), sunburn(1%), burning (<1% to 5%)

Postmarketing and/or case reports: Colitis, diarrhea, pseudomembranous colitis

Drug Interactions

Increased Effect/Toxicity: Tretinoin may cause increased adverse events with concurrent use.

Decreased Effect: Erythromycin may antagonize clindamycin's effects.

Stability

BenzaClin®: Store at room temperature of 25°C (77°F); do not freeze. Reconstitute clindamycin with purified water (5 mL per vial); shake well. Add solution to benzoyl peroxide gel and stir until homogenous in appearance. Discard unused portion after 3 months.

Duac™: Prior to dispensing, store in refrigerator, between 2°C to 8°C (36°F to 46°F). Once dispensed, may be stored by patient at room temperature of up to 25°C (77°F) if used within 60 days. Do not freeze.

Mechanism of Action Clindamycin and benzoyl peroxide have activity against *Propionibacterium acnes in vitro*. This organism has been associated with acne vulgaris. Benzoyl peroxide releases free-radical oxygen which oxidizes bacterial proteins in the sebaceous follicles decreasing the number of anaerobic bacteria and decreasing irritating-type free fatty acids. Clindamycin reversibly binds to 50S ribosomal subunits preventing peptide bond formation thus inhibiting bacterial protein synthesis; bacteriostatic or bactericidal depending on drug concentration, infection site, and organism.

Pharmacodynamics/Kinetics See individual agents.

Dosage Topical: Children ≥12 years and Adults: Apply to affected areas after skin has been cleansed and dried

BenzaClin®: Acne: Apply twice daily (morning and evening)

Duac™: Inflammatory acne: Apply once daily in the evening

Administration Skin should be clean and dry before applying. For external use only; avoid applying to inside nose, mouth, eyes, and mucous membranes

Dosage Forms Gel, topical:

BenzaClin®: Clindamycin phosphate 1% and benzoyl peroxide 5% (25 g, 50 g)

Duac™: Clindamycin phosphate 1% and benzoyl peroxide 5% (45 g)

Clindamycin Hydrochloride *see* Clindamycin *on page 752*

Clindamycin Palmitate *see* Clindamycin *on page 752*

Clindamycin Phosphate *see* Clindamycin *on page 752*

Clindamycin Phosphate and Benzoyl Peroxide *see* Clindamycin and Benzoyl Peroxide *on page 756*

Clindesse™ *see* Clindamycin *on page 752*

Clindets® *see* Clindamycin *on page 752*

Clindoxyl® (Can) *see* Clindamycin *on page 752*

Clofazimine (kloe FA zi meen)

Related Information

Tuberculosis *on page 1315*

U.S. Brand Names Lamprene® [DSC]

Canadian Brand Names Lamprene®

Synonyms Clofazimine Palmitate

Generic Available No

Use Treatment of lepromatous leprosy including dapsone-resistant leprosy and lepromatous leprosy with erythema nodosum leprosum; multibacillary leprosy

Unlabeled/Investigational Use Investigational: Multidrug-resistant tuberculosis

Restrictions Clofazimine is no longer available through most US pharmacies. Requests for clofazimine to treat leprosy should be directed to the National Hansen's Disease Program (a division of the U.S. Department of Health and Human Services), which holds the IND for this indication. The Administrative Officer may be contacted at 225-578-9861 (phone) or 225-578-9856 (fax). Requests for clofazimine to treat MDRTB must be directed to the Division of Special Pathogen and Immunologic Drug Products (HFD-590) at 301-827-2127 (phone). These requests will be distributed by single-patient INDs administered by the FDA. Physicians must register as an investigator for this indication.

Pregnancy Risk Factor C

Pregnancy Implications Teratogenic effects have been observed in some animal studies. Clofazimine crosses the human placenta; skin of infants born following *in utero* exposure may result in pigmentation changes. Use during pregnancy only if clearly needed.

Contraindications Hypersensitivity to clofazimine or any component of the formulation

Warnings/Precautions Clofazimine may crystallize and deposit in tissues, including intestinal mucosa, liver, spleen and mesenteric lymph nodes. Severe abdominal symptoms may occur and include rare reports of splenic infarction, bowel obstruction and gastrointestinal bleeding. Use with caution in patients with GI problems (ie, abdominal pain, diarrhea). Adjust dose or discontinue if abdominal symptoms occur; dosages >100 mg/day should be used for as short a duration as possible. **Note:** Clofazimine use has been associated with an adverse outcome in the treatment of MAC disease and should not be used.

Adverse Reactions

>10%:

- Dermatologic: Dry skin
- Gastrointestinal: Abdominal pain, nausea, vomiting, diarrhea
- Miscellaneous: Pink to brownish-black discoloration of the skin

1% to 10%:

- Dermatologic: Rash, pruritus
- Endocrine & metabolic: Elevated blood sugar
- Gastrointestinal: Fecal discoloration
- Genitourinary: Discoloration of urine
- Ocular: Discoloration of conjunctiva; irritation, burning, and itching of the eyes
- Miscellaneous: Discoloration of sputum, sweat

<1%: Acneiform eruptions, albumin increased, anemia, anorexia, bilirubin increased, bone pain, bowel obstruction, constipation, cystitis, depression (secondary to skin discoloration), dizziness, drowsiness, edema, eosinophilia, eosinophilic enteritis, erythroderma, fatigue, fever, gastrointestinal bleeding, giddiness, headache, hepatitis, hypokalemia, jaundice, liver enlarged, lymphadenopathy, monilial cheilosis, neuralgia, phototoxicity, SGOT increased, splenic infarction, taste disorder, thromboembolism, vascular pain, vision decreased, weight loss

Overdosage/Toxicology Following GI decontamination, treatment is supportive.

Drug Interactions

Cytochrome P450 Effect: Inhibits CYP3A4 (weak)

Decreased Effect: Combined use may decrease effect with dapsone (unconfirmed).

Ethanol/Nutrition/Herb Interactions

Food: The presence of food increases the extent of absorption.

Stability Protect from moisture

Mechanism of Action Binds preferentially to mycobacterial DNA to inhibit mycobacterial growth; also has some anti-inflammatory activity through an unknown mechanism

Pharmacodynamics/Kinetics

Absorption: Variable (45% to 62%)

Distribution: Highly lipophilic; deposited primarily in fatty tissue and cells of the reticuloendothelial system; taken up by macrophages throughout the body; distributed to

(Continued)

Clofazimine *(Continued)*

breast milk, mesenteric lymph nodes, adrenal glands, subcutaneous fat, liver, bile, gallbladder, spleen, small intestine, muscles, bones, and skin; does not appear to cross blood-brain barrier; remains in tissues for prolonged periods

Metabolism: Partially hepatic to two metabolites

Half-life elimination: Terminal: 8 days; Tissue: 70 days

Time to peak, serum: Chronic therapy: 1-6 hours

Excretion: Primarily feces; urine (negligible amounts as unchanged drug); sputum, saliva, and sweat (small amounts)

Dosage Oral:

Children: Leprosy: 1 mg/kg/day every 24 hours in combination with dapsone and rifampin

Adults:

Dapsone-resistant leprosy: 100 mg/day in combination with one or more antileprosy drugs for 3 years; then alone 100 mg/day

Dapsone-sensitive multibacillary leprosy: 100 mg/day in combination with two or more antileprosy drugs for at least 2 years and continue until negative skin smears are obtained, then institute single drug therapy with appropriate agent

Erythema nodosum leprosum: 100-200 mg/day for up to 3 months or longer then taper dose to 100 mg/day when possible

Dosing adjustment in hepatic impairment: Should be considered in severe hepatic dysfunction

Dietary Considerations Take with meals.

Patient Information Drug may cause a pink to brownish-black discoloration of the skin, conjunctiva, tears, sweat, urine, feces, and nasal secretions; although reversible, may take months to years to disappear after therapy is complete; take with meals

Dosage Forms [DSC] = Discontinued product

Capsule: 50 mg [DSC]

Selected Readings

"Drugs for AIDS and Associated Infections," *Med Lett Drugs Ther*, 1993, 35(904):79-86.

"Effect of Combined Therapy with Ansamycin, Clofazimine, Ethambutol, and Isoniazid for *Mycobacterium avium* Infection in Patients With AIDS," *J Infect Dis*, 1989, 159(4):784-7.

Hoy J, Mijch A, Sandland M, et al, "Quadruple-Drug Therapy for *Mycobacterium avium-intracellulare* Bacteremia in AIDS Patients," *J Infect Dis*, 1990, 161(4):801-5.

Kemper CA, Meng TC, Nussbaum J, et al, "Treatment of *Mycobacterium avium* Complex Bacteremia in AIDS With a Four-Drug Oral Regimen. Rifampin, Ethambutol, Clofazimine, and Ciprofloxacin" *Ann Intern Med*, 1992, 116(6):466-72.

Clofazimine Palmitate *see* Clofazimine *on page 757*

Clorpactin® WCS-90 [OTC] *see* Oxychlorosene *on page 986*

Clotrimaderm (Can) *see* Clotrimazole *on page 758*

Clotrimazole (kloe TRIM a zole)

U.S. Brand Names Cruex® Cream [OTC]; Gyne-Lotrimin® 3 [OTC]; Lotrimin® AF Athlete's Foot Cream [OTC]; Lotrimin® AF Athlete's Foot Solution [OTC]; Lotrimin® AF Jock Itch Cream [OTC]; Mycelex®; Mycelex®-7 [OTC]; Mycelex® Twin Pack [OTC]

Canadian Brand Names Canesten® Topical; Canesten® Vaginal; Clotrimaderm; Trivagizole-3®

Generic Available Yes: Cream, solution, troche

Use Treatment of susceptible fungal infections, including oropharyngeal candidiasis, dermatophytoses, superficial mycoses, and cutaneous candidiasis, as well as vulvovaginal candidiasis; limited data suggest that clotrimazole troches may be effective for prophylaxis against oropharyngeal candidiasis in neutropenic patients

Drug of Choice or Alternative for Organism(s):

Malassezia furfur on page 213

Pregnancy Risk Factor B (topical); C (troches)

Contraindications Hypersensitivity to clotrimazole or any component of the formulation

Warnings/Precautions Clotrimazole should not be used for treatment of systemic fungal infection; safety and effectiveness of clotrimazole lozenges (troches) in children <3 years of age have not been established; when using topical formulation, avoid contact with eyes

Adverse Reactions

Oral:

>10%: Hepatic: Abnormal liver function tests

1% to 10%:

Gastrointestinal: Nausea and vomiting may occur in patients on clotrimazole troches

Local: Mild burning, irritation, stinging to skin or vaginal area

Vaginal:

1% to 10%: Genitourinary: Vulvar/vaginal burning

<1% (Limited to important or life-threatening): Vulvar itching, soreness, edema, or discharge; polyuria; burning or itching of penis of sexual partner

Drug Interactions

Cytochrome P450 Effect: Inhibits CYP1A2 (weak), 2A6 (weak), 2B6 (weak), 2C8/9 (weak), 2C19 (weak), 2D6 (weak), 2E1 (weak), 3A4 (moderate)

Increased Effect/Toxicity: Clotrimazole may increase the levels/effects of selected benzodiazepines, calcium channel blockers, cisapride, cyclosporine, ergot derivatives, selected HMG-CoA reductase inhibitors, mesoridazine, mirtazapine, nateglinide, nefazodone, pimozide, quinidine, sildenafil (and other PDE-5 inhibitors), tacrolimus, thioridazine, venlafaxine, and other CYP3A4 substrates.

Mechanism of Action Binds to phospholipids in the fungal cell membrane altering cell wall permeability resulting in loss of essential intracellular elements

Pharmacodynamics/Kinetics

Absorption: Topical: Negligible through intact skin

Time to peak, serum:

Oral topical (troche): Salivary levels occur within 3 hours following 30 minutes of dissolution time

Vaginal cream: High vaginal levels: 8-24 hours

Vaginal tablet: High vaginal levels: 1-2 days

Excretion: Feces (as metabolites)

Dosage

Children >3 years and Adults:

Oral:

Prophylaxis: 10 mg troche dissolved 3 times/day for the duration of chemotherapy or until steroids are reduced to maintenance levels

Treatment: 10 mg troche dissolved slowly 5 times/day for 14 consecutive days

Topical (cream, solution): Apply twice daily; if no improvement occurs after 4 weeks of therapy, re-evaluate diagnosis

Children >12 years and Adults:

Vaginal:

Cream:

1%: Insert 1 applicatorful vaginal cream daily (preferably at bedtime) for 7 consecutive days

2%: Insert 1 applicatorful vaginal cream daily (preferably at bedtime) for 3 consecutive days

Tablet: Insert 100 mg/day for 7 days or 500 mg single dose

Topical (cream, solution): Apply to affected area twice daily (morning and evening) for 7 consecutive days

Administration

Oral (troche): Allow to dissolve slowly over 15-30 minutes.

Topical: Avoid contact with eyes. For external use only. Apply sparingly. Protect hands with latex gloves. Do not use occlusive dressings.

Monitoring Parameters Periodic liver function tests during oral therapy with clotrimazole troche

Patient Information Oral: Do not swallow oral medication whole; allow to dissolve slowly in mouth. You may experience nausea or vomiting (small frequent meals, frequent mouth care, chewing gum, or sucking lozenges may help). Report signs of opportunistic infection (eg, white plaques in mouth, fever, chills, perianal itching or vaginal discharge, fatigue, unhealed wounds or sores).

Topical: Wash hands before applying or wear gloves. Apply thin film to affected area. May apply porous dressing. Report persistent burning, swelling, itching, worsening of condition, or lack of response to therapy.

Vaginal: Wash hands before using. Insert full applicator into vagina gently and expel cream, or insert tablet into vagina, at bedtime. Wash applicator with soap and water following use. Remain lying down for 30 minutes following administration. Avoid intercourse during therapy (sexual partner may experience penile burning or itching). Report adverse reactions (eg, vulvar itching, frequent urination), worsening of condition, or lack of response to therapy. Contact prescriber if symptoms do not improve within 3 days or you do not feel well within 7 days. Do not use tampons until therapy is complete. Contact prescriber immediately if you experience abdominal pain, fever, or foul-smelling discharge.

Dosage Forms

Combination pack (Mycelex®-7): Vaginal tablet 100 mg (7s) and vaginal cream 1% (7 g)

Cream, topical: 1% (15 g, 30 g, 45 g)

Cruex®: 1% (15 g)

(Continued)

Clotrimazole *(Continued)*

- Lotrimin® AF Athlete's Foot: 1% (12 g, 24 g)
- Lotrimin® AF Jock Itch: 1% (12 g)

Cream, vaginal: 2% (21 g)

- Mycelex®-7: 1% (45 g)

Solution, topical: 1% (10 mL, 30 mL)

- Lotrimin® AF Athlete's Foot: 1% (10 mL)

Tablet, vaginal (Gyne-Lotrimin® 3): 200 mg (3s)

Troche (Mycelex®): 10 mg

Clotrimazole and Betamethasone *see* Betamethasone and Clotrimazole *on page 685*

Cloxacillin (kloks a SIL in)

Related Information

Antimicrobial Activity Against Selected Organisms *on page 1165*

Canadian Brand Names Apo-Cloxi®; Novo-Cloxin; Nu-Cloxi; Riva-Cloxacillin

Synonyms Cloxacillin Sodium

Generic Available Yes

Use Treatment of susceptible bacterial infections, notably penicillinase-producing staphylococci causing respiratory tract, skin and skin structure, bone and joint, urinary tract infections

Restrictions Not available in U.S.

Pregnancy Risk Factor B

Contraindications Hypersensitivity to cloxacillin, any component of the formulation, or penicillins

Warnings/Precautions Monitor PT if patient concurrently on warfarin, elimination of drug is slow in renally impaired; use with caution in patients allergic to cephalosporins due to a low incidence of cross-hypersensitivity

Adverse Reactions

1% to 10%: Gastrointestinal: Nausea, diarrhea, abdominal pain

<1%: Fever, seizure with extremely high doses and/or renal failure, rash (maculopapular to exfoliative), vomiting, pseudomembranous colitis, vaginitis, eosinophilia, leukopenia, neutropenia, thrombocytopenia, agranulocytosis, anemia, hemolytic anemia, prolonged PT, hepatotoxicity, transient elevated LFTs, hematuria, interstitial nephritis, increased BUN/creatinine, serum sickness-like reactions, hypersensitivity

Overdosage/Toxicology Symptoms of penicillin overdose include neuromuscular hypersensitivity (agitation, hallucinations, asterixis, encephalopathy, confusion, and seizures) and electrolyte imbalance (with potassium or sodium salts), especially in renal failure. Hemodialysis may be helpful to aid in the removal of the drug from the blood, otherwise, most treatment is supportive or symptom-directed.

Drug Interactions

Increased Effect/Toxicity: Probenecid and disulfiram may increase levels of penicillins (cloxacillin). The hypoprothrombinemic effects of warfarin may be increased. Penicillins may increase the exposure to methotrexate during concurrent therapy; monitor.

Decreased Effect: Although anecdotal reports suggest oral contraceptive efficacy could be reduced by penicillins, this has been refuted by more rigorous scientific and clinical data.

Stability Refrigerate oral solution after reconstitution; discard after 14 days; stable for 3 days at room temperature

Mechanism of Action Inhibits bacterial cell wall synthesis by binding to one or more of the penicillin-binding proteins (PBPs) which in turn inhibits the final transpeptidation step of peptidoglycan synthesis in bacterial cell walls, thus inhibiting cell wall biosynthesis. Bacteria eventually lyse due to ongoing activity of cell wall autolytic enzymes (autolysins and murein hydrolases) while cell wall assembly is arrested.

Pharmacodynamics/Kinetics

Absorption: Oral: ~50%

Distribution: Widely to most body fluids and bone; penetration into cells, into eye, and across normal meninges is poor; crosses placenta; enters breast milk; inflammation increases amount that crosses blood-brain barrier

Protein binding: 90% to 98%

Metabolism: Extensively hepatic to active and inactive metabolites

Half-life elimination: 0.5-1.5 hours; prolonged with renal impairment and in neonates

Time to peak, serum: 0.5-2 hours

Excretion: Urine and feces

Dosage Oral:

Children >1 month (<20 kg): 50-100 mg/kg/day in divided doses every 6 hours; up to a maximum of 4 g/day

Children (>20 kg) and Adults: 250-500 mg every 6 hours

Hemodialysis: Not dialyzable (0% to 5%)

Dietary Considerations Should be taken 1 hour before or 2 hours after meals with water.

Sodium content of 250 mg capsule: 13.8 mg (0.6 mEq)

Sodium content of suspension 5 mL of 125 mg/5 mL: 11 mg (0.48 mEq)

Monitoring Parameters Observe for signs and symptoms of anaphylaxis during first dose

Test Interactions May interfere with urinary glucose tests using cupric sulfate (Benedict's solution, Clinitest®); may inactivate aminoglycosides *in vitro*; false-positive urine and serum proteins; false-positive in uric acid, urinary steroids

Patient Information Take 1 hour before or 2 hours after meals; finish all medication; do not skip doses

Dosage Forms

Capsule, as sodium: 250 mg, 500 mg

Powder for oral suspension, as sodium: 125 mg/5 mL (100 mL, 200 mL)

Selected Readings

Donowitz GR and Mandell GL, "Beta-Lactam Antibiotics," *N Engl J Med*, 1988, 318(7):419-26 and 318(8):490-500.

Wright AJ, "The Penicillins," *Mayo Clin Proc*, 1999, 74(3):290-307.

Cloxacillin Sodium *see* Cloxacillin *on page 760*

CMV-IGIV *see* Cytomegalovirus Immune Globulin (Intravenous-Human) *on page 764*

CNJ-016™ *see* Vaccinia Immune Globulin (Intravenous) *on page 1139*

CO Ciprofloxacin (Can) *see* Ciprofloxacin *on page 742*

Colistimethate (koe lis ti METH ate)

U.S. Brand Names Coly-Mycin® M

Canadian Brand Names Coly-Mycin® M

Synonyms Colistimethate Sodium

Generic Available Yes

Use Treatment of infections due to sensitive strains of certain gram-negative bacilli which are resistant to other antibacterials or in patients allergic to other antibacterials

Unlabeled/Investigational Use Used as inhalation in the prevention of *Pseudomonas aeruginosa* respiratory tract infections in immunocompromised patients, and used as inhalation adjunct agent for the treatment of *P. aeruginosa* infections in patients with cystic fibrosis and other seriously ill or chronically ill patients

Pregnancy Risk Factor C

Contraindications Hypersensitivity to colistimethate or any component of the formulation

Warnings/Precautions Use with caution in patients with pre-existing renal disease

Adverse Reactions 1% to 10%:

Central nervous system: Vertigo, slurring of speech

Dermatologic: Urticaria

Gastrointestinal: GI upset

Respiratory: Respiratory arrest

Renal: Nephrotoxicity

Drug Interactions

Increased Effect/Toxicity: Other nephrotoxic drugs, neuromuscular blocking agents.

Stability Freshly prepare any infusion and use for no longer than 24 hours.

Mechanism of Action Hydrolyzed to colistin, which acts as a cationic detergent which damages the bacterial cytoplasmic membrane causing leaking of intracellular substances and cell death

Pharmacodynamics/Kinetics

Distribution: Widely, except for CNS, synovial, pleural, and pericardial fluids

Half-life elimination: 1.5-8 hours; Anuria: ≤2-3 days

Time to peak: ~2 hours

Excretion: Primarily urine (as unchanged drug)

Dosage Children and Adults:

I.M., I.V.: 2.5-5 mg/kg/day in 2-4 divided doses

Inhalation: 50-75 mg in NS (3-4 mL total) via nebulizer 2-3 times/day

Dosing interval in renal impairment: Adults:

S_{cr} 0.7-1.2 mg/dL: 100-125 mg 2-4 times/day

S_{cr} 1.3-1.5 mg/dL: 75-115 mg twice daily

S_{cr} 1.6-2.5 mg/dL: 66-150 mg once or twice daily

(Continued)

Colistimethate *(Continued)*

S_{cr} 2.6-4 mg/dL: 100-150 mg every 36 hours

Administration

Parenteral: Reconstitute vial with 2 mL SWFI resulting in a concentration of 75 mg colistin/mL; swirl gently to avoid frothing. Administer by I.M., direct I.V. injection over 3-10 minutes, intermittent infusion over 30 minutes, or by continuous I.V. infusion. For continuous I.V. infusion, one-half of the total daily dose is administered by direct I.V. injection over 3-10 minutes followed 1-2 hours later by the remaining one-half of the total daily dose diluted in a compatible I.V. solution infused over 22-23 hours. The final concentration for administration should be based on the patient's fluid needs.

Inhalation: Further dilute dose to a total volume of 3-4 mL in NS and administer via nebulizer. If patient is on a ventilator, place medicine in a T-piece at the midinspiratory circuit of the ventilator.

Dosage Forms Injection, powder for reconstitution: 150 mg

Selected Readings

Bauldoff GS, Nunley DR, Manzetti JD, et al, "Use of Aerosolized Colistin in Cystic Fibrosis Patients Awaiting Lung Transplantation," *Transplantation*, 1997, 64(5):748-52.

Conway SP, Pond MN, Watson A, et al, "Intravenous Colistin Sulphomethate in Acute Respiratory Exacerbations in Adult Patients With Cystic Fibrosis," *Thorax*, 1997, 52(11):987-93.

Jensen T, Pederson SS, Garne S, et al, "Colistin Inhalation Therapy in Cystic Fibrosis Patients with Chronic *Pseudomonas aeruginosa* Lung Infection," *J Antimicrob Chemother*, 1987, 19(6):831-8.

Zylberberg H, Vargaftig J, Barbieux C, et al, "Prolonged Efficiency of Secondary Prophylaxis with Colistin Aerosols for Respiratory Infection Due to *Pseudomonas aeruginosa* in Patients Infected With Human Immunodeficiency Virus," *Clin Infect Dis*, 1996, 23(3):641-3.

Colistimethate Sodium *see* Colistimethate *on page 761*

Coly-Mycin® M *see* Colistimethate *on page 761*

Combantrin™ (Can) *see* Pyrantel Pamoate *on page 1021*

Combivir® *see* Zidovudine and Lamivudine *on page 1162*

Compound S *see* Zidovudine *on page 1159*

Compound S, Abacavir, and Lamivudine *see* Abacavir, Lamivudine, and Zidovudine *on page 627*

Comvax® *see Haemophilus* b Conjugate and Hepatitis B Vaccine *on page 847*

Copegus® *see* Ribavirin *on page 1040*

Cortimyxin® (Can) *see* Neomycin, Polymyxin B, and Hydrocortisone *on page 966*

Cortisporin® Cream *see* Neomycin, Polymyxin B, and Hydrocortisone *on page 966*

Cortisporin® Ointment *see* Bacitracin, Neomycin, Polymyxin B, and Hydrocortisone *on page 682*

Cortisporin® Ophthalmic *see* Neomycin, Polymyxin B, and Hydrocortisone *on page 966*

Cortisporin® Otic *see* Neomycin, Polymyxin B, and Hydrocortisone *on page 966*

Cortisporin® Topical Ointment (Can) *see* Bacitracin, Neomycin, Polymyxin B, and Hydrocortisone *on page 682*

CO Terbinafine (Can) *see* Terbinafine *on page 1097*

Co-Trimoxazole *see* Sulfamethoxazole and Trimethoprim *on page 1087*

Coviracil *see* Emtricitabine *on page 799*

CP-99,219-27 *see* Trovafloxacin *on page 1134*

Crixivan® *see* Indinavir *on page 872*

Crotamiton (kroe TAM i tonn)

U.S. Brand Names Eurax®

Generic Available No

Use Treatment of scabies (*Sarcoptes scabiei*) and symptomatic treatment of pruritus

Drug of Choice or Alternative for Organism(s):

Sarcoptes scabiei on page 293

Pregnancy Risk Factor C

Pregnancy Implications Animal reproduction studies have not been conducted; use during pregnancy only if clearly needed.

Contraindications Hypersensitivity to crotamiton or any component of the formulation; patients who manifest a primary irritation response to topical medications

Warnings/Precautions Avoid contact with face, eyes, mucous membranes, and urethral meatus; do not apply to acutely inflamed or raw skin; for external use only

Adverse Reactions Frequency not defined. Topical:

Dermatologic: Pruritus, contact dermatitis, rash

Local: Local irritation

Miscellaneous: Allergic sensitivity reactions, warm sensation

Overdosage/Toxicology Symptoms of ingestion include burning sensation in mouth; irritation of the buccal, esophageal and gastric mucosa, nausea, vomiting, and abdominal pain. There is no specific antidote. General measures to eliminate the drug and reduce its absorption, combined with symptomatic treatment, are recommended.

Stability Store at room temperature.

Mechanism of Action Crotamiton has scabicidal activity against *Sarcoptes scabiei*; mechanism of action unknown

Dosage Topical:

Scabicide: Children and Adults: Wash thoroughly and scrub away loose scales, then towel dry; apply a thin layer and massage drug onto skin of the entire body from the neck to the toes (with special attention to skin folds, creases, and interdigital spaces). Repeat application in 24 hours. Take a cleansing bath 48 hours after the final application. Treatment may be repeated after 7-10 days if live mites are still present.

Pruritus: Massage into affected areas until medication is completely absorbed; repeat as necessary

Administration For external use only. Shake lotion well before using. Avoid contact with face, eyes, mucous membranes, and urethral meatus.

Patient Information For topical use only; all contaminated clothing and bed linens should be washed to avoid reinfestation

Dosage Forms

Cream: 10% (60 g)

Lotion: 10% (60 mL, 480 mL)

Selected Readings

Eichenfield LF, Honig PJ, "Blistering Disorders in Childhood," *Pediatr Clin North Am*, 1991, 38(4):959-76.

Hogan DJ, Schachner L, Tanglertsampan C, "Diagnosis and Treatment of Childhood Scabies and Pediculosis," *Pediatr Clin North Am*, 1991, 38(4):941-57.

Cruex® Cream [OTC] *see* Clotrimazole *on page 758*

Crystalline Penicillin *see* Penicillin G (Parenteral/Aqueous) *on page 993*

Crystal Violet *see* Gentian Violet *on page 845*

Cubicin™ *see* Daptomycin *on page 768*

CycloSERINE (sye kloe SER een)

Related Information

Tuberculosis *on page 1315*

U.S. Brand Names Seromycin®

Generic Available No

Use Adjunctive treatment in pulmonary or extrapulmonary tuberculosis

Unlabeled/Investigational Use Treatment of Gaucher's disease

Pregnancy Risk Factor C

Contraindications Hypersensitivity to cycloserine or any component of the formulation

Warnings/Precautions Epilepsy, depression, severe anxiety, psychosis, severe renal insufficiency, chronic alcoholism

Adverse Reactions Frequency not defined.

Cardiovascular: Cardiac arrhythmia

Central nervous system: Drowsiness, headache, dizziness, vertigo, seizure, confusion, psychosis, paresis, coma

Dermatologic: Rash

Endocrine & metabolic: Vitamin B_{12} deficiency

Hematologic: Folate deficiency

Hepatic: Liver enzymes increased

Neuromuscular & skeletal: Tremor

Overdosage/Toxicology Symptoms include confusion, agitation, CNS depression, psychosis, coma, and seizures. Decontaminate with activated charcoal. Can be hemodialyzed. Management is supportive. Administer pyridoxine 100-300 mg/day to reduce neurotoxic effects. Acute toxicity can occur with ingestions >1 g, chronic toxicity can occur with ingestions >500 mg/day.

Drug Interactions

Increased Effect/Toxicity: Alcohol, isoniazid, and ethionamide increase toxicity of cycloserine. Cycloserine inhibits the hepatic metabolism of phenytoin and may increase risk of epileptic seizures.

Ethanol/Nutrition/Herb Interactions

Ethanol: Avoid ethanol (may increase CNS depression).

Food: May increase vitamin B_{12} and folic acid dietary requirements.

Mechanism of Action Inhibits bacterial cell wall synthesis by competing with amino acid (D-alanine) for incorporation into the bacterial cell wall; bacteriostatic or bactericidal

(Continued)

CycloSERINE *(Continued)*

Pharmacodynamics/Kinetics

Absorption: ~70% to 90%

Distribution: Widely to most body fluids and tissues including CSF, breast milk, bile, sputum, lymph tissue, lungs, and ascitic, pleural, and synovial fluids; crosses placenta

Half-life elimination: Normal renal function: 10 hours

Metabolism: Hepatic

Time to peak, serum: 3-4 hours

Excretion: Urine (60% to 70% as unchanged drug) within 72 hours; feces (small amounts); remainder metabolized

Dosage Some of the neurotoxic effects may be relieved or prevented by the concomitant administration of pyridoxine

Tuberculosis: Oral:

Children: 10-20 mg/kg/day in 2 divided doses up to 1000 mg/day for 18-24 months

Adults: Initial: 250 mg every 12 hours for 14 days, then administer 500 mg to 1 g/day in 2 divided doses for 18-24 months (maximum daily dose: 1 g)

Dosing interval in renal impairment:

Cl_{cr} 10-50 mL/minute: Administer every 24 hours

Cl_{cr} <10 mL/minute: Administer every 36-48 hours

Dietary Considerations May be taken with food; may increase vitamin B_{12} and folic acid dietary requirements.

Monitoring Parameters Periodic renal, hepatic, hematological tests, and plasma cycloserine concentrations

Reference Range Toxicity is greatly increased at levels >30 mcg/mL

Patient Information May cause drowsiness; report skin rash, mental confusion, dizziness, headache, or tremors; do not skip doses; do not drink excessive amounts of alcoholic beverages

Dosage Forms Capsule: 250 mg

Selected Readings

Davidson PT and Le HQ, "Drug Treatment of Tuberculosis - 1992," *Drugs*, 1992, 43(5):651-73.

"Drugs for Tuberculosis," *Med Lett Drugs Ther*, 1993, 35(908):99-101.

Iseman MD, "Treatment of Multidrug-Resistant Tuberculosis," *N Engl J Med*, 1993, 329(11):784-91.

CytoGam® *see* Cytomegalovirus Immune Globulin (Intravenous-Human) *on page 764*

Cytomegalovirus Immune Globulin (Intravenous-Human)

(sye toe meg a low VYE rus i MYUN GLOB yoo lin in tra VEE nus HYU man)

U.S. Brand Names CytoGam®

Synonyms CMV-IGIV

Generic Available No

Use Prophylaxis of cytomegalovirus (CMV) disease associated with kidney, lung, liver, pancreas, and heart transplants; concomitant use with ganciclovir should be considered in organ transplants (other than kidney) from CMV seropositive donors to CMV seronegative recipients

Unlabeled/Investigational Use Adjunct therapy in the treatment of CMV disease in immunocompromised patients

Pregnancy Risk Factor C

Pregnancy Implications Reproduction studies have not been conducted.

Contraindications Hypersensitivity to CMV-IGIV, other immunoglobulins, or any component of the formulation; immunoglobulin A deficiency

Warnings/Precautions Monitor for anaphylactic reactions; epinephrine and diphenhydramine should be available during infusion. Made from pooled human plasma; may theoretically transmit blood-borne viruses. Human immune globulins are associated with renal dysfunction, acute renal failure, osmotic nephrosis, and death; risk is increased in products containing sucrose. Use with caution in patients with renal insufficiency, diabetes mellitus, patients >65 years of age, volume depletion, sepsis, paraproteinemia, or patients on concomitant nephrotoxic drugs. Administer only if patient is euvolemic prior to therapy. Aseptic meningitis syndrome (AMS) may occur within hours to 2 days of treatment; occurs more frequently with high-dose treatment. Stabilized with sucrose and albumin, contains no preservative.

Adverse Reactions

<6%:

Cardiovascular: Flushing

Central nervous system: Fever, chills

Gastrointestinal: Nausea, vomiting

Neuromuscular & skeletal: Arthralgia, back pain, muscle cramps

Respiratory: Wheezing

<1%: Blood pressure decreased

Postmarketing and/or case reports: Acute renal failure, acute tubular necrosis, anaphylactic shock, angioneurotic edema, anuria, aseptic meningitis syndrome (AMS), BUN increased, serum creatinine increased, oliguria, osmotic nephrosis, proximal tubular nephropathy

Overdosage/Toxicology Symptoms related to volume overload would be expected to occur with overdose. Treatment is symptom-directed and supportive.

Drug Interactions

Decreased Effect: Decreased effect of live vaccines may be seen if given within 3 months of IGIV administration. Defer vaccination or revaccinate.

Stability Store between 2°C and 8°C (35.6°F and 46.4°F). Use reconstituted product within 6 hours; do not admix with other medications; do not use if turbid. Do not shake vials. Dilution is not recommended. Infusion with other products is not recommended. If unavoidable, may be piggybacked into an I.V. line of sodium chloride, 2.5% dextrose in water, 5% dextrose in water, 10% dextrose in water, or 20% dextrose in water. Do not dilute more than 1:2.

Mechanism of Action CMV-IGIV is a preparation of immunoglobulin G derived from pooled healthy blood donors with a high titer of CMV antibodies; administration provides a passive source of antibodies against cytomegalovirus

Dosage I.V.: Adults:

Kidney transplant:

- Initial dose (within 72 hours of transplant): 150 mg/kg/dose
- 2-, 4-, 6-, and 8 weeks after transplant: 100 mg/kg/dose
- 12 and 16 weeks after transplant: 50 mg/kg/dose

Liver, lung, pancreas, or heart transplant:

- Initial dose (within 72 hours of transplant): 150 mg/kg/dose
- 2-, 4-, 6-, and 8 weeks after transplant: 150 mg/kg/dose
- 12 and 16 weeks after transplant: 100 mg/kg/dose

Severe CMV pneumonia: Various regimens have been used, including 400 mg/kg CMV-IGIV in combination with ganciclovir on days 1, 2, 7, or 8, followed by 200 mg/kg CMV-IGIV on days 14 and 21

Elderly: Use with caution in patients >65 years of age, may be at increased risk of renal insufficiency

Dosage adjustment in renal impairment: Use with caution; specific dosing adjustments are not available. Infusion rate should be the minimum practical; do not exceed 180 mg/kg/hour

Administration Administer through an I.V. line containing an in-line filter (pore size 15 micron) using an infusion pump. Do not mix with other infusions; do not use if turbid. Begin infusion within 6 hours of entering vial, complete infusion within 12 hours.

Infuse at 15 mg/kg/hour. If no adverse reactions occur within 30 minutes, may increase rate to 30 mg/kg/hour. If no adverse reactions occur within the second 30 minutes, may increase rate to 60 mg/kg/hour; maximum rate of infusion: 75 mL/hour. When infusing subsequent doses, may decrease titration interval from 30 minutes to 15 minutes. If patient develops nausea, back pain, or flushing during infusion, slow the rate or temporarily stop the infusion. Discontinue if blood pressure drops or in case of anaphylactic reaction.

Monitoring Parameters Vital signs (throughout infusion), flushing, chills, muscle cramps, back pain, fever, nausea, vomiting, wheezing, decreased blood pressure, or anaphylaxis; renal function and urine output

Dosage Forms Injection, solution [preservative free]: 50 mg ± 10 mg/mL (50 mL) [contains human albumin and sucrose]

Selected Readings

Levinson ML and Jacobson PA, "Treatment and Prophylaxis of Cytomegalovirus Disease," *Pharmacotherapy*, 1992, 12(4):300-18.

Reed EC, Bowden RA, Dandliker PS, et al, "Efficacy of Cytomegalovirus Immunoglobulin in Marrow Transplant Recipients With Cytomegalovirus Pneumonia," *J Infect Dis*, 1987, 156:641-5.

Reed EC, Bowden RA, Dandliker PS, et al, "Treatment of Cytomegalovirus Pneumonia With Ganciclovir and Intravenous Cytomegalovirus Immunoglobulin in Patients With Bone Marrow Transplants," *Ann Intern Med*, 1988, 109:783-8.

Snydman DR, "Cytomegalovirus Immunoglobulins in the Prevention and Treatment of Cytomegalovirus Disease," *Rev Infect Dis*, 1990, 12(Suppl 7):S839-48.

Cytovene® *see* Ganciclovir *on page 834*

d4T *see* Stavudine *on page 1076*

Dalacin® C (Can) *see* Clindamycin *on page 752*

Dalacin® T (Can) *see* Clindamycin *on page 752*

Dalacin® Vaginal (Can) *see* Clindamycin *on page 752*

Dapcin *see* Daptomycin *on page 768*

Dapsone (DAP sone)

Related Information

USPHS / IDSA Guidelines for the Prevention of Opportunistic Infections in Persons Infected With HIV *on page 1237*

U.S. Brand Names Aczone™

Synonyms Diaminodiphenylsulfone

Generic Available Yes: Tablet

Use Treatment of leprosy and dermatitis herpetiformis (infections caused by *Mycobacterium leprae*); treatment of acne vulgaris

Unlabeled/Investigational Use Prophylaxis of toxoplasmosis in severely-immunocompromised patients; alternative agent for *Pneumocystis carinii* pneumonia prophylaxis (monotherapy) and treatment (in combination with trimethoprim)

Drug of Choice or Alternative for Organism(s):

Pneumocystis jiroveci on page 266

Pregnancy Risk Factor C

Pregnancy Implications There are no adequate and well-controlled studies in pregnant women. Use during pregnancy when the benefit to the mother outweighs the potential risk to the fetus.

Contraindications Hypersensitivity to dapsone or any component of the formulation

Warnings/Precautions Use with caution in patients with severe anemia, G6PD, methemoglobin reductase or hemoglobin M deficiency; hypersensitivity to other sulfonamides; aplastic anemia, agranulocytosis and other severe blood dyscrasias have resulted in death; monitor carefully; treat severe anemia prior to therapy; serious dermatologic reactions (including toxic epidermal necrolysis) are rare but potential occurrences; sulfone reactions may also occur as potentially fatal hypersensitivity reactions; these, but not leprosy reactional states, require drug discontinuation; dapsone is carcinogenic in small animals. Safety and efficacy of topical dapsone has not been adequately evaluated in patient with G6PD deficiency or in patients <12 years of age.

Adverse Reactions

>10%: Hematologic: Hemolysis (dose-related; seen in patients with and without G6PD deficiency), hemoglobin decrease (1-2 g/dL — almost all patients), reticulocyte increase (2% to 12%), methemoglobinemia, red cell life span shortened

Frequency not defined.

- Cardiovascular: Tachycardia
- Central nervous system: Fever, headache, insomnia, psychosis, tonic-clonic movement (topical), vertigo
- Dermatologic: Bullous and exfoliative dermatitis, erythema nodosum, exfoliative dermatitis (oral), morbilliform and scarlatiniform reactions, phototoxicity (oral), Stevens-Johnson syndrome, toxic epidural necrolysis, urticaria
- Endocrine & metabolic: Hypoalbuminemia (without proteinuria), male infertility
- Gastrointestinal: Abdominal pain (oral, topical), nausea, pancreatitis (oral, topical), vomiting
- Hematologic: Agranulocytosis, anemia, leukopenia, pure red cell aplasia (case report)
- Hepatic: Cholestatic jaundice, hepatitis
- Neuromuscular & skeletal: Drug-induced lupus erythematosus, lower motor neuron toxicity (prolonged therapy), peripheral neuropathy (rare, nonleprosy patients)
- Ocular: Blurred vision
- Otic: Tinnitus
- Renal: Albuminuria, nephrotic syndrome, renal papillary necrosis
- Respiratory: Interstitial pneumonitis, pharyngitis (topical), pulmonary eosinophilia
- Miscellaneous: Infectious mononucleosis-like syndrome (rash, fever, lymphadenopathy, hepatic dysfunction)

Overdosage/Toxicology Symptoms include nausea, vomiting, confusion, hyperexcitability, seizures, cyanosis, hemolysis, methemoglobinemia, sulfhemoglobinemia, metabolic acidosis, hallucinations, and hepatitis. Following decontamination, methylene blue 1-2 mg/kg I.V. is the treatment of choice if MHb level is >15%; may repeat every 6-8 hours for 2-3 days if needed. If hemolysis is present, give I.V. fluids and alkalinize urine to prevent acute tubular necrosis.

Drug Interactions

Cytochrome P450 Effect: Substrate of CYP2C8/9 (minor), 2C19 (minor), 2E1 (minor), 3A4 (major)

Increased Effect/Toxicity: Folic acid antagonists (methotrexate) may increase the risk of hematologic reactions of dapsone; probenecid decreases dapsone excretion; trimethoprim with dapsone may increase toxic effects of both drugs. CYP3A4 inhibitors may increase the levels/effects of dapsone.

Decreased Effect: CYP3A4 inducers may decrease the levels/effects of dapsone. Didanosine (except enteric coated capsules) may decrease absorption of dapsone.

Ethanol/Nutrition/Herb Interactions Herb/Nutraceutical: St John's wort may decrease dapsone levels.

Stability

Gel: Store at 20°C to 25°C (68°F to 76°F); protect from freezing; protect from light. Keep tube in original box.

Tablet: Store at 20°C to 25°C (68°F to 76°F); protect from light

Mechanism of Action Competitive antagonist of para-aminobenzoic acid (PABA) and prevents normal bacterial utilization of PABA for the synthesis of folic acid

Pharmacodynamics/Kinetics

Absorption:

Oral: Well absorbed

Topical: ~1% of the absorption of 100 mg tablet

Distribution: V_d: 1.5 L/kg; throughout total body water and present in all tissues, especially liver and kidney

Metabolism: Hepatic; forms metabolite

Half-life elimination: 30 hours (range: 10-50 hours)

Excretion: Urine (~85%)

Dosage Oral:

Leprosy:

Children: 1-2 mg/kg/24 hours, up to a maximum of 100 mg/day

Adults: 50-100 mg/day for 3-10 years

Dermatitis herpetiformis: Adults: Start at 50 mg/day, increase to 300 mg/day, or higher to achieve full control, reduce dosage to minimum level as soon as possible

Pneumocystis carinii pneumonia (unlabeled use):

Prophylaxis:

Children >1 month: 2 mg/kg/day once daily (maximum dose: 100 mg/day) or 4 mg/kg/dose once weekly (maximum dose: 200 mg)

Adults: 100 mg/day

Treatment: Adults: 100 mg/day in combination with trimethoprim (15-20 mg/kg/day) for 21 days

Topical: Acne vulgaris: Children ≥12 years and Adults: Apply pea-sized amount twice daily

Dosing in renal impairment: No specific guidelines are available

Dietary Considerations Do not administer with antacids, alkaline foods, or drugs.

Administration

Oral: May give with meals if GI upset occurs.

Topical: Apply to clean, dry skin; rub in completely. Wash hands after application.

Monitoring Parameters Check G6PD levels prior to initiation

Oral: Monitor patients for signs of jaundice and hemolysis; CBC weekly for first month, monthly for 6 months and semiannually thereafter.

Topical: For patients at risk of anemia, monitor with CBC, reticulocyte counts at baseline and routinely thereafter.

Patient Information Frequent blood tests are required during early therapy. Discontinue if rash develops and report persistent sore throat, fever, malaise, or fatigue. May cause photosensitivity.

Dosage Forms

Gel, topical (Aczone™): 5% (30 g)

Tablet: 25 mg, 100 mg

Extemporaneous Preparations One report indicated that dapsone may not be well absorbed when administered to children as suspensions made from pulverized tablets

Mirochnick M, Clarke D, Brenn A, et al, "Low Serum Dapsone Concentrations in Children Receiving an Extemporaneously Prepared Oral Formulation," [Abstract Th B 365], APS-SPR, Baltimore, MD: 1992.

Jacobus Pharmaceutical Company (609) 921-7447 makes a 2 mg/mL proprietary liquid formulation available under an IND for the prophylaxis of *Pneumocystis carinii* pneumonia

Selected Readings

El-Sadr WM, Murphy RL, Yurik TM, et al, "Atovaquone Compared With Dapsone for the Prevention of *Pneumocystis carinii* in Patients With HIV Infection Who Cannot Tolerate Trimethoprim, Sulfonamides, or Both," *N Engl J Med*, 1998, 339(26):1889-95.

Medina I, Mills J, Leoung G, et al, "Oral Therapy for *Pneumocystis carinii* Pneumonia in the Acquired Immunodeficiency Syndrome. A Controlled Trial of Trimethoprim-Sulfamethoxazole Versus Trimethoprim-Dapsone," *N Engl J Med*, 1990, 323(12):776-82.

Daptacel® *see* Diphtheria, Tetanus Toxoids, and Acellular Pertussis Vaccine *on page 782*

Daptomycin (DAP toe mye sin)

Related Information

Antimicrobial Activity Against Selected Organisms *on page 1165*

U.S. Brand Names Cubicin™

Synonyms Cidecin; Dapcin; LY146032

Generic Available No

Use Treatment of complicated skin and skin structure infections caused by susceptible aerobic Gram-positive organisms

Unlabeled/Investigational Use Treatment of bacteremia, endocarditis, and other severe infections caused by MRSA or VRE

Drug of Choice or Alternative for

Disease/Syndrome(s):

Osteomyelitis, Diabetic Foot *on page 249*

Organism(s):

Staphylococcus aureus, Methicillin-Resistant *on page 304*

Pregnancy Risk Factor B

Pregnancy Implications Teratogenic effects were not observed in animal studies. There are no adequate and well-controlled studies in pregnant women; use in pregnancy only if clearly needed.

Contraindications Hypersensitivity to daptomycin or any component of the formulation

Warnings/Precautions May be associated with an increased incidence of myopathy; discontinue in patients with signs and symptoms of myopathy in conjunction with an increase in CPK (>5 times ULN or 1000 units/L) or in asymptomatic patients with a CPK ≥10 times ULN. Myopathy may occur more frequently at dose and/or frequency in excess of recommended dosages. Not indicated for the treatment of pneumonia (poor lung penetration). Use caution in patients receiving other drugs associated with myopathy (HMG-CoA reductase inhibitors). Use caution in renal impairment (dosage adjustment required). Superinfection by resistant strains and/or pseudomembranous colitis may be associated with use. Safety and efficacy in pediatric patients have not been established.

Adverse Reactions

1% to 10%:

- Cardiovascular: Hypotension (2%), hypertension (1%)
- Central nervous system: Headache (5%), insomnia (5%), dizziness (2%), fever (2%)
- Dermatologic: Rash (4%), pruritus (3%)
- Gastrointestinal: Constipation (6%), nausea (6%), diarrhea (5%), vomiting (3%), dyspepsia (1%)
- Genitourinary: Urinary tract infection (2%)
- Hematologic: Anemia (2%)
- Hepatic: Transaminases increased (3%)
- Local: Injection site reaction (6%)
- Neuromuscular & skeletal: CPK increased (3%), limb pain (2%), arthralgia (1%)
- Renal: Renal failure (2%)
- Respiratory: Dyspnea (2%)
- Miscellaneous: Infection (fungal, 3%)

<1% (Limited to significant and/or life-threatening): Abdominal distension, asthenia, eczema, eosinophilia, eye irritation, fatigue, flatulence flushing, hypomagnesemia, hypersensitivity, INR increased, LDH increased, jaundice, leukocytosis, muscle cramps, muscle weakness, myalgia, paresthesia, rigors, stomatitis, supraventricular arrhythmia, taste disturbance, thrombocytopenia, thrombocytosis, vertigo

Overdosage/Toxicology Treatment is symptomatic and supportive; hemodialysis removes approximately 15% in 4 hours.

Drug Interactions

Increased Effect/Toxicity: No clinically-significant interactions have been identified. Theoretically, concurrent use of drugs which may cause myopathy may increase the risk of these reactions. Limited clinical studies with HMG-CoA reductase inhibitors have not demonstrated an increase in adverse effects.

Stability Store under refrigeration at 2°C to 8°C (36°F to 46°F). Reconstitute vial with NS (5 mL for 250 mg vial, 10 mL for 500 mg vial). Should be further diluted following reconstitution in an appropriate volume of NS. Reconstituted solution (either in vial or in infusion bag) is stable for a cumulative time of 12 hours at room temperature and 48 hours if refrigerated (2°C to 8°C).

Mechanism of Action Daptomycin binds to components of the cell membrane of susceptible organisms and causes rapid depolarization, inhibiting intracellular synthesis of DNA, RNA, and protein. Daptomycin is bactericidal and bacterial killing is concentration-dependent.

Pharmacodynamics/Kinetics
Distribution: 0.09 L/kg
Protein binding: 92%
Half-life elimination: 8-9 hours (up to 28 hours in renal impairment)
Excretion: Urine (78%; primarily as unchanged drug); feces (6%)

Dosage I.V.: Adults:
Skin and soft tissue: 4 mg/kg once daily for 7-14 days
Bacteremia, endocarditis (unlabeled use): 6 mg/kg once daily
Dosage adjustment in renal impairment: Skin and soft tissue infections: Cl_{cr} <30 mL/minute: 4 mg/kg every 48 hours
Hemodialysis (administer after hemodialysis) and/or CAPD: Dose as in Cl_{cr} <30 mL/minute

Administration Infuse over 30 minutes.

Monitoring Parameters Monitor signs and symptoms of infection. CPK should be monitored at least weekly during therapy.

Reference Range Trough concentrations at steady-state (4 mg/kg once daily): 5.9 mcg/mL

Dosage Forms Injection, powder for reconstitution: 250 mg, 500 mg

Daraprim® *see* Pyrimethamine *on page 1025*
1-Day™ [OTC] *see* Tioconazole *on page 1119*
ddC *see* Zalcitabine *on page 1155*
ddI *see* Didanosine *on page 774*
Deca-Durabolin® (Can) *see* Nandrolone *on page 958*
Decavac™ *see* Diphtheria and Tetanus Toxoid *on page 778*
Declomycin® *see* Demeclocycline *on page 771*
Dehydral® (Can) *see* Methenamine *on page 939*
Delatestryl® *see* Testosterone *on page 1100*

Delavirdine (de la VIR deen)

Related Information
Antiretroviral Agents *on page 1206*
Antiretroviral Therapy for HIV Infection *on page 1219*
Management of Healthcare Worker Exposures to HBV, HCV, and HIV *on page 1227*

U.S. Brand Names Rescriptor®

Canadian Brand Names Rescriptor®

Synonyms U-90152S

Generic Available No

Use Treatment of HIV-1 infection in combination with at least two additional antiretroviral agents

Drug of Choice or Alternative for Organism(s):
Human Immunodeficiency Virus *on page 181*

Pregnancy Risk Factor C

Pregnancy Implications It is not known if delavirdine crosses the human placenta. Delavirdine was shown to be teratogenic in some animal studies. Health professionals are encouraged to contact the antiretroviral pregnancy registry to monitor outcomes of pregnant women exposed to antiretroviral medications (1-800-258-4263 or www.APRegistry.com).

Contraindications Hypersensitivity to delavirdine or any component of the formulation; concurrent use of alprazolam, cisapride, ergot alkaloids, midazolam, pimozide, or triazolam

Warnings/Precautions Avoid use with benzodiazepines, cisapride, clarithromycin, dapsone, enzyme-inducing anticonvulsants (carbamazepine, phenytoin, phenobarbital, rifampin, rifabutin, or St John's wort); may lead to loss of efficacy or development of resistance. Concurrent use of lovastatin or simvastatin should be avoided (use caution with other statins). Use caution with amphetamines, antacids, antiarrhythmics, benzodiazepines (alprazolam, midazolam, and triazolam are contraindicated), clarithromycin, dihydropyridine, calcium channel blockers, dapsone, immunosuppressants, methadone, oral contraceptives, or sildenafil.

Use with caution in patients with hepatic or renal dysfunction; due to rapid emergence of resistance, delavirdine should not be used as monotherapy; cross-resistance may be conferred to other non-nucleoside reverse transcriptase inhibitors, although potential for cross-resistance with protease inhibitors is low. Long-term effects of delavirdine are not known. Safety and efficacy have not been established in children. Rash, which occurs frequently, may require discontinuation of therapy; usually occurs
(Continued)

Delavirdine *(Continued)*

within 1-3 weeks and lasts <2 weeks. Most patients may resume therapy following a treatment interruption.

Adverse Reactions

>10%: Dermatologic: Rash (3.2% required discontinuation)

1% to 10%:

Central nervous system: Headache, fatigue

Dermatologic: Pruritus

Gastrointestinal: Nausea, diarrhea, vomiting

Metabolic: Increased ALT (SGPT), increased AST (SGOT)

<1%: Abnormal coordination, ethanol intolerance, allergic reaction, alopecia, anemia, angioedema, bradycardia, calculi of kidney, chest pain, confusion, dermal leukocytoblastic vasculitis, desquamation, dyspnea, ecchymosis, edema, eosinophilia, epistaxis, erythema multiforme, granulocytosis, hallucination, hematuria, hemospermia, hyperkalemia, hyperuricemia, hypocalcemia, hyponatremia, hypophosphatemia, increased lipase, increased serum alkaline phosphatase, increased serum creatine phosphokinase, increased serum creatinine, kidney pain, malaise, myalgia, neck rigidity, neuropathy, neutropenia, nonspecific hepatitis, nystagmus, palpitation, pancytopenia, paralysis, paranoid symptoms, postural hypotension, proteinuria, Stevens-Johnson syndrome, syncope, tachycardia, thrombocytopenia, vasodilation, vertigo, vesiculobullous rash

Postmarketing and/or case reports: Hepatic failure, hemolytic anemia, rhabdomyolysis, acute renal failure

Overdosage/Toxicology Human reports of overdose with delavirdine are not available. GI decontamination and supportive measures are recommended, dialysis is unlikely to be of benefit in removing the drug since it is extensively metabolized by the liver and is highly protein bound.

Drug Interactions

Cytochrome P450 Effect: Substrate of CYP2D6 (minor), 3A4 (major); **Inhibits** CYP1A2 (weak), 2C8/9 (strong), 2C19 (strong), 2D6 (strong), 3A4 (strong)

Increased Effect/Toxicity: Delavirdine has been reported to increase the serum concentrations of amprenavir, indinavir, nelfinavir, ritonavir, and saquinavir. Dose reduction of indinavir and saquinavir should be considered. Plasma concentrations of delavirdine may be increased by fluoxetine and ketoconazole. Clarithromycin and methadone serum concentrations may be increased by delavirdine.

Delavirdine may increase the levels/effects of CYP2C8/9, 2C19, or 2D6 substrates. Example substrates include amiodarone, amphetamines, selected beta-blockers, citalopram, dextromethorphan, diazepam, fluoxetine, glimepiride, glipizide, lidocaine, methsuximide, nateglinide, nefazodone, paroxetine, phenytoin, pioglitazone, propranolol, risperidone, ritonavir, rosiglitazone, sertraline, thioridazine, tricyclic antidepressants, venlafaxine, and warfarin.

Delavirdine may increase the levels/effects of CYP3A4 substrates. Example substrates include benzodiazepines, calcium channel blockers, cisapride, cyclosporine, mirtazapine, nateglinide, nefazodone, sildenafil (and other PDE-5 inhibitors), tacrolimus, and venlafaxine. Concomitant use with alprazolam, cisapride, ergot alkaloids, midazolam, pimozide, or triazolam is contraindicated. Use with lovastatin or simvastatin is not recommended.

Decreased Effect: Antacids, histamine-2 receptor antagonists, or proton pump inhibitors (omeprazole, lansoprazole) may reduce the absorption of delavirdine. Separate administration of didanosine buffered tablets or antacids and delavirdine by 1 hour. Concomitant use with histamine-2 receptor antagonists, omeprazole, or lansoprazole is not recommended.

Decreased delavirdine concentrations may occur when used with amprenavir and nelfinavir. Delavirdine decreases plasma concentrations of didanosine and didanosine may decrease plasma concentrations of delavirdine. Separate administration of didanosine buffered tablets and delavirdine by 1 hour.

Delavirdine may decrease the levels/effects of CYP2D6 prodrug substrates. Example prodrug substrates include codeine, hydrocodone, oxycodone, and tramadol. CYP3A4 inducers may decrease the levels/effects of delavirdine. Example inducers include aminoglutethimide, carbamazepine, nafcillin, nevirapine, phenobarbital, phenytoin, and rifamycins. Carbamazepine, phenobarbital, phenytoin and rifamycins should not be coadministered with delavirdine. Dexamethasone may decrease the plasma concentrations of delavirdine.

Ethanol/Nutrition/Herb Interactions Herb/Nutraceutical: Delavirdine serum concentration may be decreased by St John's wort; avoid concurrent use.

Mechanism of Action Delavirdine binds directly to reverse transcriptase, blocking RNA-dependent and DNA-dependent DNA polymerase activities

Pharmacodynamics/Kinetics

Absorption: Rapid

Distribution: Low concentration in saliva and semen; CSF 0.4% concurrent plasma concentration
Protein binding: ~98%, primarily albumin
Metabolism: Hepatic via CYP3A4 and 2D6 (**Note:** May reduce CYP3A activity and inhibit its own metabolism.)
Bioavailability: 85%
Half-life elimination: 2-11 hours
Time to peak, plasma: 1 hour
Excretion: Urine (51%, <5% as unchanged drug); feces (44%); nonlinear kinetics exhibited

Dosage Adolescents ≥16 years and Adults: Oral: 400 mg 3 times/day

Dietary Considerations May be taken without regard to food.

Administration Patients with achlorhydria should take the drug with an acidic beverage; antacids and delavirdine should be separated by 1 hour. A dispersion of delavirdine may be prepared by adding four 100 mg tablets to at least 3 oz of water. Allow to stand for a few minutes and stir until uniform dispersion. The 200 mg tablets should be taken intact.

Monitoring Parameters Liver function tests if administered with saquinavir

Patient Information Report rash or symptoms of rash with fever, blistering, oral lesions, conjunctivitis, swelling, or muscle/joint pain. Consult pharmacist or physician prior to taking any other medications (including OTC medications and herbal products) due to the potential for drug interactions.

Additional Information Potential compliance problems, frequency of administration, and adverse effects should be discussed with patients before initiating therapy to help prevent the emergence of resistance.

Dosage Forms Tablet, as mesylate: 100 mg, 200 mg

Extemporaneous Preparations A dispersion of delavirdine may be prepared by adding four 100 mg tablets to at least 3 oz of water; allow to stand for a few minutes and stir until uniform dispersion; drink immediately; rinse glass and mouth following ingestion to ensure total dose administered

Selected Readings

Havlir DV and Lange JM, "New Antiretrovirals and New Combinations," *AIDS*, 1998, 12(Suppl A):S165-74.
Scott LJ and Perry CM, "Delavirdine: A Review of Its Use in HIV Infection," *Drugs*, 2000, 60(6):1411-44.

Delta-9-tetrahydro-cannabinol *see* Dronabinol *on page 791*
Delta-9 THC *see* Dronabinol *on page 791*

Demeclocycline (dem e kloe SYE kleen)

U.S. Brand Names Declomycin®

Canadian Brand Names Declomycin®

Synonyms Demeclocycline Hydrochloride; Demethylchlortetracycline

Generic Available Yes

Use Treatment of susceptible bacterial infections (acne, gonorrhea, pertussis and urinary tract infections) caused by both gram-negative and gram-positive organisms

Unlabeled/Investigational Use Treatment of chronic syndrome of inappropriate secretion of antidiuretic hormone (SIADH)

Pregnancy Risk Factor D

Pregnancy Implications Tetracyclines cross the placenta and enter fetal circulation; may cause permanent discoloration of teeth if used during the last half of pregnancy. Related antibiotics have been associated with mutagenesis, embryotoxicity, and oncogenic activity in animals.

Contraindications Hypersensitivity to demeclocycline, tetracyclines, or any component of the formulation; children <8 years of age; concomitant use with methoxyflurane; pregnancy

Warnings/Precautions Photosensitivity reactions occur frequently with this drug, avoid prolonged exposure to sunlight, do not use tanning equipment. Use of tetracyclines during tooth development may cause permanent discoloration of the teeth and enamel, hypoplasia and retardation of skeletal development and bone growth with risk being the greatest for children <4 years and those receiving high doses; use caution in patients with renal or hepatic impairment (eg, elderly); dosage modification required in patients with renal impairment; may act as an antianabolic agent and increase BUN; pseudotumor cerebri has been reported with tetracycline use (usually resolves with discontinuation); outdated drug can cause nephropathy; superinfection possible

Adverse Reactions Frequency not defined.

Cardiovascular: Pericarditis
Central nervous system: Bulging fontanels (infants), dizziness, headache, pseudotumor cerebri (adults)
(Continued)

Demeclocycline *(Continued)*

Dermatologic: Angioneurotic edema, erythema multiforme, erythematous rash, maculopapular rash, photosensitivity, pigmentation of skin, Stevens-Johnson syndrome (rare), urticaria

Endocrine & metabolic: Discoloration of thyroid gland (brown/black), nephrogenic diabetes insipidus

Gastrointestinal: Anorexia, diarrhea, dysphagia, enterocolitis, esophageal ulcerations, glossitis, nausea, pancreatitis, vomiting

Genitourinary: Balanitis

Hematologic: Eosinophilia, neutropenia, hemolytic anemia, thrombocytopenia

Hepatic: Hepatitis (rare), hepatotoxicity (rare), liver enzymes increased, liver failure (rare)

Neuromuscular & skeletal: Myasthenic syndrome, polyarthralgia, tooth discoloration (children <8 years, rarely in adults)

Ocular: Visual disturbances

Otic: Tinnitus

Renal: Acute renal failure

Respiratory: Pulmonary infiltrates

Miscellaneous: Anaphylaxis, anaphylactoid purpura, lupus-like syndrome, systemic lupus erythematosus exacerbation

Overdosage/Toxicology Treatment is supportive.

Drug Interactions

Increased Effect/Toxicity: Methoxyflurane anesthesia may cause fatal nephrotoxicity; retinoic acid derivatives may increase adverse and toxic effects; warfarin may result in increased anticoagulation; methotrexate levels may be increased

Decreased Effect: Antacid preparations containing calcium, magnesium, aluminum bismuth, or sodium bicarbonate may decrease tetracycline absorption; bile acid sequestrants, quinapril (magnesium-containing formulation), iron, or zinc may also decrease absorption; penicillin decrease therapeutic effect of tetracyclines. Although anecdotal reports suggest oral contraceptive efficacy could be reduced by tetracyclines, this has been refuted by more rigorous scientific and clinical data.

Ethanol/Nutrition/Herb Interactions

Food: Demeclocycline serum levels may be decreased if taken with food.

Herb/Nutraceutical: Avoid dong quai, St John's wort (may also cause photosensitization).

Stability Tetracyclines form toxic products when outdated or when exposed to light, heat, or humidity (Fanconi-like syndrome)

Mechanism of Action Inhibits protein synthesis by binding with the 30S and possibly the 50S ribosomal subunit(s) of susceptible bacteria; may also cause alterations in the cytoplasmic membrane; inhibits the action of ADH in patients with chronic SIADH

Pharmacodynamics/Kinetics

Onset of action: SIADH: Several days

Absorption: ~50% to 80%; reduced by food and dairy products

Protein binding: 41% to 50%

Metabolism: Hepatic (small amounts) to inactive metabolites; undergoes enterohepatic recirculation

Half-life elimination: 10-17 hours

Time to peak, serum: 3-6 hours

Excretion: Urine (42% to 50% as unchanged drug)

Dosage Oral:

Children ≥8 years: 8-12 mg/kg/day divided every 6-12 hours

Adults: 150 mg 4 times/day or 300 mg twice daily

SIADH (unlabeled use): 900-1200 mg/day or 13-15 mg/kg/day divided every 6-8 hours initially, then decrease to 600-900 mg/day

Dosing adjustment/comments in renal/hepatic impairment: Should be avoided in patients with renal/hepatic dysfunction

Dietary Considerations Should be taken 1 hour before or 2 hours after food or milk with plenty of fluid.

Administration Administer 1 hour before or 2 hours after food or milk with plenty of fluid

Monitoring Parameters CBC, renal and hepatic function

Test Interactions May interfere with tests for urinary glucose (false-negative urine glucose using Clinistix®, Tes-Tape®)

Patient Information Avoid prolonged exposure to sunlight or sunlamps; avoid taking antacids before tetracyclines

Dosage Forms Tablet, as hydrochloride: 150 mg, 300 mg

Selected Readings

Smilack JD, Wilson WR, and Cockerill FR 3d, "Tetracyclines, Chloramphenicol, Erythromycin, Clindamycin, and Metronidazole," *Mayo Clin Proc*, 1991, 66(12):1270-80.

Demeclocycline Hydrochloride *see* Demeclocycline *on page 771*
Demethylchlortetracycline *see* Demeclocycline *on page 771*
Denavir® *see* Penciclovir *on page 990*
Depotest® 100 (Can) *see* Testosterone *on page 1100*
Depo®-Testosterone *see* Testosterone *on page 1100*
Dermasept Antifungal [OTC] *see* Tolnaftate *on page 1127*
Dermazene® *see* Iodoquinol and Hydrocortisone *on page 892*
Dermazin™ (Can) *see* Silver Sulfadiazine *on page 1065*
Dermazole (Can) *see* Miconazole *on page 945*
Dexacidin® [DSC] *see* Neomycin, Polymyxin B, and Dexamethasone *on page 965*
Dexacine™ [DSC] *see* Neomycin, Polymyxin B, and Dexamethasone *on page 965*
Dexamethasone and Ciprofloxacin *see* Ciprofloxacin and Dexamethasone *on page 748*
Dexamethasone and Neomycin *see* Neomycin and Dexamethasone *on page 963*
Dexamethasone and Tobramycin *see* Tobramycin and Dexamethasone *on page 1126*
Dexamethasone, Neomycin, and Polymyxin B *see* Neomycin, Polymyxin B, and Dexamethasone *on page 965*
Dexasporin *see* Neomycin, Polymyxin B, and Dexamethasone *on page 965*
DFMO *see* Eflornithine *on page 798*
DHPG Sodium *see* Ganciclovir *on page 834*
Diaminodiphenylsulfone *see* Dapsone *on page 766*

Dicloxacillin (dye kloks a SIL in)

Related Information

Antimicrobial Activity Against Selected Organisms *on page 1165*

Canadian Brand Names Dycill®; Pathocil®

Synonyms Dicloxacillin Sodium

Generic Available Yes

Use Treatment of systemic infections such as pneumonia, skin and soft tissue infections, and osteomyelitis caused by penicillinase-producing staphylococci

Drug of Choice or Alternative for Disease/Syndrome(s):

- Erysipelas *on page 141*
- Furunculosis *on page 151*
- Mastitis *on page 214*
- Osteomyelitis, Diabetic Foot *on page 249*

Pregnancy Risk Factor B

Contraindications Hypersensitivity to dicloxacillin, penicillin, or any component of the formulation

Warnings/Precautions Monitor PT if patient concurrently on warfarin; elimination of drug is slow in neonates; use with caution in patients allergic to cephalosporins

Adverse Reactions

1% to 10%: Gastrointestinal: Nausea, diarrhea, abdominal pain

<1%: Fever, seizure with extremely high doses and/or renal failure, rash (maculopapular to exfoliative), vomiting, pseudomembranous colitis, vaginitis, eosinophilia, leukopenia, neutropenia, thrombocytopenia, agranulocytosis, anemia, hemolytic anemia, prolonged PT, hepatotoxicity, transient elevated LFTs, hematuria, interstitial nephritis, increased BUN/creatinine, serum sickness-like reactions, hypersensitivity

Overdosage/Toxicology Symptoms of penicillin overdose include neuromuscular hypersensitivity (agitation, hallucinations, asterixis, encephalopathy, confusion, seizures) and electrolyte imbalance (with potassium or sodium salts), especially in renal failure. Hemodialysis may be helpful to aid in removal of the drug from the blood, otherwise, most treatment is supportive or symptom-directed.

Drug Interactions

Cytochrome P450 Effect: Induces CYP3A4 (weak)

Increased Effect/Toxicity: Disulfiram, probenecid may increase penicillin levels. Penicillins may increase the exposure to methotrexate during concurrent therapy; monitor.

Decreased Effect: Although anecdotal reports suggest oral contraceptive efficacy could be reduced by penicillins, this has been refuted by more rigorous scientific and clinical data. Decreased effect of (warfarin) anticoagulants.

Ethanol/Nutrition/Herb Interactions Food: Decreases drug absorption rate; decreases drug serum concentration.

Mechanism of Action Inhibits bacterial cell wall synthesis by binding to one or more of the penicillin binding proteins (PBPs); which in turn inhibits the final transpeptidation step of peptidoglycan synthesis in bacterial cell walls, thus inhibiting cell wall

(Continued)

Dicloxacillin *(Continued)*

biosynthesis. Bacteria eventually lyse due to ongoing activity of cell wall autolytic enzymes (autolysins and murein hydrolases) while cell wall assembly is arrested.

Pharmacodynamics/Kinetics

Absorption: 35% to 76%; rate and extent reduced by food

Distribution: Throughout body with highest concentrations in kidney and liver; CSF penetration is low; crosses placenta; enters breast milk

Protein binding: 96%

Half-life elimination: 0.6-0.8 hour; slightly prolonged with renal impairment

Time to peak, serum: 0.5-2 hours

Excretion: Feces; urine (56% to 70% as unchanged drug); prolonged in neonates

Dosage Oral:

Use in newborns not recommended

Children <40 kg: 12.5-25 mg/kg/day divided every 6 hours; doses of 50-100 mg/kg/day in divided doses every 6 hours have been used for therapy of osteomyelitis

Children >40 kg and Adults: 125-250 mg every 6 hours

Dosage adjustment in renal impairment: Not necessary

Hemodialysis: Not dialyzable (0% to 5%); supplemental dosage not necessary

Peritoneal dialysis: Supplemental dosage not necessary

Continuous arteriovenous or venovenous hemofiltration: Supplemental dosage not necessary

Dietary Considerations Administer on an empty stomach 1 hour before or 2 hours after meals. Sodium content of 250 mg capsule: 13 mg (0.6 mEq)

Administration Administer 1 hour before or 2 hours after meals. Administer around-the-clock to promote less variation in peak and trough serum levels.

Monitoring Parameters Monitor prothrombin time if patient concurrently on warfarin; monitor for signs of anaphylaxis during first dose

Test Interactions False-positive urine and serum proteins; false-positive in uric acid, urinary steroids; may interfere with urinary glucose tests using cupric sulfate (Benedict's solution, Clinitest®); may inactivate aminoglycosides *in vitro*

Patient Information Take all medication; take 1 hour before or 2 hours after meals, do not skip doses

Dosage Forms Capsule: 250 mg, 500 mg

Selected Readings

Donowitz GR and Mandell GL, "Beta-Lactam Antibiotics," *N Engl J Med*, 1988, 318(7):419-26 and 318(8):490-500.

Wright AJ, "The Penicillins," *Mayo Clin Proc*, 1999, 74(3):290-307.

Dicloxacillin Sodium *see* Dicloxacillin *on page 773*

Didanosine (dye DAN oh seen)

Related Information

Antiretroviral Agents *on page 1206*

Antiretroviral Therapy for HIV Infection *on page 1219*

Management of Healthcare Worker Exposures to HBV, HCV, and HIV *on page 1227*

U.S. Brand Names Videx®; Videx® EC

Canadian Brand Names Videx®; Videx® EC

Synonyms ddI; Dideoxyinosine

Generic Available Yes: Delayed release capsule

Use Treatment of HIV infection; always to be used in combination with at least two other antiretroviral agents

Drug of Choice or Alternative for Organism(s):

Human Immunodeficiency Virus *on page 181*

Pregnancy Risk Factor B

Pregnancy Implications Cases of fatal and nonfatal lactic acidosis, with or without pancreatitis, have been reported in pregnant women. It is not known if pregnancy itself potentiates this known side effect; however, pregnant women may be at increased risk of lactic acidosis and liver damage. Hepatic enzymes and electrolytes should be monitored frequently during the 3rd trimester of pregnancy. Use during pregnancy only if the potential benefit to the mother outweighs the potential risk of this complication. Didanosine has been shown to cross the placenta. Pharmacokinetics are not significantly altered during pregnancy; dose adjustments are not needed. The Perinatal HIV Guidelines Working Group considers didanosine to be an alternative NRTI in dual nucleoside combination regimens; use with stavudine only if no other alternatives are available. Health professionals are encouraged to contact the antiretroviral pregnancy registry to monitor outcomes of pregnant women exposed to antiretroviral medications (1-800-258-4263 or www.APRegistry.com).

Contraindications Hypersensitivity to didanosine or any component of the formulation

Warnings/Precautions Pancreatitis (sometimes fatal) has been reported, incidence is dose related. Risk factors for developing pancreatitis include a previous history of the condition, concurrent cytomegalovirus or *Mycobacterium avium-intracellulare* infection, and concomitant use of stavudine, pentamidine, or co-trimoxazole. Discontinue didanosine if clinical signs of pancreatitis occur. Lactic acidosis, symptomatic hyperlactatemia, and severe hepatomegaly with steatosis (sometimes fatal) have occurred with antiretroviral nucleoside analogues, including didanosine. Hepatotoxicity may occur even in the absence of marked transaminase elevations; suspend therapy in any patient developing clinical/laboratory findings which suggest hepatotoxicity. Pregnant women may be at increased risk of lactic acidosis and liver damage.

Peripheral neuropathy occurs in ~20% of patients receiving the drug. Retinal changes (including retinal depigmentation) and optic neuritis have been reported in adults and children using didanosine. Patients should undergo retinal examination every 6-12 months. Use with caution in patients with decreased renal or hepatic function, phenylketonuria, sodium-restricted diets, or with edema, CHF, or hyperuricemia. Twice-daily dosing is the preferred dosing frequency for didanosine tablets. Didanosine delayed release capsules are indicated for once-daily use.

Adverse Reactions As reported in monotherapy studies; risk of toxicity may increase when combined with other agents.

>10%:

- Gastrointestinal: Increased amylase (15% to 17%), abdominal pain (7% to 13%), diarrhea (19% to 28%)
- Neuromuscular & skeletal: Peripheral neuropathy (17% to 20%)

1% to 10%:

- Dermatologic: Rash, pruritus
- Endocrine & metabolic: Increased uric acid
- Gastrointestinal: Pancreatitis; patients >65 years of age had a higher frequency of pancreatitis than younger patients
- Hepatic: Increased SGOT, increased SGPT, increased alkaline phosphatase

Postmarketing reports: Alopecia, anaphylactoid reaction, anemia, anorexia, arthralgia, chills/fever, diabetes mellitus, dyspepsia, flatulence, granulocytopenia, hepatitis, hyperlactatemia (symptomatic), hypersensitivity, lactic acidosis/hepatomegaly, leukopenia, liver failure, myalgia, myopathy, neuritis, optic renal impairment, pain, retinal depigmentation, rhabdomyolysis, seizure, thrombocytopenia, weakness

Overdosage/Toxicology Chronic overdose may cause pancreatitis, peripheral neuropathy, diarrhea, hyperuricemia, and hepatic impairment. There is no known antidote for didanosine overdose. Treatment is symptomatic.

Drug Interactions

Increased Effect/Toxicity: Concomitant administration of other drugs which have the potential to cause peripheral neuropathy or pancreatitis may increase the risk of these toxicities Allopurinol may increase didanosine concentration; avoid concurrent use. Concomitant use of antacids with buffered tablet or pediatric didanosine solution may potentiate adverse effects of aluminum- or magnesium-containing antacids. Ganciclovir may increase didanosine concentration; monitor. Hydroxyurea may precipitate didanosine-induced pancreatitis if added to therapy; concomitant use is not recommended. Coadministration with ribavirin or tenofovir may increase exposure to didanosine and/or its active metabolite increasing the risk or severity of didanosine toxicities, including pancreatitis, lactic acidosis, and peripheral neuropathy; monitor closely and suspend therapy if signs or symptoms of toxicity are noted. Additionally, concomitant tenofovir administration has been associated with hyperglycemia, decreased CD4 cell counts, and reduced virologic response.

Decreased Effect: Didanosine buffered tablets and pediatric oral solution may decrease absorption of quinolones or tetracyclines (administer 2 hours prior to didanosine buffered formulations). Didanosine should be held during PCP treatment with pentamidine. Didanosine may decrease levels of indinavir. Drugs whose absorption depends on the level of acidity in the stomach such as ketoconazole, itraconazole, and dapsone should be administered at least 2 hours prior to the buffered formulations of didanosine (not affected by delayed release capsules). Methadone may decrease didanosine concentrations.

Ethanol/Nutrition/Herb Interactions

Ethanol: Avoid ethanol (increases risk of pancreatitis).

Food: Decreases AUC and C_{max}. Didanosine serum levels may be decreased by 55% if taken with food.

(Continued)

Didanosine *(Continued)*

Stability Tablets and delayed release capsules should be stored in tightly closed bottles at 15°C to 30°C; tablets undergo rapid degradation when exposed to an acidic environment; tablets dispersed in water are stable for 1 hour at room temperature. Reconstituted pediatric solution is stable for 30 days if refrigerated. Unbuffered powder for oral solution must be reconstituted and mixed with an equal volume of antacid at time of preparation.

Mechanism of Action Didanosine, a purine nucleoside (adenosine) analog and the deamination product of dideoxyadenosine (ddA), inhibits HIV replication *in vitro* in both T cells and monocytes. Didanosine is converted within the cell to the mono-, di-, and triphosphates of ddA. These ddA triphosphates act as substrate and inhibitor of HIV reverse transcriptase substrate and inhibitor of HIV reverse transcriptase thereby blocking viral DNA synthesis and suppressing HIV replication.

Pharmacodynamics/Kinetics

Absorption: Subject to degradation by acidic pH of stomach; some formulations are buffered to resist acidic pH; ≤50% reduction in peak plasma concentration is observed in presence of food. Delayed release capsules contain enteric-coated beadlets which dissolve in the small intestine.

Distribution: V_d: Children: 35.6 L/m²; Adults: 1.08 L/kg

Protein binding: <5%

Metabolism: Has not been evaluated in humans; studies conducted in dogs show extensive metabolism with allantoin, hypoxanthine, xanthine, and uric acid being the major metabolites found in urine

Bioavailability: 42%

Half-life elimination:

- Children and Adolescents: 0.8 hour
- Adults: Normal renal function: 1.5 hours; active metabolite, ddATP, has an intracellular half-life >12 hours *in vitro*; Renal impairment: 2.5-5 hours

Time to peak: Buffered tablets: 0.67 hours; Delayed release capsules: 2 hours

Excretion: Urine (~55% as unchanged drug)

Clearance: Total body: Averages 800 mL/minute

Dosage Treatment of HIV infection: Oral (administer on an empty stomach):

Children:

- 2 weeks to 8 months: 100 mg/m² twice daily is recommended by the manufacturer; 50 mg/m² may be considered in infants 2 weeks to 4 months
- >8 months: 120 mg/m² twice daily; dosing range: 90-150 mg/m² twice daily; patients with CNS disease may require higher dose

Note: At least 2 tablets per dose should be administered for adequate buffering and absorption; tablets should be chewed or dispersed (in 1 ounce of water).

Adolescents and Adults: Dosing based on patient weight:

Note: Preferred dosing frequency is twice daily for didanosine tablets/oral solution

Chewable tablets, powder for oral solution:

- <60 kg: 125 mg twice daily or 250 mg once daily
- ≥60 kg: 200 mg twice daily or 400 mg once daily

Note: Adults should receive 2-4 tablets per dose for adequate buffering and absorption; tablets should be chewed or dispersed (in 1 ounce of water).

Delayed release capsule (Videx® EC):

- <60 kg: 250 mg once daily
- ≥60 kg; 400 mg once daily

Dosing adjustment with tenofovir (didanosine tablets or delayed release capsules; based on tenofovir product labeling):

- <60 kg: 200 mg once daily
- ≥60 kg: 250 mg once daily

Recommended Dose (mg) of Didanosine by Body Weight

Creatinine Clearance (mL/min)	≥60 kg		<60 kg	
	Tablet[1] (mg)	Delayed Release Capsule (mg)	Tablet[1] (mg)	Delayed Release Capsule (mg)
≥60	400 daily or 200 twice daily	400 daily	250 daily or 125 twice daily	250 daily
30-59	200 daily or 100 twice daily	200 daily	150 daily or 75 twice daily	125 daily
10-29	150 daily	125 daily	100 daily	125 daily
<10	100 daily	125 daily	75 daily	See footnote 2.

[1]Chewable/dispersible buffered tablet; 2 tablets must be taken with each dose; different strengths of tablets may be combined to yield the recommended dose.

[2]Not suitable for use in patients <60 kg with Cl_{cr} <10 mL/minute; use alternate formulation.

Dosage adjustment in renal impairment: Dosing based on patient weight, creatinine clearance, and dosage form: See table on previous page.

Patients requiring hemodialysis or CAPD: Dose per Cl_{cr} <10 mL/minute

Hemodialysis: Removed by hemodialysis (40% to 60%)

Dosing adjustment in hepatic impairment: Should be considered; monitor for toxicity

Elderly patients have a higher frequency of pancreatitis (10% versus 5% in younger patients); monitor renal function and dose accordingly

Dietary Considerations

Videx® EC: Take on an empty stomach; administer at least 1 hour before or 2 hours after eating

Chewable/dispersible tablet: Take on an empty stomach, 30 minutes before or 2 hours after eating. Chew well or mix in water; if mixed in water, may add 2 tablespoons (1 oz) apple juice for flavor. Do not use other juices. Each chewable tablet contains 36.5 mg phenylalanine and 8.6 mEq magnesium. Sodium content of buffered tablets: 264.5 mg (11.5 mEq).

Administration

Chewable/dispersible buffered tablets: The 200 mg tablet should only be used in once-daily dosing. At least 2 tablets, but no more than 4 tablets, should be taken together to allow adequate buffering. Tablets may be chewed or dispersed prior to consumption. To disperse, dissolve in 1 oz water, stir until uniform dispersion is formed, and drink immediately. May also add 1 oz of clear apple juice to initial dispersion if additional flavor is needed. The apple juice dilution is stable for 1 hour at room temperature. Do not mix with other juices.

Pediatric powder for oral solution: Prior to dispensing, the powder should be mixed with purified water USP to an initial concentration of 20 mg/mL and then further diluted with an appropriate antacid suspension to a final mixture of 10 mg/mL. Shake well prior to use.

Monitoring Parameters Serum potassium, uric acid, creatinine; hemoglobin, CBC with neutrophil and platelet count, CD4 cells; viral load; liver function tests, amylase; weight gain; perform dilated retinal exam every 6 months

Patient Information Take as directed, 1 hour before or 2 hours after eating. You will be susceptible to infection; avoid crowds. Report numbness or tingling of fingers, toes, or feet; abdominal pain; or persistent nausea or vomiting. Should have a retinal exam every 6-12 months. Chew tablets thoroughly and/or dissolve in water. Pour powder into 4 oz of liquid, stir, and drink immediately; may add 1 oz of apple juice to the water for flavoring (do not mix with other fruit juice or acid-containing liquids). Sustained release capsules should be swallowed whole; do not chew, crush or open the capsule. Shake pediatric oral solution well before use; store in refrigerator; discard after 30 days.

Additional Information A high rate of early virologic nonresponse was observed when didanosine, lamivudine, and tenofovir were used as the initial regimen in treatment-naive patients. Use of this combination is not recommended; patients currently on this regimen should be closely monitored for modification of therapy. Early virologic failure was also observed with tenofovir and didanosine delayed release capsules, plus either efavirenz or nevirapine; use caution in treatment-naive patients with high baseline viral loads.

Dosage Forms

Capsule, delayed release: 200 mg, 250 mg, 400 mg

Videx® EC: 125 mg, 200 mg, 250 mg, 400 mg

Powder for oral solution, pediatric (Videx®): 2 g, 4 g [makes 10 mg/mL solution after final mixing]

Tablet, buffered, chewable/dispersible (Videx®): 25 mg, 50 mg, 100 mg, 150 mg, 200 mg [all strengths contain phenylalanine 36.5 mg/tablet; orange flavor]

Selected Readings

Hirsch MS and D'Aquila RT, "Therapy for Human Immunodeficiency Virus Infection," *N Engl J Med*, 1993, 328(23):1686-95.

Perry CM and Balfour JA, "Didanosine. An Update on Its Antiviral Activity, Pharmacokinetic Properties, and Therapeutic Efficacy in the Management of HIV Disease," *Drugs*, 1996, 52(6):928-62.

Rathbun RC and Martin ES 3d, "Didanosine Therapy in Patients Intolerant of or Failing Zidovudine Therapy," *Ann Pharmacother*, 1992, 26(11):1347-51.

Sande MA, Carpenter CC, Cobbs CG, et al, "Antiretroviral Therapy for Adult HIV-Infected Patients," *JAMA*, 1993, 270(21):2583-9.

Dideoxycytidine *see* Zalcitabine *on page 1155*

Dideoxyinosine *see* Didanosine *on page 774*

Diflucan® *see* Fluconazole *on page 819*

Diiodohydroxyquin *see* Iodoquinol *on page 891*

Diloxanide Furoate (dye LOKS ah nide FYOOR oh ate)

U.S. Brand Names Furamide®

Generic Available No

Use Treatment of amebiasis (asymptomatic cyst passers)

Drug of Choice or Alternative for

Disease/Syndrome(s):

Liver Abscess *on page 211*

Organism(s):

Entamoeba histolytica on page 130

Restrictions Not commercially available in U.S.

Additional Information Not commercially available in U.S.; available from:

The Centers for Disease Control Drug and Immunobiologic Service
1600 Clifton Road
Building 1 Room 1259
Atlanta, GA 30333
Monday-Friday 8 AM to 4:30 PM: (404) 639-3670
Nonbusiness hours (emergencies only): (404) 639-2888

Selected Readings

"Drugs for Parasitic Infections," *Med Lett Drugs Ther*, 1998, 40(1017):1-12.

Diochloram® (Can) *see* Chloramphenicol *on page 733*
Diodoquin® (Can) *see* Iodoquinol *on page 891*
Diogent® (Can) *see* Gentamicin *on page 841*
Diomycin® (Can) *see* Erythromycin *on page 807*
Dioptimyd® (Can) *see* Sulfacetamide and Prednisolone *on page 1082*
Dioptrol® (Can) *see* Neomycin, Polymyxin B, and Dexamethasone *on page 965*
Diosulf™ (Can) *see* Sulfacetamide *on page 1081*
Diotame® [OTC] *see* Bismuth *on page 686*

Diphtheria and Tetanus Toxoid

(dif THEER ee a & TET a nus TOKS oyd)

U.S. Brand Names Decavac™

Synonyms DT; Td; Tetanus and Diphtheria Toxoid

Generic Available No

Use

Diphtheria and tetanus toxoids adsorbed for pediatric use (DT): Infants and children through 6 years of age: Active immunity against diphtheria and tetanus when pertussis vaccine is contraindicated

Tetanus and diphtheria toxoids adsorbed for adult use (Td) (Decavac™): Children ≥7 years of age and Adults: Active immunity against diphtheria and tetanus; tetanus prophylaxis in wound management

Drug of Choice or Alternative for

Organism(s):

Corynebacterium diphtheriae on page 96

Pregnancy Risk Factor C

Pregnancy Implications The Advisory Committee on Immunization Practices (ACIP) recommends booster injections for previously vaccinated pregnant women who have not had Td vaccination within the past 10 years. Pregnant women who are not immunized or are only partially immunized should complete the primary series.

Contraindications Hypersensitivity to diphtheria, tetanus toxoid, or any component of the formulation

Warnings/Precautions Do not confuse pediatric diphtheria and tetanus (DT) with adult tetanus and diphtheria (Td). Immediate treatment for anaphylactic/anaphylactoid reaction should be available during administration. Patients with a history of severe local reaction (Arthus-type) or temperature of >39.4°C (103°F) following a previous dose should not be given further routine or emergency doses of Td more frequently than every 10 years. Continue use with caution if Guillain-Barré syndrome occurs within 6 weeks of prior tetanus toxoid. For I.M. administration; use caution with history of bleeding disorders or anticoagulant therapy. Defer administration during moderate or severe illness (with or without fever) or during outbreaks of poliomyelitis. Immune response may be decreased in immunocompromised patients. Safety and efficacy of DT have not been established in children <6 weeks of age; Td should be administered to children ≥7 years of age and adults.

Adverse Reactions All serious adverse reactions must be reported to the U.S. Department of Health and Human Services (DHHS) Vaccine Adverse Event Reporting System (VAERS) 1-800-822-7967.

>10%: Local: Injection site (adolescents and adults): Pain (81% to 85%), redness (5% to 21%), swelling (10% to 16%)

Frequency not defined; reactions reported with adult and pediatric preparations
- Cardiovascular: EEG disturbances
- Central nervous system: Brachial neuritis, Guillain-Barré syndrome, dizziness, paresthesia, seizure
- Dermatologic: Rash
- Gastrointestinal: Nausea, vomiting
- Local: Injection site: Persistent nodules; local reactions (erythema, cellulitis, swelling)
- Neuromuscular & skeletal: Arthralgia, myalgia
- Miscellaneous: Allergic/anaphylactic reactions, Arthus-type hypersensitivity reaction (severe local reaction starting 2-8 hours after injection)

Note: Other neurological conditions reported in temporal association with vaccine administration have not been demonstrated to be causally related to the vaccine. These have included demyelinating CNS diseases, mononeuropathies, and encephalopathy.

Drug Interactions

Decreased Effect: The effect of the vaccine may be decreased by immunosuppressant medications or therapies (antimetabolites, alkylating agents, cytotoxic drugs, corticosteroids, irradiation); consider deferring vaccination for 3 months after immunosuppressant therapy is discontinued

Stability Store at 2°C to 8°C (35°F to 46°F); do not freeze; discard if product has been frozen

Dosage I.M.:

Infants and Children ≤6 years (DT): Primary immunization:
- 6 weeks to 1 year: Three 0.5 mL doses at least 4 weeks apart; administer a reinforcing dose 6-12 months after the third injection
- 1-6 years: Two 0.5 mL doses at least 4 weeks apart; reinforcing dose 6-12 months after second injection; if final dose is given after seventh birthday, use adult preparation
- 4-6 years (booster immunization): 0.5 mL; not necessary if the fourth dose was given after fourth birthday; routinely administer booster doses at 10-year intervals with the adult preparation

Children ≥7 years and Adults:
- Primary immunization: Patients previously not immunized should receive 2 primary doses of 0.5 mL each, given at an interval of 4-6 weeks; third (reinforcing) dose of 0.5 mL 6-12 months later
- Booster immunization: 0.5 mL every 10 years; to be given to children 11-12 years of age if at least 5 years have elapsed since last dose of toxoid containing vaccine. Subsequent routine doses are not recommended more often than every 10 years.
- Tetanus prophylaxis in wound management; use of tetanus toxoid (Td*) and/or tetanus immune globulin (TIG) depends upon the number of prior tetanus toxoid doses and type of wound: See table.

Tetanus Prophylaxis in Wound Management

Number of Prior Tetanus Toxoid Doses	Clean, Minor Wounds		All Other Wounds	
	Td[1]	TIG[2]	Td[1]	TIG[2]
Unknown or <3	Yes	No	Yes	Yes
≥3[3]	No[4]	No	No[5]	No

[1]Adult tetanus and diphtheria toxoids; use pediatric preparations (DT or DTP) if the patient is <7 years old.

[2]Tetanus immune globulin.

[3]If only three doses of fluid tetanus toxoid have been received, a fourth dose of toxoid, preferably an adsorbed toxoid, should be given.

[4]Yes, if >10 years since last dose.

[5]Yes, if >5 years since last dose.

Adapted from Report of the Committee on Infectious Diseases, American Academy of Pediatrics, Elk Grove Village, IL: American Academy of Pediatrics, 1986.

Administration For I.M. administration; prior to use, shake suspension well
- Td: Administer in the deltoid muscle; do not inject in the gluteal area
- DT: Administer in the anterolateral aspect of the thigh or the deltoid muscle; do not inject in the gluteal area

For patients at risk of hemorrhage following intramuscular injection, the ACIP recommends "it should be administered intramuscularly if, in the opinion of the physician familiar with the patients bleeding risk, the vaccine can be administered with reasonable safety by this route. If the patient receives antihemophilia or other similar therapy, intramuscular vaccination can be scheduled shortly after such therapy is

(Continued)

Diphtheria and Tetanus Toxoid *(Continued)*

administered. A fine needle (23 gauge or smaller) can be used for the vaccination and firm pressure applied to the site (without rubbing) for at least 2 minutes. The patient should be instructed concerning the risk of hematoma from the injection."

Patient Information May cause mild fever or soreness, swelling, and redness/knot at the injection site; these problems usually last 1-2 days

Additional Information Pediatric dosage form should only be used in patients ≤6 years of age. Federal law requires that the date of administration, the vaccine manufacturer, lot number of vaccine, and the administering person's name, title, and address be entered into the patient's permanent medical record.

Since protective tetanus and diphtheria antibodies decline with age, only 28% of persons >70 years of age in the U.S. are believed to be immune to tetanus, and most of the tetanus-induced deaths occur in people >60 years of age, it is advisable to offer Td especially to the elderly concurrent with their influenza and other immunization programs if history of vaccination is unclear; boosters should be given at 10-year intervals; earlier for wounds

DT contains higher proportions of diphtheria toxoid than Td.

Dosage Forms

Injection, suspension, adult: Diphtheria 2 Lf units and tetanus 5 Lf units per 0.5 mL (5 mL)

Decavac™: Diphtheria 2 Lf units and tetanus 5 Lf units per 0.5 mL (0.5 mL) [latex free prefilled syringe; contains thimerosal]

Injection, suspension, pediatric [preservative free]: Diphtheria 6.7 Lf units and tetanus 5 Lf units per 0.5 mL (0.5 mL)

Diphtheria and Tetanus Toxoids and Acellular Pertussis Adsorbed, Hepatitis B (Recombinant) and Inactivated Poliovirus Vaccine Combined *see* Diphtheria, Tetanus Toxoids, Acellular Pertussis, Hepatitis B (Recombinant), and Poliovirus (Inactivated) Vaccine *on page 780*

Diphtheria Antitoxin (dif THEER ee a an tee TOKS in)

Generic Available No

Use Treatment of diphtheria (neutralizes unbound toxin, available from CDC)

Pregnancy Risk Factor D

Dosage I.M. or slow I.V. infusion: Dosage varies; range: 20,000-120,000 units

Dosage Forms Injection: ≥500 units/mL (40 mL) [20,000 units/vial]

Diphtheria CRM_{197} Protein *see* Pneumococcal Conjugate Vaccine (7-Valent) *on page 1008*

Diphtheria CRM_{197} Protein Conjugate *see Haemophilus* b Conjugate Vaccine *on page 848*

Diphtheria, Tetanus Toxoids, Acellular Pertussis, Hepatitis B (Recombinant), and Poliovirus (Inactivated) Vaccine

(dif THEER ee a, TET a nus TOKS oyds, ay CEL yoo lar per TUS sis, hep a TYE tis bee ree KOM be nant, & POE lee oh VYE rus vak SEEN, in ak ti VAY ted vak SEEN)

U.S. Brand Names Pediarix™

Synonyms Diphtheria and Tetanus Toxoids and Acellular Pertussis Adsorbed, Hepatitis B (Recombinant) and Inactivated Poliovirus Vaccine Combined

Generic Available No

Use Combination vaccine for the active immunization against diphtheria, tetanus, pertussis, hepatitis B virus (all known subtypes), and poliomyelitis (caused by poliovirus types 1, 2, and 3)

Pregnancy Risk Factor C

Pregnancy Implications Reproduction studies have not been conducted; not indicated for women of childbearing age.

Contraindications Hypersensitivity to diphtheria and tetanus toxoids, pertussis, hepatitis B, poliovirus vaccine, yeast, neomycin, polymyxin B, or any component of the vaccine; encephalopathy occurring within 7 days of a previous pertussis vaccine not (not attributable to another identifiable cause); progressive neurologic disorders (including infantile spasms, uncontrolled epilepsy, or progressive encephalopathy)

Warnings/Precautions Immediate treatment for anaphylactic/anaphylactoid reaction should be available during vaccine use. Infants born of HB_sAg-positive mothers should receive monovalent hepatitis B vaccine and hepatitis B immune globulin;

infants born of HB_sAg-unknown mothers should receive monovalent hepatitis B vaccine; use of combination product in these patients to complete the hepatitis B vaccination series has not been studied. Use caution if one or more has occurred following the use of whole-cell DTP or a vaccine containing acellular pertussis: Temperature ≥40.5°C (≥105°F) within 48 hours not due to an identifiable cause; collapse or shock-like state within 48 hours; persistent, inconsolable crying that occurs within 48 hours and lasts ≥3 hours; seizures with or without fever that occur within 3 days. Use caution if Guillain-Barré syndrome occurs within 6 weeks of prior vaccination with tetanus toxoid. Defer administration during moderate or severe illness with or without fever. Antipyretics should be administered at the time of and for 24 hours following vaccination to patients at high risk for seizures. Use caution with bleeding disorders. Not for use as a booster dose following the 3-dose primary series. Safety and efficacy have not been established for use in children <6 weeks or adults and children ≥7 years of age.

Adverse Reactions All serious adverse reactions must be reported to the U.S. Department of Health and Human Services (DHHS) Vaccine Adverse Event Reporting System (VAERS) 1-800-822-7967.

As reported in a U.S. lot Consistency Study:

>10%:

- Central nervous system:
  - Sleeping increased (28% to 47%, grade 3: <1% to 2%)
  - Restlessness (28% to 30%, grade 3: ≤1%)
  - Fever ≥100.4°F (26% to 31%); >103.1°F (<1%); incidence of fever is higher than reported with separately administered vaccines
- Gastrointestinal: Appetite decreased (19% to 22%, grade 3: <1%)
- Local: Injection site:
  - Redness (25% to 36%, >20 mm: ≤1%)
  - Pain (23% to 30%, grade 3: ≤1%)
  - Swelling (15% to 22%; >20 mm: 1%)
- Miscellaneous: Fussiness (57% to 64%; grade 3: 2% to 3%)

Refer to individual product monographs for additional adverse reactions, including postmarketing and case reports.

Drug Interactions

Decreased Effect: Immunosuppressant medications or therapies (antimetabolites, alkylating agents, cytotoxic drugs, corticosteroids, irradiation) may decrease vaccine effectiveness, consider deferring vaccination for 3 months after immunosuppressant therapy is discontinued.

Stability Store under refrigeration at 2°C to 8°C (36°F to 46°F). Do not freeze; discard if frozen.

Mechanism of Action Promotes active immunity to diphtheria, tetanus, pertussis, hepatitis B and poliovirus (types 1, 2 and 3) by inducing production of specific antibodies and antitoxins.

Pharmacodynamics/Kinetics Onset of action: Immune response observed to all components 1 month following the 3-dose series

Dosage I.M.: Children:

Immunization: 0.5 mL; repeat in 6-8 week intervals (preferably 8-week intervals) for a total of 3 doses. Vaccination usually begins at 2 months, but may be started as early as 6 weeks of age.

Use in children previously vaccinated with one or more component, and who are also scheduled to receive all vaccine components:

Hepatitis B vaccine: Infants born of HB_sAg-negative mothers who received 1 dose of hepatitis B vaccine at birth may be given Pediarix™ (safety data limited); use in infants who received more than 1 dose of hepatitis B vaccine has not been studied. Infants who received 1 or more doses of hepatitis B vaccine (recombinant) may be given Pediarix™ to complete the hepatitis B series (safety and efficacy not established).

Diphtheria and tetanus toxoids, and acellular pertussis vaccine (DTaP): Infants previously vaccinated with 1 or 2 doses of Infanrix® may use Pediarix™ to complete the first 3 doses of the series (safety and efficacy not established); use of Pediarix™ to complete DTaP vaccination started with products other than Infanrix® is not recommended.

Inactivated polio vaccine (IPV): Infants previously vaccinated with 1 or 2 doses of IPV may use Pediarix™ to complete the first 3 doses of the series (safety and efficacy not established).

Administration For I.M. use only; do not administer I.V. or SubQ. Shake well prior to use; do not use unless a homogeneous, turbid, white suspension forms. Administer in the anterolateral aspects of the thigh or the deltoid muscle of the upper arm. Do not

(Continued)

Diphtheria, Tetanus Toxoids, Acellular Pertussis, Hepatitis B (Recombinant), and Poliovirus (Inactivated) Vaccine *(Continued)*

inject in the gluteal area (suboptimal hepatitis B immune response) or where there may be a major nerve trunk. Do not administer additional vaccines or immunoglobulins at the same site, or using the same syringe.

For patients at risk of hemorrhage following intramuscular injection, the ACIP recommends "it should be administered intramuscularly if, in the opinion of the physician familiar with the patients bleeding risk, the vaccine can be administered with reasonable safety by this route. If the patient receives antihemophilia or other similar therapy, intramuscular vaccination can be scheduled shortly after such therapy is administered. A fine needle (23 gauge or smaller) can be used for the vaccination and firm pressure applied to the site (without rubbing) for at least 2 minutes. The patient should be instructed concerning the risk of hematoma from the injection."

Federal law requires that the date of administration, name of the vaccine manufacturer, lot number of vaccine, and the administering person's name, title, and address be entered into the patient's permanent medical record.

Patient Information Mild reactions include redness or soreness at the injection site, fever, fussiness, decreased appetite, or feeling tired. Contact prescriber for any of the following less common reactions: Fever of 101.3°F or higher, seizures, or if your child becomes limp, pale, or less alert. It is important that each child receive all the recommended doses in the series in order to be fully immunized. This vaccine is not used in adults or children ≥7 years or <6 weeks of age.

Additional Information Contains the following three pertussis antigens: inactivated pertussis toxin (PT), filamentous hemagglutinin (FHA) and pertactin. Contains the same diphtheria and tetanus toxoids and pertussis antigens found in Infanrix®. Contains the same hepatitis B surface antigen (HB_sAg) found in Engerix-B® (recombinant vaccine). Thimerosal is used during manufacturing, but removed to less than detectable levels in the final suspension.

Dosage Forms Injection, suspension [single-dose]: Diphtheria toxoid 25 Lf, tetanus toxoid 10 Lf, inactivated PT 25 mcg, FHA 25 mcg, pertactin 8 mcg, HB_sAg 10 mcg, poliovirus type 1 40 DU, poliovirus type 2 8 DU, and poliovirus type 3 32 DU per 0.5 mL [contains neomycin sulfate ≤0.05 ng/0.5 mL, polymyxin B ≤0.01 ng/0.5 mL, and yeast protein ≤5%; packaged in vials or prefilled syringes; the needleless prefilled syringes contain dry natural latex rubber in the tip cap and plunger]

Diphtheria, Tetanus Toxoids, and Acellular Pertussis Vaccine

(dif THEER ee a, TET a nus TOKS oyds & ay CEL yoo lar per TUS sis vak SEEN)

Related Information

Immunization Recommendations *on page 1249*

U.S. Brand Names Adacel™; Boostrix®; Daptacel®; Infanrix®; Tripedia®

Canadian Brand Names Adacel™

Synonyms DTaP; dTpa; Tdap; Tetanus Toxoid, Reduced Diphtheria Toxoid, and Acellular Pertussis, Adsorbed

Generic Available No

Use

Daptacel®, Infanrix®, Tripedia® (DTaP): Active immunization against diphtheria, tetanus, and pertussis from age 6 weeks through seventh birthday

Adacel™, Boostrix® (Tdap): Active booster immunization against diphtheria, tetanus, and pertussis

Drug of Choice or Alternative for Organism(s):

Bordetella pertussis on page 53
Corynebacterium diphtheriae on page 96

Pregnancy Risk Factor C

Pregnancy Implications

Animal reproduction studies have not been conducted. It is not known whether the vaccine can cause fetal harm when administered to a pregnant woman or can affect reproductive capacity. Daptacel®, Infanrix®, and Tripedia® are not recommended for use in a pregnant woman or any patient ≥7 years of age. A pregnancy registry has been established for women who may become exposed to Boostrix® (888-825-5249) or Adacel™ (800-822-2463) while pregnant.

Contraindications Hypersensitivity to diphtheria, tetanus toxoids, pertussis, or any component of the formulation; history of any of the following effects from previous administration of pertussis-containing vaccine — progressive neurologic disorder,

including infantile spasms, uncontrolled epilepsy or progressive epilepsy (postpone until condition stabilized); encephalopathy occurring within 7 days of administration and not attributable to another cause

Warnings/Precautions Defer administration during moderate or severe illness (with or without fever). Carefully consider use in patients with history of any of the following effects from previous administration of whole-cell DTP or acellular pertussis vaccine: Fever ≥105°F (40.5°C) within 48 hours of unknown cause; convulsions with or without fever occurring within 3 days; persistent, inconsolable crying episodes lasting ≥3 hours and occurring within 48 hours; shock or collapse within 48 hours. Carefully consider use in patients with history of Guillain-Barré syndrome occurring within 6 weeks of a vaccine containing tetanus toxoid. Td or Tdap vaccines and emergency doses of Td vaccine should not be given more frequently than every 10 years in patients who have experienced a serious Arthus-type hypersensitivity reaction following a prior use of tetanus toxoid.

Use caution in children with coagulation disorders (including thrombocytopenia) where intramuscular injections should not be used. Patients who are immunocompromised may have reduced response; may be used in patients with HIV infection. Defer immunization during outbreaks of poliomyelitis. Use caution in patients with history of seizure disorder, progressive neurologic disease, or conditions predisposing to seizures; ACIP and APP guidelines recommend deferring immunization until health status can be assessed and condition stabilized. Products may contain thimerosal; packaging may contain natural latex rubber. Immediate treatment for anaphylactic/anaphylactoid reaction should be available during vaccine use.

Adacel™ is formulated with the same antigens found in Daptacel® but with reduced quantities of tetanus and pertussis. Safety and efficacy have not been established in children <11 years or adults ≥65 years of age. Boostrix® is formulated with the same antigens found in Infanrix®, but in reduced quantities. Safety and efficacy have not been established in patients <7 years or >18 years of age. Use of Adacel™ or Boostrix® in the primary immunization series or to complete the primary series has not been evaluated.

Daptacel®, Infanrix®, Tripedia®: Safety and efficacy in children <6 weeks of age or ≥7 years of age have not been established.

Adverse Reactions All serious adverse reactions must be reported to the U.S. Department of Health and Human Services (DHHS) Vaccine Adverse Event Reporting System (VAERS) 1-800-822-7967.

Daptacel®, Infanrix®, Tripedia® (incidence of erythema, swelling, and fever increases with successive doses):

Frequency not defined:

Central nervous system: Drowsiness, fever

Gastrointestinal: Appetite decreased, vomiting

Local: Pain, redness, swelling

Miscellaneous: Prolonged or persistent crying, refusal to play

Postmarketing and/or case reports: Anaphylactic reactions, cellulitis, crying, cyanosis, diarrhea, ear pain, encephalopathy, erythema, hypersensitivity, hypotonia, hypotonic-hyporesponsive episode, idiopathic thrombocytopenic purpura, injection site reaction, intussusception, irritability, limb swelling, lymphadenopathy, pruritus, rash, respiratory tract infection, seizure, somnolence, sudden infant death syndrome, thrombocytopenia, urticaria

Adacel™, Boostrix®: Note: Ranges presented, actual percent varies by product and age group

>10%:

Central nervous system: Fatigue, tiredness (24% to 37%; grade 3/severe: 1% to 4%), headache (34% to 44%; grade 3/severe: 2% to 4%), chills (8% to 15%; severe: <1%)

Gastrointestinal: Gastrointestinal symptoms, includes abdominal pain, diarrhea, nausea and/or vomiting (3% to 26%; grade 3/severe: ≤3%)

Local: Injection site pain (66% to 78%; grade 3/severe: 1% to 5%), arm circumference increased (28%; >40 mm: 0.5%), redness (21% to 25%; ≥50 mm: 2% to 4%), swelling (21%; ≥50 mm: 3%)

Neuromuscular & skeletal: Body aches/muscle weakness (22% to 30%; severe: 1%), soreness/swollen joints (9% to 11%; severe: <1%)

1% to 10%:

Central nervous system: Fever ≥38°C (≥100.4°F: 1% to 5%)

Dermatologic: Rash (2% to 3%)

Miscellaneous: Lymph node swelling (7%; severe: <1%)

Postmarketing and/or case reports: Arthralgia, back pain, bruising, diabetes mellitus, encephalitis, exanthema, facial palsy, Henoch-Schönlein purpura, injection site

(Continued)

Diphtheria, Tetanus Toxoids, and Acellular Pertussis Vaccine *(Continued)*

reaction (induration, inflammation, mass, nodule, warmth), limb swelling (extensive), lymphadenitis, lymphadenopathy, myalgia, myocarditis, nerve compression, paresthesia, pruritus, seizure, sterile abscess, urticaria

Drug Interactions

Increased Effect/Toxicity: Increased bleeding/bruising with anticoagulants.

Decreased Effect: Vaccine effect may be decreased with corticosteroids and immunosuppressant agents. Consider deferring vaccine for 1 month after agent is discontinued.

Stability Refrigerate at 2°C to 8°C (35°F to 46°F); do not freeze

Mechanism of Action Promotes active immunity to diphtheria, tetanus, and pertussis by inducing production of specific antibodies and antitoxins.

Dosage

Primary immunization:

Children 6 weeks to <7 years: (Daptacel®, Infanrix®, Tripedia®): I.M.: 0.5 mL per dose, total of 5 doses administered as follows:

Three doses, usually given at 2-, 4-, and 6 months of age; may be given as early as 6 weeks of age and repeated every 4-8 weeks; use same product for all 3 doses

Fourth dose: Given at ~15-20 months of age, but at least 6 months after third dose

Fifth dose: Given at 5-6 years of age, prior to starting school or kindergarten; if the fourth dose is given at ≥4 years of age, the fifth dose may be omitted

Booster immunization:

Children 10-18 years (Boostrix®): I.M.: 0.5 mL as a single dose, administered 5 years after last dose of DTwP or DTaP vaccine.

Children ≥11 years and Adults ≤64 years (Adacel™): I.M.: 0.5 mL as a single dose, administered 5 years after last dose of DTwP or DTaP vaccine.

Adacel™ (in patients 11-64 years of age) or Boostrix® (in patients 10-18 years of age) may be used as an alternative to Td vaccine when a tetanus toxoid-containing vaccine is needed for wound management, and in whom the pertussis component is also indicated. Td vaccine is the preferred agent in children ≥7 years and adults.

Administration Shake suspension well.

Adacel™, Boostrix®: Administer only I.M. in deltoid muscle of upper arm.

Daptacel®, Infanrix®, Tripedia®: Administer only I.M. in anterolateral aspect of thigh or deltoid muscle of upper arm.

For patients at risk of hemorrhage following intramuscular injection, the ACIP recommends "it should be administered intramuscularly if, in the opinion of the physician familiar with the patients bleeding risk, the vaccine can be administered with reasonable safety by this route. If the patient receives antihemophilia or other similar therapy, intramuscular vaccination can be scheduled shortly after such therapy is administered. A fine needle (23 gauge or smaller) can be used for the vaccination and firm pressure applied to the site (without rubbing) for at least 2 minutes. The patient should be instructed concerning the risk of hematoma from the injection."

Patient Information A nodule may be palpable at the injection site for a few weeks. Reactions to the vaccine, if seen, usually occur within 3 days. Mild reactions include sore arm or leg, fever, fussiness, decreased appetite, tiredness, or vomiting. Contact prescriber for any of the following less common reactions: Nonstop crying for 3 hours or more, fever of 105°F or higher, seizures, or if your child becomes limp, pale, or less alert. It is important that each child receive all the recommended doses in the series in order to be fully immunized.

Additional Information DTaP may be given for the fourth and fifth doses in children who started immunization with DTP vaccine. In patients who cannot be given pertussis vaccine, DT for pediatric use should be given to complete the series.

TriHIBit® is Tripedia® vaccine used to reconstitute ActHIB® (*Haemophilus* b conjugate) vaccine. The combination can be used for the DTaP dose given at 15-18 months when Tripedia® was used for the initial doses and a primary series of HIB vaccine has been given.

Adacel™ is formulated with the same antigens found in Daptacel® but with reduced quantities of pertussis and tetanus. It is intended for use as a booster dose in children and adults, 11-64 years of age, and **not** for primary immunization.

Boostrix® is formulated with the same antigens found in Infanrix® but in reduced quantities. It is intended for use as a booster dose in children 10-18 years, and is **not** for primary immunization.

Acetaminophen or ibuprofen may reduce or prevent fever; the child's medical record should document that the small risk of postvaccination seizure and the benefits of the pertussis vaccination were discussed with the patient; parents or guardians should be questioned prior to administration of vaccine as to any adverse reactions from previous dose. Provide Vaccine Information Materials, as required by National Childhood Vaccine Injury Act of 1986, prior to immunization.

Federal law requires that the date of administration, the vaccine manufacturer, lot number of vaccine, and the administering person's name, title and address be entered into the patient's permanent medical record.

Dosage Forms

Injection, suspension:

- Adacel™: Diphtheria 2 Lf units, tetanus 5 Lf units, and acellular pertussis 2.5 mcg per 0.5 mL (0.5 mL) [vial stopper is latex free]
- Boostrix®: Diphtheria 2.5 Lf units, tetanus 5 Lf units, and acellular pertussis 8 mcg per 0.5 mL (0.5 mL) [available in vial and prefilled syringe; syringe cap and rubber plunger contain natural latex rubber]
- Daptacel®: Diphtheria 15 Lf units, tetanus 5 Lf units, and acellular pertussis 10 mcg per 0.5 mL (0.5 mL) [vial stopper contains natural latex rubber]
- Infanrix®: Diphtheria 25 Lf units, tetanus 10 Lf units, and acellular pertussis 25 mcg per 0.5 mL (0.5 mL) [available in vial and prefilled syringe; syringe cap and rubber plunger contain natural latex rubber]
- Tripedia®: Diphtheria 6.7 Lf units, tetanus 5 Lf units, and acellular pertussis 46.8 mcg per 0.5 mL (7.5 mL) [contains trace amounts of thimerosal; vial stopper contains natural latex rubber]

Note: Tripedia® vaccine is also used to reconstitute ActHIB® to prepare TriHIBit® vaccine (diphtheria, tetanus toxoids, and acellular pertussis and *Haemophilus influenzae* b conjugate vaccine combination)

Selected Readings

"Use of Diphtheria Toxoid-Tetanus Toxoid-Acellular Pertussis Vaccine as a Five-Dose Series," *MMWR*, 2000, 49(RR-13);1-8.

Diphtheria, Tetanus Toxoids, and Acellular Pertussis Vaccine and *Haemophilus influenzae* b Conjugate Vaccine

(dif THEER ee a, TET a nus TOKS oyds & ay CEL yoo lar per TUS sis vak SEEN & hem OF fi lus in floo EN za bee KON joo gate vak SEEN)

U.S. Brand Names TriHIBit®

Synonyms *Haemophilus influenzae* b Conjugate Vaccine and Diphtheria, Tetanus Toxoids, and Acellular Pertussis Vaccine

Generic Available No

Use Active immunization of children 15-18 months of age for prevention of diphtheria, tetanus, pertussis, and invasive disease caused by *H. influenzae* type b.

Drug of Choice or Alternative for Organism(s):

Bordetella pertussis on page 53
Corynebacterium diphtheriae on page 96

Contraindications Any contraindication of the component vaccines (see individual agents); contraindicated in children <15 months of age

Dosage Children >15 months of age: I.M.: 0.5 mL (as part of a general vaccination schedule; see individual vaccines). Vaccine should be used within 30 minutes of reconstitution.

Administration For patients at risk of hemorrhage following intramuscular injection, the ACIP recommends "it should be administered intramuscularly if, in the opinion of the physician familiar with the patients bleeding risk, the vaccine can be administered with reasonable safety by this route. If the patient receives antihemophilia or other similar therapy, intramuscular vaccination can be scheduled shortly after such therapy is administered. A fine needle (23 gauge or smaller) can be used for the vaccination and firm pressure applied to the site (without rubbing) for at least 2 minutes. The patient should be instructed concerning the risk of hematoma from the injection."

Additional Information TriHIBit® is Tripedia® vaccine used to reconstitute ActHIB® (*Haemophilus* b conjugate) vaccine. The combination can be used for the DTaP dose given at 15-18 months when Tripedia® was used for the initial doses and a primary series of HIB vaccine has been given. Federal law requires that the date of administration, the vaccine manufacturer, lot number of vaccine, and the administering person's name, title and address be entered into the patient's permanent medical record.

(Continued)

Diphtheria, Tetanus Toxoids, and Acellular Pertussis Vaccine and *Haemophilus influenzae* b Conjugate Vaccine *(Continued)*

Dosage Forms Injection, suspension: 5 Lf units tetanus toxoid, 6.7 Lf units diphtheria toxoid, 46.8 mcg pertussis antigens, and 10 mcg *H. influenzae* type b purified capsular polysaccharide per 0.5 mL (0.5 mL) [The combination of Tripedia® vaccine used to reconstitute ActHIB® forms TriHIBit®]

Diphtheria Toxoid Conjugate *see Haemophilus* b Conjugate Vaccine *on page 848*

Dirithromycin (dye RITH roe mye sin)

U.S. Brand Names Dynabac®

Generic Available No

Use Treatment of mild to moderate upper and lower respiratory tract infections due to *Moraxella catarrhalis, Streptococcus pneumoniae, Legionella pneumophila, H. influenzae*, or *S. pyogenes*, ie, acute exacerbation of chronic bronchitis, secondary bacterial infection of acute bronchitis, community-acquired pneumonia, pharyngitis/tonsillitis, and uncomplicated infections of the skin and skin structure due to *Staphylococcus aureus*

Pregnancy Risk Factor C

Pregnancy Implications Animal studies indicate the use of dirithromycin during pregnancy should be avoided if possible.

Contraindications Hypersensitivity to any macrolide or component of dirithromycin; use with pimozide

Warnings/Precautions Pseudomembranous colitis has been reported and should be considered in patients presenting with diarrhea subsequent to therapy with dirithromycin.

Adverse Reactions

1% to 10%:

Central nervous system: Headache, dizziness, vertigo, insomnia
Dermatologic: Rash, pruritus, urticaria
Endocrine & metabolic: Hyperkalemia
Gastrointestinal: Abdominal pain, nausea, diarrhea, vomiting, dyspepsia, flatulence
Hematologic: Thrombocytosis, eosinophilia, segmented neutrophils
Neuromuscular & skeletal: Weakness, pain, increased CPK
Respiratory: Increased cough, dyspnea

<1%: Palpitations, vasodilation, syncope, edema, anxiety, depression, somnolence, fever, malaise, dysmenorrhea, hypochloremia, hypophosphatemia, increased uric acid, dehydration, abnormal stools, anorexia, gastritis, constipation, abnormal taste, xerostomia, abdominal pain, mouth ulceration, polyuria, vaginitis, neutropenia, thrombocytopenia, decreased hemoglobin/hematocrit; increased alkaline phosphatase, bands, basophils; leukocytosis, monocytosis, Increased ALT/AST, GGT; hyperbilirubinemia, paresthesia, tremor, myalgia, amblyopia, tinnitus, increased creatinine, phosphorus, epistaxis, hemoptysis, hyperventilation, hypoalbuminemia, flu-like syndrome, diaphoresis, thirst

Overdosage/Toxicology Symptoms include nausea, vomiting, abdominal pain, and diarrhea. Treatment is supportive. Dialysis has not been found to be effective.

Drug Interactions

Cytochrome P450 Effect: Substrate of CYP3A4 (minor)

Increased Effect/Toxicity: Absorption of dirithromycin is slightly enhanced with concomitant antacids and H_2 antagonists. Dirithromycin may, like erythromycin, increase the effect of alfentanil, anticoagulants, bromocriptine, carbamazepine, cyclosporine, digoxin, disopyramide, ergots, methylprednisolone, cisapride, and triazolam.

Note: Interactions with nonsedating antihistamines (eg, astemizole) or theophylline are not known to occur; however, caution is advised with coadministration.

Mechanism of Action After being converted during intestinal absorption to its active form, erythromycylamine, dirithromycin inhibits protein synthesis by binding to the 50S ribosomal subunits of susceptible microorganisms

Pharmacodynamics/Kinetics

Absorption: Rapid
Distribution: V_d: 800 L; rapidly and widely (higher levels in tissues than plasma)
Protein binding: 14% to 30%
Metabolism: Hydrolyzed to erythromycylamine
Bioavailability: 10%
Half-life elimination: 8 hours (range: 2-36 hours)
Time to peak: 4 hours
Excretion: Feces (81% to 97%)

Dosage Adults: Oral: 500 mg once daily for 5-14 days (14 days required for treatment of community-acquired pneumonia due to *Legionella*, *Mycoplasma*, or *S. pneumoniae*; 10 days is recommended for treatment of *S. pyogenes* pharyngitis/tonsillitis)

Dosing adjustment in renal impairment: None necessary

Dosing adjustment in hepatic impairment: None needed in mild dysfunction; not studied in moderate to severe dysfunction

Dietary Considerations Should be taken with food or within 1 hour of eating. May contain up to 1.6 mg (0.07 mEq) sodium per tablet.

Administration Administer with food or within an hour following a meal. Do not alter (chew or crush) enteric coated dosage form.

Monitoring Parameters Temperature, CBC

Patient Information Take with food or within an hour following a meal; do not cut, chew, or crush tablets; entire course of medication should be taken to ensure eradication of organism

Dosage Forms Tablet, enteric coated: 250 mg

Selected Readings

"Dirithromycin," *Med Lett Drugs Ther*, 1995, 37(962):109-10.

Sharma R and Cramer M, "Focus on Dirithromycin: A New Once Daily Macrolide Antibiotic," *Formulary*, 1995, 30:769-83.

Tartaglione TA, "Therapeutic Options for the Management and Prevention of *Mycobacterium avium* Complex Infection in Patients With the Acquired Immunodeficiency Syndrome," *Pharmacotherapy*, 1996, 16(2):171-82.

Wintermeyer SM, Abdel-Rahman SM, and Nahata MC, "Dirithromycin: A New Macrolide," *Ann Pharmacother*, 1996, 30(10):1141-9.

DisperMox™ *see* Amoxicillin *on page 642*

5071-1DL(6) *see* Megestrol *on page 932*

Docosanol (doe KOE san ole)

U.S. Brand Names Abreva® [OTC]

Synonyms Behenyl Alcohol; *n*-Docosanol

Generic Available No

Use Treatment of herpes simplex of the face or lips

Contraindications Hypersensitivity to docosanol or any component of the formulation

Warnings/Precautions For external use only. Do not apply to inside of mouth or around eyes. Not for use in children <12 years of age.

Adverse Reactions Limited information; headache reported (frequency similar to placebo)

Stability Store at 20°C to 25°C (68°F to 77°F); do not freeze.

Mechanism of Action Prevents viral entry and replication at the cellular level

Dosage Children ≥12 years and Adults: Topical: Apply 5 times/day to affected area of face or lips. Start at first sign of cold sore or fever blister and continue until healed.

Patient Information Wash hands before and after applying cream. Begin treatment at first tingle of cold sore or fever blister. Rub into area gently, but completely. Do not apply directly to inside of mouth or around eyes. Contact prescriber if sore gets worse or does not heal within 10 days. Do not share this product with others, may spread infection.

Dosage Forms Cream: 10% (2 g)

Doryx® *see* Doxycycline *on page 787*

Doxy-100® *see* Doxycycline *on page 787*

Doxycin (Can) *see* Doxycycline *on page 787*

Doxycycline (doks i SYE kleen)

Related Information

Animal and Human Bites *on page 1270*

Community-Acquired Pneumonia in Adults *on page 1278*

Malaria Treatment *on page 1292*

U.S. Brand Names Adoxa™; Doryx®; Doxy-100®; Monodox®; Periostat®; Vibramycin®; Vibra-Tabs®

Canadian Brand Names Apo-Doxy®; Apo-Doxy Tabs®; Doxycin; Doxytec; Novo-Doxylin; Nu-Doxycycline; Periostat®; Vibra-Tabs®

Synonyms Doxycycline Calcium; Doxycycline Hyclate; Doxycycline Monohydrate

Generic Available Yes: Excludes powder for oral solution, syrup

Use Principally in the treatment of infections caused by susceptible *Rickettsia*, *Chlamydia*, and *Mycoplasma*; alternative to mefloquine for malaria prophylaxis; treatment for syphilis, uncomplicated *Neisseria gonorrhoeae*, *Listeria*, *Actinomyces israelii*, and *Clostridium* infections in penicillin-allergic patients; used for community-acquired pneumonia and other common infections due to susceptible organisms; anthrax due to *Bacillus anthracis*, including inhalational anthrax (postexposure); treatment of

(Continued)

Doxycycline *(Continued)*

infections caused by uncommon susceptible gram-negative and gram-positive organisms including *Borrelia recurrentis, Ureaplasma urealyticum, Haemophilus ducreyi, Yersinia pestis, Francisella tularensis, Vibrio cholerae, Campylobacter fetus, Brucella* spp, *Bartonella bacilliformis,* and *Calymmatobacterium granulomatis*

Unlabeled/Investigational Use Sclerosing agent for pleural effusion injection; vancomycin-resistant enterococci (VRE)

Drug of Choice or Alternative for

Disease/Syndrome(s):

Acne Rosacea *on page 26*
Acne Vulgaris *on page 27*
Amnionitis *on page 33*
Bronchitis *on page 60*
Cervicitis *on page 71*
Endometritis *on page 127*
Epididymitis/Orchitis *on page 138*
Impetigo *on page 193*
Pelvic Inflammatory Disease *on page 260*
Pneumonia, Community-Acquired *on page 270*
Prostatitis *on page 277*
Traveler's Diarrhea *on page 333*
Urethritis, Nongonococcal *on page 344*

Organism(s):

Actinomyces Species *on page 27*
Bartonella Species *on page 48*
Borrelia burgdorferi on page 56
Brucella Species *on page 61*
Burkholderia mallei on page 64
Calymmatobacterium granulomatis on page 65
Campylobacter jejuni on page 66
Chlamydia psittaci on page 73
Chlamydophila pneumoniae on page 78
Coxiella burnetii on page 100
Ehrlichia Species *on page 119*
Enterococcus Species *on page 134*
Francisella tularensis on page 149
Leptospira interrogans on page 205
Mycoplasma pneumoniae on page 238
Rickettsia rickettsii on page 289
Staphylococcus aureus, Methicillin-Resistant *on page 304*
Stenotrophomonas maltophilia on page 312
Treponema pallidum on page 334
Ureaplasma urealyticum on page 342
Vibrio cholerae on page 351
Yersinia pestis on page 355

Pregnancy Risk Factor D

Pregnancy Implications Exposure during the last half or pregnancy causes permanent yellow-gray-brown discoloration of the teeth. Tetracyclines also form a complex in bone-forming tissue, leading to a decreased fibula growth rate when given to premature infants.

According to the FDA, the Teratogen Information System concluded that therapeutic doses during pregnancy are unlikely to produce substantial teratogenic risk, but data are insufficient to say that there is no risk. In general, reports of exposure have been limited to short durations of therapy in the first trimester. When considering treatment for life-threatening infection and/or prolonged duration of therapy (such as in anthrax), the potential risk to the fetus must be balanced against the severity of the potential illness.

Contraindications Hypersensitivity to doxycycline, tetracycline or any component of the formulation; children <8 years of age, except in treatment of anthrax (including inhalational anthrax postexposure prophylaxis); severe hepatic dysfunction; pregnancy

Warnings/Precautions Do not use during pregnancy - use of tetracyclines during tooth development may cause permanent discoloration of the teeth and enamel hypoplasia; prolonged use may result in superinfection, including oral or vaginal candidiasis; photosensitivity reaction may occur with this drug; avoid prolonged exposure to sunlight or tanning equipment. Avoid in children ≤8 years of age.

Additional specific warnings for Periostat®: Effectiveness has not been established in patients with coexistent oral candidiasis; use with caution in patients with a history or predisposition to oral candidiasis

Adverse Reactions Frequency not defined.

Cardiovascular: Intracranial hypertension, pericarditis

Dermatologic: Angioneurotic edema, exfoliative dermatitis (rare), photosensitivity, rash, urticaria

Endocrine & metabolic: Brown/black discoloration of thyroid gland (no dysfunction reported)

Gastrointestinal: Anorexia, diarrhea, dysphagia, enterocolitis, esophagitis (rare), esophageal ulcerations (rare), glossitis, inflammatory lesions in anogenital region, tooth discoloration (children)

Hematologic: Eosinophilia, hemolytic anemia, neutropenia, thrombocytopenia

Renal: Increased BUN

Miscellaneous: Anaphylactoid purpura, anaphylaxis, bulging fontanels (infants), SLE exacerbation

Note: Adverse effects in clinical trials with Periostat® occurring at a frequency more than 1% greater than placebo included nausea, dyspepsia, joint pain, diarrhea, menstrual cramp, and pain.

Overdosage/Toxicology Symptoms include nausea, anorexia, and diarrhea. Following GI decontamination, care is supportive only. Fluid support may be required for hypotension.

Drug Interactions

Cytochrome P450 Effect: Substrate of CYP3A4 (major); **Inhibits** CYP3A4 (moderate)

Increased Effect/Toxicity: Increased digoxin toxicity when taken with digoxin. Increased prothrombin time with warfarin. Doxycycline may increase the levels/effects of selected benzodiazepines, calcium channel blockers, cyclosporine, mirtazapine, nateglinide, nefazodone, quinidine, sildenafil (and other PDE-5 inhibitors), tacrolimus, venlafaxine, and other CYP3A4 substrates. Selected benzodiazepines (midazolam, triazolam), cisapride, ergot alkaloids, selected HMG-CoA reductase inhibitors (lovastatin and simvastatin), mesoridazine, pimozide, and thioridazine are generally contraindicated with strong CYP3A4 inhibitors. When used with strong CYP3A4 inhibitors, dosage adjustment/limits are recommended

Decreased Effect: Decreased levels of doxycycline may occur when taken with antacids containing aluminum, calcium, or magnesium. Decreased levels when taken with iron, bismuth subsalicylate, barbiturates, sucralfate, didanosine, and quinapril. Concurrent use of tetracycline and Penthrane® has been reported to result in fatal renal toxicity. Although anecdotal reports suggest oral contraceptive efficacy could be reduced by tetracyclines, this has been refuted by more rigorous scientific and clinical data. The levels/effects of doxycycline may be decreased by include aminoglutethimide, carbamazepine, nafcillin, nevirapine, phenobarbital, phenytoin, rifamycins, and other CYP3A4 inducers.

Ethanol/Nutrition/Herb Interactions

Ethanol: Chronic ethanol ingestion may reduce the serum concentration of doxycycline.

Food: Doxycycline serum levels may be slightly decreased if taken with food or milk. Administration with iron or calcium may decrease doxycycline absorption. May decrease absorption of calcium, iron, magnesium, zinc, and amino acids.

Herb/Nutraceutical: St John's wort may decrease doxycycline levels. Avoid dong quai, St John's wort (may also cause photosensitization).

Stability

Capsules/tablets: Store at controlled room temperature; protect from light

I.V. infusion: Following reconstitution with sterile water for injection, dilute to a final concentration of 0.1-1 mg/mL using a compatible solution. Solutions for I.V. infusion may be prepared using 0.9% sodium chloride, D_5W, Ringer's injection, lactated Ringer's, D_5LR. Protect from light. Stability varies based on solution.

Mechanism of Action Inhibits protein synthesis by binding with the 30S and possibly the 50S ribosomal subunit(s) of susceptible bacteria; may also cause alterations in the cytoplasmic membrane

Periostat® capsules (proposed mechanism): Has been shown to inhibit collagenase activity *in vitro*. Also has been noted to reduce elevated collagenase activity in the gingival crevicular fluid of patients with periodontal disease. Systemic levels do not reach inhibitory concentrations against bacteria.

Pharmacodynamics/Kinetics

Absorption: Oral: Almost complete; reduced by food or milk by 20%

Distribution: Widely into body tissues and fluids including synovial, pleural, prostatic, seminal fluids, and bronchial secretions; saliva, aqueous humor, and CSF penetration is poor; readily crosses placenta; enters breast milk

(Continued)

Doxycycline *(Continued)*

Protein binding: 90%

Metabolism: Not hepatic; partially inactivated in GI tract by chelate formation

Half-life elimination: 12-15 hours (usually increases to 22-24 hours with multiple doses); End-stage renal disease: 18-25 hours

Time to peak, serum: 1.5-4 hours

Excretion: Feces (30%); urine (23%)

Dosage

Children:

Anthrax: Doxycycline should be used in children if antibiotic susceptibility testing, exhaustion of drug supplies, or allergic reaction preclude use of penicillin or ciprofloxacin. For treatment, the consensus recommendation does not include a loading dose for doxycycline.

Inhalational (postexposure prophylaxis) (*MMWR*, 2001, 50:889-893): Oral, I.V. (use oral route when possible):

≤8 years: 2.2 mg/kg every 12 hours for 60 days

>8 years and ≤45 kg: 2.2 mg/kg every 12 hours for 60 days

>8 years and >45 kg: 100 mg every 12 hours for 60 days

Cutaneous (treatment): Oral: See dosing for "Inhalational (postexposure prophylaxis)"

Note: In the presence of systemic involvement, extensive edema, and/or lesions on head/neck, doxycycline should initially be administered I.V.

Inhalational/gastrointestinal/oropharyngeal (treatment): I.V.: Refer to dosing for inhalational anthrax (postexposure prophylaxis); switch to oral therapy when clinically appropriate; refer to Adults dosing for "Note" on combined therapy and duration

Children ≥8 years (<45 kg): Susceptible infections: Oral, I.V.: 2-5 mg/kg/day in 1-2 divided doses, not to exceed 200 mg/day

Children >8 years (>45 kg) and Adults: Susceptible infections: Oral, I.V.: 100-200 mg/day in 1-2 divided doses

Acute gonococcal infection (PID) in combination with another antibiotic: 100 mg every 12 hours until improved, followed by 100 mg orally twice daily to complete 14 days

Community-acquired pneumonia: 100 mg twice daily

Lyme disease: Oral: 100 mg twice daily for 14-21 days

Early syphilis: 200 mg/day in divided doses for 14 days

Late syphilis: 200 mg/day in divided doses for 28 days

Uncomplicated chlamydial infections: 100 mg twice daily for ≥7 days

Endometritis, salpingitis, parametritis, or peritonitis: 100 mg I.V. twice daily with cefoxitin 2 g every 6 hours for 4 days and for ≥48 hours after patient improves; then continue with oral therapy 100 mg twice daily to complete a 10- to 14-day course of therapy

Sclerosing agent for pleural effusion injection (unlabeled use): 500 mg as a single dose in 30-50 mL of NS or SWI

Periodontitis: Oral (Periostat®): 20 mg twice daily as an adjunct following scaling and root planing; may be administered for up to 9 months. Safety beyond 12 months of treatment and efficacy beyond 9 months of treatment have not been established.

Adults:

Anthrax:

Inhalational (postexposure prophylaxis): Oral, I.V. (use oral route when possible): 100 mg every 12 hours for 60 days (*MMWR*, 2001, 50:889-93); **Note:** Preliminary recommendation, FDA review and update is anticipated.

Cutaneous (treatment): Oral: 100 mg every 12 hours for 60 days. **Note:** In the presence of systemic involvement, extensive edema, lesions on head/neck, refer to I.V. dosing for treatment of inhalational/gastrointestinal/oropharyngeal anthrax

Inhalational/gastrointestinal/oropharyngeal (treatment): I.V.: Initial: 100 mg every 12 hours; switch to oral therapy when clinically appropriate; some recommend initial loading dose of 200 mg, followed by 100 mg every 8-12 hours (*JAMA*, 1997, 278:399-411). **Note:** Initial treatment should include two or more agents predicted to be effective (per CDC recommendations). Agents suggested for use in conjunction with doxycycline or ciprofloxacin include rifampin, vancomycin, imipenem, penicillin, ampicillin, chloramphenicol, clindamycin, and clarithromycin. May switch to oral antimicrobial therapy when clinically appropriate. Continue combined therapy for 60 days

Dosing adjustment in renal impairment: No adjustment necessary

Dialysis: Not dialyzable; 0% to 5% by hemo- and peritoneal methods or by continuous arteriovenous or venovenous hemofiltration: No supplemental dosage necessary

Dietary Considerations Take with food if gastric irritation occurs. While administration with food may decrease GI absorption of doxycycline by up to 20%, administration on an empty stomach is not recommended due to GI intolerance. Of currently available tetracyclines, doxycycline has the least affinity for calcium.

Administration Oral: May give with meals to decrease GI upset. Capsule and tablet: Administer with at least 8 ounces of water and have patient sit up for at least 30 minutes after taking to reduce the risk of esophageal irritation and ulceration.

Doryx®: Capsules may be opened and contents sprinkled on applesauce. Applesauce should be swallowed immediately; do not chew. Follow with 8 ounces of water. Applesauce should not be hot and should be soft enough to swallow without chewing.

I.V.: Infuse I.V. doxycycline over 1-4 hours; avoid extravasation

Test Interactions False elevations of urine catecholamine levels; false-negative urine glucose using Clinistix®, Tes-Tape®

Patient Information Avoid unnecessary exposure to sunlight; finish all medication; do not skip doses. Consult prescriber if you are pregnant.

Dosage Forms

Capsule, as hyclate: 50 mg, 100 mg
Vibramycin®: 100 mg
Capsule, as monohydrate (Monodox®): 50 mg, 100 mg
Capsule, coated pellets, as hyclate (Doryx®): 75 mg, 100 mg
Injection, powder for reconstitution, as hyclate (Doxy-100®): 100 mg
Powder for oral suspension, as monohydrate (Vibramycin®): 25 mg/5 mL (60 mL) [raspberry flavor]
Syrup, as calcium (Vibramycin®): 50 mg/5 mL (480 mL) [contains sodium metabisulfite; raspberry-apple flavor]
Tablet, as hyclate: 100 mg
Periostat®: 20 mg
Vibra-Tabs®: 100 mg
Tablet, as monohydrate (Adoxa™): 50 mg, 75 mg, 100 mg

Extemporaneous Preparations If liquid doxycycline is unavailable for the treatment of anthrax, emergency doses may be prepared for children using the tablets.

Crush one 100 mg tablet and grind into a fine powder. Mix with 4 teaspoons of food or drink (lowfat milk, chocolate milk, chocolate pudding, or apple juice). Appropriate dose may be taken from this mixture. Mixture may be stored for up to 24 hours. Dairy mixtures should be refrigerated; apple juice may be stored at room temperature.

U.S. Food and Drug Administration, Center for Drug Evaluation and Research, "How to Prepare Emergency Dosages of Doxycycline at Home for Infants and Children," April 25, 2003, viewable at http://www.fda.gov/cder/drug/infopage/penG_doxy/doxycyclinePeds.htm, last accessed May 8, 2003.

Selected Readings

Joshi N and Miller DQ, "Doxycycline Revisited," *Arch Intern Med*, 1997, 157(13):1421-8.
Pao D, Goh BT, and Bingham JS, "Management Issues in Syphilis," *Drugs*, 2002, 62(10):1447-61.
Smilack JD, Wilson WR, and Cockerill FR 3d, "Tetracyclines, Chloramphenicol, Erythromycin, Clindamycin, and Metronidazole," *Mayo Clin Proc*, 1991, 66(12):1270-80.
US Department of Health and Human Services, "1993 Sexually Transmitted Diseases Treatment Guidelines," *MMWR*, 1993, 42(RR-14).
Wyler DJ, "Malaria: Overview and Update," *Clin Infect Dis*, 1993, 16(4):449-56.

Doxycycline Calcium *see* Doxycycline *on page 787*
Doxycycline Hyclate *see* Doxycycline *on page 787*
Doxycycline Monohydrate *see* Doxycycline *on page 787*
Doxytec (Can) *see* Doxycycline *on page 787*
Dried Smallpox Vaccine *see* Smallpox Vaccine *on page 1066*

Dronabinol (droe NAB i nol)

Related Information

AIDS Wasting Treatment *on page 1205*

U.S. Brand Names Marinol®

Canadian Brand Names Marinol®

Synonyms Delta-9-tetrahydro-cannabinol; Delta-9 THC; Tetrahydrocannabinol; THC

Generic Available No

Use Chemotherapy-associated nausea and vomiting refractory to other antiemetic; AIDS-related anorexia

Unlabeled/Investigational Use

Cancer-related anorexia

Restrictions C-III

Pregnancy Risk Factor C

(Continued)

Dronabinol *(Continued)*

Contraindications Hypersensitivity to dronabinol, cannabinoids, or any component of the formulation, or marijuana; should be avoided in patients with a history of schizophrenia

Warnings/Precautions Use with caution in patients with heart disease, hepatic disease, or seizure disorders. Reduce dosage in patients with severe hepatic impairment. May cause additive CNS effects with sedatives, hypnotics or other psychoactive agents; patients must be cautioned about performing tasks which require mental alertness (eg, operating machinery or driving).

May have potential for abuse; drug is psychoactive substance in marijuana; use caution in patients with a history of substance abuse. May cause withdrawal symptoms upon abrupt discontinuation. Use with caution in patients with mania, depression, or schizophrenia; careful psychiatric monitoring is recommended.

Adverse Reactions

>10%:

Central nervous system: Drowsiness (48%), sedation (53%), confusion (30%), dizziness (21%), detachment, anxiety, difficulty concentrating, mood change

Gastrointestinal: Appetite increased (when used as an antiemetic), xerostomia (38% to 50%)

1% to 10%:

Cardiovascular: Orthostatic hypotension, tachycardia

Central nervous system: Ataxia (4%), depression (7%), headache, vertigo, hallucinations (5%), memory lapse (4%)

Neuromuscular & skeletal: Paresthesia, weakness

<1%: Syncope, nightmares, diarrhea, myalgia, tinnitus, diaphoresis

Overdosage/Toxicology Symptoms of overdose may include tachycardia, hyper- or hypotension, behavioral disturbances, lethargy, panic reactions, seizures or motor incoordination. Benzodiazepines may be helpful for agitative behavior; Trendelenburg position and hydration may be helpful for hypotensive effects. For other manifestations, treatment should be symptom-directed and supportive.

Drug Interactions

Increased Effect/Toxicity: Sedative effects may be additive with CNS depressants (includes barbiturates, narcotic analgesics, and other sedative agents).

Ethanol/Nutrition/Herb Interactions

Ethanol: Avoid ethanol (may increase CNS depression).

Food: Administration with high-lipid meals may increase absorption.

Herb/Nutraceutical: St John's wort may decrease dronabinol levels.

Stability Store under refrigeration (or in a cool environment) between 8°C and 15°C (46°F and 59°F); protect from freezing

Mechanism of Action Unknown, may inhibit endorphins in the emetic center, suppress prostaglandin synthesis, and/or inhibit medullary activity through an unspecified cortical action

Pharmacodynamics/Kinetics

Onset of action: Within 1 hour

Peak effect: 2-4 hours

Duration: 24 hours (appetite stimulation)

Absorption: Oral: 90% to 95%; 10% to 20% of dose gets into systemic circulation

Distribution: V_d: 10 L/kg; dronabinol is highly lipophilic and distributes to adipose tissue

Protein binding: 97% to 99%

Metabolism: Hepatic to at least 50 metabolites, some of which are active; 11-hydroxy-delta-9-tetrahydrocannabinol (11-OH-THC) is the major metabolite; extensive first-pass effect

Half-life elimination: Dronabinol: 25-36 hours (terminal); Dronabinol metabolites: 44-59 hours

Time to peak, serum: 0.5-4 hours

Excretion: Feces (50% as unconjugated metabolites, 5% as unchanged drug); urine (10% to 15% as acid metabolites and conjugates)

Dosage Refer to individual protocols. Oral:

Antiemetic: Children and Adults: 5 mg/m^2 1-3 hours before chemotherapy, then 5 mg/m^2/dose every 2-4 hours after chemotherapy for a total of 4-6 doses/day; increase doses in increments of 2.5 mg/m^2 to a maximum of 15 mg/m^2/dose.

Appetite stimulant: Adults: Initial: 2.5 mg twice daily (before lunch and dinner); titrate up to a maximum of 20 mg/day.

Dietary Considerations

Capsules contain sesame oil.

Monitoring Parameters CNS effects, heart rate, blood pressure, behavioral profile

Reference Range Antinauseant effects: 5-10 ng/mL

Test Interactions Decreased FSH, LH, growth hormone, and testosterone

Patient Information Avoid activities such as driving which require motor coordination, avoid alcohol and other CNS depressants; may impair coordination and judgment

Dosage Forms Capsule, gelatin: 2.5 mg, 5 mg, 10 mg [contains sesame oil]

Selected Readings

Lane M, Smith FE, Sullivan RA, et al, "Dronabinol and Prochlorperazine Alone and in Combination as Antiemetic Agents for Cancer Chemotherapy," *Am J Clin Oncol*, 1990, 13(6):480-4.

Drotrecogin Alfa (dro TRE coe jin AL fa)

U.S. Brand Names Xigris®

Canadian Brand Names Xigris®

Synonyms Activated Protein C, Human, Recombinant; Drotrecogin Alfa, Activated; Protein C (Activated), Human, Recombinant

Generic Available No

Use Reduction of mortality from severe sepsis (associated with organ dysfunction) in adults at high risk of death (eg, APACHE II score ≥25)

Unlabeled/Investigational Use Purpura fulminans

Drug of Choice or Alternative for Disease/Syndrome(s):

Sepsis *on page 295*

Pregnancy Risk Factor C

Contraindications Hypersensitivity to drotrecogin alfa or any component of the formulation; active internal bleeding; recent hemorrhagic stroke (within 3 months); severe head trauma (within 2 months); recent intracranial or intraspinal surgery (within 2 months); intracranial neoplasm or mass lesion; evidence of cerebral herniation; presence of an epidural catheter; trauma with an increased risk of life-threatening bleeding

Warnings/Precautions Increases risk of bleeding; careful evaluation of risks and benefit is required prior to initiation (see Contraindications). Bleeding risk is increased in patients receiving concurrent therapeutic heparin, oral anticoagulants, glycoprotein IIb/IIIa antagonists, platelet aggregation inhibitors, or aspirin at a dosage of >650 mg/day (within 7 days). In addition, an increased bleeding risk is associated with prolonged INR (>3.0), gastrointestinal bleeding (within 6 weeks), decreased platelet count (<30,000/mm^3), thrombolytic therapy (within 3 days), recent ischemic stroke (within 3 months), intracranial AV malformation or aneurysm, known bleeding diathesis, severe hepatic disease (chronic), or other condition where bleeding is a significant hazard or difficult to manage due to its location. Discontinue if significant bleeding occurs (may consider continued use after stabilization). Suspend administration for 2 hours prior to invasive procedures or other procedure with significant bleeding risk; may continue treatment immediately following uncomplicated, minimally-invasive procedures, but delay for 12 hours after major invasive procedures/surgery. During treatment, aPTT cannot be used to assess coagulopathy (PT/INR not affected).

Efficacy not established in adult patients at a low risk of death (APACHE II score <25). Patients with pre-existing nonsepsis-related medical conditions with a poor prognosis (anticipated survival <28 days), patients with acute pancreatitis (no established source of infection), HIV-infected patients with a CD4 count ≤50 cells/mm^3, chronic dialysis patients, pre-existing hypercoagulable conditions, and patients who had received bone marrow, liver, lung, pancreas, or small bowel transplants were excluded from the clinical trial which established benefit. In addition, patients with a high body weight (>135 kg) were not evaluated. Safety and efficacy have not been established in pediatric patients.

Adverse Reactions As with all drugs which may affect hemostasis, bleeding is the major adverse effect associated with drotrecogin alfa. Hemorrhage may occur at virtually any site. Risk is dependent on multiple variables, including the dosage administered, concurrent use of multiple agents which alter hemostasis, and patient predisposition.

>10%:
- Dermatologic: Bruising
- Gastrointestinal: Gastrointestinal bleeding

1% to 10%: Hematologic: Bleeding (serious 2.4% during infusion vs 3.5% during 28-day study period; individual events listed as <1%)

<1%: Gastrointestinal hemorrhage, intrathoracic hemorrhage, retroperitoneal bleeding, genitourinary bleeding, intracranial hemorrhage (0.2%; frequencies up to 2% noted in a previous trial without placebo control), skin/soft tissue bleeding, immune reaction (antibody production)

Overdosage/Toxicology There has been no reported experience with overdose. Hemorrhagic complications are likely consequences of overdose. Treatment is

(Continued)

Drotrecogin Alfa *(Continued)*

supportive including immediate interruption of the infusion and monitoring for hemorrhagic complications. There is no known antidote.

Drug Interactions

Increased Effect/Toxicity: Concurrent use of antiplatelet agents, including aspirin (>650 mg/day, recent use within 7 days), cilostazol, clopidogrel, dipyridamole, ticlopidine, NSAIDs, or glycoprotein IIb/IIIa antagonists (recent use within 7 days) may increase risk of bleeding. Concurrent use of low molecular weight heparins or heparin at therapeutic rates of infusion may increase the risk of bleeding. However, the use of low-dose prophylactic heparin does not appear to affect safety. Recent use of thrombolytic agents (within 3 days) may increase the risk of bleeding. Recent use of warfarin (within 7 days or elevation of INR ≥3) may increase the risk of bleeding. Other drugs which interfere with coagulation may increase risk of bleeding (including antithrombin III, danaparoid, direct thrombin inhibitors)

Ethanol/Nutrition/Herb Interactions Herb/Nutraceutical: Recent use/intake of herbs with anticoagulant or antiplatelet activity (including cat's claw, feverfew, garlic, ginkgo, ginseng, and horse chestnut seed) may increase the risk of bleeding.

Stability Store vials under refrigeration at 2°C to 8°C (36°F to 46°F). Protect from light. Do not freeze. Reconstitute 5 mg vials with 2.5 mL and 20 mg vials with 10 mL sterile water for injection (resultant solution ~2 mg/mL). Must be further diluted (within 3 hours of reconstitution) in 0.9% sodium chloride, typically to a concentration between 100 mcg/mL and 200 mcg/mL when using infusion pump and between 100 mcg/mL and 1000 mcg/mL when infused via syringe pump. Although product information states administration must be completed within 12 hours of preparation, additional studies (data on file, Lilly Research Laboratories) show that the final solution is stable for 14 hours at 15°C to 30°C (59°F to 86°F). If not used immediately, a prepared solution may be stored in the refrigerator for up to 12 hours. The total expiration time (refrigeration and administration) should be ≤24 hours from time of preparation.

Mechanism of Action Inhibits factors Va and VIIIa, limiting thrombotic effects. Additional *in vitro* data suggest inhibition of plasminogen activator inhibitor-1 (PAF-1) resulting in profibrinolytic activity, inhibition of macrophage production of tumor necrosis factor, blocking of leukocyte adhesion, and limitation of thrombin-induced inflammatory responses. Relative contribution of effects on the reduction of mortality from sepsis is not completely understood.

Pharmacodynamics/Kinetics

Duration: Plasma nondetectable within 2 hours of discontinuation

Metabolism: Inactivated by endogenous plasma protease inhibitors; mean clearance: 40 L/hour; increased with severe sepsis (~50%)

Half-life elimination: 1.6 hours

Dosage I.V.:

Children and Adults: Purpura fulminans (unlabeled use): 24 mcg/kg/hour

Adults: Sepsis: 24 mcg/kg/hour for a total of 96 hours; stop infusion **immediately** if clinically-important bleeding is identified

Dosage adjustment in renal impairment: No specific adjustment recommended.

Administration Infuse separately from all other medications. Only dextrose, normal saline, dextrose/saline combinations, and lactated Ringer's solution may be infused through the same line. May administer via infusion pump. Administration of prepared solution must be completed within 12 hours of preparation. Suspend administration for 2 hours prior to invasive procedures or other procedure with significant bleeding risk; may continue treatment immediately following uncomplicated, minimally-invasive procedures, but delay for 12 hours after major invasive procedures/surgery.

Monitoring Parameters Monitor for signs and symptoms of bleeding, hemoglobin/hematocrit, PT/INR, platelet count

Test Interactions May interfere with one-stage coagulation assays based on the aPTT (such as factor VIII, IX, and XI assays).

Additional Information Prepared by recombinant DNA technology in human cell line

Dosage Forms Injection, powder for reconstitution [preservative free]: 5 mg [contains sucrose 31.8 mg], 20 mg [contains sucrose 124.9 mg]

Drotrecogin Alfa, Activated *see* Drotrecogin Alfa *on page 793*

Dryvax® *see* Smallpox Vaccine *on page 1066*

DT *see* Diphtheria and Tetanus Toxoid *on page 778*

DTaP *see* Diphtheria, Tetanus Toxoids, and Acellular Pertussis Vaccine *on page 782*

dTpa *see* Diphtheria, Tetanus Toxoids, and Acellular Pertussis Vaccine *on page 782*

Duac™ *see* Clindamycin and Benzoyl Peroxide *on page 756*

Durabolin® (Can) *see* Nandrolone *on page 958*

Duricef® *see* Cefadroxil *on page 698*

DW286 *see* Gemifloxacin *on page 840*

Dycill® (Can) *see* Dicloxacillin *on page 773*

Dynabac® *see* Dirithromycin *on page 786*

Dynacin® *see* Minocycline *on page 947*

Dyna-Hex® [OTC] *see* Chlorhexidine Gluconate *on page 735*

Econazole (e KONE a zole)

U.S. Brand Names Spectazole®

Canadian Brand Names Ecostatin®; Spectazole™

Synonyms Econazole Nitrate

Generic Available Yes

Use Topical treatment of tinea pedis (athlete's foot), tinea cruris (jock itch), tinea corporis (ringworm), tinea versicolor, and cutaneous candidiasis

Pregnancy Risk Factor C

Pregnancy Implications Do not use during the 1st trimester of pregnancy, unless essential to a patient's welfare; use during the second and third trimesters only if clearly needed

Contraindications Hypersensitivity to econazole or any component of the formulation

Warnings/Precautions Discontinue drug if sensitivity or chemical irritation occurs; not for ophthalmic or intravaginal use

Adverse Reactions

1% to 10%: Genitourinary: Vulvar/vaginal burning

<1% (Limited to important or life-threatening): Vulvar itching, soreness, edema, or discharge; polyuria; burning or itching of penis of sexual partner

Drug Interactions

Cytochrome P450 Effect: Inhibits CYP2E1 (weak)

Mechanism of Action Alters fungal cell wall membrane permeability; may interfere with RNA and protein synthesis, and lipid metabolism

Pharmacodynamics/Kinetics

Absorption: <10%

Metabolism: Hepatic to more than 20 metabolites

Excretion: Urine; feces (<1%)

Dosage Children and Adults: Topical:

Tinea pedis, tinea cruris, tinea corporis, tinea versicolor: Apply sufficient amount to cover affected areas once daily

Cutaneous candidiasis: Apply sufficient quantity twice daily (morning and evening)

Duration of treatment: Candidal infections and tinea cruris, versicolor, and corporis should be treated for 2 weeks and tinea pedis for 1 month; occasionally, longer treatment periods may be required

Administration

Occasionally, longer treatment periods may be required. For external use only. Avoid contact with the eyes.

Patient Information For external use only; avoid eye contact; report if condition worsens or persists, or irritation occurs

Dosage Forms Cream, topical, as nitrate: 1% (15 g, 30 g, 85 g)

Econazole Nitrate *see* Econazole *on page 795*

Ecostatin® (Can) *see* Econazole *on page 795*

E.E.S.® *see* Erythromycin *on page 807*

Efavirenz (e FAV e renz)

Related Information

Antiretroviral Agents *on page 1206*

Antiretroviral Therapy for HIV Infection *on page 1219*

Management of Healthcare Worker Exposures to HBV, HCV, and HIV *on page 1227*

U.S. Brand Names Sustiva®

Canadian Brand Names Sustiva®

Generic Available No

Use Treatment of HIV-1 infections in combination with at least two other antiretroviral agents

Drug of Choice or Alternative for Organism(s):

Human Immunodeficiency Virus *on page 181*

Pregnancy Risk Factor D

Pregnancy Implications Teratogenic effects have been observed in Primates receiving efavirenz. Severe CNS defects have been reported in infants following efavirenz exposure in the first trimester. Pregnancy should be avoided and alternate

(Continued)

Efavirenz *(Continued)*

therapy should be considered in women of childbearing potential. Women of childbearing potential should undergo pregnancy testing prior to initiation of efavirenz. Barrier contraception should be used in combination with other (hormonal) methods of contraception. If therapy with efavirenz is administered during pregnancy, avoid use during the first trimester. Health professionals are encouraged to contact the antiretroviral pregnancy registry to monitor outcomes of pregnant women exposed to antiretroviral medications (1-800-258-4263 or www.APRegistry.com).

Contraindications Clinically-significant hypersensitivity to efavirenz or any component of the formulation; concurrent use of cisapride, midazolam, triazolam, voriconazole, or ergot alkaloids (includes dihydroergotamine, ergotamine, ergonovine, methylergonovine); pregnancy

Warnings/Precautions Do not use as single-agent therapy; avoid pregnancy; women of childbearing potential should undergo pregnancy testing prior to initiation of therapy; use caution with other agents metabolized by cytochrome P450 isoenzyme 3A4 (see Contraindications); use caution with history of mental illness/drug abuse (predisposition to psychological reactions); may cause CNS and psychiatric symptoms, which include impaired concentration, dizziness or drowsiness (avoid potentially hazardous tasks such as driving or operating machinery if these effects are noted); serious psychiatric side effects have been associated with efavirenz, including severe depression, suicide, paranoia, and mania; discontinue if severe rash (involving blistering, desquamation, mucosal involvement or fever) develops. Children are more susceptible to development of rash; prophylactic antihistamines may be used. Caution in patients with known or suspected hepatitis B or C infection (monitoring of liver function is recommended); hepatic impairment. Persistent elevations of serum transaminases >5 times the upper limit of normal should prompt evaluation - benefit of continued therapy should be weighed against possible risk of hepatotoxicity. Concomitant use with St John's wort is not recommended.

Adverse Reactions

>10%:

Central nervous system: Dizziness* (2% to 28%), depression (1% to 16%), insomnia (6% to 16%), anxiety (1% to 11%), pain* (1% to 13%)

Dermatologic: Rash* (NCI grade 1: 9% to 11%, NCI grade 2: 15% to 32%, NCI grade 3 or 4: <1%); 26% experienced new rash vs 17% in control groups; up to 46% of pediatric patients experience rash (median onset: 8 days)

Endocrine & metabolic: HDL increased (25% to 35%), total cholesterol increased (20% to 40%)

Gastrointestinal: Diarrhea* (3% to 14%), nausea* (2% to 12%)

1% to 10%:

Central nervous system: Impaired concentration (2% to 8%), headache* (2% to 7%), somnolence (2% to 7%), fatigue (2% to 7%), abnormal dreams (1% to 6%), nervousness (2% to 6%), severe depression (2%), hallucinations (1%)

Dermatologic: Pruritus (1% to 9%)

Gastrointestinal: Vomiting* (6% to 7%), dyspepsia (3%), abdominal pain (1% to 3%), anorexia (1% to 2%)

Miscellaneous: Diaphoresis increased (1% to 2%)

*Adverse effect reported in ≥10% of patients 3-16 years of age

<1%: Aggressive behavior, manic reaction, rash (NCI grades 3 or 4), paranoid reaction, suicide attempts, suicidal ideation

Postmarketing and/or case reports: Allergic reaction, aggressive reaction, agitation, arthralgia, ataxia, body fat accumulation/redistribution, constipation, convulsions, coordination abnormal, delusions, dyspnea, emotional lability, erythema multiforme, flushing, gynecomastia, hepatitis, hypertriglyceridemia, hypoesthesia, liver failure, liver enzyme elevations, malabsorption, mania, myalgia, myopathy, nail disorder, neuropathy, neurosis, palpitation, paranoia, paresthesia, psychosis, skin discoloration, Stevens-Johnson syndrome, suicide, tinnitus, tremor, visual abnormality, weakness

Overdosage/Toxicology Increased central nervous system symptoms and involuntary muscle contractions have been reported in accidental overdose. Treatment is supportive. Activated charcoal may enhance elimination. Dialysis is unlikely to remove the drug.

Drug Interactions

Cytochrome P450 Effect: Substrate (major) of CYP2B6, 3A4; **Inhibits** CYP2C8/9 (moderate), 2C19 (moderate), 3A4 (moderate); **Induces** CYP2B6 (weak), 3A4 (strong)

Increased Effect/Toxicity: Coadministration with medications metabolized by these enzymes may lead to increased concentration-related effects. Cisapride, midazolam, triazolam, and ergot alkaloids may result in life-threatening toxicities; concurrent use is contraindicated. May increase (or decrease) effect of warfarin.

Decreased Effect: CYP2B6 inducers may decrease the levels/effects of efavirenz; example inducers include carbamazepine, nevirapine, phenobarbital, phenytoin, and rifampin. St John's wort may decrease serum concentrations of efavirenz. Concentrations of atazanavir, indinavir, and/or lopinavir may be reduced; dosage adjustments required. Concentrations of saquinavir may be decreased (use as sole protease inhibitor is not recommended). Serum concentrations of methadone may be decreased; monitor for withdrawal. May decrease (or increase) effect of warfarin. Serum concentrations of sertraline may be decreased by efavirenz. CYP3A4 inducers may decrease the levels/effects of efavirenz; example inducers include aminoglutethimide, carbamazepine, nafcillin, nevirapine, phenobarbital, phenytoin, and rifamycins. Voriconazole serum levels may be reduced by efavirenz (concurrent use is contraindicated).

Efavirenz may increase the levels/effects of CYP2C8/9 substrates; example substrates include fluoxetine, glimepiride, glipizide, nateglinide, phenytoin, pioglitazone, rosiglitazone, sertraline, and warfarin. Efavirenz may increase the levels/effects of CYP2C19 substrates; example substrates include citalopram, diazepam, methsuximide, phenytoin, propranolol, and sertraline. Efavirenz may alter the levels/effects of CYP3A4 substrates; example substrates include benzodiazepines, calcium channel blockers, ergot derivatives, mirtazapine, nateglinide, nefazodone, tacrolimus, and venlafaxine.

Ethanol/Nutrition/Herb Interactions

Ethanol: Avoid ethanol (hepatic and CNS adverse effects).

Food: Avoid high-fat meals (increase the absorption of efavirenz).

Herb/Nutraceutical: St John's wort may decrease efavirenz serum levels. Avoid concurrent use.

Stability Store below 25°C (77°F).

Mechanism of Action As a non-nucleoside reverse transcriptase inhibitor, efavirenz has activity against HIV-1 by binding to reverse transcriptase. It consequently blocks the RNA-dependent and DNA-dependent DNA polymerase activities including HIV-1 replication. It does not require intracellular phosphorylation for antiviral activity.

Pharmacodynamics/Kinetics

Absorption: Increased by fatty meals

Distribution: CSF concentrations exceed free fraction in serum

Protein binding: >99%, primarily to albumin

Metabolism: Hepatic via CYP3A4 and 2B6; may induce its own metabolism

Half-life elimination: Single dose: 52-76 hours; Multiple doses: 40-55 hours

Time to peak: 3-8 hours

Excretion: Feces (16% to 41% primarily as unchanged drug); urine (14% to 34% as metabolites)

Dosage Oral: Dosing at bedtime is recommended to limit central nervous system effects; should not be used as single-agent therapy

Children: Dosage is based on body weight

10 kg to <15 kg: 200 mg once daily
15 kg to <20 kg: 250 mg once daily
20 kg to <25 kg: 300 mg once daily
25 kg to <32.5 kg: 350 mg once daily
32.5 kg to <40 kg: 400 mg once daily
≥40 kg: 600 mg once daily

Adults: 600 mg once daily

Dosing adjustment in renal impairment: None recommended

Dosing comments in hepatic impairment: Limited clinical experience, use with caution

Dietary Considerations Should be taken on an empty stomach.

Administration Administer on an empty stomach. Capsules may be opened and added to liquids or small amounts of food.

Monitoring Parameters Serum transaminases (discontinuation of treatment should be considered for persistent elevations greater than five times the upper limit of normal), cholesterol, triglycerides, signs and symptoms of infection

Test Interactions False positive test for cannabinoids have been reported when the CEDIA DAU Multilevel THC assay is used. False positive results with other assays for cannabinoids have not been observed.

Patient Information Report all side effects; do not alter dose or discontinue without consulting prescriber; do not take prescription, OTC products, or herbal products without consulting prescriber; may cause dizziness, drowsiness, impaired concentration, delusions or depression; taking at bedtime may minimize these effects; caution in performing potentially hazardous tasks such as operating machinery or driving; do not get pregnant while taking this medication; avoid high-fat meals

(Continued)

Efavirenz *(Continued)*

Additional Information Efavirenz oral solution is available only through an expanded access (compassionate use) program. Enrollment information may be obtained by calling 1-877-372-7097.

Early virologic failure was observed with tenofovir and didanosine delayed release capsules, plus either efavirenz or nevirapine; use caution in treatment-naive patients with high baseline viral loads.

Dosage Forms
Capsule: 50 mg, 100 mg, 200 mg
Tablet: 600 mg

Selected Readings
"Three New Drugs for HIV Infection," *Med Lett Drugs Ther*, 1998, 40(1041):114-6.

Eflornithine (ee FLOR ni theen)

U.S. Brand Names Vaniqa™

Synonyms DFMO; Eflornithine Hydrochloride

Generic Available No

Use Cream: Females ≥12 years: Reduce unwanted hair from face and adjacent areas under the chin

Orphan status: Injection: Treatment of meningoencephalitic stage of *Trypanosoma brucei gambiense* infection (sleeping sickness)

Pregnancy Risk Factor C

Pregnancy Implications There are no adequate and well-controlled studies of topical eflornithine cream in pregnant women. The potential benefits to the mother versus the possible risks to the fetus should be considered prior to use.

Contraindications Hypersensitivity to eflornithine or any component of the formulation

Warnings/Precautions
Injection: Must be diluted before use; frequent monitoring for myelosuppression should be done; use with caution in patients with a history of seizures and in patients with renal impairment; serial audiograms should be obtained; due to the potential for relapse, patients should be followed up for at least 24 months
Cream: For topical use by females only; discontinue if hypersensitivity occurs; safety and efficacy in children <12 years has not been studied

Adverse Reactions
Injection:
>10%: Hematologic (reversible): Anemia (55%), leukopenia (37%), thrombocytopenia (14%)
1% to 10%:
Central nervous system: Seizures (may be due to the disease) (8%), dizziness
Dermatologic: Alopecia
Gastrointestinal: Vomiting, diarrhea
Hematologic: Eosinophilia
Otic: Hearing impairment
<1%: Abdominal pain, anorexia, facial edema, headache, weakness
Topical:
>10%: Dermatologic: Acne (11% to 21%), pseudofolliculitis barbae (5% to 15%)
1% to 10%:
Central nervous system: Headache (4% to 5%), dizziness (1%), vertigo (0.3% to 1%)
Dermatologic: Pruritus (3% to 4%), burning skin (2% to 4%), tingling skin (1% to 4%), dry skin (2% to 3%), rash (1% to 3%), facial edema (0.3% to 3%), alopecia (1% to 2%), skin irritation (1% to 2%), erythema (0% to 2%), ingrown hair (0.3% to 2%), folliculitis (0% to 1%)
Gastrointestinal: Dyspepsia (2%), anorexia (0.7% to 2%)
<1%: Bleeding skin, cheilitis, contact dermatitis, herpes simplex, lip swelling, nausea, numbness, rosacea, weakness

Overdosage/Toxicology There is no known antidote. Treatment is supportive. In mice and rats CNS depression, seizures, and death have occurred. Overdose with the topical product is not expected due to low percutaneous penetration.

Drug Interactions
Increased Effect/Toxicity: Cream: Possible interactions with other topical products have not been studied.
Decreased Effect: Cream: Possible interactions with other topical products have not been studied.

Stability
Injection: Must be diluted before use and used within 24 hours of preparation
Cream: Store at controlled room temperature 25°C (77°F); do not freeze

Mechanism of Action Eflornithine exerts antitumor and antiprotozoal effects through specific, irreversible ("suicide") inhibition of the enzyme ornithine decarboxylase (ODC). ODC is the rate-limiting enzyme in the biosynthesis of putrescine, spermine, and spermidine, the major polyamines in nucleated cells. Polyamines are necessary for the synthesis of DNA, RNA, and proteins and are, therefore, necessary for cell growth and differentiation. Although many microorganisms and higher plants are able to produce polyamines from alternate biochemical pathways, all mammalian cells depend on ornithine decarboxylase to produce polyamines. Eflornithine inhibits ODC and rapidly depletes animal cells of putrescine and spermidine; the concentration of spermine remains the same or may even increase. Rapidly dividing cells appear to be most susceptible to the effects of eflornithine. Topically, the inhibition of ODC in the skin leads to a decreased rate of hair growth.

Pharmacodynamics/Kinetics

Absorption: Topical: <1%

Half-life elimination: I.V.: 3-3.5 hours; Topical: 8 hours

Excretion: Primarily urine (as unchanged drug)

Dosage

Children ≥12 years and Adults: Females: Topical: Apply thin layer of cream to affected areas of face and adjacent chin twice daily, at least 8 hours apart

Adults: I.V. infusion: 100 mg/kg/dose given every 6 hours (over at least 45 minutes) for 14 days

Dosing adjustment in renal impairment: Injection: Dose should be adjusted although no specific guidelines are available

Administration

I.V.: Parenteral formulation is for I.V. use only; not for I.M. administration

Cream: Apply thin layer of eflornithine cream to affected areas of face and adjacent chin area twice daily, at least 8 hours apart. Rub in thoroughly. Hair removal techniques must still be continued; wait at least 5 minutes after removing hair to apply cream. Do not wash affected area for at least 8 hours following application.

Monitoring Parameters CBC with platelet counts

Patient Information

Injection: Report any persistent or unusual fever, sore throat, fatigue, bleeding, or bruising; frequent blood tests are needed during therapy.

Cream: For topical use only. This product will not prevent hair growth, but will decrease the rate of growth. You will still need to use hair removal techniques, such as shaving and plucking, while using eflornithine cream. Wait at least 5 minutes after removing hair to apply cream. Improvement can be seen within 4-8 weeks of use. Following discontinuation of use, pretreatment hair growth will be seen in about 8 weeks. Contact prescriber if skin irritation or intolerance develop. Do not wash affected area for at least 8 hours following application. You may apply cosmetics or make-up over the affected area once the cream has dried.

Dosage Forms

Cream, topical, as hydrochloride: 13.9% (30 g)

Injection, solution, as hydrochloride: 200 mg/mL (100 mL) [orphan drug status]

Selected Readings

"Drugs for Parasitic Infections," *Med Lett Drugs Ther*, 1998, 40(1017):1-12.

Eflornithine Hydrochloride *see* Eflornithine *on page 798*

Elimite® *see* Permethrin *on page 1001*

Emtricitabine (em trye SYE ta been)

Related Information

Antiretroviral Agents *on page 1206*

Antiretroviral Therapy for HIV Infection *on page 1219*

U.S. Brand Names Emtriva™

Synonyms BW524W91; Coviracil; FTC

Generic Available No

Use Treatment of HIV infection in combination with at least two other antiretroviral agents

Unlabeled/Investigational Use Investigational: Hepatitis B

Drug of Choice or Alternative for Organism(s):

Human Immunodeficiency Virus *on page 181*

Pregnancy Risk Factor B

Pregnancy Implications Cases of fatal and nonfatal lactic acidosis, with or without pancreatitis, have been reported in pregnant women receiving reverse transcriptase inhibitors. It is not known if pregnancy itself potentiates this known side effect; however, pregnant women may be at increased risk of lactic acidosis and liver

(Continued)

Emtricitabine *(Continued)*

damage. Hepatic enzymes and electrolytes should be monitored frequently during the 3rd trimester of pregnancy. There are no studies of emtricitabine during pregnancy. The Perinatal HIV Guidelines Working Group considers emtricitabine to be an alternative NRTI in dual nucleoside combination regimens. Health professionals are encouraged to contact the antiretroviral pregnancy registry to monitor outcomes of pregnant women exposed to antiretroviral medications (1-800-258-4263 or www.APRegistry.com).

Contraindications Hypersensitivity to emtricitabine or any component of the formulation

Warnings/Precautions Lactic acidosis, severe hepatomegaly, and hepatic failure have occurred rarely with emtricitabine (similar to other nucleoside analogues). Some cases have been fatal; stop treatment if lactic acidosis or hepatotoxicity occur. Prior liver disease, obesity, extended duration of therapy, and female gender may represent risk factors for severe hepatic reactions. Testing for hepatitis B is recommended prior to the initiation of therapy; hepatitis B may be exacerbated following discontinuation of emtricitabine. Use caution in patients with renal impairment (dosage adjustment required).

Adverse Reactions Clinical trials were conducted in patients receiving other antiretroviral agents, and it is not possible to correlate frequency of adverse events with emtricitabine alone. The range of frequencies of adverse events is generally comparable to comparator groups, with the exception of hyperpigmentation, which occurred more frequently in patients receiving emtricitabine.

>10%:
- Central nervous system: Headache (13% to 22%), dizziness (4% to 25%), insomnia (7% to 16%)
- Dermatologic: Rash (17% to 30%; includes rash, pruritus, maculopapular rash, vesiculobullous rash, pustular rash, and allergic reaction)
- Gastrointestinal: Diarrhea (23%), nausea (13% to 18%), abdominal pain (8% to 14%)
- Neuromuscular & skeletal: Weakness (12% to 16%), CPK increased (11% to 12%)
- Respiratory: Cough (14%), rhinitis (12% to 18%)

1% to 10%:
- Central nervous system: Abnormal dreams (2% to 11%), depression (6% to 9%), neuropathy/neuritis (4%)
- Dermatologic: Hyperpigmentation (2% to 6%; primarily of palms and/or soles but may include tongue, arms, lip and nails; generally mild and nonprogressive without associated local reactions such as pruritus or rash)
- Endocrine & metabolic: Serum triglycerides increased (9% to 10%), disordered glucose homeostasis (2% to 3%), serum amylase increased (2% to 5%)
- Gastrointestinal: Dyspepsia (4% to 8%), vomiting (9%)
- Hepatic: Transaminases increased (2% to 6%), bilirubin increased (1%)
- Neuromuscular & skeletal: Myalgia (4% to 6%), arthralgia (3% to 5%), paresthesia (5% to 6%)

Overdosage/Toxicology Treatment is supportive and symptom-directed. Approximately 30% of a dose is removed by hemodialysis.

Drug Interactions

Increased Effect/Toxicity: Concomitant use of ribavirin and nucleoside analogues may increase the risk of developing lactic acidosis.

Ethanol/Nutrition/Herb Interactions Food: Food decreases peak plasma concentrations, but does not alter the extent of absorption or overall systemic exposure.

Stability Store capsules at 25°C (77°F); excursions permitted to 15°C to 30°C (59°F to 86°F).

Mechanism of Action Nucleoside reverse transcriptase inhibitor; emtricitabine is a cytosine analogue which is phosphorylated intracellularly to emtricitabine 5'-triphosphate which interferes with HIV viral RNA dependent DNA polymerase resulting in inhibition of viral replication.

Pharmacodynamics/Kinetics

Absorption: Rapid, extensive
Protein binding: <4%
Metabolism: Limited, via oxidation and conjugation (not via CYP isoenzymes)
Bioavailability: 93%
Half-life elimination: Normal renal function: 10 hours
Time to peak, plasma: 1-2 hours
Excretion: Urine (86% primarily as unchanged drug, 13% as metabolites); feces (14%)

Dosage Oral: Adults: 200 mg once daily

Dosage adjustment in renal impairment:

Cl_{cr} 30-49 mL/minute: 200 mg every 48 hours

Cl_{cr} 15-29 mL/minute: 200 mg every 72 hours
Cl_{cr} <15 mL/minute (including hemodialysis patients): 200 mg every 96 hours

Dosage adjustment in hepatic impairment: No adjustment required.

Dietary Considerations May be taken with or without food.

Administration May be administered with or without food.

Monitoring Parameters Viral load, CD4, liver function tests; hepatitis B testing is recommended prior to initiation of therapy

Patient Information May cause headache, dizziness (use caution when driving or engaging in potentially hazardous tasks until response to drug is known); nausea, vomiting, (small, frequent meals, frequent mouth care, chewing gum, or sucking lozenges may help). May cause changes in skin pigmentation, especially on soles and palms. Report muscle weakness or pain; tingling, numbness, or pain in toes or fingers; weakness of extremities; chest pain, palpitations, or rapid heartbeat; swelling of extremities; weight gain or loss >5 lb/week; signs of infection (eg, fever, chills, sore throat, burning urination, fatigue); unusual bleeding (eg, tarry stools, easy bruising, or blood in stool, urine, or mouth); skin rash or irritation.

Dosage Forms Capsule: 200 mg

Emtricitabine and Tenofovir (em trye SYE ta been & te NOE fo veer)

Related Information

Antiretroviral Agents *on page 1206*
Antiretroviral Therapy for HIV Infection *on page 1219*

U.S. Brand Names Truvada™

Synonyms Tenofovir and Emtricitabine

Generic Available No

Use Treatment of HIV infection in combination with other antiretroviral agents

Drug of Choice or Alternative for Organism(s):

Human Immunodeficiency Virus *on page 181*

Pregnancy Risk Factor B

Pregnancy Implications Refer to individual agents.

Contraindications Hypersensitivity to emtricitabine, tenofovir, or any component of the formulation; severe renal impairment (Cl_{cr} <30 mL/minute).

Warnings/Precautions Not recommended as a component of a triple nucleoside regimen.

Lactic acidosis and severe hepatomegaly with steatosis have been reported with nucleoside analogues, including fatal cases; use with caution in patients with risk factors for liver disease (risk may be increased in obese patients or prolonged exposure) and suspend treatment in any patient who develops clinical or laboratory findings suggestive of lactic acidosis (transaminase elevation may/may not accompany hepatomegaly and steatosis).

Use caution in moderate renal impairment (Cl_{cr} 30-50 mL/minute); dosage adjustment required. May cause osteomalacia and/or renal toxicity; avoid concurrent therapy with other nephrotoxic drugs; monitor renal function and possible bone abnormalities during therapy. Use caution in hepatic impairment. All patients with HIV should be tested for HBV prior to initiation of treatment. Safety and efficacy during coinfection of HIV and HBV have not been established; acute, severe exacerbations of HBV have been reported following discontinuation of antiretroviral therapy. In HBV coinfected patients, monitor hepatic function closely for several months following discontinuation. Safety and efficacy have not been established in pediatric patients.

Adverse Reactions The adverse reaction profile of combination therapy has not been established. See individual agents.

Drug Interactions

Increased Effect/Toxicity: Refer to individual agents.

Ethanol/Nutrition/Herb Interactions Food: Food decreases peak plasma concentrations, but does not alter the extent of absorption or overall systemic exposure.

Stability Store tablets at 25°C (77°F); excursions permitted to 15°C to 30°C (59°F to 86°F).

Mechanism of Action Nucleoside and nucleotide reverse transcriptase inhibitor combination; emtricitabine is a cytosine analogue while tenofovir disoproxil fumarate (TDF) is an analog of adenosine 5'-monophosphate. Each drug interferes with HIV viral RNA dependent DNA polymerase resulting in inhibition of viral replication.

Pharmacodynamics/Kinetics Refer to individual monographs.

Dosage Adults: Oral: One tablet (emtricitabine 200 mg and tenofovir 300 mg) once daily

Dosage adjustment in renal impairment:

Cl_{cr} 30-49 mL/minute: Increase interval to every 48 hours.
Cl_{cr} <30 mL/minute or hemodialysis: Not recommended.

(Continued)

Emtricitabine and Tenofovir *(Continued)*

Dietary Considerations May be taken without regard to meals. Consider calcium and vitamin D supplementation in patients with history of bone fracture or osteopenia.

Administration May be administered with or without food. If used with didanosine; refer to didanosine monograph for additional information.

Monitoring Parameters CBC with differential, reticulocyte count, serum creatine kinase, CD4 count, HIV RNA plasma levels, renal and hepatic function tests, bone density (long-term), serum phosphorus; testing for HBV is recommended prior to the initiation of antiretroviral therapy

Patients with HIV and HBV coinfection should be monitored for several months following tenofovir discontinuation.

Dosage Forms Tablet, film coated: Emtricitabine 200 mg and tenofovir disoproxil fumarate 300 mg

Emtriva™ *see* Emtricitabine *on page 799*

Endantadine® (Can) *see* Amantadine *on page 636*

Enfuvirtide (en FYOO vir tide)

Related Information

Antiretroviral Agents *on page 1206*
Antiretroviral Therapy for HIV Infection *on page 1219*

U.S. Brand Names Fuzeon™

Canadian Brand Names Fuzeon™

Synonyms T-20

Generic Available No

Use Treatment of HIV-1 infection in combination with other antiretroviral agents in treatment-experienced patients with evidence of HIV-1 replication despite ongoing antiretroviral therapy

Drug of Choice or Alternative for Organism(s):

Human Immunodeficiency Virus *on page 181*

Pregnancy Risk Factor B

Pregnancy Implications Teratogenic effects were not observed in animal studies, however there are no studies in pregnant women. An antiretroviral registry has been established to monitor maternal and fetal outcomes in women receiving antiretroviral drugs. Physicians are encouraged to register patients at 1-800-258-4263 or www.APRegistry.com.

Contraindications Hypersensitivity to enfuvirtide or any component of the formulation

Warnings/Precautions Monitor closely for signs/symptoms of pneumonia; associated with an increased incidence during clinical trials, particularly in patients with a low CD4 cell count, high initial viral load, I.V. drug use, smoking, or a history of lung disease. May cause hypersensitivity reactions (symptoms may include rash, fever, nausea, vomiting, hypotension, and elevated transaminases). In addition, local injection site reactions may occur. Safety and efficacy have not been established in children <6 years of age.

Adverse Reactions

>10%:

- Central nervous system: Insomnia (11%)
- Local: Injection site reactions (98%; may include pain, erythema, induration, pruritus, ecchymosis, nodule or cyst formation)

1% to 10%:

- Central nervous system: Depression (9%), anxiety (6%)
- Dermatologic: Pruritus (5%)
- Endocrine & metabolic: Weight loss (7%), anorexia (3%)
- Gastrointestinal: Triglycerides increased (9%), appetite decreased (6%), constipation (4%), abdominal pain (3%), pancreatitis (2%), taste disturbance (2%), serum amylase increased (6%)
- Hematologic: Eosinophilia (8%), anemia (2%)
- Hepatic: Transaminases increased (4%)
- Local: Injection site infection (1%)
- Neuromuscular & skeletal: Neuropathy (9%), weakness (6%), myalgia (5%)
- Ocular: Conjunctivitis (2%)
- Respiratory: Cough (7%), pneumonia (4.7 events per 100 patient years vs 0.61 events per 100 patient years in control group), sinusitis (6%)
- Miscellaneous: Infections (4% to 6%), flu-like symptoms (2%), lymphadenopathy (2%)

<1%: Glomerulonephritis, Guillain-Barré syndrome, hepatic steatosis, hyperglycemia; hypersensitivity reactions (symptoms may include rash, fever, nausea, vomiting,

hypotension, and hepatic transaminases increased); neutropenia, renal failure, renal insufficiency, sixth nerve palsy, toxic hepatitis, tubular necrosis, worsening of abacavir hypersensitivity, thrombocytopenia

Overdosage/Toxicology No clinical experience in overdosage. Treatment is supportive.

Drug Interactions

Increased Effect/Toxicity: No significant interactions identified.

Decreased Effect: No significant interactions identified.

Stability Store powder at 25°C (77°F); excursions permitted to 15°C to 30°C (59 to 86°F). Reconstitute with 1.1 mL SWFI; tap vial for 10 seconds and roll gently to ensure contact with diluent; then allow to stand until solution is completed; may require up to 45 minutes to form solution. Reconstituted solutions should be refrigerated and must be used within 24 hours.

Mechanism of Action Binds to the first heptad-repeat (HR1) in the gp41 subunit of the viral envelope glycoprotein. Inhibits the fusion of HIV-1 virus with CD4 cells by blocking the conformational change in gp41 required for membrane fusion and entry into CD4 cells

Pharmacodynamics/Kinetics

Distribution: V_d: 5.5 L

Protein binding: 92%

Metabolism: Proteolytic hydrolysis (CYP isoenzymes do not appear to contribute to metabolism); clearance: 24.8 mL/hour/kg

Half-life elimination: 3.8 hours

Time to peak: 8 hours

Dosage SubQ:

Children ≥6 years: 2 mg/kg twice daily (maximum dose: 90 mg twice daily)

Adults: 90 mg twice daily

Dosage adjustment in renal impairment: No dosage adjustment required

Administration Inject subcutaneously into upper arm, abdomen, or anterior thigh. Do not inject into moles, scar tissue, bruises, or the navel. Rotate injection site, give injections at a site different from the preceding injection site; do not inject into any site where an injection site reaction is evident.

Patient Information Report any signs/symptoms of hypersensitivity or infection, including pneumonia (risk may be increased during therapy). Follow injection instructions closely. Rotate injection site, give injections at a site different from the preceding injection site; do not inject into any site where an injection site reaction is evident. Inject subcutaneously into upper arm, abdomen, or anterior thigh. Do not inject into moles, scar tissue, bruises, or the navel.

Dosage Forms Injection, powder for reconstitution [single-use vial]: 108 mg [90 mg/mL following reconstitution; available in convenience kit of 60 vials, SWFI, syringes, alcohol wipes, patient instructions]

Engerix-B® *see* Hepatitis B Vaccine *on page 856*

Engerix-B® and Havrix® *see* Hepatitis A Inactivated and Hepatitis B (Recombinant) Vaccine *on page 852*

Enhanced-potency Inactivated Poliovirus Vaccine *see* Poliovirus Vaccine (Inactivated) *on page 1011*

Entacyl® (Can) *see* Piperazine *on page 1006*

Entecavir

U.S. Brand Names Baraclude™

Generic Available No

Use Treatment of chronic hepatitis B infection in adults with evidence of active viral replication and either evidence of persistent transaminase elevations or histologically-active disease

Pregnancy Risk Factor C

Pregnancy Implications Teratogenic effects have been observed in animal studies. There are no adequate and well-controlled studies in pregnant women. Use only if benefit outweighs risk. Pregnant women taking entecavir should enroll in the pregnancy registry by calling 1-800-258-4263.

Contraindications Hypersensitivity to entecavir or any component of the formulation

Warnings/Precautions Cases of lactic acidosis and severe hepatomegaly with steatosis, some fatal, have been reported; severe, acute exacerbation of hepatitis B may occur upon discontinuation; monitor liver function several months after stopping treatment; reinitiation of antihepatitis B therapy may be required. Use caution in patients with renal impairment or patients receiving concomitant therapy which may reduce renal function; monitor renal function before and during treatment in liver transplant patients receiving concurrent therapy of cyclosporine or tacrolimus; entecavir dosage may need to be adjusted. Cross-resistance may develop in patients failing previous

(Continued)

Entecavir *(Continued)*

therapy with lamivudine. Entecavir does not exhibit any clinically-relevant activity against human immunodeficiency virus (HIV type 1). Safety and efficacy in pediatric patients and liver transplant patients have not been established.

Adverse Reactions

>10%: Hepatic: Alanine aminotransferase increased (2% to 12%)

1% to 10%:

- Central nervous system: Headache (2% to 4%), fatigue (1% to 3%)
- Endocrine & metabolic: Hyperglycemia (2%)
- Gastrointestinal: Lipase increased (7% to 8%), amylase increased (2% to 3%), diarrhea (≤1%), dyspepsia (≤1%)
- Hepatic: Aspartate aminotransferase increased (5%), bilirubin increased (2% to 3%)
- Renal: Hematuria (9%), glycosuria (4%), creatinine increased (1% to 2%),

<1%: Dizziness, hypoalbuminemia, insomnia, nausea, somnolence, thrombocytopenia, vomiting

Overdosage/Toxicology There have been limited reports of healthy subjects receiving single doses up to 40 mg or multiple doses up to 20 mg/day for 14 days with no adverse effects. Treatment should be symptom-directed and supportive. Hemodialysis (4 hours) will remove approximately 13% of dose.

Ethanol/Nutrition/Herb Interactions

Food: Food delays absorption and reduces AUC by 20%.

Stability Store at 15°C to 30°C (59°F to 86°F). Protect oral solution from light.

Mechanism of Action Entecavir is intracellularly phosphorylated to guanosine triphosphate which competes with natural substrates to effectively inhibit hepatitis B viral polymerase; enzyme inhibition blocks reverse transcriptase activity thereby reducing viral DNA synthesis.

Pharmacodynamics/Kinetics

Distribution: Extensive (V_d in excess of body water)

Protein binding: 13%

Metabolism: Minor hepatic glucuronide/sulfate conjugation

Half-life elimination: Terminal: 5-6 days; accumulation: 24 hours

Time to peak, plasma: 0.5-1.5 hours

Excretion: Urine (60% to 70% as unchanged drug)

Dosage Oral: Adolescents ≥16 years and Adults:

Nucleoside treatment naive: 0.5 mg daily

Lamivudine-resistant viremia (or known lamivudine-resistant mutations): 1 mg daily

Dosage adjustment in renal impairment: Cl_{cr} <50 mL/minute (including hemodialysis/CAPD):

- Cl_{cr} 30-49 mL/minute: Administer 50% of usual dose
- Cl_{cr} 10-29 mL/minute: Administer 30% of usual dose
- Cl_{cr} <10 mL/minute (including dialysis): Administer 10% of usual dose; administer after hemodialysis

Dietary Considerations Take on an empty stomach (2 hours before or after a meal).

Administration Administer on an empty stomach. Do not dilute or mix oral solution with water or other beverages; use calibrated oral dosing syringe. Oral solution and tablet are bioequivalent on a mg-to-mg basis.

Monitoring Parameters Liver function tests, renal function

Patient Information You will need periodic blood tests to monitor liver function and adjust dosage for maximum therapeutic effect. Inform your doctor if you have reduced kidney function; your dose may need to be adjusted. Inform prescriber of all prescriptions, OTC medications, or herbal products you are taking, and any allergies you have. Do not take any new medication during therapy unless approved by prescriber. Entecavir is not a cure for hepatitis B, nor has it been found to reduce transmission. Long-term effects are unknown. Take as directed; do not discontinue (even if feeling better) as worsening of hepatitis infection may occur. Take on an empty stomach (2 hours before or after a meal)

Dosage Forms

Oral solution: 0.05 mg/mL (210 mL) [orange flavor]

Tablet: 0.5 mg, 1 mg

Epaxal Berna® (Can) *see* Hepatitis A Vaccine *on page 853*

Epivir® *see* Lamivudine *on page 905*

Epivir-HBV® *see* Lamivudine *on page 905*

Epzicom™ *see* Abacavir and Lamivudine *on page 626*

Ertaczo™ *see* Sertaconazole *on page 1064*

Ertapenem (er ta PEN em)

Related Information

Community-Acquired Pneumonia in Adults *on page 1278*

U.S. Brand Names Invanz®

Canadian Brand Names Invanz®

Synonyms Ertapenem Sodium; L-749,345; MK0826

Generic Available No

Use Treatment of moderate-severe, complicated intra-abdominal infections, complicated skin and skin structure infections, complicated UTI (including pyelonephritis), acute pelvic infections, and community-acquired pneumonia. Antibacterial coverage includes aerobic gram-positive organisms, aerobic gram-negative organisms, anaerobic organisms.

Note: Methicillin-resistant *Staphylococcus*, *Enterococcus* spp, penicillin-resistant strains of *Streptococcus pneumoniae*, beta-lactamase-positive strains of *Haemophilus influenzae* are **resistant** to ertapenem, as are most *Pseudomonas aeruginosa*.

Drug of Choice or Alternative for Disease/Syndrome(s):

Cholangitis, Acute *on page 79*
Fever, Neutropenic *on page 148*
Intra-abdominal Abscess *on page 194*
Liver Abscess *on page 211*
Osteomyelitis, Diabetic Foot *on page 249*
Pancreatitis/Pancreatic Abscess *on page 253*
Peritonitis, Secondary *on page 263*
Peritonitis, Spontaneous Bacterial *on page 264*
Pneumonia, Community-Acquired *on page 270*
Pneumonia, Hospital-Acquired *on page 272*
Pneumonia, Ventilator-Associated *on page 273*

Pregnancy Risk Factor B

Pregnancy Implications There are no adequate and well-controlled studies in pregnant women. Use only if clearly needed. Ertapenem is approved for use in postpartum endomyometritis, septic abortion, and postsurgical gynecologic infections.

Contraindications Hypersensitivity to ertapenem, other carbapenems, or any component of the formulation; anaphylactic reactions to beta-lactam antibiotics. If using intramuscularly, known hypersensitivity to local anesthetics of the amide type (lidocaine is the diluent).

Warnings/Precautions Use caution with renal impairment. Dosage adjustment required in patients with moderate-to-severe renal dysfunction; elderly patients often require lower doses (based upon renal function); prolonged use may result in superinfection; has been associated with CNS adverse effects, including confusional states and seizures; use caution with CNS disorders (eg, brain lesions, history of seizures); serious hypersensitivity reactions, including anaphylaxis, have been reported (some without a history of previous allergic reactions to beta-lactams). Doses for I.M. administration are mixed with lidocaine. Safety and efficacy in patients <3 months of age have not been established.

Adverse Reactions Note: Percentages reported in adults.

1% to 10%:

- Cardiovascular: Swelling/edema (3%), chest pain (1%), hypertension (0.7% to 2%), hypotension (1% to 2%), tachycardia (1% to 2%)
- Central nervous system: Headache (6% to 7%), altered mental status (ie, agitation, confusion, disorientation, decreased mental acuity, changed mental status, somnolence, stupor) (3% to 5%), fever (2% to 5%), insomnia (3%), dizziness (2%), fatigue (1%), anxiety (0.8% to 1%)
- Dermatologic: Rash (2% to 3%), pruritus (1% to 2%), erythema (1% to 2%)
- Gastrointestinal: Diarrhea (9% to 10%), nausea (6% to 9%), abdominal pain (4%), vomiting (4%), constipation (3% to 4%), acid regurgitation (1% to 2%), dyspepsia (1%), oral candidiasis (0.1% to 1%)
- Genitourinary: Vaginitis (1% to 3%)
- Hematologic: Platelet count increased (4% to 7%), eosinophils increased (1% to 2%)
- Hepatic: Hepatic enzyme elevations (7% to 9%), alkaline phosphatase increase (4% to 7%)
- Local: Infused vein complications (5% to 7%), phlebitis/thrombophlebitis (1.5% to 2%), extravasation (0.7% to 2%)
- Neuromuscular & skeletal: Leg pain (0.4% to 1%)
- Respiratory: Dyspnea (1% to 3%), cough (1% to 2%), pharyngitis (0.7% to 1%), rales/rhonchi (0.5% to 1%), respiratory distress (0.2% to 1%)

(Continued)

Ertapenem *(Continued)*

<1%: Abdominal distention, aggressive behavior, anorexia, arrhythmia, asthma, asystole, atrial fibrillation, bicarbonate (serum) decreased, bilirubin (direct and indirect) increased, bladder dysfunction, BUN increased, bradycardia, bronchoconstriction, candidiasis, cardiac arrest, chills, cholelithiasis, *C. difficile*-associated diarrhea, dehydration, depression, dermatitis, desquamation, duodenitis, dysphagia, epistaxis, epithelial (urine) cells increased, esophagitis, facial edema, flank pain, flatulence, flushing, gastritis, gastrointestinal hemorrhage, gout, jaundice, heart failure, heart murmur, hematoma, hematuria, hemoptysis, hemorrhoids, hiccups, hypoesthesia, hypoxemia, ileus, injection site induration, injection site pain, malaise, monocytes increased, mouth ulcer, necrosis, nervousness, oliguria/anuria, pain, pancreatitis, paresthesia, PTT increased, pharyngeal discomfort, pleural effusion, pleuritic pain, pseudomembranous colitis, pyloric stenosis, renal insufficiency, seizure (0.5%), sodium (serum) increased, spasm, stomatitis, subdural hemorrhage, sweating, syncope, taste perversion, tremor, urinary retention, urticaria, vaginal candidiasis, vaginal pruritus, vulvovaginitis, weight loss, ventricular tachycardia, vertigo, voice disturbance

Postmarketing and/or case reports: Anaphylaxis, hallucinations

Drug Interactions

Increased Effect/Toxicity: Probenecid may increase serum concentrations of ertapenem; use caution.

Decreased Effect: Ertapenem may decrease valproic acid serum concentrations to subtherapeutic levels; monitor.

Stability Before reconstitution store at ≤25°C (77°F).

I.M.: Reconstitute 1 g vial with 3.2 mL of 1% lidocaine HCl injection (without epinephrine). Shake well. Use within 1 hour after preparation.

I.V.: Reconstitute 1 g vial with 10 mL of water for injection, 0.9% sodium chloride injection, or bacteriostatic water for injection. Shake well. For adults, transfer dose to 50 mL of 0.9% sodium chloride injection; for children, dilute dose with NS to a final concentration of ≤20 mg/mL. Reconstituted I.V. solution may be stored at room temperature and used within 6 hours **or** refrigerated, stored for up to 24 hours and used within 4 hours after removal from refrigerator. Do not freeze.

Mechanism of Action Inhibits bacterial cell wall synthesis by binding to one or more of the penicillin binding proteins; which in turn inhibits the final transpeptidation step of peptidoglycan synthesis in bacterial cell walls, thus inhibiting cell wall biosynthesis. Bacteria eventually lyse due to ongoing activity of cell wall autolytic enzymes (autolysins and murein hydrolases) while cell wall assembly is arrested.

Pharmacodynamics/Kinetics

Absorption: I.M.: Almost complete

Distribution: V_{dss}:

- Children 3 months to 12 years: 0.2 L/kg
- Children 13-17 years: 0.16 L/kg
- Adults: 0.12 L/kg

Protein binding (concentration dependent): 85% at 300 mcg/mL, 95% at <100 mcg/mL

Metabolism: Hydrolysis to inactive metabolite

Bioavailability: I.M.: 90%

Half-life elimination:

- Children 3 months to 12 years: 2.5 hours
- Children ≥13 years and Adults: 4 hours

Time to peak: I.M.: 2.3 hours

Excretion: Urine (80% as unchanged drug and metabolite); feces (10%)

Dosage Note: I.V. therapy may be administered for up to 14 days; I.M. therapy for up to 7 days

Children 3 months to 12 years: I.M., I.V.:

- Intra-abdominal infection: 15 mg/kg twice daily (maximum: 1 g/day) for 5-14 days
- Skin and skin structure infections: 15 mg/kg twice daily (maximum: 1 g/day) for 7-14 days
- Community-acquired pneumonia: 15 mg/kg twice daily (maximum: 1 g/day); duration of total antibiotic treatment: 10-14 days*
- Urinary tract infections/pyelonephritis: 15 mg/kg twice daily (maximum: 1 g/day); duration of total antibiotic treatment: 10-14 days*
- Acute pelvic infections: 15 mg/kg twice daily (maximum: 1 g/day) for 3-10 days

Children ≥13 years and Adults: I.M., I.V.:

- Intra-abdominal infection: 1 g/day for 5-14 days
- Skin and skin structure infections: 1 g/day for 7-14 days
- Community-acquired pneumonia: 1 g/day; duration of total antibiotic treatment: 10-14 days*

Urinary tract infections/pyelonephritis: 1 g/day; duration of total antibiotic treatment: 10-14 days*

Acute pelvic infections: 1 g/day for 3-10 days

*Duration includes possible switch to appropriate oral therapy after at least 3 days of parenteral treatment, once clinical improvement demonstrated.

Elderly: Refer to adult dosing.

Dosage adjustment in renal impairment: Adults: Cl_{cr} <30 mL/minute: 500 mg/day

Hemodialysis: Adults: When the daily dose is given within 6 hours prior to hemodialysis, a supplementary dose of 150 mg is required following hemodialysis.

Dosage adjustment in hepatic impairment: Adjustments cannot be recommended (lack of experience and research in this patient population).

Dietary Considerations Sodium content: 137 mg (~6 mEq) per gram of ertapenem

Administration

I.M.: Avoid injection into a blood vessel. Make sure patient does not have an allergy to lidocaine or another anesthetic of the amide type. Administer by deep I.M. injection into a large muscle mass (eg, gluteal muscle or lateral part of the thigh). Do not administer I.M. preparation or drug reconstituted for I.M. administration intravenously.

I.V.: Infuse over 30 minutes

Monitoring Parameters Periodic renal, hepatic, and hematopoietic assessment during prolonged therapy; neurological assessment

Patient Information Report warmth, swelling, irritation at infusion or injection site. Report unresolved nausea or vomiting (small, frequent meals may help). Report feelings of excessive dizziness, palpitations, visual disturbances, headache, diarrhea, and CNS changes. Report chills, unusual discharge, or foul-smelling urine.

Dosage Forms Injection, powder for reconstitution: 1 g [contains sodium 137 mg/g (~6 mEq/g)]

Ertapenem Sodium *see* Ertapenem *on page 805*

Erybid™ (Can) *see* Erythromycin *on page 807*

Eryc® *see* Erythromycin *on page 807*

Eryderm® *see* Erythromycin *on page 807*

Erygel® *see* Erythromycin *on page 807*

EryPed® *see* Erythromycin *on page 807*

Ery-Tab® *see* Erythromycin *on page 807*

Erythrocin® *see* Erythromycin *on page 807*

Erythromid® (Can) *see* Erythromycin *on page 807*

Erythromycin (er ith roe MYE sin)

Related Information

Animal and Human Bites *on page 1270*

Antimicrobial Activity Against Selected Organisms *on page 1165*

Community-Acquired Pneumonia in Adults *on page 1278*

U.S. Brand Names Akne-Mycin®; A/T/S®; E.E.S.®; Eryc®; Eryderm®; Erygel®; EryPed®; Ery-Tab®; Erythrocin®; PCE®; Romycin®; Staticin® [DSC]; Theramycin Z®; T-Stat® [DSC]

Canadian Brand Names Apo-Erythro Base®; Apo-Erythro E-C®; Apo-Erythro-ES®; Apo-Erythro-S®; Diomycin®; EES®; Erybid™; Eryc®; Erythromid®; Novo-Rythro Estolate; Novo-Rythro Ethylsuccinate; Nu-Erythromycin-S; PCE®; PMS-Erythromycin; Sans Acne®

Synonyms Erythromycin Base; Erythromycin Estolate; Erythromycin Ethylsuccinate; Erythromycin Gluceptate; Erythromycin Lactobionate; Erythromycin Stearate

Generic Available Yes

Use

Systemic: Treatment of susceptible bacterial infections including *S. pyogenes*, some *S. pneumoniae*, some *S. aureus*, *M. pneumoniae*, *Legionella pneumophila*, diphtheria, pertussis, chancroid, *Chlamydia*, erythrasma, *N. gonorrhoeae*, *E. histolytica*, syphilis and nongonococcal urethritis, and *Campylobacter* gastroenteritis; used in conjunction with neomycin for decontaminating the bowel

Ophthalmic: Treatment of superficial eye infections involving the conjunctiva or cornea; neonatal ophthalmia

Topical: Treatment of acne vulgaris

Unlabeled/Investigational Use Systemic: Treatment of gastroparesis

Drug of Choice or Alternative for Disease/Syndrome(s):

Acne Vulgaris *on page 27*

Blepharitis *on page 52*

Bronchitis *on page 60*

(Continued)

Erythromycin *(Continued)*

Cervicitis *on page 71*
Impetigo *on page 193*
Pharyngitis *on page 264*
Urethritis, Nongonococcal *on page 344*

Organism(s):

Bartonella Species *on page 48*
Bordetella pertussis on page 53
Calymmatobacterium granulomatis on page 65
Campylobacter jejuni on page 66
Chlamydia psittaci on page 73
Chlamydophila pneumoniae on page 78
Corynebacterium diphtheriae on page 96
Corynebacterium Species, Other Than *C. jeikeium on page 99*
Haemophilus ducreyi on page 158
Legionella pneumophila on page 202
Mycoplasma pneumoniae on page 238
Rhodococcus Species *on page 288*
Streptococcus agalactiae on page 313
Streptococcus pyogenes on page 321
Ureaplasma urealyticum on page 342

Pregnancy Risk Factor B

Contraindications Hypersensitivity to erythromycin or any component of the formulation

Systemic: Pre-existing liver disease (erythromycin estolate); concomitant use with ergot derivatives, pimozide, or cisapride

Warnings/Precautions Systemic: Use caution with hepatic impairment with or without jaundice has occurred, it may be accompanied by malaise, nausea, vomiting, abdominal colic, and fever; discontinue use if these occur; avoid using erythromycin lactobionate in neonates since formulations may contain benzyl alcohol which is associated with toxicity in neonates; observe for superinfections. Use in infants has been associated with infantile hypertrophic pyloric stenosis (IHPS). Macrolides have been associated with rare QT prolongation and ventricular arrhythmias, including torsade de pointes. Elderly may be at increased risk of adverse events, including hearing loss and/or torsade de pointes when dosage ≥4 g/day, particularly if concurrent renal/hepatic impairment.

Adverse Reactions

Systemic:

Cardiovascular: Ventricular arrhythmia, QT_c prolongation, torsade de pointes (rare), ventricular tachycardia (rare)

Central nervous system: Headache (8%), pain (2%), fever, seizure

Dermatitis: Rash (3%), pruritus (1%)

Gastrointestinal: Abdominal pain (8%), cramping, nausea (8%), oral candidiasis, vomiting (3%), diarrhea (7%), dyspepsia (2%), flatulence (2%), anorexia, pseudomembranous colitis, hypertrophic pyloric stenosis (including cases in infants or IHPS), pancreatitis

Hematologic: Eosinophilia (1%)

Hepatic: Cholestatic jaundice (most common with estolate), increased liver function tests (2%)

Local: Phlebitis at the injection site, thrombophlebitis

Neuromuscular & skeletal: Weakness (2%)

Respiratory: Dyspnea (1%), cough (3%)

Miscellaneous: Hypersensitivity reactions, allergic reactions

Topical: 1% to 10%: Dermatologic: Erythema, desquamation, dryness, pruritus

Overdosage/Toxicology Symptoms include nausea, vomiting, and diarrhea. Treatment consists of general and supportive care only.

Drug Interactions

Cytochrome P450 Effect: Substrate of CYP2B6 (minor), 3A4 (major); **Inhibits** CYP1A2 (weak), 3A4 (moderate)

Increased Effect/Toxicity: Avoid concomitant use of the following with erythromycin due to increased risk of malignant arrhythmias: Cisapride, gatifloxacin, moxifloxacin, pimozide, sparfloxacin, thioridazine. Other agents that prolong the QT_c interval, including type Ia (eg, quinidine) and type III antiarrhythmic agents, and selected antipsychotic agents (eg, mesoridazine, thioridazine) should be used with extreme caution. Concurrent use of ergot alkaloids with erythromycin is also contraindicated.

Erythromycin is a moderate CYP3A4 inhibitor, and may increase the levels/effects of selected benzodiazepines, calcium channel blockers, cyclosporine, mirtazapine,

nateglinide, nefazodone, quinidine, sildenafil (and other PDE-5 inhibitors), tacrolimus, venlafaxine, and other CYP3A4 substrates. Selected benzodiazepines (midazolam, triazolam), cisapride, ergot alkaloids, selected HMG-CoA reductase inhibitors (lovastatin and simvastatin), and pimozide are generally contraindicated with strong CYP3A4 inhibitors. When used with strong CYP3A4 inhibitors, dosage adjustment/limits are recommended for sildenafil and other PDE-5 inhibitors; refer to individual monographs. The effects of neuromuscular-blocking agents and warfarin have been potentiated by erythromycin.

The levels/effects of erythromycin may be increased by azole antifungals, ciprofloxacin, clarithromycin, diclofenac, doxycycline, imatinib, isoniazid, nefazodone, nicardipine, propofol, protease inhibitors, quinidine, telithromycin, verapamil, and other CYP3A4 inhibitors.

Decreased Effect: Erythromycin may decrease the serum concentrations of zafirlukast. Erythromycin may antagonize the therapeutic effects of clindamycin and lincomycin. The levels/effects of erythromycin may be decreased by aminoglutethimide, carbamazepine, nafcillin, nevirapine, phenobarbital, phenytoin, rifamycins, and other CYP3A4 inducers.

Ethanol/Nutrition/Herb Interactions

Ethanol: Avoid ethanol (may decrease absorption of erythromycin or enhance ethanol effects).

Food: Increased drug absorption with meals; erythromycin serum levels may be altered if taken with food.

Herb/Nutraceutical: St John's wort may decrease erythromycin levels.

Stability

Injection:

Erythromycin lactobionate should be reconstituted with sterile water for injection without preservatives to avoid gel formation; the reconstituted solution is stable for 2 weeks when refrigerated or for 24 hours at room temperature

Erythromycin I.V. infusion solution is stable at pH 6-8. Stability of lactobionate is pH dependent; I.V. form has the longest stability in 0.9% sodium chloride (NS) and should be prepared in this base solution whenever possible. Do not use D_5W as a diluent unless sodium bicarbonate is added to solution. If I.V. must be prepared in D_5W, 0.5 mL of the 8.4% sodium bicarbonate solution should be added per each 100 mL of D_5W.

Stability of parenteral admixture at room temperature (25°C) and at refrigeration temperature (4°C): 24 hours

Standard diluent: 500 mg/250 mL D_5W/NS; 750 mg/250 mL D_5W/NS; 1 g/250 mL D_5W/NS

Oral suspension:

Granules: After mixing, store under refrigeration and use within 10 days.

Powder: Refrigerate to preserve taste. Erythromycin ethylsuccinate may be stored at room temperature if used within 14 days. EryPed® drops should be used within 35 days following reconstitution; may store at room temperature or under refrigeration.

Topical and ophthalmic formulations: Store at room temperature.

Mechanism of Action Inhibits RNA-dependent protein synthesis at the chain elongation step; binds to the 50S ribosomal subunit resulting in blockage of transpeptidation

Pharmacodynamics/Kinetics

Absorption: Oral: Variable but better with salt forms than with base form; 18% to 45%; ethylsuccinate may be better absorbed with food

Distribution: Crosses placenta; enters breast milk

Relative diffusion from blood into CSF: Minimal even with inflammation

CSF:blood level ratio: Normal meninges: 1% to 12%; Inflamed meninges: 7% to 25%

Protein binding: 75% to 90%

Metabolism: Hepatic via demethylation

Half-life elimination: Peak: 1.5-2 hours; End-stage renal disease: 5-6 hours

Time to peak, serum: Base: 4 hours; Ethylsuccinate: 0.5-2.5 hours; delayed with food due to differences in absorption

Excretion: Primarily feces; urine (2% to 15% as unchanged drug)

Dosage

Neonates: Ophthalmic: Prophylaxis of neonatal gonococcal or chlamydial conjunctivitis: 0.5-1 cm ribbon of ointment should be instilled into each conjunctival sac

Infants and Children:

Treatment of susceptible infections:

Oral: (**Note:** Due to differences in absorption, 400 mg erythromycin ethylsuccinate produces the same serum levels as 250 mg erythromycin base, sterate or estolate)

Base: 30-50 mg/kg/day in 2-4 divided doses; do not exceed 2 g/day

(Continued)

Erythromycin *(Continued)*

Estolate: 30-50 mg/kg/day in 2-4 divided doses; do not exceed 2 g/day
Ethylsuccinate: 30-50 mg/kg/day in 2-4 divided doses; do not exceed 3.2 g/day
Stearate: 30-50 mg/kg/day in 2-4 divided doses; do not exceed 2 g/day
I.V.: Lactobionate: 15-50 mg/kg/day divided every 6 hours, not to exceed 4 g/day
Preop bowel preparation: 20 mg/kg erythromycin base at 1, 2, and 11 PM on the day before surgery combined with mechanical cleansing of the large intestine and oral neomycin

Children and Adults:
Ophthalmic: Instill ½" (1.25 cm) 2-6 times/day depending on the severity of the infection
Topical: Apply over the affected area twice daily after the skin has been thoroughly washed and patted dry

Adults:
Treatment of susceptible infections:
Oral:
Base: 250-500 mg every 6-12 hours
Ethylsuccinate: 400-800 mg every 6-12 hours
I.V. (lactobionate): 15-20 mg/kg/day divided every 6 hours or 500 mg to 1 g every 6 hours, or given as a continuous infusion over 24 hours (maximum: 4 g/24 hours)
Preop bowel preparation: Oral: 1 g erythromycin base at 1, 2, and 11 PM on the day before surgery combined with mechanical cleansing of the large intestine and oral neomycin
Gastrointestinal prokinetic (unlabeled use): Erythromycin has been used as a prokinetic agent to improve gastric emptying time and intestinal motility. In adults, 200 mg was infused I.V. initially followed by 250 mg orally 3 times/day 30 minutes before meals. Lower dosages have been used in some trials.

Dosage adjustment in renal impairment: Dialysis: Slightly dialyzable (5% to 20%); no supplemental dosage necessary in hemo- or peritoneal dialysis or in continuous arteriovenous or venovenous hemofiltration

Dietary Considerations Systemic: Drug may cause GI upset; may take with food.

Administration

Oral: Do not crush enteric coated drug product. GI upset, including diarrhea, is common. May be administered with food to decrease GI upset. Do not give with milk or acidic beverages.

I.V.: Infuse 1 g over 20-60 minutes. I.V. infusion may be very irritating to the vein. If phlebitis/pain occurs with used dilution, consider diluting further (eg, 1:5) if fluid status of the patient will tolerate, or consider administering in larger available vein. The addition of lidocaine or bicarbonate does not decrease the irritation of erythromycin infusions.

Ophthalmic: Avoid contact of tip of ophthalmic ointment tube with affected eye

Test Interactions False-positive urinary catecholamines

Patient Information Refrigerate after reconstitution; take entire course of medication; chewable tablets should not be swallowed whole; report if persistent diarrhea occurs; discard any unused portion after 10 days; absorption of estolate, ethylsuccinate, and base in a delayed release form are unaffected by food; take stearate salt and nondelayed release base preparations 2 hours before or after meals

Additional Information Due to differences in absorption, 400 mg erythromycin ethylsuccinate produces the same serum levels as 250 mg erythromycin base, stearate, or estolate. Do not use D_5W as a diluent unless sodium bicarbonate is added to solution; infuse over 20-60 minutes.

Dosage Forms [CAN] = Canadian brand name

Capsule, delayed release, enteric-coated pellets, as base (Eryc®): 250 mg
Gel, topical: 2% (30 g, 60 g)
A/T/S®: 2% (30 g) [contains alcohol 92%]
Erygel®: 2% (30 g, 60 g) [contains alcohol 92%]
Granules for oral suspension, as ethylsuccinate (E.E.S.®): 200 mg/5 mL (100 mL, 200 mL) [cherry flavor]
Injection, powder for reconstitution, as lactobionate (Erythrocin®): 500 mg, 1 g
Ointment, ophthalmic: 0.5% [5 mg/g] (1 g, 3.5 g)
Romycin®: 0.5% [5 mg/g] (3.5 g)
Ointment, topical (Akne-Mycin®): 2% (25 g)
Powder for oral suspension, as ethylsuccinate (EryPed®): 200 mg/5 mL (100 mL, 200 mL) [fruit flavor]; 400 mg/5 mL (100 mL, 200 mL) [banana flavor]
Powder for oral suspension, as ethylsuccinate [drops] (EryPed®): 100 mg/2.5 mL (50 mL) [fruit flavor]
Solution, topical: 2% (60 mL)

A/T/S®: 2% (60 mL) [contains alcohol 66%]
Eryderm®, T-Stat® [DSC], Theramycin Z®: 2% (60 mL) [contain alcohol]
Sans Acne® [CAN]: 2% (60 mL) [contains ethyl alcohol 44%; not available in U.S.]
Staticin®: 1.5% (60 mL) [DSC]

Suspension, oral, as estolate: 125 mg/5 mL (480 mL); 250 mg/5 mL (480 mL)

Suspension, oral, as ethylsuccinate: 200 mg/5 mL (480 mL); 400 mg/5 mL (480 mL)
E.E.S.®: 200 mg/5 mL (100 mL, 480 mL) [fruit flavor]; 400 mg/5 mL (100 mL, 480 mL) [orange flavor]

Swab (T-Stat® [DSC]): 2% (60s)

Tablet, chewable, as ethylsuccinate (EryPed®): 200 mg [fruit flavor] [DSC]

Tablet, delayed release, enteric coated, as base (Ery-Tab®): 250 mg, 333 mg, 500 mg

Tablet [film coated], as base: 250 mg, 500 mg

Tablet [film coated], as ethylsuccinate (E.E.S.®): 400 mg

Tablet [film coated], as stearate: 250 mg
Erythrocin®: 250 mg, 500 mg

Tablet [polymer-coated particles], as base (PCE®): 333 mg, 500 mg

Selected Readings

Amsden GW, "Erythromycin, Clarithromycin, and Azithromycin: Are the Differences Real?" *Clin Ther*, 1996, 18(1):56-72.

Goldman MP and Longworth DL, "The Role of Azithromycin and Clarithromycin in Clinical Practice," *Cleve Clin J Med*, 1993, 60(5):359-64.

Smilack JD, Wilson WR, and Cockerill FR 3d, "Tetracyclines, Chloramphenicol, Erythromycin, Clindamycin, and Metronidazole," *Mayo Clin Proc*, 1991, 66(12):1270-80.

Tartaglione TA, "Therapeutic Options for the Management and Prevention of *Mycobacterium avium* Complex Infection in Patients With the Acquired Immunodeficiency Syndrome," *Pharmacotherapy*, 1996, 16(2):171-82.

Erythromycin and Benzoyl Peroxide

(er ith roe MYE sin & BEN zoe il per OKS ide)

Related Information

Erythromycin *on page 807*

U.S. Brand Names Benzamycin®; Benzamycin® Pak

Synonyms Benzoyl Peroxide and Erythromycin

Generic Available No

Use Topical control of acne vulgaris

Pregnancy Risk Factor C

Drug Interactions

Cytochrome P450 Effect: Erythromycin: **Substrate** of CYP2B6 (minor), 3A4 (major); **Inhibits** CYP1A2 (weak), 3A4 (moderate)

Pharmacodynamics/Kinetics See individual agents.

Dosage Apply twice daily, morning and evening

Dosage Forms

Gel, topical:
Benzamycin®: Erythromycin 30 mg and benzoyl peroxide 50 mg per g (47 g)
Benzamycin® Pak: Erythromycin 30 mg and benzoyl peroxide 50 mg per 0.8 g packet (60s) [supplied with diluent containing alcohol]

Erythromycin and Sulfisoxazole

(er ith roe MYE sin & sul fi SOKS a zole)

Related Information

Erythromycin *on page 807*
SulfiSOXAZOLE *on page 1091*

U.S. Brand Names Pediazole®

Canadian Brand Names Pediazole®

Synonyms Sulfisoxazole and Erythromycin

Generic Available Yes

Use Treatment of susceptible bacterial infections of the upper and lower respiratory tract, otitis media in children caused by susceptible strains of *Haemophilus influenzae*, and many other infections in patients allergic to penicillin

Drug of Choice or Alternative for Disease/Syndrome(s):

Otitis Media, Acute *on page 253*

Pregnancy Risk Factor C

Contraindications Hypersensitivity to erythromycin, sulfonamides, or any component of the formulation; hepatic dysfunction; infants <2 months of age (sulfas compete with bilirubin for binding sites); porphyria; concurrent use with pimozide or cisapride

Warnings/Precautions Use with caution in patients with impaired renal or hepatic function, G6PD deficiency (hemolysis may occur). Chemical similarities are present among sulfonamides, sulfonylureas, carbonic anhydrase inhibitors, thiazides, and loop diuretics (except ethacrynic acid). In patients with allergy to one of these

(Continued)

Erythromycin and Sulfisoxazole *(Continued)*

compounds, a risk of cross-reaction exists; avoid use when previous reaction has been severe.

Adverse Reactions Frequency not defined.

Cardiovascular: Ventricular arrhythmia,
Central nervous system: Headache, fever
Dermatologic: Rash, Stevens-Johnson syndrome, toxic epidermal necrolysis
Gastrointestinal: Abdominal pain, cramping, nausea, vomiting, oral candidiasis, hypertrophic pyloric stenosis, diarrhea, pseudomembranous colitis
Hematologic: Agranulocytosis, aplastic anemia, eosinophilia
Hepatic: Hepatic necrosis, cholestatic jaundice
Local: Phlebitis at the injection site, thrombophlebitis
Renal: Toxic nephrosis, crystalluria
Miscellaneous: Hypersensitivity reactions

Overdosage/Toxicology Symptoms include nausea, vomiting, diarrhea, prostration, reversible pancreatitis, and hearing loss with or without tinnitus or vertigo. Treatment consists of general and supportive care only. Keep well hydrated.

Drug Interactions

Cytochrome P450 Effect:

Erythromycin: **Substrate** of CYP2B6 (minor), 3A4 (major); **Inhibits** CYP1A2 (weak), 3A4 (moderate)

Sulfisoxazole: **Substrate** of CYP2C8/9 (major); **Inhibits** CYP2C8/9 (strong)

Increased Effect/Toxicity: See individual agents.

Decreased Effect: See individual agents.

Stability Reconstituted suspension is stable for 14 days when refrigerated

Mechanism of Action Erythromycin inhibits bacterial protein synthesis; sulfisoxazole competitively inhibits bacterial synthesis of folic acid from para-aminobenzoic acid

Pharmacodynamics/Kinetics See individual agents.

Dosage Oral (dosage recommendation is based on the product's erythromycin content):

Children ≥2 months: 50 mg/kg/day erythromycin and 150 mg/kg/day sulfisoxazole in divided doses every 6 hours; not to exceed 2 g erythromycin/day or 6 g sulfisoxazole/day for 10 days

Adults >45 kg: 400 mg erythromycin and 1200 mg sulfisoxazole every 6 hours

Dosing adjustment in renal impairment (sulfisoxazole must be adjusted in renal impairment):

Cl_{cr} 10-50 mL/minute: Administer every 8-12 hours
Cl_{cr} <10 mL/minute: Administer every 12-24 hours

Monitoring Parameters CBC and periodic liver function test

Test Interactions False-positive urinary protein

Patient Information Maintain adequate fluid intake; avoid prolonged exposure to sunlight; discontinue if rash appears; take until gone, do not skip doses

Dosage Forms Powder for oral suspension: Erythromycin ethylsuccinate 200 mg and sulfisoxazole acetyl 600 mg per 5 mL (100 mL, 150 mL, 200 mL) [strawberry-banana flavor]

Selected Readings

Rodriguez WJ, Schwartz RH, Sait T, et al, "Erythromycin-Sulfisoxazole vs Amoxicillin in the Treatment of Acute Otitis Media in Children," *Am J Dis Child*, 1985, 139(8):766-70.

Tartaglione TA, "Therapeutic Options for the Management and Prevention of *Mycobacterium avium* Complex Infection in Patients With the Acquired Immunodeficiency Syndrome," *Pharmacotherapy*, 1996, 16(2):171-82.

Erythromycin Base *see* Erythromycin *on page 807*
Erythromycin Estolate *see* Erythromycin *on page 807*
Erythromycin Ethylsuccinate *see* Erythromycin *on page 807*
Erythromycin Gluceptate *see* Erythromycin *on page 807*
Erythromycin Lactobionate *see* Erythromycin *on page 807*
Erythromycin Stearate *see* Erythromycin *on page 807*

Ethambutol (e THAM byoo tole)

Related Information

Tuberculosis *on page 1315*
USPHS / IDSA Guidelines for the Prevention of Opportunistic Infections in Persons Infected With HIV *on page 1237*

U.S. Brand Names Myambutol®
Canadian Brand Names Etibi®
Synonyms Ethambutol Hydrochloride
Generic Available Yes

Use Treatment of tuberculosis and other mycobacterial diseases in conjunction with other antituberculosis agents

Drug of Choice or Alternative for Organism(s):

Mycobacterium avium-intracellulare (Complex) *on page 228*
Mycobacterium bovis *on page 229*
Mycobacterium kansasii *on page 231*
Mycobacterium tuberculosis *on page 234*

Pregnancy Risk Factor C

Pregnancy Implications There are no adequate and well-controlled studies in pregnant women; teratogenic effects have been seen in animals. Ethambutol has been used safely during pregnancy.

Contraindications Hypersensitivity to ethambutol or any component of the formulation; optic neuritis; use in children, unconscious patients, or any other patient who may be unable to discern and report visual changes

Warnings/Precautions May cause optic neuritis, resulting in decreased visual acuity or other vision changes. Discontinue promptly in patients with changes in vision, color blindness, or visual defects (effects normally reversible, but reversal may require up to a year). Use only in children whose visual acuity can accurately be determined and monitored (not recommended for use in children <13 years of age unless the benefit outweighs the risk). Dosage modification is required in patients with renal insufficiency. Hepatic toxicity has been reported, possibly due to concurrent therapy.

Adverse Reactions Frequency not defined.

Cardiovascular: Myocarditis, pericarditis

Central nervous system: Headache, confusion, disorientation, malaise, mental confusion, fever, dizziness, hallucinations

Dermatologic: Rash, pruritus, dermatitis, exfoliative dermatitis

Endocrine & metabolic: Acute gout or hyperuricemia

Gastrointestinal: Abdominal pain, anorexia, nausea, vomiting

Hematologic: Leukopenia, thrombocytopenia, eosinophilia, neutropenia, lymphadenopathy

Hepatic: Abnormal LFTs, hepatotoxicity (possibly related to concurrent therapy), hepatitis

Neuromuscular & skeletal: Peripheral neuritis, arthralgia

Ocular: Optic neuritis; symptoms may include decreased acuity, scotoma, color blindness, or visual defects (usually reversible with discontinuation, irreversible blindness has been described)

Renal: Nephritis

Respiratory: Infiltrates (with or without eosinophilia), pneumonitis

Miscellaneous: Anaphylaxis, anaphylactoid reaction; hypersensitivity syndrome (rash, eosinophilia, and organ-specific inflammation)

Overdosage/Toxicology Symptoms include decreased visual acuity, anorexia, joint pain, and numbness of the extremities. Following GI decontamination, treatment is supportive.

Drug Interactions

Decreased Effect: Decreased absorption with aluminum hydroxide. Avoid concurrent administration of aluminum-containing antacids for at least 4 hours following ethambutol.

Stability Store at controlled room temperature of 20°C to 25°C (68°F to 77°F).

Mechanism of Action Suppresses mycobacteria multiplication by interfering with RNA synthesis

Pharmacodynamics/Kinetics

Absorption: ~80%

Distribution: Widely throughout body; concentrated in kidneys, lungs, saliva, and red blood cells

Relative diffusion from blood into CSF: Adequate with or without inflammation (exceeds usual MICs)

CSF:blood level ratio: Normal meninges: 0%; Inflamed meninges: 25%

Protein binding: 20% to 30%

Metabolism: Hepatic (20%) to inactive metabolite

Half-life elimination: 2.5-3.6 hours; End-stage renal disease: 7-15 hours

Time to peak, serum: 2-4 hours

Excretion: Urine (~50%) and feces (20%) as unchanged drug

Dosage Oral:

Treatment of tuberculosis: **Note:** Used as part of a multidrug regimen. Treatment regimens consist of an initial 2 month phase, followed by a continuation phase of 4 or 7 additional months; frequency of dosing may differ depending on phase of therapy.

(Continued)

Ethambutol *(Continued)*

Children:
Daily therapy: 15-20 mg/kg/day (maximum: 1 g/day)
Twice weekly directly observed therapy (DOT): 50 mg/kg (maximum: 4 g/dose)
Adults (suggested doses by lean body weight):
Daily therapy: 15-25 mg/kg
40-55 kg: 800 mg
56-75 kg: 1200 mg
76-90 kg: 1600 mg (maximum dose regardless of weight)
Twice weekly directly observed therapy (DOT): 50 mg/kg
40-55 kg: 2000 mg
56-75 kg: 2800 mg
76-90 kg: 4000 mg (maximum dose regardless of weight)
Three times/week DOT: 25-30 mg/kg (maximum: 2.5 g)
40-55 kg: 1200 mg
56-75 kg: 2000 mg
76-90 kg: 2400 mg (maximum dose regardless of weight)
Disseminated *Mycobacterium avium* complex (MAC) in patients with advanced HIV infection: 15 mg/kg ethambutol in combination with azithromycin 600 mg daily

Dosing interval in renal impairment:
Cl_{cr} 10-50 mL/minute: Administer every 24-36 hours
Cl_{cr} <10 mL/minute: Administer every 48 hours
Hemodialysis: Slightly dialyzable (5% to 20%); Administer dose postdialysis
Peritoneal dialysis: Dose for Cl_{cr} <10 mL/minute
Continuous arteriovenous or venovenous hemofiltration: Administer every 24-36 hours

Dietary Considerations May be taken with food as absorption is not affected, may cause gastric irritation.

Monitoring Parameters Baseline and periodic (monthly) visual testing (each eye individually, as well as both eyes tested together) in patients receiving >15 mg/kg/day; baseline and periodic renal, hepatic, and hematopoietic tests

Patient Information Report any visual changes or rash; may cause stomach upset, take with food; do not take within 2 hours of aluminum-containing antacids. Do not discontinue medication without consulting prescriber.

Dosage Forms Tablet, as hydrochloride: 100 mg, 400 mg

Selected Readings

Davidson PT and Le HQ, "Drug Treatment of Tuberculosis - 1992," *Drugs*, 1992, 43(5):651-73.
"Drugs for Tuberculosis," *Med Lett Drugs Ther*, 1993, 35(908):99-101.
Havlir DV and Barnes PF, "Tuberculosis in Patients With Human Immunodeficiency Virus Infection," *N Engl J Med*, 1999, 340(5):367-73.
Iseman MD, "Treatment of Multidrug-Resistant Tuberculosis," *N Engl J Med*, 1993, 329(11):784-91.
"Prevention and Treatment of Tuberculosis Among Patients Infected With Human Immunodeficiency Virus: Principles of Therapy and Revised Recommendations. Centers for Disease Control and Prevention," *MMWR*, 1998, 47(RR-20):1-58.
Van Scoy RE and Wilkowske CJ, "Antituberculous Agents," *Mayo Clin Proc*, 1992, 67(2):179-87.

Ethambutol Hydrochloride *see* Ethambutol *on page 812*

Ethionamide (e thye on AM ide)

Related Information
Tuberculosis *on page 1315*

U.S. Brand Names Trecator®

Canadian Brand Names Trecator®

Generic Available No

Use Treatment of tuberculosis and other mycobacterial diseases, in conjunction with other antituberculosis agents, when first-line agents have failed or resistance has been demonstrated

Pregnancy Risk Factor C

Pregnancy Implications Ethionamide crosses the placenta; teratogenic effects were observed in animal studies. Use during pregnancy is not recommended.

Contraindications Hypersensitivity to ethionamide or any component of the formulation; severe hepatic impairment

Warnings/Precautions Use with caution in patients with diabetes mellitus; use with caution in patients receiving cycloserine or isoniazid. Use caution when switching patients from the sugar-coated tablet formulation (Trecator®-SC) to film-coated tablet (Trecator®); the dosage may need retitrated in order to avoid intolerance.

Adverse Reactions Frequency not defined.
Cardiovascular: Postural hypotension

Central nervous system: Depression, dizziness, drowsiness, headache, psychiatric disturbances, restlessness, seizure
Dermatologic: Acne, alopecia, photosensitivity, purpura, rash
Endocrine & metabolic: Gynecomastia, hypoglycemia, hypothyroidism or goiter, pellagra-like syndrome
Gastrointestinal: Abdominal pain, anorexia, diarrhea, excessive salivation, metallic taste, nausea, stomatitis, vomiting, weight loss
Genitourinary: Impotence
Hematologic: Thrombocytopenia
Hepatic: Hepatitis, jaundice, liver function tests increased
Neuromuscular & skeletal: Peripheral neuritis, weakness (common)
Ocular: Blurred vision, diplopia, optic neuritis
Respiratory: Olfactory disturbances
Miscellaneous: Hypersensitivity reaction

Overdosage/Toxicology Symptoms include peripheral neuropathy, anorexia, and joint pain. Following GI decontamination, treatment is supportive. Pyridoxine may be given to prevent peripheral neuropathy.

Ethanol/Nutrition/Herb Interactions
Ethanol: Avoid excessive ethanol ingestion; psychotic reaction may occur.

Mechanism of Action Inhibits peptide synthesis

Pharmacodynamics/Kinetics
Absorption: Rapid, complete
Distribution: Crosses placenta; V_d: 93.5 L
Protein binding: ~30%
Metabolism: Extensively hepatic to active and inactive metabolites
Bioavailability: 80%
Half-life elimination: 2-3 hours
Time to peak, serum: 1 hour
Excretion: Urine (<1% as unchanged drug; as active and inactive metabolites)

Dosage Oral:
Children: 15-20 mg/kg/day in 2-3 divided doses, not to exceed 1 g/day
Adults: 15-20 mg/kg/day; initiate dose at 250 mg/day for 1-2 days, then increase to 250 mg twice daily for 1-2 days, with gradual increases to highest tolerated dose; average adult dose: 750 mg/day (maximum: 1 g/day in 3-4 divided doses)
Dosing adjustment in renal impairment: Cl_{cr} <30 mL/minute: 250-500 mg/day

Dietary Considerations Healthcare provider may recommend an increase in dietary intake of pyridoxine to prevent neurotoxic effects of ethionamide. Avoid alcohol.

Administration Neurotoxic effects may be relieved by the administration of pyridoxine (6-100 mg daily, lower doses are more common). May be taken with or without meals. Gastrointestinal adverse effects may be decreased by administration at bedtime, decreased dose, or giving antiemetics.

Monitoring Parameters Initial and periodic serum ALT and AST; ophthalmic exams; thyroid function

Patient Information Take with meals; report persistent or severe stomach upset, loss of appetite, or metallic taste; frequent blood tests are needed for monitoring; increase dietary intake of pyridoxine

Additional Information Neurotoxic effects may be relieved by the administration of pyridoxine.

Dosage Forms Tablet: 250 mg

Selected Readings

Davidson PT and Le HQ, "Drug Treatment of Tuberculosis - 1992," *Drugs*, 1992, 43(5):651-73.
"Drugs for Tuberculosis," *Med Lett Drugs Ther*, 1993, 35(908):99-101.
Iseman MD, "Treatment of Multidrug-Resistant Tuberculosis," *N Engl J Med*, 1993, 329(11):784-91.

Ethoxynaphthamido Penicillin Sodium *see* Nafcillin *on page 955*
Etibi® (Can) *see* Ethambutol *on page 812*
Eurax® *see* Crotamiton *on page 762*
Everone® 200 (Can) *see* Testosterone *on page 1100*
Evoclin™ *see* Clindamycin *on page 752*
Exelderm® *see* Sulconazole *on page 1080*
Exsel® [DSC] *see* Selenium Sulfide *on page 1063*
F_3T *see* Trifluridine *on page 1129*
Factive® *see* Gemifloxacin *on page 840*

Famciclovir (fam SYE kloe veer)

U.S. Brand Names Famvir®

Canadian Brand Names Famvir®

Generic Available No

(Continued)

Famciclovir *(Continued)*

Use Management of acute herpes zoster (shingles) and recurrent episodes of genital herpes; treatment of recurrent herpes simplex in immunocompetent patients

Drug of Choice or Alternative for

Disease/Syndrome(s):

Esophagitis *on page 147*

Organism(s):

Herpes Simplex Virus *on page 172*

Varicella-Zoster Virus *on page 347*

Pregnancy Risk Factor B

Pregnancy Implications Use only if the benefit to the patient clearly exceeds the potential risk to the fetus.

Contraindications Hypersensitivity to famciclovir or any component of the formulation

Warnings/Precautions Has not been established for use in initial episodes of genital herpes, patients with ophthalmic or disseminated zoster, or in immunocompromised patients with herpes zoster; dosage adjustment is required in patients with renal insufficiency (Cl_{cr} <60 mL/minute) and in patients with noncompensated hepatic disease; safety and efficacy have not been established in children <18 years of age; animal studies indicated increases in incidence of carcinomas, mutagenic changes, and decreases in fertility with extremely large doses

Adverse Reactions

1% to 10%:

Central nervous system: Fatigue (4% to 6%), fever (1% to 3%), dizziness (3% to 5%), somnolence (1% to 2%), headache

Dermatologic: Pruritus (1% to 4%)

Gastrointestinal: Diarrhea (4% to 8%), vomiting (1% to 5%), constipation (1% to 5%), anorexia (1% to 3%), abdominal pain (1% to 4%), nausea

Neuromuscular & skeletal: Paresthesia (1% to 3%)

Respiratory: Sinusitis/pharyngitis (2%)

<1%: Rigors, arthralgia, upper respiratory infection

Overdosage/Toxicology Supportive and symptomatic care is recommended. Hemodialysis may enhance elimination.

Drug Interactions

Increased Effect/Toxicity:

Cimetidine: Penciclovir AUC may increase due to impaired metabolism.

Digoxin: C_{max} of digoxin increases by ~19%.

Probenecid: Penciclovir serum levels significantly increase.

Theophylline: Penciclovir AUC/C_{max} may increase and renal clearance decrease, although not clinically significant.

Ethanol/Nutrition/Herb Interactions Food: Rate of absorption and/or conversion to penciclovir and peak concentration are reduced with food, but bioavailability is not affected.

Mechanism of Action After undergoing rapid biotransformation to the active compound, penciclovir, famciclovir is phosphorylated by viral thymidine kinase in HSV-1, HSV-2, and VZV-infected cells to a monophosphate form; this is then converted to penciclovir triphosphate and competes with deoxyguanosine triphosphate to inhibit HSV-2 polymerase (ie, herpes viral DNA synthesis/replication is selectively inhibited)

Pharmacodynamics/Kinetics

Absorption: Food decreases maximum peak concentration and delays time to peak; AUC remains the same

Distribution: V_{dss}: 0.98-1.08 L/kg

Protein binding: 20%

Metabolism: Rapidly deacetylated and oxidized to penciclovir; not via CYP

Bioavailability: 77%

Half-life elimination: Penciclovir: 2-3 hours (10, 20, and 7 hours in HSV-1, HSV-2, and VZV-infected cells, respectively); prolonged with renal impairment

Time to peak: 0.9 hours; C_{max} and T_{max} are decreased and prolonged with noncompensated hepatic impairment

Excretion: Urine (>90% as unchanged drug)

Dosage Initiate therapy as soon as herpes zoster is diagnosed: Adults: Oral:

Acute herpes zoster: 500 mg every 8 hours for 7 days

Recurrent herpes simplex in immunocompetent patients: 125 mg twice daily for 5 days

Genital herpes:

First episode: 250 mg 3 times/day for 7-10 days

Recurrent episodes: 125 mg twice daily for 5 days

Prophylaxis: 250 mg twice daily
Severe (hospitalized patients): 250 mg twice daily

Dosing interval in renal impairment:

Herpes zoster:
- Cl_{cr} ≥60 mL/minute: Administer 500 mg every 8 hours
- Cl_{cr} 40-59 mL/minute: Administer 500 mg every 12 hours
- Cl_{cr} 20-39 mL/minute: Administer 500 mg every 24 hours
- Cl_{cr} <20 mL/minute: Administer 250 mg every 24 hours

Recurrent genital herpes:
- Cl_{cr} ≥40 mL/minute: Administer 125 mg every 12 hours
- Cl_{cr} 20-39 mL/minute: Administer 125 mg every 24 hours
- Cl_{cr} <20 mL/minute: Administer 125 mg every 48 hours

Suppression of recurrent genital herpes:
- Cl_{cr} ≥40 mL/minute: Administer 250 mg every 12 hours
- Cl_{cr} 20-39 mL/minute: Administer 125 mg every 12 hours
- Cl_{cr} <20 mL/minute: Administer 125 mg every 24 hours

Recurrent orolabial or genital herpes in HIV-infected patients:
- Cl_{cr} ≥40 mL/minute: Administer 500 mg every 12 hours
- Cl_{cr} 20-39 mL/minute: Administer 500 mg every 24 hours
- Cl_{cr} <20 mL/minute: Administer 250 mg every 24 hours

Dietary Considerations May be taken with food or on an empty stomach.

Monitoring Parameters Periodic CBC during long-term therapy

Patient Information Initiate therapy as soon as herpes zoster is diagnosed; may take medication with food or on an empty stomach

Additional Information Most effective if therapy is initiated within 72 hours of initial lesion.

Dosage Forms Tablet: 125 mg, 250 mg, 500 mg

Selected Readings

Alrabiah FA and Sacks SL, "New Antiherpesvirus Agents. Their Targets and Therapeutic Potential," *Drugs*, 1996, 52(1):17-32.
Luber AD and Flaherty JF Jr, "Famciclovir for Treatment of Herpesvirus Infections," *Ann Pharmacother*, 1996, 30(9):978-85.
Perry CM and Wagstaff AJ, "Famciclovir. A Review of Its Pharmacological Properties and Therapeutic Efficacy in Herpesvirus Infections," *Drugs*, 1995, 50(2):396-415.
Sacks SL, "Genital Herpes Simplex Virus and Its Treatment Focus on Famciclovir," *Semin Dermatol*, 1996, 15(2 Suppl 1):32-6.
Tyring SK, "Efficacy of Famciclovir in the Treatment of Herpes Zoster," *Semin Dermatol*, 1996, 15(2 Suppl 1):27-31.

Famvir® *see* Famciclovir *on page 815*
Fansidar® *see* Sulfadoxine and Pyrimethamine *on page 1085*
5-FC *see* Flucytosine *on page 822*
Femizol-M™ [OTC] *see* Miconazole *on page 945*
Femstat® One (Can) *see* Butoconazole *on page 691*

Filgrastim (fil GRA stim)

U.S. Brand Names Neupogen®

Canadian Brand Names Neupogen®

Synonyms G-CSF; Granulocyte Colony Stimulating Factor

Generic Available No

Use Stimulation of granulocyte production in patients with malignancies, including myeloid malignancies; receiving myelosuppressive therapy associated with a significant risk of neutropenia; severe chronic neutropenia (SCN); receiving bone marrow transplantation (BMT); undergoing peripheral blood progenitor cell (PBPC) collection

Pregnancy Risk Factor C

Contraindications Hypersensitivity to filgrastim, *E. coli*-derived proteins, or any component of the formulation; concurrent myelosuppressive chemotherapy or radiation therapy

Warnings/Precautions Do not use filgrastim in the period 24 hours before to 24 hours after administration of cytotoxic chemotherapy because of the potential sensitivity of rapidly dividing myeloid cells to cytotoxic chemotherapy. Precaution should be exercised in the usage of filgrastim in any malignancy with myeloid characteristics. Filgrastim can potentially act as a growth factor for any tumor type, particularly myeloid malignancies. Tumors of nonhematopoietic origin may have surface receptors for filgrastim.

Allergic-type reactions have occurred in patients receiving the parent compound, filgrastim (G-CSF) with first or later doses. Reactions tended to occur more frequently with intravenous administration and within 30 minutes of infusion. Rare cases of splenic rupture or adult respiratory distress syndrome have been reported in association with filgrastim; patients must be instructed to report left upper quadrant pain or

(Continued)

Filgrastim *(Continued)*

shoulder tip pain or respiratory distress. Use caution in patients with sickle cell diseases; sickle cell crises have been reported following filgrastim therapy.

Adverse Reactions

>10%:
- Cardiovascular: Chest pain
- Central nervous system: Fever
- Dermatologic: Alopecia
- Endocrine & metabolic: Fluid retention
- Gastrointestinal: Nausea, vomiting, diarrhea, mucositis; splenomegaly - up to 33% of patients with cyclic neutropenia/congenital agranulocytosis receiving filgrastim for ≥14 days; rare in other patients
- Neuromuscular & skeletal: Bone pain (24%), commonly in the lower back, posterior iliac crest, and sternum

1% to 10%:
- Cardiovascular: S-T segment depression (3%)
- Central nervous system: Headache
- Dermatologic: Rash
- Gastrointestinal: Anorexia, constipation, sore throat
- Hematologic: Leukocytosis
- Local: Pain at injection site
- Neuromuscular & skeletal: Weakness
- Respiratory: Dyspnea, cough

<1%: Transient supraventricular arrhythmia, pericarditis, hypotension, thrombophlebitis, hypersensitivity reactions

Overdosage/Toxicology No clinical adverse effects have been seen with high doses producing ANC >10,000/mm^3.

Stability Intact vials and prefilled syringes should be stored under refrigeration at 2°C to 8°C (36°F to 46°F) and protected from direct sunlight. Filgrastim should be protected from freezing and temperatures >30°C to avoid aggregation. If inadvertently frozen, thaw in a refrigerator and use within 24 hours; do not use if frozen >24 hours or frozen more than once. The solution should not be shaken since bubbles and/or foam may form. If foaming occurs, the solution should be left undisturbed for a few minutes until bubbles dissipate.

Filgrastim vials and prefilled syringes are stable for 7 days at 9°C to 30°C (47°F to 86°F), however, the manufacturer recommends discarding after 24 hours because of microbiological concerns. The product is packaged without a preservative.

Undiluted filgrastim is stable for 24 hours at 15°C to 30°C and for 2 weeks at 2°C to 8°C (36°F to 46°F) in tuberculin syringes. However, the manufacturer recommends to use immediately because of concern for bacterial contamination.

Filgrastim may be diluted in dextrose 5% in water to a concentration ≥15 mcg/mL for I.V. infusion administration. Minimum concentration is 15 mcg/mL. This diluted solution is stable for 7 days at 2°C to 8°C (36°F to 46°F). Concentrations <15 mcg/mL require addition of albumin (1 mL of 5%) to the bag to prevent absorption to plastics/PVC.

Mechanism of Action Stimulates the production, maturation, and activation of neutrophils; filgrastim activates neutrophils to increase both their migration and cytotoxicity. See table.

Comparative Effects — Filgrastim vs GM-CSF

Proliferation/Differentiation	Filgrastim	GM-CSF (Sargramostim)
Neutrophils	Yes	Yes
Eosinophils	No	Yes
Macrophages	No	Yes
Neutrophil migration	Enhanced	Inhibited

Pharmacodynamics/Kinetics

- Onset of action: ~24 hours; plateaus in 3-5 days
- Duration: ANC decreases by 50% within 2 days after discontinuing filgrastim; white counts return to the normal range in 4-7 days; peak plasma levels can be maintained for up to 12 hours
- Absorption: SubQ: 100%
- Distribution: V_d: 150 mL/kg; no evidence of drug accumulation over a 11- to 20-day period
- Metabolism: Systemically degraded

Half-life elimination: 1.8-3.5 hours
Time to peak, serum: SubQ: 2-6 hours

Dosage Refer to individual protocols.

Dosing, even in morbidly obese patients, should be based on actual body weight. Rounding doses to the nearest vial size often enhances patient convenience and reduces costs without compromising clinical response.

Myelosuppressive therapy: 5 mcg/kg/day - doses may be increased by 5 mcg/kg according to the duration and severity of the neutropenia.

Bone marrow transplantation: 5-10 mcg/kg/day - doses may be increased by 5 mcg/kg according to the duration and severity of neutropenia; recommended steps based on neutrophil response:

When ANC >1000/mm^3 for 3 consecutive days: Reduce filgrastim dose to 5 mcg/kg/day

If ANC remains >1000/mm^3 for 3 more consecutive days: Discontinue filgrastim

If ANC decreases to <1000/mm^3: Resume at 5 mcg/kg/day

If ANC decreases <1000/mm^3 during the 5 mcg/kg/day dose, increase filgrastim to 10 mcg/kg/day and follow the above steps

Peripheral blood progenitor cell (PBPC) collection: 10 mcg/kg/day **or** 5-8 mcg/kg twice daily in donors. The optimal timing and duration of growth factor stimulation has not been determined.

Severe chronic neutropenia:
Congenital: 6 mcg/kg twice daily
Idiopathic/cyclic: 5 mcg/kg/day

Not removed by hemodialysis

Dietary Considerations Injection solution contains sodium 0.035 mg/mL and sorbitol.

Administration May be administered undiluted by SubQ or by I.V. infusion over 15-60 minutes in D_5W

Monitoring Parameters WBC should be monitored 7-10 days after beginning filgrastim, then every 7-10 days until WBC recovers. Leukocytosis (white blood cell counts ≥100,000/mm^3) has been observed in ~2% of patients receiving filgrastim at doses >5 mcg/kg/day.

Reference Range No clinical benefit seen with ANC >10,000/mm^3

Patient Information Follow directions for proper storage and administration of SubQ medication. Never reuse syringes or needles. You may experience bone pain (request analgesic); nausea or vomiting (small frequent meals may help); hair loss (reversible); or sore mouth (frequent mouth care with a soft toothbrush or cotton swab may help). Report unusual fever or chills; unhealed sores; severe bone pain; pain, redness, or swelling at injection site; unusual swelling of extremities or difficulty breathing; or chest pain and palpitations.

Additional Information

Reimbursement Hotline: 1-800-272-9376
Professional Services [Amgen]: 1-800-77-AMGEN

Dosage Forms

Injection, solution [preservative free]: 300 mcg/mL (1 mL, 1.6 mL) [vial; contains sodium 0.035 mg/mL and sorbitol]

Injection, solution [preservative free]: 600 mcg/mL (0.5 mL, 0.8 mL) [prefilled Singleject® syringe; contains sodium 0.035 mg/mL and sorbitol]

First® Testosterone *see* Testosterone *on page 1100*
First® Testosterone MC *see* Testosterone *on page 1100*
Flagyl® *see* Metronidazole *on page 940*
Flagyl ER® *see* Metronidazole *on page 940*
Flagyl® I.V. RTU™ *see* Metronidazole *on page 940*
Flamazine® (Can) *see* Silver Sulfadiazine *on page 1065*
Florazole® ER (Can) *see* Metronidazole *on page 940*
Floxin® *see* Ofloxacin *on page 977*
Floxin Otic Singles *see* Ofloxacin *on page 977*

Fluconazole (floo KOE na zole)

Related Information

USPHS / IDSA Guidelines for the Prevention of Opportunistic Infections in Persons Infected With HIV *on page 1237*

U.S. Brand Names Diflucan®

Canadian Brand Names Apo-Fluconazole®; Diflucan®; Fluconazole Omega; Gen-Fluconazole; Novo-Fluconazole

Generic Available Yes

(Continued)

Fluconazole *(Continued)*

Use Treatment of candidiasis (vaginal, oropharyngeal, esophageal, urinary tract infections, peritonitis, pneumonia, and systemic infections); cryptococcal meningitis; antifungal prophylaxis in allogeneic bone marrow transplant recipients

Drug of Choice or Alternative for Disease/Syndrome(s):

Balanitis *on page 48*
Endocarditis, Prosthetic Valve, Early *on page 124*
Endocarditis, Prosthetic Valve, Late *on page 125*
Esophagitis *on page 147*
Peritonitis, CAPD-Associated *on page 262*
Thrombophlebitis, Suppurative *on page 330*

Organism(s):

Blastomyces dermatitidis on page 50
Candida Species *on page 67*
Coccidioides immitis on page 91
Cryptococcus neoformans on page 102
Dematiaceous Fungi *on page 112*
Dermatophytes *on page 114*
Histoplasma capsulatum on page 177
Malassezia furfur on page 213
Prototheca Species *on page 280*

Pregnancy Risk Factor C

Pregnancy Implications When used in high doses, fluconazole is teratogenic in animal studies. Following exposure during the first trimester, case reports have noted similar malformations in humans when used in higher doses (400 mg/day) over extended periods of time. Use of lower doses (150 mg as a single dose or 200 mg/day) may have less risk; however, additional data is needed. Use during pregnancy only if the potential benefit to the mother outweighs any potential risk to the fetus.

Contraindications Hypersensitivity to fluconazole, other azoles, or any component of the formulation; concomitant administration with cisapride

Warnings/Precautions Should be used with caution in patients with renal and hepatic dysfunction or previous hepatotoxicity from other azole derivatives. Patients who develop abnormal liver function tests during fluconazole therapy should be monitored closely and discontinued if symptoms consistent with liver disease develop. Use caution in patients at risk of proarrhythmias.

Adverse Reactions Frequency not always defined.

Cardiovascular: Angioedema, pallor, QT prolongation, torsade de pointes
Central nervous system: Headache (2% to 13%), seizure, dizziness
Dermatologic: Rash (2%), alopecia, toxic epidermal necrolysis, Stevens-Johnson syndrome
Endocrine & metabolic: Hypercholesterolemia, hypertriglyceridemia, hypokalemia
Gastrointestinal: Nausea (4% to 7%), vomiting (2%), abdominal pain (2% to 6%), diarrhea (2% to 3%), taste perversion, dyspepsia
Hematologic: Agranulocytosis, leukopenia, neutropenia, thrombocytopenia
Hepatic: Hepatic failure (rare), hepatitis, cholestasis, jaundice, increased ALT/AST, increased alkaline phosphatase
Respiratory: Dyspnea
Miscellaneous: Anaphylactic reactions (rare)

Overdosage/Toxicology Symptoms include decreased lacrimation, salivation, respiration, GI motility, urinary incontinence, and cyanosis. Treatment includes supportive measures. A 3-hour hemodialysis will remove 50% of the drug.

Drug Interactions

Cytochrome P450 Effect: Inhibits CYP1A2 (weak), 2C8/9 (strong), 2C19 (strong), 3A4 (moderate)

Increased Effect/Toxicity: Concurrent use of fluconazole with cisapride is contraindicated due to the potential for malignant arrhythmias. Fluconazole may increase the levels/effects of amiodarone, selected benzodiazepines, calcium channel blockers, cisapride, citalopram, cyclosporine, diazepam, ergot derivatives, fluoxetine, glimepiride, glipizide, HMG-CoA reductase inhibitors, methsuximide, mirtazapine, nateglinide, nefazodone, phenytoin, pioglitazone, propranolol, rosiglitazone, sertraline, sildenafil (and other PDE-5 inhibitors), tacrolimus, venlafaxine, warfarin, and other substrates of CYP2C8/9, 2C19, and 3A4.

Decreased Effect: Rifampin decreases concentrations of fluconazole.

Stability

Powder for oral suspension: Store dry powder at ≤30°C (86°F). Following reconstitution, store at 5°C to 30°C (41°F to 86°F). Discard unused portion after 2 weeks. Do not freeze.

Injection: Store injection in glass at 5°C to 30°C (41°F to 86°F). Store injection in Viaflex® at 5°C to 25°C (41°F to 77°F). Protect from freezing. Do not unwrap unit until ready for use.

Mechanism of Action Interferes with cytochrome P450 activity, decreasing ergosterol synthesis (principal sterol in fungal cell membrane) and inhibiting cell membrane formation

Pharmacodynamics/Kinetics

Distribution: Widely throughout body with good penetration into CSF, eye, peritoneal fluid, sputum, skin, and urine

Relative diffusion blood into CSF: Adequate with or without inflammation (exceeds usual MICs)

CSF:blood level ratio: Normal meninges: 70% to 80%; Inflamed meninges: >70% to 80%

Protein binding, plasma: 11% to 12%

Bioavailability: Oral: >90%

Half-life elimination: Normal renal function: ~30 hours

Time to peak, serum: Oral: 1-2 hours

Excretion: Urine (80% as unchanged drug)

Dosage The daily dose of fluconazole is the same for oral and I.V. administration

Neonates: First 2 weeks of life, especially premature neonates: Same dose as older children every 72 hours

Children: Once-daily dosing by indication: See table on next page.

Adults: Oral, I.V.: **Note:** Susceptibility for *Candida* is divided into susceptible, susceptible-dose dependent (SDD), and resistant. Increased dose (up to 400 mg/day) may be used to treat SDD strains, especially when there has been treatment failure at lower doses.

Once-daily dosing by indication: See table below.

Dosing adjustment/interval in renal impairment:

No adjustment for vaginal candidiasis single-dose therapy

For multiple dosing, administer usual load then adjust daily doses

Fluconazole Once-Daily Dosing – Adults

Indication	Day 1	Daily Therapy	Minimum Duration of Therapy
Oropharyngeal candidiasis (OPC) (long-term suppression)	200 mg	200 mg	Chronic therapy in AIDS patients with history of OPC
Esophageal candidiasis	200 mg	100-200 mg	14-21 d after clinical improvement
Prevention of candidiasis in bone marrow transplant	400 mg	400 mg	3 d before neutropenia, 7 d after neutrophils >1000 cells/mm^3
Urinary candidiasis	--	200 mg	14 d
Candidemia, primary therapy, non-neutropenic	--	400-800 mg	14 d after last positive blood culture and resolution of signs/ symptoms
Candidemia, alternative therapy, non-neutropenic	--	800 mg with AmB for 4-7 d, followed by 800 mg/ day	14 d after last positive blood culture and resolution of signs/ symptoms
Candidemia, secondary, neutropenic	--	6-12 mg/kg/ day	14 d after last positive blood culture and resolution of signs/ symptoms
Cryptococcal meningitis consolidation (after induction with amphotericin plus flucytosine)	--	400 mg	10 wk
relapse suppression (maintenance)	--	200-400 mg	N/A
Vaginal candidiasis	150 mg	Single dose	N/A

N/A = not applicable. AmB = conventional deoxycholate amphotericin B.

(Continued)

Fluconazole *(Continued)*

Fluconazole Once-Daily Dosing – Children

Indication	Day 1	Daily Therapy	Minimum Duration of Therapy
Oropharyngeal candidiasis	6 mg/kg	3 mg/kg	14 d
Esophageal candidiasis	6 mg/kg	3-12 mg/kg	21 d and for at least 2 wk following resolution of symptoms
Systemic candidiasis	—	6 mg/kg every 12 hours	28 d
Cryptococcal meningitis acute	12 mg/kg	6-12 mg/kg	10-12 wk after CSF culture becomes negative
relapse suppression	6 mg/kg	6 mg/kg	N/A

N/A = Not applicable.

Cl_{cr} ≤50 mL/minute (no dialysis): Administer 50% of recommended dose or administer every 48 hours.

Hemodialysis: 50% is removed by hemodialysis; administer 100% of daily dose (according to indication) after each dialysis treatment.

Continuous arteriovenous or venovenous hemofiltration: Dose as for Cl_{cr} 10-50 mL/minute.

Dietary Considerations Take with or without regard to food.

Administration Parenteral fluconazole must be administered by I.V. infusion over approximately 1-2 hours; do not exceed 200 mg/hour when giving I.V. infusion

Monitoring Parameters Periodic liver function tests (AST, ALT, alkaline phosphatase) and renal function tests, potassium

Patient Information May take with food; take entire course of medication; report if side effects develop

Dosage Forms

Infusion [premixed in sodium chloride]: 2 mg/mL (100 mL, 200 mL)

Diflucan® [premixed in sodium chloride or dextrose] 2 mg/mL (100 mL, 200 mL)

Powder for oral suspension (Diflucan®): 10 mg/mL (35 mL); 40 mg/mL (35 mL) [contains sodium benzoate; orange flavor]

Tablet (Diflucan®): 50 mg, 100 mg, 150 mg, 200 mg

Selected Readings

Amichai B and Grunwald MH, "Adverse Drug Reactions of the New Oral Antifungal Agents - Terbinafine, Fluconazole, and Itraconazole," *Int J Dermatol*, 1998, 37(6):410-5.

Como JA and Dismukes WE, "Oral Azole Drugs as Systemic Antifungal Therapy," *N Engl J Med*, 1993, 330(4):263-72.

Goa KL and Barradell LB, "Fluconazole. An Update of Its Pharmacodynamic and Pharmacokinetic Properties and Therapeutic Use in Major Superficial and Systemic Mycoses in Immunocompromised Patients," *Drugs*, 1995, 50(4):658-90.

Kauffman CA and Carver PL, "Antifungal Agents in the 1990s. Current Status and Future Developments," *Drugs*, 1997, 53(4):539-49.

Kowalsky SF and Dixon DM, "Fluconazole: A New Antifungal Agent," *Clin Pharm*, 1991, 10(3):179-94.

Lyman CA and Walsh TJ, "Systemically Administered Antifungal Agents. A Review of Their Clinical Pharmacology and Therapeutic Applications," *Drugs*, 1992, 44(1):9-35.

Perry CM, Whittington R, and McTavish D, "Fluconazole. An Update of Its Antimicrobial Activity, Pharmacokinetic Properties, and Therapeutic Use in Vaginal Candidiasis," *Drugs*, 1995, 49(6):984-1006.

Terrell CL, "Antifungal Agents. Part II. The Azoles," *Mayo Clin Proc*, 1999, 74(1):78-100.

Trepanier EF and Amsden GW, "Current Issues in Onchomycosis," *Ann Pharmacother*, 1998, 32(2):204-14.

Fluconazole Omega (Can) *see* Fluconazole *on page 819*

Flucytosine (floo SYE toe seen)

U.S. Brand Names Ancobon®

Canadian Brand Names Ancobon®

Synonyms 5-FC; 5-Fluorocytosine

Generic Available No

Use Adjunctive treatment of susceptible fungal infections (usually *Candida* or *Cryptococcus*); synergy with amphotericin B for certain fungal infections (*Cryptococcus* spp., *Candida* spp.)

Drug of Choice or Alternative for Organism(s):

Candida Species *on page 67*

Cryptococcus neoformans on page 102

Dematiaceous Fungi *on page 112*

Pregnancy Risk Factor C

Pregnancy Implications Teratogenic in some animal studies, however, there are no adequate and well-controlled studies in pregnant women.

Contraindications Hypersensitivity to flucytosine or any component of the formulation

Warnings/Precautions Use with extreme caution in patients with renal dysfunction; dosage adjustment required. Avoid use as monotherapy; resistance rapidly develops. Use with caution in patients with bone marrow depression; patients with hematologic disease or who have been treated with radiation or drugs that suppress the bone marrow may be at greatest risk. Bone marrow toxicity can be irreversible.

Adverse Reactions Frequency not defined.

Cardiovascular: Cardiac arrest, myocardial toxicity, ventricular dysfunction, chest pain
Central nervous system: Confusion, headache, hallucinations, dizziness, drowsiness, psychosis, parkinsonism, ataxia, sedation, pyrexia, seizure, fatigue
Dermatologic: Rash, photosensitivity, pruritus, urticaria, Lyell's syndrome
Endocrine & metabolic: Temporary growth failure, hypoglycemia, hypokalemia
Gastrointestinal: Nausea, vomiting, diarrhea, abdominal pain, loss of appetite, dry mouth, hemorrhage, ulcerative colitis
Hematologic: Bone marrow suppression, anemia, leukopenia, thrombocytopenia, agranulocytosis, aplastic anemia, eosinophilia, pancytopenia
Hepatic: Liver enzymes increased, hepatitis, jaundice, azotemia, bilirubin increased
Neuromuscular & skeletal: Peripheral neuropathy, paresthesia, weakness
Otic: Hearing loss
Renal: BUN and serum creatinine increased, renal failure, azotemia, crystalluria
Respiratory: Respiratory arrest, dyspnea
Miscellaneous: Anaphylaxis, allergic reaction

Overdosage/Toxicology Symptoms include nausea, vomiting, diarrhea, hepatitis, and bone marrow suppression. Treatment is supportive. Removed by hemodialysis.

Drug Interactions

Increased Effect/Toxicity: Increased effect with amphotericin B. Amphotericin B-induced renal dysfunction may predispose patient to flucytosine accumulation and myelosuppression.

Decreased Effect: Cytarabine may inactivate flucytosine activity.

Ethanol/Nutrition/Herb Interactions Food: Food decreases the rate, but not the extent of absorption.

Stability Store at 25°C (77°F); protect from light

Mechanism of Action Penetrates fungal cells and is converted to fluorouracil which competes with uracil interfering with fungal RNA and protein synthesis

Pharmacodynamics/Kinetics

Absorption: 75% to 90%
Distribution: Into CSF, aqueous humor, joints, peritoneal fluid, and bronchial secretions; V_d: 0.6 L/kg
Protein binding: 2% to 4%
Metabolism: Minimally hepatic; deaminated, possibly via gut bacteria, to 5-fluorouracil
Half-life elimination:
- Normal renal function: 2-5 hours
- Anuria: 85 hours (range: 30-250)
- End stage renal disease: 75-200 hours

Time to peak, serum: ~2-6 hours
Excretion: Urine (>90% as unchanged drug)

Dosage Children and Adults: Oral: 50-150 mg/kg/day in divided doses every 6 hours

Dosing interval in renal impairment: Use lower initial dose:
- Cl_{cr} 20-40 mL/minute: Administer every 12 hours
- Cl_{cr} 10-20 mL/minute: Administer every 24 hours
- Cl_{cr} <10 mL/minute: Administer every 24-48 hours

Hemodialysis: Dialyzable (50% to 100%); administer dose posthemodialysis
Peritoneal dialysis: Adults: Administer 0.5-1 g every 24 hours
Continuous arteriovenous or venovenous hemodiafiltration effects: Dose as for Cl_{cr} 10-50 mL/minute

Administration Administer around-the-clock to promote less variation in peak and trough serum levels. To avoid nausea and vomiting, administer a few capsules at a time over 15 minutes until full dose is taken.

Monitoring Parameters

Pretreatment: Electrolytes, CBC, BUN, renal function, blood culture
During treatment: CBC and LFTs frequently, serum flucytosine concentration, renal function

Reference Range

Therapeutic: 25-100 mcg/mL (peak) (SI: 195-775 μmol/L); peak levels should not exceed 100-120 mcg/mL to avoid toxic bone marrow depressive effects
Trough: Draw just prior to dose administration
(Continued)

Flucytosine *(Continued)*

Peak: Draw 2 hours after an oral dose administration

Test Interactions Flucytosine causes markedly false elevations in serum creatinine values when the Ektachem® analyzer is used

Patient Information Take capsules a few at a time with food over a 15-minute period to avoid nausea

Dosage Forms Capsule: 250 mg, 500 mg

Extemporaneous Preparations Flucytosine oral liquid has been prepared by using the contents of ten 500 mg capsules triturated in a mortar and pestle with a small amount of distilled water; the mixture was transferred to a 500 mL volumetric flask; the mortar was rinsed several times with a small amount of distilled water and the fluid added to the flask; sufficient distilled water was added to make a total volume of 500 mL of a 10 mg/mL liquid; oral liquid was stable for 70 days when stored in glass or plastic prescription bottles at 4°C or for up to 14 days at room temperature.

Wintermeyer SM and Nahata MC, "Stability of Flucytosine in an Extemporaneously Compounded Oral Liquid," *Am J Health Syst Pharm*, 1996, 53:407-9.

Selected Readings

Lyman CA and Walsh TJ, "Systemically Administered Antifungal Agents. A Review of Their Clinical Pharmacology and Therapeutic Applications," *Drugs*, 1992, 44(1):9-35.

Patel R, "Antifungal Agents. Part I. Amphotericin B Preparations and Flucytosine," *Mayo Clin Proc*, 1998, 73(12):1205-25.

Wintermeyer SM and Nahata MC, "Stability of Flucytosine in an Extemporaneously Compounded Oral Liquid," *Am J Health Syst Pharm*, 1996, 53:407-9.

Flumadine® *see* Rimantadine *on page 1054*

FluMist® *see* Influenza Virus Vaccine *on page 875*

Fluorometholone and Sulfacetamide *see* Sulfacetamide Sodium and Fluorometholone *on page 1083*

Fluoroquinolones

Refer to

Ciprofloxacin *on page 742*
Gatifloxacin *on page 837*
Gemifloxacin *on page 840*
Levofloxacin *on page 908*
Lomefloxacin *on page 917*
Moxifloxacin *on page 949*
Nalidixic Acid *on page 957*
Norfloxacin *on page 973*
Ofloxacin *on page 977*
Sparfloxacin *on page 1073*
Trovafloxacin *on page 1134*

Drug of Choice or Alternative for Disease/Syndrome(s):

Bronchitis *on page 60*
Catheter Infection, Intravascular *on page 70*
Diverticulitis *on page 116*
Endometritis *on page 127*
Epididymitis/Orchitis *on page 138*
Intra-abdominal Abscess *on page 194*
Keratitis, Bacterial and Fungal *on page 199*
Osteomyelitis, Diabetic Foot *on page 249*
Osteomyelitis, Healthy Adult *on page 250*
Pelvic Inflammatory Disease *on page 260*
Peritonitis, Secondary *on page 263*
Pneumonia, Community-Acquired *on page 270*
Prostatitis *on page 277*
Sinusitis, Community-Acquired, Acute *on page 299*
Urinary Tract Infection, Pyelonephritis *on page 346*
Urinary Tract Infection, Uncomplicated *on page 346*

Organism(s):

Aeromonas Species *on page 30*
Alcaligenes Species *on page 31*
Bordetella bronchiseptica on page 52
Campylobacter jejuni on page 66
Chlamydophila pneumoniae on page 78
Citrobacter Species *on page 81*
Coxiella burnetii on page 100
Enterobacter Species *on page 132*
Escherichia coli on page 142

Haemophilus influenzae on page 159
Klebsiella Species *on page 200*
Legionella pneumophila on page 202
Moraxella catarrhalis on page 223
Mycoplasma hominis and *Mycoplasma genitalium on page 237*
Mycoplasma pneumoniae on page 238
Neisseria meningitidis on page 245
Proteus Species *on page 278*
Pseudomonas aeruginosa on page 282
Serratia Species *on page 296*
Shigella Species *on page 297*
Staphylococcus saprophyticus on page 312
Stenotrophomonas maltophilia on page 312

Fluoxymesterone (floo oks i MES te rone)

Related Information
AIDS Wasting Treatment *on page 1205*

U.S. Brand Names Halotestin®

Canadian Brand Names Halotestin®

Generic Available Yes

Use Replacement of endogenous testicular hormone; in females, used as palliative treatment of breast cancer

Unlabeled/Investigational Use Stimulation of erythropoiesis, angioneurotic edema

Restrictions C-III

Pregnancy Risk Factor X

Contraindications Hypersensitivity to fluoxymesterone or any component of the formulation; serious cardiac disease, liver or kidney disease; pregnancy

Warnings/Precautions May accelerate bone maturation without producing compensatory gain in linear growth in children; in prepubertal children perform radiographic examination of the hand and wrist every 6 months to determine the rate of bone maturation and to assess the effect of treatment on the epiphyseal centers

Adverse Reactions

>10%:
- Male: Priapism
- Female: Menstrual problems (amenorrhea), virilism, breast soreness
- Cardiovascular: Edema
- Dermatologic: Acne

1% to 10%:
- Male: Prostatic carcinoma, hirsutism (increase in pubic hair growth), impotence, testicular atrophy
- Cardiovascular: Edema
- Gastrointestinal: GI irritation, nausea, vomiting
- Genitourinary: Prostatic hyperplasia
- Hepatic: Hepatic dysfunction

<1%:
- Male: Gynecomastia
- Female: Amenorrhea
- Hypercalcemia, leukopenia, polycythemia, hepatic necrosis, cholestatic hepatitis, hypersensitivity reactions

Overdosage/Toxicology Symptoms include abnormal liver function tests and water retention.

Drug Interactions

Increased Effect/Toxicity: Fluoxymesterone may suppress clotting factors II, V, VII, and X; therefore, bleeding may occur in patients on anticoagulant therapy May elevate cyclosporine serum levels. May enhance hypoglycemic effect of insulin therapy; may decrease blood glucose concentrations and insulin requirements in patients with diabetes. Lithium may potentiate EPS and other CNS effect. May potentiate the effects of narcotics including respiratory depression

Decreased Effect: May decrease barbiturate levels and fluphenazine effectiveness.

Stability Protect from light

Mechanism of Action Synthetic androgenic anabolic hormone responsible for the normal growth and development of male sex hormones and development of male sex organs and maintenance of secondary sex characteristics; synthetic testosterone derivative with significant androgen activity; stimulates RNA polymerase activity resulting in an increase in protein production; increases bone development; halogenated derivative of testosterone with up to 5 times the activity of methyltestosterone

Pharmacodynamics/Kinetics

Absorption: Rapid

(Continued)

Fluoxymesterone *(Continued)*

Protein binding: 98%
Metabolism: Hepatic; enterohepatic recirculation
Half-life elimination: 10-100 minutes
Excretion: Urine (90%)

Dosage Adults: Oral:
Male:
Hypogonadism: 5-20 mg/day
Delayed puberty: 2.5-20 mg/day for 4-6 months
Female: Inoperable breast carcinoma: 10-40 mg/day in divided doses for 1-3 months

Monitoring Parameters In prepubertal children, perform radiographic examination of the hand and wrist every 6 months

Test Interactions Decreased levels of thyroxine-binding globulin; decreased total T_4 serum levels; increased resin uptake of T_3 and T_4

Patient Information Take as directed; do not discontinue without consulting prescriber. Diabetics should monitor serum glucose closely and notify prescriber of changes; this medication can alter hypoglycemic requirements. You may experience acne, growth of body hair, loss of libido, impotence, or menstrual irregularity (usually reversible); nausea or vomiting (small frequent meals, frequent mouth care, sucking lozenges, or chewing gum may help). Report changes in menstrual pattern; deepening of voice or unusual growth of body hair; fluid retention (swelling of ankles, feet, or hands, difficulty breathing, or sudden weight gain); change in color of urine or stool; yellowing of eyes or skin; unusual bruising or bleeding; or other adverse reactions.

Dosage Forms [DSC] = Discontinued product
Tablet: 10 mg
Halotestin®: 2 mg, 5 mg, 10 mg [contains tartrazine; 10 mg tablet DSC]

5-Fluorocytosine *see* Flucytosine *on page 822*
Fluviral S/F® (Can) *see* Influenza Virus Vaccine *on page 875*
Fluvirin® *see* Influenza Virus Vaccine *on page 875*
Fluzone® *see* Influenza Virus Vaccine *on page 875*
FML-S® *see* Sulfacetamide Sodium and Fluorometholone *on page 1083*

Fomivirsen (foe MI vir sen)

Related Information
USPHS / IDSA Guidelines for the Prevention of Opportunistic Infections in Persons Infected With HIV *on page 1237*

U.S. Brand Names Vitravene™ [DSC]

Canadian Brand Names Vitravene™

Synonyms Fomivirsen Sodium

Generic Available No

Use Local treatment of cytomegalovirus (CMV) retinitis in patients with acquired immunodeficiency syndrome who are intolerant or insufficiently responsive to other treatments for CMV retinitis or when other treatments for CMV retinitis are contraindicated

Drug of Choice or Alternative for Organism(s):
Cytomegalovirus *on page 107*

Pregnancy Implications Studies have not been conducted in pregnant women. Should be used in pregnancy only when potential benefit to the mother outweighs the potential risk to the fetus.

Contraindications Hypersensitivity to fomivirsen or any component

Warnings/Precautions For ophthalmic use via intravitreal injection only. Uveitis occurs frequently, particularly during induction dosing. Do not use in patients who have received intravenous or intravitreal cidofovir within 2-4 weeks (risk of exaggerated inflammation is increased). Patients should be monitored for CMV disease in the contralateral eye and/or extraocular disease. Commonly increases intraocular pressure - monitoring is recommended.

Adverse Reactions
5% to 10%:
Central nervous system: Fever, headache
Gastrointestinal: Abdominal pain, diarrhea, nausea, vomiting
Hematologic: Anemia
Neuromuscular & skeletal: Asthenia
Ocular: Uveitis, abnormal vision, anterior chamber inflammation, blurred vision, cataract, conjunctival hemorrhage, decreased visual acuity, loss of color vision, eye pain, increased intraocular pressure, photophobia, retinal detachment, retinal edema, retinal hemorrhage, retinal pigment changes, vitreitis
Respiratory: Pneumonia, sinusitis

Miscellaneous: Systemic CMV, sepsis, infection

2% to 5%:

Cardiovascular: Chest pain

Central nervous system: Confusion, depression, dizziness, neuropathy, pain

Endocrine & metabolic: Dehydration

Gastrointestinal: Abnormal LFTs, pancreatitis, anorexia, weight loss

Hematologic: Thrombocytopenia, lymphoma

Neuromuscular & skeletal: Back pain, cachexia

Ocular: Application site reaction, conjunctival hyperemia, conjunctivitis, corneal edema, decreased peripheral vision, eye irritation, keratic precipitates, optic neuritis, photopsia, retinal vascular disease, visual field defect, vitreous hemorrhage, vitreous opacity

Renal: Kidney failure

Respiratory: Bronchitis, dyspnea, cough

Miscellaneous: Allergic reaction, flu-like syndrome, diaphoresis (increased)

Stability Store between 2°C to 25°C (35°F to 77°F); protect from excessive heat or light

Mechanism of Action Inhibits synthesis of viral protein by binding to mRNA which blocks replication of cytomegalovirus through an antisense mechanism

Pharmacodynamics/Kinetics Pharmacokinetic studies have not been conducted in humans. In animal models, the drug is cleared from the eye after 7-10 days. It is metabolized by sequential nucleotide removal, with a small amount of the radioactivity from a dose appearing in the urine.

Dosage Adults: Intravitreal injection: Induction: 330 mcg (0.05 mL) every other week for 2 doses, followed by maintenance dose of 330 mcg (0.05 mL) every 4 weeks

If progression occurs during maintenance, a repeat of the induction regimen may be attempted to establish resumed control. Unacceptable inflammation during therapy may be managed by temporary interruption, provided response has been established. Topical corticosteroids have been used to reduce inflammation.

Administration Administered by intravitreal injection following application of standard topical and/or local anesthetics and antibiotics.

Monitoring Parameters Immediately after injection, light perception and optic nerve head perfusion should be monitored. Anterior chamber paracentesis may be necessary if perfusion is not complete within 7-10 minutes after injection. Subsequent patient evaluation should include monitoring for contralateral CMV infection or extraocular CMV disease, and intraocular pressure prior to each injection.

Additional Information Because the mechanism of action of fomivirsen is different than other antiviral agents active against CMV, fomivirsen may be active against isolates resistant to ganciclovir, foscarnet, or cidofovir. The converse may also be true.

Dosage Forms [DSC] = Discontinued product

Injection, solution, intravitreal, as sodium: 6.6 mg/mL (0.25 mL) [DSC]

Selected Readings

Leeds JM, Henry SP, Bistner S, et al, "Pharmacokinetics of an Antisense Oligonucleotide Injected Intravitreally in Monkeys," *Drug Metab Dispos*, 1998, 26(7):670-5.

Leeds JM, Henry SP, Truong L, et al, "Pharmacokinetics of a Potential Human Cytomegalovirus Therapeutic, a Phosphorothioate Oligonucleotide, After Intravitreal Injection in the Rabbit," *Drug Metab Dispos*, 1997, 25(8):921-6.

Fomivirsen Sodium *see* Fomivirsen *on page 826*

Fortaz® *see* Ceftazidime *on page 717*

Fortovase® [DSC] *see* Saquinavir *on page 1060*

Fosamprenavir (FOS am pren a veer)

Related Information

Antiretroviral Agents *on page 1206*

Antiretroviral Therapy for HIV Infection *on page 1219*

U.S. Brand Names Lexiva™

Canadian Brand Names Telzir®

Synonyms Fosamprenavir Calcium; GW433908G

Generic Available No

Use Treatment of HIV infections in combination with at least two other antiretroviral agents

Drug of Choice or Alternative for Organism(s):

Human Immunodeficiency Virus *on page 181*

Pregnancy Risk Factor C

Pregnancy Implications It is not known if amprenavir crosses the human placenta and there are no clinical studies currently underway to evaluate its use in pregnant women. Pregnancy and protease inhibitors are both associated with an increased risk

(Continued)

Fosamprenavir *(Continued)*

of hyperglycemia. Glucose levels should be closely monitored. Health professionals are encouraged to contact the antiretroviral pregnancy registry to monitor outcomes of pregnant women exposed to antiretroviral medications (1-800-258-4263 or www.APRegistry.com).

Contraindications Hypersensitivity to amprenavir or any component of the formulation; concurrent therapy with cisapride, ergot derivatives, midazolam, pimozide, and triazolam; severe previous allergic reaction to sulfonamides

Warnings/Precautions Because of hepatic metabolism and effect on cytochrome P450 enzymes, amprenavir should be used with caution in combination with other agents metabolized by this system (see Contraindications and Drug Interactions). Avoid concurrent administration of lovastatin or simvastatin (may increase the risk of rhabdomyolysis). Avoid use of hormonal contraceptives, rifampin, and/or St John's wort (may lead to loss of virologic response and/or resistance). Use with caution in patients with diabetes mellitus, sulfonamide allergy, hepatic impairment, or hemophilia. Redistribution of fat may occur (eg, buffalo hump, peripheral wasting, cushingoid appearance). Dosage adjustment is required for combination therapies (ritonavir and/or efavirenz); in addition, the risk of hyperlipidemia may be increased during concurrent therapy. Discontinue therapy in severe or dermatologic reactions or when a moderate rash is accompanied by systemic symptoms.

Adverse Reactions

>10%:

- Central nervous system: Headache (19% to 21%), fatigue (10% to 18%)
- Dermatologic: Rash (17% to 35%; moderate to severe reactions 3% to 8%)
- Gastrointestinal: Nausea (37% to 39%), diarrhea (34% to 52%), vomiting (16% to 20%), abdominal pain (5% to 11%)

1% to 10%:

- Central nervous system: Depression (8%), fatigue, headache, paresthesia
- Dermatologic: Pruritus (3% to 8%)
- Endocrine & metabolic: Hypertriglyceridemia (0% to 11%), serum lipase increased (6% to 8%), hyperglycemia (<1% to 2%)
- Hematologic: Neutropenia (3%)
- Hepatic: Transaminases increased (4% to 8%)
- Miscellaneous: Perioral tingling/numbness (2% to 10%)

<1% (Limited to important or life-threatening): Stevens-Johnson syndrome

Drug Interactions

Cytochrome P450 Effect: As amprenavir: **Substrate** of CYP2C8/9 (minor), 3A4 (major); **Inhibits** CYP2C19 (weak), 3A4 (strong)

Increased Effect/Toxicity: Concurrent use of cisapride, midazolam, pimozide, quinidine, or triazolam is contraindicated. Concurrent use of ergot alkaloids (dihydroergotamine, ergotamine, ergonovine, methylergonovine) with amprenavir is also contraindicated (may cause vasospasm and peripheral ischemia). Concurrent use of oral solution with disulfiram or metronidazole is contraindicated, due to the risk of propylene glycol toxicity.

Serum concentrations of amiodarone, bepridil, lidocaine, quinidine and other antiarrhythmics may be increased, potentially leading to toxicity; when amprenavir is coadministered with ritonavir, flecainide and propafenone are contraindicated. HMG-CoA reductase inhibitors serum concentrations may be increased by amprenavir, increasing the risk of myopathy/rhabdomyolysis; lovastatin and simvastatin are not recommended; fluvastatin and pravastatin may be safer alternatives.

Amprenavir may increase the levels/effects of selected benzodiazepines (midazolam and triazolam are contraindicated), calcium channel blockers, cyclosporine, mirtazapine, nateglinide, nefazodone, quinidine, sildenafil (and other PDE-5 inhibitors), tacrolimus, venlafaxine, and other CYP3A4 substrates. When used with strong CYP3A4 inhibitors, dosage adjustment/limits are recommended for sildenafil and other PDE-5 inhibitors; refer to individual monographs.

Concurrent therapy with ritonavir may result in increased serum concentrations: dosage adjustment is recommended. Clarithromycin, indinavir, nelfinavir may increase serum concentrations of amprenavir.

Decreased Effect: CYP3A4 inducers may decrease the levels/effects of amprenavir; example inducers include aminoglutethimide, carbamazepine, nafcillin, nevirapine, phenobarbital, phenytoin, and rifamycins. The administration of didanosine (buffered formulation) should be separated from amprenavir by 1 hour to limit interaction between formulations. Serum concentrations of estrogen (oral contraceptives) may be decreased, use alternative (nonhormonal) forms of contraception. Dexamethasone may decrease the therapeutic effect of amprenavir. Serum concentrations of delavirdine may be decreased; may lead to loss of virologic response and possible resistance to delavirdine; concomitant use is not

recommended. Efavirenz and nevirapine may decrease serum concentrations of amprenavir (dosing for combinations not established). Avoid St John's wort (may lead to subtherapeutic concentrations of amprenavir). Effect of amprenavir may be diminished when administered with methadone (consider alternative antiretroviral); in addition, effect of methadone may be reduced (dosage increase may be required).

Ethanol/Nutrition/Herb Interactions Herb/Nutraceutical: Amprenavir serum concentration may be decreased by St John's wort; avoid concurrent use.

Stability Store at 25°C (77°F); excursions permitted to 15°C to 30°C (59°F to 86°F).

Mechanism of Action Fosamprenavir is rapidly and almost completely converted to amprenavir *in vivo*. Amprenavir binds to the protease activity site and inhibits the activity of the enzyme. HIV protease is required for the cleavage of viral polyprotein precursors into individual functional proteins found in infectious HIV. Inhibition prevents cleavage of these polyproteins, resulting in the formation of immature, noninfectious viral particles.

Pharmacodynamics/Kinetics

Absorption: 63%

Bioavailability: Not established; food does not have a significant effect on absorption

Protein-binding: 90%

Half-Life elimination: 7.7 hours

Time to peak, plasma: 1.5-4 hours

Metabolism: Fosamprenavir is rapidly and almost completely converted to amprenavir by cellular phosphatases; amprenavir is hepatically metabolized via CYP isoenzymes (primarily CYP3A4)

Excretion: Feces (75%); urine (14% as metabolites; <1% as unchanged drug)

Dosage Oral: Adults: HIV infection:

Antiretroviral therapy-naive patients:

Unboosted regimen: 1400 mg twice daily (without ritonavir)

Ritonavir-boosted regimens:

Once-daily regimen: Fosamprenavir 1400 mg plus ritonavir 200 mg once daily

Twice-daily regimen: Fosamprenavir 700 mg plus ritonavir 100 mg twice daily. **Note:** Also used in protease inhibitor-experienced patients

Protease inhibitor-experienced patients: Fosamprenavir 700 mg plus ritonavir 100 mg twice daily. **Note:** Once-daily administration is not recommended in protease inhibitor-experienced patients.

Combination therapy with efavirenz (ritonavir-boosted regimen):

Once-daily regimen: Fosamprenavir 1400 mg daily plus ritonavir 300 mg once daily

Twice-daily regimen: No dosage adjustment recommended for twice-daily regimen

Dosage adjustment in renal impairment: No dosage adjustment required.

Dosage adjustment in hepatic impairment:

Mild-to-moderate impairment (Child-Pugh score 5-8): Reduce dosage of fosamprenavir to 700 mg twice daily (without concurrent ritonavir)

Severe impairment: Use is not recommended

Note: No recommendations are available for dosage adjustment in patients receiving ritonavir and fosamprenavir.

Dietary Considerations May be taken with or without food.

Dosage Forms Tablet, as calcium: 700 mg

Fosamprenavir Calcium *see* Fosamprenavir *on page 827*

Foscarnet (fos KAR net)

U.S. Brand Names Foscavir®

Canadian Brand Names Foscavir®

Synonyms PFA; Phosphonoformate; Phosphonoformic Acid

Generic Available No

Use

Treatment of herpes virus infections suspected to be caused by acyclovir-resistant (HSV, VZV) or ganciclovir-resistant (CMV) strains; this occurs almost exclusively in immunocompromised persons (eg, with advanced AIDS) who have received prolonged treatment for a herpes virus infection

Treatment of CMV retinitis in persons with AIDS

Unlabeled/Investigational Use Other CMV infections in persons unable to tolerate ganciclovir; may be given in combination with ganciclovir in patients who relapse after monotherapy with either drug

Drug of Choice or Alternative for

Disease/Syndrome(s):

Esophagitis *on page 147*

Organism(s):

Cytomegalovirus *on page 107*

(Continued)

Foscarnet *(Continued)*

Herpes Simplex Virus *on page 172*

Pregnancy Risk Factor C

Contraindications Hypersensitivity to foscarnet or any component of the formulation; Cl_{cr} <0.4 mL/minute/kg during therapy

Warnings/Precautions Renal impairment occurs to some degree in the majority of patients treated with foscarnet; renal impairment may occur at any time and is usually reversible within 1 week following dose adjustment or discontinuation of therapy, however, several patients have died with renal failure within 4 weeks of stopping foscarnet; therefore, renal function should be closely monitored. Foscarnet is deposited in teeth and bone of young, growing animals; it has adversely affected tooth enamel development in rats; safety and effectiveness in children have not been studied. Imbalance of serum electrolytes or minerals occurs in 6% to 18% of patients (hypocalcemia, low ionized calcium, hypo- or hyperphosphatemia, hypomagnesemia or hypokalemia).

Patients with a low ionized calcium may experience perioral tingling, numbness, paresthesias, tetany, and seizures. Seizures have been experienced by up to 10% of AIDS patients. Risk factors for seizures include a low baseline absolute neutrophil count (ANC), impaired baseline renal function and low total serum calcium. Some patients who have experienced seizures have died, while others have been able to continue or resume foscarnet treatment after their mineral or electrolyte abnormality has been corrected, their underlying disease state treated, or their dose decreased. Foscarnet has been shown to be mutagenic *in vitro* and in mice at very high doses. Information on the use of foscarnet is lacking in the elderly; dose adjustments and proper monitoring must be performed because of the decreased renal function common in older patients.

Adverse Reactions

>10%:
- Central nervous system: Fever (65%), headache (26%), seizure (10%)
- Gastrointestinal: Nausea (47%), diarrhea (30%), vomiting
- Hematologic: Anemia (33%)
- Renal: Abnormal renal function/decreased creatinine clearance (27%)

1% to 10%:
- Central nervous system: Fatigue, malaise, dizziness, hypoesthesia, depression/confusion/anxiety (≥5%)
- Dermatologic: Rash
- Endocrine & metabolic: Electrolyte imbalance (especially potassium, calcium, magnesium, and phosphorus)
- Gastrointestinal: Anorexia
- Hematologic: Granulocytopenia, leukopenia (≥5%), thrombocytopenia, thrombosis
- Local: Injection site pain
- Neuromuscular & skeletal: Paresthesia, involuntary muscle contractions, rigors, neuropathy (peripheral), weakness
- Ocular: Vision abnormalities
- Respiratory: Coughing, dyspnea (≥5%)
- Miscellaneous: Sepsis, diaphoresis (increased)

<1%: Cardiac failure, bradycardia, arrhythmia, cerebral edema, leg edema, peripheral edema, syncope, substernal chest pain, hypothermia, abnormal crying, malignant hyperpyrexia, vertigo, coma, speech disorders, gynecomastia, decreased gonadotropins, cholecystitis, cholelithiasis, hepatitis, hepatosplenomegaly, ascites, abnormal gait, dyskinesia, hypertonia, nystagmus, vocal cord paralysis

Overdosage/Toxicology Symptoms include seizures, renal dysfunction, perioral or limb paresthesias, and hypocalcemia. Treatment is supportive. Administer I.V. calcium salts for hypocalcemia.

Drug Interactions

Increased Effect/Toxicity: Concurrent use with ciprofloxacin (or other fluoroquinolone) increases seizure potential. Acute renal failure (reversible) has been reported with cyclosporine due most likely to a synergistic toxic effect. Nephrotoxic drugs (amphotericin B, I.V. pentamidine, aminoglycosides, etc) should be avoided, if possible, to minimize additive renal risk with foscarnet. Concurrent use of pentamidine also increases the potential for hypocalcemia. Protease inhibitors (ritonavir, saquinavir) have been associated with an increased risk of renal impairment during concurrent use of foscarnet

Stability

Foscarnet injection is a clear, colorless solution; it should be stored at room temperature and protected from temperatures >40°C and from freezing

Foscarnet should be diluted in D_5W or NS and transferred to PVC containers; stable for 24 hours at room temperature or refrigeration

For peripheral line administration, foscarnet **must** be diluted to 12 mg/mL with D_5W or NS

For central line administration, foscarnet may be administered undiluted

Incompatible with dextrose 30%, I.V. solutions containing calcium, magnesium, vancomycin, TPN

Mechanism of Action Pyrophosphate analogue which acts as a noncompetitive inhibitor of many viral RNA and DNA polymerases as well as HIV reverse transcriptase. Similar to ganciclovir, foscarnet is a virostatic agent. Foscarnet does not require activation by thymidine kinase.

Pharmacodynamics/Kinetics

Distribution: Up to 28% of cumulative I.V. dose may be deposited in bone

Metabolism: Biotransformation does not occur

Half-life elimination: ~3 hours

Excretion: Urine (≤28% as unchanged drug)

Dosage

CMV retinitis: I.V.:

Induction treatment: 60 mg/kg/dose every 8 hours **or** 100 mg/kg every 12 hours for 14-21 days

Maintenance therapy: 90-120 mg/kg/day as a single infusion

Herpes simplex infections (acyclovir-resistant): Induction: I.V.: 40 mg/kg/dose every 8-12 hours for 14-21 days

Dosage adjustment in renal impairment:

Induction and maintenance dosing schedules based on creatinine clearance (mL/minute/kg): See tables.

Induction Dosing of Foscarnet in Patients With Abnormal Renal Function

Cl_{cr} (mL/min/kg)	HSV	HSV	CMV	CMV
	Equivalent to 40 mg/kg q12h	Equivalent to 40 mg/kg q8h	Equivalent to 60 mg/kg q8h	Equivalent to 90 mg/kg q12h
<0.4	Not recommended	Not recommended	Not recommended	Not recommended
≥0.4-0.5	20 mg/kg every 24 hours	35 mg/kg every 24 hours	50 mg/kg every 24 hours	50 mg/kg every 24 hours
>0.5-0.6	25 mg/kg every 24 hours	40 mg/kg every 24 hours	60 mg/kg every 24 hours	60 mg/kg every 24 hours
>0.6-0.8	35 mg/kg every 24 hours	25 mg/kg every 12 hours	40 mg/kg every 12 hours	80 mg/kg every 24 hours
>0.8-1.0	20 mg/kg every 12 hours	35 mg/kg every 12 hours	50 mg/kg every 12 hours	50 mg/kg every 12 hours
>1.0-1.4	30 mg/kg every 12 hours	30 mg/kg every 8 hours	45 mg/kg every 8 hours	70 mg/kg every 12 hours
>1.4	40 mg/kg every 12 hours	40 mg/kg every 8 hours	60 mg/kg every 8 hours	90 mg/kg every 12 hours

Maintenance Dosing of Foscarnet in Patients With Abnormal Renal Function

Cl_{cr} (mL/min/kg)	CMV	CMV
	Equivalent to 90 mg/kg q24h	Equivalent to 120 mg/kg q24h
<0.4	Not recommended	Not recommended
≥0.4-0.5	50 mg/kg every 48 hours	65 mg/kg every 48 hours
>0.5-0.6	60 mg/kg every 48 hours	80 mg/kg every 48 hours
>0.6-0.8	80 mg/kg every 48 hours	105 mg/kg every 48 hours
>0.8-1.0	50 mg/kg every 24 hours	65 mg/kg every 24 hours
>1.0-1.4	70 mg/kg every 24 hours	90 mg/kg every 24 hours
>1.4	90 mg/kg every 24 hours	120 mg/kg every 24 hours

Hemodialysis:

Foscarnet is highly removed by hemodialysis (30% in 4 hours HD)

Doses of 50 mg/kg/dose posthemodialysis have been found to produce similar serum concentrations as doses of 90 mg/kg twice daily in patients with normal renal function

Doses of 60-90 mg/kg/dose loading dose (posthemodialysis) followed by 45 mg/kg/dose posthemodialysis (3 times/week) with the monitoring of weekly plasma concentrations to maintain peak plasma concentrations in the range of 400-800 µMolar has been recommended by some clinicians

Continuous arteriovenous or venovenous hemodiafiltration effects: Dose as for Cl_{cr} 10-50 mL/minute

(Continued)

Foscarnet *(Continued)*

Administration Foscarnet is administered by intravenous infusion, using an infusion pump, at a rate not exceeding 1 mg/kg/minute. Undiluted (24 mg/mL) solution can be administered without further dilution when using a central venous catheter for infusion. For peripheral vein administration, the solution **must** be diluted to a final concentration **not to exceed** 12 mg/mL. The recommended dosage, frequency, and rate of infusion should not be exceeded.

Patient Information Close monitoring is important and any symptom of electrolyte abnormalities should be reported immediately; maintain adequate fluid intake and hydration; regular ophthalmic examinations are necessary. Report any numbness in the extremities, paresthesias, or perioral tingling.

Additional Information Sodium loading with 500 mL of 0.9% sodium chloride solution before and after foscarnet infusion helps to minimize the risk of nephrotoxicity.

Dosage Forms Injection, solution: 24 mg/mL (250 mL, 500 mL)

Selected Readings

Chrisp P and Clissold SP, "Foscarnet. A Review of Its Antiviral Activity, Pharmacokinetic Properties and Therapeutic Use in Immunocompromised Patients With Cytomegalovirus Retinitis," *Drugs*, 1991, 41(1):104-29.

Deray G, Martinez F, Katlama C, et al, "Foscarnet Nephrotoxicity: Mechanism, Incidence and Prevention," *Am J Nephrol*, 1989, 9:316-21.

"Drugs for Non-HIV Viral Infections," *Med Lett Drugs Ther*, 1994, 36(919):27.

Jayaweera DT, "Minimizing the Dosage-Limiting Toxicities of Foscarnet Induction Therapy," *Drug Saf*, 1997, 16(4):258-66.

Keating MR, "Antiviral Agents," *Mayo Clin Proc*, 1992, 67(2):160-78.

Whitley RJ, Jacobson MA, Friedberg DN, et al, "Guidelines for the Treatment of Cytomegalovirus Diseases in Patients With AIDS in the Era of Potent Antiretroviral Therapy: Recommendations of an International Panel. International AIDS Society-USA," *Arch Intern Med*, 1998, 158(9):957-69.

Foscavir® *see* Foscarnet *on page 829*

Fosfomycin (fos foe MYE sin)

U.S. Brand Names Monurol™

Canadian Brand Names Monurol™

Synonyms Fosfomycin Tromethamine

Generic Available No

Use Single oral dose in the treatment of uncomplicated urinary tract infections in women due to susceptible strains of *E. coli* and *Enterococcus*; may have an advantage over other agents since it maintains high concentration in the urine for up to 48 hours

Unlabeled/Investigational Use Multiple doses have been investigated for complicated urinary tract infections in men

Pregnancy Risk Factor B

Adverse Reactions

1% to 10%:

- Central nervous system: Headache (47%), dizziness (1%)
- Dermatologic: Rash (1%)
- Gastrointestinal: Diarrhea (2% to 10%), nausea (4%), epigastric discomfort (1%), abdominal pain
- Genitourinary: Vaginitis
- Neuromuscular & skeletal: Weakness (1%)

<1%: Anorexia, drowsiness, fatigue, paresthesia, pruritus, somnolence, vomiting

Postmarketing and/or case reports: Angioedema, aplastic anemia, cholestasis, hepatic necrosis, jaundice, optic neuritis, toxic megacolon

Overdosage/Toxicology Symptomatic and supportive treatment is recommended in the event of an overdose.

Drug Interactions

Decreased Effect: Antacids or calcium salts may cause precipitate formation and decrease fosfomycin absorption. Increased gastrointestinal motility due to metoclopramide may lower fosfomycin tromethamine serum concentrations and urinary excretion. This drug interaction possibly could be extrapolated to other medications which increase gastrointestinal motility.

Stability Store at 15°C to 30°C (59°F to 86°F)

Mechanism of Action As a phosphoric acid derivative, fosfomycin inhibits bacterial wall synthesis (bactericidal) by inactivating the enzyme, pyruvyl transferase, which is critical in the synthesis of cell walls by bacteria; the tromethamine salt is preferable to the calcium salt due to its superior absorption

Pharmacodynamics/Kinetics

Absorption: Well absorbed

Distribution: V_d: 2 L/kg; high concentrations in urine; well into other tissues; crosses maximally into CSF with inflamed meninges

Protein binding: <3%

Bioavailability: 34% to 58%
Half-life elimination: 4-8 hours; Cl_{cr} <10 mL/minute: 50 hours
Time to peak, serum: 2 hours
Excretion: Urine (as unchanged drug); high urinary levels (100 mcg/mL) persist for >48 hours

Dosage Adults: Oral:
Female: Uncomplicated UTI: Single dose of 3 g in 4 oz of water
Male:
Complicated UTI (unlabeled): 3 g every 2-3 days for 3 doses
Prostatitis (unlabeled): 3 g every 3 days for a total of 21 days
Dosing adjustment in renal impairment: Decrease dose; 80% removed by dialysis, repeat dose after dialysis
Dosing adjustment in hepatic impairment: No dosage decrease needed

Administration Always mix with water before ingesting; do not administer in its dry form; pour contents of envelope into 90-120 mL of water (not hot), stir to dissolve and take immediately

Monitoring Parameters Signs and symptoms of urinary tract infection; urine culture plus sensitivity

Patient Information May be taken with or without food; avoid use of antacids or calcium salts within 4 hours before or 2 hours after taking fosfomycin; report signs of allergy; if symptoms do not improve after 2-3 days, contact your prescriber

Additional Information Many gram-positive and gram-negative organisms such as staphylococci, pneumococci, *E. coli*, *Salmonella*, *Shigella*, *H. influenzae*, *Neisseria* spp, and some strains of *P. aeruginosa*, indole-negative *Proteus*, and *Providencia* are inhibited. *B. fragilis*, and anaerobic gram-negative cocci are resistant.

Dosage Forms Powder, as tromethamine: 3 g

Selected Readings

Patel SS, Balfour JA, and Bryson HM, "Fosfomycin Tromethamine. A Review of Its Antibacterial Activity, Pharmacokinetic Properties, and Therapeutic Efficacy as a Single-Dose Oral Treatment for Acute Uncomplicated Lower Urinary Tract Infections," *Drugs*, 1997, 53(4):637-56.

Fosfomycin Tromethamine *see* Fosfomycin *on page 832*
FTC *see* Emtricitabine *on page 799*
Fulvicin® U/F (Can) *see* Griseofulvin *on page 845*
Fungi-Guard [OTC] *see* Tolnaftate *on page 1127*
Fungi-Nail® [OTC] *see* Undecylenic Acid and Derivatives *on page 1139*
Fungizone® (Can) *see* Amphotericin B (Conventional) *on page 650*
Fungoid® Tincture [OTC] *see* Miconazole *on page 945*
Furadantin® *see* Nitrofurantoin *on page 971*
Furamide® *see* Diloxanide Furoate *on page 778*

Furazolidone (fyoor a ZOE li done)

Canadian Brand Names Furoxone®

Synonyms Furoxone

Generic Available No

Use Treatment of bacterial or protozoal diarrhea and enteritis caused by susceptible organisms *Giardia lamblia* and *Vibrio cholerae*

Restrictions Not available in U.S.

Pregnancy Risk Factor C

Contraindications Hypersensitivity to furazolidone or any component of the formulation; concurrent use of ethanol; infants <1 month of age because of the possibility of producing hemolytic anemia; foods high in tyramine content

Warnings/Precautions Use caution in patients with G6PD deficiency when administering large doses for prolonged periods; furazolidone inhibits monoamine oxidase

Adverse Reactions
>10%: Genitourinary: Discoloration of urine (dark yellow to brown)
1% to 10%:
Central nervous system: Headache
Gastrointestinal: Abdominal pain, diarrhea, nausea, vomiting
<1%: Agranulocytosis, arthralgia, disulfiram-like reaction after ethanol ingestion, dizziness, drowsiness, fever, hemolysis in patients with G6PD deficiency, hypoglycemia, leukopenia, malaise, orthostatic hypotension, rash

Overdosage/Toxicology Symptoms include nausea, vomiting, and serotonin crisis. Treatment is supportive care only. Serotonin crisis may require dantrolene/bromocriptine.

Drug Interactions
Increased Effect/Toxicity: Increased effect with sympathomimetic amines, tricyclic antidepressants, tyramine-containing foods, MAO inhibitors, meperidine,

(Continued)

Furazolidone *(Continued)*

anorexiants, dextromethorphan, fluoxetine, paroxetine, sertraline, and trazodone. Increased effect/toxicity of levodopa. Disulfiram-like reaction with alcohol.

Ethanol/Nutrition/Herb Interactions

Ethanol: Avoid ethanol (a disulfiram-like reaction may occur).

Food: Marked elevation of blood pressure, hypertensive crisis, or hemorrhagic stroke may occur with foods high in tyramine content.

Mechanism of Action Inhibits several vital enzymatic reactions causing antibacterial and antiprotozoal action

Pharmacodynamics/Kinetics

Absorption: Poor

Excretion: Urine (33% as active drug and metabolites)

Dosage Oral:

Children >1 month: 5-8 mg/kg/day in 4 divided doses for 7 days, not to exceed 400 mg/day or 8.8 mg/kg/day

Adults: 100 mg 4 times/day for 7 days

Monitoring Parameters CBC

Test Interactions False-positive results for urine glucose with Clinitest®

Patient Information May discolor urine to a brown tint; avoid alcohol during or for 4 days after therapy and avoid eating tyramine-containing foods; consult with physician or pharmacist for a list of these foods. Do not take any prescription or nonprescription drugs without consulting the physician or pharmacist; if result not achieved at the end of treatment contact physician.

Additional Information Not available in U.S.

Dosage Forms

Liquid: 50 mg/15 mL (60 mL, 473 mL)

Tablet: 100 mg

Selected Readings

"Drugs for Parasitic Infections," *Med Lett Drugs Ther*, 1998, 40(1017):1-12.

Furoxone® (Can) *see* Furazolidone *on page 833*

Fuzeon™ *see* Enfuvirtide *on page 802*

Gamimune® N *see* Immune Globulin (Intravenous) *on page 867*

Gamma Benzene Hexachloride *see* Lindane *on page 913*

Gammagard® Liquid *see* Immune Globulin (Intravenous) *on page 867*

Gammagard® S/D *see* Immune Globulin (Intravenous) *on page 867*

Gamma Globulin *see* Immune Globulin (Intramuscular) *on page 866*

Gammar®-P I.V. *see* Immune Globulin (Intravenous) *on page 867*

Gamunex® *see* Immune Globulin (Intravenous) *on page 867*

Ganciclovir (gan SYE kloe veer)

Related Information

USPHS / IDSA Guidelines for the Prevention of Opportunistic Infections in Persons Infected With HIV *on page 1237*

U.S. Brand Names Cytovene®; Vitrasert®

Canadian Brand Names Cytovene®; Vitrasert®

Synonyms DHPG Sodium; GCV Sodium; Nordeoxyguanosine

Generic Available Yes: Capsule

Use

Parenteral: Treatment of CMV retinitis in immunocompromised individuals, including patients with acquired immunodeficiency syndrome; prophylaxis of CMV infection in transplant patients

Oral: Alternative to the I.V. formulation for maintenance treatment of CMV retinitis in immunocompromised patients, including patients with AIDS, in whom retinitis is stable following appropriate induction therapy and for whom the risk of more rapid progression is balanced by the benefit associated with avoiding daily I.V. infusions.

Implant: Treatment of CMV retinitis

Unlabeled/Investigational Use May be given in combination with foscarnet in patients who relapse after monotherapy with either drug

Drug of Choice or Alternative for

Disease/Syndrome(s):

Esophagitis *on page 147*

Organism(s):

Cytomegalovirus *on page 107*

Herpes Simplex Virus *on page 172*

Pregnancy Risk Factor C

Contraindications Hypersensitivity to ganciclovir, acyclovir, or any component of the formulation; absolute neutrophil count <500/mm^3; platelet count <25,000/mm^3

Warnings/Precautions Hazardous agent - use appropriate precautions for handling and disposal. Dosage adjustment or interruption of ganciclovir therapy may be necessary in patients with neutropenia and/or thrombocytopenia and patients with impaired renal function. Use with extreme caution in children since long-term safety has not been determined and due to ganciclovir's potential for long-term carcinogenic and adverse reproductive effects; ganciclovir may adversely affect spermatogenesis and fertility; due to its mutagenic potential, contraceptive precautions for female and male patients need to be followed during and for at least 90 days after therapy with the drug; take care to administer only into veins with good blood flow.

Adverse Reactions

>10%:

- Central nervous system: Fever (38% to 48%)
- Dermatologic: Rash (15% oral, 10% I.V.)
- Gastrointestinal: Abdominal pain (17% to 19%), diarrhea (40%), nausea (25%), anorexia (15%), vomiting (13%)
- Hematologic: Anemia (20% to 25%), leukopenia (30% to 40%)

1% to 10%:

- Central nervous system: Confusion, neuropathy (8% to 9%), headache (4%)
- Dermatologic: Pruritus (5%)
- Hematologic: Thrombocytopenia (6%), neutropenia with ANC <500/mm^3 (5% oral, 14% I.V.)
- Neuromuscular & skeletal: Paresthesia (6% to 10%), weakness (6%)
- Ocular: Retinal detachment (8% oral, 11% I.V.; relationship to ganciclovir not established)
- Miscellaneous: Sepsis (4% oral, 15% I.V.)

<1% (Limited to important or life-threatening): Alopecia, arrhythmia, ataxia, bronchospasm, coma, dyspnea, encephalopathy, exfoliative dermatitis, extrapyramidal symptoms, nervousness, pancytopenia, psychosis, seizure, alopecia, urticaria, eosinophilia, hemorrhage, Stevens-Johnson syndrome, torsade de pointes, renal failure, SIADH, visual loss

Overdosage/Toxicology Symptoms include neutropenia, vomiting, hypersalivation, bloody diarrhea, cytopenia, and testicular atrophy. Treatment is supportive. Hemodialysis removes 50% of drug. Hydration may be of some benefit.

Drug Interactions

Increased Effect/Toxicity: Immunosuppressive agents may increase hematologic toxicity of ganciclovir. Imipenem/cilastatin may increase seizure potential. Oral ganciclovir increases blood levels of zidovudine, although zidovudine decreases steady-state levels of ganciclovir. Since both drugs have the potential to cause neutropenia and anemia, some patients may not tolerate concomitant therapy with these drugs at full dosage. Didanosine levels are increased with concurrent ganciclovir. Other nephrotoxic drugs (eg, amphotericin and cyclosporine) may have additive nephrotoxicity with ganciclovir.

Decreased Effect: A decrease in blood levels of ganciclovir AUC may occur when used with didanosine.

Stability Intact vials should be stored at room temperature and protected from temperatures >40°C Reconstitute powder with unpreserved sterile water **not** bacteriostatic water because parabens may cause precipitation; dilute in 250-1000 mL D_5W or NS to a concentration ≤10 mg/mL for infusion.

Reconstituted solution is stable for 12 hours at room temperature, however, conflicting data indicates that reconstituted solution is stable for 60 days under refrigeration (4°C). Stability of parenteral admixture at room temperature (25°C) and at refrigeration temperature (4°C) is 5 days.

Mechanism of Action Ganciclovir is phosphorylated to a substrate which competitively inhibits the binding of deoxyguanosine triphosphate to DNA polymerase resulting in inhibition of viral DNA synthesis

Pharmacodynamics/Kinetics

- Distribution: V_d: 15.26 L/1.73 m^2; widely to all tissues including CSF and ocular tissue
- Protein binding: 1% to 2%
- Bioavailability: Oral: Fasting: 5%; Following food: 6% to 9%; Following fatty meal: 28% to 31%
- Half-life elimination: 1.7-5.8 hours; prolonged with renal impairment; End-stage renal disease: 5-28 hours
- Excretion: Urine (80% to 99% as unchanged drug)

Dosage

CMV retinitis: Slow I.V. infusion (dosing is based on total body weight):

Children >3 months and Adults:

Induction therapy: 5 mg/kg/dose every 12 hours for 14-21 days followed by maintenance therapy

(Continued)

Ganciclovir *(Continued)*

Maintenance therapy: 5 mg/kg/day as a single daily dose for 7 days/week or 6 mg/kg/day for 5 days/week

CMV retinitis: Oral: 1000 mg 3 times/day with food **or** 500 mg 6 times/day with food

Prevention of CMV disease in patients with advanced HIV infection and normal renal function: Oral: 1000 mg 3 times/day with food

Prevention of CMV disease in transplant patients: Same initial and maintenance dose as CMV retinitis except duration of initial course is 7-14 days, duration of maintenance therapy is dependent on clinical condition and degree of immunosuppression

Intravitreal implant: One implant for 5- to 8-month period; following depletion of ganciclovir, as evidenced by progression of retinitis, implant may be removed and replaced

Elderly: Refer to adult dosing; in general, dose selection should be cautious, reflecting greater frequency of organ impairment

Dosing adjustment in renal impairment:

I.V. (Induction):

Cl_{cr} 50-69 mL/minute: Administer 2.5 mg/kg/dose every 12 hours

Cl_{cr} 25-49 mL/minute: Administer 2.5 mg/kg/dose every 24 hours

Cl_{cr} 10-24 mL/minute: Administer 1.25 mg/kg/dose every 24 hours

Cl_{cr} <10 mL/minute: Administer 1.25 mg/kg/dose 3 times/week following hemodialysis

I.V. (Maintenance):

Cl_{cr} 50-69 mL/minute: Administer 2.5 mg/kg/dose every 24 hours

Cl_{cr} 25-49 mL/minute: Administer 1.25 mg/kg/dose every 24 hours

Cl_{cr} 10-24 mL/minute: Administer 0.625 mg/kg/dose every 24 hours

Cl_{cr} <10 mL/minute: Administer 0.625 mg/kg/dose 3 times/week following hemodialysis

Oral:

Cl_{cr} 50-69 mL/minute: Administer 1500 mg/day or 500 mg 3 times/day

Cl_{cr} 25-49 mL/minute: Administer 1000 mg/day or 500 mg twice daily

Cl_{cr} 10-24 mL/minute: Administer 500 mg/day

Cl_{cr} <10 mL/minute: Administer 500 mg 3 times/week following hemodialysis

Hemodialysis effects: Dialyzable (50%) following hemodialysis; administer dose postdialysis. During peritoneal dialysis, dose as for Cl_{cr} <10 mL/minute. During continuous arteriovenous or venovenous hemofiltration, administer 2.5 mg/kg/dose every 24 hours.

Dietary Considerations Sodium content of 500 mg vial: 46 mg

Administration

Oral: Should be administered with food.

I.V.: Should not be administered by I.M., SubQ, or rapid IVP; administer by slow I.V. infusion over at least 1 hour

Monitoring Parameters CBC with differential and platelet count, serum creatinine, ophthalmologic exams

Patient Information Regular ophthalmologic examinations should be done; close monitoring of blood counts should be done while on therapy and dosage adjustments may need to be made; take with food to increase absorption

Dosage Forms

Capsule: 250 mg, 500 mg

Cytovene®: 250 mg, 500 mg [DSC]

Implant, intravitreal (Vitrasert®): 4.5 mg [released gradually over 5-8 months]

Injection, powder for reconstitution, as sodium (Cytovene®): 500 mg

Selected Readings

Alrabiah FA and Sacks SL, "New Antiherpesvirus Agents. Their Targets and Therapeutic Potential," *Drugs*, 1996, 52(1):17-32.

"Drugs for Non-HIV Viral Infections," *Med Lett Drugs Ther*, 1994, 36(919):27.

Keating MR, "Antiviral Agents," *Mayo Clin Proc*, 1992, 67(2):160-78.

Matthews T and Boehme R, "Antiviral Activity and Mechanism of Action of Ganciclovir," *Rev Infect Dis*, 1988, 10(Suppl 3):S490-4.

McGavin JK and Goa KL, "Ganciclovir: An Update of Its Use in the Prevention of Cytomegalovirus Infection and Disease in Transplant Recipients," *Drugs*, 2001, 61(8):1153-83.

Whitley RJ, Jacobson MA, Friedberg DN, et al, "Guidelines for the Treatment of Cytomegalovirus Diseases in Patients With AIDS in the Era of Potent Antiretroviral Therapy: Recommendations of an International Panel. International AIDS Society-USA," *Arch Intern Med*, 1998, 158(9):957-69.

Gantrisin® *see* SulfiSOXAZOLE *on page 1091*

GAR-936 *see* Tigecycline *on page 1116*

Garamycin® (Can) *see* Gentamicin *on page 841*

Gatifloxacin (gat i FLOKS a sin)

Related Information

Antimicrobial Activity Against Selected Organisms *on page 1165*
Community-Acquired Pneumonia in Adults *on page 1278*
Tuberculosis *on page 1315*

U.S. Brand Names Tequin®; Zymar™

Canadian Brand Names Tequin®; Zymar™

Generic Available No

Use

Oral, I.V.: Treatment of the following infections when caused by susceptible bacteria: Acute bacterial exacerbation of chronic bronchitis; acute sinusitis; community-acquired pneumonia including pneumonia caused by multidrug-resistant *S. pneumoniae* (MDRSP); uncomplicated skin and skin structure infection; uncomplicated urinary tract infections (cystitis); complicated urinary tract infections; pyelonephritis; uncomplicated urethral and cervical gonorrhea; acute, uncomplicated rectal infections in women

Ophthalmic: Bacterial conjunctivitis

Drug of Choice or Alternative for Disease/Syndrome(s):

Pneumonia, Community-Acquired *on page 270*

Organism(s):

Streptococcus pneumoniae, Drug-Resistant *on page 316*

Pregnancy Risk Factor C

Pregnancy Implications Reports of arthropathy (observed in immature animals and reported rarely in humans) have limited the use of fluoroquinolones during pregnancy. Gatifloxacin has been show to be fetotoxic in animal studies. There are no adequate and well-controlled studies in pregnant women. Based on limited data, quinolones are not expected to be a major human teratogen. Although quinolone antibiotics should not be used as first-line agents during pregnancy, when considering treatment for life-threatening infection and/or prolonged duration of therapy, the potential risk to the fetus must be balanced against the severity of the potential illness.

Contraindications Hypersensitivity to gatifloxacin, other quinolone antibiotics, or any component of the formulation

Warnings/Precautions Use with caution in patients with significant bradycardia or acute myocardial ischemia. May prolong QT interval (concentration related). Use caution in patients with known prolongation of QT interval, uncorrected hypokalemia, or concurrent administration of other medications known to prolong the QT interval (including Class Ia and Class III antiarrhythmics, cisapride, erythromycin, antipsychotics, and tricyclic antidepressants). May cause increased CNS stimulation, increased intracranial pressure, convulsions, or psychosis. Use with caution in individuals at risk of seizures (CNS disorders or concurrent therapy with medications which may lower seizure threshold). Discontinue in patients who experience significant CNS adverse effects (dizziness, hallucinations, suicidal ideation or actions). Use caution in renal dysfunction (dosage adjustment required) and in severe hepatic insufficiency (no data available). Serious disruptions in glucose regulation (including hyperglycemia and severe hypoglycemia) may occur, generally in patients with diabetes and typically within 1-3 days of initiation. Monitor closely and discontinue if hyper- or hypoglycemia occur. Tendon inflammation and/or rupture has been reported with this and other quinolone antibiotics. Risk may be increased with concurrent corticosteroids, particularly in the elderly. Discontinue at first signs or symptoms of tendon or pain.

Severe hypersensitivity reactions, including anaphylaxis, have occurred with quinolone therapy. If an allergic reaction occurs (itching, urticaria, dyspnea, facial edema, loss of consciousness, tingling, cardiovascular collapse) discontinue drug immediately. Prolonged use may result in superinfection; pseudomembranous colitis may occur and should be considered in all patients who present with diarrhea. Quinolones may exacerbate myasthenia gravis, use with caution (rare, potentially life-threatening weakness of respiratory muscles may occur). May cause peripheral neuropathy (rare); discontinue if symptoms of sensory or sensorimotor neuropathy occur. Do not inject ophthalmic solution subconjunctively or introduce directly into the anterior chamber of the eye.

Safety and efficacy for ophthalmic use have not been established in children <1 year of age. Safety and efficacy for systemic use have not been established in patients <18 years of age.

Adverse Reactions

Systemic therapy:

3% to 10%:

Central nervous system: Headache (3%), dizziness (3%)

(Continued)

Gatifloxacin *(Continued)*

Gastrointestinal: Nausea (8%), diarrhea (4%)
Genitourinary: Vaginitis (6%)
Local: Injection site reactions (5%)

0.1% to 3%: Abdominal pain, abnormal dreams, abnormal vision, agitation, alkaline phosphatase increased, allergic reaction, anorexia, anxiety, arthralgia, back pain, chest pain, chills, confusion, constipation, diaphoresis, dry skin, dyspepsia, dyspnea, dysuria, facial edema, fever, flatulence, gastritis, glossitis, hematuria, hyperglycemia, hypertension, insomnia, leg cramps, mouth ulceration, nervousness, oral candidiasis, palpitation, paresthesia, peripheral edema, pharyngitis, pruritus, rash, serum amylase increased, serum bilirubin increased, serum transaminases increased, somnolence, stomatitis, taste perversion, thirst, tinnitus, tremor, weakness, vasodilation, vertigo, vomiting

<0.1%: Abnormal thinking, arthritis, asthenia, ataxia, bone pain, bradycardia, breast pain, bronchospasm, cheilitis, colitis, cyanosis, depersonalization, depression, diabetes mellitus, dysphagia, ear pain, ecchymosis, edema, epistaxis, ethanol intolerance, euphoria, eye pain, gastrointestinal hemorrhage, gingivitis, halitosis, hallucination, hematemesis, hematuria, hostility, hyperesthesia, hypertonia, hyperventilation, hypoglycemia, lymphadenopathy, maculopapular rash, metrorrhagia, migraine, myalgia, myasthenia, neck pain, panic attacks, paranoia, parosmia, photophobia, pseudomembranous colitis, psychosis, ptosis, rectal hemorrhage, seizure, stress, tachycardia, taste disturbance, tongue edema, vesiculobullous rash

Postmarketing and/or case reports: Acute renal failure, anaphylactic reaction, angioneurotic edema, hepatitis, INR increased, prothrombin time increased, severe hyper-/hypoglycemia, nonketotic hyperglycemia, pancreatitis, peripheral neuropathy, Stevens-Johnson syndrome, syncope, tendon rupture, thrombocytopenia, torsade de pointes

Ophthalmic therapy:

5% to 10%: Ocular: Conjunctival irritation, keratitis, lacrimation increased, papillary conjunctivitis

1% to 4%:
Central nervous system: Headache
Gastrointestinal: Taste disturbance
Ocular: Chemosis, conjunctival hemorrhage, discharge, dry eye, edema, irritation, pain, visual acuity decreased

Overdosage/Toxicology Potential symptoms of overdose include CNS excitation, seizures, QT prolongation, and arrhythmias (including torsade de pointes). Monitor by continuous ECG in the event of an overdose. Management is supportive and symptomatic. The drug is not removed by dialysis.

Drug Interactions

Increased Effect/Toxicity: Gatifloxacin may increase the effects/toxicity of hypoglycemic agents and warfarin. Concomitant use with corticosteroids may increase the risk of tendon rupture. Concomitant use with other QT_c-prolonging agents (eg, Class Ia and Class III antiarrhythmics, erythromycin, cisapride, antipsychotics, and cyclic antidepressants) may result in arrhythmias, such as torsade de pointes. Probenecid may increase gatifloxacin levels.

Decreased Effect: Concurrent administration of metal cations, including most antacids (not calcium carbonate), oral electrolyte supplements, quinapril, sucralfate, some didanosine formulations (chewable/buffered tablets and pediatric powder for oral suspension), and other highly-buffered oral drugs, may decrease quinolone levels; separate doses.

Ethanol/Nutrition/Herb Interactions Herb/Nutraceutical: Avoid dong quai, St John's wort (may also cause photosensitization).

Stability

Ophthalmic solution: Store between 15°C to 25°C (59°F to 77°F). Do not freeze.

Solution for injection: Store at 25°C (77°F). Do not freeze. Single-use vials must be diluted to a concentration of 2 mg/mL prior to administration; may be diluted with D_5W, NS, D_5NS, D_5LR, 5% sodium bicarbonate, or Plasma-Lyte® 56 and D_5W. Do not dilute with SWFI (a hypertonic solution results). Following dilution, stable for 14 days when stored between 20°C to 25°C or 2° to 8°C. Diluted solutions (except those prepared in 5% sodium bicarbonate) may also be frozen for up to 6 months when stored at -25°C to -10°C (-13°F to 14°F). Solutions may then be thawed at room temperature and should be used within 14 days (store between 20°C to 25°C or 2°C to 8°C); do not refreeze.

Tablet: Store at 25°C (77°F).

Mechanism of Action Gatifloxacin is a DNA gyrase inhibitor, and also inhibits topoisomerase IV. DNA gyrase (topoisomerase II) is an essential bacterial enzyme that maintains the superhelical structure of DNA. DNA gyrase is required for DNA

replication and transcription, DNA repair, recombination, and transposition; inhibition is bactericidal.

Pharmacodynamics/Kinetics

Absorption: Oral: Well absorbed; Ophthalmic: Not measurable

Distribution: V_d: 1.5-2.0 L/kg; concentrates in alveolar macrophages and lung parenchyma

Protein binding: 20%

Metabolism: Only 1%; no interaction with CYP

Bioavailability: 96%

Half-life elimination: 7.1-13.9 hours; ESRD/CAPD: 30-40 hours

Time to peak: Oral: 1 hour

Excretion: Urine (70% as unchanged drug, <1% as metabolites); feces (5%)

Dosage

Children ≥1 year and Adults: Ophthalmic: Bacterial conjunctivitis:

Days 1 and 2: Instill 1 drop into affected eye(s) every 2 hours while awake (maximum: 8 times/day)

Days 3-7: Instill 1 drop into affected eye(s) up to 4 times/day while awake

Adults: Oral, I.V.:

Acute bacterial exacerbation of chronic bronchitis: 400 mg every 24 hours for 5 days

Acute sinusitis: 400 mg every 24 hours for 10 days

Community-acquired pneumonia: 400 mg every 24 hours for 7-14 days

Uncomplicated skin/skin structure infections: 400 mg every 24 hours for 7-10 days

Uncomplicated urinary tract infections (cystitis): 400 mg single dose or 200 mg every 24 hours for 3 days

Complicated urinary tract infections: 400 mg every 24 hours for 7-10 days

Acute pyelonephritis: 400 mg every 24 hours for 7-10 days

Uncomplicated urethral gonorrhea in men, cervical or rectal gonorrhea in women: 400 mg single dose

Elderly: No dosage adjustment is required based on age, however, assessment of renal function is particularly important in this population.

Dosage adjustment in renal impairment: Creatinine clearance <40 mL/minute (or patients on hemodialysis/CAPD) should receive an initial dose of 400 mg, followed by a subsequent dose of 200 mg every 24 hours. Patients receiving single-dose or 3-day therapy for appropriate indications do not require dosage adjustment. Administer after hemodialysis.

Dosage adjustment in hepatic impairment: No dosage adjustment is required in mild-moderate hepatic disease. No data are available in severe hepatic impairment (Child-Pugh Class C).

Dietary Considerations May take tablets with or without food, milk, or calcium supplements. Gatifloxacin should be taken 4 hours before supplements (including multivitamins) containing iron, zinc, or magnesium.

Administration

Oral: May be administered with or without food, milk, or calcium supplements. Gatifloxacin should be taken 4 hours before supplements (including multivitamins) containing iron, zinc, or magnesium.

I.V.: For I.V. infusion only. Concentrated injection (10 mg/mL) must be diluted to 2 mg/mL prior to administration. No further dilution is required for premixed 100 mL and 200 mL solutions. Infuse over 60 minutes. Avoid rapid or bolus infusions.

Monitoring Parameters WBC, signs of infection

Patient Information Tablets may be taken with or without food. Drink plenty of fluids. Avoid exposure to direct sunlight during therapy and for several days following. Take gatifloxacin 4 hours before antacids or mineral supplements (iron, magnesium, or zinc). Report immediately signs of allergy or signs of tendon inflammation or pain. Take entire course of medication.

Dosage Forms

Injection, infusion [premixed in D_5W] (Tequin®): 200 mg (100 mL); 400 mg (200 mL)

Injection, solution [preservative free] (Tequin®): 10 mg/mL (40 mL)

Solution, ophthalmic (Zymar™): 0.3% (2.5 mL, 5 mL) [contains benzalkonium chloride]

Tablet (Tequin®): 200 mg, 400 mg

Tequin® Teq-paq™ [unit-dose pack]: 400 mg (5s)

Selected Readings

Blondeau JM, "Expanded Activity and Utility of the New Fluoroquinolones: A Review," *Clinical Therapeutics*, 1999, 21(1):3-40.

Fish DN and North DS, "Gatifloxacin, An Advanced 8-Methoxy Fluoroquinolone," *Pharmacotherapy*, 2001, 21(1):35-59.

"Gatifloxacin and Moxifloxacin: Two New Fluoroquinolones," *Med Lett Drugs Ther*, 2000, Vol 42, 1072:15.

Perry CM, Barman Balfour JA, Lamb HM, "Gatifloxacin," *Drugs*, 1999, 58(4):683-96.

Perry CM, Ormrod D, Hurst M, et al, "Gatifloxacin: A Review of Its Use in the Management of Bacterial Infections," *Drugs*, 2002, 62(1):169-207.

G-CSF *see* Filgrastim *on page 817*

GCV Sodium *see* Ganciclovir *on page 834*

Gemifloxacin (je mi FLOKS a sin)

Related Information

Community-Acquired Pneumonia in Adults *on page 1278*

U.S. Brand Names Factive®

Synonyms DW286; Gemifloxacin Mesylate; LA 20304a; SB-265805

Generic Available No

Use Treatment of acute exacerbation of chronic bronchitis; treatment of community-acquired pneumonia, including pneumonia caused by multidrug-resistant strains of *S. pneumoniae* (MDRSP)

Unlabeled/Investigational Use Acute sinusitis, uncomplicated urinary tract infection

Pregnancy Risk Factor C

Pregnancy Implications There are no adequate and well-controlled studies in pregnant women. Reports of arthropathy (observed in immature animals and reported rarely in humans) have limited the use of fluoroquinolones in pregnancy. Reversible fetal growth retardation was observed with gemifloxacin in some animal studies. Based on limited data, quinolones are not expected to be a major human teratogen. Although quinolone antibiotics should not be used as first-line agents during pregnancy, when considering treatment for life-threatening infection and/or prolonged duration of therapy, the potential risk to the fetus must be balanced against the severity of the potential illness.

Contraindications Hypersensitivity to gemifloxacin, other fluoroquinolones, or any component of the formulation

Warnings/Precautions Fluoroquinolones may prolong QT_c interval; avoid use of gemifloxacin in patients with uncorrected hypokalemia, hypomagnesemia, or concurrent administration of other medications known to prolong the QT interval (including Class Ia and Class III antiarrhythmics, cisapride, erythromycin, antipsychotics, and tricyclic antidepressants). Use with caution in patients with significant bradycardia or acute myocardial ischemia. Use with caution in individuals at risk of seizures (CNS disorders or concurrent therapy with medications which may lower seizure threshold). Discontinue in patients who experience significant CNS adverse effects (dizziness, hallucinations, suicidal ideation or actions). Use caution in renal dysfunction (dosage adjustment required).

Severe hypersensitivity reactions, including anaphylaxis, have occurred with quinolone therapy. If an allergic reaction occurs (itching, urticaria, dyspnea or facial edema, loss of consciousness, tingling, cardiovascular collapse), discontinue drug immediately. Prolonged use may result in superinfection; pseudomembranous colitis may occur and should be considered in all patients who present with diarrhea. Tendon inflammation and/or rupture has been reported with other quinolone antibiotics; risk may increase with concurrent corticosteroids, particularly in the elderly. Discontinue at first sign of tendon inflammation or pain. Peripheral neuropathy has been linked to the use of quinolones; these cases were rare. Experience with quinolones in immature animals has resulted in permanent arthropathy. Safety and effectiveness in pediatric patients (<18 years of age) have not been established.

Adverse Reactions

1% to 10%:

Central nervous system: Headache (1%), dizziness (1%)

Dermatologic: Rash (3%)

Gastrointestinal: Diarrhea (4%), nausea (3%), abdominal pain (1%), vomiting (1%)

Hepatic: Transaminases increased (1% to 2%)

<1%: Abnormal vision, anemia, anorexia, arthralgia, asthenia, back pain, bilirubin increased, constipation, CPK increased, cramps (leg), dermatitis, dry mouth, dyspepsia, dyspnea, eczema, eosinophilia, fatigue, flatulence, fungal infection, gastritis, genital moniliasis, GGT increased, granulocytopenia, hyperglycemia, insomnia, leukopenia, moniliasis, myalgia, nervousness, pharyngitis, photosensitivity, pruritus, somnolence, taste perversion, thrombocythemia, thrombocytopenia, tremor, urticaria, vaginitis, vertigo

Important adverse effects reported with other agents in this drug class include (not reported for gemifloxacin): Allergic reactions, CNS stimulation, hepatitis, jaundice, peripheral neuropathy, pneumonitis (eosinophilic), seizure; sensorimotor-axonal neuropathy (paresthesia, hypoesthesias, dysesthesias, weakness); severe dermatologic reactions (toxic epidermal necrolysis, Stevens-Johnson syndrome); tendon rupture, torsade de pointes, vasculitis

Overdosage/Toxicology Treatment should be symptom-directed and supportive; 20% to 30% removed by hemodialysis.

Drug Interactions

Increased Effect/Toxicity: Gemifloxacin may increase the effects/toxicity of glyburide and warfarin. Concomitant use with corticosteroids may increase the risk of tendon rupture. Concomitant use with other QT_c-prolonging agents (eg, Class Ia and Class III antiarrhythmics, erythromycin, cisapride, antipsychotics, and cyclic antidepressants) may result in arrhythmias, such as torsade de pointes. Probenecid may increase gemifloxacin levels.

Decreased Effect: Concurrent administration of metal cations, including most antacids, oral electrolyte supplements, quinapril, sucralfate, some didanosine formulations (chewable/buffered tablets and pediatric powder for oral suspension), and other highly-buffered oral drugs, may decrease quinolone levels; separate doses.

Ethanol/Nutrition/Herb Interactions Herb/Nutraceutical: Avoid dong quai, St John's wort (may also cause photosensitization).

Stability Store at 25°C (77°F); excursions permitted to 15°C to 30°C (59°F to 86°F); protect from light

Mechanism of Action Gemifloxacin is a DNA gyrase inhibitor and also inhibits topoisomerase IV. DNA gyrase (topoisomerase IV) is an essential bacterial enzyme that maintains the superhelical structure of DNA. DNA gyrase is required for DNA replication and transcription, DNA repair, recombination, and transposition; bactericidal

Pharmacodynamics/Kinetics

Absorption: Well absorbed from the GI tract
Bioavailability: 71%
Metabolism: Hepatic (minor); forms metabolites (CYP isoenzymes are not involved)
Time to peak, plasma: 1-2 hours
Protein binding: 60% to 70%
Half-life elimination: 7 hours (range 4-12 hours)
Excretion: Urine (30% to 40%); feces (60%)

Dosage Oral: Adults: 320 mg once daily

Duration of therapy:
Acute exacerbations of chronic bronchitis: 5 days
Community-acquired pneumonia (mild to moderate severity): 7 days

Dosage adjustment in renal impairment: Cl_{cr} ≤40 mL/minute (or patients on hemodialysis/CAPD): 160 mg once daily (administer dose following hemodialysis)

Dosage adjustment in hepatic impairment: No adjustment required.

Dietary Considerations May take tablets with or without food, milk, or calcium supplements. Gemifloxacin should be taken 3 hours before or 2 hours after supplements (including multivitamins) containing iron, zinc, or magnesium.

Administration May be administered with or without food, milk, or calcium supplements. Gemifloxacin should be taken 3 hours before or 2 hours after supplements (including multivitamins) containing iron, zinc, or magnesium.

Monitoring Parameters WBC, signs/symptoms of infection

Dosage Forms Tablet, as mesylate: 320 mg

Gemifloxacin Mesylate *see* Gemifloxacin *on page 840*

Gen-Acyclovir (Can) *see* Acyclovir *on page 629*

Gen-Amoxicillin (Can) *see* Amoxicillin *on page 642*

Gen-Ciprofloxacin (Can) *see* Ciprofloxacin *on page 742*

Gen-Fluconazole (Can) *see* Fluconazole *on page 819*

Gen-Hydroxychloroquine (Can) *see* Hydroxychloroquine *on page 859*

Gen-Minocycline (Can) *see* Minocycline *on page 947*

Genoptic® *see* Gentamicin *on page 841*

Genotropin® *see* Somatropin *on page 1069*

Genotropin Miniquick® *see* Somatropin *on page 1069*

Gentacidin® [DSC] *see* Gentamicin *on page 841*

Gentak® *see* Gentamicin *on page 841*

Gentamicin (jen ta MYE sin)

Related Information

Aminoglycoside Dosing and Monitoring *on page 1267*
Antibiotic Treatment of Adults With Infective Endocarditis *on page 1271*
Antimicrobial Activity Against Selected Organisms *on page 1165*

U.S. Brand Names Genoptic®; Gentacidin® [DSC]; Gentak®

Canadian Brand Names Alcomicin®; Diogent®; Garamycin®; Minim's Gentamicin 0.3%; SAB-Gentamicin

Synonyms Gentamicin Sulfate

Generic Available Yes

(Continued)

Gentamicin *(Continued)*

Use Treatment of susceptible bacterial infections, normally gram-negative organisms including *Pseudomonas*, *Proteus*, *Serratia*, and gram-positive *Staphylococcus*; treatment of bone infections, respiratory tract infections, skin and soft tissue infections, as well as abdominal and urinary tract infections, endocarditis, and septicemia; used topically to treat superficial infections of the skin or ophthalmic infections caused by susceptible bacteria; prevention of bacterial endocarditis prior to dental or surgical procedures

Drug of Choice or Alternative for

Disease/Syndrome(s):

Brain Abscess *on page 58*
Endocarditis, Acute, I.V. Drug Abuse *on page 123*
Endocarditis, Acute Native Valve *on page 124*
Endocarditis, Prosthetic Valve, Early *on page 124*
Endocarditis, Prosthetic Valve, Late *on page 125*
Endocarditis, Subacute Native Valve *on page 126*
Endometritis *on page 127*
Endophthalmitis, Bacterial and Fungal *on page 128*
Meningitis, Neonatal (<1 month of age) *on page 217*
Pelvic Inflammatory Disease *on page 260*
Pneumonia, Hospital-Acquired *on page 272*
Pneumonia, Ventilator-Associated *on page 273*
Sinusitis, Hospital-Acquired *on page 300*
Urinary Tract Infection, Pyelonephritis *on page 346*

Organism(s):

Brucella Species *on page 61*
Corynebacterium jeikeium on page 98
Enterococcus Species *on page 134*
Francisella tularensis on page 149
Listeria monocytogenes on page 208
Staphylococcus epidermidis, Methicillin-Resistant *on page 309*
Streptococcus, Viridans Group *on page 326*
Yersinia pestis on page 355

Pregnancy Risk Factor C

Contraindications Hypersensitivity to gentamicin or other aminoglycosides

Warnings/Precautions Not intended for long-term therapy due to toxic hazards associated with extended administration; pre-existing renal insufficiency, vestibular or cochlear impairment, myasthenia gravis, hypocalcemia, conditions which depress neuromuscular transmission

Parenteral aminoglycosides have been associated with significant nephrotoxicity or ototoxicity; the ototoxicity may be directly proportional to the amount of drug given and the duration of treatment; tinnitus or vertigo are indications of vestibular injury and impending hearing loss; renal damage is usually reversible

Adverse Reactions

>10%:
- Central nervous system: Neurotoxicity (vertigo, ataxia)
- Neuromuscular & skeletal: Gait instability
- Otic: Ototoxicity (auditory), ototoxicity (vestibular)
- Renal: Nephrotoxicity, decreased creatinine clearance

1% to 10%:
- Cardiovascular: Edema
- Dermatologic: Skin itching, reddening of skin, rash

<1%: Drowsiness, headache, pseudomotor cerebri, photosensitivity, allergic reaction, erythema, anorexia, nausea, vomiting, weight loss, increased salivation, enterocolitis, granulocytopenia, agranulocytosis, thrombocytopenia, elevated LFTs, burning, stinging, tremor, muscle cramps, weakness, dyspnea

Overdosage/Toxicology Symptoms include ototoxicity, nephrotoxicity, and neuromuscular toxicity. Serum level monitoring is recommended. The treatment of choice, following a single acute overdose, appears to be the maintenance of urine output of at least 3 mL/kg/hour. Dialysis is of questionable value in enhancing aminoglycoside elimination. If required, hemodialysis is preferred over peritoneal dialysis in patients with normal renal function. Careful hydration may be all that is required to promote diuresis and therefore enhance the drug's elimination. Chelation with penicillins is experimental.

Drug Interactions

Increased Effect/Toxicity: Penicillins, cephalosporins, amphotericin B, loop diuretics may increase nephrotoxic potential. Aminoglycosides may potentiate the effects of neuromuscular blocking agents.

Stability

Gentamicin is a colorless to slightly yellow solution which should be stored between 2°C to 30°C, but refrigeration is not recommended

I.V. infusion solutions mixed in NS or D_5W solution are stable for 24 hours at room temperature and refrigeration

Premixed bag: Manufacturer expiration date

Out of overwrap stability: 30 days

Mechanism of Action Interferes with bacterial protein synthesis by binding to 30S and 50S ribosomal subunits resulting in a defective bacterial cell membrane

Pharmacodynamics/Kinetics

Absorption: Oral: None

Distribution: Crosses placenta

V_d: Increased by edema, ascites, fluid overload; decreased with dehydration

Neonates: 0.4-0.6 L/kg

Children: 0.3-0.35 L/kg

Adults: 0.2-0.3 L/kg

Relative diffusion from blood into CSF: Minimal even with inflammation

CSF:blood level ratio: Normal meninges: Nil; Inflamed meninges: 10% to 30%

Protein binding: <30%

Half-life elimination:

Infants: <1 week old: 3-11.5 hours; 1 week to 6 months old: 3-3.5 hours

Adults: 1.5-3 hours; End-stage renal disease: 36-70 hours

Time to peak, serum: I.M.: 30-90 minutes; I.V.: 30 minutes after 30-minute infusion

Excretion: Urine (as unchanged drug)

Clearance: Directly related to renal function

Dosage Individualization is **critical** because of the low therapeutic index.

Use of ideal body weight (IBW) for determining the mg/kg/dose appears to be more accurate than dosing on the basis of total body weight (TBW). In morbid obesity, dosage requirement may best be estimated using a dosing weight of IBW + 0.4 (TBW - IBW).

Initial and periodic plasma drug levels (eg, peak and trough with conventional dosing) should be determined, particularly in critically-ill patients with serious infections or in disease states known to significantly alter aminoglycoside pharmacokinetics (eg, cystic fibrosis, burns, or major surgery).

Infants and Children <5 years: I.M., I.V.: 2.5 mg/kg/dose every 8 hours*

Children ≥5 years: I.M., I.V.: 2-2.5 mg/kg/dose every 8 hours*

Prevention of bacterial endocarditis: Dental, oral, upper respiratory procedures, GI/GU procedures: 1.5 mg/kg with ampicillin (50 mg/kg) 30 minutes prior to procedure

***Note:** Higher individual doses and/or more frequent intervals (eg, every 6 hours) may be required in selected clinical situations (cystic fibrosis) or serum levels document the need

Children and Adults:

Intrathecal: 4-8 mg/day

Ophthalmic:

Ointment: Instill 1/2" (1.25 cm) 2-3 times/day to every 3-4 hours

Solution: Instill 1-2 drops every 2-4 hours, up to 2 drops every hour for severe infections

Topical: Apply 3-4 times/day to affected area

Adults: I.M., I.V.: Systemic infections:

Severe, life-threatening infections:

Conventional dosing: 2-2.5 mg/kg/dose every 8-12 hours; to ensure adequate peak concentrations early in therapy, higher initial dosages may be considered in selected patients when extracellular water is increased (edema, septic shock, postsurgical, or trauma)

Once-daily dosing: Some clinicians suggest a daily dose of 4-7 mg/kg once daily for all patients with normal renal function; this dose is at least as efficacious with similar, if not less, toxicity than conventional dosing.

Urinary tract infections: 1.5 mg/kg/dose every 8 hours

Synergy (for gram-positive infections): 1 mg/kg/dose

Prevention of bacterial endocarditis:

Dental, oral, or upper respiratory procedures: 1.5 mg/kg (not to exceed 80 mg) with ampicillin (1-2 g) 30 minutes prior to procedure

GI/GU surgery: 1.5 mg/kg (not to exceed 80 mg) with ampicillin (2 g) 30 minutes prior to procedure

Dosing interval in renal impairment:

Conventional dosing:

Cl_{cr} ≥60 mL/minute: Administer every 8 hours

(Continued)

Gentamicin *(Continued)*

Cl_{cr} 40-60 mL/minute: Administer every 12 hours
Cl_{cr} 20-40 mL/minute: Administer every 24 hours
Cl_{cr} <20 mL/minute: Loading dose, then monitor levels
High-dose therapy: Interval may be extended (eg, every 48 hours) in patients with moderate renal impairment (Cl_{cr} 30-59 mL/minute) and/or adjusted based on serum level determinations.

Hemodialysis: Dialyzable; removal by hemodialysis: 30% removal of aminoglycosides occurs during 4 hours of HD; administer dose after dialysis and follow levels

Removal by continuous ambulatory peritoneal dialysis (CAPD):
Administration via CAPD fluid:
Gram-negative infection: 4-8 mg/L (4-8 mcg/mL) of CAPD fluid
Gram-positive infection (eg, synergy): 3-4 mg/L (3-4 mcg/mL) of CAPD fluid
Administration via I.V., I.M. route during CAPD: Dose as for Cl_{cr} <10 mL/minute and follow levels
Removal via continuous arteriovenous or venovenous hemofiltration: Dose as for Cl_{cr} 10-40 mL/minute and follow levels

Dosing adjustment/comments in hepatic disease: Monitor plasma concentrations

Dietary Considerations Calcium, magnesium, potassium: Renal wasting may cause hypocalcemia, hypomagnesemia, and/or hypokalemia.

Administration

I.M.: Administer by deep I.M. route if possible. Slower absorption and lower peak concentrations, probably due to poor circulation in the atrophic muscle, may occur following I.M. injection; in paralyzed patients, suggest I.V. route.

I.V.: Administer other antibiotics at least 1 hour before or 1 hour after gentamicin.

Ophthalmic: Administer any other ophthalmics 10 minutes before or after gentamicin preparations.

Monitoring Parameters Urinalysis, urine output, BUN, serum creatinine; hearing should be tested before, during, and after treatment; particularly in those at risk for ototoxicity or who will be receiving prolonged therapy (>2 weeks)

Reference Range

Timing of serum samples: Draw peak 30 minutes after 30-minute infusion has been completed or 1 hour after I.M. injection; draw trough immediately before next dose

Sample size: 0.5-2 mL blood (red top tube) or 0.1-1 mL serum (separated)

Therapeutic levels:
Peak:
Serious infections: 6-8 mcg/mL (12-17 μmol/L)
Life-threatening infections: 8-10 mcg/mL (17-21 μmol/L)
Urinary tract infections: 4-6 mcg/mL
Synergy against gram-positive organisms: 3-5 mcg/mL
Trough:
Serious infections: 0.5-1 mcg/mL
Life-threatening infections: 1-2 mcg/mL

Obtain drug levels after the third dose unless renal dysfunction/toxicity suspected

Test Interactions Penicillin may decrease aminoglycoside serum concentrations *in vitro*

Patient Information Report any dizziness or sensations of ringing or fullness in ears; do not touch ophthalmics to eye; use no other eye drops within 5-10 minutes of instilling ophthalmic

Dosage Forms [DSC] = Discontinued product

Cream, topical, as sulfate: 0.1% (15 g, 30 g)

Infusion, as sulfate [premixed in NS]: 40 mg (50 mL); 60 mg (50 mL, 100 mL); 70 mg (50 mL); 80 mg (50 mL, 100 mL); 90 mg (100 mL); 100 mg (50 mL, 100 mL); 120 mg (100 mL)

Injection, solution, as sulfate [ADD-Vantage® vial]: 10 mg/mL (6 mL, 8 mL, 10 mL)

Injection, solution, as sulfate: 40 mg/mL (2 mL, 20 mL) [may contain sodium metabisulfite]

Injection, solution, pediatric, as sulfate: 10 mg/mL (2 mL) [may contain sodium metabisulfite]

Injection, solution, pediatric, as sulfate [preservative free]: 10 mg/mL (2 mL)

Ointment, ophthalmic, as sulfate (Gentak®): 0.3% [3 mg/g] (3.5 g)

Ointment, topical, as sulfate: 0.1% (15 g, 30 g)

Solution, ophthalmic, as sulfate: 0.3% (5 mL, 15 mL) [contains benzalkonium chloride]
Genoptic®: 0.3% (1 mL) [contains benzalkonium chloride]
Gentacidin®: 0.3% (5 mL) [contains benzalkonium chloride] [DSC]
Gentak®: 0.3% (5 mL, 15 mL) [contains benzalkonium chloride]

Selected Readings

Begg EJ and Barclay ML, "Aminoglycosides - 50 Years On," *Br J Clin Pharmacol*, 1995, 39(6):597-603.

Cunha BA, "Aminoglycosides: Current Role in Antimicrobial Therapy," *Pharmacotherapy*, 1988, 8(6):334-50.
Edson RS and Terrell CL, "The Aminoglycosides," *Mayo Clin Proc*, 1999, 74(5):519-28.
Gilbert DN, "Once-Daily Aminoglycoside Therapy," *Antimicrob Agents Chemother*, 1991, 35(3):399-405.
Hustinx WN, and Hoepelman IM, "Aminoglycoside Dosage Regimens. Is Once a Day Enough?" *Clin Pharmacokinet*, 1993, 25(6):427-32.
Iseman MD, "Treatment of Multidrug-Resistant Tuberculosis," *N Engl J Med*, 1993, 329(11):784-91.
Lortholary O, Tod M, Cohen Y, et al, "Aminoglycosides," *Med Clin North Am*, 1995, 79(4):761-87.
McCormack JP and Jewesson PJ, "A Critical Re-Evaluation of the "Therapeutic Range" of Aminoglycosides," *Clin Infect Dis*, 1992, 14(1):320-39.

Gentamicin and Prednisolone *see* Prednisolone and Gentamicin *on page 1018*
Gentamicin Sulfate *see* Gentamicin *on page 841*
Gen-Terbinafine (Can) *see* Terbinafine *on page 1097*

Gentian Violet (JEN shun VYE oh let)

Synonyms Crystal Violet; Methylrosaniline Chloride
Generic Available Yes
Use Treatment of cutaneous or mucocutaneous infections caused by *Candida albicans* and other superficial skin infections
Pregnancy Risk Factor C
Contraindications Hypersensitivity to gentian violet or any component of the formulation; ulcerated areas; porphyria
Warnings/Precautions Infants should be turned face down after application to minimize amount of drug swallowed; may result in tattooing of the skin when applied to granulation tissue; solution is for external use only; avoid contact with eyes
Adverse Reactions Frequency not defined.
Dermatologic: Vesicle formation
Gastrointestinal: Esophagitis, ulceration of mucous membranes
Local: Burning, irritation
Respiratory: Laryngitis, laryngeal obstruction, tracheitis
Miscellaneous: Sensitivity reactions
Overdosage/Toxicology Signs and symptoms include laryngeal obstruction.
Mechanism of Action Topical antiseptic/germicide effective against some vegetative gram-positive bacteria, particularly *Staphylococcus* sp, and some yeast; it is much less effective against gram-negative bacteria and is ineffective against acid-fast bacteria
Dosage Children and Adults: Topical: Apply 0.5% to 2% locally with cotton to lesion 2-3 times/day for 3 days, do not swallow and avoid contact with eyes
Patient Information Drug stains skin and clothing purple; do not apply to an ulcerative lesion; may result in "tattooing" of the skin.
Dosage Forms Solution, topical: 1% (30 mL); 2% (30 mL)

Geocillin® *see* Carbenicillin *on page 694*
German Measles Vaccine *see* Rubella Virus Vaccine (Live) *on page 1059*
Glycerol Triacetate *see* Triacetin *on page 1129*
Gold Bond® Antifungal [OTC] *see* Tolnaftate *on page 1127*
Gramicidin, Neomycin, and Polymyxin B *see* Neomycin, Polymyxin B, and Gramicidin *on page 965*
Granulocyte Colony Stimulating Factor *see* Filgrastim *on page 817*
Grifulvin® V *see* Griseofulvin *on page 845*

Griseofulvin (gri see oh FUL vin)

U.S. Brand Names Grifulvin® V; Gris-PEG®
Canadian Brand Names Fulvicin® U/F
Synonyms Griseofulvin Microsize; Griseofulvin Ultramicrosize
Generic Available Yes: Suspension, ultramicrosized product
Use Treatment of susceptible tinea infections of the skin, hair, and nails
Drug of Choice or Alternative for Organism(s):
Dermatophytes *on page 114*
Pregnancy Risk Factor C
Contraindications Hypersensitivity to griseofulvin or any component of the formulation; severe liver disease; porphyria (interferes with porphyrin metabolism)
Warnings/Precautions Safe use in children ≤2 years of age has not been established; during long-term therapy, periodic assessment of hepatic, renal, and hematopoietic functions should be performed; may cause fetal harm when administered to pregnant women; avoid exposure to intense sunlight to prevent photosensitivity reactions; hypersensitivity cross reaction between penicillins and griseofulvin is possible
Adverse Reactions Frequency not defined.
Central nervous system: Headache, fatigue, dizziness, insomnia, mental confusion

(Continued)

Griseofulvin *(Continued)*

Dermatologic: Rash (most common), urticaria (most common), photosensitivity, erythema multiforme, angioneurotic edema (rare)
Gastrointestinal: Nausea, vomiting, epigastric distress, diarrhea, GI bleeding
Genitourinary: Menstrual irregularities (rare)
Hematologic: Leukopenia, granulocytopenia
Neuromuscular & skeletal: Paresthesia (rare)
Renal: Hepatotoxicity, proteinuria, nephrosis
Miscellaneous: Oral thrush, drug-induced lupus-like syndrome (rare)

Overdosage/Toxicology Symptoms include lethargy, vertigo, blurred vision, nausea, vomiting, and diarrhea. Following GI decontamination, treatment is supportive.

Drug Interactions

Cytochrome P450 Effect: Induces CYP1A2 (weak), 2C8/9 (weak), 3A4 (weak)

Increased Effect/Toxicity: Increased toxicity with ethanol, may cause tachycardia and flushing.

Decreased Effect: Barbiturates may decrease levels. Decreased warfarin activity. Decreased oral contraceptive effectiveness.

Ethanol/Nutrition/Herb Interactions

Ethanol: Avoid ethanol (may increase CNS depression). Ethanol will cause "disulfiram"-type reaction consisting of flushing, headache, nausea, and in some patients, vomiting and chest and/or abdominal pain.
Food: Griseofulvin concentrations may be increased if taken with food, especially with high-fat meals.

Mechanism of Action Inhibits fungal cell mitosis at metaphase; binds to human keratin making it resistant to fungal invasion

Pharmacodynamics/Kinetics

Absorption: Ultramicrosize griseofulvin absorption is almost complete; absorption of microsize griseofulvin is variable (25% to 70% of an oral dose); enhanced by ingestion of a fatty meal (GI absorption of ultramicrosize is ~1.5 times that of microsize)
Distribution: Crosses placenta
Metabolism: Extensively hepatic
Half-life elimination: 9-22 hours
Excretion: Urine (<1% as unchanged drug); feces; perspiration

Dosage Oral:

Children >2 years:
- Microsize: 10-20 mg/kg/day in single or 2 divided doses. In the treatment of tinea capitis, higher dosages (20-25 mg/kg/day for 8-12 weeks) have been recommended by some authors (unlabeled).
- Ultramicrosize: >2 years: 5-10 mg/kg/day in single or 2 divided doses. In the treatment of tinea capitis, higher dosages (15 mg/kg/day for 8-12 weeks) have been recommended by some authors (unlabeled).

Adults:
- Microsize: 500-1000 mg/day in single or divided doses
- Ultramicrosize: 330-375 mg/day in single or divided doses; doses up to 750 mg/day have been used for infections more difficult to eradicate such as tinea unguium

Duration of therapy depends on the site of infection:
- Tinea corporis: 2-4 weeks
- Tinea capitis: 4-6 weeks or longer (up to 8-12 weeks)
- Tinea pedis: 4-8 weeks
- Tinea unguium: 3-6 months or longer

Administration Oral: Administer with a fatty meal (peanuts or ice cream) to increase absorption, or with food or milk to avoid GI upset

Monitoring Parameters Periodic renal, hepatic, and hematopoietic function tests

Test Interactions False-positive urinary VMA levels

Patient Information Avoid exposure to sunlight, take with fatty meal; headaches usually go away with continued therapy; may cause dizziness, drowsiness, and impair judgment; do not take if pregnant; if you become pregnant, discontinue immediately

Dosage Forms

Suspension, oral, microsize (Grifulvin® V): 125 mg/5 mL (120 mL) [contains alcohol 0.2%]
Tablet, microsize (Grifulvin® V): 500 mg
Tablet, ultramicrosize: 125 mg, 250 mg, 330 mg
- Gris-PEG®: 125 mg, 250 mg

Selected Readings

Trepanier EF and Amsden GW, "Current Issues in Onchomycosis," *Ann Pharmacother*, 1998, 32(2):204-14.

Griseofulvin Microsize *see* Griseofulvin *on page 845*
Griseofulvin Ultramicrosize *see* Griseofulvin *on page 845*
Gris-PEG® *see* Griseofulvin *on page 845*
GW433908G *see* Fosamprenavir *on page 827*
Gynazole-1® *see* Butoconazole *on page 691*
Gyne-Lotrimin® 3 [OTC] *see* Clotrimazole *on page 758*

Haemophilus b Conjugate and Hepatitis B Vaccine

(he MOF i lus bee KON joo gate & hep a TYE tis bee vak SEEN)

U.S. Brand Names Comvax®

Synonyms *Haemophilus* b (meningococcal protein conjugate) Conjugate Vaccine; Hepatitis b Vaccine (Recombinant); Hib

Generic Available No

Use

Immunization against invasive disease caused by *H. influenzae* type b and against infection caused by all known subtypes of hepatitis B virus in infants 6 weeks to 15 months of age born of hepatitis B surface antigen (HB_sAg) negative mothers

Infants born of HB_sAg-positive mothers or mothers of unknown HB_sAg status should receive hepatitis B immune globulin and hepatitis B vaccine (recombinant) at birth and should complete the hepatitis B vaccination series given according to a particular schedule

Pregnancy Risk Factor C

Pregnancy Implications Reproduction studies have not been conducted. This product is not indicated for use in women of childbearing age.

Contraindications Hypersensitivity to *Haemophilus* b vaccine, hepatitis B vaccine, yeast, or to any component of the formulation

Warnings/Precautions If used in persons with malignancies or those receiving immunosuppressive therapy or who are otherwise immunocompromised, the expected immune response may not be obtained; may be used in patients with HIV infection.

Patients who develop symptoms suggestive of hypersensitivity after an injection should not receive further injections of the vaccine.

The decision to administer or delay vaccination because of current or recent febrile illness depends on the severity of symptoms and the etiology of the disease. Immunization should be delayed during the course of an acute febrile illness. Use caution in children with coagulation disorders (including thrombocytopenia) where intramuscular injections should not be used. Epinephrine 1:1000 should be readily available. Packaging contains natural latex rubber.

Adverse Reactions All serious adverse reactions must be reported to the U.S. Department of Health and Human Services (DHHS) Vaccine Adverse Event Reporting System (VAERS) 1-800-822-7967.

>10%:

- Central nervous system: Irritability (32% to 57%), somnolence (21% to 50%), fever (101°F to 102.9°F: 11% to 14%), crying (unusual/high pitched: 3% to 11%)
- Local: Injection site reactions: Pain/soreness (24% to 35%), swelling/induration (<1 inch: 27% to 30%), erythema (<1 inch: 22% to 27%)

1% to 10%:

- Central nervous system: Fever (≥103°F: <1% to 3%), crying (<1% to 2%)
- Dermatologic: Rash (≤1%)
- Gastrointestinal: Anorexia (<1% to 4%), vomiting (1% to 3%), diarrhea (<1% to 2%), oral candidiasis (≤1%)
- Local: Injection site reactions: Erythema (>1 inch: 1% to 3%), swelling/induration (>1 inch: 3% to 4%)
- Otic: Otitis media (<1% to 3%)
- Respiratory: cough (≤1%), respiratory congestion (≤1%), rhinorrhea (≤1%), upper respiratory tract infection (≤1%)

Postmarketing and/or case reports: Anaphylaxis, angioedema, erythema multiforme, febrile seizure, seizure, thrombocytopenia, urticaria

Stability Store at 2°C to 8°C (36°F to 48°F); do not freeze

Mechanism of Action See individual agents.

Pharmacodynamics/Kinetics See individual agents.

Dosage Infants: I.M.: 0.5 mL at 2, 4, and 12-15 months of age (total of 3 doses)

If the recommended schedule cannot be followed, the interval between the first two doses should be at least 6 weeks and the interval between the second and third dose should be as close as possible to 8-11 months. Minimum age for first dose is 6 weeks.

(Continued)

Haemophilus b Conjugate and Hepatitis B Vaccine *(Continued)*

Modified Schedule: Children who receive one dose of hepatitis B vaccine at or shortly after birth may receive Comvax® on a schedule of 2, 4, and 12-15 months of age

Administration Shake well prior to use. Administer 0.5 mL I.M. into anterolateral thigh [data suggests that injections given in the buttocks frequently are given into fatty tissue instead of into muscle to result in lower seroconversion rates]; **do not administer intravenously, intradermally, or subcutaneously.** May be administered with DTP, DTaP, OPV, IPV, MMR-II and varicella virus vaccines, using separate injection sites and syringes (for the injectable vaccines).

For patients at risk of hemorrhage following intramuscular injection, the ACIP recommends "it should be administered intramuscularly if, in the opinion of the physician familiar with the patients bleeding risk, the vaccine can be administered with reasonable safety by this route. If the patient receives antihemophilia or other similar therapy, intramuscular vaccination can be scheduled shortly after such therapy is administered. A fine needle (23 gauge or smaller) can be used for the vaccination and firm pressure applied to the site (without rubbing) for at least 2 minutes. The patient should be instructed concerning the risk of hematoma from the injection."

Patient Information May use acetaminophen for postdose fever

Additional Information Inactivated bacterial vaccine and inactivated viral vaccine. Federal law requires that the date of administration, the vaccine manufacturer, lot number of vaccine, and the administering person's name, title, and address be entered into the patient's permanent medical record.

Dosage Forms Injection, suspension [preservative free]: *Haemophilus* b PRP 7.5 mcg and HB_sAg 5 mcg per 0.5 mL (0.5 mL) [vial stopper contains latex]

Haemophilus b Conjugate Vaccine

(he MOF fi lus bee KON joo gate vak SEEN)

Related Information

Immunization Recommendations *on page 1249*

U.S. Brand Names ActHIB®; HibTITER®; PedvaxHIB®

Canadian Brand Names ActHIB®; PedvaxHIB®

Synonyms Diphtheria CRM_{197} Protein Conjugate; Diphtheria Toxoid Conjugate; *Haemophilus* b Oligosaccharide Conjugate Vaccine; *Haemophilus* b Polysaccharide Vaccine; HbCV; HbOC; Hib Polysaccharide Conjugate; PRP-OMP; PRP-T

Generic Available No

Use Routine immunization of children 2 months to 5 years of age against invasive disease caused by *H. influenzae*

Unimmunized children ≥5 years of age with a chronic illness known to be associated with increased risk of *Haemophilus influenzae* type b disease, specifically, persons with anatomic or functional asplenia or sickle cell anemia or those who have undergone splenectomy, should receive *Haemophilus influenzae* type b (Hib) vaccine.

Haemophilus b conjugate vaccines are not indicated for prevention of bronchitis or other infections due to *H. influenzae* in adults; adults with specific dysfunction or certain complement deficiencies who are at especially high risk of *H. influenzae* type b infection (HIV-infected adults); patients with Hodgkin's disease (vaccinated at least 2 weeks before the initiation of chemotherapy or 3 months after the end of chemotherapy)

Pregnancy Risk Factor C

Pregnancy Implications Reproduction studies have not been conducted.

Contraindications Hypersensitivity to *Haemophilus* b polysaccharide vaccine or any component of the formulation

Warnings/Precautions If used in persons with malignancies or those receiving immunosuppressive therapy or who are otherwise immunocompromised, the expected immune response may not be obtained; may be used in patients with HIV infection. Patients who develop symptoms suggestive of hypersensitivity after an injection should not receive further injections of the vaccine. The decision to administer or delay vaccination because of current or recent febrile illness depends on the severity of symptoms and the etiology of the disease. Immunization should be delayed during the course of an acute febrile illness. Use caution in children with coagulation disorders (including thrombocytopenia) where intramuscular injections should not be used. Epinephrine 1:1000 should be readily available.

Children in whom DTP or DT vaccination is deferred: The carrier proteins used in HbOC and PRP-T (but not PRP-OMP) are chemically and immunologically related to toxoids contained in DTP vaccine. Earlier or simultaneous vaccination with diphtheria or tetanus toxoids may be required to elicit an optimal anti-PRP antibody response to

HbOC. In contrast, the immunogenicity of PRP-OMP is not affected by vaccination with DTP. In infants in whom DTP or DT vaccination is deferred, PRP-OMP may be advantageous for *Haemophilus influenzae* type b vaccination.

Children with immunologic impairment: Children with chronic illness associated with increased risk of *Haemophilus influenzae* type b disease may have impaired anti-PRP antibody responses to conjugate vaccination. Examples include those with HIV infection, immunoglobulin deficiency, anatomic or functional asplenia, and sickle cell disease, as well as recipients of bone marrow transplants and recipients of chemotherapy for malignancy. Some children with immunologic impairment may benefit from more doses of conjugate vaccine than normally indicated.

Adverse Reactions All serious adverse reactions must be reported to the U.S. Department of Health and Human Services (DHHS) Vaccine Adverse Event Reporting System (VAERS) 1-800-822-7967. Frequency not defined:

Central nervous system: Crying (unusual, high pitched, prolonged); fever, irritability, pain, sleepiness

Dermatologic: Rash

Gastrointestinal: Anorexia, diarrhea, vomiting

Local: Injection site: Erythema, induration, pain, soreness, swelling

Otic: Otitis media

Respiratory: Upper respiratory tract infection

Postmarketing and/or case reports: Anaphylactoid reactions, angioedema, erythema multiforme, facial edema, febrile seizures, Guillain-Barré syndrome, headache, hypersensitivity, hypotonia, inflammation, injection site abscess (sterile), lethargy, lymphadenopathy, malaise, mass, seizure, skin discoloration, urticaria

Drug Interactions

Decreased Effect: The effect of the vaccine may be decreased with immunosuppressive agents; consider deferring vaccination for 3 months after immunosuppressant therapy is discontinued.

Stability Store under refrigeration at 2°C to 8°C (36°F to 46°F); do not freeze

ActHIB®: Use within 24 hours following reconstitution with saline; use within 30 minutes following reconstitution with Tripedia®

Mechanism of Action Stimulates production of anticapsular antibodies and provides active immunity to *Haemophilus influenzae*

Pharmacodynamics/Kinetics Seroconversion following one dose of Hib vaccine for children 18 months or 24 months of age or older is 75% to 90% respectively.

Onset of action: Serum antibody response: 1-2 weeks

Duration: Immunity: 1.5 years

Dosage Children: I.M.: 0.5 mL as a single dose should be administered according to one of the following "brand-specific" schedules; do not inject I.V. (see table)

Vaccination Schedule for Haemophilus b Conjugate Vaccines

Age at 1st Dose (mo)	ActHIBHib®, HibTITER®		PedvaxHIB®	
	Primary Series	Booster	Primary Series	Booster
2-6	3 doses, 2 months apart	15 mo[1]	2 doses, 2 months apart	12-15 mo[1]
7-11	2 doses, 2 months apart	15 mo[1]	2 doses, 2 months apart	12-15 mo[1]
12-14	1 dose	15 mo[1]	1 dose	15 mo[1]
15-71	1 dose	—	1 dose	—

[1]At least 2 months after previous dose.

Note: DTaP/Hib combination vaccines should not be used for infants at ages 2, 4, or 6 months, but can be used as boosters following any Hib vaccine.

Administration For patients at risk of hemorrhage following intramuscular injection, the ACIP recommends "it should be administered intramuscularly if, in the opinion of the physician familiar with the patients bleeding risk, the vaccine can be administered with reasonable safety by this route. If the patient receives antihemophilia or other similar therapy, intramuscular vaccination can be scheduled shortly after such therapy is administered. A fine needle (23 gauge or smaller) can be used for the vaccination and firm pressure applied to the site (without rubbing) for at least 2 minutes. The patient should be instructed concerning the risk of hematoma from the injection."

Test Interactions May interfere with interpretation of antigen detection tests

Patient Information May use acetaminophen for postdose fever

Additional Information Federal law requires that the date of administration, the vaccine manufacturer, lot number of vaccine, and the administering person's name, title, and address be entered into the patient's permanent medical record.

(Continued)

Haemophilus b Conjugate Vaccine *(Continued)*

The three conjugate vaccines currently available consist of *Haemophilus influenzae* type b (Hib) capsular polysaccharide (also referred to as PRP) linked to a carrier protein. The carrier protein for HibTITER® (HbOC) is a nontoxic diphtheria toxoid. PedvaxHIB® (PRP-OMP) is linked to the outer membrane protein complex from *Neisseria meningitidis*. ActHIB® (PRP-T) uses tetanus toxoid conjugate as the carrier protein.

Dosage Forms

Injection, powder for reconstitution (ActHIB®) [preservative free]: *Haemophilus* b capsular polysaccharide 10 mcg and tetanus toxoid 24 mcg per dose [may be reconstituted with provided diluent (forms solution; vial stopper contains latex) or TriHIBit® (forms suspension)]

Injection, solution [preservative free] (HibTITER®): *Haemophilus* b saccharide 10 mcg and diphtheria CRM 197 protein 25 mcg per 0.5 mL (0.5 mL) [vial stopper contains latex]

Injection, suspension (PedvaxHIB®): *Haemophilus* b capsular polysaccharide 7.5 mcg and *Neisseria meningitidis* OMPC 125 mcg per 0.5 mL (0.5 mL) [contains aluminum 225 mcg/0.5 mL]

***Haemophilus* b (meningococcal protein conjugate) Conjugate Vaccine** *see* *Haemophilus* b Conjugate and Hepatitis B Vaccine *on page 847*

***Haemophilus* b Oligosaccharide Conjugate Vaccine** *see* *Haemophilus* b Conjugate Vaccine *on page 848*

***Haemophilus* b Polysaccharide Vaccine** *see* *Haemophilus* b Conjugate Vaccine *on page 848*

***Haemophilus influenzae* b Conjugate Vaccine and Diphtheria, Tetanus Toxoids, and Acellular Pertussis Vaccine** *see* Diphtheria, Tetanus Toxoids, and Acellular Pertussis Vaccine and *Haemophilus influenzae* b Conjugate Vaccine *on page 785*

Halofantrine (ha loe FAN trin)

Related Information

Malaria Treatment *on page 1292*

Synonyms Halofantrine Hydrochloride

Generic Available No

Use Treatment of mild to moderate acute malaria caused by susceptible strains of *Plasmodium falciparum* and *Plasmodium vivax*

Drug of Choice or Alternative for Organism(s):

Plasmodium Species *on page 265*

Restrictions Not available in U.S.

Pregnancy Risk Factor C

Pregnancy Implications There are no adequate and well-controlled trials in pregnant women; has been shown to be embryotoxic in animal tests.

Contraindications Family history of congenital QT_c prolongation; hypersensitivity to halofantrine or any component of the formulation; drugs or clinical conditions known to prolong QT_c intervals; previous treatment with mefloquine; known or suspected ventricular dysrhythmias; AV conduction abnormalities or unexplained syncope; concurrent or prior treatment with mefloquine

Warnings/Precautions Monitor closely for decreased hematocrit and hemoglobin. Use caution in chronic liver disease. May prolong QT_c at therapeutic dosages; perform baseline ECG to ensure normal QT_c prior to treatment. Safety and efficacy have not been established in pediatric patients.

Adverse Reactions

1% to 10%:

- Cardiovascular: Edema
- Central nervous system: Malaise, headache (3%), dizziness (5%)
- Dermatologic: Pruritus (3%)
- Gastrointestinal: Nausea (3%), vomiting (4%), abdominal pain (9%), diarrhea (6%), anorexia (5%)
- Hematologic: Leukocytosis
- Hepatic: Elevated LFTs
- Local: Tenderness
- Neuromuscular & skeletal: Myalgia (1%), rigors (2%)
- Respiratory: Cough
- Miscellaneous: Lymphadenopathy

<1%: Tachycardia, hypotension, hypoglycemia, sterile abscesses, asthma, anaphylactic shock, chest pain, palpitation, orthostasis, weakness, confusion, depression, paresthesia, constipation, abnormal vision, tinnitus, facial edema, urticaria

Postmarketing and/or case reports: Anaphylaxis, CVA, hemolytic anemia, hypertensive crisis, pulmonary edema, QT_c prolongation, seizure, tetany, ventricular arrhythmia

Overdosage/Toxicology GI distress with abdominal pain, vomiting, diarrhea, cramping, and palpitations have been reported at higher than recommended doses. Treatment should be symptom-directed and supportive, including ECG monitoring; vomiting should be induced.

Drug Interactions

Cytochrome P450 Effect: Substrate of CYP2C8/9 (minor), 2D6 (minor), 3A4 (major); **Inhibits** CYP2D6 (weak)

Increased Effect/Toxicity: CYP3A4 inhibitors may increase the levels/effects of halofantrine; example inhibitors include azole antifungals, ciprofloxacin, clarithromycin, diclofenac, doxycycline, erythromycin, imatinib, isoniazid, nefazodone, nicardipine, propofol, protease inhibitors, quinidine, and verapamil. Increased toxicity (QT_c interval prolongation) with other agents that cause QT_c interval prolongation, especially mefloquine.

Decreased Effect: CYP3A4 inducers may decrease the levels/effects of halofantrine; example inducers include aminoglutethimide, carbamazepine, nafcillin, nevirapine, phenobarbital, phenytoin, and rifamycins.

Ethanol/Nutrition/Herb Interactions Food: May increase absorption, increasing the risk of toxicity.

Stability Store at 20°C to 25°C (68°F to 77°F); protect from light

Mechanism of Action Exact mechanism unknown; destruction of asexual blood forms, possible inhibition of proton pump

Pharmacodynamics/Kinetics

Absorption: Erratic and variable; serum levels are proportional to dose up to 1000 mg; smaller doses should be divided; may be increased 60% with high fat meals

Distribution: V_d: 570 L/kg; widely to most tissues

Metabolism: Hepatic to active metabolite

Half-life elimination: 6-10 days; Metabolite: 3-4 days; may be prolonged in active disease

Excretion: Primarily in feces (hepatobiliary)

Clearance: Parasite: Mean: 40-84 hours

Dosage Oral:

Children (unlabeled):

<40 kg: 8 mg/kg every 6 hours for 3 doses; repeat in 1 week

≥40 kg: 500 mg every 6 hours for 3 doses; repeat in 1 week

Adults: 500 mg every 6 hours for 3 doses; repeat in 1 week

Dietary Considerations Take on an empty stomach, 1 hour before or 2 hours after food. Avoid high-fat meals.

Administration Administer on an empty stomach, 1 hour before or 2 hours after food. Avoid high-fat meals.

Monitoring Parameters CBC, LFTs, parasite counts; pretreatment ECG; monitor cardiac rhythm during and for 8-12 hours following completion of therapy

Test Interactions Increased serum transaminases, bilirubin

Patient Information Take on an empty stomach, 1 hour before or 2 hours after food; avoid high-fat meals; notify prescriber of persistent nausea, vomiting, abdominal pain, light stools, dark urine

Dosage Forms Tablet, as hydrochloride: 250 mg

Selected Readings

White NJ, "The Treatment of Malaria," *N Engl J Med*, 1996, 335(11):800-6.

Halofantrine Hydrochloride *see* Halofantrine *on page 850*

Halotestin® *see* Fluoxymesterone *on page 825*

Havrix® *see* Hepatitis A Vaccine *on page 853*

Havrix® and Engerix-B® *see* Hepatitis A Inactivated and Hepatitis B (Recombinant) Vaccine *on page 852*

HbCV *see Haemophilus* b Conjugate Vaccine *on page 848*

HBIG *see* Hepatitis B Immune Globulin *on page 855*

HbOC *see Haemophilus* b Conjugate Vaccine *on page 848*

HDCV *see* Rabies Virus Vaccine *on page 1034*

Head & Shoulders® Intensive Treatment [OTC] *see* Selenium Sulfide *on page 1063*

Helidac® *see* Bismuth Subsalicylate, Metronidazole, and Tetracycline *on page 688*

Hepatitis A Inactivated and Hepatitis B (Recombinant) Vaccine

(hep a TYE tis aye in ak ti VAY ted & hep a TYE tis bee ree KOM be nant vak SEEN)

U.S. Brand Names Twinrix®

Canadian Brand Names Twinrix®

Synonyms Engerix-B® and Havrix®; Havrix® and Engerix-B®; Hepatitis B (Recombinant) and Hepatitis A Inactivated Vaccine

Generic Available No

Use Active immunization against disease caused by hepatitis A virus and hepatitis B virus (all known subtypes) in populations desiring protection against or at high risk of exposure to these viruses.

Populations include travelers to areas of intermediate/high endemicity for **both** HAV and HBV; those at increased risk of HBV infection due to behavioral or occupational factors; patients with chronic liver disease; laboratory workers who handle live HAV and HBV; healthcare workers, police, and other personnel who render first-aid or medical assistance; workers who come in contact with sewage; employees of day care centers and correctional facilities; patients/staff of hemodialysis units; male homosexuals; patients frequently receiving blood products; military personnel; users of injectable illicit drugs; close household contacts of patients with hepatitis A and hepatitis B infection.

Pregnancy Risk Factor C

Pregnancy Implications Healthcare providers are encouraged to call the manufacturer of Twinrix® to register any patients who may have received this vaccine during pregnancy.

Contraindications Hypersensitivity to hepatitis A vaccine or hepatitis B vaccine, or any component of the formulation

Warnings/Precautions Use caution in patients on anticoagulants, with thrombocytopenia, or bleeding disorders (bleeding may occur following intramuscular injection). Treatment for anaphylactic reactions should be immediately available. Postpone vaccination in moderate to severe acute illness (minor illness is not a contraindication). May not prevent infection if adequate antibody titers are not achieved (including immunosuppressed patients, patients on immunosuppressant therapy). Safety and efficacy in patients <18 years of age have not been established.

See individual agents.

Adverse Reactions All serious adverse reactions must be reported to the U.S. Department of Health and Human Services (DHHS) Vaccine Adverse Event Reporting System (VAERS) 1-800-822-7967.

Incidence of adverse effects of the combination product were similar to those occurring after administration of hepatitis A vaccine and hepatitis B vaccine alone. (Incidence reported is not versus placebo.)

>10%:

- Central nervous system: Headache (13% to 22%), fatigue (11% to 14%)
- Local: Injection site reaction: Soreness (37% to 41%), redness (9% to 11%)

1% to 10%:

- Central nervous system: Fever (2% to 3%)
- Gastrointestinal: Diarrhea (4% to 6%), nausea (2% to 4%), vomiting (≤1%)
- Local: Injection site reaction: Swelling (4% to 6%), induration
- Respiratory: Upper respiratory tract infection
- Miscellaneous: Flu-like syndrome

<1%: Abdominal pain, agitation, anorexia, arthralgia, back pain, bruising at the injection site, diaphoresis, dizziness, erythema, flushing, insomnia, irritability, migraine, myalgia, paresthesia, petechia, pruritus at the injection site, rash, somnolence, syncope, urticaria, vertigo, vomiting, weakness

Postmarketing and/or case reports (as reported with hepatitis A vaccine and hepatitis B vaccine; also see individual agents): Allergic reactions, alopecia, anaphylaxis, anaphylactoid reactions, angioedema, arthritis, Bell's palsy, bronchospasm, congenital abnormality, conjunctivitis, convulsions, dyspepsia, dyspnea, earache, eczema, encephalopathy, erythema multiforme, erythema nodosum, Guillain-Barré syndrome, hepatitis, herpes zoster, hyperhydrosis, jaundice, keratitis, liver function test abnormalities, myelitis, neuropathy, optic neuritis, paresis, serum sickness like syndrome, Stevens-Johnson syndrome, thrombocytopenia, tinnitus, visual disturbances

Drug Interactions

Decreased Effect: Immunosuppressant agents: May decrease immune response to vaccine

Stability Store in refrigerator at 2°C to 8°C (36°F to 46°F); do not freeze (discard if frozen)

Mechanism of Action

Hepatitis A vaccine (Havrix®), an inactivated virus vaccine, offers active immunization against hepatitis A virus infection at an effective immune response rate in up to 99% of subjects.

Recombinant hepatitis B vaccine (Engerix-B®) is a noninfectious subunit viral vaccine. The vaccine is derived from hepatitis B surface antigen (HB_sAg) produced through recombinant DNA techniques from yeast cells. The portion of the hepatitis B gene which codes for HB_sAg is cloned into yeast which is then cultured to produce hepatitis B vaccine.

In immunocompetent people, Twinrix® provides active immunization against hepatitis A virus infection (at an effective immune response rate >99% of subjects) and against hepatitis B virus infection (at an effective immune response rate of 93% to 97%) 30 days after completion of the 3-dose series. This is comparable to using hepatitis A vaccine (Havrix®) and hepatitis B vaccine (Engerix-B®) concomitantly.

Pharmacodynamics/Kinetics

Onset of action: Seroconversion for antibodies against HAV and HBV were detected 1 month after completion of the 3-dose series.

Duration: Patients remained seropositive for at least 4 years during clinical studies.

Dosage I.M.: Adults: Primary immunization: Three doses (1 mL each) given on a 0-, 1-, and 6-month schedule

Administration I.M.: Shake well prior to use. Do not dilute prior to administration. Administer in the deltoid region; do not administer in the gluteal region (may give suboptimal response). Do not administer at the same site, or using the same syringe, as additional vaccines or immunoglobulins.

For patients at risk of hemorrhage following intramuscular injection, the ACIP recommends "it should be administered intramuscularly if, in the opinion of the physician familiar with the patients bleeding risk, the vaccine can be administered with reasonable safety by this route. If the patient receives antihemophilia or other similar therapy, intramuscular vaccination can be scheduled shortly after such therapy is administered. A fine needle (23 gauge or smaller) can be used for the vaccination and firm pressure applied to the site (without rubbing) for at least 2 minutes. The patient should be instructed concerning the risk of hematoma from the injection."

Additional Information Federal law requires that the date of administration, the vaccine manufacturer, lot number of vaccine, and the administering person's name, title, and address be entered into the patient's permanent medical record.

Dosage Forms Injection, suspension: Inactivated hepatitis A virus 720 ELISA units and hepatitis B surface antigen 20 mcg per mL (1 mL) [prefilled syringe; single-dose vial]

Hepatitis A Vaccine (hep a TYE tis aye vak SEEN)

Related Information

Immunization Recommendations *on page 1249*

USPHS / IDSA Guidelines for the Prevention of Opportunistic Infections in Persons Infected With HIV *on page 1237*

U.S. Brand Names Havrix®; VAQTA®

Canadian Brand Names Avaxim®; Avaxim®-Pediatric; Epaxal Berna®; Havrix®; VAQTA®

Generic Available No

Use For populations desiring protection against hepatitis A or for populations at high risk of exposure to hepatitis A virus (travelers to developing countries, household and sexual contacts of persons infected with hepatitis A), child day care employees, patients with chronic liver disease, illicit drug users, male homosexuals, institutional workers (eg, institutions for the mentally and physically handicapped persons, prisons), and healthcare workers who may be exposed to hepatitis A virus (eg, laboratory employees); protection lasts for approximately 15 years

Drug of Choice or Alternative for Organism(s):

Hepatitis A Virus *on page 164*

Pregnancy Risk Factor C

Contraindications Hypersensitivity to hepatitis A vaccine or any component of the formulation

Warnings/Precautions Use caution in patients with serious active infection, cardiovascular disease, or pulmonary disorders; treatment for anaphylactic reactions should be immediately available

(Continued)

Hepatitis A Vaccine *(Continued)*

Adverse Reactions All serious adverse reactions must be reported to the U.S. Department of Health and Human Services (DHHS) Vaccine Adverse Event Reporting System (VAERS) 1-800-822-7967.

Percentage unknown: Fatigue, fever (rare), transient LFT abnormalities

>10%:

Central nervous system: Headache

Local: Pain, tenderness, and warmth

1% to 10%:

Endocrine & metabolic: Pharyngitis (1%)

Gastrointestinal: Abdominal pain (1%)

Local: Cutaneous reactions at the injection site (soreness, edema, and redness)

Mechanism of Action As an inactivated virus vaccine, hepatitis A vaccine offers active immunization against hepatitis A virus infection at an effective immune response rate in up to 99% of subjects

Pharmacodynamics/Kinetics

Onset of action (protection): 3 weeks after a single dose

Duration: Neutralizing antibodies have persisted for >3 years; unconfirmed evidence indicates that antibody levels may persist for 5-10 years

Dosage I.M.:

Havrix®:

Children 2-18 years: 720 ELISA units (administered as 2 injections of 360 ELISA units [0.5 mL]) 15-30 days prior to travel with a booster 6-12 months following primary immunization; the deltoid muscle should be used for I.M. injection

Adults: 1440 ELISA units (1 mL) 15-30 days prior to travel with a booster 6-12 months following primary immunization; injection should be in the deltoid

VAQTA®:

Children 2-17 years: 25 units (0.5 mL) with 25 units (0.5 mL) booster to be given 6-18 months after primary immunization

Adults: 50 units (1 mL) with 50 units (1 mL) booster to be given 6 months after primary immunization

Administration For patients at risk of hemorrhage following intramuscular injection, the ACIP recommends "it should be administered intramuscularly if, in the opinion of the physician familiar with the patients bleeding risk, the vaccine can be administered with reasonable safety by this route. If the patient receives antihemophilia or other similar therapy, intramuscular vaccination can be scheduled shortly after such therapy is administered. A fine needle (23 gauge or smaller) can be used for the vaccination and firm pressure applied to the site (without rubbing) for at least 2 minutes. The patient should be instructed concerning the risk of hematoma from the injection."

Monitoring Parameters Liver function tests

Reference Range Seroconversion for Havrix®: Antibody >20 milli-international units/mL

Additional Information Some investigators suggest simultaneous or sequential administration of inactivated hepatitis A vaccine and immune globulin for postexposure protection, especially for travelers requiring rapid immunization, although a slight decrease in vaccine immunogenicity may be observed with this technique. Federal law requires that the date of administration, the vaccine manufacturer, lot number of vaccine, and the administering person's name, title and address be entered into the patient's permanent medical record.

Dosage Forms

Injection, suspension, adult [prefilled syringe; single-dose vial]:

Havrix®: Viral antigen 1440 ELISA units/mL (1 mL)

VAQTA®: HAV protein 50 units/mL (1 mL)

Injection, suspension, pediatric [prefilled syringe; single-dose vial] (Havrix®): Viral antigen 720 ELISA units/0.5 mL (0.5 mL)

Injection, suspension, pediatric/adolescent [prefilled syringe; single-dose vial] (VAQTA®): HAV protein 25 units/0.5 mL (0.5 mL)

Selected Readings

Bancroft WH, "Hepatitis A Vaccine," *N Engl J Med*, 1992, 327(7):453-7.

Koff RS, "Hepatitis A," *Lancet*, 1998, 351(9116):1643-9.

Lemon SM, "Inactivated Hepatitis A Vaccines," *JAMA*, 1994, 271(17):1363-4.

Niu MT, Salive M, Krueger C, et al, "Two-Year Review of Hepatitis A Vaccine Safety: Data From the Vaccine Adverse Event Reporting System (VAERS)," *Clin Infect Dis*, 1998, 26(6):1475-6.

Hepatitis B Immune Globulin (hep a TYE tis bee i MYUN GLOB yoo lin)

U.S. Brand Names BayHep B®; Nabi-HB®

Canadian Brand Names BayHep B®

Synonyms HBIG

Generic Available No

Use Provide prophylactic passive immunity to hepatitis B infection to those individuals exposed; newborns of mothers known to be hepatitis B surface antigen positive; hepatitis B immune globulin is not indicated for treatment of active hepatitis B infections and is ineffective in the treatment of chronic active hepatitis B infection

Drug of Choice or Alternative for Organism(s):

Hepatitis B Virus *on page 165*

Pregnancy Risk Factor C

Contraindications Hypersensitivity to hepatitis B immune globulin or any component of the formulation; allergies to gamma globulin or anti-immunoglobulin antibodies; allergies to thimerosal; IgA deficiency

Warnings/Precautions Have epinephrine 1:1000 available for anaphylactic reactions. As a product of human plasma, this product may potentially transmit disease; screening of donors, as well as testing and/or inactivation of certain viruses reduces this risk. Use caution in patients with thrombocytopenia or coagulation disorders (I.M. injections may be contraindicated), in patients with isolated IgA deficiency, or in patients with previous systemic hypersensitivity to human immunoglobulins. Not for intravenous administration.

Adverse Reactions Frequency not defined.

Central nervous system: Dizziness, malaise, fever, lethargy, chills
Dermatologic: Urticaria, angioedema, rash, erythema
Gastrointestinal: Vomiting, nausea
Genitourinary: Nephrotic syndrome
Local: Pain, tenderness, and muscular stiffness at injection site
Neuromuscular & skeletal: Arthralgia, myalgia
Miscellaneous: Anaphylaxis

Stability Refrigerate at 2°C to 8°C (36°F to 46°F); do not freeze

Mechanism of Action Hepatitis B immune globulin (HBIG) is a nonpyrogenic sterile solution containing 10% to 18% protein of which at least 80% is monomeric immunoglobulin G (IgG). HBIG differs from immune globulin in the amount of anti-HB_s. Immune globulin is prepared from plasma that is not preselected for anti-HB_s content. HBIG is prepared from plasma preselected for high titer anti-HB_s. In the U.S., HBIG has an anti-HB_s high titer >1:100,000 by IRA. There is no evidence that the causative agent of AIDS (HTLV-III/LAV) is transmitted by HBIG.

Pharmacodynamics/Kinetics

Absorption: Slow
Time to peak, serum: 1-6 days

Dosage I.M.:

Newborns: Hepatitis B: 0.5 mL as soon after birth as possible (within 12 hours); may repeat at 3 months in order for a higher rate of prevention of the carrier state to be achieved; at this time an active vaccination program with the vaccine may begin

Adults: Postexposure prophylaxis: 0.06 mL/kg as soon as possible after exposure (ie, within 24 hours of needlestick, ocular, or mucosal exposure or within 14 days of sexual exposure); usual dose: 3-5 mL; repeat at 28-30 days after exposure

Note: HBIG may be administered at the same time (but at a different site) or up to 1 month preceding hepatitis B vaccination without impairing the active immune response

Administration I.M. injection only in gluteal or deltoid region; to prevent injury from injection, care should be taken when giving to patients with thrombocytopenia or bleeding disorders; has been administered intravenously in hepatitis B-positive liver transplant patients

Additional Information Has been administered intravenously in hepatitis B-positive liver transplant patients.

Dosage Forms Note: Potency expressed in international units as compared to the WHO standard

Injection, solution [preservative free]:

BayHepB®: 217 int. units/mL (0.5 mL) [neonatal single-dose syringe]; (1 mL) [single-dose syringe or single-dose vial]; (5 mL) [single-dose vial]

Nabi-HB®: 208 int. units/mL (1 mL, 5 mL) [single-dose vial]

Hepatitis B Inactivated Virus Vaccine (plasma derived) *see* Hepatitis B Vaccine *on page 856*

Hepatitis B Inactivated Virus Vaccine (recombinant DNA) *see* Hepatitis B Vaccine *on page 856*

Hepatitis B (Recombinant) and Hepatitis A Inactivated Vaccine *see* Hepatitis A Inactivated and Hepatitis B (Recombinant) Vaccine *on page 852*

Hepatitis B Vaccine (hep a TYE tis bee vak SEEN)

Related Information

Immunization Recommendations *on page 1249*

USPHS / IDSA Guidelines for the Prevention of Opportunistic Infections in Persons Infected With HIV *on page 1237*

U.S. Brand Names Engerix-B®; Recombivax HB®

Canadian Brand Names Engerix-B®; Recombivax HB®

Synonyms Hepatitis B Inactivated Virus Vaccine (plasma derived); Hepatitis B Inactivated Virus Vaccine (recombinant DNA)

Generic Available No

Use Immunization against infection caused by all known subtypes of hepatitis B virus, in individuals considered at high risk of potential exposure to hepatitis B virus or HB_sAg-positive materials: See table.

Pre-exposure Prophylaxis for Hepatitis B
Healthcare workers[1]
Special patient groups (eg, adolescents, infants born to HB_sAg-positive mothers, children born after 11/21/91, military personnel, etc)
Hemodialysis patients[2] (see dosing recommendations)
Recipients of certain blood products[3]
Lifestyle factors
Homosexual and bisexual men
Intravenous drug abusers
Heterosexually-active persons with multiple sexual partners or recently acquired sexually-transmitted diseases
Environmental factors
Household and sexual contacts of HBV carriers
Prison inmates
Clients and staff of institutions for the mentally handicapped
Residents, immigrants, and refugees from areas with endemic HBV infection
International travelers at increased risk of acquiring HBV infection

[1]The risk of hepatitis B virus (HBV) infection for healthcare workers varies both between hospitals and within hospitals. Hepatitis B vaccination is recommended for all healthcare workers with blood exposure.

[2]Hemodialysis patients often respond poorly to hepatitis B vaccination; higher vaccine doses or increased number of doses are required. A special formulation of one vaccine is now available for such persons (Recombivax HB®, 40 mcg/mL). The anti-Hb_s (antibody to hepatitis B surface antigen) response of such persons should be tested after they are vaccinated, and those who have not responded should be revaccinated with 1-3 additional doses.

Patients with chronic renal disease should be vaccinated as early as possible, ideally before they require hemodialysis. In addition, their anti-HB_s levels should be monitored at 6- to 12-month intervals to assess the need for revaccination.

[3]Patients with hemophilia should be immunized subcutaneously, not intramuscularly.

Drug of Choice or Alternative for Organism(s):

Hepatitis B Virus *on page 165*

Pregnancy Risk Factor C

Pregnancy Implications Reproduction studies have not been conducted. The ACIP suggests vaccination should be considered if otherwise indicated.

Contraindications Hypersensitivity to yeast, hepatitis B vaccine, or any component of the formulation

Warnings/Precautions Immediate treatment for anaphylactic/anaphylactoid reaction should be available during vaccine use; consider delaying vaccination during acute febrile illness; use caution with decreased cardiopulmonary function; unrecognized hepatitis B infection may be present, immunization may not prevent infection in these patients; patients >65 years may have lower response rates

Adverse Reactions All serious adverse reactions must be reported to the U.S. Department of Health and Human Services (DHHS) Vaccine Adverse Event Reporting System (VAERS) 1-800-822-7967.

Frequency not defined. The most common adverse effects reported with both products included injection site reactions (>10%).

Cardiovascular: Hypotension

Central nervous system: Agitation, chills, dizziness, fatigue, fever (≥37.5°C/100°F), flushing, headache, insomnia, irritability, lightheadedness, malaise, vertigo

Dermatologic: Angioedema, petechiae, pruritus, rash, urticaria
Gastrointestinal: Abdominal pain, appetite decreased, cramps, diarrhea, dyspepsia, nausea, vomiting
Genitourinary: Dysuria
Local: Injection site reactions: Ecchymosis, erythema, induration, pain, nodule formation, soreness, swelling, tenderness, warmth
Neuromuscular & skeletal: Achiness, arthralgia, back pain, myalgia, neck pain, neck stiffness, paresthesia, shoulder pain, weakness
Otic: Earache
Respiratory: Cough, pharyngitis, rhinitis, upper respiratory tract infection
Miscellaneous: Lymphadenopathy, diaphoresis

Postmarketing and/or case reports: Alopecia, anaphylaxis, arthritis, Bell's palsy, bronchospasm, conjunctivitis, constipation, eczema, encephalitis, erythema nodosum, erythema multiforme, erythrocyte sedimentation rate increased, Guillain-Barré syndrome, herpes zoster, hypoesthesia, keratitis, liver enzyme elevation, migraine, multiple sclerosis, optic neuritis, palpitation, paresis, paresthesia, purpura, seizure, serum-sickness like syndrome (may be delayed days to weeks), Stevens-Johnson syndrome, syncope, tachycardia, thrombocytopenia, transverse myelitis, visual disturbances, vertigo

Drug Interactions

Decreased Effect: Decreased effect: Immunosuppressive agents

Stability Refrigerate at 2°C to 8°C (36°F to 46°F). Do not freeze.

Mechanism of Action Recombinant hepatitis B vaccine is a noninfectious subunit viral vaccine. The vaccine is derived from hepatitis B surface antigen (HB_sAg) produced through recombinant DNA techniques from yeast cells. The portion of the hepatitis B gene which codes for HB_sAg is cloned into yeast which is then cultured to produce hepatitis B vaccine.

Pharmacodynamics/Kinetics Duration of action: Following a 3-dose series, immunity lasts ~5-7 years

Dosage I.M.:

Immunization regimen: Regimen consists of 3 doses (0, 1, and 6 months): First dose given on the elected date, second dose given 1 month later, third dose given 6 months after the first dose; see table.

Routine Immunization Regimen of Three I.M. Hepatitis B Vaccine Doses

Age	Initial		1 mo		6 mo	
	Recombivax HB® (mL)	Engerix-B® (mL)	Recombivax HB® (mL)	Engerix-B® (mL)	Recombivax HB® (mL)	Engerix-B® (mL)
Birth[1] to 19 y	0.5[2]	0.5[3]	0.5[2]	0.5[3]	0.5[2]	0.5[3]
≥20 y	1[4]	1[5]	1[4]	1[5]	1[4]	1[5]
Dialysis or immunocompromised patients[6]	1[7]	2[8]	1[7]	2[8]	1[7]	2[8]

[1]Infants born of HB_sAg **negative** mothers.

[2]5 mcg/0.5 mL pediatric/adolescent formulation

[3]10 mcg/0.5 mL formulation

[4]10 mcg/mL adult formulation

[5]20 mcg/mL formulation

[6]Revaccinate if anti-HB_s <10 mIU/mL ≥1-2 months after third dose.

[7]40 mcg/mL dialysis formulation

[8]Two 1 mL doses given at different sites using the 40 mcg/2 mL dialysis formulation

Alternative dosing schedule for **Recombivax HB®:** Children 11-15 years (10 mcg/mL adult formulation): First dose of 1 mL given on the elected date, second dose given 4-6 months later

Alternative dosing schedules for **Engerix-B®:**

Children ≤10 years (10 mcg/0.5 mL formulation): High-risk children: 0.5 mL at 0, 1, 2, and 12 months; lower-risk children ages 5-10 who are candidates for an extended administration schedule may receive an alternative regimen of 0.5 mL at 0, 12, and 24 months. If booster dose is needed, revaccinate with 0.5 mL.

Adolescents 11-19 years (20 mcg/mL formulation): 1 mL at 0, 1, and 6 months. High-risk adolescents: 1 mL at 0, 1, 2, and 12 months; lower-risk adolescents 11-16 years who are candidates for an extended administration schedule may receive an alternative regimen of 0.5 mL (using the 10 mcg/0.5 mL) formulation at 0, 12, and 24 months. If booster dose is needed, revaccinate with 20 mcg.

Adults ≥20 years: High-risk adults (20 mcg/mL formulation): 1 mL at 0, 1, 2, and 12 months. If booster dose is needed, revaccinate with 1 mL.

(Continued)

Hepatitis B Vaccine *(Continued)*

Postexposure prophylaxis: See table.

Postexposure Prophylaxis Recommended Dosage for Infants Born to HB_sAg-Positive Mothers

Treatment	Birth	Within 7 d	1 mo	6 mo
Engerix-B® (pediatric formulation 10 mcg/ 0.5 mL)[1]	Note[2]	0.5 mL[2]	0.5 mL	0.5 mL
Recombivax HB® (pediatric/adolescent formulation 5 mcg/0.5 mL)	Note[2]	0.5 mL[2]	0.5 mL	0.5 mL
Hepatitis B immune globulin	0.5 mL	—	—	—

[1]An alternate regimen is administration of the vaccine at birth, within 7 days of birth, and 1, 2, and 12 months later.

[2]The first dose may be given at birth at the same time as HBIG, but give in the opposite anterolateral thigh. This may better ensure vaccine absorption.

Administration It is possible to interchange the vaccines for completion of a series or for booster doses; the antibody produced in response to each type of vaccine is comparable, however, the quantity of the vaccine will vary

I.M. injection only; in adults, the deltoid muscle is the preferred site; the anterolateral thigh is the recommended site in infants and young children. Not for gluteal administration. Shake well prior to withdrawal and use.

For patients at risk of hemorrhage following intramuscular injection, the ACIP recommends "it should be administered intramuscularly if, in the opinion of the physician familiar with the patients bleeding risk, the vaccine can be administered with reasonable safety by this route. If the patient receives antihemophilia or other similar therapy, intramuscular vaccination can be scheduled shortly after such therapy is administered. A fine needle (23 gauge or smaller) can be used for the vaccination and firm pressure applied to the site (without rubbing) for at least 2 minutes. The patient should be instructed concerning the risk of hematoma from the injection."

Federal law requires that the date of administration, the vaccine manufacturer, lot number of vaccine, and the administering person's name, title, and address be entered into the patient's permanent medical record.

Patient Information Must complete full course of injections for adequate immunization

Additional Information Inactivated virus vaccine. Federal law requires that the date of administration, the vaccine manufacturer, lot number of vaccine, and the administering person's name, title, and address be entered into the patient's permanent medical record.

Dosage Forms

Injection, suspension [recombinant DNA]:
- Engerix-B®:
  - Adult: Hepatitis B surface antigen 20 mcg/mL (1 mL) [contains trace amounts of thimerosal]
  - Pediatric/adolescent: Hepatitis B surface antigen 10 mcg/0.5 mL (0.5 mL) [contains trace amounts of thimerosal]
- Recombivax HB®:
  - Adult [preservative free]: Hepatitis B surface antigen 10 mcg/mL (1 mL, 3 mL)
  - Dialysis [preservative free]: Hepatitis B surface antigen 40 mcg/mL (1 mL)
  - Pediatric/adolescent [preservative free]: Hepatitis B surface antigen 5 mcg/0.5 mL (0.5 mL)

Hepatitis b Vaccine (Recombinant) *see Haemophilus* b Conjugate and Hepatitis B Vaccine *on page 847*

Hepsera™ *see* Adefovir *on page 633*

Heptovir® (Can) *see* Lamivudine *on page 905*

Hexachlorocyclohexane *see* Lindane *on page 913*

Hexachlorophene (heks a KLOR oh feen)

U.S. Brand Names pHisoHex®

Canadian Brand Names pHisoHex®

Generic Available No

Use Surgical scrub and as a bacteriostatic skin cleanser; control an outbreak of gram-positive infection when other procedures have been unsuccessful

Pregnancy Risk Factor C

Contraindications Hypersensitivity to halogenated phenol derivatives or hexachlorophene; use in premature infants; use on burned or denuded skin; occlusive dressing; application to mucous membranes

Warnings/Precautions Discontinue use if signs of cerebral irritability occur; exposure of preterm infants or patients with extensive burns has been associated with apnea, convulsions, agitation and coma; do not use for bathing infants, premature infants are particularly susceptible to hexachlorophene topical absorption

Adverse Reactions <1%: CNS injury, seizure, irritability, photosensitivity, dermatitis, redness, dry skin

Stability Store in nonmetallic container (**incompatible** with many metals); prolonged direct exposure to strong light may cause brownish surface discoloration, but this does not affect its action

Mechanism of Action Bacteriostatic polychlorinated biphenyl which inhibits membrane-bound enzymes and disrupts the cell membrane

Pharmacodynamics/Kinetics

Absorption: Percutaneously through inflamed, excoriated, and intact skin

Distribution: Crosses placenta

Half-life elimination: Infants: 6.1-44.2 hours

Dosage Children and Adults: Topical: Apply 5 mL cleanser and water to area to be cleansed; lather and rinse thoroughly under running water

Dosage Forms Liquid, topical (pHisoHex®): 3% (150 mL, 500 mL, 3840 mL)

Selected Readings

Halling H, "Suspected Link Between Exposure to Hexachlorophene and Malformed Infants," *Ann N Y Acad Sci*, 1979, 320:426-35.

Lester RS, "Topical Formulary for the Pediatrician," *Pediatr Clin North Am*, 1983, 30(4):749-65.

Lockhart JD, "How Toxic is Hexachlorophene?" *Pediatrics*, 1972, 50(2):229-35.

Marquardt ED, "Hexachlorophene Toxicity in a Pediatric Burn Patient," *Drug Intell Clin Pharm*, 1986, 20(7-8):624.

Nagy L and Orosz M, "Occupational Asthma Due to Hexachlorophene," *Thorax*, 1984, 39(8):630-1.

Hexamethylenetetramine *see* Methenamine *on page 939*

Hexit™ (Can) *see* Lindane *on page 913*

Hib *see Haemophilus* b Conjugate and Hepatitis B Vaccine *on page 847*

Hibiclens® [OTC] *see* Chlorhexidine Gluconate *on page 735*

Hibidil® 1:2000 (Can) *see* Chlorhexidine Gluconate *on page 735*

Hibistat® [OTC] *see* Chlorhexidine Gluconate *on page 735*

Hib Polysaccharide Conjugate *see Haemophilus* b Conjugate Vaccine *on page 848*

HibTITER® *see Haemophilus* b Conjugate Vaccine *on page 848*

Hiprex® *see* Methenamine *on page 939*

Hivid® *see* Zalcitabine *on page 1155*

HMR 3647 *see* Telithromycin *on page 1093*

Hp-PAC® (Can) *see* Lansoprazole, Amoxicillin, and Clarithromycin *on page 908*

Human Diploid Cell Cultures Rabies Vaccine *see* Rabies Virus Vaccine *on page 1034*

Human Growth Hormone *see* Somatropin *on page 1069*

Humatin® *see* Paromomycin *on page 989*

Humatrope® *see* Somatropin *on page 1069*

Hydrocortisone, Acetic Acid, and Propylene Glycol Diacetate *see* Acetic Acid, Propylene Glycol Diacetate, and Hydrocortisone *on page 629*

Hydrocortisone and Ciprofloxacin *see* Ciprofloxacin and Hydrocortisone *on page 749*

Hydrocortisone and Iodoquinol *see* Iodoquinol and Hydrocortisone *on page 892*

Hydrocortisone, Bacitracin, Neomycin, and Polymyxin B *see* Bacitracin, Neomycin, Polymyxin B, and Hydrocortisone *on page 682*

Hydrocortisone, Neomycin, and Polymyxin B *see* Neomycin, Polymyxin B, and Hydrocortisone *on page 966*

Hydrocortisone, Propylene Glycol Diacetate, and Acetic Acid *see* Acetic Acid, Propylene Glycol Diacetate, and Hydrocortisone *on page 629*

Hydroxychloroquine (hye droks ee KLOR oh kwin)

U.S. Brand Names Plaquenil®

Canadian Brand Names Apo-Hydroxyquine®; Gen-Hydroxychloroquine; Plaquenil®

Synonyms Hydroxychloroquine Sulfate

Generic Available Yes

Use Suppression and treatment of acute attacks of malaria; treatment of systemic lupus erythematosus and rheumatoid arthritis

Unlabeled/Investigational Use Porphyria cutanea tarda, polymorphous light eruptions

Drug of Choice or Alternative for Organism(s):

Coxiella burnetii on page 100

(Continued)

Hydroxychloroquine *(Continued)*

Pregnancy Risk Factor C

Contraindications Hypersensitivity to hydroxychloroquine, 4-aminoquinoline derivatives, or any component of the formulation; retinal or visual field changes attributable to 4-aminoquinolines

Warnings/Precautions Use with caution in patients with hepatic disease, G6PD deficiency, psoriasis, and porphyria; long-term use in children is not recommended; perform baseline and periodic (6 months) ophthalmologic examinations; test periodically for muscle weakness

Adverse Reactions Frequency not defined.

Cardiovascular: Cardiomyopathy (rare, relationship to hydroxychloroquine unclear)

Central nervous system: Irritability, nervousness, emotional changes, nightmares, psychosis, headache, dizziness, vertigo, seizure, ataxia, lassitude

Dermatologic: Bleaching of hair, alopecia, pigmentation changes (skin and mucosal; black-blue color), rash (urticarial, morbilliform, lichenoid, maculopapular, purpuric, erythema annulare centrifugum, Stevens-Johnson syndrome, acute generalized exanthematous pustulosis, and exfoliative dermatitis)

Endocrine & metabolic: Weight loss

Gastrointestinal: Anorexia, nausea, vomiting, diarrhea, abdominal cramping

Hematologic: Aplastic anemia, agranulocytosis, leukopenia, thrombocytopenia, hemolysis (in patients with glucose-6-phosphate deficiency)

Hepatic: Abnormal liver function/hepatic failure (isolated cases)

Neuromuscular & skeletal: Myopathy, palsy, or neuromyopathy leading to progressive weakness and atrophy of proximal muscle groups (may be associated with mild sensory changes, loss of deep tendon reflexes, and abnormal nerve conduction)

Ocular: Disturbance in accommodation, keratopathy, corneal changes/deposits (visual disturbances, blurred vision, photophobia - reversible on discontinuation), macular edema, atrophy, abnormal pigmentation, retinopathy (early changes reversible - may progress despite discontinuation if advanced), optic disc pallor/atrophy, attenuation of retinal arterioles, pigmentary retinopathy, scotoma, decreased visual acuity, nystagmus

Otic: Tinnitus, deafness

Miscellaneous: Exacerbation of porphyria and nonlight sensitive psoriasis

Overdosage/Toxicology Symptoms include headache, drowsiness, visual changes, cardiovascular collapse, and seizures, followed by respiratory and cardiac arrest. Treatment is symptomatic. Activated charcoal will bind the drug following GI decontamination. Urinary alkalinization will enhance renal elimination.

Drug Interactions

Increased Effect/Toxicity: Cimetidine increases levels of chloroquine and probably other 4-aminoquinolones.

Decreased Effect: Chloroquine and other 4-aminoquinolones absorption may be decreased due to GI binding with kaolin or magnesium trisilicate.

Ethanol/Nutrition/Herb Interactions Ethanol: Avoid ethanol (due to GI irritation).

Mechanism of Action Interferes with digestive vacuole function within sensitive malarial parasites by increasing the pH and interfering with lysosomal degradation of hemoglobin; inhibits locomotion of neutrophils and chemotaxis of eosinophils; impairs complement-dependent antigen-antibody reactions

Pharmacodynamics/Kinetics

Onset of action: Rheumatic disease: May require 4-6 weeks to respond

Absorption: Complete

Protein binding: 55%

Metabolism: Hepatic

Half-life elimination: 32-50 days

Time to peak: Rheumatic disease: Several months

Excretion: Urine (as metabolites and unchanged drug); may be enhanced by urinary acidification

Dosage Note: Hydroxychloroquine sulfate 200 mg is equivalent to 155 mg hydroxychloroquine base and 250 mg chloroquine phosphate. Oral:

Children:

Chemoprophylaxis of malaria: 5 mg/kg (base) once weekly; should not exceed the recommended adult dose; begin 2 weeks before exposure; continue for 4-6 weeks after leaving endemic area; if suppressive therapy is not begun prior to the exposure, double the initial dose and give in 2 doses, 6 hours apart

Acute attack: 10 mg/kg (base) initial dose; followed by 5 mg/kg at 6, 24, and 48 hours

JRA or SLE: 3-5 mg/kg/day divided 1-2 times/day; avoid exceeding 7 mg/kg/day

Adults:

Chemoprophylaxis of malaria: 310 mg base weekly on same day each week; begin 2 weeks before exposure; continue for 4-6 weeks after leaving endemic area; if

suppressive therapy is not begun prior to the exposure, double the initial dose and give in 2 doses, 6 hours apart

Acute attack: 620 mg first dose day 1; 310 mg in 6 hours day 1; 310 mg in 1 dose day 2; and 310 mg in 1 dose on day 3

Rheumatoid arthritis: 310-465 mg/day to start taken with food or milk; increase dose until optimum response level is reached; usually after 4-12 weeks dose should be reduced by 1/2 and a maintenance dose of 155-310 mg/day given

Lupus erythematosus: 310 mg every day or twice daily for several weeks depending on response; 155-310 mg/day for prolonged maintenance therapy

Dietary Considerations May be taken with food or milk.

Administration Administer with food or milk

Monitoring Parameters Ophthalmologic exam, CBC

Patient Information Take with food or milk; take entire course of medication; wear sunglasses in bright sunlight; report blurring or other vision changes, ringing in the ears, or hearing loss

Dosage Forms Tablet, as sulfate: 200 mg [equivalent to 155 mg base]

Extemporaneous Preparations A 25 mg/mL hydroxychloroquine sulfate suspension is made by removing the coating off of fifteen 200 mg hydroxychloroquine sulfate tablets with a towel moistened with alcohol; tablets are ground to a fine powder and levigated to a paste with 15 mL of Ora-Plus® suspending agent; add an additional 45 mL of suspending agent and levigate until a uniform mixture is obtained; qs ad to 120 mL with sterile water for irrigation; a 30 day expiration date is recommended, although stability testing has not been performed

Pesko LJ, "Compounding: Hydroxychloroquine," *Am Druggist*, 1993, 207:57.

Selected Readings

"Drugs for Parasitic Infections," *Med Lett Drugs Ther*, 1998, 40(1017):1-12.
Panisko DM and Keystone JS, "Treatment of Malaria - 1990," *Drugs*, 1990, 39(2):160-89.
White NJ, "The Treatment of Malaria," *N Engl J Med*, 1996, 335(11):800-6.

Hydroxychloroquine Sulfate *see* Hydroxychloroquine *on page 859*

IFLrA *see* Interferon Alfa-2a *on page 878*

IG *see* Immune Globulin (Intramuscular) *on page 866*

IGIM *see* Immune Globulin (Intramuscular) *on page 866*

Imipemide *see* Imipenem and Cilastatin *on page 861*

Imipenem and Cilastatin (i mi PEN em & sye la STAT in)

Related Information

Animal and Human Bites *on page 1270*
Antimicrobial Activity Against Selected Organisms *on page 1165*
Neutropenic Fever Guidelines *on page 1295*

U.S. Brand Names Primaxin®

Canadian Brand Names Primaxin®

Synonyms Imipemide

Generic Available No

Use Treatment of respiratory tract, urinary tract, intra-abdominal, gynecologic, bone and joint, skin structure, and polymicrobic infections as well as bacterial septicemia and endocarditis. Antibacterial activity includes resistant gram-negative bacilli (*Pseudomonas aeruginosa* and *Enterobacter* sp), gram-positive bacteria (methicillin-sensitive *Staphylococcus aureus* and *Streptococcus* sp) and anaerobes.

Note: I.M. administration is not intended for severe or life-threatening infections (eg, septicemia, endocarditis, shock)

Drug of Choice or Alternative for Disease/Syndrome(s):

Fever, Neutropenic *on page 148*
Intra-abdominal Abscess *on page 194*
Liver Abscess *on page 211*
Osteomyelitis, Diabetic Foot *on page 249*
Pancreatitis/Pancreatic Abscess *on page 253*
Peritonitis, Secondary *on page 263*
Peritonitis, Spontaneous Bacterial *on page 264*
Pneumonia, Community-Acquired *on page 270*
Pneumonia, Hospital-Acquired *on page 272*
Pneumonia, Ventilator-Associated *on page 273*

Organism(s):

Acinetobacter Species *on page 24*
Alcaligenes Species *on page 31*
Bordetella bronchiseptica *on page 52*
Burkholderia mallei *on page 64*
Citrobacter Species *on page 81*
Enterobacter Species *on page 132*

(Continued)

Imipenem and Cilastatin *(Continued)*

Erysipelothrix rhusiopathiae on page 141
Klebsiella Species *on page 200*
Pseudomonas aeruginosa on page 282
Rhodococcus Species *on page 288*
Serratia Species *on page 296*

Pregnancy Risk Factor C

Pregnancy Implications There are no well-controlled or adequate studies in pregnant women. Use during pregnancy only if the potential benefits outweigh the potential risks to mother and fetus.

Contraindications Hypersensitivity to imipenem/cilastatin or any component of the formulation; consult information on Lidocaine for contraindications associated with I.M. dosing

Warnings/Precautions Dosage adjustment required in patients with impaired renal function; prolonged use may result in superinfection; has been associated with CNS adverse effects, including confusional states and seizures; use with caution in patients with a history of seizures or hypersensitivity to beta-lactams (including penicillins and cephalosporins); serious hypersensitivity reactions, including anaphylaxis, have been reported (some without a history of previous allergic reactions to beta-lactams); elderly patients often require lower doses (adjust carefully to renal function); not recommended in pediatric CNS infections. Doses for I.M. administration are mixed with lidocaine, consult information on lidocaine for associated warnings/precautions. Two different imipenem/cilastin products are available; due to differences in formulation, the I.V. and I.M. preparations **cannot** be interchanged.

Adverse Reactions

1% to 10%:

Gastrointestinal: Nausea/diarrhea/vomiting (1% to 2%)

Local: Phlebitis (3%), pain at I.M. injection site (1.2%)

<1%: Abnormal urinalysis, anaphylaxis, anemia, confusion (acute), dizziness, emergence of resistant strains of *P. aeruginosa* eosinophilia, fever, hypersensitivity, hypotension, increased BUN/creatine, increased LFTs, increased PT, neutropenia (including agranulocytosis), pain at injection site, palpitation, positive Coombs' test, pruritus, pseudomembranous colitis, rash, seizure, somnolence, thrombocytopenia, urticaria

Postmarketing reports and/or case reports: Hemorrhagic colitis, hepatitis, jaundice, abdominal pain, staining of teeth, glossitis, pancytopenia, leukopenia, hemolytic anemia, encephalopathy, tremor, confusion, myoclonus, paresthesia, vertigo, headache, psychic disturbances, hallucinations, tinnitus, taste perversion, dyspnea, thoracic spine pain, tachycardia, Stevens-Johnson syndrome, toxic epidermal necrolysis, erythema multiforme, angioneurotic edema, flushing, cyanosis, hyperhidrosis, candidiasis, pruritus vulvae, polyarthralgia, drug fever, asthenia, acute renal failure, polyuria, urine discoloration

Overdosage/Toxicology Symptoms include neuromuscular hypersensitivity and seizures. Hemodialysis may be helpful to aid in removal of the drug from the blood, otherwise most treatment is supportive or symptom-directed.

Drug Interactions

Decreased Effect: Imipenem may decrease valproic acid concentrations to subtherapeutic levels; monitor.

Stability

Imipenem/cilastatin powder for injection should be stored at <25°C (77°F).

I.M.: Prepare 500 mg vial with 2 mL 1% lidocaine (do not use lidocaine with epinephrine). The I.V. formulation does not form a stable suspension in lidocaine and cannot be used to prepare an I.M dose. The I.M. suspension should be used within 1 hour of reconstitution.

I.V.: Prior to use, dilute dose into 100 mL of an appropriate solution. Imipenem is inactivated at acidic or alkaline pH. Final concentration should not exceed 5 mg/mL. The I.M. formulation is not buffered and cannot be used to prepare I.V. solutions. Reconstituted I.V. solutions are stable for 4 hours at room temperature and 24 hours when refrigerated.

Mechanism of Action Inhibits bacterial cell wall synthesis by binding to one or more of the penicillin binding proteins (PBPs); which in turn inhibits the final transpeptidation step of peptidoglycan synthesis in bacterial cell walls, thus inhibiting cell wall biosynthesis. Bacteria eventually lyse due to ongoing activity of cell wall autolytic enzymes (autolysins and murein hydrolases) while cell wall assembly is arrested. Cilastatin prevents renal metabolism of imipenem by competitive inhibition of dehydropeptidase along the brush border of the renal tubules.

Pharmacodynamics/Kinetics

Absorption: I.M.: Imipenem: 60% to 75%; cilastatin: 95% to 100%

Distribution: Rapidly and widely to most tissues and fluids including sputum, pleural fluid, peritoneal fluid, interstitial fluid, bile, aqueous humor, reproductive organs, and bone; highest concentrations in pleural fluid, interstitial fluid, peritoneal fluid, and reproductive organs; low concentrations in CSF; crosses placenta; enters breast milk

Metabolism: Renally by dehydropeptidase; activity is blocked by cilastatin; cilastatin is partially metabolized renally

Half-life elimination: Both drugs: 60 minutes; prolonged with renal impairment

Excretion: Both drugs: Urine (~70% as unchanged drug)

Dosage Dosage based on **imipenem** content:

Neonates: Non-CNS infections: I.V.:

- <1 week: 25 mg/kg every 12 hours
- 1-4 weeks: 25 mg/kg every 8 hours
- 4 weeks to 3 months: 25 mg/kg every 6 hours

Children: >3 months: Non-CNS infections: I.V.: 15-25 mg/kg every 6 hours

Maximum dosage: Susceptible infections: 2 g/day; moderately susceptible organisms: 4 g/day

Children: Cystic fibrosis: I.V.: Doses up to 90 mg/kg/day have been used

Imipenem and Cilastatin Dosage in Renal Impairment

Reduced I.V. Dosage Regimen Based on Creatinine Clearance (mL/minute/1.73 m²) and/or Body Weight <70 kg					
	Body Weight (kg)				
	≥70	60	50	40	30
Total daily dose for normal renal function: 1 g/day					
Cl_{cr} ≥71	250 mg q6h	250 mg q8h	125 mg q6h	125 mg q6h	125 mg q8h
Cl_{cr} 41-70	250 mg q8h	125 mg q6h	125 mg q6h	125 mg q8h	125 mg q8h
Cl_{cr} 21-40	250 mg q12h	250 mg q12h	125 mg q8h	125 mg q12h	125 mg q12h
Cl_{cr} 6-20	250 mg q12h	125 mg q12h	125 mg q12h	125 mg q12h	125 mg q12h
Total daily dose for normal renal function: 1.5 g/day					
Cl_{cr} ≥71	500 mg q8h	250 mg q6h	250 mg q6h	250 mg q8h	125 mg q6h
Cl_{cr} 41-70	250 mg q6h	250 mg q8h	250 mg q8h	125 mg q6h	125 mg q8h
Cl_{cr} 21-40	250 mg q8h	250 mg q8h	250 mg q12h	125 mg q8h	125 mg q8h
Cl_{cr} 6-20	250 mg q12h	250 mg q12h	250 mg q12h	125 mg q12h	125 mg q12h
Total daily dose for normal renal function: 2 g/day					
Cl_{cr} ≥71	500 mg q6h	500 mg q8h	250 mg q6h	250 mg q6h	250 mg q8h
Cl_{cr} 41-70	500 mg q8h	250 mg q6h	250 mg q6h	250 mg q8h	125 mg q6h
Cl_{cr} 21-40	250 mg q6h	250 mg q8h	250 mg q8h	250 mg q12h	125 mg q8h
Cl_{cr} 6-20	250 mg q12h	250 mg q12h	250 mg q12h	250 mg q12h	125 mg q12h
Total daily dose for normal renal function: 3 g/day					
Cl_{cr} ≥71	1000 mg q8h	750 mg q8h	500 mg q6h	500 mg q8h	250 mg q6h
Cl_{cr} 41-70	500 mg q6h	500 mg q8h	500 mg q8h	250 mg q6h	250 mg q8h
Cl_{cr} 21-40	500 mg q8h	500 mg q8h	250 mg q6h	250 mg q8h	250 mg q8h
Cl_{cr} 6-20	500 mg q12h	500 mg q12h	250 mg q12h	250 mg q12h	250 mg q12h
Total daily dose for normal renal function: 4 g/day					
Cl_{cr} ≥71	1000 mg q6h	1000 mg q8h	750 mg q8h	500 mg q6h	500 mg q8h
Cl_{cr} 41-70	750 mg q8h	750 mg q8h	500 mg q6h	500 mg q8h	250 mg q6h
Cl_{cr} 21-40	500 mg q6h	500 mg q8h	500 mg q8h	250 mg q6h	250 mg q8h
Cl_{cr} 6-20	500 mg q12h	500 mg q12h	500 mg q12h	250 mg q12h	250 mg q12h

(Continued)

Imipenem and Cilastatin *(Continued)*

Adults: **Note:** For adults weighing <70 kg, refer to Dosing Adjustment in Renal Impairment:
- Moderate infections:
  - I.M.: 750 mg every 12 hours
  - I.V.:
    - Fully-susceptible organisms: 500 mg every 6-8 hours (1.5-2 g/day)
    - Moderately-susceptible organisms: 500 mg every 6 hours or 1 g every 8 hours (2-3 g/day)
- Severe infections: I.V.: **Note:** I.M. administration is not intended for severe or life-threatening infections (eg, septicemia, endocarditis, shock):
  - Fully-susceptible organisms: 500 mg every 6 hours (2 g/day)
  - Moderately-susceptible organisms: 1 g every 6-8 hours (3-4 g/day)
  - Maximum daily dose should not exceed 50 mg/kg or 4 g/day, whichever is lower
- Urinary tract infection, uncomplicated: I.V.: 250 mg every 6 hours (1 g/day)
- Urinary tract infection, complicated: I.V.: 500 mg every 6 hours (2 g/day)
- Mild infections: **Note:** Rarely a suitable option in mild infections; normally reserved for moderate-severe cases:
  - I.M.: 500 mg every 12 hours; intra-abdominal infections: 750 mg every 12 hours
  - I.V.:
    - Fully-susceptible organisms: 250 mg every 6 hours (1g/day)
    - Moderately-susceptible organisms: 500 mg every 6 hours (2 g/day)

Dosage adjustment in renal impairment: I.V.: **Note:** Adjustments have not been established for I.M. dosing:
- Patients with a Cl_{cr} <5 mL/minute/1.73 m^2 should not receive imipenem/cilastatin unless hemodialysis is instituted within 48 hours.
- Patients weighing <30 kg with impaired renal function should not receive imipenem/cilastatin.
- Hemodialysis: Use the dosing recommendation for patients with a Cl_{cr} 6-20 mL/minute
- Peritoneal dialysis: Dose as for Cl_{cr} <10 mL/minute
- Continuous arteriovenous or venovenous hemofiltration: Dose as for Cl_{cr} 20-30 mL/minute; monitor for seizure activity; imipenem is well removed by CAVH but cilastatin is not; removes 20 mg of imipenem per liter of filtrate per day

See table on previous page.

Dietary Considerations Sodium content of 500 mg injection:
- I.M.: 32 mg (1.4 mEq)
- I.V.: 37.5 mg (1.6 mEq)

Administration
- I.M.: Administer by deep injection into a large muscle (gluteal or lateral thigh). Aspiration is necessary to avoid inadvertent injection into a blood vessel. **Only the I.M. formulation can be used for I.M. administration.**
- I.V.: Do not administer I.V. push. Infuse doses ≤500 mg over 20-30 minutes; infuse doses ≥750 mg over 40-60 minutes. **Only the I.V. formulation can be used for I.V. administration.**

Monitoring Parameters Periodic renal, hepatic, and hematologic function tests; monitor for signs of anaphylaxis during first dose

Test Interactions Interferes with urinary glucose determination using Clinitest®

Dosage Forms
- Injection, powder for reconstitution [I.M.]: Imipenem 500 mg and cilastatin 500 mg [contains sodium 32 mg (1.4 mEq)]
- Injection, powder for reconstitution [I.V.]: Imipenem 250 mg and cilastatin 250 mg [contains sodium 18.8 mg (0.8 mEq)]; imipenem 500 mg and cilastatin 500 mg [contains sodium 37.5 mg (1.6 mEq)]

Selected Readings

Balfour JA, Bryson HM, and Brogden RN, "Imipenem/Cilastatin: An Update of Its Antibacterial Activity, Pharmacokinetics, and Therapeutic Efficacy in the Treatment of Serious Infections," *Drugs*, 1996, 51(1):99-136.

Barza M, "Imipenem: First of a New Class of Beta-Lactam Antibiotics," *Ann Intern Med*, 1985, 103(4):552-60.

Donowitz GR and Mandell GL, "Beta-Lactam Antibiotics," *N Engl J Med*, 1988, 318(7):419-26 and 318(8):490-500.

Hellinger WC and Brewer NS, "Carbapenems and Monobactams: Imipenem, Meropenem, and Aztreonam," *Mayo Clin Proc*, 1999, 74(4):420-34.

Imiquimod (i mi KWI mod)

U.S. Brand Names Aldara™

Canadian Brand Names Aldara™

Generic Available No

Use Treatment of external genital and perianal warts/condyloma acuminata in children ≥12 years of age and adults; nonhyperkeratotic, nonhypertrophic actinic keratosis; superficial basal cell carcinoma (SBCC)

Unlabeled/Investigational Use Treatment of common warts

Pregnancy Risk Factor C

Contraindications Hypersensitivity to imiquimod or any component of the formulation

Warnings/Precautions Imiquimod has not been evaluated for the treatment of urethral, intravaginal, cervical, rectal, or intra-anal human papilloma viral disease and is not recommended for these conditions. Topical imiquimod is not intended for ophthalmic use. Topical imiquimod administration is not recommended until genital/perianal tissue is healed from any previous drug or surgical treatment. Imiquimod has the potential to exacerbate inflammatory conditions of the skin. May increase sunburn susceptibility; patients should protect themselves from the sun. Use in basal cell carcinoma should be limited to superficial carcinomas with a maximum diameter of 2 cm. Efficacy in treatment of SBCC lesions of the face, head, and anogenital area, or other subtypes of basal cell carcinoma, have not been established. Safety and efficacy in immunosuppressed patients have not been established. Safety and efficacy in patients <12 years of age have not been established.

Adverse Reactions

>10%:

- Local, mild/moderate: Erythema (54% to 61%), itching (22% to 32%), erosion (21% to 32%), burning (9% to 26%), excoriation/flaking (18% to 25%), edema (12% to 17%), scabbing (9% to 13%), fungal infection (2% to 11%)
- Respiratory: Upper respiratory infection (15%)

1% to 10%:

- Cardiovascular: Atrial fibrillation (1%)
- Central nervous system: Pain (2% to 8%), headache (4% to 5%), fatigue (actinic keratosis 1%), fever (actinic keratosis 1%), dizziness (1%)
- Endocrine & metabolic: Hypercholesterolemia (2%)
- Gastrointestinal: Diarrhea (3%), dyspepsia (3%)
- Local:
  - Severe: Hyperkeratosis (actinic keratosis 9%), erythema (4%), eczema (2%), erosion (1%), edema (1%), alopecia (actinic keratosis 1%)
  - Mild/moderate: Pain, induration, ulceration (5% to 7%), vesicles (2% to 3%), soreness (<1% to 3%)
- Neuromuscular & skeletal: Myalgia (1%), back pain (actinic keratosis 1%)
- Respiratory: Sinusitis (7%), pharyngitis (2%)
- Miscellaneous: Influenza-like symptoms (1% to 3%), squamous cell carcinoma (4%)

Overdosage/Toxicology Overdosage is unlikely because of minimal percutaneous absorption. Persistent topical overdosing of imiquimod could result in severe local skin reactions. The most clinically serious adverse event reported, following multiple oral imiquimod doses of ≥200 mg, was hypotension which resolved following oral or I.V. fluid administration. Treat symptomatically.

Drug Interactions

Cytochrome P450 Effect: Substrate (minor) of CYP1A2, 3A4

Stability Do not store at <25°C (77°F); avoid freezing

Mechanism of Action Mechanism of action is unknown; however, induces cytokines, including interferon-alpha and others

Pharmacodynamics/Kinetics

Absorption: Minimal

Excretion: Urine and feces (<0.9%)

Dosage Topical:

Children ≥12 years and Adults: Perianal warts/condyloma acuminata: Apply 3 times/week prior to bedtime and leave on skin for 6-10 hours. Remove with mild soap and water. Examples of 3 times/week application schedules are: Monday, Wednesday, Friday; or Tuesday, Thursday, Saturday. Continue imiquimod treatment until there is total clearance of the genital/perianal warts for ≤16 weeks. A rest period of several days may be taken if required by the patient's discomfort or severity of the local skin reaction. Treatment may resume once the reaction subsides.

Adults:

- Actinic keratosis: Apply twice weekly for 16 weeks to a treatment area on face or scalp; apply prior to bedtime and leave on skin for 8 hours. Remove with mild soap and water.
- Common oral worts (dental use): Apply once daily prior to bedtime
- Common warts (unlabeled use): Apply once daily prior to bedtime
- Superficial basal cell carcinoma: Apply once daily prior to bedtime, 5 days/week for 6 weeks. Treatment area should include a 1 cm margin of skin around the tumor. Leave on skin for 8 hours.

(Continued)

Imiquimod *(Continued)*

Administration Nonocclusive dressings such as cotton gauze or cotton underwear may be used in the management of skin reactions. Handwashing before and after cream application is recommended. Imiquimod is packaged in single-use packets that contain sufficient cream to cover a wart area of up to 20 cm^2; avoid use of excessive amounts of cream. Instruct patients to apply imiquimod to external or perianal warts; not for vaginal use. Apply a thin layer to the wart area and rub in until the cream is no longer visible. Do not occlude the application site.

Monitoring Parameters Reduction in wart size is indicative of a therapeutic response; patients should be monitored for signs and symptoms of hypersensitivity to imiquimod

Patient Information Imiquimod is not a cure; new warts may develop during therapy. May also be used to treat sun-damaged skin. Imiquimod may weaken condoms and vaginal diaphragms; therefore, concurrent use is not recommended. This medication is for external use only; avoid contact with eyes. Do not occlude the treatment area with bandages or other covers or wraps. Avoid sexual (genital, anal, oral) contact while the cream is on the skin. (Females: Do not apply in the vagina.) Wash the treatment area with mild soap and water 6-10 hours following application of imiquimod. Patients commonly experience local skin reactions such as erythema, erosion, excoriation/flaking, and edema at the site of application or surrounding areas. Most skin reactions are mild to moderate. Severe skin reactions can occur; promptly report severe reactions. Uncircumcised males treating warts under the foreskin should retract the foreskin and clean the area daily.

Dosage Forms Cream: 5% (12s) [contains benzyl alcohol; single-dose packets]

ImmuCyst® (Can) *see* BCG Vaccine *on page 683*

Immune Globulin (Intramuscular)

(i MYUN GLOB yoo lin, IN tra MUS kyoo ler)

U.S. Brand Names BayGam®

Canadian Brand Names BayGam®

Synonyms Gamma Globulin; IG; IGIM; Immune Serum Globulin; ISG

Generic Available No

Use Household and sexual contacts of persons with hepatitis A, measles, varicella, and possibly rubella; travelers to high-risk areas outside tourist routes; staff, attendees, and parents of diapered attendees in day-care center outbreaks

For travelers, IG is not an alternative to careful selection of foods and water; immune globulin can interfere with the antibody response to parenterally administered live virus vaccines. Frequent travelers should be tested for hepatitis A antibody, immune hemolytic anemia, and neutropenia (with ITP, I.V. route is usually used).

Drug of Choice or Alternative for Organism(s):

Hepatitis A Virus *on page 164*
Measles Virus *on page 215*

Pregnancy Risk Factor C

Contraindications Hypersensitivity to immune globulin, thimerosal, or any component of the formulation; IgA deficiency; I.M. injections in patients with thrombocytopenia or coagulation disorders

Warnings/Precautions Skin testing should not be performed as local irritation can occur and be misinterpreted as a positive reaction; IG should **not** be used to control outbreaks of measles. As a product of human plasma, this product may potentially transmit disease; screening of donors, as well as testing and/or inactivation of certain viruses reduces this risk. Epidemiologic and laboratory data indicate current IMIG products do not have a discernible risk of transmitting HIV. Use caution in patients with thrombocytopenia or coagulation disorders (I.M. injections may be contraindicated). Not for I.V. administration.

Adverse Reactions Frequency not defined.

Cardiovascular: Flushing, angioedema
Central nervous system: Chills, lethargy, fever
Dermatologic: Urticaria, erythema
Gastrointestinal: Nausea, vomiting
Local: Pain, tenderness, muscle stiffness at I.M. site
Neuromuscular & skeletal: Myalgia
Miscellaneous: Hypersensitivity reactions

Drug Interactions

Increased Effect/Toxicity: Increased toxicity: Live virus, vaccines (measles, mumps, rubella); do not administer within 3 months after administration of these vaccines.

Stability Keep in refrigerator; do not freeze

Mechanism of Action Provides passive immunity by increasing the antibody titer and antigen-antibody reaction potential

Pharmacodynamics/Kinetics

Duration: Immune effect: Usually 3-4 weeks

Half-life elimination: 23 days

Time to peak, serum: I.M.: ~24-48 hours

Dosage I.M.:

Hepatitis A:

Pre-exposure prophylaxis upon travel into endemic areas (hepatitis A vaccine preferred):

0.02 mL/kg for anticipated risk 1-3 months

0.06 mL/kg for anticipated risk >3 months

Repeat approximate dose every 4-6 months if exposure continues

Postexposure prophylaxis: 0.02 mL/kg given within 7 days of exposure

Measles:

Prophylaxis: 0.25 mL/kg/dose (maximum dose: 15 mL) given within 6 days of exposure followed by live attenuated measles vaccine in 3 months or at 15 months of age (whichever is later)

For patients with leukemia, lymphoma, immunodeficiency disorders, generalized malignancy, or receiving immunosuppressive therapy: 0.5 mL/kg (maximum dose: 15 mL)

Poliomyelitis: Prophylaxis: 0.3 mL/kg/dose as a single dose

Rubella: Prophylaxis: 0.55 mL/kg/dose within 72 hours of exposure

Varicella: Prophylaxis: 0.6-1.2 mL/kg (varicella zoster immune globulin preferred) within 72 hours of exposure

IgG deficiency: 1.3 mL/kg, then 0.66 mL/kg in 3-4 weeks

Hepatitis B: Prophylaxis: 0.06 mL/kg/dose (HBIG preferred)

Administration Intramuscular injection only

Test Interactions Skin tests should **not** be done

Dosage Forms Injection, solution [preservative free]: 15% to 18% (2 mL, 10 mL)

Selected Readings

ASHP Commission on Therapeutics, "ASHP Therapeutic Guidelines for Intravenous Immune Globulin," *Clin Pharm*, 1992, 11(2):117-36.

Berkman SA, Lee ML, and Gale RP, "Clinical Uses of Intravenous Immunoglobulins," *Ann Intern Med*, 1990, 112(4):278-92.

Immune Globulin (Intravenous)

(i MYUN GLOB yoo lin, IN tra VEE nus)

U.S. Brand Names Carimune™ [DSC]; Carimune™ NF; Gamimune® N; Gammagard® Liquid; Gammagard® S/D; Gammar®-P I.V.; Gamunex®; Iveegam EN; Octagam®; Panglobulin® NF; Polygam® S/D

Canadian Brand Names Gamimune® N; Gammagard® S/D; Gamunex®; Iveegam Immuno®

Synonyms IVIG

Generic Available No

Use

Treatment of primary immunodeficiency syndromes (congenital agammaglobulinemia, severe combined immunodeficiency syndromes [SCIDS], common variable immunodeficiency, X-linked immunodeficiency, Wiskott-Aldrich syndrome); idiopathic thrombocytopenic purpura (ITP); Kawasaki disease (in combination with aspirin)

Prevention of bacterial infection in B-cell chronic lymphocytic leukemia (CLL); pediatric HIV infection; bone marrow transplant (BMT)

Unlabeled/Investigational Use Autoimmune diseases (myasthenia gravis, SLE, bullous pemphigoid, severe rheumatoid arthritis), Guillain-Barré syndrome; used in conjunction with appropriate anti-infective therapy to prevent or modify acute bacterial or viral infections in patients with iatrogenically-induced or disease-associated immunodepression; autoimmune hemolytic anemia or neutropenia, refractory dermatomyositis/polymyositis

Pregnancy Risk Factor C

Pregnancy Implications Immune globulins cross the placenta in increased amounts after 30 weeks gestation.

Contraindications Hypersensitivity to immune globulin or any component of the formulation; selective IgA deficiency

Warnings/Precautions Anaphylactic hypersensitivity reactions can occur, especially in IgA-deficient patients; studies indicate that the currently available products have no discernible risk of transmitting HIV or hepatitis B; aseptic meningitis may occur with high doses (≥2 g/kg). Use with caution in the elderly, patients with renal disease,

(Continued)

Immune Globulin (Intravenous) *(Continued)*

diabetes mellitus, volume depletion, sepsis, paraproteinemia, and nephrotoxic medications due to risk of renal dysfunction. Patients should be adequately hydrated prior to therapy. Acute renal dysfunction (increased serum creatinine, oliguria, acute renal failure) can rarely occur; usually within 7 days of use (more likely with products stabilized with sucrose). Use caution in patients with a history of thrombotic events or cardiovascular disease; there is clinical evidence of a possible association between thrombotic events and administration of intravenous immune globulin. For intravenous administration only.

Adverse Reactions Frequency not defined.

Cardiovascular: Flushing of the face, tachycardia, hyper-/hypotension, chest tightness, angioedema, lightheadedness, chest pain, MI, CHF, pulmonary embolism

Central nervous system: Anxiety, chills, dizziness, drowsiness, fatigue, fever, headache, irritability, lethargy, malaise, aseptic meningitis syndrome

Dermatologic: Pruritus, rash, urticaria

Gastrointestinal: Abdominal cramps, diarrhea, nausea, sore throat, vomiting

Hematologic: Autoimmune hemolytic anemia, hematocrit decreased, leukopenia, mild hemolysis

Hepatic: Liver function test increased

Local: Pain or irritation at the infusion site

Neuromuscular & skeletal: Arthralgia, back or hip pain, myalgia, nuchal rigidity

Ocular: Photophobia, painful eye movements

Renal: Acute renal failure, acute tubular necrosis, anuria, BUN increased, creatinine increased, nephrotic syndrome, oliguria, proximal tubular nephropathy, osmotic nephrosis

Respiratory: Cough, dyspnea, wheezing, nasal congestion, pharyngeal pain, rhinorrhea, sinusitis

Miscellaneous: Diaphoresis, hypersensitivity reactions, anaphylaxis

Postmarketing and/or case reports: Abdominal pain, apnea, ARDS, bronchospasm, bullous dermatitis, cardiac arrest, Coombs' test positive, cyanosis, epidermolysis, erythema multiforme, hepatic dysfunction, hypoxemia, leukopenia, loss of consciousness, pancytopenia, pulmonary edema, rigors, seizure, Stevens-Johnson syndrome, thromboembolism, transfusion-related acute lung injury (TRALI), tremor, vascular collapse

Drug Interactions

Decreased Effect: Decreased effect of live virus vaccines (eg, measles, mumps, rubella); separate administration by at least 3 months

Stability Stability and dilution is dependent upon the manufacturer and brand; do not mix with other drugs; do not freeze; do not shake, avoid foaming; discard unused portion:

Carimune™ NF, Panglobulin® NF: Prior to reconstitution, store at or below 30°C (86°F). Reconstitute with NS, D_5W, or SWFI. Following reconstitution, store under refrigeration; use within 24 hours. Do not freeze.

Gamimune® N: Store at 2°C to 8°C (36°F to 46°F).

Gammagard® Liquid: May be stored for up to 9 months at room temperature of 25°C (77°F) within 24 months of manufacture date. May be stored for up to 36 months under refrigeration at 2°C to 8°C (36°F to 46°F). May dilute in D_5W only. Do not freeze.

Gammagard® S/D, Polygam® S/D: Store below 25°C (77°F). Reconstitute with SWFI; when diluted aseptically in a sterile laminar air flow hood, may store diluted solution under refrigeration for up to 24 hours. If reconstituted outside of laminar flow hood, use within 2 hours.

Gammar®-P I.V.: Store below 25°C (77°F). Reconstitute with SWFI.

Gamunex®: May be stored for up to 5 months at room temperature up to 25°C (up to 77°F) within 18 months of manufacture date.

Iveegam EN: Store at 2°C to 8°C (36°F to 46°F). Reconstitute with SWFI; use immediately after reconstitution.

Octagam®: Store at 2°C to 8°C (36°F to 46°F) for 24 months or ≤25°C (77°F) for 18 months.

Polygam® S/D: Store at room temperature at or below 25°C (77°F). Do not freeze.

Mechanism of Action Replacement therapy for primary and secondary immunodeficiencies; interference with F_c receptors on the cells of the reticuloendothelial system for autoimmune cytopenias and ITP; possible role of contained antiviral-type antibodies

Pharmacodynamics/Kinetics

Onset of action: I.V.: Provides immediate antibody levels

Duration: Immune effect: 3-4 weeks (variable)

Distribution: V_d: 0.09-0.13 L/kg

Intravascular portion: Healthy subjects: 41% to 57%; Patients with congenital humoral immunodeficiencies: ~70%

Half-life elimination: IgG (variable among patients): Healthy subjects: 14-24 days; Patients with congenital humoral immunodeficiencies: 26-40 days; hypermetabolism associated with fever and infection have coincided with a shortened half-life

Dosage Approved doses and regimens may vary between brands; check manufacturer guidelines. **Note:** Some clinicians dose IVIG on ideal body weight or an adjusted ideal body weight in morbidly obese patients. The volume of distribution of IVIG preparations in healthy subjects is similar to that observed with endogenous IgG. IVIG remains primarily in the intravascular space. Patients with congenital humoral immunodeficiencies appear to have about 70% of the IVIG available in the intravascular space.

Infants and Children: Prevention of gastroenteritis (unlabeled use): Oral: 50 mg/kg/day divided every 6 hours

Children: I.V.:

- Pediatric HIV: 400 mg/kg every 28 days
- Severe systemic viral and bacterial infections (unlabeled use): 500-1000 mg/kg/week

Children and Adults: I.V.:

- Primary immunodeficiency disorders: 200-400 mg/kg every 4 weeks or as per monitored serum IgG concentrations
  - Gammagard® Liquid, Gamunex®, Octagam®: 300-600 mg/kg every 3-4 weeks; adjusted based on dosage and interval in conjunction with monitored serum IgG concentrations.
- B-cell chronic lymphocytic leukemia (CLL): 400 mg/kg/dose every 3 weeks
- Idiopathic thrombocytopenic purpura (ITP):
  - Acute: 400 mg/kg/day for 5 days or 1000 mg/kg/day for 1-2 days
  - Chronic: 400 mg/kg as needed to maintain platelet count >30,000/mm^3; may increase dose to 800 mg/kg (1000 mg/kg if needed)
- Kawasaki disease: Initiate therapy within 10 days of disease onset: 2 g/kg as a single dose administered over 10 hours, or 400 mg/kg/day for 4 days. **Note:** Must be used in combination with aspirin: 80-100 mg/kg/day in 4 divided doses for 14 days; when fever subsides, dose aspirin at 3-5 mg/kg once daily for ≥6-8 weeks
- Acquired immunodeficiency syndrome (patients must be symptomatic) (unlabeled use): Various regimens have been used, including:
  - 200-250 mg/kg/dose every 2 weeks
  - **or**
  - 400-500 mg/kg/dose every month or every 4 weeks
- Autoimmune hemolytic anemia and neutropenia (unlabeled use): 1000 mg/kg/dose for 2-3 days
- Autoimmune diseases (unlabeled use): 400 mg/kg/day for 4 days
- Bone marrow transplant: 500 mg/kg beginning on days 7 and 2 pretransplant, then 500 mg/kg/week for 90 days post-transplant
- Adjuvant to severe cytomegalovirus infections (unlabeled use): 500 mg/kg/dose every other day for 7 doses
- Guillain-Barré syndrome (unlabeled use): Various regimens have been used, including:
  - 400 mg/kg/day for 4 days
  - **or**
  - 1000 mg/kg/day for 2 days
  - **or**
  - 2000 mg/kg/day for one day
- Refractory dermatomyositis (unlabeled use): 2 g/kg/dose every month x 3-4 doses
- Refractory polymyositis (unlabeled use): 1 g/kg/day x 2 days every month x 4 doses
- Chronic inflammatory demyelinating polyneuropathy (unlabeled use): Various regimens have been used, including:
  - 400 mg/kg/day for 5 doses once each month
  - **or**
  - 800 mg/kg/day for 3 doses once each month
  - **or**
  - 1000 mg/kg/day for 2 days once each month

Dosing adjustment/comments in renal impairment: Cl_{cr} <10 mL/minute: Avoid use; in patients at risk of renal dysfunction, consider infusion at a rate less than maximum.

Dietary Considerations Octagam® contains sodium 30 mmol/L

Administration I.V. use only; for initial treatment, a lower concentration and/or a slower rate of infusion should be used. Administer in separate infusion line from other medications; if using primary line, flush with saline prior administration. Refrigerated product should be warmed to room temperature prior to infusion. Decrease dose, rate

(Continued)

Immune Globulin (Intravenous) *(Continued)*

and/or concentration of infusion in patients who may be at risk of renal failure. Decreasing the rate or stopping the infusion may help relieve some adverse effects (flushing, changes in pulse rate, changes in blood pressure). Epinephrine should be available during administration. The lot number and expiration date of vials used should be recorded.

Monitoring Parameters Renal function, urine output, hemoglobin and hematocrit, infusion-related adverse reactions, anaphylaxis

Test Interactions Octagam® contains maltose which may interfere with blood and urine glucose tests.

Additional Information

Intravenous Immune Globulin Product Comparison:

Carimune™ NF, Panglobulin® NF:

FDA indication: Primary immunodeficiency, ITP
Contraindication: IgA deficiency
IgA content: 720 mcg/mL
Plasma source: Pooled donors
Half-life: 23 days
IgG subclass (%):
  IgG1 (60-70): 60.5
  IgG2 (19-31): 30.2
  IgG3 (5-8.4): 6.6
  IgG4 (0.7-4): 2.8
Storage: Room temperature at or below 30°C (86°F); refrigerate after reconstitution
Recommendations for **initial** infusion rate: 0.5-1 mL/minute
Maximum infusion rate: 2 mg/kg/minute

Gamimune® N:

FDA indication: Primary immunodeficiency, ITP
Contraindication: IgA deficiency
IgA content: 270 mcg/mL
Adverse reactions (%): 5.2
Plasma source: >2000 paid donors
Half-life: 21 days
IgG subclass (%):
  IgG_1 (60-70): 60
  IgG_2 (19-31): 29.4
  IgG_3 (5-8.4): 6.5
  IgG_4 (0.7-4): 4.1
Monomers (%): >95
Gamma globulin (%): >98
Storage: Refrigerate
Recommendations for **initial** infusion rate: 0.01-0.02 mL/kg/minute
Maximum infusion rate: 0.08 mL/kg/minute
Maximum concentration for infusion (%): 10

Gammagard® Liquid:

FDA indication: Primary immunodeficiency
Contraindication: IgA deficiency, history of anaphylaxis with immune globulin
IgA content: 37 mcg/mL
Half-life: 35 days
Storage: Room temperature (stable for 9 months) or refrigeration (stable for 36 months)
Recommendations for **initial** infusion rate: 0.5 mL/kg/hour
Maximum infusion rate: 5 mL/kg/hour; <2 mL/kg/hour in patients at risk for renal impairment or thrombosis

Gammagard® SD:

FDA indication: Primary immunodeficiency, ITP, CLL prophylaxis
Contraindication: None (caution with IgA deficiency)
IgA content: 0.92-1.6 mcg/mL
Adverse reactions (%): 6
Plasma source: 4000-5000 paid donors
Half-life: 24 days
IgG subclass (%):
  IgG_1 (60-70): 67 (66.8)
  IgG_2 (19-31): 25 (25.4)
  IgG_3 (5-8.4): 5 (7.4)
  IgG_4 (0.7-4): 3 (0.3)
Monomers (%): >95
Gamma globulin (%): >90

Storage: Room temperature
Recommendations for **initial** infusion rate: 0.5 mL/kg/hour
Maximum infusion rate: 4 mL/kg/hour
Maximum concentration for infusion (%): 5

Gammar®-P I.V.:
FDA indication: Primary immunodeficiency
Contraindication: IgA deficiency
IgA content: <20 mcg/mL
Adverse reactions (%): 15
Plasma source: >8000 paid donors
Half-life: 21-24 days
IgG subclass (%):
IgG_1 (60-70): 69
IgG_2 (19-31): 23
IgG_3 (5-8.4): 6
IgG_4 (0.7-4): 2
Monomers (%): >98
Gamma globulin (%): >98
Storage: Room temperature
Recommendations for **initial** infusion rate: 0.01-0.02 mL/kg/minute
Maximum infusion rate: 0.06 mL/kg/minute
Maximum concentration for infusion (%): 5

Gamunex®:
FDA indication: Primary immunodeficiency, ITP
Contraindication: Caution in severe, selective IgA deficiency
IgA content: 40 mcg/mL
IgM content: <2 mcg/mL
Plasma source: Pooled donors
Half-life: 36 days
IgG subclass (%):
IgG_1 (60-70): 65
IgG_2 (19-31): 26
IgG_3 (5-8.4): 5.6
IgG_4 (0.7-4): 2.6
Monomer + dimer (%): 100
Gamma globulin (%): >98
Storage: 2°C to 8°C; may be stored at room temperature for 5 months (only during first 18 months after manufacture)
Recommendations for **initial** infusion rate: 0.01 mL/kg/minute
Maximum infusion rate: 0.08 mL/kg/minute
Maximum concentration for infusion (%): 10

Octagam®:
FDA indication: Primary immunodeficiency
Contraindications: IgA deficiency
IgA content: 100 mcg/mL
Half-life: Immunodeficiency: 40 days
IgG subclass (%):
IgG_1 (60-70): 65
IgG_2 (19-31): 30
IgG_3 (5-8.4): 3
IgG_4 (0.7-4): 2
Monomers (%): ≥90
Gamma globulin (%): 96
Storage: Refrigerated or room temperature
Recommendations for initial infusion rate: 0.6 mL/kg/hour
Maximum infusion rate: 4 mL/kg/hour
Maximum concentration for infusion: 5%

Polygam®:
FDA indication: Primary immunodeficiency, ITP, CLL
Contraindication: None (caution with IgA deficiency)
IgA content: 0.74 ± 0.33 mcg/mL
Adverse reactions (%): 6
Plasma source: 50,000 voluntary donors
Half-life: 21-25 days
IgG subclass (%):
IgG_1 (60-70): 67
IgG_2 (19-31): 25
IgG_3 (5-8.4): 5

(Continued)

Immune Globulin (Intravenous) *(Continued)*

IgG_4 (0.7-4): 3
Monomers (%): >95
Gamma globulin (%): >90
Storage: Room temperature
Recommendations for **initial** infusion rate: 0.5 mL/kg/hour
Maximum infusion rate: 4 mL/kg/hour
Maximum concentration for infusion (%): 10

Dosage Forms [DSC] = Discontinued product

Injection, powder for reconstitution [preservative free]:
Carimune™: 1 g, 3 g, 6 g, 12 g [contains sucrose] [DSC]
Gammar®-P I.V.: 5 g, 10 g [stabilized with human albumin and sucrose]
Iveegam EN: 5 g [stabilized with glucose]

Injection, powder for reconstitution [preservative free, nanofiltered]:
Carimune™ NF: 3 g, 6 g, 12 g [contains sucrose]
Panglobulin® NF: 6 g, 12 g [contains sucrose]

Injection, powder for reconstitution [preservative free, solvent detergent treated]
Gammagard® S/D: 2.5 g, 5 g, 10 g [stabilized with human albumin, glycine, glucose, and polyethylene glycol]
Polygam® S/D: 5 g, 10 g [stabilized with human albumin, glycine, glucose, and polyethylene glycol]

Injection, solution [preservative free; solvent detergent-treated]:
Gamimune® N: 10% [100 mg/mL] (10 mL, 25 mL, 50 mL, 100 mL, 200 mL)
Gammagard® Liquid: 10% [100 mg/mL] (10 mL, 25 mL, 50 mL, 100 mL, 200 mL) [latex free, sucrose free; stabilized with glycine]
Octagam®: 5% [50 mg/mL] (20 mL, 50 mL, 100 mL, 200 mL) [sucrose free; contains sodium 30 mmol/L and maltose]

Injection, solution [preservative free] (Gamunex®): 10% (10 mL, 25 mL, 50 mL, 100 mL, 200 mL) [caprylate/chromatography purified]

Immune Serum Globulin *see* Immune Globulin (Intramuscular) *on page 866*

Imogam® Rabies-HT *see* Rabies Immune Globulin (Human) *on page 1034*

Imogam® Rabies Pasteurized (Can) *see* Rabies Immune Globulin (Human) *on page 1034*

Imovax® Rabies *see* Rabies Virus Vaccine *on page 1034*

Indinavir (in DIN a veer)

Related Information

Antiretroviral Agents *on page 1206*
Antiretroviral Therapy for HIV Infection *on page 1219*
Management of Healthcare Worker Exposures to HBV, HCV, and HIV *on page 1227*

U.S. Brand Names Crixivan®

Canadian Brand Names Crixivan®

Synonyms Indinavir Sulfate

Generic Available No

Use Treatment of HIV infection; should always be used as part of a multidrug regimen (at least three antiretroviral agents)

Drug of Choice or Alternative for Organism(s):

Human Immunodeficiency Virus *on page 181*

Pregnancy Risk Factor C

Pregnancy Implications Plasma levels of indinavir were 74% lower at weeks 30-32 of gestation when compared to the same women at 14-28 weeks of gestation. Plasma levels were not measurable in some patients 8 hours post dose. Hyperbilirubinemia may be exacerbated in neonates. Pregnancy and protease inhibitors are both associated with an increased risk of hyperglycemia. Glucose levels should be closely monitored. Until optimal dosing during pregnancy has been established, the manufacturer does not recommend indinavir use in pregnant patients. Healthcare professionals are encouraged to contact the antiretroviral pregnancy registry to monitor outcomes of pregnant women exposed to antiretroviral medications (1-800-258-4263 or www.APRegistry.com).

Contraindications Hypersensitivity to indinavir or any component of the formulation; concurrent use of amiodarone, cisapride, triazolam, midazolam, pimozide, or ergot alkaloids

Warnings/Precautions Because indinavir may cause nephrolithiasis/urolithiasis the drug should be discontinued if signs and symptoms occur; risk is substantially higher in pediatric patients versus adults. Adequate hydration is recommended. May cause

tubulointerstitial nephritis (rare); severe asymptomatic leukocyturia may warrant evaluation. Indinavir should not be administered concurrently with lovastatin or simvastatin (caution with atorvastatin and cerivastatin) because of competition for metabolism of these drugs through the CYP3A4 system, and potential serious or life-threatening events. Use caution with other drugs metabolized by this enzyme (particular caution with phosphodiesterase-5 inhibitors, including sildenafil). Avoid concurrent use of St John's wort (may lead to loss of virologic response and/or resistance). Patients with hepatic insufficiency due to cirrhosis should have dose reduction. Warn patients about fat redistribution that can occur. Indinavir has been associated with hemolytic anemia (discontinue if diagnosed), hepatitis, and hyperglycemia (exacerbation or new-onset diabetes). Treatment may result in immune reconstitution syndrome (acute inflammatory response to indolent or residual opportunistic infections). Use caution in patients with hemophilia; spontaneous bleeding has been reported.

Adverse Reactions Protease inhibitors cause dyslipidemia which includes elevated cholesterol and triglycerides and a redistribution of body fat centrally to cause increased abdominal girth, buffalo hump, facial atrophy, and breast enlargement. These agents also cause hyperglycemia (exacerbation or new-onset diabetes).

>10%:

Gastrointestinal: Nausea (12%)

Hepatic: Hyperbilirubinemia (14%)

Renal: Nephrolithiasis/urolithiasis (29%, pediatric patients; 12% adult patients)

1% to 10%:

Central nervous system: Headache (6%), insomnia (3%)

Gastrointestinal: Abdominal pain (9%), diarrhea/vomiting (4% to 5%), taste perversion (3%)

Neuromuscular & skeletal: Weakness (4%), flank pain (3%)

Renal: Hematuria

<1%: Malaise, dizziness, somnolence, anorexia, xerostomia, decreased hemoglobin, pancreatitis, urticaria, depression, increased serum cholesterol, fever, MI, angina

Postmarketing and/or case reports: Acute renal failure, alopecia, anaphylactoid reactions, bleeding (spontaneous in patients with hemophilia A or B), crystalluria, depression, dysuria, erythema multiforme, hemolytic anemia, hepatic failure, hepatitis, hyperglycemia, immune reconstitution syndrome, interstitial nephritis (with medullary calcification and cortical atrophy), leukocyturia (severe and asymptomatic), MI, new-onset diabetes, paresthesia (oral), pruritus, pyelonephritis, Stevens-Johnson syndrome, vasculitis

Drug Interactions

Cytochrome P450 Effect: Substrate of CYP2D6 (minor), 3A4 (major); **Inhibits** CYP2C8/9 (weak), 2C19 (weak), 2D6 (weak), 3A4 (strong)

Increased Effect/Toxicity: Indinavir may increase the levels/effects of selected benzodiazepines, calcium channel blockers, cyclosporine, mirtazapine, nateglinide, nefazodone, quinidine, sildenafil (and other PDE-5 inhibitors), tacrolimus, venlafaxine, and other CYP3A4 substrates. Selected benzodiazepines (midazolam, triazolam), cisapride, ergot alkaloids, selected HMG-CoA reductase inhibitors (lovastatin and simvastatin), mesoridazine, pimozide, and thioridazine are generally contraindicated with strong CYP3A4 inhibitors. When used with strong CYP3A4 inhibitors, dosage adjustment/limits are recommended for sildenafil and other PDE-5 inhibitors; refer to individual monographs.

Itraconazole or ketoconazole may increase the serum concentrations of indinavir; dosage adjustment is recommended. The levels/effects of indinavir may be increased by azole antifungals, ciprofloxacin, clarithromycin, diclofenac, doxycycline, erythromycin, imatinib, isoniazid, nefazodone, nicardipine, propofol, protease inhibitors, quinidine, verapamil, and other CYP3A4 inhibitors.

When used with delavirdine, serum levels of indinavir are increased; dosage adjustment of indinavir may be required for this combination. Serum levels of both nelfinavir and indinavir are increased with concurrent use. Serum concentrations of indinavir may be increased by ritonavir; serum levels of ritonavir and saquinavir may be increased; dosage adjustments of indinavir are required during concurrent therapy. Rifabutin serum concentrations has been increased when coadministered with indinavir; dosage adjustments of both agents required. Concurrent use or atazanavir with indinavir may increase the risk of hyperbilirubinemia.

Decreased Effect: The levels/effects of indinavir may be decreased by aminoglutethimide, carbamazepine, nafcillin, nevirapine, phenobarbital, phenytoin, rifamycins, and other CYP3A4 inducers; dosage adjustment may be recommended (see individual agents). Rifampin and/or St John's wort (*Hypericum perforatum*); should not be used with indinavir.

(Continued)

Indinavir *(Continued)*

Ethanol/Nutrition/Herb Interactions

Food: Indinavir bioavailability may be decreased if taken with food. Meals high in calories, fat, and protein result in a significant decrease in drug levels. Indinavir serum concentrations may be decreased by grapefruit juice.

Herb/Nutraceutical: St John's wort *(Hypericum)* appears to induce CYP3A enzymes and has lead to 57% reductions in indinavir AUCs and 81% reductions in trough serum concentrations, which may lead to treatment failures; should not be used concurrently with indinavir.

Stability Capsules are sensitive to moisture; medication should be stored and used in the original container and the desiccant should remain in the bottle

Mechanism of Action Indinavir is a human immunodeficiency virus protease inhibitor, binding to the protease activity site and inhibiting the activity of this enzyme. HIV protease is an enzyme required for the cleavage of viral polyprotein precursors into individual functional proteins found in infectious HIV. Inhibition prevents cleavage of these polyproteins resulting in the formation of immature noninfectious viral particles.

Pharmacodynamics/Kinetics

Absorption: Administration with a high fat, high calorie diet resulted in a reduction in AUC and in maximum serum concentration (77% and 84% respectively); lighter meal resulted in little or no change in these parameters.

Protein binding, plasma: 60%

Metabolism: Hepatic via CYP3A4; seven metabolites of indinavir identified

Bioavailability: Good

Half-life elimination: 1.8 ± 0.4 hour

Time to peak: 0.8 ± 0.3 hour

Excretion: Urine and feces

Dosage

Children 4-15 years (investigational): 500 mg/m^2 every 8 hours

Adults: Oral:

Unboosted regimen: 800 mg every 8 hours

Ritonavir-boosted regimens:

Ritonavir 100-200 mg twice daily plus indinavir 800 mg twice daily **or**

Ritonavir 400 mg twice daily plus indinavir 400 mg twice daily

Dosage adjustments for indinavir when administered in combination therapy:

Delavirdine, itraconazole, or ketoconazole: Reduce indinavir dose to 600 mg every 8 hours

Efavirenz: Increase indinavir dose to 1000 mg every 8 hours

Lopinavir and ritonavir (Kaletra™): Indinavir 600 mg twice daily

Nelfinavir: Increase indinavir dose to 1200 mg twice daily

Nevirapine: Increase indinavir dose to 1000 mg every 8 hours

Rifabutin: Reduce rifabutin to ½ the standard dose plus increase indinavir to 1000 mg every 8 hours

Dosage adjustment in hepatic impairment: Mild-moderate impairment due to cirrhosis: 600 mg every 8 hours or with ketoconazole coadministration

Dietary Considerations Should be taken without food but with water 1 hour before or 2 hours after a meal. Administration with lighter meals (eg, dry toast, skim milk, corn flakes) resulted in little/no change in indinavir concentration. If taking with ritonavir, may take with food. Patient should drink at least 48 oz of water daily. May be taken with food when administered in combination with ritonavir.

Administration Drink at least 48 oz of water daily. Administer with water, 1 hour before or 2 hours after a meal. Administer around-the-clock to avoid significant fluctuation in serum levels. May be taken with food when administered in combination with ritonavir.

Monitoring Parameters Monitor viral load, CD4 count, triglycerides, cholesterol, glucose, liver function tests, CBC, urinalysis (severe leukocyturia should be monitored frequently).

Patient Information Take with a full glass of water; if any symptoms of kidney stones (eg, flank pain, dysuria), contact prescriber. Drug should be administered on an empty stomach 1 hour before or 2 hours after a large meal. May take with a small, light meal. Do not use prescription medications, OTC products, or herbal products without consulting prescriber. Indinavir should be stored and used in the original container.

Dosage Forms Capsule: 100 mg, 200 mg, 333 mg, 400 mg

Selected Readings

Deeks SG, Smith M, Holodniy M, et al, "HIV-1 Protease Inhibitors. A Review for Clinicians," *JAMA*, 1997, 277(2):145-53.

Kakuda TN, Struble KA, and Piscitelli SC, "Protease Inhibitors for the Treatment of Human Immunodeficiency Virus Infection," *Am J Health Syst Pharm*, 1998, 55(3):233-54.

Kaul DR, Cinti SK, Carver PL, et al, "HIV Protease Inhibitors: Advances in Therapy and Adverse Reactions, Including Metabolic Complications," *Pharmacotherapy*, 1999, 19(3):281-98.

McDonald CK and Kuritzkes DR, "Human Immunodeficiency Virus Type 1 Protease Inhibitors," *Arch Intern Med*, 1997, 157(9):951-9.

Indinavir Sulfate *see* Indinavir *on page 872*

INF-alpha 2 *see* Interferon Alfa-2b *on page 881*

Infanrix® *see* Diphtheria, Tetanus Toxoids, and Acellular Pertussis Vaccine *on page 782*

Infergen® *see* Interferon Alfacon-1 *on page 889*

Influenza Virus Vaccine (in floo EN za VYE rus vak SEEN)

Related Information

Immunization Recommendations *on page 1249*

U.S. Brand Names FluMist®; Fluvirin®; Fluzone®

Canadian Brand Names Fluviral S/F®; Fluzone®; Vaxigrip®

Synonyms Influenza Virus Vaccine (Purified Surface Antigen); Influenza Virus Vaccine (Split-Virus); Influenza Virus Vaccine (Trivalent, Live)

Generic Available No

Use Provide active immunity to influenza virus strains contained in the vaccine

Groups at Increased Risk for Influenza-Related Complications: Recommendations for vaccination:

- Persons ≥65 years of age
- Residents of nursing homes and other chronic-care facilities that house persons of any age with chronic medical conditions
- Adults and children with chronic disorders of the pulmonary or cardiovascular systems, including children with asthma
- Adults and children who have required regular medical follow-up or hospitalization during the preceding year because of chronic metabolic diseases (including diabetes mellitus), renal dysfunction, hemoglobinopathies, or immunosuppression (including immunosuppression caused by medications or HIV)
- Adults and children with conditions which may compromise respiratory function, the handling of respiratory secretions, or that can increase the risk of aspiration (eg, cognitive dysfunction, spinal; cord injuries, seizure disorders, other neuromuscular disorders)
- Children and adolescents (6 months to 18 years of age) who are receiving long-term aspirin therapy and therefore, may be at risk for developing Reye's syndrome after influenza
- Women who will be pregnant during the influenza season
- Children 6-23 months of age

Vaccination is also recommended for persons 50-64 years of age, close contacts of children 0-23 months of age, and healthy persons who may transmit influenza to those at risk and all healthcare workers.

Pregnancy Risk Factor C

Pregnancy Implications Reproduction studies have not been conducted. Case reports and limited studies suggest pregnancy may increase the risk of serious medical complications from influenza infection. Vaccination is recommended regardless of stage of pregnancy.

Contraindications Hypersensitivity to influenza virus vaccine, or any component of the formulation; presence of acute respiratory disease or other active infections or illnesses; active neurological disorder (immunization should be delayed)

In addition, for nasal spray: Patients at increased risk for influenza-related complications (see Use); history of Guillain-Barré syndrome; history of asthma or reactive airway disease; children 5-17 years of age receiving aspirin therapy; underlying medical conditions such as diabetes, renal dysfunction, cardiovascular disease, hemoglobinopathies; immunosuppressed or concomitant immunosuppressant therapy; pregnancy

Warnings/Precautions Antigenic response may not be as great as expected in patients requiring immunosuppressive drug or HIV-infected persons with <100 CD4 cells and with >30,000 viral copies of HIV type 1/mL; some products contain thimerosal or are manufactured with eggs and/or gentamicin; hypersensitivity reactions (presumably to egg proteins) may occur; because of potential for febrile reactions, risks and benefits must carefully be considered in patients with history of febrile convulsions; influenza vaccines from previous seasons must not be used. Inactivated vaccine is preferred over live virus vaccine for household members, healthcare workers and others coming in close contact with severely-immunosuppressed persons requiring care in a protected environment. Treatment for anaphylactic reactions (including epinephrine) should be readily available.

(Continued)

Influenza Virus Vaccine *(Continued)*

Injection: For I.M. use only; use caution with thrombocytopenia or any coagulation disorder. Safety and efficacy for use in children <6 months of age have not been established. Use caution with history of Guillain-Barré syndrome (GBS).

Nasal spray: For intranasal use only. **Avoid contact with severely immunocompromised individuals for at least 7 days following vaccination.** For use in healthy children and adults 5-49 years of age only; safety and efficacy for use in children <5 years or adults ≥50 years of age have not been established. Defer immunization if nasal congestion is present which may impede delivery of vaccine.

Adverse Reactions All serious adverse reactions must be reported to the U.S. Department of Health and Human Services (DHHS) Vaccine Adverse Event Reporting System (VAERS) 1-800-822-7967.

Injection: Frequency not defined:

- Central nervous system: Fever and malaise (may start within 6-12 hours and last 1-2 days; incidence equal to placebo in adults; occurs more frequently than placebo in children); GBS (previously reported with older vaccine formulations; relationship to current formulations not known, however, patients with history of GBS have a greater likelihood of developing GBS than those without)
- Dermatologic: Angioedema, urticaria
- Local: Tenderness, redness, or induration at the site of injection (10% to 64%; may last up to 2 days)
- Neuromuscular & skeletal: Myalgia (may start within 6-12 hours and last 1-2 days; incidence equal to placebo in adults; occurs more frequently than placebo in children)
- Miscellaneous: Allergic or anaphylactoid reactions (most likely to residual egg protein; includes allergic asthma, angioedema, hives, systemic anaphylaxis)

Nasal spray: **Note:** Frequency of events reported within 10 days

>10%:

- Central nervous system: Headache (children 18% after first dose, < placebo after second dose; adults 40%) irritability (children 10% to 19%)
- Neuromuscular & skeletal: Tiredness/weakness (adults 26%), muscle aches (children 5% to 6%; adults 17%)
- Respiratory: Cough, nasal congestion/ runny nose (children 46% to 48%; adults 9% to 45%), sore throat (children < placebo; adults 28%)
- Miscellaneous: Activity decreased (children 14% after first dose, < placebo after second dose)

1% to 10%:

- Central nervous system: Chills,
- Gastrointestinal: Abdominal pain, diarrhea, vomiting
- Otic: Otitis media

Drug Interactions

Increased Effect/Toxicity: Concomitant use of aspirin and the nasal spray formulation may increase the risk of Reye syndrome in patients 5-17 years; concomitant use in this age group is contraindicated.

Decreased Effect: Decreased effect with immunosuppressive agents; some manufacturers and clinicians recommend that the flu vaccine not be administered concomitantly with DTP due to the potential for increased febrile reactions (specifically whole-cell pertussis) and that one should wait at least 3 days. However, ACIP recommends that children at high risk for influenza may get the vaccine concomitantly with DTP. Safety and efficacy of nasal spray with other vaccines have not been established; do not give within 1 month of other live virus vaccines or within 2 weeks of inactivated or subunit vaccines.

Stability

Injection: Store between 2°C to 8°C (36°F to 46°F). Potency is destroyed by freezing; do not use if product has been frozen.

Nasal spray: Store in a freezer at or below -15°C (5°F); may thaw in refrigerator and store at 2°C to 8°C (36°F to 46°F) ≤60 hours; must be used within 24 hours after removal from the freezer; do not refreeze after thawing.

Mechanism of Action Promotes immunity to influenza virus by inducing specific antibody production. Each year the formulation is standardized according to the U.S. Public Health Service. Preparations from previous seasons must not be used.

Pharmacodynamics/Kinetics

Onset: Protective antibody levels achieved ~2 weeks after vaccination

Duration: Protective antibody levels persist approximately ≥6 months

Dosage Optimal time to receive vaccine is October-November, prior to exposure to influenza; however, vaccination can continue into December and later as long as vaccine is available.

I.M.:
- Fluzone®:
  - Children 6-35 months: 0.25 mL/dose (1 or 2 doses per season; see **Note**)
  - Children 3-8 years: 0.5 mL/dose (1 or 2 doses per season; see **Note**)
  - Children ≥9 years and Adults: 0.5 mL/dose (1 dose per season)
- Fluvirin®:
  - Children 4-8 years: 0.5 mL/dose (1 or 2 doses per season; see **Note**)
  - Children ≥9 years and Adults: 0.5 mL/dose (1 dose per season)

Note: Previously unvaccinated children <9 years should receive 2 doses, given >1 month apart in order to achieve satisfactory antibody response.

Intranasal (FluMist®):
- Children 5-8 years, previously **not vaccinated** with influenza vaccine: Initial season: Two 0.5 mL doses separated by 6-10 weeks
- Children 5-8 years, previously **vaccinated** with influenza vaccine: 0.5 mL/dose (1 dose per season)
- Children ≥9 years and Adults ≤49 years: 0.5 mL/dose (1 dose per season)

Administration

Injection: For I.M. administration only. Inspect for particulate matter and discoloration prior to administration. Adults and older children should be vaccinated in the deltoid muscle. Infants and young children should be vaccinated in the anterolateral aspect of the thigh. Suspensions should be shaken well prior to use. **Note:** For patients at risk of hemorrhage following intramuscular injection, the ACIP recommends "it should be administered intramuscularly if, in the opinion of the physician familiar with the patients bleeding risk, the vaccine can be administered with reasonable safety by this route. If the patient receives antihemophilia or other similar therapy, intramuscular vaccination can be scheduled shortly after such therapy is administered. A fine needle (23 gauge or smaller) can be used for the vaccination and firm pressure applied to the site (without rubbing) for at least 2 minutes. The patient should be instructed concerning the risk of hematoma from the injection."

Intranasal: Must be thawed prior to administration. May thaw in refrigerator and store at 2°C to 8°C (36°F to 46°F) ≤60 hours; must be used within 24 hours after removal from the freezer. May also be thawed by holding sprayer in the palm of the hand and supporting the plunger rod with thumb; use immediately. Half the dose (0.25 mL) is administered to each nostril; patient should be in upright position. A dose divider clip is provided. Severely-immunocompromised persons should not administer the live vaccine. If recipient sneezes following administration, the dose should not be repeated.

Patient Information You may experience the following: Soreness or swelling in the area where the shot is given, fever, aches. Some effects may last 1-2 days. Notify your prescriber immediately if these effects continue or are severe, or for a high fever, seizures, or allergic reaction (difficulty breathing, hives, weakness, dizziness, fast heart beat). Prior to vaccination, notify prescriber if you are allergic to eggs (develop hives, swelling of lip and/or tongue, or if you having trouble breathing after eating eggs).

Additional Information Pharmacies will stock the formulations(s) standardized according to the USPHS requirements for the season. Influenza vaccines from previous seasons must not be used. Federal law requires that the date of administration, the vaccine manufacturer, lot number of vaccine, and the administering person's name, title, and address be entered into the patient's permanent medical record.

During periods of inactivated influenza vaccine shortage, the CDC and ACIP have recommended vaccination be prioritized based on the following three tiers. The grouping is based on influenza associated mortality and hospitalization rates. Those listed in group 1 should be vaccinated first, followed by persons in group 2, and then group 3. If the vaccine supply is extremely limited, group 1 has also been subdivided in three tiers, where those in group 1A should be vaccinated first, followed by 1B, then 1C. When inactivated influenza vaccine is in limited supply, eligible persons should be encouraged to receive live, attenuated vaccine.

Priority groups for vaccination with inactivated influenza vaccine during periods of vaccine shortage:

- Tier 1A:
  - Persons ≥65 years with comorbid conditions
  - Residents of long-term-care facilities
- Tier 1B:
  - Persons 2-64 years with comorbid conditions
  - Persons ≥65 years without comorbid conditions
  - Children 6-23 months
  - Pregnant women
- Tier 1C:
  - Healthcare personnel
  - Household contacts and out-of-home caregivers of children <6 months

(Continued)

Influenza Virus Vaccine *(Continued)*

Tier 2:

Household contacts of children and adults at increased risk of influenza associated complications

Healthy persons 50-64 years

Tier 3:

Persons 2-49 years without high-risk conditions

Further information available at http://www.cdc.gov/mmwr/preview/mmwrhtml/mm5430a4.htm

Dosage Forms

Injection, solution, purified split-virus surface antigen [preservative free] (Fluvirin®): (0.5 mL) [prefilled syringe; contains thimerosal (trace amounts); manufactured using neomycin and polymyxin]; (5 mL) [multidose vial; contains thimerosal; manufactured using neomycin and polymyxin]

Injection, suspension, purified split-virus [produced in chick embryo cell culture]

Fluzone®: (5 mL) [vial; contains thimerosal]

Fluzone® [preservative free]: (0.25 mL) [prefilled syringe]; (0.5 mL) [vial]

Solution, nasal spray, trivalent, live virus [preservative free] (FluMist®): (0.5 mL) [manufactured using eggs and gentamicin]

Influenza Virus Vaccine (Purified Surface Antigen) *see* Influenza Virus Vaccine *on page 875*

Influenza Virus Vaccine (Split-Virus) *see* Influenza Virus Vaccine *on page 875*

Influenza Virus Vaccine (Trivalent, Live) *see* Influenza Virus Vaccine *on page 875*

INH *see* Isoniazid *on page 893*

α-2-interferon *see* Interferon Alfa-2b *on page 881*

Interferon Alfa-2a (in ter FEER on AL fa too aye)

U.S. Brand Names Roferon-A®

Canadian Brand Names Roferon-A®

Synonyms IFLrA; rIFN-A

Generic Available No

Use

Patients >18 years of age: Hairy cell leukemia, AIDS-related Kaposi's sarcoma, chronic hepatitis C

Children and Adults: Chronic myelogenous leukemia (CML), Philadelphia chromosome positive, within 1 year of diagnosis (limited experience in children)

Unlabeled/Investigational Use Adjuvant therapy for malignant melanoma, AIDS-related thrombocytopenia, cutaneous ulcerations of Behçet's disease, brain tumors, metastatic ileal carcinoid tumors, cervical and colorectal cancers, genital warts, idiopathic mixed cryoglobulinemia, hemangioma, hepatitis D, hepatocellular carcinoma, idiopathic hypereosinophilic syndrome, mycosis fungoides, Sézary syndrome, low-grade non-Hodgkin's lymphoma, macular degeneration, multiple myeloma, renal cell carcinoma, basal and squamous cell skin cancer, essential thrombocythemia, cutaneous T-cell lymphoma

Restrictions An FDA-approved medication guide is available at www.fda.gov/cder/Offices/ODS/labeling.htm; distribute to each patient to whom this medication is dispensed.

Pregnancy Risk Factor C

Pregnancy Implications Safety and efficacy for use during pregnancy have not been established. Interferon alpha has been shown to decrease serum estradiol and progesterone levels in humans. Menstrual irregularities and abortion have been reported in animals. Effective contraception is recommended during treatment.

Warnings/Precautions Use caution in patients with a history of depression. May cause severe psychiatric adverse events (psychosis, mania, depression, suicidal behavior/ideation) in patients with and without previous psychiatric symptoms; careful neuropsychiatric monitoring is required during therapy. Use with caution in patients with seizure disorders, brain metastases, or compromised CNS function. Higher doses in the elderly or in malignancies other than hairy cell leukemia may result in severe obtundation.

Use caution in patients with autoimmune diseases; development or exacerbation of autoimmune diseases has been reported. Use caution in patients with pre-existing cardiac disease (ischemic or thromboembolic), arrhythmias, renal impairment (Cl_{cr} <50 mL/minute), mild hepatic impairment, or myelosuppression. Also use caution in patients receiving therapeutic immunosuppression. May cause thyroid dysfunction or hyperglycemia, use caution in patients with diabetes or pre-existing thyroid disease.

Pulmonary dysfunction may be induced or aggravated by interferon alpha; discontinue if persistent unexplained pulmonary infiltrates are noted. Gastrointestinal ischemia, ulcerative colitis and hemorrhage have been associated rarely with alpha interferons; some cases are severe and life-threatening. Ophthalmologic disorders (including retinal hemorrhages, cotton wool spots, and retinal artery or vein obstruction) have occurred in patients receiving alpha interferons; close monitoring is warranted.

Treatment should be discontinued in patients with worsening or persistently severe signs/symptoms of autoimmune, infectious, ischemic, or neuropsychiatric disorders (including depression and/or suicidal thoughts/behavior). Discontinue treatment if neutrophils <0.5 x 10^9/L or platelets <25 x 10^9/L. **Due to differences in dosage, patients should not change brands of interferons.** Injection solution contains benzyl alcohol; do not use in neonates or infants. Safety and efficacy in children <18 years of age have not been established.

Adverse Reactions Note: A flu-like syndrome (fever, chills, tachycardia, malaise, myalgia, arthralgia, headache) occurs within 1-2 hours of administration; may last up to 24 hours and may be dose-limiting (symptoms in up to 92% of patients). For the listing below, the percentage of incidence noted generally corresponds to highest reported ranges. Incidence depends upon dosage and indication.

>10%:

Cardiovascular: Chest pain (4% to 11%), edema (11%), hypertension (11%)

Central nervous system: Psychiatric disturbances (including depression and suicidal behavior/ideation; reported incidence highly variable, generally >15%), fatigue (90%), headache (52%), dizziness (21%), irritability (15%), insomnia (14%), somnolence, lethargy, confusion, mental impairment, and motor weakness (most frequently seen at high doses [>100 million units], usually reverses within a few days); vertigo (19%); mental status changes (12%)

Dermatologic: Rash (usually maculopapular) on the trunk and extremities (7% to 18%), alopecia (19% to 22%), pruritus (13%), dry skin

Endocrine & metabolic: Hypocalcemia (10% to 51%), hyperglycemia (33% to 39%), transaminases increased (25% to 30%), alkaline phosphatase increased (48%)

Gastrointestinal: Loss of taste, anorexia (30% to 70%), nausea (28% to 53%), vomiting (10% to 30%, usually mild), diarrhea (22% to 34%, may be severe), taste change (13%), dry throat, xerostomia, abdominal cramps, abdominal pain

Hematologic (often due to underlying disease): Myelosuppression; neutropenia (32% to 70%); thrombocytopenia (22% to 70%); anemia (24% to 65%, may be dose-limiting, usually seen only during the first 6 months of therapy)

Onset: 7-10 days

Nadir: 14 days, may be delayed 20-40 days in hairy cell leukemia

Recovery: 21 days

Hepatic: Elevation of AST (SGOT) (77% to 80%), LDH (47%), bilirubin (31%)

Local: Injection site reaction (29%)

Neuromuscular & skeletal: Weakness (may be severe at doses >20,000,000 units/day); arthralgia and myalgia (5% to 73%, usually during the first 72 hours of treatment); rigors

Renal: Proteinuria (15% to 25%)

Respiratory: Cough (27%), irritation of oropharynx (14%)

Miscellaneous: Flu-like syndrome (up to 92% of patients), diaphoresis (15%)

1% to 10%:

Cardiovascular: Hypotension (6%), supraventricular tachyarrhythmia, palpitation (<3%), acute MI (<1% to 1%)

Central nervous system: Confusion (10%), delirium

Dermatologic: Erythema (diffuse), urticaria

Endocrine & metabolic: Hyperphosphatemia (2%)

Gastrointestinal: Stomatitis, pancreatitis (<5%), flatulence, liver pain

Genitourinary: Impotence (6%), menstrual irregularities

Neuromuscular & skeletal: Leg cramps; peripheral neuropathy, paresthesia (7%), and numbness (4%) are more common in patients previously treated with vinca alkaloids or receiving concurrent vinblastine

Ocular: Conjunctivitis (4%)

Respiratory: Dyspnea (7.5%), epistaxis (4%), rhinitis (3%)

Miscellaneous: Antibody production to interferon (10%)

<1%: Abdominal fullness, angioedema, aplastic anemia, arthritis, ascites, autoimmune reaction with worsening of liver disease, bronchospasm, bronchiolitis obliterans, BUN/creatinine increased, cardiomyopathy, coagulopathy, coma, CHF, cutaneous eruptions, distal cyanosis, diffuse encephalopathy, dysphasia, eczema, EEG abnormalities, hallucinations, hemolytic anemia, hyper-/hypothyroidism, hypermotility, hypertriglyceridemia, hyponatremia (SIADH), mania, gait disturbance, gastrointestinal hemorrhage, hepatic failure, idiopathic thrombocytopenia

(Continued)

Interferon Alfa-2a *(Continued)*

purpura, interstitial nephritis, interstitial pneumonitis, ischemic colitis, leukopenia, libido decreased, lupus erythematosus syndrome, myositis, nasal congestion, nephrotic syndrome, optic neuritis, pneumonia, pneumonitis, presenile dementia, proteinuria, psoriasis, psychotic episodes, Raynaud's phenomenon, renal failure (acute), rhabdomyolysis, sarcoidosis, seborrhea, seizure, stroke, syncope, tachypnea, ulcerative colitis, urticaria, vasculitis, visual acuity decreased

Overdosage/Toxicology Symptoms include CNS depression, obtundation, flu-like symptoms, and myelosuppression. Treatment is supportive.

Drug Interactions

Cytochrome P450 Effect: Inhibits CYP1A2 (weak)

Increased Effect/Toxicity: Note: May exacerbate the toxicity of other agents with respect to CNS, myelotoxicity, or cardiotoxicity. Theophylline clearance has been reported to be decreased in hepatitis patients receiving interferon. Interferons may increase the adverse/toxic effects of ACE inhibitors, specifically the development of granulocytopenia. Agranulocytosis has been reported with concurrent use of clozapine (case report). Interferons may increase the anticoagulant effects of warfarin, and interferons may increase serum levels of zidovudine.

Decreased Effect: Prednisone may decrease the therapeutic effects of interferon alpha. A decreased response to erythropoietin has been reported (case reports) in patients receiving interferons. Interferon alpha may decrease the serum concentrations of melphalan (may or may not decrease toxicity of melphalan).

Stability Refrigerate (2°C to 8°C/36°F to 46°F); do not freeze; do not shake. Reconstitute vial with the diluent provided, or SWFI, NS, or D_5W; concentrations ≥3 x 10^6 units/mL are hypertonic. After reconstitution, the solution is stable for 24 hours at room temperature and for 1 month when refrigerated.

Mechanism of Action Following activation, multiple effects can be detected including induction of gene transcription. Inhibits cellular growth, alters the state of cellular differentiation, interferes with oncogene expression, alters cell surface antigen expression, increases phagocytic activity of macrophages, and augments cytotoxicity of lymphocytes for target cells

Pharmacodynamics/Kinetics

Absorption: Filtered and absorbed at the renal tubule

Distribution: V_d: 0.223-0.748 L/kg

Metabolism: Primarily renal; filtered through glomeruli and undergoes rapid proteolytic degradation during tubular reabsorption

Bioavailability: I.M.: 83%; SubQ: 90%

Half-life elimination: I.V.: 3.7-8.5 hours (mean ~5 hours)

Time to peak, serum: I.M., SubQ: ~6-8 hours

Dosage Refer to individual protocols

Children (limited data):

Chronic myelogenous leukemia (CML): I.M.: 2.5-5 million units/m²/day; **Note:** In juveniles, higher dosages (30 million units/m²/day) have been associated with severe adverse events, including death

Adults:

Hairy cell leukemia: SubQ, I.M.: 3 million units/day for 16-24 weeks, then 3 million units 3 times/week for up to 6-24 months

Chronic myelogenous leukemia (CML): SubQ, I.M.: 9 million units/day, continue treatment until disease progression

AIDS-related Kaposi's sarcoma: SubQ, I.M.: 36 million units/day for 10-12 weeks, then 36 million units 3 times/week; to minimize adverse reactions, can use escalating dose (3-, 9-, then 18 million units each day for 3 days, then 36 million units daily thereafter).

Hepatitis C: SubQ, I.M.: 3 million units 3 times/week for 12 months

Dosage adjustment in renal impairment: Not removed by hemodialysis

Administration SubQ administration is suggested for those who are at risk for bleeding or are thrombocytopenic; rotate SubQ injection site; patient should be well hydrated

Monitoring Parameters Baseline ophthalmologic exam should be performed in all patients, with periodic reassessment in patients with impairment. Patients with thyroid dysfunction should be monitored by TSH levels at baseline and every 3 months during therapy.

Chronic hepatitis C: Monitor ALT (at baseline, after 2 weeks, and monthly thereafter) and HCV-RNA (particularly in first 3 months of therapy)

CML/hairy cell leukemia: Hematologic monitoring should be performed monthly

Patient Information Use as directed; do not change dosage or schedule of administration without consulting prescriber. Maintain adequate hydration (2-3 L/day of fluids unless instructed to restrict fluid intake). You may experience flu-like syndrome (acetaminophen may help); this syndrome subsides after several weeks of continuous

dosing, but usually recurs during each cycle of intermittent therapy. You may also experience nausea, vomiting, dry mouth, or metallic taste (frequent small meals, frequent mouth care, sucking lozenges, or chewing gum may help); drowsiness, dizziness, agitation, abnormal thinking (use caution when driving or engaging in tasks requiring alertness until response to drug is known). Inform prescriber **immediately** if you feel depressed or have any thoughts of suicide. Report unusual bruising or bleeding; persistent abdominal disturbances; unusual fatigue; muscle pain or tremors; chest pain or palpitation; swelling of extremities or unusual weight gain; difficulty breathing; pain, swelling, or redness at injection site; or other unusual symptoms.

Dosage Forms Injection, solution, [single-dose prefilled syringe; SubQ use only]: 3 million units/0.5 mL (0.5 mL); 6 million units/0.5 mL (0.5 mL); 9 million units/0.5 mL (0.5 mL) [contains benzyl alcohol]

Selected Readings

Barreca T, Corsini G, Franceschini R, et al, "Lichen Planus Induced by Interferon-Alpha-2a Therapy for Chronic Active Hepatitis C," *Eur J Gastroenterol Hepatol*, 1995, 7(4):367-8.

Fukumoto Y, Shigemitsu T, Kajii N, et al, "Abducent Nerve Paralysis During Interferon Alpha-2a Therapy in a Case of Chronic Active Hepatitis C," *Intern Med*, 1994, 33(10):637-40.

Haria M and Benfield P, "Interferon-Alpha-2a. A Review of Its Pharmacological Properties and Therapeutic Use in the Management of Viral Hepatitis," *Drugs*, 1995, 50(5):873-96.

Hoofnagle JH, "Alpha-Interferon Therapy of Chronic Hepatitis B, Current Status and Recommendations," *J Hepatol*, 1990, 11(Suppl 1):S100-7.

Morris DJ, "Adverse Effects and Drug Interactions of Clinical Importance With Antiviral Drugs," *Drug Saf*, 1994, 10(4):281-91.

Vial T and Descotes J, "Clinical Toxicity of the Interferons," *Drug Saf*, 1994, 10(2):115-50.

Interferon Alfa-2b (in ter FEER on AL fa too bee)

U.S. Brand Names Intron® A

Canadian Brand Names Intron® A

Synonyms α-2-interferon; INF-alpha 2; rLFN-α2

Generic Available No

Use

Patients ≥1 year of age: Chronic hepatitis B

Patients ≥18 years of age: Condyloma acuminata, chronic hepatitis C, hairy cell leukemia, malignant melanoma, AIDS-related Kaposi's sarcoma, follicular non-Hodgkin's lymphoma

Unlabeled/Investigational Use AIDS-related thrombocytopenia, cutaneous ulcerations of Behçet's disease, carcinoid syndrome, cervical cancer, lymphomatoid granulomatosis, genital herpes, hepatitis D, chronic myelogenous leukemia (CML), non-Hodgkin's lymphomas (other than follicular lymphoma, see approved use), polycythemia vera, medullary thyroid carcinoma, multiple myeloma, renal cell carcinoma, basal and squamous cell skin cancers, essential thrombocytopenia, thrombocytopenic purpura

Investigational: West Nile virus

Drug of Choice or Alternative for Organism(s):

Hepatitis B Virus *on page 165*

Hepatitis C Virus *on page 167*

Pregnancy Risk Factor C

Pregnancy Implications Safety and efficacy for use during pregnancy have not been established. Interferon alpha has been shown to decrease serum estradiol and progesterone levels in humans. Menstrual irregularities and abortion have been reported in animals. Effective contraception is recommended during treatment.

Contraindications Hypersensitivity to interferon alfa or any component of the formulation; patients with visceral AIDS-related Kaposi's sarcoma associated with rapidly-progressing or life-threatening disease; decompensated liver disease; autoimmune hepatitis; history of autoimmune disease; immunosuppressed transplant patients

Warnings/Precautions Suicidal ideation or attempts may occur more frequently in pediatric patients when compared to adults. May cause severe psychiatric adverse events (psychosis, mania, depression, suicidal behavior/ideation) in patients with and without previous psychiatric symptoms, avoid use in severe psychiatric disorders or in patients with a history of depression; careful neuropsychiatric monitoring is required during therapy. Use with caution in patients with a history of seizures, brain metastases, multiple sclerosis, cardiac disease (ischemic or thromboembolic), arrhythmias, myelosuppression, hepatic impairment, or renal dysfunction (use is not recommended if Cl_{cr}<50 mL/minute). Use caution in patients with a history of pulmonary disease, coagulopathy, thyroid disease (monitor thyroid function), hypertension, or diabetes mellitus (particularly if prone to DKA). Caution in patients receiving drugs that may cause lactic acidosis (eg, nucleoside analogues).

(Continued)

Interferon Alfa-2b *(Continued)*

Avoid use in patients with autoimmune disorders; worsening of psoriasis and/or development of autoimmune disorders has been associated with alpha interferons. Higher doses in elderly patients, or diseases other than hairy cell leukemia, may result in increased CNS toxicity. Treatment should be discontinued in patients who develop severe pulmonary symptoms with chest x-ray changes, autoimmune disorders, worsening of hepatic function, psychiatric symptoms (including depression and/or suicidal thoughts/behaviors), ischemic and/or infectious disorders. Ophthalmologic disorders (including retinal hemorrhages, cotton wool spots and retinal artery or vein obstruction) have occurred in patients receiving alpha interferons. Hypertriglyceridemia has been reported (discontinue if severe).

Safety and efficacy in children <1 year of age have not been established. Do not treat patients with visceral AIDS-related Kaposi's sarcoma associated with rapidly-progressing or life-threatening disease. A transient increase in SGOT (>2x baseline) is common in patients treated with interferon alfa-2b for chronic hepatitis. Therapy generally may continue, however, functional indicators (albumin, prothrombin time, bilirubin) should be monitored at 2-week intervals. **Due to differences in dosage, patients should not change brands of interferons.**

Intron® A may cause bone marrow suppression, including very rarely, aplastic anemia. Hemolytic anemia (hemoglobin <10 g/dL) was observed in 10% of treated patients in clinical trials; anemia occurred within 1-2 weeks of initiation of therapy.

Adverse Reactions Note: In a majority of patients, a flu-like syndrome (fever, chills, tachycardia, malaise, myalgia, headache), occurs within 1-2 hours of administration; may last up to 24 hours and may be dose-limiting.

>10%:
- Cardiovascular: Chest pain (2% to 28%)
- Central nervous system: Fatigue (8% to 96%), headache (21% to 62%), fever (34% to 94%), depression (4% to 40%), somnolence (1% to 33%), irritability (1% to 22%), paresthesia (1% to 21%, more common in patients previously treated with vinca alkaloids or receiving concurrent vinblastine), dizziness (7% to 23%), confusion (1% to 12%), malaise (3% to 14%), pain (3% to 15%), insomnia (1% to 12%), impaired concentration (1% to 14%, usually reverses within a few days), amnesia (1% to 14%), chills (45% to 54%)
- Dermatologic: Alopecia (8% to 38%), rash (usually maculopapular) on the trunk and extremities (1% to 25%), pruritus (3% to 11%), dry skin (1% to 10%)
- Endocrine & metabolic: Alkaline phosphatase increased (48%), hypocalcemia (10% to 51%), hyperglycemia (33% to 39%), amenorrhea (up to 12% in lymphoma)
- Gastrointestinal: Anorexia (1% to 69%), nausea (19% to 66%), vomiting (2% to 32%, usually mild), diarrhea (2% to 45%, may be severe), taste change (2% to 24%), xerostomia (1% to 28%), abdominal pain (2% to 23%), gingivitis (2% to 14%), constipation (1% to 14%)
- Hematologic: Myelosuppression; neutropenia (30% to 66%); thrombocytopenia (5% to 15%); anemia (15% to 32%, may be dose-limiting, usually seen only during the first 6 months of therapy)
  - Onset: 7-10 days
  - Nadir: 14 days, may be delayed 20-40 days in hairy cell leukemia
  - Recovery: 21 days
- Hepatic: Right upper quadrant pain (15% in hepatitis C), transaminases increased (increased SGOT in up to 63%)
- Local: Injection site reaction (1% to 20%)
- Neuromuscular & skeletal: Weakness (5% to 63%) may be severe at doses >20,000,000 units/day; mild arthralgia and myalgia (5% to 75% - usually during the first 72 hours of treatment), rigors (2% to 42%), back pain (1% to 19%), musculoskeletal pain (1% to 21%), paresthesia (1% to 21%)
- Renal: Urinary tract infection (up to 5% in hepatitis C)
- Respiratory: Dyspnea (1% to 34%), cough (1% to 31%), pharyngitis (1% to 31%),
- Miscellaneous: Loss of smell, flu-like symptoms (5% to 79%), diaphoresis (2% to 21%)

5% to 10%:
- Cardiovascular: Hypertension (9% in hepatitis C)
- Central nervous system: Anxiety (1% to 9%), nervousness (1% to 3%), vertigo (up to 8% in lymphoma)
- Dermatologic: Dermatitis (1% to 8%)
- Endocrine & metabolic: Decreased libido (1% to 5%)
- Gastrointestinal: Loose stools (1% to 21%), dyspepsia (2% to 8%)
- Neuromuscular & skeletal: Hypoesthesia (1% to 10%)
- Respiratory: Nasal congestion (1% to 10%)

<5% (Limited to important or life-threatening):
- Cardiovascular: Angina, arrhythmia, atrial fibrillation, bradycardia, tachycardia, vasculitis, CHF, cardiomegaly, cardiomyopathy, hypotension, Raynaud's phenomenon, thrombosis, pulmonary embolism, MI
- Central nervous system: Abnormal coordination, aggravated depression, aphasia, ataxia, Bell's palsy, coma, seizure, dysphonia, extrapyramidal disorder, flushing, hallucinations, manic reaction, migraine, neuropathy, paranoia, psychosis, stroke, suicidal ideation, suicide attempt, syncope, tremor
- Dermatologic: Diffuse erythema, eczema, epidermal necrolysis, hirsutism, psoriasis, urticaria
- Endocrine & metabolic: Diabetes mellitus, hyperthyroidism, hypothyroidism, hypertriglyceridemia, hyperglycemia, goiter, pancreatitis
- Gastrointestinal: Ascites, colitis, esophagitis, gastritis, gastrointestinal hemorrhage, gingival hyperplasia, mucositis, rectal hemorrhage, stomatitis, taste loss
- Genitourinary: Cystitis, incontinence, dysuria
- Hematologic: Anemia, granulocytopenia, leukopenia, hemolytic anemia, thrombocytopenic purpura
- Hepatic: Hyperbilirubinemia, jaundice, hepatic encephalopathy (rare), hepatic failure (rare), hepatotoxic reaction
- Neuromuscular & skeletal: Arthritis, leg cramps, polyarteritis nodosa, tendonitis, rheumatoid arthritis, spondylitis, lupus erythematosus
- Ocular: Abnormal vision, nystagmus
- Renal: Proteinuria, hematuria, increased BUN, nephrotic syndrome, renal failure
- Respiratory: Asthma, bronchospasm, hemoptysis, hypoventilation, pulmonary fibrosis, pleural effusion, pneumonitis, respiratory insufficiency
- Miscellaneous: Acute hypersensitivity reactions, allergic reactions

Overdosage/Toxicology Symptoms include CNS depression, obtundation, flu-like symptoms, and myelosuppression. Treatment is supportive.

Drug Interactions

Cytochrome P450 Effect: Inhibits CYP1A2 (weak)

Increased Effect/Toxicity: Theophylline clearance has been reported to be decreased in hepatitis patients receiving interferon. Interferons may increase the adverse/toxic effects of ACE inhibitors, specifically the development of granulocytopenia. Agranulocytosis has been reported with concurrent use of clozapine (case report). Interferons may increase the anticoagulant effects of warfarin, and interferons may increase serum levels of zidovudine.

Stability Store powder and solution for injection (vials and pens) under refrigeration (2°C to 8°C). The manufacturer recommends reconstituting vial with the diluent provided (SWFI). To prepare solution for infusion, further dilute appropriate dose in NS 100 mL. Final concentration should not be <10 million units/100 mL.

Powder for injection: Following reconstitution, should be used immediately, but may be stored under refrigeration for up to 24 hours.

Prefilled pens: After first use, discard unused portion after 1 month.

Mechanism of Action Following activation, multiple effects can be detected including induction of gene transcription. Inhibits cellular growth, alters the state of cellular differentiation, interferes with oncogene expression, alters cell surface antigen expression, increases phagocytic activity of macrophages, and augments cytotoxicity of lymphocytes for target cells

Pharmacodynamics/Kinetics

Distribution: V_d: 31 L; but has been noted to be much greater (370-720 L) in leukemia patients receiving continuous infusion IFN; IFN does not penetrate the CSF

Metabolism: Primarily renal

Bioavailability: I.M.: 83%; SubQ: 90%

Half-life elimination: I.M., I.V.: 2 hours; SubQ: 3 hours

Time to peak, serum: I.M., SubQ: ~3-12 hours

Dosage Refer to individual protocols

Children 1-17 years: Chronic hepatitis B: SubQ: 3 million units/m^2 3 times/week for 1 week; then 6 million units/m^2 3 times/week; maximum: 10 million units 3 times/week; total duration of therapy 16-24 weeks

Adults:
- Hairy cell leukemia: I.M., SubQ: 2 million units/m^2 3 times/week for 2-6 months
- Lymphoma (follicular): SubQ: 5 million units 3 times/week for up to 18 months
- Malignant melanoma: 20 million units/m^2 I.V. for 5 consecutive days per week for 4 weeks, then 10 million units/m^2 SubQ 3 times/week for 48 weeks
- AIDS-related Kaposi's sarcoma: I.M., SubQ: 30 million units/m^2 3 times/week
- Chronic hepatitis B: I.M., SubQ: 5 million units/day or 10 million units 3 times/week for 16 weeks
- Chronic hepatitis C: I.M., SubQ: 3 million units 3 times/week for 16 weeks. In patients with normalization of ALT at 16 weeks, continue treatment for 18-24 months; consider discontinuation if normalization does not occur at 16 weeks.

(Continued)

Interferon Alfa-2b *(Continued)*

Note: May be used in combination therapy with ribavirin in previously untreated patients or in patients who relapse following alpha interferon therapy; refer to Interferon Alfa-2b and Ribavirin Combination Pack monograph.

Condyloma acuminata: Intralesionally: 1 million units/lesion (maximum: 5 lesions/treatment) 3 times/week (on alternate days) for 3 weeks; may administer a second course at 12-16 weeks

Dosage adjustment in renal impairment: Combination therapy with ribavirin (hepatitis C) should not be used in patients with reduced renal function (Cl_{cr} <50 mL/minute).

Not removed by peritoneal or hemodialysis

Dosage adjustment for toxicity: Manufacturer-recommended adjustments, listed according to indication:

Lymphoma (follicular):

Severe toxicity (neutrophils <1000 cells/mm^3 or platelets <50,000 cells/mm^3): Reduce dose by 50% or temporarily discontinue

AST/ALT >5 times ULN: Permanently discontinue

Hairy cell leukemia:

Severe toxicity: Reduce dose by 50% or temporarily discontinue; permanently discontinue if persistent or recurrent severe toxicity is noted

Hepatitis B or C:

WBC <1500 cells/mm^3, granulocytes <750 cells/mm^3, or platelet count <50,000 cells/mm^3: Reduce dose by 50%

WBC <1000 cells/mm^3, granulocytes <500 cells/mm^3, or platelet count <25,000 cells/mm^3: Permanently discontinue

Kaposi sarcoma: Severe toxicity: Reduce dose by 50% or temporarily discontinue

Malignant melanoma:

Severe toxicity (neutrophils <500 cells/mm^3 or AST/ALT >5 times ULN): Reduce dose by 50% or temporarily discontinue

Neutrophils <250 cells/mm^3 or AST/ALT >10 times ULN: Permanently discontinue

Administration SubQ: Suggested for those who are at risk for bleeding or are thrombocytopenic. Rotate SubQ injection site. Patient should be well hydrated. Reconstitute with recommended amount of SWFI and agitate gently; do not shake. **Note:** Different vial strengths require different amounts of diluent. Not every dosage form is appropriate for every indication; refer to manufacturer's labeling.

Monitoring Parameters Baseline chest x-ray, ECG, CBC with differential, liver function tests, electrolytes, thyroid function tests, platelets, weight; patients with pre-existing cardiac abnormalities, or in advanced stages of cancer should have ECGs taken before and during treatment.

Patient Information Without the advice of prescriber, do not change brands of interferon as changes in dosage may result; do not operate heavy machinery while on therapy since changes in mental status may occur; report any persistent or severe sore throat, fever, fatigue, unusual bleeding, or bruising. You may experience flu-like syndrome (acetaminophen may help); this syndrome subsides after several weeks of continuous dosing, but usually recurs during each cycle of intermittent therapy.

Dosage Forms

Injection, powder for reconstitution: 10 million units; 18 million units; 50 million units [contains human albumin]

Injection, solution [multidose prefilled pen]:

Delivers 3 million units/0.2 mL (1.5 mL) [delivers 6 doses; 18 million units]

Delivers 5 million units/0.2 mL (1.5 mL) [delivers 6 doses; 30 million units]

Delivers 10 million units/0.2 mL (1.5 mL) [delivers 6 doses; 60 million units]

Injection, solution [multidose vial]: 6 million units/mL (3 mL); 10 million units/mL (2.5 mL)

Injection, solution [single-dose vial]: 10 million units/ mL (1 mL)

See also Interferon Alfa-2b and Ribavirin Combination Pack monograph.

Selected Readings

Davis GL, Esteban-Mur R, Rustgi V, et al, "Interferon Alfa-2b Alone or in Combination With Ribavirin for the Treatment of Relapse of Chronic Hepatitis C," *N Engl J Med*, 1998, 339(21):1493-9.

"Drugs for Non-HIV Viral Infections," *Med Lett Drugs Ther*, 1994, 36(919):27.

McHutchison JG, Gordon SC, Schiff ER, et al, "Interferon Alfa-2b Alone or in Combination With Ribavirin as Initial Treatment for Chronic Hepatitis C," *N Engl J Med*, 1998, 339(21):1485-92.

Interferon Alfa-2b and Ribavirin

(in ter FEER on AL fa too bee & rye ba VYE rin)

Related Information

Interferon Alfa-2b *on page 881*

Ribavirin *on page 1040*

U.S. Brand Names Rebetron®

Canadian Brand Names Rebetron®

Synonyms Interferon Alfa-2b and Ribavirin Combination Pack; Ribavirin and Interferon Alfa-2b Combination Pack

Generic Available No

Use Combination therapy for the treatment of chronic hepatitis C in patients with compensated liver disease previously untreated with alpha interferon or who have relapsed after alpha interferon therapy

Drug of Choice or Alternative for Organism(s):

Hepatitis C Virus *on page 167*

Restrictions An FDA-approved medication guide is available at www.fda.gov/cder/Offices/ODS/labeling.htm; distribute to each patient to whom this medication is dispensed.

Pregnancy Risk Factor X

Pregnancy Implications Abortifacient and teratogenic effects have been reported with ribavirin. Negative pregnancy test is required before initiation and monthly thereafter. Avoid pregnancy in female patients and female partners of patients during therapy by using two effective forms of contraception; continue contraceptive measures for at least 6 months after completion of therapy. If patient or female partner becomes pregnant during treatment, she should be counseled about potential risks of exposure. Pregnancies that occur during use, or within 6 months after treatment, should be reported to the manufacturer (800-593-2214).

Contraindications Hypersensitivity to interferon alfa-2b, ribavirin, or any component of the formulation; autoimmune hepatitis; males with a pregnant female partner; pregnancy

Warnings/Precautions

Interferon alfa-2b: Suicidal ideation or attempts may occur more frequently in pediatric patients when compared to adults. May cause severe psychiatric adverse events (psychosis, mania, depression, suicidal behavior/ideation) in patients with and without previous psychiatric symptoms, avoid use in severe psychiatric disorders or in patients with a history of depression; careful neuropsychiatric monitoring is required during therapy. Use with caution in patients with a history of seizures, brain metastases, multiple sclerosis, cardiac disease (ischemic or thromboembolic), arrhythmias, myelosuppression, hepatic impairment, or renal dysfunction (use is not recommended if Cl_{cr}<50 mL/minute). Use caution in patients with a history of pulmonary disease, coagulopathy, thyroid disease (monitor thyroid function), hypertension, or diabetes mellitus (particularly if prone to DKA). Caution in patients receiving drugs that may cause lactic acidosis (eg, nucleoside analogues). Avoid use in patients with autoimmune disorders; worsening of psoriasis and/or development of autoimmune disorders has been associated with alpha interferons. Higher doses in elderly patients, or diseases other than hairy cell leukemia, may result in increased CNS toxicity. Treatment should be discontinued in patients who develop severe pulmonary symptoms with chest x-ray changes, autoimmune disorders, worsening of hepatic function, psychiatric symptoms (including depression and/or suicidal thoughts/behaviors), ischemic and/or infectious disorders. Ophthalmologic disorders (including retinal hemorrhages, cotton wool spots and retinal artery or vein obstruction) have occurred in patients receiving alpha interferons. Hypertriglyceridemia has been reported (discontinue if severe).

Safety and efficacy in children <3 years of age have not been established. Do not treat patients with visceral AIDS-related Kaposi's sarcoma associated with rapidly-progressing or life-threatening disease. A transient increase in SGOT (>2x baseline) is common in patients treated with interferon alfa-2b for chronic hepatitis. Therapy generally may continue, however, functional indicators (albumin, prothrombin time, bilirubin) should be monitored at 2-week intervals. **Due to differences in dosage, patients should not change brands of interferons.**

Intron® A may cause bone marrow suppression, including very rarely, aplastic anemia. Hemolytic anemia (hemoglobin <10 g/dL) was observed in 10% of treated patients in clinical trials; anemia occurred within 1-2 weeks of initiation of therapy.

Ribavirin: Oral: Anemia has been observed in patients receiving the interferon/ribavirin combination. Severe psychiatric events have also occurred including depression and suicidal behavior during combination therapy; avoid use in patients with a psychiatric history. Hemolytic anemia is a significant toxicity; usually occurring within 1-2 weeks. Assess cardiac disease before initiation. Anemia may worsen underlying cardiac disease; use caution. If any deterioration in cardiovascular status occurs, discontinue therapy. Use caution in pulmonary disease; pulmonary symptoms have been associated with administration. Use caution in patients with sarcoidosis (exacerbation reported). Negative pregnancy test is required before initiation and monthly thereafter. Avoid pregnancy in female patients and female partners of patients during

(Continued)

Interferon Alfa-2b and Ribavirin *(Continued)*

therapy. Discontinue therapy in suspected/confirmed pancreatitis. Use caution in elderly patients; higher frequency of anemia; take renal function into consideration before initiating. Safety and efficacy have not been established in organ transplant patients, decompensated liver disease, concurrent hepatitis B virus or HIV exposure, or pediatric patients <3 years of age. Use caution in patients receiving concurrent medications which may cause lactic acidosis (eg, nucleoside analogues).

Adverse Reactions Note: Adverse reactions listed are specific to combination regimen in previously untreated hepatitis patients. See individual agents for additional adverse reactions reported with each agent during therapy for other diseases.

>10%:

Central nervous system: Fatigue (children 61%; adults 68%), headache (63%), insomnia (children 14%; adults 39%), fever (children 61%; adults 37%), depression (children 13%; adults 32% to 36%), irritability (children 10%; adults 23% to 32%), dizziness (17% to 23%), emotional lability (children 16%; adults 7% to 11%), impaired concentration (5% to 14%)

Dermatologic: Alopecia (23% to 32%), pruritus (children 12%; adults 19% to 21%), rash (17% to 28%)

Gastrointestinal: Nausea (33% to 46%), anorexia (children 51%; adults 25% to 27%), dyspepsia (children <1%; adults 14% to 16%), vomiting (children 42%; adults 9% to 11%)

Hematologic: Leukopenia, neutropenia (usually recovers within 4 weeks of treatment discontinuation), anemia

Hepatic: Hyperbilirubinemia (27%; only 0.9% to 2% >3.0-6 mg/dL)

Local: Injection site inflammation (13%)

Neuromuscular & skeletal: Myalgia (children 32%; adults 61% to 64%), rigors (40%), arthralgia (children 15%; adults 30% to 33%), musculoskeletal pain (20% to 28%)

Respiratory: Dyspnea (children 5%; adults 18% to 19%)

Miscellaneous: Flu-like syndrome (children 31%; adults 14% to 18%)

1% to 10%:

Cardiovascular: Chest pain (5% to 9%)

Central nervous system: Nervousness (3% to 4%)

Endocrine & metabolic: Thyroid abnormalities (hyper- or hypothyroidism), serum uric acid increased, hyperglycemia

Gastrointestinal: Taste perversion (children <1%; adults 7% to 8%)

Hematologic: Hemolytic anemia (10%), thrombocytopenia

Local: Injection site reaction (7%)

Neuromuscular & skeletal: Weakness (5% to 9%)

Respiratory: Sinusitis (children <1%; adults 9% to 10%)

<1%: Acute hypersensitivity reactions, anaphylaxis, angioedema, aplastic anemia (very rare), arrhythmia, bronchoconstriction, cardiomyopathy, cotton wool spots, diabetes, hearing loss, hepatotoxic reactions, hypotension, MI, pneumonia, pneumonitis, retinal hemorrhages, retinal artery or vein obstruction, severe psychiatric reactions, suicidal behavior, suicidal ideation, tinnitus, urticaria; rare cases of autoimmune diseases including vasculitis, polyarteritis reaction, rheumatoid arthritis, lupus erythematosus, and Raynaud's phenomenon

Postmarketing and/or case reports: Hypertriglyceridemia, nephrotic syndrome, pancreatitis, hallucinations, renal failure, sarcoidosis (including exacerbations of sarcoidosis)

Drug Interactions

Cytochrome P450 Effect: Interferon Alfa-2b: **Inhibits** CYP1A2 (weak)

Increased Effect/Toxicity: Interferon alpha: Cimetidine may augment the antitumor effects of interferon in melanoma. Theophylline clearance has been reported to be decreased in hepatitis patients receiving interferon. Vinblastine enhances interferon toxicity in several patients; increased incidence of paresthesia has also been noted. Interferons may increase the adverse/toxic effects of ACE inhibitors, specifically the development of granulocytopenia. Agranulocytosis has been reported with concurrent use of clozapine (case report). Interferons may increase the anticoagulant effects of warfarin, and interferons may increase serum levels of zidovudine. Concomitant use of ribavirin and nucleoside analogues may increase the risk of developing lactic acidosis.

Decreased Effect:

Interferon alpha: Prednisone may decrease the therapeutic effects of interferon alpha. A decreased response to erythropoietin has been reported (case reports) in patients receiving interferons. Interferon alpha may decrease the serum concentrations of melphalan (may or may not decrease toxicity of melphalan). Thyroid dysfunction has been reported during treatment; monitor response to thyroid hormones.

Ribavirin: Decreased effect of stavudine and zidovudine.

Stability Store the Rebetol® capsules plus Intron® A injection combination package refrigerated between 2°C and 8°C (36°F and 46°F)

When separated, the individual carton of Rebetol® capsules should be stored refrigerated between 2°C and 8°C (36°F and 46°F) or at 25°C (77°F); excursions are permitted between 15°C and 30°C (59°F and 86°F)

When separated, the individual carton or vial of Intron® A injection and the Intron® A multidose pen should be stored refrigerated between 2°C and 8°C (36°F and 46°F)

Mechanism of Action

Interferon Alfa-2b: Alpha interferons are a family of proteins, produced by nucleated cells, that have antiviral, antiproliferative, and immune-regulating activity. There are 16 known subtypes of alpha interferons. Interferons interact with cells through high affinity cell surface receptors. Following activation, multiple effects can be detected including induction of gene transcription. Inhibits cellular growth, alters the state of cellular differentiation, interferes with oncogene expression, alters cell surface antigen expression, increases phagocytic activity of macrophages, and augments cytotoxicity of lymphocytes for target cells

Ribavirin: Inhibits replication of RNA and DNA viruses; inhibits influenza virus RNA polymerase activity and inhibits the initiation and elongation of RNA fragments resulting in inhibition of viral protein synthesis

Pharmacodynamics/Kinetics See individual agents.

Dosage

Children ≥3 years: Chronic hepatitis C: **Note:** Duration of therapy: genotype 1: 48 weeks; genotype 2 or 3: 24 weeks. Discontinue treatment in any patient if HCV-RNA is not below the limits of detection of the assay after 24 weeks of therapy. Combination therapy:
- Intron® A: SubQ:
  - 25-61 kg: 3 million int. units/m^2 3 times/week
  - >61 kg: Refer to Adults dosing
- Rebetol®: Oral: **Note:** Oral solution should be used in children 3-5 years of age, children ≤25 kg, or those unable to swallow capsules.
  - Capsule/solution: 15 mg/kg/day in 2 divided doses (morning and evening)
  - Capsule dosing recommendations:
    - 25-36 kg: 400 mg/day (200 mg morning and evening)
    - 37-49 kg: 600 mg/day (200 mg in the morning and two 200 mg capsules in the evening)
    - 50-61 kg: 800 mg/day (two 200 mg capsules morning and evening)
    - >61 kg: Refer to Adults dosing

Adults: Chronic hepatitis C: Recommended dosage of combination therapy:
- Intron® A: SubQ: 3 million int. units 3 times/week **and**
- Rebetol® capsule: Oral:
  - ≤75 kg (165 lb): 1000 mg/day (two 200 mg capsules in the morning and three 200 mg capsules in the evening)
  - >75 kg: 1200 mg/day (three 200 mg capsules in the morning and three 200 mg capsules in the evening)

Treatment duration recommendations:
- Following relapse after alpha interferon monotherapy: 24 weeks
- Previously untreated: 24-48 weeks (individualized based on response, tolerance, and baseline characteristics)
- Consider discontinuing therapy in any patient not achieving HCV-RNA below the limit of assay detection by 24 weeks.

Dosing adjustment for toxicity: Note: Recommendations (per manufacturer labeling):

Anemia (RBC depression):
- Patient **without** cardiac history:
  - Hemoglobin <10 g/dL:
    - Children: Decrease dose by 1/2
    - Adults: Decrease dose to 600 mg/day
  - Hemoglobin <8.5 g/dL: Permanently discontinue treatment
- Patient **with** cardiac history:
  - Hemoglobin has ≥2 g/dL decrease during any 4-week period of treatment:
    - Children: Decrease ribavirin dose by 1/2 **and** decrease interferon alfa-2b to 1.5 million int. units 3 times/week
    - Adults: Decrease dose to ribavirin to 600 mg/day **and** decrease interferon-alfa 2b dose to 1.5 million int. units 3 times/week.
  - Hemoglobin <12 g/dL after 4 weeks of reduced dose: Permanently discontinue treatment

(Continued)

Interferon Alfa-2b and Ribavirin *(Continued)*

WBC, neutrophil, or platelet depression:

WBC <1500 cells/mm^3, neutrophils <750 cells/mm^3, or platelet count <50,000 cells/mm^3 (<80,000 cells/ mm^3 in children): Reduce interferon alfa-2b dose to 1.5 million int. units 3 times/week (50% reduction)

WBC <1000 cells/mm^3, neutrophils <500 cells/mm^3, or platelet count <25,000 cells/mm^3 (<50,000 cells/mm^3 in children): Permanently discontinue therapy

Dosage adjustment in renal impairment: Patients with Cl_{cr} <50 mL/minutes should not receive ribavirin.

Dietary Considerations Take oral formulation without regard to food, but always in a consistent manner with respect to food intake (ie, always take with food or always take on an empty stomach).

Administration Capsule should not be opened, crushed, chewed, or broken. Capsules are not for use in children <5 years of age. Use oral solution for children 3-5 years, those ≤25 kg, or those who cannot swallow capsules.

Monitoring Parameters Obtain pretreatment CBC, liver function tests, TSH, and electrolytes and monitor routinely throughout therapy (at 2 weeks and 4 weeks, more frequently if indicated); discontinue if WBC <1.0 x 10^9/L, neutrophils <0.5 x 10^9/L, platelets <25 x 10^9/L, or if hemoglobin <8.5 g/dL (in cardiac patients, discontinue if hemoglobin <12 g/dL after 4 weeks of dosage reduction). Pretreatment and monthly pregnancy test for women of childbearing age. Baseline chest x-ray, ECG, weight; patients with pre-existing cardiac abnormalities, or in advanced stages of cancer should have ECGs taken before and during treatment; reticulocyte count, serum HCV RNA levels; I & O

Reference Range Peak serum level after I.V. infusion of 10 million units: 546 units/mL

Dosage Forms Combination package:

For patients ≤75 kg [contains single-dose vials]:

Injection, solution: Interferon alfa-2b (Intron® A): 3 million int. units/0.5 mL (0.5 mL) [6 vials (3 million int. units/vial), 6 syringes, and alcohol swabs]

Capsules: Ribavirin (Rebetol®): 200 mg (70s)

For patients ≤75 kg [contains multidose vials]:

Injection, solution: Interferon alfa-2b (Intron® A): 3 million int. units/0.5 mL (3.8 mL) [1 multidose vial (18 million int. units/vial), 6 syringes, and alcohol swabs]

Capsules: Ribavirin (Rebetol®): 200 mg (70s)

For patients ≤75 kg [contains multidose pen]:

Injection, solution: Interferon alfa-2b (Intron® A): 3 million int. units/0.2 mL (1.5 mL) [1 multidose pen (18 million int. units/pen), 6 needles, and alcohol swabs]

Capsules: Ribavirin (Rebetol®): 200 mg (70s)

For patients >75 kg [contains single-dose vials]:

Injection, solution: Interferon alfa-2b (Intron® A): 3 million int. units/0.5 mL (0.5 mL) [6 vials (3 million int. units/vial), 6 syringes, and alcohol swabs]

Capsules: Ribavirin (Rebetol®): 200 mg (84s)

For patients >75 kg [contains multidose vials]:

Injection, solution: Interferon alfa-2b (Intron® A): 3 million int. units/0.5 mL (3.8 mL) [1 multidose vial (18 million int. units/vial), 6 syringes, and alcohol swabs]

Capsules: Ribavirin (Rebetol®): 200 mg (84s)

For patients >75 kg [contains multidose pen]:

Injection, solution: Interferon alfa-2b (Intron® A): 3 million int. units/0.2 mL (1.5 mL) [1 multidose pen (18 million int. units/pen), 6 needles, and alcohol swabs]

Capsules: Ribavirin (Rebetol®): 200 mg (84s)

For Rebetol® dose reduction [contains single-dose vials]:

Injection, solution: Interferon alfa-2b (Intron® A): 3 million int. units/0.5 mL (0.5 mL) [6 vials (3 million int. units/vial), 6 syringes, and alcohol swabs]

Capsules: Ribavirin (Rebetol®): 200 mg (42s)

For Rebetol® dose reduction [contains multidose vials]:

Injection, solution: Interferon alfa-2b (Intron® A): 3 million int. units/0.5 mL (3.8 mL) [1 multidose vial (18 million int. units/vial), 6 syringes, and alcohol swabs]

Capsules: Ribavirin (Rebetol®): 200 mg (42s)

For Rebetol® dose reduction [contains multidose pen]:

Injection, solution: Interferon alfa-2b (Intron® A): 3 million int. units/0.2 mL (1.5 mL) [1 multidose pen (18 million int. units/pen), 6 needles, and alcohol swabs]

Capsules: Ribavirin (Rebetol®): 200 mg (42s)

Interferon Alfa-2b and Ribavirin Combination Pack *see* Interferon Alfa-2b and Ribavirin *on page 884*

Interferon Alfacon-1 (in ter FEER on AL fa con one)

U.S. Brand Names Infergen®

Canadian Brand Names Infergen®

Generic Available No

Use Treatment of chronic hepatitis C virus (HCV) infection in patients ≥18 years of age with compensated liver disease and anti-HCV serum antibodies or HCV RNA.

Restrictions An FDA-approved medication guide is available at www.fda.gov/cder/Offices/ODS/labeling.htm; distribute to each patient to whom this medication is dispensed.

Pregnancy Risk Factor C

Pregnancy Implications There have been no well-controlled studies in pregnant women. Animal studies have shown embryolethal or abortifacient effects. Males and females who are being treated with interferon alfacon-1 should use effective contraception.

Contraindications Hypersensitivity to interferon alfacon-1 or any component of the formulation, other alpha interferons, or *E. coli*-derived products

Warnings/Precautions Severe psychiatric adverse effects, including depression, suicidal ideation, and suicide attempt, may occur. Avoid use in severe psychiatric disorders. Use with caution in patients with a history of depression. Use with caution in patients with prior cardiac disease (ischemic or thromboembolic), arrhythmias, patients who are chronically immunosuppressed, and patients with endocrine disorders. Do not use in patients with hepatic decompensation. Ophthalmologic disorders (including retinal hemorrhages, cotton wool spots and retinal artery or vein obstruction) have occurred in patients using other alpha interferons. Prior to start of therapy, visual exams are recommended for patients with diabetes mellitus or hypertension. Treatment should be discontinued in patients with worsening or persistently severe signs/symptoms of autoimmune, infectious, ischemic (including radiographic changes or worsening hepatic function), or neuropsychiatric disorders (including depression and/or suicidal thoughts/behavior). Use caution in patients with autoimmune disorders; type-1 interferon therapy has been reported to exacerbate autoimmune diseases. Do not use interferon alfacon-1 in patients with autoimmune hepatitis. Use caution in patients with low peripheral blood counts or myelosuppression, including concurrent use of myelosuppressive therapy. Safety and efficacy have not been determined for patients <18 years of age.

Adverse Reactions Adverse reactions reported using 9 mcg/dose interferon alfacon-1 3 times/week. Reactions listed were reported in ≥5% of patients treated.

>10%:

- Central nervous system: Headache (82%), fatigue (69%), fever (61%), insomnia (39%), nervousness (31%), depression (26%), dizziness (22%), anxiety (19%), noncardiac chest pain (13%), emotional lability (12%), malaise (11%)
- Dermatologic: Alopecia (14%), pruritus (14%), rash (13%)
- Endocrine & metabolic: Hot flashes (13%)
- Gastrointestinal: Abdominal pain (41%), nausea (40%), diarrhea (29%), anorexia (24%), dyspepsia (21%), vomiting (12%)
- Hematologic: Granulocytopenia (23%), thrombocytopenia (19%), leukopenia (15%)
- Local: Injection site erythema (23%)
- Neuromuscular & skeletal: Myalgia (58%), body pain (54%), arthralgia (51%), back pain (42%), limb pain (26%), neck pain (14%), skeletal pain (14%), paresthesia (13%)
- Respiratory: Pharyngitis (34%), upper respiratory tract infection (31%), cough (22%), sinusitis (17%), rhinitis (13%), respiratory tract congestion (12%)
- Miscellaneous: Flu-like syndrome (15%), diaphoresis increased (12%)

1% to 10%:

- Cardiovascular: Peripheral edema (9%), hypertension (5%), tachycardia (4%), palpitation (3%)
- Central nervous system: Amnesia (10%), hypoesthesia (10%), abnormal thinking (8%), agitation (6%), confusion (4%), somnolence (4%)
- Dermatologic: Bruising (6%), erythema (6%), dry skin (6%), wound (4%)
- Endocrine & metabolic: Thyroid test abnormalities (9%), dysmenorrhea (9%), increased triglycerides (6%), menstrual disorder (6%), decreased libido (5%), hypothyroidism (4%)
- Gastrointestinal: Constipation (9%), flatulence (8%), toothache (7%), decreased salivation (6%), hemorrhoids (6%), weight loss (5%), taste perversion (3%)
- Genitourinary: Vaginitis (8%), genital moniliasis (2%)
- Hepatic: Hepatomegaly (5%), liver tenderness (5%), increased prothrombin time (3%)
- Local: Injection site pain (9%), access pain (8%), injection site bruising (6%)
- Neuromuscular & skeletal: Weakness (9%), hypertonia (7%), musculoskeletal disorder (4%)

(Continued)

Interferon Alfacon-1 *(Continued)*

Ocular: Conjunctivitis (8%), eye pain (5%), vision abnormalities (3%)
Otic: Tinnitus (6%), earache (5%), otitis (2%)
Respiratory: Upper respiratory tract congestion (10%), epistaxis (8%), dyspnea (7%), bronchitis (6%)
Miscellaneous: Allergic reaction (7%), lymphadenopathy (6%), lymphocytosis (5%), infection (3%)

Flu-like symptoms (which included headache, fatigue, fever, myalgia, rigors, arthralgia, and increased diaphoresis) were the most commonly reported adverse reaction. This was reported separately from flu-like syndrome. Most patients were treated symptomatically.

Other adverse reactions associated with interferon therapy include arrhythmia, autoimmune disorders, chest pain, hepatotoxic reactions, lupus erythematosus, MI, neuropsychiatric disorders (including suicidal thoughts/behavior), pneumonia, pneumonitis, severe hypersensitivity reactions (rare), vasculitis

Overdosage/Toxicology One overdose has been reported. A patient received ten times the prescribed dose (150 mcg) for 3 days. In addition to an increase in anorexia, chills, fever, and myalgia, there was also an increase in ALT, AST, and LDH. Laboratory values reportedly returned to baseline within 30 days.

Drug Interactions

Increased Effect/Toxicity: Cimetidine may augment the antitumor effects of interferon in melanoma. Theophylline clearance has been reported to be decreased in hepatitis patients receiving interferon. Vinblastine enhances interferon toxicity in several patients; increased incidence of paresthesia has also been noted. Interferons may increase the adverse/toxic effects of ACE inhibitors, specifically the development of granulocytopenia. Agranulocytosis has been reported with concurrent use of clozapine (case report). Interferons may increase the anticoagulant effects of warfarin, and interferons may increase serum levels of zidovudine.

Decreased Effect: Prednisone may decrease the therapeutic effects of interferon alpha. A decreased response to erythropoietin has been reported (case reports) in patients receiving interferons. Interferon alpha may decrease the serum concentrations of melphalan (may or may not decrease toxicity of melphalan).

Stability Store in refrigerator 2°C to 8°C (36°F to 46°F). Do not freeze. Avoid exposure to direct sunlight. Do not shake vigorously.

Mechanism of Action Alpha interferons are a family of proteins, produced by nucleated cells, that have antiviral, antiproliferative, and immune-regulating activity. There are at least 25 alpha interferons identified. Interferons interact with cells through high affinity cell surface receptors. Following activation, multiple effects can be detected. Interferons induce gene transcription, inhibit cellular growth, alter the state of cellular differentiation, interfere with oncogene expression, alter cell surface antigen expression, increase phagocytic activity of macrophages, and augment cytotoxicity of lymphocytes for target cells. Although all alpha interferons share similar properties, the actual biological effects vary between subtypes.

Pharmacodynamics/Kinetics Pharmacokinetic studies have not been conducted on patients with chronic hepatitis C.

Time to peak: Healthy volunteers: 24-36 hours

Dosage Adults ≥18 years: SubQ:

Chronic HCV infection: 9 mcg 3 times/week for 24 weeks; allow 48 hours between doses

Patients who have previously tolerated interferon therapy but did not respond or relapsed: 15 mcg 3 times/week for 6 months

Dose reduction for toxicity: Dose should be held in patients who experience a severe adverse reaction, and treatment should be stopped or decreased if the reaction does not become tolerable.

Doses were reduced from 9 mcg to 7.5 mcg in the pivotal study.

For patients receiving 15 mcg/dose, doses were reduced in 3 mcg increments. Efficacy is decreased with doses <7.5 mcg

Dosage adjustment in renal impairment: No information available.

Dosage adjustment in hepatic impairment: Avoid use in decompensated hepatic disease.

Elderly: No information available.

Administration Interferon alfacon-1 is administered by SubQ injection, 3 times/week, with at least 48 hours between doses

Monitoring Parameters

Hemoglobin and hematocrit; white blood cell count; platelets; triglycerides; thyroid function. Laboratory tests should be taken 2 weeks prior to therapy, after therapy has begun, and periodically during treatment. HCV RNA, ALT to determine success/response to therapy.

The following guidelines were used during the clinical studies as acceptable baseline values:
Platelet count ≥75 x 10^9/L
Hemoglobin ≥100 g/L
ANC ≥1500 x 10^6/L
S_{cr} <180 µmol/L (<2 mg/dL) or Cl_{cr} >0.83 mL/second (>50 mL/minute)
Serum albumin ≥25 g/L
Bilirubin WNL
TSH and T_4 WNL

Patients should also be monitored for signs of depression. Patients with pre-existing diabetes mellitus or hypertension should have an ophthalmologic exam prior to treatment.

Patient Information There are many different types of interferon products. Do not change brands or change your dose without consulting with your prescriber. Promptly report any adverse effects to your prescriber, including flu-like symptoms, signs of infection, signs of depression, suicidal thoughts, or visual complaints. Flu-like symptoms include fatigue, fever, rigors, headache, arthralgia, myalgia, and increased sweating. Because interferon alfacon-1 may have hazardous effects to a fetus, males and females using this medication should use effective contraception. You will need periodic laboratory tests while on this medication. If you have diabetes or hypertension you should also have an eye exam prior to starting therapy. If self-administering this medication at home, follow procedures for proper disposal of your syringes and needles.

Dosage Forms Injection, solution [preservative free]: 30 mcg/mL (0.3 mL, 0.5 mL)

Intron® A *see* Interferon Alfa-2b *on page 881*
Invanz® *see* Ertapenem *on page 805*
Invirase® *see* Saquinavir *on page 1060*

Iodoquinol (eye oh doe KWIN ole)

U.S. Brand Names Yodoxin®
Canadian Brand Names Diodoquin®
Synonyms Diiodohydroxyquin
Generic Available No
Use Treatment of acute and chronic intestinal amebiasis; asymptomatic cyst passers; *Blastocystis hominis* infections; ineffective for amebic hepatitis or hepatic abscess
Drug of Choice or Alternative for Disease/Syndrome(s):
Liver Abscess *on page 211*
Organism(s):
Entamoeba histolytica on page 130
Pregnancy Risk Factor C
Contraindications Hypersensitivity to iodine or iodoquinol or any component of the formulation; hepatic damage; pre-existing optic neuropathy
Warnings/Precautions Optic neuritis, optic atrophy, and peripheral neuropathy have occurred following prolonged use; avoid long-term therapy
Adverse Reactions Frequency not defined.
Central nervous system: Fever, chills, agitation, retrograde amnesia, headache
Dermatologic: Rash, urticaria, pruritus
Endocrine & metabolic: Thyroid gland enlargement
Gastrointestinal: Diarrhea, nausea, vomiting, stomach pain, abdominal cramps
Neuromuscular & skeletal: Peripheral neuropathy, weakness
Ocular: Optic neuritis, optic atrophy, visual impairment
Miscellaneous: Itching of rectal area
Overdosage/Toxicology Chronic overdose can result in vomiting, diarrhea, abdominal pain, metallic taste, paresthesias, paraplegia, and loss of vision. Can lead to destruction of the long fibers of the spinal cord and optic nerve. Acute overdose symptoms includes delirium, stupor, coma, and amnesia. Following GI decontamination, treatment is symptomatic.
Mechanism of Action Contact amebicide that works in the lumen of the intestine by an unknown mechanism
Pharmacodynamics/Kinetics
Absorption: Poor and erratic
Metabolism: Hepatic
Excretion: Feces (high percentage)
Dosage Oral:
Children: 30-40 mg/kg/day (maximum: 650 mg/dose) in 3 divided doses for 20 days; not to exceed 1.95 g/day
Adults: 650 mg 3 times/day after meals for 20 days; not to exceed 1.95 g/day
(Continued)

Iodoquinol *(Continued)*

Dietary Considerations Should be taken after meals.

Administration Tablets may be crushed and mixed with applesauce or chocolate syrup. May take with food or milk to reduce stomach upset. Complete full course of therapy.

Monitoring Parameters Ophthalmologic exam

Test Interactions May increase protein-bound serum iodine concentrations reflecting a decrease in ^{131}I uptake; false-positive ferric chloride test for phenylketonuria

Patient Information May take with food or milk to reduce stomach upset; take entire course of medication

Dosage Forms Tablet: 210 mg, 650 mg

Selected Readings

"Drugs for Parasitic Infections," *Med Lett Drugs Ther*, 1998, 40(1017):1-12.

Iodoquinol and Hydrocortisone

(eye oh doe KWIN ole & hye droe KOR ti sone)

U.S. Brand Names Dermazene®; Vytone®

Synonyms Hydrocortisone and Iodoquinol

Generic Available Yes

Use Treatment of eczema; infectious dermatitis; chronic eczematoid otitis externa; mycotic dermatoses

Pregnancy Risk Factor C

Contraindications

Based on **iodoquinol** component: Hypersensitivity to iodine or iodoquinol or any component of the formulation; hepatic damage; pre-existing optic neuropathy

Based on **hydrocortisone** component: Hypersensitivity to hydrocortisone or any component of the formulation; serious infections, except septic shock or tuberculous meningitis; viral, fungal, or tubercular skin lesions

Warnings/Precautions

Based on **iodoquinol** component: Optic neuritis, optic atrophy, and peripheral neuropathy have occurred following prolonged use; avoid long-term therapy

Based on **hydrocortisone** component:

- Use with caution in patients with hyperthyroidism, cirrhosis, nonspecific ulcerative colitis, hypertension, osteoporosis, thromboembolic tendencies, CHF, convulsive disorders, myasthenia gravis, thrombophlebitis, peptic ulcer, diabetes
- Acute adrenal insufficiency may occur with abrupt withdrawal (depending on degree of systemic absorption) after long-term therapy or with stress; young pediatric patients may be more susceptible to adrenal axis suppression from topical therapy

Adverse Reactions

Based on **iodoquinol** component:

- Central nervous system: Fever, chills, agitation, retrograde amnesia, headache
- Dermatologic: Rash, urticaria, pruritus
- Endocrine & metabolic: Thyroid gland enlargement
- Gastrointestinal: Diarrhea, nausea, vomiting, stomach pain, abdominal cramps
- Neuromuscular & skeletal: Peripheral neuropathy, weakness
- Ocular: Optic neuritis, optic atrophy, visual impairment
- Miscellaneous: Itching of rectal area

Based on **hydrocortisone** component:

>10%:

- Central nervous system: Insomnia, nervousness
- Gastrointestinal: Increased appetite, indigestion

1% to 10%:

- Dermatologic: Hirsutism
- Endocrine & metabolic: Diabetes mellitus
- Neuromuscular & skeletal: Arthralgia
- Ocular: Cataracts
- Respiratory: Epistaxis

<1%: Hypertension, edema, euphoria, headache, delirium, hallucinations, seizure, mood swings, acne, dermatitis, skin atrophy, bruising, hyperpigmentation, hypokalemia, hyperglycemia, Cushing's syndrome, sodium and water retention, bone growth suppression, amenorrhea, peptic ulcer, abdominal distention, ulcerative esophagitis, pancreatitis, muscle wasting, hypersensitivity reactions, immunosuppression

Drug Interactions

Cytochrome P450 Effect: Hydrocortisone: **Substrate** of CYP3A4 (minor); **Induces** CYP3A4 (weak)

Pharmacodynamics/Kinetics See individual agents.

Dosage Apply 3-4 times/day

Additional Information Complete prescribing information for this medication should be consulted for additional detail.

Dosage Forms Cream: Iodoquinol 1% and hydrocortisone acetate 1% (30 g)

Dermazene®: Iodoquinol 1% and hydrocortisone acetate 1% (30 g, 45 g)

Vytone®: Iodoquinol 1% and hydrocortisone acetate 1% (30 g)

Iosat™ [OTC] *see* Potassium Iodide *on page 1014*

IPOL® *see* Poliovirus Vaccine (Inactivated) *on page 1011*

IPV *see* Poliovirus Vaccine (Inactivated) *on page 1011*

Iquix® *see* Levofloxacin *on page 908*

ISG *see* Immune Globulin (Intramuscular) *on page 866*

Isoniazid (eye soe NYE a zid)

Related Information

Tuberculosis *on page 1315*

USPHS / IDSA Guidelines for the Prevention of Opportunistic Infections in Persons Infected With HIV *on page 1237*

U.S. Brand Names Nydrazid® [DSC]

Canadian Brand Names Isotamine®; PMS-Isoniazid

Synonyms INH; Isonicotinic Acid Hydrazide

Generic Available Yes

Use Treatment of susceptible tuberculosis infections; treatment of latent tuberculosis infection (LTBI)

Drug of Choice or Alternative for Organism(s):

Mycobacterium bovis on page 229

Mycobacterium kansasii on page 231

Mycobacterium tuberculosis on page 234

Pregnancy Risk Factor C

Pregnancy Implications Isoniazid was found to be embryocidal in animal studies; teratogenic effects were not noted. Isoniazid crosses the human placenta. Due to the risk of tuberculosis to the fetus, treatment is recommended when the probability of maternal disease is moderate to high. Pyridoxine supplementation is recommended (25 mg/day).

Contraindications Hypersensitivity to isoniazid or any component of the formulation; acute liver disease; previous history of hepatic damage during isoniazid therapy

Warnings/Precautions Use with caution in patients with renal impairment and chronic liver disease. Severe and sometimes fatal hepatitis may occur or develop even after many months of treatment; patients must report any prodromal symptoms of hepatitis, such as fatigue, weakness, malaise, anorexia, nausea, or vomiting. Malnourished patients should receive concomitant pyridoxine therapy. Periodic ophthalmic examinations are recommended even when usual symptoms do not occur; pyridoxine (10-50 mg/day) is recommended in individuals likely to develop peripheral neuropathies.

Adverse Reactions Frequency not defined.

Cardiovascular: Hypertension, palpitation, tachycardia, vasculitis

Central nervous system: Dizziness, encephalopathy, memory impairment, slurred speech, lethargy, fever, depression, psychosis, seizure

Dermatologic: Rash (morbilliform, maculopapular, pruritic, or exfoliative), flushing

Endocrine & metabolic: Hyperglycemia, metabolic acidosis, gynecomastia, pellagra, pyridoxine deficiency

Gastrointestinal: Anorexia, nausea, vomiting, stomach pain

Hematologic: Agranulocytosis, anemia (sideroblastic, hemolytic, or aplastic), thrombocytopenia, eosinophilia, lymphadenopathy

Hepatic: LFTs mildly increased (10% to 20%); hyperbilirubinemia, jaundice, hepatitis (may involve progressive liver damage; risk increases with age; 2.3% in patients >50 years)

Neuromuscular & skeletal: Weakness, peripheral neuropathy (dose-related incidence, 10% to 20% incidence with 10 mg/kg/day), hyper-reflexia, arthralgia, lupus-like syndrome

Ocular: Blurred vision, loss of vision, optic neuritis and atrophy

Overdosage/Toxicology Symptoms generally occur within 30 minutes to 3 hours, and may include nausea, vomiting, slurred speech, dizziness, blurred vision, metabolic acidosis, hallucinations, stupor, coma, and intractable seizures. Because of severe morbidity and high mortality rates associated with isoniazid overdose, patients who are asymptomatic after an overdose should be monitored for 4-6 hours. Pyridoxine has been shown to be effective in the treatment of intoxication, especially when seizures occur. Pyridoxine I.V. is administered on a milligram to milligram dose.

(Continued)

Isoniazid *(Continued)*

If the amount of isoniazid ingested is unknown, 5 g of pyridoxine should be given over 3-5 minutes and may be followed by an additional 5 g in 30 minutes. Treatment is supportive. Airway protection and ventilation may be required, with diazepam for seizures, and sodium bicarbonate for acidosis. Forced diuresis and hemodialysis can result in more rapid removal.

Drug Interactions

Cytochrome P450 Effect: Substrate of CYP2E1 (major); **Inhibits** CYP1A2 (weak), 2A6 (moderate), 2C8/9 (moderate), 2C19 (strong), 2D6 (moderate), 2E1 (moderate), 3A4 (strong); **Induces** CYP2E1 (after discontinuation) (weak)

Increased Effect/Toxicity: Concurrent use of disulfiram may result in acute intolerance reactions. Isoniazid may increase the levels/effects of amiodarone, amphetamines, benzodiazepines, beta-blockers, calcium channel blockers, citalopram, dexmedetomidine, dextromethorphan, diazepam, fluoxetine, glimepiride, glipizide, ifosfamide, inhalational anesthetics, lidocaine, mesoridazine, methsuximide, mirtazapine, nateglinide, nefazodone, paroxetine, phenytoin, pioglitazone, propranolol, risperidone, ritonavir, rosiglitazone, sertraline, sildenafil (and other PDE-5 inhibitors) tacrolimus, theophylline, thioridazine, tricyclic antidepressants, trimethadione, venlafaxine. warfarin, and other substrates of CYP2A6, 2C8/9, 2C19, 2D6, 2E1, or 3A4. Selected benzodiazepines (midazolam and triazolam), cisapride, ergot alkaloids, selected HMG-CoA reductase inhibitors (lovastatin and simvastatin), and pimozide are generally contraindicated with strong CYP3A4 inhibitors. Mesoridazine and thioridazine are generally contraindicated with strong CYP2D6 inhibitors. When used with strong CYP3A4 inhibitors, dosage adjustment/limits are recommended for sildenafil and other PDE-5 inhibitors; consult individual monographs.

Decreased Effect: Decreased effect/levels of isoniazid with aluminum salts or antacids. Isoniazid may decrease the levels/effects of CYP2D6 prodrug substrates (eg, codeine, hydrocodone, oxycodone, tramadol).

Ethanol/Nutrition/Herb Interactions

Ethanol: Avoid ethanol (increases the risk of hepatitis).

Food: Isoniazid serum levels may be decreased if taken with food. Has some ability to inhibit tyramine metabolism; several case reports of mild reactions (flushing, palpitations) after ingestion of cheese with or without wine. Isoniazid decreases folic acid absorption. Isoniazid alters pyridoxine metabolism.

Stability Protect oral dosage forms from light

Mechanism of Action Unknown, but may include the inhibition of myocolic acid synthesis resulting in disruption of the bacterial cell wall

Pharmacodynamics/Kinetics

Absorption: Rapid and complete; rate can be slowed with food

Distribution: All body tissues and fluids including CSF; crosses placenta; enters breast milk

Protein binding: 10% to 15%

Metabolism: Hepatic with decay rate determined genetically by acetylation phenotype

Half-life elimination: Fast acetylators: 30-100 minutes; Slow acetylators: 2-5 hours; may be prolonged with hepatic or severe renal impairment

Time to peak, serum: 1-2 hours

Excretion: Urine (75% to 95%); feces; saliva

Dosage Recommendations often change due to resistant strains and newly-developed information; consult *MMWR* for current CDC recommendations:

Oral (injectable is available for patients who are unable to either take or absorb oral therapy):

Infants and Children:

Treatment of latent TB infection (LTBI): 10-20 mg/kg/day in 1-2 divided doses (maximum: 300 mg/day) or 20-40 mg/kg (maximum: 900 mg/dose) twice weekly for 9 months

Treatment of active TB infection:

Daily therapy: 10-15 mg/kg/day in 1-2 divided doses (maximum: 300 mg/day)

Twice weekly directly observed therapy (DOT): 20-30 mg/kg (maximum: 900 mg)

Adults:

Treatment of latent tuberculosis infection (LTBI): 300 mg/day or 900 mg twice weekly for 6-9 months in patients who do not have HIV infection (9 months is optimal, 6 months may be considered to reduce costs of therapy) and 9 months in patients who have HIV infection. Extend to 12 months of therapy if interruptions in treatment occur.

Treatment of active TB infection (drug susceptible):

Daily therapy: 5 mg/kg/day given daily (usual dose: 300 mg/day); 10 mg/kg/day in 1-2 divided doses in patients with disseminated disease

Twice weekly directly observed therapy (DOT): 15 mg/kg (maximum: 900 mg); 3 times/week therapy: 15 mg/kg (maximum: 900 mg)

Note: Treatment may be defined by the number of doses administered (eg, "six-month" therapy involves 192 doses of INH and rifampin, and 56 doses of pyrazinamide). Six months is the shortest interval of time over which these doses may be administered, assuming no interruption of therapy.

Note: Concomitant administration of 6-50 mg/day pyridoxine is recommended in malnourished patients or those prone to neuropathy (eg, alcoholics, diabetics)

Dosing adjustment in renal impairment:

Cl_{cr} <10 mL/minute: Administer 50% of normal dose

Hemodialysis: Dialyzable (50% to 100%)

Administer dose postdialysis

Peritoneal dialysis, continuous arteriovenous or venovenous hemofiltration: Dose for Cl_{cr} <10 mL/minute

Dosing adjustment in hepatic impairment: Dose should be reduced in severe hepatic disease

Dietary Considerations Should be taken 1 hour before or 2 hours after meals on an empty stomach; increase dietary intake of folate, niacin, magnesium. No need to restrict tyramine-containing foods.

Administration Should be administered 1 hour before or 2 hours after meals on an empty stomach.

Monitoring Parameters Periodic liver function tests; sputum cultures monthly (until 2 consecutive negative cultures reported); monitoring for prodromal signs of hepatitis

Reference Range Therapeutic: 1-7 mcg/mL (SI: 7-51 µmol/L); Toxic: 20-710 mcg/mL (SI: 146-5176 µmol/L)

Test Interactions False-positive urinary glucose with Clinitest®

Patient Information Report any symptoms of hepatitis (fatigue, weakness, nausea, vomiting, dark urine, or yellowing of eyes) or any burning, tingling, or numbness in the extremities. Do not discontinue medication without consulting prescriber.

Additional Information The AAP recommends that pyridoxine supplementation (1-2 mg/kg/day) should be administered to malnourished patients, children or adolescents on meat or milk-deficient diets, breast-feeding infants, and those predisposed to neuritis to prevent peripheral neuropathy; administration of isoniazid syrup has been associated with diarrhea

Dosage Forms

Injection, solution (Nydrazid®): 100 mg/mL (10 mL) [DSC]

Syrup: 50 mg/5 mL (473 mL) [orange flavor]

Tablet: 100 mg, 300 mg

Extemporaneous Preparations A 10 mg/mL oral suspension was stable for 21 days when refrigerated when compounded as follows:

Triturate ten 100 mg tablets in a mortar, reduce to a fine powder, then add 10 mL of purified water U.S.P. to make a paste; then transfer to a graduate and qs to 100 mL with sorbitol (do not use sugar-based solutions)

Shake well before using and keep in refrigerator

Nahata MC and Hipple TF, *Pediatric Drug Formulations*, 3rd ed, Cincinnati, OH: Harvey Whitney Books Co, 1997.

Selected Readings

Davidson PT and Le HQ, "Drug Treatment of Tuberculosis - 1992," *Drugs*, 1992, 43(5):651-73.

Havlir DV and Barnes PF, "Tuberculosis in Patients With Human Immunodeficiency Virus Infection," *N Engl J Med*, 1999, 340(5):367-73.

"Drugs for Tuberculosis," *Med Lett Drugs Ther*, 1993, 35(908):99-101.

Iseman MD, "Treatment of Multidrug-Resistant Tuberculosis," *N Engl J Med*, 1993, 329(11):784-91.

"Prevention and Treatment of Tuberculosis Among Patients Infected With Human Immunodeficiency Virus: Principles of Therapy and Revised Recommendations. Centers for Disease Control and Prevention," *MMWR*, 1998, 47(RR-20):1-58.

Van Scoy RE and Wilkowske CJ, "Antituberculosis Agents," *Mayo Clin Proc*, 1992, 67(2):179-87.

Isoniazid and Rifampin *see* Rifampin and Isoniazid *on page 1050*

Isoniazid, Rifampin, and Pyrazinamide *see* Rifampin, Isoniazid, and Pyrazinamide *on page 1050*

Isonicotinic Acid Hydrazide *see* Isoniazid *on page 893*

Isotamine® (Can) *see* Isoniazid *on page 893*

Itraconazole (i tra KOE na zole)

Related Information

USPHS / IDSA Guidelines for the Prevention of Opportunistic Infections in Persons Infected With HIV *on page 1237*

U.S. Brand Names Sporanox®

Canadian Brand Names Sporanox®

Generic Available No

(Continued)

Itraconazole *(Continued)*

Use Treatment of susceptible fungal infections in immunocompromised and immunocompetent patients including blastomycosis and histoplasmosis; indicated for aspergillosis, and onychomycosis of the toenail; treatment of onychomycosis of the fingernail without concomitant toenail infection via a pulse-type dosing regimen; has activity against *Aspergillus, Candida, Coccidioides, Cryptococcus, Sporothrix*, tinea unguium

Oral: Useful in superficial mycoses including dermatophytoses (eg, tinea capitis), pityriasis versicolor, sebopsoriasis, vaginal and chronic mucocutaneous candidiases; systemic mycoses including candidiasis, meningeal and disseminated cryptococcal infections, paracoccidioidomycosis, coccidioidomycoses; miscellaneous mycoses such as sporotrichosis, chromomycosis, leishmaniasis, fungal keratitis, alternariosis, zygomycosis

Oral solution: Treatment of oral and esophageal candidiasis

Intravenous solution: Indicated in the treatment of blastomycosis, histoplasmosis (nonmeningeal), and aspergillosis (in patients intolerant or refractory to amphotericin B therapy); empiric therapy of febrile neutropenic fever

Drug of Choice or Alternative for Disease/Syndrome(s):

Esophagitis *on page 147*

Organism(s):

Aspergillus Species *on page 38*
Blastomyces dermatitidis on page 50
Candida Species *on page 67*
Coccidioides immitis on page 91
Cryptococcus neoformans on page 102
Dematiaceous Fungi *on page 112*
Dermatophytes *on page 114*
Histoplasma capsulatum on page 177
Malassezia furfur on page 213
Penicillium marneffei on page 260

Pregnancy Risk Factor C

Pregnancy Implications Should not be used to treat onychomycosis during pregnancy. Effective contraception should be used during treatment and for 2 months following treatment. Congenital abnormalities have been reported during postmarketing surveillance, but a causal relationship has not been established.

Contraindications Hypersensitivity to itraconazole, any component of the formulation, or to other azoles; concurrent administration with cisapride, dofetilide, ergot derivatives, levomethadyl, lovastatin, midazolam, pimozide, quinidine, simvastatin, or triazolam; treatment of onychomycosis in patients with evidence of left ventricular dysfunction, CHF, or a history of CHF

Warnings/Precautions Discontinue if signs or symptoms of CHF or neuropathy occur during treatment. Rare cases of serious cardiovascular adverse events (including death), ventricular tachycardia, and torsade de pointes have been observed due to increased cisapride concentrations induced by itraconazole. Use with caution in patients with left ventricular dysfunction or a history of CHF. Not recommended for use in patients with active liver disease, elevated liver enzymes, or prior hepatotoxic reactions to other drugs. Itraconazole has been associated with rare cases of serious hepatotoxicity (including fatal cases and cases within the first week of treatment); treatment should be discontinued in patients who develop clinical symptoms of liver dysfunction or abnormal liver function tests during itraconazole therapy except in cases where expected benefit exceeds risk. Large differences in itraconazole pharmacokinetic parameters have been observed in cystic fibrosis patients receiving the solution; if a patient with cystic fibrosis does not respond to therapy, alternate therapies should be considered. **Due to differences in bioavailability, oral capsules and oral solution cannot be used interchangeably.** Intravenous formulation should be used with caution in renal impairment; consider conversion to oral therapy if renal dysfunction/toxicity is noted. Initiation of treatment with oral solution is not recommended in patients at immediate risk for systemic candidiasis (eg, patients with severe neutropenia).

Adverse Reactions Listed incidences are for higher doses appropriate for systemic fungal infection.

>10%: Gastrointestinal: Nausea (11%)

1% to 10%:

Cardiovascular: Edema (4%), hypertension (3%)

Central nervous system: Headache (4%), fatigue (2% to 3%), malaise (1%), fever (3%), dizziness (2%)

Dermatologic: Rash (9%), pruritus (3%)

Endocrine & metabolic: Decreased libido (1%), hypertriglyceridemia, hypokalemia (2%)

Gastrointestinal: Abdominal pain (2%), anorexia (1%), vomiting (5%), diarrhea (3%)

Hepatic: Abnormal LFTs (3%), hepatitis

Renal: Albuminuria (1%)

<1%: Adrenal suppression, constipation, gastritis, gynecomastia, impotence, somnolence, tinnitus

Postmarketing and/or case reports: Allergic reactions (urticaria, angioedema); alopecia, anaphylactoid reactions, anaphylaxis, arrhythmia, CHF, hepatic failure, menstrual disorders, neutropenia, peripheral neuropathy, photosensitivity, pulmonary edema, Stevens-Johnson syndrome

Overdosage/Toxicology Overdoses are well tolerated. Following decontamination, if possible, supportive measures only are required. Dialysis is not effective.

Drug Interactions

Cytochrome P450 Effect: Substrate of CYP3A4 (major); **Inhibits** CYP3A4 (strong)

Increased Effect/Toxicity: Itraconazole is a strong inhibitor of CYP3A4, and is contraindicated with cisapride, dofetilide, ergot derivatives, lovastatin, midazolam, pimozide, quinidine, simvastatin, and triazolam. Itraconazole may also increase the levels of alfentanil, benzodiazepines (alprazolam, diazepam, and others), buspirone, busulfan, calcium channel blockers (felodipine, nifedipine, verapamil), carbamazepine, corticosteroids, cyclosporine, digoxin, docetaxel, eletriptan, HMG-CoA reductase inhibitors (except fluvastatin, pravastatin), indinavir, oral hypoglycemics (sulfonylureas), phenytoin, rifabutin, ritonavir, saquinavir, sirolimus, tacrolimus, trimetrexate, vincristine, vinblastine, warfarin, and zolpidem. Other medications metabolized by CYP3A4 should be used with caution. Serum concentrations of itraconazole may be increased by strong CYP3A4 inhibitors. Serum concentrations of PDE-5 inhibitors (sildenafil, tadalafil, and vardenafil) are increased by itraconazole; specific dosage reductions/limitations are recommended.

Decreased Effect: Absorption of itraconazole requires gastric acidity; therefore, antacids, H_2 antagonists (cimetidine, famotidine, nizatidine, and ranitidine), proton pump inhibitors (omeprazole, lansoprazole, rabeprazole), and sucralfate may significantly reduce bioavailability resulting in treatment failures and should not be administered concomitantly. Antacids may decrease serum concentration of itraconazole; administer antacids 1 hour before or 2 hours after itraconazole capsules. Serum levels of itraconazole may be decreased with didanosine, isoniazid, and nevirapine. The levels/effects of itraconazole may be reduced by aminoglutethimide, carbamazepine, nafcillin, phenobarbital, phenytoin, rifamycins, and other CYP3A4 inducers. Oral contraceptive efficacy may be reduced (limited data).

Ethanol/Nutrition/Herb Interactions

Food:

Capsules: Enhanced by food and possibly by gastric acidity. cola drinks have been shown to increase the absorption of the capsules in patients with achlorhydria or those taking H_2-receptor antagonists or other gastric acid suppressors. Avoid grapefruit juice.

Solution: Decreased by food, time to peak concentration prolonged by food.

Herb/Nutraceutical: St John's wort may decrease itraconazole levels.

Stability

Capsule: Store at room temperature, 15°C to 25°C (59°F to 77°F); protect from light and moisture

Oral solution: Store at ≤25°C (77°F); do not freeze

Solution for injection: Store at ≤25°C (77°F); protect from light; do not freeze. Dilute with 0.9% sodium chloride. Stable for 48 hours at room temperature or under refrigeration. A precise mixing ratio is required to maintain stability (3.33:1) and avoid precipitate formation. Add 25 mL (1 ampul) to 50 mL 0.9% sodium chloride. Mix and withdraw 15 mL of solution before infusing.

Mechanism of Action Interferes with cytochrome P450 activity, decreasing ergosterol synthesis (principal sterol in fungal cell membrane) and inhibiting cell membrane formation

Pharmacodynamics/Kinetics

Absorption: Requires gastric acidity; capsule better absorbed with food, solution better absorbed on empty stomach

Distribution: V_d (average): 796 ± 185 L or 10 L/kg; highly lipophilic and tissue concentrations are higher than plasma concentrations. The highest concentrations: adipose, omentum, endometrium, cervical and vaginal mucus, and skin/nails. Aqueous fluids (eg, CSF and urine) contain negligible amounts.

Protein binding, plasma: 99.9%; metabolite hydroxy-itraconazole: 99.5%

(Continued)

Itraconazole *(Continued)*

Metabolism: Extensively hepatic via CYP3A4 into >30 metabolites including hydroxy-itraconazole (major metabolite); appears to have *in vitro* antifungal activity. Main metabolic pathway is oxidation; may undergo saturation metabolism with multiple dosing.

Bioavailability: Variable, ~55% (oral solution) in 1 small study; **Note:** Oral solution has a higher degree of bioavailability (149% ± 68%) relative to oral capsules; should not be interchanged

Half-life elimination: Oral: After single 200 mg dose: 21 ± 5 hours; 64 hours at steady-state; I.V.: steady-state: 35 hours; steady-state concentrations are achieved in 13 days with multiple administration of itraconazole 100-400 mg/day.

Excretion: Feces (~3% to 18%); urine (~0.03% as parent drug, 40% as metabolites)

Dosage Note: Capsule: Absorption is best if taken with food, therefore, it is best to administer itraconazole after meals; Solution: Should be taken on an empty stomach.

Children: Efficacy and safety have not been established; a small number of patients 3-16 years of age have been treated with 100 mg/day for systemic fungal infections with no serious adverse effects reported. A dose of 5 mg/kg once daily was used in a pharmacokinetic study using the oral solution in patients 6 months to 12 years; duration of study was 2 weeks.

Adults:

Oral:

Blastomycosis/histoplasmosis: 200 mg once daily, if no obvious improvement or there is evidence of progressive fungal disease, increase the dose in 100 mg increments to a maximum of 400 mg/day; doses >200 mg/day are given in 2 divided doses; length of therapy varies from 1 day to >6 months depending on the condition and mycological response

Aspergillosis: 200-400 mg/day

Onychomycosis: 200 mg once daily for 12 consecutive weeks

Life-threatening infections: Loading dose: 200 mg 3 times/day (600 mg/day) should be given for the first 3 days of therapy

Oropharyngeal candidiasis: Oral solution: 200 mg once daily for 1-2 weeks; in patients unresponsive or refractory to fluconazole: 100 mg twice daily (clinical response expected in 1-2 weeks)

Esophageal candidiasis: Oral solution: 100-200 mg once daily for a minimum of 3 weeks; continue dosing for 2 weeks after resolution of symptoms

I.V.: 200 mg twice daily for 4 doses, followed by 200 mg daily

Dosing adjustment in renal impairment: Not necessary; itraconazole injection is not recommended in patients with Cl_{cr} <30 mL/minute; hydroxypropyl-β-cyclodextrin (the excipient) is eliminated primarily by the kidneys.

Hemodialysis: Not dialyzable

Dosing adjustment in hepatic impairment: May be necessary, but specific guidelines are not available. Risk-to-benefit evaluation should be undertaken in patients who develop liver function abnormalities during treatment.

Dietary Considerations

Capsule: Administer with food.

Solution: Take without food, if possible.

Administration

Oral: Doses >200 mg/day are given in 2 divided doses; do not administer with antacids. Capsule absorption is best if taken with food, therefore, it is best to administer itraconazole after meals; solution should be taken on an empty stomach. When treating oropharyngeal and esophageal candidiasis, solution should be swished vigorously in mouth, then swallowed.

I.V.: Infuse 60 mL of the dilute solution (3.33 mg/mL = 200 mg itraconazole, pH ~4.8) over 60 minutes; flush with 15-20 mL of 0.9% sodium chloride over 30 seconds to 15 minutes

Monitoring Parameters Liver function in patients with pre-existing hepatic dysfunction, and in all patients being treated for longer than 1 month

Patient Information Take capsule with food; take solution on an empty stomach; stop therapy and report any signs and symptoms that may suggest liver dysfunction immediately so that the appropriate laboratory testing can be done; signs and symptoms may include unusual fatigue, anorexia, nausea and/or vomiting, jaundice, dark urine, or pale stool

Additional Information Due to potential toxicity, the manufacturer recommends confirmation of diagnosis testing of nail specimens prior to treatment of onychomycosis.

Dosage Forms

Capsule: 100 mg

Injection, solution: 10 mg/mL (25 mL) [packaged in a kit containing sodium chloride 0.9% (50 mL); filtered infusion set (1)]

Solution, oral: 100 mg/10 mL (150 mL) [cherry flavor]

Selected Readings

Amichai B and Grunwald MH, "Adverse Drug Reactions of the New Oral Antifungal Agents - Terbinafine, Fluconazole, and Itraconazole," *Int J Dermatol*, 1998, 37(6):410-5.

Cleary JD, Taylor JW, and Chapman SW, "Itraconazole in Antifungal Therapy," *Ann Pharmacother*, 1992, 26(4):502-9.

Grant SM and Clissold SP, "Itraconazole. A Review of Its Pharmacodynamic and Pharmacokinetic Properties, and Therapeutic Use in Superficial and Systemic Mycoses," *Drugs*, 1989, 37(3):310-44.

Haria M, Bryson HM, and Goa KL, "Itraconazole: A Reappraisal of Its Pharmacological Properties and Therapeutic Use in the Management of Superficial Fungal Infections," *Drugs*, 1996, 51(4):585-620.

Jennings TS and Hardin TC, "Treatment of Aspergillosis With Itraconazole," *Ann Pharmacother*, 1993, 27(10):1206-11.

Kauffman CA and Carver PL, "Antifungal Agents in the 1990s. Current Status and Future Developments," *Drugs*, 1997, 53(4):539-49.

Lyman CA and Walsh TJ, "Systemically Administered Antifungal Agents. A Review of Their Clinical Pharmacology and Therapeutic Applications," *Drugs*, 1992, 44(1):9-35.

Slain D, Rogers PD, Cleary JD, et al, "Intravenous Itraconazole," *Ann Pharmacother*, 2001, 35(6):720-9.

Terrell CL, "Antifungal Agents. Part II. The Azoles," *Mayo Clin Proc*, 1999, 74(1):78-100.

Trepanier EF and Amsden GW, "Current Issues in Onchomycosis," *Ann Pharmacother*, 1998, 32(2):204-14.

Iveegam EN *see* Immune Globulin (Intravenous) *on page 867*

Iveegam Immuno® (Can) *see* Immune Globulin (Intravenous) *on page 867*

Ivermectin (eye ver MEK tin)

U.S. Brand Names Stromectol®

Generic Available No

Use Treatment of the following infections: Strongyloidiasis of the intestinal tract due to the nematode parasite *Strongyloides stercoralis*. Onchocerciasis due to the nematode parasite *Onchocerca volvulus*. Ivermectin is only active against the immature form of *Onchocerca volvulus*, and the intestinal forms of *Strongyloides stercoralis*.

Unlabeled/Investigational Use Has been used for other parasitic infections including *Ascaris lumbricoides*, Bancroftian filariasis, *Brugia malayi*, scabies, *Enterobius vermicularis*, *Mansonella ozzardi*, *Trichuris trichiura*.

Drug of Choice or Alternative for Organism(s):

Strongyloides stercoralis *on page 328*

Pregnancy Risk Factor C

Pregnancy Implications Safety and efficacy have not been established in pregnant women. The WHO considers use after the first trimester as "probably acceptable."

Contraindications Hypersensitivity to ivermectin or any component of the formulation

Warnings/Precautions Data have shown that antihelmintic drugs like ivermectin may cause cutaneous and/or systemic reactions (Mazzoti reaction) of varying severity including ophthalmological reactions in patients with onchocerciasis. These reactions are probably due to allergic and inflammatory responses to the death of microfilariae. Patients with hyper-reactive onchodermatitis may be more likely than others to experience severe adverse reactions, especially edema and aggravation of the onchodermatitis. Repeated treatment may be required in immunocompromised patients (eg, HIV); control of extraintestinal strongyloidiasis may necessitate suppressive (once monthly) therapy. Pretreatment assessment for *Loa loa* infection is recommended in any patient with significant exposure to endemic areas (West and Central Africa); serious and/or fatal encephalopathy has been reported during treatment in patients with loiasis. Safety and efficacy in children <15 kg have not be established.

Adverse Reactions Frequency not defined.

Cardiovascular: Hypotension, mild ECG changes, orthostasis, peripheral and facial edema, transient tachycardia

Central nervous system: Dizziness, headache, hyperthermia, insomnia, somnolence, vertigo

Dermatologic: Pruritus, rash, urticaria, toxic epidermal necrolysis, Stevens-Johnson syndrome

Gastrointestinal: Abdominal pain, anorexia, constipation, diarrhea, nausea, vomiting

Hematologic: Anemia, eosinophilia, leukopenia

Hepatic: ALT/AST increased

Neuromuscular & skeletal: Limbitis, myalgia, tremor, weakness

Ocular: Blurred vision, mild conjunctivitis, punctate opacity

Respiratory: Asthma exacerbation

Mazzotti reaction (with onchocerciasis): Arthralgia, edema, fever, lymphadenopathy, ocular damage, pruritus, rash, synovitis

Overdosage/Toxicology Accidental intoxication with, or significant exposure to unknown quantities of veterinary formulations of ivermectin in humans, either by ingestion, inhalation, injection, or exposure to body surfaces, has resulted in the following adverse effects: rash, edema, headache, dizziness, asthenia, nausea, vomiting, and diarrhea. Other adverse effects that have been reported include seizure

(Continued)

Ivermectin *(Continued)*

and ataxia. Treatment is supportive. The usual methods for decontamination are recommended.

Drug Interactions

Cytochrome P450 Effect: Substrate of CYP3A4 (minor)

Ethanol/Nutrition/Herb Interactions

Food: Bioavailability is increased 2.5-fold when administered following a high-fat meal.

Mechanism of Action Ivermectin is a semisynthetic antihelminthic agent; it binds selectively and with strong affinity to glutamate-gated chloride ion channels which occur in invertebrate nerve and muscle cells. This leads to increased permeability of cell membranes to chloride ions then hyperpolarization of the nerve or muscle cell, and death of the parasite.

Pharmacodynamics/Kinetics

Onset of action: Peak effect: 3-6 months

Absorption: Well absorbed

Distribution: Does not cross blood-brain barrier

Half-life elimination: 16-35 hours

Metabolism: Hepatic (>97%)

Excretion: Urine (<1%); feces

Dosage Oral: Children ≥15 kg and Adults:

Strongyloidiasis: 200 mcg/kg as a single dose; follow-up stool examinations

Onchocerciasis: 150 mcg/kg as a single dose; retreatment may be required every 3-12 months until the adult worms die

Dietary Considerations Take on an empty stomach with water.

Administration Administer on an empty stomach with water.

Monitoring Parameters Skin and eye microfilarial counts, periodic ophthalmologic exams

Patient Information If infected with strongyloidiasis, repeated stool examinations are required to document clearance of the organisms; repeated follow-up and retreatment is usually required in the treatment of onchocerciasis

Dosage Forms Tablet [scored]: 3 mg

Selected Readings

de Silva N, Guyatt H, and Bundy D, "Anthelmintics. A Comparative Review of Their Clinical Pharmacology," *Drugs*, 1997, 53(5):769-88.

"Drugs for Parasitic Infections," *Med Lett Drugs Ther*, 1998, 40(1017):1-12.

IVIG *see* Immune Globulin (Intravenous) *on page 867*

Japanese Encephalitis Virus Vaccine (Inactivated)

(jap a NEESE en sef a LYE tis VYE rus vak SEEN, in ak ti VAY ted)

Related Information

Immunization Recommendations *on page 1249*

U.S. Brand Names JE-VAX®

Canadian Brand Names JE-VAX®

Generic Available No

Use Active immunization against Japanese encephalitis for persons 1 year of age and older who plan to spend 1 month or more in endemic areas in Asia, especially persons traveling during the transmission season or visiting rural areas; consider vaccination for shorter trips to epidemic areas or extensive outdoor activities in rural endemic areas; elderly (>55 years of age) individuals should be considered for vaccination, since they have increased risk of developing symptomatic illness after infection; those planning travel to or residence in endemic areas should consult the Travel Advisory Service (Central Campus) for specific advice

Pregnancy Risk Factor C

Contraindications Serious adverse reaction (generalized urticaria or angioedema) to a prior dose of this vaccine; proven or suspected hypersensitivity to proteins or rodent or neural origin; hypersensitivity to thimerosal (used as a preservative). *CDC recommends that the following should not generally receive the vaccine, unless benefit to the individual clearly outweighs the risk*:

- those acutely ill or with active infections
- persons with heart, kidney, or liver disorders
- persons with generalized malignancies such as leukemia or lymphoma
- persons with a history of multiple allergies or hypersensitivity to components of the vaccine
- pregnant women, unless there is a very high risk of Japanese encephalitis during the woman's stay in Asia

Warnings/Precautions Severe adverse reactions manifesting as generalized urticaria or angioedema may occur within minutes following vaccination, or up to 17 days later; most reactions occur within 10 days, with the majority within 48 hours; observe vaccinees for 30 minutes after vaccination; warn them of the possibility of delayed generalized urticaria and to remain where medical care is readily available for 10 days following any dose of the vaccine; because of the potential for severe adverse reactions, Japanese encephalitis vaccine is **not** recommended for all persons traveling to or residing in Asia; safety and efficacy in infants <1 year of age have not been established; therefore, immunization of infants should be deferred whenever possible; it is not known whether the vaccine is excreted in breast milk

Adverse Reactions Report allergic or unusual adverse reactions to the Vaccine Adverse Event Reporting System (VAERS) 1-800-822-7967.

Frequency not defined, common:

- Cardiovascular: Hypotension
- Central nervous system: Fever, headache, malaise, chills, dizziness
- Dermatologic: Rash, urticaria, itching with or without accompanying rash
- Gastrointestinal: Nausea, vomiting, abdominal pain
- Local: Tenderness, redness, and swelling at injection site
- Neuromuscular & skeletal: Myalgia

Frequency not defined, rare:

- Cardiovascular: Angioedema
- Central nervous system: Seizure, encephalitis, encephalopathy
- Dermatologic: Erythema multiforme, erythema nodosum
- Neuromuscular & skeletal: Peripheral neuropathy, joint swelling
- Respiratory: Dyspnea
- Miscellaneous: Anaphylactic reaction

Stability Refrigerate, discard 8 hours after reconstitution

Dosage U.S. recommended primary immunization schedule:

Children 1-3 years: SubQ: Three 0.5 mL doses given on days 0, 7, and 30; abbreviated schedules should be used only when necessary due to time constraints

Children >3 years and Adults: SubQ: Three 1 mL doses given on days 0, 7, and 30. Give third dose on day 14 when time does not permit waiting; 2 doses a week apart produce immunity in about 80% of recipients; the longest regimen yields highest titers after 6 months.

Booster dose: Give after 2 years, or according to current recommendation

Note: Travel should not commence for at least 10 days after the last dose of vaccine, to allow adequate antibody formation and recognition of any delayed adverse reaction

Advise concurrent use of other means to reduce the risk of mosquito exposure when possible, including bed nets, insect repellents, protective clothing, avoidance of travel in endemic areas, and avoidance of outdoor activity during twilight and evening periods

Administration The single-dose vial should only be reconstituted with the full 1.3 mL of diluent supplied; administer 1 mL of the resulting liquid as one standard adult dose; discard the unused portion

Patient Information Adverse reactions may occur shortly after vaccination or up to 17 days (usually within 10 days) after vaccination

Additional Information Japanese encephalitis vaccine is currently available only from the Centers for Disease Control. Contact Centers for Disease Control at (404) 639-6370 (Mon-Fri) or (404) 639-2888 (nights, weekends, or holidays). Federal law requires that the date of administration, the vaccine manufacturer, lot number of vaccine, and the administering person's name, title and address be entered into the patient's permanent medical record.

Dosage Forms Injection, powder for reconstitution: 1 mL, 10 mL

JE-VAX® *see* Japanese Encephalitis Virus Vaccine (Inactivated) *on page 900*
Kaletra® *see* Lopinavir and Ritonavir *on page 919*

Kanamycin (kan a MYE sin)

Related Information

Tuberculosis *on page 1315*

U.S. Brand Names Kantrex®

Canadian Brand Names Kantrex®

Synonyms Kanamycin Sulfate

Generic Available No

Use Treatment of serious infections caused by susceptible strains of *E. coli, Proteus* species, *Enterobacter aerogenes, Klebsiella pneumoniae, Serratia marcescens,* and *Acinetobacter* species; second-line treatment of *Mycobacterium tuberculosis*

Pregnancy Risk Factor D

(Continued)

Kanamycin *(Continued)*

Pregnancy Implications Aminoglycosides cross the placenta and may cause congenital deafness; other teratogenic effects have not been reported.

Contraindications Hypersensitivity to kanamycin, any component of the formulation, or other aminoglycosides; pregnancy

Warnings/Precautions Use with caution in patients with pre-existing renal insufficiency, vestibular or cochlear impairment, myasthenia gravis, conditions which depress neuromuscular transmission. Parenteral aminoglycosides are associated with nephrotoxicity or ototoxicity; the ototoxicity may be proportional to the amount of drug given and the duration of treatment; tinnitus or vertigo are indications of vestibular injury and impending hearing loss; renal damage is usually reversible.

Adverse Reactions Frequency not defined.

Cardiovascular: Edema

Central nervous system: Neurotoxicity, drowsiness, headache, pseudomotor cerebri

Dermatologic: Skin itching, redness, rash, photosensitivity, erythema

Gastrointestinal: Nausea, vomiting, diarrhea, malabsorption syndrome (with prolonged and high-dose therapy of hepatic coma), anorexia, weight loss, salivation increased, enterocolitis

Hematologic: Granulocytopenia, agranulocytosis, thrombocytopenia

Local: Burning, stinging

Neuromuscular & skeletal: Weakness, tremor, muscle cramps

Otic: Ototoxicity (auditory), ototoxicity (vestibular)

Renal: Nephrotoxicity

Respiratory: Dyspnea

Overdosage/Toxicology Symptoms of overdose include ototoxicity, nephrotoxicity, and neuromuscular toxicity. The treatment of choice following a single acute overdose appears to be the maintenance of good urine output of at least 3 mL/kg/hour. Hemodialysis or peritoneal dialysis may enhance kanamycin elimination; exchange transfusion may also be considered in the newborn infant.

Drug Interactions

Increased Effect/Toxicity: Increased toxicity may occur with amphotericin B, cisplatin, loop diuretics, neuromuscular-blocking agents. Use with bisphosphonate derivatives may lead to hypocalcemia.

Stability Store vial at controlled room temperature. Darkening of vials does not indicate loss of potency.

I.V.: Must be further diluted prior to I.V. infusion. For adults, dilute 500 mg in 100-200 mL of appropriate solution or 1 g in 200-400 mL; for pediatric patients, use sufficient amount to infuse solution over 30-60 minutes.

Intraperitoneal: Dilute dose in 20 mL sterile distilled water.

Aerosol: Dilute 250 mg in 3 mL normal saline.

Mechanism of Action Interferes with protein synthesis in bacterial cell by binding to ribosomal subunit

Pharmacodynamics/Kinetics

Distribution:

Relative diffusion from blood into CSF: Good only with inflammation (exceeds usual MICs)

CSF:blood level ratio: Normal meninges: Nil; Inflamed meninges: 43%

Half-life elimination: 2-4 hours; Anuria: 80 hours; End-stage renal disease: 40-96 hours

Time to peak, serum: I.M.: 1-2 hours (decreased in burn patients)

Excretion: Urine (entire amount)

Dosage Note: Dosing should be based on ideal body weight

Children: Infections: I.M., I.V.: 15 mg/kg/day in divided doses every 8-12 hours

Adults:

Infections: I.M., I.V.: 5-7.5 mg/kg/dose in divided doses every 8-12 hours (<15 mg/kg/day)

Intraperitoneal: After contamination in surgery: 500 mg

Irrigating solution: 0.25%; maximum 1.5 g/day (via all administration routes)

Aerosol: 250 mg 2-4 times/day

Dosing adjustment/interval in renal impairment:

Cl_{cr} 50-80 mL/minute: Administer 60% to 90% of dose or administer every 8-12 hours

Cl_{cr} 10-50 mL/minute: Administer 30% to 70% of dose or administer every 12 hours

Cl_{cr} <10 mL/minute: Administer 20% to 30% of dose or administer every 24-48 hours

Administration

I.M.: Administer deeply in upper outer quadrant of the gluteal muscle.

I.V.: Infuse over 30-60 minutes.

Monitoring Parameters Serum creatinine and BUN every 2-3 days; peak and trough concentrations; hearing

Reference Range Therapeutic: Peak: 15-30 mcg/mL; Trough: 5-10 mcg/mL; Toxic: Peak: >35 mcg/mL; Trough: >10 mcg/mL

Patient Information Report any dizziness or sensations of ringing or fullness in ears

Dosage Forms Injection, solution, as sulfate: 1 g/3 mL (3 mL) [contains sodium bisulfate]

Selected Readings

Begg EJ and Barclay ML, "Aminoglycosides - 50 Years On," *Br J Clin Pharmacol*, 1995, 39(6):597-603.

Cunha BA, "Aminoglycosides: Current Role in Antimicrobial Therapy," *Pharmacotherapy*, 1988, 8(6):334-50.

"Drugs for Tuberculosis," *Med Lett Drugs Ther*, 1993, 35(908):99-101.

Iseman MD, "Treatment of Multidrug-Resistant Tuberculosis," *N Engl J Med*, 1993, 329(11):784-91.

Kanamycin Sulfate *see* Kanamycin *on page 901*

Kantrex® *see* Kanamycin *on page 901*

Kaopectate® [OTC] *see* Bismuth *on page 686*

Kaopectate® Extra Strength [OTC] *see* Bismuth *on page 686*

Kaopectolin *(new formulation)* [OTC] *see* Bismuth *on page 686*

Keflex® *see* Cephalexin *on page 727*

Keftab® (Can) *see* Cephalexin *on page 727*

Kefurox® (Can) *see* Cefuroxime *on page 725*

Ketek® *see* Telithromycin *on page 1093*

Ketoconazole (kee toe KOE na zole)

U.S. Brand Names Nizoral®; Nizoral® A-D [OTC]

Canadian Brand Names Apo-Ketoconazole®; Ketoderm®; Nizoral®; Novo-Ketoconazole

Generic Available Yes

Use Treatment of susceptible fungal infections, including candidiasis, oral thrush, blastomycosis, histoplasmosis, paracoccidioidomycosis, coccidioidomycosis, chromomycosis, candiduria, chronic mucocutaneous candidiasis, as well as certain recalcitrant cutaneous dermatophytoses; used topically for treatment of tinea corporis, tinea cruris, tinea versicolor, and cutaneous candidiasis, seborrheic dermatitis

Unlabeled/Investigational Use Treatment of prostate cancer (androgen synthesis inhibitor)

Drug of Choice or Alternative for Organism(s):

Blastomyces dermatitidis on page 50
Candida Species *on page 67*
Coccidioides immitis on page 91
Dematiaceous Fungi *on page 112*
Dermatophytes *on page 114*
Histoplasma capsulatum on page 177
Malassezia furfur on page 213
Prototheca Species *on page 280*

Pregnancy Risk Factor C

Contraindications Hypersensitivity to ketoconazole or any component of the formulation; CNS fungal infections (due to poor CNS penetration); coadministration with ergot derivatives or cisapride is contraindicated due to risk of potentially fatal cardiac arrhythmias

Warnings/Precautions Use with caution in patients with impaired hepatic function; has been associated with hepatotoxicity, including some fatalities; perform periodic liver function tests; high doses of ketoconazole may depress adrenocortical function.

Adverse Reactions

Oral:

1% to 10%:

Dermatologic: Pruritus (2%)

Gastrointestinal: Nausea/vomiting (3% to 10%), abdominal pain (1%)

<1%: Headache, dizziness, somnolence, fever, chills, bulging fontanelles, depression, gynecomastia, diarrhea, impotence, thrombocytopenia, leukopenia, hemolytic anemia, hepatotoxicity, photophobia

Cream: Severe irritation, pruritus, stinging (~5%)

Shampoo: Increases in normal hair loss, irritation (<1%), abnormal hair texture, scalp pustules, mild dryness of skin, itching, oiliness/dryness of hair

Overdosage/Toxicology Symptoms include dizziness, headache, nausea, vomiting, and diarrhea. Overdoses are well tolerated. Treatment includes supportive measures and gastric decontamination.

(Continued)

Ketoconazole *(Continued)*

Drug Interactions

Cytochrome P450 Effect: Substrate of CYP3A4 (major); **Inhibits** CYP1A2 (strong), 2A6 (moderate), 2B6 (weak), 2C8/9 (strong), 2C19 (moderate), 2D6 (moderate), 3A4 (strong)

Increased Effect/Toxicity: Due to inhibition of hepatic CYP3A4, ketoconazole use is contraindicated with cisapride, lovastatin, midazolam, simvastatin, and triazolam due to large substantial increases in the toxicity of these agents. Ketoconazole may increase the serum levels/effects of amiodarone, amphetamines, benzodiazepines, beta-blockers, buspirone, busulfan, calcium channel blockers, citalopram, dexmedetomidine, dextromethorphan, diazepam, digoxin, docetaxel, fluoxetine, fluvoxamine, glimepiride, glipizide, ifosfamide, inhalational anesthetics, lidocaine, mesoridazine, methsuximide, mexiletine, mirtazapine, nateglinide, nefazodone, paroxetine, phenytoin, pioglitazone, propranolol, risperidone, ritonavir, ropinirole, rosiglitazone, sertraline, sirolimus, tacrolimus, theophylline, thioridazine, tricyclic antidepressants, trifluoperazine, trimetrexate, venlafaxine, vincristine, vinblastine, warfarin, zolpidem, and other substrates of CYP1A2, 2A6, 2C8/9, 2C19, 2D6, or 3A4. Selected benzodiazepines (midazolam and triazolam), cisapride, ergot alkaloids, selected HMG-CoA reductase inhibitors (lovastatin and simvastatin), and pimozide are generally contraindicated with strong CYP3A4 inhibitors. Mesoridazine and thioridazine are generally contraindicated with strong CYP2D6 inhibitors. When used with strong CYP3A4 inhibitors, dosage adjustment/limits are recommended for sildenafil and other PDE-5 inhibitors; consult individual monographs.

Decreased Effect: Oral: Absorption requires gastric acidity; therefore, antacids, H_2 antagonists (cimetidine, famotidine, nizatidine, and ranitidine), proton pump inhibitors (omeprazole, lansoprazole, rabeprazole), and sucralfate may significantly reduce bioavailability resulting in treatment failures and should not be administered concomitantly. Decreased serum levels with didanosine and isoniazid. The levels/effects of ketoconazole may be decreased by aminoglutethimide, carbamazepine, nafcillin, nevirapine, phenobarbital, phenytoin, rifamycins, or other CYP3A4 inducers. **Should not be administered concomitantly with rifampin.** Oral contraceptive efficacy may be reduced (limited data). Ketoconazole may decrease the levels/effects of CYP2D6 prodrug substrates (eg, codeine, hydrocodone, oxycodone, tramadol).

Ethanol/Nutrition/Herb Interactions

Food: Ketoconazole peak serum levels may be prolonged if taken with food.

Herb/Nutraceutical: St John's wort may decrease ketoconazole levels.

Mechanism of Action Alters the permeability of the cell wall by blocking fungal cytochrome P450; inhibits biosynthesis of triglycerides and phospholipids by fungi; inhibits several fungal enzymes that results in a build-up of toxic concentrations of hydrogen peroxide; also inhibits androgen synthesis

Pharmacodynamics/Kinetics

Absorption: Oral: Rapid (~75%); Shampoo: None

Distribution: Well into inflamed joint fluid, saliva, bile, urine, breast milk, sebum, cerumen, feces, tendons, skin and soft tissues, and testes; crosses blood-brain barrier poorly; only negligible amounts reach CSF

Protein binding: 93% to 96%

Metabolism: Partially hepatic via CYP3A4 to inactive compounds

Bioavailability: Decreases as gastric pH increases

Half-life elimination: Biphasic: Initial: 2 hours; Terminal: 8 hours

Time to peak, serum: 1-2 hours

Excretion: Feces (57%); urine (13%)

Dosage

Fungal infections:

Oral:

Children ≥2 years: 3.3-6.6 mg/kg/day as a single dose for 1-2 weeks for candidiasis, for at least 4 weeks in recalcitrant dermatophyte infections, and for up to 6 months for other systemic mycoses

Adults: 200-400 mg/day as a single daily dose for durations as stated above

Shampoo: Apply twice weekly for 4 weeks with at least 3 days between each shampoo

Topical: Rub gently into the affected area once daily to twice daily

Prostate cancer (unlabeled use): Oral: Adults: 400 mg 3 times/day

Dosing adjustment in hepatic impairment: Dose reductions should be considered in patients with severe liver disease

Hemodialysis: Not dialyzable (0% to 5%)

Dietary Considerations May be taken with food or milk to decrease GI adverse effects.

Administration Administer tablets 2 hours prior to antacids to prevent decreased absorption due to the high pH of gastric contents.

Monitoring Parameters Liver function tests

Patient Information Cream is for topical application to the skin only; avoid contact with the eye; avoid taking antacids at the same time as ketoconazole; may take with food; may cause drowsiness, impair judgment or coordination. Report unusual fatigue, anorexia, vomiting, dark urine, or pale stools.

Dosage Forms

Cream, topical: 2% (15 g, 30 g, 60 g)

Shampoo, topical (Nizoral® A-D): 1% (6 mL, 120 mL, 210 mL)

Tablet (Nizoral®): 200 mg

Extemporaneous Preparations A 20 mg/mL suspension may be made by pulverizing twelve 200 mg ketoconazole tablets to a fine powder; add 40 mL Ora-Plus® in small portions with thorough mixing; incorporate Ora-Sweet® to make a final volume of 120 mL and mix thoroughly; refrigerate (no stability information is available)

Allen LV, "Ketoconazole Oral Suspension," *US Pharm*, 1993, 18(2):98-9, 101.

Selected Readings

Como JA and Dismukes WE, "Oral Azole Drugs as Systemic Antifungal Therapy," *N Engl J Med*, 1993, 330(4):263-72.

Lyman CA and Walsh TJ, "Systemically Administered Antifungal Agents. A Review of Their Clinical Pharmacology and Therapeutic Applications," *Drugs*, 1992, 44(1):9-35.

Terrell CL, "Antifungal Agents. Part II. The Azoles," *Mayo Clin Proc*, 1999, 74(1):78-100.

Ketoderm® (Can) *see* Ketoconazole *on page 903*

KI *see* Potassium Iodide *on page 1014*

Klaron® *see* Sulfacetamide *on page 1081*

Kwellada-P™ (Can) *see* Permethrin *on page 1001*

L-749,345 *see* Ertapenem *on page 805*

LA 20304a *see* Gemifloxacin *on page 840*

L-AmB *see* Amphotericin B (Liposomal) *on page 655*

Lamisil® *see* Terbinafine *on page 1097*

Lamisil® AT™ [OTC] *see* Terbinafine *on page 1097*

Lamivudine (la MI vyoo deen)

Related Information

Antiretroviral Agents *on page 1206*

Antiretroviral Therapy for HIV Infection *on page 1219*

Management of Healthcare Worker Exposures to HBV, HCV, and HIV *on page 1227*

U.S. Brand Names Epivir®; Epivir-HBV®

Canadian Brand Names Heptovir®; 3TC®

Synonyms 3TC

Generic Available No

Use

Epivir®: Treatment of HIV infection when antiretroviral therapy is warranted; should always be used as part of a multidrug regimen (at least three antiretroviral agents)

Epivir-HBV®: Treatment of chronic hepatitis B associated with evidence of hepatitis B viral replication and active liver inflammation

Unlabeled/Investigational Use Prevention of HIV following needlesticks (with or without protease inhibitor)

Drug of Choice or Alternative for Organism(s):

Hepatitis B Virus *on page 165*

Human Immunodeficiency Virus *on page 181*

Pregnancy Risk Factor C

Pregnancy Implications Lamivudine crosses the placenta. The pharmacokinetics of lamivudine during pregnancy are not significantly altered and dosage adjustment is not required. The Perinatal HIV Guidelines Working Group recommends lamivudine for use during pregnancy; the combination of lamivudine with zidovudine is the recommended dual combination NRTI in pregnancy. It may also be used in combination with zidovudine in HIV-infected women who are in labor, but have had no prior antiretroviral therapy, in order to reduce the maternal-fetal transmission of HIV. Cases of lactic acidosis/hepatic steatosis syndrome have been reported in pregnant women receiving nucleoside analogues. It is not known if pregnancy itself potentiates this known side effect; however, pregnant women may be at increased risk of lactic acidosis and liver damage. Hepatic enzymes and electrolytes should be monitored frequently during the 3rd trimester of pregnancy in women receiving nucleoside analogues. Health professionals are encouraged to contact the antiretroviral pregnancy registry to monitor outcomes of pregnant women exposed to antiretroviral medications (1-800-258-4263 or www.APRegistry.com).

(Continued)

Lamivudine *(Continued)*

Contraindications Hypersensitivity to lamivudine or any component of the formulation

Warnings/Precautions A decreased dosage is recommended in patients with renal dysfunction since AUC, C_{max}, and half-life increased with diminishing renal function; use with extreme caution in children with history of pancreatitis or risk factors for development of pancreatitis. Do not use as monotherapy in treatment of HIV. Treatment of HBV in patients with unrecognized/untreated HIV may lead to rapid HIV resistance. In addition, treatment of HIV in patients with unrecognized/untreated HBV may lead to rapid HBV resistance. Patients with HIV infection should receive only dosage forms appropriate for treatment of HIV.

Lactic acidosis and severe hepatomegaly with steatosis have been reported, including fatal cases. Use caution in hepatic impairment. Pregnancy, obesity, and/or prolonged therapy may increase the risk of lactic acidosis and liver damage.

Monitor patients closely for several months following discontinuation of therapy for chronic hepatitis B; clinical exacerbations may occur.

Adverse Reactions (As reported in adults treated for HIV infection)

>10%:
- Central nervous system: Headache, fatigue
- Gastrointestinal: Nausea, diarrhea, vomiting, pancreatitis (range: 0.5% to 18%; higher percentage in pediatric patients)
- Neuromuscular & skeletal: Peripheral neuropathy, paresthesia, musculoskeletal pain

1% to 10%:
- Central nervous system: Dizziness, depression, fever, chills, insomnia
- Dermatologic: Rash
- Gastrointestinal: Anorexia, abdominal pain, heartburn, elevated amylase
- Hematologic: Neutropenia
- Hepatic: Elevated AST, ALT
- Neuromuscular & skeletal: Myalgia, arthralgia
- Respiratory: Nasal signs and symptoms, cough

<1%, postmarketing, and/or case reports: Alopecia, anaphylaxis, anemia, hepatomegaly, hyperbilirubinemia, hyperglycemia, increased CPK, lactic acidosis, lymphadenopathy, peripheral neuropathy, pruritus, red cell aplasia, rhabdomyolysis, splenomegaly, steatosis, stomatitis, thrombocytopenia, urticaria, weakness

Overdosage/Toxicology Very limited information is available, although there have been no clinical signs or symptoms noted in overdose, and hematologic tests have remained normal as well. No antidote is available. Limited (negligible) removal following 4-hour hemodialysis. It is not known if continuous 24-hour hemodialysis would be effective.

Drug Interactions

Increased Effect/Toxicity: Zidovudine concentrations increase significantly (~39%) with lamivudine coadministration. sulfamethoxazole/trimethoprim increases lamivudine's blood levels. Concomitant use of ribavirin and nucleoside analogues may increase the risk of developing lactic acidosis (includes adefovir, didanosine, lamivudine, stavudine, zalcitabine, zidovudine). Trimethoprim (and other drugs excreted by organic cation transport) may increase serum levels/effects of lamivudine.

Decreased Effect: Zalcitabine and lamivudine may inhibit the intracellular phosphorylation of each other; concomitant use should be avoided.

Ethanol/Nutrition/Herb Interactions Food: Food decreases the rate of absorption and C_{max}; however, there is no change in the systemic AUC. Therefore, may be taken with or without food.

Stability Store at 2°C to 25°C (68°F to 77°F) tightly closed.

Mechanism of Action Lamivudine is a cytosine analog. After lamivudine is triphosphorylated, the principle mode of action is inhibition of HIV reverse transcription via viral DNA chain termination; inhibits RNA- and DNA-dependent DNA polymerase activities of reverse transcriptase. The monophosphate form of lamivudine is incorporated into the viral DNA by hepatitis B virus polymerase, resulting in DNA chain termination.

Pharmacodynamics/Kinetics

Absorption: Rapid
Distribution: V_d: 1.3 L/kg
Protein binding, plasma: <36%
Metabolism: 5.6% to trans-sulfoxide metabolite
Bioavailability: Absolute; Cp_{max} decreased with food although AUC not significantly affected
  Children: 66%

Adults: 87%
Half-life elimination: Children: 2 hours; Adults: 5-7 hours
Excretion: Primarily urine (as unchanged drug)

Dosage Note: The formulation and dosage of Epivir-HBV® are not appropriate for patients infected with both HBV and HIV. Use with at least two other antiretroviral agents when treating HIV

Oral:
- Children 3 months to 16 years: HIV: 4 mg/kg twice daily (maximum: 150 mg twice daily)
- Children 2-17 years: Treatment of hepatitis B (Epivir-HBV®): 3 mg/kg once daily (maximum: 100 mg/day)
- Adolescents and Adults: Prevention of HIV following needlesticks (unlabeled use): 150 mg twice daily (with zidovudine with or without a protease inhibitor, depending on risk)
- Adults:
  - HIV: 150 mg twice daily **or** 300 mg once daily
    - <50 kg: 4 mg/kg twice daily (maximum: 150 mg twice daily)
  - Treatment of hepatitis B (Epivir-HBV®): 100 mg/day

Dosing interval in renal impairment in pediatric patients: Insufficient data; however, dose reduction should be considered.

Dosing interval in renal impairment in patients >16 years for HIV:
- Cl_{cr} 30-49 mL/minute: Administer 150 mg once daily
- Cl_{cr} 15-29 mL/minute: Administer 150 mg first dose, then 100 mg once daily
- Cl_{cr} 5-14 mL/minute: Administer 150 mg first dose, then 50 mg once daily
- Cl_{cr} <5 mL/minute: Administer 50 mg first dose, then 25 mg once daily

Dosing interval in renal impairment in adult patients with hepatitis B:
- Cl_{cr} 30-49: Administer 100 mg first dose then 50 mg once daily
- Cl_{cr} 15-29: Administer 100 mg first dose then 25 mg once daily
- Cl_{cr} 5-14: Administer 35 mg first dose then 15 mg once daily
- Cl_{cr} <5: Administer 35 mg first dose then 10 mg once daily

Dialysis: Negligible amounts are removed by 4-hour hemodialysis or peritoneal dialysis. Supplemental dosing is not required.

Dietary Considerations May be taken with or without food. Each 5 mL of oral solution contains 1 g of sucrose.

Administration May be taken with or without food. Adjust dosage in renal failure.

Monitoring Parameters Amylase, bilirubin, liver enzymes, hematologic parameters, viral load, and CD4 count; signs and symptoms of pancreatitis

Patient Information Take exactly as prescribed; children should be monitored for symptoms of pancreatitis

Additional Information Lamivudine has been well studied in the treatment of chronic hepatitis B infection. Potential compliance problems, frequency of administration, and adverse effects should be discussed with patients before initiating therapy to help prevent the emergence of resistance.

A high rate of early virologic nonresponse was observed when abacavir, lamivudine and tenofovir were used as the initial regimen in treatment-naive patients. A high rate of early virologic nonresponse was also observed when didanosine, lamivudine, and tenofovir were used as the initial regimen in treatment-naive patients. Use of either of these combinations is not recommended; patients currently on either of these regimens should be closely monitored for modification of therapy.

Dosage Forms

Solution, oral:
- Epivir®: 10 mg/mL (240 mL) [strawberry-banana flavor]
- Epivir-HBV®: 5 mg/mL (240 mL) [strawberry-banana flavor]

Tablet:
- Epivir®: 150 mg, 300 mg
- Epivir-HBV®: 100 mg

Selected Readings

Dienstag JL, Perrillo, RP, Schiff, ER, et al, "A Preliminary Trial of Lamivudine for Chronic Hepatitis B Infection," *N Engl J Med*, 1995, 333(25):1657-61.

Eron JJ, Benoit SL, Jemsek J, et al, "Treatment with Lamivudine, Zidovudine, or Both in HIV-Positive Patients with 200 to 500 CD4+ Cells per Cubic Millimeter," *N Engl J Med*, 1995, 333(25):1662-9.

Lai CL, Chien RN, Leung NW, et al, "A One-Year Trial of Lamivudine for Chronic Hepatitis B," *N Engl J Med*, 1998, 339(2):61-8.

Perry CM and Faulds D, "Lamivudine. A Review of Its Antiviral Activity, Pharmacokinetic Properties and Therapeutic Efficacy in the Management of HIV Infection," *Drugs*, 1997, 53(4):657-80.

Lamivudine, Abacavir, and Zidovudine *see* Abacavir, Lamivudine, and Zidovudine *on page 627*

Lamivudine and Abacavir *see* Abacavir and Lamivudine *on page 626*

Lamivudine and Zidovudine *see* Zidovudine and Lamivudine *on page 1162*

Lamprene® **[DSC]** *see* Clofazimine *on page 757*

Lansoprazole, Amoxicillin, and Clarithromycin

(lan SOE pra zole, a moks i SIL in, & kla RITH roe mye sin)

U.S. Brand Names Prevpac®

Canadian Brand Names Hp-PAC®; Prevpac®

Synonyms Amoxicillin, Lansoprazole, and Clarithromycin; Clarithromycin, Lansoprazole, and Amoxicillin

Generic Available No

Use Eradication of *H. pylori* to reduce the risk of recurrent duodenal ulcer

Pregnancy Risk Factor C (clarithromycin)

Pregnancy Implications See individual agents.

Contraindications Hypersensitivity to lansoprazole, amoxicillin (or any penicillin), clarithromycin (or erythromycin), or any component of the formulation; concurrent use with pimozide or cisapride

Warnings/Precautions

Based on **lansoprazole** component: Severe liver dysfunction may require dosage reductions.

Based on **amoxicillin** component: In patients with renal impairment, doses and/or frequency of administration should be modified in response to the degree of renal impairment; a high percentage of patients with infectious mononucleosis have developed rash during therapy with amoxicillin; a low incidence of cross-allergy with other beta-lactams and cephalosporins exists

Based on **clarithromycin** component: Dosage adjustment required with severe renal impairment, decreased dosage or prolonged dosing interval may be appropriate; antibiotic-associated colitis has been reported with use of clarithromycin. Macrolides (including clarithromycin) have been associated with rare QT prolongation and ventricular arrhythmias, including torsade de pointes.

Adverse Reactions Note: Frequencies noted refer to experience with combination therapy for 14 days with all components. Refer to individual monographs for more extensive information on adverse reactions reported with each component.

3% to 10%:

Central nervous system: Headache (6%)

Gastrointestinal: Diarrhea (7%), taste perversion (5%)

<3%: Abdominal pain, candidiasis (oral), confusion, dark stools, dermatologic reactions, dizziness, dry mouth, glossitis, myalgia, nausea, rectal itching, thirst, tongue discoloration, vaginitis, vomiting

Overdosage/Toxicology

See individual agents.

Drug Interactions

Cytochrome P450 Effect:

Lansoprazole: **Substrate** of CYP2C8/9 (minor), 2C19 (major), 3A4 (major); **Inhibits** CYP2C8/9 (weak), 2C19 (moderate), 2D6 (weak), 3A4 (weak); **Induces** CYP1A2 (weak)

Clarithromycin: **Substrate** of CYP3A4 (major); **Inhibits** CYP1A2 (weak), 3A4 (strong)

Increased Effect/Toxicity: See individual agents.

Decreased Effect: See individual agents.

Stability

Store at controlled room temperature of 20°C to 25°C (68°F to 77°F); protect from light and moisture

Pharmacodynamics/Kinetics See individual agents.

Dosage Oral: Adults: Lansoprazole 30 mg, amoxicillin 1 g, and clarithromycin 500 mg taken together twice daily for 10 or 14 days

Dosage adjustment in renal impairment: Cl_{cr} <30 mL/minute: Use is not recommended

Additional Information Complete prescribing information for this medication should be consulted for additional detail.

Dosage Forms Combination package (Prevpac®) [each administration card contains]:

Capsule (Trimox®): Amoxicillin 500 mg (4 capsules/day)

Capsule, delayed release (Prevacid®): Lansoprazole 30 mg (2 capsules/day)

Tablet (Biaxin®): Clarithromycin 500 mg (2 tablets/day)

Lariam® *see* Mefloquine *on page 929*

Levaquin® *see* Levofloxacin *on page 908*

Levofloxacin (lee voe FLOKS a sin)

Related Information

Antimicrobial Activity Against Selected Organisms *on page 1165*

Community-Acquired Pneumonia in Adults *on page 1278*
Tuberculosis *on page 1315*

U.S. Brand Names Iquix®; Levaquin®; Quixin™

Canadian Brand Names Levaquin®; Novo-Levofloxacin

Generic Available No

Use

Systemic: Treatment of mild, moderate, or severe infections caused by susceptible organisms. Includes the treatment of community-acquired pneumonia, including multidrug resistant strains of *S. pneumoniae* (MDRSP); nosocomial pneumonia; chronic bronchitis (acute bacterial exacerbation); acute bacterial sinusitis; urinary tract infection (uncomplicated or complicated), including acute pyelonephritis caused by *E. coli*; prostatitis (chronic bacterial); skin or skin structure infections (uncomplicated or complicated); prevention of inhalational anthrax (postexposure)

Ophthalmic: Treatment of bacterial conjunctivitis caused by susceptible organisms (Quixin™ 0.5% ophthalmic solution); treatment of corneal ulcer caused by susceptible organisms (Iquix® 1.5% ophthalmic solution)

Drug of Choice or Alternative for

Disease/Syndrome(s):

Cervicitis *on page 71*
Osteomyelitis, Diabetic Foot *on page 249*
Pneumonia, Community-Acquired *on page 270*
Pneumonia, Hospital-Acquired *on page 272*
Pneumonia, Ventilator-Associated *on page 273*
Traveler's Diarrhea *on page 333*

Organism(s):

Neisseria gonorrhoeae on page 244
Streptococcus pneumoniae, Drug-Resistant *on page 316*

Pregnancy Risk Factor C

Pregnancy Implications Reports of arthropathy (observed in immature animals and reported rarely in humans) have limited the use of fluoroquinolones in pregnancy. Teratogenic effects were not observed with levofloxacin in animal studies; however, decreased body weight and increased fetal mortality were reported. Based on limited data, quinolones are not expected to be a major human teratogen. Although quinolone antibiotics should not be used as first-line agents during pregnancy, when considering treatment for life-threatening infection and/or prolonged duration of therapy, the potential risk to the fetus must be balanced against the severity of the potential illness.

Contraindications Hypersensitivity to levofloxacin, any component of the formulation, or other quinolones

Warnings/Precautions

Systemic: Not recommended in children <18 years of age; CNS stimulation may occur (tremor, restlessness, confusion, and very rarely hallucinations or seizures); use with caution in patients with known or suspected CNS disorders or renal dysfunction; use caution to avoid possible photosensitivity reactions during and for several days following fluoroquinolone therapy

Rare cases of torsade de pointes have been reported in patients receiving levofloxacin. Risk may be minimized by avoiding use in patients with known prolongation of QT interval, bradycardia, hypokalemia, hypomagnesemia, cardiomyopathy, or in those receiving concurrent therapy with Class Ia or Class III antiarrhythmics.

Severe hypersensitivity reactions, including anaphylaxis, have occurred with quinolone therapy. If an allergic reaction occurs (itching, urticaria, dyspnea or facial edema, loss of consciousness, tingling, cardiovascular collapse), discontinue drug immediately. Prolonged use may result in superinfection; pseudomembranous colitis may occur and should be considered in all patients who present with diarrhea. Tendon inflammation and/or rupture has been reported; risk may be increased with concurrent corticosteroids, particularly in the elderly. Discontinue at first sign of tendon inflammation or pain. Peripheral neuropathies have been linked to levofloxacin use; discontinue if numbness, tingling, or weakness develops. Quinolones may exacerbate myasthenia gravis; use with caution (rare, potentially life-threatening weakness of respiratory muscles may occur).

Ophthalmic solution: For topical use only. Do not inject subconjunctivally or introduce into anterior chamber of the eye. Contact lenses should not be worn during treatment for bacterial conjunctivitis. Safety and efficacy in children <1 year of age (Quixin™) or <6 years of age (Iquix®) have not been established. **Note:** Indications for ophthalmic solutions are product concentration-specific and should not be used interchangeably.

Adverse Reactions

1% to 10%:

Cardiovascular: Chest pain (1%)

(Continued)

Levofloxacin *(Continued)*

Central nervous system: Headache (6%), insomnia (5%), dizziness (2%), fatigue (1%), pain (1%), fever

Dermatologic: Pruritus (1%), rash (1%)

Gastrointestinal: Nausea (7%), diarrhea (5%), abdominal pain (3%), constipation (3%), dyspepsia (2%), vomiting (2%), flatulence (1%)

Genitourinary: Vaginitis (1%)

Hematologic: Lymphopenia (2%)

Ocular (with ophthalmic solution use): Decreased vision (transient), foreign body sensation, transient ocular burning, ocular pain or discomfort, photophobia

Respiratory: Pharyngitis (4%), dyspnea (1%), rhinitis (1%), sinusitis (1%)

<1% (Limited to important or life-threatening):

Systemic: Acute renal failure; allergic reaction (including pneumonitis rash, pneumonitis, and anaphylaxis); agranulocytosis, anaphylactoid reaction, anorexia, anxiety, arrhythmia (including atrial/ventricular tachycardia/fibrillation and torsade de pointes), arthralgia, ascites, bradycardia, bronchospasm, carcinoma, cardiac failure, cerebrovascular disorder, cholecystitis, cholelithiasis, confusion, conjunctivitis, dehydration, depression, ear disorder, edema, EEG abnormalities, electrolyte abnormality, encephalopathy, eosinophilia, erythema multiforme, gangrene, GI hemorrhage, granulocytopenia, hallucination, heart block, hematoma, hemolytic anemia, hemoptysis, hepatic failure, hyper-/hypotension, infection, INR increased, intestinal obstruction, intracranial hypertension, involuntary muscle contractions, jaundice, leukocytosis, leukopenia, leukorrhea, lymphadenopathy, MI, migraine, multiple organ failure, pancreatitis, paralysis, paresthesia, peripheral neuropathy, phlebitis, photosensitivity (<0.1%), pleural effusion, postural hypotension, prothrombin time increased/decreased, pseudomembraneous colitis, pulmonary edema,pulmonary embolism, purpura, QT_c prolongation, respiratory depression, respiratory disorder, rhabdomyolysis, seizure, skin disorder, somnolence,speech disorder, Stevens-Johnson syndrome, stupor, syncope, taste perversion, tendon rupture, tongue edema, transaminases increased, thrombocythemia, thrombocytopenia, tremor, WBC abnormality

Ophthalmic solution: Allergic reaction, lid edema, ocular dryness, ocular itching

Overdosage/Toxicology Symptoms include acute renal failure and seizures. Treatment should include GI decontamination and supportive care. Not removed by peritoneal or hemodialysis.

Drug Interactions

Increased Effect/Toxicity: Levofloxacin may increase the effects/toxicity of glyburide and warfarin. Concomitant use with corticosteroids may increase the risk of tendon rupture. Concomitant use with other QT_c-prolonging agents (eg, Class Ia and Class III antiarrhythmics, erythromycin, cisapride, antipsychotics, and cyclic antidepressants) may result in arrhythmias, such as torsade de pointes. Probenecid may increase levofloxacin levels.

Decreased Effect: Concurrent administration of metal cations, including most antacids, oral electrolyte supplements, quinapril, sucralfate, some didanosine formulations (chewable/buffered tablets and pediatric powder for oral suspension), and other highly-buffered oral drugs, may decrease quinolone levels; separate doses.

Stability

Solution for injection:

Vial: Store at room temperature; protect from light. When diluted to 5 mg/mL in a compatible I.V. fluid, solution is stable for 72 hours when stored at room temperature; stable for 14 days when stored under refrigeration. When frozen, stable for 6 months; do not refreeze. Do not thaw in microwave or by bath immersion.

Premixed: Store at ≤25°C (77°F); brief exposure to 40°C (104°F) does not affect product; protect from freezing and light.

Tablet, oral solution: Store at 25°C (77°F); excursions permitted to 15°C to 25°C (59°F to 77°F).

Ophthalmic solution: Store at 15°C to 25°C (59°F to 77°F).

Mechanism of Action As the S (-) enantiomer of the fluoroquinolone, ofloxacin, levofloxacin, inhibits DNA-gyrase in susceptible organisms thereby inhibits relaxation of supercoiled DNA and promotes breakage of DNA strands. DNA gyrase (topoisomerase II), is an essential bacterial enzyme that maintains the superhelical structure of DNA and is required for DNA replication and transcription, DNA repair, recombination, and transposition.

Pharmacodynamics/Kinetics

Absorption: Rapid and complete

Distribution: V_d: 1.25 L/kg; CSF concentrations ~15% of serum levels; high concentrations are achieved in prostate, lung, and gynecological tissues, sinus, saliva

Protein binding: 50%

Metabolism: Minimally hepatic
Bioavailability: 99%
Half-life elimination: 6-8 hours
Time to peak, serum: 1-2 hours
Excretion: Primarily urine (as unchanged drug)

Dosage

Oral, I.V.: Adults:

Note: Sequential therapy (intravenous to oral) may be instituted based on prescriber's discretion.

Bacterial sinusitis (acute): 500 mg every 24 hours for 10-14 days or 750 mg every 24 hours for 5 days

Chronic bronchitis (acute bacterial exacerbation): 500 mg every 24 hours for at least 7 days

Inhalational anthrax: 500 mg every 24 hours for 60 days, beginning as soon as possible after exposure

Pneumonia:

Community-acquired: 500 mg every 24 hours for 7-14 days or 750 mg every 24 hours for 5 days (efficacy of 5-day regimen for MDRSP not established)

Nosocomial: 750 mg every 24 hours for 7-14 days

Prostatitis (chronic bacterial): 500 mg every 24 hours for 28 days

Skin infections:

Uncomplicated: 500 mg every 24 hours for 7-10 days

Complicated: 750 mg every 24 hours for 7-14 days

Urinary tract infections:

Uncomplicated: 250 mg once daily for 3 days

Complicated, including acute pyelonephritis: 250 mg every 24 hours for 10 days

Ophthalmic:

Conjunctivitis (0.5% ophthalmic solution): Children ≥1 year and Adults:

Treatment day 1 and day 2: Instill 1-2 drops into affected eye(s) every 2 hours while awake, up to 8 times/day

Treatment day 3 through day 7: Instill 1-2 drops into affected eye(s) every 4 hours while awake, up to 4 times/day

Corneal ulceration (1.5% ophthalmic solution): Children ≥6 years and Adults:

Treatment day 1 through day 3: Instill 1-2 drops into affected eye(s) every 30 minutes to 2 hours while awake and ~4-6 hours after retiring.

Treatment day 4 to treatment completion: Instill 1-2 drops into affected eye(s) every 1-4 hours while awake.

Dosing adjustment in renal impairment:

Chronic bronchitis, acute bacterial sinusitis, uncomplicated skin infection, community-acquired pneumonia, chronic bacterial prostatitis, or inhalational anthrax: Initial: 500 mg, then as follows:

Cl_{cr} 20-49 mL/minute: 250 mg every 24 hours

Cl_{cr} 10-19 mL/minute: 250 mg every 48 hours

Hemodialysis/CAPD: 250 mg every 48 hours

Uncomplicated UTI: No dosage adjustment required

Complicated UTI, acute pyelonephritis: Cl_{cr} 10-19 mL/minute: 250 mg every 48 hours

Complicated skin infection, acute bacterial sinusitis, community-acquired pneumonia, or nosocomial pneumonia: Initial: 750 mg, then as follows:

Cl_{cr} 20-49 mL/minute: 750 mg every 48 hours

Cl_{cr} 10-19 mL/minute: 500 mg every 48 hours

Hemodialysis/CAPD: 500 mg every 48 hours

Dietary Considerations Tablets may be taken without regard to meals. Oral solution should be administered on an empty stomach (1 hour before or 2 hours after a meal).

Administration

Oral: Tablets may be administered without regard to meals. Oral solution should be administered 1 hour before or 2 hours after meals.

I.V.: Infuse 250-500 mg I.V. solution over 60 minutes; infuse 750 mg I.V. solution over 90 minutes. Too rapid of infusion can lead to hypotension. Avoid administration through an intravenous line with a solution containing multivalent cations (eg, magnesium, calcium).

Monitoring Parameters Evaluation of organ system functions (renal, hepatic, ophthalmologic, and hematopoietic) is recommended periodically during therapy; the possibility of crystalluria should be assessed; WBC and signs of infection

Patient Information

Oral: Take per recommended schedule, preferably on an empty stomach (1 hour before or 2 hours after meals). Maintain adequate hydration (2-3 L/day of fluids unless instructed to restrict fluid intake). Take entire course of medication. Do not

(Continued)

Levofloxacin *(Continued)*

take with antacids; separate by 2 hours. You may experience dizziness, lightheadedness, or confusion; use caution when driving or engaging in tasks that require alertness until response to drug is known. Small frequent meals and frequent mouth care may reduce nausea or vomiting. You may experience photosensitivity; use sunscreen, wear protective clothing and eyewear, and avoid direct sunlight. Report palpitations or chest pain, persistent diarrhea, GI disturbances or abdominal pain, muscle tremor or pain, yellowing of eyes or skin, easy bruising or bleeding, unusual fatigue, fever, chills, signs of infection, or worsening of condition. Report immediately any rash, itching, unusual CNS changes, or any facial swelling. Report immediately any pain, inflammation, or rupture of tendon.

Ophthalmic: Wash hands before instilling solution. Sit or lie down to instill. Open eye, look at ceiling, and instill prescribed amount of solution. Close eye and roll eye in all directions, and apply gentle pressure to inner corner of eye. Do not let tip of applicator touch eye or contaminate tip of applicator. Temporary stinging or blurred vision may occur. Report persistent pain, burning, vision disturbances, swelling, itching, or worsening of condition. Discontinue medication and contact prescriber immediately if you develop a rash or allergic reaction. Do not wear contact lenses.

Dosage Forms

Infusion [premixed in D_5W] (Levaquin®): 250 mg (50 mL); 500 mg (100 mL); 750 mg (150 mL)

Injection, solution [preservative free] (Levaquin®): 25 mg/mL (20 mL, 30 mL)

Solution, ophthalmic:
- Iquix®: 1.5% (5 mL)
- Quixin™: 0.5% (5 mL) [contains benzalkonium chloride]

Solution, oral (Levaquin®): 25 mg/mL (480 mL) [contains benzyl alcohol]

Tablet (Levaquin®): 250 mg, 500 mg, 750 mg
- Levaquin® Leva-Pak: 750 mg (5s)

Selected Readings

Ernst ME, Ernst EJ, and Klepser ME, "Levofloxacin and Trovafloxacin: The Next Generation of Fluoroquinolones?" *Am J Health Syst Pharm*, 1997, 54(22):2569-84.

Hoogkamp-Korstanje JA, "*In vitro* Activities of Ciprofloxacin, Levofloxacin, Lomefloxacin, Ofloxacin, Pefloxacin, Sparfloxacin, and Trovafloxacin Against Gram-Positive and Gram-Negative Pathogens From Respiratory Tract Infections," *J Antimicrob Chemother*, 1997, 40(3):427-31.

Martin SJ, Meyer JM, Chuck SK, et al, "Levofloxacin and Sparfloxacin: New Quinolone Antibiotics," *Ann Pharmacother*, 1998, 32(3):320-36.

North DS, Fish DN, and Redington JJ, "Levofloxacin, A Second-Generation Fluoroquinolone," *Pharmacotherapy*, 1998, 18(5):915-35.

Pfaller MA and Jones RN, "Comparative Antistreptococcal Activity of Two Newer Fluoroquinolones, Levofloxacin and Sparfloxacin," *Diagn Microbiol Infect Dis*, 1997, 29(3):199-201.

"Sparfloxacin and Levofloxacin," *Med Lett Drugs Ther*, 1997, 39(999):41-3.

Lexiva™ *see* Fosamprenavir *on page 827*

Lice-Aid [OTC] *see* Pyrethrins and Piperonyl Butoxide *on page 1023*

Licide® [OTC] *see* Pyrethrins and Piperonyl Butoxide *on page 1023*

LID-Pack® (Can) *see* Bacitracin and Polymyxin B *on page 681*

Lin-Amox (Can) *see* Amoxicillin *on page 642*

Lincocin® *see* Lincomycin *on page 912*

Lincomycin (lin koe MYE sin)

U.S. Brand Names Lincocin®

Canadian Brand Names Lincocin®

Synonyms Lincomycin Hydrochloride

Generic Available No

Use Treatment of susceptible bacterial infections, mainly those caused by streptococci and staphylococci resistant to other agents

Pregnancy Risk Factor B

Contraindications Hypersensitivity to lincomycin, any component of the formulation, or clindamycin; minor bacterial infections or viral infections

Adverse Reactions Frequency not defined.

Central nervous system: Vertigo
Dermatologic: Vesiculobullous dermatitis (rare)
Gastrointestinal: Nausea, vomiting, diarrhea
Hematologic: Pancytopenia (rare)
Miscellaneous: Serum sickness (rare)

Drug Interactions

Increased Effect/Toxicity: Increased activity/toxicity of neuromuscular blocking agents.

Decreased Effect: Decreased effect with erythromycin.

Ethanol/Nutrition/Herb Interactions Food: May decrease absorption of lincomycin.

Stability Store capsules in a lightproof container.

Mechanism of Action Lincosamide antibiotic which was isolated from a strain of *Streptomyces lincolnensis*; lincomycin, like clindamycin, inhibits bacterial protein synthesis by specifically binding on the 50S subunit and affecting the process of peptide chain initiation. Other macrolide antibiotics (erythromycin) also bind to the 50S subunit. Since only one molecule of antibiotic can bind to a single ribosome, the concomitant use of erythromycin and lincomycin is not recommended.

Pharmacodynamics/Kinetics

Absorption: Oral: ~20% to 30%

Half-life elimination, serum: 2-11.5 hours

Time to peak, serum: Oral: 2-4 hours; I.M.: 1 hour

Dosage

Children >1 month:

Oral: 30-60 mg/kg/day in divided doses every 8 hours

I.M.: 10 mg/kg every 8-12 hours

I.V.: 10-20 mg/kg/day in divided doses every 8-12 hours

Adults:

Oral: 500 mg every 6-8 hours

I.M.: 600 mg every 12-24 hours

I.V.: 600-1 g every 8-12 hours up to 8 g/day

Dosing interval in renal impairment:

Cl_{cr} 10-50 mL/minute: Administer every 6-12 hours

Cl_{cr} <10 mL/minute: Administer every 12 hours

Dosing adjustment in hepatic impairment: Reductions are indicated; however, no specific guidelines are available

Dietary Considerations Should be taken on empty stomach with water.

Administration Administer oral dosage form with a full glass of water to minimize esophageal ulceration; administer around-the-clock to promote less variation in peak and trough serum levels

Dosage Forms Injection, solution, as hydrochloride: 300 mg/mL (2 mL, 10 mL) [contains benzyl alcohol]

Lincomycin Hydrochloride *see* Lincomycin *on page 912*

Lindane (LIN dane)

Canadian Brand Names Hexit™; PMS-Lindane

Synonyms Benzene Hexachloride; Gamma Benzene Hexachloride; Hexachlorocyclohexane

Generic Available Yes

Use Treatment of *Sarcoptes scabiei* (scabies), *Pediculus capitis* (head lice), and *Phthirus pubis* (crab lice); FDA recommends reserving lindane as a second-line agent or with inadequate response to other therapies

Drug of Choice or Alternative for Organism(s):

Lice *on page 207*

Sarcoptes scabiei on page 293

Restrictions An FDA-approved medication guide is available at www.fda.gov/cder/Offices/ODS/labeling.htm; distribute to each patient to whom this medication is dispensed.

Pregnancy Risk Factor C

Pregnancy Implications There are no well-controlled studies in pregnant women.

Contraindications Hypersensitivity to lindane or any component of the formulation; uncontrolled seizure disorders; crusted (Norwegian) scabies, acutely-inflamed skin or raw, weeping surfaces or other skin conditions which may increase systemic absorption

Warnings/Precautions Not considered a drug of first choice; seizures and death have been reported with use; use with caution in infants, small children, patients <50 kg, or patients with a history of seizures; use caution with conditions which may increase risk of seizures or medications which decrease seizure threshold; use caution with hepatic impairment; avoid contact with face, eyes, mucous membranes, and urethral meatus. Because of the potential for systemic absorption and CNS side effects, lindane should be used with caution; consider permethrin or crotamiton agent first. Oil-based hair dressing may increase toxic potential. A lindane medication use guide must be given to all patients along with instructions for proper use. Should be used as a part of an overall lice management program.

Adverse Reactions Frequency not defined (includes postmarketing and/or case reports).

Cardiovascular: Cardiac arrhythmia

Central nervous system: Ataxia, dizziness, headache, restlessness, seizure, pain

(Continued)

Lindane *(Continued)*

Dermatologic: Alopecia, contact dermatitis, skin and adipose tissue may act as repositories, eczematous eruptions, pruritus, urticaria
Gastrointestinal: Nausea, vomiting
Hematologic: Aplastic anemia
Hepatic: Hepatitis
Local: Burning and stinging
Neuromuscular & skeletal: Paresthesias
Renal: Hematuria
Respiratory: Pulmonary edema

Overdosage/Toxicology Symptoms include vomiting, restlessness, ataxia, seizures, arrhythmias, pulmonary edema, hematuria, and hepatitis. The drug is absorbed through skin, mucous membranes, and the GI tract. When used excessively for prolonged periods or when accidental ingestion has occurred, the drug has occasionally caused serious CNS, hepatic, and renal toxicity. If ingested, perform gastric lavage and general supportive measures. Diazepam 0.01 mg/kg can be used to control seizures.

Drug Interactions

Increased Effect/Toxicity: Increased toxicity: Drugs which lower seizure threshold

Mechanism of Action Directly absorbed by parasites and ova through the exoskeleton; stimulates the nervous system resulting in seizures and death of parasitic arthropods

Pharmacodynamics/Kinetics

Absorption: ≤13% systemically
Distribution: Stored in body fat; accumulates in brain; skin and adipose tissue may act as repositories
Metabolism: Hepatic
Half-life elimination: Children: 17-22 hours
Time to peak, serum: Children: 6 hours
Excretion: Urine and feces

Dosage Children and Adults: Topical:

Scabies: Apply a thin layer of lotion and massage it on skin from the neck to the toes; after 8-12 hours, bathe and remove the drug
Head lice, crab lice: Apply shampoo to dry hair and massage into hair for 4 minutes; add small quantities of water to hair until lather forms, then rinse hair thoroughly and comb with a fine tooth comb to remove nits. Amount of shampoo needed is based on length and density of hair; most patients will require 30 mL (maximum: 60 mL).

Administration For topical use only; never administer orally. Caregivers should apply with gloves (avoid natural latex, may be permeable to lindane). Rinse off with warm (not hot) water.

Lotion: Apply to dry, cool skin; do not apply to face or eyes. Wait at least 1 hour after bathing or showering (wet or warm skin increases absorption). Skin should be clean and free of any other lotions, creams, or oil prior to lindane application.
Shampoo: Apply to clean, dry hair. Wait at least 1 hour after washing hair before applying lindane shampoo. Hair should be washed with a shampoo not containing a conditioner; hair and skin of head and neck should be free of any lotions, oils, or creams prior to lindane application.

Patient Information Topical use only, do not apply to face, avoid getting in eyes; do **not** apply lotion immediately after a hot, soapy bath. For scabies, Apply from neck to toes. Bathe to remove drug after 8-12 hours. For head lice or crab lice, massage into dry hair for 4 minutes; add water to hair to form lather, then rinse thoroughly. Clothing and bedding should be washed in hot water or by dry cleaning to kill the scabies mite. Combs and brushes may be washed with lindane shampoo then thoroughly rinsed with water. Notify prescriber if condition worsens; treat sexual contact simultaneously.

Dosage Forms

Lotion, topical: 1% (60 mL)
Shampoo, topical: 1% (60 mL) [contains alcohol 0.5%]

Selected Readings

Liu LX and Weller PF, "Antiparasitic Drugs," *N Engl J Med*, 1996, 334(18):1178-84.

Linezolid (li NE zoh lid)

Related Information

Antimicrobial Activity Against Selected Organisms *on page 1165*
Community-Acquired Pneumonia in Adults *on page 1278*

U.S. Brand Names Zyvox™

Canadian Brand Names Zyvoxam®

Generic Available No

Use Treatment of vancomycin-resistant *Enterococcus faecium* (VRE) infections, nosocomial pneumonia caused by *Staphylococcus aureus* including MRSA or *Streptococcus pneumoniae* (including multidrug-resistant strains [MDRSP]), complicated and uncomplicated skin and skin structure infections (including diabetic foot infections without concomitant osteomyelitis), and community-acquired pneumonia caused by susceptible gram-positive organisms

Drug of Choice or Alternative for Disease/Syndrome(s):

Osteomyelitis, Diabetic Foot *on page 249*
Pneumonia, Hospital-Acquired *on page 272*
Pneumonia, Ventilator-Associated *on page 273*

Organism(s):

Enterococcus Species *on page 134*
Staphylococcus aureus, Methicillin-Resistant *on page 304*
Staphylococcus aureus, Methicillin-Susceptible *on page 307*

Pregnancy Risk Factor C

Pregnancy Implications Teratogenic effects were not observed in animal studies. There are no adequate and well-controlled studies in pregnant women. Should be used in pregnancy only if the potential benefit justifies the risk to the fetus.

Contraindications Hypersensitivity to linezolid or any other component of the formulation

Warnings/Precautions Myelosuppression has been reported and may be dependent on duration of therapy (generally >2 weeks of treatment); use with caution in patients with pre-existing myelosuppression, in patients receiving other drugs which may cause bone marrow suppression, or in chronic infection (previous or concurrent antibiotic therapy). Weekly CBC monitoring is recommended. Discontinue linezolid in patients developing myelosuppression (or in whom myelosuppression worsens during treatment).

Lactic acidosis has been reported with use. Patients who develop recurrent nausea and vomiting, unexplained acidosis, or low bicarbonate levels need immediate evaluation.

Linezolid exhibits mild MAO inhibitor properties and has the potential to have the same interactions as other MAO inhibitors; use with caution in uncontrolled hypertension, pheochromocytoma, carcinoid syndrome, or untreated hyperthyroidism; avoid use with serotonergic agents such as TCAs, venlafaxine, trazodone, sibutramine, meperidine, dextromethorphan, and SSRIs; concomitant use has been associated with the development of serotonin syndrome. Unnecessary use may lead to the development of resistance to linezolid; consider alternatives before initiating outpatient treatment,

Peripheral and optic neuropathy (with vision loss) has been reported and may occur primarily with extended courses of therapy >28 days; any symptoms of visual change or impairment warrant immediate ophthalmic evaluation and possible discontinuation of therapy.

Adverse Reactions Percentages as reported in adults; frequency similar in pediatric patients

>10%:

Central nervous system: Headache (<1% to 11%)
Gastrointestinal: Diarrhea (3% to 11%)

1% to 10%:

Central nervous system: Insomnia (3%), dizziness (0.4% to 2%), fever (2%)
Dermatologic: Rash (2%)
Gastrointestinal: Nausea (3% to 10%), vomiting (1% to 4%), pancreatic enzymes increased (<1% to 4%), constipation (2%), taste alteration (1% to 2%), tongue discoloration (0.2% to 1%), oral moniliasis (0.4% to 1%), pancreatitis
Genitourinary: Vaginal moniliasis (1% to 2%)
Hematologic: Thrombocytopenia (0.3% to 10%), hemoglobin decreased (0.9% to 7%), anemia, leukopenia, neutropenia; **Note:** Myelosuppression (including anemia, leukopenia, pancytopenia, and thrombocytopenia; may be more common in patients receiving linezolid for >2 weeks)
Hepatic: Abnormal LFTs (0.4% to 1%)
Renal: BUN increased (<1% to 2%)
Miscellaneous: Fungal infection (0.1% to 2%), lactate dehydrogenase increased (<1% to 2%)

<1% or frequency not defined: Blurred vision, *C. difficile*-related complications, creatinine increased, dyspepsia, hypertension, localized abdominal pain, pruritus

Postmarketing and/or case reports: Lactic acidosis, peripheral neuropathy, optic neuropathy, serotonin syndrome (with concurrent use of other serotonergic agents)

(Continued)

Linezolid *(Continued)*

Overdosage/Toxicology Treatment is supportive. Hemodialysis may improve elimination (30% of a dose is removed during a 3-hour hemodialysis session).

Drug Interactions

Increased Effect/Toxicity: Linezolid is a reversible, nonselective inhibitor of MAO. Serotonergic agents (eg, TCAs, venlafaxine, trazodone, sibutramine, meperidine, dextromethorphan, and SSRIs) may cause a serotonin syndrome (eg, hyperpyrexia, cognitive dysfunction) when used concomitantly. Adrenergic agents (eg, phenylpropanolamine, pseudoephedrine, sympathomimetic agents, vasopressor or dopaminergic agents) may cause hypertension. Tramadol may increase the risk of seizures when used concurrently with linezolid. Myelosuppressive medications may increase risk of myelosuppression when used concurrently with linezolid.

Ethanol/Nutrition/Herb Interactions

Ethanol: Avoid ethanol (may contain tyramine, hypertensive crisis may result).

Food: Avoid foods (eg, cheese) and beverages containing tyramine in patients receiving linezolid (hypertensive crisis may result).

Stability

Infusion: Store at 25°C (77°F). Protect from light. Keep infusion bags in overwrap until ready for use. Protect infusion bags from freezing.

Oral suspension: Following reconstitution, store at room temperature; use reconstituted suspension within 21 days

Mechanism of Action Inhibits bacterial protein synthesis by binding to bacterial 23S ribosomal RNA of the 50S subunit. This prevents the formation of a functional 70S initiation complex that is essential for the bacterial translation process. Linezolid is bacteriostatic against enterococci and staphylococci and bactericidal against most strains of streptococci.

Pharmacodynamics/Kinetics

Absorption: Rapid and extensive

Distribution: V_{dss}: Adults: 40-50 L

Protein binding: Adults: 31%

Metabolism: Hepatic via oxidation of the morpholine ring, resulting in two inactive metabolites (aminoethoxyacetic acid, hydroxyethyl glycine); does not involve CYP

Bioavailability: 100%

Half-life elimination: Children ≥1 week (full-term) to 11 years: 1.5-3 hours; Adults: 4-5 hours

Time to peak: Adults: Oral: 1-2 hours

Excretion: Urine (30% as parent drug, 50% as metabolites); feces (9% as metabolites)

Nonrenal clearance: 65%; increased in children ≥1 week to 11 years

Dosage

VRE infections: Oral, I.V.:

Preterm neonates (<34 weeks gestational age): 10 mg/kg every 12 hours; neonates with a suboptimal clinical response can be advanced to 10 mg/kg every 8 hours. By day 7 of life, all neonates should receive 10 mg/kg every 8 hours.

Infants (excluding preterm neonates <1 week) and Children ≤11 years: 10 mg/kg every 8 hours for 14-28 days

Children ≥12 years and Adults: 600 mg every 12 hours for 14-28 days

Nosocomial pneumonia, complicated skin and skin structure infections, community acquired pneumonia including concurrent bacteremia: Oral, I.V.:

Infants (excluding preterm neonates <1 week) and Children ≤11 years: 10 mg/kg every 8 hours for 10-14 days

Children ≥12 years and Adults: 600 mg every 12 hours for 10-14 days

Uncomplicated skin and skin structure infections: Oral:

Infants (excluding preterm neonates <1 week) and Children <5 years: 10 mg/kg every 8 hours for 10-14 days

Children 5-11 years: 10 mg/kg every 12 hours for 10-14 days

Children ≥12-18 years: 600 mg every 12 hours for 10-14 days

Adults: 400 mg every 12 hours for 10-14 days

Elderly: No dosage adjustment required

Dosage adjustment in renal impairment: No adjustment is recommended. The two primary metabolites may accumulate in patients with renal impairment but the clinical significance is unknown. Weigh the risk of accumulation of metabolites versus the benefit of therapy. Both linezolid and the two metabolites are eliminated by dialysis. Linezolid should be given after hemodialysis.

Dosage adjustment in hepatic impairment: No dosage adjustment required for mild to moderate hepatic insufficiency (Child-Pugh Class A or B). Use in severe hepatic insufficiency has not been adequately evaluated.

Dietary Considerations Take with or without food. Avoid foods with high tyramine content (eg, pickled or fermented foods, cheese, beer and wine). Suspension

contains 20 mg phenylalanine per teaspoonful. Sodium content: 0.1 mEq/tablet; 0.4 mEq/5 mL; 1.7 mEq/100 mL infusion; 3.3 mEq/200 mL infusion; 5 mEq/300 mL infusion

Administration

I.V.: Administer intravenous infusion over 30-120 minutes. Do not mix or infuse with other medications. When the same intravenous line is used for sequential infusion of other medications, flush line with D_5W, NS, or LR before and after infusing linezolid. The yellow color of the injection may intensify over time without affecting potency.

Oral suspension: Invert gently to mix prior to administration, do not shake.

Monitoring Parameters Weekly CBC and platelet counts, particularly in patients at increased risk of bleeding, with pre-existing myelosuppression, on concomitant medications that cause bone marrow suppression, in those who require >2 weeks of therapy, or in those with chronic infection who have received previous or concomitant antibiotic therapy; visual function with extended therapy (≥3 months) or in patients with new onset visual symptoms, regardless of therapy length

Patient Information Take with or without food. Take with food if medicine causes stomach upset. Tell your prescriber if you have hypertension or are taking any cold remedy or decongestant. Limit quantities of tyramine-containing foods. Gently mix suspension. Store at room temperature. Notify your prescriber if you feel very weak, have any bleeding problems, bruising, new signs/symptoms of infection, shortness of breath, rapid heartbeats, or weight loss.

Dosage Forms

Infusion [premixed]: 200 mg (100 mL) [contains sodium 1.7 mEq]; 400 mg (200 mL) [contains sodium 3.3 mEq]; 600 mg (300 mL) [contains sodium 5 mEq]

Powder for oral suspension: 20 mg/mL (150 mL) [contains phenylalanine 20 mg/5 mL, sodium benzoate, and sodium 0.4 mEq/5 mL; orange flavor]

Tablet: 600 mg [contains sodium 0.1 mEq/tablet]

Selected Readings

Bain KT and Wittbrodt ET, "Linezolid for the Treatment of Resistant Gram-Positive Cocci," *Ann Pharmacother*, 2001, 35(5):566-75.

Ford C, Hamel J, Stapert D, et al, "Oxazolidinones: A New Class of Antimicrobials," *Infect Med*, 1999, 16:435-45.

Perry CM and Jarvis B, "Linezolid: A Review of Its Use in the Management of Serious Gram-Positive Infections," *Drugs*, 2001, 61(4):525-51.

Sisson TL, Jungbluth GL, and Hopkins NK, "A Pharmacokinetic Evaluation of Concomitant Administration of Linezolid and Aztreonam," *J Clin Pharmacol*, 1999, 39(12):1277-82.

Lin-Megestrol (Can) *see* Megestrol *on page 932*

Lomefloxacin (loe me FLOKS a sin)

Related Information

Antimicrobial Activity Against Selected Organisms *on page 1165*

U.S. Brand Names Maxaquin®

Synonyms Lomefloxacin Hydrochloride

Generic Available No

Use Acute bacterial exacerbation of chronic bronchitis caused by susceptible gram-negative organisms; urinary tract infections (uncomplicated and complicated) caused by susceptible organisms; surgical prophylaxis (transrectal prostate biopsy or transurethral procedures)

Pregnancy Risk Factor C

Pregnancy Implications Reports of arthropathy (observed in immature animals and reported rarely in humans) have limited the use of fluoroquinolones in pregnancy. Teratogenic effects were not observed with lomefloxacin in animal studies; however, an increase in fetal loss was observed in one species. Based on limited data, quinolones are not expected to be a major human teratogen. Although quinolone antibiotics should not be used as first-line agents during pregnancy, when considering treatment for life-threatening infection and/or prolonged duration of therapy, the potential risk to the fetus must be balanced against the severity of the potential illness.

Contraindications Hypersensitivity to lomefloxacin, any component of the formulation, or other members of the quinolone group (such as, nalidixic acid, oxolinic acid, cinoxacin, norfloxacin, and ciprofloxacin); avoid use in children <18 years of age due to association of other quinolones with transient arthropathies

Warnings/Precautions CNS stimulation may occur (tremor, restlessness, confusion, and very rarely hallucinations or seizures); use with caution in patients with known or suspected CNS disorders; use caution to avoid possible photosensitivity reactions during and for several days following fluoroquinolone therapy. Use caution in renal impairment; may require dosage adjustment. Severe hypersensitivity reactions, including anaphylaxis, have occurred with quinolone therapy. If an allergic reaction occurs (itching, urticaria, dyspnea or facial edema, loss of consciousness, tingling, cardiovascular collapse), discontinue drug immediately. Prolonged use may result in

(Continued)

Lomefloxacin *(Continued)*

superinfection; pseudomembranous colitis may occur and should be considered in all patients who present with diarrhea.

Rare incidence of peripheral neuropathy has been documented; discontinue if patient experiences symptoms of neuropathy including pain, burning, tingling, weakness or other sensory abnormalities. Tendon inflammation and/or rupture has been reported. Risk may be increased with concurrent corticosteroids, particularly in the elderly. Discontinue at first sign of tendon inflammation or pain. Quinolones may exacerbate myasthenia gravis; use with caution (rare, potentially life-threatening weakness of respiratory muscles may occur); avoid use in children <18 years of age due to association of other quinolones with transient arthropathies. Safety and efficacy has not been established in pediatric patients and adolescents <18 years of age, pregnant or lactating women.

Adverse Reactions

1% to 10%:

Central nervous system: Headache (4%), dizziness (2%)

Dermatologic: Photosensitivity (2%)

Gastrointestinal: Nausea (4%), abdominal pain (1%), diarrhea (1%)

<1% (Limited to important or life-threatening): Agranulocytosis, allergic reaction, anaphylaxis, angioedema, anemia, angina pectoris, anuria, arrhythmia, bradycardia, bronchospasm, BUN increased, cardiac failure, cardiomyopathy, cerebrovascular disorder, chest pain, coma, convulsions, creatinine increased, cyanosis, dyspnea, dysuria, electrolyte disturbances, eosinophilia, extrasystoles, fibrinolysis increased, hematuria, hepatitis, hepatic necrosis, hyper-/hypotension, hyper-/hypoglycemia, intestinal perforation, leukocytosis, leukopenia, liver function tests increased, MI, moniliasis, monocytosis, myasthenia gravis (exacerbation), paresthesia, peripheral neuropathy, pseudomembranous colitis, psychiatric disturbances, pulmonary edema, pulmonary embolism, purpura, QT_c prolongation, renal failure, stridor, Stevens-Johnson syndrome, syncope, tachycardia, thrombocythemia, thrombocytopenia, torsade de pointes, toxic epidermal necrolysis, urinary disorders, tendon rupture, tendonitis

Overdosage/Toxicology Symptoms include acute renal failure and seizures. Treatment consists of GI decontamination and supportive care. Administer diazepam for the treatment of seizures. Not removed by peritoneal or hemodialysis.

Drug Interactions

Cytochrome P450 Effect: Inhibits CYP1A2 (weak)

Increased Effect/Toxicity: Concomitant use with corticosteroids may increase the risk of tendon rupture. Probenecid may increase lomefloxacin levels.

Decreased Effect: Concurrent administration of metal cations, including most antacids, oral electrolyte supplements, quinapril, sucralfate, some didanosine formulations (chewable/buffered tablets and pediatric powder for oral suspension), and other highly-buffered oral drugs, may decrease quinolone level; separate doses.

Ethanol/Nutrition/Herb Interactions

Food: Lomefloxacin peak serum levels may be prolonged if taken with food.

Herb/Nutraceutical: Avoid dong quai, St John's wort (may cause photosensitization).

Mechanism of Action Inhibits DNA-gyrase in susceptible organisms thereby inhibits relaxation of supercoiled DNA and promotes breakage of DNA strands. DNA gyrase (topoisomerase II), is an essential bacterial enzyme that maintains the superhelical structure of DNA and is required for DNA replication and transcription, DNA repair, recombination, and transposition.

Pharmacodynamics/Kinetics

Absorption: Well absorbed (95% to 98%)

Distribution: V_d: 2.4-3.5 L/kg; into bronchus, prostatic tissue, and urine

Protein binding: 10%

Half-life elimination: 7.8 hours

Time to peak, plasma: 1.5 hours

Excretion: Urine (65% as unchanged drug, 9% as metabolite); feces (10% as unchanged drug)

Dosage Oral: Adults:

Acute bacterial exacerbation of chronic bronchitis: 400 mg once daily for 10 days

Urinary tract infection (UTI) due to susceptible organisms:

Uncomplicated cystitis caused by *Escherichia coli*: 400 mg once daily for 3 successive days

Uncomplicated cystitis caused by *Klebsiella pneumoniae*, *Proteus mirabilis*, or *Staphylococcus saprophyticus*: 400 mg once daily for 10 successive days

Complicated UTI caused by *Escherichia coli*, *Klebsiella pneumoniae*, *Proteus mirabilis*, or *Pseudomonas aeruginosa*: 400 mg once daily for 14 successive days

Urologic surgical prophylaxis:

Transrectal prostate biopsy: 400 mg as a single dose, 1-6 hours before procedure

Transurethral surgical procedure: 400 mg as a single dose, 2-6 hours before procedure

Elderly: Refer to Adults dosing

Dosing adjustment in renal impairment:

Cl_{cr} 11-39 mL/minute: Loading dose: 400 mg, then 200 mg every day

Hemodialysis: Same as for renal impairment

Dietary Considerations May be taken without regard to meals.

Administration Take 1 hour before or 2 hours after meals.

Dosage Forms Tablet: 400 mg

Selected Readings

Hooper DC and Wolfson JS, "Fluoroquinolone Antimicrobial Agents," *N Engl J Med*, 1991, 324(6):384-94.
Lomaestro BM and Bailie GR, "Quinolone-Cation Interactions: A Review," *DICP*, 1991, 25(11):1249-58.
Stein GE, "The 4-Quinolone Antibiotics: Past, Present, and Future," *Pharmacotherapy*, 1988, 8(6):301-14.
Walker RC and Wright AJ, "The Fluoroquinolones," *Mayo Clin Proc*, 1991, 66(12):1249-59.

Lomefloxacin Hydrochloride *see* Lomefloxacin *on page 917*

Lopinavir and Ritonavir (loe PIN a veer & rit ON uh veer)

Related Information

Antiretroviral Agents *on page 1206*
Antiretroviral Therapy for HIV Infection *on page 1219*
Management of Healthcare Worker Exposures to HBV, HCV, and HIV *on page 1227*

U.S. Brand Names Kaletra®

Canadian Brand Names Kaletra®

Synonyms Ritonavir and Lopinavir

Generic Available No

Use Treatment of HIV infection in combination with other antiretroviral agents

Drug of Choice or Alternative for Organism(s):

Human Immunodeficiency Virus *on page 181*

Pregnancy Risk Factor C

Pregnancy Implications Safety and pharmacokinetic studies in pregnant women are not completed. Preliminary information suggests increased dosage may be needed during pregnancy, although specific recommendations are not yet available. The Perinatal HIV Guidelines Working Group considers this combination an alternative PI agent for use during pregnancy. Pregnancy and protease inhibitors are both associated with an increased risk of hyperglycemia. Glucose levels should be closely monitored. Health professionals are encouraged to contact the antiretroviral pregnancy registry to monitor outcomes of pregnant women exposed to antiretroviral medications (1-800-258-4263 or www.APRegistry.com).

Contraindications Hypersensitivity to lopinavir, ritonavir, or any component of the formulation; administration with medications highly dependent upon CYP3A or CYP2D6 for clearance for which increased levels are associated with serious and/or life-threatening events; concomitant use with cisapride, dihydroergotamine, ergonovine, ergotamine, methylergonovine, midazolam, pimozide, triazolam, or voriconazole

Warnings/Precautions Associated with many potential drug interactions; concurrent use of azole antifungals (high dose), lovastatin, rifampin, and simvastatin is not recommended (per manufacturer). Avoid concurrent use of St John's wort (may lead to loss of virologic response and/or resistance). Cases of pancreatitis, some fatal, have been associated with lopinavir/ritonavir; use caution in patients with a history of pancreatitis. Patients with signs or symptoms of pancreatitis should be evaluated and therapy suspended as clinically appropriate. Diabetes mellitus and exacerbation of diabetes mellitus have been reported in patients taking protease inhibitors. Use caution in patients with hepatic impairment; patients with hepatitis or elevations in transaminases prior to the start of therapy may be at increased risk for further increases in transaminases or hepatic dysfunction (rare fatalities reported in postmarketing). Large increases in total cholesterol and triglycerides have been reported; screening should be done prior to therapy and periodically throughout treatment. Increased bleeding may be seen in patients with hemophilia A or B who are taking protease inhibitors. Redistribution or accumulation of body fat has been observed in patients using antiretroviral therapy. An inflammatory response to indolent or residual opportunistic infections (referred to as immune reconstitution syndrome) has occurred with the use of combination retroviral therapy, including Kaletra™; further evaluation and treatment may be required. The potential for cross-resistance with other protease inhibitors is currently under study. Safety and efficacy have not been established for children <6 months of age.

(Continued)

Lopinavir and Ritonavir *(Continued)*

Adverse Reactions Protease inhibitors cause dyslipidemia which includes elevated cholesterol and triglycerides and a redistribution of body fat centrally to cause increased abdominal girth, buffalo hump, facial atrophy, and breast enlargement. These agents also cause hyperglycemia.

>10%:

- Endocrine & metabolic: Hypercholesterolemia (9% to 39%), triglycerides increased (9% to 36%)
- Gastrointestinal: Diarrhea (5% to 27%), nausea (5% to 16%)
- Hepatic: GGT increased (6% to 29%)

2% to 10%:

- Central nervous system: Headache (2% to 7%), fever (2%), chills (up to 2%), depression (up to 2%), pain (up to 2%), insomnia (up to 2%)
- Dermatologic: Rash (up to 4%)
- Endocrine & metabolic: Hyperglycemia (1% to 5%), hyperuricemia (up to 3%), sodium decreased (3% children), inorganic phosphorus decreased (up to 2%), amylase increased (3% to 8%), libido decreased (2%)
- Gastrointestinal: Abnormal stools (up to 6%), abdominal pain (2% to 10%), vomiting (2% to 6%), dyspepsia (up to 5%), flatulence (1% to 4%), weight loss (up to 3%), dysphagia (up to 2%)
- Hematologic: Platelets decreased (4% children), neutrophils decreased (1% to 5%)
- Hepatic: AST increased (2% to 9%), ALT increased (4% to 10%), bilirubin increased (children 3%)
- Neuromuscular & skeletal: Weakness (up to 9%)
- Respiratory: Bronchitis (2%)

<2%:

- Cardiovascular: Atrial fibrillation, chest pain, cerebral infarction, deep vein thrombosis, edema, facial edema, palpitation, peripheral edema, varicose veins, vasculitis,
- Central nervous system: Abnormal dreams, abnormal thinking, agitation, amnesia, anxiety, apathy, ataxia, confusion, dizziness, emotional lability, encephalopathy, facial paralysis, malaise, migraine, nervousness, neuropathy, paresthesia, peripheral neuritis, seizure, somnolence, tremor, vertigo
- Dermatologic: Acne, alopecia, benign neoplasm, dry skin, exfoliative dermatitis, furunculosis, maculopapular rash, nail disorder, pruritus, seborrhea, skin discoloration, skin ulcer
- Endocrine & metabolic: Amenorrhea, breast enlargement, Cushing's syndrome, dehydration, diabetes mellitus, glucose intolerance, gynecomastia, hypothyroidism, lactic acidosis, weight gain
- Gastrointestinal: Anorexia, appetite increased, constipation, dry mouth, enteritis, enterocolitis, eructation, esophagitis, fecal incontinence, gastritis, gastroenteritis, gastrointestinal disorder, hemorrhagic colitis, pancreatitis, periodontitis, sialadenitis, stomatitis, taste perversion, ulcerative stomatitis
- Genitourinary: Abnormal ejaculation
- Hematologic: Anemia, leukopenia, lymphadenopathy
- Hepatic: Cholangitis, cholecystitis, hepatic dysfunction, jaundice
- Local: Thrombophlebitis
- Neuromuscular & skeletal: Arthralgia, arthrosis, back pain, dyskinesia, hypertonia, myalgia
- Ocular: Abnormal vision, eye disorder
- Otic: Otitis media, tinnitus
- Renal: Kidney calculus, nephritis, urine abnormality
- Respiratory: Asthma, dyspnea, lung edema, pharyngitis, rhinitis, sinusitis
- Miscellaneous: Avitaminosis, bacterial infection, bone necrosis, cyst, diaphoresis, flu-like syndrome, hypertrophy, obesity, viral infection

Postmarketing and/or case reports: Bradyarrhythmia, erythema multiforme, Stevens-Johnson syndrome

Overdosage/Toxicology The solution contains 42.4% alcohol. Overdosage in a child may cause alcohol-related toxicity and may be potentially lethal. Treatment should be symptomatic and supportive. Activated charcoal may aid in the removal of unabsorbed medication. Given extensive protein binding, hemodialysis is unlikely to be effective.

Drug Interactions

Cytochrome P450 Effect:

Lopinavir: **Substrate** of 3A4 (minor)

Ritonavir: **Substrate** of CYP1A2 (minor), 2B6 (minor), 2D6 (major), 3A4 (major); **Inhibits** CYP2C8/9 (weak), 2C19 (weak), 2D6 (strong), 2E1 (weak), 3A4 (strong); **Induces** CYP1A2 (weak), 2C8/9 (weak), 3A4 (weak)

Increased Effect/Toxicity: Concurrent use of cisapride, ergot alkaloids, (dihydroergotamine, ergonovine, methylergonovine), lovastatin, midazolam, pimozide, simvastatin, and triazolam is contraindicated. Alfuzosin serum level may be increased by ritonavir; concurrent use is contraindicated (by the manufacturer of ritonavir). Antiarrhythmic agents (including amiodarone, bepridil, flecainide, propafenone, lidocaine (systemic), and quinidine) should be used with caution; life-threatening arrhythmias may result from concurrent use.

Ritonavir may increase the levels/effects of amphetamines, selected beta-blockers, selected benzodiazepines (midazolam and triazolam contraindicated), calcium channel blockers, dextromethorphan, fluoxetine, lidocaine, HMG-CoA reductase inhibitors (lovastatin and simvastatin are not recommended), mesoridazine, mirtazapine, nateglinide, nefazodone, paroxetine, risperidone, sildenafil (and other PDE-5 inhibitors), thioridazine, tricyclic antidepressants, venlafaxine, and other substrates of CYP2D6 or 3A4. Mesoridazine and thioridazine are generally contraindicated with strong CYP2D6 inhibitors. When used with strong CYP3A4 inhibitors, dosage adjustment/limits are recommended for sildenafil and other PDE-5 inhibitors; refer to individual monographs. Warfarin levels/effects may also be increased. High dosages of itraconazole or ketoconazole (>200 mg/day) are not recommended.

Serum levels of protease inhibitors may be altered during concurrent therapy. Ritonavir may increase serum concentrations of amprenavir, indinavir, or saquinavir. Delavirdine increases levels of lopinavir; dosing recommendations are not yet established. Serum concentrations of corticosteroids (eg, budesonide, dexamethasone, fluticasone, prednisone) may be increased by lopinavir/ritonavir, resulting in decreased serum cortisol, HPA axis suppression; concurrent use is not recommended.

Lopinavir/ritonavir solution contains alcohol, concurrent use with disulfiram or metronidazole should be avoided. May cause disulfiram-like reaction. Serum concentrations of meperidine's neuroexcitatory metabolite (normeperidine) are increased by ritonavir, which may increase the risk of CNS toxicity/seizures. Rifabutin and rifabutin metabolite serum concentrations may be increased by ritonavir; reduce rifabutin dose to 150 mg every other day. Tenofovir serum concentration/effects may be increased by lopinavir/ritonavir. Trazodone serum concentration/effects may be increased by lopinavir/ritonavir; use caution and reduce trazodone dose.

Decreased Effect: The levels/effects of ritonavir may be decreased by aminoglutethimide, carbamazepine, nafcillin, nevirapine, phenobarbital, phenytoin, rifamycins, and other CYP3A4 inducers. Concurrent use of rifampin is not recommended. Ritonavir may decrease the levels/effects of CYP2D6 prodrug substrates (eg, codeine, hydrocodone, oxycodone, tramadol). Non-nucleoside reverse transcriptase inhibitors (efavirenz, nevirapine) may decrease levels of lopinavir. To avoid incompatibility with didanosine, administer didanosine 1 hour before or 2 hours after lopinavir/ritonavir. Decreased levels of ethinyl estradiol may result from concurrent use (alternative contraception is recommended). Lopinavir/ritonavir may decrease levels of abacavir, atovaquone, or zidovudine. Voriconazole serum levels are reduced by ritonavir (concurrent use is contraindicated; effect of lopinavir/ritonavir has not been evaluated). Lopinavir/ritonavir may decrease the concentration and effect of amprenavir when administered as fosamprenavir.

Ethanol/Nutrition/Herb Interactions Herb/Nutraceutical: St John's wort may decrease levels of protease inhibitors and lead to possible resistance; concurrent use in not recommended.

Stability Oral solution and gelatin capsules: Store at 2°C to 8°C (36°F to 46°F). Avoid exposure to excessive heat. If stored at room temperature (25°C or 77°F), use within 2 months.

Mechanism of Action A coformulation of lopinavir and ritonavir. The lopinavir component is the active inhibitor of HIV protease. Lopinavir inhibits HIV protease and renders the enzyme incapable of processing polyprotein precursor which leads to production of noninfectious immature HIV particles. The ritonavir component inhibits the CYP3A metabolism of lopinavir, allowing increased plasma levels of lopinavir.

Pharmacodynamics/Kinetics

Ritonavir: See Ritonavir monograph.

Lopinavir:

Protein binding: 98% to 99%; decreased with mild-to-moderate hepatic dysfunction

Metabolism: Hepatic via CYP3A; 13 metabolites identified

Half-life elimination: 5-6 hours

Excretion: Feces (83%, 20% as unchanged drug); urine (2%)

(Continued)

Lopinavir and Ritonavir *(Continued)*

Dosage Oral (take with food):

Children 6 months to 12 years: Dosage based on weight, presented based on mg of lopinavir (maximum dose: Lopinavir 400 mg/ritonavir 100 mg)

7-<15 kg: 12 mg/kg twice daily

15-40 kg: 10 mg/kg twice daily

>40 kg: Refer to adult dosing. **Note:** Once-daily dosing regimen has not been evaluated in pediatric patients.

Children >12 years and Adults:

Therapy-naive: Lopinavir 800 mg/ritonavir 200 mg once daily **or** lopinavir 400 mg/ritonavir 100 mg twice daily

Therapy-experienced: Lopinavir 400 mg/ritonavir 100 mg twice daily

Note: Once-daily dosing regimen has not been evaluated with concurrent indinavir or saquinavir and should not be used with concomitant phenytoin, carbamazepine, or phenobarbital therapy.

Dosage adjustment when taken with amprenavir, efavirenz, nelfinavir, or nevirapine:

Note: Once-daily dosing regimen should not be used when concomitantly taking amprenavir, efavirenz, nelfinavir, or nevirapine therapy.

Children 6 months to 12 years:

7-<15 kg: 13 mg/kg twice daily

15-45 kg: 11 mg/kg twice daily

>45 kg: Refer to adult dosing

Note: In the USHHS guidelines, the cutoff for adult dosing is 50 kg. (Pediatric Guidelines - March 24, 2005, are available at http://www.aidsinfo.nih.gov)

Children >12 years and Adults: Lopinavir 533 mg/ritonavir 133 mg twice daily

Elderly: Initial studies did not include enough elderly patients to determine effects based on age. Use with caution due to possible decreased hepatic, renal, and cardiac function.

Dosage adjustment in renal impairment: Has not been studied in patients with renal impairment; however, a decrease in clearance is not expected

Dosage adjustment in hepatic impairment: Plasma levels may be increased in patients with mild-to-moderate hepatic impairment. Lopinavir's AUC may be increased by 30%.

Dietary Considerations Should be taken with food.

Administration Administer with food; if using didanosine, take didanosine 1 hour before or 2 hours after lopinavir/ritonavir

Monitoring Parameters Triglycerides, cholesterol, LFTs, electrolytes, basic HIV monitoring, viral load and CD4 count, glucose

Patient Information This medication will be used with other medications to treat HIV infection. Take medication daily as prescribed. Take with food. Do not change doses or discontinue without contacting prescriber. It is important to find out what other medications cannot be taken with this medication. Do not take any prescription medications, over-the-counter products or herbal products, especially St John's wort, without consulting prescriber. May interfere with certain oral contraceptives; alternate contraceptive measures may be needed.

Dosage Forms

Capsule: Lopinavir 133.3 mg and ritonavir 33.3 mg

Solution, oral: Lopinavir 80 mg and ritonavir 20 mg per mL (160 mL) [contains alcohol 42.4%]

Selected Readings

Mangum EM and Graham KK, "Lopinavir-Ritonavir: A New Protease Inhibitor," *Pharmacotherapy*, 2001, 21(11):1352-63.

Loprox® *see* Ciclopirox *on page 739*

Lorabid® *see* Loracarbef *on page 922*

Loracarbef (lor a KAR bef)

Related Information

Antimicrobial Activity Against Selected Organisms *on page 1165*

U.S. Brand Names Lorabid®

Canadian Brand Names Lorabid®

Generic Available No

Use Infections caused by susceptible organisms involving the respiratory tract, acute otitis media, sinusitis, skin and skin structure, bone and joint, and urinary tract and gynecologic

Pregnancy Risk Factor B

Contraindications Hypersensitivity to loracarbef, any component of the formulation, or cephalosporins

Warnings/Precautions Modify dosage in patients with severe renal impairment; prolonged use may result in superinfection; use with caution in patients with a previous history of hypersensitivity to other beta-lactam antibiotics (eg, penicillins, cephalosporins)

Adverse Reactions

≥1%:

Central nervous system: Headache (1% to 3%), somnolence (<2%)

Dermatologic: Rash (1% to 3%)

Gastrointestinal: Diarrhea (4% to 6%), nausea (2%), vomiting (1% to 3%), anorexia (<2%), abdominal pain (1%)

Genitourinary: Vaginitis (1%)

Respiratory: Rhinitis (2% to 6%)

<1%: Anaphylaxis, arthralgia, candidiasis, cholestasis, eosinophilia, hemolytic anemia, interstitial nephritis, jaundice, nephrotoxicity with transient elevations of BUN/creatinine, nervousness, neutropenia, positive Coombs' test, pruritus, pseudomembranous colitis, seizure (with high doses and renal dysfunction), serum sickness-like reaction, slightly increased AST/ALT, Stevens-Johnson syndrome, thrombocytopenia, urticaria

Overdosage/Toxicology Symptoms include abdominal discomfort and diarrhea. Treatment is supportive only.

Drug Interactions

Increased Effect/Toxicity: Loracarbef serum levels are increased with coadministered probenecid.

Ethanol/Nutrition/Herb Interactions Food: Administration with food decreases and delays the peak plasma concentration.

Stability Suspension may be kept at room temperature for 14 days

Mechanism of Action Inhibits bacterial cell wall synthesis by binding to one or more of the penicillin binding proteins (PBPs); inhibits the final transpeptidation step of peptidoglycan synthesis in bacterial cell walls, thus inhibiting cell wall biosynthesis. It is thought that beta-lactam antibiotics inactivate transpeptidase via acylation of the enzyme with cleavage of the CO-N bond of the beta-lactam ring. Upon exposure to beta-lactam antibiotics, bacteria eventually lyse due to ongoing activity of cell wall autolytic enzymes (autolysins and murein hydrolases) while cell wall assembly is arrested.

Pharmacodynamics/Kinetics

Absorption: Rapid

Half-life elimination: ~1 hour

Time to peak, serum: ~1 hour

Excretion: Clearance: Plasma: ~200-300 mL/minute

Dosage Oral:

Children:

Acute otitis media: 15 mg/kg twice daily for 10 days

Pharyngitis and impetigo: 7.5-15 mg/kg twice daily for 10 days

Adults:

Uncomplicated urinary tract infections: 200 mg once daily for 7 days

Skin and soft tissue: 200-400 mg every 12-24 hours

Uncomplicated pyelonephritis: 400 mg every 12 hours for 14 days

Upper/lower respiratory tract infection: 200-400 mg every 12-24 hours for 7-14 days

Dosing comments in renal impairment:

Cl_{cr} 10-49 mL/minute: 50% of usual dose at usual interval or usual dose given half as often

Cl_{cr} <10 mL/minute: Administer usual dose every 3-5 days

Hemodialysis: Doses should be administered after dialysis sessions

Dietary Considerations Should be taken on an empty stomach at least 1 hour before or 2 hours after meals.

Administration Take on an empty stomach at least 1 hour before or 2 hours after meals. Finish all medication. Shake suspension well before using.

Patient Information Take as directed, preferably on an empty stomach (1 hour before or 2 hours after meals). Take entire prescription even if feeling better. Shake suspension well before using. Maintain adequate hydration (2-3 L/day of fluids unless instructed to restrict fluid intake). Report immediately any signs of skin rash, joint or back pain, or difficulty breathing. Report unusual fever, chills, vaginal itching or foul-smelling vaginal discharge, or easy bruising or bleeding.

Dosage Forms

Capsule: 200 mg, 400 mg

Powder for oral suspension: 100 mg/5 mL (100 mL); 200 mg/5 mL (100 mL) [strawberry bubble gum flavor]

(Continued)

Loracarbef *(Continued)*

Selected Readings

Force RW and Nahata MC, "Loracarbef: A New Orally Administered Carbacephem Antibiotic," *Ann Pharmacother*, 1993, 27(3):321-9.

Marshall WF and Blair JE, "The Cephalosporins," *Mayo Clin Proc*, 1999, 74(2):187-95.

Schatz BS, Karavokiros KT, Taeubel MA, et al, "Comparison of Cefprozil, Cefpodoxime Proxetil, Loracarbef, Cefixime, and Ceftibuten," *Ann Pharmacother*, 1996, 30(3):258-68.

Lotriderm® (Can) *see* Betamethasone and Clotrimazole *on page 685*

Lotrimin® AF Athlete's Foot Cream [OTC] *see* Clotrimazole *on page 758*

Lotrimin® AF Athlete's Foot Solution [OTC] *see* Clotrimazole *on page 758*

Lotrimin® AF Jock Itch Cream [OTC] *see* Clotrimazole *on page 758*

Lotrimin® AF Powder/Spray [OTC] *see* Miconazole *on page 945*

Lotrimin® Ultra™ [OTC] *see* Butenafine *on page 691*

Lotrisone® *see* Betamethasone and Clotrimazole *on page 685*

LY146032 *see* Daptomycin *on page 768*

M-M-R® II *see* Measles, Mumps, and Rubella Vaccines (Combined) *on page 926*

Macrobid® *see* Nitrofurantoin *on page 971*

Macrodantin® *see* Nitrofurantoin *on page 971*

Macrolides

Refer to

Azithromycin *on page 674*
Clarithromycin *on page 749*
Dirithromycin *on page 786*
Erythromycin and Sulfisoxazole *on page 811*
Erythromycin *on page 807*
Lansoprazole, Amoxicillin, and Clarithromycin *on page 908*
Lincomycin *on page 912*
Troleandomycin *on page 1133*

Drug of Choice or Alternative for

Disease/Syndrome(s):

Pneumonia, Community-Acquired *on page 270*
Sinusitis, Community-Acquired, Acute *on page 299*
Sinusitis, Community-Acquired, Chronic *on page 299*
Sinusitis, Hospital-Acquired *on page 300*

Organism(s):

Coxiella burnetii on page 100
Mycoplasma hominis and *Mycoplasma genitalium on page 237*
Streptococcus pneumoniae, Drug-Susceptible *on page 319*

Mafenide (MA fe nide)

U.S. Brand Names Sulfamylon®

Synonyms Mafenide Acetate

Generic Available No

Use Adjunct in the treatment of second- and third-degree burns to prevent septicemia caused by susceptible organisms such as *Pseudomonas aeruginosa*

Orphan drug: Prevention of graft loss of meshed autografts on excised burn wounds

Pregnancy Risk Factor C

Contraindications Hypersensitivity to mafenide, sulfites, or any component of the formulation

Warnings/Precautions Use with caution in patients with renal impairment and in patients with G6PD deficiency; prolonged use may result in superinfection

Adverse Reactions Frequency not defined.

Cardiovascular: Facial edema
Central nervous system: Pain
Dermatologic: Rash, erythema
Endocrine & metabolic: Hyperchloremia, metabolic acidosis
Hematologic: Porphyria, bone marrow suppression, hemolytic anemia, bleeding
Local: Burning sensation, excoriation
Respiratory: Hyperventilation, tachypnea, dyspnea
Miscellaneous: Hypersensitivity

Stability

Mafenide 5% topical solution preparation:

Dissolve the 50 g mafenide acetate (Sulfamylon®) packet in 200 mL of either sterile water for irrigation or sterile saline for irrigation (minimum solubility of 50 g of mafenide is in 200 mL of either solution)

Sterilize this solution by pushing through a 0.22 micron filter

Further dissolve this 200 mL of sterile Sulfamylon® solution in 800 mL of the initial diluent (either sterile water for irrigation or normal saline for irrigation)

This solution is stable and sterile for a total of 48 hours at room temperature

Note: Mafenide acetate topical solution CANNOT be mixed with nystatin due to reduced activity of mafenide

Note: Pilot *in vitro* studies: Silvadene® and Furacin® cream combined with nystatin cream were equally effective against the microorganisms as were the individual drugs. However, Sulfamylon® cream combined with nystatin lost its antimicrobial capability (*J Burn Care Rehabil*, 1989, 109:508-11).

Mechanism of Action Interferes with bacterial folic acid synthesis through competitive inhibition of para-aminobenzoic acid

Pharmacodynamics/Kinetics

Absorption: Diffuses through devascularized areas and is rapidly absorbed from burned surface

Metabolism: To para-carboxybenzene sulfonamide, a carbonic anhydrase inhibitor

Time to peak, serum: 2-4 hours

Excretion: Urine (as metabolites)

Dosage Children and Adults: Topical: Apply once or twice daily with a sterile gloved hand; apply to a thickness of approximately 16 mm; the burned area should be covered with cream at all times

Monitoring Parameters Acid base balance

Patient Information Discontinue and report immediately if rash, blisters, or swelling appear while using cream; discontinue if condition persists or worsens while using this product; for external use only

Dosage Forms

Cream, topical, as acetate: 85 mg/g (60 g, 120 g, 454 g) [contains sodium metabisulfite]

Powder, for topical solution: 5% (5s) [50 g/packet]

Mafenide Acetate *see* Mafenide *on page 924*

Malarone® *see* Atovaquone and Proguanil *on page 672*

Malathion (mal a THYE on)

U.S. Brand Names Ovide®

Generic Available No

Use Treatment of head lice and their ova

Pregnancy Risk Factor B

Pregnancy Implications No evidence of teratogenicity in animal models. There are no adequate and well-controlled studies in pregnant women. Use (or handle) during pregnancy only if clearly needed.

Contraindications Hypersensitivity to malathion or any component of the formulation; use in neonates and/or infants

Warnings/Precautions For topical use only; avoid contact with eyes. Lotion is flammable; do not expose to open flames; patients should avoid electric heat sources (eg, hair dryers, curling irons). Safety and efficacy in children <6 years of age have not been established.

Adverse Reactions Frequency not defined.

Dermatologic: Skin/scalp irritation

Ocular: Conjunctivitis (following contact with eyes)

Dosage Sprinkle Ovide® lotion on dry hair and rub gently until the scalp is thoroughly moistened; pay special attention to the back of the head and neck. Allow to dry naturally - use no heat and leave uncovered. After 8-12 hours, the hair should be washed with a nonmedicated shampoo; rinse and use a fine-toothed comb to remove dead lice and eggs. If required, repeat with second application in 7-9 days. Further treatment is generally not necessary. Other family members should be evaluated to determine if infested and if so, receive treatment.

Administration Refer to Dosing.

Patient Information For topical use only; avoid contact with eyes. Lotion is flammable; do not expose to open flames; patients should avoid electric heat sources (eg, hair dryers, curling irons).

Dosage Forms Lotion: 0.5% (59 mL) [contains isopropyl alcohol 78%]

Selected Readings

"Drugs for Parasitic Infections," *Med Lett Drugs Ther*, 1998, 40(1017):1-12.

Mandelamine® *see* Methenamine *on page 939*

Mantoux *see* Tuberculin Tests *on page 1136*

Marinol® *see* Dronabinol *on page 791*

3M™ Avagard™ [OTC] *see* Chlorhexidine Gluconate *on page 735*

Maxaquin® *see* Lomefloxacin *on page 917*

Maxipime® *see* Cefepime *on page 705*

Maxitrol® *see* Neomycin, Polymyxin B, and Dexamethasone *on page 965*

MCV4 *see* Meningococcal Polysaccharide (Groups A / C / Y and W-135) Diphtheria Toxoid Conjugate Vaccine *on page 933*

Measles, Mumps, and Rubella Vaccines (Combined)

(MEE zels, mumpz & roo BEL a vak SEENS, kom BINED)

Related Information

Immunization Recommendations *on page 1249*

U.S. Brand Names M-M-R® II

Canadian Brand Names M-M-R® II; Priorix™

Synonyms MMR; Mumps, Measles and Rubella Vaccines, Combined; Rubella, Measles and Mumps Vaccines, Combined

Generic Available No

Use Measles, mumps, and rubella prophylaxis

Drug of Choice or Alternative for Organism(s):

Measles Virus *on page 215*

Mumps Virus *on page 226*

Pregnancy Risk Factor C

Pregnancy Implications Animal reproduction studies have not been conducted. It is not known whether the drug can cause fetal harm or affect reproduction capacity (contracting natural measles during pregnancy can increase fetal risk). Do not administer to pregnant females, and avoid pregnancy for 28 days following vaccination.

Contraindications Hypersensitivity to measles, mumps, and rubella vaccine or any component of the formulation; hypersensitivity to neomycin or gelatin; current febrile respiratory illness or other febrile infection; severely-immunocompromised persons; blood dyscrasias, cancers affecting the bone marrow or lymphatic systems; children with active untreated tuberculosis

Warnings/Precautions

Females should not become pregnant within 28 days of vaccination.

MMR vaccine should not be given within 3 months of immune globulin or whole blood.

Immediate treatment for anaphylactic/anaphylactoid reaction should be available during vaccine use. Use extreme caution in patients with immediate-type hypersensitivity reactions to eggs.

MMR vaccine should not be administered to severely immunocompromised persons with the exception of asymptomatic children with HIV (ACIP and AAP recommendation).

Severely immunocompromised patients and symptomatic HIV-infected patients who are exposed to measles should receive immune globulin, regardless of prior vaccination status.

The immunogenicity of measles virus vaccine is decreased if vaccine is administered <6 months after immune globulin.

Patients with minor illnesses (diarrhea, mild upper respiratory tract infection with or without low grade fever or other illnesses with low-grade fever) may receive vaccine. Leukemia patients who are in remission and who have not received chemotherapy for at least 3 months may be vaccinated.

Use caution with history of cerebral injury, convulsions, or other conditions where stress due to fever should be avoided. Use caution in patients with thrombocytopenia and those who develop thrombocytopenia after first dose; thrombocytopenia may worsen.

Adverse Reactions All serious adverse reactions must be reported to the U.S. Department of Health and Human Services (DHHS) Vaccine Adverse Event Reporting System (VAERS) 1-800-822-7967.

Frequency not defined:

Cardiovascular: Syncope, vasculitis

Central nervous system: Ataxia, dizziness, febrile convulsions, fever, encephalitis, encephalopathy, Guillain-Barré syndrome, headache, irritability, malaise, measles inclusion body encephalitis, polyneuritis, polyneuropathy, seizure, subacute sclerosing panencephalitis

Dermatologic: Angioneurotic edema, erythema multiforme, purpura, rash, Stevens-Johnson syndrome, urticaria

Endocrine & metabolic: Diabetes mellitus, parotitis

Gastrointestinal: Diarrhea, nausea, pancreatitis, sore throat, vomiting

Genitourinary: Orchitis

Hematologic: Leukocytosis, thrombocytopenia

Local: Injection site reactions which include burning, induration, redness, stinging, swelling, tenderness, wheal and flare, vesiculation

Neuromuscular & skeletal: Arthralgia/arthritis (variable; highest rates in women, 12% to 26% versus children, up to 3%), myalgia, paresthesia

Ocular: Ocular palsies

Otic: Otitis media

Renal: Conjunctivitis, retinitis, optic neuritis, papillitis, retrobulbar neuritis

Respiratory: Bronchospasm, cough, pneumonitis, rhinitis

Miscellaneous: Anaphylactoid reactions, anaphylaxis, atypical measles, panniculitis, regional lymphadenopathy

Postmarketing and/or case reports: Aseptic meningitis (associated with Urabe strain of mumps vaccine)

Drug Interactions

Decreased Effect: The effect of the vaccine may be decreased in individuals who are receiving immunosuppressant drugs (including high dose systemic corticosteroids). Effect of vaccine may be decreased when given with immune globulin; do not administer with vaccine. Effectiveness of MMR may be decreased if given within 30 days of varicella vaccine (effectiveness not decreased when administered simultaneously).

Stability Prior to reconstitution, store the powder at 2°C to 8°C (36°F to 46°F) or colder (freezing does not affect potency). Protect from light. Diluent may be stored with powder or at room temperature. Use entire contents of the provided diluent to reconstitute vaccine. Gently agitate to mix thoroughly. Discard if powder does not dissolve. Use as soon as possible following reconstitution (may be stored at 2°C to 8°C/36°F to 46°F; protect from light); discard if not used within 8 hours.

Mechanism of Action As a live, attenuated vaccine, MMR vaccine offers active immunity to disease caused by the measles, mumps, and rubella viruses.

Dosage SubQ:

Infants <12 months: If there is risk of exposure to measles, single-antigen measles vaccine should be administered at 6-11 months of age with a second dose (of MMR) at >12 months of age.

Children ≥12 months: 0.5 mL at 12 months and then repeated at 4-6 years of age. If the second dose was not received, the schedule should be completed by the 11- to 12-year old visit. Administer in outer aspect of the upper arm. Recommended age of primary immunization is 12-15 months; revaccination is recommended prior to elementary school.

Administration Administer SubQ in outer aspect of the upper arm. **Not for I.V. administration.** Federal law requires that the date of administration, the vaccine manufacturer, lot number of vaccine, and the administering person's name, title and address be entered into the patient's permanent medical record.

Test Interactions Temporary suppression of TB skin test reactivity with onset approximately 3 days after administration

Patient Information Females should not become pregnant within 28 days of vaccination

Additional Information Adults born before 1957 are generally considered to be immune to measles and mumps; all born in or after 1957 without documentation of live vaccine on or after first birthday, physician-diagnosed measles or mumps, or laboratory evidence of immunity should be vaccine with two doses separated by no less than 1 month; for those previously vaccinated with one dose of measles vaccine, revaccination is indicated for students entering institutions of higher learning, health-care workers at time of employment, and for travelers to endemic areas. Guidelines for rubella vaccination are the same with the exception of birth year; all adults should be vaccinated against rubella. Booster doses of mumps and rubella are not necessary; women who are pregnant when vaccinated or become pregnant within 28 days should be counseled on the risks to the fetus; although the risks appear negligible.

Using separate sites and syringes, MMR may be administered concurrently with DTaP or *Haemophilus* b conjugate vaccine (PedvaxHIB®). Varicella vaccine may be administered with MMR using separate sites and syringes; however, if not administered simultaneously, doses should be separated by at least 30 days. Unless otherwise specified, MMR should be given 1 month before or 1 month after live viral vaccines.

Dosage Forms Injection, powder for reconstitution [preservative free]: Measles virus 1000 $TCID_{50}$, rubella virus 1000 $TCID_{50}$, and mumps virus 20,000 $TCID_{50}$ [contains neomycin 25 mcg, gelatin, human albumin, and bovine serum; produced in chick embryo cell culture]

Measles Virus Vaccine (Live) (MEE zels VYE rus vak SEEN, live)

Related Information

Immunization Recommendations *on page 1249*

(Continued)

Measles Virus Vaccine (Live) *(Continued)*

U.S. Brand Names Attenuvax®

Synonyms More Attenuated Enders Strain; Rubeola Vaccine

Generic Available No

Use Adults born before 1957 are generally considered to be immune. All those born in or after 1957 without documentation of live vaccine on or after first birthday, physician-diagnosed measles, or laboratory evidence of immunity should be vaccinated, ideally with two doses of vaccine separated by no less than 1 month. For those previously vaccinated with one dose of measles vaccine, revaccination is recommended for students entering colleges and other institutions of higher education, for healthcare workers at the time of employment, and for international travelers who visit endemic areas.

MMR is the vaccine of choice if recipients are likely to be susceptible to rubella and/or mumps as well as to measles. Persons vaccinated between 1963 and 1967 with a killed measles vaccine, followed by live vaccine within 3 months, or with a vaccine of unknown type should be revaccinated with live measles virus vaccine.

Drug of Choice or Alternative for Organism(s):

Measles Virus *on page 215*

Pregnancy Risk Factor X

Contraindications Hypersensitivity to neomycin or any component of the formulation; acute respiratory infections, activated tuberculosis, immunosuppressed patients; pregnancy; known anaphylactoid reaction to eggs

Warnings/Precautions Avoid use in immunocompromised patients; defer administration in presence of acute respiratory or other active infections or inactive, untreated tuberculosis; avoid pregnancy for 3 months following vaccination; history of febrile seizures, hypersensitivity reactions may occur

Adverse Reactions All serious adverse reactions must be reported to the U.S. Department of Health and Human Services (DHHS) Vaccine Adverse Event Reporting System (VAERS) 1-800-822-7967.

>10%:
- Cardiovascular: Edema
- Central nervous system: Fever (<100°F)
- Local: Burning or stinging, induration

1% to 10%:
- Central nervous system: Fever between 100°F and 103°F usually between 5th and 12th days postvaccination
- Dermatologic: Rash (rarely generalized)

<1%: Fatigue, convulsions, encephalitis, confusion, severe headache, fever (>103°F - prolonged), palsies, Guillain-Barré syndrome, ataxia, urticaria, itching, reddening of skin (especially around ears and eyes), erythema multiforme, vomiting, sore throat, diarrhea, thrombocytopenic purpura, diplopia, stiff neck, dyspnea, cough, rhinitis, lymphadenopathy, coryza, allergic reactions

Stability Refrigerate at 2°C to 8°C (36°F to 46°F); discard if left at room temperature for over 8 hours; protect from light

Mechanism of Action Promotes active immunity to measles virus by inducing specific measles IgG and IgM antibodies.

Dosage Children ≥15 months and Adults: SubQ: 0.5 mL in outer aspect of the upper arm, no routine boosters

Administration Vaccine should not be administered I.V.; SubQ injection preferred with a 25-gauge 5/8" needle

Test Interactions May temporarily depress tuberculin skin test sensitivity

Patient Information Parents should monitor children closely for fever for 5-11 days after vaccination; females should not become pregnant within 3 months of vaccination

Additional Information Contains 25 mcg neomycin per dose. Federal law requires that the date of administration, the vaccine manufacturer, lot number of vaccine, and the administering person's name, title, and address be entered into the patient's permanent medical record.

Dosage Forms Injection, powder for reconstitution [preservative free]: 1000 $TCID_{50}$ [contains human albumin, bovine serum, and neomycin; produced in chick embryo cell culture]

Mebendazole (me BEN da zole)

U.S. Brand Names Vermox® [DSC]

Canadian Brand Names Vermox®

Generic Available Yes

Use Treatment of pinworms (*Enterobius vermicularis*), whipworms (*Trichuris trichiura*), roundworms (*Ascaris lumbricoides*), and hookworms (*Ancylostoma duodenale*)

Drug of Choice or Alternative for Organism(s):

Ancylostoma duodenale on page 34
Ascaris on page 37
Enterobius vermicularis on page 133
Trichinella spiralis on page 338

Pregnancy Risk Factor C

Contraindications Hypersensitivity to mebendazole or any component of the formulation

Warnings/Precautions Pregnancy and children <2 years of age are relative contraindications since safety has not been established; not effective for hydatid disease

Adverse Reactions Frequency not defined.

Cardiovascular: Angioedema
Central nervous system: Fever, dizziness, headache, seizure
Dermatologic: Rash, itching, alopecia (with high doses)
Gastrointestinal: Abdominal pain, diarrhea, nausea, vomiting
Hematologic: Neutropenia (sore throat, unusual fatigue)
Neuromuscular & skeletal: Unusual weakness

Overdosage/Toxicology Symptoms include abdominal pain and altered mental status. Treatment is GI decontamination and supportive care.

Drug Interactions

Decreased Effect: Anticonvulsants such as carbamazepine and phenytoin may increase metabolism of mebendazole

Ethanol/Nutrition/Herb Interactions Food: Mebendazole serum levels may be increased if taken with food.

Mechanism of Action Selectively and irreversibly blocks glucose uptake and other nutrients in susceptible adult intestine-dwelling helminths

Pharmacodynamics/Kinetics

Absorption: 2% to 10%
Distribution: To serum, cyst fluid, liver, omental fat, and pelvic, pulmonary, and hepatic cysts; highest concentrations found in liver; relatively high concentrations found in muscle-encysted *Trichinella spiralis* larvae; crosses placenta
Protein binding: 95%
Metabolism: Extensively hepatic
Half-life elimination: 1-11.5 hours
Time to peak, serum: 2-4 hours
Excretion: Primarily feces; urine (5% to 10%)

Dosage Children and Adults: Oral:

Pinworms: 100 mg as a single dose; may need to repeat after 2 weeks; treatment should include family members in close contact with patient
Whipworms, roundworms, hookworms: One tablet twice daily, morning and evening on 3 consecutive days; if patient is not cured within 3-4 weeks, a second course of treatment may be administered
Capillariasis: 200 mg twice daily for 20 days
Dosing adjustment in hepatic impairment: Dosage reduction may be necessary in patients with liver dysfunction
Hemodialysis: Not dialyzable (0% to 5%)

Dietary Considerations Tablet can be crushed and mixed with food, swallowed whole, or chewed.

Administration Tablets may be chewed, swallowed whole, or crushed and mixed with food.

Monitoring Parameters Check for helminth ova in feces within 3-4 weeks following the initial therapy

Patient Information Tablets may be chewed, swallowed whole, or crushed and mixed with food; hygienic precautions should be taken to prevent reinfection such as wearing shoes and washing hands

Dosage Forms Tablet, chewable: 100 mg

Selected Readings

de Silva N, Guyatt H, and Bundy D, "Anthelmintics. A Comparative Review of Their Clinical Pharmacology," *Drugs*, 1997, 53(5):769-88.
"Drugs for Parasitic Infections," *Med Lett Drugs Ther*, 1998, 40(1017):1-12.

Mefloquine (ME floe kwin)

Related Information

Malaria Treatment *on page 1292*
(Continued)

Mefloquine *(Continued)*

U.S. Brand Names Lariam®

Canadian Brand Names Apo-Mefloquine®; Lariam®

Synonyms Mefloquine Hydrochloride

Generic Available Yes

Use Treatment of acute malarial infections and prevention of malaria

Drug of Choice or Alternative for Organism(s):

Plasmodium Species *on page 265*

Restrictions A medication guide and wallet card must be provided to patients when mefloquine is dispensed for malaria. An FDA-approved medication guide is available at www.fda.gov/cder/Offices/ODS/labeling.htm.

Pregnancy Risk Factor C

Pregnancy Implications Mefloquine crosses the placenta and is teratogenic in animals. There are no adequate and well-controlled studies in pregnant women, however, clinical experience has not shown teratogenic or embryotoxic effects; use with caution during pregnancy if travel to endemic areas cannot be postponed. Nonpregnant women of childbearing potential are advised to use contraception and avoid pregnancy during malaria prophylaxis and for 3 months thereafter. In case of an unplanned pregnancy, treatment with mefloquine is not considered a reason for pregnancy termination.

Contraindications Hypersensitivity mefloquine, related compounds (such as quinine and quinidine), or any component of the formulation; history of convulsions; cardiac conduction abnormalities; severe psychiatric disorder (including active or recent history of depression, generalized anxiety disorder, psychosis, or schizophrenia); use with halofantrine

Warnings/Precautions Use with caution in patients with a previous history of depression (see Contraindications regarding severe psychiatric illness, including active/recent depression). May cause a range of psychiatric symptoms (anxiety, paranoia, depression, hallucinations and psychosis). Occasionally, symptoms have been reported to persist long after mefloquine has been discontinued. Rare cases of suicidal ideation and suicide have been reported (no causal relationship established). The appearance of psychiatric symptoms such as acute anxiety, depression, restlessness or confusion may be considered a prodrome to more serious events. When used as prophylaxis, substitute an alternative medication. Discontinue if unexplained neuropsychiatric disturbances occur. Use caution in patients with significant cardiac disease. If mefloquine is to be used for a prolonged period, periodic evaluations including liver function tests and ophthalmic examinations should be performed. (Retinal abnormalities have not been observed with mefloquine in humans; however, it has with long-term administration to rats.) In cases of life-threatening, serious, or overwhelming malaria infections due to *Plasmodium falciparum*, patients should be treated with intravenous antimalarial drug. Mefloquine may be given orally to complete the course. Dizziness, loss of balance, and other CNS disorders have been reported; due to long half-life, effects may persist after mefloquine is discontinued. Use caution in activities requiring alertness and fine motor coordination (driving, piloting planes, operating machinery, deep sea diving, etc).

Adverse Reactions

Frequency not defined: Neuropsychiatric events

1% to 10%:

- Central nervous system: Headache, fever, chills, fatigue
- Dermatologic: Rash
- Gastrointestinal: Vomiting (3%), diarrhea, stomach pain, nausea, appetite decreased
- Neuromuscular & skeletal: Myalgia
- Otic: Tinnitus

<1%: Alopecia, bradycardia, dizziness, emotional lability, extrasystoles, pruritus, seizure, syncope, weakness

Postmarketing and/or case reports: Abnormal dreams, ataxia, aggressive behavior, agitation, anaphylaxis, anxiety, arthralgia, AV block, chest pain, conduction abnormalities (transient), confusion, convulsions, depression, diaphoresis (increased), dyspepsia, dyspnea, edema, encephalopathy, erythema multiforme, exanthema, hallucinations, hearing impairment, hypotension, insomnia, leukocytosis, malaise, mood changes, muscle cramps/weakness, palpitation, panic attacks, paranoia, paresthesia, psychosis, somnolence, Stevens-Johnson syndrome, suicidal ideation and behavior (causal relationship not established), tachycardia, thrombocytopenia, tremor, urticaria, vertigo, visual disturbances

Overdosage/Toxicology Following GI contamination, care is supportive only. Monitor cardiac function and psychiatric status for at least 24 hours.

Drug Interactions

Cytochrome P450 Effect: Substrate of CYP3A4 (major); **Inhibits** CYP2D6 (weak), 3A4 (weak)

Increased Effect/Toxicity: Use caution with drugs that alter cardiac conduction; increased toxicity with chloroquine, quinine, and quinidine (hold treatment until at least 12 hours after these later drugs); increased toxicity with halofantrine (concurrent use is contraindicated). CYP3A4 inhibitors may increase the levels/effects of mefloquine; example inhibitors include azole antifungals, ciprofloxacin, clarithromycin, diclofenac, doxycycline, erythromycin, imatinib, isoniazid, nefazodone, nicardipine, propofol, protease inhibitors, quinidine, and verapamil.

Decreased Effect: Mefloquine may decrease the effect of valproic acid, carbamazepine, phenobarbital, and phenytoin. CYP3A4 inducers may decrease the levels/effects of mefloquine; example inducers include aminoglutethimide, carbamazepine, nafcillin, nevirapine, phenobarbital, phenytoin, and rifamycins.

Ethanol/Nutrition/Herb Interactions Food: Food increases bioavailability by ~40%.

Stability Store at 25°C (77°F); excursions permitted to 15°C to 30°C (59°F to 86°F)

Mechanism of Action Mefloquine is a quinoline-methanol compound structurally similar to quinine; mefloquine's effectiveness in the treatment and prophylaxis of malaria is due to the destruction of the asexual blood forms of the malarial pathogens that affect humans, *Plasmodium falciparum, P. vivax, P. malariae, P. ovale*

Pharmacodynamics/Kinetics

Absorption: Well absorbed

Distribution: V_d: 19 L/kg; blood, urine, CSF, tissues; enters breast milk

Protein binding: 98%

Metabolism: Extensively hepatic; main metabolite is inactive

Bioavailability: Increased by food

Half-life elimination: 21-22 days

Time to peak, plasma: 6-24 hours (median: ~17 hours)

Excretion: Primarily bile and feces; urine (9% as unchanged drug, 4% as primary metabolite)

Dosage Oral (dose expressed as mg of mefloquine hydrochloride):

Children ≥6 months and >5 kg:

Malaria treatment: 20-25 mg/kg in 2 divided doses, taken 6-8 hours apart (maximum: 1250 mg) Take with food and an ample amount of water. If clinical improvement is not seen within 48-72 hours, an alternative therapy should be used for retreatment.

Malaria prophylaxis: 5 mg/kg/once weekly (maximum dose: 250 mg) starting 1 week before, arrival in endemic area, continuing weekly during travel and for 4 weeks after leaving endemic area. Take with food and an ample amount of water.

Adults:

Malaria treatment (mild to moderate infection): 5 tablets (1250 mg) as a single dose. Take with food and at least 8 oz of water. If clinical improvement is not seen within 48-72 hours, an alternative therapy should be used for retreatment.

Malaria prophylaxis: 1 tablet (250 mg) weekly starting 1 week before, arrival in endemic area, continuing weekly during travel and for 4 weeks after leaving endemic area. Take with food and at least 8 oz of water.

Dosage adjustment in renal impairment: No dosage adjustment needed in patients with renal impairment or on dialysis.

Dosage adjustment in hepatic impairment: Half-life may be prolonged and plasma levels may be higher.

Dietary Considerations Take with food and with at least 8 oz of water.

Administration Administer with food and with at least 8 oz of water. When used for malaria prophylaxis, dose should be taken once weekly on the same day each week. If vomiting occurs within 30-60 minutes after dose, an additional half-dose should be given. Tablets may be crushed and suspended in a small amount of water, milk, or another beverage for persons unable to swallow tablets.

Monitoring Parameters LFTS; ocular examination

Patient Information Begin therapy before trip and continue after; do not take drug on empty stomach; take with food and at least 8 oz of water; women of childbearing age should use reliable contraception during prophylaxis treatment and for 3 months after the last dose; be aware of signs and symptoms of malaria when traveling to an endemic area. Caution should be exercised with regard to driving, piloting airplanes, and operating machines since dizziness, disturbed sense of balance, or neuropsychiatric reactions have been reported with mefloquine. Report any symptoms of anxiety, confusion, depression, or restlessness immediately; if mefloquine is being used as malaria prophylaxis, drug should be discontinued (alternative therapy substituted).

Dosage Forms Tablet, as hydrochloride: 250 mg [equivalent to 228 mg base]

(Continued)

Mefloquine *(Continued)*

Selected Readings

Panisko DM and Keystone JS, "Treatment of Malaria - 1990," *Drugs*, 1990, 39(2):160-89.
White NJ, "The Treatment of Malaria," *N Engl J Med*, 1996, 335(11):800-6.
Wyler DJ, "Malaria Chemoprophylaxis for the Traveler," *N Engl J Med*, 1993, 329(1):31-7.

Mefloquine Hydrochloride *see* Mefloquine *on page 929*

Mefoxin® *see* Cefoxitin *on page 712*

Megace® *see* Megestrol *on page 932*

Megace® ES *see* Megestrol *on page 932*

Megace® OS (Can) *see* Megestrol *on page 932*

Megestrol (me JES trole)

Related Information

AIDS Wasting Treatment *on page 1205*

U.S. Brand Names Megace®; Megace® ES

Canadian Brand Names Apo-Megestrol®; Lin-Megestrol; Megace®; Megace® OS; Nu-Megestrol

Synonyms 5071-1DL(6); Megestrol Acetate; NSC-10363

Generic Available Yes

Use Palliative treatment of breast and endometrial carcinoma; treatment of anorexia, cachexia, or unexplained significant weight loss in patients with AIDS

Pregnancy Risk Factor X

Contraindications Hypersensitivity to megestrol or any component of the formulation; pregnancy

Warnings/Precautions Use with caution in patients with a history of thrombophlebitis. Elderly females may have vaginal bleeding or discharge. May suppress hypothalamic-pituitary-adrenal (HPA) axis during chronic administration. Consider the possibility of adrenal suppression in any patient receiving or being withdrawn from chronic therapy when signs/symptoms suggestive of hypoadrenalism are noted (during stress or in unstressed state). Laboratory evaluation and replacement/stress doses of rapid-acting glucocorticoid should be considered.

Adverse Reactions

Cardiovascular: Edema, hypertension (≤8%), cardiomyopathy, palpitation

Central nervous system: Insomnia, fever (2% to 6%), headache (≤10%), pain (≤6%, similar to placebo), confusion (1% to 3%), convulsions (1% to 3%), depression (1% to 3%)

Dermatologic: Allergic rash (2% to 12%) with or without pruritus, alopecia

Endocrine & metabolic: Breakthrough bleeding and amenorrhea, spotting, changes in menstrual flow, changes in cervical erosion and secretions, increased breast tenderness, changes in vaginal bleeding pattern, edema, fluid retention, hyperglycemia (≤6%), diabetes, HPA axis suppression, adrenal insufficiency, Cushing's syndrome

Gastrointestinal: Weight gain (not attributed to edema or fluid retention), nausea, vomiting (7%), diarrhea (8% to 15%, similar to placebo), flatulence (≤10%), constipation (1% to 3%)

Genitourinary: Impotence (4% to 14%), decreased libido (≤5%)

Hepatic: Cholestatic jaundice, hepatotoxicity, hepatomegaly (1% to 3%)

Local: Thrombophlebitis

Neuromuscular & skeletal: Carpal tunnel syndrome, weakness, paresthesia (1% to 3%)

Respiratory: Hyperpnea, dyspnea (1% to 3%), cough (1% to 3%)

Miscellaneous: Diaphoresis

Overdosage/Toxicology Toxicity is unlikely following single exposures of excessive doses.

Ethanol/Nutrition/Herb Interactions Herb/Nutraceutical: Avoid black cohosh, dong quai in estrogen-dependent tumors.

Stability Store at 25°C (77°F); excursions permitted at 15°C to 30°C (59°F to 86°F)

Mechanism of Action A synthetic progestin with antiestrogenic properties which disrupt the estrogen receptor cycle. Megestrol interferes with the normal estrogen cycle and results in a lower LH titer. May also have a direct effect on the endometrium. Megestrol is an antineoplastic progestin thought to act through an antileutenizing effect mediated via the pituitary. May stimulate appetite by antagonizing the metabolic effects of catabolic cytokines.

Pharmacodynamics/Kinetics

Absorption: Well absorbed orally

Metabolism: Completely hepatic to free steroids and glucuronide conjugates

Time to peak, serum: 1-3 hours

Half-life elimination: 15-100 hours

Excretion: Urine (57% to 78% as steroid metabolites and inactive compound); feces (8% to 30%)

Dosage Adults: Oral:

Female (refer to individual protocols):

Breast carcinoma: 40 mg 4 times/day

Endometrial carcinoma: 40-320 mg/day in divided doses; use for 2 months to determine efficacy; maximum doses used have been up to 800 mg/day

Male/Female: HIV-related cachexia:

Megace®: Initial dose: 800 mg/day; daily doses of 400 and 800 mg/day were found to be clinically effective

Megace ES®: 625 mg/day

Dosing adjustment in renal impairment: No data available; however, the urinary excretion of megestrol acetate administered in doses of 4-90 mg ranged from 56% to 78% within 10 days

Hemodialysis: Megestrol acetate has not been tested for dialyzability; however, due to its low solubility, it is postulated that dialysis would not be an effective means of treating an overdose

Administration Megestrol acetate (Megace®) oral suspension is compatible with water, orange juice, apple juice, or Sustacal H.C. for immediate consumption.

Monitoring Parameters Observe for signs of thromboembolic phenomena

Test Interactions Altered thyroid and liver function tests

Patient Information Follow dosage schedule and do not take more than prescribed. You may experience sensitivity to sunlight (use sunblock, wear protective clothing, and avoid extended exposure to direct sunlight); dizziness, anxiety, depression (use caution when driving or engaging in tasks that require alertness until response to drug is known); change in appetite (maintain adequate hydration and diet - 2-3 L/day of fluids unless instructed to restrict fluid intake); decreased libido or increased body hair (reversible when drug is discontinued); hot flashes (cool clothes and environment may help). Report swelling of face, lips, or mouth; absence or altered menses; abdominal pain; vaginal itching, irritation, or discharge; heat, warmth, redness, or swelling of extremities; or sudden onset change in vision.

Dosage Forms

Suspension, oral, as acetate: 40 mg/mL (240 mL, 480 mL)

Megace®: 40 mg/mL (240 mL) [contains alcohol 0.06% and sodium benzoate; lemon-lime flavor]

Megace® ES: 125 mg/mL (150 mL) [contains alcohol 0.06% and sodium benzoate; lemon-lime flavor]

Tablet, as acetate: 20 mg, 40 mg

Selected Readings

Jeffrey LP, Chairman, National Study Commission on Cytotoxic Exposure. Position Statement. "The Handling of Cytotoxic Agents by Women Who Are Pregnant, Attempting to Conceive, or Breast-Feeding," January 12, 1987.

Megestrol Acetate *see* Megestrol *on page 932*

Menactra™ *see* Meningococcal Polysaccharide (Groups A / C / Y and W-135) Diphtheria Toxoid Conjugate Vaccine *on page 933*

Meningitec® (Can) *see* Meningococcal Polysaccharide (Groups A / C / Y and W-135) Diphtheria Toxoid Conjugate Vaccine *on page 933*

Meningococcal Polysaccharide (Groups A / C / Y and W-135) Diphtheria Toxoid Conjugate Vaccine

(me NIN joe kok al pol i SAK a ride groops aye, see, why & dubl yoo won thur tee fyve dif THEER ee a TOKS oyds KON joo gate vak SEEN)

Related Information

Immunization Recommendations *on page 1249*

U.S. Brand Names Menactra™

Canadian Brand Names Meningitec®

Synonyms MCV4

Generic Available No

Use Provide active immunization of adolescents and adults (11-55 years of age) against invasive meningococcal disease caused by *N. meningitidis* serogroups A, C, Y and W-135

The ACIP recommends routine vaccination of all adolescents at age 11-12 years. For adolescents not previously vaccinated, vaccine should be administered prior to high school entry (~15 years of age).

(Continued)

Meningococcal Polysaccharide (Groups A / C / Y and W-135) Diphtheria Toxoid Conjugate Vaccine *(Continued)*

The ACIP also recommends routine vaccination for persons at increased risk for meningococcal disease. (MCV4 is preferred for persons aged 11-55 years; MPSV4 may be used if MCV4 is not available). Persons at increased risk include:

College freshmen living in dormitories

Microbiologists routinely exposed to isolates of *N. meningitides*

Military recruits

Persons traveling to or who reside in countries where *N. meningitides* is hyperendemic or epidemic, particularly if contact with local population will be prolonged

Persons with terminal complement component deficiencies

Persons with anatomic or functional asplenia

Use is also recommended during meningococcal outbreaks caused by vaccine preventable serogroups.

Drug of Choice or Alternative for Organism(s):

Neisseria meningitidis on page 245

Pregnancy Risk Factor C

Pregnancy Implications Teratogenic effects were observed in animal studies. Carcinogenic or mutagenic studies have not been performed. There are no adequate and well-controlled studies in pregnant women. Patients should contact the Aventis Pasteur Inc vaccine registry at 1-800-822-2463 if they are pregnant or become aware they were pregnant at the time of Menactra™ vaccination.

Contraindications Hypersensitivity to any component of the formulation, including diphtheria toxoid; latex hypersensitivity

Warnings/Precautions Due to risk of hemorrhage, avoid using in patients with any bleeding disorder, such as thrombocytopenia or hemophilia. Consider risk-to-benefit in patients receiving anticoagulant therapy. Defer vaccination until improvement from moderate to severe acute illness. Menactra™ is not to be used to treat meningococcal infections or to provide immunity against *N. meningitidis* serogroup B or diphtheria. Response may not be as great as desired in immunosuppressed patients. Vial stopper contains latex. Safety and efficacy have not been established in children <11 years of age or adults >55 years.

Adverse Reactions All serious adverse reactions must be reported to the U.S. Department of Health and Human Services Vaccine Adverse Event Reporting System (VAERS) 1-800-822-7967 or www.vaers.org.

>10%:

Central nervous system: Pain (59%), headache (41%), fatigue (35%), malaise (24%)

Gastrointestinal: Diarrhea (16%), anorexia (12%)

Local: Redness (14%), swelling (13%), induration (17%)

Neuromuscular & skeletal: Arthralgia (20%)

1% to 10%:

Central nervous system: Chills (10%), fever (5%)

Gastrointestinal: Vomiting (2%)

Local: Rash (2%)

Stability Store between 2°C to 8°C (35°F to 46°F). Do not freeze; discard product exposed to freezing. Do not mix with other vaccines in the same syringe.

Mechanism of Action Induces immunity against meningococcal disease via the formation of bactericidal antibodies directed toward the polysaccharide capsular components of *Neisseria meningitidis* serogroups A, C, Y and W-135.

Pharmacodynamics/Kinetics

Onset: Protective antibody levels achieved within 7-10 days of vaccination.

Dosage I.M.:

Adolescents 11-18 years and Adults ≤55 years: 0.5 mL

NOTE: Revaccination: May be indicated in patients previously vaccinated with MPSV4 who remain at increased risk for infection. The ACIP recommends the use of MCV4 for revaccination in patients 11-55 years, however use of MPSV4 is also acceptable. Consider revaccination after 3-5 years. The need for revaccination in patients previously vaccinated with MCV4 is currently under study.

Elderly: Safety and efficacy not established in patients >55 years

Administration Administer by I.M. route, preferably into the upper deltoid region. Do not administer via I.V., SubQ or I.D. route. For patients at risk of hemorrhage, the ACIP recommends "it should be administered intramuscularly if, in the opinion of a physician familiar with the patient's bleeding risk, the vaccine can be administered

with reasonable safety by this route. If the patient receives antihemophilia or other similar therapy, intramuscular vaccination can be scheduled shortly after such therapy is administered. A fine needle (≤23 gauge) can be used for the vaccination and firm pressure applied to the site (without rubbing) for at least 2 minutes. The patient or family should be instructed concerning the risk of hematoma from the injection."

Patient Information Refer to the Vaccine Information Statement (VIS) provided by the Centers for Disease Control (www.cdc.gov); contact prescriber regarding any unusual condition, such as a severe allergic reaction, high fever, or unusual behavior. If a serious allergic reaction occurred, it would happen within a few minutes to a few hours after the shot. Signs of a serious allergic reaction may include difficulty breathing, weakness, hoarseness or wheezing, a fast heart beat, hives, dizziness, paleness, or swelling of the throat.

Additional Information Federal law requires that the date of administration, the vaccine manufacturer, lot number of vaccine, and the administering person's name, title and address be entered into the patient's permanent medical record.

Dosage Forms Injection, solution: 4 mcg each of polysaccharide antigen groups A, C, Y and W-135 per 0.5 mL [conjugated to 48 mcg diphtheria toxoid protein; adjuvant and preservative free; vial stopper contains dry, natural latex rubber]

Meningococcal Polysaccharide Vaccine (Groups A / C / Y and W-135)

(me NIN joe kok al pol i SAK a ride vak SEEN groops aye, see, why & dubl yoo won thur tee fyve)

Related Information

Immunization Recommendations *on page 1249*

U.S. Brand Names Menomune®-A/C/Y/W-135

Synonyms MPSV4

Generic Available No

Use Provide active immunity to meningococcal serogroups contained in the vaccine

The ACIP recommends routine vaccination for persons at increased risk for meningococcal disease. (Use of MPSV4 is recommended in children 2-10 years and adults > 55 years. MCV4 is preferred for persons aged 11-55 years; MPSV4 may be used if MCV4 is not available). Persons at increased risk include:

- College freshmen living in dormitories
- Microbiologists routinely exposed to isolates of *N. meningitides*
- Military recruits
- Persons traveling to or who reside in countries where *N. meningitides* is hyperendemic or epidemic, particularly if contact with local population will be prolonged
- Persons with terminal complement component deficiencies
- Persons with anatomic or functional asplenia

Use is also recommended during meningococcal outbreaks caused by vaccine preventable serogroups.

Drug of Choice or Alternative for Organism(s):

Neisseria meningitidis on page 245

Pregnancy Risk Factor C

Pregnancy Implications Animal studies have not been conducted. Based on limited data, teratogenic effects have not been reported when used during pregnancy. Pregnancy should not preclude vaccination with MPSV4 if indicated. Patients may contact the Aventis Pasteur Inc vaccine registry at 1-800-822-2463 if they are pregnant or become aware they were pregnant at the time of vaccination.

Contraindications Hypersensitivity to any component of the formulation; defer immunization during acute illness

Warnings/Precautions Patients who undergo splenectomy secondary to trauma or nonlymphoid tumors respond well; however, those asplenic patients with lymphoid tumors who receive either chemotherapy or irradiation respond poorly. Response may not be as great as desired in immunosuppressed patients. Use in pediatric patients <2 years of age is usually not recommended. Use with caution in patients with latex sensitivity; the stopper to the vial contains dry, natural latex rubber. Some dosage forms contain thimerosal.

Adverse Reactions All serious adverse reactions must be reported to the U.S. Department of Health and Human Services (DHHS) Vaccine Adverse Event Reporting System (VAERS) 1-800-822-7967. Percentages reported in adults; incidence of erythema, swelling, or tenderness may be higher in children

>10%: Local: Tenderness (9% to 36%)

(Continued)

Meningococcal Polysaccharide Vaccine (Groups A / C / Y and W-135) *(Continued)*

1% to 10%:

Central nervous system: Headache (2% to 5%), malaise (2%), fever (100°F to 106°F: 3%), chills (2%)

Local: Pain at injection site (2% to 3%), erythema (1% to 4%), induration (1% to 4%)

Drug Interactions

Increased Effect/Toxicity: Should not be administered with whole-cell pertussis or whole-cell typhoid vaccines due to combined endotoxin content.

Decreased Effect: Decreased effect with administration of immunoglobulin within 1 month.

Stability Prior to and following reconstitution, store at 2°C to 8°C (35°F to 46°F). Reconstitute using provided diluent; shake well. Use single-dose vial within 30 minutes of reconstitution. Use multidose vial within 35 days of reconstitution.

Mechanism of Action Induces the formation of bactericidal antibodies to meningococcal antigens; the presence of these antibodies is strongly correlated with immunity to meningococcal disease caused by *Neisseria meningitidis* groups A, C, Y and W-135.

Pharmacodynamics/Kinetics

Onset of action: Antibody levels: 7-10 days

Duration: Antibodies against group A and C polysaccharides decline markedly (to prevaccination levels) over the first 3 years following a single dose of vaccine, especially in children <4 years of age

Dosage SubQ:

Children <2 years: Not usually recommended. Two doses (0.5 mL/dose), 3 months apart, may be considered in children 3-18 months to elicit short-term protection against serogroup A disease. A single dose may be considered in children 19-23 months.

Children ≥2 years and Adults: 0.5 mL

Note: Revaccination: May be indicated in patients previously vaccinated with MPSV4 who remain at increased risk for infection. The ACIP recommends the use of MCV4 for revaccination in patients 11-55 years, however use of MPSV4 is also acceptable.

Children first vaccinated at <4 years: Revaccinate after 2-3 years.

Adults: Not determined, consider revaccination after 3-5 years.

Administration Administer by SubQ injection; do not administer intradermally, I.M., or I.V.

Additional Information Federal law requires that the date of administration, the vaccine manufacturer, lot number of vaccine, and the administering person's name, title and address be entered into the patient's permanent medical record.

Dosage Forms Injection, powder for reconstitution: 50 mcg each of polysaccharide antigen groups A, C, Y, and W-135 [contains lactose; packaged with 0.78 mL preservative free diluent or 6 mL diluent containing thimerosal; vial stoppers contain dry, natural latex rubber]

Menomune®-A/C/Y/W-135 *see* Meningococcal Polysaccharide Vaccine (Groups A / C / Y and W-135) *on page 935*

Mentax® *see* Butenafine *on page 691*

Mepron® *see* Atovaquone *on page 670*

Meropenem (mer oh PEN em)

Related Information

Antimicrobial Activity Against Selected Organisms *on page 1165*

Neutropenic Fever Guidelines *on page 1295*

U.S. Brand Names Merrem® I.V.

Canadian Brand Names Merrem®

Generic Available No

Use Treatment of intra-abdominal infections (complicated appendicitis and peritonitis); treatment of bacterial meningitis in pediatric patients ≥3 months of age caused by *S. pneumoniae*, *H. influenzae*, and *N. meningitidis*; treatment of complicated skin and skin structure infections caused by susceptible organisms

Unlabeled/Investigational Use

Febrile neutropenia, urinary tract infections

Drug of Choice or Alternative for Disease/Syndrome(s):

Fever, Neutropenic *on page 148*

Intra-abdominal Abscess *on page 194*

Liver Abscess *on page 211*
Meningitis, Pediatric (>1 month of age) *on page 218*
Meningitis, Postsurgical *on page 218*
Meningitis, Post-traumatic *on page 219*
Pancreatitis/Pancreatic Abscess *on page 253*
Peritonitis, Secondary *on page 263*
Peritonitis, Spontaneous Bacterial *on page 264*
Pneumonia, Community-Acquired *on page 270*
Pneumonia, Hospital-Acquired *on page 272*
Pneumonia, Ventilator-Associated *on page 273*

Organism(s):

Acinetobacter Species *on page 24*
Alcaligenes Species *on page 31*
Citrobacter Species *on page 81*
Enterobacter Species *on page 132*
Klebsiella Species *on page 200*
Neisseria meningitidis on page 245
Pseudomonas aeruginosa on page 282
Serratia Species *on page 296*

Pregnancy Risk Factor B

Pregnancy Implications Teratogenic effects have not been found in animal studies; use during pregnancy only if clearly indicated.

Contraindications Hypersensitivity to meropenem, any component of the formulation, or other carbapenems (eg, imipenem); patients who have experienced anaphylactic reactions to other beta-lactams

Warnings/Precautions

Hypersensitivity reactions, including anaphylaxis, have occurred and often require immediate drug discontinuation. Seizures and other CNS adverse reactions have occurred, most commonly in patients with renal impairment and/or underlying neurologic disorders (less frequent than with Primaxin®). Thrombocytopenia has been reported in patients with significant renal dysfunction. Pseudomembranous colitis has been associated with meropenem use. Superinfection is possible with long courses of therapy. Safety and efficacy have not been established for children <3 months of age

Adverse Reactions

1% to 10%:

Cardiovascular: Peripheral vascular disorder (<1%)

Central nervous system: Headache (2% to 8%), pain (5%)

Dermatologic: Rash (2% to 3%, includes diaper-area moniliasis in pediatrics), pruritus (1%)

Gastrointestinal: Diarrhea (4% to 5%), nausea/vomiting (1% to 8%), constipation (1% to 7%), oral moniliasis (up to 2% in pediatric patients), glossitis

Hematologic: Anemia (up to 6%)

Local: Inflammation at the injection site (2%), phlebitis/thrombophlebitis (1%), injection site reaction (1%)

Respiratory: Apnea (1%)

Miscellaneous: Sepsis (2%), septic shock (1%)

<1%: Abdominal enlargement, abdominal pain, agitation/delirium, anemia, anorexia, anxiety, arrhythmia, asthma, back pain, bilirubin increased, bradycardia, BUN increased, chest pain, chills, cholestatic jaundice/jaundice, confusion, cough, creatinine increased, decreased platelets, decreased prothrombin time, depression, diaphoresis, dizziness, dyspepsia, dyspnea, dysuria, edema, eosinophilia, epistaxis (0.2%), fever, flatulence, gastrointestinal hemorrhage (0.5%), hallucinations, hearing loss, heart failure, hemoperitoneum (0.2%), hepatic failure, hypertension, hypokalemia, hypotension, ileus, insomnia, intestinal obstruction, leukocytosis, melena (0.3%), MI, nervousness, paresthesia, pelvic pain, pleural effusion, pulmonary edema, pulmonary embolism, renal failure, seizure, skin ulcer, somnolence, syncope, tachycardia, thrombocytopenia, thrombocytosis, urinary incontinence, urticaria, vaginal moniliasis, weakness, whole body pain

Postmarketing and/or case reports: Agranulocytosis, angioedema, erythema multiforme, leukopenia, neutropenia, Stevens-Johnson syndrome, toxic epidermal necrolysis

Overdosage/Toxicology No cases of acute overdosage are reported which have resulted in symptoms. Supportive therapy is recommended. Meropenem and its metabolite are removable by dialysis.

Drug Interactions

Increased Effect/Toxicity: Probenecid may increase meropenem serum concentrations.

(Continued)

Meropenem *(Continued)*

Decreased Effect: Meropenem may decrease valproic acid serum concentrations to subtherapeutic levels.

Stability Dry powder should be stored at controlled room temperature 20°C to 25°C (68°F to 77°F). Meropenem infusion vials may be reconstituted with SWFI or a compatible diluent (eg, NS). The 500 mg vials should be reconstituted with 10 mL, and 1 g vials with 20 mL. May be further diluted with compatible solutions for infusion. Consult detailed reference/product labeling for compatibility.

Injection reconstitution: SWFI: Stable for up to 2 hours at room temperature and for up to 12 hours under refrigeration

Infusion reconstitution:

- Sodium chloride: Stable for up to 2 hours at room temperature or for up to 18 hours under refrigeration
- SWFI: Stable for up to 2 hours at room temperature or for up to 12 hours under refrigeration
- Dextrose 5% injection: Stable for 1 hour at room temperature or for 8 hours under refrigeration

Mechanism of Action Inhibits bacterial cell wall synthesis by binding to several of the penicillin-binding proteins, which in turn inhibit the final transpeptidation step of peptidoglycan synthesis in bacterial cell walls, thus inhibiting cell wall biosynthesis; bacteria eventually lyse due to ongoing activity of cell wall autolytic enzymes (autolysins and murein hydrolases) while cell wall assembly is arrested

Pharmacodynamics/Kinetics

Distribution: V_d: Adults: ~0.3 L/kg, Children: 0.4-0.5 L/kg; penetrates well into most body fluids and tissues; CSF concentrations approximate those of the plasma

Protein binding: 2%

Metabolism: Hepatic; metabolized to open beta-lactam form (inactive)

Half-life elimination:

- Normal renal function: 1-1.5 hours
- Cl_{cr} 30-80 mL/minute: 1.9-3.3 hours
- Cl_{cr} 2-30 mL/minute: 3.82-5.7 hours

Time to peak, tissue: 1 hour following infusion

Excretion: Urine (~25% as inactive metabolites)

Dosage I.V.:

Children >3 months (<50 kg):

- Complicated skin and skin structure infections: 10 mg/kg every 8 hours (maximum dose: 500 mg every 8 hours)
- Intra-abdominal infections: 20 mg/kg every 8 hours (maximum dose: 1 g every 8 hours)
- Meningitis: 40 mg/kg every 8 hours (maximum dose: 2 g every 8 hours)
- Febrile neutropenia (unlabeled use): 20 mg/kg every 8 hours (maximum dose: 1 g every 8 hours)

Children >50 kg and Adults:

- Complicated skin and skin structure infections: 500 mg every 8 hours
- Intra-abdominal infections: 1 g every 8 hours
- Meningitis: 2 g every 8 hours
- Febrile neutropenia, pneumonia, other severe infections (unlabeled use): 1 g every 8 hours
- Urinary tract infections, complicated (unlabeled use): 500 mg to 1 g every 8 hours

Dosing adjustment in renal impairment: Adults:

- Cl_{cr} 26-50 mL/minute: Administer recommended dose based on indication every 12 hours
- Cl_{cr} 10-25 mL/minute: Administer one-half recommended dose every 12 hours
- Cl_{cr} <10 mL/minute: Administer one-half recommended dose every 24 hours

Dialysis: Meropenem and its metabolites are readily dialyzable

Continuous arteriovenous or venovenous hemodiafiltration effects: Dose as Cl_{cr} 10-50 mL/minute

Dietary Considerations 1 g of meropenem contains 90.2 mg of sodium as sodium carbonate (3.92 mEq)

Administration Administer I.V. infusion over 15-30 minutes; I.V. bolus injection over 3-5 minutes

Monitoring Parameters Monitor for signs of anaphylaxis during first dose

Dosage Forms Injection, powder for reconstitution: 500 mg [contains sodium 45.1 mg as sodium carbonate (1.96 mEq)]; 1 g [contains sodium 90.2 mg as sodium carbonate (3.92 mEq)]

Selected Readings

Fish DN and Singletary TJ, "Meropenem, A New Carbapenem Antibiotic," *Pharmacotherapy*, 1997, 17(4):644-69.

Hellinger WC and Brewer NS, "Carbapenems and Monobactams: Imipenem, Meropenem, and Aztreonam," *Mayo Clin Proc*, 1999, 74(4):420-34.

Lowe MN and Lamb HM, "Meropenem: An Updated Review of Its Use in the Management of Intra-abdominal Infections," *Drugs*, 2000, 60(3):619-46.
Wiseman LR, Wagstaff AJ, Brogden RN, et al, "Meropenem. A Review of Its Antibacterial Activity, Pharmacokinetic Properties, and Clinical Efficacy," *Drugs*, 1995, 50(1):73-101.

Merrem® (Can) *see* Meropenem *on page 936*
Merrem® I.V. *see* Meropenem *on page 936*
Meruvax® II *see* Rubella Virus Vaccine (Live) *on page 1059*
Methadex *see* Neomycin, Polymyxin B, and Dexamethasone *on page 965*

Methenamine (meth EN a meen)

U.S. Brand Names Hiprex®; Mandelamine®; Urex®

Canadian Brand Names Dehydral®; Hiprex®; Mandelamine®; Urasal®; Urex®

Synonyms Hexamethylenetetramine; Methenamine Hippurate; Methenamine Mandelate

Generic Available Yes

Use Prophylaxis or suppression of recurrent urinary tract infections; urinary tract discomfort secondary to hypermotility

Pregnancy Risk Factor C

Pregnancy Implications Following a single 1 g dose of methenamine hippurate given prior to delivery, methenamine was found to slowly pass through the placental barrier. There were no signs of accumulation in the fetal circulation. Actual concentrations in the amniotic fluid varied. Methenamine has been considered to be "probably safe" for use during pregnancy. Methenamine has been shown to interfere with urine oestriol concentrations during pregnancy; serum levels are not affected.

Contraindications Hypersensitivity to methenamine or any component of the formulation; severe dehydration, renal insufficiency, hepatic insufficiency in patients receiving hippurate salt; concurrent treatment with sulfonamides

Warnings/Precautions Methenamine should not be used to treat infections outside of the lower urinary tract. Use with caution in patients with hepatic disease, gout, and the elderly; doses of 8 g/day for 3-4 weeks may cause bladder irritation. Use care to maintain an acid pH of the urine, especially when treating infections due to urea splitting organisms (eg, *Proteus* and strains of *Pseudomonas*); reversible increases in LFTs have occurred during therapy especially in patients with hepatic dysfunction. Hiprex® contains tartrazine dye.

Adverse Reactions

1% to 10%:
- Dermatologic: Rash (<4%)
- Gastrointestinal: Nausea, dyspepsia (<4%)
- Genitourinary: Dysuria (<4%)

<1%: Bladder irritation, crystalluria (especially with large doses), increased AST/ALT (reversible, rare)

Overdosage/Toxicology Well tolerated. Treatment includes GI decontamination, if possible, and supportive care.

Drug Interactions

Increased Effect/Toxicity: Sulfonamides may precipitate in the urine; concurrent use is contraindicated.

Decreased Effect: Sodium bicarbonate and acetazolamide will decrease effect secondary to alkalinization of urine.

Ethanol/Nutrition/Herb Interactions Food: Foods/diets which alkalinize urine pH >5.5 decrease therapeutic effect of methenamine.

Stability Protect from excessive heat

Mechanism of Action Methenamine is hydrolyzed to formaldehyde and ammonia in acidic urine; formaldehyde has nonspecific bactericidal action

Pharmacodynamics/Kinetics

Absorption: Readily
Metabolism: Gastric juices: Hydrolyze 10% to 30% unless protected via enteric coating; Hepatic: ~10% to 25%
Half-life elimination: 3-6 hours
Excretion: Urine (~70% to 90% as unchanged drug) within 24 hours

Dosage Oral:

Children:
- >2-6 years: *Mandelate:* 50-75 mg/kg/day in 3-4 doses or 0.25 g/30 lb 4 times/day
- 6-12 years:
  - *Hippurate:* 0.5-1 g twice daily
  - *Mandelate:* 50-75 mg/kg/day in 3-4 doses or 0.5 g 4 times/day

>12 years and Adults:
- *Hippurate:* 0.5-1 g twice daily
- *Mandelate:* 1 g 4 times/day after meals and at bedtime

Dosing adjustment/comments in renal impairment: Cl_{cr} <50 mL/minute: Avoid use

(Continued)

Methenamine *(Continued)*

Dietary Considerations Foods/diets which alkalinize urine pH >5.5 decrease activity of methenamine; cranberry juice can be used to acidify urine and increase activity of methenamine. Hiprex® contains tartrazine dye.

Administration Administer around-the-clock to promote less variation in effect. Foods/diets which alkalinize urine pH >5.5 decrease activity of methenamine.

Monitoring Parameters Urinalysis, periodic liver function tests

Test Interactions Increased catecholamines and VMA (U); decreased HIAA (U)

Patient Information Take with food to minimize GI upset; take with ascorbic acid to acidify urine; drink sufficient fluids to ensure adequate urine flow. Avoid excessive intake of alkalinizing foods (citrus fruits and milk products) or medication (bicarbonate, acetazolamide); report skin rash, painful urination or excessive abdominal pain.

Additional Information Should not be used to treat infections outside of the lower urinary tract. Methenamine has little, if any, role in the treatment or prevention of infections in patients with indwelling urinary (Foley) catheters. Furthermore, in noncatheterized patients, more effective antibiotics are available for the prevention or treatment of urinary tract infections. The influence of decreased renal function on the pharmacologic effects of methenamine results are unknown.

Dosage Forms

Tablet, as hippurate (Hiprex®, Urex®): 1 g [Hiprex® contains tartrazine dye]

Tablet, enteric coated, as mandelate (Mandelamine®): 500 mg, 1 g

Methenamine Hippurate *see* Methenamine *on page 939*

Methenamine Mandelate *see* Methenamine *on page 939*

Methylphenyl Isoxazolyl Penicillin *see* Oxacillin *on page 983*

Methylrosaniline Chloride *see* Gentian Violet *on page 845*

MetroCream® *see* Metronidazole *on page 940*

MetroGel® *see* Metronidazole *on page 940*

MetroGel-Vaginal® *see* Metronidazole *on page 940*

MetroLotion® *see* Metronidazole *on page 940*

Metronidazole (me troe NI da zole)

Related Information

Antimicrobial Activity Against Selected Organisms *on page 1165*

Helicobacter pylori Treatment *on page 1288*

U.S. Brand Names Flagyl®; Flagyl ER®; Flagyl® I.V. RTU™; MetroCream®; MetroGel®; MetroGel-Vaginal®; MetroLotion®; Noritate®

Canadian Brand Names Apo-Metronidazole®; Flagyl®; Florazole® ER; MetroCream®; Metrogel®; Nidagel™; Noritate®; Novo-Nidazol; Trikacide

Synonyms Metronidazole Hydrochloride

Generic Available Yes: Cream, infusion, tablet

Use Treatment of susceptible anaerobic bacterial and protozoal infections in the following conditions: Amebiasis, symptomatic and asymptomatic trichomoniasis; skin and skin structure infections; CNS infections; intra-abdominal infections (as part of combination regimen); systemic anaerobic infections; treatment of antibiotic-associated pseudomembranous colitis (AAPC), bacterial vaginosis; as part of a multidrug regimen for *H. pylori* eradication to reduce the risk of duodenal ulcer recurrence

Topical: Treatment of inflammatory lesions and erythema of rosacea

Unlabeled/Investigational Use Crohn's disease

Drug of Choice or Alternative for Disease/Syndrome(s):

Acne Rosacea *on page 26*

Brain Abscess *on page 58*

Cervicitis *on page 71*

Cholangitis, Acute *on page 79*

Diverticulitis *on page 116*

Endometritis *on page 127*

Intra-abdominal Abscess *on page 194*

Liver Abscess *on page 211*

Lung Abscess *on page 212*

Mastitis *on page 214*

Osteomyelitis, Diabetic Foot *on page 249*

Pelvic Inflammatory Disease *on page 260*

Peritonitis, Secondary *on page 263*

Peritonitis, Spontaneous Bacterial *on page 264*

Vaginosis, Bacterial *on page 347*

Organism(s):

Bacteroides and *Prevotella* Species *on page 46*
Blastocystis hominis on page 49
Clostridium difficile on page 85
Clostridium perfringens on page 88
Clostridium tetani on page 90
Entamoeba histolytica on page 130
Gardnerella vaginalis on page 153
Giardia lamblia on page 155
Helicobacter pylori on page 162
Microsporidia *on page 220*
Mobiluncus Species *on page 221*
Trichomonas vaginalis on page 339

Pregnancy Risk Factor B (may be contraindicated in 1st trimester)

Pregnancy Implications Crosses the placenta (carcinogenic in rats); contraindicated for the treatment of trichomoniasis during the first trimester of pregnancy, unless alternative treatment is inadequate. Until safety and efficacy for other indications have been established, use only during pregnancy when the benefit to the mother outweighs the potential risk to the fetus.

Contraindications Hypersensitivity to metronidazole, nitroimidazole derivatives, or any component of the formulation; pregnancy (1st trimester - found to be carcinogenic in rats)

Warnings/Precautions Use with caution in patients with liver impairment due to potential accumulation, blood dyscrasias; history of seizures, CHF, or other sodium retaining states; reduce dosage in patients with severe liver impairment, CNS disease, and severe renal failure (Cl_{cr} <10 mL/minute); if *H. pylori* is not eradicated in patients being treated with metronidazole in a regimen, it should be assumed that metronidazole-resistance has occurred and it should not again be used; seizures and neuropathies have been reported especially with increased doses and chronic treatment; if this occurs, discontinue therapy

Adverse Reactions

Systemic: Frequency not defined:

Cardiovascular: Flattening of the T-wave, flushing
Central nervous system: Ataxia, confusion, coordination impaired, dizziness, fever, headache, insomnia, irritability, seizure, vertigo
Dermatologic: Erythematous rash, urticaria
Endocrine & metabolic: Disulfiram-like reaction, dysmenorrhea, libido decreased
Gastrointestinal: Nausea (~12%), anorexia, abdominal cramping, constipation, diarrhea, furry tongue, glossitis, proctitis, stomatitis, unusual/metallic taste, vomiting, xerostomia
Genitourinary: Cystitis, darkened urine (rare), dysuria, incontinence, polyuria, vaginitis
Hematologic: Neutropenia (reversible), thrombocytopenia (reversible, rare)
Neuromuscular & skeletal: Peripheral neuropathy, weakness
Respiratory: Nasal congestion, rhinitis, sinusitis, pharyngitis
Miscellaneous: Flu-like syndrome, moniliasis

Topical: Frequency not defined:

Central nervous system: Headache
Dermatologic: Burning, contact dermatitis, dryness, erythema, irritation, pruritus, rash
Gastrointestinal: Unusual/metallic taste, nausea, constipation
Local: Local allergic reaction
Neuromuscular & skeletal: Tingling/numbness of extremities
Ocular: Eye irritation

Vaginal:

>10%: Genitourinary: Vaginal discharge (12%)

1% to 10%:

Central nervous system: Headache (5%), dizziness (2%)
Gastrointestinal: Gastrointestinal discomfort (7%), nausea and/or vomiting (4%), unusual/metallic taste (2%), diarrhea (1%)
Genitourinary: Vaginitis (10%), vulva/vaginal irritation (9%), pelvic discomfort (3%)
Hematologic: WBC increased (2%)

<1%: Abdominal bloating, abdominal gas, darkened urine, depression, fatigue, itching, rash, thirst, xerostomia

Overdosage/Toxicology Symptoms include nausea, vomiting, ataxia, seizures, and peripheral neuropathy. Treatment is symptomatic and supportive.

(Continued)

Metronidazole *(Continued)*

Drug Interactions

Cytochrome P450 Effect: Inhibits CYP2C8/9 (weak), 3A4 (moderate)

Increased Effect/Toxicity: Ethanol may cause a disulfiram-like reaction. Warfarin and metronidazole may increase bleeding times (PT) which may result in bleeding. Cimetidine may increase metronidazole levels. Metronidazole may inhibit metabolism of cisapride, causing potential arrhythmias; avoid concurrent use. Metronidazole may increase lithium levels/toxicity. Metronidazole may increase the levels/effects of selected benzodiazepines, calcium channel blockers, cyclosporine, ergot derivatives, selected HMG-CoA reductase inhibitors, mirtazapine, nateglinide, nefazodone, sildenafil (and other PDE-5 inhibitors), tacrolimus, venlafaxine, and other CYP3A4 substrates.

Decreased Effect: Phenytoin, phenobarbital (potentially other enzyme inducers) may decrease metronidazole half-life and effects.

Ethanol/Nutrition/Herb Interactions

Ethanol: The manufacturer recommends to avoid all ethanol or any ethanol-containing drugs (may cause disulfiram-like reaction characterized by flushing, headache, nausea, vomiting, sweating or tachycardia).

Food: Peak antibiotic serum concentration lowered and delayed, but total drug absorbed not affected.

Stability Metronidazole injection should be stored at 15°C to 30°C and protected from light. Product may be refrigerated but crystals may form; crystals redissolve on warming to room temperature. Prolonged exposure to light will cause a darkening of the product. However, short-term exposure to normal room light does not adversely affect metronidazole stability. Direct sunlight should be avoided. Stability of parenteral admixture at room temperature (25°C): Out of overwrap stability: 30 days.

Standard diluent: 500 mg/100 mL NS

Mechanism of Action After diffusing into the organism, interacts with DNA to cause a loss of helical DNA structure and strand breakage resulting in inhibition of protein synthesis and cell death in susceptible organisms

Pharmacodynamics/Kinetics

Absorption: Oral: Well absorbed; Topical: Concentrations achieved systemically after application of 1 g topically are 10 times less than those obtained after a 250 mg oral dose

Distribution: To saliva, bile, seminal fluid, breast milk, bone, liver, and liver abscesses, lung and vaginal secretions; crosses placenta and blood-brain barrier

CSF:blood level ratio: Normal meninges: 16% to 43%; Inflamed meninges: 100%

Protein binding: <20%

Metabolism: Hepatic (30% to 60%)

Half-life elimination: Neonates: 25-75 hours; Others: 6-8 hours, prolonged with hepatic impairment; End-stage renal disease: 21 hours

Time to peak, serum: Oral: Immediate release: 1-2 hours

Excretion: Urine (20% to 40% as unchanged drug); feces (6% to 15%)

Dosage

Infants and Children:

- Amebiasis: Oral: 35-50 mg/kg/day in divided doses every 8 hours for 10 days
- Trichomoniasis: Oral: 15-30 mg/kg/day in divided doses every 8 hours for 7 days
- Anaerobic infections:
  - Oral: 15-35 mg/kg/day in divided doses every 8 hours
  - I.V.: 30 mg/kg/day in divided doses every 6 hours
- *Clostridium difficile* (antibiotic-associated colitis): Oral: 20 mg/kg/day divided every 6 hours
  - Maximum dose: 2 g/day

Adults:

- Amebiasis: Oral: 500-750 mg every 8 hours for 5-10 days
- Trichomoniasis: Oral: 250 mg every 8 hours for 7 days **or** 375 mg twice daily for 7 days **or** 2 g as a single dose
- Anaerobic infections: Oral, I.V.: 500 mg every 6-8 hours, not to exceed 4 g/day
- Antibiotic-associated pseudomembranous colitis: Oral: 250-500 mg 3-4 times/day for 10-14 days
- *Helicobacter pylori* eradication: Oral: 250-500 mg with meals and at bedtime for 14 days; requires combination therapy with at least one other antibiotic and an acid-suppressing agent (proton pump inhibitor or H_2 blocker)
- Bacterial vaginosis:
  - Oral: 750 mg (extended release tablet) once daily for 7 days
  - Vaginal: 1 applicatorful (~37.5 mg metronidazole) intravaginally once or twice daily for 5 days; apply once in morning and evening if using twice daily, if daily, use at bedtime

Acne rosacea: Topical:

0.75%: Apply and rub a thin film twice daily, morning and evening, to entire affected areas after washing. Significant therapeutic results should be noticed within 3 weeks. Clinical studies have demonstrated continuing improvement through 9 weeks of therapy.

1%: Apply thin film to affected area once daily

Elderly: Use lower end of dosing recommendations for adults, do not administer as a single dose

Dosing adjustment in renal impairment: Cl_{cr} <10 mL/minute: Administer 50% of dose or every 12 hours

Hemodialysis: Extensively removed by hemodialysis and peritoneal dialysis (50% to 100%); administer dose posthemodialysis

Peritoneal dialysis: Dose as for Cl_{cr} <10 mL/minute

Continuous arteriovenous or venovenous hemofiltration: Administer usual dose

Dosing adjustment/comments in hepatic disease: Unchanged in mild liver disease; reduce dosage in severe liver disease

Dietary Considerations Take on an empty stomach. Drug may cause GI upset; if GI upset occurs, take with food. Extended release tablets should be taken on an empty stomach (1 hour before or 2 hours after meals). Sodium content of 500 mg (I.V.): 322 mg (14 mEq). The manufacturer recommends that ethanol be avoided during treatment and for 3 days after therapy is complete.

Administration

Oral: May be taken with food to minimize stomach upset. Extended release tablets should be taken on an empty stomach (1 hour before or 2 hours after meals).

Topical: No disulfiram-like reactions have been reported after **topical** application, although metronidazole can be detected in the blood. Apply to clean, dry skin. Cosmetics may be used after application (wait at least 5 minutes after using lotion).

Test Interactions May interfere with AST, ALT, triglycerides, glucose, and LDH testing

Patient Information Urine may be discolored to a dark or reddish-brown; do not take alcohol for at least 24 hours after the last dose; avoid beverage alcohol or any topical products containing alcohol during therapy; may cause metallic taste; may be taken with food to minimize stomach upset; report numbness or tingling in extremities; avoid contact of the topical product with the eyes; cleanse areas to be treated well before application

Dosage Forms

Capsule (Flagyl®): 375 mg

Cream, topical: 0.75% (45 g)

MetroCream®: 0.75% (45 g) [contains benzyl alcohol]

Noritate®: 1% (60 g)

Gel, topical (MetroGel®): 0.75% (45 g), 1% (45 g)

Gel, vaginal (MetroGel-Vaginal®): 0.75% (70 g)

Infusion (Flagyl® I.V. RTU™) [premixed iso-osmotic sodium chloride solution]: 500 mg (100 mL) [contains sodium 14 mEq]

Lotion, topical (MetroLotion®): 0.75% (60 mL) [contains benzyl alcohol]

Tablet (Flagyl®): 250 mg, 500 mg

Tablet, extended release (Flagyl® ER): 750 mg

Extemporaneous Preparations A 20 mg/mL oral suspension can be prepared by crushing ten 250 mg tablets in a mortar, and then adding 10 mL purified water USP to create a uniform paste. Add a small quantity of syrup, then transfer to a graduate and add a sufficient quantity of syrup to make 125 mL. Label "shake well" and "refrigerate." Refrigerated stability is 10 days.

Irwin DB, Dupuis LL, Prober CG, et al, "The Acceptability, Stability, and Relative Bioavailability of an Extemporaneous Metronidazole Suspension," *Can J Hosp Pharm*, 1987, 40:42-6.

Nahata MC, Morosco RS, and Hipple TF, 4th ed, *Pediatric Drug Formulations*, Cincinnati, OH: Harvey Whitney Books Co, 2000.

Selected Readings

Falagas ME and Gorbach SL, "Clindamycin and Metronidazole," *Med Clin North Am*, 1995, 79(4):845-67.

Fekety R and Shah AB, "Diagnosis and Treatment of *Clostridium difficile* Colitis," *JAMA*, 1993, 269(1):71-5.

Freeman CD, Klutman NE, and Lamp KC, "Metronidazole. A Therapeutic Review and Update," *Drugs*, 1997, 54(5):679-708.

Kelly CP, Pothoulakis C, and LaMont JT, "*Clostridium difficile* Colitis," *N Engl J Med*, 1994, 330(4):257-62.

Smilack JD, Wilson WR, and Cockerill FR 3d, "Tetracyclines, Chloramphenicol, Erythromycin, Clindamycin, and Metronidazole," *Mayo Clin Proc*, 1991, 66(12):1270-80.

Metronidazole, Bismuth Subsalicylate, and Tetracycline *see* Bismuth Subsalicylate, Metronidazole, and Tetracycline *on page 688*

Metronidazole Hydrochloride *see* Metronidazole *on page 940*

Metronidazole, Tetracycline, and Bismuth Subsalicylate *see* Bismuth Subsalicylate, Metronidazole, and Tetracycline *on page 688*

Micaderm® [OTC] *see* Miconazole *on page 945*

Micafungin (mi ka FUN gin)

U.S. Brand Names Mycamine™

Synonyms Micafungin Sodium

Use Esophageal candidiasis; *Candida* prophylaxis in patients undergoing hematopoietic stem cell transplant

Unlabeled/Investigational Use Treatment of infections due to *Aspergillus* spp; prophylaxis of HIV-related esophageal candidiasis

Drug of Choice or Alternative for Organism(s):

Candida Species *on page 67*

Pregnancy Risk Factor C

Pregnancy Implications Visceral teratogenic and abortifacient effects were noted in animal studies. There are no adequate and well-controlled studies in pregnant women. Use only if benefit outweighs risk.

Contraindications Hypersensitivity to micafungin or any component of the formulation

Warnings/Precautions Anaphylactic reactions, including shock, have been reported. New onset or worsening hepatic failure has been reported; use caution in pre-existing mild-moderate hepatic impairment; safety in severe liver failure has not been evaluated. Hemolytic anemia and hemoglobinuria have been reported. Safety and efficacy in pediatric patients have not been established.

Adverse Reactions

1% to 10%:

Cardiovascular: Phlebitis (2%), hypertension (1%), flushing (1%)

Central nervous system: Headache (2%), pyrexia (2%), delirium (1%), dizziness (1%), somnolence (1%)

Dermatologic: Rash (2%), pruritus (1%), febrile neutropenia (1%)

Endocrine & metabolic: Hypokalemia (1%), hypocalcemia (1%), hypomagnesemia (1%), hypophosphatemia (1%)

Gastrointestinal: Nausea (3%), diarrhea (2%), vomiting (2%), abdominal pain (1%), appetite decreased (1%), dysgeusia (1%), dyspepsia (1%)

Hematologic: Leukopenia (2%), neutropenia (1%), thrombocytopenia (1%), anemia (1%), lymphopenia (1%), eosinophilia (1%)

Hepatic: Transaminase increased (2% to 3%), serum alkaline phosphatase increased (2%), hyperbilirubinemia (1%)

Local: Infusion site inflammation (1%)

Neuromuscular & skeletal: Rigors (1%), lactate dehydrogenase increased (1%)

Renal: Serum creatinine increased (1%), serum urea increased (1%)

<1%, postmarketing and/or case reports, or frequency not defined: Acidosis, anorexia, anuria, apnea, arrhythmia, arthralgia, cardiac arrest, coagulopathy, constipation, convulsions, cyanosis, dyspnea, deep vein thrombosis, hypoxia, encephalopathy, erythema multiforme, facial edema, hemoglobinuria, hemolysis, hemolytic anemia, hepatic failure, hepatocellular damage, hepatomegaly, hiccups, hyponatremia, hypotension, infection, injection site necrosis, intracranial hemorrhage, jaundice, MI, mycosal inflammation, oliguria, pancytopenia, pneumonia, pulmonary embolism, renal failure, renal tubular necrosis, sepsis, shock, tachycardia, skin necrosis, thrombotic thrombocytopenia purpura, thrombophlebitis, urticaria, vasodilatation

Overdosage/Toxicology Treatment should be symptom-directed and supportive. Not removed by dialysis.

Drug Interactions

Cytochrome P450 Effect:

Substrate of CYP3A4 (minor); **Inhibits** CYP3A4 (weak)

Increased Effect/Toxicity:

No clinically-significant interactions have been identified.

Decreased Effect:

No clinically-signficant interactions have been identified.

Stability Store at 25°C (77°F); reconstituted and diluted solutions are stable for 24 hours at room temperature; protect from light. Aseptically add 5 mL of NS (preservative-free) to each 50 mg vial; swirl to dissolve; do not shake. Further dilute 50-150 mg in 100 mL NS; protect from light. Alternatively, D_5W may be used for reconstitution and dilution.

Mechanism of Action Concentration-dependent inhibition of 1,3-beta-D-glucan synthase resulting in reduced formation of 1,3-beta-D-glucan, an essential polysaccharide comprising 30% to 60% of *Candida* cell walls (absent in mammalian cells); decreased glucan content leads to osmotic instability and cellular lysis

Pharmacodynamics/Kinetics

Distribution: 0.28-0.5 L/kg

Protein binding: >99%

Metabolism: Hepatic; forms M-1 (catechol) and M-2 (methoxy) metabolites (activity unknown)

Half-life elimination: 11-21 hours

Excretion: Primarily feces (71%), urine (<15%, unchanged drug)

Dosage I.V.: Adults:

Esophageal candidiasis: 150 mg daily; median duration of therapy (from clinical trials) was 14 days

Prophylaxis of *Candida* infection in hematopoietic stem cell transplantation: 50 mg daily; median duration of therapy (from clinical trials) was 18 days

Administration For intravenous use only; infuse over 1 hour

Monitoring Parameters Liver function tests

Patient Information Inform prescriber of all prescriptions, OTC medications, or herbal products you are taking, and any allergies you have. This medication can only be administered by infusion. Report immediately any pain, burning, or swelling at infusion site, or any signs of allergic reaction (eg, respiratory difficulty or swallowing, back pain, chest tightness, rash, hives, or swelling of lips or mouth). Report nausea, vomiting, abdominal pain, or diarrhea.

Dosage Forms Injection, powder for reconstitution, as sodium [preservative-free]: Micafungin 50 mg [contains lactose]

Micafungin Sodium *see* Micafungin *on page 944*

Micatin® [OTC] *see* Miconazole *on page 945*

Miconazole (mi KON a zole)

U.S. Brand Names Aloe Vesta® 2-n-1 Antifungal [OTC]; Baza® Antifungal [OTC]; Carrington Antifungal [OTC]; Femizol-M™ [OTC]; Fungoid® Tincture [OTC]; Lotrimin® AF Powder/Spray [OTC]; Micaderm® [OTC]; Micatin® [OTC]; Micro-Guard® [OTC]; Mitrazol™ [OTC]; Monistat® 1 Combination Pack [OTC]; Monistat® 3 [OTC]; Monistat® 7 [OTC]; Monistat-Derm®; Triple Care® Antifungal [OTC]; Zeasorb®-AF [OTC]

Canadian Brand Names Dermazole; Micatin®; Micozole; Monistat®; Monistat® 3

Synonyms Miconazole Nitrate

Generic Available Yes

Use Treatment of vulvovaginal candidiasis and a variety of skin and mucous membrane fungal infections

Drug of Choice or Alternative for Organism(s):

Malassezia furfur on page 213

Pregnancy Risk Factor C

Contraindications Hypersensitivity to miconazole or any component of the formulation

Warnings/Precautions For external use only; discontinue if sensitivity or irritation develop. Petrolatum-based vaginal products may damage rubber or latex condoms or diaphragms. Separate use by 3 days.

Adverse Reactions Frequency not defined.

Topical: Allergic contact dermatitis, burning, maceration

Vaginal: Abdominal cramps, burning, irritation, itching

Drug Interactions

Cytochrome P450 Effect: Substrate of CYP3A4 (major); **Inhibits** CYP1A2 (moderate), 2A6 (strong), 2B6 (weak), 2C8/9 (strong), 2C19 (strong), 2D6 (strong), 2E1 (moderate), 3A4 (strong)

Increased Effect/Toxicity: Note: The majority of reported drug interactions were observed following intravenous miconazole administration. Although systemic absorption following topical and/or vaginal administration is low, potential interactions due to CYP isoenzyme inhibition may occur (rarely). This may be particularly true in situations where topical absorption may be increased (ie, inflamed tissue).

Miconazole coadministered with warfarin has increased the anticoagulant effect of warfarin (including reports associated with vaginal miconazole therapy of as little as 3 days). Concurrent administration of cisapride is contraindicated due to an increased risk of cardiotoxicity. Miconazole may increase the serum levels/effects of amiodarone, amphetamines, benzodiazepines, beta-blockers, buspirone, busulfan, calcium channel blockers, citalopram, dexmedetomidine, dextromethorphan, diazepam, digoxin, docetaxel, fluoxetine, fluvoxamine, glimepiride, glipizide,

(Continued)

Miconazole *(Continued)*

ifosfamide, inhalational anesthetics, lidocaine, mesoridazine, methsuximide, mexiletine, mirtazapine, nateglinide, nefazodone, paroxetine, phenytoin, pioglitazone, propranolol, risperidone, ritonavir, ropinirole, rosiglitazone, sertraline, sirolimus, tacrolimus, theophylline, thioridazine, tricyclic antidepressants, trifluoperazine, trimetrexate, venlafaxine, vincristine, vinblastine, warfarin, zolpidem, and other substrates of CYP1A2, 2A6, 2C8/9, 2C19, 2D6, or 3A4. Selected benzodiazepines (midazolam and triazolam), cisapride, ergot alkaloids, selected HMG-CoA reductase inhibitors (lovastatin and simvastatin), and pimozide are generally contraindicated with strong CYP3A4 inhibitors. Mesoridazine and thioridazine are generally contraindicated with strong CYP2D6 inhibitors. When used with strong CYP3A4 inhibitors, dosage adjustment/limits are recommended for sildenafil and other PDE-5 inhibitors; consult individual monographs.

Decreased Effect: Amphotericin B may decrease antifungal effect of both agents. The levels/effects of miconazole may be decreased by aminoglutethimide, carbamazepine, nafcillin, nevirapine, phenobarbital, phenytoin, rifamycins or other CYP3A4 inducers. Miconazole may decrease the levels/effects of CYP2D6 prodrug substrates (eg, codeine, hydrocodone, oxycodone, tramadol).

Ethanol/Nutrition/Herb Interactions Herb/Nutraceutical: St John's wort may decrease miconazole levels.

Mechanism of Action Inhibits biosynthesis of ergosterol, damaging the fungal cell wall membrane, which increases permeability causing leaking of nutrients

Pharmacodynamics/Kinetics

Absorption: Topical: Negligible

Distribution: Widely to body tissues; penetrates well into inflamed joints, vitreous humor of eye, and peritoneal cavity, but poorly into saliva and sputum; crosses blood-brain barrier but only to a small extent

Protein binding: 91% to 93%

Metabolism: Hepatic

Half-life elimination: Multiphasic: Initial: 40 minutes; Secondary: 126 minutes; Terminal: 24 hours

Excretion: Feces (~50%); urine (<1% as unchanged drug)

Dosage

Topical: Children and Adults: **Note:** Not for OTC use in children <2 years:
- Tinea pedis and tinea corporis: Apply twice daily for 4 weeks
- Tinea cruris: Apply twice daily for 2 weeks

Vaginal: Adults: Vulvovaginal candidiasis:
- Cream, 2%: Insert 1 applicatorful at bedtime for 7 days
- Cream, 4%: Insert 1 applicatorful at bedtime for 3 days
- Suppository, 100 mg: Insert 1 suppository at bedtime for 7 days
- Suppository, 200 mg: Insert 1 suppository at bedtime for 3 days
- Suppository, 1200 mg: Insert 1 suppository (a one-time dose); may be used at bedtime or during the day

Note: Many products are available as a combination pack, with a suppository for vaginal instillation and cream to relieve external symptoms. External cream may be used twice daily, as needed, for up to 7 days.

Patient Information Take full course of therapy as directed; do not discontinue without consulting prescriber. Some infections may require long periods of therapy. Practice good hygiene measures to prevent reinfection. If you are diabetic, you should test serum glucose regularly at the same time of day. You may experience nausea and vomiting (small, frequent meals may help) or headache, dizziness (use caution when driving). Report unresolved headache, rash, burning, itching, anorexia, unusual fatigue, diarrhea, nausea, or vomiting.

Topical: Wash and dry area before applying medication; apply thinly. Do not get in or near eyes.

Vaginal: Insert high in vagina. Refrain from intercourse during treatment. OTC products, even if administered topically, may not mix well with certain prescription medications (which may lead to drug interactions). Consult with your prescriber. Deodorant-free pads or panty shields may be used to protect clothing during use.

Dosage Forms

[DSC] = Discontinued product

Combination products: Miconazole nitrate vaginal suppository 200 mg (3s) and miconazole nitrate external cream 2%; Miconazole nitrate vaginal suppository 100 mg (7s) and miconazole nitrate external cream 2%

Monistat® 1 Combination Pack: Miconazole nitrate vaginal insert 1200 mg (1) and miconazole external cream 2% (5 g) [Note: Do not confuse with 1-Day™ (formerly Monistat® 1) which contains tioconazole]

Monistat® 3 Combination Pack: Miconazole nitrate vaginal suppository 200 mg (3s) and miconazole nitrate external cream 2%
Monistat® 3 Cream Combination Pack: Miconazole nitrate vaginal cream 4% and miconazole nitrate external cream 2%
Monistat® 7 Combination Pack:
Miconazole nitrate vaginal suppository 100 mg (7s) and miconazole nitrate external cream 2%
Miconazole nitrate vaginal cream 2% (7 prefilled applicators) and miconazole nitrate external cream 2%
Cream, topical, as nitrate: 2% (15 g, 30 g, 45 g)
Baza® Antifungal: 2% (4 g, 57 g, 142 g) [zinc oxide based formula]
Carrington Antifungal: 2% (150 g)
Micaderm®: 2% (30 g)
Micatin®: 2% (15 g)
Micro-Guard®, Mitrazol™: 2% (60 g)
Monistat-Derm®: 2% (15 g, 30 g, 85 g)
Triple Care® Antifungal: 2% (60 g, 98 g)
Cream, vaginal, as nitrate [prefilled or with single refillable applicator]: 2% (45 g)
Femizol-M™: 2% (47 g)
Monistat® 3: 4% (15 g, 25 g)
Monistat® 7: 2% (45 g)
Liquid, spray, as nitrate (Micatin®): 2% (90 mL, 105 mL)
Lotion, powder, as nitrate (Zeasorb®-AF): 2% (56 g) [contains alcohol 70%]
Ointment, topical, as nitrate: (Aloe Vesta® 2-n-1 Antifungal): 2% (60 g, 150 g)
Powder, topical, as nitrate:
Lotrimin® AF, Micatin®, Micro-Guard®: 2% (90 g)
Mitrazol™: 2% (30 g)
Zeasorb®-AF: 2% (70 g)
Powder spray, topical, as nitrate (Lotrimin® AF): 2% (100 g)
Suppository, vaginal, as nitrate: 100 mg (7s); 200 mg (3s)
Monistat® 3: 200 mg (3s) [DSC]
Monistat® 7: 100 mg (7s)
Tincture, topical, as nitrate (Fungoid®): 2% (30 mL, 473 mL) [contains isopropyl alcohol 30%]

Miconazole Nitrate *see* Miconazole *on page 945*

Micozole (Can) *see* Miconazole *on page 945*

MICRhoGAM® *see* Rh_o(D) Immune Globulin *on page 1038*

Micro-Guard® [OTC] *see* Miconazole *on page 945*

Minidyne® [OTC] *see* Povidone-Iodine *on page 1016*

Minim's Gentamicin 0.3% (Can) *see* Gentamicin *on page 841*

Minocin® *see* Minocycline *on page 947*

Minocycline (mi noe SYE kleen)

U.S. Brand Names Dynacin®; Minocin®; myrac™

Canadian Brand Names Alti-Minocycline; Apo-Minocycline®; Gen-Minocycline; Minocin®; Novo-Minocycline; PMS-Minocycline; Rhoxal-minocycline

Synonyms Minocycline Hydrochloride

Generic Available Yes

Use Treatment of susceptible bacterial infections of both gram-negative and gram-positive organisms; treatment of anthrax (inhalational, cutaneous, and gastrointestinal); acne; meningococcal carrier state; Rickettsial diseases (including Rocky Mountain spotted fever, Q fever); nongonococcal urethritis, gonorrhea; acute intestinal amebiasis

Drug of Choice or Alternative for Disease/Syndrome(s):

Acne Vulgaris *on page 27*

Organism(s):

Burkholderia cepacia on page 62
Burkholderia mallei on page 64
Nocardia Species *on page 247*
Stenotrophomonas maltophilia on page 312

Pregnancy Risk Factor D

Pregnancy Implications May cause permanent discoloration (brown-gray) of teeth. Animal studies indicate possible tumorigenicity and impairment of fertility. Congenital anomalies have been reported postmarketing.

Contraindications Hypersensitivity to minocycline, other tetracyclines, or any component of the formulation; pregnancy
(Continued)

Minocycline *(Continued)*

Warnings/Precautions May cause permanent tooth discoloration; avoid use during tooth development (children ≤8 years of age) unless other drugs are not likely to be effective or are contraindicated. May be associated with increases in BUN secondary to antianabolic effects; use caution in patients with renal or hepatic insufficiency. CNS effects (lightheadedness, vertigo) may occur; patients must be cautioned about performing tasks which require mental alertness (eg, operating machinery or driving). Has been associated (rarely) with pseudotumor cerebri. May cause photosensitivity; discontinue if skin erythema occurs. May cause overgrowth of nonsusceptible organisms, including fungi; discontinue if superinfection occurs. Avoid use in children ≤8 years of age.

Adverse Reactions Frequency not defined.

Cardiovascular: Myocarditis, pericarditis, vasculitis

Central Nervous System: Bulging fontanels, convulsions, dizziness, fever, headache, hypoesthesia, paresthesia, pseudotumor cerebri, sedation, vertigo

Dermatologic: Alopecia, angioedema, epidermal necrolysis, erythema nodosum, erythematous rash, exfoliative dermatitis, hyperpigmentation of nails, maculopapular rash, photosensitivity, pigmentation of the skin and mucous membranes, pruritus, Stevens-Johnson syndrome, toxic erythema multiforme, urticaria

Endocrine & metabolic: Thyroid dysfunction

Gastrointestinal: Anorexia, diarrhea, dyspepsia, dysphagia, enamel hypoplasia, enterocolitis, esophageal ulcerations, esophagitis, glossitis, inflammatory lesions (oral/anogenital), moniliasis, nausea, oral cavity discoloration, pancreatitis, pseudomembranous colitis, stomatitis, tooth discoloration, vomiting

Genitourinary: Balanitis, vulvovaginitis

Hematologic: Agranulocytosis, eosinophilia, hemolytic anemia, leukopenia, neutropenia, pancytopenia, thrombocytopenia

Hepatic: Hepatic cholestasis, hepatic failure, hepatitis, hyperbilirubinemia, jaundice, liver enzyme increases

Neuromuscular & skeletal: Arthralgia, arthritis, bone discoloration, joint stiffness, joint swelling, myalgia

Otic: Hearing loss, tinnitus

Renal: Acute renal failure, BUN increased, interstitial nephritis

Respiratory: Asthma, bronchospasm, cough, dyspnea, pneumonitis, pulmonary infiltrate

Miscellaneous: Anaphylaxis, lupus erythematosus

Overdosage/Toxicology Symptoms include diabetes insipidus, nausea, anorexia, dizziness, vomiting, and diarrhea. Following GI decontamination, care is supportive only. Fluid support may be required. Not dialyzable (0% to 5%).

Drug Interactions

Increased Effect/Toxicity: Minocycline may increase the effect of warfarin. Retinoic acid derivatives may increase risk of pseudotumor cerebri.

Decreased Effect: Although anecdotal reports suggest oral contraceptive efficacy could be reduced by tetracyclines, this has been refuted by more rigorous scientific and clinical data. Calcium-, magnesium-, or aluminum-containing antacids, bile acid sequestrants, bismuth, oral contraceptives, iron, zinc, sodium bicarbonate, penicillins, cimetidine, quinapril may decrease absorption of tetracyclines. Methoxyflurane anesthesia (when concurrent with tetracyclines) may cause fatal nephrotoxicity. Tetracyclines may reduce bactericidal efficacy of penicillins and cephalosporins.

Ethanol/Nutrition/Herb Interactions

Food: Minocycline serum concentrations are not significantly altered if taken with food or dairy products.

Herb/Nutraceutical: Avoid dong quai, St John's wort (may also cause photosensitization).

Mechanism of Action Inhibits bacterial protein synthesis by binding with the 30S and possibly the 50S ribosomal subunit(s) of susceptible bacteria; cell wall synthesis is not affected

Pharmacodynamics/Kinetics

Absorption: Well absorbed

Distribution: Majority deposits for extended periods in fat; crosses placenta; enters breast milk

Protein binding: 70% to 75%

Half-life elimination: 16 hours (range: 11-23 hours)

Excretion: Urine

Dosage Oral:

Children >8 years: Initial: 4 mg/kg followed by 2 mg/kg/dose every 12 hours

Adults:

Susceptible infections: 200 mg initially, followed by 100 mg every 12 hours, not to exceed 400 mg/24 hours

Acne: 50-100 mg daily
Chlamydial or *Ureaplasma urealyticum* infection, uncomplicated: Urethral, endocervical, or rectal: 100 mg every 12 hours for at least 7 days
Gonococcal infection, uncomplicated (males): Without urethritis or anorectal infection: 200 mg initially, followed by 100 mg every 12 hours for at least 4 days (cultures 2-3 days post-therapy)
Gonococcal infection, uncomplicated urethritis: 100 mg every 12 hours for 5 days
Meningococcal carrier state: 100 mg every 12 hours for 5 days
Mycobacterium marinum: 100 mg every 12 hours for 6-8 weeks (**Note:** Optimal doses have not been established)
Syphilis: 200 mg initially, followed by 100 mg every 12 hours for 10-15 days

Dosage adjustment in renal impairment: Consider decreasing dose or increasing dosing interval; total daily dose should not exceed 200 mg

Dietary Considerations May be taken with food or milk.

Administration

Oral: May be taken with food or milk. Administer with adequate fluid to decrease the risk of esophageal irritation and ulceration.

I.V.: Infuse slowly, usually over a 4- to 6-hour period.

Test Interactions May cause interference with fluorescence test for urinary catecholamines (false elevations)

Patient Information Avoid unnecessary exposure to sunlight; do not take with antacids or iron products; finish all medication; do not skip doses; take 1 hour before or 2 hours after meals; take with adequate fluids to decrease risk of irritation

Dosage Forms [DSC] = Discontinued product

Capsule: 50 mg, 75 mg, 100 mg
Dynacin®: 50 mg [DSC], 75 mg, 100 mg
Capsule, pellet-filled (Minocin®): 50 mg, 100 mg
Tablet (Dynacin®, myrac™): 50 mg, 75 mg, 100 mg

Selected Readings

Smilack JD, Wilson WR, and Cockerill FR 3d, "Tetracyclines, Chloramphenicol, Erythromycin, Clindamycin, and Metronidazole," *Mayo Clin Proc*, 1991, 66(12):1270-80.

Minocycline Hydrochloride *see* Minocycline *on page 947*
Mintezol® *see* Thiabendazole *on page 1111*
Mitrazol™ [OTC] *see* Miconazole *on page 945*
MK0826 *see* Ertapenem *on page 805*
MMR *see* Measles, Mumps, and Rubella Vaccines (Combined) *on page 926*
Monistat® (Can) *see* Miconazole *on page 945*
Monistat® 1 Combination Pack [OTC] *see* Miconazole *on page 945*
Monistat® 3 [OTC] *see* Miconazole *on page 945*
Monistat® 7 [OTC] *see* Miconazole *on page 945*
Monistat-Derm® *see* Miconazole *on page 945*
Monodox® *see* Doxycycline *on page 787*
Monurol™ *see* Fosfomycin *on page 832*
More Attenuated Enders Strain *see* Measles Virus Vaccine (Live) *on page 927*

Moxifloxacin (moxs i FLOKS a sin)

Related Information

Antimicrobial Activity Against Selected Organisms *on page 1165*
Community-Acquired Pneumonia in Adults *on page 1278*
Tuberculosis *on page 1315*

U.S. Brand Names Avelox®; Avelox® I.V.; Vigamox™

Canadian Brand Names Avelox®; Vigamox™

Synonyms Moxifloxacin Hydrochloride

Generic Available No

Use Treatment of mild-to-moderate community-acquired pneumonia, including multidrug-resistant *Streptococcus pneumoniae* (MDRSP); acute bacterial exacerbation of chronic bronchitis; acute bacterial sinusitis; complicated and uncomplicated skin and skin structure infections; bacterial conjunctivitis (ophthalmic formulation)

Drug of Choice or Alternative for Disease/Syndrome(s):

Cholangitis, Acute *on page 79*
Peritonitis, Spontaneous Bacterial *on page 264*
Pneumonia, Community-Acquired *on page 270*
Pneumonia, Hospital-Acquired *on page 272*
Pneumonia, Ventilator-Associated *on page 273*

Organism(s):

Streptococcus pneumoniae, Drug-Resistant *on page 316*
(Continued)

Moxifloxacin *(Continued)*

Pregnancy Risk Factor C

Pregnancy Implications Reports of arthropathy (observed in immature animals and reported rarely in humans) have limited the use of fluoroquinolones during pregnancy. Teratogenic effects were not observed with moxifloxacin in animal studies; however, delayed skeletal development and smaller fetuses were observed in some species. There are no adequate and well-controlled studies in pregnant women. Based on limited data, quinolones are not expected to be a major human teratogen. Although quinolone antibiotics should not be used as first-line agents during pregnancy, when considering treatment for life-threatening infection and/or prolonged duration of therapy, the potential risk to the fetus must be balanced against the severity of the potential illness.

Contraindications Hypersensitivity to moxifloxacin, other quinolone antibiotics, or any component of the formulation

Warnings/Precautions Use with caution in patients with significant bradycardia or acute myocardial ischemia. Moxifloxacin causes a concentration-dependent QT prolongation. Do not exceed recommended dose or infusion rate. Avoid use with uncorrected hypokalemia, with other drugs that prolong the QT interval or induce bradycardia, or with class IA or III antiarrhythmic agents. Use with caution in individuals at risk of seizures (CNS disorders or concurrent therapy with medications which may lower seizure threshold). Discontinue in patients who experience significant CNS adverse effects (dizziness, hallucinations, suicidal ideation or actions). Not recommended in patients with moderate to severe hepatic insufficiency. Use with caution in diabetes; glucose regulation may be altered. Tendon inflammation and/or rupture have been reported with quinolone antibiotics. Risk may be increased with concurrent corticosteroids, particularly in the elderly. Discontinue at first signs or symptoms of tendon pain.

Severe hypersensitivity reactions, including anaphylaxis, have occurred with quinolone therapy. If an allergic reaction occurs (itching, urticaria, dyspnea or facial edema, loss of consciousness, tingling, cardiovascular collapse) discontinue drug immediately. Prolonged use may result in superinfection; pseudomembranous colitis may occur and should be considered in all patients who present with diarrhea. Quinolones may exacerbate myasthenia gravis, use with caution (rare, potentially life-threatening weakness of respiratory muscles may occur). Peripheral neuropathy may rarely occur. Safety and efficacy of systemically administered moxifloxacin (oral, intravenous) in patients <18 years of age have not been established.

Ophthalmic: Eye drops should not be injected subconjunctivally or introduced directly into the anterior chamber of the eye. Contact lenses should not be worn during therapy.

Adverse Reactions

Systemic:

3% to 10%: Gastrointestinal: Nausea (6%), diarrhea (5%)

0.1% to 3%:

- Cardiovascular: Hypertension, palpitation, QT_c prolongation, tachycardia, vasodilation
- Central nervous system: Anxiety, chills, dizziness, headache, insomnia, nervousness, pain, somnolence, tremor, vertigo
- Dermatologic: Dry skin, pruritus, rash (maculopapular, purpuric, pustular)
- Endocrine & metabolic: Serum chloride increased (≥2%), serum ionized calcium increased (≥2%), serum glucose decreased (≥2%)
- Gastrointestinal: Abdominal pain, amylase increased, amylase decreased (≥2%), anorexia, constipation, dry mouth, dyspepsia, flatulence, glossitis, lactic dehydrogenase increased, stomatitis, taste perversion, vomiting
- Genitourinary: Vaginal moniliasis, vaginitis
- Hematologic: Anemia, eosinophilia, leukopenia, prothrombin time prolonged, increased INR, thrombocythemia
  - Increased serum levels of the following (≥2%): MCH, neutrophils, WBC
  - Decreased serum levels of the following (≥2%): Basophils, eosinophils, hemoglobin, RBC, neutrophils
- Hepatic: Bilirubin decreased or increased (≥2%), GGTP increased, liver function test abnormal
- Local: Injection site reaction
- Neuromuscular & skeletal: Arthralgia, myalgia, weakness
- Renal: Kidney function abnormal, serum albumin increased (≥2%)
- Respiratory: Pharyngitis, pneumonia, rhinitis, sinusitis, pO_2 increased (≥2%)
- Miscellaneous: Allergic reaction, infection, diaphoresis

<0.1%, postmarketing, and/or case reports: Abnormal dreams, agitation, amblyopia, amnesia, anaphylactic reaction, anaphylactic shock, anemia, angioedema,

aphasia, arthritis, asthma, atrial fibrillation, back pain, *C. difficile*-positive diarrhea, chest pain, cholestasis, confusion, convulsions, depersonalization, depression, dysphagia, dyspnea, ECG abnormalities, emotional lability, face edema, gastritis, hallucinations, hepatitis, hyperglycemia, hyperlipidemia, hypertonia, hyperuricemia, hypoesthesia, hypotension, incoordination, jaundice (cholestatic), laryngeal edema, leg pain, malaise, parsthesia, parosmia, pelvic pain, peripheral edema, peripheral neuropathy, prothrombin time decreased, pseudomembranous colitis, psychotic reaction, sleep disorder, speech disorder, Stevens-Johnson syndrome, supraventricular tachycardia, taste loss, tendon disorder or rupture, thinking abnormal, thrombocytopenia, thromboplastin decreased, tinnitus, tongue discoloration, urticaria, ventricular tachycardia, vision abnormalities; torsade de pointes and cardiac arrest (usually in patients with concurrent, severe proarrhythmic conditions)

Additional reactions with **ophthalmic** preparation: 1% to 6%: Conjunctivitis, dry eye, ocular discomfort, ocular hyperemia, ocular pain, ocular pruritus, subconjunctival hemorrhage, tearing, visual acuity decreased

Overdosage/Toxicology Potential symptoms of overdose may include CNS excitation, seizures, QT prolongation, and arrhythmias (including torsade de pointes). Patients should be monitored by continuous ECG in the event of an overdose. Management is supportive and symptomatic.

Drug Interactions

Increased Effect/Toxicity: Moxifloxacin may increase the effects/toxicity of glyburide and warfarin. Concomitant use with corticosteroids may increase the risk of tendon rupture. Concomitant use with other QT_c-prolonging agents (eg, Class Ia and Class III antiarrhythmics, erythromycin, cisapride, antipsychotics, and cyclic antidepressants) may result in arrhythmias, such as torsade de pointes.

Decreased Effect: Concurrent administration of metal cations, including most antacids, oral electrolyte supplements, quinapril, sucralfate, some didanosine formulations (chewable/buffered tablets and pediatric powder for oral suspension), and other higly-buffered oral drugs, may decrease quinolone levels; separate doses.

Ethanol/Nutrition/Herb Interactions Food: Absorption is not affected by administration with a high-fat meal or yogurt.

Stability Store at 15°C to 30°C (59°F to 86°F). Do not refrigerate infusion solution.

Mechanism of Action Moxifloxacin is a DNA gyrase inhibitor, and also inhibits topoisomerase IV. DNA gyrase (topoisomerase II) is an essential bacterial enzyme that maintains the superhelical structure of DNA. DNA gyrase is required for DNA replication and transcription, DNA repair, recombination, and transposition; inhibition is bactericidal.

Pharmacodynamics/Kinetics

Absorption: Well absorbed; not affected by high fat meal or yogurt

Distribution: V_d: 1.7 to 2.7 L/kg; tissue concentrations often exceed plasma concentrations in respiratory tissues, alveolar macrophages, and sinus tissues

Protein binding: 50%

Metabolism: Hepatic (52% of dose) via glucuronide (14%) and sulfate (38%) conjugation

Bioavailability: 90%

Half-life elimination: Oral: 12 hours; I.V.: 15 hours

Excretion: Approximately 45% of a dose is excreted in feces (25%) and urine (20%) as unchanged drug

Metabolites: Sulfate conjugates in feces, glucuronide conjugates in urine

Dosage

Ophthalmic: Children ≥1 year and Adults: Instill 1 drop into affected eye(s) 3 times/day for 7 days

Oral, I.V.: Adults:

Acute bacterial sinusitis: 400 mg every 24 hours for 10 days

Chronic bronchitis, acute bacterial exacerbation: 400 mg every 24 hours for 5 days

Note: Avelox® ABC Pack™ (Avelox® Bronchitis Course) contains five tablets of 400 mg each.

Community-acquired pneumonia (including MDRSP): 400 mg every 24 hours for 7-14 days

Complicated skin and skin structure infections: 400 mg every 24 hours for 7-21 days

Uncomplicated skin and skin structure infections: 400 mg every 24 hours for 7 days

Elderly: No dosage adjustments are required based on age

Dosage adjustment in renal impairment: No dosage adjustment is required, including patients on hemodialysis or CAPD

Dosage adjustment in hepatic impairment: No dosage adjustment is required in mild to moderate hepatic insufficiency (Child-Pugh Class A and B). Not recommended in patients with severe hepatic insufficiency.

(Continued)

Moxifloxacin *(Continued)*

Dietary Considerations May be taken with or without food. Take 4 hours before or 8 hours after multiple vitamins, antacids, or other products containing magnesium, aluminum, iron, or zinc.

Administration I.V.: Infuse over 60 minutes; do not infuse by rapid or bolus intravenous infusion

Monitoring Parameters WBC, signs of infection

Patient Information Tablet: May be taken with or without food; drink plenty of fluids; do not take antacids within 4 hours before or 8 hours after dosing. Contact your prescriber immediately if signs of allergy occur. Contact your prescriber immediately if signs of tendon inflammation or pain occur. Do not discontinue therapy until your course has been completed. Take a missed dose as soon as possible, unless it is almost time for your next dose.

Dosage Forms

Infusion [premixed in sodium chloride 0.8%] (Avelox® I.V.): 400 mg (250 mL)
Solution, ophthalmic (Vigamox™): 0.5% (3 mL)
Tablet [film coated]:
Avelox®: 400 mg
Avelox® ABC Pack [unit-dose pack]: 400 mg (5s)

Selected Readings

Balfour JA and Wiseman LR, "Moxifloxacin," *Drugs*, 1999, 57(3):363-73.
Blondeau JM, "Expanded Activity and Utility of the New Fluoroquinolones: A Review," *Clinical Therapeutics*, 1999, 21(1):3-40.
"Gatifloxacin and Moxifloxacin: Two New Fluoroquinolones," *Med Lett Drugs Ther*, 2000, Vol 42, 1072:15.
Nightingale CH, "Moxifloxacin, a New Antibiotic Designed to Treat Community-Acquired Respiratory Tract Infections: A Review of Microbiologic and Pharmacokinetic-Pharmacodynamic Characteristics," *Pharmacotherapy*, 2000, 20(3):245-56.

Moxifloxacin Hydrochloride *see* Moxifloxacin *on page 949*

Moxilin® *see* Amoxicillin *on page 642*

MPSV4 *see* Meningococcal Polysaccharide Vaccine (Groups A / C / Y and W-135) *on page 935*

Mumps, Measles and Rubella Vaccines, Combined *see* Measles, Mumps, and Rubella Vaccines (Combined) *on page 926*

Mumpsvax® *see* Mumps Virus Vaccine (Live/Attenuated) *on page 952*

Mumps Virus Vaccine (Live/Attenuated)

(mumpz VYE rus vak SEEN, live, a ten YOO ate ed)

Related Information

Immunization Recommendations *on page 1249*

U.S. Brand Names Mumpsvax®

Canadian Brand Names Mumpsvax®

Generic Available No

Use Mumps prophylaxis by promoting active immunity

Note: Trivalent measles-mumps-rubella (MMR) vaccine is the preferred agent for most children and many adults; persons born prior to 1957 are generally considered immune and need not be vaccinated

Drug of Choice or Alternative for

Organism(s):

Mumps Virus *on page 226*

Pregnancy Risk Factor C

Pregnancy Implications Reproduction studies have not been conducted. Rates of spontaneous abortion may be increased if mumps infection occurs during the first trimester. Although mumps vaccine virus can infect the placenta and fetus, there is not good evidence that it causes congenital malformations. Pregnancy should be avoided for 3 months following vaccination.

Contraindications

Hypersensitivity to mumps vaccine or any component of the formulation, including gelatin; febrile respiratory illness or active febrile infection; immunosuppressant therapy; primary or acquired immunodeficiency states; blood dyscrasias, leukemia, lymphoma or other malignant neoplasm affecting bone marrow or lymphatic systems; untreated tuberculosis; pregnancy

Warnings/Precautions Use caution with hypersensitivity to eggs or neomycin; patients with history of anaphylactic reaction may be at increased risk of immediate-type hypersensitivity reaction. Patients with minor illnesses (diarrhea, mild upper respiratory tract infection with or without low grade fever or other illnesses with low-grade fever) may receive vaccine. Leukemia patients who are in remission and who have not received chemotherapy for at least 3 months may be vaccinated. Patients with a history of congenital or hereditary immunodeficiency should not receive immunization until immune competence is demonstrated. Do not administer

to severely immunocompromised persons with the exception of asymptomatic children with HIV. Corticosteroid replacement therapy is not a contraindication for vaccination. Use caution in patients with thrombocytopenia and those who develop thrombocytopenia after first dose; thrombocytopenia may worsen. Immediate treatment for anaphylactic/anaphylactoid reaction should be available during vaccine use. Safety and efficacy in children <12 months of age have not been established.

Adverse Reactions All serious adverse reactions must be reported to the U.S. Department of Health and Human Services (DHHS) Vaccine Adverse Event Reporting System (VAERS) 1-800-822-7967.

Frequency not defined.

Cardiovascular: Syncope, vasculitis

Central nervous system: Encephalitis, febrile seizures, fever, Guillain-Barré syndrome, irritability

Dermatologic: Angioneurotic edema, erythema multiforme, purpura, Stevens-Johnson syndrome, urticaria

Endocrine & metabolic: Diabetes mellitus, parotitis

Gastrointestinal: Diarrhea, pancreatitis

Genitourinary: Orchitis

Hematologic: Leukocytosis, thrombocytopenia

Local: Burning/stinging at injection site, wheal and flare at injection site

Ocular: Conjunctivitis, ocular palsies, optic neuritis, papillitis, retrobulbar neuritis

Otic: Nerve deafness, otitis media

Respiratory: Bronchial spasm, cough, rhinitis

Miscellaneous: Anaphylaxis, anaphylactoid reactions, lymphadenopathy

Drug Interactions

Decreased Effect:

In patients receiving high doses of systemic corticosteroids for ≥14 days, wait at least 1 month between discontinuing steroid therapy and administering vaccine. Do not administer this vaccine with Immune globulin, whole blood, plasma; immune response may be compromised (defer vaccine administration for ≥3 months). The effect of the vaccine may be decreased with Immunosuppressant medications. Do not give within 1 month of other live virus vaccine.

Stability

Product is shipped at ≤10°C (50°F); prior to reconstitution, vaccine must be stored at ≤2°C to 8°C (36°F to 46°F). Reconstitute using entire contents of one vial of provided preservative free diluent. Following reconstitution, use as soon as possible, but may be stored at 2°C to 8°C (36°F to 46°F) for up to 8 hours. Protect from light prior to and after reconstitution.

Mechanism of Action Promotes active immunity to mumps virus by inducing specific antibodies.

Dosage Children ≥12-15 months and Adults: SubQ: 0.5 mL as a single dose

Administration For SubQ administration in outer aspect of the upper arm using a 25G 5/8' needle

Test Interactions Temporary suppression of tuberculosis skin test

Patient Information Pregnancy should be avoided for 3 months following vaccination; a little swelling of the glands in the cheeks and under the jaw may occur that lasts for a few days; this could happen from 1-2 weeks after getting the mumps vaccine; this happens rarely

Additional Information Federal law requires that the date of administration, the vaccine manufacturer, lot number of vaccine, and the administering person's name, title, and address be entered into the patient's permanent medical record. All adults without documentation of live vaccine on or after the first birthday or physician-diagnosed mumps, or laboratory evidence or immunity (particularly males and young adults who work in or congregate in hospitals, colleges, and on military bases) should be vaccinated. It is reasonable to consider persons born before 1957 immune, but there is no contraindication to vaccination of older persons. Susceptible travelers should be vaccinated.

Dosage Forms Injection, powder for reconstitution [preservative free]: 20,000 $TCID_{50}$ [contains human albumin, bovine serum, gelatin, neomycin; packaged with diluent]

Mupirocin (myoo PEER oh sin)

U.S. Brand Names Bactroban®; Bactroban® Nasal; Centany™

Canadian Brand Names Bactroban®

Synonyms Mupirocin Calcium; Pseudomonic Acid A

Generic Available Yes: Topical ointment

Use

Intranasal: Eradication of nasal colonization with MRSA in adult patients and health-care workers

(Continued)

Mupirocin *(Continued)*

Topical treatment of impetigo due to *Staphylococcus aureus*, beta-hemolytic *Streptococcus*, and *S. pyogenes*

Unlabeled/Investigational Use Intranasal: Surgical prophylaxis to prevent wound infections

Drug of Choice or Alternative for Disease/Syndrome(s):

Impetigo *on page 193*

Pregnancy Risk Factor B

Pregnancy Implications There are no adequate and well-controlled studies in pregnant women; use during pregnancy only if clearly needed.

Contraindications Hypersensitivity to mupirocin, polyethylene glycol, or any component of the formulation

Warnings/Precautions Potentially toxic amounts of polyethylene glycol contained in the vehicle may be absorbed percutaneously in patients with extensive burns or open wounds; prolonged use may result in over growth of nonsusceptible organisms; for external use only; not for treatment of pressure sores

Adverse Reactions Frequency not defined.

Central nervous system: Dizziness, headache
Dermatologic: Pruritus, rash, erythema, dry skin, cellulitis, dermatitis
Gastrointestinal: Nausea, taste perversion
Local: Burning, stinging, tenderness, edema, pain
Respiratory: Rhinitis, upper respiratory tract infection, pharyngitis, cough

Stability Do not mix with Aquaphor®, coal tar solution, or salicylic acid

Mechanism of Action Binds to bacterial isoleucyl transfer-RNA synthetase resulting in the inhibition of protein and RNA synthesis

Pharmacodynamics/Kinetics

Absorption: Topical: Penetrates outer layers of skin; systemic absorption minimal through intact skin
Protein binding: 95%
Metabolism: Skin: 3% to monic acid
Half-life elimination: 17-36 minutes
Excretion: Urine

Dosage

Children ≥12 years and Adults: Intranasal: Approximately one-half of the ointment from the single-use tube should be applied into one nostril and the other half into the other nostril twice daily for 5 days
Children ≥3 months and Adults: Topical: Apply small amount to affected area 2-5 times/day for 5-14 days

Administration For external use only.

Patient Information For topical use only; do not apply into the eye; discontinue if rash, itching, or irritation occurs; improvement should be seen in 5 days

Additional Information Not for treatment of pressure sores; contains polyethylene glycol vehicle.

Dosage Forms

Cream, topical, as calcium (Bactroban®): 2% (15 g, 30 g) [contains benzyl alcohol]
Ointment, intranasal, topical, as calcium (Bactroban® Nasal): 2% (1 g) [single-use tube]
Ointment, topical: 2% (22 g)
  Bactroban®: 2% (22 g)
  Centany™: 2% (15 g, 30 g)

Mupirocin Calcium *see* Mupirocin *on page 953*
Myambutol® *see* Ethambutol *on page 812*
Mycamine™ *see* Micafungin *on page 944*
Mycelex® *see* Clotrimazole *on page 758*
Mycelex®-3 [OTC] *see* Butoconazole *on page 691*
Mycelex®-7 [OTC] *see* Clotrimazole *on page 758*
Mycelex® Twin Pack [OTC] *see* Clotrimazole *on page 758*
Mycobutin® *see* Rifabutin *on page 1045*
Mycolog®-II [DSC] *see* Nystatin and Triamcinolone *on page 977*
Myco-Nail [OTC] *see* Triacetin *on page 1129*
Mycostatin® *see* Nystatin *on page 976*
myrac™ *see* Minocycline *on page 947*
Nabi-HB® *see* Hepatitis B Immune Globulin *on page 855*
Nadopen-V® (Can) *see* Penicillin V Potassium *on page 998*

Nafcillin (naf SIL in)

Related Information

Antibiotic Treatment of Adults With Infective Endocarditis *on page 1271*
Antimicrobial Activity Against Selected Organisms *on page 1165*

Canadian Brand Names Nallpen®; Unipen®

Synonyms Ethoxynaphthamido Penicillin Sodium; Nafcillin Sodium; Nallpen; Sodium Nafcillin

Generic Available Yes

Use Treatment of infections such as osteomyelitis, septicemia, endocarditis, and CNS infections caused by susceptible strains of staphylococci species

Drug of Choice or Alternative for Disease/Syndrome(s):

Brain Abscess *on page 58*
Mastitis *on page 214*

Pregnancy Risk Factor B

Contraindications Hypersensitivity to nafcillin, or any component of the formulation, or penicillins

Warnings/Precautions Extravasation of I.V. infusions should be avoided; modification of dosage is necessary in patients with both severe renal and hepatic impairment; elimination rate will be slow in neonates; use with caution in patients with cephalosporin hypersensitivity

Adverse Reactions Frequency not defined.

Central nervous system: Pain, fever
Dermatologic: Rash
Gastrointestinal: Nausea, diarrhea
Hematologic: Agranulocytosis, bone marrow depression, neutropenia
Local: Pain, swelling, inflammation, phlebitis, skin sloughing, and thrombophlebitis at the injection site; oxacillin (less likely to cause phlebitis) is often preferred in pediatric patients
Renal: Interstitial nephritis (acute)
Miscellaneous: Hypersensitivity reactions

Overdosage/Toxicology Symptoms of penicillin overdose include neuromuscular hypersensitivity (agitation, hallucinations, asterixis, encephalopathy, confusion, and seizures) and electrolyte imbalance (with potassium or sodium salts), especially in renal failure. Treatment is supportive or symptom-directed.

Drug Interactions

Cytochrome P450 Effect: Induces CYP3A4 (strong)

Increased Effect/Toxicity: Probenecid may cause an increase in nafcillin levels. Penicillins may increase the exposure to methotrexate during concurrent therapy; monitor.

Decreased Effect: Chloramphenicol may decrease nafcillin efficacy. If taken concomitantly with warfarin, nafcillin may inhibit the anticoagulant response to warfarin. This effect may persist for up to 30 days after nafcillin has been discontinued. Subtherapeutic cyclosporine levels may result when taken concomitantly with nafcillin. Although anecdotal reports suggest oral contraceptive efficacy could be reduced by penicillins, this has been refuted by more rigorous scientific and clinical data. Nafcillin may decrease the levels/effects of benzodiazepines, calcium channel blockers, clarithromycin, cyclosporine, erythromycin, estrogens, mirtazapine, nateglinide, nefazodone, nevirapine, protease inhibitors, tacrolimus, venlafaxine, and other CYP3A4 substrates.

Stability Reconstituted parenteral solution is stable for 3 days at room temperature and 7 days when refrigerated or 12 weeks when frozen; for I.V. infusion in NS or D_5W, solution is stable for 24 hours at room temperature and 96 hours when refrigerated

Mechanism of Action Interferes with bacterial cell wall synthesis during active multiplication, causing cell wall death and resultant bactericidal activity against susceptible bacteria

Pharmacodynamics/Kinetics

Distribution: Widely distributed; CSF penetration is poor but enhanced by meningeal inflammation; crosses placenta
Protein binding: 70% to 90%
Metabolism: Primarily hepatic; undergoes enterohepatic recirculation
Half-life elimination:
- Neonates: <3 weeks: 2.2-5.5 hours; 4-9 weeks: 1.2-2.3 hours
- Children 3 months to 14 years: 0.75-1.9 hours
- Adults: 30 minutes to 1.5 hours with normal renal and hepatic function

Time to peak, serum: I.M.: 30-60 minutes
Excretion: Primarily feces; urine (10% to 30% as unchanged drug)

(Continued)

Nafcillin *(Continued)*

Dosage

Neonates:
- <2000 g, <7 days: 50 mg/kg/day divided every 12 hours
- <2000 g, >7 days: 75 mg/kg/day divided every 8 hours
- >2000 g, <7 days: 50 mg/kg/day divided every 8 hours
- >2000 g, >7 days: 75 mg/kg/day divided every 6 hours

Children:
- I.M.: 25 mg/kg twice daily
- I.V.:
  - Mild to moderate infections: 50-100 mg/kg/day in divided doses every 6 hours
  - Severe infections: 100-200 mg/kg/day in divided doses every 4-6 hours
- Maximum dose: 12 g/day

Adults:
- I.M.: 500 mg every 4-6 hours
- I.V.: 500-2000 mg every 4-6 hours

Dosing adjustment in renal impairment: Not necessary

Dosing adjustment in hepatic impairment: In patients with both hepatic and renal impairment, modification of dosage may be necessary; no data available.

Dialysis: Not dialyzable (0% to 5%) via hemodialysis; supplemental dosage not necessary with hemo- or peritoneal dialysis or continuous arteriovenous or venovenous hemofiltration

Dietary Considerations Sodium content of 1 g: 76.6 mg (3.33 mEq)

Administration

I.M.: Rotate injection sites

I.V.: Vesicant. Administer around-the-clock to promote less variation in peak and trough serum levels; infuse over 30-60 minutes

Extravasation management: Use cold packs. Hyaluronidase: Add 1 mL NS to 150 unit vial to make 150 units/mL of concentration; mix 0.1 mL of above with 0.9 mL NS in 1 mL syringe to make final concentration = 15 units/mL.

Monitoring Parameters Periodic CBC, urinalysis, BUN, serum creatinine, AST and ALT; observe for signs and symptoms of anaphylaxis during first dose

Test Interactions Positive Coombs' test (direct), false-positive urinary and serum proteins; may inactivate aminoglycosides *in vitro*

Dosage Forms

Infusion [premixed iso-osmotic dextrose solution]: 1 g (50 mL); 2 g (100 mL)

Injection, powder for reconstitution, as sodium: 1 g, 2 g, 10 g

Selected Readings

Donowitz GR and Mandell GL, "Beta-Lactam Antibiotics," *N Engl J Med*, 1988, 318(7):419-26 and 318(8):490-500.

Wright AJ, "The Penicillins," *Mayo Clin Proc*, 1999, 74(3):290-307.

Nafcillin Sodium *see* Nafcillin *on page 955*

Naftifine (NAF ti feen)

U.S. Brand Names Naftin®

Synonyms Naftifine Hydrochloride

Generic Available No

Use Topical treatment of tinea cruris (jock itch), tinea corporis (ringworm), and tinea pedis (athlete's foot)

Pregnancy Risk Factor B

Contraindications Hypersensitivity to any component

Warnings/Precautions For external use only

Adverse Reactions

>10%: Local: Burning, stinging

1% to 10%:
- Dermatologic: Erythema, itching
- Local: Dryness, irritation

Mechanism of Action Synthetic, broad-spectrum antifungal agent in the allylamine class; appears to have both fungistatic and fungicidal activity. Exhibits antifungal activity by selectively inhibiting the enzyme squalene epoxidase in a dose-dependent manner which results in the primary sterol, ergosterol, within the fungal membrane not being synthesized.

Pharmacodynamics/Kinetics

Absorption: Systemic: Cream: 6%; Gel: ≤4%

Half-life elimination: 2-3 days

Excretion: Urine and feces (as metabolites)

Dosage Adults: Topical: Apply cream once daily and gel twice daily (morning and evening) for up to 4 weeks

Patient Information External use only; avoid eyes, mouth, and other mucous membranes; do not use occlusive dressings unless directed to do so; discontinue if irritation or sensitivity develops; wash hands after application

Dosage Forms

Cream, as hydrochloride: 1% (15 g, 30 g, 60 g) [contains benzyl alcohol]

Gel, as hydrochloride: 1% (20 g, 40 g, 60 g) [contains alcohol 52%]

Naftifine Hydrochloride *see* Naftifine *on page 956*

Naftin® *see* Naftifine *on page 956*

Nalidixic Acid (nal i DIKS ik AS id)

U.S. Brand Names NegGram®

Canadian Brand Names NegGram®

Synonyms Nalidixinic Acid

Generic Available No

Use Treatment of urinary tract infections

Pregnancy Risk Factor C

Pregnancy Implications Teratogenic and embryocidal effects were observed in animal studies. One study suggests that use late in pregnancy may increase the risk of infantile pyloric stenosis in the newborn. However, this finding was based on a small number of cases and other causes such as chance could not be excluded. Other authors suggest that nalidixic acid is unlikely to be teratogenic at therapeutic doses, but that there is not enough data to state there is no risk.

Contraindications Hypersensitivity to nalidixic acid or any component of the formulation; infants <3 months of age; porphyria, seizures; concurrent melphalan or other alkylating agent; breast-feeding

Warnings/Precautions Use with caution in patients with impaired hepatic or renal function and prepubertal children; has been shown to cause cartilage degeneration in immature animals; may induce hemolysis in patients with G6PD deficiency; use caution in patients with seizure disorder. Tendon inflammation and/or rupture have been reported. Risk may be increased with concurrent corticosteroids, particularly in the elderly. Discontinue at first sign of tendon inflammation or pain. Peripheral neuropathy may rarely occur; prompt discontinuation is recommended in patients with signs and symptoms of neuropathy.

Severe hypersensitivity reactions, including anaphylaxis, have occurred with quinolone therapy. If an allergic reaction occurs (itching, urticaria, dyspnea, facial edema, loss of consciousness, tingling, cardiovascular collapse), discontinue drug immediately. Prolonged use may result in superinfection; pseudomembranous colitis may occur and should be considered in all patients who present with diarrhea. Quinolones may exacerbate myasthenia gravis, use with caution (rare, potentially life-threatening weakness of respiratory muscles may occur).

Adverse Reactions Frequency not defined.

Central nervous system: Chills, confusion, dizziness, drowsiness, fever, headache, intracranial pressure increased, malaise, seizure, toxic psychosis, vertigo

Dermatologic: Erythema multiforme, photosensitivity reactions, pruritus, rash, Stevens-Johnson syndrome, urticaria

Endocrine & metabolic: Metabolic acidosis

Gastrointestinal: Nausea, vomiting

Hematologic: Eosinophilia, hemolytic anemia, leukopenia, thrombocytopenia

Hepatic: Cholestasis, hepatotoxicity

Neuromuscular and skeletal: Arthralgias, neuropathy, paresthesia, weakness

Ocular: Visual disturbances

Miscellaneous: Anaphylactic shock, anaphylactoid reaction, angioedema, tendon rupture and tendonitis

Overdosage/Toxicology Symptoms include nausea, vomiting, toxic psychosis, convulsions, increased intracranial pressure, and metabolic acidosis. Severe overdose, intracranial hypertension, increased pressure, and seizures have occurred. After GI decontamination, treatment is symptomatic.

Drug Interactions

Cytochrome P450 Effect: Inhibits CYP1A2 (weak)

Increased Effect/Toxicity: Nalidixic acid increases the effect of caffeine and warfarin. Serum levels of some quinolones are increased by probenecid. This effect may be more important for quinolones with high percentage of renal elimination than with nalidixic acid. Concurrent use of corticosteroids may increase risk of tendon rupture. Concomitant use of I.V. melphalan may cause serious GI toxicity.

Decreased Effect: Concurrent administration of metal cations, including most antacids, oral electrolyte supplements, quinapril, sucralfate, some didanosine formulations (chewable/buffered tablets and pediatric powder for oral suspension),

(Continued)

Nalidixic Acid *(Continued)*

and other highly-buffered oral drugs, may decrease quinolone levels; separate doses.

Ethanol/Nutrition/Herb Interactions Food: Enteral feedings may decrease plasma concentrations of nalidixic acid probably by >30% inhibition of absorption.

Stability Store at room temperature.

Mechanism of Action Inhibits DNA polymerization in late stages of chromosomal replication

Pharmacodynamics/Kinetics

Distribution: Achieves significant antibacterial concentrations only in the urinary tract; crosses placenta; enters breast milk

Protein binding: 90%

Metabolism: Partially hepatic; active metabolite, hydroxynalidixic acid

Half-life elimination: 6-7 hours; significantly prolonged with renal impairment

Time to peak, serum: 1-2 hours

Excretion: Urine (as unchanged drug, 80% as metabolites); feces (small amounts)

Dosage Oral:

Children 3 months to 12 years: 55 mg/kg/day divided every 6 hours; suppressive therapy is 33 mg/kg/day divided every 6 hours

Adults: 1 g 4 times/day for 2 weeks; then suppressive therapy of 500 mg 4 times/day

Dosing comments in renal impairment: Cl_{cr} <50 mL/minute: Avoid use

Dietary Considerations May administer with food to minimize GI upset.

Administration May be administered with or without food; drink fluids liberally

Monitoring Parameters Urinalysis, urine culture; CBC, renal, and hepatic function tests

Test Interactions False-positive urine glucose with Clinitest®, false increase in urinary VMA

Patient Information Avoid undue exposure to direct sunlight or use a sunscreen; finish all medication, do not skip doses

Dosage Forms [DSC] = Discontinued product

Suspension, oral: 250 mg/5 mL (473 mL) [raspberry flavor]

Tablet: 250 mg [DSC], 500 mg, 1 g [DSC]

Nalidixinic Acid *see* Nalidixic Acid *on page 957*

Nallpen® (Can) *see* Nafcillin *on page 955*

Nandrolone (NAN droe lone)

Related Information

AIDS Wasting Treatment *on page 1205*

Canadian Brand Names Deca-Durabolin®; Durabolin®

Synonyms Nandrolone Decanoate; Nandrolone Phenpropionate

Generic Available Yes

Use Control of metastatic breast cancer; management of anemia of renal insufficiency

Restrictions C-III

Pregnancy Risk Factor X

Contraindications Hypersensitivity to nandrolone or any component of the formulation; carcinoma of breast or prostate; nephrosis; pregnancy; not for use in infants

Warnings/Precautions Monitor diabetic patients carefully; anabolic steroids may cause peliosis hepatis, liver cell tumors, and blood lipid changes with increased risk of arteriosclerosis; use with caution in elderly patients, they may be at greater risk for prostatic hyperplasia; use with caution in patients with cardiac, renal, or hepatic disease or epilepsy

Adverse Reactions

Male:

Postpubertal:

>10%:

Dermatologic: Acne

Endocrine & metabolic: Gynecomastia

Genitourinary: Bladder irritability, priapism

1% to 10%:

Central nervous system: Insomnia, chills

Endocrine & metabolic: Decreased libido, hepatic dysfunction

Gastrointestinal: Nausea, diarrhea

Genitourinary: Prostatic hyperplasia (elderly)

Hematologic: Iron-deficiency anemia, suppression of clotting factors

<1%: Hepatic necrosis, hepatocellular carcinoma

Prepubertal:

>10%:

Dermatologic: Acne

Endocrine & metabolic: Virilism

1% to 10%:

Central nervous system: Chills, insomnia

Dermatologic: Hyperpigmentation

Gastrointestinal: Diarrhea, nausea

Hematologic: Iron deficiency anemia, suppression of clotting

<1%: Hepatocellular carcinoma, necrosis

Female:

>10%: Endocrine & metabolic: Virilism

1% to 10%:

Central nervous system: Chills, insomnia

Endocrine & metabolic: Hypercalcemia

Gastrointestinal: Nausea, diarrhea

Hematologic: Iron deficiency anemia, suppression of clotting factors

Hepatic: Hepatic dysfunction

<1%: Hepatic necrosis, hepatocellular carcinoma

Drug Interactions

Increased Effect/Toxicity: Nandrolone may increase the effect of oral anticoagulants, insulin, oral hypoglycemic agents, adrenal steroids, or ACTH when taken together.

Mechanism of Action Promotes tissue-building processes, increases production of erythropoietin, causes protein anabolism; increases hemoglobin and red blood cell volume

Pharmacodynamics/Kinetics

Onset of action: 3-6 months

Duration: Up to 30 days

Absorption: I.M.: 77%

Metabolism: Hepatic

Excretion: Urine

Dosage Deep I.M. (into gluteal muscle):

Children 2-13 years (decanoate): 25-50 mg every 3-4 weeks

Adults:

Male:

Breast cancer (phenpropionate): 50-100 mg/week

Anemia of renal insufficiency (decanoate): 100-200 mg/week

Female: 50-100 mg/week

Breast cancer (phenpropionate): 50-100 mg/week

Anemia of renal insufficiency (decanoate): 50-100 mg/week

Administration Inject deeply I.M., preferably into the gluteal muscle

Test Interactions Altered glucose tolerance tests

Patient Information Virilization may occur in female patients; report menstrual irregularities; male patients report persistent penile erections; all patients should report persistent GI distress, diarrhea, dark urine, pale stools, yellow coloring of skin or sclera; diabetic patients should monitor glucose closely

Additional Information Both phenpropionate and decanoate are injections in oil.

Dosage Forms Injection, solution, as decanoate [in sesame oil]: 100 mg/mL (2 mL); 200 mg/mL (1 mL) [contains benzyl alcohol]

Nandrolone Decanoate *see* Nandrolone *on page 958*

Nandrolone Phenpropionate *see* Nandrolone *on page 958*

Natacyn® *see* Natamycin *on page 959*

Natamycin (na ta MYE sin)

U.S. Brand Names Natacyn®

Canadian Brand Names Natacyn®

Synonyms Pimaricin

Generic Available No

Use Treatment of blepharitis, conjunctivitis, and keratitis caused by susceptible fungi (*Aspergillus*, *Candida*), *Cephalosporium*, *Curvularia*, *Fusarium*, *Penicillium*, *Microsporum*, *Epidermophyton*, *Blastomyces dermatitidis*, *Coccidioides immitis*, *Cryptococcus neoformans*, *Histoplasma capsulatum*, *Sporothrix schenckii*, and *Trichomonas vaginalis*

Pregnancy Risk Factor C

Contraindications Hypersensitivity to natamycin or any component of the formulation

(Continued)

Natamycin *(Continued)*

Warnings/Precautions Failure to improve (keratitis) after 7-10 days of administration suggests infection caused by a microorganism not susceptible to natamycin; inadequate as a single agent in fungal endophthalmitis

Adverse Reactions Frequency not defined: Ocular: Blurred vision, photophobia, eye pain, eye irritation not present before therapy

Drug Interactions

Increased Effect/Toxicity: Topical corticosteroids (concomitant use contraindicated).

Stability Store at room temperature (8°C to 24°C/46°F to 75°F); protect from excessive heat and light; do not freeze

Mechanism of Action Increases cell membrane permeability in susceptible fungi

Pharmacodynamics/Kinetics

Absorption: Ophthalmic: Systemic, <2%

Distribution: Adheres to cornea, retained in conjunctival fornices

Dosage Adults: Ophthalmic: Instill 1 drop in conjunctival sac every 1-2 hours, after 3-4 days reduce to one drop 6-8 times/day; usual course of therapy is 2-3 weeks.

Administration Ophthalmic: Shake well before using, do not touch dropper to eye.

Patient Information Shake well before using, do not touch dropper to eye; notify prescriber if condition worsens or does not improve after 3-4 days

Dosage Forms Suspension, ophthalmic: 5% (15 mL) [contains benzalkonium chloride]

***n*-Docosanol** *see* Docosanol *on page 787*

Nebcin® (Can) *see* Tobramycin *on page 1122*

NebuPent® *see* Pentamidine *on page 999*

NegGram® *see* Nalidixic Acid *on page 957*

Nelfinavir (nel FIN a veer)

Related Information

Antiretroviral Agents *on page 1206*

Antiretroviral Therapy for HIV Infection *on page 1219*

Management of Healthcare Worker Exposures to HBV, HCV, and HIV *on page 1227*

U.S. Brand Names Viracept®

Canadian Brand Names Viracept®

Synonyms NFV

Generic Available No

Use In combination with other antiretroviral therapy in the treatment of HIV infection

Drug of Choice or Alternative for Organism(s):

Human Immunodeficiency Virus *on page 181*

Pregnancy Risk Factor B

Pregnancy Implications The Perinatal HIV Guidelines Working Group recommends nelfinavir as the preferred PI in combination regimens during pregnancy, especially with HAART for perinatal prophylaxis. A dose of 1250 mg twice daily has been shown to provide adequate plasma levels; 750 mg 3 times/day produced low and variable levels. Pregnancy and protease inhibitors are both associated with an increased risk of hyperglycemia. Glucose levels should be closely monitored. Health professionals are encouraged to contact the antiretroviral pregnancy registry to monitor outcomes of pregnant women exposed to antiretroviral medications (1-800-258-4263 or www.APRegistry.com).

Contraindications Hypersensitivity to nelfinavir or any component of the formulation; concurrent therapy with amiodarone, ergot derivatives, midazolam, pimozide, quinidine, triazolam; additional medications which should not be coadministered (per manufacturer) include lovastatin and simvastatin

Warnings/Precautions Nelfinavir is hepatically metabolized and has multiple drug interactions. A listing of medications that should not be used is available with each bottle and patients should be provided with this information. Use caution with hepatic impairment. Warn patients that redistribution of body fat can occur. New onset diabetes mellitus, exacerbation of diabetes, and hyperglycemia have been reported in HIV-infected patients receiving protease inhibitors. The oral powder contains phenylalanine; use caution in patients with phenylketonuria.

Adverse Reactions

>10%: Gastrointestinal: Diarrhea

2% to 10%:

Dermatologic: Rash

Gastrointestinal: Nausea, flatulence

Hematologic: Abnormal creatine kinase, hemoglobin, lymphocytes, neutrophils
Hepatic: Abnormal ALT, AST

<2% (Limited to important or life-threatening): Acute iritis, allergic reaction, amylase increased, anemia, anorexia, anxiety, arthralgia, back pain, body fat redistribution/accumulation, creatinine phosphokinase increased, dehydration, depression, diaphoresis, dizziness, dyspepsia, dyspnea, epigastric pain, fever, folliculitis, gamma glutamyl transpeptidase increased, gastrointestinal bleeding, headache, hepatitis, hyperkinesia, hyperglycemia, hyperlipemia, hyperuricemia, hypoglycemia, insomnia, kidney calculus, lactic dehydrogenase increased, leukopenia, maculopapular rash, myalgia, myasthenia, myopathy, pain, pancreatitis, paresthesia, pruritus, seizure, sexual dysfunction, sleep disorder, somnolence, suicidal ideation, thrombocytopenia, urticaria, vomiting, weakness

Postmarketing and/or case reports: Bilirubinemia; hypersensitivity reaction (bronchospasm, rash, edema); jaundice, metabolic acidosis, QT_c prolongation, torsade de pointes

Overdosage/Toxicology Limited data are available. However, unabsorbed drug should be removed via gastric lavage and activated charcoal. Significant symptoms beyond gastrointestinal disturbances are likely following acute overdose. Hemodialysis will not be effective due to the high protein binding of nelfinavir.

Drug Interactions

Cytochrome P450 Effect: Substrate of CYP2C8/9 (minor), 2C19 (major), 2D6 (minor), 3A4 (major); **Inhibits** CYP1A2 (weak), 2B6 (weak), 2C8/9 (weak), 2C19 (weak), 2D6 (weak), 3A4 (strong)

Increased Effect/Toxicity: Nelfinavir effects may be increased by azithromycin, delavirdine, and protease inhibitors. Nelfinavir may increase the levels/effects of selected benzodiazepines, calcium channel blockers, cyclosporine, mirtazapine, nateglinide, nefazodone, quinidine, sildenafil (and other PDE-5 inhibitors), tacrolimus, venlafaxine, and other CYP3A4 substrates. Selected benzodiazepines (midazolam, triazolam), cisapride, ergot alkaloids, selected HMG-CoA reductase inhibitors (lovastatin and simvastatin), and pimozide are generally contraindicated with strong CYP3A4 inhibitors. When used with strong CYP3A4 inhibitors, dosage adjustment/limits are recommended for sildenafil and other PDE-5 inhibitors; refer to individual monographs.

Decreased Effect: The levels/effects of nelfinavir may be decreased by aminoglutethimide, carbamazepine, nafcillin, nevirapine, phenobarbital, phenytoin, rifamycins, or other inducers of CYP2C19 or 3A4. Nelfinavir effects may be decreased by St John's wort. Nelfinavir may decrease the effects of delavirdine, methadone, and oral contraceptives

Ethanol/Nutrition/Herb Interactions

Food: Nelfinavir taken with food increases plasma concentration time curve (AUC) by two- to threefold. Do not administer with acidic food or juice (orange juice, apple juice, or applesauce) since the combination may have a bitter taste.

Herb/Nutraceutical: St John's wort may decrease nelfinavir serum concentrations; avoid concurrent use.

Stability Store at room temperature. Oral powder (or dissolved tablets) diluted in nonacidic liquid is stable for 6 hours under refrigeration.

Mechanism of Action Inhibits the HIV-1 protease; inhibition of the viral protease prevents cleavage of the gag-pol polyprotein resulting in the production of immature, noninfectious virus

Pharmacodynamics/Kinetics

Absorption: Food increases plasma concentration-time curve (AUC) by two- to threefold

Distribution: V_d: 2-7 L/kg

Protein binding: 98%

Metabolism: Hepatic via CYP2C19 and 3A4; major metabolite has activity comparable to parent drug

Half-life elimination: 3.5-5 hours

Time to peak, serum: 2-4 hours

Excretion: Feces (98% to 99%, 78% as metabolites, 22% as unchanged drug); urine (1% to 2%)

Dosage Oral:

Children 2-13 years: 45-55 mg/kg twice daily **or** 25-35 mg/kg 3 times/day (maximum: 2500 mg/day); all doses should be taken with a meal. If tablets are unable to be taken, use oral powder in small amount of water, milk, formula, or dietary supplements; do not use acidic food/juice or store for >6 hours.

Adults: 750 mg 3 times/day with meals or 1250 mg twice daily with meals in combination with other antiretroviral therapies

Note: Dosage adjustments for nelfinavir when administered in combination with ritonavir: Nelfinavir 500-750 mg twice daily plus ritonavir 400 mg twice daily

(Continued)

Nelfinavir *(Continued)*

Dosing adjustment in renal impairment: No adjustment needed

Dosing adjustment in hepatic impairment: Use caution

Dietary Considerations Should be taken as scheduled with food. Oral powder contains phenylalanine 11.2 mg/g.

Administration Mix powder or tablets in a small amount of water, milk, formula, soy milk, soy formula, or dietary supplement. Be sure entire contents is consumed to receive full dose. Do not use acidic food/juice to dilute due to bitter taste. One mixed, solution should be used immediately, but may be stored for up to 6 hours if refrigerated.

Monitoring Parameters Liver function tests, viral load, CD4 count, triglycerides, cholesterol, blood glucose, CBC with differential

Patient Information Nelfinavir should be taken with food to increase its absorption; it is not a cure for HIV infection and the long-term effects of the drug are unknown at this time; the drug has not demonstrated a reduction in the risk of transmitting HIV to others. Take the drug as prescribed; if you miss a dose, take it as soon as possible and then return to your usual schedule (never double a dose, however). If tablets are unable to be taken, use oral powder in small amount of water, milk, formula, or dietary supplement; do not use acidic food/juice or store dilution for >6 hours. Do not take any prescription medications, over-the-counter products or herbal products, especially St John's wort, without consulting prescriber. Nelfinavir has many drug interactions. A listing of medications that should not be used is available and should be reviewed with every prescription refill. Use an alternative method of contraception from birth control pills during nelfinavir therapy.

Dosage Forms

Powder, oral: 50 mg/g (144 g) [contains phenylalanine 11.2 mg/g]

Tablet [film coated]: 250 mg, 625 mg

Selected Readings

Bardsley-Elliot A and Plosker GL, "Nelfinavir: An Update on Its Use in HIV Infection," *Drugs*, 2000, 59(3):581-620.

Deeks SG, Smith M, Holodniy M, et al, "HIV-1 Protease Inhibitors. A Review for Clinicians," *JAMA*, 1997, 277(2):145-53.

Havlir DV and Lange JM, "New Antiretrovirals and New Combinations," *AIDS*, 1998, 12(Suppl A):S165-74.

Kakuda TN, Struble KA, and Piscitelli SC, "Protease Inhibitors for the Treatment of Human Immunodeficiency Virus Infection," *Am J Health Syst Pharm*, 1998, 55(3):233-54.

Kaul DR, Cinti SK, Carver PL, et al, "HIV Protease Inhibitors: Advances in Therapy and Adverse Reactions, Including Metabolic Complications," *Pharmacotherapy*, 1999, 19(3):281-98.

McDonald CK and Kuritzkes DR, "Human Immunodeficiency Virus Type 1 Protease Inhibitors," *Arch Intern Med*, 1997, 157(9):951-9.

Perry CM and Benfield P, "Nelfinavir," *Drugs*, 1997, 54(1):81-7.

Nemasol® Sodium (Can) *see* Aminosalicylic Acid *on page 641*

NeoDecadron® *see* Neomycin and Dexamethasone *on page 963*

Neo-Fradin™ *see* Neomycin *on page 962*

Neomycin (nee oh MYE sin)

U.S. Brand Names Neo-Fradin™; Neo-Rx

Synonyms Neomycin Sulfate

Generic Available Yes

Use Orally to prepare GI tract for surgery; topically to treat minor skin infections; treatment of diarrhea caused by *E. coli*; adjunct in the treatment of hepatic encephalopathy; bladder irrigation; ocular infections

Drug of Choice or Alternative for Disease/Syndrome(s):

Otitis Externa, Mild *on page 252*

Pregnancy Risk Factor C

Contraindications Hypersensitivity to neomycin or any component of the formulation, or other aminoglycosides; intestinal obstruction

Warnings/Precautions Use with caution in patients with renal impairment, pre-existing hearing impairment, neuromuscular disorders; neomycin is more toxic than other aminoglycosides when given parenterally; **do not administer parenterally**; topical neomycin is a contact sensitizer with sensitivity occurring in 5% to 15% of patients treated with the drug; symptoms include itching, reddening, edema, and failure to heal; **do not use as peritoneal lavage** due to significant systemic adsorption of the drug

Adverse Reactions

Oral:

>10%: Gastrointestinal: Nausea, diarrhea, vomiting, irritation or soreness of the mouth or rectal area

<1% (Limited to important or life-threatening): Dyspnea, eosinophilia, nephrotoxicity, neurotoxicity, ototoxicity (auditory), ototoxicity (vestibular)

Topical: >10%: Dermatologic: Contact dermatitis

Overdosage/Toxicology Symptoms of overdose are rare, due to poor oral bioavailability, but include ototoxicity, nephrotoxicity, and neuromuscular toxicity. The treatment of choice following a single acute overdose appears to be the maintenance of urine output of at least 3 mL/kg/hour. Dialysis is of questionable value in enhancing aminoglycoside elimination. If required, hemodialysis is preferred over peritoneal dialysis in patients with normal renal function. Chelation with penicillin may be of benefit.

Drug Interactions

Increased Effect/Toxicity: Oral neomycin may potentiate the effects of oral anticoagulants. Neomycin may increase the adverse effects with other neurotoxic, ototoxic, or nephrotoxic drugs.

Decreased Effect: May decrease GI absorption of digoxin and methotrexate.

Mechanism of Action Interferes with bacterial protein synthesis by binding to 30S ribosomal subunits

Pharmacodynamics/Kinetics

Absorption: Oral, percutaneous: Poor (3%)

Distribution: V_d: 0.36 L/kg

Metabolism: Slightly hepatic

Half-life elimination (age and renal function dependent): 3 hours

Time to peak, serum: Oral: 1-4 hours

Excretion: Feces (97% of oral dose as unchanged drug); urine (30% to 50% of absorbed drug as unchanged drug)

Dosage

Children: Oral:

Preoperative intestinal antisepsis: 90 mg/kg/day divided every 4 hours for 2 days; or 25 mg/kg at 1 PM, 2 PM, and 11 PM on the day preceding surgery as an adjunct to mechanical cleansing of the intestine and in combination with erythromycin base

Hepatic encephalopathy: 50-100 mg/kg/day in divided doses every 6-8 hours or 2.5-7 g/m^2/day divided every 4-6 hours for 5-6 days not to exceed 12 g/day

Children and Adults: Topical: Topical solutions containing 0.1% to 1% neomycin have been used for irrigation

Adults: Oral:

Preoperative intestinal antisepsis: 1 g each hour for 4 doses then 1 g every 4 hours for 5 doses; or 1 g at 1 PM, 2 PM, and 11 PM on day preceding surgery as an adjunct to mechanical cleansing of the bowel and oral erythromycin; or 6 g/day divided every 4 hours for 2-3 days

Hepatic encephalopathy: 500-2000 mg every 6-8 hours or 4-12 g/day divided every 4-6 hours for 5-6 days

Chronic hepatic insufficiency: 4 g/day for an indefinite period

Monitoring Parameters Renal function tests, audiometry in symptomatic patients

Patient Information Report redness, burning, itching, ringing in the ears, hearing impairment, or dizziness or if condition does not improve in 3-4 days

Dosage Forms

Powder, micronized, as sulfate [for prescription compounding] (Neo-Rx): (10 g, 100 g)

Solution, oral, as sulfate (Neo-Fradin™): 125 mg/5 mL (60 mL, 480 mL) [contains benzoic acid; cherry flavor]

Tablet, as sulfate: 500 mg

Selected Readings

Begg EJ and Barclay ML, "Aminoglycosides - 50 Years On," *Br J Clin Pharmacol*, 1995, 39(6):597-603.

Edson RS and Terrell CL, "The Aminoglycosides," *Mayo Clin Proc*, 1999, 74(5):519-28.

Neomycin and Dexamethasone

(nee oh MYE sin & deks a METH a sone)

Related Information

Neomycin *on page 962*

U.S. Brand Names NeoDecadron®

Synonyms Dexamethasone and Neomycin

Generic Available No

Use Treatment of steroid responsive inflammatory conditions of the palpebral and bulbar conjunctiva, lid, cornea, and anterior segment of the globe

Pregnancy Risk Factor C

Contraindications

Based on **neomycin** component: Hypersensitivity to neomycin or any component of the formulation, or other aminoglycosides; intestinal obstruction

(Continued)

Neomycin and Dexamethasone *(Continued)*

Based on **dexamethasone** component: Hypersensitivity to dexamethasone or any component of the formulation; active untreated infections; ophthalmic use in viral, fungal, or tuberculosis diseases of the eye

Warnings/Precautions See individual agents.

Adverse Reactions <1%: Burning, local irritation or transient stinging; epithelial punctate keratitis, increased intraocular pressure, mydriasis, ptosis, and possible corneal or scleral malacia can occur

Drug Interactions

Cytochrome P450 Effect: Dexamethasone: **Substrate** of CYP3A4 (minor); **Induces** CYP2A6 (weak), 2B6 (weak), 2C8/9 (weak), 3A4 (weak)

Stability Store in tight, light-resistant container

Pharmacodynamics/Kinetics See individual agents.

Dosage Ophthalmic: Instill 1-2 drops in eye(s) every 3-4 hours

Dosage Forms Solution, ophthalmic: Neomycin sulfate 0.35% [3.5 mg/mL] and dexamethasone sodium phosphate 0.1% [1 mg/mL] (5 mL) [contains benzalkonium chloride and sodium bisulfite]

Neomycin and Polymyxin B (nee oh MYE sin & pol i MIKS in bee)

Related Information

Neomycin *on page 962*

Polymyxin B *on page 1012*

U.S. Brand Names Neosporin® G.U. Irrigant

Canadian Brand Names Neosporin® Irrigating Solution

Synonyms Polymyxin B and Neomycin

Generic Available No

Use Short-term as a continuous irrigant or rinse in the urinary bladder to prevent bacteriuria and gram-negative rod septicemia associated with the use of indwelling catheters; to help prevent infection in minor cuts, scrapes, and burns

Pregnancy Risk Factor C/D (for G.U. irrigant)

Contraindications Hypersensitivity to neomycin, polymyxin B, or any component of the formulation; pregnancy (GU irrigant)

Adverse Reactions Frequency not defined.

Dermatologic: Contact dermatitis, erythema, rash, urticaria

Genitourinary: Bladder irritation

Local: Burning

Neuromuscular & skeletal: Neuromuscular blockade

Otic: Ototoxicity

Renal: Nephrotoxicity

Stability Store irrigation solution in refrigerator; aseptic prepared dilutions (1 mL/1 L) should be stored in the refrigerator and discarded after 48 hours

Mechanism of Action See individual agents.

Pharmacodynamics/Kinetics

Absorption: Topical: Not absorbed following application to intact skin; absorbed through denuded or abraded skin, peritoneum, wounds, or ulcers

See individual agents.

Dosage Children and Adults: Bladder irrigation: **Not for injection**; add 1 mL irrigant to 1 liter isotonic saline solution and connect container to the inflow of lumen of 3-way catheter. Continuous irrigant or rinse in the urinary bladder for up to a maximum of 10 days with administration rate adjusted to patient's urine output; usually no more than 1 L of irrigant is used per day.

Administration Bladder irrigant: Do not inject irrigant solution; concentrated irrigant solution must be diluted in 1 L normal saline before administration; connect irrigation container to the inflow lumen of a 3-way catheter to permit continuous irrigation of the urinary bladder

Dosage Forms Solution, irrigant: Neomycin 40 mg and polymyxin B sulfate 200,000 units per mL (1 mL, 20 mL)

Neomycin, Bacitracin, and Polymyxin B *see* Bacitracin, Neomycin, and Polymyxin B *on page 681*

Neomycin, Bacitracin, Polymyxin B, and Hydrocortisone *see* Bacitracin, Neomycin, Polymyxin B, and Hydrocortisone *on page 682*

Neomycin, Bacitracin, Polymyxin B, and Pramoxine *see* Bacitracin, Neomycin, Polymyxin B, and Pramoxine *on page 683*

Neomycin, Polymyxin B, and Dexamethasone

(nee oh MYE sin, pol i MIKS in bee, & deks a METH a sone)

Related Information

Neomycin *on page 962*
Polymyxin B *on page 1012*

U.S. Brand Names AK-Trol®; Dexacidin® [DSC]; Dexacine™ [DSC]; Dexasporin; Maxitrol®; Methadex

Canadian Brand Names Dioptrol®; Maxitrol®

Synonyms Dexamethasone, Neomycin, and Polymyxin B; Polymyxin B, Neomycin, and Dexamethasone

Generic Available Yes

Use Steroid-responsive inflammatory ocular conditions in which a corticosteroid is indicated and where bacterial infection or a risk of bacterial infection exists

Pregnancy Risk Factor C

Pregnancy Implications See individual agents.

Contraindications Hypersensitivity to neomycin, polymyxin B, dexamethasone, or any component of the formulation; viral, fungal, or tuberculosis diseases of the eye

Warnings/Precautions Sensitivity to neomycin may develop; discontinue if sensitivity reaction occurs. Prolonged use of corticosteroids may result in glaucoma; damage to the optic nerve, defects in visual acuity and fields of vision, and posterior subcapsular cataract formation may occur. Prolonged use of corticosteroids may increase the incidence of secondary ocular infection or mask acute infection (including fungal infections); may prolong or exacerbate ocular viral infections; use following cataract surgery may delay healing or increase the incidence of bleb formation. A maximum of 8 g of ointment or 20 mL of suspension should be prescribed initially; patients should be evaluated prior to additional refills. Suspension contains benzalkonium chloride which may be adsorbed by contact lenses; contact lenses should not be worn during treatment of ophthalmic infections.

Adverse Reactions Frequency not defined: Ocular: Allergic sensitivity, cutaneous sensitization, eye pain, development of glaucoma, cataract, increased intraocular pressure, optic nerve damage, wound healing delayed

Drug Interactions

Cytochrome P450 Effect: Dexamethasone: **Substrate** of CYP3A4 (minor); **Induces** CYP2A6 (weak), 2B6 (weak), 2C8/9 (weak), 3A4 (weak)

Mechanism of Action See individual agents.

Pharmacodynamics/Kinetics See individual agents.

Dosage Children and Adults: Ophthalmic:

Ointment: Place a small amount (~½") in the affected eye 3-4 times/day or apply at bedtime as an adjunct with drops

Suspension: Instill 1-2 drops into affected eye(s) every 3-4 hours; in severe disease, drops may be used hourly and tapered to discontinuation

Administration Contact lenses should not be worn during therapy.

Ointment: Do not touch tip of tube to eye. Instill ointment into pocket between eyeball and lower lid; patient should look downward before closing eye.

Suspension: Shake suspension before use. Tilt head back, instill suspension in conjunctival sac and close eye(s). Do not touch dropper to eye. Apply light finger pressure on lacrimal sac for 1 minute following instillation.

Monitoring Parameters Monitor intraocular pressure with use longer than 10 days

Dosage Forms [DSC] = Discontinued product

Ointment, ophthalmic (Dexacine™ [DSC], Maxitrol®): Neomycin 3.5 mg, polymyxin B sulfate 10,000 units, and dexamethasone 0.1% per g (3.5 g)

Suspension, ophthalmic (AK-Trol®, Dexacidin® [DSC], Dexasporin, Maxitrol®, Methadex): Neomycin 3.5 mg, polymyxin B sulfate 10,000 units, and dexamethasone 0.1% per mL (5 mL) [contains benzalkonium chloride]

Neomycin, Polymyxin B, and Gramicidin

(nee oh MYE sin, pol i MIKS in bee, & gram i SYE din)

Related Information

Neomycin *on page 962*
Polymyxin B *on page 1012*

U.S. Brand Names Neosporin® Ophthalmic Solution

Canadian Brand Names Neosporin®; Optimyxin Plus®

Synonyms Gramicidin, Neomycin, and Polymyxin B; Polymyxin B, Neomycin, and Gramicidin

Generic Available Yes

Use Treatment of superficial ocular infection

Pregnancy Risk Factor C

(Continued)

Neomycin, Polymyxin B, and Gramicidin *(Continued)*

Contraindications Hypersensitivity to neomycin, polymyxin B, gramicidin or any component of the formulation

Warnings/Precautions Symptoms of neomycin sensitization include itching, reddening, edema, failure to heal; prolonged use may result in glaucoma, defects in visual acuity, posterior subcapsular cataract formation, and secondary ocular infections

Adverse Reactions Frequency not defined: Ocular: Transient irritation, burning, stinging, itching, inflammation, angioneurotic edema, urticaria, vesicular and maculopapular dermatitis

Drug Interactions

Increased Effect/Toxicity: See individual agents.

Decreased Effect: See individual agents.

Mechanism of Action Interferes with bacterial protein synthesis by binding to 30S ribosomal subunits; binds to phospholipids, alters permeability, and damages the bacterial cytoplasmic membrane permitting leakage of intracellular constituents

Dosage Children and Adults: Ophthalmic: Instill 1-2 drops 4-6 times/day or more frequently as required for severe infections

Patient Information Tilt head back, place medication in conjunctival sac, and close eyes; apply finger pressure on lacrimal sac for 1 minute following instillation

Dosage Forms Solution, ophthalmic: Neomycin 1.75 mg, polymyxin B 10,000 units, and gramicidin 0.025 mg per mL (10 mL) [contains alcohol 0.5% and thimerosal]

Neomycin, Polymyxin B, and Hydrocortisone

(nee oh MYE sin, pol i MIKS in bee, & hye droe KOR ti sone)

Related Information

Neomycin *on page 962*

Polymyxin B *on page 1012*

U.S. Brand Names AntibiOtic® Ear; Cortisporin® Cream; Cortisporin® Ophthalmic; Cortisporin® Otic; PediOtic®

Canadian Brand Names Cortimyxin®; Cortisporin® Otic

Synonyms Hydrocortisone, Neomycin, and Polymyxin B; Polymyxin B, Neomycin, and Hydrocortisone

Generic Available Yes

Use Steroid-responsive inflammatory condition for which a corticosteroid is indicated and where bacterial infection or a risk of bacterial infection exists

Pregnancy Risk Factor C

Contraindications Hypersensitivity to neomycin, polymyxin B, hydrocortisone, or any component of the formulation

Adverse Reactions Frequency not defined.

Dermatologic: Contact dermatitis, erythema, rash, urticaria

Local: Burning, itching, swelling, pain, stinging

Ocular: Intraocular pressure increased, glaucoma, cataracts, conjunctival erythema, transient irritation, burning, stinging, itching, inflammation, angioneurotic edema, urticaria, vesicular and maculopapular dermatitis

Otic: Ototoxicity

Miscellaneous: Hypersensitivity, sensitization to neomycin, secondary infection

Drug Interactions

Cytochrome P450 Effect: Hydrocortisone: **Substrate** of CYP3A4 (minor); **Induces** CYP3A4 (weak)

Mechanism of Action See individual agents.

Pharmacodynamics/Kinetics See individual agents.

Dosage Duration of use should be limited to 10 days unless otherwise directed by the physician

Otic solution is used **only** for swimmer's ear (infections of external auditory canal)

Otic:

- Children: Instill 3 drops into affected ear 3-4 times/day
- Adults: Instill 4 drops 3-4 times/day; otic suspension is the preferred otic preparation

Children and Adults:

- Ophthalmic: Drops: Instill 1-2 drops 2-4 times/day, or more frequently as required for severe infections; in acute infections, instill 1-2 drops every 15-30 minutes gradually reducing the frequency of administration as the infection is controlled
- Topical: Apply a thin layer 1-4 times/day. Therapy should be discontinued when control is achieved; if no improvement is seen, reassessment of diagnosis may be necessary.

Administration Shake suspension well before using. Otic solution should not be used when the integrity of the tympanic membrane is in question.

Dosage Forms

Cream, topical (Cortisporin®): Neomycin 3.5 mg, polymyxin B 10,000 units, and hydrocortisone 5 mg per g (7.5 g)

Solution, otic (AntibiOtic® Ear; Cortisporin®): Neomycin 3.5 mg, polymyxin B 10,000 units, and hydrocortisone 10 mg per mL (10 mL) [contains potassium metabisulfite]

Suspension, ophthalmic (Cortisporin®): Neomycin 3.5 mg, polymyxin B 10,000 units, and hydrocortisone 10 mg per mL (7.5 mL) [contains thimerosal]

Suspension, otic: Neomycin 3.5 mg, polymyxin B 10,000 units, and hydrocortisone 10 mg per mL (10 mL)

AntibiOtic® Ear, Cortisporin®: Neomycin 3.5 mg, polymyxin B 10,000 units, and hydrocortisone 10 mg per mL (10 mL) [contains thimerosal]

PediOtic®: Neomycin 3.5 mg, polymyxin B 10,000 units, and hydrocortisone 10 mg per mL (7.5 mL) [contains thimerosal]

Neomycin, Polymyxin B, and Prednisolone

(nee oh MYE sin, pol i MIKS in bee, & pred NIS oh lone)

Related Information

Neomycin *on page 962*

Polymyxin B *on page 1012*

U.S. Brand Names Poly-Pred®

Synonyms Polymyxin B, Neomycin, and Prednisolone; Prednisolone, Neomycin, and Polymyxin B

Generic Available No

Use Steroid-responsive inflammatory ocular condition in which bacterial infection or a risk of bacterial ocular infection exists

Pregnancy Risk Factor C

Contraindications Hypersensitivity to neomycin, polymyxin B, prednisolone, or any component of the formulation

Adverse Reactions Frequency not defined.

Dermatologic: Cutaneous sensitization, skin rash, delayed wound healing

Ocular: Increased intraocular pressure, glaucoma, optic nerve damage, cataracts, conjunctival sensitization, transient irritation, burning, stinging, itching, inflammation, angioneurotic edema, urticaria, vesicular and maculopapular dermatitis

Drug Interactions

Cytochrome P450 Effect: Prednisolone: **Substrate** of CYP3A4 (minor); **Inhibits** CYP3A4 (weak)

Mechanism of Action See individual agents.

Pharmacodynamics/Kinetics See individual agents.

Dosage Children and Adults: Ophthalmic: Instill 1-2 drops every 3-4 hours; acute infections may require every 30-minute instillation initially with frequency of administration reduced as the infection is brought under control. To treat the lids: Instill 1-2 drops every 3-4 hours, close the eye and rub the excess on the lids and lid margins.

Administration Shake suspension before use.

Dosage Forms Suspension, ophthalmic: Neomycin 0.35%, polymyxin B 10,000 units per mL, and prednisolone acetate 0.5% (5 mL; 10 mL [DSC]) [contains thimerosal]

Neomycin Sulfate *see* Neomycin *on page 962*

Neo-Rx *see* Neomycin *on page 962*

Neosporin® (Can) *see* Neomycin, Polymyxin B, and Gramicidin *on page 965*

Neosporin® G.U. Irrigant *see* Neomycin and Polymyxin B *on page 964*

Neosporin® Irrigating Solution (Can) *see* Neomycin and Polymyxin B *on page 964*

Neosporin® Neo To Go® [OTC] *see* Bacitracin, Neomycin, and Polymyxin B *on page 681*

Neosporin® Ophthalmic Ointment *see* Bacitracin, Neomycin, and Polymyxin B *on page 681*

Neosporin® Ophthalmic Solution *see* Neomycin, Polymyxin B, and Gramicidin *on page 965*

Neosporin® + Pain Ointment [OTC] *see* Bacitracin, Neomycin, Polymyxin B, and Pramoxine *on page 683*

Neosporin® Topical [OTC] *see* Bacitracin, Neomycin, and Polymyxin B *on page 681*

Neotopic® (Can) *see* Bacitracin, Neomycin, and Polymyxin B *on page 681*

Neupogen® *see* Filgrastim *on page 817*

NeuTrexin® *see* Trimetrexate Glucuronate *on page 1132*

Nevirapine (ne VYE ra peen)

Related Information

Antiretroviral Agents *on page 1206*

Antiretroviral Therapy for HIV Infection *on page 1219*

(Continued)

Nevirapine *(Continued)*

Management of Healthcare Worker Exposures to HBV, HCV, and HIV *on page 1227*

U.S. Brand Names Viramune®

Canadian Brand Names Viramune®

Synonyms NVP

Generic Available No

Use In combination therapy with other antiretroviral agents for the treatment of HIV-1

Drug of Choice or Alternative for Organism(s):

Human Immunodeficiency Virus *on page 181*

Restrictions An FDA-approved medication guide is available at www.fda.gov/cder/Offices/ODS/labeling.htm.

Pregnancy Risk Factor C

Pregnancy Implications Nevirapine crosses the placenta. Pharmacokinetics are not altered during pregnancy and dose adjustment is not needed. The Perinatal HIV Guidelines Working Group recommends nevirapine as the NNRTI for use during pregnancy. When used to prevent perinatal transmission in women who do not need therapy for their own health, use is not recommended if CD4⁺ lymphocyte counts >250/mm^3 (monitor for liver toxicity during first 18 weeks of therapy). It may also be used in combination with zidovudine in HIV-infected women who are in labor, but have had no prior antiretroviral therapy, in order to reduce the maternal-fetal transmission of HIV. Health professionals are encouraged to contact the antiretroviral pregnancy registry to monitor outcomes of pregnant women exposed to antiretroviral medications (1-800-258-4263 or www.APRegistry.com).

Contraindications Hypersensitivity to nevirapine or any component of the formulation

Warnings/Precautions Severe hepatotoxic reactions may occur (fulminant and cholestatic hepatitis, hepatic necrosis) and, in some cases, have resulted in hepatic failure and death. Intensive monitoring is required during the initial 18 weeks of therapy to detect potentially life-threatening dermatologic, hypersensitivity, and hepatic reactions. The greatest risk of these reactions is within the initial 6 weeks of treatment. Patients with a history of chronic hepatitis (B or C) or increased baseline transaminase levels may be at increased risk of hepatotoxic reactions. Female gender and patients with increased $CD4^+$-cell counts may be at substantially greater risk of hepatic events (often associated with rash). Therapy should not be started with elevated $CD4^+$-cell counts unless the benefit of therapy outweighs the risk of serious hepatotoxicity (adult females: $CD4^+$-cell counts >250 cells/mm^3; adult males: $CD4^+$-cell counts >400 cells/mm^3).

Severe life-threatening skin reactions (eg, Stevens-Johnson syndrome, toxic epidermal necrolysis, hypersensitivity reactions with rash and organ dysfunction) have occurred. Nevirapine must be initiated with a 14-day lead-in dosing period to decrease the incidence of adverse effects.

If a severe dermatologic or hypersensitivity reaction occurs, or if signs and symptoms of hepatitis occur, nevirapine should be permanently discontinued. These may include a severe rash, or a rash associated with fever, blisters, oral lesions, conjunctivitis, facial edema, muscle or joint aches, general malaise, hepatitis, eosinophilia, granulocytopenia, lymphadenopathy, or renal dysfunction.

Consider alteration of antiretroviral therapies if disease progression occurs while patients are receiving nevirapine. Safety and efficacy have not been established in neonates.

Adverse Reactions Note: Potentially life-threatening nevirapine-associated adverse effects may present with the following symptoms: Abrupt onset of flu-like symptoms, abdominal pain, jaundice, or fever with or without rash; may progress to hepatic failure with encephalopathy. Skin rash is present in ~50% of cases.

Percentages of adverse effects vary by clinical trial:

>10%:

- Dermatologic: Rash (grade 1/2: 13%; grade 3/4: 1.5%) is the most common toxicity; occurs most frequently within the first 6 weeks of therapy; women may be at higher risk than men
- Hepatic: ALT >250 units/L (5% to 14%); symptomatic hepatic events (4%, range: up to 11%) are more common in women, women with $CD4^+$ cell counts >250 cells/mm^3, and men with $CD4^+$ cell counts >400 cells/mm^3

1% to 10%:

- Central nervous system: Headache (1% to 4%), fatigue (up to 5%)
- Gastrointestinal: Nausea (<1% to 9%), abdominal pain (<1% to 2%), diarrhea (up to 2%)

Hepatic: AST >250 units/L (4% to 8%); coinfection with hepatitis B or C and/or increased liver function tests at the beginning of therapy are associated with a greater risk of asymptomatic transaminase elevations (ALT or AST >5 times ULN: 6%, range: up to 9%) or symptomatic events occurring ≥6 weeks after beginning treatment

Postmarketing and/or case reports: Allergic reactions, anaphylaxis, anemia, angioedema, arthralgia, blisters, bullous eruptions, conjunctivitis, eosinophilia, facial edema, fever, fulminant and cholestatic hepatitis, granulocytopenia, hepatic failure, hepatic necrosis, hypersensitivity syndrome, jaundice, lymphadenopathy, malaise, neutropenia, oral lesions, paresthesia, redistribution/accumulation of body fat, renal dysfunction, Stevens-Johnson syndrome, somnolence, toxic epidermal necrolysis, ulcerative stomatitis, urticaria, vomiting

Overdosage/Toxicology Edema, erythema nodosum, fatigue, fever, headache, insomnia, nausea, pulmonary infiltrates, rash, vertigo, and weight loss have been reported following large doses.

Drug Interactions

Cytochrome P450 Effect: Substrate of CYP2B6 (minor), 2D6 (minor), 3A4 (major); **Inhibits** CYP1A2 (weak), 2D6 (weak), 3A4 (weak); **Induces** CYP2B6 (strong), 3A4 (strong)

Increased Effect/Toxicity: Cimetidine, itraconazole, ketoconazole, and some macrolide antibiotics may increase nevirapine plasma concentrations. Concurrent administration of prednisone for the initial 14 days of nevirapine therapy was associated with an increased incidence and severity of rash. Rifabutin concentrations are increased by nevirapine.

Decreased Effect: The levels/effects of nevirapine may be decreased by aminoglutethimide, carbamazepine, nafcillin, nevirapine, phenobarbital, phenytoin, and rifamycins, and other CYP3A4 inducers; avoid concurrent use. Nevirapine may decrease the levels/effects of benzodiazepines, bupropion, calcium channel blockers, clarithromycin, cyclosporine, efavirenz, erythromycin, estrogens, mirtazapine, nateglinide, nefazodone, promethazine, selegiline, sertraline, tacrolimus, venlafaxine, and other CYP2B6 or 3A4 substrates. Nevirapine may decrease serum concentrations of some protease inhibitors (AUC of indinavir, lopinavir, nelfinavir, and saquinavir may be decreased, however, no effect noted with ritonavir); specific dosage adjustments have not been recommended; no adjustment recommended for ritonavir, unless combined with lopinavir (Kaletra™). Nevirapine may decrease the effectiveness of oral contraceptives; suggest alternate method or additional form of birth control. Nevirapine also decreases the effect of ketoconazole and methadone.

Ethanol/Nutrition/Herb Interactions Herb/Nutraceutical: Nevirapine serum concentration may be decreased by St John's wort; avoid concurrent use.

Stability Store at room temperature

Mechanism of Action As a non-nucleoside reverse transcriptase inhibitor, nevirapine has activity against HIV-1 by binding to reverse transcriptase. It consequently blocks the RNA-dependent and DNA-dependent DNA polymerase activities including HIV-1 replication. It does not require intracellular phosphorylation for antiviral activity.

Pharmacodynamics/Kinetics

Absorption: >90%

Distribution: Widely; V_d: 1.2-1.4 L/kg; CSF penetration approximates 40% to 50% of plasma

Protein binding, plasma: 60%

Metabolism: Extensively hepatic via CYP3A4 (hydroxylation to inactive compounds); may undergo enterohepatic recycling

Half-life elimination: Decreases over 2- to 4-week time with chronic dosing due to autoinduction (ie, half-life = 45 hours initially and decreases to 25-30 hours)

Time to peak, serum: 2-4 hours

Excretion: Urine (~81%, primarily as metabolites, <3% as unchanged drug); feces (~10%)

Dosage Oral:

Children 2 months to <8 years: Initial: 4 mg/kg/dose once daily for 14 days; increase dose to 7 mg/kg/dose every 12 hours if no rash or other adverse effects occur; maximum dose: 200 mg/dose every 12 hours

Children ≥8 years: Initial: 4 mg/kg/dose once daily for 14 days; increase dose to 4 mg/kg/dose every 12 hours if no rash or other adverse effects occur; maximum dose: 200 mg/dose every 12 hours

Note: Alternative pediatric dosing (AIDSinfo guidelines): 120-200 mg/m^2 every 12 hours; this dosing has been proposed due to the fact that dosing based on mg/kg may result in an abrupt decrease in dose at the 8th birthday, which may be inappropriate.

(Continued)

Nevirapine *(Continued)*

Adults: Initial: 200 mg once daily for 14 days; maintenance: 200 mg twice daily (in combination with an additional antiretroviral agent)

Note: If patient experiences a rash during the 14-day lead-in period, dose should not be increased until the rash has resolved. Discontinue if severe rash, or rash with constitutional symptoms, is noted. If therapy is interrupted for >7 days, restart with initial dose for 14 days. Use of prednisone to prevent nevirapine-associated rash is not recommended. Permanently discontinue if symptomatic hepatic events occur.

Dosage adjustment in renal impairment:

Cl_{cr} ≥20 mL/minute: No adjustment required

Hemodialysis: An additional 200 mg dose is recommended following dialysis.

Dosage adjustment in hepatic impairment: Use not recommended with moderate-to-severe hepatic impairment. Permanently discontinue if symptomatic hepatic events occur.

Administration Oral: May be administered with or without food; may be administered with an antacid or didanosine; shake suspension gently prior to administration

Monitoring Parameters Liver function tests should be monitored at baseline, and intensively during the first 18 weeks of therapy (optimal frequency not established, some practitioners recommend more often than once a month, including prior to dose escalation, and at 2 weeks following dose escalation), then periodically throughout therapy; observe for CNS side effects. Assess/evaluate AST/ALT in any patients with a rash. Permanently discontinue if patient experiences severe rash, constitutional symptoms associated with rash, rash with elevated AST/ALT, or clinical hepatitis, Mild-to-moderate rash without AST/ALT elevation may continue treatment per discretion of prescriber. If mild-to-moderate urticarial rash, do not restart if treatment is interrupted.

Patient Information Report any right upper quadrant pain, jaundice, or rash immediately

Additional Information Potential compliance problems, frequency of administration, and adverse effects should be discussed with patients before initiating therapy to help prevent the emergence of resistance. Early virologic failure was observed with tenofovir and didanosine delayed release capsules, plus either efavirenz or nevirapine; use caution in treatment-naive patients with high baseline viral loads.

Dosage Forms

Suspension, oral: 50 mg/5 mL (240 mL)

Tablet: 200 mg

Selected Readings

D'Aquila RT, Hughes MD, Johnson VA, et al, "Nevirapine, Zidovudine, and Didanosine Compared With Zidovudine and Didanosine in Patients With HIV-1 Infection," *Ann Intern Med*, 1996, 124:1019-30.

Hammer SM, Kessler HA, and Saag MS, "Issues in Combination Antiretroviral Therapy: A Review," *J Acquir Immune Defic Syndr*, 1994, 7(Suppl 2):S24-37.

Havlir DV and Lange JM, "New Antiretrovirals and New Combinations," *AIDS*, 1998, 12(Suppl A):S165-74.

Weverling GJ, Lange JM, Jurriaans S, et al, "Alternative Multidrug Regimen Provides Improved Suppression of HIV-1 Replication Over Triple Therapy," *AIDS*, 1998, 12(11):F117-22.

NFV *see* Nelfinavir *on page 960*

Nidagel™ (Can) *see* Metronidazole *on page 940*

Nilstat (Can) *see* Nystatin *on page 976*

Nitazoxanide (nye ta ZOX a nide)

U.S. Brand Names Alinia®

Synonyms NTZ

Generic Available No

Use Treatment of diarrhea caused by *Cryptosporidium parvum* or *Giardia lamblia*

Pregnancy Risk Factor B

Pregnancy Implications Teratogenic effects were not observed in animal studies. There are no adequate and well-controlled studies in pregnant women.

Contraindications Hypersensitivity to nitazoxanide or any component of the formulation

Warnings/Precautions Use caution with renal or hepatic impairment. Safety and efficacy have not been established with HIV infection, immunodeficiency, or in children <1 year of age.

Adverse Reactions Rates of adverse effects were similar to those reported with placebo.

1% to 10%:

Central nervous system: Headache (1% to 3%)

Gastrointestinal: Abdominal pain (7% to 8%), diarrhea (2% to 4%), nausea (3%), vomiting (1%)

<1% (Limited to important or life-threatening): Allergic reaction, ALT increased, anemia, anorexia, appetite increased, creatinine increased, diaphoresis, dizziness, eye discoloration (pale yellow), fever, flatulence, hypertension, infection, malaise, nausea, pruritus, rhinitis, salivary glands enlarged, tachycardia, urine discoloration

Overdosage/Toxicology Treatment should be symptomatic and supportive.

Ethanol/Nutrition/Herb Interactions Food: Food increases AUC.

Stability

Suspension: Prior to and following reconstitution, store at room temperature of 15°C to 30°C (59°F to 86°F). For preparation at time of dispensing, add 48 mL incrementally to 60 mL bottle; shake vigorously; resulting suspension is 20 mg/mL (100 mg per 5 mL). Following reconstitution, discard unused portion of suspension after 7 days.

Tablet: Store at room temperature.

Mechanism of Action Nitazoxanide is rapidly metabolized to the active metabolite tizoxanide *in vivo*. Activity may be due to interference with the pyruvate:ferredoxin oxidoreductase (PFOR) enzyme-dependent electron transfer reaction which is essential to anaerobic metabolism. *In vitro*, nitazoxanide and tizoxanide inhibit the growth of sporozoites and oocysts of *Cryptosporidium parvum* and trophozoites of *Giardia lamblia*.

Pharmacodynamics/Kinetics

Protein binding: Tizoxanide: >99%

Bioavailability: Relative bioavailability of suspension compared to tablet: 70%

Metabolism: Hepatic, to an active metabolite, tizoxanide. Tizoxanide undergoes conjugation to form tizoxanide glucuronide. Nitazoxanide is not detectable in the serum following oral administration.

Time to peak, plasma: Tizoxanide and tizoxanide glucuronide: 1-4 hours

Excretion: Tizoxanide: Urine, bile, and feces; Tizoxanide glucuronide: Urine and bile

Dosage Diarrhea caused by *Cryptosporidium parvum* or *Giardia lamblia*:

Children 1-3 years: 100 mg every 12 hours for 3 days

Children 4-11 years: 200 mg every 12 hours for 3 days

Children ≥12 years and Adults: 500 mg every 12 hours for 3 days

Dosage adjustment in renal/hepatic impairment: Specific recommendations are not available; use with caution

Dietary Considerations Should be taken with food. Suspension contains sucrose 1.48 g/5 mL.

Administration Administer with food. Shake suspension well prior to administration.

Patient Information Take with food; shake suspension well prior to using. May discolor eyes or urine.

Dosage Forms

Powder for oral suspension: 100 mg/5 mL (60 mL) [contains sucrose 1.48 g/5 mL, sodium benzoate; strawberry flavor]

Tablet: 500 mg

Alinia® 3-Day Therapy Packs™ [unit-dose pack]: 500 mg (6s)

Nitrofurantoin (nye troe fyoor AN toyn)

Related Information

Antimicrobial Activity Against Selected Organisms *on page 1165*

U.S. Brand Names Furadantin®; Macrobid®; Macrodantin®

Canadian Brand Names Apo-Nitrofurantoin®; Macrobid®; Macrodantin®; Novo-Furantoin

Generic Available Yes: Excludes suspension

Use Prevention and treatment of urinary tract infections caused by susceptible gram-negative and some gram-positive organisms; *Pseudomonas*, *Serratia*, and most species of *Proteus* are generally resistant to nitrofurantoin

Drug of Choice or Alternative for

Disease/Syndrome(s):

Asymptomatic Bacteriuria *on page 39*

Urinary Tract Infection, Pyelonephritis *on page 346*

Organism(s):

Staphylococcus saprophyticus on page 312

Pregnancy Risk Factor B (contraindicated at term)

Pregnancy Implications Teratogenic effects have not been observed, however, may cause hemolytic anemia in infants. Use of nitrofurantoin is contraindicated at term (38-42 weeks gestation), during labor and delivery, or when the onset of labor is imminent.

Contraindications Hypersensitivity to nitrofurantoin or any component of the formulation; renal impairment (anuria, oliguria, significantly elevated serum creatinine, or Cl_{cr}< 60 mL/minute); infants <1 month (due to the possibility of hemolytic anemia);

(Continued)

Nitrofurantoin *(Continued)*

pregnancy at term (38-42 weeks gestation), during labor and delivery, or when the onset of labor is imminent

Warnings/Precautions Use with caution in patients with G6PD deficiency or in patients with anemia. Therapeutic concentrations of nitrofurantoin are not attained in urine of patients with Cl_{cr}<60 mL/minute. Use with caution if prolonged therapy is anticipated due to possible pulmonary toxicity. Acute, subacute, or chronic (usually after 6 months of therapy) pulmonary reactions have been observed in patients treated with nitrofurantoin; if these occur, discontinue therapy immediately; monitor closely for malaise, dyspnea, cough, fever, radiologic evidence of diffuse interstitial pneumonitis or fibrosis. Rare, but severe hepatic reactions have been associated with nitrofurantoin (onset may be insidious); discontinue immediately if hepatitis occurs. Has been associated with peripheral neuropathy (rare); risk may be increased by renal impairment, diabetes, vitamin B deficiency, or electrolyte imbalance; use caution.

Adverse Reactions Frequency not defined.

Cardiovascular: Chest pain, cyanosis, ECG changes (associated with pulmonary toxicity)

Central nervous system: Chills, depression, dizziness, drowsiness, fatigue, fever, headache, pseudotumor cerebri, psychotic reaction

Dermatologic: Alopecia, erythema multiforme, exfoliative dermatitis, pruritus, rash, Stevens-Johnson syndrome

Gastrointestinal: Abdominal pain, *C. difficile*-colitis, constipation, diarrhea, dyspepsia, loss of appetite, nausea (most common), pancreatitis, sore throat, vomiting

Hematologic: Agranulocytosis, aplastic anemia, eosinophilia, hemolytic anemia, methemoglobinemia, thrombocytopenia

Hepatic: Cholestasis, hepatitis, hepatic necrosis, transaminases increased, jaundice (cholestatic)

Neuromuscular & skeletal: Arthralgia, numbness, paresthesia, peripheral neuropathy, weakness

Ocular: Amblyopia, nystagmus, optic neuritis (rare)

Respiratory: Cough, dyspnea, pneumonitis, pulmonary fibrosis

Miscellaneous: Hypersensitivity (including acute pulmonary hypersensitivity), lupus-like syndrome

Overdosage/Toxicology Symptoms include vomiting. Treatment is supportive care only.

Drug Interactions

Increased Effect/Toxicity: Probenecid decreases renal excretion of nitrofurantoin.

Decreased Effect: Antacids decrease absorption of nitrofurantoin.

Ethanol/Nutrition/Herb Interactions

Ethanol: Avoid ethanol (may increase CNS depression).

Food: Nitrofurantoin serum concentrations may be increased if taken with food.

Stability Store at room temperature 15°C to 30°C (59°F to 86°F).

Mechanism of Action Inhibits several bacterial enzyme systems including acetyl coenzyme A interfering with metabolism and possibly cell wall synthesis

Pharmacodynamics/Kinetics

Absorption: Well absorbed; macrocrystalline form absorbed more slowly due to slower dissolution (causes less GI distress)

Distribution: V_d: 0.8 L/kg; crosses placenta; enters breast milk

Protein binding: 60% to 90%

Metabolism: Body tissues (except plasma) metabolize 60% of drug to inactive metabolites

Bioavailability: Increased with food

Half-life elimination: 20-60 minutes; prolonged with renal impairment

Excretion:

Suspension: Urine (40%) and feces (small amounts) as metabolites and unchanged drug

Macrocrystals: Urine (20% to 25% as unchanged drug)

Dosage Oral:

Children >1 month: 5-7 mg/kg/day in divided doses every 6 hours; maximum: 400 mg/day

UTI prophylaxis (chronic): 1-2 mg/kg/day in divided doses every 12-24 hours; maximum: 100 mg/day

Adults: 50-100 mg/dose every 6 hours

Macrocrystal/monohydrate: 100 mg twice daily

UTI prophylaxis (chronic): 50-100 mg/dose at bedtime

Dosing adjustment in renal impairment: Cl_{cr} <60 mL/minute: Contraindicated

Contraindicated in hemo- and peritoneal dialysis and continuous arteriovenous or venovenous hemofiltration

Administration Administer with meals to slow the rate of absorption and decrease adverse effects; suspension may be mixed with water, milk, fruit juice, or infant formula

Monitoring Parameters Signs of pulmonary reaction, signs of numbness or tingling of the extremities, periodic liver function tests

Test Interactions False-positive urine glucose (Benedict's and Fehling's methods); no false positives with enzymatic tests

Patient Information Take with food or milk; may discolor urine to a dark yellow or brown color; report fever, chest pain, persistent, nonproductive cough, or difficulty breathing; avoid alcohol

Dosage Forms

Capsule, macrocrystal: 50 mg, 100 mg

Macrodantin®: 25 mg, 50 mg, 100 mg

Capsule, macrocrystal/monohydrate (Macrobid®): 100 mg

Suspension, oral (Furadantin®): 25 mg/5 mL (470 mL)

Nix® [OTC] *see* Permethrin *on page 1001*

Nizoral® *see* Ketoconazole *on page 903*

Nizoral® A-D [OTC] *see* Ketoconazole *on page 903*

Nordeoxyguanosine *see* Ganciclovir *on page 834*

Norditropin® *see* Somatropin *on page 1069*

Norditropin® NordiFlex® *see* Somatropin *on page 1069*

Norfloxacin (nor FLOKS a sin)

Related Information

Antimicrobial Activity Against Selected Organisms *on page 1165*

U.S. Brand Names Noroxin®

Canadian Brand Names Apo-Norflox®; Norfloxacine®; Novo-Norfloxacin; PMS-Norfloxacin; Riva-Norfloxacin

Generic Available No

Use Uncomplicated urinary tract infections and cystitis caused by susceptible gram-negative and gram-positive bacteria; sexually-transmitted disease (eg, uncomplicated urethral and cervical gonorrhea) caused by *N. gonorrhoeae*; prostatitis due to *E. coli*

Drug of Choice or Alternative for Organism(s):

Neisseria gonorrhoeae on page 244

Pregnancy Risk Factor C

Pregnancy Implications Reports of arthropathy (observed in immature animals and reported rarely in humans) have limited the use of fluoroquinolones in pregnancy. Teratogenic effects have not been reported with norfloxacin in animal studies; however, embryonic loss has been reported with one species. Norfloxacin crosses the placenta. The Teratogen Information System concluded that therapeutic doses during pregnancy are unlikely to produce substantial teratogenic risk, but data are insufficient to say that there is no risk. There are no adequate and well-controlled studies in pregnant women. When considering treatment for life-threatening infection and/or prolonged duration of therapy, the potential risk to the fetus must be balanced against the severity of the potential illness.

Contraindications Hypersensitivity to norfloxacin, quinolones, or any component of the formulation

Warnings/Precautions

Concurrent disease:

- Renal impairment: Use caution with renal impairment.
- Myasthenia gravis: Quinolones may exacerbate myasthenia gravis, use with caution (rare, potentially life-threatening weakness of respiratory muscles may occur).
- G6PD deficiency: Use caution in patients with glucose-6-phosphate dehydrogenase deficiency.

Key adverse reactions:

- Allergic reactions: Severe hypersensitivity reactions, including anaphylaxis, have occurred with quinolone therapy. If an allergic reaction occurs (itching, urticaria, dyspnea, facial edema, loss of consciousness, tingling, cardiovascular collapse), discontinue drug immediately.
- Tendon rupture: Tendon inflammation and/or rupture have been reported with norfloxacin and other quinolone antibiotics. Risk may be increased with concurrent corticosteroids, particularly in the elderly. Discontinue at first sign of tendon inflammation or pain.
- CNS effects: CNS stimulation may occur which may lead to tremor, restlessness, confusion, and very rarely to hallucinations or convulsive seizures.

(Continued)

Norfloxacin *(Continued)*

- QT_c prolongation: Use may be associated (rarely) with prolongation of QT_c interval; avoid concurrent use with class Ia and class III antiarrhythmics; use caution with other drugs which may cause QT_c prolongation.
- Photosensitization: Avoid excessive exposure to sunlight; other quinolones have been associated with phototoxicity.
- Neuropathy/paresthesia: May be associated with the development of peripheral neuropathy and/or paresthesias; discontinue in patients who develop symptoms consistent with neuropathy.
- Developmental effects: Not recommended in children <18 years of age; other quinolones have caused transient arthropathy in children; use with caution in patients with known or suspected CNS disorders.
- Superinfection: Prolonged use may result in superinfection; pseudomembranous colitis may occur and should be considered in all patients who present with diarrhea.

Adverse Reactions

1% to 10%:

Central nervous system: Headache (3%), dizziness (3%)

Gastrointestinal: Nausea (4%)

Neuromuscular & skeletal: Weakness (1%)

<1%, postmarketing, and/or case reports: Abdominal pain, acute renal failure, agranulocytosis, anaphylaxis, anaphylactoid reactions, angioedema, anorexia, anxiety, arthralgia, arthritis, ataxia, back pain, bitter taste, cholestatic jaundice, confusion, constipation, CPK increased, depression, diarrhea, diplopia, dysgeusia, dyspepsia, dyspnea, erythema multiforme, erythema, exacerbation of myasthenia gravis, exfoliative dermatitis, fever, flatulence, GI bleeding, Guillain-Barré syndrome, hearing loss, heartburn, hemolytic anemia (sometimes associated with G6PD deficiency), hepatitis, hyperhidrosis, insomnia, jaundice, leukopenia, loose stools, myalgia, myoclonus, neutropenia, pancreatitis, paresthesia, peripheral neuropathy, photosensitivity, pruritus, pseudomembraneous colitis, psychotic reactions, QT_c prolongation, rash, seizure, serum creatinine/BUN increased, somnolence, Stevens-Johnson syndrome, thrombocytopenia, tinnitus, torsade de pointes, toxic epidermal necrolysis, transaminases increased, tremor, urticaria, vasculitis, vomiting, weakness, ventricular arrhythmia, xerostomia

Overdosage/Toxicology Symptoms include acute renal failure and seizures. Following GI decontamination, use supportive measures.

Drug Interactions

Cytochrome P450 Effect: Inhibits CYP1A2 (strong), 3A4 (moderate)

Increased Effect/Toxicity: Norfloxacin may increase the effects/toxicity of cyclosporine, CYP1A2 substrates (eg, aminophylline, fluvoxamine, mexiletine, mirtazapine, ropinirole, and trifluoperazine), CYP3A4 substrates (such as benzodiazepines, calcium channel blockers, cisapride, ergot alkaloids, selected HMG-CoA reductase inhibitors, mirtazapine, nateglinide, nefazodone, pimozide, sildenafil (and other PDE-5 inhibitors), tacrolimus, and venlafaxine), glyburide, theophylline, and warfarin. Concomitant use with corticosteroids may increase the risk of tendon rupture. Concomitant use with other QT_c-prolonging agents (eg, Class Ia and Class III antiarrhythmics, erythromycin, cisapride, antipsychotics, and cyclic antidepressants) may result in arrhythmias such as torsade de pointes. Probenecid may increase norfloxacin levels.

Decreased Effect: Concurrent administration of metal cations, including most antacids, oral electrolyte supplements, quinapril, sucralfate, some didanosine formulations (chewable/buffered tablets and pediatric powder for oral suspension), and other highly-buffered oral drugs, may decrease quinolone levels; separate doses.

Ethanol/Nutrition/Herb Interactions

Food: Norfloxacin average peak serum concentrations may be decreased if taken with dairy products.

Herb/Nutraceutical: Avoid dong quai, St John's wort (may also cause photosensitization).

Stability Store at 25°C (77°F); keep container tightly closed

Mechanism of Action Norfloxacin is a DNA gyrase inhibitor. DNA gyrase is an essential bacterial enzyme that maintains the superhelical structure of DNA. DNA gyrase is required for DNA replication and transcription, DNA repair, recombination, and transposition; bactericidal

Pharmacodynamics/Kinetics

Absorption: Oral: Rapid, up to 40%

Distribution: Crosses placenta; small amounts enter breast milk

Protein binding: 15%

Metabolism: Hepatic

Half-life elimination: 3-4 hours; Renal impairment (Cl_{cr} ≤30 mL/minute): 6.5 hours; Elderly: 4 hours

Time to peak, serum: 1-2 hours

Excretion: Urine (26% to 36%); feces (30%)

Dosage Oral: Adults:

Urinary tract infections: 400 mg twice daily for 3-21 days depending on severity of infection or organism sensitivity; maximum: 800 mg/day

Uncomplicated gonorrhea: 800 mg as a single dose (CDC recommends as an alternative regimen to ciprofloxacin or ofloxacin)

Prostatitis: 400 mg every 12 hours for 4 weeks

Dosing interval in renal impairment: Cl_{cr} 10-30 mL/minute: Urinary tract infections: Administer 400 mg every 24 hours

Dietary Considerations Oral formulations should be administered on an empty stomach with water (1 hour before or 2 hours after meals, milk, or other dairy products).

Administration Hold antacids or sucralfate for 3-4 hours after giving norfloxacin; do not administer together. Best taken on an empty stomach with water (1 hour before or 2 hours after meals, milk, or other dairy products).

Patient Information Tablets should be taken at least 1 hour before or at least 2 hours after a meal with a glass of water; patients receiving norfloxacin should be well hydrated; take all the medication, do not skip doses; do not take with antacids; contact your prescriber immediately with inflammation or tendon pain

Dosage Forms Tablet: 400 mg

Selected Readings

Hooper DC and Wolfson JS, "Fluoroquinolone Antimicrobial Agents," *N Engl J Med*, 1991, 324(6):384-94.
Lomaestro BM and Bailie GR, "Quinolone-Cation Interactions: A Review," *DICP*, 1991, 25(11):1249-58.
Stein GE, "The 4-Quinolone Antibiotics: Past, Present, and Future," *Pharmacotherapy*, 1988, 8(6):301-14.
Walker RC and Wright AJ, "The Fluoroquinolones," *Mayo Clin Proc*, 1991, 66(12):1249-59.

NTZ *see* Nitazoxanide *on page 970*
Nu-Acyclovir (Can) *see* Acyclovir *on page 629*
Nu-Amoxi (Can) *see* Amoxicillin *on page 642*
Nu-Ampi (Can) *see* Ampicillin *on page 657*
Nu-Cefaclor (Can) *see* Cefaclor *on page 697*
Nu-Cephalex (Can) *see* Cephalexin *on page 727*
Nu-Cloxi (Can) *see* Cloxacillin *on page 760*
Nu-Cotrimox (Can) *see* Sulfamethoxazole and Trimethoprim *on page 1087*
Nu-Doxycycline (Can) *see* Doxycycline *on page 787*
Nu-Erythromycin-S (Can) *see* Erythromycin *on page 807*
Nu-Megestrol (Can) *see* Megestrol *on page 932*
Nu-Pen-VK (Can) *see* Penicillin V Potassium *on page 998*
Nu-Tetra (Can) *see* Tetracycline *on page 1106*
Nutropin® *see* Somatropin *on page 1069*
Nutropin AQ® *see* Somatropin *on page 1069*
Nutropine® (Can) *see* Somatropin *on page 1069*
NVP *see* Nevirapine *on page 967*
Nyaderm (Can) *see* Nystatin *on page 976*
Nyamyc™ *see* Nystatin *on page 976*
Nydrazid® [DSC] *see* Isoniazid *on page 893*

Nystatin (nye STAT in)

U.S. Brand Names Bio-Statin®; Mycostatin®; Nyamyc™; Nystat-Rx®; Nystop®; Pedi-Dri®

Canadian Brand Names Candistatin®; Mycostatin®; Nilstat; Nyaderm; PMS-Nystatin

Generic Available Yes: Cream, ointment, powder, suspension, tablet

Use Treatment of susceptible cutaneous, mucocutaneous, and oral cavity fungal infections normally caused by the *Candida* species

Pregnancy Risk Factor B/C (oral)

Contraindications Hypersensitivity to nystatin or any component of the formulation

Adverse Reactions

Frequency not defined: Dermatologic: Contact dermatitis, Stevens-Johnson syndrome

1% to 10%: Gastrointestinal: Nausea, vomiting, diarrhea, stomach pain

<1%: Hypersensitivity reactions

Overdosage/Toxicology Symptoms include nausea, vomiting, and diarrhea. Treatment is supportive.

Stability

Vaginal insert: Store in refrigerator; protect from temperature extremes, moisture, and light

Oral tablet, ointment, topical powder, and oral suspension: Store at controlled room temperature of 15°C to 25°C (59°F to 77°F)

Mechanism of Action Binds to sterols in fungal cell membrane, changing the cell wall permeability allowing for leakage of cellular contents

Pharmacodynamics/Kinetics

Onset of action: Symptomatic relief from candidiasis: 24-72 hours

Absorption: Topical: None through mucous membranes or intact skin; Oral: Poorly absorbed

Excretion: Feces (as unchanged drug)

Dosage

Oral candidiasis:

Suspension (swish and swallow orally):

Premature infants: 100,000 units 4 times/day

Infants: 200,000 units 4 times/day or 100,000 units to each side of mouth 4 times/day

Children and Adults: 400,000-600,000 units 4 times/day

Powder for compounding: Children and Adults: 1/8 teaspoon (500,000 units) to equal approximately 1/2 cup of water; give 4 times/day

Mucocutaneous infections: Children and Adults: Topical: Apply 2-3 times/day to affected areas; very moist topical lesions are treated best with powder

Intestinal infections: Adults: Oral: 500,000-1,000,000 units every 8 hours

Vaginal infections: Adults: Vaginal tablets: Insert 1 tablet/day at bedtime for 2 weeks

Administration Suspension: Shake well before using. Should be swished about the mouth and retained in the mouth for as long as possible (several minutes) before swallowing.

Patient Information The oral suspension should be swished about the mouth and retained in the mouth for as long as possible (several minutes) before swallowing. For

neonates and infants, paint nystatin suspension into recesses of the mouth. Troches must be allowed to dissolve slowly and should not be chewed or swallowed whole. If topical irritation occurs, discontinue; for external use only; do not discontinue therapy even if symptoms are gone

Dosage Forms

Capsule (Bio-Statin®): 500,000 units, 1 million units
Cream: 100,000 units/g (15 g, 30 g)
Mycostatin®: 100,000 units/g (30 g)
Ointment, topical: 100,000 units/g (15 g, 30 g)
Powder, for prescription compounding: 50 million units (10 g); 150 million units (30 g); 500 million units (100 g); 2 billion units (400 g)
Nystat-Rx®: 50 million units (10 g); 150 million units (30 g); 500 million units (100 g); 1 billion units (190 g); 2 billion units (350 g)
Powder, topical:
Mycostatin®: 100,000 units/g (15 g)
Nyamyc™: 100,000 units/g (15 g, 30 g)
Nystop®: 100,000 units/g (15 g, 30 g, 60 g)
Pedi-Dri®: 100,000 units/g (56.7 g)
Suspension, oral: 100,000 units/mL (5 mL, 60 mL, 480 mL)
Tablet: 500,000 units
Tablet, vaginal: 100,000 units (15s) [packaged with applicator]

Nystatin and Triamcinolone (nye STAT in & trye am SIN oh lone)

Related Information

Nystatin *on page 976*

U.S. Brand Names Mycolog®-II [DSC]

Synonyms Triamcinolone and Nystatin

Generic Available Yes

Use Treatment of cutaneous candidiasis

Pregnancy Risk Factor C

Contraindications Hypersensitivity to nystatin, triamcinolone, or any component of the formulation

Warnings/Precautions Avoid use of occlusive dressings; limit therapy to least amount necessary for effective therapy, pediatric patients may be more susceptible to HPA axis suppression due to larger BSA to weight ratio

Adverse Reactions 1% to 10%:

Dermatologic: Dryness, folliculitis, hypertrichosis, acne, hypopigmentation, allergic dermatitis, maceration of the skin, skin atrophy
Local: Burning, itching, irritation
Miscellaneous: Increased incidence of secondary infection

Mechanism of Action Nystatin is an antifungal agent that binds to sterols in fungal cell membrane, changing the cell wall permeability allowing for leakage of cellular contents. Triamcinolone is a synthetic corticosteroid; it decreases inflammation by suppression of migration of polymorphonuclear leukocytes and reversal of increased capillary permeability. It suppresses the immune system reducing activity and volume of the lymphatic system. It suppresses adrenal function at high doses.

Pharmacodynamics/Kinetics See individual agents.

Dosage Children and Adults: Topical: Apply sparingly 2-4 times/day. Therapy should be discontinued when control is achieved; if no improvement is seen, reassessment of diagnosis may be necessary.

Administration External use only; do not use on open wounds; apply sparingly to occlusive dressings; should not be used in the presence of open or weeping lesions

Dosage Forms [DSC] = Discontinued product

Cream (Mycolog®-II [DSC]): Nystatin 100,000 units and triamcinolone acetonide 0.1% (15 g, 30 g, 60 g)
Ointment: Nystatin 100,000 units and triamcinolone acetonide 0.1% (15 g, 30 g, 60 g)
Mycolog®-II: Nystatin 100,000 units and triamcinolone acetonide 0.1% (15 g, 30 g, 60 g) [DSC]

Nystat-Rx® *see* Nystatin *on page 976*
Nystop® *see* Nystatin *on page 976*
Octagam® *see* Immune Globulin (Intravenous) *on page 867*
Ocuflox® *see* Ofloxacin *on page 977*

Ofloxacin (oh FLOKS a sin)

Related Information

Antimicrobial Activity Against Selected Organisms *on page 1165*
Tuberculosis *on page 1315*
(Continued)

Ofloxacin *(Continued)*

U.S. Brand Names Floxin®; Ocuflox®

Canadian Brand Names Apo-Oflox®; Apo-Ofloxacin®; Floxin®; Novo-Ofloxacin; Ocuflox®; pms-Ofloxacin

Synonyms Floxin Otic Singles

Generic Available Yes: Tablet, ophthalmic solution

Use Quinolone antibiotic for the treatment of acute exacerbations of chronic bronchitis, community-acquired pneumonia, skin and skin structure infections (uncomplicated), urethral and cervical gonorrhea (acute, uncomplicated), urethritis and cervicitis (nongonococcal), mixed infections of the urethra and cervix, pelvic inflammatory disease (acute), cystitis (uncomplicated), urinary tract infections (complicated), prostatitis

Ophthalmic: Treatment of superficial ocular infections involving the conjunctiva or cornea due to strains of susceptible organisms

Otic: Otitis externa, chronic suppurative otitis media, acute otitis media

Unlabeled/Investigational Use Epididymitis (gonorrhea)

Drug of Choice or Alternative for

Disease/Syndrome(s):

Cervicitis *on page 71*
Epididymitis/Orchitis *on page 138*
Prostatitis *on page 277*
Traveler's Diarrhea *on page 333*

Organism(s):

Neisseria gonorrhoeae on page 244

Pregnancy Risk Factor C

Pregnancy Implications Reports of arthropathy (observed in immature animals and reported rarely in humans) have limited the use of fluoroquinolones in pregnancy. Teratogenic effects were not observed with ofloxacin in animal studies; however, decreased fetal body weight and increased fetal mortality were observed in some species. Ofloxacin crosses the placenta. Although quinolone antibiotics should not be used as first-line agents during pregnancy, when considering treatment for life-threatening infection and/or prolonged duration of therapy, the potential risk to the fetus must be balanced against the severity of the potential illness.

Contraindications Hypersensitivity to ofloxacin or other members of the quinolone group such as nalidixic acid, oxolinic acid, cinoxacin, norfloxacin, and ciprofloxacin; hypersensitivity to any component of the formulation

Warnings/Precautions Use with caution in patients with epilepsy or other CNS diseases which could predispose seizures; use with caution in patients with renal or hepatic impairment. Tendon inflammation and/or rupture have been reported with quinolone antibiotics, including ofloxacin. Risk may be increased with concurrent corticosteroids, particularly in the elderly. Discontinue at first sign of tendon inflammation or pain. Peripheral neuropathies have been linked to ofloxacin use; discontinue if numbness, tingling, or weakness develops.

Rare cases of torsade de pointes have been reported in patients receiving ofloxacin and other quinolones. Risk may be minimized by avoiding use in patients with known prolongation of the QT interval, bradycardia, hypokalemia, hypomagnesemia, cardiomyopathy, or in those receiving concurrent therapy with Class Ia or Class III antiarrhythmics.

Severe hypersensitivity reactions, including anaphylaxis, have occurred with quinolone therapy. If an allergic reaction occurs (itching, urticaria, dyspnea, facial edema, loss of consciousness, tingling, cardiovascular collapse), discontinue drug immediately. Prolonged use may result in superinfection; pseudomembranous colitis may occur and should be considered in all patients who present with diarrhea. Quinolones may exacerbate myasthenia gravis, use with caution (rare, potentially life-threatening weakness of respiratory muscles may occur).

Adverse Reactions

Systemic:

1% to 10%:

Cardiovascular: Chest pain (1% to 3%)

Central nervous system: Headache (1% to 9%), insomnia (3% to 7%), dizziness (1% to 5%), fatigue (1% to 3%), somnolence (1% to 3%), sleep disorders (1% to 3%), nervousness (1% to 3%), pyrexia (1% to 3%)

Dermatologic: Rash/pruritus (1% to 3%)

Gastrointestinal: Diarrhea (1% to 4%), vomiting (1% to 4%), GI distress (1% to 3%), abdominal cramps (1% to 3%), flatulence (1% to 3%), abnormal taste (1% to 3%), xerostomia (1% to 3%), decreased appetite (1% to 3%), nausea (3% to 10%), constipation (1% to 3%)

Genitourinary: Vaginitis (1% to 5%), external genital pruritus in women (1% to 3%)

Ocular: Visual disturbances (1% to 3%)
Respiratory: Pharyngitis (1% to 3%)
Miscellaneous: Trunk pain

<1%, postmarketing, and/or case reports (limited to important or life-threatening): Anaphylaxis reactions, anxiety, blurred vision, chills, cognitive change, cough, depression, dream abnormality, ecchymosis, edema, erythema nodosum, euphoria, extremity pain, hallucinations, hearing acuity decreased, hepatic dysfunction, hepatitis, hyper/hypoglycemia, hypertension, interstitial nephritis, lightheadedness, malaise, myasthenia gravis exacerbation, palpitation, paresthesia, peripheral neuropathy, photophobia, photosensitivity, psychotic reactions, rhabdomyolysis, seizure, Stevens-Johnson syndrome, syncope, tendonitis and tendon rupture, thirst, tinnitus, torsade de pointes, Tourette's syndrome, toxic epidermal necrolysis, vasculitis, vasodilation, vertigo, weakness, weight loss

Ophthalmic: Frequency not defined:
Central nervous system: Dizziness
Gastrointestinal: Nausea
Ocular: Blurred vision, burning, chemical conjunctivitis/keratitis, discomfort, dryness, edema, eye pain, foreign body sensation, itching, photophobia, redness, stinging, tearing

Otic:
>10%: Local: Application site reaction (<1% to 17%)
1% to 10%:
Central nervous system: Dizziness (≤1%), vertigo (≤1%)
Dermatologic: Pruritus (1% to 4%), rash (1%)
Gastrointestinal: Taste perversion (7%)
Neuromuscular & skeletal: Paresthesia (1%)

<1% (Limited to important or life-threatening): Diarrhea, fever, headache, hearing loss, hypertension, nausea, otorrhagia, tinnitus, tremor, vomiting, xerostomia

Postmarketing and/case reports: Transient neuropsychiatric disturbances

Overdosage/Toxicology Symptoms include acute renal failure, seizures, nausea, and vomiting. Treatment includes GI decontamination, if possible, and supportive care.

Drug Interactions

Cytochrome P450 Effect: Inhibits CYP1A2 (strong)

Increased Effect/Toxicity: Ofloxacin may increase the effects/toxicity of CYP1A2 substrates (eg, aminophylline, fluvoxamine, mexiletine, mirtazapine, ropinirole, and trifluoperazine), glyburide, theophylline and warfarin. Concomitant use with corticosteroids may increase the risk of tendon rupture. Concomitant use with other QT_c-prolonging agents (eg, Class Ia and Class III antiarrhythmics, erythromycin, cisapride, antipsychotics, and cyclic antidepressants) may result in arrhythmias such as torsade de pointes. Probenecid may increase ofloxacin levels.

Decreased Effect: Concurrent administration of metal cations, including most antacids, oral electrolyte supplements, quinapril, sucralfate, some didanosine formulations (chewable/buffered tablets and pediatric powder for oral suspension), and other highly-buffered oral drugs, may decrease quinolone levels; separate doses.

Ethanol/Nutrition/Herb Interactions

Food: Ofloxacin average peak serum concentrations may be decreased by 20% if taken with food.

Herb/Nutraceutical: Avoid dong quai, St John's wort (may also cause photosensitization).

Stability

Ophthalmic and otic solution: Store at 15°C to 25°C (59°F to 77°F)

Otic Singles™: Store at 15°C to 30°C (59°F to 86°F); store in pouch to protect from light

Tablet: Store below 30°C (86°F)

Mechanism of Action Ofloxacin is a DNA gyrase inhibitor. DNA gyrase is an essential bacterial enzyme that maintains the superhelical structure of DNA. DNA gyrase is required for DNA replication and transcription, DNA repair, recombination, and transposition; bactericidal

Pharmacodynamics/Kinetics

Absorption: Well absorbed; food causes only minor alterations
Distribution: V_d: 2.4-3.5 L/kg
Protein binding: 20%
Bioavailability: Oral: 98%
Half-life elimination: Biphasic: 5-7.5 hours and 20-25 hours (accounts for <5%); prolonged with renal impairment
Excretion: Primarily urine (as unchanged drug)
(Continued)

Ofloxacin *(Continued)*

Dosage

Oral: Adults:

Chronic bronchitis (acute exacerbation), community-acquired pneumonia, skin and skin structure infections (uncomplicated): 400 mg every 12 hours for 10 days

Urethral and cervical gonorrhea (acute, uncomplicated): 400 mg as a single dose

Cervicitis/urethritis (nongonococcal) due to *C. trachomatis*, mixed infection of urethra and cervix due to *C. trachomatis* and *N. gonorrhoea*: 300 mg every 12 hours for 7 days

Pelvic inflammatory disease (acute): 400 mg every 12 hours for 10-14 days

Cystitis (uncomplicated):

Due to *E. coli* or *K. pneumoniae*: 200 mg every 12 hours for 3 days

Due to other organisms: 200 mg every 12 hours for 7 days

UTI (complicated): 200 mg every 12 hours for 10 days

Prostatitis: 200 mg every 12 hours for 6 weeks

Epididymitis (gonorrhea; unlabeled use): 300 mg twice daily for 10 days

Ophthalmic: Children >1 year and Adults:

Conjunctivitis: Instill 1-2 drops in affected eye(s) every 2-4 hours for the first 2 days, then use 4 times/day for an additional 5 days

Corneal ulcer: Instill 1-2 drops every 30 minutes while awake and every 4-6 hours after retiring for the first 2 days; beginning on day 3, instill 1-2 drops every hour while awake for 4-6 additional days; thereafter, 1-2 drops 4 times/day until clinical cure.

Otic:

Acute otitis media with tympanostomy tubes: Children 1-12 years: Instill 5 drops (or the contents of 1 single-dose container) into affected ear(s) twice daily for 10 days

Chronic suppurative otitis media with perforated tympanic membranes: Children >12 years and Adults: Instill 10 drops (or the contents of 2 single-dose containers) into affected ear twice daily for 14 days

Otitis externa:

Children 6 months to 13 years: Instill 5 drops (or the contents of 1 single-dose container) into affected ear(s) once daily for 7 days

Children ≥13 years and Adults: Instill 10 drops (or the contents of 2 single-dose containers) into affected ear(s) once daily for 7 days

Dosing adjustment/interval in renal impairment: Adults: Oral: After a normal initial dose, adjust as follows:

Cl_{cr} 20-50 mL/minute: Administer usual dose every 24 hours

Cl_{cr} <20 mL/minute: Administer half the usual dose every 24 hours

Continuous arteriovenous or venovenous hemodiafiltration effects: Administer 300 mg every 24 hours

Dosing adjustment in hepatic impairment: Severe impairment: Maximum dose: 400 mg/day

Administration

Ophthalmic: For ophthalmic use only; avoid touching tip of applicator to eye or other surfaces.

Oral: Do not take within 2 hours of food or any antacids which contain zinc, magnesium, or aluminum.

Otic: Prior to use, warm solution by holding container in hands for 1-2 minutes. Patient should lie down with affected ear upward and medication instilled. Pump tragus 4 times to ensure penetration of medication. Patient should remain in this position for 5 minutes.

Patient Information Report any skin rash or other allergic reactions; avoid excessive sunlight; do not take with food; do not take within 2 hours of any products including antacids which contain calcium, magnesium, or aluminum; contact your prescriber immediately with signs of inflammation or tendon pain

Dosage Forms

Solution, ophthalmic (Ocuflox®): 0.3% (5 mL, 10 mL) [contains benzalkonium chloride]

Solution, otic:

Floxin®: 0.3% (5 mL, 10 mL) [contains benzalkonium chloride]

Floxin® Otic Singles™: 0.3% (0.25 mL) [contains benzalkonium chloride; packaged as 2 single-dose containers per pouch, 10 pouches per carton, total net volume 5 mL]

Tablet (Floxin®): 200 mg, 300 mg, 400 mg

Selected Readings

Hooper DC and Wolfson JS, "Fluoroquinolone Antimicrobial Agents," *N Engl J Med*, 1991, 324(6):384-94.

Lomaestro BM and Bailie GR, "Quinolone-Cation Interactions: A Review," *DICP*, 1991, 25(11):1249-58.

Monk JP and Campoli-Richards DM, "Ofloxacin. A Review of Its Antibacterial Activity, Pharmacokinetic Properties and Therapeutic Use," *Drugs*, 1987, 33(4):346-91.

Stein GE, "The 4-Quinolone Antibiotics: Past, Present, and Future," *Pharmacotherapy*, 1988, 8(6):301-14.
US Department of Health and Human Services, "1993 Sexually Transmitted Diseases Treatment Guidelines," *MMWR*, 1993, 42(RR-14).
Walker RC and Wright AJ, "The Fluoroquinolones," *Mayo Clin Proc*, 1991, 66(12):1249-59.

Omnicef® *see* Cefdinir *on page 702*

Oncotice™ (Can) *see* BCG Vaccine *on page 683*

Operand® [OTC] *see* Povidone-Iodine *on page 1016*

Operand® Chlorhexidine Gluconate [OTC] *see* Chlorhexidine Gluconate *on page 735*

Ophthalmics, Bacterial

Refer to

Bacitracin and Polymyxin B *on page 681*
Bacitracin, Neomycin, Polymyxin B, and Hydrocortisone *on page 682*
Bacitracin, Neomycin, and Polymyxin B *on page 1054*
Bacitracin *on page 1034*
Ciprofloxacin *on page 742*
Erythromycin *on page 807*
Gatifloxacin *on page 837*
Gentamicin *on page 841*
Moxifloxacin *on page 949*
Neomycin, Polymyxin B, and Dexamethasone *on page 965*
Neomycin, Polymyxin B, and Gramicidin *on page 965*
Neomycin, Polymyxin B, and Hydrocortisone *on page 966*
Neomycin, Polymyxin B, and Prednisolone *on page 967*
Oxytetracycline and Polymyxin B *on page 987*
Sulfacetamide Sodium and Fluorometholone *on page 1083*
Sulfacetamide *on page 1081*
Tobramycin and Dexamethasone *on page 1126*
Tobramycin *on page 1122*
Trimethoprim and Polymyxin B *on page 1131*

Ophthalmics, Viral

Refer to

Fomivirsen *on page 826*
Trifluridine *on page 1129*

Optimyxin® (Can) *see* Bacitracin and Polymyxin B *on page 681*

Optimyxin Plus® (Can) *see* Neomycin, Polymyxin B, and Gramicidin *on page 965*

ORO-Clense (Can) *see* Chlorhexidine Gluconate *on page 735*

Oseltamivir (oh sel TAM i vir)

Related Information

USPHS / IDSA Guidelines for the Prevention of Opportunistic Infections in Persons Infected With HIV *on page 1237*

U.S. Brand Names Tamiflu®

Canadian Brand Names Tamiflu®

Generic Available No

Use Treatment of uncomplicated acute illness due to influenza (A or B) infection in adults and children >1 year of age who have been symptomatic for no more than 2 days; prophylaxis against influenza (A or B) infection in adults and adolescents ≥13 years of age

Drug of Choice or Alternative for Organism(s):

Influenza Virus *on page 193*

Pregnancy Risk Factor C

Pregnancy Implications There are insufficient human data to determine the risk to a pregnant woman or developing fetus. Studies evaluating the effects on embryo-fetal development in rats and rabbits showed a dose-dependent increase in the rates of minor skeleton abnormalities in exposed offspring. The rate of each abnormality remained within the background rate of occurrence in the species studied.

Contraindications Hypersensitivity to oseltamivir or any component of the formulation

Warnings/Precautions Oseltamivir is not a substitute for the flu shot. Dosage adjustment is required for creatinine clearance between 10-30 mL/minute. Safety and efficacy in children (<1 year of age) have not been established for treatment regimens. Safety and efficacy have not been established for prophylactic use in patients <13 years of age. Also consider primary or concomitant bacterial infections. Safety and efficacy for treatment or prophylaxis in immunocompromised patients have not been established.

(Continued)

Oseltamivir *(Continued)*

Adverse Reactions

As seen with **treatment** doses: 1% to 10%:

Central nervous system: Insomnia (adults 1%), vertigo (adults 1%)

Gastrointestinal: Nausea (adults 10%), vomiting (adults 9%, children 15%), abdominal pain (children 5%)

Ocular: Conjunctivitis (children 1%)

Otic: Ear disorder (children 2%)

Respiratory: Epistaxis (children 3%)

Similar adverse effects were seen in **prophylactic** use, however, the incidence was generally less. The following reactions were seen more commonly with prophylactic use: Headache (20%), fatigue (8%), diarrhea (3%)

<1% and case reports (any indication): Aggravation of diabetes, anemia, arrhythmia, confusion, hepatitis, humerus fracture, peritonsillar abscess, pneumonia, pseudomembranous colitis, pyrexia, rash, seizure, transaminases increased, toxic epidermal necrolysis, unstable angina, swelling of face or tongue

Overdosage/Toxicology Single doses of 1000 mg resulted in nausea and vomiting.

Drug Interactions

Increased Effect/Toxicity: Cimetidine and amoxicillin have no effect on plasma concentrations. Probenecid increases oseltamivir carboxylate serum concentration by twofold. Dosage adjustments are not required.

Stability

Capsules: Store at 25°C (77°F).

Oral suspension: Store powder for suspension at 25°C (77°F). Reconstitute with 23 mL of water (to make 25 mL total suspension). Once reconstituted, store suspension under refrigeration at 2°C to 8°C (36°F to 46°F); do not freeze. Use within 10 days of preparation.

Mechanism of Action Oseltamivir, a prodrug, is hydrolyzed to the active form, oseltamivir carboxylate. It is thought to inhibit influenza virus neuraminidase, with the possibility of alteration of virus particle aggregation and release. In clinical studies of the influenza virus, 1.3% of post-treatment isolates had decreased neuraminidase susceptibility to oseltamivir carboxylate.

Pharmacodynamics/Kinetics

Absorption: Well absorbed

Distribution: V_d: 23-26 L (oseltamivir carboxylate)

Protein binding, plasma: Oseltamivir carboxylate: 3%; Oseltamivir: 42%

Metabolism: Hepatic (90%) to oseltamivir carboxylate; neither the parent drug nor active metabolite has any effect on CYP

Bioavailability: 75% reaches systemic circulation in active form

Half-life elimination: Oseltamivir carboxylate: 6-10 hours; similar in geriatrics (68-78 years)

Time to peak: C_{max}: Oseltamivir: 65 ng/mL; Oseltamivir carboxylate: 348 ng/mL

Excretion: Urine (as carboxylate metabolite)

Dosage Oral:

Treatment: Initiate treatment within 2 days of onset of symptoms; duration of treatment: 5 days:

Children: 1-12 years:

- ≤15 kg: 30 mg twice daily
- >15 kg - ≤23 kg: 45 mg twice daily
- >23 kg - ≤40 kg: 60 mg twice daily
- >40 kg: 75 mg twice daily

Adolescents ≥13 years and Adults: 75 mg twice daily

Prophylaxis: Adolescents ≥13 years and Adults: 75 mg once daily for at least 7 days; treatment should begin within 2 days of contact with an infected individual. During community outbreaks, dosing is 75 mg once daily. May be used for up to 6 weeks; duration of protection lasts for length of dosing period

Dosage adjustment in renal impairment:

Cl_{cr} 10-30 mL/minute:

Treatment: Reduce dose to 75 mg once daily for 5 days

Prophylaxis: 75 mg every other day

Cl_{cr} <10 mL/minute: Has not been studied

Dosage adjustment in hepatic impairment: Has not been evaluated

Elderly: No adjustments required

Dietary Considerations Take with or without food; take with food to improve tolerance.

Patient Information When used as treatment of influenza infection, take within 2 days of onset of flu symptoms (fever, cough, headache, fatigue, muscular weakness, and sore throat). When used as prevention of influenza infection, take every day

during the "flu season" as instructed by your prescriber. This is not a substitute for the flu shot. Not recommended for pregnant or nursing women. For best results, do not miss doses.

Suspension: Shake well before using; may be stored under refrigeration or at room temperature. Use the oral syringe provided to measure appropriate dose.

Dosage Forms

Capsule, as phosphate: 75 mg

Powder for oral suspension: 12 mg/mL (25 mL) [contains sodium benzoate; tutti-frutti flavor]

Selected Readings

Anonymous, "Neuraminidase Inhibitors for Treatment of Influenza A and B Infections," *MMWR*, 1999, 48(RR-14):1-9.

Bardsley-Elliot A and Noble S, "Oseltamivir," *Drugs*, 1999, 58(5):851-60.

Hayden FG, Atmar RL, Schilling M, et al, "Use of the Selective Oral Neuraminidase Inhibitor Oseltamivir to Prevent Influenza," *N Engl J Med*, 1999, 341(18):1387-8.

He G, Massarella J, and Ward P, "Clinical Pharmacokinetics of the Prodrug Oseltamivir and Its Active Metabolite Ro 64-0802," 1999, 37(6):471-84.

JAMA, 1999, 282:1240-6.

McClellan K and Perry CM, "Oseltamivir: A Review of Its Use in Influenza," *Drugs*, 2001, 61(2):263-83.

McNicholl IR and McNicholl JJ, "Neuraminidase Inhibitors: Zanamivir and Oseltamivir," *Ann Pharmacother*, 2001, 35(1):57-70.

Ovace™ *see* Sulfacetamide *on page 1081*

Ovide® *see* Malathion *on page 925*

Oxacillin (oks a SIL in)

Related Information

Antibiotic Treatment of Adults With Infective Endocarditis *on page 1271*

Antimicrobial Activity Against Selected Organisms *on page 1165*

Synonyms Methylphenyl Isoxazolyl Penicillin; Oxacillin Sodium

Generic Available Yes

Use Treatment of infections such as osteomyelitis, septicemia, endocarditis, and CNS infections caused by susceptible strains of *Staphylococcus*

Drug of Choice or Alternative for Disease/Syndrome(s):

Arthritis, Septic *on page 36*

Mastitis *on page 214*

Pregnancy Risk Factor B

Pregnancy Implications Teratogenicity not observed in animal studies.

Contraindications Hypersensitivity to oxacillin or other penicillins or any component of the formulation

Warnings/Precautions Elimination rate will be slow in neonates; modify dosage in patients with renal impairment and in the elderly; use with caution in patients with cephalosporin hypersensitivity

Adverse Reactions Frequency not defined.

Central nervous system: Fever

Dermatologic: Rash

Gastrointestinal: Nausea, diarrhea, vomiting

Hematologic: Eosinophilia, leukopenia, neutropenia, thrombocytopenia, agranulocytosis

Hepatic: Hepatotoxicity, AST increased

Renal: Acute interstitial nephritis, hematuria

Miscellaneous: Serum sickness-like reactions

Overdosage/Toxicology Symptoms of penicillin overdose include neuromuscular hypersensitivity (agitation, hallucinations, asterixis, encephalopathy, confusion, and seizures) and electrolyte imbalance (with potassium or sodium salts), especially in renal failure. Hemodialysis may be helpful to aid in the removal of the drug from the blood, otherwise most treatment is supportive or symptom-directed.

Drug Interactions

Increased Effect/Toxicity: Probenecid increases penicillin levels. Penicillins and anticoagulants may increase the effect of anticoagulants. Penicillins may increase the exposure to methotrexate during concurrent therapy; monitor.

Decreased Effect: Although anecdotal reports suggest oral contraceptive efficacy could be reduced by penicillins, this has been refuted by more rigorous scientific and clinical data.

Stability Reconstituted parenteral solution is stable for 3 days at room temperature and 7 days when refrigerated; for I.V. infusion in NS or D_5W, solution is stable for 24 hours at room temperature

Mechanism of Action Inhibits bacterial cell wall synthesis by binding to one or more of the penicillin binding proteins (PBPs); which in turn inhibits the final transpeptidation step of peptidoglycan synthesis in bacterial cell walls, thus inhibiting cell wall

(Continued)

Oxacillin *(Continued)*

biosynthesis. Bacteria eventually lyse due to ongoing activity of cell wall autolytic enzymes (autolysins and murein hydrolases) while cell wall assembly is arrested.

Pharmacodynamics/Kinetics

Distribution: Into bile, synovial and pleural fluids, bronchial secretions, peritoneal, and pericardial fluids; crosses placenta; enters breast milk; penetrates the blood-brain barrier only when meninges are inflamed

Protein binding: ~94%

Metabolism: Hepatic to active metabolites

Half-life elimination: Children 1 week to 2 years: 0.9-1.8 hours; Adults: 23-60 minutes; prolonged in neonates and with renal impairment

Time to peak, serum: I.M.: 30-60 minutes

Excretion: Urine and feces (small amounts as unchanged drug and metabolites)

Dosage I.M., I.V.:

Infants and Children:

Mild-to-moderate infections: 100-150 mg/kg/day in divided doses every 6 hours (maximum: 4 g/day)

Severe infections: 150-200 mg/kg/day in divided doses every 6 hours (maximum: 12 g/day)

Adults:

Mild-to-moderate infections: 250-500 mg every 4-6 hours

Severe infections: 1-2 g every 4-6 hours

Dosing adjustment in renal impairment: Cl_{cr} <10 mL/minute: Use lower range of the usual dosage

Hemodialysis: Not dialyzable (0% to 5%)

Dietary Considerations Sodium content of 1 g: 92.4 mg (4.02 mEq)

Administration Administer around-the-clock to promote less variation in peak and trough serum levels. Administer IVP over 10 minutes. Administer IVPB over 30 minutes.

Monitoring Parameters Observe for signs and symptoms of anaphylaxis during first dose; monitor periodic CBC, urinalysis, BUN, serum creatinine, AST and ALT

Test Interactions May interfere with urinary glucose tests using cupric sulfate (Benedict's solution, Clinitest®); may inactivate aminoglycosides *in vitro*; false-positive urinary and serum proteins

Dosage Forms

Infusion [premixed iso-osmotic dextrose solution]: 1 g (50 mL); 2 g (50 mL)

Injection, powder for reconstitution, as sodium: 1 g, 2 g, 10 g

Selected Readings

Donowitz GR and Mandell GL, "Beta-Lactam Antibiotics," *N Engl J Med*, 1988, 318(7):419-26 and 318(8):490-500.

Wright AJ, "The Penicillins," *Mayo Clin Proc*, 1999, 74(3):290-307.

Oxacillin Sodium *see* Oxacillin *on page 983*

Oxandrin® *see* Oxandrolone *on page 984*

Oxandrolone (oks AN droe lone)

Related Information

AIDS Wasting Treatment *on page 1205*

U.S. Brand Names Oxandrin®

Generic Available No

Use Adjunctive therapy to promote weight gain after weight loss following extensive surgery, chronic infections, or severe trauma, and in some patients who, without definite pathophysiologic reasons, fail to gain or to maintain normal weight; to offset protein catabolism with prolonged corticosteroid administration; relief of bone pain associated with osteoporosis

Restrictions C-III

Pregnancy Risk Factor X

Pregnancy Implications Masculinization of the fetus has been reported.

Contraindications Hypersensitivity to oxandrolone or any component of the formulation; nephrosis; carcinoma of breast or prostate; hypercalcemia; pregnancy

Warnings/Precautions Anabolic steroids may cause peliosis hepatis or liver cell tumors which may not be apparent until liver failure or intra-abdominal hemorrhage develop. Discontinue in case of cholestatic hepatitis with jaundice or abnormal liver function tests. Use caution with concomitant warfarin therapy; warfarin dose may need significantly decreased. May cause blood lipid changes with increased risk of arteriosclerosis. Use with caution in elderly patients, they may be at greater risk for prostatic hyperplasia, fluid retention, and transaminase elevations. Use with caution in patients with cardiac, renal, or hepatic disease, COPD, diabetes or epilepsy.

Discontinue with evidence of mild virilization in women. May stunt bone growth in children.

Adverse Reactions Frequency not defined.

Cardiovascular: Edema

Central nervous system: Depression, excitation, insomnia

Dermatologic: Acne (females and prepubertal males)

Also reported in females: Hirsutism, male-pattern baldness

Endocrine & metabolic: Electrolyte imbalances, glucose intolerance, gonadotropin secretion inhibited, gynecomastia, HDL decreased, LDL increased

Also reported in females: Clitoral enlargement, menstrual irregularities

Genitourinary:

Prepubertal males: Increased or persistent erections, penile enlargement

Postpubertal males: Bladder irritation, epididymitis, impotence, oligospermia, priapism (chronic), testicular atrophy, testicular function inhibited

Hepatic: Alkaline phosphatase increased, ALT/AST increased, bilirubin increased, cholestatic jaundice, hepatic necrosis (rare), hepatocellular neoplasms, peliosis hepatitis (with long-term therapy)

Neuromuscular & skeletal: CPK increased, premature closure of epiphyses (in children)

Renal: Creatinine excretion increased

Miscellaneous: Bromsulfophthalein retention, habituation, voice alteration (deepening, in females)

Drug Interactions

Increased Effect/Toxicity: ACTH, adrenal steroids may increase risk of edema and acne. Oxandrolone enhances the hypoprothrombinemic effects of oral anticoagulants, and enhances the hypoglycemic effects of insulin and sulfonylureas (oral hypoglycemics).

Mechanism of Action Synthetic testosterone derivative with similar androgenic and anabolic actions

Pharmacodynamics/Kinetics Half-life elimination: 10-13 hours

Dosage

Children: Total daily dose: ≤0.1 mg/kg **or** ≤0.045 mg/lb

Adults: 2.5-20 mg in divided doses 2-4 times/day based on individual response; a course of therapy of 2-4 weeks is usually adequate. This may be repeated intermittently as needed.

Elderly: 5 mg twice daily

Dosing adjustment in renal impairment: Caution is recommended because of the propensity of oxandrolone to cause edema and water retention

Dosing adjustment in hepatic impairment: Caution is advised but there are not specific guidelines for dosage reduction

Monitoring Parameters Liver function tests, cholesterol profile, hemoglobin/hematocrit; INR/PT in patients on anticoagulant therapy

Children: Radiographs of left wrist every 6 months (to assess bone maturation)

Adult females: Signs of virilization (deepening voice, hirsutism, acne, clitoromegaly); urine and serum calcium in women with breast cancer

Test Interactions May suppress factors II, V, VII, and X; may increase PT; may decrease thyroxine-binding globulin and radioactive iodine uptake

Patient Information High protein, high caloric diet is suggested, restrict salt intake; glucose tolerance may be altered in diabetics

Dosage Forms Tablet: 2.5 mg, 10 mg

Oxiconazole (oks i KON a zole)

U.S. Brand Names Oxistat®

Canadian Brand Names Oxistat®; Oxizole®

Synonyms Oxiconazole Nitrate

Generic Available No

Use Treatment of tinea pedis (athlete's foot), tinea cruris (jock itch), and tinea corporis (ringworm)

Pregnancy Risk Factor B

Pregnancy Implications Teratogenic effects were not observed in animal studies. There are no adequate or well-controlled studies in pregnant women.

Contraindications Hypersensitivity to oxiconazole or any component of the formulation; not for ophthalmic use

Warnings/Precautions May cause irritation during therapy; if a sensitivity to oxiconazole occurs, therapy should be discontinued; avoid contact with eyes or vagina

Adverse Reactions 1% to 10%:

Dermatologic: Itching, erythema

Local: Transient burning, local irritation, stinging, dryness

Stability Store between 15°C to 30°C (59°F to 86°F). Shake lotion well before use.

(Continued)

Oxiconazole *(Continued)*

Mechanism of Action The cytoplasmic membrane integrity of fungi is destroyed by oxiconazole which exerts a fungicidal activity through inhibition of ergosterol synthesis. Effective for treatment of tinea pedis, tinea cruris, tinea corporis, and tinea versicolor. Active against *Trichophyton rubrum*, *Trichophyton mentagrophytes*, *Trichophyton violaceum*, *Microsporum canis*, *Microsporum audouinii*, *Microsporum gypseum*, *Epidermophyton floccosum*, *Candida albicans*, and *Malassezia furfur*.

Pharmacodynamics/Kinetics

Absorption: In each layer of the dermis; very little systemically after one topical dose

Distribution: To each layer of the dermis; enters breast milk

Excretion: Urine (<0.3%)

Dosage Topical:

Children and Adults:

Tinea corporis/tinea cruris: Cream, lotion: Apply to affected areas 1-2 times daily for 2 weeks

Tinea pedis: Cream, lotion: Apply to affected areas 1-2 times daily for 1 month

Adults: Tinea versicolor: Cream: Apply to affected areas once daily for 2 weeks

Patient Information External use only; discontinue if sensitivity or chemical irritation occurs, contact prescriber if condition fails to improve in 3-4 days

Dosage Forms

Cream: 1% (15 g, 30 g, 60 g) [contains benzoic acid]

Lotion: 1% (30 mL) [contains benzoic acid]

Oxiconazole Nitrate *see* Oxiconazole *on page 985*

Oxistat® *see* Oxiconazole *on page 985*

Oxizole® (Can) *see* Oxiconazole *on page 985*

Oxychlorosene (oks i KLOR oh seen)

U.S. Brand Names Clorpactin® WCS-90 [OTC]

Synonyms Oxychlorosene Sodium

Generic Available No

Use Treatment of localized infections

Contraindications Hypersensitivity to oxychlorosene or any component of the formulation; site of infection not exposed to direct contact with the solution

Stability Refrigerate

Dosage Topical (0.1% to 0.5% solutions): Apply by irrigation, instillation, spray, soaks, or wet compresses

Dosage Forms Powder for solution, as sodium: 2 g

Oxychlorosene Sodium *see* Oxychlorosene *on page 986*

Oxymetholone (oks i METH oh lone)

Related Information

AIDS Wasting Treatment *on page 1205*

U.S. Brand Names Anadrol®

Generic Available No

Use Treatment of anemias caused by deficient red cell production

Restrictions C-III

Pregnancy Risk Factor X

Pregnancy Implications Oligospermia or amenorrhea may occur resulting in an impairment of fertility.

Contraindications Hypersensitivity to oxymetholone or any component of the formulation; breast cancer in men; breast cancer in women with hypercalcemia; prostate cancer; severe liver dysfunction; nephrosis; pregnancy

Warnings/Precautions Anabolic steroids may cause peliosis hepatis, liver cell tumors, and blood lipid changes with increased risk of arteriosclerosis; monitor diabetic patients carefully. Use with caution in elderly men; they may be at greater risk for prostate hyperplasia and cancer. Use caution with cardiac, renal, or hepatic disease; may develop edema. In breast cancer, may cause hypercalcemia by stimulating osteolysis. Use caution in children; may accelerate epiphyseal maturation thereby compromising adult height.

Adverse Reactions Frequency not defined.

Cardiovascular: Coronary artery disease, peripheral edema

Central nervous system: Excitation, insomnia

Dermatologic: Acne (prepubertal males, women); hirsutism (women), hypercalcemia, hyperchloremia, hyperkalemia, hyperphosphatemia, hyperpigmentation; male-pattern baldness (postpubertal males, women)

Endocrine & metabolic: Amenorrhea, cholesterol increased, clitoromegaly, creatinine phosphokinase increased, glucose tolerance decreased, gynecomastia,

HDL-cholesterol decreased, hoarseness (women), hypernatremia, impotence (postpubertal males), LDL-cholesterol decreased, libido increased/decreased, menstrual irregularities, oligospermia, phallic enlargement (prepubertal males), priapism (postpubertal males), testicular atrophy (postpubertal males), testicular dysfunction (postpubertal males); virilism (women, high dose); voice deepening (women)

Gastrointestinal: Diarrhea, nausea, vomiting

Genitourinary: Bladder irritability (postpubertal males), epididymitis (postpubertal males), prostatic hyperplasia (elderly males), seminal volume decreased (postpubertal males)

Hematologic: Iron-deficiency anemia, polycythemia, suppression of clotting factors

Hepatic: Cholestatic hepatitis, hepatic necrosis, hepatocellular carcinoma jaundice, liver cell tumors, peliosis hepatic, transaminases increased

Neuromuscular & skeletal: Premature closure of epiphysis (children)

Drug Interactions

Increased Effect/Toxicity: Androgens may enhance the hepatotoxic effect of cyclosporine; may enhance the anticoagulant effect of warfarin

Stability Store at 15°C to 30°C (59°F to 86°F).

Mechanism of Action Enhances the production and urinary excretion of erythropoietin in patients with anemias due to bone marrow failure; stimulates erythropoiesis in anemias due to deficient red cell production.

Dosage Children and Adults: Erythropoietic effects: Oral: 1-5 mg/kg/day in one daily dose; usual effective dose: 1-2 mg/kg/day; give for a minimum trial of 3-6 months because response may be delayed

Dosing adjustment in hepatic impairment:

Mild to moderate hepatic impairment: Oxymetholone should be used with caution in patients with liver dysfunction because of its hepatotoxic potential

Severe hepatic impairment: Oxymetholone should **not** be used

Monitoring Parameters Liver function, blood sugars, lipid profile, iron studies, hemoglobin/hematocrit, x-ray of bones every 6 months (prepubertal patients); signs of virilization (females)

Test Interactions Decreased thyroxine-binding globulin, T_4; increased resin uptake of T_3 and T_4

Dosage Forms Tablet: 50 mg

Oxytetracycline (oks i tet ra SYE kleen)

U.S. Brand Names Terramycin® I.M.

Canadian Brand Names Terramycin®

Synonyms Oxytetracycline Hydrochloride

Generic Available No

Use Treatment of susceptible bacterial infections; both gram-positive and gram-negative, as well as, *Rickettsia* and *Mycoplasma* organisms

Pregnancy Risk Factor D

Contraindications Hypersensitivity to tetracycline or any component of the formulation

Warnings/Precautions Avoid in children ≤8 years of age, pregnant and nursing women; photosensitivity can occur with oxytetracycline

Adverse Reactions Frequency not defined; also refer to Tetracycline monograph

Cardiovascular: Pericarditis

Central nervous system: Bulging fontanels (infants), intracranial hypertension (adults)

Dermatologic: Angioneurotic edema, erythematous rash, exfoliative dermatitis (uncommon), maculopapular rash, photosensitivity, urticaria

Gastrointestinal: Anogenital inflammatory lesions, diarrhea, dysphagia, enamel hyperplasia, enterocolitis, glossitis, nausea, tooth discoloration, vomiting

Hematologic: Anemia, eosinophilia, neutropenia, thrombocytopenia

Local: Irritation

Renal: BUN increased

Miscellaneous: Anaphylactoid purpura, anaphylaxis, hypersensitivity reaction, SLE exacerbation

Overdosage/Toxicology Symptoms include nausea, anorexia, and diarrhea. Treatment following GI decontamination is supportive care only.

Drug Interactions

Increased Effect/Toxicity: Oral anticoagulant (warfarin) effects may be increased.

Decreased Effect: Barbiturates, phenytoin, and carbamazepine decrease serum levels of tetracyclines. Although anecdotal reports suggest oral contraceptive efficacy could be reduced by tetracyclines, this has been refuted by more rigorous scientific and clinical data.

(Continued)

Oxytetracycline *(Continued)*

Mechanism of Action Inhibits bacterial protein synthesis by binding with the 30S and possibly the 50S ribosomal subunit(s) of susceptible bacteria, cell wall synthesis is not affected

Pharmacodynamics/Kinetics

Absorption: Poor

Distribution: Crosses placenta

Metabolism: Hepatic (small amounts)

Half-life elimination: 8.5-9.6 hours; prolonged with renal impairment

Excretion: Urine; feces

Dosage I.M.:

Children >8 years: 15-25 mg/kg/day (maximum: 250 mg/dose) in divided doses every 8-12 hours

Adults: 250 mg every 24 hours or 300 mg/day divided every 8-12 hours

Dosing interval in renal impairment: Cl_{cr} <10 mL/minute: Administer every 24 hours or avoid use if possible

Dosing adjustment/comments in hepatic impairment: Avoid use in patients with severe liver disease

Administration Injection for intramuscular use only.

Patient Information Avoid unnecessary exposure to sunlight.

Dosage Forms Injection, solution: 5% [50 mg/mL] (10 mL) [contains lidocaine hydrochloride 2%]

Oxytetracycline and Polymyxin B

(oks i tet ra SYE kleen & pol i MIKS in bee)

Related Information

Oxytetracycline *on page 987*

Polymyxin B *on page 1012*

U.S. Brand Names Terak™

Synonyms Polymyxin B and Oxytetracycline

Generic Available No

Use Treatment of superficial ocular infections involving the conjunctiva and/or cornea

Pregnancy Risk Factor D

Drug Interactions

Increased Effect/Toxicity: See individual agents.

Decreased Effect: See individual agents.

Pharmacodynamics/Kinetics See individual agents.

Dosage Topical: Apply ½" of ointment onto the lower lid of affected eye 2-4 times/day

Dosage Forms Ointment, ophthalmic: Oxytetracycline 5 mg and polymyxin B sulfate 10,000 units per g (3.5 g)

Oxytetracycline Hydrochloride *see* Oxytetracycline *on page 987*

Pacis™ (Can) *see* BCG Vaccine *on page 683*

Palivizumab (pah li VIZ u mab)

U.S. Brand Names Synagis®

Canadian Brand Names Synagis®

Generic Available No

Use Prevention of serious lower respiratory tract disease caused by respiratory syncytial virus (RSV) in infants and children <2 years of age at high risk of RSV disease

Pregnancy Risk Factor C

Pregnancy Implications Not for adult use; reproduction studies have not been conducted

Contraindications History of severe prior reaction to palivizumab or any component of the formulation

Warnings/Precautions Very rare cases of anaphylaxis have been observed following palivizumab. Rare cases of severe acute hypersensitivity reactions have also been reported. Safety and efficacy of palivizumab have not been demonstrated in the treatment of established RSV disease. Use with caution in patients with thrombocytopenia or any coagulation disorder.

Adverse Reactions The incidence of adverse events was similar between the palivizumab and placebo groups.

>1%:

Central nervous system: Nervousness, fever

Dermatologic: Fungal dermatitis, eczema, seborrhea, rash

Gastrointestinal: Diarrhea, vomiting, gastroenteritis

Hematologic: Anemia

Hepatic: ALT increase, abnormal LFTs

Local: Injection site reaction, erythema, induration
Ocular: Conjunctivitis
Otic: Otitis media
Respiratory: Cough, wheezing, bronchiolitis, pneumonia, bronchitis, asthma, croup, dyspnea, sinusitis, apnea, upper respiratory infection, rhinitis
Miscellaneous: Oral moniliasis, failure to thrive, viral infection, flu syndrome

Postmarketing and/or case reports: Hypersensitivity reactions, anaphylaxis (very rare)

Overdosage/Toxicology No data from clinical studies are available.

Stability Store in refrigerator at a temperature between 2°C to 8°C (35.6°F to 46.4°F) in original container; do not freeze

Powder for injection: Use aseptic technique when reconstituting; add 1 mL of sterile water for injection to a 100 mg vial; swirl vial gently for 30 seconds to avoid foaming. Do not shake vial. Allow to stand at room temperature for 20 minutes until the solution clarifies; solution should be administered within 6 hours of reconstitution.

Mechanism of Action Exhibits neutralizing and fusion-inhibitory activity against RSV; these activities inhibit RSV replication in laboratory and clinical studies

Pharmacodynamics/Kinetics

Half-life elimination: Children <24 months: 20 days; Adults: 18 days
Time to peak, serum: 48 hours

Dosage I.M.: Infants and Children: 15 mg/kg of body weight, monthly throughout RSV season (First dose administered prior to commencement of RSV season)

Administration Injection should (preferably) be in the anterolateral aspect of the thigh; gluteal muscle should not be used routinely; injection volume over 1 mL should be administered as divided doses

Additional Information RSV prophylaxis should be initiated at the onset of the RSV season. In most areas of the United States, onset of RSV outbreaks is October to December, and termination is March to May, but regional differences occur.

Dosage Forms

Injection, powder for reconstitution: 50 mg, 100 mg
Injection, solution [preservative free]: 50 mg/0.5 mL (0.5 mL); 100 mg/mL (1 mL)

Selected Readings

Johnson S, Oliver C, Prince GA, et al, "Development of a Humanized Monoclonal Antibody (MEDI-493) With Potent *In Vitro* and *In Vivo* Activity Against Respiratory Syncytial Virus," *J Infect Dis*, 1997, 176(5):1215-24.

"Prevention of Respiratory Syncytial Virus Infections: Indications for the Use of Palivizumab and Update on the Use of RSV-IGIV. American Academy of Pediatrics Committee on Infectious Diseases and Committee of Fetus and Newborn," *Pediatrics*, 1998, 102(5):1211-6.

Simoes EA, Sondheimer HM, Top FH Jr, et al, "Respiratory Syncytial Virus Immune Globulin for Prophylaxis Against Respiratory Syncytial Virus Disease in Infants and Children With Congential Heart Disease. The Cardiac Study Group," *J Pediatr*, 1998, 133(4):492-9.

Subramanian KN, Weisman, LE, Rhodes T, et al, "Safety, Tolerance and Pharmacokinetics of a Humanized Monoclonal Antibody to Respiratory Syncytial Virus in Premature Infants With Bronchopulmonary Dysplasia. MEDI-493 Study Group," *Pediatr Infect Dis J*, 1998, 17(2):110-5.

Wandstrat TL, "Respiratory Syncytial Virus Immune Globulin Intravenous," *Ann Pharmacother*, 1997, 31(1):83-8.

Welliver RC, "Respiratory Syncytial Virus Immunoglobulin and Monoclonal Antibodies in the Prevention and Treatment of Respiratory Syncytial Virus Infection," *Semin Perinatol*, 1998, 22(1):87-95.

Pamix™ [OTC] *see* Pyrantel Pamoate *on page 1021*
Panglobulin® NF *see* Immune Globulin (Intravenous) *on page 867*
Panixine DisperDose™ *see* Cephalexin *on page 727*
Para-Aminosalicylate Sodium *see* Aminosalicylic Acid *on page 641*

Paromomycin (par oh moe MYE sin)

U.S. Brand Names Humatin®

Canadian Brand Names Humatin®

Synonyms Paromomycin Sulfate

Generic Available Yes

Use Treatment of acute and chronic intestinal amebiasis; hepatic coma

Unlabeled/Investigational Use Treatment of cryptosporidiosis

Drug of Choice or Alternative for

Disease/Syndrome(s):

Liver Abscess *on page 211*

Organism(s):

Entamoeba histolytica on page 130
Giardia lamblia on page 155

Pregnancy Risk Factor C

Contraindications Hypersensitivity to paromomycin or any component of the formulation; intestinal obstruction, renal failure

(Continued)

Paromomycin *(Continued)*

Warnings/Precautions Use with caution in patients with impaired renal function or possible or proven ulcerative bowel lesions

Adverse Reactions

1% to 10%: Gastrointestinal: Diarrhea, abdominal cramps, nausea, vomiting, heartburn

<1%: Headache, vertigo, exanthema, rash, pruritus, steatorrhea, secondary enterocolitis, eosinophilia, ototoxicity

Overdosage/Toxicology Symptoms include nausea, vomiting, and diarrhea. Treatment following GI decontamination, if possible, is supportive and symptomatic.

Ethanol/Nutrition/Herb Interactions Food: Paromomycin may cause malabsorption of xylose, sucrose, and fats.

Mechanism of Action Acts directly on ameba; has antibacterial activity against normal and pathogenic organisms in the GI tract; interferes with bacterial protein synthesis by binding to 30S ribosomal subunits

Pharmacodynamics/Kinetics

Absorption: None

Excretion: Feces (100% as unchanged drug)

Dosage Oral:

Intestinal amebiasis: Children and Adults: 25-35 mg/kg/day in 3 divided doses for 5-10 days

Dientamoeba fragilis: Children and Adults: 25-30 mg/kg/day in 3 divided doses for 7 days

Cryptosporidium (unlabeled use): Adults with AIDS: 1.5-2.25 g/day in 3-6 divided doses for 10-14 days (occasionally courses of up to 4-8 weeks may be needed)

Tapeworm (fish, dog, bovine, porcine):

- Children: 11 mg/kg every 15 minutes for 4 doses
- Adults: 1 g every 15 minutes for 4 doses

Hepatic coma: Adults: 4 g/day in 2-4 divided doses for 5-6 days

Dwarf tapeworm: Children and Adults: 45 mg/kg/dose every day for 5-7 days

Patient Information Take full course of therapy; do not skip doses; report ringing in ears, hearing loss, or dizziness

Dosage Forms Capsule: 250 mg

Selected Readings

Danziger LH, Kanyok TP, and Novak RM, "Treatment of Cryptosporidial Diarrhea in an AIDS Patient With Paromomycin," *Ann Pharmacother*, 1993, 27(12):1460-2.

"Drugs for Parasitic Infections," *Med Lett Drugs Ther*, 1998, 40(1017):1-12.

Paromomycin Sulfate *see* Paromomycin *on page 989*

PAS *see* Aminosalicylic Acid *on page 641*

Paser® *see* Aminosalicylic Acid *on page 641*

Pathocil® (Can) *see* Dicloxacillin *on page 773*

PCE® *see* Erythromycin *on page 807*

PCEC *see* Rabies Virus Vaccine *on page 1034*

PCV7 *see* Pneumococcal Conjugate Vaccine (7-Valent) *on page 1008*

Pediarix™ *see* Diphtheria, Tetanus Toxoids, Acellular Pertussis, Hepatitis B (Recombinant), and Poliovirus (Inactivated) Vaccine *on page 780*

Pediazole® *see* Erythromycin and Sulfisoxazole *on page 811*

Pedi-Dri® *see* Nystatin *on page 976*

PediOtic® *see* Neomycin, Polymyxin B, and Hydrocortisone *on page 966*

PedvaxHIB® *see Haemophilus* b Conjugate Vaccine *on page 848*

Penciclovir (pen SYE kloe veer)

U.S. Brand Names Denavir®

Generic Available No

Use Topical treatment of herpes simplex labialis (cold sores)

Pregnancy Risk Factor B

Contraindications Hypersensitivity to the penciclovir or any component of the formulation; previous and significant adverse reactions to famciclovir

Warnings/Precautions Penciclovir should only be used on herpes labialis on the lips and face; because no data are available, application to mucous membranes is not recommended. Avoid application in or near eyes since it may cause irritation. The effect of penciclovir has not been established in immunocompromised patients.

Adverse Reactions

>10%: Dermatologic: Mild erythema (50%)

1% to 10%: Central nervous system: Headache (5.3%)

<1%: Local anesthesia (0.9%)

Postmarketing and/or case reports: Application site reaction, local edema, urticaria, pain, pruritus, paresthesia, skin discoloration, erythematous rash, oropharyngeal edema, parosmia

Stability Store at controlled room temperature of 20°C to 25°C (68°F to 77°F).

Mechanism of Action In cells infected with HSV-1 or HSV-2, viral thymidine kinase phosphorylates penciclovir to a monophosphate form which, in turn, is converted to penciclovir triphosphate by cellular kinases. Penciclovir triphosphate inhibits HSV polymerase competitively with deoxyguanosine triphosphate. Consequently, herpes viral DNA synthesis and, therefore, replication are selectively inhibited

Pharmacodynamics/Kinetics Absorption: Topical: None

Dosage Children ≥12 years and Adults: Topical: Apply cream at the first sign or symptom of cold sore (eg, tingling, swelling); apply every 2 hours during waking hours for 4 days

Monitoring Parameters Reduction in virus shedding, negative cultures for herpes virus; resolution of pain and healing of cold sore lesion

Patient Information Report if you experience significant burning, itching, stinging, or redness when using this medication

Additional Information Penciclovir is the active metabolite of the prodrug famciclovir. Penciclovir is an alternative to topical acyclovir for HSV-1 and HSV-2 infections. Neither drug will prevent recurring HSV attacks.

Dosage Forms Cream: 1% (1.5 g)

Selected Readings

Alrabiah FA and Sacks SL, "New Antiherpesvirus Agents. Their Targets and Therapeutic Potential," *Drugs*, 1996, 52(1):17-32.

Penicillin G Benzathine (pen i SIL in jee BENZ a theen)

U.S. Brand Names Bicillin® L-A

Synonyms Benzathine Benzylpenicillin; Benzathine Penicillin G; Benzylpenicillin Benzathine

Generic Available No

Use Active against some gram-positive organisms, few gram-negative organisms such as *Neisseria gonorrhoeae*, and some anaerobes and spirochetes; used in the treatment of syphilis; used only for the treatment of mild to moderately severe infections caused by organisms susceptible to low concentrations of penicillin G or for prophylaxis of infections caused by these organisms

Drug of Choice or Alternative for

Disease/Syndrome(s):

Pharyngitis *on page 264*

Organism(s):

Treponema pallidum on page 334

Pregnancy Risk Factor B

Contraindications Hypersensitivity to penicillin or any component of the formulation

Warnings/Precautions Use with caution in patients with impaired renal function, seizure disorder, or history of hypersensitivity to other beta-lactams; CDC and AAP do not currently recommend the use of penicillin G benzathine to treat congenital syphilis or neurosyphilis due to reported treatment failures and lack of published clinical data on its efficacy

Adverse Reactions Frequency not defined.

Central nervous system: Convulsions, confusion, drowsiness, myoclonus, fever

Dermatologic: Rash

Endocrine & metabolic: Electrolyte imbalance

Hematologic: Positive Coombs' reaction, hemolytic anemia

Local: Pain, thrombophlebitis

Renal: Acute interstitial nephritis

Miscellaneous: Anaphylaxis, hypersensitivity reactions, Jarisch-Herxheimer reaction

Overdosage/Toxicology Symptoms of penicillin overdose include neuromuscular hypersensitivity (agitation, hallucinations, asterixis, encephalopathy, confusion, seizures) and electrolyte imbalance with potassium or sodium salts, especially in renal failure. Hemodialysis may be helpful to aid in removal of the drug from the blood, otherwise, most treatment is supportive or symptom-directed.

Drug Interactions

Increased Effect/Toxicity: Probenecid increases penicillin levels. Aminoglycosides may lead to synergistic efficacy. Penicillins may increase the exposure to methotrexate during concurrent therapy; monitor.

Decreased Effect: Tetracyclines may decrease penicillin effectiveness. Although anecdotal reports suggest oral contraceptive efficacy could be reduced by penicillins, this has been refuted by more rigorous scientific and clinical data.

Stability Store in refrigerator

(Continued)

Penicillin G Benzathine *(Continued)*

Mechanism of Action Interferes with bacterial cell wall synthesis during active multiplication, causing cell wall death and resultant bactericidal activity against susceptible bacteria

Pharmacodynamics/Kinetics

Duration: 1-4 weeks (dose dependent); larger doses result in more sustained levels

Absorption: I.M.: Slow

Time to peak, serum: 12-24 hours

Dosage I.M.: Administer undiluted injection; higher doses result in more sustained rather than higher levels. Use a penicillin G benzathine-penicillin G procaine combination to achieve early peak levels in acute infections.

Infants and Children:

- Group A streptococcal upper respiratory infection: 25,000-50,000 units/kg as a single dose; maximum: 1.2 million units
- Prophylaxis of recurrent rheumatic fever: 25,000-50,000 units/kg every 3-4 weeks; maximum: 1.2 million units/dose
- Early syphilis: 50,000 units/kg as a single injection; maximum: 2.4 million units
- Syphilis of more than 1-year duration: 50,000 units/kg every week for 3 doses; maximum: 2.4 million units/dose

Adults:

- Group A streptococcal upper respiratory infection: 1.2 million units as a single dose
- Prophylaxis of recurrent rheumatic fever: 1.2 million units every 3-4 weeks or 600,000 units twice monthly
- Early syphilis: 2.4 million units as a single dose in 2 injection sites
- Syphilis of more than 1-year duration: 2.4 million units in 2 injection sites once weekly for 3 doses
- Not indicated as single drug therapy for neurosyphilis, but may be given 1 time/week for 3 weeks following I.V. treatment; refer to Penicillin G Parenteral/Aqueous monograph for dosing

Administration Administer by deep I.M. injection in the upper outer quadrant of the buttock do **not** administer I.V., intra-arterially, or SubQ; in children <2 years of age, I.M. injections should be made into the midlateral muscle of the thigh, not the gluteal region; when doses are repeated, rotate the injection site

Monitoring Parameters Observe for signs and symptoms of anaphylaxis during first dose

Test Interactions Positive Coombs' [direct], false-positive urinary and/or serum proteins; false-positive or negative urinary glucose using Clinitest®

Patient Information Report any rash

Dosage Forms Injection, suspension [prefilled syringe] (Bicillin® L-A): 600,000 units/mL (1 mL, 2 mL, 4 mL)

Selected Readings

Pao D, Goh BT, and Bingham JS, "Management Issues in Syphilis," *Drugs*, 2002, 62(10):1447-61.

US Department of Health and Human Services, "1993 Sexually Transmitted Diseases Treatment Guidelines," *MMWR*, 1993, 42(RR-14).

Wright AJ, "The Penicillins," *Mayo Clin Proc*, 1999, 74(3):290-307.

Penicillin G Benzathine and Penicillin G Procaine

(pen i SIL in jee BENZ a theen & pen i SIL in jee PROE kane)

Related Information

Penicillin G Benzathine *on page 991*

Penicillin G Procaine *on page 995*

U.S. Brand Names Bicillin® C-R; Bicillin® C-R 900/300

Synonyms Penicillin G Procaine and Benzathine Combined

Generic Available No

Use May be used in specific situations in the treatment of streptococcal infections

Drug of Choice or Alternative for Disease/Syndrome(s):

Pharyngitis *on page 264*

Pregnancy Risk Factor B

Contraindications Hypersensitivity to penicillin or any component of the formulation

Warnings/Precautions Use with caution in patients with impaired renal function, impaired cardiac function or seizure disorder

Adverse Reactions Frequency not defined.

Central nervous system: CNS toxicity (convulsions, confusion, drowsiness, myoclonus)

Hematologic: Positive Coombs' reaction, hemolytic anemia

Renal: Interstitial nephritis

Miscellaneous: Hypersensitivity reactions, Jarisch-Herxheimer reaction

Overdosage/Toxicology Many beta-lactam-containing antibiotics have the potential to cause neuromuscular hyperirritability or convulsive seizures. Hemodialysis may be helpful to aid in removal of the drug from the blood, otherwise, most treatment is supportive or symptom-directed.

Drug Interactions

Increased Effect/Toxicity: Probenecid increases penicillin levels. Aminoglycosides may lead to synergistic efficacy. Warfarin effects may be increased. Penicillins may increase the exposure to methotrexate during concurrent therapy; monitor.

Decreased Effect: Tetracyclines may decrease penicillin effectiveness. Although anecdotal reports suggest oral contraceptive efficacy could be reduced by penicillins, this has been refuted by more rigorous scientific and clinical data.

Stability Store in refrigerator.

Mechanism of Action Inhibits bacterial cell wall synthesis by binding to one or more of the penicillin binding proteins (PBPs); which in turn inhibits the final transpeptidation step of peptidoglycan synthesis in bacterial cell walls, thus inhibiting cell wall biosynthesis. Bacteria eventually lyse due to ongoing activity of cell wall autolytic enzymes (autolysins and murein hydrolases) while cell wall assembly is arrested.

Dosage I.M.:

Children:

- <30 lb: 600,000 units in a single dose
- 30-60 lb: 900,000 units to 1.2 million units in a single dose

Children >60 lb and Adults: 2.4 million units in a single dose

Administration Administer by deep I.M. injection in the upper outer quadrant of the buttock; administered around-the-clock rather than 4 times/day, 3 times/day, etc (ie, 12-6-12-6, not 9-1-5-9) to promote less variation in peak and trough serum levels; do **not** administer I.V., intravascularly, or intra-arterially. In infants and children, I.M. injections should be made into the midlateral muscle of the thigh.

Monitoring Parameters Observe for signs and symptoms of anaphylaxis during first dose

Test Interactions May interfere with urinary glucose tests using cupric sulfate (Benedict's solution, Clinitest®); may inactivate aminoglycosides *in vitro*; positive Coombs' [direct], increased protein

Dosage Forms Injection, suspension [prefilled syringe]:

Bicillin® C-R:

- 600,000 units: Penicillin G benzathine 300,000 units and penicillin G procaine 300,000 units per 1 mL (1 mL)
- 1,200,000 units: Penicillin G benzathine 600,000 units and penicillin G procaine 600,000 units per 2 mL (2 mL)
- 2,400,000 units: Penicillin G benzathine 1,200,000 units and penicillin G procaine 1,200,000 units per 4 mL (4 mL)

Bicillin® C-R 900/300: 1,200,000 units: Penicillin G benzathine 900,000 units and penicillin G procaine 300,000 units per 2 mL (2 mL)

Penicillin G (Parenteral/Aqueous)

(pen i SIL in jee, pa REN ter al, AYE kwee us)

Related Information

Antimicrobial Activity Against Selected Organisms *on page 1165*

U.S. Brand Names Pfizerpen®

Canadian Brand Names Pfizerpen®

Synonyms Benzylpenicillin Potassium; Benzylpenicillin Sodium; Crystalline Penicillin; Penicillin G Potassium; Penicillin G Sodium

Generic Available Yes

Use Active against some gram-positive organisms, generally not *Staphylococcus aureus*; some gram-negative organisms such as *Neisseria gonorrhoeae*, and some anaerobes and spirochetes

Drug of Choice or Alternative for

Disease/Syndrome(s):

- Brain Abscess *on page 58*
- Keratitis, Bacterial and Fungal *on page 199*
- Lung Abscess *on page 212*
- Myositis *on page 242*
- Necrotizing Fasciitis *on page 243*

Organism(s):

- *Actinomyces* Species *on page 27*
- *Borrelia burgdorferi on page 56*
- *Clostridium perfringens on page 88*
- *Clostridium tetani on page 90*
- *Corynebacterium jeikeium on page 98*
- *Corynebacterium* Species, Other Than *C. jeikeium on page 99*

(Continued)

Penicillin G (Parenteral/Aqueous) *(Continued)*

Enterococcus Species *on page 134*
Erysipelothrix rhusiopathiae on page 141
Leptospira interrogans on page 205
Listeria monocytogenes on page 208
Neisseria meningitidis on page 245
Pasteurella multocida on page 258
Streptococcus agalactiae on page 313
Streptococcus bovis on page 315
Streptococcus pneumoniae, Drug-Susceptible *on page 319*
Streptococcus pyogenes on page 321
Streptococcus-Related Gram-Positive Cocci *on page 325*
Streptococcus, Viridans Group *on page 326*
Treponema pallidum on page 334

Pregnancy Risk Factor B

Contraindications Hypersensitivity to penicillin or any component of the formulation

Warnings/Precautions Avoid intra-arterial administration or injection into or near major peripheral nerves or blood vessels since such injections may cause severe and/or permanent neurovascular damage; use with caution in patients with renal impairment (dosage reduction required), pre-existing seizure disorders, or with a history of hypersensitivity to cephalosporins

Adverse Reactions Frequency not defined.

Central nervous system: Convulsions, confusion, drowsiness, myoclonus, fever
Dermatologic: Rash
Endocrine & metabolic: Electrolyte imbalance
Hematologic: Positive Coombs' reaction, hemolytic anemia
Local: Injection site reaction, thrombophlebitis
Renal: Acute interstitial nephritis
Miscellaneous: Anaphylaxis, hypersensitivity reactions, Jarisch-Herxheimer reaction

Overdosage/Toxicology Symptoms of penicillin overdose include neuromuscular hypersensitivity (agitation, hallucinations, asterixis, encephalopathy, confusion, seizures) and electrolyte imbalance with potassium or sodium salts, especially in renal failure. Hemodialysis may be helpful to aid in removal of the drug from the blood, otherwise, most treatment is supportive or symptom-directed.

Drug Interactions

Increased Effect/Toxicity: Probenecid increases penicillin levels. Aminoglycosides may lead to synergistic efficacy. Penicillins may increase the exposure to methotrexate during concurrent therapy; monitor.

Decreased Effect: Tetracyclines may decrease penicillin effectiveness. Although anecdotal reports suggest oral contraceptive efficacy could be reduced by penicillins, this has been refuted by more rigorous scientific and clinical data.

Stability

Penicillin G potassium is stable at room temperature
Reconstituted parenteral solution is stable for 7 days when refrigerated (2°C to 15°C)
Penicillin G potassium for I.V. infusion in NS or D_5W, solution is stable for 24 hours at room temperature

Incompatible with aminoglycosides; inactivated in acidic or alkaline solutions

Mechanism of Action Interferes with bacterial cell wall synthesis during active multiplication, causing cell wall death and resultant bactericidal activity against susceptible bacteria

Pharmacodynamics/Kinetics

Distribution: Poor penetration across blood-brain barrier, despite inflamed meninges; crosses placenta; enters breast milk
Relative diffusion from blood into CSF: Good only with inflammation (exceeds usual MICs)
CSF:blood level ratio: Normal meninges: <1%; Inflamed meninges: 3% to 5%
Protein binding: 65%
Metabolism: Hepatic (30%) to penicilloic acid
Half-life elimination:
Neonates: <6 days old: 3.2-3.4 hours; 7-13 days old: 1.2-2.2 hours; >14 days old: 0.9-1.9 hours
Children and Adults: Normal renal function: 20-50 minutes
End-stage renal disease: 3.3-5.1 hours
Time to peak, serum: I.M.: ~30 minutes; I.V. ~1 hour
Excretion: Urine

Dosage I.M., I.V.:

Infants:
<7 days, <2000 g: 50,000 units/kg/day in divided doses every 12 hours
<7 days, >2000 g: 50,000 units/kg/day in divided doses every 8 hours

>7 days, <2000 g: 75,000 units/kg/day in divided doses every 8 hours
>7 days, >2000 g: 100,000 units/kg/day in divided doses every 6 hours

Infants and Children (sodium salt is preferred in children): 100,000-250,000 units/kg/day in divided doses every 4 hours

Severe infections: Up to 400,000 units/kg/day in divided doses every 4 hours; maximum dose: 24 million units/day

Congenital syphilis:

Newborns: 50,000 units/kg/day I.V. every 8-12 hours for 10-14 days

Infants: 50,000 units/kg every 4-6 hours for 10-14 days

Disseminated gonococcal infections or gonococcus ophthalmia (if organism proven sensitive): 100,000 units/kg/day in 2 equal doses (4 equal doses/day for infants >1 week)

Gonococcal meningitis: 150,000 units/kg in 2 equal doses (4 doses/day for infants >1 week)

Adults: 2-24 million units/day in divided doses every 4 hours depending on sensitivity of the organism and severity of the infection

Neurosyphilis: 18-24 million units/day in divided doses every 3-4 hours for 10-14 days

Dosing interval in renal impairment:

Cl_{cr} 30-50 mL/minute: Administer every 6 hours

Cl_{cr} 10-30 mL/minute: Administer every 8 hours

Cl_{cr} <10 mL/minute: Administer every 12 hours

Hemodialysis: Moderately dialyzable (20% to 50%)

Continuous arteriovenous or venovenous hemodiafiltration effects: Dose as for Cl_{cr} 10-50 mL/minute

Dietary Considerations

Injection powder for reconstitution as potassium contains sodium 6.8 mg (0.3 mEq) and potassium 65.6 mg (1.68 mEq) per 1 million units

Administration Administer I.M. by deep injection in the upper outer quadrant of the buttock

Monitoring Parameters Observe for signs and symptoms of anaphylaxis during first dose

Test Interactions False-positive or negative urinary glucose determination using Clinitest®; positive Coombs' [direct]; false-positive urinary and/or serum proteins

Patient Information Report any rash or shortness of breath

Additional Information 1 million units is approximately equal to 625 mg.

Penicillin G potassium injection:

Potassium content per million units: 65.6 mg (1.7 mEq)

Sodium content per million units: 23.5 mg (1.02 mEq)

Dosage Forms

Infusion, as potassium [premixed iso-osmotic dextrose solution, frozen]: 1 million units (50 mL), 2 million units (50 mL), 3 million units (50 mL)

Injection, powder for reconstitution, as potassium (Pfizerpen®): 5 million units, 20 million units [contains sodium 6.8 mg (0.3 mEq) and potassium 65.6 mg (1.68 mEq) per 1 million units]

Injection, powder for reconstitution, as sodium: 5 million units

Selected Readings

Donowitz GR and Mandell GL, "Beta-Lactam Antibiotics," *N Engl J Med*, 1988, 318(7):419-26 and 318(8):490-500.

Wright AJ, "The Penicillins," *Mayo Clin Proc*, 1999, 74(3):290-307.

Penicillin G Potassium *see* Penicillin G (Parenteral/Aqueous) *on page 993*

Penicillin G Procaine (pen i SIL in jee PROE kane)

Related Information

Antimicrobial Activity Against Selected Organisms *on page 1165*

Canadian Brand Names Pfizerpen-AS®; Wycillin®

Synonyms APPG; Aqueous Procaine Penicillin G; Procaine Benzylpenicillin; Procaine Penicillin G; Wycillin [DSC]

Generic Available Yes

Use Moderately severe infections due to *Treponema pallidum* and other penicillin G-sensitive microorganisms that are susceptible to low, but prolonged serum penicillin concentrations; anthrax due to *Bacillus anthracis* (postexposure) to reduce the incidence or progression of disease following exposure to aerolized *Bacillus anthracis*

Drug of Choice or Alternative for Organism(s):

Corynebacterium diphtheriae on page 96

Treponema pallidum on page 334

Pregnancy Risk Factor B

(Continued)

Penicillin G Procaine *(Continued)*

Contraindications Hypersensitivity to penicillin, procaine, or any component of the formulation

Warnings/Precautions May need to modify dosage in patients with severe renal impairment, seizure disorders, or history of hypersensitivity to cephalosporins; avoid I.V., intravascular, or intra-arterial administration of penicillin G procaine since severe and/or permanent neurovascular damage may occur; use of penicillin for longer than 2 weeks may be associated with an increased risk for some adverse reactions (neutropenia, serum sickness)

Adverse Reactions Frequency not defined.

Cardiovascular: Myocardial depression, vasodilation, conduction disturbances

Central nervous system: Confusion, drowsiness, myoclonus, CNS stimulation, seizure

Hematologic: Positive Coombs' reaction, hemolytic anemia, neutropenia

Local: Pain at injection site, thrombophlebitis, sterile abscess at injection site

Renal: Interstitial nephritis

Miscellaneous: Pseudoanaphylactic reactions, hypersensitivity reactions, Jarisch-Herxheimer reaction, serum sickness

Overdosage/Toxicology Symptoms of penicillin overdose include neuromuscular hypersensitivity (agitation, hallucinations, asterixis, encephalopathy, confusion, seizures) and electrolyte imbalance with potassium or sodium salts, especially in renal failure. Hemodialysis may be helpful to aid in removal of the drug from the blood, otherwise, most treatment is supportive or symptom-directed.

Drug Interactions

Increased Effect/Toxicity: Probenecid increases penicillin levels. Aminoglycosides may lead to synergistic efficacy. Penicillins may increase the exposure to methotrexate during concurrent therapy; monitor.

Decreased Effect: Tetracyclines may decrease penicillin effectiveness. Although anecdotal reports suggest oral contraceptive efficacy could be reduced by penicillins, this has been refuted by more rigorous scientific and clinical data.

Stability Store in refrigerator

Mechanism of Action Inhibits bacterial cell wall synthesis by binding to one or more of the penicillin binding proteins (PBPs); which in turn inhibits the final transpeptidation step of peptidoglycan synthesis in bacterial cell walls, thus inhibiting cell wall biosynthesis. Bacteria eventually lyse due to ongoing activity of cell wall autolytic enzymes (autolysins and murein hydrolases) while cell wall assembly is arrested.

Pharmacodynamics/Kinetics

Duration: Therapeutic: 15-24 hours

Absorption: I.M.: Slow

Distribution: Penetration across the blood-brain barrier is poor, despite inflamed meninges; enters breast milk

Protein binding: 65%

Metabolism: ~30% hepatically inactivated

Time to peak, serum: 1-4 hours

Excretion: Urine (60% to 90% as unchanged drug)

Clearance: Renal: Delayed in neonates, young infants, and with impaired renal function

Dosage I.M.:

Children: 25,000-50,000 units/kg/day in divided doses 1-2 times/day; not to exceed 4.8 million units/24 hours

Anthrax, inhalational (postexposure prophylaxis): 25,000 units/kg every 12 hours (maximum: 1,200,000 units every 12 hours); see "Note" in Adults dosing

Congenital syphilis: 50,000 units/kg/day for 10-14 days

Adults: 0.6-4.8 million units/day in divided doses every 12-24 hours

Anthrax:

Inhalational (postexposure prophylaxis): 1,200,000 units every 12 hours

Note: Overall treatment duration should be 60 days. Available safety data suggest continued administration of penicillin G procaine for longer than 2 weeks may incur additional risk for adverse reactions. Clinicians may consider switching to effective alternative treatment for completion of therapy beyond 2 weeks.

Cutaneous (treatment): 600,000-1,200,000 units/day; alternative therapy is recommended in severe cutaneous or other forms of anthrax infection

Endocarditis caused by susceptible viridans *Streptococcus* (when used in conjunction with an aminoglycoside): 1.2 million units every 6 hours for 2-4 weeks

Neurosyphilis: I.M.: 2-4 million units/day with 500 mg probenecid by mouth 4 times/day for 10-14 days; **penicillin G aqueous I.V. is the preferred agent**

Hemodialysis: Moderately dialyzable (20% to 50%)

Administration Procaine suspension for deep I.M. injection only; do not inject in gluteal muscle in children <2 years of age; rotate the injection site; avoid I.V., intravascular, or intra-arterial administration of penicillin G procaine since severe and/or permanent neurovascular damage may occur

Monitoring Parameters Periodic renal and hematologic function tests with prolonged therapy; fever, mental status, WBC count

Test Interactions Positive Coombs' [direct], false-positive urinary and/or serum proteins

Patient Information Report skin rash, itching, hives, or severe diarrhea.

Dosage Forms Injection, suspension: 600,000 units/mL (1 mL, 2 mL)

Selected Readings

Donowitz GR and Mandell GL, "Beta-Lactam Antibiotics," *N Engl J Med*, 1988, 318(7):419-26 and 318(8):490-500.

Pao D, Goh BT, and Bingham JS, "Management Issues in Syphilis," *Drugs*, 2002, 62(10):1447-61.

Wright AJ, "The Penicillins," *Mayo Clin Proc*, 1999, 74(3):290-307.

Penicillin G Procaine and Benzathine Combined *see* Penicillin G Benzathine and Penicillin G Procaine *on page 992*

Penicillin G Sodium *see* Penicillin G (Parenteral/Aqueous) *on page 993*

Penicillins, Extended-Spectrum

Refer to

Piperacillin and Tazobactam Sodium *on page 1003*
Piperacillin *on page 1002*
Ticarcillin and Clavulanate Potassium *on page 1114*
Ticarcillin *on page 1113*

Drug of Choice or Alternative for Disease/Syndrome(s):

Catheter Infection, Intravascular *on page 70*
Fever, Neutropenic *on page 148*
Meningitis, Postsurgical *on page 218*
Meningitis, Post-traumatic *on page 219*
Otitis Externa, Severe (Malignant) *on page 252*
Sepsis *on page 295*
Sinusitis, Hospital-Acquired *on page 300*
Wound Infection, Surgical *on page 354*

Organism(s):

Acinetobacter Species *on page 24*
Bordetella bronchiseptica on page 52
Burkholderia cepacia on page 62
Burkholderia mallei on page 64
Citrobacter Species *on page 81*
Klebsiella Species *on page 200*
Proteus Species *on page 278*
Providencia Species *on page 281*
Pseudomonas aeruginosa on page 282
Serratia Species *on page 296*

Penicillins, Penicillinase-Resistant

Refer to

Cloxacillin *on page 760*
Dicloxacillin *on page 773*
Nafcillin *on page 955*
Oxacillin *on page 983*

Drug of Choice or Alternative for Disease/Syndrome(s):

Catheter Infection, Intravascular *on page 70*
Joint Replacement, Early Infection *on page 197*
Joint Replacement, Late Infection *on page 198*
Osteomyelitis, Healthy Adult *on page 250*
Osteomyelitis, Pediatric *on page 251*
Skin and Soft Tissue *on page 300*
Thrombophlebitis, Suppurative *on page 330*
Toxic Shock Syndrome *on page 331*
Wound Infection, Surgical *on page 354*

Organism(s):

Staphylococcus aureus, Methicillin-Susceptible *on page 307*
Staphylococcus epidermidis, Methicillin-Susceptible *on page 310*

Penicillin V Potassium (pen i SIL in vee poe TASS ee um)

Related Information

Antimicrobial Activity Against Selected Organisms *on page 1165*

U.S. Brand Names Veetids®

Canadian Brand Names Apo-Pen VK®; Nadopen-V®; Novo-Pen-VK; Nu-Pen-VK; PVF® K

Synonyms Pen VK; Phenoxymethyl Penicillin

Generic Available Yes

Use Treatment of infections caused by susceptible organisms involving the respiratory tract, otitis media, sinusitis, skin, and urinary tract; prophylaxis in rheumatic fever

Drug of Choice or Alternative for

Disease/Syndrome(s):

Erysipelas *on page 141*
Impetigo *on page 193*
Pharyngitis *on page 264*

Organism(s):

Capnocytophaga Species *on page 69*
Erysipelothrix rhusiopathiae on page 141
Pasteurella multocida on page 258

Pregnancy Risk Factor B

Contraindications Hypersensitivity to penicillin or any component of the formulation

Warnings/Precautions Use with caution in patients with severe renal impairment (modify dosage), history of seizures, or hypersensitivity to cephalosporins

Adverse Reactions

>10%: Gastrointestinal: Mild diarrhea, vomiting, nausea, oral candidiasis

<1%: Convulsions, fever, hemolytic anemia, positive Coombs' reaction, acute interstitial nephritis, hypersensitivity reactions, anaphylaxis

Overdosage/Toxicology Symptoms of penicillin overdose include neuromuscular hypersensitivity (agitation, hallucinations, asterixis, encephalopathy, confusion, seizures) and electrolyte imbalance with potassium or sodium salts, especially in renal failure. Hemodialysis may be helpful to aid in removal of the drug from the blood, otherwise, most treatment is supportive or symptom-directed.

Drug Interactions

Increased Effect/Toxicity: Probenecid increases penicillin levels. Aminoglycosides may cause synergistic efficacy. Penicillins may increase the exposure to methotrexate during concurrent therapy; monitor.

Decreased Effect: Tetracyclines may decrease penicillin effectiveness. Although anecdotal reports suggest oral contraceptive efficacy could be reduced by penicillins, this has been refuted by more rigorous scientific and clinical data.

Ethanol/Nutrition/Herb Interactions Food: Decreases drug absorption rate; decreases drug serum concentration.

Stability Refrigerate suspension after reconstitution; discard after 14 days

Mechanism of Action Inhibits bacterial cell wall synthesis by binding to one or more of the penicillin binding proteins (PBPs); which in turn inhibits the final transpeptidation step of peptidoglycan synthesis in bacterial cell walls, thus inhibiting cell wall biosynthesis. Bacteria eventually lyse due to ongoing activity of cell wall autolytic enzymes (autolysins and murein hydrolases) while cell wall assembly is arrested.

Pharmacodynamics/Kinetics

Absorption: 60% to 73%
Distribution: Enters breast milk
Protein binding, plasma: 80%
Half-life elimination: 30 minutes; prolonged with renal impairment
Time to peak, serum: 0.5-1 hour
Excretion: Urine (as unchanged drug and metabolites)

Dosage Oral:

Systemic infections:

Children <12 years: 25-50 mg/kg/day in divided doses every 6-8 hours; maximum dose: 3 g/day
Children ≥12 years and Adults: 125-500 mg every 6-8 hours

Prophylaxis of pneumococcal infections:

Children <5 years: 125 mg twice daily
Children ≥5 years and Adults: 250 mg twice daily

Prophylaxis of recurrent rheumatic fever:

Children <5 years: 125 mg twice daily
Children ≥5 years and Adults: 250 mg twice daily

Dosing interval in renal impairment: Cl_{cr} <10 mL/minute: Administer 250 mg every 6 hours

Dietary Considerations Take on an empty stomach 1 hour before or 2 hours after meals.

Administration Administer on an empty stomach to increase oral absorption

Monitoring Parameters Periodic renal and hematologic function tests during prolonged therapy; monitor for signs of anaphylaxis during first dose

Test Interactions False-positive or negative urinary glucose determination using Clinitest®; positive Coombs' [direct]; false-positive urinary and/or serum proteins

Patient Information Take on an empty stomach 1 hour before or 2 hours after meals, take until gone, do not skip doses, report any rash or shortness of breath; shake liquid well before use

Additional Information 0.7 mEq of potassium per 250 mg penicillin V; 250 mg equals 400,000 units of penicillin

Dosage Forms Note: 250 mg = 400,000 units

Powder for oral solution: 125 mg/5 mL (100 mL, 200 mL); 250 mg/5 mL (100 mL, 200 mL)

Tablet: 250 mg, 500 mg

Penlac® *see* Ciclopirox *on page 739*

Pentacarinat® (Can) *see* Pentamidine *on page 999*

Pentam-300® *see* Pentamidine *on page 999*

Pentamidine (pen TAM i deen)

Related Information

USPHS / IDSA Guidelines for the Prevention of Opportunistic Infections in Persons Infected With HIV *on page 1237*

U.S. Brand Names NebuPent®; Pentam-300®

Canadian Brand Names Pentacarinat®

Synonyms Pentamidine Isethionate

Generic Available No

Use Treatment and prevention of pneumonia caused by *Pneumocystis carinii* (PCP)

Unlabeled/Investigational Use Treatment of trypanosomiasis and visceral leishmaniasis

Drug of Choice or Alternative for Organism(s):

Pneumocystis jiroveci on page 266

Pregnancy Risk Factor C

Contraindications Hypersensitivity to pentamidine isethionate or any component of the formulation (inhalation and injection)

Warnings/Precautions Use with caution in patients with diabetes mellitus, renal or hepatic dysfunction, hyper-/hypotension, leukopenia, thrombocytopenia, asthma, or hypo-/hyperglycemia.

Adverse Reactions Injection (I); Aerosol (A)

>10%:

- Cardiovascular: Chest pain (A - 10% to 23%)
- Central nervous system: Fatigue (A - 50% to 70%); dizziness (A - 31% to 47%)
- Dermatologic: Rash (31% to 47%)
- Endocrine & metabolic: Hyperkalemia
- Gastrointestinal: Anorexia (A - 50% to 70%), nausea (A - 10% to 23%)
- Local: Local reactions at injection site
- Renal: Increased creatinine (I - 23%)
- Respiratory: Wheezing (A - 10% to 23%), dyspnea (A - 50% to 70%), cough (A - 31% to 47%), pharyngitis (10% to 23%)

1% to 10%:

- Cardiovascular: Hypotension (I - 4%)
- Central nervous system: Confusion/hallucinations (1% to 2%), headache (A - 1% to 5%)
- Dermatologic: Rash (I - 3.3%)
- Endocrine & metabolic: Hypoglycemia <25 mg/dL (I - 2.4%)
- Gastrointestinal: Nausea/anorexia (I - 6%), diarrhea (A - 1% to 5%), vomiting
- Hematologic: Severe leukopenia (I - 2.8%), thrombocytopenia <20,000/mm^3 (I - 1.7%), anemia (A - 1% to 5%)
- Hepatic: Increased LFTs (I - 8.7%)

<1%: Hypotension <60 mm Hg systolic (I - 0.9%), tachycardia, arrhythmia, dizziness (I), fever, fatigue (I), hyperglycemia or hypoglycemia, hypocalcemia, pancreatitis, megaloblastic anemia, granulocytopenia, leukopenia, renal insufficiency, extrapulmonary pneumocystosis, irritation of the airway, pneumothorax, Jarisch-Herxheimer-like reaction, mild renal or hepatic injury

Overdosage/Toxicology Symptoms include hypotension, hypoglycemia, and cardiac arrhythmias. Treatment is supportive.

(Continued)

Pentamidine *(Continued)*

Drug Interactions

Cytochrome P450 Effect: Substrate of CYP2C19 (major); **Inhibits** CYP2C8/9 (weak), 2C19 (weak), 2D6 (weak), 3A4 (weak)

Increased Effect/Toxicity: CYP2C19 inhibitors may increase the levels/effects of pentamidine; example inhibitors include delavirdine, fluconazole, fluvoxamine, gemfibrozil, isoniazid, omeprazole, and ticlopidine. Pentamidine may potentiate the effect of other drugs which prolong QT interval (cisapride, sparfloxacin, gatifloxacin, moxifloxacin, pimozide, and type Ia and type III antiarrhythmics).

Decreased Effect: CYP2C19 inducers may decrease the levels/effects of pentamidine; example inducers include aminoglutethimide, carbamazepine, phenytoin, and rifampin.

Ethanol/Nutrition/Herb Interactions Ethanol: Avoid ethanol (may increase CNS depression or aggravate hypoglycemia).

Stability Store intact vials at controlled room temperature and protect from light. Do not refrigerate due to the possibility of crystallization. Powder for inhalation should be reconstituted with sterile water for injection. Powder for injection may be reconstituted with sterile water for injection or D_5W. **Do not use NS as a diluent.** Precipitation may occur if products are reconstituted with NS. Following reconstitution, solution for injection may be diluted. Solutions for injection (1-2.5 mg/mL) in D_5W are stable for at least 24 hours at room temperature. The manufacturer's labeling recommends D_5W, however, stability in NS has also been documented; in addition, light protection is recommended by the manufacturer, but stability has been documented without protection from light.

Mechanism of Action Interferes with RNA/DNA, phospholipids and protein synthesis, through inhibition of oxidative phosphorylation and/or interference with incorporation of nucleotides and nucleic acids into RNA and DNA, in protozoa

Pharmacodynamics/Kinetics

Absorption: I.M.: Well absorbed; Inhalation: Limited systemic absorption

Half-life elimination: Terminal: 6.4-9.4 hours; may be prolonged with severe renal impairment

Excretion: Urine (33% to 66% as unchanged drug)

Dosage

Children:

- Treatment of PCP pneumonia: I.M., I.V. (I.V. preferred): 4 mg/kg/day once daily for 10-14 days
- Prevention of PCP pneumonia:
  - I.M., I.V.: 4 mg/kg monthly or every 2 weeks
  - Inhalation (aerosolized pentamidine in children ≥5 years): 300 mg/dose given every 3-4 weeks via Respirgard® II inhaler (8 mg/kg dose has also been used in children <5 years)
- Treatment of trypanosomiasis (unlabeled use): I.V.: 4 mg/kg/day once daily for 10 days

Adults:

- Treatment: I.M., I.V. (I.V. preferred): 4 mg/kg/day once daily for 14-21 days
- Prevention: Inhalation: 300 mg every 4 weeks via Respirgard® II nebulizer

Dialysis: Not removed by hemo or peritoneal dialysis or continuous arteriovenous or venovenous hemofiltration; supplemental dosage is not necessary

Dosing adjustment in renal impairment: Adults: I.V.:

- Cl_{cr} 10-50 mL/minute: Administer 4 mg/kg every 24-36 hours
- Cl_{cr} <10 mL/minute: Administer 4 mg/kg every 48 hours

Administration Infuse I.V. slowly over a period of at least 60 minutes or administer deep I.M.; patients receiving I.V. or I.M. pentamidine should be lying down and blood pressure should be monitored closely during administration of drug and several times thereafter until it is stable

Monitoring Parameters Liver function tests, renal function tests, blood glucose, serum potassium and calcium, ECG, blood pressure

Patient Information PCP pneumonia may still occur despite pentamidine use; report fever, shortness of breath, or coughing up blood; maintain adequate fluid intake

Additional Information Virtually undetectable amounts are transferred to healthcare personnel during aerosol administration.

Dosage Forms

Injection, powder for reconstitution, as isethionate (Pentam-300®): 300 mg

Powder for nebulization, as isethionate (NebuPent®): 300 mg

Selected Readings

Goa KL and Campoli-Richards DM, "Pentamidine Isethionate. A Review of Its Antiprotozoal Activity, Pharmacokinetic Properties and Therapeutic Use in *Pneumocystis carinii* Pneumonia," *Drugs*, 1987, 33(3):242-58.

Masur H, "Prevention and Treatment of *Pneumocystis* Pneumonia," *N Engl J Med*, 1992, 327(26):1853-60.
Monk JP and Benfield P, "Inhaled Pentamidine. An Overview of Its Pharmacological Properties and a Review of Its Therapeutic Use in *Pneumocystis carinii* Pneumonia," *Drugs*, 1990, 39(5):741-56.
Sattler FR, Cowan R, Nielsen DM, et al, " Trimethoprim-Sulfamethoxazole Compared With Pentamidine for Treatment of *Pneumocystis carinii* Pneumonia in the Acquired Immunodeficiency Syndrome," *Ann Intern Med*, 1988, 109(4):280-7.

Pentamidine Isethionate *see* Pentamidine *on page 999*
Pentamycetin® (Can) *see* Chloramphenicol *on page 733*
Pen VK *see* Penicillin V Potassium *on page 998*
Pepto-Bismol® [OTC] *see* Bismuth *on page 686*
Pepto-Bismol® Maximum Strength [OTC] *see* Bismuth *on page 686*
Peridex® *see* Chlorhexidine Gluconate *on page 735*
PerioChip® *see* Chlorhexidine Gluconate *on page 735*
PerioGard® *see* Chlorhexidine Gluconate *on page 735*
Periostat® *see* Doxycycline *on page 787*

Permethrin (per METH rin)

U.S. Brand Names A200® Lice [OTC]; Acticin®; Elimite®; Nix® [OTC]; Rid® Spray [OTC]

Canadian Brand Names Kwellada-P™; Nix®

Generic Available Yes: Excludes spray

Use Single-application treatment of infestation with *Pediculus humanus capitis* (head louse) and its nits or *Sarcoptes scabiei* (scabies); indicated for prophylactic use during epidemics of lice

Drug of Choice or Alternative for Organism(s):
Lice *on page 207*
Sarcoptes scabiei on page 293

Pregnancy Risk Factor B

Contraindications Hypersensitivity to pyrethyroid, pyrethrin, chrysanthemums, or any component of the formulation; lotion is contraindicated for use in infants <2 months of age

Warnings/Precautions Treatment may temporarily exacerbate the symptoms of itching, redness, swelling; for external use only; use during pregnancy only if clearly needed

Adverse Reactions 1% to 10%:
Dermatologic: Pruritus, erythema, rash of the scalp
Local: Burning, stinging, tingling, numbness or scalp discomfort, edema

Mechanism of Action Inhibits sodium ion influx through nerve cell membrane channels in parasites resulting in delayed repolarization and thus paralysis and death of the pest

Pharmacodynamics/Kinetics
Absorption: <2%
Metabolism: Hepatic via ester hydrolysis to inactive metabolites
Excretion: Urine

Dosage Topical:
Head lice: Children >2 months and Adults: After hair has been washed with shampoo, rinsed with water, and towel dried, apply a sufficient volume of topical liquid (lotion or cream rinse) to saturate the hair and scalp. Leave on hair for 10 minutes before rinsing off with water; remove remaining nits; may repeat in 1 week if lice or nits still present.
Scabies: Apply cream from head to toe; leave on for 8-14 hours before washing off with water; for infants, also apply on the hairline, neck, scalp, temple, and forehead; may reapply in 1 week if live mites appear
Permethrin 5% cream was shown to be safe and effective when applied to an infant <1 month of age with neonatal scabies; time of application was limited to 6 hours before rinsing with soap and water

Administration Because scabies and lice are so contagious, use caution to avoid spreading or infecting oneself; wear gloves when applying
Cream: Apply from neck to toes. Bathe to remove drug after 8-14 hours. Repeat in 7 days if lice or nits are still present. Report if condition persists or infection occurs.
Cream rinse/lotion: Apply immediately after hair is shampooed, rinsed, and towel-dried. Apply enough to saturate hair and scalp (especially behind ears and on nape of neck). Leave on hair for 10 minutes before rinsing with water. Remove nits with fine-tooth comb. May repeat in 1 week if lice or nits are still present.

Patient Information Avoid contact with eyes and mucous membranes during application; shake well before using; notify prescriber if irritation persists; clothing and bedding should be washed in hot water or dry cleaned to kill the scabies mite

(Continued)

Permethrin *(Continued)*

Dosage Forms

Cream, topical (Acticin®, Elimite®): 5% (60 g) [contains coconut oil]

Liquid, topical [creme rinse formulation] (Nix®): 1% (60 mL) [contains isopropyl alcohol 20%]

Lotion, topical: 1% (59 mL)

Solution, spray [for bedding and furniture]:

A200® Lice: 0.5% (180 mL)

Nix®: 0.25% (148 mL)

Rid®: 0.5% (150 mL)

Selected Readings

"Drugs for Parasitic Infections," *Med Lett Drugs Ther*, 1998, 40(1017):1-12.

Liu LX and Weller PF, "Antiparasitic Drugs," *N Engl J Med*, 1996, 334(18):1178-84.

PFA *see* Foscarnet *on page 829*

Pfizerpen® *see* Penicillin G (Parenteral/Aqueous) *on page 993*

Pfizerpen-AS® (Can) *see* Penicillin G Procaine *on page 995*

Phenoxymethyl Penicillin *see* Penicillin V Potassium *on page 998*

pHisoHex® *see* Hexachlorophene *on page 858*

Phosphonoformate *see* Foscarnet *on page 829*

Phosphonoformic Acid *see* Foscarnet *on page 829*

***p*-Hydroxyampicillin** *see* Amoxicillin *on page 642*

Pima® *see* Potassium Iodide *on page 1014*

Pimaricin *see* Natamycin *on page 959*

Pin-X® [OTC] *see* Pyrantel Pamoate *on page 1021*

Pink Bismuth *see* Bismuth *on page 686*

Piperacillin (pi PER a sil in)

Related Information

Antimicrobial Activity Against Selected Organisms *on page 1165*

Synonyms Piperacillin Sodium

Generic Available Yes

Use Treatment of susceptible infections such as septicemia, acute and chronic respiratory tract infections, skin and soft tissue infections, and urinary tract infections due to susceptible strains of *Pseudomonas*, *Proteus*, and *Escherichia coli* and *Enterobacter*, active against some streptococci and some anaerobic bacteria; febrile neutropenia (as part of combination regimen)

Drug of Choice or Alternative for Disease/Syndrome(s):

Cholangitis, Acute *on page 79*

Keratitis, Bacterial and Fungal *on page 199*

Pneumonia, Community-Acquired *on page 270*

Organism(s):

Alcaligenes Species *on page 31*

Pregnancy Risk Factor B

Contraindications Hypersensitivity to piperacillin, other penicillins, or any component of the formulation

Warnings/Precautions Dosage modification required in patients with impaired renal function; history of seizure activity; use with caution in patients with a history of beta-lactam allergy

Adverse Reactions Frequency not defined.

Central nervous system: Confusion, convulsions, drowsiness, fever, Jarisch-Herxheimer reaction

Dermatologic: Rash

Endocrine & metabolic: Electrolyte imbalance

Hematologic: Abnormal platelet aggregation and prolonged PT (high doses), hemolytic anemia, Coombs' reaction (positive)

Local: Thrombophlebitis

Neuromuscular & skeletal: Myoclonus

Renal: Acute interstitial nephritis

Miscellaneous: Anaphylaxis, hypersensitivity reactions

Overdosage/Toxicology Symptoms of penicillin overdose include neuromuscular hypersensitivity (agitation, hallucinations, asterixis, encephalopathy, confusion, and seizures) and electrolyte imbalance (with potassium or sodium salts), especially in renal failure. Hemodialysis may be helpful to aid in the removal of the drug from the blood, otherwise, most treatment is supportive or symptom-directed.

Drug Interactions

Increased Effect/Toxicity: Probenecid may increase penicillin levels. Neuromuscular blockers may increase duration of blockade. Penicillins may increase the exposure to methotrexate during concurrent therapy; monitor.

Decreased Effect: Tetracyclines may decrease penicillin effectiveness. High concentrations of piperacillin may cause physical inactivation of aminoglycosides and lead to potential toxicity in patients with mild-moderate renal dysfunction. Although anecdotal reports suggest oral contraceptive efficacy could be reduced by penicillins, this has been refuted by more rigorous scientific and clinical data.

Stability Reconstituted solution is stable (I.V. infusion) in NS or D_5W for 24 hours at room temperature, 7 days when refrigerated or 4 weeks when frozen; after freezing, thawed solution is stable for 24 hours at room temperature or 48 hours when refrigerated; 40 g bulk vial should **not** be frozen after reconstitution; **incompatible** with aminoglycosides

Mechanism of Action Inhibits bacterial cell wall synthesis by binding to one or more of the penicillin binding proteins (PBPs); which in turn inhibits the final transpeptidation step of peptidoglycan synthesis in bacterial cell walls, thus inhibiting cell wall biosynthesis. Bacteria eventually lyse due to ongoing activity of cell wall autolytic enzymes (autolysins and murein hydrolases) while cell wall assembly is arrested.

Pharmacodynamics/Kinetics

Absorption: I.M.: 70% to 80%

Distribution: Crosses placenta; low concentrations enter breast milk

Protein binding: 22%

Half-life elimination (dose dependent; prolonged with moderately severe renal or hepatic impairment):

- Neonates: 1-5 days old: 3.6 hours; >6 days old: 2.1-2.7 hours
- Children: 1-6 months: 0.79 hour; 6 months to 12 years: 0.39-0.5 hour
- Adults: 36-80 minutes

Time to peak, serum: I.M.: 30-50 minutes

Excretion: Primarily urine; partially feces

Dosage

Neonates: 100 mg/kg every 12 hours

Infants and Children: I.M., I.V.: 200-300 mg/kg/day in divided doses every 4-6 hours

- Higher doses have been used in cystic fibrosis: 350-500 mg/kg/day in divided doses every 4-6 hours

Adults: I.M., I.V.:

- Moderate infections (urinary tract infections): 2-3 g/dose every 6-12 hours; maximum: 2 g I.M./site
- Serious infections: 3-4 g/dose every 4-6 hours; maximum: 24 g/24 hours
- Uncomplicated gonorrhea: 2 g I.M. in a single dose accompanied by 1 g probenecid 30 minutes prior to injection

Dosing adjustment in renal impairment: Adults: I.V.:

- Cl_{cr} 20-40 mL/minute: Administer 3-4 g every 8 hours
- Cl_{cr} <20 mL/minute: Administer 3-4 g every 12 hours

Moderately dialyzable (20% to 50%)

Continuous arteriovenous or venovenous hemodiafiltration effects: Dose as for Cl_{cr} 10-50 mL/minute

Dietary Considerations Sodium content of 1 g: 1.85 mEq

Administration Administer around-the-clock to promote less variation in peak and trough serum levels. Give at least 1 hour apart from aminoglycosides. Rapid administration can lead to seizures. Administer direct I.V. over 3-5 minutes. Intermittently infusion over 30 minutes. Do not administer more than 2 g per I.M. injection site.

Monitoring Parameters Observe for signs and symptoms of anaphylaxis during first dose

Test Interactions May interfere with urinary glucose tests using cupric sulfate (Benedict's solution, Clinitest®); may inactivate aminoglycosides *in vitro*; false-positive urinary and serum proteins, positive Coombs' test [direct]

Additional Information As of September 2002, piperacillin is not available from the manufacturer. This product is anticipated to return to the market in 2003.

Dosage Forms Injection, powder for reconstitution: 2 g, 3 g, 4 g, 40 g

Selected Readings

Donowitz GR and Mandell GL, "Beta-Lactam Antibiotics," *N Engl J Med*, 1988, 318(7):419-26 and 318(8):490-500.

Tan JS and File TM Jr, "Antipseudomonal Penicillins," *Med Clin North Am*, 1995, 79(4):679-93.

Wright AJ, "The Penicillins," *Mayo Clin Proc*, 1999, 74(3):290-307.

Piperacillin and Tazobactam Sodium

(pi PER a sil in & ta zoe BAK tam SOW dee um)

Related Information

Antimicrobial Activity Against Selected Organisms *on page 1165*

(Continued)

Piperacillin and Tazobactam Sodium *(Continued)*

U.S. Brand Names Zosyn®

Canadian Brand Names Tazocin®

Synonyms Piperacillin Sodium and Tazobactam Sodium

Generic Available No

Use Treatment of infections caused by susceptible organisms, including infections of the lower respiratory tract (community-acquired pneumonia, nosocomial pneumonia); urinary tract; skin and skin structures; gynecologic (endometritis, pelvic inflammatory disease); bone and joint infections; intra-abdominal infections (appendicitis with rupture/abscess, peritonitis); and septicemia. Tazobactam expands activity of piperacillin to include beta-lactamase producing strains of *S. aureus*, *H. influenzae*, *Bacteroides*, and other gram-negative bacteria.

Drug of Choice or Alternative for Disease/Syndrome(s):

Amnionitis *on page 33*
Cholangitis, Acute *on page 79*
Diverticulitis *on page 116*
Endocarditis, Acute, I.V. Drug Abuse *on page 123*
Endometritis *on page 127*
Epididymitis/Orchitis *on page 138*
Intra-abdominal Abscess *on page 194*
Liver Abscess *on page 211*
Lung Abscess *on page 212*
Osteomyelitis, Diabetic Foot *on page 249*
Pancreatitis/Pancreatic Abscess *on page 253*
Peritonitis, Secondary *on page 263*
Pneumonia, Community-Acquired *on page 270*

Organism(s):

Bacteroides and *Prevotella* Species *on page 46*
Enterobacter Species *on page 132*

Pregnancy Risk Factor B

Pregnancy Implications Piperacillin and tazobactam were not teratogenic in animal studies. Both piperacillin and tazobactam cross the human placenta.

Contraindications Hypersensitivity to penicillins, beta-lactamase inhibitors, or any component of the formulation

Warnings/Precautions Due to sodium load and to the adverse effects of high serum concentrations of penicillins, dosage modification is required in patients with impaired or underdeveloped renal function; use with caution in patients with seizures or in patients with history of beta-lactam allergy; safety and efficacy have not been established in children <12 years of age

Adverse Reactions

>10%: Gastrointestinal: Diarrhea (11%)

1% to 10%:

- Cardiovascular: Hypertension (2%)
- Central nervous system: Insomnia (7%), headache (7% to 8%), agitation (2%), fever (2%), dizziness (1%)
- Dermatologic: Rash (4%), pruritus (3%)
- Gastrointestinal: Constipation (7% to 8%), nausea (7%), vomiting/dyspepsia (3%)
- Hepatic: Transaminases increased
- Respiratory: Rhinitis/dyspnea (~1%)
- Miscellaneous: Serum sickness-like reaction

<1%: Bronchospasm, *Clostridium difficile* colitis, confusion, edema, hepatitis, hepatotoxicity, hypotension, leukopenia, pseudomembranous colitis, seizure, thrombocytopenia

Postmarketing and/or case reports: Agranulocytosis, anaphylaxis, anaphylactoid reactions, cholestatic jaundice, erythema multiforme, hemolytic anemia, hypersensitivity, interstitial nephritis, pancytopenia, Stevens-Johnson syndrome, toxic epidermal necrolysis

Several laboratory abnormalities have rarely been associated with piperacillin/tazobactam including reversible eosinophilia, and neutropenia (associated most often with prolonged therapy), positive direct Coombs' test, prolonged PT and aPTT, transient elevations of LFT, increases in creatinine

Overdosage/Toxicology Symptoms of penicillin overdose include neuromuscular hypersensitivity (agitation, hallucinations, asterixis, encephalopathy, confusion, and seizures) and electrolyte imbalance (with potassium or sodium salts), especially in renal dysfunction. Hemodialysis may be helpful to aid in the removal of the drug from the blood, otherwise, most treatment is supportive or symptom-directed.

Drug Interactions

Increased Effect/Toxicity: Probenecid may increase penicillin levels. Neuromuscular blockers may increase duration of blockade. Penicillins may increase methotrexate exposure; clinical significance has not been established.

Decreased Effect: Tetracyclines may decrease penicillin effectiveness. Aminoglycosides may cause physical inactivation of aminoglycosides in the presence of high concentrations of piperacillin and potential toxicity in patients with mild-moderate renal dysfunction. Although anecdotal reports suggest oral contraceptive efficacy could be reduced by penicillins, this has been refuted by more rigorous scientific and clinical data.

Stability Store at controlled room temperature; after reconstitution, solution is stable in NS or D_5W for 24 hours at room temperature and 7 days when refrigerated; use single-dose vials immediately after reconstitution (discard unused portions after 24 hours at room temperature and 48 hours if refrigerated)

Mechanism of Action Inhibits bacterial cell wall synthesis by binding to one or more of the penicillin binding proteins (PBPs); which in turn inhibits the final transpeptidation step of peptidoglycan synthesis in bacterial cell walls, thus inhibiting cell wall biosynthesis. Bacteria eventually lyse due to ongoing activity of cell wall autolytic enzymes (autolysins and murein hydrolases) while cell wall assembly is arrested. Tazobactam inhibits many beta-lactamases, including staphylococcal penicillinase and Richmond and Sykes types II, III, IV, and V, including extended spectrum enzymes; it has only limited activity against class I beta-lactamases other than class Ic types.

Pharmacodynamics/Kinetics Both AUC and peak concentrations are dose proportional; hepatic impairment does not affect kinetics

Distribution: Well into lungs, intestinal mucosa, skin, muscle, uterus, ovary, prostate, gallbladder, and bile; penetration into CSF is low in subject with noninflamed meninges

Protein binding: Piperacillin: ~26% to 33%; Tazobactam: 31% to 32%

Metabolism: Piperacillin: 6% to 9%; Tazobactam: ~26%

Half-life elimination: Piperacillin: 1 hour; Metabolite: 1-1.5 hours; Tazobactam: 0.7-0.9 hour

Excretion: Both piperacillin and tazobactam are directly proportional to renal function
- Piperacillin: Urine (50% to 70%); feces (10% to 20%)
- Tazobactam: Urine (26% as inactive metabolite) within 24 hours

Dosage

Infants and Children ≥6 months: **Note:** Not FDA-approved for use in children <12 years of age:
- I.V.: 240 mg of piperacillin component/kg/day in divided doses every 8 hours; higher doses have been used for serious pseudomonal infections: 300-400 mg of piperacillin component/kg/day in divided doses every 6 hours.

Children >12 years and Adults:
- Nosocomial pneumonia: I.V.: Piperacillin/tazobactam 4/0.5 g every 6 hours for 7-14 days (when used empirically, combination with an aminoglycoside is recommended; consider discontinuation of aminoglycoside if *P. aeruginosa* is not isolated)
- Severe infections: I.V.: Piperacillin/tazobactam 4/0.5 g every 8 hours or 3/0.375 g every 6 hours for 7-10 days
- Moderate infections: I.M.: Piperacillin/tazobactam 2/0.25 g every 6-8 hours; treatment should be continued for ≥7-10 days depending on severity of disease (**Note:** I.M. route not FDA-approved)

Dosing interval in renal impairment:
- Cl_{cr} 20-40 mL/minute: Administer 2/0.25 g every 6 hours (3/0.375 g every 6 hours for nosocomial pneumonia)
- Cl_{cr} <20 mL/minute: Administer 2/0.25 g every 8 hours (2/0.25 g every 6 hours for nosocomial pneumonia)

Hemodialysis: Administer 2/0.25 g every 12 hours (every 8 hours for nosocomial pneumonia) with an additional dose of 0.75 g after each dialysis

Continuous arteriovenous or venovenous hemodiafiltration effects: Dose as for Cl_{cr} 10-50 mL/minute

Dietary Considerations

Infusion, premixed: 2.25 g contains sodium 5.7 mEq (131 mg); 3.375 g contains sodium 8.6 mEq (197 mg); 4.5 g contains sodium 11.4 mEq (263 mg)

Injection, powder for reconstitution: 2.25 g contains sodium 4.69 mEq (108 mg); 3.375 g contains sodium 7.04 mEq (162 mg); 4.5 g contains sodium 9.39 mEq (216 mg); 40.5 g contains sodium 84.5 mEq (1944 mg, bulk pharmacy vial)

Administration Administer by I.V. infusion over 30 minutes; reconstitute with 5 mL of diluent per 1 g of piperacillin and then further dilute; **compatible** diluents include NS, SW, dextran 6%, D_5W, D_5W with potassium chloride 40 mEq, bacteriostatic saline

(Continued)

Piperacillin and Tazobactam Sodium *(Continued)*

and water; **incompatible** with lactated Ringer's solution; discontinue primary infusion, if possible, during infusion and administer aminoglycosides separately from Zosyn®.

Monitoring Parameters LFTs, creatinine, BUN, CBC with differential, serum electrolytes, urinalysis, PT, PTT; monitor for signs of anaphylaxis during first dose

Test Interactions Positive Coombs' [direct] test 3.8%, ALT, AST, bilirubin, and LDH; may result in false positive results with the Platelia® *Aspergillus* enzyme immunoassay (EIA)

Dosage Forms Note: 8:1 ratio of piperacillin sodium/tazobactam sodium:

Infusion [premixed iso-osmotic solution, frozen]:

- 2.25 g: Piperacillin 2 g and tazobactam 0.25 g (50 mL) [contains sodium 5.7 mEq (131 mg)]
- 3.375 g: Piperacillin 3 g and tazobactam 0.375 g (50 mL) [contains sodium 8.6 mEq (197 mg)]
- 4.5 g: Piperacillin 4 g and tazobactam 0.5 g (50 mL) [contains sodium 11.4 mEq (263 mg)]

Injection, powder for reconstitution:

- 2.25 g: Piperacillin 2 g and tazobactam 0.25 g [contains sodium 4.69 mEq (108 mg)]
- 3.375 g: Piperacillin 3 g and tazobactam 0.375 g [contains sodium 7.04 mEq (162 mg)]
- 4.5 g: Piperacillin 4 g and tazobactam 0.5 g [contains sodium 9.39 mEq (216 mg)]
- 40.5 g: Piperacillin 36 g and tazobactam 4.5 g [contains sodium 84.5 mEq (1944 mg); bulk pharmacy vial]

Selected Readings

"Piperacillin/Tazobactam," *Med Lett Drugs Ther*, 1994, 36(914):7-9.

Sanders WE Jr and Sanders CC, "Piperacillin/Tazobactam: A Critical Review of the Evolving Clinical Literature," *Clin Infect Dis*, 1996, 22(1):107-23.

Schoonover LL, Occhipinti DJ, Rodvold KA, et al, "Piperacillin/Tazobactam: A New Beta-Lactam/Beta-Lactamase Inhibitor Combination," *Ann Pharmacother*, 1995, 29(5):501-14.

Piperacillin Sodium *see* Piperacillin *on page 1002*

Piperacillin Sodium and Tazobactam Sodium *see* Piperacillin and Tazobactam Sodium *on page 1003*

Piperazine (PI per a zeen)

Canadian Brand Names Entacyl®

Synonyms Piperazine Citrate

Generic Available Yes

Use Treatment of pinworm and roundworm infections (used as an alternative to first-line agents, mebendazole, or pyrantel pamoate)

Pregnancy Risk Factor B

Contraindications Hypersensitivity to piperazine or any component of the formulation; seizure disorders; liver or kidney impairment

Warnings/Precautions Use with caution in patients with anemia or malnutrition; avoid prolonged use especially in children

Adverse Reactions <1%: Bronchospasms, diarrhea, dizziness, EEG changes, headache, hemolytic anemia, hypersensitivity reactions, nausea, seizure, vertigo, visual impairment, vomiting, weakness

Drug Interactions

Decreased Effect: Pyrantel pamoate (antagonistic mode of action).

Mechanism of Action Causes muscle paralysis of the roundworm by blocking the effects of acetylcholine at the neuromuscular junction

Pharmacodynamics/Kinetics

Absorption: Well absorbed

Time to peak, serum: 1 hour

Excretion: Urine (as unchanged drug and metabolites)

Dosage Oral:

Pinworms: Children and Adults: 65 mg/kg/day (not to exceed 2.5 g/day) as a single daily dose for 7 days; in severe infections, repeat course after a 1-week interval

Roundworms:

- Children: 75 mg/kg/day as a single daily dose for 2 days; maximum: 3.5 g/day
- Adults: 3.5 g/day for 2 days (in severe infections, repeat course, after a 1-week interval)

Monitoring Parameters Stool exam for worms and ova

Dosage Forms Piperazine citrate is available from Panorama Pharmacy (1-800-247-9767).

Piperazine Citrate *see* Piperazine *on page 1006*

Piperonyl Butoxide and Pyrethrins *see* Pyrethrins and Piperonyl Butoxide *on page 1023*

Pitrex (Can) *see* Tolnaftate *on page 1127*

Plague Vaccine (plaig vak SEEN)

Generic Available No

Use Selected travelers to countries reporting cases for whom avoidance of rodents and fleas is impossible; all laboratory and field personnel working with *Yersinia pestis* organisms possibly resistant to antimicrobials; those engaged in *Yersinia pestis* aerosol experiments or in field operations in areas with enzootic plague where regular exposure to potentially infected wild rodents, rabbits, or their fleas cannot be prevented. Prophylactic antibiotics may be indicated following definite exposure, whether or not the exposed persons have been vaccinated.

Pregnancy Risk Factor C

Contraindications Hypersensitivity to any of the vaccine constituents (see manufacturer's label); patients who have had severe local or systemic reactions to a previous dose; defer immunization in patients with a febrile illness until resolved

Warnings/Precautions Pregnancy, unless there is substantial and unavoidable risk of exposure; the expected immune response may not be obtained if plague vaccine is administered to immunosuppressed persons or patients receiving immunosuppressive therapy; be prepared with epinephrine injection (1:1000) in cases of anaphylaxis

Adverse Reactions All serious adverse reactions must be reported to the U.S. Department of Health and Human Services (DHHS) Vaccine Adverse Event Reporting System (VAERS) 1-800-822-7967.

1% to 10%:

- Central nervous system: Malaise (10%), fever, headache (7% to 20%)
- Dermatologic: Tenderness (20% to 80%)

<1%: Local erythema (5%), nausea (3% to 13%), sterile abscess, tachycardia, vomiting

Mechanism of Action Promotes active immunity to plague in high-risk individuals.

Dosage Three I.M. doses: First dose 1 mL, second dose (0.2 mL) 1 month later, third dose (0.2 mL) 5 months after the second dose; booster doses (0.2 mL) at 1- to 2-year intervals if exposure continues

Administration For patients at risk of hemorrhage following intramuscular injection, the ACIP recommends "it should be administered intramuscularly if, in the opinion of the physician familiar with the patients bleeding risk, the vaccine can be administered with reasonable safety by this route. If the patient receives antihemophilia or other similar therapy, intramuscular vaccination can be scheduled shortly after such therapy is administered. A fine needle (23 gauge or smaller) can be used for the vaccination and firm pressure applied to the site (without rubbing) for at least 2 minutes. The patient should be instructed concerning the risk of hematoma from the injection."

Test Interactions Temporary suppression of tuberculosis skin test

Additional Information Federal law requires that the date of administration, the vaccine manufacturer, lot number of vaccine, and the administering person's name, title, and address be entered into the patient's permanent medical record.

Dosage Forms Injection: 2 mL, 20 mL

Plaquenil® *see* Hydroxychloroquine *on page 859*

PMPA *see* Tenofovir *on page 1095*

PMS-Amantadine (Can) *see* Amantadine *on page 636*

PMS-Amoxicillin (Can) *see* Amoxicillin *on page 642*

PMS-Cefaclor (Can) *see* Cefaclor *on page 697*

PMS-Ciprofloxacin (Can) *see* Ciprofloxacin *on page 742*

PMS-Erythromycin (Can) *see* Erythromycin *on page 807*

PMS-Isoniazid (Can) *see* Isoniazid *on page 893*

PMS-Lindane (Can) *see* Lindane *on page 913*

PMS-Minocycline (Can) *see* Minocycline *on page 947*

PMS-Norfloxacin (Can) *see* Norfloxacin *on page 973*

PMS-Nystatin (Can) *see* Nystatin *on page 976*

PMS-Ofloxacin (Can) *see* Ofloxacin *on page 977*

PMS-Polytrimethoprim (Can) *see* Trimethoprim and Polymyxin B *on page 1131*

PMS-Terbinafine (Can) *see* Terbinafine *on page 1097*

PMS-Tobramycin (Can) *see* Tobramycin *on page 1122*

Pneumo 23™ (Can) *see* Pneumococcal Polysaccharide Vaccine (Polyvalent) *on page 1010*

Pneumococcal 7-Valent Conjugate Vaccine *see* Pneumococcal Conjugate Vaccine (7-Valent) *on page 1008*

Pneumococcal Conjugate Vaccine (7-Valent)

(noo moe KOK al KON ju gate vak SEEN, seven vay lent)

U.S. Brand Names Prevnar®

Canadian Brand Names Prevnar®

Synonyms Diphtheria CRM_{197} Protein; PCV7; Pneumococcal 7-Valent Conjugate Vaccine

Generic Available No

Use Immunization of infants and toddlers against *Streptococcus pneumoniae* infection caused by serotypes included in the vaccine

Advisory Committee on Immunization Practices (ACIP) guidelines also recommend PCV7 for use in:

- All children 2-23 months
- Children ≥2-59 months with cochlear implants
- Children ages 24-59 months with: Sickle cell disease (including other sickle cell hemoglobinopathies, asplenia, splenic dysfunction), HIV infection, immunocompromising conditions (congenital immunodeficiencies, renal failure, nephrotic syndrome, diseases associated with immunosuppressive or radiation therapy, solid organ transplant), chronic illnesses (cardiac disease, cerebrospinal fluid leaks, diabetes mellitus, pulmonary disease excluding asthma unless on high dose corticosteroids)
- Consider use in all children 24-59 months with priority given to:
  - Children 24-35 months
  - Children 24-59 months who are of Alaska native, American Indian, or African-American descent
  - Children 24-59 months who attend group day care centers

Pregnancy Risk Factor C

Pregnancy Implications

Reproduction studies have not been conducted. This product is indicated for use in infants and toddlers.

Contraindications Hypersensitivity to pneumococcal vaccine or any component of the formulation, including diphtheria toxoid; current or recent severe or moderate febrile illness

Warnings/Precautions Use caution in latex sensitivity. Children with impaired immune responsiveness may have a reduced response to active immunization. The decision to administer or delay vaccination because of current or recent febrile illness depends on the severity of symptoms and the etiology of the disease. Immunization should be delayed during the course of an acute febrile illness. Use caution in children with coagulation disorders (including thrombocytopenia) where intramuscular injections should not be used. Epinephrine 1:1000 should be readily available. Use of pneumococcal conjugate vaccine does not replace use of the 23-valent pneumococcal polysaccharide vaccine in children ≥24 months of age with sickle cell disease, asplenia, HIV infection, chronic illness or if immunocompromised. Safety and efficacy have not been established in children <6 weeks or ≥10 years of age. Not for I.V. use.

Adverse Reactions All serious adverse reactions must be reported to the U.S. Department of Health and Human Services (DHHS) Vaccine Adverse Event Reporting System (VAERS) 1-800-822-7967.

>10%:

- Central nervous system: Fever, irritability, drowsiness, restlessness
- Dermatologic: Erythema
- Gastrointestinal: Decreased appetite, vomiting, diarrhea
- Local: Induration, tenderness, nodule

1% to 10%: Dermatologic: Rash

Postmarketing and/or case reports: Anaphylactic reaction, anaphylactoid reaction, angioneurotic edema, apnea, bronchospasm, dyspnea, erythema multiforme, facial edema, febrile seizure, hypersensitivity reaction, injection site reaction (eg, dermatitis, lymphadenopathy, pruritus, urticaria, shock)

Overdosage/Toxicology

Higher than recommended doses, and doses administered closer than the recommended interval, have been reported. Adverse events were similar to those reported with single doses; most patients were asymptomatic.

Drug Interactions

Decreased Effect: Immunosuppressants may decrease response to active immunizations.

Stability Store refrigerated at 2°C to 8°C (36°F to 46°F).

Mechanism of Action Promotes active immunization against invasive disease caused by *S. pneumoniae* capsular serotypes 4, 6B, 9V, 18C, 19F, and 23F, all which are individually conjugated to CRM197 protein

Dosage I.M.:

Infants: 2-6 months: 0.5 mL at approximately 2-month intervals for 3 consecutive doses, followed by a fourth dose of 0.5 mL at 12-15 months of age; first dose may be given as young as 6 weeks of age, but is typically given at 2 months of age. In case of a moderate shortage of vaccine, defer the fourth dose until shortage is resolved; in case of a severe shortage of vaccine, defer third and fourth doses until shortage is resolved.

Previously Unvaccinated Older Infants and Children:

7-11 months: 0.5 mL for a total of 3 doses; 2 doses at least 4 weeks apart, followed by a third dose after the 1-year birthday (12-15 months), separated from the second dose by at least 2 months. In case of a severe shortage of vaccine, defer the third dose until shortage is resolved.

12-23 months: 0.5 mL for a total of 2 doses, separated by at least 2 months. In case of a severe shortage of vaccine, defer the second dose until shortage is resolved.

24-59 months:

Healthy Children: 0.5 mL as a single dose. In case of a severe shortage of vaccine, defer dosing until shortage is resolved.

Children with sickle cell disease, asplenia, HIV infection, chronic illness or immunocompromising conditions (not including bone marrow transplants - results pending; use PPV23 [pneumococcal polysaccharide vaccine, polyvalent] at 12- and 24-months until studies are complete): 0.5 mL for a total of 2 doses, separated by 2 months

Previously Vaccinated Children with a lapse in vaccine administration:

7-11 months: Previously received 1 or 2 doses PCV7: 0.5 mL dose at 7-11 months of age, followed by a second dose ≥2 months later at 12-15 months of age

12-23 months:

Previously received 1 dose before 12 months of age: 0.5 mL dose, followed by a second dose ≥2 months later

Previously received 2 doses before age 12 months: 0.5 mL dose ≥2 months after the most recent dose

24-59 months: Any incomplete schedule: 0.5 mL as a single dose; **Note:** Patients with chronic diseases or immunosuppressing conditions should receive 2 doses ≥2 months apart

Administration Shake well prior to use. Do not inject I.V.; avoid intradermal route; administer I.M. (deltoid muscle for toddlers and young children or lateral midthigh in infants)

For patients at risk of hemorrhage following intramuscular injection, the ACIP recommends "it should be administered intramuscularly if, in the opinion of the physician familiar with the patients bleeding risk, the vaccine can be administered with reasonable safety by this route. If the patient receives antihemophilia or other similar therapy, intramuscular vaccination can be scheduled shortly after such therapy is administered. A fine needle (23 gauge or smaller) can be used for the vaccination and firm pressure applied to the site (without rubbing) for at least 2 minutes. The patient should be instructed concerning the risk of hematoma from the injection."

Additional Information Children 24-59 months of age at high risk for pneumococcal disease but that have already received pneumococcal polysaccharide vaccine (PPV23) may benefit from the immunologic response induced by PCV7. Suggested dosing: Starting ≥2 months after last PPV23 dose: 0.5 mL dose of PCV7, followed by a second dose ≥2 months later. (**Note:** Although it is believed that this will provide additional protection, safety data is limited.)

Federal law requires that the date of administration, the vaccine manufacturer, lot number of vaccine, and the administering person's name, title and address be entered into the patient's permanent medical record.

Dosage Forms Injection, suspension: 2 mcg of each saccharide for serotypes 4, 9V, 14, 18C, 19F, and 23F, and 4 mcg of serotype 6B per 0.5 mL (0.5 mL) [contains 16 mcg total saccharide; also contains diphtheria CRM197 carrier protein ~20 mcg/0.5 mL and aluminum 0.125 mg/0.5 mL (as aluminum phosphate adjuvant); serotypes grown in soy peptone broth; vial stopper contains latex]

Selected Readings

Butler JC, Hoffman J, Cetron MS, et al, "The Continued Emergence of Drug-Resistant *Streptococcus pneumoniae* in the United Staes. An Update from the Centers for Disease Control and Prevention's Pneumococcal Sentinel Surveillance System," *J Infect Dis*, 1996, 174:986-93.

"Preventing Pneumococcal Disease Among Infants and Young Children: Recommendations of the Advisory Committee on Immunization Practices (ACIP), Centers for Disease Control and Prevention," *MMWR*, 2000, 49(RR-9):1-35.

(Continued)

Pneumococcal Conjugate Vaccine (7-Valent) *(Continued)*

Rennels MD, Edward KM, Keyscrling HL, et al, "Safety and Immunogenicity of Heptavalent Pneumococcal Vaccine Conjugated to CRM_{197} in U.S. Infants," *Pediatrics*, 1998, 101(4):604-11.

Sheinfield HR, Black S, and Ray P, "Safety and Immunogenicity of Heptavalent Pneumococcal CRM_{197} Conjugate Vaccine in Infants and Toddlers," *Pediatr Infect Dis J*, 1999, 18:757-62.

Pneumococcal Polysaccharide Vaccine (Polyvalent)

(noo moe KOK al pol i SAK a ride vak SEEN, pol i VAY lent)

Related Information

Immunization Recommendations *on page 1249*

U.S. Brand Names Pneumovax® 23

Canadian Brand Names Pneumo 23™; Pneumovax® 23

Synonyms PPV23; 23PS; 23-Valent Pneumococcal Polysaccharide Vaccine

Generic Available No

Use Children ≥2 years of age and adults who are at increased risk of pneumococcal disease and its complications because of underlying health conditions (including patients with cochlear implants); routine use in older adults >50 years of age, including all those ≥65 years

Current Advisory Committee on Immunization Practices (ACIP) guidelines recommend **pneumococcal 7-valent conjugate vaccine (PCV7)** be used for children 2-23 months of age and, in certain situations, children up to 59 months of age

Pregnancy Risk Factor C

Pregnancy Implications The safety of vaccine in pregnant women has not been evaluated; it should not be given during pregnancy unless the risk of infection is high

Contraindications Hypersensitivity to pneumococcal vaccine or any component of the formulation

Warnings/Precautions Use caution in patients with severe cardiovascular or pulmonary disease where a systemic reaction may pose a significant risk. Use caution and consider delay of vaccination in any active infection. Use caution in individuals who have had episodes of pneumococcal infection within the preceding 3 years (pre-existing pneumococcal antibodies may result in increased reactions to vaccine); may cause relapse in patients with stable idiopathic thrombocytopenia purpura. Epinephrine injection (1:1000) must be immediately available in the case of anaphylaxis.

Patients who will be receiving immunosuppressive therapy (including Hodgkin's disease, cancer chemotherapy, or transplantation) should be vaccinated at least 2 weeks prior to the initiation of therapy. Immune responses may be impaired for several months following intensive immunosuppressive therapy (up to 2 years in Hodgkin's disease patients). Patients who will undergo splenectomy should also be vaccinated 2 weeks prior to surgery, if possible. Patients with HIV should be vaccinated as soon as possible (following confirmation of the diagnosis). Not recommended in children <2 years of age.

Adverse Reactions All serious adverse reactions must be reported to the U.S. Department of Health and Human Services (DHHS) Vaccine Adverse Event Reporting System (VAERS) 1-800-822-7967.

Frequency not defined.

- Cardiovascular: Malaise
- Central nervous system: Guillain-Barré syndrome, fever ≤102°F*, fever >102°F, headache, radiculoneuropathy
- Dermatologic: Angioneurotic edema, cellulitis, rash, urticaria
- Gastrointestinal: Nausea, vomiting
- Hematologic: Hemolytic anemia (in patients with other hematologic disorders), thrombocytopenia (in patients with stabilized ITP)
- Local: Injection site reaction* (erythema, induration, swelling, soreness, warmth)
- Neuromuscular & skeletal: Arthralgia, arthritis, myalgia, paresthesia, weakness
- Miscellaneous: Anaphylactoid reaction, lymphadenitis, serum sickness

*Reactions most commonly reported in clinical trials.

Drug Interactions

Decreased Effect: The effect of the vaccine may be decreased with immunosuppressant medications.

Stability Store under refrigeration at 2°C to 8°C (36°F to 46°F).

Mechanism of Action Although there are more than 80 known pneumococcal capsular types, pneumococcal disease is mainly caused by only a few types of pneumococci. Pneumococcal vaccine contains capsular polysaccharides of 23 pneumococcal types of *Streptococcal pneumoniae* which represent at least 85% to 90% of pneumococcal disease isolates in the United States. The pneumococcal vaccine with 23 pneumococcal capsular polysaccharide types became available in 1983. The 23

capsular pneumococcal vaccine contains purified capsular polysaccharides of pneumococcal types 1, 2, 3, 4, 5, 6B, 7F, 8, 9N, 9V, 10A, 11A, 12F, 14, 15B, 17F, 18C, 19F, 19A, 20, 22F, 23F, and 33F. These are the main pneumococcal types associated with serious infections in the United States.

Dosage I.M., SubQ:

Children >2 years and Adults: 0.5 mL

Previously vaccinated with PCV7 vaccine: Children ≥2 years and Adults:

With sickle cell disease, asplenia, immunocompromised or HIV infection: 0.5 mL at ≥2 years of age and ≥2 months after last dose of PCV7; revaccination with PPV23 should be given ≥5 years for children >10 years of age and every 3-5 years for children ≤10 years of age; revaccination should not be administered <3 years after the previous PPV23 dose

With chronic illness: 0.5 mL at ≥2 years of age and ≥2 months after last dose of PCV7; revaccination with PPV23 is not recommended

Following bone marrow transplant (use of PCV7 under study): Administer one dose PPV23 at 12- and 24-months following BMT

Revaccination should be considered:

1. If ≥6 years since initial vaccination has elapsed, or
2. In patients who received 14-valent pneumococcal vaccine and are at highest risk (asplenic) for fatal infection or
3. At ≥6 years in patients with nephrotic syndrome, renal failure, or transplant recipients, or
4. 3-5 years in children with nephrotic syndrome, asplenia, or sickle cell disease

Administration Do not inject I.V., avoid intradermal, administer SubQ or I.M. (deltoid muscle or lateral midthigh)

For patients at risk of hemorrhage following intramuscular injection, the ACIP recommends "it should be administered intramuscularly if, in the opinion of the physician familiar with the patients bleeding risk, the vaccine can be administered with reasonable safety by this route. If the patient receives antihemophilia or other similar therapy, intramuscular vaccination can be scheduled shortly after such therapy is administered. A fine needle (23 gauge or smaller) can be used for the vaccination and firm pressure applied to the site (without rubbing) for at least 2 minutes. The patient should be instructed concerning the risk of hematoma from the injection."

Additional Information Inactivated bacteria vaccine. Federal law requires that the date of administration, the vaccine manufacturer, lot number of vaccine, and the administering person's name, title, and address be entered into the patient's permanent medical record.

Dosage Forms Injection, solution: 25 mcg each of 23 polysaccharide isolates/0.5 mL (0.5 mL, 2.5 mL)

Selected Readings

"Preventing Pneumococcal Disease Among Infants and Young Children: Recommendations of the Advisory Committee on Immunization Practices (ACIP), Centers for Disease Control and Prevention," *MMWR*, 2000, 49(RR-9):1-35.

Pneumovax® 23 *see* Pneumococcal Polysaccharide Vaccine (Polyvalent) *on page 1010*

Poliovirus Vaccine (Inactivated)

(POE lee oh VYE rus vak SEEN, in ak ti VAY ted)

Related Information

Immunization Recommendations *on page 1249*

U.S. Brand Names IPOL®

Canadian Brand Names IPOL®

Synonyms Enhanced-potency Inactivated Poliovirus Vaccine; IPV; Salk Vaccine

Generic Available No

Use

As the global eradication of poliomyelitis continues, the risk for importation of wild-type poliovirus into the United States decreases dramatically. To eliminate the risk for vaccine-associated paralytic poliomyelitis (VAPP), an all-IPV schedule is recommended for routine childhood vaccination in the United States. All children should receive four doses of IPV (at age 2 months, age 4 months, between ages 6-18 months, and between ages 4-6 years). Oral poliovirus vaccine (OPV), if available, may be used only for the following special circumstances:

Mass vaccination campaigns to control outbreaks of paralytic polio

Unvaccinated children who will be traveling within 4 weeks to areas where polio is endemic or epidemic

Children of parents who do not accept the recommended number of vaccine injections; these children may receive OPV only for the third or fourth dose or both. In this situation, healthcare providers should administer OPV only after discussing the risk for VAPP with parents or caregivers.

(Continued)

Poliovirus Vaccine (Inactivated) *(Continued)*

OPV supplies are expected to be very limited in the United States after inventories are depleted. ACIP reaffirms its support for the global eradication initiative and use of OPV as the vaccine of choice to eradicate polio where it is endemic.

Pregnancy Risk Factor C

Contraindications Hypersensitivity to any component including neomycin, streptomycin, or polymyxin B; defer vaccination for persons with acute febrile illness until recovery

Warnings/Precautions Although there is no convincing evidence documenting adverse effects of either OPV or E-IPV on the pregnant woman or developing fetus, it is prudent on theoretical grounds to avoid vaccinating pregnant women. However, if immediate protection against poliomyelitis is needed, OPV is recommended. OPV should not be given to immunocompromised individuals or to persons with known or possibly immunocompromised family members; E-IPV is recommended in such situations.

Adverse Reactions All serious adverse reactions must be reported to the U.S. Department of Health and Human Services (DHHS) Vaccine Adverse Event Reporting System (VAERS) 1-800-822-7967.

1% to 10%:

- Central nervous system: Fever (>101.3°F)
- Dermatologic: Rash
- Local: Tenderness or pain at injection site

<1%: Crying, decreased appetite, dyspnea, erythema, fatigue, fussiness, Guillain-Barré, reddening of skin, sleepiness, weakness

Stability Refrigerate

Dosage SubQ: **Enhanced-potency inactivated poliovirus vaccine (E-IPV) is preferred for primary vaccination of adults**, two doses SubQ 4-8 weeks apart, a third dose 6-12 months after the second. For adults with a completed primary series and for whom a booster is indicated, either OPV or E-IPV can be given (E-IPV preferred). If immediate protection is needed, either OPV or E-IPV is recommended.

Administration Do not administer I.V.

Additional Information Federal law requires that the date of administration, the vaccine manufacturer, lot number of vaccine, and the administering person's name, title, and address be entered into the patient's permanent medical record.

Dosage Forms Injection, suspension: Type 1 poliovirus 40 D antigen units/0.5 mL, Type 2 poliovirus 8 D antigen units/0.5 mL, and Type 3 poliovirus 32 D antigen units/0.5 mL (5 mL) [contains calf serum protein, neomycin, streptomycin, and polymyxin B]

Polycidin® Ophthalmic Ointment (Can) *see* Bacitracin and Polymyxin B *on page 681*

Polygam® S/D *see* Immune Globulin (Intravenous) *on page 867*

Polymyxin B (pol i MIKS in bee)

U.S. Brand Names Poly-Rx

Synonyms Polymyxin B Sulfate

Generic Available Yes

Use Treatment of acute infections caused by susceptible strains of *Pseudomonas aeruginosa*; used occasionally for gut decontamination; parenteral use of polymyxin B has mainly been replaced by less toxic antibiotics, reserved for life-threatening infections caused by organisms resistant to the preferred drugs (eg, pseudomonal meningitis - intrathecal administration)

Drug of Choice or Alternative for Disease/Syndrome(s):

Otitis Externa, Mild *on page 252*

Pregnancy Risk Factor B (per expert opinion)

Pregnancy Implications Safety and efficacy for use in pregnant women have not been established.

Contraindications Hypersensitivity to polymyxin B or any component of the formulation; concurrent use of neuromuscular blockers

Warnings/Precautions Use with caution in patients with impaired renal function (modify dosage); polymyxin B-induced nephrotoxicity may be manifested by albuminuria, cellular casts, and azotemia. Discontinue therapy with decreasing urinary output and increasing BUN; neurotoxic reactions are usually associated with high serum levels, often in patients with renal dysfunction. Avoid concurrent or sequential use of other nephrotoxic and neurotoxic drugs (eg, aminoglycosides). The drug's neurotoxicity can result in respiratory paralysis from neuromuscular blockade, especially when the drug is given soon after anesthesia or muscle relaxants. Polymyxin B sulfate is most toxic when given parenterally; avoid parenteral use whenever possible.

Adverse Reactions Frequency not defined.

Cardiovascular: Facial flushing

Central nervous system: Neurotoxicity (irritability, drowsiness, ataxia, perioral paresthesia, numbness of the extremities, and blurred vision); dizziness, drug fever, meningeal irritation with intrathecal administration

Dermatologic: Urticarial rash

Endocrine & metabolic: Hypocalcemia, hyponatremia, hypokalemia, hypochloremia

Local: Pain at injection site

Neuromuscular & skeletal: Neuromuscular blockade, weakness

Renal: Nephrotoxicity

Respiratory: Respiratory arrest

Miscellaneous: Anaphylactoid reaction

Overdosage/Toxicology Symptoms include respiratory paralysis, ototoxicity, and nephrotoxicity. Supportive care is indicated. Ventilatory support may be necessary.

Drug Interactions

Increased Effect/Toxicity: Increased/prolonged effect of neuromuscular blocking agents.

Stability Prior to reconstitution, store at room temperature of 15°C to 30°C (59°F to 86°F); protect from light. After reconstitution, store under refrigeration at 2°C to 8°C (36°F to 46°F); discard any unused solution after 72 hours. **Incompatible** with strong acids/alkalies, calcium, magnesium, cephalothin, cefazolin, chloramphenicol, heparin, penicillins.

Mechanism of Action Binds to phospholipids, alters permeability, and damages the bacterial cytoplasmic membrane permitting leakage of intracellular constituents

Pharmacodynamics/Kinetics

Absorption: Well absorbed from peritoneum; minimal from GI tract (except in neonates) from mucous membranes or intact skin

Distribution: Minimal into CSF; does not cross placenta

Half-life elimination: 4.5-6 hours; prolonged with renal impairment

Time to peak, serum: I.M.: ~2 hours

Excretion: Urine (>60% primarily as unchanged drug)

Dosage

Otic (in combination with other drugs): 1-2 drops, 3-4 times/day; should be used sparingly to avoid accumulation of excess debris

Infants <2 years:

I.M.: Up to 40,000 units/kg/day divided every 6 hours (not routinely recommended due to pain at injection sites)

I.V.: Up to 40,000 units/kg/day divided every 12 hours

Intrathecal: 20,000 units/day for 3-4 days, then 25,000 units every other day for at least 2 weeks after CSF cultures are negative and CSF (glucose) has returned to within normal limits

Children ≥2 years and Adults:

I.M.: 25,000-30,000 units/kg/day divided every 4-6 hours (not routinely recommended due to pain at injection sites)

I.V.: 15,000-25,000 units/kg/day divided every 12 hours

Intrathecal: 50,000 units/day for 3-4 days, then every other day for at least 2 weeks after CSF cultures are negative and CSF (glucose) has returned to within normal limits

Total daily dose should not exceed 2,000,000 units/day

Bladder irrigation: Continuous irrigant or rinse in the urinary bladder for up to 10 days using 20 mg (equal to 200,000 units) added to 1 L of normal saline; usually no more than 1 L of irrigant is used per day unless urine flow rate is high; administration rate is adjusted to patient's urine output

Topical irrigation or topical solution: 500,000 units/L of normal saline; topical irrigation should not exceed 2 million units/day in adults

Gut sterilization: Oral: 15,000-25,000 units/kg/day in divided doses every 6 hours

Clostridium difficile enteritis: Oral: 25,000 units every 6 hours for 10 days

Ophthalmic: A concentration of 0.1% to 0.25% is administered as 1-3 drops every hour, then increasing the interval as response indicates to 1-2 drops 4-6 times/day

Dosing adjustment/interval in renal impairment:

Cl_{cr} 20-50 mL/minute: Administer 75% to 100% of normal dose every 12 hours

Cl_{cr} 5-20 mL/minute: Administer 50% of normal dose every 12 hours

Cl_{cr} <5 mL/minute: Administer 15% of normal dose every 12 hours

Administration Dissolve 500,000 units in 300-500 mL D_5W for continuous I.V. drip; dissolve 500,000 units in 2 mL water for injection, saline, or 1% procaine solution for I.M. injection; dissolve 500,000 units in 10 mL physiologic solution for intrathecal administration

(Continued)

Polymyxin B *(Continued)*

Extravasation management: Monitor I.V. site closely; extravasation may cause serious injury with possible necrosis and tissue sloughing. Rotate infusion site frequently.

Monitoring Parameters Neurologic symptoms and signs of superinfection; renal function (decreasing urine output and increasing BUN may require discontinuance of therapy)

Reference Range Serum concentrations >5 mcg/mL are toxic in adults

Patient Information Report any dizziness or sensations of ringing in the ear, loss of hearing, or any muscle weakness

Additional Information 1 mg = 10,000 units

Dosage Forms

Injection, powder for reconstitution: 500,000 units

Powder [for prescription compounding] (Poly-Rx): 100 million units (13 g)

Polymyxin B and Bacitracin *see* Bacitracin and Polymyxin B *on page 681*

Polymyxin B and Neomycin *see* Neomycin and Polymyxin B *on page 964*

Polymyxin B and Oxytetracycline *see* Oxytetracycline and Polymyxin B *on page 988*

Polymyxin B and Trimethoprim *see* Trimethoprim and Polymyxin B *on page 1131*

Polymyxin B, Bacitracin, and Neomycin *see* Bacitracin, Neomycin, and Polymyxin B *on page 681*

Polymyxin B, Bacitracin, Neomycin, and Hydrocortisone *see* Bacitracin, Neomycin, Polymyxin B, and Hydrocortisone *on page 682*

Polymyxin B, Neomycin, and Dexamethasone *see* Neomycin, Polymyxin B, and Dexamethasone *on page 965*

Polymyxin B, Neomycin, and Gramicidin *see* Neomycin, Polymyxin B, and Gramicidin *on page 965*

Polymyxin B, Neomycin, and Hydrocortisone *see* Neomycin, Polymyxin B, and Hydrocortisone *on page 966*

Polymyxin B, Neomycin, and Prednisolone *see* Neomycin, Polymyxin B, and Prednisolone *on page 967*

Polymyxin B, Neomycin, Bacitracin, and Pramoxine *see* Bacitracin, Neomycin, Polymyxin B, and Pramoxine *on page 683*

Polymyxin B Sulfate *see* Polymyxin B *on page 1012*

Poly-Pred® *see* Neomycin, Polymyxin B, and Prednisolone *on page 967*

Poly-Rx *see* Polymyxin B *on page 1012*

Polysporin® Ophthalmic *see* Bacitracin and Polymyxin B *on page 681*

Polysporin® Topical [OTC] *see* Bacitracin and Polymyxin B *on page 681*

Polytrim® *see* Trimethoprim and Polymyxin B *on page 1131*

Potassium Iodide (poe TASS ee um EYE oh dide)

U.S. Brand Names Iosat™ [OTC]; Pima®; SSKI®; ThyroSafe™ [OTC]; ThyroShield™ [OTC]

Synonyms KI

Use Expectorant for the symptomatic treatment of chronic pulmonary diseases complicated by mucous; reduce thyroid vascularity prior to thyroidectomy and management of thyrotoxic crisis; block thyroidal uptake of radioactive isotopes of iodine in a radiation emergency or other exposure to radioactive iodine

Unlabeled/Investigational Use Lymphocutaneous and cutaneous sporotrichosis

Drug of Choice or Alternative for Organism(s):

Sporothrix schenckii on page 302

Pregnancy Risk Factor D

Pregnancy Implications Iodide crosses the placenta (may cause hypothyroidism and goiter in fetus/newborn). Use as an expectorant during pregnancy is contraindicated by the AAP. Use for protection against thyroid cancer secondary to radioactive iodine exposure is considered acceptable based upon risk/benefit, keeping in mind the dose and duration. Repeat dosing should be avoided if possible.

Contraindications Hypersensitivity to iodine or any component of the formulation; hyperkalemia; pulmonary edema; impaired renal function; hyperthyroidism; iodine-induced goiter; dermatitis herpetiformis; hypocomplementemic vasculitis

Warnings/Precautions Prolonged use can lead to hypothyroidism; cystic fibrosis patients have an exaggerated response; can cause acne flare-ups, can cause dermatitis; use with caution in patients with a history of thyroid disease, Addison's disease, cardiac disease, myotonia congenita, tuberculosis, acute bronchitis

Adverse Reactions Frequency not defined.

Cardiovascular: Irregular heart beat
Central nervous system: Confusion, tiredness, fever
Dermatologic: Skin rash
Endocrine & metabolic: Goiter, salivary gland swelling/tenderness, thyroid adenoma, swelling of neck/throat, myxedema, lymph node swelling, hyper-/hypothyroidism
Gastrointestinal: Diarrhea, gastrointestinal bleeding, metallic taste, nausea, stomach pain, stomach upset, vomiting
Neuromuscular & skeletal: Numbness, tingling, weakness, joint pain
Miscellaneous: Chronic iodine poisoning (with prolonged treatment/high doses); iodism, hypersensitivity reactions (angioedema, cutaneous and mucosal hemorrhage, serum sickness-like symptoms)

Overdosage/Toxicology Symptoms include angioedema, laryngeal edema in patients with hypersensitivity; muscle weakness, paralysis, peaked T waves, flattened P waves, prolongation of QRS complex, ventricular arrhythmias. Removal of potassium can be accomplished by various means such as through the GI tract with Kayexalate® administration, by way of the kidney through diuresis, mineralocorticoid administration or increased sodium intake, by hemodialysis or peritoneal dialysis, or by shifting potassium back into the cells by insulin and glucose infusion.

Drug Interactions

Increased Effect/Toxicity: Lithium may cause additive hypothyroid effects; ACE inhibitors, potassium-sparing diuretics, and potassium/potassium-containing products may lead to hyperkalemia, cardiac arrhythmias, or cardiac arrest

Stability Store at controlled room temperature of 25°C (77°F) excursions permitted to 15°C to 30°C (59°F to 86°F); protect from light, keep tightly closed.

SSKI®: If exposed to cold, crystallization may occur. Warm and shake to redissolve. If solution becomes brown/yellow, it should be discarded. May be mixed in water, fruit juice, or milk.

Preparation of oral solution:

Concentration of 16.25 mg/5 mL oral solution: Crush one 130 mg tablet into a fine powder. Add 20 mL of water and mix until powder is dissolved. Add an additional 20 mL of low-fat milk (white or chocolate), orange juice, flat soda, raspberry syrup or infant formula. Final concentration will be 16.25 mg/5 mL. Stable for 7 days under refrigeration.

Concentration of 8.125 mg/5 mL oral solution: Crush one 65 mg tablet into a fine powder. Add 20 mL of water and mix until powder is dissolved. Add an additional 20 mL of low-fat milk (white or chocolate), orange juice, flat soda, raspberry syrup, or infant formula. Final concentration will be 8.125 mg/5 mL. Stable for 7 days under refrigeration.

Mechanism of Action Reduces viscosity of mucus by increasing respiratory tract secretions; inhibits secretion of thyroid hormone, fosters colloid accumulation in thyroid follicles. Following radioactive iodine exposure, potassium iodide blocks uptake of radioiodine by the thyroid, reducing the risk of thyroid cancer.

Pharmacodynamics/Kinetics

Onset of action: Hyperthyroidism: 24-48 hours
Peak effect: 10-15 days after continuous therapy
Duration: Radioactive iodine exposure: ~ 24 hours

Dosage Oral:

Adults: RDA: 150 mcg (iodine)
Expectorant:
Children (Pima®):
<3 years: 162 mg 3 times day
>3 years: 325 mg 3 times/day
Adults:
Pima®: 325-650 mg 3 times/day
SSKI®: 300-600 mg 3-4 times/day
Preoperative thyroidectomy: Children and Adults: 50-250 mg (1-5 drops SSKI®) 3 times/day; administer for 10 days before surgery
Radiation protectant to radioactive isotopes of iodine (Pima®):
Children:
Infants up to 1 year: 65 mg once daily for 10 days; start 24 hours prior to exposure
>1 year: 130 mg once daily for 10 days; start 24 hours prior to exposure
Adults: 195 mg once daily for 10 days; start 24 hours prior to exposure 7
To reduce risk of thyroid cancer following nuclear accident (Iosat™, ThyroSafe™, ThyroShield™): Dosing should continue until risk of exposure has passed or other measures are implemented:
Children (see adult dose for children >68 kg):
Infants <1 month: 16.25 mg once daily
1 month to 3 years: 32.5 mg once daily
3-18 years: 65 mg once daily
(Continued)

Potassium Iodide *(Continued)*

Children >68 kg and Adults (including pregnant/lactating women): 130 mg once daily

Thyrotoxic crisis:

Infants <1 year: 150-250 mg (3-5 drops SSKI®) 3 times/day

Children and Adults: 300-500 mg (6-10 drops SSKI®) 3 times/day

Sporotrichosis (cutaneous, lymphocutaneous; unlabeled use): Adults: Oral: Initial: 5 drops (SSKI®) 3 times/day; increase to 40-50 drops (SSKI®) 3 times/day as tolerated for 3-6 months

Dietary Considerations SSKI®: Take with food to decrease gastric irritation.

Administration

Pima®: When used as an expectorant, take each dose with at least 4-6 ounces of water

SSKI®: Dilute in a glassful of water, fruit juice or milk. Take with food to decrease gastric irritation

Monitoring Parameters Thyroid function tests, signs/symptoms of hyperthyroidism; thyroid function should be monitored in pregnant women, neonates, and young infants if repeat doses are required following radioactive iodine exposure

Test Interactions May alter thyroid function tests.

Patient Information SSKI®: Take after meals. Dilute in 6 oz of water, fruit juice, or milk. Do not exceed recommended dosage. You may experience a metallic taste. Discontinue use and report stomach pain, severe nausea or vomiting, black or tarry stools, or unresolved weakness.

Additional Information 10 drops of SSKI® = potassium iodide 500 mg

Dosage Forms

Solution, oral:

SSKI®: 1 g/mL (30 mL, 240 mL) [contains sodium thiosulfate]

ThyroShield™: 65 mg/mL (30 mL) [black raspberry flavor]

Syrup (Pima®): 325 mg/5 mL (473 mL) [equivalent to iodide 249 mg/5 mL; black raspberry flavor]

Tablet:

Iosat™: 130 mg

ThyroSafe™: 65 mg [equivalent to iodine 50 mg]

Extemporaneous Preparations Preparation of oral solution:

Concentration of 16.25 mg/5 mL oral solution: Crush one 130 mg tablet into a fine powder. Add 20 mL of water and mix until powder is dissolved. Add an additional 20 mL of low-fat milk (white or chocolate), orange juice, flat soda, raspberry syrup or infant formula. Final concentration will be 16.25 mg/5 mL.

Concentration of 8.125 mg/5 mL oral solution: Crush one 65 mg tablet into a fine powder. Add 20 mL of water and mix until powder is dissolved. Add an additional 20 mL of low-fat milk (white or chocolate), orange juice, flat soda, raspberry syrup, or infant formula. Final concentration will be 8.125 mg/5 mL.

Povidone-Iodine (POE vi done EYE oh dyne)

U.S. Brand Names ACU-dyne® [OTC]; Betadine® [OTC]; Betadine® Ophthalmic; Minidyne® [OTC]; Operand® [OTC]; Summer's Eve® Medicated Douche [OTC]; Vagi-Gard® [OTC]

Canadian Brand Names Betadine®; Proviodine

Generic Available Yes

Use External antiseptic with broad microbicidal spectrum against bacteria, fungi, viruses, protozoa, and yeasts

Pregnancy Risk Factor D

Contraindications Hypersensitivity to iodine or any component of the formulation; pregnancy

Warnings/Precautions Highly toxic if ingested; sodium thiosulfate is the most effective chemical antidote; avoid contact with eyes; use with caution in infants and nursing women

Adverse Reactions

1% to 10%:

Dermatologic: Rash, pruritus

Local: Local edema

<1%: Systemic absorption in extensive burns causing iododerma, metabolic acidosis, renal impairment

Mechanism of Action Povidone-iodine is known to be a powerful broad spectrum germicidal agent effective against a wide range of bacteria, viruses, fungi, protozoa, and spores.

Pharmacodynamics/Kinetics Absorption: Topical: Healthy volunteers: Little systemic absorption; Vaginal: Rapid, serum concentrations of total iodine and inorganic iodide are increased significantly

Dosage

Shampoo: Apply 2 teaspoons to hair and scalp, lather and rinse; repeat application 2 times/week until improvement is noted, then shampoo weekly

Topical: Apply as needed for treatment and prevention of susceptible microbial infections

Patient Information Do not swallow; avoid contact with eyes

Dosage Forms

- Gel, topical (Operand®): 10% (120 g)
- Liquid, topical: 7.5% (120 mL)
  - ACU-dyne®: 7.5% (60 mL, 240 mL, 480 mL, 960 mL, 3840 mL)
  - Betadine®: 7.5% (120 mL)
- Liquid, topical scrub: 7.5% (120 mL)
  - Betadine®: 7.5% (120 mL, 480 mL, 960 mL, 3840 mL)
  - Operand®: 7.5% (960 mL)
- Ointment, topical: 10% (1 g, 3.5 g, 30 g)
  - Betadine®: 10% (0.9 g, 3.7 g, 30 g)
- Pad [prep pads]: 10% (200s)
- Solution, ophthalmic (Betadine®): 5% (50 mL)
- Solution, perineal (Betadine®, Operand®): 10% (240 mL)
- Solution, topical: 10% (30 mL, 120 mL, 240 mL, 480 mL, 3840 mL)
  - Betadine®: 10% (15 mL, 120 mL, 240 mL, 480 mL, 960 mL, 3840 mL)
  - Minidyne®: 10% (15 mL)
  - Operand®: 10% (60 mL, 120 mL, 240 mL, 480 mL, 960 mL, 3840 mL)
- Solution, topical scrub: 7.5% (120 mL, 240 mL, 480 mL, 3840 mL)
  - Operand®: 7.5% (60 mL, 120 mL, 240 mL, 480 mL, 960 mL, 3840 mL)
- Solution, topical spray (Betadine®): 5% (90 mL)
- Solution, vaginal douche: 10% (240 mL) [concentrate]
  - Betadine®: 10% (180 mL, 240 mL) [concentrate]
  - Operand®: 10% (240 mL) [concentrate]
  - Summer's Eve® Medicated Douche: 0.3% (135 mL)
  - Vagi-Gard®: 10% (240 mL) [concentrate]
- Solution, whirlpool: 10% (3840 mL) [concentrate]
  - Operand®: 1% (3840 mL)
- Swabsticks: 7.5% (25s, 50s); 10% (25s, 50s)
  - Betadine®: 10% (50s, 150s, 200s, 1000s)

PPD *see* Tuberculin Tests *on page 1136*

PPV23 *see* Pneumococcal Polysaccharide Vaccine (Polyvalent) *on page 1010*

Pramoxine, Neomycin, Bacitracin, and Polymyxin B *see* Bacitracin, Neomycin, Polymyxin B, and Pramoxine *on page 683*

Praziquantel (pray zi KWON tel)

U.S. Brand Names Biltricide®

Canadian Brand Names Biltricide®

Generic Available No

Use All stages of schistosomiasis caused by all *Schistosoma* species pathogenic to humans; clonorchiasis and opisthorchiasis

Unlabeled/Investigational Use Cysticercosis and many intestinal tapeworms

Drug of Choice or Alternative for Organism(s):

Cestodes *on page 72*

Schistosoma mansoni on page 294

Pregnancy Risk Factor B

Contraindications Hypersensitivity to praziquantel or any component of the formulation; ocular cysticercosis

Warnings/Precautions Use caution in patients with severe hepatic disease; patients with cerebral cysticercosis require hospitalization

Adverse Reactions

1% to 10%:

- Central nervous system: Dizziness, drowsiness, headache, malaise, CSF reaction syndrome in patients being treated for neurocysticercosis
- Gastrointestinal: Abdominal pain, loss of appetite, nausea, vomiting
- Miscellaneous: Diaphoresis

<1%: Diarrhea, fever, itching, rash, urticaria

(Continued)

Praziquantel *(Continued)*

Overdosage/Toxicology Symptoms include dizziness, drowsiness, headache, and liver function impairment. Treatment is supportive following GI decontamination. Administer fast-acting laxative.

Drug Interactions

Cytochrome P450 Effect: Inhibits CYP2D6 (weak)

Mechanism of Action Increases the cell permeability to calcium in schistosomes, causing strong contractions and paralysis of worm musculature leading to detachment of suckers from the blood vessel walls and to dislodgment

Pharmacodynamics/Kinetics

Absorption: Oral: ~80%

Distribution: CSF concentration is 14% to 20% of plasma concentration; enters breast milk

Protein binding: ~80%

Metabolism: Extensive first-pass effect

Half-life elimination: Parent drug: 0.8-1.5 hours; Metabolites: 4.5 hours

Time to peak, serum: 1-3 hours

Excretion: Urine (99% as metabolites)

Dosage Children >4 years and Adults: Oral:

Schistosomiasis: 20 mg/kg/dose 2-3 times/day for 1 day at 4- to 6-hour intervals

Flukes (unlabeled use): 25 mg/kg/dose every 8 hours for 1-2 days

Cysticercosis (unlabeled use): 50 mg/kg/day divided every 8 hours for 14 days

Tapeworms (unlabeled use): 10-20 mg/kg as a single dose (25 mg/kg for *Hymenolepis nana*)

Clonorchiasis/opisthorchiasis: 3 doses of 25 mg/kg as a 1-day treatment

Patient Information Do not chew tablets due to bitter taste; take with food; caution should be used when performing tasks requiring mental alertness, may impair judgment and coordination

Dosage Forms Tablet [tri-scored]: 600 mg

Selected Readings

de Silva N, Guyatt H, and Bundy D, "Anthelmintics. A Comparative Review of Their Clinical Pharmacology," *Drugs*, 1997, 53(5):769-88.

"Drugs for Parasitic Infections," *Med Lett Drugs Ther*, 1998, 40(1017):1-12.

Pred-G® *see* Prednisolone and Gentamicin *on page 1018*

Prednisolone and Gentamicin (pred NIS oh lone & jen ta MYE sin)

Related Information

Gentamicin *on page 841*

U.S. Brand Names Pred-G®

Synonyms Gentamicin and Prednisolone

Generic Available No

Use Treatment of steroid responsive inflammatory conditions and superficial ocular infections due to microorganisms susceptible to gentamicin

Pregnancy Risk Factor C

Contraindications Hypersensitivity to gentamicin, prednisolone, other aminoglycosides or corticosteroids, or any component of the formulation; viral disease of the cornea and conjunctiva (including epithelia herpes simplex keratitis, vaccinia, varicella); mycobacterial or fungal infection of the eye; uncomplicated removal of a corneal foreign body

Warnings/Precautions Prolonged use of corticosteroids may result in glaucoma; damage to the optic nerve, defects in visual acuity and fields of vision, and posterior subcapsular cataract formation may occur. Prolonged use of corticosteroids may increase the incidence of secondary ocular infection or mask acute infection (including fungal infections); may prolong or exacerbate ocular viral infections; use following cataract surgery may delay healing or increase the incidence of bleb formation.

Adverse Reactions Frequency not defined.

Dermatologic: Delayed wound healing

Local: Burning, stinging

Ocular: Intraocular pressure increased, glaucoma, superficial punctate keratitis, optic nerve damage (infrequent), posterior subcapsular cataract formation

Miscellaneous: Secondary infection

Drug Interactions

Cytochrome P450 Effect: Prednisolone: **Substrate** of CYP3A4 (minor); **Inhibits** CYP3A4 (weak)

Pharmacodynamics/Kinetics See individual agents.

Dosage Ophthalmic: Children and Adults:

Ointment: Apply ½ inch ribbon in the conjunctival sac 1-3 times/day

Suspension: 1 drop 2-4 times/day; during the initial 24-48 hours, the dosing frequency may be increased if necessary up to 1 drop every hour

Administration Ophthalmic:

Ointment: For topical application into the conjunctival sac

Suspension: For topical application to the eye only; shake suspension well before using; do not inject subconjunctivally or introduce into the anterior chamber of the eye

Patient Information Shake suspension well; to avoid contamination, do not touch tip of container to any surface

Dosage Forms

Ointment, ophthalmic: Prednisolone acetate 0.6% and gentamicin sulfate 0.3% (3.5 g)

Suspension, ophthalmic: Prednisolone acetate 1% and gentamicin sulfate 0.3% (2 mL, 5 mL, 10 mL) [contains benzalkonium chloride]

Prednisolone and Sulfacetamide *see* Sulfacetamide and Prednisolone *on page 1082*

Prednisolone, Neomycin, and Polymyxin B *see* Neomycin, Polymyxin B, and Prednisolone *on page 967*

Prevnar® *see* Pneumococcal Conjugate Vaccine (7-Valent) *on page 1008*

Prevpac® *see* Lansoprazole, Amoxicillin, and Clarithromycin *on page 908*

Priftin® *see* Rifapentine *on page 1051*

Primaquine (PRIM a kween)

Related Information

Malaria Treatment *on page 1292*

Synonyms Primaquine Phosphate; Prymaccone

Generic Available Yes

Use Treatment of malaria

Unlabeled/Investigational Use Prevention of malaria; treatment *Pneumocystis carinii* pneumonia

Pregnancy Risk Factor C

Contraindications Hypersensitivity to primaquine, similar alkaloids, or any component of the formulation; acutely ill patients who have a tendency to develop granulocytopenia (rheumatoid arthritis, SLE); patients receiving other drugs capable of depressing the bone marrow (eg, quinacrine and primaquine)

Warnings/Precautions Use with caution in patients with G6PD deficiency, NADH methemoglobin reductase deficiency; do not exceed recommended dosage

Adverse Reactions Frequency not defined.

Cardiovascular: Arrhythmias

Central nervous system: Headache

Dermatologic: Pruritus

Gastrointestinal: Abdominal pain, nausea, vomiting

Hematologic: Agranulocytosis, hemolytic anemia in G6PD deficiency, leukopenia, leukocytosis, methemoglobinemia in NADH-methemoglobin reductase-deficient individuals

Ocular: Interference with visual accommodation

Overdosage/Toxicology Symptoms of acute overdose include abdominal cramps, vomiting, cyanosis, methemoglobinemia (possibly severe), leukopenia, acute hemolytic anemia (often significant), and granulocytopenia. With chronic overdose, symptoms include ototoxicity and retinopathy. Following GI decontamination, treatment is supportive (fluids, anticonvulsants, blood transfusions, methylene blue if methemoglobinemia is severe - 1-2 mg/kg over several minutes).

Drug Interactions

Cytochrome P450 Effect: Substrate of CYP3A4 (major); **Inhibits** CYP1A2 (strong), 2D6 (weak), 3A4 (weak); **Induces** CYP1A2 (weak)

Increased Effect/Toxicity: Increased toxicity/levels with quinacrine. Primaquine may increase the levels/effects of aminophylline, fluvoxamine, mexiletine, mirtazapine, ropinirole, theophylline, trifluoperazine, and other CYP1A2 substrates.

Decreased Effect: The levels/effects of primaquine may be decreased by aminoglutethimide, carbamazepine, nafcillin, nevirapine, phenobarbital, phenytoin, rifamycins, and other CYP3A4 inducers.

Ethanol/Nutrition/Herb Interactions Ethanol: Avoid ethanol (due to GI irritation).

Mechanism of Action Eliminates the primary tissue exoerythrocytic forms of *P. falciparum*; disrupts mitochondria and binds to DNA

Pharmacodynamics/Kinetics

Absorption: Well absorbed

Metabolism: Hepatic to carboxyprimaquine (active)

Half-life elimination: 3.7-9.6 hours

Time to peak, serum: 1-2 hours

(Continued)

Primaquine *(Continued)*

Excretion: Urine (small amounts as unchanged drug)

Dosage Oral: Dosage expressed as mg of base (15 mg base = 26.3 mg primaquine phosphate)

Treatment of malaria (decrease risk of delayed primary attacks and prevent relapse):

Children: 0.3 mg base/kg/day once daily for 14 days (not to exceed 15 mg/day) or 0.9 mg base/kg once weekly for 8 weeks not to exceed 45 mg base/week

Adults: 15 mg/day (base) once daily for 14 days or 45 mg base once weekly for 8 weeks

CDC treatment recommendations: Begin therapy during last 2 weeks of, or following a course of, suppression with chloroquine or a comparable drug

Note: A second course (30 mg/day) for 14 days may be required in patients with relapse. Higher initial doses (30 mg/day) have also been used following exposure in S.E. Asia or Somalia.

Prevention of malaria (unlabeled use): Initiate prior to travel and continue for 7 days after departure from malaria-endemic area:

Children: 0.5 mg/kg once daily

Adults: 30 mg once daily

Pneumocystis carinii pneumonia (unlabeled use): Adults: 30 mg once daily for 21 days (in conjunction with clindamycin)

Administration Take with meals to decrease adverse GI effects. Drug has a bitter taste.

Monitoring Parameters Periodic CBC, visual color check of urine, glucose, electrolytes; if hemolysis suspected, monitor CBC, haptoglobin, peripheral smear, urinalysis dipstick for occult blood

Patient Information Take with meals to decrease adverse GI effects; drug has a bitter taste; report if darkening of urine occurs or if shortness of breath, weakness or skin discoloration (chocolate cyanosis) occurs; complete full course of therapy

Dosage Forms Tablet, as phosphate: 26.3 mg [15 mg base]

Selected Readings

Panisko DM and Keystone JS, "Treatment of Malaria - 1990," *Drugs*, 1990, 39(2):160-89.
White NJ, "The Treatment of Malaria," *N Engl J Med*, 1996, 335(11):800-6.
Wyler DJ, "Malaria Chemoprophylaxis for the Traveler," *N Engl J Med*, 1993, 329(1):31-7.

Primaquine Phosphate *see* Primaquine *on page 1019*
Primaxin® *see* Imipenem and Cilastatin *on page 861*
Primsol® *see* Trimethoprim *on page 1130*
Principen® *see* Ampicillin *on page 657*
Priorix™ (Can) *see* Measles, Mumps, and Rubella Vaccines (Combined) *on page 926*
Pristinamycin *see* Quinupristin and Dalfopristin *on page 1032*
Procaine Benzylpenicillin *see* Penicillin G Procaine *on page 995*
Procaine Penicillin G *see* Penicillin G Procaine *on page 995*
Proguanil and Atovaquone *see* Atovaquone and Proguanil *on page 672*
Proloprim® *see* Trimethoprim *on page 1130*
Pronto® Complete Lice Killing Kit [OTC] *see* Pyrethrins and Piperonyl Butoxide *on page 1023*
Pronto® Lice Control (Can) *see* Pyrethrins and Piperonyl Butoxide *on page 1023*
Pronto® Plus Hair and Scalp Masque [OTC] *see* Pyrethrins and Piperonyl Butoxide *on page 1023*
Pronto® Plus Mousse [OTC] *see* Pyrethrins and Piperonyl Butoxide *on page 1023*
Pronto® Plus Warm Oil Treatment and Conditioner [OTC] *see* Pyrethrins and Piperonyl Butoxide *on page 1023*
Pronto® Plus with Natural Extracts and Oils [OTC] *see* Pyrethrins and Piperonyl Butoxide *on page 1023*
Propylene Glycol Diacetate, Acetic Acid, and Hydrocortisone *see* Acetic Acid, Propylene Glycol Diacetate, and Hydrocortisone *on page 629*
Propylene Glycol Diacetate, Hydrocortisone, and Acetic Acid *see* Acetic Acid, Propylene Glycol Diacetate, and Hydrocortisone *on page 629*
Proquin® XR *see* Ciprofloxacin *on page 742*

Protease Inhibitors

Refer to

Amprenavir *on page 662*
Atazanavir *on page 668*
Fosamprenavir *on page 827*
Indinavir *on page 872*
Lopinavir and Ritonavir *on page 919*
Nelfinavir *on page 960*

Ritonavir *on page 1055*
Saquinavir *on page 1060*
Tipranavir *on page 1120*

Protein C (Activated), Human, Recombinant *see* Drotrecogin Alfa *on page 793*
Protropine® (Can) *see* Somatropin *on page 1069*
Proviodine (Can) *see* Povidone-Iodine *on page 1016*
PRP-OMP *see Haemophilus* b Conjugate Vaccine *on page 848*
PRP-T *see Haemophilus* b Conjugate Vaccine *on page 848*
Prymaccone *see* Primaquine *on page 1019*
23PS *see* Pneumococcal Polysaccharide Vaccine (Polyvalent) *on page 1010*
Pseudomonic Acid A *see* Mupirocin *on page 953*
Purified Chick Embryo Cell *see* Rabies Virus Vaccine *on page 1034*
PVF® K (Can) *see* Penicillin V Potassium *on page 998*

Pyrantel Pamoate (pi RAN tel PAM oh ate)

U.S. Brand Names Pamix™ [OTC]; Pin-X® [OTC]; Reese's® Pinworm Medicine [OTC]
Canadian Brand Names Combantrin™
Generic Available No
Use Treatment of pinworms (*Enterobius vermicularis*) and roundworms (*Ascaris lumbricoides*)
Unlabeled/Investigational Use Treatment of whipworms (*Trichuris trichiura*) and hookworms (*Ancylostoma duodenale*)
Drug of Choice or Alternative for Organism(s):
Ancylostoma duodenale on page 34
Ascaris on page 37
Enterobius vermicularis on page 133
Pregnancy Risk Factor C
Contraindications Hypersensitivity to pyrantel pamoate or any component of the formulation
Warnings/Precautions Use with caution in patients with liver impairment, anemia, malnutrition, or pregnancy. Since pinworm infections are easily spread to others, treat all family members in close contact with the patient.
Adverse Reactions Frequency not defined.
Central nervous system: Dizziness, drowsiness, insomnia, headache
Dermatologic: Rash
Gastrointestinal: Anorexia, nausea, vomiting, abdominal cramps, diarrhea, tenesmus
Hepatic: Elevated liver enzymes
Neuromuscular & skeletal: Weakness
Overdosage/Toxicology Symptoms include anorexia, nausea, vomiting, cramps, diarrhea, and ataxia. Treatment is supportive following GI decontamination.
Drug Interactions
Decreased Effect: Decreased effect with piperazine
Stability Protect from light
Mechanism of Action Causes the release of acetylcholine and inhibits cholinesterase; acts as a depolarizing neuromuscular blocker, paralyzing the helminths
Pharmacodynamics/Kinetics
Absorption: Oral: Poor
Metabolism: Partially hepatic
Time to peak, serum: 1-3 hours
Excretion: Feces (50% as unchanged drug); urine (7% as unchanged drug)
Dosage Children and Adults (purgation is not required prior to use): Oral:
Roundworm, pinworm, or trichostrongyliasis: 11 mg/kg administered as a single dose; maximum dose: 1 g. (**Note:** For pinworm infection, dosage should be repeated in 2 weeks and all family members should be treated).
Hookworm (unlabeled use): 11 mg/kg administered once daily for 3 days
Administration May be mixed with milk or fruit juice
Monitoring Parameters Stool for presence of eggs, worms, and occult blood, serum AST and ALT
Patient Information May mix drug with milk or fruit juice; strict hygiene is essential to prevent reinfection
Dosage Forms
Suspension, oral as pamoate:
Pamix™: 144 mg/mL (30 mL, 60 mL, 240 mL) [equivalent to pyrantel base 50 mg/mL; contains sodium benzoate]
Pin-X®: 144 mg/mL (30 mL, 60 mL) [equivalent to pyrantel base 50 mg/mL; contains sodium benzoate; caramel flavor]
(Continued)

Pyrantel Pamoate *(Continued)*

Reese's® Pinworm Medicine: 144 mg/mL (30 mL) [equivalent to pyrantel base 50 mg/mL]

Tablet, as pamoate (Reese's® Pinworm Medicine): 180 mg [equivalent to pyrantel base 62.5 mg/tablet]

Selected Readings

"Drugs for Parasitic Infections," *Med Lett Drugs Ther*, 1998, 40(1017):1-12.

Pyrazinamide (peer a ZIN a mide)

Related Information

Tuberculosis *on page 1315*

Canadian Brand Names Tebrazid™

Synonyms Pyrazinoic Acid Amide

Generic Available Yes

Use Adjunctive treatment of tuberculosis in combination with other antituberculosis agents

Drug of Choice or Alternative for Organism(s):

Mycobacterium tuberculosis on page 234

Pregnancy Risk Factor C

Contraindications Hypersensitivity to pyrazinamide or any component of the formulation; acute gout; severe hepatic damage

Warnings/Precautions Use with caution in patients with renal failure, chronic gout, diabetes mellitus, or porphyria. Use with caution in patients receiving concurrent medications associated with hepatotoxicity (particularly with rifampin), or in patients with a history of alcoholism (even if ethanol consumption is discontinued during therapy).

Adverse Reactions

1% to 10%:

- Central nervous system: Malaise
- Gastrointestinal: Nausea, vomiting, anorexia
- Neuromuscular & skeletal: Arthralgia, myalgia

<1%: Acne, angioedema (rare), anticoagulant effect, dysuria, fever, gout, hepatotoxicity, interstitial nephritis, itching, photosensitivity, porphyria, rash, sideroblastic anemia, thrombocytopenia, urticaria

Overdosage/Toxicology Symptoms include gout, gastric upset, and hepatic damage (mild). Treatment following GI decontamination is supportive.

Drug Interactions

Increased Effect/Toxicity: Combination therapy with rifampin and pyrazinamide has been associated with severe and fatal hepatotoxic reactions.

Mechanism of Action Converted to pyrazinoic acid in susceptible strains of *Mycobacterium* which lowers the pH of the environment; exact mechanism of action has not been elucidated

Pharmacodynamics/Kinetics Bacteriostatic or bactericidal depending on drug's concentration at infection site

Absorption: Well absorbed

Distribution: Widely into body tissues and fluids including liver, lung, and CSF

- Relative diffusion from blood into CSF: Adequate with or without inflammation (exceeds usual MICs)
- CSF:blood level ratio: Inflamed meninges: 100%

Protein binding: 50%

Metabolism: Hepatic

Half-life elimination: 9-10 hours

Time to peak, serum: Within 2 hours

Excretion: Urine (4% as unchanged drug)

Dosage Oral: Treatment of tuberculosis:

Note: Used as part of a multidrug regimen. Treatment regimens consist of an initial 2-month phase, followed by a continuation phase of 4 or 7 additional months; frequency of dosing may differ depending on phase of therapy.

Children:

- Daily therapy: 15-30 mg/kg/day (maximum: 2 g/day)
- Twice weekly directly observed therapy (DOT): 50 mg/kg/dose (maximum: 4 g/dose)

Adults (dosing is based on lean body weight):

- Daily therapy: 15-30 mg/kg/day
  - 40-55 kg: 1000 mg
  - 56-75 kg: 1500 mg
  - 76-90 kg: 2000 mg (maximum dose regardless of weight)

Twice weekly directly observed therapy (DOT): 50 mg/kg
40-55 kg: 2000 mg
56-75 kg: 3000 mg
76-90 kg: 4000 mg (maximum dose regardless of weight)
Three times/week DOT: 25-30 mg/kg (maximum: 2.5 g)
40-55 kg: 1500 mg
56-75 kg: 2500 mg
76-90 kg: 3000 mg (maximum dose regardless of weight)

Elderly: Start with a lower daily dose (15 mg/kg) and increase as tolerated.

Dosing adjustment in renal impairment: Cl_{cr} <50 mL/minute: Avoid use or reduce dose to 12-20 mg/kg/day

Avoid use in hemo- and peritoneal dialysis as well as continuous arteriovenous or venovenous hemofiltration.

Dosing adjustment in hepatic impairment: Reduce dose

Monitoring Parameters Periodic liver function tests, serum uric acid, sputum culture, chest x-ray 2-3 months into treatment and at completion

Test Interactions Reacts with Acetest® and Ketostix® to produce pinkish-brown color

Patient Information Report fever, loss of appetite, malaise, nausea, vomiting, darkened urine, pale stools; do not stop taking without consulting a physician

Dosage Forms Tablet: 500 mg

Extemporaneous Preparations Pyrazinamide suspension can be compounded with simple syrup or 0.5% methylcellulose with simple syrup at a concentration of 100 mg/mL; the suspension is stable for 2 months at 4°C or 25°C when stored in glass or plastic bottles

To prepare pyrazinamide suspension in 0.5% methylcellulose with simple syrup: Crush 200 pyrazinamide 500 mg tablets and mix with a suspension containing 500 mL of 1% methylcellulose and 500 mL simple syrup. Add to this a suspension containing 140 crushed pyrazinamide tablets in 350 mL of 1% methylcellulose and 350 mL of simple syrup to make 1.7 L of suspension containing pyrazinamide 100 mg/mL in 0.5% methylcellulose with simple syrup.

Nahata MC, Morosco RS, and Peritre SP, "Stability of Pyrazinamide in Two Suspensions," *Am J Health Syst Pharm*, 1995, 52:1558-60.

Selected Readings

Davidson PT and Le HQ, "Drug Treatment of Tuberculosis - 1992," *Drugs*, 1992, 43(5):651-73.
"Drugs for Tuberculosis," *Med Lett Drugs Ther*, 1993, 35(908):99-101.
Havlir DV and Barnes PF, "Tuberculosis in Patients With Human Immunodeficiency Virus Infection," *N Engl J Med*, 1999, 340(5):367-73.
Iseman MD, "Treatment of Multidrug-Resistant Tuberculosis," *N Engl J Med*, 1993, 329(11):784-91.
"Prevention and Treatment of Tuberculosis Among Patients Infected With Human Immunodeficiency Virus: Principles of Therapy and Revised Recommendations. Centers for Disease Control and Prevention," *MMWR*, 1998, 47(RR-20):1-58.
Van Scoy RE and Wilkowske CJ, "Antituberculous Agents," *Mayo Clin Proc*, 1992, 67(2):179-87.

Pyrazinamide, Rifampin, and Isoniazid *see* Rifampin, Isoniazid, and Pyrazinamide *on page 1050*

Pyrazinoic Acid Amide *see* Pyrazinamide *on page 1022*

Pyrethrins and Piperonyl Butoxide

(pye RE thrins & pi PER oh nil byo TOKS ide)

U.S. Brand Names A-200® Maximum Strength [OTC]; Lice-Aid [OTC]; Licide® [OTC]; Pronto® Complete Lice Killing Kit [OTC]; Pronto® Plus Hair and Scalp Masque [OTC]; Pronto® Plus Mousse [OTC]; Pronto® Plus Warm Oil Treatment and Conditioner [OTC]; Pronto® Plus with Natural Extracts and Oils [OTC]; Pyrinyl Plus® [OTC]; RID® Maximum Strength [OTC]; Tisit® [OTC]; Tisit® Blue Gel [OTC]

Canadian Brand Names Pronto® Lice Control; R & C™ II; R & C™ Shampoo/Conditioner; RID® Mousse

Synonyms Piperonyl Butoxide and Pyrethrins

Generic Available Yes: Shampoo

Use Treatment of *Pediculus humanus* infestations (head lice, body lice, pubic lice and their eggs)

Drug of Choice or Alternative for Organism(s):

Lice *on page 207*

Pregnancy Risk Factor C

Contraindications Hypersensitivity to pyrethrins, ragweed, chrysanthemums, or any component of the formulation

Warnings/Precautions For external use only; do not use near the eye, in eyelashes or eyebrows. Avoid contact with mucosal tissues (nasal, oral, or genital).

Adverse Reactions Frequency not defined.

Dermatologic: Pruritus

(Continued)

Pyrethrins and Piperonyl Butoxide *(Continued)*

Local: Burning, stinging, irritation with repeat use

Stability Store at room temperature of 20°C to 25°C (68°F to 77°F); do not puncture or incinerate mousse container

Mechanism of Action Pyrethrins are derived from flowers that belong to the chrysanthemum family. The mechanism of action on the neuronal membranes of lice is similar to that of DDT. Piperonyl butoxide is usually added to pyrethrin to enhance the product's activity by decreasing the metabolism of pyrethrins in arthropods.

Pharmacodynamics/Kinetics

Onset of action: ~30 minutes

Absorption: Minimal

Metabolism: Via ester hydrolysis and hydroxylation

Dosage Application of pyrethrins:

Topical products:

Apply enough solution to completely wet infested area, including hair

Allow to remain on area for 10 minutes

Wash and rinse with large amounts of warm water.

Use fine-toothed comb to remove lice and eggs from hair

Shampoo hair to restore body and luster

Treatment may be repeated if necessary once in a 24-hour period

Repeat treatment in 7-10 days to kill newly hatched lice

Note: Keep out of eyes when rinsing hair; protect eyes with a wash cloth or towel

Solution for furniture, bedding: Spray on entire area to be treated; allow to dry before use. Intended for use on items which cannot be laundered or dry cleaned. **Not for use on humans or animals.**

Administration For external use only; avoid touching eyes, mouth, or other mucous membranes.

Patient Information For external use only; avoid touching eyes, mouth, or other mucous membranes; do not use in eyelashes or eyebrows; contact prescriber if irritation occurs or if condition does not improve in 2-3 days

Dosage Forms

Cream, topical (Pronto® Plus Hair and Scalp Masque): Pyrethrins 0.33% and piperonyl butoxide 4% (60 g) [green cream shampoo; contains coconut and sesame oil; apple herb scent; packaged with nit removal comb]

Foam, topical [mousse] (RID® Maximum Strength): Pyrethrins 0.33% and piperonyl butoxide 4% (156 g) [packaged with nit removal comb]

Gel (Tisit® Blue Gel): Pyrethrins 0.33% and piperonyl butoxide 3% (30 g)

Liquid, topical (Tisit®): Pyrethrins 0.33% and piperonyl butoxide 2% (60 mL, 120 mL) [packaged with nit removal comb]

Oil, topical (Pronto® Plus Warm Oil Treatment and Conditioner): Pyrethrins 0.33% and piperonyl butoxide 4% (36 mL) [fruity herbal scent; packaged with nit removal comb]

Shampoo: Pyrethrins 0.33% and piperonyl butoxide 4% (60 mL, 120 mL)

A-200® Maximum Strength: Pyrethrins 0.33% and piperonyl butoxide 4% (60 mL, 120 mL) [contains benzyl alcohol; packaged with nit removal comb]

Lice-Aid: Pyrethrins 0.33% and piperonyl butoxide 4% (120 mL)

Licide®: Pyrethrins 0.33% and piperonyl butoxide 4% (120 mL) [packaged with nit removal comb; also available in a kit containing shampoo, household spray and nit removal comb]

Pronto® Complete Lice Killing kit: Pyrethrins 0.33% and piperonyl butoxide 4% (120 mL) [contains benzyl alcohol; packaged in a kit containing shampoo, creme rinse, hair separators, nit removal comb, magnifying glass, and furniture spray]

Pronto® Plus Mousse: Pyrethrins 0.33% and piperonyl butoxide 4% (120 mL) [blue mousse shampoo; contains vitamin E; packaged with nit removal comb]

Pronto® Plus with Natural Extracts and Oils: Pyrethrins 0.33% and piperonyl butoxide 4% (60 mL) [orange scent; packaged with metal nit removal comb; also available in a kit packaged with lice/egg remover and household spray]

Pyrinyl Plus®: Pyrethrins 0.33% and piperonyl butoxide 4% (60 mL) [contains benzyl alcohol; packaged with nit removal comb]

RID® Maximum Strength: Pyrethrins 0.33% and piperonyl butoxide 4% (60 mL, 120 mL, 180 mL, 240 mL) [packaged with nit removal comb; also available in a kit containing shampoo, gel, and furniture spray]

Tisit®: Pyrethrins 0.33% and piperonyl butoxide 3% (60 mL, 120 mL) [also available in a kit containing shampoo, nit removal comb, and furniture spray]

Solution, spray [for furniture, garments, bedding; not for human or animal use] (Tisit®): Pyrethrins 0.4% and piperonyl butoxide 2% (150 mL)

Selected Readings

"Drugs for Parasitic Infections," *Med Lett Drugs Ther*, 1998, 40(1017):1-12.

Liu LX and Weller PF, "Antiparasitic Drugs," *N Engl J Med*, 1996, 334(18):1178-84.

Pyrimethamine (peer i METH a meen)

Related Information

USPHS / IDSA Guidelines for the Prevention of Opportunistic Infections in Persons Infected With HIV *on page 1237*

U.S. Brand Names Daraprim®

Canadian Brand Names Daraprim®

Generic Available No

Use Prophylaxis of malaria due to susceptible strains of plasmodia; used in conjunction with quinine and sulfadiazine for the treatment of uncomplicated attacks of chloroquine-resistant *P. falciparum* malaria; used in conjunction with fast-acting schizonticide to initiate transmission control and suppression cure; synergistic combination with sulfonamide in treatment of toxoplasmosis

Drug of Choice or Alternative for Disease/Syndrome(s):

Brain Abscess *on page 58*

Organism(s):

Toxoplasma gondii on page 331

Pregnancy Risk Factor C

Pregnancy Implications There are no adequate or well-controlled studies in pregnant women. Teratogenicity has been reported in animal studies. If administered during pregnancy (ie, for toxoplasmosis), supplementation of folate is strongly recommended. Pregnancy should be avoided during therapy.

Contraindications Hypersensitivity to pyrimethamine or any component of the formulation; chloroguanide; resistant malaria; megaloblastic anemia secondary to folate deficiency

Warnings/Precautions When used for more than 3-4 days, it may be advisable to administer leucovorin to prevent hematologic complications; monitor CBC and platelet counts every 2 weeks; use with caution in patients with impaired renal or hepatic function or with possible G6PD. Use caution in patients with seizure disorders or possible folate deficiency (eg, malabsorption syndrome, pregnancy, alcoholism).

Adverse Reactions Frequency not defined.

Cardiovascular: Arrhythmias (large doses)

Central nervous system: Depression, fever, insomnia, lightheadedness, malaise, seizure

Dermatologic: Abnormal skin pigmentation, dermatitis, erythema multiforme, rash, Stevens-Johnson syndrome, toxic epidermal necrolysis

Gastrointestinal: Anorexia, abdominal cramps, vomiting, diarrhea, xerostomia, atrophic glossitis

Hematologic: Megaloblastic anemia, leukopenia, pancytopenia, thrombocytopenia, pulmonary eosinophilia

Genitourinary: Hematuria

Miscellaneous: Anaphylaxis

Overdosage/Toxicology Symptoms include megaloblastic anemia, leukopenia, thrombocytopenia, anorexia, CNS stimulation, seizures, nausea, vomiting, and hematemesis. Following GI decontamination, leucovorin should be administered in a dosage of 5-15 mg/day I.M., I.V., or oral for 5-7 days, or as required to reverse symptoms of folic acid deficiency. Diazepam 0.1-0.25 mg/kg can be used to treat seizures.

Drug Interactions

Cytochrome P450 Effect: Inhibits CYP2C8/9 (moderate), 2D6 (moderate)

Increased Effect/Toxicity: Serum levels of antipsychotic agents may be increased by pyrimethamine. Sulfonamides (synergy), methotrexate, TMP/SMZ, and zidovudine may increase the risk of bone marrow suppression. Pyrimethamine may increase the levels/effects of amiodarone, amphetamines, selected beta-blockers, dextromethorphan, fluoxetine, glimepiride, glipizide, lidocaine, mirtazapine, nateglinide, nefazodone, paroxetine, phenytoin, pioglitazone, risperidone, ritonavir, rosiglitazone, sertraline, thioridazine, tricyclic antidepressants, venlafaxine, warfarin, and other CYP2C8/9 or 2D6 substrates.

Decreased Effect: Pyrimethamine may decrease the levels/effects of CYP2D6 prodrug substrates (eg, codeine, hydrocodone, oxycodone, tramadol).

Stability Store at 15°C to 25°C (59°F to 77°F); protect from light

Mechanism of Action Inhibits parasitic dihydrofolate reductase, resulting in inhibition of vital tetrahydrofolic acid synthesis

Pharmacodynamics/Kinetics

Onset of action: ~1 hour

Absorption: Well absorbed

Distribution: Widely, mainly in blood cells, kidneys, lungs, liver, and spleen; crosses into CSF; crosses placenta; enters breast milk

(Continued)

Pyrimethamine *(Continued)*

Protein binding: 80% to 87%
Metabolism: Hepatic
Half-life elimination: 80-95 hours
Time to peak, serum: 1.5-8 hours
Excretion: Urine (20% to 30% as unchanged drug)

Dosage

Malaria chemoprophylaxis (for areas where chloroquine-resistant *P. falciparum* exists): Begin prophylaxis 2 weeks before entering endemic area:
- Children: 0.5 mg/kg once weekly; not to exceed 25 mg/dose

or

- Children:
  - <4 years: 6.25 mg once weekly
  - 4-10 years: 12.5 mg once weekly
- Children >10 years and Adults: 25 mg once weekly
- Dosage should be continued for all age groups for at least 6-10 weeks after leaving endemic areas

Chloroquine-resistant *P. falciparum* malaria (when used in conjunction with quinine and sulfadiazine):
- Children:
  - <10 kg: 6.25 mg/day once daily for 3 days
  - 10-20 kg: 12.5 mg/day once daily for 3 days
  - 20-40 kg: 25 mg/day once daily for 3 days
- Adults: 25 mg twice daily for 3 days

Toxoplasmosis:
- Infants (congenital toxoplasmosis): Oral: 1 mg/kg once daily for 6 months with sulfadiazine then every other month with sulfa, alternating with spiramycin.
- Children: Loading dose: 2 mg/kg/day divided into 2 equal daily doses for 1-3 days (maximum: 100 mg/day) followed by 1 mg/kg/day divided into 2 doses for 4 weeks; maximum: 25 mg/day
  - With sulfadiazine or trisulfapyrimidines: 2 mg/kg/day divided every 12 hours for 3 days, followed by 1 mg/kg/day once daily or divided twice daily for 4 weeks given with trisulfapyrimidines or sulfadiazine
- Adults: 50-75 mg/day together with 1-4 g of a sulfonamide for 1-3 weeks depending on patient's tolerance and response, then reduce dose by 50% and continue for 4-5 weeks **or** 25-50 mg/day for 3-4 weeks

Prophylaxis for first episode of *Toxoplasma gondii*:
- Children ≥1 month of age: 1 mg/kg/day once daily with dapsone, plus oral folinic acid 5 mg every 3 days
- Adolescents and Adults: 50 mg once weekly with dapsone, plus oral folinic acid 25 mg once weekly

Prophylaxis to prevent recurrence of *Toxoplasma gondii*:
- Children ≥1 month of age: 1 mg/kg/day once daily given with sulfadiazine or clindamycin, plus oral folinic acid 5 mg every 3 days
- Adolescents and Adults: 25-50 mg once daily in combination with sulfadiazine or clindamycin, plus oral folinic acid 10-25 mg daily; atovaquone plus oral folinic acid has also been used in combination with pyrimethamine.

Administration Administer with meals to minimize GI distress.

Monitoring Parameters CBC, including platelet counts

Patient Information Take with meals to minimize vomiting; begin malaria prophylaxis at least 1-2 weeks prior to departure; discontinue at first sign of skin rash; report persistent fever, sore throat, bleeding or bruising; regular blood work may be necessary in patients taking high doses

Additional Information Leucovorin may be administered in a dosage of 3-9 mg/day for 3 days or 5 mg every 3 days or as required to reverse symptoms of or to prevent hematologic problems due to folic acid deficiency

Dosage Forms Tablet: 25 mg

Extemporaneous Preparations Pyrimethamine tablets may be crushed to prepare oral suspensions of the drug in water, cherry syrup or sucrose-containing solutions at a concentration of 1 mg/mL; stable at room temperature for 5-7 days

AHFS Drug Information, McEvoy G, ed, Bethesda, MD: American Society of Health-System Pharmacists, 1996.

Selected Readings

"Drugs for Parasitic Infections," *Med Lett Drugs Ther*, 1998, 40(1017):1-12.
Porter SB and Sande MA, "Toxoplasmosis of the Central Nervous System in the Acquired Immunodeficiency Syndrome," *N Engl J Med*, 1992, 327(23):1643-8.
White NJ, "The Treatment of Malaria," *N Engl J Med*, 1996, 335(11):800-6.

Pyrimethamine and Sulfadoxine *see* Sulfadoxine and Pyrimethamine *on page 1085*
Pyrinyl Plus® [OTC] *see* Pyrethrins and Piperonyl Butoxide *on page 1023*

Quinate® (Can) *see* Quinidine *on page 1027*

Quinidine (KWIN i deen)

Related Information

Malaria Treatment *on page 1292*

Canadian Brand Names Apo-Quin-G®; Apo-Quinidine®; BioQuin® Durules™; Novo-Quinidin; Quinate®

Synonyms Quinidine Gluconate; Quinidine Polygalacturonate; Quinidine Sulfate

Generic Available Yes

Use Prophylaxis after cardioversion of atrial fibrillation and/or flutter to maintain normal sinus rhythm; prevent recurrence of paroxysmal supraventricular tachycardia, paroxysmal AV junctional rhythm, paroxysmal ventricular tachycardia, paroxysmal atrial fibrillation, and atrial or ventricular premature contractions; has activity against *Plasmodium falciparum* malaria

Drug of Choice or Alternative for Organism(s):

Plasmodium Species *on page 265*

Pregnancy Risk Factor C

Contraindications Hypersensitivity to quinidine or any component of the formulation; thrombocytopenia; thrombocytopenic purpura; myasthenia gravis; heart block greater than first degree; idioventricular conduction delays (except in patients with a functioning artificial pacemaker); those adversely affected by anticholinergic activity; concurrent use of quinolone antibiotics which prolong QT interval, cisapride, amprenavir, or ritonavir

Warnings/Precautions Monitor and adjust dose to prevent QT_c prolongation. Watch for proarrhythmic effects. May precipitate or exacerbate CHF. Reduce dosage in hepatic impairment. In patients with atrial fibrillation or flutter, block the AV node before initiating. Correct hypokalemia before initiating therapy. Hypokalemia may worsen toxicity. Use may cause digoxin-induced toxicity (adjust digoxin's dose). Use caution with concurrent use of other antiarrhythmics. Hypersensitivity reactions can occur. Can unmask sick sinus syndrome (causes bradycardia). Has been associated with severe hepatotoxic reactions, including granulomatous hepatitis. Hemolysis may occur in patients with G6PD (glucose-6-phosphate dehydrogenase) deficiency. Different salt products are not interchangeable.

Adverse Reactions

Frequency not defined: Hypotension, syncope

>10%:

- Cardiovascular: QT_c prolongation (modest prolongation is common, however, excessive prolongation is rare and indicates toxicity)
- Central nervous system: Lightheadedness (15%)
- Gastrointestinal: Diarrhea (35%), upper GI distress, bitter taste, diarrhea, anorexia, nausea, vomiting, stomach cramping (22%)

1% to 10%:

- Cardiovascular: Angina (6%), palpitation (7%), new or worsened arrhythmia (proarrhythmic effect)
- Central nervous system: Syncope (1% to 8%), headache (7%), fatigue (7%), sleep disturbance (3%), tremor (2%), nervousness (2%), incoordination (1%)
- Dermatologic: Rash (5%)
- Neuromuscular & skeletal: Weakness (5%)
- Ocular: Blurred vision
- Otic: Tinnitus
- Respiratory: Wheezing

<1% (Limited to important or life-threatening): Tachycardia, QT_c prolongation (excessive), torsade de pointes, heart block, ventricular fibrillation, ventricular tachycardia, paradoxical increase in ventricular rate during atrial fibrillation/flutter, exacerbated bradycardia (in sick sinus syndrome), vascular collapse, confusion, delirium, vertigo, impaired hearing, respiratory depression, pneumonitis, bronchospasm, fever, urticaria, flushing, exfoliative rash, psoriaform rash, pruritus, lymphadenopathy, hemolytic anemia, vasculitis, thrombocytopenic purpura, thrombocytopenia, pancytopenia, uveitis, angioedema, agranulocytosis, sicca syndrome, arthralgia, myalgia, increased CPK, drug-induced lupus-like syndrome, cerebral hypoperfusion (possibly resulting in ataxia, apprehension, and seizure), acute psychotic reactions, depression, hallucinations, mydriasis, disturbed color perception, night blindness, scotoma, optic neuritis, visual field loss, photosensitivity, abnormal pigmentation, granulomatous hepatitis, hepatotoxic reaction (rare), eczematous dermatitis, livedo reticularis

Postmarketing and/or case reports: Melanin pigmentation of the hard palate, esophagitis, nephropathy, cholestasis, pneumonitis, lichen planus

(Continued)

Quinidine *(Continued)*

Note: Cinchonism, a syndrome which may include tinnitus, high-frequency hearing loss, deafness, vertigo, blurred vision, diplopia, photophobia, headache, confusion, and delirium has been associated with quinidine use. Usually associated with chronic toxicity, this syndrome has also been described after brief exposure to a moderate dose in sensitive patients. Vomiting and diarrhea may also occur as isolated reactions to therapeutic quinidine levels.

Overdosage/Toxicology

Has a low toxic:therapeutic ratio and may easily produce fatal intoxication (acute toxic dose: 1 g in adults); symptoms include sinus bradycardia, sinus node arrest or asystole, PR, QRS, or QT interval prolongation, torsade de pointes (polymorphous ventricular tachycardia) and depressed myocardial contractility, which along with alpha-adrenergic or ganglionic blockade, may result in hypotension and pulmonary edema. Other effects are anticholinergic (dry mouth, dilated pupils, and delirium) as well as seizures, coma and respiratory arrest.

Treatment is primarily symptomatic and effects usually respond to conventional therapies (fluids, positioning, vasopressors, anticonvulsants, antiarrhythmics). **Note:** Do not use other type 1a or 1c antiarrhythmic agents to treat ventricular tachycardia. Sodium bicarbonate may treat wide QRS intervals or hypotension. Markedly impaired conduction or high degree AV block, unresponsive to bicarbonate, indicates consideration of a pacemaker is needed.

Drug Interactions

Cytochrome P450 Effect: Substrate of CYP2C8/9 (minor), 2E1 (minor), 3A4 (major); **Inhibits** CYP2C8/9 (weak), 2D6 (strong), 3A4 (strong)

Increased Effect/Toxicity: Effects may be additive with drugs which prolong the QT interval, including amiodarone, amitriptyline, bepridil, cisapride (use is contraindicated), disopyramide, erythromycin, haloperidol, imipramine, pimozide, procainamide, sotalol, thioridazine, and some quinolones (sparfloxacin, gatifloxacin, moxifloxacin - concurrent use is contraindicated). Concurrent use of amprenavir, or ritonavir is contraindicated. Quinidine increases digoxin serum concentrations; digoxin dosage may need to be reduced (by 50%) when quinidine is initiated; new steady-state digoxin plasma concentrations occur in 5-7 days.

Quinidine may increase the levels/effects of amphetamines, selected beta-blockers, selected benzodiazepines, calcium channel blockers, cisapride, cyclosporine, dextromethorphan, ergot alkaloids, fluoxetine, selected HMG-CoA reductase inhibitors, lidocaine, mesoridazine, mirtazapine, nateglinide, nefazodone, paroxetine, risperidone, ritonavir, sildenafil (and other PDE-5 inhibitors), tacrolimus, thioridazine, tricyclic antidepressants, venlafaxine, and other substrates of CYP2D6 or 3A4. Selected benzodiazepines (midazolam and triazolam), cisapride, ergot alkaloids, selected HMG-CoA reductase inhibitors (lovastatin and simvastatin), mesoridazine, pimozide, and thioridazine are generally contraindicated with strong CYP3A4 inhibitors. When used with strong CYP3A4 inhibitors, dosage adjustment/limits are recommended for sildenafil and other PDE-5 inhibitors; refer to individual monographs.

The levels/effects of quinidine may be increased by azole antifungals, ciprofloxacin, clarithromycin, diclofenac, doxycycline, erythromycin, imatinib, isoniazid, nefazodone, nicardipine, propofol, protease inhibitors (amprenavir and ritonavir are contraindicated), verapamil, and other CYP3A4 inhibitors. Quinidine potentiates nondepolarizing and depolarizing muscle relaxants. When combined with quinidine, amiloride may cause prolonged ventricular conduction leading to arrhythmias. Urinary alkalinizers (antacids, sodium bicarbonate, acetazolamide) increase quinidine blood levels. Warfarin effects may be increased by quinidine.

Decreased Effect: The levels/effects of quinidine may be decreased by aminoglutethimide, carbamazepine, nafcillin, nevirapine, phenobarbital, phenytoin, rifamycins, and other CYP3A4 inducers. Quinidine may decrease the levels/effects of CYP2D6 prodrug substrates (eg, codeine, hydrocodone, oxycodone, tramadol).

Ethanol/Nutrition/Herb Interactions

Food: Dietary salt intake may alter the rate and extent of quinidine absorption. A decrease in dietary salt may lead to an increase in quinidine serum concentrations. Avoid changes in dietary salt intake. Quinidine serum levels may be increased if taken with food. Food has a variable effect on absorption of sustained release formulation. The rate of absorption of quinidine may be decreased following the ingestion of grapefruit juice. In addition, CYP3A4 metabolism of quinidine may be reduced by grapefruit juice. Grapefruit juice should be avoided. Excessive intake of fruit juices or vitamin C may decrease urine pH and result in increased clearance of quinidine with decreased serum concentration. Alkaline foods may result in increased quinidine serum concentrations.

Herb/Nutraceutical: St John's wort may decrease quinidine levels. Avoid ephedra (may worsen arrhythmia).

Stability Do not use discolored parenteral solution.

Mechanism of Action Class 1a antiarrhythmic agent; depresses phase O of the action potential; decreases myocardial excitability and conduction velocity, and myocardial contractility by decreasing sodium influx during depolarization and potassium efflux in repolarization; also reduces calcium transport across cell membrane

Pharmacodynamics/Kinetics

Distribution: V_d: Adults: 2-3.5 L/kg, decreased with congestive heart failure, malaria; increased with cirrhosis; crosses placenta; enters breast milk

Protein binding:

Newborns: 60% to 70%; decreased protein binding with cyanotic congenital heart disease, cirrhosis, or acute myocardial infarction

Adults: 80% to 90%

Metabolism: Extensively hepatic (50% to 90%) to inactive compounds

Bioavailability: Sulfate: 80%; Gluconate: 70%

Half-life elimination, plasma: Children: 2.5-6.7 hours; Adults: 6-8 hours; prolonged with elderly, cirrhosis, and congestive heart failure

Excretion: Urine (15% to 25% as unchanged drug)

Dosage Dosage expressed in terms of the salt: 267 mg of quinidine gluconate = 200 mg of quinidine sulfate.

Children: Test dose for idiosyncratic reaction (sulfate, oral or gluconate, I.M.): 2 mg/kg or 60 mg/m^2

Oral (quinidine sulfate): 15-60 mg/kg/day in 4-5 divided doses or 6 mg/kg every 4-6 hours; usual 30 mg/kg/day or 900 mg/m^2/day given in 5 daily doses

I.V. **not** recommended (quinidine gluconate): 2-10 mg/kg/dose given at a rate ≤10 mg/minute every 3-6 hours as needed

Adults: Test dose: Oral, I.M.: 200 mg administered several hours before full dosage (to determine possibility of idiosyncratic reaction)

Oral (for malaria):

Sulfate: 100-600 mg/dose every 4-6 hours; begin at 200 mg/dose and titrate to desired effect (maximum daily dose: 3-4 g)

Gluconate: 324-972 mg every 8-12 hours

I.M.: 400 mg/dose every 2-6 hours; initial dose: 600 mg (gluconate)

I.V.: 200-400 mg/dose diluted and given at a rate ≤10 mg/minute; may require as much as 500-750 mg

Dosing adjustment in renal impairment: Cl_{cr} <10 mL/minute: Administer 75% of normal dose.

Hemodialysis: Slightly hemodialyzable (5% to 20%); 200 mg supplemental dose posthemodialysis is recommended.

Peritoneal dialysis: Not dialyzable (0% to 5%)

Dosing adjustment/comments in hepatic impairment: Larger loading dose may be indicated, reduce maintenance doses by 50% and monitor serum levels closely.

Dietary Considerations Administer with food or milk to decrease gastrointestinal irritation. Avoid changes in dietary salt intake.

Administration Administer around-the-clock to promote less variation in peak and trough serum levels

Oral: Do not crush, chew, or break sustained release dosage forms.

Parenteral: When injecting I.M., aspirate carefully to avoid injection into a vessel; maximum I.V. infusion rate: 10 mg/minute

Monitoring Parameters Cardiac monitor required during I.V. administration; CBC, liver and renal function tests, should be routinely performed during long-term administration

Reference Range Therapeutic: 2-5 mcg/mL (SI: 6.2-15.4 μmol/L). Patient dependent therapeutic response occurs at levels of 3-6 mcg/mL (SI: 9.2-18.5 μmol/L). Optimal therapeutic level is method dependent; >6 mcg/mL (SI: >18 μmol/L).

Patient Information Do not crush or chew sustained release preparations. Report rash, fever, unusual bleeding or bruising, ringing in the ears, visual disturbances, or syncope; seek emergency help if palpitations occur.

Dosage Forms

Injection, solution, as gluconate: 80 mg/mL (10 mL) [equivalent to quinidine base 50 mg]

Tablet, as sulfate: 200 mg, 300 mg

Tablet, extended release, as gluconate: 324 mg [equivalent to quinidine base 202 mg]

Tablet, extended release, as sulfate: 300 mg [equivalent to quinidine base 249 mg]

Extemporaneous Preparations A 10 mg/mL oral liquid preparation made from tablets and 3 different vehicles (cherry syrup, a 1:1 mixture of Ora-Sweet® and Ora-Plus®, or a 1:1 mixture of Ora-Sweet® SF and Ora-Plus®) was stable for 60 days

(Continued)

Quinidine *(Continued)*

when stored in amber plastic prescription bottles in the dark at room temperature (25°C) or under refrigeration (5°C); Grind six 200 mg tablets in a mortar into a fine powder; add 15 mL of the vehicle and mix well to form a uniform paste; mix while adding the vehicle in geometric proportions to **almost** 120 mL; transfer to a calibrated bottle and qsad to 120 mL; label "shake well" and "protect from light" (Allen 1998).

Allen LV and Erickson MA, "Stability of Bethanechol Chloride, Pyrazinamide, Quinidine Sulfate, Rifampin, and Tetracycline in Extemporaneously Compounded Oral Liquids," *Am J Health Syst Pharm*, 1998, 55(17):1804-9.

Selected Readings

Panisko DM and Keystone JS, "Treatment of Malaria - 1990," *Drugs*, 1990, 39(2):160-89.
Wyler DJ, "Malaria Chemoprophylaxis for the Traveler," *N Engl J Med*, 1993, 329(1):31-7.
Wyler DJ, "Malaria: Overview and Update," *Clin Infect Dis*, 1993, 16(4):449-56.

Quinidine Gluconate *see* Quinidine *on page 1027*

Quinidine Polygalacturonate *see* Quinidine *on page 1027*

Quinidine Sulfate *see* Quinidine *on page 1027*

Quinine (KWYE nine)

Related Information

Malaria Treatment *on page 1292*

Canadian Brand Names Apo-Quinine®; Novo-Quinine; Quinine-Odan™

Synonyms Quinine Sulfate

Generic Available Yes

Use In conjunction with other antimalarial agents, suppression or treatment of chloroquine-resistant *P. falciparum* malaria; treatment of *Babesia microti* infection in conjunction with clindamycin

Unlabeled/Investigational Use Prevention and treatment of nocturnal recumbency leg muscle cramps

Drug of Choice or Alternative for Organism(s):

Babesia microti on page 40

Pregnancy Risk Factor X

Contraindications Hypersensitivity to quinine or any component of the formulation; tinnitus, optic neuritis, G6PD deficiency; history of black water fever; thrombocytopenia with quinine or quinidine; pregnancy

Warnings/Precautions Use with caution in patients with cardiac arrhythmias (quinine has quinidine-like activity) and in patients with myasthenia gravis

Adverse Reactions

Frequency not defined:

- Central nervous system: Severe headache
- Gastrointestinal: Nausea, vomiting, diarrhea
- Ocular: Blurred vision
- Otic: Tinnitus
- Miscellaneous: Cinchonism (risk of cinchonism is directly related to dose and duration of therapy)

<1%: Flushing of the skin, anginal symptoms, fever, rash, pruritus, hypoglycemia, epigastric pain, hemolysis in G6PD deficiency, thrombocytopenia, hepatitis, nightblindness, diplopia, optic atrophy, impaired hearing, hypersensitivity reactions

Overdosage/Toxicology Symptoms of mild toxicity include nausea, vomiting, and cinchonism. Severe intoxication may cause ataxia, obtundation, convulsions, coma, and respiratory arrest. With massive intoxication quinidine-like cardiotoxicity (hypotension, QRS and QT interval prolongation, AV block, and ventricular arrhythmias) may be fatal. Retinal toxicity occurs 9-10 hours after ingestion (blurred vision, impaired color perception, constriction of visual fields, blindness). Other toxic effects include hypokalemia, hypoglycemia, hemolysis, and congenital malformations when taken during pregnancy. Treatment includes symptomatic therapy with conventional agents (anticonvulsants, fluids, positioning, vasoconstrictors, antiarrhythmias). **Note:** Avoid type 1a and 1c antiarrhythmic drugs. Treat cardiotoxicity with sodium bicarbonate. Dialysis and hemoperfusion procedures are ineffective in enhancing elimination.

Drug Interactions

Cytochrome P450 Effect: Substrate (minor) of CYP1A2, 2C19, 3A4; **Inhibits** CYP2C8/9 (moderate), 2D6 (strong), 3A4 (weak)

Increased Effect/Toxicity: Quinine may increase the levels/effects of CYP2D6 substrates (eg, amphetamines, selected beta-blockers, dextromethorphan, fluoxetine, lidocaine, mirtazapine, nefazodone, paroxetine, risperidone, ritonavir, thioridazine, tricyclic antidepressants, venlafaxine). Beta-blockers with quinine may increase bradycardia. Quinine may enhance warfarin anticoagulant effect. Quinine

potentiates nondepolarizing and depolarizing muscle relaxants. Quinine may increase plasma concentration of digoxin. Closely monitor digoxin concentrations. Digoxin dosage may need to be reduced (by one-half) when quinine is initiated. New steady-state digoxin plasma concentrations occur in 5-7 days. Verapamil, amiodarone, alkalinizing agents, and cimetidine may increase quinine serum concentrations.

Decreased Effect: Phenobarbital, phenytoin, and rifampin may decrease quinine serum concentrations. Quinine may decrease the levels/effects of CYP2D6 prodrug substrates (eg, codeine, hydrocodone, oxycodone, tramadol).

Ethanol/Nutrition/Herb Interactions Herb/Nutraceutical: St John's wort may decrease quinine levels.

Stability Protect from light

Mechanism of Action Depresses oxygen uptake and carbohydrate metabolism; intercalates into DNA, disrupting the parasite's replication and transcription; affects calcium distribution within muscle fibers and decreases the excitability of the motor end-plate region; cardiovascular effects similar to quinidine

Pharmacodynamics/Kinetics

Absorption: Readily, mainly from upper small intestine

Protein binding: 70% to 95%

Metabolism: Primarily hepatic

Half-life elimination: Children: 6-12 hours; Adults: 8-14 hours

Time to peak, serum: 1-3 hours

Excretion: Feces and saliva; urine (<5% as unchanged drug)

Dosage Oral:

Children:

Treatment of chloroquine-resistant malaria: 25-30 mg/kg/day in divided doses every 8 hours for 3-7 days with tetracycline (consider risk versus benefit in children <8 years of age)

Babesiosis: 25 mg/kg/day divided every 8 hours for 7 days

Adults:

Treatment of chloroquine-resistant malaria: 650 mg every 8 hours for 3-7 days with tetracycline

Suppression of malaria: 325 mg twice daily and continued for 6 weeks after exposure

Babesiosis: 650 mg every 6-8 hours for 7 days

Leg cramps: 200-300 mg at bedtime

Dosing interval/adjustment in renal impairment:

Cl_{cr} 10-50 mL/minute: Administer every 8-12 hours or 75% of normal dose

Cl_{cr} <10 mL/minute: Administer every 24 hours or 30% to 50% of normal dose

Dialysis: Not removed

Peritoneal dialysis: Dose as for Cl_{cr} <10 mL/minute

Continuous arteriovenous or venovenous hemodiafiltration effects: Dose for Cl_{cr} 10-50 mL/minute

Dietary Considerations May be taken with food.

Administration Avoid use of aluminum-containing antacids because of drug absorption problems. Swallow dose whole to avoid bitter taste. May be administered with food.

Monitoring Parameters

Monitor CBC with platelet count, liver function tests, blood glucose, ophthalmologic examination

Reference Range Toxic: >10 mcg/mL

Test Interactions Positive Coombs' [direct]; false elevation of urinary steroids and catecholamines

Patient Information Avoid use of aluminum-containing antacids because of drug absorption problems; swallow dose whole to avoid bitter taste; may cause night blindness. Report rash, fever, unusual bleeding or bruising, ringing in the ears, visual disturbances, or syncope; seek emergency help if palpitations occur.

Dosage Forms

Capsule, as sulfate: 200 mg, 325 mg

Tablet, as sulfate: 260 mg

Selected Readings

Panisko DM and Keystone JS, "Treatment of Malaria - 1990," *Drugs*, 1990, 39(2):160-89.

White NJ, "The Treatment of Malaria," *N Engl J Med*, 1996, 335(11):800-6.

Wyler DJ, "Malaria Chemoprophylaxis for the Traveler," *N Engl J Med*, 1993, 329(1):31-7.

Wyler DJ, "Malaria: Overview and Update," *Clin Infect Dis*, 1993, 16(4):449-56.

Quinine-Odan™ (Can) *see* Quinine *on page 1030*

Quinine Sulfate *see* Quinine *on page 1030*

Quinupristin and Dalfopristin (kwi NYOO pris tin & dal FOE pris tin)

Related Information

Antimicrobial Activity Against Selected Organisms *on page 1165*

U.S. Brand Names Synercid®

Canadian Brand Names Synercid®

Synonyms Pristinamycin; RP-59500

Generic Available No

Use Treatment of serious or life-threatening infections associated with vancomycin-resistant *Enterococcus faecium* bacteremia; treatment of complicated skin and skin structure infections caused by methcillin-susceptible *Staphylococcus aureus* or *Streptococcus pyogenes*

Has been studied in the treatment of a variety of infections caused by *Enterococcus faecium* (not *E. fecalis*) including vancomycin-resistant strains. May also be effective in the treatment of serious infections caused by *Staphylococcus* species including those resistant to methicillin.

Drug of Choice or Alternative for Organism(s):

Enterococcus Species *on page 134*
Staphylococcus aureus, Methicillin-Resistant *on page 304*
Staphylococcus aureus, Methicillin-Susceptible *on page 307*

Pregnancy Risk Factor B

Pregnancy Implications No evidence of impaired fertility or harm to the fetus in animal reproductive studies.

Contraindications Hypersensitivity to quinupristin, dalfopristin, pristinamycin, or virginiamycin, or any component of the formulation

Warnings/Precautions May cause pain and phlebitis when infused through a peripheral line (not relieved by hydrocortisone or diphenhydramine). Superinfection may occur. As with many antibiotics, antibiotic-associated colitis and pseudomembranous colitis may occur. May cause arthralgias, myalgias, and hyperbilirubinemia. May inhibit the metabolism of many drugs metabolized by CYP3A4. Concurrent therapy with cisapride (which may prolong QT_c interval and lead to arrhythmias) should be avoided.

Adverse Reactions

>10%:
- Hepatic: Hyperbilirubinemia (3% to 35%)
- Local: Inflammation at infusion site (38% to 42%), local pain (40% to 44%), local edema (17% to 18%), infusion site reaction (12% to 13%)
- Neuromuscular & skeletal: Arthralgia (up to 47%), myalgia (up to 47%)

1% to 10%:
- Central nervous system: Pain (2% to 3%), headache (2%)
- Dermatologic: Pruritus (2%), rash (3%)
- Endocrine & metabolic: Hyperglycemia (1%)
- Gastrointestinal: Nausea (3% to 5%), diarrhea (3%), vomiting (3% to 4%)
- Hematologic: Anemia (3%)
- Hepatic: GGT increased (2%), LDH increased (3%)
- Local: Thrombophlebitis (2%)
- Neuromuscular & skeletal: CPK increased (2%)

<1%: Abdominal pain, allergic reaction, anaphylactoid reaction, anxiety, apnea, arrhythmia, bone pain, BUN increased, cardiac arrest, chest pain, coagulation disorder, confusion, constipation, creatinine increased, diaphoresis, dizziness, dysautonomia, dyspepsia, dyspnea, encephalopathy, fever, gastrointestinal hemorrhage, gout, hematuria, hemolysis, hemolytic anemia, hepatitis, hyperkalemia, hypertonia, hypoglycemia, hyponatremia, hypotension, hypoventilation, hypovolemia, infection, insomnia, leg cramps, maculopapular rash, mesenteric artery occlusion, myasthenia, neck rigidity, neuropathy, oral candidiasis, palpitation, pancreatitis, pancytopenia, paraplegia, paresthesia, pericarditis, peripheral edema, phlebitis, pleural effusion, pseudomembranous colitis, respiratory distress, seizure, shock, skin ulcer, stomatitis, syncope, thrombocytopenia, tremor, transaminases increased, urticaria, vaginitis, vasodilation

Overdosage/Toxicology Symptoms may include dyspnea, emesis, tremors, and ataxia. Treatment is supportive. Not removed by hemodialysis or peritoneal dialysis.

Drug Interactions

Cytochrome P450 Effect: Quinupristin: **Inhibits** CYP3A4 (weak)

Increased Effect/Toxicity: The manufacturer states that quinupristin/dalfopristin may increase cisapride concentrations and cause QT_c prolongation, and recommends to avoid concurrent use with cisapride. Quinupristin/dalfopristin may increase cyclosporine concentrations; monitor.

Stability Store unopened vials under refrigeration (2°C to 8°C/36°F to 46°F). Reconstitute single dose vial with 5 mL of 5% dextrose in water or sterile water for injection. Swirl gently to dissolve, do not shake (to limit foam formation). The reconstituted solution should be diluted within 30 minutes. Stability of the diluted solution prior to the infusion is established as 5 hours at room temperature or 54 hours if refrigerated at 2°C to 8°C. Reconstituted solution should be added to at least 250 mL of 5% dextrose in water for peripheral administration (increase to 500 mL or 750 mL if necessary to limit venous irritation). An infusion volume of 100 mL may be used for central line infusions. Do not freeze solution.

Mechanism of Action Quinupristin/dalfopristin inhibits bacterial protein synthesis by binding to different sites on the 50S bacterial ribosomal subunit thereby inhibiting protein synthesis

Pharmacodynamics/Kinetics

Distribution: Quinupristin: 0.45 L/kg; Dalfopristin: 0.24 L/kg

Protein binding: Moderate

Metabolism: To active metabolites via nonenzymatic reactions

Half-life elimination: Quinupristin: 0.85 hour; Dalfopristin: 0.7 hour (mean elimination half-lives, including metabolites: 3 and 1 hours, respectively)

Excretion: Feces (75% to 77% as unchanged drug and metabolites); urine (15% to 19%)

Dosage I.V.:

Children (limited information): Dosages similar to adult dosing have been used in the treatment of complicated skin/soft tissue infections and infections caused by vancomycin-resistant *Enterococcus faecium*

CNS shunt infection due to vancomycin-resistant *Enterococcus faecium*: 7.5 mg/kg/dose every 8 hours; concurrent intrathecal doses of 1-2 mg/day have been administered for up to 68 days

Adults:

Vancomycin-resistant *Enterococcus faecium*: 7.5 mg/kg every 8 hours

Complicated skin and skin structure infection: 7.5 mg/kg every 12 hours

Dosage adjustment in renal impairment: No adjustment required in renal failure, hemodialysis, or peritoneal dialysis

Dosage adjustment in hepatic impairment: Pharmacokinetic data suggest dosage adjustment may be necessary; however, specific recommendations have not been proposed

Elderly: No dosage adjustment is required

Administration Line should be flushed with 5% dextrose in water prior to and following administration. Incompatible with saline. Infusion should be completed over 60 minutes (toxicity may be increased with shorter infusion). Compatible (Y-site injection) with aztreonam, ciprofloxacin, haloperidol, metoclopramide or potassium chloride when admixed in 5% dextrose in water. Also compatible (Y-site injection) with fluconazole (used as undiluted solution). If severe venous irritation occurs following peripheral administration of quinupristin/dalfopristin diluted in 250 mL 5% dextrose in water, consideration should be given to increasing the infusion volume to 500 mL or 750 mL, changing the infusion site, or infusing by a peripherally inserted central catheter (PICC) or a central venous catheter.

Dosage Forms

Injection, powder for reconstitution:

500 mg: Quinupristin 150 mg and dalfopristin 350 mg

600 mg: Quinupristin 180 mg and dalfopristin 420 mg

Selected Readings

Bryson HM and Spencer CM, "Quinupristin/Dalfopristin," *Drugs*, 1996, 52(3):406-15.

Chant C and Rybak MH, "Quinupristin/Dalfopristin (RP 59500): A New Streptogramin Antibiotic," *Ann Pharmacother*, 1995, 29(10):1022-7.

Delgado G Jr, Neuhauser MM, Bearden DT, et al, "Quinupristin-Dalfopristin: An Overview," *Pharmacotherapy*, 2000, 20(12):1469-85.

Griswold MW, Lomaestro BM, and Briceland LL, "Quinupristin-Dalfopristin (RP 59500): An Injectable Streptogramin Combination," *Am J Health Syst Pharm*, 1996, 53:2045-53.

Nadler H, Dowzicky MJ, Feger C, et al, "Quinupristin/Dalfopristin: A Novel Selective-Spectrum Antibiotic for the Treatment of Multiresistant and Other Gram-Positive Pathogens," *Clin Microbiol Newslett*, 1999, 21(13):103-12.

Quixin™ *see* Levofloxacin *on page 908*

R & C™ II (Can) *see* Pyrethrins and Piperonyl Butoxide *on page 1023*

R & C™ Shampoo/Conditioner (Can) *see* Pyrethrins and Piperonyl Butoxide *on page 1023*

RabAvert® *see* Rabies Virus Vaccine *on page 1034*

Rabies Immune Globulin (Human)

(RAY beez i MYUN GLOB yoo lin, HYU man)

U.S. Brand Names BayRab®; Imogam® Rabies-HT

Canadian Brand Names BayRab™; Imogam® Rabies Pasteurized

Synonyms RIG

Generic Available No

Use Part of postexposure prophylaxis of persons with rabies exposure who lack a history of pre-exposure or postexposure prophylaxis with rabies vaccine or a recently documented neutralizing antibody response to previous rabies vaccination; although it is preferable to administer RIG with the first dose of vaccine, it can be given up to 8 days after vaccination

Drug of Choice or Alternative for Organism(s):

Rabies Virus *on page 283*

Pregnancy Risk Factor C

Contraindications Hypersensitivity to thimerosal or any component of the formulation

Warnings/Precautions Have epinephrine 1:1000 available for anaphylactic reactions. As a product of human plasma, this product may potentially transmit disease; screening of donors, as well as testing and/or inactivation of certain viruses reduces this risk. Use caution in patients with thrombocytopenia or coagulation disorders (I.M. injections may be contraindicated), in patients with isolated IgA deficiency, or in patients with previous systemic hypersensitivity to human immunoglobulins. Not for intravenous administration.

Adverse Reactions

1% to 10%:

Central nervous system: Fever (mild)

Local: Soreness at injection site

<1%: Urticaria, angioedema, stiffness, soreness of muscles, anaphylactic shock

Stability Refrigerate

Mechanism of Action Rabies immune globulin is a solution of globulins dried from the plasma or serum of selected adult human donors who have been immunized with rabies vaccine and have developed high titers of rabies antibody. It generally contains 10% to 18% of protein of which not less than 80% is monomeric immunoglobulin G.

Dosage Children and Adults: I.M.: 20 units/kg in a single dose (RIG should always be administered as part of rabies vaccine (HDCV)) regimen (as soon as possible after the first dose of vaccine, up to 8 days); infiltrate $^1/_2$ of the dose locally around the wound; administer the remainder I.M.

Note: Persons known to have an adequate titer or who have been completely immunized with rabies vaccine should not receive RIG, only booster doses of HDCV

Administration Intramuscular injection only; injection should be made into the gluteal muscle

Dosage Forms Injection, solution:

BayRab®: 150 int. units/mL (2 mL, 10 mL) [solvent/detergent treated]

Imogam® Rabies-HT: 150 int. units/mL (2 mL, 10 mL) [heat treated]

Selected Readings

"A New Rabies Vaccine," *Med Lett Drugs Ther*, 1998, 40(1029):64-5.

Dreesen DW and Hanlon CA, "Current Recommendations for the Prophylaxis and Treatment of Rabies," *Drugs*, 1998, 56(5):801-9.

Lang J and Plotkin SA, "Rabies Risk and Immunoprophylaxis in Children," *Adv Pediatr Infect Dis*, 1997, 13:219-55.

Strady A, Lang J, Lienard M, et al, "Antibody Persistence Following Pre-exposure Regimens of Cell-Culture Rabies Vaccines: 10-Year Follow-up and Proposal for a New Booster Policy," *J Infect Dis*, 1998, 177(5):1290-5.

Rabies Virus Vaccine (RAY beez VYE rus vak SEEN)

Related Information

Immunization Recommendations *on page 1249*

U.S. Brand Names Imovax® Rabies; RabAvert®

Canadian Brand Names Imovax® Rabies; RabAvert®

Synonyms HDCV; Human Diploid Cell Cultures Rabies Vaccine; PCEC; Purified Chick Embryo Cell

Generic Available No

Use Pre-exposure immunization: Vaccinate persons with greater than usual risk due to occupation or avocation including veterinarians, rangers, animal handlers, certain laboratory workers, and persons living in or visiting countries for longer than 1 month where rabies is a constant threat.

Postexposure prophylaxis: If a bite from a carrier animal is unprovoked, if it is not captured and rabies is present in that species and area, administer rabies immune globulin (RIG) and the vaccine as indicated

Drug of Choice or Alternative for Organism(s):
Rabies Virus *on page 283*

Pregnancy Risk Factor C

Pregnancy Implications Pregnancy is not a contraindication to postexposure prophylaxis. Pre-exposure prophylaxis during pregnancy may also be considered if risk of rabies is great.

Contraindications Hypersensitivity to any component of the formulation; developing febrile illness (during pre-exposure therapy only); life-threatening allergic reactions to rabies vaccine or any components of the formulation (however, carefully consider a patient's risk of rabies before continuing therapy)

Warnings/Precautions Report serious reactions to the State Health Department or the manufacturer/distributor, an immune complex reaction is possible 2-21 days following booster doses of HDCV; hypersensitivity reactions may be treated with antihistamines or epinephrine, if severe. Immune response may be decreased in immunosuppressed patients. Imovax® Rabies contains albumin and neomycin. RabAvert® contains amphotericin B, bovine gelatin, chicken protein, chlortetracycline, and neomycin. For I. M. administration only.

Adverse Reactions All serious adverse reactions must be reported to the U.S. Department of Health and Human Services (DHHS) Vaccine Adverse Event Reporting System (VAERS) 1-800-822-7967.

Frequency not defined.

Cardiovascular: Edema

Central nervous system: Dizziness, malaise, encephalomyelitis, transverse myelitis, fever, pain, headache, neuroparalytic reactions

Gastrointestinal: Nausea, abdominal pain

Local: Local discomfort, pain at injection site, itching, erythema, swelling or pain

Neuromuscular & skeletal: Myalgia

Postmarketing and/or case reports: Anaphylaxis, encephalitis, Guillain-Barré syndrome, meningitis, transient paralysis, urticaria pigmentosa

Stability Store under refrigeration at 2°C to 8°C (36°F to 46°F); protect from light; do not freeze

Mechanism of Action Rabies vaccine is an inactivated virus vaccine which promotes immunity by inducing an active immune response. The production of specific antibodies requires about 7-10 days to develop. Rabies immune globulin or antirabies serum, equine (ARS) is given in conjunction with rabies vaccine to provide immune protection until an antibody response can occur.

Pharmacodynamics/Kinetics

Onset of action: I.M.: Rabies antibody: ~7-10 days

Peak effect: ~30-60 days

Duration: ≥1 year

Dosage

Pre-exposure prophylaxis: 1 mL I.M. on days 0, 7, and 21 to 28. **Note:** Prolonging the interval between doses does not interfere with immunity achieved after the concluding dose of the basic series.

Postexposure prophylaxis: All postexposure treatment should begin with immediate cleansing of the wound with soap and water

Persons not previously immunized as above: I.M.: 5 doses (1 mL each) on days 0, 3, 7, 14, 28. In addition, patients should receive rabies immune globulin 20 units/kg body weight, half infiltrated at bite site if possible, remainder I.M.)

Persons who have previously received postexposure prophylaxis with rabies vaccine, received a recommended I.M. pre-exposure series of rabies vaccine or have a previously documented rabies antibody titer considered adequate: 1 mL of either vaccine I.M. only on days 0 and 3; do not administer RIG

Booster (for occupational or other continuing risk): 1 mL I.M. every 2-5 years or based on antibody titers

Administration For I.M. administration only; this rabies vaccine product must not be administered intradermally; in adults and children, administer I.M. injections in the deltoid muscle, not the gluteal; for younger children, use the outer aspect of the thigh.

For patients at risk of hemorrhage following intramuscular injection, the ACIP recommends "it should be administered intramuscularly if, in the opinion of the physician familiar with the patients bleeding risk, the vaccine can be administered with reasonable safety by this route. If the patient receives antihemophilia or other similar therapy, intramuscular vaccination can be scheduled shortly after such therapy is administered. A fine needle (23 gauge or smaller) can be used for the vaccination and firm pressure applied to the site (without rubbing) for at least 2 minutes. The patient should be instructed concerning the risk of hematoma from the injection."

Monitoring Parameters Serum rabies antibody every 6 months to 2 years in patients at high risk for exposure

(Continued)

Rabies Virus Vaccine *(Continued)*

Reference Range Antibody titers ≥115 as determined by rapid fluorescent-focus inhibition test are indicative of adequate response; collect titers on day 28 postexposure

Additional Information Federal law requires that the date of administration, the vaccine manufacturer, lot number of vaccine, and the administering person's name, title, and address be entered into the patient's permanent medical record.

Dosage Forms

Injection, powder for reconstitution:

Imovax® Rabies: 2.5 int. units [HDCV; grown in human diploid cell culture; contains albumin <100 mg, neomycin <150 mcg]

RabAvert®: 2.5 int. units [PCEC; grown in chicken fibroblasts; contains amphotericin <2 ng, chlortetracycline <20 ng, and neomycin <1 mcg]

Selected Readings

"A New Rabies Vaccine," *Med Lett Drugs Ther*, 1998, 40(1029):64-5.

Dreesen DW and Hanlon CA, "Current Recommendations for the Prophylaxis and Treatment of Rabies," *Drugs*, 1998, 56(5):801-9.

Lang J and Plotkin SA, "Rabies Risk and Immunoprophylaxis in Children," *Adv Pediatr Infect Dis*, 1997, 13:219-55.

Strady A, Lang J, Lienard M, et al, "Antibody Persistence Following Pre-exposure Regimens of Cell-Culture Rabies Vaccines: 10-Year Follow-up and Proposal for a New Booster Policy," *J Infect Dis*, 1998, 177(5):1290-5.

Raniclor™ *see* Cefaclor *on page 697*

ratio-Aclavulanate (Can) *see* Amoxicillin and Clavulanate Potassium *on page 645*

ratio-Acyclovir (Can) *see* Acyclovir *on page 629*

ratio-Cefuroxime (Can) *see* Cefuroxime *on page 725*

ratio-Ciprofloxacin (Can) *see* Ciprofloxacin *on page 742*

ratio-Clarithromycin (Can) *see* Clarithromycin *on page 749*

Rebetol® *see* Ribavirin *on page 1040*

Rebetron® *see* Interferon Alfa-2b and Ribavirin *on page 884*

Recombivax HB® *see* Hepatitis B Vaccine *on page 856*

Reese's® Pinworm Medicine [OTC] *see* Pyrantel Pamoate *on page 1021*

Rejuva-A® (Can) *see* Tretinoin (Topical) *on page 1127*

Relenza® *see* Zanamivir *on page 1157*

Renova® *see* Tretinoin (Topical) *on page 1127*

Rescriptor® *see* Delavirdine *on page 769*

RespiGam® [DSC] *see* Respiratory Syncytial Virus Immune Globulin (Intravenous) *on page 1036*

Respiratory Syncytial Virus Immune Globulin (Intravenous)

(RES peer rah tor ee sin SISH al VYE rus i MYUN GLOB yoo lin in tra VEE nus)

U.S. Brand Names RespiGam® [DSC]

Synonyms RSV-IGIV

Generic Available No

Use Orphan drug: Prevention of serious lower respiratory infection caused by respiratory syncytial virus (RSV) in children <24 months of age with bronchopulmonary dysplasia (BPD) or a history of premature birth (≤35 weeks gestation)

Pregnancy Risk Factor C

Contraindications Hypersensitivity to any component of the formulation; selective IgA deficiency; history of severe prior reaction to any immunoglobulin preparation

Warnings/Precautions Use caution to avoid fluid overload in patients, particularly infants with bronchopulmonary dysplasia (BPD), when administering RSV-IGIV; hypersensitivity including anaphylaxis or angioneurotic edema may occur; keep epinephrine 1:1000 readily available during infusion; rare occurrences of aseptic meningitis syndrome have been associated with IGIV treatment, particularly with high doses; observe carefully for signs and symptoms and treat promptly.

RespiGam® contains sucrose. Renal dysfunction and /or acute renal failure has been reported with the administration of IVIG; the majority of cases were associated with sucrose-containing IVIG products. Use caution in patients at increased risk of renal failure (including pre-existing renal insufficiency, volume depletion, or concurrent treatment with nephrotoxic drugs). Ensure adequate hydration prior to infusion.

Adverse Reactions

1% to 10%:

Cardiovascular: Tachycardia (1%), hypertension (1%), hypotension

Central nervous system: Fever (6%)

Dermatologic: Rash (1%)
Endocrine & metabolic: Fluid overload (1%)
Gastrointestinal: Vomiting (2%), diarrhea (1%), gastroenteritis (1%)
Local: Injection site inflammation (1%)
Respiratory: Respiratory distress (2%), wheezing (2%), rales, hypoxia (1%), tachypnea (1%)

<1%: Edema, pallor, heart murmur, cyanosis, flushing, palpitation, chest tightness, dizziness, anxiety, eczema, pruritus, abdominal cramps, myalgia, arthralgia, cough, rhinorrhea, dyspnea

Overdosage/Toxicology Likely symptoms of overdose include those associated with fluid overload. Treatment is supportive (eg, diuretics).

Stability Store between 2°C and 8°C; do not freeze or shake vial; avoid foaming; discard after single use since it is preservative free

Mechanism of Action RSV-IGIV is a sterile liquid immunoglobulin G containing neutralizing antibody to respiratory syncytial virus. It is effective in reducing the incidence and duration of RSV hospitalization and the severity of RSV illness in high risk infants.

Dosage I.V.: Children <24 months of age: Prevention of respiratory syncytial virus (RSV) infection: 750 mg/kg/month according to the following infusion schedule:

Initial infusion rate for the first 15 minutes: 1.5 mL/kg/hour; after 15 minutes increase to 3.6 mL/kg/hour (maximum infusion rate: 3.6 mL/kg/hour); rate should be decreased in patients at risk of renal dysfunction

Dietary Considerations Contains sodium 1-1.5 mEq per 50 mL, sucrose 50 mg, human albumin 10 mg

Administration Begin infusion within 6 hours and complete within 12 hours after entering vial. Observe for signs of intolerance during and after infusion; administer through an I.V. line using a constant infusion pump and through a separate I.V. line, if possible; if needed, RSV-IGIV may be "piggybacked" into dextrose with or without saline solutions, avoiding dilutions >2:1 with such line configurations. An in-line filter with a pore size >15 micrometers may be used.

Monitoring Parameters Monitor for symptoms of allergic reaction; check vital signs, cardiopulmonary status after each rate increase and thereafter at 30-minute intervals until 30 minutes following completion of the infusion

Dosage Forms [DSC] = Discontinued product

Injection, solution [preservative free]: 50 mg/mL (50 mL) [contains sodium 1-1.5 mEq per 50 mL, sucrose 50 mg, human albumin 10 mg] [DSC]

Selected Readings

American Academy of Pediatrics Committee on Infectious Diseases, Committee on Fetus and Newborn, "Respiratory Syncytial Virus Immune Globulin Intravenous: Indications for Use," *Pediatrics*, 1997, 99(4):645-50.

Ellenberg SS, Epstein JS, Fratantoni JC, et al, "A Trial of RSV Immune Globulin in Infants and Young Children: The FDA's View," *N Engl J Med*, 1994, 331(3):203-5.

Groothius JR, Simoes EA, Levin MJ, et al, "Prophylactic Administration of Respiratory Syncytial Virus Immune Globulin to High-Risk Infants and Young Children. The Respiratory Syncytial Virus Immune Globulin Study Group," *N Engl J Med*, 1993, 329(21):1524-30.

Ottolini MG and Hemming VG, "Prevention and Treatment Recommendations for Respiratory Syncytial Virus Infection. Background and Clinical Experience 40 Years After Discovery," *Drugs*, 1997, 54(6):867-84.

"Prevention of Respiratory Syncytial Virus Infections: Indications for the Use of Palivizumab and Update on the Use of RSV-IGIV. American Academy of Pediatrics Committee on Infectious Diseases and Committee of Fetus and Newborn," *Pediatrics*, 1998, 102(5):1211-6.

Simoes EA, Sondheimer HM, Top FH Jr, et al, "Respiratory Syncytial Virus Immune Globulin for Prophylaxis Against Respiratory Syncytial Virus Disease in Infants and Children With Congenital Heart Disease. The Cardiac Study Group," *J Pediatr*, 1998, 133(4):492-9.

Wandstrat TL, "Respiratory Syncytial Virus Immune Globulin Intravenous," *Ann Pharmacother*, 1997, 31(1):83-8.

Retin-A® *see* Tretinoin (Topical) *on page 1127*

Retin-A® Micro *see* Tretinoin (Topical) *on page 1127*

Retinoic Acid *see* Tretinoin (Topical) *on page 1127*

Retinova® (Can) *see* Tretinoin (Topical) *on page 1127*

Retrovir® *see* Zidovudine *on page 1159*

Reverse Transcriptase Inhibitors

Refer to

Abacavir and Lamivudine *on page 626*
Abacavir, Lamivudine, and Zidovudine *on page 627*
Abacavir *on page 624*
Delavirdine *on page 769*
Didanosine *on page 774*
Efavirenz *on page 795*
Emtricitabine and Tenofovir *on page 801*
Emtricitabine *on page 799*
(Continued)

Reverse Transcriptase Inhibitors *(Continued)*

Lamivudine *on page 905*
Nevirapine *on page 967*
Stavudine *on page 1076*
Zalcitabine *on page 1155*
Zidovudine and Lamivudine *on page 1162*
Zidovudine *on page 1159*

Reyataz® *see* Atazanavir *on page 668*
RhIG *see* Rh_0(D) Immune Globulin *on page 1038*

Rh_0(D) Immune Globulin (ar aych oh (dee) i MYUN GLOB yoo lin)

U.S. Brand Names BayRho-D® Full-Dose; BayRho-D® Mini-Dose; MICRhoGAM®; RhoGAM®; Rhophylac®; WinRho SDF®

Canadian Brand Names BayRho-D® Full-Dose

Synonyms RhIG; Rho(D) Immune Globulin (Human); RhoIGIV; RhoIVIM

Generic Available No

Use

Suppression of Rh isoimmunization: Use in the following situations when an Rh_0(D)-negative individual is exposed to Rh_0(D)-positive blood: During delivery of an Rh_0(D)-positive infant; abortion; amniocentesis; chorionic villus sampling; ruptured tubal pregnancy; abdominal trauma; transplacental hemorrhage. Used when the mother is Rh_0(D) negative, the father of the child is either Rh_0(D) positive or Rh_0(D) unknown, the baby is either Rh_0(D) positive or Rh_0(D) unknown.

Transfusion: Suppression of Rh isoimmunization in Rh_0(D)-negative female children and female adults in their childbearing years transfused with Rh_0(D) antigen-positive RBCs or blood components containing Rh_0(D) antigen-positive RBCs

Treatment of idiopathic thrombocytopenic purpura (ITP): Used in the following nonsplenectomized Rh_0(D) positive individuals: Children with acute or chronic ITP, adults with chronic ITP, children and adults with ITP secondary to HIV infection

Pregnancy Risk Factor C

Pregnancy Implications Animal studies have not been conducted. Available evidence suggests that Rh_0(D) immune globulin administration during pregnancy does not harm the fetus or affect future pregnancies.

Contraindications Hypersensitivity to immune globulins or any component of the formulation; prior sensitization to Rh_0(D)

Warnings/Precautions As a product of human plasma, may potentially transmit disease; screening of donors, as well as testing and/or inactivation of certain viruses reduces this risk. Not for replacement therapy in immune globulin deficiency syndromes. Use caution with IgA deficiency, may contain trace amounts of IgA; patients who are IgA deficient may have the potential for developing IgA antibodies, anaphylactic reactions may occur. Administer I.M. injections with caution in patients with thrombocytopenia or coagulation disorders.

ITP: Do not administer I.M. or SubQ; administer dose I.V. only. Safety and efficacy not established in Rh_0(D) negative or splenectomized patients. Decrease dose with hemoglobin <10 g/dL; use with extreme caution if hemoglobin <8 g/dL

Rh_0(D) suppression: For use in the mother; do not administer to the neonate.

Adverse Reactions Frequency not defined.

Cardiovascular: Hypotension, pallor, tachycardia, vasodilation
Central nervous system: Chills, dizziness, fever, headache, malaise, somnolence
Dermatologic: Pruritus, rash
Gastrointestinal: Abdominal pain, diarrhea, nausea, vomiting
Hematologic: Hemoglobin decreased (patients with ITP), intravascular hemolysis (patients with ITP)
Hepatic: LDH increased
Local: Injection site reaction: Discomfort, induration, mild pain, redness, swelling
Neuromuscular & skeletal: Back pain, hyperkinesia, myalgia, weakness
Miscellaneous: Anaphylaxis, diaphoresis

Overdosage/Toxicology No symptoms are likely, however, high doses have been associated with a mild, transient hemolytic anemia. Treatment is supportive.

Drug Interactions

Decreased Effect: Rh_0(D) immune globulin may interfere with the response of live vaccines; vaccines should not be administered within 3 months after Rh_0(D)

Stability Store at 2°C to 8°C (35°F to 46°F); do not freeze

Rhophylac®: Stored at this temperature, Rhophylac® has a shelf life of 36 months. Protect from light.

WinRho SDF®: Dilute with provided NS only. Inject diluent slowly into vial and gently swirl until dissolved; do not shake. Following reconstitution, may store at room temperature for up to 12 hours.

Mechanism of Action

Rh suppression: Suppresses the immune response and antibody formation of Rh_o(D) negative individuals to Rh_o(D) positive red blood cells.

ITP: Coats the patients Rh_o(D) positive red blood cells with antibody, so that as they are cleared by the spleen, the spleens ability to clear antibody-coated cells is saturated, sparing the platelets.

Pharmacodynamics/Kinetics

Onset of platelet increase: ITP: 1-3 days

Duration: Suppression of Rh isoimmunization: ~12 weeks; Treatment of ITP: 3-4 weeks

Distribution: V_d: I.M.: 8.59 L

Half-life elimination: 21-30 days

Time to peak, plasma: I.M.: 5-10 days

Dosage

ITP: Children and Adults: WinRho SDF®: I.V.:

Initial: 50 mcg/kg as a single injection, or can be given as a divided dose on separate days. If hemoglobin is <10 g/dL: Dose should be reduced to 25-40 mcg/kg.

Subsequent dosing: 25-60 mcg/kg can be used if required to elevate platelet count

Maintenance dosing if patient **did respond** to initial dosing: 25-60 mcg/kg based on platelet and hemoglobin levels:

Maintenance dosing if patient **did not respond** to initial dosing:

Hemoglobin 8-10 g/dL: Redose between 25-40 mcg/kg

Hemoglobin >10 g/dL: Redose between 50-60 mcg/kg

Hemoglobin <8 g/dL: Use with caution

Rh_o(D) suppression: Adults: **Note:** One "full dose" (300 mcg) provides enough antibody to prevent Rh sensitization if the volume of RBC entering the circulation is ≤15 mL. When >15 mL is suspected, a fetal red cell count should be performed to determine the appropriate dose.

Pregnancy:

Antepartum prophylaxis: In general, dose is given at 28 weeks. If given early in pregnancy, administer every 12 weeks to ensure adequate levels of passively acquired anti-Rh

BayRho-D® Full Dose, RhoGAM®: I.M.: 300 mcg

Rhophylac®, WinRho SDF®: I.M., I.V.: 300 mcg

Postpartum prophylaxis: In general, dose is administered as soon as possible after delivery, preferably within 72 hours. Can be given up to 28 days following delivery

BayRho-D® Full Dose, RhoGAM®: I.M.: 300 mcg

Rhophylac®: I.M., I.V.: 300 mcg

WinRho SDF®: I.M., I.V.: 120 mcg

Threatened abortion, any time during pregnancy (with continuation of pregnancy):

BayRho-D® Full Dose, RhoGAM®: I.M.: 300 mcg; administer as soon as possible

Rhophylac®, WinRho SDF®: I.M., I.V.: 300 mcg; administer as soon as possible

Abortion, miscarriage, termination of ectopic pregnancy:

BayRho-D®, RhoGAM®: I.M.: ≥13 weeks gestation: 300 mcg.

BayRho-D® Mini Dose, MICRhoGAM®: <13 weeks gestation: I.M.: 50 mcg

Rhophylac®: I.M., I.V.: 300 mcg

WinRho SDF®: I.M., I.V.: After 34 weeks gestation: 120 mcg; administer immediately or within 72 hours

Amniocentesis, chorionic villus sampling:

BayRho-D®, RhoGAM®: I.M.: At 15-18 weeks gestation or during the 3rd trimester: 300 mcg. If dose is given between 13-18 weeks, repeat at 26-28 weeks and within 72 hours of delivery.

Rhophylac®: I.M., I.V.: 300 mcg

WinRho SDF®: I.M., I.V.: Before 34 weeks gestation: 300 mcg; administer immediately, repeat dose every 12 weeks during pregnancy; After 34 weeks gestation: 120 mcg, administered immediately or within 72 hours

Abdominal trauma, manipulation:

BayRho-D®, RhoGAM®: I.M.: 2nd or 3rd trimester: 300 mcg. If dose is given between 13-18 weeks, repeat at 26-28 weeks and within 72 hours of delivery

WinRho SDF®: I.M./I.V.: After 34 weeks gestation: 120 mcg; administer immediately or within 72 hours

Transfusion:

Children and Adults: WinRho SDF®: Administer within 72 hours after exposure of incompatible blood transfusions or massive fetal hemorrhage.

(Continued)

Rh_o(D) Immune Globulin *(Continued)*

I.V.: Calculate dose as follows; administer 600 mcg every 8 hours until the total dose is administered:
Exposure to Rh_o(D) positive whole blood: 9 mcg/mL blood
Exposure to Rh_o(D) positive red blood cells: 18 mcg/mL cells

I.M.: Calculate dose as follows; administer 1200 mcg every 12 hours until the total dose is administered:
Exposure to Rh_o(D) positive whole blood: 12 mcg/mL blood
Exposure to Rh_o(D) positive red blood cells: 24 mcg/mL cells

Adults:
BayRho-D®, RhoGAM®: I.M.: Multiply the volume of Rh positive whole blood administered by the hematocrit of the donor unit to equal the volume of RBCs transfused. The volume of RBCs is then divided by 15 mL, providing the number of 300 mcg doses (vials/syringes) to administer. If the dose calculated results in a fraction, round up to the next higher whole 300 mcg dose (vial/syringe).
Rhophylac®: I.M., I.V.: 20 mcg/2 mL transfused blood or 20 mcg/mL erythrocyte concentrate

Administration The total volume can be administered in divided doses at different sites at one time or may be divided and given at intervals, provided the total dosage is given within 72 hours of the fetomaternal hemorrhage or transfusion.
I.M.: Administer into the deltoid muscle of the upper arm or anterolateral aspect of the upper thigh; avoid gluteal region due to risk of sciatic nerve injury. If large doses (>5 mL) are needed, administration in divided doses at different sites is recommended.
I.V.: WinRho SDF®: Infuse over 3-5 minutes; do not administer with other medications

Monitoring Parameters Signs and symptoms of intravascular hemolysis (IVH), anemia, and renal insufficiency; observe patient for side effects for at least 20 minutes following administration

Test Interactions Some infants born to women given Rh_o(D) antepartum have a weakly positive Coombs' test at birth. Fetal-maternal hemorrhage may cause false blood-typing result in the mother; when there is any doubt to the patients' Rh type, Rh_o(D) immune globulin should be administered

Patient Information This medication is only given by injection. It may be given as a one-time dose, or may need repeated. You may experience pain at the injection site. Notify prescriber if you experience chills, headache, dizziness, fever or rash.

Additional Information A "full dose" of Rh_o(D) immune globulin has previously been referred to as a 300 mcg dose. It is not the actual anti-D content. Although dosing has traditionally been expressed in mcg, potency is listed in int. units.

Dosage Forms
Injection, solution [preservative free]:
BayRho-D® Full-Dose, RhoGAM®: 300 mcg [for I.M. use only]
BayRho-D® Mini-Dose, MICRhoGAM®: 50 mcg [for I.M. use only]
Rhophylac®: 300 mcg/2 mL (2 mL) [1500 int. units; for I.M. or I.V. use]
Injection, powder for reconstitution [preservative free] (WinRho SDF®): 120 mcg [600 int. units], 300 mcg [1500 int. units], 1000 mcg [5000 int. units] [for I.M. or I.V. use]

Selected Readings

Hartwell EA, "Use of Rh Immune Globulin: ASCP Practice Parameter. American Society of Clinical Pathologists," *Am J Clin Pathol*, 1998, 110(3):281-92.
"Rh_o(D) Immune Globulin I.V. for Prevention of Rh Isoimmunization and for Treatment of ITP," *Med Lett Drugs Ther*, 1996, 38(966):6-8.
Simpson KN, Coughlin CM, Eron J, et al, "Idiopathic Thrombocytopenia Purpura: Treatment Patterns and an Analysis of Cost Associated With Intravenous Immunoglobulin and Anti-D Therapy," *Semin Hematol*, 1998, 35(1 Suppl 1):58-64.
Ware RE and Zimmerman SA, "Anti-D: Mechanisms of Action," *Semin Hematol*, 1998, 35(1 Suppl 1):14-22.

Rho(D) Immune Globulin (Human) *see* Rh_o(D) Immune Globulin *on page 1038*
RhoGAM® *see* Rh_o(D) Immune Globulin *on page 1038*
RhoIGIV *see* Rh_o(D) Immune Globulin *on page 1038*
RhoIVIM *see* Rh_o(D) Immune Globulin *on page 1038*
Rhophylac® *see* Rh_o(D) Immune Globulin *on page 1038*
Rhoxal-ciprofloxacin (Can) *see* Ciprofloxacin *on page 742*
Rhoxal-minocycline (Can) *see* Minocycline *on page 947*
Ribasphere™ *see* Ribavirin *on page 1040*

Ribavirin (rye ba VYE rin)

U.S. Brand Names Copegus®; Rebetol®; Ribasphere™; Virazole®
Canadian Brand Names Virazole®
Synonyms RTCA; Tribavirin
Generic Available Yes: Capsule

Use

Inhalation: Treatment of patients with respiratory syncytial virus (RSV) infections; specially indicated for treatment of severe lower respiratory tract RSV infections in patients with an underlying compromising condition (prematurity, bronchopulmonary dysplasia and other chronic lung conditions, congenital heart disease, immunodeficiency, immunosuppression), and recent transplant recipients

Oral capsule:

In combination with interferon alfa-2b (Intron® A) injection for the treatment of chronic hepatitis C in patients with compensated liver disease who have relapsed after alpha interferon therapy or were previously untreated with alpha interferons

In combination with peginterferon alfa-2b (PEG-Intron®) injection for the treatment of chronic hepatitis C in patients with compensated liver disease who were previously untreated with alpha interferons

Oral solution: In combination with interferon alfa 2b (Intron® A) injection for the treatment of chronic hepatitis C in patients ≥3 years of age with compensated liver disease who were previously untreated with alpha interferons or patients ≥18 years of age who have relapsed after alpha interferon therapy

Oral tablet: In combination with peginterferon alfa-2a (Pegasys®) injection for the treatment of chronic hepatitis C in patients with compensated liver disease who were previously untreated with alpha interferons (includes patients with histological evidence of cirrhosis [Child-Pugh class A] and patients with clinically-stable HIV disease)

Unlabeled/Investigational Use Used in other viral infections including influenza A and B and adenovirus

Drug of Choice or Alternative for Organism(s):

Respiratory Syncytial Virus *on page 285*

Restrictions An FDA-approved medication guide is available at www.fda.gov/cder/Offices/ODS/labeling.htm; distribute to each patient to whom this medication is dispensed for the treatment of hepatitis C.

Pregnancy Risk Factor X

Pregnancy Implications Produced significant embryocidal and/or teratogenic effects in all animal studies at ~0.01 times the maximum recommended daily human dose. Use is contraindicated in pregnancy. Negative pregnancy test is required before initiation and monthly thereafter. Avoid pregnancy in female patients and female partners of male patients during therapy by using two effective forms of contraception; continue contraceptive measures for at least 6 months after completion of therapy. If patient or female partner becomes pregnant during treatment, she should be counseled about potential risks of exposure. If pregnancy occurs during use or within 6 months after treatment, report to company (800-593-2214).

Contraindications Hypersensitivity to ribavirin or any component of the formulation; women of childbearing age who will not use contraception reliably; pregnancy

Additional contraindications for oral formulation: Male partners of pregnant women; Cl_{cr}< 50 mL/minute; hemoglobinopathies (eg, thalassemia major, sickle cell anemia); as monotherapy for treatment of chronic hepatitis C; patients with autoimmune hepatitis, anemia, severe heart disease

Refer to individual monographs for Interferon Alfa-2b (Intron® A) and Peginterferon Alfa-2a (Pegasys®) for additional contraindication information.

Warnings/Precautions Negative pregnancy test is required before initiation and monthly thereafter. Avoid pregnancy in female patients and female partners of male patients, during therapy, and for at least 6 months after treatment; two forms of contraception should be used. Elderly patients are more susceptible to adverse effects; use caution. Safety and efficacy have not been established in patients who have failed other alpha interferon therapy, received organ transplants, or been coinfected with hepatitis B or HIV (Copegus® may be used in HIV coinfected patients unless CD4+ cell count is <100 cells/microL). Safety and efficacy have not been established in patients <3 years of age.

Inhalation: Use with caution in patients requiring assisted ventilation because precipitation of the drug in the respiratory equipment may interfere with safe and effective patient ventilation; monitor carefully in patients with COPD and asthma for deterioration of respiratory function. Ribavirin is potentially mutagenic, tumor-promoting, and gonadotoxic. Although anemia has not been reported with inhalation therapy, consider monitoring for anemia 1-2 weeks post-treatment. Pregnant healthcare workers may consider unnecessary occupational exposure; ribavirin has been detected in healthcare workers' urine. Healthcare professionals or family members who are pregnant (or may become pregnant) should be counseled about potential risks of exposure and counseled about risk reduction strategies.

(Continued)

Ribavirin *(Continued)*

Oral: Severe psychiatric events have occurred including depression and suicidal behavior during combination therapy. Avoid use in patients with a psychiatric history; discontinue if severe psychiatric symptoms occur. Hemolytic anemia is a significant toxicity; usually occurring within 1-2 weeks. Assess cardiac disease before initiation. Anemia may worsen underlying cardiac disease; use caution. If any deterioration in cardiovascular status occurs, discontinue therapy. Use caution in pulmonary disease; pulmonary symptoms have been associated with administration. Discontinue therapy in suspected/confirmed pancreatitis or if hepatic decompensation occurs. Use caution in patients with sarcoidosis (exacerbation reported).

Adverse Reactions

Inhalation:

1% to 10%:

Central nervous system: Fatigue, headache, insomnia
Gastrointestinal: Nausea, anorexia
Hematologic: Anemia

<1%: Hypotension, cardiac arrest, digitalis toxicity, conjunctivitis, mild bronchospasm, worsening of respiratory function, apnea

Note: Incidence of adverse effects (approximate) in healthcare workers: Headache (51%); conjunctivitis (32%); rhinitis, nausea, rash, dizziness, pharyngitis, and lacrimation (10% to 20%)

Oral (all adverse reactions are documented while receiving combination therapy with interferon alpha-2b or interferon alpha-2a; percentages as reported in adults):

>10%:

Central nervous system: Fatigue (60% to 70%)*, headache (43% to 66%)*, fever (32% to 46%)*, insomnia (26% to 41%), depression (20% to 36%)*, irritability (23% to 32%), dizziness (14% to 26%), impaired concentration (10% to 14%)*, emotional lability (7% to 12%)*

Dermatologic: Alopecia (27% to 36%), pruritus (13% to 29%), dry skin (13% to 24%), rash (5% to 28%), dermatitis (up to 16%)

Gastrointestinal: Nausea (33% to 47%), anorexia (21% to 32%), weight decrease (10% to 29%), diarrhea (10% to 22%), dyspepsia (8% to 16%), vomiting (9% to 14%)*, abdominal pain (8% to 13%), xerostomia (up to 12%), RUQ pain (up to 12%)

Hematologic: Neutropenia (8% to 27%; 40% with HIV coinfection), hemoglobin decreased (25% to 36%), hyperbilirubinemia (24% to 34%), anorexia (24% to 26%), anemia (11% to 17%), lymphopenia (12% to 14%), absolute neutrophil count <0.5 x 10^9/L (5% to 11%), thrombocytopenia (<1% to 14%), hemolytic anemia (10% to 13%), WBC decreased

Neuromuscular & skeletal: Myalgia (40% to 64%)*, rigors (40% to 48%), arthralgia (22% to 34%)*, musculoskeletal pain (19% to 28%)

Respiratory: Dyspnea (13% to 26%), cough (7% to 23%), pharyngitis (up to 13%), sinusitis (up to 12%)*, nasal congestion

Miscellaneous: Flu-like syndrome (13% to 18%)*, viral infection (up to 12%), diaphoresis increased (up to 11%)

*Similar to interferon alone

1% to 10%:

Cardiovascular: Chest pain (5% to 9%)*, flushing (up to 4 %)
Central nervous system: Mood alteration (up to 6%; 9% with HIV coinfection), memory impairment (up to 6%), malaise (up to 6%), nervousness (~5%)*
Dermatologic: Eczema (4% to 5%)
Endocrine & metabolic: Hypothyroidism (up to 5%)
Gastrointestinal: Taste perversion (4% to 9%), constipation (up to 5%)
Genitourinary: Menstrual disorder (up to 7%)
Hematologic: Hepatomegaly (up to 4%)
Neuromuscular & skeletal: Weakness (9% to 10%), back pain (5%)
Optic: Conjunctivitis (up to 6%), blurred vision (up to 5%)
Respiratory: Rhinitis (up to 8%), exertional dyspnea (up to 7%)
Miscellaneous: Fungal infection (up to 6%)
*Similar to interferon alone

<1%: Diabetes mellitus, gout, pancreatitis, pulmonary dysfunction, suicidal ideation, thyroid function test abnormalities

Postmarketing and/or case reports: Hearing disorder, vertigo, sarcoidosis (including exacerbations of sarcoidosis)

Incidence of anorexia, headache, fever, suicidal ideation, and vomiting are higher in children.

Drug Interactions

Increased Effect/Toxicity: Concomitant use of ribavirin and nucleoside analogues may increase the risk of developing lactic acidosis (includes adefovir, didanosine,

lamivudine, stavudine, zalcitabine, zidovudine). Concurrent therapy of zidovudine with ribavirin/interferon alfa-2a may cause increased risk of severe anemia and/or severe neutropenia. Concurrent use with didanosine has been noted to increase the risk of pancreatitis and/or peripheral neuropathy in addition to lactic acidosis. Suspend therapy if signs/symptoms of toxicity are present.

Decreased Effect: Decreased effect of lamivudine, stavudine, and zidovudine (*in vitro*).

Ethanol/Nutrition/Herb Interactions Food: Oral: High-fat meal increases the AUC and C_{max}.

Stability

Inhalation: Store vials in a dry place at 15°C to 25°C (59°F to 78°F). Do not use any water containing an antimicrobial agent to reconstitute drug; reconstituted solution is stable for 24 hours at room temperature. Should not be mixed with other aerosolized medication.

Oral: Store at 15°C to 30°C (59°F to 86°F). Solution may also be refrigerated at 2°C to 8°C (36°F to 46°F).

Mechanism of Action Inhibits replication of RNA and DNA viruses; inhibits influenza virus RNA polymerase activity and inhibits the initiation and elongation of RNA fragments resulting in inhibition of viral protein synthesis

Pharmacodynamics/Kinetics

Absorption: Inhalation: Systemic; dependent upon respiratory factors and method of drug delivery; maximal absorption occurs with the use of aerosol generator via endotracheal tube; highest concentrations in respiratory tract and erythrocytes

Distribution: Oral capsule: Single dose: V_d 2825 L; distribution significantly prolonged in the erythrocyte (16-40 days), which can be used as a marker for intracellular metabolism

Protein binding: Oral: None

Metabolism: Hepatically and intracellularly (forms active metabolites); may be necessary for drug action

Bioavailability: Oral: 64%

Half-life elimination, plasma:

- Children: Inhalation: 6.5-11 hours
- Adults: Oral:
  - Capsule, single dose (Rebetol®, Ribasphere™): 24 hours in healthy adults, 44 hours with chronic hepatitis C infection (increases to ~298 hours at steady state)
  - Tablet, single dose (Copegus®): 120-170 hours

Time to peak, serum: Inhalation: At end of inhalation period; Oral capsule: Multiple doses: 3 hours

Excretion: Inhalation: Urine (40% as unchanged drug and metabolites); Oral capsule: Urine (61%), feces (12%)

Dosage

Aerosol inhalation: Infants and children: Use with Viratek® small particle aerosol generator (SPAG-2) at a concentration of 20 mg/mL (6 g reconstituted with 300 mL of sterile water without preservatives). Continuous aerosol administration: 12-18 hours/day for 3 days, up to 7 days in length

Oral capsule or solution: Children ≥3 years: Chronic hepatitis C (in combination with interferon alfa-2b):

- Rebetol®: Oral: **Note:** Oral solution should be used in children 3-5 years of age, children ≤25 kg, or those unable to swallow capsules.
  - Capsule/solution: 15 mg/kg/day in 2 divided doses (morning and evening)
  - Capsule dosing recommendations:
    - 25-36 kg: 400 mg/day (200 mg morning and evening)
    - 37-49 kg: 600 mg/day (200 mg in the morning and two 200 mg capsules in the evening)
    - 50-61 kg: 800 mg/day (two 200 mg capsules morning and evening)
    - >61 kg: Refer to Adults dosing
  - **Note:** Duration of therapy is 48 weeks in pediatric patients with genotype 1 and 24 weeks in patients with genotype 2,3. Discontinue treatment in any patient if HCV-RNA is not below the limit of detection of the assay after 24 weeks of therapy.
  - **Note:** Also refer to Interferon Alfa-2b/Ribavirin combination pack monograph.

Oral capsule (Rebetol®, Ribasphere™): Adults:

- Chronic hepatitis C (in combination with interferon alfa-2b):
  - ≤75 kg: 400 mg in the morning, then 600 mg in the evening
  - >75 kg: 600 mg in the morning, then 600 mg in the evening
  - **Note:** If HCV-RNA is undetectable at 24 weeks, duration of therapy is 48 weeks. In patients who relapse following interferon therapy, duration of dual therapy is 24 weeks.
  - **Note:** Also refer to Interferon Alfa-2b/Ribavirin combination pack monograph.

(Continued)

Ribavirin *(Continued)*

Chronic hepatitis C (in combination with peginterferon alfa-2b): 400 mg twice daily; duration of therapy is 1 year; after 24 weeks of treatment, if serum HCV-RNA is not below the limit of detection of the assay, consider discontinuation.

Oral tablet (Copegus®, in combination with peginterferon alfa-2b): Adults: Chronic hepatitis C:

Monoinfection, genotype 1,4:

<75kg: 1000 mg/day in 2 divided doses for 48 weeks

≥75kg: 1200 mg/day in 2 divided doses for 48 weeks

Monoinfection, genotype 2,3: 800 mg/day in 2 divided doses for 24 weeks

Coinfection with HIV: 800 mg/day in 2 divided doses for 48 weeks

Note: Also refer to Peginterferon Alfa-2a monograph.

Dosage adjustment in renal impairment: Cl_{cr} <50 mL/minute: Oral route is contraindicated

Dosage adjustment for toxicity: Oral: Capsule, solution, tablet:

Patient **without** cardiac history:

Hemoglobin <10 g/dL:

Children: 7.5 mg/kg/day

Adults: Decrease dose to 600 mg/day

Hemoglobin <8.5 g/dL: Children and Adults: Permanently discontinue treatment

Patient **with** cardiac history:

Hemoglobin has decreased ≥2 g/dL during any 4-week period of treatment:

Children: 7.5 mg/kg/day

Adults: Decrease dose to 600 mg/day

Hemoglobin <12 g/dL after 4 weeks of reduced dose: Children and Adults: Permanently discontinue treatment

Dietary Considerations When used in combination with interferon alfa-2b, capsules and solution may be taken with or without food, but always in a consistent manner in regard to food intake (ie, always take with food or always take on an empty stomach). When used in combination with peginterferon alfa 2b, capsules should be taken with food. Tablets should be taken with food.

Administration

Inhalation: Ribavirin should be administered in well-ventilated rooms (at least 6 air changes/hour). In mechanically-ventilated patients, ribavirin can potentially be deposited in the ventilator delivery system depending on temperature, humidity, and electrostatic forces; this deposition can lead to malfunction or obstruction of the expiratory valve, resulting in inadvertently high positive end-expiratory pressures. The use of one-way valves in the inspiratory lines, a breathing circuit filter in the expiratory line, and frequent monitoring and filter replacement have been effective in preventing these problems. Solutions in SPAG-2 unit should be discarded at least every 24 hours and when the liquid level is low before adding newly reconstituted solution. Should not be mixed with other aerosolized medication.

Oral: Administer concurrently with interferon alfa injection. Capsule should not be opened, crushed, chewed, or broken. Capsules are not for use in children <5 years of age. Use oral solution for children 3-5 years, those ≤25 kg, or those who cannot swallow capsules.

Capsule, in combination with interferon alfa-2b: May be administered with or without food, but always in a consistent manner in regard to food intake.

Capsule, in combination with peginterferon alfa 2b: Administer with food.

Solution, in combination with interferon alfa-2b: May be administered with or without food, but always in a consistent manner in regard to food intake.

Tablet: Should be administered with food.

Monitoring Parameters

Inhalation: Respiratory function, hemoglobin, reticulocyte count, CBC, I & O

Oral: CBC with differential (pretreatment, 2- and 4 weeks after initiation); pretreatment and monthly pregnancy test for women of childbearing age; LFTs, TSH, HCV-RNA after 24 weeks of therapy; ECG in patients with pre-existing cardiac disease

Patient Information Do not use if you are pregnant.

Dosage Forms

Capsule (Rebetol®, Ribasphere™): 200 mg

Powder for aerosol (Virazole®): 6 g

Powder for solution, inhalation [for aerosol administration] (Virazole®): 6 g [reconstituted product provides 20 mg/mL]

Tablet (Copegus®): 200 mg

Selected Readings

Davis GL, Esteban-Mur R, Rustgi V, et al, "Interferon Alfa-2b Alone or in Combination With Ribavirin for the Treatment of Relapse of Chronic Hepatitis C. International Hepatitis Interventional Therapy Group," *N Engl J Med*, 1998, 339(21):1493-9.

"Drugs for Non-HIV Viral Infections," *Med Lett Drugs Ther*, 1994, 36(919):27.

Keating MR, "Antiviral Agents," *Mayo Clin Proc*, 1992, 67(2):160-78.
McHutchison JG, Gordon SC, Schiff ER, et al, "Interferon Alfa-2b Alone or in Combination With Ribavirin as Initial Treatment for Chronic Hepatitis C. Hepatitis Interventional Therapy Group," *N Engl J Med*, 1998, 339(21):1485-92.
Ottolini MG and Hemming VG, "Prevention and Treatment Recommendations for Respiratory Syncytial Virus Infection. Background and Clinical Experience 40 Years After Discovery," *Drugs*, 1997, 54(6):867-84.

Ribavirin and Interferon Alfa-2b Combination Pack *see* Interferon Alfa-2b and Ribavirin *on page 884*

RID® Maximum Strength [OTC] *see* Pyrethrins and Piperonyl Butoxide *on page 1023*

RID® Mousse (Can) *see* Pyrethrins and Piperonyl Butoxide *on page 1023*

Rid® Spray [OTC] *see* Permethrin *on page 1001*

Rifabutin (rif a BYOO tin)

Related Information

USPHS / IDSA Guidelines for the Prevention of Opportunistic Infections in Persons Infected With HIV *on page 1237*

U.S. Brand Names Mycobutin®

Canadian Brand Names Mycobutin®

Synonyms Ansamycin

Generic Available No

Use Prevention of disseminated *Mycobacterium avium* complex (MAC) in patients with advanced HIV infection

Unlabeled/Investigational Use Utilized in multidrug regimens for treatment of MAC

Drug of Choice or Alternative for Organism(s):

Mycobacterium avium-intracellulare (Complex) *on page 228*
Mycobacterium kansasii on page 231

Pregnancy Risk Factor B

Contraindications Hypersensitivity to rifabutin, any other rifamycins, or any component of the formulation; rifabutin is contraindicated in patients with a WBC <1000/mm³ or a platelet count <50,000/mm³

Warnings/Precautions Rifabutin as a single agent must not be administered to patients with active tuberculosis since its use may lead to the development of tuberculosis that is resistant to both rifabutin and rifampin; rifabutin should be discontinued in patients with AST >500 units/L or if total bilirubin is >3 mg/dL. Use with caution in patients with liver impairment; modification of dosage should be considered in patients with renal impairment.

Adverse Reactions

>10%:
- Dermatologic: Rash (11%)
- Genitourinary: Discoloration of urine (30%)
- Hematologic: Neutropenia (25%), leukopenia (17%)

1% to 10%:
- Central nervous system: Headache (3%)
- Gastrointestinal: Vomiting/nausea (3%), abdominal pain (4%), diarrhea (3%), anorexia (2%), flatulence (2%), eructation (3%)
- Hematologic: Anemia, thrombocytopenia (5%)
- Hepatic: Increased AST/ALT (7% to 9%)
- Neuromuscular & skeletal: Myalgia

<1%: Chest pain, fever, insomnia, dyspepsia, dyspnea, taste perversion, uveitis

Overdosage/Toxicology Symptoms include nausea, vomiting, hepatotoxicity, lethargy, and CNS depression. Treatment is supportive. Hemodialysis will remove rifabutin, its effect on outcome is unknown.

Drug Interactions

Cytochrome P450 Effect: Substrate (major) of CYP1A2, 3A4; **Induces** CYP3A4 (strong)

Increased Effect/Toxicity: Rifabutin may increase the therapeutic effect of clopidogrel; concurrent use with isoniazid may increase risk of hepatotoxicity; the levels/toxicity of rifabutin may be increased by imidazole antifungals, macrolide antibiotics, and protease inhibitors

Decreased Effect: Rifabutin may decrease the levels/effects of alfentanil, amiodarone, angiotensin II receptor blockers (irbesartan, losartan), CYP3A4 substrates (eg, clarithromycin, erythromycin, mirtazapine, nefazodone, venlafaxine), 5-HT_3 antagonists, imidazole antifungals, aprepitant, barbiturates, benzodiazepines (metabolized by oxidation), beta blockers, buspirone, calcium channel blockers, chloramphenicol, corticosteroids, cyclosporine, dapsone, disopyramide, estrogen and progestin contraceptives, fluconazole, gefitinib, HMG-CoA reductase inhibitors, methadone, morphine, phenytoin, propafenone, protease inhibitors, quinidine,

(Continued)

Rifabutin *(Continued)*

repaglinide, reverse transcriptase inhibitors (non-nucleoside), tacrolimus, tamoxifen, terbinafine, tocainide, tricyclic antidepressants, warfarin, zaleplon, zolpidem. The effects of rifabutin may be decreased by CYP3A4 inducers (eg, aminoglutethimide, carbamazepine, nafcillin, nevirapine, phenobarbital, phenytoin).

Ethanol/Nutrition/Herb Interactions Food: High-fat meal may decrease the rate but not the extent of absorption.

Mechanism of Action Inhibits DNA-dependent RNA polymerase at the beta subunit which prevents chain initiation

Pharmacodynamics/Kinetics

Absorption: Readily, 53%

Distribution: V_d: 9.32 L/kg; distributes to body tissues including the lungs, liver, spleen, eyes, and kidneys

Protein binding: 85%

Metabolism: To active and inactive metabolites

Bioavailability: Absolute: HIV: 20%

Half-life elimination: Terminal: 45 hours (range: 16-69 hours)

Time to peak, serum: 2-4 hours

Excretion: Urine (10% as unchanged drug, 53% as metabolites); feces (10% as unchanged drug, 30% as metabolites)

Dosage Oral:

Children >1 year:

Prophylaxis: 5 mg/kg daily; higher dosages have been used in limited trials

Treatment (unlabeled use): Patients not receiving NNRTIs or protease inhibitors:

Initial phase (2 weeks to 2 months): 10-20 mg/kg daily (maximum: 300 mg).

Second phase: 10-20 mg/kg daily (maximum: 300 mg) or twice weekly

Adults:

Prophylaxis: 300 mg once daily (alone or in combination with azithromycin)

Treatment (unlabeled use):

Patients not receiving NNRTIs or protease inhibitors:

Initial phase: 5 mg/kg daily (maximum: 300 mg)

Second phase: 5 mg/kg daily or twice weekly

Patients receiving nelfinavir, amprenavir, indinavir: Reduce dose to 150 mg/day; no change in dose if administered twice weekly

Dosage adjustment in renal impairment: Cl_{cr} <30 mL/minute: Reduce dose by 50%

Dietary Considerations May be taken with meals or without food or mix with applesauce.

Administration Should be administered on an empty stomach, but may be taken with meals to minimize nausea or vomiting.

Monitoring Parameters Periodic liver function tests, CBC with differential, platelet count

Patient Information May discolor urine, tears, sweat, or other body fluids to a red-orange color; take 1 hour before or 2 hours after a meal on an empty stomach; soft contact lenses may be permanently stained; report any severe or persistent flu-like symptoms, nausea, vomiting, dark urine or pale stools, unusual bleeding or bruising, or any eye problems; can be taken with meals or sprinkled on applesauce

Dosage Forms Capsule: 150 mg

Selected Readings

Agins BD, Berman DS, Spicehandler D, et al, "Effect of Combined Therapy with Ansamycin, Clofazimine, Ethambutol, and Isoniazid for *Mycobacterium avium* Infection in Patients With AIDS," *J Infect Dis*, 1989, 159(4):784-7.

"Drugs for AIDS and Associated Infections," *Med Lett Drugs Ther*, 1993, 35(904):79-86.

Hoy J, Mijch A, Sandland M, et al, "Quadruple-Drug Therapy for *Mycobacterium avium-intracellulare* Bacteremia in AIDS Patients," *J Infect Dis*, 1990, 161(4):801-5.

Nightingale SD, Cameron DW, Gordin FM, et al, "Two Controlled Trials of Rifabutin Prophylaxis Against *Mycobacterium avium* Complex Infection in AIDS," *N Engl J Med*, 1993, 329(12):828-33.

Tseng AL and Walmsley SL, "Rifabutin-Associated Uveitis," *Ann Pharmacother*, 1995, 29(11):1149-55.

Rifadin® *see* Rifampin *on page 1046*

Rifamate® *see* Rifampin and Isoniazid *on page 1050*

Rifampicin *see* Rifampin *on page 1046*

Rifampin (RIF am pin)

Related Information

Antibiotic Treatment of Adults With Infective Endocarditis *on page 1271*

Antimicrobial Activity Against Selected Organisms *on page 1165*

Tuberculosis *on page 1315*

USPHS / IDSA Guidelines for the Prevention of Opportunistic Infections in Persons Infected With HIV *on page 1237*

U.S. Brand Names Rifadin®

Canadian Brand Names Rifadin®; Rofact™

Synonyms Rifampicin

Generic Available Yes

Use Management of active tuberculosis in combination with other agents; elimination of meningococci from the nasopharynx in asymptomatic carriers

Unlabeled/Investigational Use Prophylaxis of *Haemophilus influenzae* type b infection; *Legionella* pneumonia; used in combination with other anti-infectives in the treatment of staphylococcal infections; treatment of *M. leprae* infections

Drug of Choice or Alternative for

Disease/Syndrome(s):

Endocarditis, Acute, I.V. Drug Abuse *on page 123*
Endocarditis, Prosthetic Valve, Early *on page 124*
Endocarditis, Prosthetic Valve, Late *on page 125*
Epididymitis/Orchitis *on page 138*
Joint Replacement, Early Infection *on page 197*
Joint Replacement, Late Infection *on page 198*

Organism(s):

Brucella Species *on page 61*
Legionella pneumophila on page 202
Mycobacterium bovis on page 229
Mycobacterium kansasii on page 231
Mycobacterium tuberculosis on page 234
Rhodococcus Species *on page 288*
Staphylococcus epidermidis, Methicillin-Resistant *on page 309*
Streptococcus pneumoniae, Drug-Resistant *on page 316*

Pregnancy Risk Factor C

Pregnancy Implications Teratogenic effects have bee reported in animal studies. Rifampin crosses the human placenta. Due to the risk of tuberculosis to the fetus, treatment is recommended when the probability of maternal disease is moderate to high. Postnatal hemorrhages have been reported in the infant and mother with isoniazid administration during the last few weeks of pregnancy.

Contraindications Hypersensitivity to rifampin, any rifamycins, or any component of the formulation; concurrent use of amprenavir, saquinavir/ritonavir (possibly other protease inhibitors)

Warnings/Precautions Use with caution and modify dosage in patients with liver impairment; observe for hyperbilirubinemia; discontinue therapy if this in conjunction with clinical symptoms or any signs of significant hepatocellular damage develop; since rifampin has enzyme-inducing properties, porphyria exacerbation is possible; use with caution in patients with porphyria; do not use for meningococcal disease, only for short-term treatment of asymptomatic carrier states. Use with caution in patients receiving concurrent medications associated with hepatotoxicity (particularly with pyrazinamide), or in patients with a history of alcoholism (even if ethanol consumption is discontinued during therapy).

Monitor for compliance and effects including hypersensitivity, thrombocytopenia in patients on intermittent therapy; urine, feces, saliva, sweat, tears, and CSF may be discolored to red/orange; do not administer I.V. form via I.M. or SubQ routes; restart infusion at another site if extravasation occurs; remove soft contact lenses during therapy since permanent staining may occur; regimens of 600 mg once or twice weekly have been associated with a high incidence of adverse reactions including a flu-like syndrome

Adverse Reactions

Frequency not defined:

- Cardiovascular: Edema, flushing
- Central nervous system: Ataxia, behavioral changes, concentration impaired, confusion, dizziness, drowsiness, fatigue, fever, headache, numbness, psychosis
- Dermatologic: Pemphigoid reaction, pruritus, urticaria
- Endocrine & metabolic: Adrenal insufficiency, menstrual disorders
- Hematologic: Agranulocytosis (rare), DIC, eosinophilia, hemoglobin decreased, hemolysis, hemolytic anemia, leukopenia, thrombocytopenia (especially with high-dose therapy)
- Hepatic: Hepatitis (rare), jaundice
- Neuromuscular & skeletal: Myalgia, osteomalacia, weakness
- Ocular: Exudative conjunctivitis, visual changes
- Renal: Acute renal failure, BUN increased, hemoglobinuria, hematuria, interstitial nephritis, uric acid increased
- Miscellaneous: Flu-like syndrome

1% to 10%:

- Dermatologic: Rash (1% to 5%)

(Continued)

Rifampin *(Continued)*

Gastrointestinal (1% to 2%): Anorexia, cramps, diarrhea, epigastric distress, flatulence, heartburn, nausea, pseudomembranous colitis, pancreatitis vomiting

Hepatic: LFTs increased (up to 14%)

Overdosage/Toxicology Symptoms include nausea, vomiting, discoloration of bodily fluids, skin, and/or feces, and hepatotoxicity. Treatment is supportive. Lavage with activated charcoal is preferred to ipecac, as emesis is frequently present with overdose. Hemodialysis will remove rifampin, but its effect on outcome is unknown.

Drug Interactions

Cytochrome P450 Effect: Substrate (major) of CYP2A6, 2C8/9, 3A4; **Induces** CYP1A2 (strong), 2A6 (strong), 2B6 (strong), 2C8/9 (strong), 2C19 (strong), 3A4 (strong)

Increased Effect/Toxicity: Rifampin may increase the therapeutic effect of clopidogrel; concurrent use with isoniazid, pyrazinamide, or protease inhibitors (amprenavir, saquinavir/ritonavir) may increase risk of hepatotoxicity; macrolide antibiotics may increase levels/toxicity of rifampin

Decreased Effect: Rifampin may decrease the levels/effects of the following drugs: Acetaminophen, alfentanil, amiodarone, angiotensin II receptor blockers (irbesartan and losartan), 5-HT_3 antagonists, imidazole antifungals, aprepitant, barbiturates, benzodiazepines (metabolized by oxidation), beta blockers, buspirone, calcium channel blockers, chloramphenicol, corticosteroids, cyclosporine; CYP1A2, 2A6, 2B6, 2C8/9, 2C19, and 3A4 substrates (eg, aminophylline, amiodarone, bupropion, fluoxetine, fluvoxamine, ifosfamide, methsuximide, mirtazapine, nateglinide, pioglitazone, promethazine, proton pump inhibitors, ropinirole, rosiglitazone, selegiline, sertraline, theophylline, venlafaxine, and zafirlukast); dapsone, disopyramide, estrogen and progestin contraceptives, fexofenadine, fluconazole, fusidic acid, gefitinib, HMG-CoA reductase inhibitors, methadone, morphine, phenytoin, propafenone, protease inhibitors, quinidine, repaglinide, reverse transcriptase inhibitors (non-nucleoside), sulfonylureas, tacrolimus, tamoxifen, terbinafine, tocainide, tricyclic antidepressants, warfarin, zaleplon, zidovudine, zolpidem. The effects of rifampin may be decreased by CYP2A6, 2C8/9, and 3A4 inducers (eg, aminoglutethimide, barbiturates, carbamazepine, nafcillin, nevirapine, and phenytoin).

Ethanol/Nutrition/Herb Interactions

Ethanol: Avoid ethanol (may increase risk of hepatotoxicity).

Food: Food decreases the extent of absorption; rifampin concentrations may be decreased if taken with food.

Herb/Nutraceutical: St John's wort may decrease rifampin levels.

Stability Rifampin powder is reddish brown. Intact vials should be stored at room temperature and protected from excessive heat and light. Reconstitute powder for injection with SWFI; prior to injection, dilute in appropriate volume of compatible diluent (eg, 100 mL D_5W). Reconstituted vials are stable for 24 hours at room temperature

Stability of parenteral admixture at room temperature (25°C) is 4 hours for D_5W and 24 hours for NS

Mechanism of Action Inhibits bacterial RNA synthesis by binding to the beta subunit of DNA-dependent RNA polymerase, blocking RNA transcription

Pharmacodynamics/Kinetics

Duration: ≤24 hours

Absorption: Oral: Well absorbed; food may delay or slightly reduce peak

Distribution: Highly lipophilic; crosses blood-brain barrier well

Relative diffusion from blood into CSF: Adequate with or without inflammation (exceeds usual MICs)

CSF:blood level ratio: Inflamed meninges: 25%

Protein binding: 80%

Metabolism: Hepatic; undergoes enterohepatic recirculation

Half-life elimination: 3-4 hours; prolonged with hepatic impairment; End-stage renal disease: 1.8-11 hours

Time to peak, serum: Oral: 2-4 hours

Excretion: Feces (60% to 65%) and urine (~30%) as unchanged drug

Dosage Oral (I.V. infusion dose is the same as for the oral route):

Tuberculosis therapy (drug susceptible): Note: A four-drug regimen (isoniazid, rifampin, pyrazinamide, and ethambutol) is preferred for the initial, empiric treatment of TB. When the drug susceptibility results are available, the regimen should be altered as appropriate.

Infants and Children <12 years:

Daily therapy: 10-20 mg/kg/day usually as a single dose (maximum: 600 mg/day)

Twice weekly directly observed therapy (DOT): 10-20 mg/kg (maximum: 600 mg)

Adults:

Daily therapy: 10 mg/kg/day (maximum: 600 mg/day)

Twice weekly directly observed therapy (DOT): 10 mg/kg (maximum: 600 mg); 3 times/week: 10 mg/kg (maximum: 600 mg)

Latent tuberculosis infection (LTBI): As an alternative to isoniazid:

Children: 10-20 mg/kg/day (maximum: 600 mg/day) for 6 months

Adults: 10 mg/kg/day (maximum: 600 mg/day) for 4 months. **Note:** Combination with pyrazinamide should not generally be offered (*MMWR*, Aug 8, 2003).

***H. influenzae* prophylaxis (unlabeled use):**

Infants and Children: 20 mg/kg/day every 24 hours for 4 days, not to exceed 600 mg/dose

Adults: 600 mg every 24 hours for 4 days

Leprosy (unlabeled use): Adults:

Multibacillary: 600 mg once monthly for 24 months in combination with ofloxacin and minocycline

Paucibacillary: 600 mg once monthly for 6 months in combination with dapsone

Single lesion: 600 mg as a single dose in combination with ofloxacin 400 mg and minocycline 100 mg

Meningococcal meningitis prophylaxis:

Infants <1 month: 10 mg/kg/day in divided doses every 12 hours for 2 days

Infants ≥1 month and Children: 20 mg/kg/day in divided doses every 12 hours for 2 days (maximum: 600 mg/dose)

Adults: 600 mg every 12 hours for 2 days

Nasal carriers of *Staphylococcus aureus* (unlabeled use):

Children: 15 mg/kg/day divided every 12 hours for 5-10 days in combination with other antibiotics

Adults: 600 mg/day for 5-10 days in combination with other antibiotics

Synergy for *Staphylococcus aureus* infections (unlabeled use): Adults: 300-600 mg twice daily with other antibiotics

Dosing adjustment in hepatic impairment: Dose reductions may be necessary to reduce hepatotoxicity

Hemodialysis or peritoneal dialysis: Plasma rifampin concentrations are not significantly affected by hemodialysis or peritoneal dialysis.

Dietary Considerations Rifampin should be taken on an empty stomach.

Administration

I.V.: Administer I.V. preparation once daily by slow I.V. infusion over 30 minutes to 3 hours at a final concentration not to exceed 6 mg/mL.

Oral: Administer on an empty stomach (ie, 1 hour prior to, or 2 hours after meals or antacids) to increase total absorption. The compounded oral suspension must be shaken well before using. May mix contents of capsule with applesauce or jelly.

Monitoring Parameters Periodic (baseline and every 2-4 weeks during therapy) monitoring of liver function (AST, ALT, bilirubin), CBC; hepatic status and mental status, sputum culture, chest x-ray 2-3 months into treatment

Test Interactions Positive Coombs' reaction [direct], rifampin inhibits standard assay's ability to measure serum folate and B_{12}; transient increase in LFTs and decreased biliary excretion of contrast media

Patient Information May discolor urine, tears, sweat, or other body fluids to a red-orange color; take 1 hour before or 2 hours after a meal on an empty stomach; soft contact lenses may be permanently stained; report any severe or persistent flu-like symptoms, nausea, vomiting, dark urine or pale stools, or unusual bleeding or bruising; utilize an alternate form from oral/other systemic contraceptives during therapy; compliance and completion with course of therapy is very important; if you are a diabetic taking oral medications or if you regularly take oral anticoagulant therapy, your medication may need special and careful adjustment.

Dosage Forms

Capsule (Rifadin®): 150 mg, 300 mg

Injection, powder for reconstitution (Rifadin®): 600 mg

Extemporaneous Preparations For pediatric and adult patients with difficulty swallowing or where lower doses are needed, the package insert lists an extemporaneous liquid suspension as follows:

Rifampin 1% w/v suspension (10 mg/mL) can be compounded using one of four syrups (Syrup NF, simple syrup, Syrpalta® syrup, or raspberry syrup)

Empty contents of four 300 mg capsules or eight 150 mg capsules onto a piece of weighing paper

If necessary, crush contents to produce a fine powder

Transfer powder blend to a 4 oz amber glass or plastic prescription bottle

Rinse paper and spatula with 20 mL of syrup and add the rinse to bottle; shake vigorously

Add 100 mL of syrup to the bottle and shake vigorously

(Continued)

Rifampin *(Continued)*

This compounding procedure results in a 1% w/v suspension containing 10 mg rifampin/mL; stability studies indicate suspension is stable at room temperature (25°C ± 3°C) or in refrigerator (2°C to 8°C) for 4 weeks; shake well prior to administration

Selected Readings

Davidson PT and Le HQ, "Drug Treatment of Tuberculosis - 1992," *Drugs*, 1992, 43(5):651-73.
"Drugs for Tuberculosis," *Med Lett Drugs Ther*, 1993, 35(908):99-101.
Havlir DV and Barnes PF, "Tuberculosis in Patients With Human Immunodeficiency Virus Infection," *N Engl J Med*, 1999, 340(5):367-73.
Iseman MD, "Treatment of Multidrug-Resistant Tuberculosis," *N Engl J Med*, 1993, 329(11):784-91.
Lundstrom TS and Sobel JD, "Vancomycin, Trimethoprim-Sulfamethoxazole, and Rifampin," *Infect Dis Clin North Am*, 1995, 9(3):747-67.
"Prevention and Treatment of Tuberculosis Among Patients Infected With Human Immunodeficiency Virus: Principles of Therapy and Revised Recommendations. Centers for Disease Control and Prevention," *MMWR*, 1998, 47(RR-20):1-58.
Van Scoy RE and Wilkowske CJ, "Antituberculosis Agents," *Mayo Clin Proc*, 1992, 67(2):179-87.
Vesely JJ, Pien FD, and Pien BC, "Rifampin, a Useful Drug for Nonmycobacterial Infections," *Pharmacotherapy*, 1998, 18(2):345-57.

Rifampin and Isoniazid (RIF am pin & eye soe NYE a zid)

Related Information

Isoniazid *on page 893*
Rifampin *on page 1046*

U.S. Brand Names Rifamate®

Canadian Brand Names Rifamate®

Synonyms Isoniazid and Rifampin

Generic Available No

Use Management of active tuberculosis; see individual agents for additional information

Drug of Choice or Alternative for Organism(s):

Mycobacterium tuberculosis on page 234

Pregnancy Risk Factor C

Pregnancy Implications Refer to Rifampin monograph.

Drug Interactions

Cytochrome P450 Effect:

Rifampin: **Substrate** (major) of CYP2A6, 2C8/9, 3A4; **Induces** CYP1A2 (strong), 2A6 (strong), 2B6 (strong), 2C8/9 (strong), 2C19 (strong), 3A4 (strong)

Isoniazid: **Substrate** of CYP2E1 (major); **Inhibits** CYP1A2 (weak), 2A6 (moderate), 2C8/9 (moderate), 2C19 (strong), 2D6 (moderate), 2E1 (moderate), 3A4 (strong); **Induces** CYP2E1 (after discontinuation) (weak)

Pharmacodynamics/Kinetics See individual agents.

Dosage Oral: 2 capsules/day

Dosage Forms Capsule: Rifampin 300 mg and isoniazid 150 mg

Rifampin, Isoniazid, and Pyrazinamide

(RIF am pin, eye soe NYE a zid, & peer a ZIN a mide)

Related Information

Isoniazid *on page 893*
Pyrazinamide *on page 1022*
Rifampin *on page 1046*

U.S. Brand Names Rifater®

Canadian Brand Names Rifater®

Synonyms Isoniazid, Rifampin, and Pyrazinamide; Pyrazinamide, Rifampin, and Isoniazid

Generic Available No

Use Initial phase, short-course treatment of pulmonary tuberculosis; see individual agents for additional information

Pregnancy Risk Factor C

Pregnancy Implications See individual agents.

Contraindications

Hypersensitivity to rifampin, isoniazid, pyrazinamide, or any component of the formulation; acute or chronic liver disease; gout; concurrent use with amprenavir or saquinavir/ritonavir (and possibly other protease inhibitors); severe fever, chills, or arthritis

Warnings/Precautions

Rifampin, isoniazid, and pyrazinamide can each cause liver impairment; use with caution and modify dosage in patients with acute or chronic liver impairment of any origin; dosage reduction may be necessary. Baseline serum uric acid and LFTs are recommended; monitor for hyperbilirubinemia and discontinue therapy if this occurs

in conjunction with clinical symptoms or any signs of significant hepatocellular damage. Severe and sometimes fatal hepatitis may occur or develop even after many months of treatment; patients must report any prodromal symptoms of hepatitis, such as fatigue, weakness, malaise, anorexia, nausea, or vomiting. Use with caution in patients with porphyria since exacerbations have been reported. Do not use for meningococcal disease, only for short-term treatment of asymptomatic carrier states. Use with caution in patients receiving concurrent medications associated with hepatotoxicity, or in patients with a history of alcoholism (even if ethanol consumption is discontinued during therapy).

Monitor for compliance and effects including hypersensitivity or thrombocytopenia; urine, feces, saliva, sweat, tears, and CSF may be discolored to red/orange. Regimens of rifampin 600 mg once or twice weekly have been associated with a high incidence of adverse reactions including a flu-like syndrome.

Use with caution in patients with renal impairment and chronic liver disease. Malnourished patients or individuals likely to develop peripheral neuropathies should receive concomitant pyridoxine therapy (10-50 mg/day). Periodic ophthalmic examinations are recommended even when usual symptoms do not occur. Use with caution in patients with diabetes mellitus. Fixed combination product should not be used in children <15 years of age.

Adverse Reactions Note: During clinical trial evaluation, the frequency of cardiorespiratory events (eg, chest pain, hemoptysis, palpitation, chest tightness, and pneumothorax) was higher with the combination product (7%) that that reported with individual agents (2%). Also see individual agents.

Drug Interactions

Cytochrome P450 Effect:

Rifampin: **Substrate** (major) of CYP2A6, 2C8/9, 3A4; **Induces** CYP1A2 (strong), 2A6 (strong), 2B6 (strong), 2C8/9 (strong), 2C19 (strong), 3A4 (strong)

Isoniazid: **Substrate** of CYP2E1 (major); **Inhibits** CYP1A2 (weak), 2A6 (moderate), 2C8/9 (moderate), 2C19 (strong), 2D6 (moderate), 2E1 (moderate), 3A4 (strong); CYP2E1 (after discontinuation) (weak)

Increased Effect/Toxicity: Increased effect/toxicity: Combination therapy with rifampin and pyrazinamide has been associated with severe and fatal hepatotoxic reactions.

Based on **rifampin** component: Rifampin levels may be increased when given with co-trimoxazole, probenecid, or ritonavir. Rifampin given with halothane or isoniazid increases the potential for hepatotoxicity.

Ethanol/Nutrition/Herb Interactions

See individual agents.

Pharmacodynamics/Kinetics See individual agents.

Dosage Adults: Oral: Patients weighing:

≤44 kg: 4 tablets

45-54 kg: 5 tablets

≥55 kg: 6 tablets

Doses should be administered in a single daily dose

Dietary Considerations Administer dose either 1 hour before or 2 hours after a meal with a full glass of water.

Dosage Forms Tablet: Rifampin 120 mg, isoniazid 50 mg, and pyrazinamide 300 mg

Rifapentine (RIF a pen teen)

Related Information

Tuberculosis *on page 1315*

U.S. Brand Names Priftin®

Canadian Brand Names Priftin®

Generic Available No

Use Treatment of pulmonary tuberculosis; rifapentine must always be used in conjunction with at least one other antituberculosis drug to which the isolate is susceptible; it may also be necessary to add a third agent (either streptomycin or ethambutol) until susceptibility is known.

Pregnancy Risk Factor C

Pregnancy Implications Has been shown to be teratogenic in rats and rabbits. Rat offspring showed cleft palates, right aortic arch, and delayed ossification and increased number of ribs. Rabbits displayed ovarian agenesis, pes varus, arhinia, microphthalmia, and irregularities of the ossified facial tissues. Rat studies also show decreased fetal weight, increased number of stillborns, and decreased gestational survival. There are no adequate and well-controlled studies in pregnant women. Rifapentine should be used during pregnancy only if the potential benefits justifies the potential risk to the fetus.

Contraindications Hypersensitivity to rifapentine, rifampin, rifabutin, any rifamycin analog, or any component of the formulation

(Continued)

Rifapentine *(Continued)*

Warnings/Precautions Compliance with dosing regimen is absolutely necessary for successful drug therapy. Patients with abnormal liver tests and/or liver disease should only be given rifapentine when absolutely necessary and under strict medical supervision. Monitoring of liver function tests should be carried out prior to therapy and then every 2-4 weeks during therapy if signs of liver disease occur or worsen, rifapentine should be discontinued. Porphyria exacerbation is possible. Pseudomembranous colitis has been reported to occur with various antibiotics including other rifamycins. If this is suspected, rifapentine should be stopped and the patient treated with specific and supportive treatment. Experience in treating TB in HIV-infected patients is limited.

Rifapentine may produce a red-orange discoloration of body tissues/fluids including skin, teeth, tongue, urine, feces, saliva, sputum, tears, sweat, and cerebral spinal fluid. Contact lenses may become permanently stained. All patients treated with rifapentine should have baseline measurements of liver function tests and enzymes, bilirubin, and a complete blood count. patients should be seen monthly and specifically questioned regarding symptoms associated with adverse reactions. Routine laboratory monitoring in people with normal baseline measurements is generally not necessary.

Adverse Reactions

>10%: Endocrine & metabolic: Hyperuricemia (most likely due to pyrazinamide from initiation phase combination therapy)

1% to 10%:

- Cardiovascular: Hypertension
- Central nervous system: Headache, dizziness
- Dermatologic: Rash, pruritus, acne
- Gastrointestinal: Anorexia, nausea, vomiting, dyspepsia, diarrhea
- Hematologic: Neutropenia, lymphopenia, anemia, leukopenia, thrombocytosis
- Hepatic: Increased ALT/AST
- Neuromuscular & skeletal: Arthralgia, pain
- Renal: Pyuria, proteinuria, hematuria, urinary casts
- Respiratory: Hemoptysis

<1%: Peripheral edema, aggressive reaction, fatigue, urticaria, skin discoloration, hyperkalemia, hypovolemia, increased alkaline phosphatase, increased LDH, constipation, esophagitis, gastritis, pancreatitis, thrombocytopenia, neutrophilia, leukocytosis, purpura, hematoma, bilirubinemia, hepatitis, gout, arthrosis

Postmarketing and/or case reports: Rifampin has been associated with exacerbation of porphyria. Rifapentine is assumed to share this potential.

Overdosage/Toxicology There is no experience with treatment of acute overdose. Experience with other rifamycins suggests that gastric lavage, followed by activated charcoal, may help adsorb any remaining drug from the GI tract. Hemodialysis or forced diuresis is not expected to enhance elimination of unchanged rifapentine in an overdose.

Drug Interactions

Cytochrome P450 Effect: Induces CYP2C8/9 (strong), 3A4 (strong)

Increased Effect/Toxicity: Rifapentine may increase the therapeutic effect of clopidogrel; concurrent use with isoniazid may increase risk of hepatotoxicity

Decreased Effect: Rifapentine may decrease the levels/effects of the following drugs: alfentanil, amiodarone, angiotensin II receptor blockers (irbesartan, losartan), 5-HT_3 antagonists, imidazole antifungals, aprepitant, barbiturates, benzodiazepines (metabolized by oxidation), beta blockers, buspirone, calcium channel blockers, corticosteroids, cyclosporine; CYP2C8/9 and 3A4 substrates (eg, amiodarone, clarithromycin, erythromycin, fluoxetine, mirtazapine, nateglinide, nefazodone, nevirapine, pioglitazone, rosiglitazone, sertraline, venlafaxine, and zafirlukast); dapsone, disopyramide, estrogen and progestin contraceptives, fluconazole, gefitinib, HMG-CoA reductase inhibitors, methadone, morphine, phenytoin, propafenone, protease inhibitors, quinidine, repaglinide, reverse transcriptase inhibitors (non-nucleoside), tacrolimus, tamoxifen, terbinafine, tocainide, tricyclic antidepressants, warfarin, zaleplon, zidovudine, and zolpidem.

Ethanol/Nutrition/Herb Interactions Food: Food increases AUC and maximum serum concentration by 43% and 44% respectively as compared to fasting conditions.

Stability Store at room temperature (15°C to 30°C; 59°F to 86°F); protect from excessive heat and humidity

Mechanism of Action Inhibits DNA-dependent RNA polymerase in susceptible strains of *Mycobacterium tuberculosis* (but not in mammalian cells). Rifapentine is bactericidal against both intracellular and extracellular MTB organisms. MTB resistant to other rifamycins including rifampin are likely to be resistant to rifapentine. Cross-resistance does not appear between rifapentine and other nonrifamycin antimycobacterial agents.

Pharmacodynamics/Kinetics

Absorption: Food increases AUC and C_{max} by 43% and 44% respectively.

Distribution: V_d: ~70.2 L; rifapentine and metabolite accumulate in human monocyte-derived macrophages with intracellular/extracellular ratios of 24:1 and 7:1 respectively

Protein binding: Rifapentine and 25-desacetyl metabolite: 97.7% and 93.2%, primarily to albumin

Metabolism: Hepatic; hydrolyzed by an esterase and esterase enzyme to form the active metabolite 25-desacetyl rifapentine

Bioavailability: ~70%

Half-life elimination: Rifapentine: 14-17 hours; 25-desacetyl rifapentine: 13 hours

Time to peak, serum: 5-6 hours

Excretion: Urine (17% primarily as metabolites)

Dosage

Children: No dosing information available

Adults: **Rifapentine should not be used alone**; initial phase should include a 3- to 4-drug regimen

Intensive phase (initial 2 months) of short-term therapy: 600 mg (four 150 mg tablets) given twice weekly (with an interval of not less than 72 hours between doses); following the intensive phase, treatment should continue with rifapentine 600 mg once weekly for 4 months in combination with INH or appropriate agent for susceptible organisms

Dosing adjustment in renal or hepatic impairment: Unknown

Monitoring Parameters Patients with pre-existing hepatic problems should have liver function tests monitored every 2-4 weeks during therapy

Test Interactions Rifampin has been shown to inhibit standard microbiological assays for serum folate and vitamin B_{12}; this should be considered for rifapentine; therefore, alternative assay methods should be considered.

Patient Information May produce a reddish coloration of urine, sweat, sputum, tears, and contact lenses may be permanently stained. Oral or other systemic hormonal contraceptives may not be effective while taking rifapentine; alternative contraceptive measures should be used. Administration of rifapentine with food may decrease GI intolerance. Report fever, decreased appetite, malaise, nausea/vomiting, darkened urine, yellowish discoloration of skin or eyes, chest pain, palpitations, and pain or swelling of the joints. Adherence with the full course of therapy is essential; no doses of therapy should be missed.

Additional Information Rifapentine has only been studied in patients with tuberculosis receiving a 6-month short-course intensive regimen approval. Outcomes have been based on 6-month follow-up treatment observed in clinical trial 008 as a surrogate for the 2-year follow-up generally accepted as evidence for efficacy in the treatment of pulmonary tuberculosis.

Dosage Forms Tablet [film coated]: 150 mg

Selected Readings

Grosser J, Lounis N, Truffot-Pernot C, et al, "Once Weekly Rifapentine-Containing Regimens for Treatment of Tuberculosis in Mice," *Am J Respir Crit Care Med*, 1998, 157:1436-40.

Jarvis B and Lamb HM, "Rifapentine," *Drugs*, 1998, 56(4):607-16.

Keung AC, Eller MG, and Weir SJ, "Pharmacokinetics of Rifapentine in Patients With Varying Degrees of Hepatic Dysfunction," *J Clin Pharmacol*, 1998, 38:517-24.

Moghazeh SI, Pan X, Arain T, et al, "Comparative Antimycobacterial Activities of Rifampin, Rifapentine, and KRM-1648 Against a Collection of Rifampin-Resistant *Mycobacterium* Tuberculosis Isolates With Known rpoβ Mutations," *Antimicrob Agents Chemother*, 1996, 40:265-7.

Tam CM, Chan SL, Lam CW, et al, "Rifapentine and Isoniazid in the Continuation Phase of Treating Pulmonary Tuberculosis, Initial Report," *Am J Respir Crit Care Med*, 1998, 157:1726-33.

Rifater® *see* Rifampin, Isoniazid, and Pyrazinamide *on page 1050*

Rifaximin (rif AX i min)

U.S. Brand Names Xifaxan™

Generic Available No

Use Treatment of travelers' diarrhea caused by noninvasive strains of *E. coli*

Pregnancy Risk Factor C

Pregnancy Implications Teratogenic effects were observed in animal studies. There are no adequate and well-controlled studies in pregnant women.

Contraindications Hypersensitivity to rifaximin, other rifamycin antibiotics, or any component of the formulation; diarrhea with fever or blood in the stool

Warnings/Precautions Efficacy has not been established for the treatment of diarrhea due to pathogens other than *E. coli*, including *C. jejuni*, *Shigella*, and *Salmonella*. Consider alternative therapy if symptoms persist or worsen after 24-48 hours of treatment. Not for treatment of systemic infections; <1% is absorbed orally. Safety and efficacy have not been established in children <12 years of age.

(Continued)

Rifaximin *(Continued)*

Adverse Reactions Incidence of adverse effects reported as ≥2% occurred more in the placebo group than the rifaximin group except for headache.

2% to 10%: Central nervous system: Headache (10%; placebo 9%)

<2%, postmarketing, and/or case reports (limited to important or life-threatening): Abnormal dreams, allergic dermatitis, angioneurotic edema, fatigue, hypersensitivity reactions, insomnia, motion sickness, pruritus, rash, sunburn, tinnitus, urticaria

Overdosage/Toxicology Specific information not available. Treatment should be symptom-directed and supportive.

Drug Interactions

Cytochrome P450 Effect: Induces CYP3A4 (minor)

Stability Store at controlled room temperature of 20°C to 25°C (68°F to 77°F).

Mechanism of Action Rifaximin inhibits bacterial RNA synthesis by binding to bacterial DNA-dependent RNA polymerase.

Pharmacodynamics/Kinetics

Absorption: Oral: <0.4%

Distribution: 80% to 90% in the gut

Half-life elimination: ~6 hours

Excretion: Feces (~97% as unchanged drug); urine (<1%)

Dosage Oral: Children ≥12 years and Adults: Travelers' diarrhea: 200 mg 3 times/day for 3 days

Dietary Considerations May be taken with or without food.

Administration May be administered with or without food.

Monitoring Parameters Temperature, blood in stool, change in symptoms

Dosage Forms Tablet: 200 mg

rIFN-A *see* Interferon Alfa-2a *on page 878*

RIG *see* Rabies Immune Globulin (Human) *on page 1034*

Rimantadine (ri MAN ta deen)

Related Information

USPHS / IDSA Guidelines for the Prevention of Opportunistic Infections in Persons Infected With HIV *on page 1237*

U.S. Brand Names Flumadine®

Canadian Brand Names Flumadine®

Synonyms Rimantadine Hydrochloride

Generic Available Yes: Tablet

Use Prophylaxis (adults and children >1 year of age) and treatment (adults) of influenza A viral infection

Unlabeled/Investigational Use Treatment of influenza A viral infection in children ≥13 years of age

Drug of Choice or Alternative for Organism(s):

Influenza Virus *on page 193*

Pregnancy Risk Factor C

Pregnancy Implications Embryotoxic in high dose rat studies.

Contraindications Hypersensitivity to drugs of the adamantine class, including rimantadine and amantadine, or any component of the formulation

Warnings/Precautions Use with caution in patients with renal and hepatic dysfunction; avoid use, if possible, in patients with recurrent and eczematoid dermatitis, uncontrolled psychosis, or severe psychoneurosis. An increase in seizure incidence may occur in patients with seizure disorders; discontinue drug if seizures occur; resistance may develop during treatment; viruses exhibit cross-resistance between amantadine and rimantadine.

Adverse Reactions

1% to 10%:

Central nervous system: Dizziness (2%), insomnia (2%), anxiety (1%), fatigue (1%), headache (1%), nervousness (1%)

Gastrointestinal: Nausea (3%), anorexia (2%), vomiting (2%), xerostomia (2%), abdominal pain (1%)

Neuromuscular and skeletal: Weakness (1%)

<1%: Agitation, ataxia, bronchospasm, cardiac failure, concentration impaired, confusion, convulsions, cough, depression, diarrhea, dyspepsia, dyspnea, euphoria, gait abnormality, hallucinations, heart block, hyperkinesias, hypertension, lactation, palpitation, pallor, parosmia, pedal edema, rash, somnolence, syncope, tachycardia, taste alteration, tinnitus, tremor

Overdosage/Toxicology Agitation, hallucinations, ventricular cardiac arrhythmias (torsade de pointes and PVCs), slurred speech, anticholinergic effects (dry mouth, urinary retention and mydriasis), ataxia, tremor, myoclonus, seizures, and death have been reported with amantadine (a related drug). Treatment is symptomatic (do not use physostigmine). Tachyarrhythmias may be treated with beta-blockers such as propranolol. Dialysis is not recommended except possibly in renal failure.

Drug Interactions

Increased Effect/Toxicity: Cimetidine increases blood levels/toxicity of rimantadine.

Decreased Effect: Acetaminophen may cause a small reduction in AUC and peak concentration of rimantadine. Peak plasma and AUC concentrations of rimantadine are slightly reduced by aspirin.

Ethanol/Nutrition/Herb Interactions Food: Food does not affect rate or extent of absorption

Mechanism of Action Exerts its inhibitory effect on three antigenic subtypes of influenza A virus (H1N1, H2N2, H3N2) early in the viral replicative cycle, possibly inhibiting the uncoating process; it has no activity against influenza B virus and is two- to eightfold more active than amantadine

Pharmacodynamics/Kinetics

Onset of action: Antiviral activity: No data exist establishing a correlation between plasma concentration and antiviral effect

Absorption: Tablet and syrup formulations are equally absorbed

Metabolism: Extensively hepatic

Half-life elimination: 25.4 hours; prolonged in elderly

Time to peak: 6 hours

Excretion: Urine (<25% as unchanged drug)

Clearance: Hemodialysis does not contribute to clearance

Dosage Oral:

Prophylaxis:

Children 1-10 years or <40 kg: 5 mg/kg/day in 2 divided doses; maximum: 150 mg/day

Children >10 years and Adults: 100 mg twice daily

Elderly: 100 mg/day in nursing home patients or all elderly patients who may experience adverse effects using the adult dose

Treatment:

Children ≥13 years (unlabeled use): 100 mg twice daily; children <40 kg should receive 5 mg/kg/day in divided doses, maximum dose 200 mg/day

Adults: 100 mg twice daily

Elderly: 100 mg once daily in patients ≥65 years

Dosage adjustment in renal impairment:

Cl_{cr} >10 mL/minute: Dose adjustment not required

Cl_{cr} ≤10 mL/minute: 100 mg/day

Dosage adjustment in hepatic impairment: Severe dysfunction: 100 mg/day

Administration Initiation of rimantadine within 48 hours of the onset of influenza A illness halves the duration of illness and significantly reduces the duration of viral shedding and increased peripheral airways resistance; continue therapy for 5-7 days after symptoms begin

Monitoring Parameters Monitor for CNS or GI effects in elderly or patients with renal or hepatic impairment

Dosage Forms

Syrup, as hydrochloride: 50 mg/5 mL (240 mL) [raspberry flavor]

Tablet, as hydrochloride: 100 mg

Selected Readings

Dolin R, Reichman RC, Madore HP, et al, "A Controlled Trial of Amantadine and Rimantadine in the Prophylaxis of Influenza A Infection," *N Engl J Med*, 1982, 307(10):580-4.

"Drugs for Non-HIV Viral Infections," *Med Lett Drugs Ther*, 1994, 36(919):27.

Keating MR, "Antiviral Agents," *Mayo Clin Proc*, 1992, 67(2):160-78.

Wintermeyer SM and Nahata MC, "Rimantadine: A Clinical Perspective," *Ann Pharmacother*, 1995, 29(3):299-310.

Rimantadine Hydrochloride *see* Rimantadine *on page 1054*

Ritonavir (ri TOE na veer)

Related Information

Antiretroviral Agents *on page 1206*

Antiretroviral Therapy for HIV Infection *on page 1219*

Management of Healthcare Worker Exposures to HBV, HCV, and HIV *on page 1227*

U.S. Brand Names Norvir®

Canadian Brand Names Norvir®; Norvir® SEC

Generic Available No

(Continued)

Ritonavir *(Continued)*

Use Treatment of HIV infection; should always be used as part of a multidrug regimen (at least three antiretroviral agents); may be used as a pharmacokinetic 'booster' for other protease inhibitors

Drug of Choice or Alternative for Organism(s):

Human Immunodeficiency Virus *on page 181*

Pregnancy Risk Factor B

Pregnancy Implications Early studies have shown lower plasma levels during pregnancy compared to postpartum. If needed during pregnancy, use in combination with another PI to boost levels of second PI. Pregnancy and protease inhibitors are both associated with an increased risk of hyperglycemia. Glucose levels should be closely monitored. The Perinatal HIV Guidelines Working Group considers ritonavir to be an alternative PI for use during pregnancy. Healthcare professionals are encouraged to contact the antiretroviral pregnancy registry to monitor outcomes of pregnant women exposed to antiretroviral medications (1-800-258-4263 or www.APRegistry.com).

Contraindications Hypersensitivity to ritonavir or any component of the formulation; concurrent alfuzosin, amiodarone, bepridil, cisapride, dihydroergotamine, ergonovine, ergotamine, flecainide, lovastatin, methylergonovine, midazolam, pimozide, propafenone, quinidine, simvastatin, St John's wort, triazolam, and voriconazole

Warnings/Precautions Use caution in patients with hepatic insufficiency; safety and efficacy have not been established in children <2 years of age; use caution with benzodiazepines, rifabutin, sildenafil, and certain analgesics (meperidine, piroxicam, propoxyphene). Selected HMG-CoA reductase inhibitors are contraindicated (see Contraindications); atorvastatin should be used at the lowest possible dose, while fluvastatin or pravastatin may be safer alternatives. Ritonavir may interact with many medications. Careful review is required. Cushing's syndrome and adrenal suppression have been reported in patients receiving concomitant ritonavir and fluticasone; avoid concurrent use unless benefit outweighs risk. Dosage adjustment is required for combination therapy with amprenavir and ritonavir; in addition, the risk of hyperlipidemia may be increased during concurrent therapy. Warn patients that redistribution of fat may occur.

Adverse Reactions Protease inhibitors cause dyslipidemia which includes elevated cholesterol and triglycerides and a redistribution of body fat centrally to cause increased abdominal girth, buffalo hump, facial atrophy, and breast enlargement. These agents also cause hyperglycemia.

>10%:
- Endocrine & metabolic: Triglycerides increased
- Gastrointestinal: Diarrhea, nausea, vomiting, taste perversion
- Hematologic: Anemia, WBCs decreased
- Hepatic: GGT increased
- Neuromuscular & skeletal: Weakness

1% to 10%:
- Cardiovascular: Vasodilation
- Central nervous system: Fever, headache, malaise, dizziness, insomnia, somnolence, thinking abnormally
- Dermatologic: Rash
- Endocrine & metabolic: Hyperlipidemia, uric acid increased, glucose increased
- Gastrointestinal: Abdominal pain, anorexia, constipation, dyspepsia, flatulence, local throat irritation
- Hematologic: Neutropenia, eosinophilia, neutrophilia, prolonged PT, leukocytosis
- Hepatic: LFTs increased
- Neuromuscular & skeletal: CPK increased, myalgia, paresthesia
- Respiratory: Pharyngitis
- Miscellaneous: Diaphoresis, potassium increased, calcium increased

<1%: Abnormal vision, adrenal insufficiency, allergic reactions, cerebral ischemia, cerebral venous thrombosis, cholestatic jaundice, dementia, diabetes mellitus, dyspnea, erythema multiforme, exfoliative dermatitis, gastrointestinal hemorrhage, hallucinations, hepatitis, interstitial pneumonitis, MI, migraine, neuropathy, pancreatitis, paralysis, photosensitivity, renal failure (acute), vertigo

Postmarketing and/or case reports: Adrenal suppression (coadministration with fluticasone), Cushing's syndrome, dehydration, orthostatic hypotension, redistribution of body fat, seizure, syncope, vasospasm (coadministration with ergot alkaloids)

Overdosage/Toxicology Human experience is limited. There is no specific antidote for overdose with ritonavir. The oral solution contains 43% ethanol by volume, potentially causing significant ethanol-related toxicity in younger patients. Dialysis is unlikely to be beneficial in significant removal of the drug. Charcoal or gastric lavage may be useful to remove unabsorbed drug.

Drug Interactions

Cytochrome P450 Effect: Substrate of CYP1A2 (minor), 2B6 (minor), 2D6 (minor), 3A4 (major); **Inhibits** CYP2C8/9 (weak), 2C19 (weak), 2D6 (strong), 2E1 (weak), 3A4 (strong); **Induces** CYP1A2 (weak), 2C8/9 (weak), 3A4 (weak)

Increased Effect/Toxicity: Concurrent use of alfuzosin, amiodarone, bepridil, cisapride, ergot alkaloids (dihydroergotamine, ergonovine, methylergonovine), flecainide, lovastatin, midazolam, pimozide, propafenone, quinidine, simvastatin, and triazolam is contraindicated.

Saquinavir's serum concentrations are increased by ritonavir; the dosage of both agents should be reduced to 400 mg twice daily. Concurrent therapy with amprenavir may result in increased serum concentrations: dosage adjustment is recommended. Metronidazole or disulfiram may cause disulfiram reaction (oral solution contains 43% ethanol). Serum levels/effects of corticosteroids (eg, budesonide, dexamethasone, fluticasone, prednisone) and immunosuppressants (cyclosporine, sirolimus, tacrolimus; monitor) may be increased by ritonavir. Serum concentrations of meperidine's neuroexcitatory metabolite (normeperidine) are increased by ritonavir, which may increase the risk of CNS toxicity/seizures. Rifabutin and rifabutin metabolite serum concentrations may be increased by ritonavir; reduce rifabutin dose to 150 mg every other day.

Ritonavir may increase the levels/effects of amphetamines, selected beta-blockers, selected benzodiazepines (midazolam and triazolam contraindicated), calcium channel blockers (bepridil contraindicated), cisapride (contraindicated), dextromethorphan, ergot alkaloids (contraindicated), fluoxetine, lidocaine, HMG-CoA reductase inhibitors (lovastatin and simvastatin are contraindicated), mesoridazine, mirtazapine, nateglinide, nefazodone, paroxetine, pimozide (contraindicated), propafenone (contraindicated), risperidone, sildenafil (and other PDE-5 inhibitors), thioridazine, trazodone, tricyclic antidepressants, venlafaxine, and other substrates of CYP2D6 or 3A4. Mesoridazine and thioridazine are generally contraindicated with strong CYP2D6 inhibitors. When used with strong CYP3A4 inhibitors, dosage adjustment/limits are recommended for sildenafil and other PDE-5 inhibitors; refer to individual monographs.

Decreased Effect: The administration of didanosine (buffered formulation) should be separated from ritonavir by 2.5 hours to limit interaction with ritonavir. Concurrent use of rifampin, rifabutin, dexamethasone, and many anticonvulsants may lower serum concentration of ritonavir. Ritonavir may reduce the concentration of ethinyl estradiol which may result in loss of contraception (including combination products). Theophylline concentrations may be reduced in concurrent therapy. Levels of didanosine and zidovudine may be decreased by ritonavir, however, no dosage adjustment is necessary. Voriconazole serum levels are reduced by ritonavir (concurrent use is contraindicated). In addition, ritonavir may decrease the serum concentrations of the following drugs: Atovaquone, divalproex, lamotrigine, methadone, phenytoin, warfarin. The levels/effects of ritonavir may be decreased by aminoglutethimide, carbamazepine, nafcillin, nevirapine, phenobarbital, phenytoin, rifamycins, and other CYP3A4 inducers. Ritonavir may decrease the levels/effects of CYP2D6 prodrug substrates (eg, codeine, hydrocodone, oxycodone, tramadol).

Ethanol/Nutrition/Herb Interactions

Food: Food enhances absorption.

Herb/Nutraceutical: St John's wort may decrease ritonavir serum levels. Avoid use.

Stability

Capsule: Store under refrigeration at 2°C to 8°C (36°F to 46°F); may be left out at room temperature of <25°C (<77°F) if used within 30 days. Protect from light. Avoid exposure to excessive heat.

Solution: Store at room temperature at 20°C to 25°C (68°F to 77°F). Do not refrigerate.

Mechanism of Action Ritonavir inhibits HIV protease and renders the enzyme incapable of processing of polyprotein precursor which leads to production of noninfectious immature HIV particles

Pharmacodynamics/Kinetics

Absorption: Variable, with or without food

Distribution: High concentrations in serum and lymph nodes

Protein binding: 98% to 99%

Metabolism: Hepatic; five metabolites, low concentration of an active metabolite achieved in plasma (oxidative); see Drug Interactions

Half-life elimination: 3-5 hours

Excretion: Urine (negligible amounts)

Dosage Treatment of HIV infection: Oral:

Children ≥2 years: 250 mg/m^2 twice daily; titrate dose upward to 400 mg/m^2 twice daily (maximum: 600 mg twice daily)

(Continued)

Ritonavir *(Continued)*

Adults: 600 mg twice daily; dose escalation tends to avoid nausea that many patients experience upon initiation of full dosing. Escalate the dose as follows: 300 mg twice daily for 1 day, 400 mg twice daily for 2 days, 500 mg twice daily for 1 day, then 600 mg twice daily. Ritonavir may be better tolerated when used in combination with other antiretrovirals by initiating the drug alone and subsequently adding the second agent within 2 weeks.

Pharmacokinetic "booster" in combination with other protease inhibitors: 100-400 mg/day

Refer to individual monographs; specific dosage recommendations often require adjustment of both agents.

Note: Dosage adjustments for ritonavir when administered in combination therapy:

Amprenavir: Adjustments necessary for each agent:

Amprenavir 1200 mg with ritonavir 200 mg once daily **or**

Amprenavir 600 mg with ritonavir 100 mg twice daily

Amprenavir plus efavirenz (3-drug regimen): Amprenavir 1200 mg twice daily plus ritonavir 200 mg twice daily plus efavirenz at standard dose

Indinavir: Adjustments necessary for both agents:

Indinavir 800 mg twice daily plus ritonavir 100-200 mg twice daily **or**

Indinavir 400 mg twice daily plus ritonavir 400 mg twice daily

Nelfinavir or saquinavir: Ritonavir 400 mg twice daily

Rifabutin: Decrease rifabutin dose to 150 mg every other day

Dosing adjustment in renal impairment: None necessary

Dosing adjustment in hepatic impairment: No adjustment required in mild or moderate impairment; however, careful monitoring is required in moderate hepatic impairment (levels may be decreased); caution advised with severe impairment (no data available)

Dietary Considerations Should be taken with food. Oral solution contains 43% ethanol by volume.

Administration Administer with food. Liquid formulations usually have an unpleasant taste. Consider mixing it with chocolate milk or a liquid nutritional supplement.

Monitoring Parameters Triglycerides, cholesterol, CBC, LFTs, CPK, uric acid, basic HIV monitoring, viral load, and CD4 count, glucose

Patient Information Take with food. Mix liquid formulation with chocolate milk or liquid nutritional supplement. You may experience headache or confusion; if these persist notify prescriber. Diarrhea may be moderate to severe. Notify prescriber if problematic. Report swelling, numbness of tongue, mouth, lips, unresolved vomiting, fever, chills, or extreme fatigue. Do not take any prescription medications, over-the-counter products or herbal products, especially St John's wort, without consulting prescriber.

Additional Information Potential compliance problems, frequency of administration and adverse effects should be discussed with patients before initiating therapy to help prevent the emergence of resistance.

Dosage Forms

Capsule: 100 mg [contains ethanol and polyoxyl 35 castor oil]

Solution: 80 mg/mL (240 mL) [contains ethanol and polyoxyl 35 castor oil; peppermint and caramel flavor]

Selected Readings

Deeks SG, Smith M, Holodniy M, et al, "HIV-1 Protease Inhibitors. A Review for Clinicians," *JAMA*, 1997, 277(2):145-53.

Hsu A, Granneman GR, Cao G, et al, "Pharmacokinetic Interactions Between Two Human Immunodeficiency Virus Protease Inhibitors, Ritonavir and Saquinavir," *Clin Pharmacol Ther*, 1998, 63(4):453-64.

Kakuda TN, Struble KA, and Piscitelli SC, "Protease Inhibitors for the Treatment of Human Immunodeficiency Virus Infection," *Am J Health Syst Pharm*, 1998, 55(3):233-54.

Kaul DR, Cinti SK, Carver PL, et al, "HIV Protease Inhibitors: Advances in Therapy and Adverse Reactions, Including Metabolic Complications," *Pharmacotherapy*, 1999, 19(3):281-98.

Lea AP and Faulds D, "Ritonavir," *Drugs*, 1996, 52(4):541-6.

McDonald CK and Kuritzkes DR, "Human Immunodeficiency Virus Type 1 Protease Inhibitors," *Arch Intern Med*, 1997, 157(9):951-9.

Rathbun RC and Rossi DR, "Low-Dose Ritonavir for Protease Inhibitor Pharmacokinetic Enhancement," *Ann Pharmacother*, 2002, 36(4):702-6.

Ritonavir and Lopinavir *see* Lopinavir and Ritonavir *on page 919*

Riva-Cloxacillin (Can) *see* Cloxacillin *on page 760*

Riva-Norfloxacin (Can) *see* Norfloxacin *on page 973*

rLFN-α2 *see* Interferon Alfa-2b *on page 881*

Rocephin® *see* Ceftriaxone *on page 722*

Rofact™ (Can) *see* Rifampin *on page 1046*

Roferon-A® *see* Interferon Alfa-2a *on page 878*

Romycin® *see* Erythromycin *on page 807*

RP-59500 *see* Quinupristin and Dalfopristin *on page 1032*

RSV-IGIV *see* Respiratory Syncytial Virus Immune Globulin (Intravenous) *on page 1036*

RTCA *see* Ribavirin *on page 1040*

Rubella, Measles and Mumps Vaccines, Combined *see* Measles, Mumps, and Rubella Vaccines (Combined) *on page 926*

Rubella Virus Vaccine (Live) (rue BEL a VYE rus vak SEEN, live)

U.S. Brand Names Meruvax® II

Synonyms German Measles Vaccine

Generic Available No

Use Selective active immunization against rubella; vaccination is routinely recommended for persons from 12 months of age to puberty. All adults, both male and female, lacking documentation of live vaccine on or after first birthday, or laboratory evidence of immunity (particularly women of childbearing age and young adults who work in or congregate in hospitals, colleges, and on military bases) should be vaccinated. Susceptible travelers should be vaccinated.

Note: Trivalent measles - mumps - rubella (MMR) vaccine is the preferred immunizing agent for most children and many adults.

Pregnancy Risk Factor C

Pregnancy Implications Women who are pregnant when vaccinated or who become pregnant within 28 days of vaccination should be counseled on the theoretical risks to the fetus. The risk of rubella-associated malformations in these women is so small as to be negligible. MMR is the vaccine of choice if recipients are likely to be susceptible to measles or mumps as well as to rubella.

Contraindications Hypersensitivity to gelatin or any other component of the vaccine; history of anaphylactic reactions to neomycin; individuals with blood dyscrasias, leukemia, lymphomas, or other malignant neoplasms affecting the bone marrow or lymphatic systems; concurrent immunosuppressive therapy; primary and acquired immunodeficiency states; family history of congenital or hereditary immunodeficiency; active/untreated tuberculosis; current febrile illness or active febrile infection; pregnancy

Warnings/Precautions Immediate treatment for anaphylactic/anaphylactoid reaction should be available during vaccine use. Use with caution in patients with thrombocytopenia and those who develop thrombocytopenia after first dose; thrombocytopenia may worsen. Defer vaccine following blood, plasma, or immune globulin (human) administration; children with HIV infection, who are asymptomatic and not immunosuppressed may be vaccinated. Patients with minor illnesses (diarrhea, mild upper respiratory tract infection with or without low-grade fever or other illnesses with low-grade fever) may receive vaccine.

Adverse Reactions All serious adverse reactions must be reported to the U.S. Department of Health and Human Services (DHHS) Vaccine Adverse Event Reporting System (VAERS) 1-800-822-7967.

Frequency not defined.

Cardiovascular: Syncope, vasculitis

Central nervous system: Dizziness, encephalitis, fever, Guillain-Barré syndrome, headache, irritability, malaise, polyneuritis, polyneuropathy

Dermatologic: Angioneurotic edema, erythema multiforme, purpura, rash, Stevens-Johnson syndrome, urticaria

Gastrointestinal: Diarrhea, nausea, sore throat, vomiting

Hematologic: Leukocytosis, thrombocytopenia

Local: Injection site reactions which include burning, induration, pain, redness, stinging, wheal and flare

Neuromuscular & skeletal: Arthralgia/arthritis (variable; highest rates in women, 12% to 26% versus children, up to 3%), myalgia, paresthesia

Ocular: Conjunctivitis, optic neuritis, papillitis, retrobulbar neuritis

Otic: Nerve deafness, otitis media

Respiratory: Bronchial spasm, cough, rhinitis

Miscellaneous: Anaphylactoid reactions, anaphylaxis, regional lymphadenopathy

Drug Interactions

Decreased Effect: The effect of the vaccine may be decreased in individuals who are receiving immunosuppressant drugs (including high-dose systemic corticosteroids). Effect of vaccine may be decreased in given with immune globulin, whole blood or plasma; do not administer with vaccine. Effectiveness may be decreased if given within 30 days of varicella vaccine (effectiveness not decreased when administered simultaneously).

Stability Refrigerate, discard reconstituted vaccine after 8 hours; store at 2°C to 8°C (36°F to 46°F); ship vaccine at 10°C; may use dry ice, protect from light

Mechanism of Action Rubella vaccine is a live attenuated vaccine that contains the Wistar Institute RA 27/3 strain, which is adapted to and propagated in human diploid

(Continued)

Rubella Virus Vaccine (Live) *(Continued)*

cell culture. Promotes active immunity by inducing rubella hemagglutination-inhibiting antibodies.

Pharmacodynamics/Kinetics Onset of action: Antibodies to vaccine: 2-4 weeks

Dosage Children ≥12 months and Adults: SubQ: 0.5 mL in outer aspect of upper arm; children vaccinated before 12 months of age should be revaccinated. Recommended age for primary immunization is 12-15 months; revaccination with MMR-II is recommended prior to elementary school.

Administration SubQ injection only in outer aspect of upper arm; avoid injection into blood vessel. **Not for I.V. administration.** Federal law requires that the date of administration, the vaccine manufacturer, lot number of vaccine, and the administering person's name, title and address be entered into the patient's permanent medical record.

Test Interactions May depress tuberculin skin test sensitivity

Patient Information Patient may experience burning or stinging at the injection site; joint pain usually occurs 1-10 weeks after vaccination and persists 1-3 days

Additional Information Live virus vaccine. Federal law requires that the date of administration, the vaccine manufacturer, lot number of vaccine, and the administering person's name, title, and address be entered into the patient's permanent record.

Using separate sites and syringes, rubella virus vaccine may be administered concurrently with DTaP, *Haemophilus* b conjugate vaccine (PedvaxHIB®), or hepatitis B vaccine. Unless otherwise specified, rubella virus vaccine should be given 1 month before or 1 month after other live viral vaccines. OPV and rubella virus vaccines may be administered together. Rubella virus vaccine and varicella virus vaccine may be administered together (using separate sites and syringes); however, if vaccines are not administered simultaneously, doses should be separated by at least 30 days.

Dosage Forms Injection, powder for reconstitution [single dose]: 1000 $TCID_{50}$ (Wistar RA 27/3 Strain) [contains gelatin, human albumin, and neomycin]

Rubeola Vaccine *see* Measles Virus Vaccine (Live) *on page 927*
SAB-Gentamicin (Can) *see* Gentamicin *on page 841*
SAB-Trifluridine (Can) *see* Trifluridine *on page 1129*
Saizen® *see* Somatropin *on page 1069*
Salk Vaccine *see* Poliovirus Vaccine (Inactivated) *on page 1011*
Sans Acne® (Can) *see* Erythromycin *on page 807*

Saquinavir (sa KWIN a veer)

Related Information

Antiretroviral Agents *on page 1206*
Antiretroviral Therapy for HIV Infection *on page 1219*

U.S. Brand Names Fortovase® [DSC]; Invirase®

Canadian Brand Names Fortovase®; Invirase®

Synonyms Saquinavir Mesylate

Generic Available No

Use Treatment of HIV infection; used in combination with at least two other antiretroviral agents

Drug of Choice or Alternative for Organism(s):

Human Immunodeficiency Virus *on page 181*

Pregnancy Risk Factor B

Pregnancy Implications Saquinavir soft gelatin capsules (Fortovase®) provide adequate levels when used in normal doses during pregnancy; pharmacokinetic data not available for Invirase®. The Perinatal HIV Guidelines Working Group considers Fortovase® and ritonavir to be a preferred combination for use during pregnancy. Pregnancy and protease inhibitors are both associated with an increased risk of hyperglycemia. Glucose levels should be closely monitored. Health professionals are encouraged to contact the antiretroviral pregnancy registry to monitor outcomes of pregnant women exposed to antiretroviral medications (1-800-258-4263 or www.APRegistry.com).

Contraindications Hypersensitivity to saquinavir or any component of the formulation; exposure to direct sunlight without sunscreen or protective clothing; severe hepatic impairment; coadministration with amiodarone, bepridil, cisapride, flecainide, midazolam, pimozide, propafenone, quinidine, rifampin, triazolam, or ergot derivatives

Warnings/Precautions Use caution in patients with hepatic insufficiency. May exacerbate pre-existing hepatic dysfunction; use with caution in patients with hepatitis B or C and in cirrhosis. May be associated with fat redistribution (buffalo hump, increased

abdominal girth, breast engorgement, facial atrophy). Use caution in hemophilia. May increase cholesterol and/or triglycerides; hypertriglyceridemia may increase risk of pancreatitis.

Saquinavir interacts with multiple medications (including herbal products) when given concurrently; refer to Drug Interactions. Fortovase® and Invirase® are not bioequivalent and should not be used interchangeably; only Fortovase® should be used to initiate therapy. Fortovase® is recommended when saquinavir will be given as the sole protease inhibitor; Invirase® may be used only if combined with ritonavir. Safety and efficacy have not been established in children <16 years of age.

Adverse Reactions Protease inhibitors cause dyslipidemia which includes elevated cholesterol and triglycerides and a redistribution of body fat centrally to cause increased abdominal girth, buffalo hump, facial atrophy, and breast enlargement. These agents also cause hyperglycemia.

10%: Gastrointestinal: Diarrhea, nausea

1% to 10%:

- Cardiovascular: Chest pain
- Central nervous system: Anxiety, depression, fatigue, headache, insomnia, pain
- Dermatologic: Rash, verruca
- Endocrine & metabolic: Hyperglycemia, hypoglycemia, hyperkalemia, libido disorder, serum amylase increased
- Gastrointestinal: Abdominal discomfort, abdominal pain, appetite decreased, buccal mucosa ulceration, constipation, dyspepsia, flatulence, taste alteration, vomiting
- Hepatic: AST increased, ALT increased, bilirubin increased
- Neuromuscular & skeletal: Paresthesia, weakness, CPK increased
- Renal: Creatinine kinase increased

<1% (Limited to important or life-threatening): Acute myeloblastic leukemia, alkaline phosphatase increased, allergic reaction, ascites, ataxia, bullous skin eruption, calcium increased, cholangitis, chronic liver disease exacerbation, confusion, hemoglobin decreased, hemolytic anemia, hepatitis, hypokalemia, jaundice, LFTs increased, neuropathy, pain, pancreatitis, polyarthritis, portal hypertension, seizure, serum phosphate decreased, Stevens-Johnson syndrome, syncope, thrombocytopenia, thrombophlebitis, triglycerides increased, upper quadrant abdominal pain

Drug Interactions

Cytochrome P450 Effect: Substrate of CYP2D6 (minor), 3A4 (major); **Inhibits** CYP2C8/9 (weak), 2C19 (weak), 2D6 (weak), 3A4 (moderate)

Increased Effect/Toxicity: Concurrent use of amiodarone, bepridil, cisapride, flecainide, midazolam, pimozide, propafenone, quinidine, rifampin, triazolam, or ergot derivatives is contraindicated.

Saquinavir may increase the levels/effects of selected benzodiazepines, calcium channel blockers, cisapride, cyclosporine, ergot alkaloids, selected HMG-CoA reductase inhibitors, mirtazapine, nateglinide, nefazodone, pimozide, quinidine, sildenafil (and other PDE-5 inhibitors), tacrolimus, venlafaxine, and other CYP3A4 substrates. The effects of warfarin may also be increased.

Serum concentrations of saquinavir may be increased by azole antifungals (itraconazole, ketoconazole); dose adjustment was not needed at the study dose when used for a limited time (ketoconazole 400 mg once daily and Fortovase® 1200 mg 3 times/day). Saquinavir serum concentrations may be increased by delavirdine. Indinavir and ritonavir may increase serum levels of saquinavir. Serum levels of saquinavir and nelfinavir may be increased with concurrent use. Lopinavir/ritonavir (combination product) may increase serum levels of saquinavir. Refer to Dosage.

Serum concentrations of saquinavir and clarithromycin may both be increased. Dose adjustment not was not needed at the study dose when used for 7 days (clarithromycin 500 mg twice daily and Fortovase® 1200 mg 3 times/day); dosage adjustment of clarithromycin is recommended in patients with renal impairment.

Serum concentrations of saquinavir are decreased and levels of rifabutin are increased when used together. Saquinavir should not be used as the sole protease inhibitor when given with rifabutin.

Decreased Effect: The levels/effects of saquinavir may be reduced by aminoglutethimide, carbamazepine, nafcillin, nevirapine, phenobarbital, phenytoin, rifamycins, and other CYP3A4 inducers. Loss of efficacy and potential resistance may occur. Concurrent use with rifampin is contraindicated.

Serum concentrations of methadone may be decreased; an increased dose may be needed when administered with saquinavir. Serum levels of the hormones in oral contraceptives may decrease significantly with administration of saquinavir.

(Continued)

Saquinavir *(Continued)*

Patients should use alternative methods of contraceptives during saquinavir therapy.

Serum levels of saquinavir and efavirenz may be decreased with concurrent use; saquinavir should not be used as the sole protease inhibitor with efavirenz or nevirapine.

Dexamethasone may decrease serum concentrations of saquinavir; use with caution. Serum concentrations of saquinavir are decreased and levels of rifabutin are increased when used together. Saquinavir should not be used as the sole protease inhibitor when given with rifabutin.

Ethanol/Nutrition/Herb Interactions

Food: A high-fat meal maximizes bioavailability. Saquinavir levels may increase if taken with grapefruit juice.

Herb/Nutraceutical: Saquinavir serum concentrations may be decreased by St John's wort; avoid concurrent use. Garlic capsules may decrease saquinavir serum concentrations; avoid use if saquinavir is the only protease inhibitor.

Stability

Fortovase®: Store in refrigerator. Stable for 3 months when stored at room temperature.

Invirase®: Store at room temperature.

Mechanism of Action As an inhibitor of HIV protease, saquinavir prevents the cleavage of viral polyprotein precursors which are needed to generate functional proteins in and maturation of HIV-infected cells

Pharmacodynamics/Kinetics

Absorption: Poor; increased with high fat meal; Fortovase® has improved absorption over Invirase®

Distribution: V_d: 700 L; does not distribute into CSF

Protein binding, plasma: ~98%

Metabolism: Extensively hepatic via CYP3A4; extensive first-pass effect

Bioavailability: Invirase®: ~4%; Fortovase®: 12% to 15%

Excretion: Feces (81% to 88%), urine (1% to 3%) within 5 days

Dosage Oral: Children ≥16 years and Adults: **Note:** Fortovase® and Invirase® are not bioequivalent and should not be used interchangeably; only Fortovase® should be used to initiate therapy:

Unboosted regimen: Fortovase®: 1200 mg (six 200 mg capsules) 3 times/day or 1600 mg twice daily within 2 hours after a meal in combination with a nucleoside analog **Note:** Saquinavir hard-gel capsules (Invirase®) should not be used in 'unboosted regimens.'

Ritonavir-boosted regimens:

Fortovase®: 1000 mg (five 200 mg capsules) twice daily in combination with ritonavir 100 mg twice daily

Invirase®: 1000 mg (five 200 mg capsules or two 500 mg tablets) twice daily given in combination with ritonavir 100 mg twice daily. This combination should be given together and within 2 hours after a full meal in combination with a nucleoside analog.

Dosage adjustments of Fortovase® when administered in combination therapy:

Delavirdine: Fortovase® 800 mg 3 times/day

Lopinavir and ritonavir (Kaletra™): Fortovase® or Invirase® 1000 mg twice daily

Nelfinavir: Fortovase®: 1200 mg twice daily

Elderly: Clinical studies did not include sufficient numbers of patients ≥65 years of age; use caution due to increased frequency of organ dysfunction

Dietary Considerations Administer within 2 hours of a meal. Invirase® capsules contain lactose 63.3 mg/capsule (not expected to induce symptoms of intolerance).

Administration Take saquinavir within 2 hours after a full meal. Avoid direct sunlight when taking saquinavir. When used with ritonavir, saquinavir and ritonavir should be administered at the same time.

Monitoring Parameters Monitor viral load, CD4 count, triglycerides, cholesterol, glucose

Patient Information Saquinavir is not a cure for HIV infection nor has it been found to reduce the transmission of HIV; opportunistic infections and other illnesses associated with AIDS may still occur; take saquinavir within 2 hours after a full meal; avoid direct sunlight when taking saquinavir. Do not take any prescription medications, over-the-counter products or herbal products, especially St John's wort, without consulting prescriber.

Additional Information The indication for saquinavir for the treatment of HIV infection is based on changes in surrogate markers. At present, there are no results from controlled clinical trials evaluating the effect of regimens containing saquinavir on patient survival or the clinical progression of HIV infection, such as the occurrence of

opportunistic infections or malignancies; in cell culture, saquinavir is additive to synergistic with AZT, ddC, and DDI without enhanced toxicity. According to the manufacturer, Invirase® will be phased out over time and completely replaced by Fortovase®. Potential compliance problems, frequency of administration and adverse effects should be discussed with patients before initiating therapy to help prevent the emergence of resistance.

Dosage Forms Note: Strength expressed as base; [DSC] = Discontinued product

Capsule, as mesylate (Invirase®): 200 mg [contains lactose 63.3 mg/capsule]

Capsule, soft gelatin, as base (Fortovase®): 200 mg [DSC]

Tablet, as base (Invirase®): 500 mg

Selected Readings

Deeks SG, Smith M, Holodniy M, et al, "HIV-1 Protease Inhibitors. A Review for Clinicians," *JAMA*, 1997, 277(2):145-53.

Figgitt DP and Plosker GL, "Saquinavir Soft-Gel Capsule: An Updated Review of Its Use in the Management of HIV Infection," *Drugs*, 2000, 60(2):481-516.

Hsu A, Granneman GR, Cao G, et al, "Pharmacokinetic Interactions Between Two Human Immunodeficiency Virus Protease Inhibitors, Ritonavir and Saquinavir," *Clin Pharmacol Ther*, 1998, 63(4):453-64.

Kakuda TN, Struble KA, and Piscitelli SC, "Protease Inhibitors for the Treatment of Human Immunodeficiency Virus Infection," *Am J Health Syst Pharm*, 1998, 55(3):233-54.

Kaul DR, Cinti SK, Carver PL, et al, "HIV Protease Inhibitors: Advances in Therapy and Adverse Reactions, Including Metabolic Complications," *Pharmacotherapy*, 1999, 19(3):281-98.

McDonald CK and Kuritzkes DR, "Human Immunodeficiency Virus Type 1 Protease Inhibitors," *Arch Intern Med*, 1997, 157(9):951-9.

Noble S and Faulds D, "Saquinavir: A Review of Its Pharmacology and Clinical Potential in the Management of HIV Infection," *Drugs*, 1996, 52(1):93-112.

Perry CM and Noble S, "Saquinavir Soft-Gel Capsule Formulation. A Review of Its Use in Patients With HIV Infection," *Drugs*, 1998, 55(3):461-86.

Vella S and Floridia M, "Saquinavir. Clinical Pharmacology and Efficacy," *Clin Pharmacokinet*, 1998, 34(3):189-201.

Saquinavir Mesylate *see* Saquinavir *on page 1060*

SB-265805 *see* Gemifloxacin *on page 840*

Selenium Sulfide (se LEE nee um SUL fide)

U.S. Brand Names Exsel® [DSC]; Head & Shoulders® Intensive Treatment [OTC]; Selsun®; Selsun Blue® 2-in-1 Treatment [OTC]; Selsun Blue® Balanced Treatment [OTC]; Selsun Blue® Medicated Treatment [OTC]; Selsun Blue® Moisturizing Treatment [OTC]

Canadian Brand Names Versel®

Generic Available Yes

Use Treatment of itching and flaking of the scalp associated with dandruff, to control scalp seborrheic dermatitis; treatment of tinea versicolor

Drug of Choice or Alternative for Organism(s):

Malassezia furfur on page 213

Pregnancy Risk Factor C

Pregnancy Implications Animal studies have not been conducted.

Contraindications Hypersensitivity to selenium or any component of the formulation

Warnings/Precautions Do not use on damaged skin to avoid any systemic toxicity; avoid topical use in very young children; safety of topical in infants has not been established

Adverse Reactions Frequency not defined.

Central nervous system: Lethargy

Dermatologic: Alopecia or hair discoloration, unusual dryness or oiliness of scalp

Gastrointestinal: Vomiting following long-term use on damaged skin, abdominal pain, garlic breath

Local: Irritation

Neuromuscular & skeletal: Tremor

Miscellaneous: Diaphoresis

Overdosage/Toxicology Symptoms include nausea, vomiting, and diarrhea.

Mechanism of Action May block the enzymes involved in growth of epithelial tissue

Pharmacodynamics/Kinetics

Absorption: Topical: None through intact skin, but can be absorbed through damaged skin

Excretion: Urine, feces, lungs, skin

Dosage Topical:

Dandruff, seborrhea: Massage 5-10 mL into wet scalp, leave on scalp 2-3 minutes, rinse thoroughly

Tinea versicolor: Apply the 2.5% lotion to affected area and lather with small amounts of water; leave on skin for 10 minutes, then rinse thoroughly; apply every day for 7 days

Administration Shake well before using. May damage jewelry; remove before treatment. For external use only; do not apply to broken or inflamed skin.

(Continued)

Selenium Sulfide *(Continued)*

Patient Information Topical formulations are for external use only; notify prescriber if condition persists or worsens; avoid contact with eyes; thoroughly rinse after application. May damage jewelry; remove before treatment. If used before or after bleaching, tinting, or permanent waving of the hair, rinse hair thoroughly (at least 5 minutes) to avoid or decrease hair discoloration.

Dosage Forms [DSC] = Discontinued product

Lotion, topical: 2.5% (120 mL)

Shampoo, topical: 1% (210 mL)

Exsel® [DSC], Selsun®: 2.5% (120 mL)

Head & Shoulders® Intensive Treatment: 1% (400 mL)

Selsun Blue® Balanced Treatment, Selsun Blue® Medicated Treatment, Selsun Blue® Moisturizing Treatment, Selsun Blue® 2-in-1 Treatment: 1% (120 mL, 210 mL, 330 mL)

Selsun® *see* Selenium Sulfide *on page 1063*

Selsun Blue® 2-in-1 Treatment [OTC] *see* Selenium Sulfide *on page 1063*

Selsun Blue® Balanced Treatment [OTC] *see* Selenium Sulfide *on page 1063*

Selsun Blue® Medicated Treatment [OTC] *see* Selenium Sulfide *on page 1063*

Selsun Blue® Moisturizing Treatment [OTC] *see* Selenium Sulfide *on page 1063*

Septra® *see* Sulfamethoxazole and Trimethoprim *on page 1087*

Septra® DS *see* Sulfamethoxazole and Trimethoprim *on page 1087*

Septra® Injection (Can) *see* Sulfamethoxazole and Trimethoprim *on page 1087*

Seromycin® *see* CycloSERINE *on page 763*

Serostim® *see* Somatropin *on page 1069*

Sertaconazole (ser ta KOE na zole)

U.S. Brand Names Ertaczo™

Synonyms Sertaconazole Nitrate

Generic Available No

Use Topical treatment of tinea pedis (athlete's foot)

Pregnancy Risk Factor C

Pregnancy Implications There are no adequate or well-controlled studies in pregnant women. Use during pregnancy only if clearly needed.

Contraindications Hypersensitivity to sertaconazole, other imidazoles (manufacturer-based contraindication), or any component of the formulation

Warnings/Precautions Discontinue drug if sensitivity or chemical irritation occurs. For external use only; not for ophthalmic or intravaginal use. Hypersensitivity to one imidazole antifungal may result in cross-reactivity with another. Safety and efficacy have not been established in pediatric patients <12 years of age.

Adverse Reactions

1% to 10%: Dermatologic: Burning, contact dermatitis, dry skin, tenderness

Postmarketing and/or case reports: Desquamation, erythema, hyperpigmentation, pruritus, vesiculation

Stability Store at 25°C (77°F).

Mechanism of Action Alters fungal cell wall membrane permeability; inhibits the CYP450-dependent synthesis of ergosterol

Pharmacodynamics/Kinetics

Absorption: Topical: Minimal

Dosage Topical: Children ≥12 years and Adults: Apply between toes and to surrounding healthy skin twice daily for 4 weeks

Administration For external use only. Apply to affected area between toes and to surrounding healthy skin. Make sure skin is dry before applying. Avoid use of occlusive dressing. Avoid contact with eyes, nose, mouth, and other mucous membranes.

Monitoring Parameters Reassess diagnosis if no clinical improvement after 2 weeks.

Dosage Forms Cream, topical, as nitrate: 2% (30 g)

Sertaconazole Nitrate *see* Sertaconazole *on page 1064*

Silvadene® *see* Silver Sulfadiazine *on page 1065*

Silver Nitrate (SIL ver NYE trate)

Synonyms $AgNO_3$

Generic Available Yes

Use Cauterization of wounds and sluggish ulcers, removal of granulation tissue and warts; aseptic prophylaxis of burns

Pregnancy Risk Factor C

Contraindications Hypersensitivity to silver nitrate or any component of the formulation; not for use on broken skin, cuts, or wounds

Warnings/Precautions Do not use applicator sticks on the eyes. Prolonged use may result in skin discoloration.

Adverse Reactions Frequency not defined.

Dermatologic: Burning and skin irritation, staining of the skin
Endocrine & metabolic: Hyponatremia
Hematologic: Methemoglobinemia

Overdosage/Toxicology Symptoms include pain and burning of the mouth, salivation, vomiting, diarrhea, shock, coma, convulsions, death and blackening of skin and mucous membranes. Absorbed nitrate can cause methemoglobinemia. Fatal dose is as low as 2 g. Administer sodium chloride in water (10 g/L) to cause precipitation of silver.

Stability Must be stored in a dry place. Store in a tight, light-resistant container. Exposure to light causes silver to oxidize and turn brown, dipping in water causes oxidized film to readily dissolve.

Mechanism of Action Free silver ions precipitate bacterial proteins by combining with chloride in tissue forming silver chloride; coagulates cellular protein to form an eschar; silver ions or salts or colloidal silver preparations can inhibit the growth of both gram-positive and gram-negative bacteria. This germicidal action is attributed to the precipitation of bacterial proteins by liberated silver ions. Silver nitrate coagulates cellular protein to form an eschar, and this mode of action is the postulated mechanism for control of benign hematuria, rhinitis, and recurrent pneumothorax.

Pharmacodynamics/Kinetics

Absorption: Because silver ions readily combine with protein, there is minimal GI and cutaneous absorption of the 0.5% and 1% preparations

Excretion: Highest amounts of silver noted on autopsy have been in kidneys, excretion in urine is minimal

Dosage Children and Adults:

Sticks: Apply to mucous membranes and other moist skin surfaces only on area to be treated 2-3 times/week for 2-3 weeks

Topical solution: Apply a cotton applicator dipped in solution on the affected area 2-3 times/week for 2-3 weeks

Administration Applicators are **not** for ophthalmic use.

Monitoring Parameters With prolonged use, monitor methemoglobin levels

Patient Information Discontinue topical preparation if redness or irritation develop

Additional Information Silver nitrate solutions stain skin and utensils.

Dosage Forms

Applicator sticks, topical: Silver nitrate 75% and potassium nitrate 25% (6", 12", 18")
Solution, topical: 10% (30 mL); 25% (30 mL); 50% (30 mL)

Selected Readings

US Department of Health and Human Services, "1993 Sexually Transmitted Diseases Treatment Guidelines," *MMWR*, 1993, 42(RR-14).

Silver Sulfadiazine (SIL ver sul fa DYE a zeen)

U.S. Brand Names Silvadene®; SSD®; SSD® AF; Thermazene®

Canadian Brand Names Dermazin™; Flamazine®; SSD™

Generic Available Yes

Use Prevention and treatment of infection in second and third degree burns

Pregnancy Risk Factor B

Contraindications Hypersensitivity to silver sulfadiazine or any component of the formulation; premature infants or neonates <2 months of age (sulfonamides may displace bilirubin and cause kernicterus); pregnancy (approaching or at term)

Warnings/Precautions Use with caution in patients with G6PD deficiency, renal impairment, or history of allergy to other sulfonamides; sulfadiazine may accumulate in patients with impaired hepatic or renal function; fungal superinfection may occur; use of analgesic might be needed before application; systemic absorption is significant and adverse reactions may occur

Adverse Reactions Frequency not defined.

Dermatologic: Itching, rash, erythema multiforme, discoloration of skin, photosensitivity
Hematologic: Hemolytic anemia, leukopenia, agranulocytosis, aplastic anemia
Hepatic: Hepatitis
Renal: Interstitial nephritis
Miscellaneous: Allergic reactions may be related to sulfa component

Drug Interactions

Decreased Effect: Topical proteolytic enzymes are inactivated by silver sulfadiazine.

(Continued)

Silver Sulfadiazine *(Continued)*

Stability Silvadene® cream will occasionally darken either in the jar or after application to the skin. This color change results from a light catalyzed reaction which is a common characteristic of all silver salts. A similar analogy is the oxidation of silverware. The product of this color change reaction is silver oxide which ranges in color from gray to black. Silver oxide has rarely been associated with permanent skin discoloration. Additionally, the antimicrobial activity of the product is not substantially diminished because the color change reaction involves such a small amount of the active drug and is largely a surface phenomenon.

Mechanism of Action Acts upon the bacterial cell wall and cell membrane. Bactericidal for many gram-negative and gram-positive bacteria and is effective against yeast. Active against *Pseudomonas aeruginosa*, *Pseudomonas maltophilia*, *Enterobacter* species, *Klebsiella* species, *Serratia* species, *Escherichia coli*, *Proteus mirabilis*, *Morganella morganii*, *Providencia rettgeri*, *Proteus vulgaris*, *Providencia* species, *Citrobacter* species, *Acinetobacter calcoaceticus*, *Staphylococcus aureus*, *Staphylococcus epidermidis*, *Enterococcus* species, *Candida albicans*, *Corynebacterium diphtheriae*, and *Clostridium perfringens*

Pharmacodynamics/Kinetics

Absorption: Significant percutaneous absorption of silver sulfadiazine can occur especially when applied to extensive burns

Half-life elimination: 10 hours; prolonged with renal impairment

Time to peak, serum: 3-11 days of continuous therapy

Excretion: Urine (~50% as unchanged drug)

Dosage Children and Adults: Topical: Apply once or twice daily with a sterile-gloved hand; apply to a thickness of $^1/_{16}$"; burned area should be covered with cream at all times

Administration Apply with a sterile-gloved hand. Apply to a thickness $^1/_{16}$". Burned area should be covered with cream at all times.

Monitoring Parameters Serum electrolytes, urinalysis, renal function tests, CBC in patients with extensive burns on long-term treatment

Patient Information For external use only; bathe daily to aid in debridement (if not contraindicated); apply liberally to burned areas; for external use only; notify prescriber if condition persists or worsens

Additional Information Contains methylparaben and propylene glycol

Dosage Forms Cream, topical: 1% (25 g, 50 mg, 85 g, 400 g)

Silvadene®, Thermazene®: 1% (20 g, 50 g, 85 g, 400 g, 1000 g)

SSD®: 1% (25 g, 50 g, 85 g, 400 g)

SSD® AF: 1% (50 g, 400 g)

Selected Readings

Kulick MI, Wong R, Okarma TB, et al, "Prospective Study of Side Effects Associated With the Use of Silver Sulfadiazine in Severely Burned Patients," *Ann Plast Surg*, 1985, 14(5):407-18.

Lockhart SP, Rushworth A, Azmy AA, et al, "Topical Silver Sulfadiazine: Side Effects and Urinary Excretion," *Burns Incl Therm Inj*, 1983, 10(1):9-12.

Smallpox Vaccine (SMAL poks vak SEEN)

U.S. Brand Names Dryvax®

Synonyms Dried Smallpox Vaccine; Vaccinia Vaccine

Generic Available No

Use Active immunization against vaccinia virus, the causative agent of smallpox in persons determined to be at risk for smallpox infection. The ACIP recommends vaccination of laboratory workers at risk of exposure from cultures or contaminated animals which may be a source of vaccinia or related Orthopoxviruses capable of causing infections in humans (monkeypox, cowpox, or variola). The ACIP also recommends that consideration be given for vaccination in healthcare workers having contact with clinical specimens, contaminated material, or patients receiving vaccinia or recombinant vaccinia viruses. Revaccination is recommended every 10 years. The Armed Forces recommend vaccination of certain personnel categories. Recommendations for use in response to bioterrorism are regularly updated by the CDC, and may be found at www.cdc.gov.

Restrictions FDA Licenses Vaccinia Vaccine

In October 2002, the FDA approved the licensing of the current stockpile of smallpox vaccine. This approval allows the vaccine to be distributed and administered in the event of a smallpox attack. The bulk of current supplies have been designated for use by the U.S. military. Additionally, laboratory workers who may be at risk of exposure may require vaccination. Bioterrorism experts have proposed immunization of first responders (including police, fire, and emergency workers), but these plans may not be implemented until additional stocks of vaccine are licensed.

Pregnancy Risk Factor C

Pregnancy Implications Animal reproduction studies have not been conducted. Vaccinia vaccine has not been associated with the development of congenital malformations. On rare occasions, vaccination has been reported to cause fetal infection. Fetal vaccina infection is associated with stillbirth or neonatal mortality. Pregnancy should be avoided for at least 28 days following vaccination. Healthcare providers may enroll pregnant women who were inadvertently vaccinated during pregnancy (or within 42 days prior to conception) in the CDC pregnancy registry by calling 404-639-8253 or 877-554-4625. Military cases should be reported to the Department of Defense.

Contraindications Hypersensitivity to the vaccine or any component, including polymyxin B, dihydrostreptomycin, chlortetracycline, and neomycin; patients with a history of eczema or patients whose household contacts have acute or chronic exfoliative skin conditions (atopic dermatitis, eczema, burns, impetigo, Varicella zoster, or wounds); immunosuppressed patients and their household contacts, including patients with congenital or acquired immune deficiencies (including HIV, agammaglobulinemia, leukemia, lymphoma, neoplastic disease of the bone marrow or lymphatic system), patients receiving radiation, immunosuppressive drugs, or systemic corticosteroids ≥20 mg/day or ≥2 mg/kg body weight of prednisone for >2 weeks; patients using ocular steroid medications; moderate to severe intercurrent illness; history of Darier disease (or if household contact has active disease); pregnancy or suspected pregnancy (including household contacts of pregnant women); breast-feeding

Note: There are no absolute contraindications regarding vaccination of individuals with a high-risk exposure to smallpox. The decision to vaccinate in an emergency situation must be based on a careful analysis of potential benefits and possible risks.

Warnings/Precautions For vaccination by scarification (multiple punctures into superficial layers of the skin) only. Not for I.M., I.V., or SubQ injection. Packaging contains latex, which may cause hypersensitivity reactions in allergic individuals. Materials used to prepare and vaccinate should be disposed of per manufacturer's recommendations. Virus may be cultured from vaccination sites until scab separates from lesion. Individuals should be instructed to avoid contact with patients at high risk of transmission/adverse effects, including patients with eczema or immunodeficiency during this time. Patients should be advised not to donate blood for 21 days or until the scab has separated; contacts who have inadvertently contracted vaccinia should avoid donating blood for 14 days. Acute myopericarditis and encephalitis have been observed following vaccination. Progressive vaccinia may occur in the immunocompromised. Severe skin infections may occur in patients with eczema. Immunocompromised patients or those with eczema or cardiovascular disease should not be vaccinated in nonemergency situations. Not for use in infants <12 months of age (in emergency conditions) or for use in pediatric patients <18 years of age (nonemergency conditions). May not protect all individuals receiving the vaccine.

Adverse Reactions All serious adverse reactions must be reported to the U.S. Department of Health and Human Services (DHHS) Vaccine Adverse Event Reporting System (VAERS) 1-800-822-7967. In addition, clinicians may enroll patients with adverse reactions in the CDC Registry at 877-554-4625.

Frequency not established for all reactions. Most severe reactions are rare.

Cardiovascular: Myopericarditis, ischemic cardiac events, dilated cardiomyopathy

Central nervous system: Headache, fatigue, chills, fever (up to 70%; may be ≥102°F in up to 20% in children; frequency in adults may be lower). Rare reactions include: Encephalitis, encephalomyelitis, and encephalopathy

Dermatologic: Rash, secondary pyogenic infection, erythema multiforme

Adverse reactions requiring evaluation or possible treatment: Inadvertent inoculation, generalized vaccinia, eczema vaccinatum, progressive vaccinia, postvaccinial CNS disease, fetal vaccinia

Rare reactions include: Stevens-Johnson syndrome (rare); generalized vaccinia; secondary inoculation of eyelid, face, nose, mouth, genitalia, or rectum (often from autoinoculation from the site of the vaccination and occasionally from contact spread from recently immunized individuals); and rare progressive vaccinia or eczema vaccinatum

Local: Pain at the injection site, satellite lesions, inflammation, lymphadenopathy

Neuromuscular & skeletal: Myalgia

Overdosage/Toxicology No specific experience in overdose. Symptoms may include headache, nausea, vomiting, and hypotension. Treatment is supportive.

Drug Interactions

Decreased Effect: Smallpox vaccine may suppress tuberculin (PPD) skin test; avoid skin test for ≥1 month after vaccine to prevent false-negative reactions.

Stability Store at 2°C to 8°C (36°F to 46°F). May be stored for no longer than 15 days following reconstitution. Do not freeze.

(Continued)

Smallpox Vaccine *(Continued)*

Release vacuum in vial prior to reconstitution by inserting a sterile 21-gauge needle (or smaller) through the stopper. Do not use this needle to reconstitute vaccine. Use the vented needle (provided with kit) to reconstitute solution. Solution should be reconstituted with the diluent provided (to reduce viscosity, this solution may require warming in hands prior to drawing into the syringe). Reconstitute with entire volume of diluent. Following reconstitution, allow to stand for 3-5 minutes, then swirl gently (if necessary) to effect complete reconstitution. Restoppered vial of vaccine is stable for up to 90 days when refrigerated at 2°C to 8°C (36°F to 46°F).

Mechanism of Action Live vaccinia virus at a concentration of ~100 million infectious particles per mL. Vaccination results in viral replication, production of neutralizing antibodies, immunity, and cellular hypersensitivity.

Pharmacodynamics/Kinetics Onset: Neutralizing antibodies appear 10-13 days after vaccination.

Dosage Not for I.M., I.V., or SubQ injection: Vaccination by scarification (multiple-puncture technique) only: **Note:** A trace of blood should appear at vaccination site after 15-20 seconds; if no trace of blood is visible, an additional 3 insertions should be made using the same needle, without reinserting the needle into the vaccine bottle.

Adults (children ≥12 months in emergency conditions only):

Primary vaccination: Use a single drop of vaccine suspension and 2 or 3 needle punctures (using the same needle) into the superficial skin

Revaccination: Use a single drop of vaccine suspension and 15 needle punctures (using the same needle) into the superficial skin

Dosage adjustment in renal impairment: No dosage adjustment required

Administration Using a bifurcated needle, 1 drop of vaccine is introduced into the superficial layers of the skin using a multiple-puncture technique. The skin over the insertion of the deltoid muscle or the posterior aspect of the arm over the triceps are the preferred sites for vaccination.

A single-use bifurcated needle should be dipped carefully into the reconstituted vaccine (following removal of rubber stopper). Visually confirm that the needle picks up a drop of vaccine solution. Deposit the drop of vaccine onto clean, dry skin at the vaccination site. Holding the bifurcated needle perpendicular to the skin, punctures are to be made rapidly into the superficial skin of the vaccination site. The puncture strokes should be vigorous enough to allow a trace of blood to appear after approximately 15-20 seconds. Wipe off any remaining vaccine with dry sterile gauze. Dispose of all materials in a biohazard waste container. All materials must be burned, boiled, or autoclaved. If no evidence of vaccine take is apparent after 7 days, the individual may be vaccinated again.

To prevent transmission of the virus, cover vaccination site with gauze and cover gauze with a semipermeable barrier or clothing. Good handwashing prevents inadvertent inoculation. Vaccinees should change bandages away from others and launder their own linens to prevent transmission.

Monitoring Parameters Monitor vaccination site; inspect after 6-8 days. Evidence of a major reaction (vesicular or pustular lesion or an area of palpable induration surrounding a central lesion) confirms success of vaccination. An equivocal reaction (all responses other than a major reaction) requires revaccination (preferably with another vial or vaccine lot, if available). Consult CDC or state or local health department if response to a second vaccination is equivocal.

Patient Information To avoid transmitting virus, wash hands with soapy water or hand rubs containing ≥60% alcohol immediately after touching vaccination site or after changing vaccination bandages. Place used bandages in sealed plastic bag before disposing.

Additional Information Initial reaction of the vaccine includes formation of a papule (2-5 days following vaccination). The papule forms a vesicle on day 5 or day 6, which becomes pustular, with surrounding erythema and induration. The maximal area of erythema usually occurs around day 10, and crusting of the lesion normally occurs between day 12 and day 21. At the peak of the reaction, systemic symptoms (fever, malaise) and lymphadenopathy may occur. All materials used in vaccination must be burned, boiled, or autoclaved. Vaccination can decrease the rate of severe or fatal smallpox if administered during the first 4 days of exposure.

Dosage Forms Injection, powder for reconstitution [calf liver source]: ~100 million vaccinia virions per mL following reconstitution [contains polymyxin B, neomycin, dihydrostreptomycin sulfate, and chlortetracycline (trace amounts); packed with diluent, venting needle, and 100 bifurcated needles]

SMZ-TMP *see* Sulfamethoxazole and Trimethoprim *on page 1087*

Sodium Nafcillin *see* Nafcillin *on page 955*

Sodium PAS *see* Aminosalicylic Acid *on page 641*
Sodium Sulamyd® (Can) *see* Sulfacetamide *on page 1081*
Sodium Sulfacetamide *see* Sulfacetamide *on page 1081*
Somatrem *see* Somatropin *on page 1069*

Somatropin (soe ma TROE pin)

U.S. Brand Names Genotropin®; Genotropin Miniquick®; Humatrope®; Norditropin®; Norditropin® NordiFlex®; Nutropin®; Nutropin AQ®; Saizen®; Serostim®; Tev-Tropin™; Zorbtive™

Canadian Brand Names Humatrope®; Nutropin® AQ; Nutropine®; Protropine®; Saizen®; Serostim®

Synonyms Human Growth Hormone; Somatrem

Generic Available No

Use

Children:

- Long-term treatment of growth failure due to inadequate endogenous growth hormone secretion (Genotropin®, Humatrope®, Norditropin®, Nutropin®, Nutropin AQ®, Saizen®, Tev-Tropin™)
- Long-term treatment of short stature associated with Turner syndrome (Humatrope®, Nutropin®, Nutropin AQ®)
- Treatment of Prader-Willi syndrome (Genotropin®)
- Treatment of growth failure associated with chronic renal insufficiency (CRI) up until the time of renal transplantation (Nutropin®, Nutropin AQ®)
- Long-term treatment of growth failure in children born small for gestational age who fail to manifest catch-up growth by 2 years of age (Genotropin®)
- Long-term treatment of idiopathic short stature (nongrowth hormone-deficient short stature) defined by height standard deviation score (SDS) less than or equal to -2.25 and growth rate not likely to attain normal adult height (Humatrope®)

Adults:

- AIDS-wasting or cachexia with concomitant antiviral therapy (Serostim®)
- Replacement of endogenous growth hormone in patients with adult growth hormone deficiency who meet both of the following criteria (Genotropin®, Humatrope®, Norditropin®, Nutropin®, Nutropin AQ®, Saizen®):
  - Biochemical diagnosis of adult growth hormone deficiency by means of a subnormal response to a standard growth hormone stimulation test (peak growth hormone ≤5 mcg/L)

    and
  - Adult-onset: Patients who have adult growth hormone deficiency whether alone or with multiple hormone deficiencies (hypopituitarism) as a result of pituitary disease, hypothalamic disease, surgery, radiation therapy, or trauma

    or
  - Childhood-onset: Patients who were growth hormone deficient during childhood, confirmed as an adult before replacement therapy is initiated
- Treatment of short-bowel syndrome (Zorbtive™)

Unlabeled/Investigational Use Investigational: Congestive heart failure; AIDS-wasting/cachexia in children (Serostim®)

Pregnancy Risk Factor B/C (depending upon manufacturer)

Contraindications Hypersensitivity to growth hormone or any component of the formulation; growth promotion in pediatric patients with closed epiphyses; progression of any underlying intracranial lesion or actively growing intracranial tumor; acute critical illness due to complications following open heart or abdominal surgery; multiple accidental trauma or acute respiratory failure; evidence of active malignancy; use in patients with Prader-Willi syndrome **without** growth hormone deficiency (except Genotropin®) or in patients with Prader-Willi syndrome **with** growth hormone deficiency who are severely obese or have severe respiratory impairment. Saizen® and Norditropin® are contraindicated with proliferative or preproliferative retinopathy.

Warnings/Precautions Use with caution in patients with diabetes or with risk factors for glucose intolerance. Intracranial hypertension has been reported with growth hormone product, funduscopic examinations are recommended; progression of scoliosis may occur in children experiencing rapid growth; patients with growth hormone deficiency may develop slipped capital epiphyses more frequently, evaluate any child with new onset of a limp or with complaints of hip or knee pain; patients with Turner syndrome are at increased risk for otitis media and other ear/hearing disorders, cardiovascular disorders (including stroke, aortic aneurysm, hypertension), and thyroid disease, monitor carefully. Concurrent glucocorticoid therapy may inhibit growth promotion effects; may require dosage adjustment or replacement glucocorticoid therapy in patients with ACTH deficiency. Products may contain benzyl alcohol, m-Cresol or glycerin, some products may be manufactured by recombinant DNA

(Continued)

Somatropin *(Continued)*

technology using *E. coli* as a host, consult specific product labeling. When administering to newborns, reconstitute with sterile water or saline for injection. Not for I.V. injection.

Fatalities have been reported in pediatric patients with Prader-Willi syndrome following the use of growth hormone. The reported fatalities occurred in patients with one or more risk factors, including severe obesity, sleep apnea, respiratory impairment, or unidentified respiratory infection; male patients with one or more of these factors may be at greater risk. Treatment interruption is recommended in patients who show signs of upper airway obstruction, including the onset of, or increased, snoring. In addition, evaluation of and/or monitoring for sleep apnea and respiratory infections are recommended.

Adverse Reactions

Growth hormone deficiency: Antigrowth hormone antibodies, carpal tunnel syndrome (rare), fluid balance disturbances, glucosuria, gynecomastia (rare), headache, hematuria, hyperglycemia (mild), hypoglycemia, hypothyroidism, leukemia, lipoatrophy, muscle pain, increased growth of pre-existing nevi (rare), pain/ local reactions at the injection site, pancreatitis (rare), peripheral edema, exacerbation of psoriasis, rash, seizure, weakness

Idiopathic short stature: Humatrope®: Myalgia (24%), scoliosis (19%), otitis media (16%), arthralgia (11%), arthrosis (11%), hyperlipidemia (8%), gynecomastia (5%), hip pain (3%), hypertension (3%)

Prader-Willi syndrome: Genotropin®: Aggressiveness, arthralgia, edema, hair loss, headache, benign intracranial hypertension, myalgia; fatalities associated with use in this population have been reported

Turner syndrome: Humatrope®: Surgical procedures (45%), otitis media (43%), ear disorders (18%), hypothyroidism (13%), increased nevi (11%), peripheral edema (7%)

Adult growth hormone replacement: ALT/AST increased, arthralgia, back pain, carpal tunnel syndrome, diabetes mellitus, fatigue, flu-like syndrome, gastritis, gastroenteritis, generalized edema, glucose intolerance, gynecomastia (rare), headache, hypertension, hypoesthesia, hypothyroidism, infection (nonviral), insomnia, joint disorder, laryngitis, myalgia, nausea, increased growth of pre-existing nevi, pain, pancreatitis (rare), paresthesia, peripheral edema, pharyngitis, rhinitis, stiffness in extremities, weakness

AIDS wasting or cachexia (limited): Serostim®: Musculoskeletal discomfort (54%), increased tissue turgor (27%), diarrhea (26%), neuropathy (26%), nausea (26%), fatigue (17%), albuminuria (15%), diaphoresis increased (14%), anorexia (12%), anemia (12%), increased AST (12%), insomnia (11%), tachycardia (11%), hyperglycemia (10%), increased ALT (10%)

Postmarketing and/or case reports: Diabetes, diabetic ketoacidosis, glucose intolerance

Short-bowel syndrome: Zorbtive™: Peripheral edema (69% to 81%), edema (facial: 44% to 50%; peripheral 13%), arthralgia (13% to 44%), injection site reaction (19% to 31%), flatulence (25%), abdominal pain (20% to 25%), vomiting (19%), malaise (13%), nausea (13%), diaphoresis increased (13%), rhinitis (7%), dizziness (6%)

Postmarketing and/or case reports: Carpal tunnel syndrome

Small for gestational age: Genotropin®: Mild, transient hyperglycemia; benign intracranial hypertension (rare); central precocious puberty; jaw prominence (rare); aggravation of pre-existing scoliosis (rare); injection site reactions; progression of pigmented nevi

Overdosage/Toxicology Symptoms of acute overdose may include initial hypoglycemia (with subsequent hyperglycemia), fluid retention, headache, nausea, and vomiting. Long-term overdose may result in signs and symptoms of acromegaly.

Drug Interactions

Decreased Effect: Glucocorticoid therapy may inhibit growth-promoting effects. Growth hormone may induce insulin resistance in patients with diabetes mellitus; monitor glucose and adjust insulin dose as necessary.

Stability

Genotropin®: Store at 2°C to 8°C (36°F to 46°F), do not freeze, protect from light

1.5 mg cartridge: Following reconstitution, store under refrigeration and use within 24 hours; discard unused portion

5.8 mg and 13.8 mg cartridge: Following reconstitution, store under refrigeration and use within 21 days

Miniquick®: Store in refrigerator prior to dispensing, but may be stored ≤25°C (77°F) for up to 3 months after dispensing; once reconstituted, solution must be refrigerated and used within 24 hours; discard unused portion

Humatrope®:

Vial: Before and after reconstitution, store at 2°C to 8°C (36°F to 46°F), avoid freezing; when reconstituted with bacteriostatic water for injection, use within 14 days; when reconstituted with sterile water for injection, use within 24 hours and discard unused portion

Cartridge: Before and after reconstitution, store at 2°C to 8°C (36°F to 46°F), avoid freezing; following reconstitution, stable for 14 days under refrigeration. Dilute with solution provided with cartridges **ONLY**; do not use diluent provided with vials

Norditropin®: Store at 2°C to 8°C (36°F to 46°F), do not freeze; avoid direct light

Cartridge: Must be used within 4 weeks once inserted into pen

Prefilled pen: Must be used within 4 weeks after initial injection

Nutropin®: Before and after reconstitution, store at 2°C to 8°C (36°F to 46°F), avoid freezing

Vial: Reconstitute with bacteriostatic water for injection; use reconstituted vials within 14 days; when reconstituted with sterile water for injection, use immediately and discard unused portion

AQ formulation: Use within 28 days following initial use

Saizen®: Prior to reconstitution, store at room temperature 15°C to 30°C (59°F to 86°F). Following reconstitution with bacteriostatic water for injection, reconstituted solution should be refrigerated and used within 14 days; when reconstituted with sterile water for injection, use immediately and discard unused portion.

5 mg vial: Reconstitute with 1-3 mL bacteriostatic water for injection or sterile water for injection; gently swirl; do not shake.

8.8 mg vial: Reconstitute with 2-3 mL bacteriostatic water for injection or sterile water for injection; gently swirl; do not shake.

Serostim®: Prior to reconstitution, store at room temperature 15°C to 30°C (59°F to 86°F); reconstitute with sterile water for injection; store reconstituted solution under refrigeration and use within 24 hours, avoid freezing. Do not use if cloudy

Tev-Tropin™: Prior to reconstitution, store at 2°C to 8°C (36°F to 46°F). Reconstitute with 1-5 mL of diluent provided. Gently swirl; do not shake. May use preservative free NS for use in newborns. Following reconstitution with bacteriostatic NS, solution should be refrigerated and used within 14 days. Some cloudiness may occur; do not use if cloudiness persists after warming to room temperature.

Zorbtive™: Store unopened vials and diluent at room temperature of 15°C to 30°C (59°F to 86°F).

8.8 mg vial: Reconstitute with 1-2 mL bacteriostatic water for injection, use within 14 days; store under refrigeration at 2°C to 8°C (36°F to 46°F); avoid freezing

Mechanism of Action Somatropin is a purified polypeptide hormones of recombinant DNA origin; somatropin contains the identical sequence of amino acids found in human growth hormone; human growth hormone stimulates growth of linear bone, skeletal muscle, and organs; stimulates erythropoietin which increases red blood cell mass; exerts both insulin-like and diabetogenic effects; enhances the transmucosal transport of water, electrolytes, and nutrients across the gut

Pharmacodynamics/Kinetics

Duration: Maintains supraphysiologic levels for 18-20 hours

Absorption: I.M., SubQ: Well absorbed

Metabolism: Hepatic and renal (~90%)

Half-life elimination: Preparation and route of administration dependent

Excretion: Urine

Dosage

Children (individualize dose):

Growth hormone deficiency:

Genotropin®: SubQ: Weekly dosage: 0.16-0.24 mg/kg divided into 6-7 doses

Humatrope®: I.M., SubQ: Weekly dosage: 0.18 mg/kg; maximum replacement dose: 0.3 mg/kg/week; dosing should be divided into equal doses given 3 times/week on alternating days, 6 times/week, or daily

Norditropin®: SubQ: Weekly dosage: 0.024-0.034 mg/kg administered in the evening, divided into doses 6-7 times/week; cartridge and vial formulations are bioequivalent; cartridge formulation does not need to be reconstituted prior to use

Nutropin®, Nutropin® AQ: SubQ: Weekly dosage: 0.3 mg/kg divided into daily doses; pubertal patients: ≤0.7 mg/kg/week divided daily

Tev-Tropin™: SubQ: Up to 0.1 mg/kg administered 3 times/week

Saizen®: I.M., SubQ: 0.06 mg/kg/dose administered 3 times/week

Note: Therapy should be discontinued when patient has reached satisfactory adult height, when epiphyses have fused, or when the patient ceases to respond. Growth of 5 cm/year or more is expected, if growth rate does not exceed 2.5 cm in a 6-month period, double the dose for the next 6 months; if there is still no satisfactory response, discontinue therapy

(Continued)

Somatropin *(Continued)*

Chronic renal insufficiency (CRI): Nutropin®, Nutropin® AQ: SubQ: Weekly dosage: 0.35 mg/kg divided into daily injections; continue until the time of renal transplantation

Dosage recommendations in patients treated for CRI who require dialysis:

Hemodialysis: Administer dose at night prior to bedtime or at least 3-4 hours after hemodialysis to prevent hematoma formation from heparin

CCPD: Administer dose in the morning following dialysis

CAPD: Administer dose in the evening at the time of overnight exchange

Turner syndrome: Humatrope®, Nutropin®, Nutropin® AQ: SubQ: Weekly dosage: ≤0.375 mg/kg divided into equal doses 3-7 times per week

Prader-Willi syndrome: Genotropin®: SubQ: Weekly dosage: 0.24 mg/kg divided into 6-7 doses

Small for gestational age: Genotropin®: SubQ: Weekly dosage: 0.48 mg/kg divided into 6-7 doses

Idiopathic short stature: Humatrope®: SubQ: Weekly dosage: 0.37 mg/kg divided into equal doses 6-7 times per week

AIDS-wasting or cachexia (unlabeled use): Serostim®: SubQ: Limited data; doses of 0.04 mg/kg/day were reported in five children, 6-17 years of age; doses of 0.07 mg/kg/day were reported in six children, 8-14 years of age

Adults:

Growth hormone deficiency: To minimize adverse events in older or overweight patients, reduced dosages may be necessary. During therapy, dosage should be decreased if required by the occurrence of side effects or excessive IGF-I levels.

Norditropin®: SubQ: Initial dose ≤0.004 mg/kg/day; after 6 weeks of therapy, may increase dose to 0.016 mg/kg/day

Nutropin®, Nutropin® AQ: SubQ: ≤0.006 mg/kg/day; dose may be increased according to individual requirements, up to a maximum of 0.025 mg/kg/day in patients <35 years of age, or up to a maximum of 0.0125 mg/kg/day in patients ≥35 years of age

Humatrope®: SubQ: ≤0.006 mg/kg/day; dose may be increased according to individual requirements, up to a maximum of 0.0125 mg/kg/day

Genotropin®: SubQ: Weekly dosage: ≤0.04 mg/kg divided into 6-7 doses; dose may be increased at 4- to 8-week intervals according to individual requirements, to a maximum of 0.08 mg/kg/week

Saizen®: SubQ: ≤0.005 mg/kg/day; dose may be increased to not more than 0.01 mg/kg/day after 4 weeks, based on individual requirements.

AIDS-wasting or cachexia:

Serostim®: SubQ: Dose should be given once daily at bedtime; patients who continue to lose weight after 2 weeks should be re-evaluated for opportunistic infections or other clinical events; rotate injection sites to avoid lipodystrophy

Daily dose based on body weight:

<35 kg: 0.1 mg/kg
35-45 kg: 4 mg
45-55 kg: 5 mg
>55 kg: 6 mg

Short-bowel syndrome (Zorbtive™): SubQ: 0.1 mg/kg once daily for 4 weeks (maximum: 8 mg/day)

Fluid retention (moderate) or arthralgias: Treat symptomatically or reduce dose by 50%

Severe toxicity: Discontinue therapy for up to 5 days; when symptoms resolve, restart at 50% of dose. If severe toxicity recurs or does not disappear within 5 days after discontinuation, permanently discontinue treatment.

Elderly: Patients ≥65 years of age may be more sensitive to the action of growth hormone and more prone to adverse effects; in general, dosing should be cautious, beginning at low end of dosing range

Dosage adjustment in renal impairment Reports indicate patients with chronic renal failure tend to have decreased clearance; specific dosing suggestions not available

Dosage adjustment in hepatic impairment: Clearance may be reduced in patients with severe hepatic dysfunction; specific dosing suggestions not available

Dietary Considerations

Prader-Willi syndrome: All patients should have effective weight control (use is contraindicated in severely-obese patients).

Short-bowel syndrome: Intravenous parenteral nutrition requirements may need reassessment as gastrointestinal absorption improves.

Administration Do not shake; administer SubQ or I.M. (rotate administration sites to avoid tissue atrophy); refer to product labeling; when administering to newborns,

reconstitute with sterile water for injection; cartridge must be administered using the corresponding color-coded NordiPen® injection pen

Monitoring Parameters Growth curve, periodic thyroid function tests, bone age (annually), periodical urine testing for glucose, somatomedin C (IGF-I) levels; funduscopic examinations at initiation of therapy and periodically during treatment; serum phosphorus, alkaline phosphatase and parathyroid hormone. If growth deceleration is observed in children treated for growth hormone deficiency, and not due to other causes, evaluate for presence of antibody formation. Strict blood glucose monitoring in diabetic patients.

Prader-Willi syndrome: Monitor for sleep apnea, respiratory infections, snoring (onset of or increased)

Patient Information This medication can only be given by injection. You will be instructed how to prepare and administer the medication. Use a small enough syringe so that the prescribed dose can be drawn from the vial with reasonable accuracy; for I.M. injections, use a needle of sufficient length (≥1") to ensure that the injection reaches the muscle layer. Rotate injection sites. Dispose of needles and syringes properly. Follow storage instructions. Report the development of a severe headache, acute visual changes, a limp, or complaints of hip or knee pain to your prescriber.

Dosage Forms

[DSC] = Discontinued product

Injection, powder for reconstitution [rDNA origin]:

- Genotropin® [preservative free]: 1.5 mg [4 int. units/mL] [delivers 1.3 mg/mL] [DSC]
- Genotropin® [with preservative]:
  - 5.8 mg [15 int. units/mL] [delivers 5 mg/mL]
  - 13.8 mg [36 int. units/mL] [delivers 12 mg/mL]
- Genotropin Miniquick® [preservative free]: 0.2 mg, 0.4 mg, 0.6 mg, 0.8 mg, 1 mg, 1.2 mg, 1.4 mg, 1.6 mg, 1.8 mg, 2 mg [each strength delivers 0.25 mL]
- Humatrope®: 5 mg [~15 int. units], 6 mg [18 int. units], 12 mg [36 int. units], 24 mg [72 int. units]
- Nutropin® [diluent contains benzyl alcohol]: 5 mg [~15 int. units]; 10 mg [~30 int. units]
- Tev-Tropin™: 5 mg [15 int. units/mL] [diluent contains benzyl alcohol]
- Saizen® [diluent contains benzyl alcohol]: 5 mg [~15 int. units; contains sucrose 34.2 mg]; 8.8 mg [~26.4 int. units; contains sucrose 60.2 mg]
- Serostim®: 4 mg [12 int. units; contains sucrose 27.3 mg]; 5 mg [15 int. units; contains sucrose 34.2 mg]; 6 mg [18 int. units; contains sucrose 41 mg]
- Zorbtive™: 8.8 mg [~26.4 int. units; contains sucrose 60.19 mg; packaged with diluent containing benzyl alcohol]

Injection, solution [rDNA origin]:

- Norditropin®: 5 mg/1.5 mL (1.5 mL); 15 mg/1.5 mL (1.5 mL) [cartridge]
- Norditropin® NordiFlex®: 5 mg/1.5 mL (1.5 mL); 15 mg/1.5 mL (1.5 mL) [prefilled pen]
- Nutropin AQ®: 5 mg/mL [~15 int. units/mL] (2 mL) [vial or cartridge]

Selected Readings

Howrie DL, "Growth Hormone for the Treatment of Growth Failure in Children," *Clin Pharm*, 1987, 6(4):283-91.

Sparfloxacin (spar FLOKS a sin)

Related Information

Antimicrobial Activity Against Selected Organisms *on page 1165*

U.S. Brand Names Zagam® [DSC]

Generic Available No

Use Treatment of adults with community-acquired pneumonia caused by *C. pneumoniae, H. influenzae, H. parainfluenzae, M. catarrhalis, M. pneumoniae* or *S. pneumoniae*; treatment of acute bacterial exacerbations of chronic bronchitis caused by *C. pneumoniae, E. cloacae, H. influenzae, H. parainfluenzae, K. pneumoniae, M. catarrhalis, S. aureus* or *S. pneumoniae*

Pregnancy Risk Factor C

Pregnancy Implications Reports of arthropathy (observed in immature animals and reported rarely in humans) have limited the use of fluoroquinolones in pregnancy. Teratogenic effects were not reported with sparfloxacin in animal studies. Based on limited data, quinolones are not expected to be a major human teratogen. Although quinolone antibiotics should not be used as first-line agents during pregnancy, when considering treatment for life-threatening infection and/or prolonged duration of therapy, the potential risk to the fetus must be balanced against the severity of the potential illness.

Contraindications Hypersensitivity to sparfloxacin, any component of the formulation, or other quinolones; a concurrent administration with drugs which increase the (Continued)

Sparfloxacin *(Continued)*

QT interval including amiodarone, bepridil, bretylium, cisapride, disopyramide, furosemide, procainamide, quinidine, sotalol, albuterol, chloroquine, halofantrine, phenothiazines, prednisone, and tricyclic antidepressants

Warnings/Precautions Not recommended in children <18 years of age, other quinolones have caused transient arthropathy in children; CNS stimulation may occur (tremor, restlessness, confusion, and very rarely hallucinations or seizures); use with caution in patients with known or suspected CNS disorder or renal dysfunction; prolonged use may result in superinfection. Moderate to severe photosensitivity reactions may occur in patients exposed to direct or indirect sunlight, or to artificial ultraviolet light. Patients should avoid unnecessary sunlight exposure during treatment and for 5 days following therapy. Pseudomembranous colitis may occur and should be considered in patients who present with diarrhea. Tendon inflammation and/or rupture have been reported with other quinolone antibiotics. Risk may be increased with concurrent corticosteroids, particularly in the elderly. Discontinue at first sign of tendon inflammation or pain.

Severe hypersensitivity reactions, including anaphylaxis, have occurred with quinolone therapy. If an allergic reaction occurs (itching, urticaria, dyspnea, facial edema, loss of consciousness, tingling, cardiovascular collapse), discontinue drug immediately. Although quinolones may exacerbate myasthenia gravis, sparfloxacin appears to be an exception; caution is still warranted.

Adverse Reactions

1% to 10%:

Cardiovascular: QT_c interval prolongation (1%), vasodilation (1%)
Central nervous system: Insomnia (2%), dizziness (2%), headache (4%)
Dermatologic: Photosensitivity reaction (8%; severe <1%), pruritus (2%)
Gastrointestinal: Diarrhea (5%), dyspepsia (2%), nausea (4%), abdominal pain (2%), vomiting (1%), flatulence (1%), taste perversion (2%)
Hepatic: Increased LFTs

<1% (Limited to important or life-threatening): Allergic reaction, anaphylactoid reaction, anemia, angina pectoris, angioedema, anxiety, arrhythmia, asthma, atrial fibrillation, atrial flutter, complete AV block, confusion, dry mouth, dyspnea, ecchymosis, eosinophilia, exfoliative dermatitis, hallucinations, leukopenia, migraine, postural hypotension, rash, sleep disorder, vertigo

Postmarketing and/or case reports: Agranulocytosis, anaphylactic shock, cerebral thrombosis, erythema nodosum, hepatic failure, hepatic necrosis, interstitial pneumonia, manic reaction, myasthenia gravis (exacerbation), pancytopenia, psychosis, renal failure, rhabdomyolysis, seizure, Stevens-Johnson syndrome, tendon rupture, tendonitis, torsade de pointes, toxic epidermal necrolysis, vasculitis

Overdosage/Toxicology Symptoms include acute renal failure and seizures. Treatment consists of GI decontamination and supportive care; it is not known if sparfloxacin is dialyzable.

Drug Interactions

Increased Effect/Toxicity: Sparfloxacin may increase the effects/toxicity of glyburide and warfarin. Concomitant use with corticosteroids may increase the risk of tendon rupture. Concomitant use with other QT_c-prolonging agents (eg, Class Ia and Class III antiarrhythmics, erythromycin, cisapride, antipsychotics, and cyclic antidepressants) may result in arrhythmias such as torsade de pointes. Probenecid may increase sparfloxacin levels.

Decreased Effect: Concurrent administration of metal cations, including most antacids, oral electrolyte supplements, quinapril, sucralfate, some didanosine formulations (chewable/buffered tablets and pediatric powder for oral suspension), and other highly-buffered oral drugs, may decrease quinolone levels; separate doses.

Ethanol/Nutrition/Herb Interactions Herb/Nutraceutical: Avoid dong quai, St John's wort (may also cause photosensitization).

Mechanism of Action Inhibits DNA-gyrase in susceptible organisms; inhibits relaxation of supercoiled DNA and promotes breakage of double-stranded DNA

Pharmacodynamics/Kinetics

Absorption: Unaffected by food or milk; reduced ~50% by concurrent administration of aluminum- and magnesium-containing antacids
Distribution: Widely throughout the body; V_d: 3.9 L/kg
Protein binding: 45%
Metabolism: Hepatic, primarily by phase II glucuronidation
Half-life elimination: Mean terminal: 20 hours (range: 16-30 hours)
Time to peak, serum: 3-5 hours
Excretion: Urine (50%; ~10% as unchanged drug); feces (50%)

Dosage Adults: Oral:

Loading dose: 400 mg on day 1
Maintenance: 200 mg/day for 10 days total therapy
Dosing adjustment in renal impairment: Cl_{cr} <50 mL/minute: Administer 400 mg on day 1, then 200 mg every 48 hours for a total of 9 days of therapy (total 6 tablets)

Dietary Considerations May be taken without regard to meals; should be taken at the same time each day.

Administration May be taken without regard to meals, however, should be administered at the same time each day. Antacids containing aluminum or magnesium; products containing iron, zinc, or calcium; and sucralfate and didanosine should all be given >4 hours after sparfloxacin.

Monitoring Parameters Evaluation of organ system functions (renal, hepatic, ophthalmologic, and hematopoietic) is recommended periodically during therapy; the possibility of crystalluria should be assessed; WBC and signs and symptoms of infection

Patient Information May take with or without food (should be taken at the same time each day). Antacids containing aluminum or magnesium; products containing iron, zinc, or calcium; and sucralfate and didanosine should all be given >4 hours after sparfloxacin. Drink with plenty of fluids; may cause photosensitivity reactions (use sunscreen, wear protective clothing and eyewear, and avoid prolonged or unnecessary exposure to direct sunlight during and for 5 days following therapy); contact your prescriber immediately if signs of allergy occur; do not discontinue therapy until your course has been completed; take a missed dose as soon as possible, unless it is almost time for your next dose

Dosage Forms [DSC] = Discontinued product
Tablet [film coated]: 200 mg [DSC]

Spectazole® *see* Econazole *on page 795*

Spectinomycin (spek ti noe MYE sin)

U.S. Brand Names Trobicin®

Synonyms Spectinomycin Hydrochloride

Generic Available No

Use Treatment of uncomplicated gonorrhea

Drug of Choice or Alternative for Organism(s):
Neisseria gonorrhoeae on page 244

Pregnancy Risk Factor B

Contraindications Hypersensitivity to spectinomycin or any component of the formulation

Warnings/Precautions Since spectinomycin is ineffective in the treatment of syphilis and may mask symptoms, all patients should be tested for syphilis at the time of diagnosis and 3 months later.

Adverse Reactions <1%: Chills, dizziness, headache, nausea, pain at injection site, pruritus, rash, urticaria, vomiting

Overdosage/Toxicology Symptoms include paresthesias, dizziness, blurred vision, ototoxicity, renal damage, nausea, sleeplessness, and decreased hemoglobin.

Stability Use reconstituted solutions within 24 hours; reconstitute with supplied diluent only

Mechanism of Action A bacteriostatic antibiotic that selectively binds to the 30s subunits of ribosomes, and thereby inhibiting bacterial protein synthesis

Pharmacodynamics/Kinetics
Duration: Up to 8 hours
Absorption: I.M.: Rapid and almost complete
Distribution: Concentrates in urine; does not distribute well into the saliva
Half-life elimination: 1.7 hours
Time to peak: ~1 hour
Excretion: Urine (70% to 100% as unchanged drug)

Dosage I.M.:
Children:
<45 kg: 40 mg/kg/dose 1 time (ceftriaxone preferred)
≥45 kg: Refer to adult dosing.
Children >8 years who are allergic to PCNS/cephalosporins may be treated with oral tetracycline
Adults:
Uncomplicated urethral, cervical, pharyngeal, or rectal gonorrhea: 2 g deep I.M. or 4 g where antibiotic resistance is prevalent 1 time; 4 g (10 mL) dose should be given as two 5 mL injections, followed by adequate chlamydial treatment (doxycycline 100 mg twice daily for 7 days)
Disseminated gonococcal infection: 2 g every 12 hours
(Continued)

Spectinomycin *(Continued)*

Dosing adjustment in renal impairment: None necessary

Hemodialysis: 50% removed by hemodialysis

Administration For I.M. use only

Dosage Forms Injection, powder for reconstitution, as hydrochloride: 2 g [diluent contains benzyl alcohol]

Selected Readings

US Department of Health and Human Services, "1993 Sexually Transmitted Diseases Treatment Guidelines," *MMWR*, 1993, 42(RR-14).

Spectinomycin Hydrochloride *see* Spectinomycin *on page 1075*

Spectracef™ *see* Cefditoren *on page 703*

Spectrocin Plus™ [OTC] *see* Bacitracin, Neomycin, Polymyxin B, and Pramoxine *on page 683*

SpectroGram 2™ (Can) *see* Chlorhexidine Gluconate *on page 735*

Sporanox® *see* Itraconazole *on page 895*

SSD® *see* Silver Sulfadiazine *on page 1065*

SSD® AF *see* Silver Sulfadiazine *on page 1065*

SSKI® *see* Potassium Iodide *on page 1014*

Staticin® [DSC] *see* Erythromycin *on page 807*

Stavudine (STAV yoo deen)

Related Information

Antiretroviral Agents *on page 1206*

Antiretroviral Therapy for HIV Infection *on page 1219*

Management of Healthcare Worker Exposures to HBV, HCV, and HIV *on page 1227*

U.S. Brand Names Zerit®

Canadian Brand Names Zerit®

Synonyms d4T

Generic Available No

Use Treatment of HIV infection in combination with other antiretroviral agents

Drug of Choice or Alternative for Organism(s):

Human Immunodeficiency Virus *on page 181*

Pregnancy Risk Factor C

Pregnancy Implications Cases of fatal and nonfatal lactic acidosis, with or without pancreatitis, have been reported in pregnant women. It is not known if pregnancy itself potentiates this known side effect; however, pregnant women may be at increased risk of lactic acidosis and liver damage. Hepatic enzymes and electrolytes should be monitored frequently during the 3rd trimester of pregnancy. Pharmacokinetics of stavudine are not significantly altered during pregnancy; dose adjustments are not needed. The Perinatal HIV Guidelines Working Group considers stavudine to be an alternative NRTI in dual nucleoside combination regimens; use with didanosine only if no alternatives are available, do not use with zidovudine. Health professionals are encouraged to contact the antiretroviral pregnancy registry to monitor outcomes of pregnant women exposed to antiretroviral medications (1-800-258-4263 or www.APRegistry.com).

Contraindications Hypersensitivity to stavudine or any component of the formulation

Warnings/Precautions Use with caution in patients who demonstrate previous hypersensitivity to zidovudine, didanosine, zalcitabine, pre-existing bone marrow suppression, renal insufficiency, or peripheral neuropathy. Peripheral neuropathy may be the dose-limiting side effect. Zidovudine should not be used in combination with stavudine. Lactic acidosis and severe hepatomegaly with steatosis have been reported with stavudine use, including fatal cases. Risk may be increased in obesity, prolonged nucleoside exposure, or in female patients. Suspend therapy in patients with suspected lactic acidosis; consider discontinuation of stavudine if lactic acidosis is confirmed. Pregnant women may be at increased risk of lactic acidosis and liver damage. Severe motor weakness (resembling Guillain-Barré syndrome) has also been reported (including fatal cases, usually in association with lactic acidosis); manufacturer recommends discontinuation if motor weakness develops (with or without lactic acidosis). Pancreatitis (including some fatal cases) has occurred during combination therapy (didanosine with or without hydroxyurea). Risk increased when used in combination regimen with didanosine and hydroxyurea. Suspend therapy with agents toxic to the pancreas (including stavudine, didanosine, or hydroxyurea) in patients with suspected pancreatitis.

Adverse Reactions All adverse reactions reported below were similar to comparative agent, zidovudine, except for peripheral neuropathy, which was greater for stavudine. Selected adverse events reported as monotherapy or in combination therapy include:

>10%:

- Central nervous system: Headache
- Dermatologic: Rash
- Gastrointestinal: Nausea, vomiting, diarrhea
- Hepatic: Transaminases increased
- Neuromuscular & skeletal: Peripheral neuropathy
- Miscellaneous: Amylase increased

1% to 10%: Hepatic: Bilirubin increased

Postmarketing and/or case reports: Abdominal pain, allergic reaction, anemia, anorexia, chills, fever, hepatitis, hepatomegaly, hepatic failure, hepatic steatosis, insomnia, lactic acidosis, leukopenia, motor weakness (severe), myalgia, pancreatitis, redistribution/accumulation of body fat, thrombocytopenia

Overdosage/Toxicology Acute toxicity was not reported following administration of 12-24 times the recommended dose in adults. Peripheral neuropathy and hepatic toxicity have been reported following chronic overdose. Stavudine may be removed by hemodialysis.

Drug Interactions

Increased Effect/Toxicity: Risk of pancreatitis may be increased with concurrent didanosine use; cases of fatal lactic acidosis have been reported with this combination when used during pregnancy (use only if clearly needed). Risk of hepatotoxicity or pancreatitis may be increased with concurrent hydroxyurea use. Zalcitabine may increase risk of peripheral neuropathy; concurrent use not recommended.

Decreased Effect: Zidovudine inhibits intracellular phosphorylation of stavudine; concurrent use not recommended. Doxorubicin may inhibit intracellular phosphorylation of stavudine; use with caution. Ribavirin may inhibit intracellular phosphorylation of stavudine; use with caution.

Stability Capsules and powder for reconstitution may be stored at room temperature. Reconstituted oral solution should be refrigerated and is stable for 30 days.

Mechanism of Action Stavudine is a thymidine analog which interferes with HIV viral DNA dependent DNA polymerase resulting in inhibition of viral replication; nucleoside reverse transcriptase inhibitor

Pharmacodynamics/Kinetics

- Distribution: V_d: 0.5 L/kg
- Bioavailability: 86.4%
- Metabolism: Undergoes intracellular phosphorylation to an active metabolite
- Half-life elimination: 1-1.6 hours
- Time to peak, serum: 1 hour
- Excretion: Urine (40% as unchanged drug)

Dosage Oral:

Newborns (Birth to 13 days): 0.5 mg/kg every 12 hours

Children:

- >14 days and <30 kg: 1 mg/kg every 12 hours
- ≥30 kg: Refer to Adults dosing

Adults:

- ≥60 kg: 40 mg every 12 hours
- <60 kg: 30 mg every 12 hours

Dosing adjustment for toxicity: If symptoms of peripheral neuropathy occur, discontinue until symptoms resolve. Treatment may then be resumed at 50% the recommended dose. If symptoms recur at lower dose, permanent discontinuation should be considered.

Dosing adjustment in renal impairment:

Children: Specific recommendations not available. Reduction in dose or increase in dosing interval should be considered.

Adults:

Cl_{cr} >50 mL/minute:
- ≥60 kg: 40 mg every 12 hours
- <60 kg: 30 mg every 12 hours

Cl_{cr} 26-50 mL/minute:
- ≥60 kg: 20 mg every 12 hours
- <60 kg: 15 mg every 12 hours

Cl_{cr} 10-25 mL/minute, hemodialysis (administer dose after hemodialysis on day of dialysis):
- ≥60 kg: 20 mg every 24 hours
- <60 kg: 15 mg every 24 hours

Elderly: Older patients should be closely monitored for signs and symptoms of peripheral neuropathy; dosage should be carefully adjusted to renal function

(Continued)

Stavudine *(Continued)*

Dietary Considerations May be taken without regard to meals.

Administration May be administered without regard to meals. Oral solution should be shaken vigorously prior to use.

Monitoring Parameters Monitor liver function tests and signs and symptoms of peripheral neuropathy; monitor viral load and CD4 count

Patient Information Take as directed; take for full length of prescription. Maintain adequate hydration and nutrition. Report immediately any tingling, unusual pain, or numbness in extremities. Report fever, chills, unusual fatigue or acute depression, acute abdominal or back pain, persistent muscle pain or weakness, nausea, vomiting, or unusual bruising or bleeding. Risk of adverse reactions may be increased with some combination therapies.

Additional Information Potential compliance problems, frequency of administration and adverse effects should be discussed with patients before initiating therapy to help prevent the emergence of resistance.

Dosage Forms

Capsule: 15 mg, 20 mg, 30 mg, 40 mg

Powder, for oral solution: 1 mg/mL (200 mL) [dye-free; fruit flavor]

Selected Readings

Dudley MN, Graham KK, Kaul S, et al, "Pharmacokinetics of Stavudine in Patients With AIDS and AIDS-Related Complex," *J Infect Dis*, 1992, 166(3):480-5.

Lea AP and Faulds D, "Stavudine: A Review of Its Pharmacodynamic and Pharmacokinetic Properties and Clinical Potential in HIV Infection," *Drugs*, 1996, 51(5):846-64.

Streptomycin (strep toe MYE sin)

Related Information

Antimicrobial Activity Against Selected Organisms *on page 1165*

Tuberculosis *on page 1315*

Synonyms Streptomycin Sulfate

Generic Available Yes

Use Part of combination therapy of active tuberculosis; used in combination with other agents for treatment of streptococcal or enterococcal endocarditis, mycobacterial infections, plague, tularemia, and brucellosis

Drug of Choice or Alternative for Organism(s):

Enterococcus Species *on page 134*

Francisella tularensis on page 149

Mycobacterium bovis on page 229

Mycobacterium tuberculosis on page 234

Yersinia pestis on page 355

Pregnancy Risk Factor D

Contraindications Hypersensitivity to streptomycin or any component of the formulation; pregnancy

Warnings/Precautions Use with caution in patients with pre-existing vertigo, tinnitus, hearing loss, neuromuscular disorders, or renal impairment; modify dosage in patients with renal impairment; aminoglycosides are associated with significant nephrotoxicity or ototoxicity; the ototoxicity is directly proportional to the amount of drug given and the duration of treatment; tinnitus or vertigo are indications of vestibular injury and impending bilateral irreversible damage; renal damage is usually reversible

Adverse Reactions Frequency not defined.

Cardiovascular: Hypotension

Central nervous system: Neurotoxicity, drowsiness, headache, drug fever, paresthesia

Dermatologic: Skin rash

Gastrointestinal: Nausea, vomiting

Hematologic: Eosinophilia, anemia

Neuromuscular & skeletal: Arthralgia, weakness, tremor

Otic: Ototoxicity (auditory), ototoxicity (vestibular)

Renal: Nephrotoxicity

Respiratory: Difficulty in breathing

Overdosage/Toxicology Symptoms include ototoxicity, nephrotoxicity, and neuromuscular toxicity. The treatment of choice following a single acute overdose appears to be the maintenance of urine output of at least 3 mL/kg/hour. Dialysis is of questionable value in the enhancement of aminoglycoside elimination. If required, hemodialysis is preferred over peritoneal dialysis in patients with normal renal function. Careful hydration may be all that is required to promote diuresis and therefore enhance elimination.

Drug Interactions

Increased Effect/Toxicity: Increased/prolonged effect with depolarizing and nondepolarizing neuromuscular blocking agents. Concurrent use with amphotericin or loop diuretics may increase nephrotoxicity.

Stability Depending upon manufacturer, reconstituted solution remains stable for 2-4 weeks when refrigerated; exposure to light causes darkening of solution without apparent loss of potency

Mechanism of Action Inhibits bacterial protein synthesis by binding directly to the 30S ribosomal subunits causing faulty peptide sequence to form in the protein chain

Pharmacodynamics/Kinetics

Absorption: I.M.: Well absorbed

Distribution: To extracellular fluid including serum, abscesses, ascitic, pericardial, pleural, synovial, lymphatic, and peritoneal fluids; crosses placenta; small amounts enter breast milk

Protein binding: 34%

Half-life elimination: Newborns: 4-10 hours; Adults: 2-4.7 hours, prolonged with renal impairment

Time to peak: Within 1 hour

Excretion: Urine (90% as unchanged drug); feces, saliva, sweat, and tears (<1%)

Dosage

Children:

Tuberculosis:

Daily therapy: 20-40 mg/kg/day (maximum: 1 g/day)

Directly observed therapy (DOT): Twice weekly: 20-40 mg/kg (maximum: 1 g)

DOT: 3 times/week: 25-30 mg/kg (maximum: 1 g)

Adults:

Tuberculosis:

Daily therapy: 15 mg/kg/day (maximum: 1 g)

Directly observed therapy (DOT): Twice weekly: 25-30 mg/kg (maximum: 1.5 g)

DOT: 3 times/week: 25-30 mg/kg (maximum: 1 g)

Enterococcal endocarditis: 1 g every 12 hours for 2 weeks, 500 mg every 12 hours for 4 weeks in combination with penicillin

Streptococcal endocarditis: 1 g every 12 hours for 1 week, 500 mg every 12 hours for 1 week

Tularemia: 1-2 g/day in divided doses for 7-10 days or until patient is afebrile for 5-7 days

Plague: 2-4 g/day in divided doses until the patient is afebrile for at least 3 days

Elderly: 10 mg/kg/day, not to exceed 750 mg/day; dosing interval should be adjusted for renal function; some authors suggest not to give more than 5 days/week or give as 20-25 mg/kg/dose twice weekly

Dosing interval in renal impairment:

Cl_{cr} 10-50 mL/minute: Administer every 24-72 hours

Cl_{cr} <10 mL/minute: Administer every 72-96 hours

Removed by hemo and peritoneal dialysis: Administer dose postdialysis

Administration Inject deep I.M. into large muscle mass; may be administered I.V. over 30-60 minutes

Monitoring Parameters Hearing (audiogram), BUN, creatinine; serum concentration of the drug should be monitored in all patients; eighth cranial nerve damage is usually preceded by high-pitched tinnitus, roaring noises, sense of fullness in ears, or impaired hearing and may persist for weeks after drug is discontinued

Reference Range Therapeutic: Peak: 20-30 mcg/mL; Trough: <5 mcg/mL; Toxic: Peak: >50 mcg/mL; Trough: >10 mcg/mL

Test Interactions False-positive urine glucose with Benedict's solution or Clinitest®; penicillin may decrease aminoglycoside serum concentrations *in vitro*

Patient Information Report any unusual symptom of hearing loss, dizziness, roaring noises, or fullness in ears

Dosage Forms Injection, powder for reconstitution: 1 g

Selected Readings

Begg EJ and Barclay ML, "Aminoglycosides - 50 Years On," *Br J Clin Pharmacol*, 1995, 39(6):597-603.

Cunha BA, "Aminoglycosides: Current Role in Antimicrobial Therapy," *Pharmacotherapy*, 1988, 8(6):334-50.

Davidson PT and Le HQ, "Drug Treatment of Tuberculosis - 1992," *Drugs*, 1992, 43(5):651-73.

"Drugs for Tuberculosis," *Med Lett Drugs Ther*, 1993, 35(908):99-101.

Edson RS and Terrell CL, "The Aminoglycosides," *Mayo Clin Proc*, 1999, 74(5):519-28.

Havlir DV and Barnes PF, "Tuberculosis in Patients With Human Immunodeficiency Virus Infection," *N Engl J Med*, 1999, 340(5):367-73.

Iseman MD, "Treatment of Multidrug-Resistant Tuberculosis," *N Engl J Med*, 1993, 329(11):784-91.

Kim-Sing A, Kays MB, Vivien EJ, et al, "Intravenous Streptomycin Use in a Patient Infected With High-Level Gentamicin-Resistant *Streptococcus faecalis*," *Ann Pharmacother*, 1993, 27(6):712-4.

Morris JT and Cooper RH, "Intravenous Streptomycin: A Useful Route of Administration," *Clin Infect Dis*, 1994, 19(6):1150-1.

(Continued)

Streptomycin *(Continued)*

"Prevention and Treatment of Tuberculosis Among Patients Infected With Human Immunodeficiency Virus: Principles of Therapy and Revised Recommendations. Centers for Disease Control and Prevention," *MMWR*, 1998, 47(RR-20):1-58.

Van Scoy RE and Wilkowske CJ, "Antituberculous Agents," *Mayo Clin Proc*, 1992, 67(2):179-87.

Streptomycin Sulfate *see* Streptomycin *on page 1078*

Striant® *see* Testosterone *on page 1100*

Stromectol® *see* Ivermectin *on page 899*

Sulbactam and Ampicillin *see* Ampicillin and Sulbactam *on page 660*

Sulconazole (sul KON a zole)

U.S. Brand Names Exelderm®

Canadian Brand Names Exelderm®

Synonyms Sulconazole Nitrate

Generic Available No

Use Treatment of superficial fungal infections of the skin, including tinea cruris (jock itch), tinea corporis (ringworm), tinea versicolor, and possibly tinea pedis (athlete's foot, cream only)

Pregnancy Risk Factor C

Contraindications Hypersensitivity to sulconazole or any component of the formulation

Warnings/Precautions Use with caution in nursing mothers; for external use only

Adverse Reactions 1% to 10%:

Dermatologic: Itching

Local: Burning, stinging, redness

Drug Interactions

Cytochrome P450 Effect: Inhibits CYP1A2 (weak), 2A6 (weak), 2C8/9 (weak), 2C19 (weak), 2D6 (weak), 2E1 (weak), 3A4 (weak)

Mechanism of Action Substituted imidazole derivative which inhibits metabolic reactions necessary for the synthesis of ergosterol, an essential membrane component. The end result is usually fungistatic; however, sulconazole may act as a fungicide in *Candida albicans* and *Candida parapsilosis* during certain growth phases.

Pharmacodynamics/Kinetics

Absorption: Topical: ~8.7% percutaneously

Excretion: Primarily urine

Dosage Adults: Topical: Apply a small amount to the affected area and gently massage once or twice daily for 3 weeks (tinea cruris, tinea corporis, tinea versicolor) to 4 weeks (tinea pedis).

Patient Information For external use only; avoid contact with eyes; if burning or irritation develops, notify prescriber

Dosage Forms

Cream, as nitrate: 1% (15 g, 30 g, 60 g)

Solution, topical, as nitrate: 1% (30 mL)

Sulconazole Nitrate *see* Sulconazole *on page 1080*

Sulfabenzamide, Sulfacetamide, and Sulfathiazole

(sul fa BENZ a mide, sul fa SEE ta mide, & sul fa THYE a zole)

U.S. Brand Names V.V.S.®

Synonyms Triple Sulfa

Generic Available Yes

Use Treatment of *Haemophilus vaginalis* vaginitis

Pregnancy Risk Factor C (avoid if near term)

Contraindications Hypersensitivity to sulfabenzamide, sulfacetamide, sulfathiazole, or any component of the formulation; renal dysfunction; pregnancy (if near term)

Warnings/Precautions Associated with Stevens-Johnson syndrome; if local irritation or systemic toxicity develops, discontinue therapy

Adverse Reactions Frequency not defined.

Dermatologic: Pruritus, urticaria, Stevens-Johnson syndrome

Local: Local irritation

Miscellaneous: Allergic reactions

Mechanism of Action Interferes with microbial folic acid synthesis and growth via inhibition of para-aminobenzoic acid metabolism

Pharmacodynamics/Kinetics

Absorption: Absorption from vagina is variable and unreliable

Metabolism: Primarily via acetylation

Excretion: Urine

Dosage Intravaginal: Adults: Female: Cream: Insert one applicatorful into vagina twice daily for 4-6 days; dosage may then be decreased to ½ to ¼ of an applicatorful twice daily

Patient Information Complete full course of therapy; notify prescriber if burning, irritation, or signs of a systemic allergic reaction occur

Dosage Forms Cream, vaginal: Sulfabenzamide 3.7%, sulfacetamide 2.86%, and sulfathiazole 3.42% (78 g with applicator)

Sulfacetamide (sul fa SEE ta mide)

U.S. Brand Names Bleph®-10; Carmol® Scalp; Klaron®; Ovace™

Canadian Brand Names Cetamide™; Diosulf™; Sodium Sulamyd®

Synonyms Sodium Sulfacetamide; Sulfacetamide Sodium

Generic Available Yes: Ointment, solution

Use

Ophthalmic: Treatment and prophylaxis of conjunctivitis due to susceptible organisms; corneal ulcers; adjunctive treatment with systemic sulfonamides for therapy of trachoma

Dermatologic: Scaling dermatosis (seborrheic); bacterial infections of the skin; acne vulgaris

Pregnancy Risk Factor C

Pregnancy Implications Animal reproduction studies have not been conducted and there are no adequate and well-controlled studies in pregnant women. Use of systemic sulfonamides during pregnancy may cause kernicterus in the newborn; the amount of systemic absorption following topical administration is not known. Use during pregnancy only if clearly needed.

Contraindications Hypersensitivity to sulfacetamide, sulfonamides, or any component of the formulation

Warnings/Precautions Severe reactions to sulfonamides have been reported, regardless of route of administration; reactions may include Stevens-Johnson syndrome, toxic epidermal necrolysis, fulminant hepatic necrosis, or blood dyscrasias. Chemical similarities are present among sulfonamides, sulfonylureas, carbonic anhydrase inhibitors, thiazides, and loop diuretics (except ethacrynic acid). Use in patients with sulfonamide allergy is specifically contraindicated in product labeling; however, a risk of cross-reaction exists in patients with allergy to any of these compounds; avoid use when previous reaction has been severe.

Ophthalmic: Inactivated by purulent exudates containing PABA; use with caution in severe dry eye; ointment may retard corneal epithelial healing. For topical application to the eye only; not for injection. Safety and efficacy have not been established in children <2 months of age.

Dermatologic: Use caution if applied to denuded or abraded skin. Some products contain sodium metabisulfite which may cause allergic reactions in certain individuals. For external use only; avoid contact with eyes. Safety and efficacy have not been established in children <12 years of age.

Adverse Reactions Frequency not defined.

Cardiovascular: Edema

Dermatologic: Burning, erythema, irritation, itching, stinging, Stevens-Johnson syndrome

Ocular (following ophthalmic application): Burning, conjunctivitis, conjunctival hyperemia, corneal ulcers, irritation, stinging

Miscellaneous: Allergic reactions, systemic lupus erythematosus

Drug Interactions

Decreased Effect: Silver containing products are incompatible with sulfacetamide solutions.

Stability Store at controlled room temperature.

Ophthalmic solution: Solution may be used if yellow; do not use if darkened.

Carmol® Scalp treatment: Do not freeze; may be used if slightly discolored.

Mechanism of Action Interferes with bacterial growth by inhibiting bacterial folic acid synthesis through competitive antagonism of PABA

Pharmacodynamics/Kinetics

Half-life elimination: 7-13 hours

Excretion: When absorbed, primarily urine (as unchanged drug)

Dosage

Children >2 months and Adults: Ophthalmic:

Ointment: Apply to lower conjunctival sac 1-4 times/day and at bedtime

Solution: Instill 1-2 drops several times daily up to every 2-3 hours in lower conjunctival sac during waking hours and less frequently at night; increase dosing interval as condition responds. Usual duration of treatment: 7-10 days

(Continued)

Sulfacetamide *(Continued)*

Trachoma: Instill 2 drops into the conjunctival sac every 2 hours; must be used in conjunction with systemic therapy

Children >12 years and Adults: Topical:

Acne: Apply thin film to affected area twice daily

Seborrheic dermatitis: Apply at bedtime and allow to remain overnight; in severe cases, may apply twice daily. Duration of therapy is usually 8-10 applications; dosing interval may be increased as eruption subsides. Applications once or twice weekly, or every other week may be used to prevent eruptions.

Secondary cutaneous bacterial infections: Apply 2-4 times/day until infection clears

Administration Topical:

Scalp lotion: Shampoo hair with a nonirritating shampoo prior to application. Part hair in sections and apply small quantities of lotion to scalp; rub in gently. Brush hair for 2-3 minutes. May discolor white fabric.

Acne lotion: Shake well before using.

Monitoring Parameters Response to therapy

Patient Information Eye drops will burn upon instillation; wait at least 10 minutes before using another eye preparation; may sting eyes when first applied; do not touch container to eye, ointment will cause blurred vision; notify prescriber if condition does not improve in 3-4 days; may cause sensitivity to sunlight

Dosage Forms

[DSC] = Discontinued product

Cream, topical, as sodium (Ovace™): 10% (30 g, 60 g)

Foam, topical, as sodium (Ovace™): 10% (50 g, 100 g)

Gel, topical, as sodium (Ovace™): 10% (30 g, 60 g)

Lotion, as sodium:

Carmol® Scalp: 10% (85 g) [contains urea 10%]

Klaron®: 10% (120 mL) [contains sodium metabisulfite]

Ovace™: 10% (180 mL, 360 mL)

Ointment, ophthalmic, as sodium: 10% (3.5 g)

Solution, ophthalmic, as sodium: 10% (15 mL)

Bleph®-10: 10% (5 mL; 15 mL [DSC]) [contains benzalkonium chloride]

Selected Readings

Lohr JA, Austin RD, Grossman M, et al, "Comparison of Three Topical Antimicrobials for Acute Bacterial Conjunctivitis," *Pediatr Infect Dis J*, 1988, 7(9):626-9.

Sulfacetamide and Prednisolone

(sul fa SEE ta mide & pred NIS oh lone)

U.S. Brand Names Blephamide®

Canadian Brand Names Blephamide®; Dioptimyd®; Vasocidin®

Synonyms Prednisolone and Sulfacetamide

Generic Available Yes: Solution

Use Steroid-responsive inflammatory ocular conditions where infection is present or there is a risk of infection; ophthalmic suspension may be used as an otic preparation

Pregnancy Risk Factor C

Pregnancy Implications Refer to Sulfacetamide monograph.

Adverse Reactions

1% to 10%: Local: Burning, stinging

<1%: Cataracts, Cushing's syndrome, fractures, glaucoma, growth suppression, headache, muscle weakness, nausea, osteoporosis, peptic ulcer, pituitary-adrenal axis suppression, pseudotumor cerebri, psychoses, seizure, skin atrophy, Stevens-Johnson syndrome, vertigo, vomiting

Drug Interactions

Cytochrome P450 Effect: Prednisolone: **Substrate** of CYP3A4 (minor); **Inhibits** CYP3A4 (weak)

Mechanism of Action Interferes with bacterial growth by inhibiting bacterial folic acid synthesis through competitive antagonism of PABA; decreases inflammation by suppression of migration of polymorphonuclear leukocytes and reversal of increased capillary permeability; suppresses the immune system by reducing activity and volume of the lymphatic system

Pharmacodynamics/Kinetics See individual agents.

Dosage Children >2 months and Adults: Ophthalmic:

Ointment: Apply to lower conjunctival sac 1-4 times/day

Solution, suspension: Instill 1-3 drops every 2-3 hours while awake

Administration Suspension: Shake well before use.

Dosage Forms

Ointment, ophthalmic (Blephamide®): Sulfacetamide sodium 10% and prednisolone acetate 0.2% (3.5 g)

Solution, ophthalmic: Sulfacetamide sodium 10% and prednisolone sodium phosphate 0.25% (5 mL, 10 mL)

Suspension, ophthalmic (Blephamide®): Sulfacetamide sodium 10% and prednisolone acetate 0.2% (5 mL, 10 mL) [contains benzalkonium chloride]

Sulfacetamide Sodium *see* Sulfacetamide *on page 1081*

Sulfacetamide Sodium and Fluorometholone

(sul fa SEE ta mide SOW dee um & flure oh METH oh lone)

Related Information

Sulfacetamide *on page 1081*

U.S. Brand Names FML-S®

Synonyms Fluorometholone and Sulfacetamide

Generic Available No

Use Steroid-responsive inflammatory ocular conditions where infection is present or there is a risk of infection

Pregnancy Risk Factor C

Pregnancy Implications

There are no adequate and well-controlled studies in pregnant women. Use only if the potential benefit to the mother outweighs the potential risk to the fetus.

Contraindications

Hypersensitivity to fluorometholone, sulfacetamide sodium, sulfonamides, other corticosteroids, or any component of the formulation; viral diseases of the cornea and conjunctiva (including epithelial herpes simplex keratitis, vaccinia and varicella); mycobacterial or fungal infections of the eye

Warnings/Precautions

Not for intraocular injection; should not be administered directly into the anterior chamber of the eye. Many staphylococcal isolates are resistant to sulfa drugs. Severe reactions to sulfonamides have been reported and cross-sensitivity to other corticosteroids has occurred; discontinue if sensitivity reaction occurs.

Long-term use of corticosteroids and various ocular diseases have caused corneal and scleral thinning; corticosteroid use with thin corneal or scleral tissue may cause perforation. Prolonged use of corticosteroids may increase the incidence of secondary ocular infection, mask acute infection (including fungal infections), or prolong or exacerbate ocular viral infections; exposure to herpes simplex should be avoided.

Use following cataract surgery may delay healing or increase the incidence of bleb formation. Damage to the optic nerve, defects in visual acuity and fields of vision, and formation of posterior subcapsular cataract may occur. Prolonged use of corticosteroids may result in glaucoma. Use in glaucoma, or for periods extending beyond 10 days should be done cautiously and include frequent monitoring of intraocular pressure. Eye exams using magnification should be done prior to initial use, and prior to renewals of medication exceeding 20 mL. Re-evaluation should be done if signs and symptoms do not improve after 2 days of use.

Safety and efficacy in pediatric patients <2 years of age have not been established.

Adverse Reactions

Incidence of adverse events are not available; see individual agents

Stability

Store at 15°C to 30°C (59°F to 86°F); protect from light; do not freeze

Mechanism of Action

See individual agents.

Pharmacodynamics/Kinetics See individual agents.

Dosage Ophthalmic: Children >2 years and Adults: Instill 1 drop into affected eye(s) 4 times/day

Note: Dose may be decreased but should not be discontinued prematurely; re-evaluation should occur if improvement is not seen within 2 days; in chronic conditions, dosing frequency should be gradually decreased prior to discontinuing treatment

Monitoring Parameters

Intraocular pressure in patients with glaucoma or when used for ≥10 days; presence of secondary infections (including the development of fungal infections and exacerbation of viral infections); persistent pain or inflammation beyond 48 hours of use (re-evaluate)

Dosage Forms Suspension, ophthalmic: Sulfacetamide sodium 10% and fluorometholone 0.1% (5 mL, 10 mL) [contains benzalkonium chloride]

SulfaDIAZINE (sul fa DYE a zeen)

Related Information

USPHS / IDSA Guidelines for the Prevention of Opportunistic Infections in Persons Infected With HIV *on page 1237*

(Continued)

SulfaDIAZINE *(Continued)*

Generic Available Yes

Use Treatment of urinary tract infections and nocardiosis; adjunctive treatment in toxoplasmosis; uncomplicated attack of malaria

Unlabeled/Investigational Use Rheumatic fever prophylaxis

Drug of Choice or Alternative for

Disease/Syndrome(s):

Brain Abscess *on page 58*

Organism(s):

Nocardia Species *on page 247*

Toxoplasma gondii on page 331

Pregnancy Risk Factor B/D (at term)

Contraindications Hypersensitivity to any sulfa drug or any component of the formulation; porphyria; children <2 months of age unless indicated for the treatment of congenital toxoplasmosis; sunscreens containing PABA; pregnancy (at term)

Warnings/Precautions Use with caution in patients with impaired hepatic function or impaired renal function, G6PD deficiency; dosage modification required in patients with renal impairment; fluid intake should be maintained ≥1500 mL/day, or administer sodium bicarbonate to keep urine alkaline; more likely to cause crystalluria because it is less soluble than other sulfonamides. Chemical similarities are present among sulfonamides, sulfonylureas, carbonic anhydrase inhibitors, thiazides, and loop diuretics (except ethacrynic acid). Use in patients with sulfonamide allergy is specifically contraindicated in product labeling, however, a risk of cross-reaction exists in patients with allergy to any of these compounds; avoid use when previous reaction has been severe.

Adverse Reactions Frequency not defined.

Central nervous system: Fever, dizziness, headache

Dermatologic: Lyell's syndrome, Stevens-Johnson syndrome, itching, rash, photosensitivity

Endocrine & metabolic: Thyroid function disturbance

Gastrointestinal: Anorexia, nausea, vomiting, diarrhea

Genitourinary: Crystalluria

Hematologic: Granulocytopenia, leukopenia, thrombocytopenia, aplastic anemia, hemolytic anemia

Hepatic: Hepatitis, jaundice

Renal: Hematuria, acute nephropathy, interstitial nephritis

Miscellaneous: Serum sickness-like reactions

Overdosage/Toxicology Symptoms include drowsiness, dizziness, anorexia, abdominal pain, nausea, vomiting, hemolytic anemia, acidosis, jaundice, fever, and agranulocytosis. Doses of as little as 2-6 g/day in divided doses every 6 hours may produce toxicity. The aniline radical is responsible for hematologic toxicity. High volume diuresis may aid in elimination and prevention of renal failure.

Drug Interactions

Cytochrome P450 Effect: Substrate of CYP2C8/9 (major), 2E1 (minor), 3A4 (minor); **Inhibits** CYP2C8/9 (strong)

Increased Effect/Toxicity: Increased effect of oral anticoagulants and oral hypoglycemic agents. Sulfadiazine may increase the levels/effects of amiodarone, fluoxetine, glimepiride, glipizide, nateglinide, phenytoin, pioglitazone, rosiglitazone, sertraline, warfarin, and other CYP2C8/9 substrates.

Decreased Effect: The levels/effects of sulfadiazine may be decreased by carbamazepine, phenobarbital, phenytoin, rifampin, rifapentine, secobarbital, and other CYP2C8/9 inducers. Decreased effect with PABA or PABA metabolites of drugs (eg, procaine, proparacaine, tetracaine, sunblock).

Ethanol/Nutrition/Herb Interactions

Food: Avoid large quantities of vitamin C or acidifying agents (cranberry juice) to prevent crystalluria.

Herb/Nutraceutical: Avoid dong quai, St John's wort (may also cause photosensitization).

Stability Tablets may be crushed to prepare oral suspension of the drug in water or with a sucrose-containing solution; aqueous suspension with concentrations of 100 mg/mL should be stored in the refrigerator and used within 7 days

Mechanism of Action Interferes with bacterial growth by inhibiting bacterial folic acid synthesis through competitive antagonism of PABA

Pharmacodynamics/Kinetics

Absorption: Well absorbed

Distribution: Throughout body tissues and fluids including pleural, peritoneal, synovial, and ocular fluids; throughout total body water; readily diffused into CSF; enters breast milk

Metabolism: Via N-acetylation
Half-life elimination: 10 hours
Time to peak: Within 3-6 hours
Excretion: Urine (43% to 60% as unchanged drug, 15% to 40% as metabolites)

Dosage Oral:

Asymptomatic meningococcal carriers:
- Infants 1-12 months: 500 mg once daily for 2 days
- Children 1-12 years: 500 mg twice daily for 2 days
- Adults: 1 g twice daily for 2 days

Congenital toxoplasmosis:
- Newborns and Children <2 months: 100 mg/kg/day divided every 6 hours in conjunction with pyrimethamine 1 mg/kg/day once daily and supplemental folinic acid 5 mg every 3 days for 6 months
- Children >2 months: 25-50 mg/kg/dose 4 times/day

Nocardiosis: 4-8 g/day for a minimum of 6 weeks

Toxoplasmosis:
- Children >2 months: Loading dose: 75 mg/kg; maintenance dose: 120-150 mg/kg/day, maximum dose: 6 g/day; divided every 4-6 hours in conjunction with pyrimethamine 2 mg/kg/day divided every 12 hours for 3 days followed by 1 mg/kg/day once daily with supplemental folinic acid
- Adults: 2-6 g/day in divided doses every 6 hours in conjunction with pyrimethamine 50-75 mg/day and with supplemental folinic acid

Prevention of recurrent attacks of rheumatic fever (unlabeled use):
- >30 kg: 1 g/day
- <30 kg: 0.5 g/day

Dietary Considerations Supplemental folinic acid should be administered to reverse symptoms or prevent problems due to folic acid deficiency.

Administration Tablets may be crushed to prepare oral suspension of the drug in water or with a sucrose-containing solution. Aqueous suspension with concentrations of 100 mg/mL should be stored in the refrigerator and used within 7 days. Administer around-the-clock to promote less variation in peak and trough serum levels.

Patient Information Drink plenty of fluids; take on an empty stomach; avoid prolonged exposure to sunlight or wear protective clothing and sunscreen; report rash, difficulty breathing, severe or persistent fever, or sore throat

Dosage Forms Tablet: 500 mg

Selected Readings

Porter SB and Sande MA, "Toxoplasmosis of the Central Nervous System in the Acquired Immunodeficiency Syndrome," *N Engl J Med*, 1992, 327(23):1643-8.

Sulfadoxine and Pyrimethamine

(sul fa DOKS een & peer i METH a meen)

Related Information

Malaria Treatment *on page 1292*

U.S. Brand Names Fansidar®

Synonyms Pyrimethamine and Sulfadoxine

Generic Available No

Use Treatment of *Plasmodium falciparum* malaria in patients in whom chloroquine resistance is suspected; malaria prophylaxis for travelers to areas where chloroquine-resistant malaria is endemic

Drug of Choice or Alternative for Organism(s):

Isospora belli on page 196
Plasmodium Species *on page 265*

Pregnancy Risk Factor C/D (at term)

Contraindications Hypersensitivity to any sulfa drug, pyrimethamine, or any component of the formulation; porphyria, megaloblastic anemia; repeated prophylactic use is contraindicated in patients with renal failure, hepatic failure, or blood dyscrasias; children <2 months of age due to competition with bilirubin for protein binding sites; pregnancy (at term)

Warnings/Precautions Use with caution in patients with renal or hepatic impairment, patients with possible folate deficiency, and patients with seizure disorders, increased adverse reactions are seen in patients also receiving chloroquine; fatalities associated with sulfonamides, although rare, have occurred due to severe reactions including Stevens-Johnson syndrome, toxic epidermal necrolysis, hepatic necrosis, agranulocytosis, aplastic anemia and other blood dyscrasias; discontinue use at first sign of rash or any sign of adverse reaction; hemolysis occurs in patients with G6PD deficiency; leucovorin should be administered to reverse signs and symptoms of folic acid deficiency. May cause photosensitivity.

(Continued)

Sulfadoxine and Pyrimethamine *(Continued)*

Chemical similarities are present among sulfonamides, sulfonylureas, carbonic anhydrase inhibitors, thiazides, and loop diuretics (except ethacrynic acid). Use in patients with sulfonamide allergy is specifically contraindicated in product labeling, however, a risk of cross-reaction exists in patients with allergy to any of these compounds; avoid use when previous reaction has been severe.

Adverse Reactions Frequency not defined.

Cardiovascular: Myocarditis (allergic), pericarditis (allergic), periorbital edema
Central nervous system: Ataxia, hallucinations, headache, polyneuritis, seizure
Dermatologic: Photosensitivity, Stevens-Johnson syndrome, erythema multiforme, toxic epidermal necrolysis, rash
Endocrine & metabolic: Thyroid function dysfunction
Gastrointestinal: Anorexia, atrophic glossitis, gastritis, pancreatitis, vomiting
Genitourinary: Crystalluria
Hematologic: Megaloblastic anemia, leukopenia, thrombocytopenia, pancytopenia
Hepatic: Hepatic necrosis, hepatitis
Neuromuscular & skeletal: Tremors
Renal: BUN increased, interstitial nephritis, renal failure, serum creatinine increased
Respiratory: Respiratory failure, alveolitis (resembling eosinophilic or allergic)
Miscellaneous: Anaphylactoid reaction, drug fever, hypersensitivity, Lupus-like syndrome, periarteritis nodosum

Overdosage/Toxicology Symptoms include anorexia, vomiting, CNS stimulation including seizures, megaloblastic anemia, leukopenia, thrombocytopenia, and crystalluria. Leucovorin should be administered in a dosage of 3-9 mg/day for 3 days or as required to reverse symptoms of folic acid deficiency. Doses of as little as 2-5 g/day may produce toxicity. The aniline radical is responsible for hematologic toxicity. High volume diuresis may aid in elimination and prevention of renal failure. Diazepam can be used to control seizures.

Drug Interactions

Cytochrome P450 Effect: Pyrimethamine: **Inhibits** CYP2C8/9 (moderate), 2D6 (moderate)

Increased Effect/Toxicity: Effect of oral hypoglycemics (rare, but severe) may occur. Combination with methenamine may result in crystalluria; avoid use. May increase methotrexate-induced bone marrow suppression. NSAIDs and salicylates may increase sulfonamide concentrations. Pyrimethamine may increase the levels/effects of amiodarone, amphetamines, selected beta-blockers, dextromethorphan, fluoxetine, glimepiride, glipizide, lidocaine, mirtazapine, nateglinide, nefazodone, paroxetine, phenytoin, pioglitazone, risperidone, ritonavir, rosiglitazone, sertraline, thioridazine, tricyclic antidepressants, venlafaxine, warfarin, and other CYP2C8/9 and 2D6 substrates.

Decreased Effect: Cyclosporine concentrations may be decreased; monitor levels and renal function. PABA (para-aminobenzoic acid - may be found in some vitamin supplements): interferes with the antibacterial activity of sulfonamides; avoid concurrent use. Pyrimethamine may decrease the levels/effects of CYP2D6 prodrug substrates (eg, codeine, hydrocodone, oxycodone, tramadol).

Stability Protect from light

Mechanism of Action Sulfadoxine interferes with bacterial folic acid synthesis and growth via competitive inhibition of para-aminiobenzoic acid; pyrimethamine inhibits microbial dihydrofolate reductase, resulting in inhibition of tetrahydrofolic acid synthesis

Pharmacodynamics/Kinetics

Absorption: Well absorbed
Distribution: Sulfadoxine: Well distributed like other sulfonamides; Pyrimethamine: Widely distributed, mainly in blood cells, kidneys, lungs, liver, and spleen
Metabolism: Pyrimethamine: Hepatic; Sulfadoxine: None
Half-life elimination: Pyrimethamine: 80-95 hours; Sulfadoxine: 5-8 days
Time to peak, serum: 2-8 hours
Excretion: Urine (as unchanged drug and several unidentified metabolites)

Dosage Children and Adults: Oral:

Treatment of acute attack of malaria: A single dose of the following number of Fansidar® tablets is used in sequence with quinine or alone:
- 2-11 months: 1/4 tablet
- 1-3 years: 1/2 tablet
- 4-8 years: 1 tablet
- 9-14 years: 2 tablets
- >14 years: 3 tablets

Malaria prophylaxis: A single dose should be carried for self-treatment in the event of febrile illness when medical attention is not immediately available:
- 2-11 months: 1/4 tablet

1-3 years: ½ tablet
4-8 years: 1 tablet
9-14 years: 2 tablets
>14 years and Adults: 3 tablets

Monitoring Parameters CBC, including platelet counts, and urinalysis should be performed periodically

Patient Information Begin prophylaxis at least 2 days before departure; drink plenty of fluids; avoid prolonged exposure to the sun; report rash, sore throat, pallor, or glossitis

Dosage Forms Tablet: Sulfadoxine 500 mg and pyrimethamine 25 mg

Selected Readings

Panisko DM and Keystone JS, "Treatment of Malaria - 1990," *Drugs*, 1990, 39(2):160-89.
Wyler DJ, "Malaria Chemoprophylaxis for the Traveler," *N Engl J Med*, 1993, 329(1):31-7.
Wyler DJ, "Malaria: Overview and Update," *Clin Infect Dis*, 1993, 16(4):449-56.

Sulfamethoxazole and Trimethoprim

(sul fa meth OKS a zole & trye METH oh prim)

Related Information

Animal and Human Bites *on page 1270*
Antimicrobial Activity Against Selected Organisms *on page 1165*

U.S. Brand Names Bactrim™; Bactrim™ DS; Septra®; Septra® DS

Canadian Brand Names Apo-Sulfatrim®; Novo-Trimel; Novo-Trimel D.S.; Nu-Cotrimox; Septra®; Septra® DS; Septra® Injection

Synonyms Co-Trimoxazole; SMZ-TMP; Sulfatrim; TMP-SMZ; Trimethoprim and Sulfamethoxazole

Generic Available Yes

Use

Oral treatment of urinary tract infections due to *E. coli*, *Klebsiella* and *Enterobacter* sp, *M. morganii*, *P. mirabilis* and *P. vulgaris*; acute otitis media in children; acute exacerbations of chronic bronchitis in adults due to susceptible strains of *H. influenzae* or *S. pneumoniae*; treatment and prophylaxis of *Pneumocystis carinii* pneumonitis (PCP); traveler's diarrhea due to enterotoxigenic *E. coli*; treatment of enteritis caused by *Shigella flexneri* or *Shigella sonnei*

I.V. treatment or severe or complicated infections when oral therapy is not feasible, for documented PCP, empiric treatment of PCP in immune compromised patients; treatment of documented or suspected shigellosis, typhoid fever, *Nocardia asteroides* infection, or other infections caused by susceptible bacteria

Unlabeled/Investigational Use Cholera and *Salmonella*-type infections and nocardiosis; chronic prostatitis; as prophylaxis in neutropenic patients with *P. carinii* infections, in leukemics, and in patients following renal transplantation, to decrease incidence of PCP; treatment of *Cyclospora* infection, typhoid fever, *Nocardia asteroides* infection

Drug of Choice or Alternative for Disease/Syndrome(s):

Acne Vulgaris *on page 27*
Asymptomatic Bacteriuria *on page 39*
Brain Abscess *on page 58*
Bronchitis *on page 60*
Furunculosis *on page 151*
Gastroenteritis, Bacterial *on page 154*
Meningitis, Community-Acquired, Adult *on page 216*
Osteomyelitis, Diabetic Foot *on page 249*
Otitis Media, Acute *on page 253*
Prostatitis *on page 277*
Sinusitis, Community-Acquired, Acute *on page 299*
Traveler's Diarrhea *on page 333*
Urinary Tract Infection, Perinephric Abscess *on page 345*
Urinary Tract Infection, Pyelonephritis *on page 346*
Urinary Tract Infection, Uncomplicated *on page 346*

Organism(s):

Aeromonas Species *on page 30*
Bartonella Species *on page 48*
Bordetella pertussis on page 53
Brucella Species *on page 61*
Burkholderia cepacia on page 62
Burkholderia mallei on page 64
Calymmatobacterium granulomatis on page 65
Coxiella burnetii on page 100
Cyclospora cayetanensis on page 105
Escherichia coli on page 142

(Continued)

Sulfamethoxazole and Trimethoprim *(Continued)*

Haemophilus influenzae on page 159
Isospora belli on page 196
Listeria monocytogenes on page 208
Moraxella catarrhalis on page 223
Nocardia Species *on page 247*
Pneumocystis jiroveci on page 266
Providencia Species *on page 281*
Salmonella Species *on page 291*
Shigella Species *on page 297*
Staphylococcus aureus, Methicillin-Resistant *on page 304*
Staphylococcus epidermidis, Methicillin-Resistant *on page 309*
Staphylococcus saprophyticus on page 312
Stenotrophomonas maltophilia on page 312
Toxoplasma gondii on page 331
Vibrio cholerae on page 351

Pregnancy Risk Factor C/D (at term - expert analysis)

Pregnancy Implications Do not use at term to avoid kernicterus in the newborn; use during pregnancy only if risks outweigh the benefits since folic acid metabolism may be affected.

Contraindications Hypersensitivity to any sulfa drug, trimethoprim, or any component of the formulation; porphyria; megaloblastic anemia due to folate deficiency; infants <2 months of age; marked hepatic damage; severe renal disease; pregnancy (at term)

Warnings/Precautions Use with caution in patients with G6PD deficiency, impaired renal or hepatic function or potential folate deficiency (malnourished, chronic anticonvulsant therapy, or elderly); maintain adequate hydration to prevent crystalluria; adjust dosage in patients with renal impairment. Injection vehicle contains benzyl alcohol and sodium metabisulfite.

Chemical similarities are present among sulfonamides, sulfonylureas, carbonic anhydrase inhibitors, thiazides, and loop diuretics (except ethacrynic acid). Use in patients with sulfonamide allergy is specifically contraindicated in product labeling, however, a risk of cross-reaction exists in patients with allergy to any of these compounds; avoid use when previous reaction has been severe.

Fatalities associated with severe reactions including Stevens-Johnson syndrome, toxic epidermal necrolysis, hepatic necrosis, agranulocytosis, aplastic anemia and other blood dyscrasias; discontinue use at first sign of rash. Elderly patients appear at greater risk for more severe adverse reactions. May cause hypoglycemia, particularly in malnourished, or patients with renal or hepatic impairment. Use with caution in patients with porphyria or thyroid dysfunction. Slow acetylators may be more prone to adverse reactions. Caution in patients with allergies or asthma. May cause hyperkalemia (associated with high doses of trimethoprim). Incidence of adverse effects appears to be increased in patients with AIDS.

Adverse Reactions The most common adverse reactions include gastrointestinal upset (nausea, vomiting, anorexia) and dermatologic reactions (rash or urticaria). Rare, life-threatening reactions have been associated with co-trimoxazole, including severe dermatologic reactions and hepatotoxic reactions. Most other reactions listed are rare, however, frequency cannot be accurately estimated.

Cardiovascular: Allergic myocarditis

Central nervous system: Confusion, depression, hallucinations, seizure, aseptic meningitis, peripheral neuritis, fever, ataxia, kernicterus in neonates

Dermatologic: Rashes, pruritus, urticaria, photosensitivity; rare reactions include erythema multiforme, Stevens-Johnson syndrome, toxic epidermal necrolysis, exfoliative dermatitis, and Henoch-Schönlein purpura

Endocrine & metabolic: Hyperkalemia (generally at high dosages), hypoglycemia

Gastrointestinal: Nausea, vomiting, anorexia, stomatitis, diarrhea, pseudomembranous colitis, pancreatitis

Hematologic: Thrombocytopenia, megaloblastic anemia, granulocytopenia, eosinophilia, pancytopenia, aplastic anemia, methemoglobinemia, hemolysis (with G6PD deficiency), agranulocytosis

Hepatic: Hepatotoxicity (including hepatitis, cholestasis, and hepatic necrosis), hyperbilirubinemia, transaminases increased

Neuromuscular & skeletal: Arthralgia, myalgia, rhabdomyolysis

Renal: Interstitial nephritis, crystalluria, renal failure, nephrotoxicity (in association with cyclosporine), diuresis

Respiratory: Cough, dyspnea, pulmonary infiltrates

Miscellaneous: Serum sickness, angioedema, periarteritis nodosa (rare), systemic lupus erythematosus (rare)

Overdosage/Toxicology Symptoms of acute overdose include nausea, vomiting, GI distress, hematuria, and crystalluria. Following GI decontamination, treatment is supportive. Adequate fluid intake is essential. Peritoneal dialysis is not effective and hemodialysis is only moderately effective in removing sulfamethoxazole and trimethoprim.

Drug Interactions

Cytochrome P450 Effect:

Sulfamethoxazole: **Substrate** of CYP2C8/9 (major), 3A4 (minor); **Inhibits** CYP2C8/9 (moderate)

Trimethoprim: **Substrate** (major) of CYP2C8/9, 3A4; **Inhibits** CYP2C8/9 (moderate)

Increased Effect/Toxicity: Sulfamethoxazole/trimethoprim may increase toxicity of methotrexate. Sulfamethoxazole/trimethoprim may increase the serum levels of procainamide. Concurrent therapy with pyrimethamine (in doses >25 mg/week) may increase the risk of megaloblastic anemia. Sulfamethoxazole/trimethoprim may increase the levels/effects of amiodarone, fluoxetine, glimepiride, glipizide, nateglinide, phenytoin, pioglitazone, rosiglitazone, sertraline, warfarin, and other CYP2C8/9 substrates.

ACE Inhibitors, angiotensin receptor antagonists, or potassium-sparing diuretics may increase the risk of hyperkalemia. Concurrent use with cyclosporine may result in an increased risk of nephrotoxicity when used with sulfamethoxazole/trimethoprim. Trimethoprim may increase the serum concentration of dapsone.

Decreased Effect: The levels/effects of sulfamethoxazole may be decreased by carbamazepine, phenobarbital, phenytoin, rifampin, rifapentine, secobarbital, and other CYP2C8/9 inducers. Although occasionally recommended to limit or reverse hematologic toxicity of high-dose sulfamethoxazole/trimethoprim, concurrent use has been associated with a decreased effectiveness in treating *Pneumocystis carinii*.

Ethanol/Nutrition/Herb Interactions Herb/Nutraceutical: Avoid dong quai, St John's wort (may also cause photosensitization).

Stability

Injection: Store at room temperature; do not refrigerate. Less soluble in more alkaline pH. Protect from light. Solution must be diluted prior to administration. Following dilution, store at room temperature; do not refrigerate. Manufacturer recommended dilutions and stability of parenteral admixture at room temperature (25°C):

5 mL/125 mL D_5W; stable for 6 hours

5 mL/100 mL D_5W; stable for 4 hours

5 mL/75 mL D_5W; stable for 2 hours

Studies have also confirmed limited stability in NS; detailed references should be consulted.

Suspension, tablet: Store at room temperature; protect from light

Mechanism of Action Sulfamethoxazole interferes with bacterial folic acid synthesis and growth via inhibition of dihydrofolic acid formation from para-aminobenzoic acid; trimethoprim inhibits dihydrofolic acid reduction to tetrahydrofolate resulting in sequential inhibition of enzymes of the folic acid pathway

Pharmacodynamics/Kinetics

Absorption: Oral: Almost completely, 90% to 100%

Protein binding: SMX: 68%, TMP: 45%

Metabolism: SMX: N-acetylated and glucuronidated; TMP: Metabolized to oxide and hydroxylated metabolites

Half-life elimination: SMX: 9 hours, TMP: 6-17 hours; both are prolonged in renal failure

Time to peak, serum: Within 1-4 hours

Excretion: Both are excreted in urine as metabolites and unchanged drug

Effects of aging on the pharmacokinetics of both agents has been variable; increase in half-life and decreases in clearance have been associated with reduced creatinine clearance

Dosage Dosage recommendations are based on the trimethoprim component. Double-strength tablets are equivalent to sulfamethoxazole 800 mg and trimethoprim 160 mg.

Children >2 months:

General dosing guidelines:

Mild-to-moderate infections: Oral: 8-12 mg TMP/kg/day in divided doses every 12 hours

Serious infection:

Oral: 20 mg TMP/kg/day in divided doses every 6 hours

I.V.: 8-12 mg TMP/kg/day in divided doses every 6 hours

Acute otitis media: Oral: 8 mg TMP/kg/day in divided doses every 12 hours for 10 days

(Continued)

Sulfamethoxazole and Trimethoprim *(Continued)*

Urinary tract infection:
Treatment:
Oral: 6-12 mg TMP/kg/day in divided doses every 12 hours
I.V.: 8-10 mg TMP/kg/day in divided doses every 6, 8, or 12 hours for up to 4 days with serious infections
Prophylaxis: Oral: 2 mg TMP/kg/dose daily or 5 mg TMP/kg/dose twice weekly
Pneumocystis:
Treatment: Oral, I.V.: 15-20 mg TMP/kg/day in divided doses every 6-8 hours
Prophylaxis: Oral, 150 mg TMP/m^2/day in divided doses every 12 hours for 3 days/week; dose should not exceed trimethoprim 320 mg and sulfamethoxazole 1600 mg daily
Alternative prophylaxis dosing schedules include:
150 mg TMP/m^2/day as a single daily dose 3 times/week on consecutive days
or
150 mg TMP/m^2/day in divided doses every 12 hours administered 7 days/week
or
150 mg TMP/m^2/day in divided doses every 12 hours administered 3 times/week on alternate days
Shigellosis:
Oral: 8 mg TMP/kg/day in divided doses every 12 hours for 5 days
I.V.: 8-10 mg TMP/kg/day in divided doses every 6, 8, or 12 hours for up to 5 days
Cyclospora (unlabeled use): Oral, I.V.: 5 mg TMP/kg twice daily for 7-10 days
Adults:
Urinary tract infection:
Oral: One double-strength tablet every 12 hours for 10-14 days
I.V.: 8-10 mg TMP/kg/day in divided doses every 6, 8, or 12 hours for up to 14 days with severe infections
Chronic bronchitis: Oral: One double-strength tablet every 12 hours for 10-14 days
Shigellosis:
Oral: One double strength tablet every 12 hours for 5 days
I.V.: 8-10 mg TMP/kg/day in divided doses every 6, 8, or 12 hours for up to 5 days
Travelers' diarrhea: Oral: One double strength tablet every 12 hours for 5 days
Sepsis: I.V.: 20 TMP/kg/day divided every 6 hours
Pneumocystis carinii:
Prophylaxis: Oral: 1 double strength tablet daily or 3 times/week
Treatment: Oral, I.V.: 15-20 mg TMP/kg/day in 3-4 divided doses
Cyclospora (unlabeled use): Oral, I.V.: 160 mg TMP twice daily for 7-10 days
Nocardia (unlabeled use): Oral, I.V.:
Cutaneous infections: 5 mg TMP/kg/day in 2 divided doses
Severe infections (pulmonary/cerebral): 10-15 mg TMP/kg/day in 2-3 divided doses. Treatment duration is controversial; an average of 7 months has been reported.

Dosing adjustment in renal impairment: Oral, I.V.:
Cl_{cr} 15-30 mL/minute: Administer 50% of recommended dose
Cl_{cr} <15 mL/minute: Use is not recommended

Dietary Considerations Should be taken with 8 oz of water on empty stomach.

Administration
I.V.: Infuse over 60-90 minutes, must dilute well before giving; may be given less diluted in a central line; not for I.M. injection
Oral: May be taken with food and water.

Test Interactions Increased creatinine (Jaffé alkaline picrate reaction); increased serum methotrexate by dihydrofolate reductase method

Patient Information Take oral medication with 8 oz of water on an empty stomach (1 hour before or 2 hours after meals) for best absorption; report any skin rashes immediately; finish all medication, do not skip doses

Dosage Forms Note: The 5:1 ratio (SMX:TMP) remains constant in all dosage forms.
Injection, solution: Sulfamethoxazole 80 mg and trimethoprim 16 mg per mL (5 mL, 10 mL, 30 mL) [contains propylene glycol ~400 mg/mL, alcohol, benzyl alcohol, and sodium metabisulfite]
Suspension, oral: Sulfamethoxazole 200 mg and trimethoprim 40 mg per 5 mL (480 mL) [contains alcohol]
Septra®: Sulfamethoxazole 200 mg and trimethoprim 40 mg per 5 mL (480 mL) [contains alcohol 0.26% and sodium benzoate; cherry and grape flavors]
Tablet: Sulfamethoxazole 400 mg and trimethoprim 80 mg
Bactrim™: Sulfamethoxazole 400 mg and trimethoprim 80 mg [contains sodium benzoate]
Septra®: Sulfamethoxazole 400 mg and trimethoprim 80 mg
Tablet, double strength: Sulfamethoxazole 800 mg and trimethoprim 160 mg

Bactrim™ DS: Sulfamethoxazole 800 mg and trimethoprim 160 mg [contains sodium benzoate]

Septra® DS: Sulfamethoxazole 800 mg and trimethoprim 160 mg

Selected Readings

Cockerill FR and Edson RS, "Trimethoprim-Sulfamethoxazole," *Mayo Clin Proc*, 1991, 66(12):1260-9.

Fischl MA, Dickinson GM, and La Voie L, "Safety and Efficacy of Sulfamethoxazole and Trimethoprim Chemoprophylaxis for *Pneumocystis carinii* Pneumonia in AIDS," *JAMA*, 1988, 259(8):1185-9.

Hughes W, Leoung G, Kramer F, et al, "Comparison of Atovaquone (566C80) With Trimethoprim-Sulfamethoxazole to Treat *Pneumocystis carinii* Pneumonia in Patients With AIDS," *N Engl J Med*, 1993, 328(21):1521-7.

Lundstrom TS and Sobel JD, "Vancomycin, Trimethoprim-Sulfamethoxazole, and Rifampin," *Infect Dis Clin North Am*, 1995, 9(3):747-67.

Masur H, "Prevention and Treatment of *Pneumocystis* Pneumonia," *N Engl J Med*, 1992, 327(26):1853-60.

Sattler FR, Cowan R, Nielsen DM, et al, " Trimethoprim-Sulfamethoxazole Compared With Pentamidine for Treatment of *Pneumocystis carinii* Pneumonia in the Acquired Immunodeficiency Syndrome," *Ann Intern Med*, 1988, 109(4):280-7.

Sulfamylon® *see* Mafenide *on page 924*

Sulfatrim *see* Sulfamethoxazole and Trimethoprim *on page 1087*

SulfiSOXAZOLE (sul fi SOKS a zole)

U.S. Brand Names Gantrisin®

Canadian Brand Names Novo-Soxazole; Sulfizole®

Synonyms Sulfisoxazole Acetyl; Sulphafurazole

Generic Available Yes: Tablet

Use Treatment of urinary tract infections, otitis media, *Chlamydia*; nocardiosis

Drug of Choice or Alternative for Organism(s):

Nocardia Species *on page 247*

Pregnancy Risk Factor B/D (near term)

Contraindications Hypersensitivity to sulfisoxazole, any sulfa drug, or any component of the formulation; porphyria; infants <2 months of age (sulfas compete with bilirubin for protein binding sites); patients with urinary obstruction; sunscreens containing PABA; pregnancy (at term)

Warnings/Precautions Use with caution in patients with G6PD deficiency (hemolysis may occur), hepatic or renal impairment; dosage modification required in patients with renal impairment; risk of crystalluria should be considered in patients with impaired renal function. Chemical similarities are present among sulfonamides, sulfonylureas, carbonic anhydrase inhibitors, thiazides, and loop diuretics (except ethacrynic acid). Use in patients with sulfonamide allergy is specifically contraindicated in product labeling, however, a risk of cross-reaction exists in patients with allergy to any of these compounds; avoid use when previous reaction has been severe.

Adverse Reactions Frequency not defined.

Cardiovascular: Vasculitis

Central nervous system: Fever, dizziness, headache

Dermatologic: Itching, rash, photosensitivity, Lyell's syndrome, Stevens-Johnson syndrome

Endocrine & metabolic: Thyroid function disturbance

Gastrointestinal: Anorexia, nausea, vomiting, diarrhea

Genitourinary: Crystalluria, hematuria

Hematologic: Granulocytopenia, leukopenia, thrombocytopenia, aplastic anemia, hemolytic anemia

Hepatic: Jaundice, hepatitis

Renal: Interstitial nephritis

Miscellaneous: Serum sickness-like reactions

Overdosage/Toxicology Symptoms include drowsiness, dizziness, anorexia, abdominal pain, nausea, vomiting, hemolytic anemia, acidosis, jaundice, fever, and agranulocytosis. Doses of as little as 2-5 g/day may produce toxicity. The aniline radical is responsible for hematologic toxicity. High volume diuresis may aid in elimination and prevention of renal failure.

Drug Interactions

Cytochrome P450 Effect: Substrate of CYP2C8/9 (major); **Inhibits** CYP2C8/9 (strong)

Increased Effect/Toxicity: Sulfisoxazole may increase the levels/effects of amiodarone, fluoxetine, glimepiride, glipizide, nateglinide, phenytoin, pioglitazone, rosiglitazone, sertraline, warfarin, and other CYP2C8/9 substrates. May increase the effect of methotrexate. Risk of adverse reactions (thrombocytopenia purpura) may be increased by thiazide diuretics.

Decreased Effect: Decreased effect with PABA or PABA metabolites of drugs (eg, procaine, proparacaine, tetracaine), thiopental. May decrease cyclosporine levels.

(Continued)

SulfiSOXAZOLE *(Continued)*

Ethanol/Nutrition/Herb Interactions

Food: Interferes with folate absorption.

Herb/Nutraceutical: Avoid dong quai, St John's wort (may also cause photosensitization).

Stability Protect from light

Mechanism of Action Interferes with bacterial growth by inhibiting bacterial folic acid synthesis through competitive antagonism of PABA

Pharmacodynamics/Kinetics

Absorption: Sulfisoxazole acetyl is hydrolyzed in GI tract to sulfisoxazole which is readily absorbed

Distribution: Crosses placenta; enters breast milk

CSF:blood level ratio: Normal meninges: 50% to 80%; Inflamed meninges: 80+%

Protein binding: 85% to 88%

Metabolism: Hepatic via acetylation and glucuronide conjugation to inactive compounds

Half-life elimination: 4-7 hours; prolonged with renal impairment

Time to peak, serum: 2-3 hours

Excretion: Urine (95%, 40% to 60% as unchanged drug) within 24 hours

Dosage Oral: Not for use in patients <2 months of age:

Children >2 months: Initial: 75 mg/kg, followed by 120-150 mg/kg/day in divided doses every 4-6 hours; not to exceed 6 g/day

Adults: Initial: 2-4 g, then 4-8 g/day in divided doses every 4-6 hours

Dosing interval in renal impairment:

Cl_{cr} 10-50 mL/minute: Administer every 8-12 hours

Cl_{cr} <10 mL/minute: Administer every 12-24 hours

Hemodialysis: >50% removed by hemodialysis

Dietary Considerations Should be taken with a glass of water on an empty stomach.

Administration Administer around-the-clock to promote less variation in peak and trough serum levels.

Monitoring Parameters CBC, urinalysis, renal function tests, temperature

Test Interactions False-positive protein in urine; false-positive urine glucose with Clinitest®

Patient Information Take with a glass of water on an empty stomach; avoid prolonged exposure to sunlight; report any sore throat, mouth sores, rash, unusual bleeding, or fever; complete full course of therapy

Dosage Forms

Suspension, oral, pediatric, as acetyl (Gantrisin®): 500 mg/5 mL (480 mL) [contains alcohol 0.3%; raspberry flavor]

Tablet: 500 mg

Sulfisoxazole Acetyl *see* SulfiSOXAZOLE *on page 1091*

Sulfisoxazole and Erythromycin *see* Erythromycin and Sulfisoxazole *on page 811*

Sulfizole® (Can) *see* SulfiSOXAZOLE *on page 1091*

Sulphafurazole *see* SulfiSOXAZOLE *on page 1091*

Summer's Eve® Medicated Douche [OTC] *see* Povidone-Iodine *on page 1016*

Sumycin® *see* Tetracycline *on page 1106*

Suprax® *see* Cefixime *on page 707*

Sustiva® *see* Efavirenz *on page 795*

Symmetrel® *see* Amantadine *on page 636*

Synagis® *see* Palivizumab *on page 988*

Synercid® *see* Quinupristin and Dalfopristin *on page 1032*

T-20 *see* Enfuvirtide *on page 802*

Tamiflu® *see* Oseltamivir *on page 981*

Tao® *see* Troleandomycin *on page 1133*

Tazicef® *see* Ceftazidime *on page 717*

Tazocin® (Can) *see* Piperacillin and Tazobactam Sodium *on page 1003*

3TC® (Can) *see* Lamivudine *on page 905*

3TC, Abacavir, and Zidovudine *see* Abacavir, Lamivudine, and Zidovudine *on page 627*

TCN *see* Tetracycline *on page 1106*

Td *see* Diphtheria and Tetanus Toxoid *on page 778*

Tdap *see* Diphtheria, Tetanus Toxoids, and Acellular Pertussis Vaccine *on page 782*

TDF *see* Tenofovir *on page 1095*

Tebrazid™ (Can) *see* Pyrazinamide *on page 1022*

Telithromycin (tel ith roe MYE sin)

Related Information

Community-Acquired Pneumonia in Adults *on page 1278*

U.S. Brand Names Ketek®

Canadian Brand Names Ketek®

Synonyms HMR 3647

Generic Available No

Use Treatment of community-acquired pneumonia (mild-to-moderate) caused by susceptible strains of *Streptococcus pneumoniae* (including multidrug-resistant isolates), *Haemophilus influenzae, Chlamydia pneumoniae, Moraxella catarrhalis,* and *Mycoplasma pneumoniae*; treatment of bacterial exacerbation of chronic bronchitis caused by susceptible strains of *S. pneumoniae*, *H. influenzae* and *Moraxella catarrhalis*; treatment of acute bacterial sinusitis caused by *Streptococcus pneumoniae*, *Haemophilus influenzae*, *Moraxella catarrhalis*, and *Staphylococcus aureus*

Unlabeled/Investigational Use Approved in Canada for use in the treatment of tonsillitis/pharyngitis due to *S. pyogenes* (as an alternative to beta-lactam antibiotics when necessary/appropriate)

Drug of Choice or Alternative for Organism(s):

Mycoplasma pneumoniae on page 238

Pregnancy Risk Factor C

Pregnancy Implications Teratogenic effects were not observed in animal studies. There are no adequate or well-controlled studies in pregnant women.

Contraindications Hypersensitivity to telithromycin, macrolide antibiotics, or any component of the formulation; concurrent use of cisapride or pimozide

Warnings/Precautions May prolong QT_c interval, leading to a risk of ventricular arrhythmias; closely-related antibiotics have been associated with malignant ventricular arrhythmias and torsade de pointes. Avoid in patients with prolongation of QT_c interval due to congenital causes, history of long QT syndrome, uncorrected electrolyte disturbances (hypokalemia or hypomagnesemia), significant bradycardia (<50 bpm), or concurrent therapy with QT_c-prolonging drugs (eg, class Ia and class III antiarrhythmics). Avoid use in patients with a prior history of confirmed cardiogenic syncope or ventricular arrhythmias while receiving macrolide antibiotics or other QT_c-prolonging drugs. Use caution in renal impairment. Use caution in patients with myasthenia gravis (use only if suitable alternatives are not available). Inform patients of potential for blurred vision, which may interfere with ability to operate machinery or drive; use caution until effects are known. Safety and efficacy not established in pediatric patients <13 years of age per Canadian approved labeling and <18 years of age per U.S. approved labeling. Pseudomembranous colitis has been reported.

Adverse Reactions

2% to 10%:

- Central nervous system: Headache (2% to 6%), dizziness (3% to 4%)
- Gastrointestinal: Diarrhea (10%), nausea (7% to 8%), vomiting (2% to 3%), loose stools (2%), dysgeusia (2%)

≥0.2% to <2%:

- Central nervous system: Vertigo, fatigue, somnolence, insomnia
- Dermatologic: Rash
- Gastrointestinal: Abdominal distension, abdominal pain, anorexia, constipation, dyspepsia, flatulence, gastritis, gastroenteritis, GI upset, glossitis, stomatitis, watery stools, xerostomia
- Genitourinary: Vaginal candidiasis
- Hematologic: Platelets increased
- Hepatic: Transaminases increased, hepatitis
- Ocular: Blurred vision, accommodation delayed, diplopia
- Miscellaneous: Candidiasis, diaphoresis increased, exacerbation of myasthenia gravis (rare)

<0.2%: Alkaline phosphatase increased, anxiety, bilirubin increased, bradycardia, eczema, eosinophilia, erythema multiforme, flushing, hypotension, paresthesia, pruritus, urticaria

Postmarketing and/or case reports: Anaphylaxis, angioedema, arrhythmia, edema (facial), hepatocellular injury, muscle cramps

Additional effects also reported with telithromycin:

- Cardiovascular: Bundle branch block, palpitation, QT_c prolongation, vasculitis
- Central nervous system: Abnormal dreams, nervousness, tremor
- Endocrine & metabolic: Appetite decreased, hypokalemia, hyperkalemia
- Gastrointestinal: Esophagitis, pharyngolaryngeal pain, pseudomembranous colitis, reflux esophagitis, tooth discoloration
- Genitourinary: Vaginal irritation, urine discoloration, polyuria

(Continued)

Telithromycin *(Continued)*

Hematologic: Anemia, coagulation disorder, leukopenia, neutropenia, thrombocytopenia, lymphopenia
Hepatic: Cholestasis
Neuromuscular & skeletal: Weakness
Renal: Serum creatinine increased
Miscellaneous: Hypersensitivity

Overdosage/Toxicology Treatment should be symptomatic and supportive. ECG and electrolytes should be monitored.

Drug Interactions

Cytochrome P450 Effect: Substrate of CYP1A2 (minor), 3A4 (major); **Inhibits** CYP2D6 (weak), 3A4 (strong)

Increased Effect/Toxicity: Concurrent use of cisapride or pimozide is contraindicated. Concurrent use with antiarrhythmics (eg, class Ia and class III) or other drugs which prolong QT_c (eg, gatifloxacin, mesoridazine, moxifloxacin, pimozide, sparfloxacin, thioridazine) may be additive; serious arrhythmias may occur. Neuromuscular-blocking agents may be potentiated by telithromycin.

Telithromycin may increase the levels/effects of selected benzodiazepines, calcium channel blockers, cyclosporine, ergot alkaloids, selected HMG-CoA reductase inhibitors, mirtazapine, nateglinide, nefazodone, pimozide, quinidine, sildenafil (and other PDE-5 inhibitors), tacrolimus, venlafaxine, warfarin (monitor), and other CYP3A4 substrates. Selected benzodiazepines (midazolam, triazolam), and selected HMG-CoA reductase inhibitors (atorvastatin, lovastatin and simvastatin) are generally contraindicated with strong CYP3A4 inhibitors. When used with strong CYP3A4 inhibitors, dosage adjustment/limits are recommended for sildenafil and other PDE-5 inhibitors; refer to individual monographs.

The levels/effects of telithromycin may be increased by azole antifungals, ciprofloxacin, clarithromycin, diclofenac, doxycycline, erythromycin, imatinib, isoniazid, nefazodone, nicardipine, propofol, protease inhibitors, quinidine, verapamil, and other CYP3A4 inhibitors.

Decreased Effect: The levels/effects of telithromycin may be decreased by aminoglutethimide, carbamazepine, nafcillin, nevirapine, phenobarbital, phenytoin, rifamycins, and other CYP3A4 inducers; avoid concurrent use.

Stability Store at room temperature between 15°C and 30°C.

Mechanism of Action Inhibits bacterial protein synthesis by binding to two sites on the 50S ribosomal subunit. Telithromycin has also been demonstrated to alter secretion of IL-1alpha and TNF-alpha; the clinical significance of this immunomodulatory effect has not been evaluated.

Pharmacodynamics/Kinetics

Absorption: Rapid
Distribution: 2.9 L/kg
Protein binding: 60% to 70%
Metabolism: Hepatic, via CYP3A4 (50%) and non-CYP-mediated pathways
Bioavailability: 57% (significant first-pass metabolism)
Half-life elimination: 10 hours
Time to peak, plasma: 1 hour
Excretion: Urine (13% unchanged drug, remainder as metabolites); feces (7%)

Dosage Oral:

Children ≥13 years and Adults: Tonsillitis/pharyngitis (unlabeled U.S. indication): 800 mg once daily for 5 days

Adults:

Acute exacerbation of chronic bronchitis, acute bacterial sinusitis: 800 mg once daily for 5 days

Community-acquired pneumonia: 800 mg once daily for 7-10 days

Dosage adjustment in renal impairment:

U.S. product labeling: Cl_{cr} <30 mL/minute: 600 mg once daily; when renal impairment is accompanied by hepatic impairment, reduce dosage to 400 mg once daily

Canadian product labeling: Cl_{cr} <30 mL/minute: Reduce dose to 400 mg once daily

Hemodialysis: Administer following dialysis

Dosage adjustment in hepatic impairment: No adjustment recommended, unless concurrent severe renal impairment is present

Dietary Considerations May be taken with or without food.

Administration May be administered with or without food.

Dosage Forms

Tablet [film coated]: 300 mg [not available in Canada], 400 mg

Ketek Pak™ [blister pack]: 400 mg (10s) [packaged as 10 tablets/card; 2 tablets/blister]

Telzir® (Can) *see* Fosamprenavir *on page 827*

Tenofovir (te NOE fo veer)

Related Information

Antiretroviral Agents *on page 1206*
Antiretroviral Therapy for HIV Infection *on page 1219*

U.S. Brand Names Viread®

Canadian Brand Names Viread®

Synonyms PMPA; TDF; Tenofovir Disoproxil Fumarate

Generic Available No

Use Management of HIV infections in combination with at least two other antiretroviral agents

Drug of Choice or Alternative for Organism(s):

Human Immunodeficiency Virus *on page 181*

Pregnancy Risk Factor B

Pregnancy Implications There are no adequate and well-controlled studies in pregnant women. Animal studies have shown decreased fetal growth and reduced fetal bone porosity. Clinical studies in children have shown bone demineralization with chronic use. Use in pregnancy only if clearly needed. Cases of lactic acidosis/hepatic steatosis syndrome have been reported in pregnant women receiving nucleoside analogues. It is not known if pregnancy itself potentiates this known side effect; however, pregnant women may be at increased risk of lactic acidosis and liver damage. Hepatic enzymes and electrolytes should be monitored frequently during the 3rd trimester of pregnancy in women receiving nucleoside analogues. Health professionals are encouraged to contact the Antiretroviral Pregnancy Registry to monitor outcomes of pregnant women exposed to antiretroviral medications (1-800-258-4263 or www.APRegistry.com).

Contraindications Hypersensitivity to tenofovir or any component of the formulation

Warnings/Precautions Lactic acidosis and severe hepatomegaly with steatosis have been reported with nucleoside analogues, including fatal cases; use with caution in patients with risk factors for liver disease (risk may be increased in obese patients or prolonged exposure) and suspend treatment in any patient who develops clinical or laboratory findings suggestive of lactic acidosis (transaminase elevation may/may not accompany hepatomegaly and steatosis). Immune reconstitution syndrome may develop resulting in the occurrence of an inflammatory response to an indolent or residual opportunistic infection; further evaluation and treatment may be required.

Increased biochemical markers of bone metabolism, serum parathyroid hormone levels and 1,25 vitamin D levels have been noted with tenofovir use. A 5% to 7 % loss of bone mineral density (BMD) has been reported in some patients. BMD monitoring should be considered in patients with a history of bone fracture or risk factors for osteopenia.

Use caution in renal impairment (Cl_{cr} <50 mL/minute); dosage adjustment required. May cause osteomalacia and/or renal toxicity; monitor renal function and possible bone abnormalities during therapy. Use caution in hepatic impairment. All patients with HIV should be tested for HBV prior to initiation of treatment. Safety and efficacy of tenofovir during coinfection of HIV and HBV have not been established; acute, severe exacerbations of HBV have been reported following tenofovir discontinuation. In HBV coinfected patients, monitor hepatic function closely for several months following discontinuation. Safety and efficacy have not been established in pediatric patients.

Adverse Reactions Percentages listed were from clinical trials with tenofovir addition to prior antiretroviral therapy. Only adverse events from treatment naïve patient studies which varied significantly were noted (eg, rash event). Frequencies listed are treatment-emergent adverse effects noted at higher frequency than in the placebo group.

>10%:

Gastrointestinal: Diarrhea (11% to 16%), nausea (8% to 11%),
Neuromuscular & skeletal: Weakness (7% to 11%)

1% to 10%:

- Central nervous system: Headache (5% to 8%), depression (4% to 8%; treatment naïve 11%), dizziness (1% to 3%)
- Dermatologic: Rash event (maculopapular, pustular, or vesiculobullous rash, pruritus or urticaria 5% to 7%; treatment naïve 18%)
- Endocrine & metabolic: Amylase increased (9%, treatment naïve)
- Gastrointestinal: Vomiting (4% to 7%), abdominal pain (4% to 7%), flatulence (3% to 4%), anorexia (3% to 4%)
- Hematologic: Neutropenia (1% to 2%)

(Continued)

Tenofovir *(Continued)*

Hepatic: Transaminases increased (2% to 4%)

Neuromuscular & skeletal: Back pain (3% to 4%; treatment naïve 9%), myalgia (3% to 4%), neuropathy (peripheral 1% to 3%)

Respiratory: Pneumonia (2% to 3%)

Postmarketing and/or case reports: Acute tubular necrosis, allergic reaction, serum creatinine increased, dyspnea, Fanconi syndrome, hepatitis, hypophosphatemia, immune reconstitution syndrome, lactic acidosis, liver enzymes increased, nephrogenic diabetes insipidus, pancreatitis, proteinuria, proximal tubulopathy, rash, renal failure

Note: Uncommon, but significant adverse reactions reported with other reverse transcriptase inhibitors include pancreatitis, peripheral neuropathy, and myopathy.

Overdosage/Toxicology Limited experience with overdose. Treatment is supportive. Hemodialysis may be beneficial; reportedly 10% of an administered single dose of 300 mg was removed during a 4-hour session.

Drug Interactions

Cytochrome P450 Effect: Inhibits CYP1A2 (weak)

Increased Effect/Toxicity: Concurrent use has been noted to increase serum concentrations/exposure to didanosine and its metabolites, potentially increasing the risk of didanosine toxicity (hyperglycemia, pancreatitis, peripheral neuropathy, or lactic acidosis); decreased CD4 cell counts and decreased virologic response have been reported. Use caution and monitor closely; suspend therapy if signs/symptoms of toxicity are present. Drugs which may compete for renal tubule secretion (including acyclovir, cidofovir, ganciclovir, valacyclovir, valganciclovir) may increase the serum concentrations of tenofovir. Drugs causing nephrotoxicity may reduce elimination of tenofovir. Lopinavir/ritonavir may increase serum concentrations of tenofovir.

Decreased Effect: Serum levels of lopinavir and/or ritonavir may be decreased by tenofovir. Tenofovir may decrease serum concentrations of atazanavir, resulting in a loss of virologic response (specific atazanavir dosing recommendations provided by manufacturer).

Ethanol/Nutrition/Herb Interactions Food: Fatty meals may increase the bioavailability of tenofovir. Tenofovir may be taken with or without food.

Stability Store at 25°C (77°F); excursions permitted to 15°C to 30°C (59°F to 86°F).

Mechanism of Action Tenofovir disoproxil fumarate (TDF) is an analog of adenosine 5'-monophosphate; it interferes with the HIV viral RNA dependent DNA polymerase resulting in inhibition of viral replication. TDF is first converted intracellularly by hydrolysis to tenofovir and subsequently phosphorylated to the active tenofovir diphosphate; nucleotide reverse transcriptase inhibitor.

Pharmacodynamics/Kinetics

Distribution: 1.2-1.3 L/kg

Protein binding: 7% to serum proteins

Metabolism: Tenofovir disoproxil fumarate (TDF) is converted intracellularly by hydrolysis (by non-CYP enzymes) to tenofovir, then phosphorylated to the active tenofovir diphosphate

Bioavailability: 25% (fasting); increases ~40% with high-fat meal

Half-life elimination: 17 hours

Time to peak, serum: Fasting: 36-84 minutes; With food: 96-144 minutes

Excretion: Urine (70% to 80%) via filtration and active secretion, primarily as unchanged tenofovir

Dosage Oral: Adults: HIV infection: 300 mg once daily

Dosage adjustment in renal impairment:

Cl_{cr} 30-49 mL/minute: 300 mg every 48 hours

Cl_{cr} 10-29 mL/minute: 300 mg twice weekly

Cl_{cr} <10 mL/minute without dialysis: No recommendation available.

Hemodialysis: 300 mg every 7 days or after a total of 12 hours of dialysis (usually once weekly assuming 3 dialysis sessions lasting about 4 hours each)

Dosage adjustment in hepatic impairment: No dosage adjustment required.

Dietary Considerations May be taken with or without food. Consider calcium and vitamin D supplementation in patients with history of bone fracture or osteopenia.

Administration May be administered with or without food.

Monitoring Parameters CBC with differential, reticulocyte count, serum creatine kinase, CD4 count, HIV RNA plasma levels, renal and hepatic function tests, bone density (long-term), serum phosphorus; testing for HBV is recommended prior to the initiation of antiretroviral therapy

Patients with HIV and HVB coinfection should be monitored for several months following tenofovir discontinuation.

Patient Information Tenofovir is not a cure for AIDS. Take as directed, with or without food. Do not take with other medications. Take precautions to avoid transmission to others. Report unresolved nausea or vomiting; abdominal pain; tingling, numbness, or pain of toes or fingers; skin rash or irritation; or muscle weakness or tremors. Notify prescriber if you are pregnant or plan to be pregnant. HIV infected mothers are discouraged from breast-feeding to prevent potential transmission of HIV.

Additional Information Approval was based on two clinical trials involving patients who were previously treated with antiretrovirals with continued evidence of HIV replication despite therapy. The risk:benefit ratio for untreated patients has not been established (studies currently ongoing), however, patients who received tenofovir showed significant decreases in HIV replication as compared to continuation of standard therapy.

A high rate of early virologic nonresponse was observed when abacavir, lamivudine, and tenofovir were used as the initial regimen in treatment-naïve patients. A high rate of early virologic nonresponse was also observed when didanosine, lamivudine, and tenofovir were used as the initial regimen in treatment-naïve patients. Use of either of these combinations is not recommended; patients currently on either of these regimens should be closely monitored for modification of therapy. Early virologic failure was also observed with tenofovir and didanosine delayed release capsules, plus either efavirenz or nevirapine; use caution in treatment-naïve patients with high baseline viral loads.

Dosage Forms Tablet, as disoproxil fumarate: 300 mg [equivalent to 245 mg tenofovir disoproxil]

Tenofovir and Emtricitabine *see* Emtricitabine and Tenofovir *on page 801*

Tenofovir Disoproxil Fumarate *see* Tenofovir *on page 1095*

Tequin® *see* Gatifloxacin *on page 837*

Terak™ *see* Oxytetracycline and Polymyxin B *on page 988*

Terazol® (Can) *see* Terconazole *on page 1099*

Terazol® 3 *see* Terconazole *on page 1099*

Terazol® 7 *see* Terconazole *on page 1099*

Terbinafine (TER bin a feen)

U.S. Brand Names Lamisil®; Lamisil® AT™ [OTC]

Canadian Brand Names Apo-Terbinafine®; CO Terbinafine; Gen-Terbinafine; Lamisil®; Novo-Terbinafine; PMS-Terbinafine

Synonyms Terbinafine Hydrochloride

Generic Available No

Use Active against most strains of *Trichophyton mentagrophytes*, *Trichophyton rubrum*; may be effective for infections of *Microsporum gypseum* and *M. nanum*, *Trichophyton verrucosum*, *Epidermophyton floccosum*, *Candida albicans*, and *Scopulariopsis brevicaulis*

Oral: Onychomycosis of the toenail or fingernail due to susceptible dermatophytes

Topical: Antifungal for the treatment of tinea pedis (athlete's foot), tinea cruris (jock itch), and tinea corporis (ringworm) [OTC/prescription formulations]; tinea versicolor [prescription formulations]

Drug of Choice or Alternative for Organism(s):

Dematiaceous Fungi *on page 112*
Dermatophytes *on page 114*
Malassezia furfur on page 213

Pregnancy Risk Factor B

Pregnancy Implications Avoid use in pregnancy since treatment of onychomycosis is postponable.

Contraindications Hypersensitivity to terbinafine, naftifine, or any component of the formulation

Warnings/Precautions While rare, the following complications have been reported and may require discontinuation of therapy: Changes in the ocular lens and retina, pancytopenia, neutropenia, Stevens-Johnson syndrome, toxic epidermal necrolysis. Rare cases of hepatic failure (including fatal cases) have been reported following oral treatment of onychomycosis. Not recommended for use in patients with active or chronic liver disease. Discontinue if symptoms or signs of hepatobiliary dysfunction or cholestatic hepatitis develop. If irritation/sensitivity develop with topical use, discontinue therapy. Oral products are not recommended for use with pre-existing liver or renal disease (≤50 mL/minute GFR). **Use caution in writing and/or filling prescription/orders. Confusion between Lamictal® (lamotrigine) and Lamisil® (terbinafine) has occurred.**

(Continued)

Terbinafine *(Continued)*

Adverse Reactions

Oral:

1% to 10%:

- Central nervous system: Headache, dizziness, vertigo
- Dermatologic: Rash, pruritus, urticaria
- Gastrointestinal: Diarrhea, dyspepsia, abdominal pain, appetite decrease, taste disturbance
- Hematologic: Lymphocytopenia
- Hepatic: Liver enzymes increased
- Ocular: Visual disturbance

<1%, postmarketing and/or case reports: Angioedema, agranulocytosis, allergic reactions, alopecia, anaphylaxis, arthralgia, changes in ocular lens and retina, fatigue, hepatic failure, malaise, myalgia, neutropenia, precipitation/exacerbation of cutaneous and systemic lupus erythematosus, Stevens-Johnson syndrome, thrombocytopenia, toxic epidermal necrolysis, vomiting

Topical: 1% to 10%:

- Dermatologic: Pruritus, contact dermatitis, irritation, burning, dryness
- Local: Irritation, stinging

Drug Interactions

Cytochrome P450 Effect: Substrate (minor) of 1A2, 2C8/9, 2C19, 3A4; **Inhibits** CYP2D6 (strong); **Induces** CYP3A4 (weak)

Increased Effect/Toxicity: Terbinafine may increase the levels/effects of amphetamines, beta-blockers, dextromethorphan, fluoxetine, lidocaine, mirtazapine, nefazodone, paroxetine, risperidone, ritonavir, thioridazine, tricyclic antidepressants, venlafaxine, and other CYP2D6 substrates. The effects of warfarin may be increased.

Decreased Effect: Terbinafine may decrease the levels/effects of CYP2D6 prodrug substrates (eg, codeine, hydrocodone, oxycodone, tramadol).

Stability

Cream: Store at 5°C to 30°C (41°F to 86°F).

Solution: Store at 5°C to 25°C (41°F to 77°F); do not refrigerate

Tablet: Store below 25°C (77°F); protect from light

Mechanism of Action Synthetic allylamine derivative which inhibits squalene epoxidase, a key enzyme in sterol biosynthesis in fungi. This results in a deficiency in ergosterol within the fungal cell wall and results in fungal cell death.

Pharmacodynamics/Kinetics

Absorption: Topical: Limited (<5%); Oral: >70%

Distribution: V_d: 2000 L; distributed to sebum and skin predominantly

Protein binding, plasma: >99%

Metabolism: Hepatic; no active metabolites; first-pass effect; little effect on CYP

Bioavailability: Oral: 40%

Half-life elimination:

- Topical: 22-26 hours
- Oral: Terminal half-life: 200-400 hours; very slow release of drug from skin and adipose tissues occurs; effective half-life: ~36 hours

Time to peak, plasma: 1-2 hours

Excretion: Urine (70% to 75%)

Dosage

Children ≥12 years and Adults:

- Topical cream, solution:
  - Athlete's foot (tinea pedis): Apply to affected area twice daily for at least 1 week, not to exceed 4 weeks [OTC/prescription formulations]
  - Ringworm (tinea corporis) and jock itch (tinea cruris): Apply cream to affected area once or twice daily for at least 1 week, not to exceed 4 weeks; apply solution once daily for 7 days [OTC formulations]

Adults:

- Oral:
  - Superficial mycoses: Fingernail: 250 mg/day for up to 6 weeks; toenail: 250 mg/day for 12 weeks; doses may be given in two divided doses
  - Systemic mycosis: 250-500 mg/day for up to 16 months
- Topical solution: Tinea versicolor: Apply to affected area twice daily for 1 week [prescription formulation]

Children: Oral (unlabeled use in children):

- 10-20 kg: 62.5 mg/day
- 20-40 kg: 125 mg/day
- >40 kg: 250 mg/day

Treatment duration:
- Tinea pedis: 2 weeks
- Tinea capitis: 2-4 weeks
- Onychomycosis: Fingernails: 6 weeks; Toenails: 12 weeks

Dosing adjustment in renal impairment: GFR <50 mL/minute: Oral administration is not recommended.

Dosing adjustment in hepatic impairment: Clearance is decreased by ~50% with hepatic cirrhosis; use is not recommended.

Monitoring Parameters CBC and LFTs at baseline and repeated if use is for >6 weeks

Patient Information Topical: Avoid contact with eyes, nose, or mouth during treatment; nursing mothers should not use on breast tissue; advise physician if eyes or skin becomes yellow or if irritation, itching, or burning develops. Do not use occlusive dressings concurrent with therapy. Full clinical effect may require several months due to the time required for a new nail to grow.

Additional Information Due to potential toxicity, the manufacturer recommends confirmation of diagnosis testing of nail specimens prior to treatment of onychomycosis. Patients should not be considered therapeutic failures until they have been symptom-free for 2-4 weeks off following a course of treatment; GI complaints usually subside with continued administration.

A meta-analysis of efficacy studies for toenail infections revealed that weighted average mycological cure rates for continuous therapy were 36.7% (griseofulvin), 54.7% (itraconazole), and 77% (terbinafine). Cure rate for 4-month pulse therapy for itraconazole and terbinafine were 73.3% and 80%. Additionally, the final outcome measure of final costs per cured infections for continuous therapy was significantly lower for terbinafine.

Dosage Forms

Cream, as hydrochloride (Lamisil® AT™): 1% (12 g) [contains benzyl alcohol]
Solution, as hydrochloride [topical spray] (Lamisil®, Lamisil® AT™): 1% (30 mL)
Tablet (Lamisil®): 250 mg

Selected Readings

Abdel-Rahman SM and Nahata MC, "Oral Terbinafine: A New Antifungal Agent," *Ann Pharmacother*, 1997, 31(4):445-56.

Amichai B and Grunwald MH, "Adverse Drug Reactions of the New Oral Antifungal Agents - Terbinafine, Fluconazole, and Itraconazole," *Int J Dermatol*, 1998, 37(6):410-5.

Angello JT, et al, "A Cost/Efficacy Analysis of Oral Antifungals Indicated for the Treatment of Onychomycosis: Griseofulvin, Itraconazole, and Terbinafine," *Am J Manage Care*, 1997, 3:443-50.

Dwyer CM, White MI, and Sinclair TS, "Cholestatic Jaundice Due to Terbinafine," *Br J Dermatol*, 1997, 136(6):976-7.

Gupta AK and Shear NH, "Terbinafine: An Update," *J Am Acad Dermatol*, 1997, 37(6):979-88.

Gupta AK, Sibbald RG, Knowles SR, et al, "Terbinafine Therapy May Be Associated With the Development of Psoriasis De Novo or Its Exacerbation: Four Case Reports and a Review of Drug Induced Psoriasis," *J Am Acad Dermatol*, 1997, 36(5 Part 2):858-62.

Jones TC, "Overview of the Use of Terbinafine in Children," *Br J Dermatol*, 1995, 132(5):683-9.

Trepanier EF and Amsden GW, "Current Issues in Onchomycosis," *Ann Pharmacother*, 1998, 32(2):204-14.

Terbinafine Hydrochloride *see* Terbinafine *on page 1097*

Terconazole (ter KONE a zole)

U.S. Brand Names Terazol® 3; Terazol® 7

Canadian Brand Names Terazol®

Synonyms Triaconazole

Generic Available Yes: Cream

Use Local treatment of vulvovaginal candidiasis

Pregnancy Risk Factor C

Contraindications Hypersensitivity to terconazole or any component of the formulation

Warnings/Precautions Should be discontinued if sensitization or irritation occurs. Microbiological studies (KOH smear and/or cultures) should be repeated in patients not responding to terconazole in order to confirm the diagnosis and rule out other pathogens.

Adverse Reactions

1% to 10%:
- Central nervous system: Fever, chills
- Gastrointestinal: Abdominal pain
- Genitourinary: Vulvar/vaginal burning, dysmenorrhea

<1% (Limited to important or life-threatening): Vulvar itching, soreness, edema, or discharge; polyuria; burning or itching of penis of sexual partner; flu-like syndrome

Stability Store at room temperature of 13°C to 30°C (59°F to 86°F).

Mechanism of Action Triazole ketal antifungal agent; involves inhibition of fungal cytochrome P450. Specifically, terconazole inhibits cytochrome P450-dependent

(Continued)

Terconazole *(Continued)*

14-alpha-demethylase which results in accumulation of membrane disturbing 14-alpha-demethylsterols and ergosterol depletion.

Pharmacodynamics/Kinetics Absorption: Extent of systemic absorption after vaginal administration may be dependent on presence of a uterus; 5% to 8% in women who had a hysterectomy versus 12% to 16% in nonhysterectomy women

Dosage Adults: Female:

Terazol® 3 vaginal cream: Insert 1 applicatorful intravaginally at bedtime for 3 consecutive days

Terazol® 7 vaginal cream: Insert 1 applicatorful intravaginally at bedtime for 7 consecutive days

Terazol® 3 vaginal suppository: Insert 1 suppository intravaginally at bedtime for 3 consecutive days

Patient Information Insert high into vagina; complete full course of therapy; contact prescriber if itching or burning occurs

Additional Information Watch for local irritation; assist patient in administration, if necessary; assess patient's ability to self-administer, may be difficult in patients with arthritis or limited range of motion

Dosage Forms

Cream, vaginal:

Terazol® 7: 0.4% (45 g) [packaged with measured-dose applicator]

Terazol® 3: 0.8% (20 g) [packaged with measured-dose applicator]

Suppository, vaginal (Terazol® 3): 80 mg (3s) [may contain coconut and/or palm kernel oil]

Selected Readings

Drug Facts and Comparisons, St Louis, MO: 1989, 528-9.

Terramycin® (Can) *see* Oxytetracycline *on page 987*

Terramycin® I.M. *see* Oxytetracycline *on page 987*

Testim® *see* Testosterone *on page 1100*

Testopel® *see* Testosterone *on page 1100*

Testosterone (tes TOS ter one)

Related Information

AIDS Wasting Treatment *on page 1205*

U.S. Brand Names Androderm®; AndroGel®; Delatestryl®; Depo®-Testosterone; First® Testosterone; First® Testosterone MC; Striant®; Testim®; Testopel®

Canadian Brand Names Andriol®; Androderm®; AndroGel®; Andropository; Delatestryl®; Depotest® 100; Everone® 200; Virilon® IM

Synonyms Testosterone Cypionate; Testosterone Enanthate

Generic Available Yes: Injection

Use

Injection: Androgen replacement therapy in the treatment of delayed male puberty; male hypogonadism (primary or hypogonadotropic); inoperable female breast cancer (enanthate only)

Pellet: Androgen replacement therapy in the treatment of delayed male puberty; male hypogonadism (primary or hypogonadotropic)

Buccal, topical: Male hypogonadism (primary or hypogonadotropic)

Restrictions C-III

Pregnancy Risk Factor X

Pregnancy Implications Testosterone may cause adverse effects, including masculinization of the female fetus, if used during pregnancy. Females who are or may become pregnant should also avoid skin-to-skin contact to areas where testosterone has been applied topically on another person.

Contraindications Hypersensitivity to testosterone or any component of the formulation (including soy); severe renal or cardiac disease; benign prostatic hyperplasia with obstruction; undiagnosed genital bleeding; males with carcinoma of the breast or prostate; pregnancy

Warnings/Precautions When used to treat delayed male puberty, perform radiographic examination of the hand and wrist every 6 months to determine the rate of bone maturation. May accelerate bone maturation without producing compensating gain in linear growth. Has both androgenic and anabolic activity, the anabolic action may enhance hypoglycemia. Use caution in elderly patients or patients with other demographic factors which may increase the risk of prostatic carcinoma; careful monitoring is required. May cause fluid retention; use caution in patients with cardiovascular disease or other edematous conditions. Prolonged use has been associated with serious hepatic effects (hepatitis, hepatic neoplasms, cholestatic hepatitis, jaundice). May potentiate sleep apnea in some male patients (obesity or chronic lung disease). Transdermal patch may contain conducting metal (eg, aluminum); remove

patch prior to MRI. Gels and buccal system have not been evaluated in males <18 years of age; safety and efficacy of injection have not been established in males <12 years of age.

Adverse Reactions Frequency not always defined.

Cardiovascular: Flushing, edema, hypertension, vasodilation

Central nervous system: Aggressive behavior, amnesia, anxiety, dizziness, emotional lability, excitation, headache, mental depression, nervousness, sleeplessness

Dermatologic: Acne, allergic contact dermatitis (transdermal 4%), alopecia, burn-like blisters (transdermal 12%), dry skin, erythema (transdermal 7%), hirsutism (increase in pubic hair growth), pruritus

Endocrine & metabolic: Breast soreness, gynecomastia, hypercalcemia, hypoglycemia, menstrual problems (amenorrhea), virilism

Gastrointestinal: GI irritation, nausea, vomiting

Following buccal administration: Bitter taste, gum edema, gum or mouth irritation, gum tenderness, taste perversion

Genitourinary: Bladder irritability, epididymitis, impotence, priapism, prostatic carcinoma, prostatic hyperplasia, testicular atrophy, urination impaired

Hepatic: Cholestatic hepatitis, hepatic dysfunction, hepatic necrosis

Hematologic: Leukopenia, polycythemia, suppression of clotting factors

Neuromuscular & skeletal: Paresthesias, weakness

Miscellaneous: Diaphoresis, hypersensitivity reactions

Drug Interactions

Cytochrome P450 Effect: Substrate (minor) of CYP2B6, 2C8/9, 2C19, 3A4; **Inhibits** CYP3A4 (weak)

Increased Effect/Toxicity: Warfarin and testosterone: Effects of oral anticoagulants may be enhanced. Testosterone may increase levels of oxyphenbutazone. May enhance fluid retention from corticosteroids.

Ethanol/Nutrition/Herb Interactions Herb/Nutraceutical: St John's wort may decrease testosterone levels.

Stability

Androderm®: Store at room temperature; do not store outside of pouch. Excessive heat may cause system to burst.

AndroGel®, Delatestryl®, Striant™, Testim™: Store at room temperature.

Depo® Testosterone: Store at room temperature; protect from light.

Testopel®: Store in a cool location.

Mechanism of Action Principal endogenous androgen responsible for promoting the growth and development of the male sex organs and maintaining secondary sex characteristics in androgen-deficient males

Pharmacodynamics/Kinetics

Duration (route and ester dependent): I.M.: Cypionate and enanthate esters have longest duration, ≤2-4 weeks

Absorption: Transdermal gel: ~10% of dose

Distribution: Crosses placenta; enters breast milk

Protein binding: 98% bound to sex hormone-binding globulin (40%) and albumin

Metabolism: Hepatic; forms metabolites

Half-life elimination: 10-100 minutes

Excretion: Urine (90%); feces (6%)

Dosage

Adolescents: I.M.:

Male hypogonadism:

Initiation of pubertal growth: 40-50 mg/m^2/dose (cypionate or enanthate ester) monthly until the growth rate falls to prepubertal levels

Terminal growth phase: 100 mg/m^2/dose (cypionate or enanthate ester) monthly until growth ceases

Maintenance virilizing dose: 100 mg/m^2/dose (cypionate or enanthate ester) twice monthly

Delayed male puberty: 40-50 mg/m^2/dose monthly (cypionate or enanthate ester) for 6 months

Adolescents and Adults: Pellet (for subcutaneous implantation): Delayed male puberty, male hypogonadism: 150-450 mg every 3-6 months

Adults:

I.M.:

Female: Inoperable breast cancer: Testosterone enanthate: 200-400 mg every 2-4 weeks

Male: Long-acting formulations: Testosterone enanthate (in oil)/testosterone cypionate (in oil):

Hypogonadism: 50-400 mg every 2-4 weeks

Delayed puberty: 50-200 mg every 2-4 weeks for a limited duration

(Continued)

Testosterone *(Continued)*

Transdermal: Primary male hypogonadism **or** hypogonadotropic hypogonadism:

Androderm®: Initial: Apply 5 mg/day once nightly to clean, dry area on the back, abdomen, upper arms, or thighs (do **not** apply to scrotum); dosing range: 2.5-7.5 mg/day; in nonvirilized patients, dose may be initiated at 2.5 mg/day

AndroGel®, Testim™: 5 g (to deliver 50 mg of testosterone with 5 mg systemically absorbed) applied once daily (preferably in the morning) to clean, dry, intact skin of the shoulder and upper arms. AndroGel® may also be applied to the abdomen. Dosage may be increased to a maximum of 10 g (100 mg). **Do not apply testosterone gel to the genitals.**

Oral (buccal): Hypogonadism or hypogonadotropic hypogonadism: 30 mg twice daily (every 12 hours) applied to the gum region above the incisor tooth

Dosing adjustment/comments in hepatic disease: Reduce dose

Dietary Considerations Testosterone USP may be synthesized from soy. Food and beverages have not been found to interfere with buccal system; ensure system is in place following eating, drinking, or brushing teeth.

Administration

I.M.: Warm to room temperature; shaking vial will help redissolve crystals that have formed after storage. Administer by deep I.M. injection into the upper outer quadrant of the gluteus maximus.

Oral: Striant™: One mucoadhesive for buccal application (buccal system) should be applied to a comfortable area above the incisor tooth. Apply flat side of system to gum. Rotate to alternate sides of mouth with each application. Hold buccal system firmly in place for 30 seconds to ensure adhesion. The buccal system should adhere to gum for 12 hours. If the buccal system falls out, replace with a new system. If the system falls out within 4 hours of next dose, the new buccal system should remain in place until the time of the following scheduled dose. System will soften and mold to shape of gum as it absorbs moisture from mouth. Do not chew or swallow the buccal system. The buccal system will not dissolve; gently remove by sliding downwards from gum; avoid scratching gum.

Transdermal (Androderm®): Apply patch to clean, dry area of skin on the arm, back, or upper buttocks. Following patch removal, mild skin irritation may be treated with OTC hydrocortisone cream. A small amount of triamcinolone acetonide 0.1% cream may be applied under the system to decrease irritation; do not use ointment. Patch should be applied nightly. Rotate administration sites, allowing 7 days between applying to the same site.

Gel: AndroGel®, Testim™: Apply (preferably in the morning) to clean, dry, intact skin of the shoulder and upper arms (AndroGel® may also be applied to the abdomen). Upon opening the packet(s), the entire contents should be squeezed into the palm of the hand and immediately applied to the application site(s). Alternatively, a portion may be squeezed onto palm of hand and applied, repeating the process until entire packet has been applied. Application sites should be allowed to dry for a few minutes prior to dressing. Hands should be washed with soap and water after application. **Do not apply testosterone gel to the genitals.**

Monitoring Parameters Periodic liver function tests, PSA, cholesterol, hemoglobin and hematocrit; radiologic examination of wrist and hand every 6 months (when using in prepubertal children)

Androderm®: Morning serum testosterone levels following application the previous evening

Gel: Morning serum testosterone levels 14 days after start of therapy

Reference Range Testosterone, urine: Male: 100-1500 ng/24 hours; Female: 100-500 ng/24 hours

Test Interactions May cause a decrease in creatinine and creatine excretion and an increase in the excretion of 17-ketosteroids, thyroid function tests

Patient Information Virilization may occur in female patients; report menstrual irregularities; male patients report persistent penile erections. All patients should report persistent GI distress, diarrhea, or jaundice. Gels are flammable; avoid smoking or exposure to fire/flame during use.

Dosage Forms

Gel, topical:

AndroGel®:

1.25 g/actuation (75 g) [1% metered-dose pump; delivers 5 g/4 actuations; provides 60 1.25 g actuations; contains ethanol]

2.5 g (30s) [1% unit dose packets; contains ethanol]

5 g (30s) [1% unit dose packets; contains ethanol]

Testim®: 5 g (30s) [1% unit-dose tube; contains ethanol]

Injection, in oil, as cypionate: 200 mg/mL (10 mL)

Depo® Testosterone: 100 mg/mL (10 mL); 200 mg/mL (1 mL, 10 mL) [contains benzyl alcohol, benzyl benzoate, and cottonseed oil]

Injection, in oil, as enanthate: 200 mg/mL (5 mL)

Delatestryl®: 200 mg/mL (1 mL [prefilled syringe; contains sesame oil]; 5 mL [multidose vial; contains sesame oil])

Kit [for prescription compounding testosterone 2%; kits also contain mixing jar and stirrer]:

First® Testosterone:

Injection, in oil: Testosterone propionate 100 mg/mL (12 mL) [contains sesame oil and benzyl alcohol]

Ointment: White petroleum (48 g)

First® Testosterone MC:

Injection, in oil: Testosterone propionate 100 mg/mL (12 mL) [contains sesame oil and benzyl alcohol]

Cream: Moisturizing cream (48 g)

Mucoadhesive, for buccal application [buccal system] (Striant®): 30 mg (10s)

Pellet, for subcutaneous implantation (Testopel®): 75 mg (1 pellet/vial)

Transdermal system (Androderm®): 2.5 mg/day (60s); 5 mg/day (30s) [contains ethanol]

Selected Readings

Borhan-Manesh F and Farnum JB, "Methyltestosterone-Induced Cholestasis. The Importance of Disproportionately Low Serum Alkaline Phosphatase Level," *Arch Intern Med*, 1989, 149(9):2127-9.

Cunningham GR, Cordero E, and Thornby JI, "Testosterone Replacement With Transdermal Therapeutic Systems. Physiological Serum Testosterone and Elevated Dihydrotestosterone Levels," *JAMA*, 1989, 261(17):2525-30.

Daigle RD, "Anabolic Steroids," *J Psychoactive Drugs*, 1990, 22(1):77-80.

Moller BB and Ekelund B, "Toxicity of Cyclosporine During Treatment With Androgens," *N Engl J Med*, 1985, 313(22):1416.

Ruch W and Jenny P, "Priapism Following Testosterone Administration for Delayed Male Puberty," *Am J Med*, 1989, 86(2):256.

Testosterone Cypionate *see* Testosterone *on page 1100*

Testosterone Enanthate *see* Testosterone *on page 1100*

Tetanus and Diphtheria Toxoid *see* Diphtheria and Tetanus Toxoid *on page 778*

Tetanus Immune Globulin (Human)

(TET a nus i MYUN GLOB yoo lin HYU man)

U.S. Brand Names BayTet™

Canadian Brand Names BayTet™

Synonyms TIG

Generic Available No

Use Passive immunization against tetanus; tetanus immune globulin is preferred over tetanus antitoxin for treatment of active tetanus; part of the management of an unclean, wound in a person whose history of previous receipt of tetanus toxoid is unknown or who has received less than three doses of tetanus toxoid; elderly may require TIG more often than younger patients with tetanus infection due to declining antibody titers with age

Drug of Choice or Alternative for Organism(s):

Clostridium tetani on page 90

Pregnancy Risk Factor C

Contraindications Hypersensitivity to tetanus immune globulin, thimerosal, or any component of the formulation

Warnings/Precautions Have epinephrine 1:1000 available for anaphylactic reactions. Use caution in patients with isolated immunoglobulin A deficiency or a history of systemic hypersensitivity to human immunoglobulins. As a product of human plasma, this product may potentially transmit disease; screening of donors, as well as testing and/or inactivation of certain viruses reduces this risk. Use caution in patients with thrombocytopenia or coagulation disorders (I.M. injections may be contraindicated). Not for intravenous administration.

Adverse Reactions

>10%: Local: Pain, tenderness, erythema at injection site

1% to 10%:

Central nervous system: Fever (mild)

Dermatologic: Urticaria, angioedema

Neuromuscular & skeletal: Muscle stiffness

Miscellaneous: Anaphylaxis reaction

<1%: Sensitization to repeated injections

Stability Refrigerate

Mechanism of Action Passive immunity toward tetanus

Pharmacodynamics/Kinetics Absorption: Well absorbed

(Continued)

Tetanus Immune Globulin (Human) *(Continued)*

Dosage I.M.:

Prophylaxis of tetanus:

Children: 4 units/kg; some recommend administering 250 units to small children

Adults: 250 units

Treatment of tetanus:

Children: 500-3000 units; some should infiltrate locally around the wound

Adults: 3000-6000 units

Administration Do not administer I.V.; I.M. use only

Additional Information Tetanus immune globulin (TIG) must not contain <50 units/mL. Protein makes up 10% to 18% of TIG preparations. The great majority of this (≥90%) is IgG. TIG has almost no color or odor and it is a sterile, nonpyrogenic, concentrated preparation of immunoglobulins that has been derived from the plasma of adults hyperimmunized with tetanus toxoid. The pooled material from which the immunoglobulin is derived may be from fewer than 1000 donors. This plasma has been shown to be free of hepatitis B surface antigen.

Dosage Forms Injection, solution [preservative free]: 250 units/mL (1 mL) [prefilled syringe]

Tetanus Toxoid (Adsorbed) (TET a nus TOKS oyd, ad SORBED)

Generic Available No

Use Active immunization against tetanus when combination antigen preparations are not indicated. **Note:** Tetanus and diphtheria toxoids for adult use (Td) is the preferred immunizing agent for most adults and for children after their seventh birthday. Young children should receive trivalent DTaP (diphtheria/tetanus/acellular pertussis), as part of their childhood immunization program, unless pertussis is contraindicated, then TD is warranted.

Pregnancy Risk Factor C

Pregnancy Implications Animal studies have not been conducted. The ACIP recommends vaccination in previously unvaccinated women or in women with an incomplete vaccination series, whose child may be born in unhygienic conditions. Vaccination using Td is preferred.

Contraindications Hypersensitivity to tetanus toxoid or any component of the formulation

Warnings/Precautions Not equivalent to tetanus toxoid fluid; the tetanus toxoid adsorbed is the preferred toxoid for immunization and Td, TD or DTaP are the preferred adsorbed forms; avoid injection into a blood vessel; allergic reactions may occur; epinephrine 1:1000 must be available; elderly may not mount adequate antibody titers following immunization. Patients who are immunocompromised may have reduced response; may be used in patients with HIV infection. May defer elective immunization during febrile illness or acute infection; defer elective immunization during outbreaks of poliomyelitis. In patients with a history of severe local reaction (Arthus-type) or temperature of >39.4°C (>103°F) following previous dose, do not give further routine or emergency doses of tetanus and diphtheria toxoids for 10 years. Use caution in patients on anticoagulants, with thrombocytopenia, or bleeding disorders (bleeding may occur following intramuscular injection). Contains thimerosal; vial stopper contains natural latex rubber. This product is not indicated for use in children <7 years of age.

Adverse Reactions All serious adverse reactions must be reported to the U.S. Department of Health and Human Services (DHHS) Vaccine Adverse Event Reporting System (VAERS) 1-800-822-7967.

Frequency not defined.

Cardiovascular: Hypotension

Central nervous system: Brachial neuritis, fever, malaise, pain

Gastrointestinal: Nausea

Local: Edema, induration (with or without tenderness), rash, redness, urticaria, warmth

Neuromuscular: Arthralgia, Guillain-Barré syndrome

Miscellaneous: Anaphylactic reaction, Arthus-type hypersensitivity reaction

Drug Interactions

Decreased Effect: When used in greater than physiologic doses, corticosteroids lead to decreased effect of vaccine (consider deferring immunization for 1 month after steroid is discontinued). Consider deferring immunization for 1 month after immunosuppressive agent is discontinued (decreased response to vaccine).

Stability Refrigerate, do not freeze

Mechanism of Action Tetanus toxoid preparations contain the toxin produced by virulent tetanus bacilli (detoxified growth products of *Clostridium tetani*). The toxin has been modified by treatment with formaldehyde so that it has lost toxicity but still

retains ability to act as antigen and produce active immunity; the aluminum salt, a mineral adjuvant, delays the rate of absorption and prolongs and enhances its properties; duration ~10 years.

Pharmacodynamics/Kinetics Duration: Primary immunization: ~10 years

Dosage Children ≥7 years and Adults: I.M.:

Primary immunization: 0.5 mL; repeat 0.5 mL at 4-8 weeks after first dose and at 6-12 months after second dose

Routine booster dose: Recommended every 10 years

Note: In most patients, Td is the recommended product for primary immunization, booster doses, and tetanus immunization in wound management (refer to Diphtheria and Tetanus Toxoid *on page 778* monograph)

Administration Inject intramuscularly in the area of the vastus lateralis (midthigh laterally) or deltoid. Do not inject into gluteal area. Shake well prior to withdrawing dose; do not use if product does not form a suspension.

For patients at risk of hemorrhage following intramuscular injection, the ACIP recommends "it should be administered intramuscularly if, in the opinion of the physician familiar with the patients bleeding risk, the vaccine can be administered with reasonable safety by this route. If the patient receives antihemophilia or other similar therapy, intramuscular vaccination can be scheduled shortly after such therapy is administered. A fine needle (23 gauge or smaller) can be used for the vaccination and firm pressure applied to the site (without rubbing) for at least 2 minutes. The patient should be instructed concerning the risk of hematoma from the injection."

Patient Information A nodule may be palpable at the injection site for a few weeks. DT, Td and T vaccines cause few problems; they may cause mild fever or soreness, swelling, and redness where the shot was given. These problems usually last 1-2 days, but this does not happen nearly as often as with DTP vaccine. Sometimes, adults who get these vaccines can have a lot of soreness and swelling where the shot was given.

Additional Information Federal law requires that the date of administration, the vaccine manufacturer, lot number of vaccine, and the administering person's name, title and address be entered into the patient's permanent medical record.

Dosage Forms Injection, suspension: Tetanus 5 Lf units per 0.5 mL (5 mL) [contains thimerosal; vial stopper contains latex]

Selected Readings

Bentley DW, "Vaccinations," *Clin Geriatr Med*, 1992, 8(4):745-60.
Gardner P and Schaffner W, "Immunization of Adults," *N Engl J Med*, 1993, 328(17):1252-8.

Tetanus Toxoid (Fluid) (TET a nus TOKS oyd FLOO id)

Synonyms Tetanus Toxoid Plain

Generic Available No

Use Indicated as booster dose in the active immunization against tetanus in the rare adult or child who is allergic to the aluminum adjuvant (a product containing adsorbed tetanus toxoid is preferred); not indicated for primary immunization

Unlabeled/Investigational Use Anergy testing (no longer recommended)

Pregnancy Risk Factor C

Pregnancy Implications Reproduction studies have not been conducted and effects to the fetus are not known. Deferring immunization until the 2nd trimester may be considered.

Contraindications Hypersensitivity to tetanus toxoid or any component of the formulation

Warnings/Precautions Epinephrine 1:1000 should be readily available; skin test responsiveness may be delayed or reduced in elderly patients. Patients who are immunocompromised may have reduced response; may be used in patients with HIV infection. May defer elective immunization during febrile illness or acute infection; defer elective immunization during outbreaks of poliomyelitis. In patients with a history of severe local reaction (Arthus-type) following previous dose, do not give further routine or emergency doses of tetanus and diphtheria toxoids for 10 years. Use caution in patients on anticoagulants, with thrombocytopenia, or bleeding disorders (bleeding may occur following intramuscular injection). Contains thimerosal; vial stopper contains natural latex rubber. Safety and efficacy in children <6 weeks of age have not been established; this product is not indicated for use in children <7 years of age.

Adverse Reactions All serious adverse reactions must be reported to the U.S. Department of Health and Human Services (DHHS) Vaccine Adverse Event Reporting System (VAERS) 1-800-822-7967.

Frequency not defined.

Cardiovascular: Hypotension

Central nervous system: Brachial neuritis, fever, Guillain-Barré syndrome, malaise

Dermatologic: Rash, urticaria

(Continued)

Tetanus Toxoid (Fluid) *(Continued)*

Gastrointestinal: Nausea

Local: Edema, induration (with or without tenderness), redness, warmth

Neuromuscular & skeletal: Arthralgia

Miscellaneous: Anaphylaxis, Arthus-type hypersensitivity reactions (severe local reaction developing 2-8 hours following injection)

Drug Interactions

Increased Effect/Toxicity: Increased bleeding and bruising may occur from I.M. injection in patients on anticoagulants.

Decreased Effect: Decreased effect of vaccine may occur with corticosteroids (greater than physiologic doses) or immunosuppressive agents

Stability Refrigerate 2°C to 8°C (35°F to 46°F); do not freeze

Mechanism of Action Tetanus toxoid preparations contain the toxin produced by virulent tetanus bacilli (detoxified growth products of *Clostridium tetani*). The toxin has been modified by treatment with formaldehyde so that is has lost toxicity but still retains ability to act as antigen and produce active immunity.

Dosage

Primary immunization: Not indicated for this use.

Booster doses: I.M., SubQ: 0.5 mL every 10 years

Anergy testing (unlabeled use; no longer recommended for this indication): Intradermal: 0.1 mL; doses that have been used range from 0.1 mL of a 1:10 dilution to 0.1 mL of the undiluted product

Administration

I.M. Shake well prior to use. Administer I.M. in lateral aspect of midthigh or deltoid muscle of upper arm

For patients at risk of hemorrhage following intramuscular injection, the ACIP recommends "it should be administered intramuscularly if, in the opinion of the physician familiar with the patients bleeding risk, the vaccine can be administered with reasonable safety by this route. If the patient receives antihemophilia or other similar therapy, intramuscular vaccination can be scheduled shortly after such therapy is administered. A fine needle (23 gauge or smaller) can be used for the vaccination and firm pressure applied to the site (without rubbing) for at least 2 minutes. The patient should be instructed concerning the risk of hematoma from the injection."

SubQ: Shake well prior to use. Administer in area of the lateral aspect of midthigh or deltoid. SubQ route may be preferred in patients with thrombocytopenia or coagulation disorders.

Additional Information Federal law requires that the date of administration, the vaccine manufacturer, lot number of vaccine, and the administering person's name, title and address be entered into the patient's permanent medical record.

Dosage Forms Injection, solution: Tetanus 4 Lf units per 0.5 mL (7.5 mL) [contains thimerosal; vial stopper contains dry natural latex rubber]

Selected Readings

Gardner P and Schaffner W, "Immunization of Adults," *N Engl J Med*, 1993, 328(17):1252-8.

Tetanus Toxoid Plain *see* Tetanus Toxoid (Fluid) *on page 1105*

Tetanus Toxoid, Reduced Diphtheria Toxoid, and Acellular Pertussis, Adsorbed *see* Diphtheria, Tetanus Toxoids, and Acellular Pertussis Vaccine *on page 782*

Tetracycline (tet ra SYE kleen)

Related Information

Antimicrobial Activity Against Selected Organisms *on page 1165*

Malaria Treatment *on page 1292*

Helicobacter pylori Treatment *on page 1288*

U.S. Brand Names Sumycin®

Canadian Brand Names Apo-Tetra®; Novo-Tetra; Nu-Tetra

Synonyms Achromycin; TCN; Tetracycline Hydrochloride

Generic Available Yes: Capsule

Use Treatment of susceptible bacterial infections of both gram-positive and gram-negative organisms; also infections due to *Mycoplasma*, *Chlamydia*, and *Rickettsia*; indicated for acne, exacerbations of chronic bronchitis, and treatment of gonorrhea and syphilis in patients that are allergic to penicillin; as part of a multidrug regimen for *H. pylori* eradication to reduce the risk of duodenal ulcer recurrence

Drug of Choice or Alternative for

Disease/Syndrome(s):

Blepharitis *on page 52*

Urethritis, Nongonococcal *on page 344*

Organism(s):

Bordetella pertussis on page 53

Chlamydophila pneumoniae on page 78
Ehrlichia Species *on page 119*
Helicobacter pylori on page 162
Leptospira interrogans on page 205
Mycoplasma hominis and *Mycoplasma genitalium on page 237*
Rickettsia rickettsii on page 289
Ureaplasma urealyticum on page 342
Vibrio cholerae on page 351
Yersinia pestis on page 355

Pregnancy Risk Factor D

Pregnancy Implications Tetracyclines cross the placenta and enter fetal circulation; may cause permanent discoloration of teeth if used during the last half of pregnancy.

Contraindications Hypersensitivity to tetracycline or any component of the formulation; do not administer to children ≤8 years of age; pregnancy

Warnings/Precautions Use of tetracyclines during tooth development may cause permanent discoloration of the teeth and enamel, hypoplasia and retardation of skeletal development and bone growth with risk being the greatest for children <4 years and those receiving high doses; use with caution in patients with renal or hepatic impairment (eg, elderly); dosage modification required in patients with renal impairment since it may increase BUN as an antianabolic agent; pseudotumor cerebri has been reported with tetracycline use (usually resolves with discontinuation); outdated drug can cause nephropathy; superinfection possible; use protective measure to avoid photosensitivity

Adverse Reactions Frequency not defined.

Cardiovascular: Pericarditis

Central nervous system: Intracranial pressure increased, bulging fontanels in infants, pseudotumor cerebri, paresthesia

Dermatologic: Photosensitivity, pruritus, pigmentation of nails, exfoliative dermatitis

Endocrine & metabolic: Diabetes insipidus syndrome

Gastrointestinal: Discoloration of teeth and enamel hypoplasia (young children), nausea, diarrhea, vomiting, esophagitis, anorexia, abdominal cramps, antibiotic-associated pseudomembranous colitis, staphylococcal enterocolitis, pancreatitis

Hematologic: Thrombophlebitis

Hepatic: Hepatotoxicity

Renal: Acute renal failure, azotemia, renal damage

Miscellaneous: Superinfection, anaphylaxis, hypersensitivity reactions, candidal superinfection

Overdosage/Toxicology Symptoms include nausea, anorexia, and diarrhea. Following GI decontamination, supportive care only.

Drug Interactions

Cytochrome P450 Effect: Substrate of CYP3A4 (major); **Inhibits** CYP3A4 (moderate)

Increased Effect/Toxicity: Methoxyflurane anesthesia when concurrent with tetracycline may cause fatal nephrotoxicity. Warfarin with tetracyclines may cause increased anticoagulation. Tetracycline may increase the levels/effects of selected benzodiazepines, calcium channel blockers, cisapride, cyclosporine, ergot alkaloids, selected HMG-CoA reductase inhibitors, mirtazapine, nateglinide, nefazodone, pimozide, quinidine, sildenafil (and other PDE-5 inhibitors), tacrolimus, venlafaxine, and other CYP3A4 substrates.

Decreased Effect: Calcium, magnesium- or aluminum-containing antacids, iron, zinc, sodium bicarbonate, sucralfate, didanosine, or quinapril may decrease tetracycline absorption. Therapeutic effect of penicillins may be reduced with coadministration of tetracycline. Although anecdotal reports suggest oral contraceptive efficacy could be reduced by tetracyclines, this has been refuted by more rigorous scientific and clinical data. The levels/effects of tetracycline may be decreased by aminoglutethimide, carbamazepine, nafcillin, nevirapine, phenobarbital, phenytoin, rifamycins, and other CYP3A4 inducers.

Ethanol/Nutrition/Herb Interactions

Food: Tetracycline serum concentrations may be decreased if taken with dairy products.

Herb/Nutraceutical: Avoid dong quai, St John's wort (may also cause photosensitization)

Stability Outdated tetracyclines have caused a Fanconi-like syndrome; protect oral dosage forms from light

Mechanism of Action Inhibits bacterial protein synthesis by binding with the 30S and possibly the 50S ribosomal subunit(s) of susceptible bacteria; may also cause alterations in the cytoplasmic membrane

(Continued)

Tetracycline *(Continued)*

Pharmacodynamics/Kinetics

Absorption: Oral: 75%

Distribution: Small amount appears in bile

Relative diffusion from blood into CSF: Good only with inflammation (exceeds usual MICs)

CSF:blood level ratio: Inflamed meninges: 25%

Protein binding: ~65%

Half-life elimination: Normal renal function: 8-11 hours; End-stage renal disease: 57-108 hours

Time to peak, serum: Oral: 2-4 hours

Excretion: Urine (60% as unchanged drug); feces (as active form)

Dosage Oral:

Children >8 years: 25-50 mg/kg/day in divided doses every 6 hours

Adults: 250-500 mg/dose every 6 hours

Helicobacter pylori eradication: 500 mg 2-4 times/day depending on regimen; requires combination therapy with at least one other antibiotic and an acid-suppressing agent (proton pump inhibitor or H_2 blocker)

Dosing interval in renal impairment:

Cl_{cr} 50-80 mL/minute: Administer every 8-12 hours

Cl_{cr} 10-50 mL/minute: Administer every 12-24 hours

Cl_{cr} <10 mL/minute: Administer every 24 hours

Dialysis: Slightly dialyzable (5% to 20%) via hemo- and peritoneal dialysis or via continuous arteriovenous or venovenous hemofiltration; no supplemental dosage necessary

Dosing adjustment in hepatic impairment: Avoid use or maximum dose is 1 g/day

Administration Should be administered on an empty stomach (ie, 1 hour prior to, or 2 hours after meals) to increase total absorption. Administer at least 1-2 hours prior to, or 4 hours after antacid because aluminum and magnesium cations may chelate with tetracycline and reduce its total absorption.

Monitoring Parameters Renal, hepatic, and hematologic function test, temperature, WBC, cultures and sensitivity, appetite, mental status

Test Interactions False-negative urine glucose with Clinistix®

Patient Information Take 1 hour before or 2 hours after meals with adequate amounts of fluid; avoid prolonged exposure to sunlight or sunlamps; avoid taking antacids, iron, or dairy products within 2 hours of taking tetracyclines; report persistent nausea, vomiting, yellow coloring of skin or eyes, dark urine, or pale stools

Dosage Forms

Capsule, as hydrochloride: 250 mg, 500 mg

Suspension, oral, as hydrochloride (Sumycin®): 125 mg/5 mL (480 mL) [contains sodium benzoate and sodium metabisulfite; fruit flavor]

Tablet, as hydrochloride (Sumycin®): 250 mg, 500 mg

Selected Readings

Smilack JD, Wilson WR, and Cockerill FR 3d, "Tetracyclines, Chloramphenicol, Erythromycin, Clindamycin, and Metronidazole," *Mayo Clin Proc*, 1991, 66(12):1270-80.

Tetracycline, Bismuth Subsalicylate, and Metronidazole *see* Bismuth Subsalicylate, Metronidazole, and Tetracycline *on page 688*

Tetracycline Hydrochloride *see* Tetracycline *on page 1106*

Tetracycline, Metronidazole, and Bismuth Subsalicylate *see* Bismuth Subsalicylate, Metronidazole, and Tetracycline *on page 688*

Tetrahydrocannabinol *see* Dronabinol *on page 791*

Tev-Tropin™ *see* Somatropin *on page 1069*

Thalidomide (tha LI doe mide)

Related Information

AIDS Wasting Treatment *on page 1205*

U.S. Brand Names Thalomid®

Canadian Brand Names Thalomid®

Generic Available No

Use Treatment and maintenance of cutaneous manifestations of erythema nodosum leprosum

Unlabeled/Investigational Use Treatment of multiple myeloma; Crohn's disease; graft-versus-host reactions after bone marrow transplantation; AIDS-related aphthous stomatitis; Behçet's syndrome; Waldenström's macroglobulinemia; Langerhans cell histiocytosis; may be effective in rheumatoid arthritis, discoid lupus erythematosus, and erythema multiforme

Restrictions Thalidomide is approved for marketing only under a special distribution program. This program, called the "System for Thalidomide Education and

Prescribing Safety" (STEPS 1-888-423-5436), has been approved by the FDA. No more than a 4-week supply should be dispensed. Blister packs should be dispensed intact (do not repackage capsules). Prescriptions must be filled within 7 days.

Pregnancy Risk Factor X

Pregnancy Implications Embryotoxic with limb defects noted from the 27th to 40th gestational day of exposure; all cases of phocomelia occur from the 27th to 42nd gestational day; fetal cardiac, gastrointestinal, and genitourinary tract abnormalities have also been described. Effective contraception must be used for at least 4 weeks before initiating therapy, during therapy, and for 4 weeks following discontinuation of thalidomide. Males (even those vasectomized) must use a latex condom during any sexual contact with women of childbearing age. Risk to the fetus from semen of male patients is unknown.

Contraindications Hypersensitivity to thalidomide or any component of the formulation; neuropathy (peripheral); pregnancy or women in childbearing years unless alternative therapies are inappropriate and adequate precautions are taken to avoid pregnancy; patient unable to comply with STEPS™ program.

Warnings/Precautions Effective contraception must be used for at least 4 weeks before initiating therapy, during therapy, and for 4 weeks following discontinuation of thalidomide. May cause sedation; patients must be warned to use caution when performing tasks which require alertness. Use caution in patients with renal or hepatic impairment, neurological disorders, cardiovascular disease, or constipation.

Thalidomide has been associated with the development of peripheral neuropathy, which may be irreversible. Consider immediate discontinuation (if clinically appropriate) in patients who develop neuropathy. Use caution in patients with a history of seizures, concurrent therapy with drugs which alter seizure threshold, or conditions which predispose to seizures. May cause neutropenia; discontinue therapy if absolute neutrophil count decreases to $<750/mm^3$. Use caution in patients with HIV infection; has been associated with increased viral loads.

May cause orthostasis and/or bradycardia; use with caution in patients with cardiovascular disease or in patients who would not tolerate transient hypotensive episodes. Thrombotic events have been reported (generally in patients with other risk factors for thrombosis [neoplastic disease, inflammatory disease, or concurrent therapy with other drugs which may cause thrombosis]). Safety and efficacy have not been established in children <12 years of age.

Adverse Reactions

Controlled clinical trials: ENL:

- >10%:
  - Central nervous system: Somnolence (37.5%), headache (12.5%)
  - Dermatologic: Rash (20.8%)
- 1% to 10%:
  - Cardiovascular: Peripheral edema
  - Central nervous system: Dizziness (4.2%), vertigo (8.3%), chills, malaise (8.3%)
  - Dermatologic: Dermatitis (fungal) (4.2%), nail disorder (4.2%), pruritus (8.3%), rash (maculopapular) (4.2%)
  - Gastrointestinal (4.2%): Constipation, diarrhea, nausea, moniliasis, tooth pain, abdominal pain
  - Genitourinary: Impotence (8.2%)
  - Neuromuscular & skeletal: Asthenia (8.3%), pain (8.3%), back pain (4.2%), neck pain (4.2%), neck rigidity (4.2%), tremor (4.2%)
  - Respiratory (4.2%): Pharyngitis, rhinitis, sinusitis

HIV-seropositive:

- General: An increased viral load has been noted in patients treated with thalidomide. This is of uncertain clinical significance - see Monitoring Parameters
- >10%:
  - Central nervous system: Somnolence (36% to 37%), dizziness (18.7% to 19.4%), fever (19.4% to 21.9%), headache (16.7% to 18.7%)
  - Dermatologic: Rash (25%), maculopapular rash (16.7% to 18.7%), acne (3.1% to 11.1%)
  - Gastrointestinal: AST increase (2.8% to 12.5%), diarrhea (11.1% to 18.7%), nausea (≤12.5%), oral moniliasis (6.3% to 11.1%)
  - Hematologic: Leukopenia (16.7% to 25%), anemia (5.6% to 12.5%)
  - Neuromuscular & skeletal: Paresthesia (may be severe and/or irreversible) (5.6% to 15.6%), weakness (5.6% to 21.9%)
  - Miscellaneous: Diaphoresis (≤12.5%), lymphadenopathy (5.6% to 12.5%)
- 1% to 10%:
  - Cardiovascular: Peripheral edema (3.1% to 8.3%)
  - Central nervous system: Nervousness (2.8% to 9.4%), insomnia (≤9.4%), agitation (≤9.4%), chills (≤9.4%), neuropathy (up to 8% in HIV-seropositive patients)

(Continued)

Thalidomide *(Continued)*

Dermatologic: Dermatitis (fungal) (5.6% to 9.4%), nail disorder (≤3.1%), pruritus (2.8% to 6.3%)

Gastrointestinal: Anorexia (2.8% to 9.4%), constipation (2.8% to 9.4%), dry mouth (8.3% to 9.4%), flatulence (8.3% to 9.4%), multiple abnormalities LFTs (≤9.4%), abdominal pain (2.8% to 3.1%)

Neuromuscular & skeletal: Back pain (≤5%), pain (≤3.1%)

Respiratory: Pharyngitis (6.3% to 8.3%), sinusitis (3.1% to 8.3%)

Miscellaneous: Accidental injury (≤5.6%), infection (6.3% to 8.3%)

Postmarketing and/or case reports (limited to important or life-threatening): Acute renal failure, arrhythmia, bradycardia, CML, dyspnea, electrolyte imbalances, erythema multiforme, erythema nodosum, Hodgkin's disease, hypersensitivity, hyperthyroidism, intestinal perforation, lethargy, lymphopenia, mental status changes, myxedema, neutropenia, orthostatic hypotension, pancytopenia, paresthesia, peripheral neuritis, photosensitivity, pleural effusion, psychosis, Raynaud's syndrome, seizure, Stevens-Johnson syndrome, suicide attempt, syncope, thrombosis, toxic epidermal necrolysis, tumor lysis syndrome

Drug Interactions

Increased Effect/Toxicity: Thalidomide may enhance the sedative activity of other drugs such as ethanol, barbiturates, reserpine, and chlorpromazine. Drugs which may cause peripheral neuropathy should be used with caution in patients receiving thalidomide. Women using any drug which may decrease the serum concentrations and/or efficacy of hormonal contraceptives must use 2 other methods of contraception or abstain from heterosexual contact. Thalidomide may be associated with increased risk of serious infection when used in combination with anakinra.

Ethanol/Nutrition/Herb Interactions

Ethanol: Avoid ethanol (may increase sedation).

Herb/Nutraceutical: Avoid cat's claw (has immunostimulant properties).

Stability Store at 15°C to 30°C (50°F to 86°F). Protect from light. Keep in original package.

Mechanism of Action A derivative of glutethimide; mode of action for immunosuppression is unclear; inhibition of neutrophil chemotaxis and decreased monocyte phagocytosis may occur; may cause 50% to 80% reduction of tumor necrosis factor - alpha

Pharmacodynamics/Kinetics

Distribution: V_d: 120 L

Protein binding: 55% to 66%

Metabolism: Nonenzymatic hydrolysis in plasma; forms multiple metabolites

Half-life elimination: 5-7 hours

Time to peak, plasma: 2-6 hours

Excretion: Urine (<1%)

Dosage Oral:

Cutaneous ENL:

Initiate dosing at 100-300 mg/day taken once daily at bedtime with water (at least 1 hour after evening meal)

Patients weighing <50 kg: Initiate at lower end of the dosing range

Severe cutaneous reaction or previously requiring high dose may be initiated at 400 mg/day; doses may be divided, but taken 1 hour after meals

Dosing should continue until active reaction subsides (usually at least 2 weeks), then tapered in 50 mg decrements every 2-4 weeks

Patients who flare during tapering or with a history or requiring prolonged maintenance should be maintained on the minimum dosage necessary to control the reaction. Efforts to taper should be repeated every 3-6 months, in increments of 50 mg every 2-4 weeks.

Behçet's syndrome (unlabeled use): 100-400 mg/day

Graft-vs-host reactions (unlabeled use): 100-1600 mg/day; usual initial dose: 200 mg 4 times/day for use up to 700 days

AIDS-related aphthous stomatitis (unlabeled use): 200 mg twice daily for 5 days, then 200 mg/day for up to 8 weeks

Discoid lupus erythematosus (unlabeled use): 100-400 mg/day; maintenance dose: 25-50 mg

Dietary Considerations Should be taken at least 1 hour after the evening meal.

Administration Oral: Avoid extensive handling of capsules; capsules should remain in blister pack until ingestion. If exposed to the powder content from broken capsules or body fluids from patients receiving thalidomide, the exposed area should be washed with soap and water.

Monitoring Parameters WBC with differential; signs of neuropathy monthly for the first 3 months, then periodically during treatment; consider monitoring of sensory

nerve application potential amplitudes (at baseline and every 6 months) to detect asymptomatic neuropathy. In HIV-seropositive patients: viral load after 1 and 3 months, then every 3 months. Pregnancy testing is required within 24 hours of initiation of therapy, weekly during the first 4 weeks, then every 4 weeks in women with regular menstrual cycles or every 2 weeks in women with irregular menstrual cycles.

Reference Range Therapeutic plasma thalidomide levels in graft-vs-host reactions are 5-8 mcg/mL, although it has been suggested that lower plasma levels (0.5-1.5 mcg/mL) may be therapeutic; peak serum thalidomide level after a 200 mg dose: 1.2 mcg/mL

Patient Information Thalidomide must be obtained via "STEPS™ Program" (1-888-423-5436). Effective contraception must be used for at least 1 month prior to beginning therapy, during therapy, and continued for 1 month after thalidomide has been discontinued. Two reliable forms of contraception must be used. Males must use a latex condom during sexual contact with women of childbearing age. Thalidomide may cause drowsiness and/or orthostatic hypotension. Patients should not donate blood. Patients should report signs of tingling, numbness, or pain in hands or feet.

Dosage Forms Capsule: 50 mg, 100 mg, 200 mg

Selected Readings

Beckman DA and Brent RL, "Mechanism of Known Environmental Teratogens: Drugs and Chemicals," *Clin Perinatol*, 1986, 13(3):649-87.

Gunzler V, "Thalidomide in Human Immunodeficiency Virus (HIV) Patients. A Review of Safety Considerations," *Drug Saf*, 1992, 7(2):116-34.

Jacobson JM, Greenspan JS, Spritzler J, et al, "Thalidomide for the Treatment of Oral Aphthous Ulcers in Patients With Human Immunodeficiency Virus Infection. National Institute of Allergy and Infectious Diseases AIDS Clinical Trials Group," *N Engl J Med*, 1997, 336(21):1487-93.

Levien T, Baker DE, and Ballasiotes AA, "Reviews of Dexrazoxane and Thalidomide," *Hosp Pharm*, 1996, 31(5):487-8, 493-4, 499-500, 504, 508, 510.

Schuler U and Ehninger G, "Thalidomide: Rationale for Renewed Use in Immunological Disorders," *Drug Saf*, 1995, 12(6):364-9.

"Thalidomide," *Med Lett Drugs Ther*, 1998, 40(1038):103-4.

Thalomid® *see* Thalidomide *on page 1108*

THC *see* Dronabinol *on page 791*

TheraCys® *see* BCG Vaccine *on page 683*

Theramycin Z® *see* Erythromycin *on page 807*

Thermazene® *see* Silver Sulfadiazine *on page 1065*

Thiabendazole (thye a BEN da zole)

U.S. Brand Names Mintezol®

Synonyms Tiabendazole

Generic Available No

Use Treatment of strongyloidiasis, cutaneous larva migrans, visceral larva migrans, dracunculiasis, trichinosis, and mixed helminthic infections

Unlabeled/Investigational Use Cutaneous larva migrans (topical application)

Drug of Choice or Alternative for

Organism(s):

Ancylostoma duodenale on page 34
Strongyloides stercoralis on page 328
Trichinella spiralis on page 338

Pregnancy Risk Factor C

Pregnancy Implications Cleft palate and skeletal defects were observed in some animal studies. There are no adequate and well-controlled studies in pregnant women.

Contraindications Hypersensitivity to thiabendazole or any component of the formulation; not for use as prophylactic treatment of enterobiasis (pinworm) infestation

Warnings/Precautions Use with caution in patients with renal or hepatic impairment, malnutrition or anemia, or dehydration. Causes sedation; caution must be used in performing tasks which require alertness. Not suitable treatment for mixed infections with *Ascaris*. Ophthalmic changes may occur and persist >1 year. Safety and efficacy are limited in children <14 kg (30 lb).

Adverse Reactions Frequency not defined.

Central nervous system: Seizures, hallucinations, delirium, dizziness, drowsiness, headache, chills

Dermatologic: Rash, Stevens-Johnson syndrome, pruritus, angioedema

Endocrine & metabolic: Hyperglycemia

Gastrointestinal: Anorexia, diarrhea, nausea, vomiting, drying of mucous membranes, abdominal pain

Genitourinary: Malodor of urine, hematuria, crystalluria, enuresis

Hematologic: Leukopenia

(Continued)

Thiabendazole *(Continued)*

Hepatic: Jaundice, cholestasis, hepatic failure, hepatotoxicity
Neuromuscular & skeletal: Numbness, incoordination
Ocular: Abnormal sensation in eyes, blurred vision, dry eyes, Sicca syndrome, vision decreased, xanthopsia
Otic: Tinnitus
Renal: Nephrotoxicity
Miscellaneous: Anaphylaxis, hypersensitivity reactions, lymphadenopathy

Overdosage/Toxicology Symptoms include altered mental status and visual problems. Supportive care only following GI decontamination.

Drug Interactions

Cytochrome P450 Effect: Substrate of CYP1A2 (minor); **Inhibits** CYP1A2 (strong)

Increased Effect/Toxicity: Thiabendazole may increase the levels/effects of aminophylline, fluvoxamine, mexiletine, mirtazapine, ropinirole, theophylline, trifluoperazine, and other CYP1A2 substrates.

Mechanism of Action Inhibits helminth-specific mitochondrial fumarate reductase

Pharmacodynamics/Kinetics

Absorption: Rapid and well absorbed
Metabolism: Rapidly hepatic; metabolized to 5-hydroxy form
Half-life elimination: 1.2 hours
Time to peak, plasma: Oral suspension: Within 1-2 hours
Excretion: Urine (90%) and feces (5%) primarily as conjugated metabolites

Dosage Purgation is not required prior to use; drinking of fruit juice aids in expulsion of worms by removing the mucous to which the intestinal tapeworms attach themselves.

Children and Adults:

Oral: 50 mg/kg/day divided every 12 hours (if >68 kg: 1.5 g/dose); maximum dose: 3 g/day

Treatment duration:

Strongyloidiasis, ascariasis, uncinariasis: For 2 consecutive days

Cutaneous larva migrans: For 2 consecutive days; if active lesions are still present 2 days after completion, a second course of treatment is recommended.

Visceral larva migrans: For 7 consecutive days

Trichinosis: For 2-4 consecutive days; optimal dosage not established

Dracunculosis: 50-75 mg/kg/day divided every 12 hours for 3 days

Topical (unlabeled): Cutaneous larva migrans: Apply directly to larval tracks 2-3 times/day for up to 2 weeks; application frequencies may range from 2-6 times/day. **Note:** Not available as a topical formulation; oral suspension (10% to 15%) has been used topically, as well as a number of extemporaneous formulations.

Dosing comments in renal/hepatic impairment: Use with caution

Monitoring Parameters Periodic renal and hepatic function tests

Patient Information Take after meals, chew chewable tablet well; may decrease alertness, avoid driving or operating machinery; drinking of fruit juice aids in expulsion of worms by removing the mucous to which the intestinal tapeworms attach themselves

Dosage Forms [DSC] = Discontinued product

Suspension, oral: 500 mg/5 mL (120 mL) [DSC]
Tablet, chewable: 500 mg [orange flavor]

Extemporaneous Preparations Topical application of thiabendazole has been recommended for the treatment of cutaneous larva migrans (*Redbook*, 2003; *Med Letter*, 2002). In some cases, the commercially-available 10% oral suspension has been used for topical application. Alternatively, a number of extemporaneous preparations have used crushed tablets to prepare distinct formulations. These include a 10% ointment (in white petrolatum), a 15% topical lotion (suspended with compound tragacanth powder 250 mg/40 mL), a 15% cream (in either hydrophilic or fat-based creams), and topical solutions (2% to 4% in DMSO). The stability of these formulations has not been established, and there are no comparative studies evaluating different formulations. All preparations have been applied between 2-6 times daily for up to 2 weeks.

Selected Readings

"Drugs for Parasitic Infections," *Med Lett Drugs Ther*, 1998, 40(1017):1-12.

ThyroSafe™ [OTC] *see* Potassium Iodide *on page 1014*

ThyroShield™ [OTC] *see* Potassium Iodide *on page 1014*

Tiabendazole *see* Thiabendazole *on page 1111*

Ticar® *see* Ticarcillin *on page 1113*

Ticarcillin (tye kar SIL in)

Related Information

Antimicrobial Activity Against Selected Organisms *on page 1165*

U.S. Brand Names Ticar®

Synonyms Ticarcillin Disodium

Generic Available No

Use Treatment of susceptible infections such as septicemia, acute and chronic respiratory tract infections, skin and soft tissue infections, and urinary tract infections due to susceptible strains of *Pseudomonas*, and other gram-negative bacteria

Drug of Choice or Alternative for Disease/Syndrome(s):

Keratitis, Bacterial and Fungal *on page 199*

Pregnancy Risk Factor B

Contraindications Hypersensitivity to ticarcillin, any component of the formulation, or penicillins

Warnings/Precautions Due to sodium load and adverse effects (anemia, neuropsychological changes), use with caution and modify dosage in patients with renal impairment; serious and occasionally severe or fatal hypersensitivity (anaphylactoid) reactions have been reported in patients on penicillin therapy (especially with a history of beta-lactam hypersensitivity and/or a history of sensitivity to multiple allergens); use with caution in patients with seizures

Adverse Reactions Frequency not defined.

Central nervous system: Confusion, convulsions, drowsiness, fever, Jarisch-Herxheimer reaction

Dermatologic: Rash

Endocrine & metabolic: Electrolyte imbalance

Gastrointestinal: *Clostridium difficile* colitis

Hematologic: Bleeding, eosinophilia, hemolytic anemia, leukopenia, neutropenia, positive Coombs' reaction, thrombocytopenia

Hepatic: Hepatotoxicity, jaundice

Local: Thrombophlebitis

Neuromuscular & skeletal: Myoclonus

Renal: Interstitial nephritis (acute)

Miscellaneous: Anaphylaxis, hypersensitivity reactions

Overdosage/Toxicology Symptoms of penicillin overdose include neuromuscular hypersensitivity (agitation, hallucinations, asterixis, encephalopathy, confusion, and seizures) and electrolyte imbalance (with potassium or sodium salts), especially in renal failure. Hemodialysis may be helpful to aid in the removal of the drug from the blood, otherwise most treatment is supportive or symptom-directed.

Drug Interactions

Increased Effect/Toxicity: Probenecid may increase penicillin levels. Neuromuscular blockers may have an increased duration of action (neuromuscular blockade). Penicillins may increase the exposure to methotrexate during concurrent therapy; monitor.

Decreased Effect: Tetracyclines may decrease penicillin effectiveness. Aminoglycosides may cause physical inactivation of aminoglycosides in the presence of high concentrations of ticarcillin and potential toxicity in patients with mild-moderate renal dysfunction. Although anecdotal reports suggest oral contraceptive efficacy could be reduced by penicillins, this has been refuted by more rigorous scientific and clinical data.

Stability Reconstituted solution is stable for 72 hours at room temperature and 14 days when refrigerated; for I.V. infusion in NS or D_5W solution is stable for 72 hours at room temperature, 14 days when refrigerated or 30 days when frozen; after freezing, thawed solution is stable for 72 hours at room temperature or 14 days when refrigerated; **incompatible** with aminoglycosides

Mechanism of Action Inhibits bacterial cell wall synthesis by binding to one or more of the penicillin binding proteins (PBPs); which in turn inhibits the final transpeptidation step of peptidoglycan synthesis in bacterial cell walls, thus inhibiting cell wall biosynthesis. Bacteria eventually lyse due to ongoing activity of cell wall autolytic enzymes (autolysins and murein hydrolases) while cell wall assembly is arrested.

Pharmacodynamics/Kinetics

Absorption: I.M.: 86%

Distribution: Blister fluid, lymph tissue, and gallbladder; low concentrations into CSF increasing with inflamed meninges, otherwise widely distributed; crosses placenta; enters breast milk (low concentrations)

Protein binding: 45% to 65%

Half-life elimination:

Neonates: <1 week old: 3.5-5.6 hours; 1-8 weeks old: 1.3-2.2 hours

(Continued)

Ticarcillin *(Continued)*

Children 5-13 years: 0.9 hour
Adults: 66-72 minutes; prolonged with renal and/or hepatic impairment
Time to peak, serum: I.M.: 30-75 minutes
Excretion: Almost entirely urine (as unchanged drug and metabolites); feces (3.5%)

Dosage Ticarcillin is generally given I.V., I.M. injection is only for the treatment of uncomplicated urinary tract infections and dose should not exceed 2 g/injection when administered I.M.

Neonates: I.M., I.V.:
Postnatal age <7 days:
<2000 g: 75 mg/kg/dose every 12 hours
>2000 g: 75 mg/kg/dose every 8 hours
Postnatal age >7 days:
<1200 g: 75 mg/kg/dose every 12 hours
1200-2000 g: 75 mg/kg/dose every 8 hours
>2000 g: 75 mg/kg/dose every 6 hours
Infants and Children:
Systemic infections: I.V.: 200-300 mg/kg/day in divided doses every 4-6 hours
Urinary tract infections: I.M., I.V.: 50-100 mg/kg/day in divided doses every 6-8 hours
Maximum dose: 24 g/day
Adults: I.M., I.V.: 1-4 g every 4-6 hours, usual dose: 3 g I.V. every 4-6 hours
Dosing adjustment in renal impairment: Adults:
Cl_{cr} 30-60 mL/minute: 2 g every 4 hours or 3 g every 8 hours
Cl_{cr} 10-30 mL/minute: 2 g every 8 hours or 3 g every 12 hours
Cl_{cr} <10 mL/minute: 2 g every 12 hours
Moderately dialyzable (20% to 50%)
Continuous arteriovenous or venovenous hemodiafiltration effects: Dose as for Cl_{cr} 10-50 mL/minute

Dietary Considerations Sodium content of 1 g: 119.6-149.5 mg (5.2-6.5 mEq)

Administration Administer 1 hour apart from aminoglycosides

Monitoring Parameters Serum electrolytes, bleeding time, and periodic tests of renal, hepatic, and hematologic function; monitor for signs of anaphylaxis during first dose

Test Interactions May interfere with urinary glucose tests using cupric sulfate (Benedict's solution, Clinitest®); may inactivate aminoglycosides *in vitro*; false-positive urinary or serum protein

Dosage Forms Injection, powder for reconstitution, as disodium: 3 g

Selected Readings

Donowitz GR and Mandell GL, "Beta-Lactam Antibiotics," *N Engl J Med*, 1988, 318(7):419-26 and 318(8):490-500.
Tan JS and File TM Jr, "Antipseudomonal Penicillins," *Med Clin North Am*, 1995, 79(4):679-93.
Wright AJ, "The Penicillins," *Mayo Clin Proc*, 1999, 74(3):290-307.

Ticarcillin and Clavulanate Potassium

(tye kar SIL in & klav yoo LAN ate poe TASS ee um)

Related Information
Antimicrobial Activity Against Selected Organisms *on page 1165*

U.S. Brand Names Timentin®

Canadian Brand Names Timentin®

Synonyms Ticarcillin and Clavulanic Acid

Generic Available No

Use Treatment of infections of lower respiratory tract, urinary tract, skin and skin structures, bone and joint, and septicemia caused by susceptible organisms. Clavulanate expands activity of ticarcillin to include beta-lactamase producing strains of *S. aureus*, *H. influenzae*, *Bacteroides* species, and some other gram-negative bacilli

Drug of Choice or Alternative for Disease/Syndrome(s):
Amnionitis *on page 33*
Cholangitis, Acute *on page 79*
Diverticulitis *on page 116*
Endometritis *on page 127*
Intra-abdominal Abscess *on page 194*
Liver Abscess *on page 211*
Lung Abscess *on page 212*
Osteomyelitis, Diabetic Foot *on page 249*
Pancreatitis/Pancreatic Abscess *on page 253*
Peritonitis, Spontaneous Bacterial *on page 264*

Organism(s):

Bacteroides and *Prevotella* Species *on page 46*
Enterobacter Species *on page 132*
Stenotrophomonas maltophilia on page 312

Pregnancy Risk Factor B

Contraindications Hypersensitivity to ticarcillin, clavulanate, any penicillin, or any component of the formulation

Warnings/Precautions Not approved for use in children <12 years of age; use with caution and modify dosage in patients with renal impairment; use with caution in patients with a history of allergy to cephalosporins and in patients with CHF due to high sodium load

Adverse Reactions Frequency not defined.

Central nervous system: Confusion, convulsions, drowsiness, fever, Jarisch-Herxheimer reaction
Dermatologic: Rash, erythema multiforme, toxic epidermal necrolysis, Stevens-Johnson syndrome
Endocrine & metabolic: Electrolyte imbalance
Gastrointestinal: *Clostridium difficile* colitis
Hematologic: Bleeding, hemolytic anemia, leukopenia, neutropenia, positive Coombs' reaction, thrombocytopenia
Hepatic: Hepatotoxicity, jaundice
Local: Thrombophlebitis
Neuromuscular & skeletal: Myoclonus
Renal: Interstitial nephritis (acute)
Miscellaneous: Anaphylaxis, hypersensitivity reactions

Overdosage/Toxicology Symptoms include neuromuscular hypersensitivity and seizures. Many beta-lactam containing antibiotics have the potential to cause neuromuscular hyperirritability or convulsive seizures. Hemodialysis may be helpful to aid in removal of the drug from the blood, otherwise most treatment is supportive or symptom-directed.

Drug Interactions

Increased Effect/Toxicity: Probenecid may increase penicillin levels. Neuromuscular blockers may have an increased duration of action (neuromuscular blockade). Penicillins may increase the exposure to methotrexate during concurrent therapy; monitor.

Decreased Effect: Tetracyclines may decrease penicillin effectiveness. Aminoglycosides may cause physical inactivation of aminoglycosides in the presence of high concentrations of ticarcillin and potential toxicity in patients with mild-moderate renal dysfunction. Although anecdotal reports suggest oral contraceptive efficacy could be reduced by penicillins, this has been refuted by more rigorous scientific and clinical data.

Stability Reconstituted solution is stable for 6 hours at room temperature and 72 hours when refrigerated; for I.V. infusion in NS is stable for 24 hours at room temperature, 7 days when refrigerated or 30 days when frozen; after freezing, thawed solution is stable for 8 hours at room temperature; for I.V. infusion in D_5W solution is stable for 24 hours at room temperature, 3 days when refrigerated or 7 days when frozen; after freezing, thawed solution is stable for 8 hours at room temperature; darkening of drug indicates loss of potency of clavulanate potassium; **incompatible** with sodium bicarbonate, aminoglycosides

Mechanism of Action Inhibits bacterial cell wall synthesis by binding to one or more of the penicillin binding proteins (PBPs); which in turn inhibits the final transpeptidation step of peptidoglycan synthesis in bacterial cell walls, thus inhibiting cell wall biosynthesis. Bacteria eventually lyse due to ongoing activity of cell wall autolytic enzymes (autolysins and murein hydrolases) while cell wall assembly is arrested.

Pharmacodynamics/Kinetics

Ticarcillin: See Ticarcillin monograph.

Clavulanic acid:

Protein binding: 9% to 30%
Metabolism: Hepatic
Half-life elimination: 66-90 minutes
Excretion: Urine (45% as unchanged drug)
Clearance: Does not affect clearance of ticarcillin

Dosage I.V.:

Children and Adults <60 kg: 200-300 mg of ticarcillin component/kg/day in divided doses every 4-6 hours
Children >60 kg and Adults: 3.1 g (ticarcillin 3 g plus clavulanic acid 0.1 g) every 4-6 hours; maximum: 24 g/day
Urinary tract infections: 3.1 g every 6-8 hours

(Continued)

Ticarcillin and Clavulanate Potassium *(Continued)*

Dosing adjustment in renal impairment:

Cl_{cr} 30-60 mL/minute: Administer 2 g every 4 hours or 3.1 g every 8 hours
Cl_{cr} 10-30 mL/minute: Administer 2 g every 8 hours or 3.1 g every 12 hours
Cl_{cr} <10 mL/minute: Administer 2 g every 12 hours

Moderately dialyzable (20% to 50%)

Continuous arteriovenous or venovenous hemodiafiltration effects: Dose as for Cl_{cr} 10-50 mL/minute

Peritoneal dialysis: 3.1 g every 12 hours

Hemodialysis: 2 g every 12 hours; supplemented with 3.1 g after each dialysis

Dosing adjustment in hepatic dysfunction: Cl_{cr} <10 mL/minute: 2 g every 24 hours

Dietary Considerations Sodium content of 1 g: 4.51 mEq; potassium content of 1 g: 0.15 mEq

Administration Infuse over 30 minutes; administer 1 hour apart from aminoglycosides

Monitoring Parameters Observe for signs and symptoms of anaphylaxis during first dose.

Test Interactions Positive Coombs' test, false-positive urinary proteins

Dosage Forms

Infusion [premixed, frozen]: Ticarcillin 3 g and clavulanic acid 0.1 g (100 mL) [contains sodium 4.51 mEq and potassium 0.15 mEq per g]

Injection, powder for reconstitution: Ticarcillin 3 g and clavulanic acid 0.1 g (3.1 g, 31 g) [contains sodium 4.51 mEq and potassium 0.15 mEq per g]

Selected Readings

Donowitz GR and Mandell GL, "Beta-Lactam Antibiotics," *N Engl J Med*, 1988, 318(7):419-26 and 318(8):490-500.

Itokazu GS and Danziger LH, "Ampicillin-Sulbactam and Ticarcillin-Clavulanic Acid: A Comparison of Their *In Vitro* Activity and Review of Their Clinical Efficacy," *Pharmacotherapy*, 1991, 11(5):382-414.

Wright AJ, "The Penicillins," *Mayo Clin Proc*, 1999, 74(3):290-307.

Ticarcillin and Clavulanic Acid *see* Ticarcillin and Clavulanate Potassium *on page 1114*

Ticarcillin Disodium *see* Ticarcillin *on page 1113*

TICE® BCG *see* BCG Vaccine *on page 683*

TIG *see* Tetanus Immune Globulin (Human) *on page 1103*

Tigecycline (tye ge SYE kleen)

Related Information

Antimicrobial Activity Against Selected Organisms *on page 1165*

U.S. Brand Names Tygacil™

Synonyms GAR-936

Generic Available No

Use Treatment of complicated skin and skin structure infections caused by susceptible organisms, including methicillin-resistant *Staphylococcus aureus* and vancomycin-sensitive *Enterococcus faecalis*; treatment of complicated intra-abdominal infections

Drug of Choice or Alternative for Disease/Syndrome(s):

Liver Abscess *on page 211*
Peritonitis, Secondary *on page 263*
Peritonitis, Spontaneous Bacterial *on page 264*

Pregnancy Risk Factor D

Pregnancy Implications Tigecycline has been shown to cross the placenta in animal studies. Decreased fetal weight, minor skeletal abnormalities, and increased fetal loss were observed. There are no adequate and well-controlled studies in pregnant women. Due to structural similarity to tetracyclines, permanent discoloration of the teeth (brown-gray) may occur if used during tooth development (fetal stage through children up to 8 years of age). Should only be used in pregnancy if the potential benefit to the mother justifies risk to the fetus.

Contraindications Hypersensitivity to tigecycline or any component of the formulation

Warnings/Precautions Due to structural similarity with tetracyclines, use caution in patients with prior hypersensitivity and/or severe adverse reactions associated with tetracycline use. Due to structural similarities with tetracyclines, may be associated with photosensitivity, pseudotumor cerebri, pancreatitis, and antianabolic effects observed with this class. May cause fetal harm if used during pregnancy; patients should be advised of potential risks associated with use. Permanent discoloration of the teeth may occur if used during tooth development (fetal stage through children up to 8 years of age). Use caution in hepatic impairment; dosage adjustment may be required.

Tigecycline may be associated with the development of *C. difficile* colitis. Use caution in intestinal perforation (in the small sample of available cases, septic shock occurred more frequently than patients treated with imipenem/cilastatin comparator). Safety and efficacy in children <18 years of age have not been established.

Adverse Reactions Note: Frequencies relative to placebo are not available; some frequencies are lower than those experienced with comparator drugs.

>10%: Gastrointestinal: Nausea (25% to 30%; severe in 1%), vomiting (20%; severe in 1%), diarrhea (13%)

2% to 10%:

Cardiovascular: Hypertension (5%), peripheral edema (3%), hypotension (2%), phlebitis (2%)

Central nervous system: Fever (7%), headache (6%), dizziness (4%), pain (4%), insomnia (2%)

Dermatologic: Pruritus (3%), rash (2%)

Endocrine & metabolic: Hypoproteinemia (5%), hyperglycemia (2%), hypokalemia (2%)

Gastrointestinal: Abdominal pain (7%), constipation (3%), dyspepsia (3%)

Hematologic: Thrombocythemia (6%), anemia (4%), leukocytosis (4%)

Hepatic: SGPT increased (6%), SGOT increased (4%), alkaline phosphatase increased (4%), amylase increased (3%), bilirubin increased (2%), LDH increased (4%)

Local: Reaction to procedure (9%)

Neuromuscular & skeletal: Weakness (3%)

Renal: BUN increased (2%)

Respiratory: Cough increased (4%), dyspnea (3%), pulmonary physical finding (2%)

Miscellaneous: Abnormal healing (4%), infection (8%), abscess (3%), diaphoresis increased (2%)

<2%: Abnormal stools, allergic reaction, anorexia, aPTT prolonged, back pain, bradycardia, chills, creatinine increased, dry mouth, eosinophilia, hypocalcemia, hypoglycemia, hyponatremia, injection site edema, injection site inflammation, injection site pain, injection site phlebitis, injection site reaction, INR increased, jaundice, leukorrhea, PT prolonged, septic shock, tachycardia, taste perversion, thrombocytopenia, thrombophlebitis, vaginal moniliasis, vaginitis, vasodilatation

Overdosage/Toxicology No specific experience in overdose. May experience increased nausea/vomiting. Not significantly removed by hemodialysis.

Drug Interactions

Increased Effect/Toxicity: Retinoic acid derivatives may increase risk of pseudotumor cerebri (reported with tetracyclines). Hypoprothrombinemic response of warfarin may be increased with tigecycline; monitor INR closely during initiation or discontinuation.

Decreased Effect: Anecdotal reports of oral contraceptives suggesting decreased contraceptive efficacy with tetracyclines have been refuted by more rigorous scientific and clinical data.

Stability Store at 20°C to 25°C prior to reconstitution, excursions permitted to 15°C to 30°C. Add 5.3 mL NS or D_5W to each 50 mg vial. Swirl gently to dissolve. Resulting solution is 10 mg/mL. Reconstituted solution must be immediately transferred (and further diluted) to allow I.V. administration; Transfer immediately to 100 mL I.V. bag for infusion (final concentration should not exceed 1 mg/mL).Following dilution, may be stored at room temperature for up to 6 hours, or up to 24 hours under refrigeration. Reconstituted solution is red-orange.

Mechanism of Action

Binds to the 30S ribosomal subunit of susceptible bacteria, inhibiting protein synthesis. Generally considered bacteriostatic. Tigecycline is a derivative of minocycline (9-t-butylglycylamido minocycline), but is not classified as a tetracycline. It has demonstrated activity against a variety of Gram-positive and -negative bacterial pathogens.

Glycylcyclines demonstrate antibacterial activity which is similar to tetracyclines, however they are more potent against tetracycline-resistant organisms with efflux and ribosomal protection mechanisms of resistance. The glycylcyclines are active against several resistant pathogens including methicillin-resistant staphylococci.

Pharmacodynamics/Kinetics Note: Systemic clearance is reduced by 55% and half-life increased by 43% in moderate hepatic impairment.

Distribution: V_d: 7-9 L/kg; extensive tissue distribution

Protein binding: 71% to 89%

Metabolism: Hepatic, via glucuronidation, N-acetylation, and epimerization to several metabolites, each <10% of the dose

Half-life elimination: Single dose: 27 hours; following multiple doses: 42 hours

Excretion: Urine (33%; with 22% as unchanged drug); feces (59%; primarily as unchanged drug)

(Continued)

Tigecycline *(Continued)*

Dosage I.V.: Adults:

Initial: 100 mg as a single dose

Maintenance dose: 50 mg every 12 hours

Recommended duration of therapy: Intra-abdominal infections or complicated skin/skin structure infections: 5-14 days.

Dosage adjustment in renal impairment: No dosage adjustment required

Dosage adjustment in hepatic impairment:

Mild-to-moderate hepatic disease: No dosage adjustment required

Severe hepatic impairment (Child-Pugh class C): Initial dose of 100 mg should be followed with 25 mg every 12 hours

Administration

Infuse over 30-60 minutes through dedicated line or via Y-site

Dosage Forms Injection, powder for reconsitution: 50 mg

Timentin® *see* Ticarcillin and Clavulanate Potassium *on page 1114*

Tinactin® Antifungal [OTC] *see* Tolnaftate *on page 1127*

Tinactin® Antifungal Jock Itch [OTC] *see* Tolnaftate *on page 1127*

Tinaderm [OTC] *see* Tolnaftate *on page 1127*

Tindamax™ *see* Tinidazole *on page 1118*

Tine Test *see* Tuberculin Tests *on page 1136*

Ting® [OTC] *see* Tolnaftate *on page 1127*

Tinidazole (tye NI da zole)

U.S. Brand Names Tindamax™

Generic Available No

Use Treatment of trichomoniasis caused by *T. vaginalis*; treatment of giardiasis caused by *G. duodenalis* (*G. lamblia*); treatment of intestinal amebiasis and amebic liver abscess caused by *E. histolytica*

Drug of Choice or Alternative for Organism(s):

Giardia lamblia on page 155

Pregnancy Risk Factor C

Pregnancy Implications Tinidazole crosses the placenta and enters the fetal circulation. Use during the first trimester is contraindicated.

Contraindications Hypersensitivity to tinidazole, nitroimidazole derivatives (including metronidazole), or any component of the formulation; pregnancy (1st trimester); breast-feeding

Warnings/Precautions Use caution with CNS diseases; seizures and peripheral neuropathy have been reported with tinidazole and other nitroimidazole derivatives. Use caution with current or history of blood dyscrasias or hepatic impairment. When used for amebiasis, not indicated for the treatment of asymptomatic cyst passage. Safety and efficacy have not been established in children ≤3 years of age.

Adverse Reactions

1% to 10%:

Central nervous system: Fatigue/malaise (1% to 2%), dizziness (≤1%), headache (≤1%)

Gastrointestinal: Metallic/bitter taste (4% to 6%), nausea (3% to 5%), anorexia (2% to 3%), dyspepsia/cramps/epigastric discomfort (1% to 2%), vomiting (1% to 2%), constipation (≤1%)

Neuromuscular & skeletal: Weakness (1% to 2%)

Frequency not defined.

Cardiovascular: Flushing, palpitation

Central nervous system: Ataxia, coma, confusion, convulsions, depression, drowsiness, fever, giddiness, insomnia, vertigo

Dermatologic: Angioedema, pruritus, rash, urticaria

Gastrointestinal: Diarrhea, furry tongue, oral candidiasis, salivation, stomatitis, thirst, tongue discoloration, xerostomia

Genitourinary: Urine darkened, vaginal discharge increased

Hematologic: Leukopenia (transient), neutropenia (transient), thrombocytopenia (reversible)

Hepatic: Transaminases increased

Neuromuscular & skeletal: Arthralgia, arthritis, myalgia, peripheral neuropathy (transient, includes numbness and paresthesia)

Respiratory: Bronchospasm, dyspnea, pharyngitis

Miscellaneous: Burning sensation, *Candida* overgrowth, diaphoresis

Overdosage/Toxicology Treatment should be symptomatic and supportive. Hemodialysis may be considered (43% removed during a 6-hour session).

Drug Interactions

Cytochrome P450 Effect: Substrate of CYP3A4 (minor)

Increased Effect/Toxicity: Specific interaction studies have not been conducted. Refer to Metronidazole monograph *on page 940.*

Decreased Effect: Specific interaction studies have not been conducted. Refer to Metronidazole monograph *on page 940.*

Ethanol/Nutrition/Herb Interactions

Ethanol: The manufacturer recommends to avoid all ethanol or any ethanol-containing drugs (may cause disulfiram-like reaction characterized by flushing, headache, nausea, vomiting, sweating or tachycardia).

Food: Peak antibiotic serum concentration lowered and delayed, but total drug absorbed not affected.

Stability Store at controlled room temperature of 20°C to 25°C (68°F to 77°F); protect from light

Mechanism of Action After diffusing into the organism, it is proposed that tinidazole causes cytotoxicity by damaging DNA and preventing further DNA synthesis.

Pharmacodynamics/Kinetics

Absorption: Rapid and complete

Distribution: V_d: 50 L

Protein binding: 12%

Metabolism: Hepatic via CYP3A4 (primarily); undergoes oxidation, hydroxylation and conjugation; forms a metabolite

Half-life elimination: 13 hours

Excretion: Urine (20% to 25%); feces (12%)

Dosage Oral:

Children >3 years:

- Amebiasis, intestinal: 50 mg/kg/day for 3 days (maximum dose: 2 g/day)
- Amebiasis, liver abscess: 50 mg/kg/day for 3-5 days (maximum dose: 2 g/day)
- Giardiasis: 50 mg/kg as a single dose (maximum dose: 2 g)

Adults:

- Amebiasis, intestinal: 2 g/day for 3 days
- Amebiasis, liver abscess: 2 g/day for 3-5 days
- Giardiasis: 2 g as a single dose
- Trichomoniasis: Oral: 2 g as a single dose; sexual partners should be treated at the same time

Dosage adjustment in renal impairment: Not necessary

Hemodialysis: An additional dose equal to ½ the usual dose, should be administered at the end of hemodialysis if tinidazole is administered on a day hemodialysis occurs

Dosage adjustment in hepatic impairment: Specific recommendations are not available; use with caution

Dietary Considerations Take with food. The manufacturer recommends that ethanol be avoided during treatment and for 3 days after therapy is complete.

Administration Administer with food

Test Interactions May interfere with AST, ALT, triglycerides, glucose, and LDH testing

Dosage Forms Tablet, scored: 250 mg, 500 mg

Extemporaneous Preparations To prepare an oral suspension: Grind four 500 mg tablets to a fine powder. Add cherry syrup 10 mL and mix until smooth. Transfer to a graduated container, rinsing mortar with a small amount of cherry syrup to remove any remaining medication. Add additional cherry syrup to q.s. to 30 mL. Suspension is stable for 7 days at room temperature. Shake well before using.

Tioconazole (tye oh KONE a zole)

U.S. Brand Names 1-Day™ [OTC]; Vagistat®-1 [OTC]

Generic Available No

Use Local treatment of vulvovaginal candidiasis

Pregnancy Risk Factor C

Contraindications Hypersensitivity to tioconazole or any component of the formulation

Warnings/Precautions For vaginal use only. Petrolatum-based vaginal products may damage rubber or latex condoms or diaphragms. Separate use by 3 days.

Adverse Reactions Frequency not defined.

Central nervous system: Headache

Gastrointestinal: Abdominal pain

Dermatologic: Burning, desquamation

Genitourinary: Discharge, dyspareunia, dysuria, irritation, itching, nocturia, vaginal pain, vaginitis, vulvar swelling

(Continued)

Tioconazole *(Continued)*

Drug Interactions

Cytochrome P450 Effect: Inhibits CYP1A2 (weak), 2A6 (weak), 2C8/9 (weak), 2C19 (weak), 2D6 (weak), 2E1 (weak)

Stability Store at room temperature.

Mechanism of Action A 1-substituted imidazole derivative with a broad antifungal spectrum against a wide variety of dermatophytes and yeasts, including *Trichophyton mentagrophytes, T. rubrum, T. erinacei, T. tonsurans, Microsporum canis, Microsporum gypseum,* and *Candida albicans.* Both agents appear to be similarly effective against *Epidermophyton floccosum.*

Pharmacodynamics/Kinetics

Onset of action: Some improvement: Within 24 hours; Complete relief: Within 7 days
Absorption: Intravaginal: Systemic (small amounts)
Distribution: Vaginal fluid: 24-72 hours
Excretion: Urine and feces

Dosage Adults: Vaginal: Insert 1 applicatorful in vagina, just prior to bedtime, as a single dose

Administration Insert high into vagina

Patient Information Insert high into vagina; contact prescriber if itching or burning continues; May interact with condoms and vaginal contraceptive diaphragms (ie, weaken latex); do not rely on these products for 3 days following treatment

Dosage Forms Ointment, vaginal: 6.5% (4.6 g) [with applicator]

Tipranavir (tip RA na veer)

U.S. Brand Names Aptivus®

Synonyms TPV; PNU-140690E

Generic Available No

Use Treatment of HIV-1 infections in combination with ritonavir and other antiretroviral agents; limited to highly treatment experienced or multi-protease inhibitor resistant patients.

Drug of Choice or Alternative for Organism(s):

Human Immunodeficiency Virus *on page 181*

Pregnancy Risk Factor C

Pregnancy Implications It is not known if tipranavir crosses the human placenta. Pregnancy and protease inhibitors are both associated with an increased risk of hyperglycemia. Glucose levels should be closely monitored. Women receiving estrogen (as hormonal contraception or replacement therapy) have an increased incidence of rash. Alternative forms of contraception may be needed. Health professionals are encouraged to contact the antiretroviral pregnancy registry to monitor outcomes of pregnant women exposed to antiretroviral medications (1-800-258-4263 or www.APRegistry.com).

Contraindications Hypersensitivity to tipranavir or any component of the formulation or any contraindication to ritonavir therapy; concurrent therapy of tipranavir/ritonavir with alfuzosin, amiodarone, bepridil, cisapride, dihydroergotamine, ergonovine, ergotamine, flecainide, lovastatin, methylergonovine, midazolam, pimozide, propafenone, quinidine, simvastatin, St John's wort, triazolam, and voriconazole; patients with hepatic insufficiency (Child-Pugh Class B and C)

Warnings/Precautions Coadministration with ritonavir is required. May cause hepatitis or exacerbate pre-existing hepatic dysfunction; use with caution in patients with hepatitis B or C and in hepatic disease. May be associated with fat redistribution (buffalo hump, increased abdominal girth, breast engorgement, facial atrophy). Use caution in hemophilia. May increase cholesterol and/or triglycerides; hypertriglyceridemia may increase risk of pancreatitis. May cause hyperglycemia. Use with caution in patients with sulfonamide allergy or hemophilia. Tipranavir has been associated with dermatological adverse effects, including rash (sometimes accompanied by joint pain, throat tightness, or generalized pruritus) and photosensitivity. Immune reconstitution syndrome, including inflammatory responses to indolent infections, has been associated with antiretroviral therapy; additional evaluation and treatment may be required.

Tipranavir should be used with caution in combination with other agents metabolized by CYP3A4. Avoid concurrent use of lovastatin or simvastatin (risk of rhabdomyolysis may be increased). Avoid concurrent use of hormonal contraceptives, rifampin, and/or St John's wort (may lead to loss of virologic response and/or resistance). Use with caution with metronidazole or disulfiram (due to ethanol content of formulation). Safety and efficacy have not been established in children.

Adverse Reactions Protease inhibitors cause dyslipidemia which includes elevated cholesterol and triglycerides and a redistribution of body fat centrally to cause

increased abdominal girth, buffalo hump, facial atrophy, and breast enlargement. These agents also cause hyperglycemia.

>10%:

Endocrine & mMetabolic: Hypercholesterolemia (>300 mg/dL: 11%), hypertriglyceridemia (>400 mg/dL: 26%)

Gastrointestinal: Diarrhea (11%)

Hepatic: Transaminase increased (ALT or AST: 24%)

2% to 10%:

Central nervous system: Fever (5%), fatigue (4%), headache (3%), depression (2%)

Dermatologic: Rash (2%)

Endocrine & metabolic: Amylase increased (3%)

Gastrointestinal: Nausea (7%), vomiting (3%), abdominal pain (3%), amylase increased (3%)

Hematologic: WBC decreased (grade 3-4: 4%)

Neuromuscular & skeletal: Weakness (2%)

Respiratory: Bronchitis (3%)

<2%: Abdominal distension, anemia, anorexia, appetite decreased, cough, dehydration, diabetes mellitus, dizziness, dyspepsia, dyspnea, exanthem, facial wasting, flatulence, gastroesophageal reflux, hepatic failure, hepatitis, hyperglycemia, hypersensitivity, insomnia, lipase increased, lipoatrophy, lipodystrophy (acquired), lipohypertrophy, muscle cramp, myalgia, neuropathy (peripheral), neutropenia, pancreatitis, pruritus, renal insufficiency, sleep disorder, somnolence, thrombocytopenia, viral infection (reactivation of herpes/varicella infection), weight loss

Drug Interactions

Cytochrome P450 Effect:

Substrate of CYP3A4 (major; minimal metabolism when coadministered with ritonavir)

Ritonavir: **Inhibits**CYP3A4 (strong) and 2D6

Increased Effect/Toxicity: Note: Listed interactions include interactions resulting from coadministration with ritonavir. Refer to Ritonavir *on page 1055* monograph for additional interaction concerns. The serum concentrations of tipranavir may be increased by ritonavir. This combination is recommended to enhance the effect ("boost") tipranavir.

Tipranavir/ritonavir may increase the levels/effects of CYP3A4 substrates. Tipranavir/ritonavir may increase the toxicity of benzodiazepines; concurrent use of midazolam and triazolam is specifically contraindicated. Tipranavir may increase serum concentrations of cisapride, increasing the risk of malignant arrhythmias; use is contraindicated. Toxicity of pimozide is significantly increased by tipranavir/ritonavir; concurrent use is contraindicated. Tipranavir/ritonavir may increase serum concentrations/toxicity of several antiarrhythmic agents; contraindicated with amiodarone, bepridil, flecainide, propafenone, and quinidine (use extreme caution with lidocaine). Tipranavir/ritonavir may also increase serum concentrations/effects of calcium channel blockers and immunosuppressants (cyclosporine, sirolimus, tacrolimus).

Serum concentrations of HMG-CoA reductase inhibitors (atorvastatin, cerivastatin, lovastatin, simvastatin) may be increased by tipranavir/ritonavir, increasing the risk of myopathy/rhabdomyolysis. Lovastatin and simvastatin are not recommended. Use lowest possible dose of atorvastatin. Fluvastatin and pravastatin may be safer alternatives. Serum concentrations of rifabutin may be increased by tipranavir/ritonavir; dosage adjustment of rifabutin is required.

The toxicity of ergot alkaloids (dihydroergotamine, ergotamine, ergonovine, methylergonovine) is increased by tipranavir; concurrent use is contraindicated. Effects of hypoglycemic agents may be altered by tipranavir/ritonavir. Concurrent therapy with tipranavir may increase serum concentrations of normeperidine, and decrease serum concentrations of meperidine. The serum concentrations of sildenafil, tadalafil, and vardenafil may be increased by tipranavir/ritonavir; dose adjustment and limitations related to ritonavir coadministration must be recognized.

Concurrent use of disulfiram with tipranavir oral solution is contraindicated due to risk of adverse reaction (due to alcohol content of formulation). Clarithromycin may increase serum concentrations of tipranavir. Tipranavir/ritonavir may increase serum concentrations of clarithromycin. Use with caution and adjust dose of clarithromycin during concurrent therapy in renally impaired patients.

Decreased Effect: CYP3A4 inducers may decrease the levels/effects of tipranavir. Example inducers include aminoglutethimide, carbamazepine, nafcillin, nevirapine, phenobarbital, phenytoin, and rifamycins. When coadministered with ritonavir, reduction of tipranavir serum concentrations is unlikely. Rifampin may decrease

(Continued)

Tipranavir *(Continued)*

serum concentrations of tipranavir. Concurrent use of rifampin is not recommended. The effect of methadone may be reduced by tipranavir (dosage increase may be required).

Serum concentrations of protease inhibitors may be decreased by tipranavir. Concurrent therapy with amprenavir, lopinavir, or saquinavir is not recommended. Tipranavir/ritonavir may decrease serum concentrations of nucleoside reverse transcriptase inhibitors (NRTIs, including abacavir, didanosine, and zidovudine); administer tipranavir/ritonavir 2 hours before or after didanosine.

Ethanol/Nutrition/Herb Interactions

Ethanol: Capsules contain dehydrated alcohol 7% w/w (0.1g per capsule)
Food: Bioavailability is increased with a high-fat meal.

Stability Prior to opening bottle, store under refrigeration at 2°C to 8°C (36°F to 46°F). After bottle is opened, may be stored at 25°C (77°F), with excursions permitted to 15°C to 30°C (59°F to 86°F) for up to 60 days.

Mechanism of Action Tipranavir is a nonpeptide inhibitor of HIV-1 protease. It binds to the protease activity site and inhibits the activity of the enzyme. HIV protease is required for the cleavage of viral polyprotein precursors into individual functional proteins found in infectious HIV. Inhibition prevents cleavage of these polyproteins, resulting in the formation of immature, noninfectious viral particles.

Pharmacodynamics/Kinetics

Absorption: Incomplete (percentage not established)
Protein binding: 99%
Metabolism: Hepatic, via CYP3A4 (minimal when coadministered with ritonavir)
Bioavailability: Not established
Half-life elimination: 6 hours
Excretion: Feces (82%); urine (4%); primarily as unchanged drug (when coadministered with ritonavir)

Dosage Oral: Adults: 500 mg twice daily with a high-fat meal. **Note:** Coadministration with ritonavir (200 mg twice daily) is required.

Dosage adjustment in renal impairment: No adjustment required

Dietary Considerations Contains dehydrated alcohol 7% w/w (0.1 g per capsule)

Administration Should be administered with food (bioavailability is increased); coadministration with ritonavir is standard

Monitoring Parameters Viral load, CD4, serum glucose, liver function tests, bilirubin

Dosage Forms Capsule, gelatin: 250 mg [contains dehydrated ethanol 7% per capsule]

TipTapToe [OTC] *see* Tolnaftate *on page 1127*
Tisit® [OTC] *see* Pyrethrins and Piperonyl Butoxide *on page 1023*
Tisit® Blue Gel [OTC] *see* Pyrethrins and Piperonyl Butoxide *on page 1023*
TMP *see* Trimethoprim *on page 1130*
TMP-SMZ *see* Sulfamethoxazole and Trimethoprim *on page 1087*
TOBI® *see* Tobramycin *on page 1122*
TobraDex® *see* Tobramycin and Dexamethasone *on page 1126*

Tobramycin (toe bra MYE sin)

Related Information

Aminoglycoside Dosing and Monitoring *on page 1267*
Antimicrobial Activity Against Selected Organisms *on page 1165*

U.S. Brand Names AKTob®; TOBI®; Tobrex®

Canadian Brand Names Apo-Tobramycin®; Nebcin®; PMS-Tobramycin; TOBI®; Tobrex®; Tomycine™

Synonyms Tobramycin Sulfate

Generic Available Yes; Excludes ophthalmic ointment, solution for nebulization

Use Treatment of documented or suspected infections caused by susceptible gram-negative bacilli including *Pseudomonas aeruginosa*; topically used to treat superficial ophthalmic infections caused by susceptible bacteria. Tobramycin solution for inhalation is indicated for the management of cystic fibrosis patients (>6 years of age) with *Pseudomonas aeruginosa*.

Drug of Choice or Alternative for Disease/Syndrome(s):

Endophthalmitis, Bacterial and Fungal *on page 128*
Meningitis, Postsurgical *on page 218*
Pneumonia, Hospital-Acquired *on page 272*
Pneumonia, Ventilator-Associated *on page 273*

Organism(s):

Burkholderia cepacia on page 62

Pregnancy Risk Factor D (injection, inhalation); B (ophthalmic)

Pregnancy Implications Aminoglycosides, including tobramycin, cross the placenta. The manufacturers of Nebcin® and TOBI® have a labeled pregnancy category of D based on reports of bilateral congenital deafness in children whose mothers used streptomycin during pregnancy. The risk of teratogenic effects and deafness following *in utero* exposure to tobramycin is considered to be small and some resources consider the pregnancy risk factor to be C. The manufacturer of Tobrex® states that animal studies have not shown harm to the fetus; however, no adequate and well-controlled studies have been conducted in pregnant women.

Contraindications Hypersensitivity to tobramycin, other aminoglycosides, or any component of the formulation; pregnancy (injection/inhalation)

Warnings/Precautions Use with caution in patients with renal impairment; pre-existing auditory or vestibular impairment; and in patients with neuromuscular disorders. Dosage modification required in patients with impaired renal function (I.M. & I.V.). Aminoglycosides are associated with significant nephrotoxicity or ototoxicity; the ototoxicity is directly proportional to the amount of drug given and the duration of treatment. Tinnitus or vertigo are indications of vestibular injury. Ototoxicity is often irreversible. Renal damage is usually reversible.

Adverse Reactions

Injection: Frequency not defined:

- Central nervous system: Confusion, disorientation, dizziness, fever, headache, lethargy, vertigo
- Dermatologic: Exfoliative dermatitis, itching, rash, urticaria
- Endocrine & metabolic: Serum calcium, magnesium, potassium, and/or sodium decreased
- Gastrointestinal: Diarrhea, nausea, vomiting
- Hematologic: Anemia, eosinophilia, granulocytopenia, leukocytosis, leukopenia, thrombocytopenia
- Hepatic: ALT, AST, bilirubin, and/or LDH increased
- Local: Pain at the injection site
- Otic: Hearing loss, tinnitus, ototoxicity (auditory), ototoxicity (vestibular), roaring in the ears
- Renal: BUN increased, cylindruria, serum creatinine increased, oliguria, proteinuria

Inhalation:

- >10%:
  - Gastrointestinal: Sputum discoloration (21%)
  - Respiratory: Voice alteration (13%)
- 1% to 10%:
  - Central nervous system: Malaise (6%)
  - Otic: Tinnitus (3%)
- Postmarketing and/or case reports: Hearing loss

Ophthalmic: <1%: Ocular: Conjunctival erythema, lid itching, lid swelling

Overdosage/Toxicology Symptoms include ototoxicity, nephrotoxicity, and neuromuscular toxicity. The treatment of choice following a single acute overdose appears to be the maintenance of urine output of at least 3 mL/kg/hour. Dialysis is of questionable value in the enhancement of aminoglycoside elimination. If required, hemodialysis is preferred over peritoneal dialysis in patients with normal renal function. Careful hydration may be all that is required to promote diuresis and therefore enhance elimination.

Drug Interactions

Increased Effect/Toxicity: Increased antimicrobial effect of tobramycin with extended spectrum penicillins (synergistic). Neuromuscular blockers may have an increased duration of action (neuromuscular blockade). Amphotericin B, cephalosporins, and loop diuretics may increase the risk of nephrotoxicity.

Stability

Injection: Stable at room temperature both as the clear, colorless solution and as the dry powder. Stability of parenteral admixture at room temperature (25°C) and at refrigeration temperature (4°C) is 48 hours. Reconstituted solutions remain stable for 24 hours at room temperature and 96 hours when refrigerated.

Separate administration of extended-spectrum penicillins (eg, carbenicillin, ticarcillin, piperacillin) from tobramycin in patients with severe renal impairment; tobramycin's efficacy may be reduced if given concurrently.

Ophthalmic solution: Store at 8°C to 27°C (46°F to 80°F).

Solution, for inhalation (TOBI®): Store under refrigeration at 2°C to 8°C (36°F to 46°F); may be stored in foil pouch at room temperature of 25°C (77°F) for up to 28 days. Avoid intense light. Solution may darken over time; however, do not use if cloudy or contains particles.

Mechanism of Action Interferes with bacterial protein synthesis by binding to 30S and 50S ribosomal subunits resulting in a defective bacterial cell membrane

(Continued)

Tobramycin *(Continued)*

Pharmacodynamics/Kinetics

Absorption: I.M.: Rapid and complete

Distribution: V_d: 0.2-0.3 L/kg; Pediatrics: 0.2-0.7 L/kg; to extracellular fluid including serum, abscesses, ascitic, pericardial, pleural, synovial, lymphatic, and peritoneal fluids; crosses placenta; poor penetration into CSF, eye, bone, prostate

Protein binding: <30%

Half-life elimination:

- Neonates: ≤1200 g: 11 hours; >1200 g: 2-9 hours
- Adults: 2-3 hours; directly dependent upon glomerular filtration rate
- Adults with impaired renal function: 5-70 hours

Time to peak, serum: I.M.: 30-60 minutes; I.V.: ~30 minutes

Excretion: Normal renal function: Urine (~90% to 95%) within 24 hours

Dosage

Individualization is **critical** because of the low therapeutic index.

Use of ideal body weight (IBW) for determining the mg/kg/dose appears to be more accurate than dosing on the basis of total body weight (TBW). In morbid obesity, dosage requirement may best be estimated using a dosing weight of IBW + 0.4 (TBW - IBW).

Initial and periodic plasma drug levels (eg, peak and trough with conventional dosing) should be determined, particularly in critically-ill patients with serious infections or in disease states known to significantly alter aminoglycoside pharmacokinetics (eg, cystic fibrosis, burns, or major surgery).

I.M., I.V.:

- Infants and Children <5 years: 2.5 mg/kg/dose every 8 hours
- Children >5 years: 2-2.5 g/kg/dose every 8 hours
  - Cystic fibrosis: 2.5-3.3 mg/kg every 6-8 hours
- **Note:** Some patients may require larger or more frequent doses if serum levels document the need (eg, cystic fibrosis or febrile granulocytopenic patients). Also see "Note" on monitoring and adjustment.
- Adults:
  - Severe life-threatening infections:
    - Conventional dosing: 2-2.5 mg/kg/dose every 8-12 hours; to ensure adequate peak concentrations early in therapy, higher initial dosages may be considered in selected patients (eg, edema, septic shock, postsurgery, and/or trauma).
    - Once-daily dosing: Some clinicians suggest a daily dose of 4-7 mg/kg for all patients with normal renal function; this dose is at least as efficacious with similar, if not less, toxicity than conventional dosing.
  - Urinary tract infection: 1.5 mg/kg/dose
  - Synergy (for gram-positive infections): 1 mg/kg/dose

Ophthalmic: Children ≥2 months and Adults:

- Ointment: Apply 2-3 times/day; for severe infections, apply every 3-4 hours
- Solution: Instill 1-2 drops every 4 hours; for severe infections, instill 2 drops every 30-60 minutes initially, then reduce to less frequent intervals

Inhalation: Pulmonary infections:

- Standard aerosolized tobramycin:
  - Children: 40-80 mg 2-3 times/day
  - Adults: 60-80 mg 3 times/day
- High-dose regimen: Children ≥6 years and Adults: 300 mg every 12 hours (do not administer doses <6 hours apart); administer in repeated cycles of 28 days on drug followed by 28 days off drug

Dosing interval in renal impairment: I.M., I.V.:

- Conventional dosing:
  - Cl_{cr} ≥60 mL/minute: Administer every 8 hours
  - Cl_{cr} 40-60 mL/minute: Administer every 12 hours
  - Cl_{cr} 20-40 mL/minute: Administer every 24 hours
  - Cl_{cr} 10-20 mL/minute: Administer every 48 hours
  - Cl_{cr} <10 mL/minute: Administer every 72 hours
- High-dose therapy: Interval may be extended (eg, every 48 hours) in patients with moderate renal impairment (Cl_{cr} 30-59 mL/minute) and/or adjusted based on serum level determinations.

Hemodialysis: Dialyzable; 30% removal of aminoglycosides occurs during 4 hours of HD - administer dose after dialysis and follow levels

Continuous arteriovenous or venovenous hemofiltration: Dose as for Cl_{cr} of 10-40 mL/minute and follow levels

- Administration in CAPD fluid:
  - Gram-negative infection: 4-8 mg/L (4-8 mcg/mL) of CAPD fluid
  - Gram-positive infection (ie, synergy): 3-4 mg/L (3-4 mcg/mL) of CAPD fluid

Administration IVPB/I.M.: Dose as for Cl_{cr} <10 mL/minute and follow levels

Dosing adjustment/comments in hepatic disease: Monitor plasma concentrations

Dietary Considerations May require supplementation of calcium, magnesium, potassium.

Administration

I.V.: Infuse over 30-60 minutes; give penicillins or cephalosporins at least 1 hour apart from tobramycin. Flush with saline before and after administration.

Inhalation (TOBI®): To be inhaled over ~15 minutes using a handheld nebulizer.

Ophthalmic: Contact lenses should not be worn during treatment of ophthalmic infections.

Ointment: Do not touch tip of tube to eye. Instill ointment into pocket between eyeball and lower lid; patient should look downward before closing eye.

Solution: Allow 5 minutes between application of "multiple-drop" therapy.

Suspension: Shake well before using; Tilt head back, instill suspension in conjunctival sac and close eye(s). Do not touch dropper to eye. Apply light finger pressure on lacrimal sac for 1 minute following instillation.

Monitoring Parameters Urinalysis, urine output, BUN, serum creatinine, peak and trough plasma tobramycin levels; be alert to ototoxicity; hearing should be tested before and during treatment

Reference Range

Timing of serum samples: Draw peak 30 minutes after 30-minute infusion has been completed or 1 hour following I.M. injection or beginning of infusion; draw trough immediately before next dose

Therapeutic levels:

Peak:

- Serious infections: 6-8 mcg/mL (SI: 12-17 mg/L)
- Life-threatening infections: 8-10 mcg/mL (SI: 17-21 mg/L)
- Urinary tract infections: 4-6 mcg/mL (SI: 7-12 mg/L)
- Synergy against gram-positive organisms: 3-5 mcg/mL

Trough:

- Serious infections: 0.5-1 mcg/mL
- Life-threatening infections: 1-2 mcg/mL
- Monitor serum creatinine and urine output; obtain drug levels after the third dose unless otherwise directed

Inhalation: Serum levels are ~1 mcg/mL one hour following a 300 mg dose in patients with normal renal function.

Patient Information Report symptoms of superinfection; for eye drops - no other eye drops 5-10 minutes before or after tobramycin; report any dizziness or sensations of ringing or fullness in ears

Additional Information Once-daily dosing: Higher peak serum drug concentration to MIC ratios, demonstrated aminoglycoside postantibiotic effect, decreased renal cortex drug uptake, and improved cost-time efficiency are supportive reasons for the use of once daily dosing regimens for aminoglycosides. Current research indicates these regimens to be as effective for nonlife-threatening infections, with no higher incidence of nephrotoxicity, than those requiring multiple daily doses. Doses are determined by calculating the entire day's dose via usual multiple dose calculation techniques and administering this quantity as a single dose. Doses are then adjusted to maintain mean serum concentrations above the MIC(s) of the causative organism(s). (Example: 2.5-5 mg/kg as a single dose; expected Cp_{max}: 10-20 mcg/mL and Cp_{min}: <1 mcg/mL). Further research is needed for universal recommendation in all patient populations and gram-negative disease; exceptions may include those with known high clearance (eg, children, patients with cystic fibrosis, or burns who may require shorter dosage intervals) and patients with renal function impairment for whom longer than conventional dosage intervals are usually required.

Dosage Forms

Infusion []premixed in NS]: 60 mg (50 mL); 80 mg (100 mL)

Injection, powder for reconstitution: 1.2 g

Injection, solution: 10 mg/mL (2 mL, 8 mL); 40 mg/mL (2 mL, 30 mL, 50 mL) [may contain sodium metabisulfite]

Ointment, ophthalmic (Tobrex®): 0.3% (3.5 g)

Solution for nebulization [preservative free] (TOBI®): 60 mg/mL (5 mL)

Solution, ophthalmic (AKTob®, Tobrex®): 0.3% (5 mL) [contains benzalkonium chloride]

Selected Readings

Begg EJ and Barclay ML, "Aminoglycosides - 50 Years On," *Br J Clin Pharmacol*, 1995, 39(6):597-603.

Cunha BA, "Aminoglycosides: Current Role in Antimicrobial Therapy," *Pharmacotherapy*, 1988, 8(6):334-50.

Edson RS and Terrell CL, "The Aminoglycosides," *Mayo Clin Proc*, 1999, 74(5):519-28.

Gilbert DN, "Once-Daily Aminoglycoside Therapy," *Antimicrob Agents Chemother*, 1991, 35(3):399-405.

(Continued)

Tobramycin *(Continued)*

Hustinx WN, and Hoepelman IM, "Aminoglycoside Dosage Regimens. Is Once a Day Enough?" *Clin Pharmacokinet*, 1993, 25(6):427-32.
Lortholary O, Tod M, Cohen Y, et al, "Aminoglycosides," *Med Clin North Am*, 1995, 79(4):761-87.
McCormack JP and Jewesson PJ, "A Critical Re-evaluation of the "Therapeutic Range" of Aminoglycosides," *Clin Infect Dis*, 1992, 14(1):320-39.

Tobramycin and Dexamethasone

(toe bra MYE sin & deks a METH a sone)

Related Information

Tobramycin *on page 1122*

U.S. Brand Names TobraDex®

Canadian Brand Names Tobradex®

Synonyms Dexamethasone and Tobramycin

Generic Available No

Use Treatment of external ocular infection caused by susceptible gram-negative bacteria and steroid responsive inflammatory conditions of the palpebral and bulbar conjunctiva, lid, cornea, and anterior segment of the globe

Pregnancy Risk Factor C

Pregnancy Implications See individual agents.

Contraindications Hypersensitivity to tobramycin, dexamethasone, or any component of the formulation; viral, fungal, or tuberculosis diseases of the eye

Warnings/Precautions Sensitivity to tobramycin may develop; discontinue if sensitivity reaction occurs. Prolonged use of corticosteroids may result in glaucoma; damage to the optic nerve, defects in visual acuity and fields of vision, and posterior subcapsular cataract formation may occur. Prolonged use of corticosteroids may increase the incidence of secondary ocular infection or mask acute infection (including fungal infections); may prolong or exacerbate ocular viral infections; use following cataract surgery may delay healing or increase the incidence of bleb formation. A maximum of 8 g of ointment or 20 mL of suspension should be prescribed initially; patients should be evaluated prior to additional refills. Suspension contains benzalkonium chloride which may be adsorbed by contact lenses; contact lenses should not be worn during treatment of ophthalmic infections. Safety and efficacy have not been established in patients <2 years of age.

Adverse Reactions Unless otherwise noted, frequency not defined.

Dermatologic: Allergic contact dermatitis, delayed wound healing

Ocular: Cataract formation, conjunctival erythema (<4%), glaucoma, intraocular pressure increased, keratitis, lacrimation, lid itching (<4%), lid swelling (<4%), optic nerve damage, secondary infection

Drug Interactions

Cytochrome P450 Effect: Dexamethasone: **Substrate** of CYP3A4 (minor); **Induces** CYP2A6 (weak), 2B6 (weak), 2C8/9 (weak), 3A4 (weak)

Increased Effect/Toxicity: See individual agents.

Decreased Effect: See individual agents.

Mechanism of Action Refer to individual monographs for Dexamethasone and Tobramycin

Pharmacodynamics/Kinetics

Absorption: Into aqueous humor

Time to peak, serum: 1-2 hours in the cornea and aqueous humor

Dosage Children and Adults: Ophthalmic: Instill 1-2 drops of solution every 4 hours; apply ointment 2-3 times/day; for severe infections apply ointment every 3-4 hours, or solution 2 drops every 30-60 minutes initially, then reduce to less frequent intervals

Administration Contact lenses should not be worn during therapy.

Ointment: Do not touch tip of tube to eye. Instill ointment into pocket between eyeball and lower lid; patient should look downward before closing eye.

Suspension: Shake well before using; Tilt head back, instill suspension in conjunctival sac and close eye(s). Do not touch dropper to eye. Apply light finger pressure on lacrimal sac for 1 minute following instillation.

Monitoring Parameters Intraocular pressure and secondary infection with prolonged use

Additional Information Complete prescribing information for this medication should be consulted for additional detail.

Dosage Forms

Ointment, ophthalmic: Tobramycin 0.3% and dexamethasone 0.1% (3.5 g)

Suspension, ophthalmic: Tobramycin 0.3% and dexamethasone 0.1% (2.5 mL, 5 mL, 10 mL) [contains benzalkonium chloride]

Tobramycin Sulfate *see* Tobramycin *on page 1122*

Tobrex® *see* Tobramycin *on page 1122*

Tolnaftate (tole NAF tate)

U.S. Brand Names Absorbine Jr.® Antifungal [OTC]; Aftate® Antifungal [OTC]; Blis-To-Sol® [OTC]; Dermasept Antifungal [OTC]; Fungi-Guard [OTC]; Gold Bond® Antifungal [OTC]; Tinactin® Antifungal [OTC]; Tinactin® Antifungal Jock Itch [OTC]; Tinaderm [OTC]; Ting® [OTC]; TipTapToe [OTC]

Canadian Brand Names Pitrex

Generic Available Yes: Cream, powder, solution, swabs

Use Treatment of tinea pedis, tinea cruris, tinea corporis

Pregnancy Risk Factor C

Contraindications Hypersensitivity to tolnaftate or any component of the formulation; nail and scalp infections

Warnings/Precautions For external use only; apply to clean, dry skin; keep away from eyes

Adverse Reactions Frequency not defined.

Dermatologic: Pruritus, contact dermatitis

Local: Irritation, stinging

Mechanism of Action Distorts the hyphae and stunts mycelial growth in susceptible fungi

Pharmacodynamics/Kinetics Onset of action: 24-72 hours

Dosage Children ≥2 years and Adults: Topical: Wash and dry affected area; spray aerosol or apply 1-3 drops of solution or a small amount of cream, gel, or powder and rub into the affected areas 2 times/day

Note: May use for up to 4 weeks for tinea pedis or tinea corporis, and up to 2 weeks for tinea cruris

Patient Information Avoid contact with the eyes; apply to clean dry area; consult the prescriber if a skin irritation develops or if the skin infection worsens or does not improve after 10 days of therapy; does not stain skin or clothing

Dosage Forms

Aerosol, liquid, topical:
- Aftate®: 1% (120 mL) [contains alcohol]
- Tinactin® Antifungal: 1% (120 mL) [contains alcohol]
- Ting®: 1% (90 mL)

Aerosol, powder, topical:
- Aftate®: 1% (105 g) [contains alcohol]
- Tinactin® Antifungal: 1% (45 g, 90 g, 100 g, 150 g) [contains alcohol]
- Tinactin® Antifungal Jock Itch: 1% (100 g) [contains alcohol]
- Ting®: 1% (90 g)

Cream, topical: 1% (15 g, 30 g)
- Fungi-Guard: 1% (15 g)
- Tinactin® Antifungal: 1% (15 g, 30 g)
- Tinactin® Antifungal Jock Itch: 1% (15 g)

Gel, topical (Absorbine Jr.® Antifungal): 1% (21 g)

Liquid, topical:
- Blis-To-Sol®: 1% (30 mL, 55 mL)
- Dermasept Antifungal: 1% (30 mL) [contains benzyl alcohol and benzoic acid]

Powder, topical: 1% (45 g)

Solution, topical: 1% (10 mL)
- Absorbine Jr.® Antifungal: 1% (60 mL)
- Tinaderm: 1% (10 mL)

Swab, topical [liquid-filled swabstick]: 1% (36s)
- Gold Bond® Antifungal: 1% (24s)
- TipTapToe: 1% (72s)

Tomycine™ (Can) *see* Tobramycin *on page 1122*

TPV; PNU-140690E *see* Tipranavir *on page 1120*

***trans*-Retinoic Acid** *see* Tretinoin (Topical) *on page 1127*

Trecator® *see* Ethionamide *on page 814*

Tretinoin (Topical) (TRET i noyn, TOP i kal)

U.S. Brand Names Avita®; Renova®; Retin-A®; Retin-A® Micro

Canadian Brand Names Rejuva-A®; Retin-A®; Retin-A® Micro; Retinova®

Synonyms Retinoic Acid; *trans*-Retinoic Acid; Vitamin A Acid

Generic Available Yes: Cream, gel

Use Treatment of acne vulgaris; photodamaged skin; palliation of fine wrinkles, mottled hyperpigmentation, and tactile roughness of facial skin as part of a comprehensive skin care and sun avoidance program

Unlabeled/Investigational Use Some skin cancers

(Continued)

Tretinoin (Topical) *(Continued)*

Drug of Choice or Alternative for Disease/Syndrome(s):

Acne Vulgaris *on page 27*

Pregnancy Risk Factor C

Pregnancy Implications Oral tretinoin is teratogenic and fetotoxic in rats at doses 1000 and 500 times the topical human dose, respectively. Tretinoin does not appear to be teratogenic when used topically since it is rapidly metabolized by the skin; however, there are rare reports of fetal defects. Use for acne only if benefit to mother outweighs potential risk to fetus. During pregnancy, do not use for palliation of fine wrinkles, mottled hyperpigmentation, and tactile roughness of facial skin.

Contraindications Hypersensitivity to tretinoin or any component of the formulation; sunburn

Warnings/Precautions Use with caution in patients with eczema; avoid excessive exposure to sunlight and sunlamps; avoid contact with abraded skin, mucous membranes, eyes, mouth, angles of the nose. Palliation of fine wrinkles, mottled hyperpigmentation, and tactile roughness of facial skin: Do not use the 0.05% cream for longer than 48 weeks or the 0.02% cream for longer than 52 weeks. Not for use on moderate- to heavily-pigmented skin. Gel is flammable; do not expose to high temperatures or flame.

Adverse Reactions

>10%: Dermatologic: Excessive dryness, erythema, scaling of the skin, pruritus

1% to 10%:

Dermatologic: Hyperpigmentation or hypopigmentation, photosensitivity, initial acne flare-up

Local: Edema, blistering, stinging

Overdosage/Toxicology Excessive application may lead to marked redness, peeling or discomfort. Oral ingestion of the topical product may lead to the same adverse reactions seen with excessive vitamin A intake (increased intracranial pressure, jaundice, ascites, cutaneous desquamation; symptoms of acute overdose [12,000 units/kg] include nausea, vomiting, and diarrhea). Toxic signs of an overdose commonly respond to drug discontinuation, and generally return to normal spontaneously within a few days to weeks. When confronted with signs of increased intracranial pressure, treatment with mannitol (0.25 g/kg I.V. up to 1 g/kg/dose repeated every 5 minutes as needed), dexamethasone (1.5 mg/kg I.V. load followed with 0.375 mg/kg every 6 hours for 5 days), and/or hyperventilation should be employed.

Drug Interactions

Cytochrome P450 Effect: Substrate (minor) of CYP2A6, 2B6, 2C8/9; **Inhibits** CYP2C8/9 (weak); **Induces** CYP2E1 (weak)

Increased Effect/Toxicity: Topical application of sulfur, benzoyl peroxide, salicylic acid, resorcinol, or any product with strong drying effects potentiates adverse reactions with tretinoin.

Photosensitizing medications (thiazides, tetracyclines, fluoroquinolones, phenothiazines, sulfonamides) augment phototoxicity and should not be used when treating palliation of fine wrinkles, mottled hyperpigmentation, and tactile roughness of facial skin.

Ethanol/Nutrition/Herb Interactions

Food: Avoid excessive intake of vitamin A (cod liver oil, halibut fish oil).

Herb/Nutraceutical: Avoid dong quai, St John's wort (may also cause photosensitization). Avoid excessive amounts of vitamin A supplements.

Stability Store at 25°C (77°F); gel is flammable, keep away from heat and flame

Mechanism of Action Keratinocytes in the sebaceous follicle become less adherent which allows for easy removal; inhibits microcomedone formation and eliminates lesions already present

Pharmacodynamics/Kinetics

Absorption: Minimal

Metabolism: Hepatic for the small amount absorbed

Excretion: Urine and feces

Dosage Topical:

Children >12 years and Adults: Acne vulgaris: Begin therapy with a weaker formulation of tretinoin (0.025% cream, 0.04% microsphere gel, or 0.01% gel) and increase the concentration as tolerated; apply once daily to acne lesions before retiring or on alternate days; if stinging or irritation develop, decrease frequency of application

Adults ≥18: Palliation of fine wrinkles, mottled hyperpigmentation, and tactile roughness of facial skin: Pea-sized amount of the 0.02% or 0.05% cream applied to entire face once daily in the evening

Elderly: Use of the 0.02% cream in patients 65-71 years of age showed similar improvement in fine wrinkles as seen in patients <65 years. Safety and efficacy of the 0.02% cream have not been established in patients >71 years of age. Safety and efficacy of the 0.05% cream have not been established in patients >50 years of age.

Administration Palliation of fine wrinkles, mottled hyperpigmentation, and tactile roughness of facial skin: Cream: Prior to application, gently wash face with a mild soap. Pat dry. Wait 20-30 minutes to apply cream. Avoid eyes, ears, nostrils, and mouth.

Patient Information For once-daily use, do not overuse. Avoid increased intake of vitamin A. Thoroughly wash hands before applying. Wash area to be treated at least 30 minutes before applying. Do not wash face more frequently than 2-3 times a day. Avoid using topical preparations that contain alcohol or harsh chemicals during treatment. You may experience increased sensitivity to sunlight; protect skin with sunblock (minimum SPF 15), wear protective clothing, or avoid direct sunlight. Stop treatment and inform prescriber if rash, skin irritation, redness, scaling, or excessive dryness occurs. When used for hyperpigmentation and tactile redness of facial skin, wrinkles will not be eliminated. Must be used in combination with a comprehensive skin care program.

Gel: Flammable; do not expose to flame and do not smoke during use.

Dosage Forms [DSC] = Discontinued product

Cream, topical: 0.025% (20 g, 45 g); 0.05% (20 g, 45 g); 0.1% (20 g, 45 g)
- Avita®: 0.025% (20 g, 45 g)
- Renova®: 0.02% (40 g); 0.05% (40 g, 60 g)
- Retin-A®: 0.025% (20 g, 45 g); 0.05% (20 g, 45 g); 0.1% (20 g, 45 g)

Gel, topical: 0.025% (15 g, 45 g)
- Avita®: 0.025% (20 g, 45 g) [contains ethanol 83%]
- Retin-A®: 0.01% (15 g, 45 g); 0.025% (15 g, 45 g) [contains alcohol 90%]
- Retin-A® Micro [microsphere gel]: 0.04% (20 g, 45 g); 0.1% (20 g, 45 g) [contains benzyl alcohol]

Liquid, topical (Retin-A®): 0.05% (28 mL) [contains alcohol 55%] [DSC]

Selected Readings

Winston MH, Shalita AR, "Acne Vulgaris, Pathogenesis and Treatment," *Pediatr Clin North Am*, 1991, 38(4):889-903.

Triacetin (trye a SEE tin)

U.S. Brand Names Myco-Nail [OTC]

Synonyms Glycerol Triacetate

Generic Available No

Use Fungistat for athlete's foot and other superficial fungal infections

Dosage Apply twice daily, cleanse areas with dilute alcohol or mild soap and water before application; continue treatment for 7 days after symptoms have disappeared

Dosage Forms Liquid, topical: 25% (30 mL)

Triacetyloleandomycin *see* Troleandomycin *on page 1133*

Triaconazole *see* Terconazole *on page 1099*

Triamcinolone and Nystatin *see* Nystatin and Triamcinolone *on page 977*

Tribavirin *see* Ribavirin *on page 1040*

Trifluorothymidine *see* Trifluridine *on page 1129*

Trifluridine (trye FLURE i deen)

U.S. Brand Names Viroptic®

Canadian Brand Names SAB-Trifluridine; Viroptic®

Synonyms F_3T; Trifluorothymidine

Generic Available Yes

Use Treatment of primary keratoconjunctivitis and recurrent epithelial keratitis caused by herpes simplex virus types I and II

Pregnancy Risk Factor C

Contraindications Hypersensitivity to trifluridine or any component of the formulation

Warnings/Precautions Mild local irritation of conjunctival and cornea may occur when instilled but usually transient effects

Adverse Reactions

1% to 10%: Local: Burning, stinging

<1%: Hyperemia, palpebral edema, epithelial keratopathy, keratitis, stromal edema, increased intraocular pressure, hypersensitivity reactions

Stability Refrigerate at 2°C to 8°C (36°F to 46°F); storage at room temperature may result in a solution altered pH which could result in ocular discomfort upon administration and/or decreased potency

(Continued)

Trifluridine *(Continued)*

Mechanism of Action Interferes with viral replication by incorporating into viral DNA in place of thymidine, inhibiting thymidylate synthetase resulting in the formation of defective proteins

Pharmacodynamics/Kinetics Absorption: Ophthalmic: Systemic absorption negligible, corneal penetration adequate

Dosage Adults: Instill 1 drop into affected eye every 2 hours while awake, to a maximum of 9 drops/day, until re-epithelialization of corneal ulcer occurs; then use 1 drop every 4 hours for another 7 days; do **not** exceed 21 days of treatment; if improvement has not taken place in 7-14 days, consider another form of therapy

Monitoring Parameters Ophthalmologic exam (test for corneal staining with fluorescein or rose bengal)

Patient Information Notify prescriber if improvement is not seen after 7 days, condition worsens, or if irritation occurs; do not discontinue without notifying the physician, do not exceed recommended dosage

Dosage Forms Solution, ophthalmic: 1% (7.5 mL)

TriHIBit® *see* Diphtheria, Tetanus Toxoids, and Acellular Pertussis Vaccine and *Haemophilus influenzae* b Conjugate Vaccine *on page 785*

Trikacide (Can) *see* Metronidazole *on page 940*

Trimethoprim (trye METH oh prim)

U.S. Brand Names Primsol®; Proloprim®

Canadian Brand Names Apo-Trimethoprim®; Proloprim®

Synonyms TMP

Generic Available Yes: Tablet

Use Treatment of urinary tract infections due to susceptible strains of *E. coli*, *P. mirabilis*, *K. pneumoniae*, *Enterobacter* sp and coagulase-negative *Staphylococcus* including *S. saprophyticus*; acute otitis media in children; acute exacerbations of chronic bronchitis in adults; in combination with other agents for treatment of toxoplasmosis, *Pneumocystis carinii*; treatment of superficial ocular infections involving the conjunctiva and cornea

Drug of Choice or Alternative for Disease/Syndrome(s):

Asymptomatic Bacteriuria *on page 39*

Organism(s):

Pneumocystis jiroveci on page 266

Pregnancy Risk Factor C

Pregnancy Implications There are no well-controlled studies on the use of trimethoprim during pregnancy. Because trimethoprim may interfere with folic acid metabolism, consider using only if the potential benefit to the mother outweighs the possible risk to the fetus.

Contraindications Hypersensitivity to trimethoprim or any component of the formulation; megaloblastic anemia due to folate deficiency

Warnings/Precautions Use with caution in patients with impaired renal or hepatic function or with possible folate deficiency

Adverse Reactions Frequency not defined.

Central nervous system: Aseptic meningitis (rare), fever

Dermatologic: Maculopapular rash (3% to 7% at 200 mg/day; incidence higher with larger daily doses), erythema multiforme (rare), exfoliative dermatitis (rare), pruritus (common), phototoxic skin eruptions, Stevens-Johnson syndrome (rare), toxic epidermal necrolysis (rare)

Endocrine & metabolic: Hyperkalemia, hyponatremia

Gastrointestinal: Epigastric distress, glossitis, nausea, vomiting

Hematologic: Leukopenia, megaloblastic anemia, methemoglobinemia, neutropenia, thrombocytopenia

Hepatic: Liver enzyme elevation, cholestatic jaundice (rare)

Renal: BUN and creatinine increased

Miscellaneous: Anaphylaxis, hypersensitivity reactions

Overdosage/Toxicology Symptom of acute toxicity includes nausea, vomiting, confusion, and dizziness. Chronic overdose results in bone marrow suppression. Treatment of acute overdose is supportive following GI decontamination. Treatment of chronic overdose includes the use of oral leucovorin 5-15 mg/day. Hemodialysis is only moderately effective in eliminating drug.

Drug Interactions

Cytochrome P450 Effect: Substrate (major) of CYP2C8/9, 3A4; **Inhibits** CYP2C8/9 (moderate)

Increased Effect/Toxicity: Increased effect/toxicity/levels of phenytoin. Concurrent use with ACE inhibitors increases risk of hyperkalemia. Increased myelosuppression with methotrexate. May increase levels of digoxin. Concurrent use with dapsone may increase levels of dapsone and trimethoprim. Concurrent use with procainamide may increase levels of procainamide and trimethoprim. Trimethoprim may increase the levels/effects of amiodarone, fluoxetine, glimepiride, glipizide, nateglinide, phenytoin, pioglitazone, rosiglitazone, sertraline, warfarin, and other CYP2C8/9 substrates.

Decreased Effect: The levels/effects of trimethoprim may be decreased by aminoglutethimide, carbamazepine, nafcillin, nevirapine, phenobarbital, phenytoin, rifampin, rifapentine, secobarbital, and other CYP2C8/9 or 3A4 inducers.

Stability Protect the 200 mg tablet from light.

Mechanism of Action Inhibits folic acid reduction to tetrahydrofolate, and thereby inhibits microbial growth

Pharmacodynamics/Kinetics

Absorption: Readily and extensive

Distribution: Widely into body tissues and fluids (middle ear, prostate, bile, aqueous humor, CSF); crosses placenta; enters breast milk

Protein binding: 42% to 46%

Metabolism: Partially hepatic

Half-life elimination: 8-14 hours; prolonged with renal impairment

Time to peak, serum: 1-4 hours

Excretion: Urine (60% to 80%) as unchanged drug

Dosage Oral:

Children: 4 mg/kg/day in divided doses every 12 hours

Adults: 100 mg every 12 hours or 200 mg every 24 hours for 10 days; longer treatment periods may be necessary for prostatitis (ie, 4-16 weeks); in the treatment of *Pneumocystis carinii* pneumonia; dose may be as high as 15-20 mg/kg/day in 3-4 divided doses

Dosing interval in renal impairment:

Cl_{cr} 15-30 mL/minute: Administer 100 mg every 18 hours or 50 mg every 12 hours

Cl_{cr} <15 mL/minute: Administer 100 mg every 24 hours or avoid use

Hemodialysis: Moderately dialyzable (20% to 50%)

Dietary Considerations May cause folic acid deficiency, supplements may be needed. Should be taken with milk or food.

Administration Administer with milk or food.

Reference Range Therapeutic: Peak: 5-15 mg/L; Trough: 2-8 mg/L

Patient Information Take with milk or food; report any skin rash, persistent or severe fatigue, fever, sore throat, or unusual bleeding or bruising; complete full course of therapy

Dosage Forms

[DSC] = Discontinued product

Solution, oral (Primsol®): 50 mg (base)/5 mL (480 mL) [contains sodium benzoate; bubble gum flavor]

Tablet: 100 mg

Proloprim®: 100 mg, 200 mg [DSC]

Trimethoprim and Polymyxin B

(trye METH oh prim & pol i MIKS in bee)

Related Information

Polymyxin B *on page 1012*

Trimethoprim *on page 1130*

U.S. Brand Names Polytrim®

Canadian Brand Names PMS-Polytrimethoprim; Polytrim™

Synonyms Polymyxin B and Trimethoprim

Generic Available Yes

Use Treatment of surface ocular bacterial conjunctivitis and blepharoconjunctivitis

Pregnancy Risk Factor C

Contraindications Hypersensitivity to trimethoprim, polymyxin B, or any component of the formulation

Adverse Reactions 1% to 10%: Local: Burning, stinging, itching, increased redness

Drug Interactions

Cytochrome P450 Effect: Trimethoprim: **Substrate** (major) of CYP2C8/9, 3A4; **Inhibits** CYP2C8/9 (moderate)

Pharmacodynamics/Kinetics See individual agents.

Dosage Instill 1-2 drops in eye(s) every 4-6 hours

Elderly: No overall differences observed between elderly and other adults

Administration Avoid contamination of the applicator tip.

(Continued)

Trimethoprim and Polymyxin B *(Continued)*

Additional Information Complete prescribing information for this medication should be consulted for additional detail.

Dosage Forms Solution, ophthalmic: Trimethoprim 1 mg and polymyxin B sulfate 10,000 units per mL (10 mL) [contains benzalkonium chloride]

Trimethoprim and Sulfamethoxazole *see* Sulfamethoxazole and Trimethoprim *on page 1087*

Trimetrexate Glucuronate (tri me TREKS ate gloo KYOOR oh nate)

U.S. Brand Names NeuTrexin®

Synonyms NSC-352122

Generic Available No

Use Alternative therapy for the treatment of moderate-to-severe *Pneumocystis carinii* pneumonia (PCP) in immunocompromised patients, including patients with acquired immunodeficiency syndrome (AIDS), who are intolerant of, or are refractory to, co-trimoxazole therapy or for whom co-trimoxazole and pentamidine are contraindicated. **Concurrent folinic acid (leucovorin) must always be administered.**

Unlabeled/Investigational Use Treatment of nonsmall cell lung cancer, metastatic colorectal cancer, metastatic head and neck cancer, pancreatic adenocarcinoma

Pregnancy Risk Factor D

Contraindications Hypersensitivity to trimetrexate, methotrexate, leucovorin, or any component of the formulation; severe existing myelosuppression; pregnancy

Warnings/Precautions The U.S. Food and Drug Administration (FDA) currently recommends that procedures for proper handling and disposal of antineoplastic agents be considered. Appropriate safety equipment is recommended for preparation, administration, and disposal of antineoplastics. If trimetrexate contacts the skin, immediately wash with soap and water. **Must be administered with concurrent leucovorin to avoid potentially serious or life-threatening toxicities.** Leucovorin therapy must extend for 72 hours past the last dose of trimetrexate. Hypersensitivity/allergic-type reactions have been reported, primarily when given as a bolus infusion, at higher than recommended doses for PCP, or in combination with fluorouracil or leucovorin. Use with caution in patients with mild myelosuppression, severe hepatic or renal dysfunction, hypoproteinemia, hypoalbuminemia, or previous extensive myelosuppressive therapies.

Adverse Reactions

>10%:
- Hematologic: Neutropenia
- Hepatic: LFTs increased

1% to 10%:
- Central nervous system: Seizures, fever
- Dermatologic: Rash
- Gastrointestinal: Stomatitis, nausea, vomiting
- Hematologic: Thrombocytopenia, anemia
- Neuromuscular & skeletal: Peripheral neuropathy
- Renal: Increased serum creatinine
- Miscellaneous: Flu-like illness, hypersensitivity reactions, anaphylactoid reactions

Drug Interactions

Increased Effect/Toxicity: Cimetidine, clotrimazole, and ketoconazole may decrease trimetrexate metabolism, resulting in increased serum levels. Trimetrexate may increase toxicity (infections) of live virus vaccines.

Stability Prior to reconstitution, vials should stored at controlled room temperature of 20°C to 25°C (68°F to 77°F). Protect from light. Reconstitute with D_5W or SWFI to a concentration of 12.5 mg/mL. Do not use if cloudy or if precipitate forms. Following reconstitution, the solution should be used immediately, but is stable for 6 hours at room temperature or 24 hours under refrigeration. Prior to administration, solution should be further diluted with D_5W to a concentration of 0.25 mg/mL to 2 mg/mL. This final diluted solution is stable under refrigeration or at room temperature for 24 hours.

Mechanism of Action Trimetrexate is a folate antimetabolite that inhibits DNA synthesis by inhibition of dihydrofolate reductase (DHFR); DHFR inhibition reduces the formation of reduced folates and thymidylate synthetase, resulting in inhibition of purine and thymidylic acid synthesis.

Pharmacodynamics/Kinetics

Distribution: V_d: 0.62 L/kg

Metabolism: Extensively hepatic

Half-life elimination: 15-17 hours

Dosage Note: Concurrent leucovorin 20 mg/m^2 every 6 hours must be administered daily (oral or I.V.) during treatment and for 72 hours past the last dose of trimetrexate glucuronate.

Adults: I.V.:

Pneumocystis carinii: 45 mg/m² once daily for 21 days; **alternative dosing based on weight:**

<50 kg:Trimetrexate glucuronate 1.5 mg/kg/day; leucovorin 0.6 mg/kg 4 times/day

50-80 kg:Trimetrexate glucuronate 1.2 mg/kg/day; leucovorin 0.5 mg/kg/4 times/day

>80 kg: Trimetrexate glucuronate 1 mg/kg/day; leucovorin 0.5 mg/kg/4 times/day

Note: Oral doses of leucovorin should be rounded up to the next higher 25 mg increment.

Antineoplastic (unlabeled use): 6-16 mg/m² once daily for 5 days every 21-28 days **or** 150-200 mg/m² every 2 weeks

Dosage adjustment in hepatic impairment: Although it may be necessary to reduce the dose in patients with liver dysfunction, no specific recommendations exist.

Administration Reconstituted solution should be filtered (0.22 μM) prior to further dilution; final solution should be clear, hue will range from colorless to pale yellow; trimetrexate forms a precipitate instantly upon contact with chloride ion or leucovorin, therefore it should not be added to solutions containing sodium chloride or other anions; trimetrexate and leucovorin solutions **must** be administered separately; intravenous lines should be flushed with at least 10 mL of D_5W between trimetrexate and leucovorin

Monitoring Parameters Check and record patient's temperature daily; absolute neutrophil counts (ANC), platelet count, renal function tests (serum creatinine, BUN), hepatic function tests (ALT, AST, alkaline phosphatase)

Patient Information Report promptly any fever, rash, flu-like symptoms, numbness or tingling in the extremities, nausea, vomiting, abdominal pain, mouth sores, increased bruising or bleeding, black tarry stools

Additional Information Not a vesicant; methotrexate derivative

Dosage Forms Injection, powder for reconstitution [preservative free]: 25 mg, 200 mg

Selected Readings

Fulton B, Wagstaff AJ, and McTavish D, "Trimetrexate. A Review of Its Pharmacodynamic and Pharmacokinetic Properties and Therapeutic Potential in the Treatment of *Pneumocystis carinii* Pneumonia," *Drugs*, 1995, 49(4):563-76.

Marshall JL and De Lap RJ, "Clinical Pharmacokinetics and Pharmacology of Trimetrexate," *Clin Pharmacokinet*, 1994, 26(3):190-200.

Masur H, "Prevention and Treatment of *Pneumocystis* Pneumonia," *N Engl J Med*, 1992, 327(26):1853-60.

Trimox® *see* Amoxicillin *on page 642*

Tripedia® *see* Diphtheria, Tetanus Toxoids, and Acellular Pertussis Vaccine *on page 782*

Triple Antibiotic *see* Bacitracin, Neomycin, and Polymyxin B *on page 681*

Triple Care® Antifungal [OTC] *see* Miconazole *on page 945*

Triple Sulfa *see* Sulfabenzamide, Sulfacetamide, and Sulfathiazole *on page 1080*

Trivagizole-3® (Can) *see* Clotrimazole *on page 758*

Trizivir® *see* Abacavir, Lamivudine, and Zidovudine *on page 627*

Trobicin® *see* Spectinomycin *on page 1075*

Troleandomycin (troe lee an doe MYE sin)

U.S. Brand Names Tao®

Synonyms Triacetyloleandomycin

Generic Available No

Use Antibiotic with spectrum of activity similar to erythromycin

Pregnancy Risk Factor C

Contraindications Hypersensitivity to troleandomycin, other macrolides, or any component of the formulation; concomitant use with ergot derivatives, pimozide, or cisapride

Warnings/Precautions Use with caution in patients with impaired hepatic function; chronic hepatitis may occur in patients with long or repetitive courses

Adverse Reactions Frequency not defined.

Gastrointestinal: Abdominal cramping and discomfort (dose related), nausea, vomiting, diarrhea, rectal burning

Dermatologic: Urticaria, rash

Hepatic: Cholestatic jaundice

Overdosage/Toxicology Symptoms include nausea, vomiting, diarrhea, and hearing loss. Following GI decontamination, treatment is supportive.

Drug Interactions

Cytochrome P450 Effect: Substrate of CYP3A4 (major); **Inhibits** CYP3A4 (moderate)

(Continued)

Troleandomycin *(Continued)*

Increased Effect/Toxicity: Avoid concomitant use of the following with troleandomycin due to increased risk of malignant arrhythmias: Cisapride, gatifloxacin, moxifloxacin, pimozide, sparfloxacin, thioridazine. Other agents that prolong the QT_c interval, including type Ia (eg, quinidine) and type III antiarrhythmic agents, and selected antipsychotic agents (eg, mesoridazine, thioridazine) should be used with extreme caution.

The effects of neuromuscular-blocking agents and warfarin have been potentiated by troleandomycin. Troleandomycin serum concentrations may be increased by amprenavir (and possibly other protease inhibitors).

Troleandomycin may increase the levels/effects of selected benzodiazepines, calcium channel blockers, cyclosporine, ergot alkaloids, HMG-CoA reductase inhibitors, mirtazapine, nateglinide, nefazodone, quinidine, sildenafil (and other PDE-5 inhibitors), tacrolimus, venlafaxine, and other CYP3A4 substrates.

Decreased Effect: Troleandomycin may decrease the serum concentrations of zafirlukast. Troleandomycin may antagonize the therapeutic effects of clindamycin and lincomycin. The levels/effects of troleandomycin may be decreased by aminoglutethimide, carbamazepine, nafcillin, nevirapine, phenobarbital, phenytoin, rifamycins, and other CYP3A4 inducers.

Ethanol/Nutrition/Herb Interactions Food: Presence of food delays absorption, but has no effect on the extent of absorption.

Mechanism of Action Decreases methylprednisolone clearance from a linear first order decline to a nonlinear decline in plasma concentration. Troleandomycin also has an undefined action independent of its effects on steroid elimination. Inhibits RNA-dependent protein synthesis at the chain elongation step; binds to the 50S ribosomal subunit resulting in blockage of transpeptidation.

Pharmacodynamics/Kinetics

Time to peak, serum: ~2 hours

Excretion: Urine (10% to 25% as active drug); feces

Dosage Oral:

Children 7-13 years: 25-40 mg/kg/day divided every 6 hours (125-250 mg every 6 hours)

Adults: 250-500 mg 4 times/day (around-the-clock every 6 hours)

Dietary Considerations May be taken with food.

Administration Administer around-the-clock every 6 hours.

Monitoring Parameters Hepatic function tests

Patient Information Complete full course of therapy; report persistent or severe abdominal pain, nausea, vomiting, jaundice, darkened urine, or fever

Dosage Forms Capsule: 250 mg

Selected Readings

Tartaglione TA, "Therapeutic Options for the Management and Prevention of *Mycobacterium avium* Complex Infection in Patients With the Acquired Immunodeficiency Syndrome," *Pharmacotherapy*, 1996, 16(2):171-82.

Trovafloxacin (TROE va floks a sin)

Related Information

Antimicrobial Activity Against Selected Organisms *on page 1165*

U.S. Brand Names Trovan® [DSC]

Synonyms Alatrofloxacin Mesylate; CP-99,219-27

Generic Available No

Use Should be used only in life- or limb-threatening infections

Treatment of nosocomial pneumonia, community-acquired pneumonia, complicated intra-abdominal infections, gynecologic/pelvic infections, complicated skin and skin structure infections

Pregnancy Risk Factor C

Pregnancy Implications Reports of arthropathy (observed in immature animals and reported rarely in humans) have limited the use of fluoroquinolones in pregnancy. Skeletal variations and fetotoxicity were reported with trovafloxacin in animal studies. Based on limited data, quinolones are not expected to be a major human teratogen. Although quinolone antibiotics should not be used as first-line agents during pregnancy, when considering treatment for life-threatening infection and/or prolonged duration of therapy, the potential risk to the fetus must be balanced against the severity of the potential illness.

Contraindications History of hypersensitivity to trovafloxacin, alatrofloxacin, quinolone antimicrobial agents, or any component of the formulation

Warnings/Precautions For use only in serious life- or limb-threatening infections. Initiation of therapy must occur in an inpatient healthcare facility. May alter GI flora resulting in pseudomembranous colitis due to *Clostridium difficile*; use with caution in

patients with seizure disorders or severe cerebral atherosclerosis; photosensitivity; CNS stimulation may occur which may lead to tremor, restlessness, confusion, hallucinations, paranoia, depression, nightmares, insomnia, or lightheadedness. Hepatic reactions have resulted in death. Risk of hepatotoxicity is increased if therapy exceeds 14 days. Tendon inflammation and/or rupture have been reported with other quinolone antibiotics. Risk may be increased with concurrent corticosteroids, particularly in the elderly. Discontinue at first sign of tendon inflammation or pain.

Severe hypersensitivity reactions, including anaphylaxis, have occurred with quinolone therapy. If an allergic reaction occurs (itching, urticaria, dyspnea, facial edema, loss of consciousness, tingling, cardiovascular collapse), discontinue drug immediately. Prolonged use may result in superinfection; pseudomembranous colitis may occur and should be considered in all patients who present with diarrhea. Quinolones may exacerbate myasthenia gravis, use with caution (rare, potentially life-threatening weakness of respiratory muscles may occur).

Adverse Reactions Note: Fatalities have occurred in patients developing hepatic necrosis.

1% to 10% (range reported in clinical trials):

- Central nervous system: Dizziness (2% to 11%), lightheadedness (<1% to 4%), headache (1% to 5%)
- Dermatologic: Rash (<1% to 2%), pruritus (<1% to 2%)
- Gastrointestinal: Nausea (4% to 8%), abdominal pain (<1% to 1%), vomiting, diarrhea
- Genitourinary: Vaginitis (<1% to 1%)
- Hepatic: Increased LFTs
- Local: Injection site reaction, pain, or inflammation

<1%: Phototoxicity, convulsions, dyskinesia, pseudomembranous colitis, allergic/anaphylactoid reaction, tendonitis, bronchospasm, interstitial nephritis, anaphylaxis, hepatic necrosis, pancreatitis, Stevens-Johnson syndrome; quinolones have been associated with tendon rupture

Overdosage/Toxicology Empty the stomach by vomiting or gastric lavage. Observe carefully and give symptomatic and supportive treatment. Maintain adequate hydration.

Drug Interactions

Increased Effect/Toxicity: Trovafloxacin may increase the effects/toxicity of glyburide and warfarin. Concomitant use with corticosteroids may increase the risk of tendon rupture. Probenecid may increase trovafloxacin levels.

Decreased Effect: Concurrent administration of metal cations, including most antacids, oral electrolyte supplements, quinapril, sucralfate, some didanosine formulations (chewable/buffered tablets and pediatric powder for oral suspension), and other highly-buffered oral drugs, may decrease quinolone levels; separate doses.

Ethanol/Nutrition/Herb Interactions

Food: Dairy products such as milk or yogurt may reduce absorption of oral trovafloxacin; avoid concurrent use. Enteral feedings may also limit absorption.

Herb/Nutraceutical: Avoid dong quai, St John's wort (may also cause photosensitization).

Stability Store undiluted vials of solution at 15°C to 30°C (50°F to 86°F). Diluted solutions are stable for up to 7 days when refrigerated and up to 3 days at room temperature. Trovan® I.V. should not be diluted with 0.9% sodium chloride injection, USP (normal saline), alone or in combination with other diluents. A precipitate may form under these conditions. In addition, Trovan® I.V. should not be diluted with lactated Ringer's, USP.

Dilute to a concentration of 0.5-2 mg/mL in dextrose 5% in water, 0.45% sodium chloride, dextrose 5% in water and 0.45% sodium chloride, dextrose 5% in water and 0.2% sodium chloride, or lactated Ringer's in dextrose 5% in water.

Mechanism of Action Inhibits DNA-gyrase in susceptible organisms; inhibits relaxation of supercoiled DNA and promotes breakage of double-stranded DNA

Pharmacodynamics/Kinetics

Distribution: Concentration in most tissues greater than plasma or serum
Protein binding: 76%
Metabolism: Hepatic conjugation; glucuronidation 13%, acetylation 9%
Bioavailability: 88%
Half-life elimination: 9-12 hours
Time to peak, serum: Oral: Within 2 hours
Excretion: Feces (43% as unchanged drug); urine (6% as unchanged drug)

Dosage Adults:

Nosocomial pneumonia: I.V.: 300 mg single dose followed by 200 mg/day orally for a total duration of 10-14 days

Community-acquired pneumonia: Oral, I.V.: 200 mg/day for 7-14 days

(Continued)

Trovafloxacin *(Continued)*

Complicated intra-abdominal infections, including postsurgical infections/gynecologic and pelvic infections: I.V.: 300 mg as a single dose followed by 200 mg/day orally for a total duration of 7-14 days

Skin and skin structure infections, complicated, including diabetic foot infections: Oral, I.V.: 200 mg/day for 10-14 days

Dosage adjustment in renal impairment: No adjustment is necessary

Dosage adjustment for hemodialysis: None required; trovafloxacin not sufficiently removed by hemodialysis

Dosage adjustment in hepatic impairment:

Mild to moderate cirrhosis:

Initial dose for normal hepatic function: 300 mg I.V.; 200 mg I.V. or oral; 100 mg oral

Reduced dose: 200 mg I.V.; 100 mg I.V. or oral; 100 mg oral

Severe cirrhosis: No data available

Administration

Oral: Administer without regard to meals.

I.V.: Not for I.M. or SubQ; administer IVPB over 60 minutes

Monitoring Parameters Periodic assessment of liver function tests should be considered

Patient Information Drink fluids liberally; do not take antacids containing magnesium or aluminum or products containing iron or zinc simultaneously or within 4 hours before or 2 hours after taking dose. May cause dizziness or lightheadedness; observe caution while driving or performing other tasks requiring alertness, coordination, or physical dexterity. CNS stimulation may occur (eg, tremor, restlessness, confusion). Avoid excessive sunlight/artificial ultraviolet light; discontinue drug if phototoxicity occurs. Avoid re-exposure to ultraviolet light. Reactions may recur up to several weeks after stopping therapy.

Dosage Forms

Injection, solution, as mesylate [alatrofloxacin]: 5 mg/mL (40 mL, 60 mL)

Tablet, as mesylate [trovafloxacin]: 100 mg, 200 mg

Selected Readings

Ernst ME, Ernst EJ, and Klepser ME, "Levofloxacin and Trovafloxacin: The Next Generation of Fluoroquinolones?" *Am J Health Syst Pharm*, 1997, 54(22):2569-84.

Garey KW and Amsden GW, "Trovafloxacin: An Overview," *Pharmacotherapy*, 1999, 19(1):21-34.

Haria M and Lamb HA, "Trovafloxacin," *Drugs*, 1997, 54(3):435-45.

Hecht DW and Osmolski JR, "Comparison of Activities of Trovafloxacin (CP-99,219) and Five Other Agents Against 585 Anaerobes With Use of Three Media," *Clin Infect Dis*, 1996, 23(Suppl 1):S44-50.

"Trovafloxacin," *Med Lett Drugs Ther*, 1998, 40(1022):30-1.

Trovan® [DSC] *see* Trovafloxacin *on page 1134*

Truvada™ *see* Emtricitabine and Tenofovir *on page 801*

TST *see* Tuberculin Tests *on page 1136*

T-Stat® [DSC] *see* Erythromycin *on page 807*

Tuberculin Purified Protein Derivative *see* Tuberculin Tests *on page 1136*

Tuberculin Skin Test *see* Tuberculin Tests *on page 1136*

Tuberculin Tests (too BER kyoo lin tests)

U.S. Brand Names Aplisol®; Tubersol®

Synonyms Mantoux; PPD; Tine Test; TST; Tuberculin Purified Protein Derivative; Tuberculin Skin Test

Generic Available No

Use Skin test in diagnosis of tuberculosis, cell-mediated immunodeficiencies

Pregnancy Risk Factor C

Contraindications 250 TU strength should not be used for initial testing

Warnings/Precautions Do not administer I.V. or SubQ; epinephrine (1:1000) should be available to treat possible allergic reactions

Adverse Reactions Frequency not defined.

Dermatologic: Ulceration, necrosis, vesiculation

Local: Pain at injection site

Stability Refrigerate; Tubersol® opened vials are stable for up to 24 hours at <75°F

Mechanism of Action Tuberculosis results in individuals becoming sensitized to certain antigenic components of the *M. tuberculosis* organism. Culture extracts called tuberculins are contained in tuberculin skin test preparations. Upon intracutaneous injection of these culture extracts, a classic delayed (cellular) hypersensitivity reaction occurs. This reaction is characteristic of a delayed course (peak occurs >24 hours after injection, induration of the skin secondary to cell infiltration, and occasional vesiculation and necrosis). Delayed hypersensitivity reactions to tuberculin may indicate infection with a variety of nontuberculosis mycobacteria, or vaccination with the

live attenuated mycobacterial strain of *M. bovis* vaccine, BCG, in addition to previous natural infection with *M. tuberculosis*.

Pharmacodynamics/Kinetics

Onset of action: Delayed hypersensitivity reactions: 5-6 hours

Peak effect: 48-72 hours

Duration: Reactions subside over a few days

Dosage Children and Adults: Intradermal: 0.1 mL about 4" below elbow; use 1/4" to 1/2" or 26- or 27-gauge needle; significant reactions are ≥5 mm in diameter

Interpretation of induration of tuberculin skin test injections: Positive: ≥10 mm; inconclusive: 5-9 mm; negative: <5 mm

Interpretation of induration of Tine test injections: Positive: >2 mm and vesiculation present; inconclusive: <2 mm (give patient Mantoux test of 5 TU/0.1 mL - base decisions on results of Mantoux test); negative: <2 mm or erythema of any size (no need for retesting unless person is a contact of a patient with tuberculosis or there is clinical evidence suggestive of the disease)

Administration Select a site without acne or hair

Patient Information Return to physician for reaction interpretation at 48-72 hours

Additional Information Whenever tuberculin is administered, a record should be made of the administration technique (Mantoux method, disposable multiple-puncture device), tuberculin used (OT or PPD), manufacturer and lot number of tuberculin used, date of administration, date of test reading, and the size of the reaction in millimeters (mm).

Dosage Forms Injection, solution: 5 TU/0.1 mL (1 mL, 5 mL)

Selected Readings

Dutt AK and Stead WW, "Tuberculosis," *Clin Geriatr Med*, 1992, 8(4):761-75.

Tubersol® *see* Tuberculin Tests *on page 1136*

Twinrix® *see* Hepatitis A Inactivated and Hepatitis B (Recombinant) Vaccine *on page 852*

Tygacil™ *see* Tigecycline *on page 1116*

Typhim Vi® *see* Typhoid Vaccine *on page 1137*

Typhoid Vaccine (TYE foid vak SEEN)

Related Information

Immunization Recommendations *on page 1249*

U.S. Brand Names Typhim Vi®; Vivotif Berna®

Canadian Brand Names Vivotif Berna®

Synonyms Typhoid Vaccine Live Oral Ty21a

Generic Available No

Use Typhoid vaccine: Live, attenuated Ty21a typhoid vaccine should not be administered to immunocompromised persons, including those known to be infected with HIV. Parenteral inactivated vaccine is a theoretically safer alternative for this group.

Parenteral: Promotes active immunity to typhoid fever for patients intimately exposed to a typhoid carrier or foreign travel to a typhoid fever endemic area

Oral: For immunization of children >6 years of age and adults who expect intimate exposure of or household contact with typhoid fever, travelers to areas of world with risk of exposure to typhoid fever, and workers in microbiology laboratories with expected frequent contact with *S. typhi*

Pregnancy Risk Factor C

Contraindications Acute respiratory or other active infections, previous sensitivity to typhoid vaccine, congenital or acquired immunodeficient state, acute febrile illness, acute GI illness (oral), other active infection, persistent diarrhea or vomiting (oral)

Warnings/Precautions Postpone use in presence of acute infection; use during pregnancy only when clearly needed, immune deficiency conditions; not all recipients of typhoid vaccine will be fully protected against typhoid fever. Travelers should take all necessary precautions to avoid contact or ingestion of potentially contaminated food or water sources. Unless a complete immunization schedule is followed, an optimum immune response may not be achieved.

Adverse Reactions All serious adverse reactions must be reported to the U.S. Department of Health and Human Services (DHHS) Vaccine Adverse Event Reporting System (VAERS) 1-800-822-7967.

Oral:

1% to 10%:

Central nervous system: Headache, fever

Dermatologic: Rash

Gastrointestinal: Abdominal discomfort, stomach cramps, diarrhea, nausea, vomiting

<1%: Anaphylactic reaction

(Continued)

Typhoid Vaccine *(Continued)*

Injection:

>10%:

Central nervous system: Headache (13% to 20%), fever (3% to 11%), malaise (4% to 24%)

Dermatologic: Local tenderness (13% to 98%), induration (5% to 15%), pain at injection site (7% to 41%)

1% to 10%:

Central nervous system: Fever ≥100°F (2%)

Gastrointestinal: Nausea (2% to 8%), diarrhea (3% to 4%), vomiting (2%)

Local: Erythema at injection site (4% to 5%)

Neuromuscular & skeletal: Myalgia (3% to 7%)

<1%: Hypotension, allergic reactions

Stability

Typhim Vi®: Store between 2°C to 8°C (35°F to 46°F); do not freeze

Vivotif Berna®: Store between 2°C to 8°C (35°F to 46°F)

Mechanism of Action Virulent strains of *Salmonella typhi* cause disease by penetrating the intestinal mucosa and entering the systemic circulation via the lymphatic vasculature. One possible mechanism of conferring immunity may be the provocation of a local immune response in the intestinal tract induced by oral ingesting of a live strain with subsequent aborted infection. The ability of *Salmonella typhi* to produce clinical disease (and to elicit an immune response) is dependent on the bacteria having a complete lipopolysaccharide. The live attenuate Ty21a strain lacks the enzyme UDP-4-galactose epimerase so that lipopolysaccharide is only synthesized under conditions that induce bacterial autolysis. Thus, the strain remains avirulent despite the production of sufficient lipopolysaccharide to evoke a protective immune response. Despite low levels of lipopolysaccharide synthesis, cells lyse before gaining a virulent phenotype due to the intracellular accumulation of metabolic intermediates.

Pharmacodynamics/Kinetics

Onset of action: Immunity to *Salmonella typhi*: Oral: ~1 week

Duration: Immunity: Oral: ~5 years; Parenteral: ~3 years

Dosage Immunization:

Oral: Children ≥6 years and Adults:

Primary immunization: One capsule on alternate days (day 1, 3, 5, and 7) for a total of 4 doses; all doses should be complete at least 1 week prior to potential exposure

Booster immunization: Repeat full course of primary immunization every 5 years

I.M. (Typhim Vi®): Children ≥2 years and Adults: 0.5 mL given at least 2 weeks prior to expected exposure

Reimmunization: 0.5 mL; optimal schedule has not been established; a single dose every 2 years is currently recommended for repeated or continued exposure

Administration Typhim Vi® may be given I.M. and is indicated for children ≥2 years of age; administer as a single 0.5 mL (25 mcg) injection in deltoid muscle

Patient Information Oral capsule should be taken 1 hour before a meal with cold or lukewarm drink, (swallow capsule whole, do not chew); systemic adverse effects may persist for 1-2 days. Take all 4 doses exactly as directed on alternate days to obtain a maximal response.

Additional Information Federal law requires that the date of administration, the vaccine manufacturer, lot number of vaccine, and the administering person's name, title, and address be entered into the patient's permanent medical record.

Dosage Forms

Capsule, enteric coated (Vivotif Berna®): Viable *S. typhi* Ty21a colony-forming units 2-6 x 10^9 and nonviable *S. typhi* Ty21a colony-forming units 5-50 x 10^9 [contains lactose]

Injection, solution (Typhim Vi®): Purified Vi capsular polysaccharide 25 mcg/0.5 mL (0.5 mL, 10 mL)

Selected Readings

Gardner P and Schaffner W, "Immunization of Adults," *N Engl J Med*, 1993, 328(17):1252-8.

Typhoid Vaccine Live Oral Ty21a *see* Typhoid Vaccine *on page 1137*

U-90152S *see* Delavirdine *on page 769*

UK109496 *see* Voriconazole *on page 1151*

Unasyn® *see* Ampicillin and Sulbactam *on page 660*

Undecylenic Acid and Derivatives

(un de sil EN ik AS id & dah RIV ah tivs)

U.S. Brand Names Fungi-Nail® [OTC]

Synonyms Zinc Undecylenate

Generic Available No

Use Treatment of athlete's foot (tinea pedis); ringworm (except nails and scalp)

Contraindications Hypersensitivity to undecylenic acid or any component of the formulation

Warnings/Precautions Discontinue if no improvement within 4 weeks. Safety and efficacy for OTC use have not been established for children <2 years of age.

Dosage Children and Adults: Topical: Apply twice daily to affected area for 4 weeks; apply to clean, dry area

Dosage Forms Solution, topical: Undecylenic acid 25% (29.57 mL)

Unipen® (Can) *see* Nafcillin *on page 955*
Urasal® (Can) *see* Methenamine *on page 939*
Urex® *see* Methenamine *on page 939*

Vaccinia Immune Globulin (Intravenous)

(vax IN ee a i MYUN GLOB yoo lin IN tra VEE nus)

U.S. Brand Names CNJ-016™

Synonyms VIGIV

Generic Available No

Use Treatment of infectious complications of smallpox (vaccinia virus) vaccination, such as eczema vaccinatum, progressive vaccinia, and severe generalized vaccinia; vaccinia infections in individuals with concurrent skin conditions or accidental virus exposure to eyes (except vaccinia keratitis), mouth, or other areas where viral infection would pose significant risk

Pregnancy Risk Factor C

Pregnancy Implications Immune globulins cross the placenta in increased amounts after 30 weeks gestation. There are no adequate and well-controlled studies in pregnant women; use only if benefits outweigh the risks.

Contraindications Hypersensitivity to immune globulin or any component of the formulation; isolated vaccinia keratitis; selective IgA deficiency

Warnings/Precautions Acute renal dysfunction (increased serum creatinine, oliguria, acute renal failure) may rarely occur, usually within 7 days of use (more likely with products stabilized with sucrose); patients should be adequately hydrated prior to therapy. Contains trace amounts of IgA. Anaphylactic hypersensitivity reactions may occur, especially in IgA-deficient patients; epinephrine 1:1000 should be readily available. Studies indicate that the currently available product has no discernible risk of transmitting HIV or hepatitis A, B, or C; aseptic meningitis, which may rarely occur, is more likely with higher doses (≥2 g/kg). It is unknown whether variant CJD can be transmitted via plasma-derived products. Use with caution in the elderly, patients with renal disease, diabetes mellitus, volume depletion, sepsis, paraproteinemia, and nephrotoxic medications due to risk of renal dysfunction. Immune globulin use may be associated with thrombotic events; use caution in patients with a history of thrombotic events or cardiovascular disease. Intravenous immune globulin has been associated with antiglobulin hemolysis, monitor for signs of hemolytic anemia; monitor for transfusion-related, noncardiogenic pulmonary edema. Not effective for use in postvaccinial encephalitis. Safety and efficacy in pediatric or geriatric populations has not been determined. For intravenous administration only.

Adverse Reactions Note: Actual frequency varies by dose, rate of infusion and specific product used

Cardiovascular: Flushing

Central nervous system: Cold or hot feeling, dizziness, fatigue, headache, pain, pallor, pyrexia

Dermatologic: Erythema, urticaria

Gastrointestinal: Abdominal pain, appetite decreased, nausea, vomiting

Local: Injection site reaction

Neuromuscular & skeletal: Arthralgia, back pain, paraesthesia, muscle cramp, rigors, tremor, weakness

Miscellaneous: Diaphoresis

Postmarketing and/or case reports (as reported with other IVIG products): Apnea, acute respiratory distress syndrome, bronchospasm, bullous dermatitis, cardiac arrest, coma, Coombs' test positive, cyanosis, dyspnea, epidermolysis, erythema multiforme, hemolysis, hepatic dysfunction, hypoxemia, hypotension, leukopenia, loss of consciousness, lung injury (transfusion-associated), pancytopenia, pulmonary edema, seizure, Stevens-Johnson syndrome, syncope, thromboembolism, vascular collapse

(Continued)

Vaccinia Immune Globulin (Intravenous) *(Continued)*

Overdosage/Toxicology Symptoms primarily related to volume overload; treatment should be supportive

Drug Interactions

Decreased Effect: Vaccina immune globulin may interfere with immune response to live virus vaccines (eg, polio, measles, mumps, and rubella); live virus vaccinations should be deferred until 6 months after administration of VIGIV; if given shortly before receiving VIGIV, revaccination with the live virus may be necessary (consult individual products for guidance)

Stability Store between 2°C and 8°C (35.6°F to 46.4°F).

CNJ-016™ (Cangene product): If frozen, use within 60 days of thawing at 2°C and 8°C. Infusion should begin within 4 hours after entering vial.

DynPort product: Use within 6 hours of piercing vial stopper; complete infusion within 12 hours of spiking vial.

Mechanism of Action Antibodies obtained from pooled human plasma of individuals immunized with the smallpox vaccine provide passive immunity

Pharmacodynamics/Kinetics

Distribution: V_d: CNJ-016™ (Cangene product): 6630 L

Half-life elimination:

CNJ-016™ (Cangene product): 30 days (range 13-67 days)

DynPort product: 22 days

Dosage I.V.:

Adults:

CNJ-016™ (Cangene product): 6000 units/kg; 9000 units/kg may be considered if patient does not respond to initial dose.

DynPort product: Total dose: 2 mL/kg (100 mg/kg); higher doses (200-500 mg/kg) may be considered if patient does not respond to initial recommended dose (sucrose-related renal impairment is worsened at doses ≥400 mg/kg)

Elderly: Safety and efficacy have not been established

Dosage adjustment in renal impairment: Use caution. Dose ≥400 mg/kg of the DynPort product are not recommended.

Dietary Considerations DynPort solution for injection contains sodium 0.02-0.03 mEq/mL.

Administration Do not shake; avoid foaming. For intravenous use only. Predilution not recommended; if dedicated line not available, flush with NS prior to administration of VIGIV. Do not exceed recommended rates of infusion.

CNJ-016™ (Cangene product): Patients ≥50 kg: Infuse at ≤2 mL/minute; Patients < 50 kg: Infuse at 0.04 mL/kg/minute. Maximum assessed rate of infusion: 4 mL/minute. Decrease rate of infusion if minor adverse reactions develop, in patients with risk factors for thrombosis/thromboembolism, and/or renal insufficiency.

DynPort product: Infuse at 1 mL/kg/hour for 30 minutes, then 2 mL/kg/hour for 30 minutes, then 3 mL/kg/hour until complete. Administer through 0.22 micron filtered set; use of infusion pump recommended.

Monitoring Parameters During infusion, monitor patient for signs of infusion-related reactions, including (but not limited to) flushing, fever, chills, respiratory distress, blood pressure or heart rate changes

Patient Information This medication can only be administered by infusion. You will be monitored closely during the infusion. If you experience nausea ask for assistance, do not get up alone. Do not have any vaccinations for the next 6 months without consulting prescriber. Immediately report chills; chest pain, tightness, or rapid heartbeat, acute back pain, or respiratory difficulty.

Dosage Forms Injection, solution [preservative free; solvent-detergent treated]:

CNJ-016™ (Cangene product): ≥50,000 units/15 mL (15 mL) [contains maltose 10% and polysorbate 80 0.03%]

DynPort product: 50 mg/mL (50 mL) [contains sucrose 50 mg/mL, human albumin 10 mg/mL, sodium 0.02-0.03 mEq/mL]

Vaccinia Vaccine *see* Smallpox Vaccine *on page 1066*

Vagi-Gard® [OTC] *see* Povidone-Iodine *on page 1016*

Vagistat®-1 [OTC] *see* Tioconazole *on page 1119*

Valacyclovir (val ay SYE kloe veer)

U.S. Brand Names Valtrex®

Canadian Brand Names Valtrex®

Synonyms Valacyclovir Hydrochloride

Generic Available No

Use Treatment of herpes zoster (shingles) in immunocompetent patients; treatment of first-episode genital herpes; episodic treatment of recurrent genital herpes; suppression of recurrent genital herpes and reduction of heterosexual transmission of genital herpes in immunocompetent patients; suppression of genital herpes in HIV-infected individuals; treatment of herpes labialis (cold sores)

Drug of Choice or Alternative for

Disease/Syndrome(s):

Esophagitis *on page 147*

Organism(s):

Cytomegalovirus *on page 107*
Herpes Simplex Virus *on page 172*
Varicella-Zoster Virus *on page 347*

Pregnancy Risk Factor B

Pregnancy Implications Teratogenicity registry has shown no increased rate of birth defects than that of the general population; however, the registry is small and use during pregnancy is only warranted if the potential benefit to the mother justifies the risk of the fetus.

Contraindications Hypersensitivity to valacyclovir, acyclovir, or any component of the formulation

Warnings/Precautions Thrombotic thrombocytopenic purpura/hemolytic uremic syndrome has occurred in immunocompromised patients (at doses of 8 g/day); use caution and adjust the dose in elderly patients or those with renal insufficiency and in patients receiving concurrent nephrotoxic agents. For genital herpes, treatment should begin as soon as possible after the first signs and symptoms (within 72 hours of onset of first diagnosis or within 24 hours of onset of recurrent episodes). For herpes zoster, treatment should begin within 72 hours of onset of rash. For cold sores, treatment should begin at with earliest symptom (tingling, itching, burning). Safety and efficacy in prepubertal patients have not been established.

Adverse Reactions

>10%: Central nervous system: Headache (14% to 35%)

1% to 10%:

- Central nervous system: Dizziness (2% to 4%), depression (0% to 7%)
- Endocrine: Dysmenorrhea (≤1% to 8%)
- Gastrointestinal: Abdominal pain (2% to 11%), nausea (6% to 15%), vomiting (<1% to 6%)
- Hematologic: Leukopenia (≤1%), thrombocytopenia (≤1%)
- Hepatic: AST increased (1% to 4%)
- Neuromuscular & skeletal: Arthralgia (≤1 to 6%)

<1%: Anemia

Postmarketing and/or case reports: Acute hypersensitivity reactions (angioedema, anaphylaxis, dyspnea, pruritus, rash, urticaria); aggression, agitation, alopecia, aplastic anemia, ataxia, creatinine increased, coma, confusion, consciousness decreased, diarrhea, dysarthria, encephalopathy, facial edema, erythema multiforme, hallucinations (auditory and visual), hemolytic uremic syndrome (HUS), hepatitis, hypertension, leukocytoclastic vasculitis, mania, photosensitivity reaction, psychosis, rash, renal failure, seizure, tachycardia, thrombotic thrombocytopenic purpura/hemolytic uremic syndrome, tremor, visual disturbances

Overdosage/Toxicology Symptoms include elevated serum creatinine, renal failure, encephalitis, and precipitation in renal tubules. Hemodialysis has resulted in up to 60% reduction in serum acyclovir levels after administration of acyclovir.

Drug Interactions

Increased Effect/Toxicity: Valacyclovir and acyclovir have increased CNS side effects with zidovudine and probenecid.

Decreased Effect: Cimetidine and/or probenecid has decreased the rate but not the extent of valacyclovir conversion to acyclovir leading to decreased effectiveness of valacyclovir.

Stability Store at 15°C to 25°C (59°F to 77°F).

Mechanism of Action Valacyclovir is rapidly and nearly completely converted to acyclovir by intestinal and hepatic metabolism. Acyclovir is converted to acyclovir monophosphate by virus-specific thymidine kinase then further converted to acyclovir triphosphate by other cellular enzymes. Acyclovir triphosphate inhibits DNA synthesis and viral replication by competing with deoxyguanosine triphosphate for viral DNA polymerase and being incorporated into viral DNA.

Pharmacodynamics/Kinetics

Absorption: Rapid

Distribution: Acyclovir is widely distributed throughout the body including brain, kidney, lungs, liver, spleen, muscle, uterus, vagina, and CSF

Protein binding: 13.5% to 17.9%

(Continued)

Valacyclovir *(Continued)*

Metabolism: Hepatic; valacyclovir is rapidly and nearly completely converted to acyclovir and L-valine by first-pass effect; acyclovir is hepatically metabolized to a very small extent by aldehyde oxidase and by alcohol and aldehyde dehydrogenase (inactive metabolites)

Bioavailability: ~55% once converted to acyclovir

Half-life elimination: Normal renal function: Adults: Acyclovir: 2.5-3.3 hours, Valacyclovir: ~30 minutes; End-stage renal disease: Acyclovir: 14-20 hours

Excretion: Urine, primarily as acyclovir (88%); **Note:** Following oral administration of radiolabeled valacyclovir, 46% of the label is eliminated in the feces (corresponding to nonabsorbed drug), while 47% of the radiolabel is eliminated in the urine.

Dosage Oral:

Adolescents and Adults: Herpes labialis (cold sores): 2 g twice daily for 1 day (separate doses by ~12 hours)

Adults:

- Herpes zoster (shingles): 1 g 3 times/day for 7 days
- Genital herpes:
  - Initial episode: 1 g twice daily for 10 days
  - Recurrent episode: 500 mg twice daily for 3 days
  - Reduction of transmission: 500 mg once daily (source partner)
  - Suppressive therapy:
    - Immunocompetent patients: 1000 mg once daily (500 mg once daily in patients with <9 recurrences per year)
    - HIV-infected patients (CD4 ≥100 cells/mm^3): 500 mg twice daily

Dosing interval in renal impairment:

- Herpes zoster: Adults:
  - Cl_{cr} 30-49 mL/minute: 1 g every 12 hours
  - Cl_{cr} 10-29 mL/minute: 1 g every 24 hours
  - Cl_{cr} <10 mL/minute: 500 mg every 24 hours
- Genital herpes: Adults:
  - Initial episode:
    - Cl_{cr} 10-29 mL/minute: 1 g every 24 hours
    - Cl_{cr} <10 mL/minute: 500 mg every 24 hours
  - Recurrent episode: Cl_{cr} <10-29 mL/minute: 500 mg every 24 hours
  - Suppressive therapy: Cl_{cr} <10-29 mL/minute:
    - For usual dose of 1 g every 24 hours, decrease dose to 500 mg every 24 hours
    - For usual dose of 500 mg every 24 hours, decrease dose to 500 mg every 48 hours
    - HIV-infected patients: 500 mg every 24 hours
- Herpes labialis: Adolescents and Adults:
  - Cl_{cr} 30-49 mL/minute: 1 g every 12 hours for 2 doses
  - Cl_{cr} 10-29 mL/minute: 500 mg every 12 hours for 2 doses
  - Cl_{cr} <10 mL/minute: 500 mg as a single dose

Hemodialysis: Dialyzable (~33% removed during 4-hour session); administer dose postdialysis

Chronic ambulatory peritoneal dialysis/continuous arteriovenous hemofiltration dialysis: Pharmacokinetic parameters are similar to those in patients with ESRD; supplemental dose not needed following dialysis

Dietary Considerations May be taken with or without food.

Administration If GI upset occurs, administer with meals.

Monitoring Parameters Urinalysis, BUN, serum creatinine, liver enzymes, and CBC

Patient Information

Herpes zoster: Therapy is most effective when started within 48 hours of onset of zoster rash

Recurrent genital herpes: Therapy should be initiated within 24 hours after the onset of signs or symptoms

Dosage Forms Caplet: 500 mg, 1000 mg

Selected Readings

Acosta EP and Fletcher CV, "Valacyclovir," *Ann Pharmacother,* 1997, 31(2):185-91.

Alrabiah FA and Sacks SL, "New Antiherpesvirus Agents. Their Targets and Therapeutic Potential," *Drugs,* 1996, 52(1):17-32.

Ormrod D and Goa K, "Valacyclovir: A Review of Its Use in the Management of Herpes Zoster," *Drugs,* 2000, 59(6):1317-40.

Perry CM and Faulds D, "Valacyclovir. A Review of Its Antiviral Activity, Pharmacokinetic Properties and Therapeutic Efficacy in Herpesvirus Infections," *Drugs,* 1996, 52(5):754-72.

"Valacyclovir," *Med Lett Drugs Ther,* 1996, 38(965):3-4.

Weller S, Blum MR, Doucette M, et al, "Pharmacokinetics of the Acyclovir Prodrug Valacyclovir After Escalating Single- and Multiple-Dose Administration to Normal Volunteers," *Clin Pharmacol Ther,* 1993, 54(6):595-605.

Valacyclovir Hydrochloride *see* Valacyclovir *on page 1140*

Valcyte™ *see* Valganciclovir *on page 1143*

23-Valent Pneumococcal Polysaccharide Vaccine *see* Pneumococcal Polysaccharide Vaccine (Polyvalent) *on page 1010*

Valganciclovir (val gan SYE kloh veer)

U.S. Brand Names Valcyte™

Canadian Brand Names Valcyte™

Synonyms Valganciclovir Hydrochloride

Generic Available No

Use Treatment of cytomegalovirus (CMV) retinitis in patients with acquired immunodeficiency syndrome (AIDS); prevention of CMV disease in high-risk patients (donor CMV positive/recipient CMV negative) undergoing kidney, heart, or kidney/pancreas transplantation

Drug of Choice or Alternative for

Disease/Syndrome(s):

Esophagitis *on page 147*

Organism(s):

Cytomegalovirus *on page 107*
Herpes Simplex Virus *on page 172*

Pregnancy Risk Factor C

Pregnancy Implications Valganciclovir is converted to ganciclovir and shares its reproductive toxicity. Ganciclovir may adversely affect spermatogenesis and fertility; due to its mutagenic potential, contraceptive precautions for female and male patients need to be followed during and for at least 90 days after therapy with this drug.

Contraindications Hypersensitivity to valganciclovir, ganciclovir, acyclovir, or any component of the formulation; absolute neutrophil count <500/mm^3; platelet count <25,000/mm^3; hemoglobin <8 g/dL

Warnings/Precautions Dosage adjustment or interruption of valganciclovir therapy may be necessary in patients with neutropenia and/or thrombocytopenia; use with caution in patients with pre-existing bone marrow suppression, cytopenias, or in those receiving myelosuppressive drugs/irradiation. Use with caution in patients with impaired renal function (dosage adjustment required). Ganciclovir may adversely affect spermatogenesis and fertility; due to its mutagenic potential, contraceptive precautions for female and male patients need to be followed during and for at least 90 days after therapy with the drug. Due to differences in bioavailability, valganciclovir tablets cannot be substituted for ganciclovir capsules on a one-to-one basis. Not indicated for use in liver transplant patients (higher incidence of tissue-invasive CMV relative to oral ganciclovir was observed in trials). Safety and efficacy have not been established in pediatric patients.

Adverse Reactions

>10%:

- Central nervous system: Fever (31%), headache (9% to 22%), insomnia (16%)
- Gastrointestinal: Diarrhea (16% to 41%), nausea (8% to 30%), vomiting (21%), abdominal pain (15%)
- Hematologic: Granulocytopenia (11% to 27%), anemia (8% to 26%)
- Ocular: Retinal detachment (15%)

1% to 10%:

- Central nervous system: Peripheral neuropathy (9%), paresthesia (8%), seizure (<5%), psychosis, hallucinations (<5%), confusion (<5%), agitation (<5%)
- Hematologic: Thrombocytopenia (8%), pancytopenia (<5%), bone marrow depression (<5%), aplastic anemia (<5%), bleeding (potentially life-threatening due to thrombocytopenia <5%)
- Renal: Decreased renal function (<5%)
- Miscellaneous: Local and systemic infection, including sepsis (<5%); allergic reaction (<5%)

<1%: Valganciclovir is expected to share the toxicities which may occur at a low incidence or due to idiosyncratic reactions which have been associated with ganciclovir

Overdosage/Toxicology Symptoms of overdose with ganciclovir include neutropenia, vomiting, hypersalivation, bloody diarrhea, cytopenia, and testicular atrophy. Treatment is supportive. Hemodialysis removes 50% of the drug. Hydration may be of some benefit.

Drug Interactions

Increased Effect/Toxicity: Reported for ganciclovir: Immunosuppressive agents may increase hematologic toxicity of ganciclovir. Imipenem/cilastatin may increase seizure potential. Oral ganciclovir increases blood levels of zidovudine, although zidovudine decreases steady-state levels of ganciclovir. Since both drugs have the potential to cause neutropenia and anemia, some patients may not tolerate concomitant therapy with these drugs at full dosage. Didanosine levels are

(Continued)

Valganciclovir *(Continued)*

increased with concurrent ganciclovir. Other nephrotoxic drugs (eg, amphotericin and cyclosporine) may have additive nephrotoxicity with ganciclovir.

Decreased Effect: Reported for ganciclovir: A decrease in blood levels of ganciclovir AUC may occur when used with didanosine.

Ethanol/Nutrition/Herb Interactions Food: Coadministration with a high-fat meal increased AUC by 30%.

Stability Store at 25°C (77°F), excursions permitted to 15°C to 30°C (59°F to 86°F).

Mechanism of Action Valganciclovir is rapidly converted to ganciclovir in the body. The bioavailability of ganciclovir from valganciclovir is increased 10-fold compared to the oral ganciclovir. A dose of 900 mg achieved systemic exposure of ganciclovir comparable to that achieved with the recommended doses of intravenous ganciclovir of 5 mg/kg. Ganciclovir is phosphorylated to a substrate which competitively inhibits the binding of deoxyguanosine triphosphate to DNA polymerase resulting in inhibition of viral DNA synthesis.

Pharmacodynamics/Kinetics

Absorption: Well absorbed; high-fat meal increases AUC by 30%

Distribution: Ganciclovir: V_d: 15.26 L/1.73 m^2; widely to all tissues including CSF and ocular tissue

Protein binding: 1% to 2%

Metabolism: Converted to ganciclovir by intestinal mucosal cells and hepatocytes

Bioavailability: With food: 60%

Half-life elimination: Ganciclovir: 4.08 hours; prolonged with renal impairment; Severe renal impairment: Up to 68 hours

Excretion: Urine (primarily as ganciclovir)

Dosage Oral: Adults:

CMV retinitis:

Induction: 900 mg twice daily for 21 days (with food)

Maintenance: Following induction treatment, or for patients with inactive CMV retinitis who require maintenance therapy: Recommended dose: 900 mg once daily (with food)

Prevention of CMV disease following transplantation: 900 mg once daily (with food) beginning within 10 days of transplantation; continue therapy until 100 days post-transplantation

Dosage adjustment in renal impairment:

Induction dose:

Cl_{cr} 40-59 mL/minute: 450 mg twice daily

Cl_{cr} 25-39 mL/minute: 450 mg once daily

Cl_{cr} 10-24 mL/minute: 450 mg every 2 days

Maintenance dose:

Cl_{cr} 40-59 mL/minute: 450 mg once daily

Cl_{cr} 25-39 mL/minute: 450 mg every 2 days

Cl_{cr} 10-24 mL/minute: 450 mg twice weekly

Note: Valganciclovir is not recommended in patients receiving hemodialysis. For patients on hemodialysis (Cl_{cr} <10 mL/minute), it is recommended that ganciclovir be used (dose adjusted as specified for ganciclovir).

Dietary Considerations Should be taken with meals.

Administration Avoid direct contact with broken or crushed tablets. Consideration should be given to handling and disposal according to guidelines issued for antineoplastic drugs. However, there is no consensus on the need for these precautions.

Monitoring Parameters Retinal exam (at least every 4-6 weeks), CBC, platelet counts, serum creatinine

Patient Information Valganciclovir is not a cure for CMV retinitis; for oral administration, take as directed (with food) and maintain adequate hydration (2-3 L/day of fluids unless instructed to restrict fluid intake). Swallow tablets whole, do not break or crush. Avoid handling broken or crushed tablets. Wash area thoroughly if contact occurs. Report fever, chills, unusual bleeding or bruising, infection, or unhealed sores or white plaques in mouth.

Dosage Forms Tablet, as hydrochloride: 450 mg [valganciclovir hydrochloride 496.3 mg equivalent to valganciclovir 450 mg]

Valganciclovir Hydrochloride *see* Valganciclovir *on page 1143*

Valtrex® *see* Valacyclovir *on page 1140*

Vancocin® *see* Vancomycin *on page 1144*

Vancomycin (van koe MYE sin)

Related Information

Antibiotic Treatment of Adults With Infective Endocarditis *on page 1271*

Antimicrobial Activity Against Selected Organisms *on page 1165*

Neutropenic Fever Guidelines *on page 1295*

U.S. Brand Names Vancocin®

Canadian Brand Names Vancocin®

Synonyms Vancomycin Hydrochloride

Generic Available Yes: Injection

Use Treatment of patients with infections caused by staphylococcal species and streptococcal species; used orally for staphylococcal enterocolitis or for antibiotic-associated pseudomembranous colitis produced by *C. difficile*

Drug of Choice or Alternative for

Disease/Syndrome(s):

Brain Abscess *on page 58*
Catheter Infection, Intravascular *on page 70*
Endocarditis, Acute, I.V. Drug Abuse *on page 123*
Endocarditis, Acute Native Valve *on page 124*
Endocarditis, Prosthetic Valve, Early *on page 124*
Endocarditis, Prosthetic Valve, Late *on page 125*
Endocarditis, Subacute Native Valve *on page 126*
Endophthalmitis, Bacterial and Fungal *on page 128*
Epididymitis/Orchitis *on page 138*
Fever, Neutropenic *on page 148*
Joint Replacement, Early Infection *on page 197*
Joint Replacement, Late Infection *on page 198*
Keratitis, Bacterial and Fungal *on page 199*
Mastitis *on page 214*
Meningitis, Community-Acquired, Adult *on page 216*
Meningitis, Neonatal (<1 month of age) *on page 217*
Meningitis, Pediatric (>1 month of age) *on page 218*
Meningitis, Postsurgical *on page 218*
Meningitis, Post-traumatic *on page 219*
Osteomyelitis, Diabetic Foot *on page 249*
Osteomyelitis, Healthy Adult *on page 250*
Osteomyelitis, Pediatric *on page 251*
Peritonitis, CAPD-Associated *on page 262*
Pneumonia, Hospital-Acquired *on page 272*
Pneumonia, Ventilator-Associated *on page 273*
Sepsis *on page 295*
Sinusitis, Hospital-Acquired *on page 300*
Skin and Soft Tissue *on page 300*
Thrombophlebitis, Suppurative *on page 330*
Toxic Shock Syndrome *on page 331*
Urinary Tract Infection, Catheter-Associated *on page 345*
Wound Infection, Surgical *on page 354*

Organism(s):

Bacillus cereus on page 44
Clostridium difficile on page 85
Corynebacterium jeikeium on page 98
Enterococcus Species *on page 134*
Rhodococcus Species *on page 288*
Staphylococcus aureus, Methicillin-Resistant *on page 304*
Staphylococcus aureus, Methicillin-Susceptible *on page 307*
Staphylococcus epidermidis, Methicillin-Resistant *on page 309*
Staphylococcus epidermidis, Methicillin-Susceptible *on page 310*
Streptococcus agalactiae on page 313
Streptococcus bovis on page 315
Streptococcus pneumoniae, Drug-Resistant *on page 316*
Streptococcus pneumoniae, Drug-Susceptible *on page 319*
Streptococcus pyogenes on page 321
Streptococcus-Related Gram-Positive Cocci *on page 325*
Streptococcus, Viridans Group *on page 326*

Pregnancy Risk Factor C

Contraindications Hypersensitivity to vancomycin or any component of the formulation; avoid in patients with previous severe hearing loss

Warnings/Precautions Use with caution in patients with renal impairment or those receiving other nephrotoxic or ototoxic drugs; dosage modification required in patients with impaired renal function (especially elderly)

Adverse Reactions

Oral:

>10%: Gastrointestinal: Bitter taste, nausea, vomiting

(Continued)

Vancomycin *(Continued)*

1% to 10%:
- Central nervous system: Chills, drug fever
- Hematologic: Eosinophilia

<1%: Vasculitis, thrombocytopenia, ototoxicity, renal failure, interstitial nephritis

Parenteral:

>10%:
- Cardiovascular: Hypotension accompanied by flushing
- Dermatologic: Erythematous rash on face and upper body (red neck or red man syndrome - infusion rate related)

1% to 10%:
- Central nervous system: Chills, drug fever
- Dermatologic: Rash
- Hematologic: Eosinophilia, reversible neutropenia

<1%: Vasculitis, Stevens-Johnson syndrome, ototoxicity (especially with large doses), thrombocytopenia, renal failure (especially with renal dysfunction or pre-existing hearing loss)

Overdosage/Toxicology Symptoms include ototoxicity and nephrotoxicity. There is no specific therapy for vancomycin overdose. Care is symptomatic and supportive. Peritoneal filtration and hemofiltration (not dialysis) have been shown to reduce the serum concentration of vancomycin. High flux dialysis may remove up to 25%.

Drug Interactions

Increased Effect/Toxicity: Increased toxicity with other ototoxic or nephrotoxic drugs. Increased neuromuscular blockade with most neuromuscular blocking agents.

Stability

Vancomycin reconstituted intravenous solutions are stable for 14 days at room temperature or refrigeration

Stability of parenteral admixture at room temperature (25°C) or refrigeration temperature (4°C): 7 days

Standard diluent: 500 mg/150 mL D_5W; 750 mg/250 mL D_5W; 1 g/250 mL D_5W

Minimum volume: Maximum concentration is 5 mg/mL to minimize thrombophlebitis

Mechanism of Action Inhibits bacterial cell wall synthesis by blocking glycopeptide polymerization through binding tightly to D-alanyl-D-alanine portion of cell wall precursor

Pharmacodynamics/Kinetics

Absorption: Oral: Poor; I.M.: Erratic; Intraperitoneal: ~38%

Distribution: Widely in body tissues and fluids. except for CSF
- Relative diffusion from blood into CSF: Good only with inflammation (exceeds usual MICs)
- CSF:blood level ratio: Normal meninges: Nil; Inflamed meninges: 20% to 30%

Protein binding: 10% to 50%

Half-life elimination: Biphasic: Terminal:
- Newborns: 6-10 hours
- Infants and Children 3 months to 4 years: 4 hours
- Children >3 years: 2.2-3 hours
- Adults: 5-11 hours; significantly prolonged with renal impairment
- End-stage renal disease: 200-250 hours

Time to peak, serum: I.V.: 45-65 minutes

Excretion: I.V.: Urine (80% to 90% as unchanged drug); Oral: Primarily feces

Dosage Initial dosage recommendation:

Neonates: I.V.:
- Postnatal age ≤7 days:
  - <1200 g: 15 mg/kg/dose every 24 hours
  - 1200-2000 g: 10 mg/kg/dose every 12 hours
  - >2000 g: 15 mg/kg/dose every 12 hours
- Postnatal age >7 days:
  - <1200 g: 15 mg/kg/dose every 24 hours
  - ≥1200 g: 10 mg/kg/dose divided every 8 hours

Infants >1 month and Children: I.V.:
- 40 mg/kg/day in divided doses every 6 hours
- Prophylaxis for bacterial endocarditis:
  - Dental, oral, or upper respiratory tract surgery: 20 mg/kg 1 hour prior to the procedure
  - GI/GU procedure: 20 mg/kg plus gentamicin 2 mg/kg 1 hour prior to surgery

Infants >1 month and Children with staphylococcal central nervous system infection:
- I.V.: 60 mg/kg/day in divided doses every 6 hours

Adults: I.V.:
- With normal renal function: 1 g **or** 10-15 mg/kg/dose every 12 hours

Prophylaxis for bacterial endocarditis:
Dental, oral, or upper respiratory tract surgery: 1 g 1 hour before surgery
GI/GU procedure: 1 g plus 1.5 mg/kg gentamicin 1 hour prior to surgery

Dosing interval in renal impairment (vancomycin levels should be monitored in patients with any renal impairment):
Cl_{cr} >60 mL/minute: Start with 1 g or 10-15 mg/kg/dose every 12 hours
Cl_{cr} 40-60 mL/minute: Start with 1 g or 10-15 mg/kg/dose every 24 hours
Cl_{cr} <40 mL/minute: Will need longer intervals; determine by serum concentration monitoring

Hemodialysis: Not dialyzable (0% to 5%); generally not removed; exception minimal-moderate removal by some of the newer high-flux filters; dose may need to be administered more frequently; monitor serum concentrations
Continuous ambulatory peritoneal dialysis (CAPD): Not significantly removed; administration via CAPD fluid: 15-30 mg/L (15-30 mcg/mL) of CAPD fluid
Continuous arteriovenous hemofiltration: Dose as for Cl_{cr} 10-40 mL/minute

Antibiotic lock technique (for catheter infections): 2 mg/mL in SWI/NS or D_5W; instill 3-5 mL into catheter port as a flush solution instead of heparin lock (**Note:** Do not mix with any other solutions)

Intrathecal: Vancomycin is available as a powder for injection and may be diluted to 1-5 mg/mL concentration in preservative-free 0.9% sodium chloride for administration into the CSF
Neonates: 5-10 mg/day
Children: 5-20 mg/day
Adults: Up to 20 mg/day

Oral: Pseudomembranous colitis produced by *C. difficile*:
Neonates: 10 mg/kg/day in divided doses
Children: 40 mg/kg/day in divided doses, added to fluids
Adults: 125 mg 4 times/day for 10 days

Dietary Considerations May be taken with food.

Administration Administer vancomycin by I.V. intermittent infusion over at least 60 minutes at a final concentration not to exceed 5 mg/mL. If a maculopapular rash appears on the face, neck, trunk, and/or upper extremities (Red man syndrome), slow the infusion rate to over 1½ to 2 hours and increase the dilution volume. Hypotension, shock, and cardiac arrest (rare) have also been reported with too rapid of infusion. Reactions are often treated with antihistamines and possibly steroids.

Extravasation treatment: Monitor I.V. site closely; extravasation will cause serious injury with possible necrosis and tissue sloughing. Rotate infusion site frequently.

Monitoring Parameters Periodic renal function tests, urinalysis, serum vancomycin concentrations, WBC, audiogram

Reference Range
Timing of serum samples: Draw peak 1 hour after 1-hour infusion has completed; draw trough just before next dose
Therapeutic levels: Peak: 25-40 mcg/mL; Trough: 5-12 mcg/mL
Toxic: >80 mcg/mL (SI: >54 μmol/L)

Patient Information Report pain at infusion site, dizziness, fullness or ringing in ears with I.V. use; nausea or vomiting with oral use

Additional Information Because of its long half-life, vancomycin should be dosed on an every 12 hour basis; monitoring of peak and trough serum levels is advisable. The "red man syndrome" characterized by skin rash and hypotension is not an allergic reaction but rather is associated with too rapid infusion of the drug. To alleviate or prevent the reaction, infuse vancomycin at a rate of ≥30 minutes for each 500 mg of drug being administered (eg, 1 g over ≥60 minutes); 1.5 g over ≥90 minutes.

Dosage Forms
Capsule (Vancocin®): 125 mg, 250 mg
Infusion [premixed in iso-osmotic dextrose] (Vancocin®): 500 mg (100 mL); 1 g (200 mL)
Injection, powder for reconstitution: 500 mg, 1 g, 5 g, 10 g

Selected Readings

Cantù TG, Yamanaka-Yuen NA, and Lietman PS, "Serum Vancomycin Concentrations: Reappraisal of Their Clinical Value," *Clin Infect Dis*, 1994, 18(4):533-43.
Cunha BA, "Vancomycin," *Med Clin North Am*, 1995, 79(4):817-31.
French GL, "Enterococci and Vancomycin Resistance," *Clin Infect Dis*, 1998, 27(Suppl 1):S75-83.
Kelly CP, Pothoulakis C, and LaMont JT, "*Clostridium difficile* colitis," *N Engl J Med*, 1994, 330(4):257-62.
Lundstrom TS and Sobel JD, "Vancomycin, Trimethoprim-Sulfamethoxazole, and Rifampin," *Infect Dis Clin North Am*, 1995, 9(3):747-67.
Wilhelm MP, "Vancomycin," *Mayo Clin Proc*, 1991, 66(11):1165-70.

Vancomycin Hydrochloride *see* Vancomycin *on page 1144*
Vaniqa™ *see* Eflornithine *on page 798*
Vantin® *see* Cefpodoxime *on page 714*
VAQTA® *see* Hepatitis A Vaccine *on page 853*

Varicella Virus Vaccine (var i SEL a VYE rus vak SEEN)

Related Information

Immunization Recommendations *on page 1249*

U.S. Brand Names Varivax®

Canadian Brand Names Varilrix®; Varivax®

Synonyms Chicken Pox Vaccine; Varicella-Zoster Virus (VZV) Vaccine

Generic Available No

Use Immunization against varicella in children ≥12 months of age and adults

Drug of Choice or Alternative for

Organism(s):

Varicella-Zoster Virus *on page 347*

Pregnancy Risk Factor C

Pregnancy Implications Animal reproduction studies have not been conducted. Varivax® should not be administered to pregnant females and pregnancy should be avoided for 3 months following vaccination. A pregnancy registry has been established for pregnant women exposed to varicella virus vaccine (800-986-8999).

Contraindications Hypersensitivity gelatin, neomycin, or any component of the vaccine;individuals with blood dyscrasias, leukemia, lymphomas, or other malignant neoplasms affecting the bone marrow or lymphatic systems; those receiving immunosuppressive therapy; primary and acquired immunodeficiency states; a family history of congenital or hereditary immunodeficiency; active untreated tuberculosis; current febrile illness; pregnancy

Warnings/Precautions Immediate treatment for anaphylactoid reaction should be available during vaccine use. Defer vaccination for at least 5 months following blood or plasma transfusions, immune globulin (IgG), or VZIG (avoid IgG or IVIG use for 2 months following vaccination); salicylates should be avoided for 6 weeks after vaccination. Vaccinated individuals should not have close association with susceptible high risk individuals (newborns, pregnant women, immunocompromised persons) for 6 weeks following vaccination. Children with HIV infection, who are asymptomatic and not immunosuppressed (CDC immunologic category 1) may receive live attenuated varicella vaccine at 12-15 months of age or older. No recommendations available for adults.

Adverse Reactions All serious adverse reactions must be reported to the U.S. Department of Health and Human Services (DHHS) Vaccine Adverse Event Reporting System (VAERS) 1-800-822-7967.

>10%:

- Central nervous system: Fever (10% to 15%)
- Local: Injection site reaction (19% to 33%)

1% to 10%:

- Central nervous system: Chills, fatigue, headache, irritability, malaise, nervousness, sleep disturbance
- Dermatologic: Generalized varicella-like rash (1% to 6%), contact rash, dermatitis, diaper rash, dry skin, eczema, heat rash, itching
- Gastrointestinal: Abdominal pain, appetite decreased, cold/canker sore, constipation, diarrhea, nausea, vomiting
- Hematologic: Lymphadenopathy
- Local: Varicella-like rash at the injection site (1% to 3%)
- Neuromuscular & skeletal: Arthralgia, myalgia, stiff neck
- Otic: Otitis
- Respiratory: Cough, lower/upper respiratory illness
- Miscellaneous: Allergic reactions, teething

<1%: Febrile seizure, pneumonitis

Postmarketing/case reports: Anaphylaxis, ataxia, Bell's palsy, cellulitis, cerebrovascular accident, dizziness, encephalitis, erythema multiforme, Guillain-Barré syndrome, Henoch-Schönlein purpura, herpes zoster, impetigo, nonfebrile seizure, paresthesia, pharyngitis, pneumonia, secondary skin infection, Stevens-Johnson syndrome, thrombocytopenia, transverse myelitis

Drug Interactions

Increased Effect/Toxicity: Salicylates may increase the risk of Reye's following varicella vaccination (avoid salicylate use for 6 weeks following vaccination).

Decreased Effect: The effect of the vaccine may be decreased and the risk of varicella disease in individuals who are receiving immunosuppressant drugs (including high dose systemic corticosteroids) may be increased. Effect of vaccine may be decreased in given within 5 months of immune globulins. Effectiveness of varicella vaccine may be decreased if given within 30 days of MMR vaccine (effectiveness not decreased when administered simultaneously).

Stability Store powder in freezer at -15°C (5°F) or colder, protect from light; store diluent separately at room temperature or in refrigerator. Powder may be stored under refrigeration for up to 72 continuous hours prior to reconstitution; if not used

within 72 hours, vaccine should be discarded. Use 0.7 mL of the provided diluent to reconstitute vaccine. Gently agitate to mix thoroughly. (Total volume of reconstituted vaccine will be ~0.5 mL.) Following reconstitution, discard if not used within 30 minutes. Do not freeze reconstituted vaccine.

Mechanism of Action As a live, attenuated vaccine, varicella virus vaccine offers active immunity to disease caused by the varicella-zoster virus

Pharmacodynamics/Kinetics

Onset of action: Seroconversion: ~4-6 weeks

Duration: Antibody titers detectable at 10 years post-vaccination

Dosage SubQ:

Children 12 months to 12 years: 0.5 mL; a second dose may be administered ≥3 months later

Children ≥13 years to Adults: 2 doses of 0.5 mL separated by 4-8 weeks

Administration Do not administer I.V.; inject immediately after reconstitution; inject SubQ into the outer aspect of the upper arm, if possible. Federal law requires that the date of administration, the vaccine manufacturer, lot number of vaccine, and the administering person's name, title and address be entered into the patient's permanent medical record.

Monitoring Parameters Rash, fever

Patient Information Report any adverse reactions to the prescriber or Vaccine Adverse Event Reporting System (1-800-822-7967). Some side effects may occur 1-6 weeks after the shot. Common side effects include soreness or swelling in the area where the shot is given, mild rash, fever. Do not take aspirin for 6 weeks after getting the vaccine. Do not use in pregnancy and do not get pregnant for 3 months after getting this vaccine.

Additional Information

Federal law requires that the date of administration, the vaccine manufacturer, lot number of vaccine, and the administering person's name, title and address be entered into the patient's permanent medical record.

Dosage Forms Injection, powder for reconstitution [preservative free; single-dose vial]: 1350 plaque-forming units (PFU) [contains gelatin and trace amounts of neomycin]

Varicella-Zoster Immune Globulin (Human)

(var i SEL a- ZOS ter i MYUN GLOB yoo lin HYU man)

Related Information

USPHS / IDSA Guidelines for the Prevention of Opportunistic Infections in Persons Infected With HIV *on page 1237*

Synonyms VZIG

Generic Available No

Use Passive immunization of susceptible patients who are at a greater risk of complications following significant exposure to varicella

Restrict administration to those patients meeting the following criteria:

Immunocompromised children including those with neoplastic disease (eg, leukemia or lymphoma); congenital or acquired immunodeficiency; immunosuppressive therapy with steroids, antimetabolites or other immunosuppressive treatment regimens

Newborn of mother who had onset of varicella (chickenpox) within 5 days before delivery or within 48 hours after delivery (not indicated if the mother has zoster)

Premature infants (≥28 weeks gestation) whose mother has no history of chickenpox

Premature infants (<28 weeks gestation or ≤1000 g) regardless of maternal history

Immunocompromised adults

Significant exposure includes:

Continuous household contact

Playmate contact (>1 hour play indoors)

Hospital contact (in same 2-4 bedroom or adjacent beds in a large ward or prolonged face-to-face contact with an infectious staff member or patient)

Pregnancy Risk Factor C

Pregnancy Implications Reproduction studies have not been conducted. Clinical use of other immunoglobulins suggest that there are no adverse effects on the fetus. Pregnant women may be at increased risk of complications from chickenpox. Use of VZIG in pregnant women should be evaluated as in other adults. VZIG administration during pregnancy does not prevent intrauterine infection, but is used to prevent complications in the mother.

Contraindications Severe reaction associated with past human immune globulin administration; prophylactic use in immunodeficient patients with history of varicella, unless immunosuppression is associated with bone marrow transplantation (BMT);

(Continued)

Varicella-Zoster Immune Globulin (Human) *(Continued)*

nonimmunodeficient patients, including pregnant women; persons with IgA deficiency; severe thrombocytopenia

Warnings/Precautions

VZIG is not indicated for prophylaxis or therapy of normal adults who are exposed to or who develop varicella; it is not indicated for treatment of herpes zoster. Do not inject I.V. There is no evidence VZIG modifies established varicella-zoster infections. Administer as soon as possible following exposure. Administration within 96 hours of exposure is advised; use >96 hours after exposure has not been evaluated. BMT recipients should not be considered immune unless varicella develops following transplant. Anaphylactic hypersensitivity reactions may occur; epinephrine 1:1000 should be readily available.

Adverse Reactions

1%: Local: Discomfort at the site of injection (pain, redness, edema)

<1%: Malaise, headache, rash, angioedema, GI symptoms, respiratory symptom, anaphylactic shock

Drug Interactions

Decreased Effect:

VZIG may interfere with the immune response; do not administer live virus vaccines within 5 months of VZIG administration

Stability Refrigerate at 2°C to 8°C (36°F to 46°F); do not freeze

Mechanism of Action Antibodies obtained from pooled human plasma of individuals with high titers of varicella-zoster provide passive immunity

Pharmacodynamics/Kinetics Duration: ~3 weeks

Dosage Note: High risk susceptible patients who are exposed again more than 3 weeks after a prior dose of VZIG should receive another full dose.

I.M.: 125 units/10 kg (22 lb); maximum dose: 625 units (5 vials); minimum dose: 125 units; do not administer fractional doses

Weight-based VZIG dosing: See table.

VZIG Dose Based on Weight

Weight of Patient		Dose	
kg	lb	Units	No. of Vials (125 units/vial)
0-10	0-22	125	1
10.1-20	22.1-44	250	2
20.1-30	44.1-66	375	3
30.1-40	66.1-88	500	4
>40	>88	625	5 (or one 625 unit vial)

Administration Administer as soon as possible after presumed exposure. Administer by deep injection in the gluteal muscle or in another large muscle mass. Do not inject I.V. Administer within 96 hours of exposure. No more than 2.5 mL should be administered into a single injection site.

Test Interactions May show false positive for immunity to VZV for ~2 months following VZIG administration.

Additional Information

Age is the most important risk factor for reactivation of varicella zoster; persons <50 years of age have incidence of 2.5 cases per 1000, whereas those 60-79 years have 6.5 cases per 1000 and those >80 years have 10 cases per 1000

Dosage Forms Injection, solution [preservative free]: 125 units (1.25 mL); 625 units (6.25 mL)

Varicella-Zoster Virus (VZV) Vaccine *see* Varicella Virus Vaccine *on page 1148*
Varilrix® (Can) *see* Varicella Virus Vaccine *on page 1148*
Varivax® *see* Varicella Virus Vaccine *on page 1148*
Vasocidin® (Can) *see* Sulfacetamide and Prednisolone *on page 1082*
Vaxigrip® (Can) *see* Influenza Virus Vaccine *on page 875*
Veetids® *see* Penicillin V Potassium *on page 998*
Velosef® *see* Cephradine *on page 731*
Vermox® [DSC] *see* Mebendazole *on page 928*
Versel® (Can) *see* Selenium Sulfide *on page 1063*
VFEND® *see* Voriconazole *on page 1151*
Vibramycin® *see* Doxycycline *on page 787*

Vibra-Tabs® *see* Doxycycline *on page 787*
Videx® *see* Didanosine *on page 774*
Videx® EC *see* Didanosine *on page 774*
Vigamox™ *see* Moxifloxacin *on page 949*
VIGIV *see* Vaccinia Immune Globulin (Intravenous) *on page 1139*
Viracept® *see* Nelfinavir *on page 960*
Viramune® *see* Nevirapine *on page 967*
Virazole® *see* Ribavirin *on page 1040*
Viread® *see* Tenofovir *on page 1095*
Virilon® IM (Can) *see* Testosterone *on page 1100*
Viroptic® *see* Trifluridine *on page 1129*
Vistide® *see* Cidofovir *on page 740*
Vitamin A Acid *see* Tretinoin (Topical) *on page 1127*
Vitrasert® *see* Ganciclovir *on page 834*
Vitravene™ [DSC] *see* Fomivirsen *on page 826*
Vivotif Berna® *see* Typhoid Vaccine *on page 1137*

Voriconazole (vor i KOE na zole)

U.S. Brand Names VFEND®

Canadian Brand Names VFEND®

Synonyms UK109496

Generic Available No

Use Treatment of invasive aspergillosis; treatment of esophageal candidiasis; treatment of candidemia (in non-neutropenic patients); treatment of *Candida* deep tissue infections; treatment of serious fungal infections caused by *Scedosporium apiospermum* and *Fusarium* spp (including *Fusarium solani*) in patients intolerant of, or refractory to, other therapy

Drug of Choice or Alternative for Disease/Syndrome(s):

Endophthalmitis, Bacterial and Fungal *on page 128*
Esophagitis *on page 147*

Organism(s):

Aspergillus Species *on page 38*
Candida Species *on page 67*
Dematiaceous Fungi *on page 112*
Fusarium Species *on page 151*
Mucor Species *on page 225*

Pregnancy Risk Factor D

Pregnancy Implications Voriconazole can cause fetal harm when administered to a pregnant woman. Voriconazole was teratogenic in animal studies, and lowered plasma estradiol in animal models. Should be used in pregnant woman only if benefit to mother justifies potential risk to the fetus.

Contraindications Hypersensitivity to voriconazole or any component of the formulation (cross-reaction with other azole antifungal agents may occur but has not been established, use caution); coadministration of CYP3A4 substrates which may lead to QT_c prolongation (cisapride, pimozide, or quinidine); coadministration with barbiturates (long acting), carbamazepine, efavirenz, ergot alkaloids, rifampin, rifabutin, ritonavir, and sirolimus; pregnancy (unless risk:benefit justifies use)

Warnings/Precautions Visual changes are commonly associated with treatment, including blurred vision, changes in visual acuity, color changes, and photophobia. Patients should be warned to avoid tasks which depend on vision, including operating machinery or driving. Changes are reversible on discontinuation following brief exposure/treatment regimens (≤28 days); reversibility following long-term administration has not been evaluated.

Serious hepatic reactions (including hepatitis, cholestasis, and fulminant hepatic failure) have occurred during treatment, primarily in patients with serious concomitant medical conditions, including hematological malignancy. However, hepatotoxicity has occurred in patients with no identifiable risk factors. Use caution in patients with pre-existing hepatic impairment (dose adjustment required).

Voriconazole tablets contain lactose; avoid administration in hereditary galactose intolerance, Lapp lactase deficiency, or glucose-galactose malabsorption. Suspension contains sucrose; use caution with fructose intolerance, sucrose-isomaltase deficiency, or glucose-galactose malabsorption. Avoid/limit use of intravenous formulation in patients with renal impairment; intravenous formulation contains excipient (Continued)

Voriconazole *(Continued)*

sulfobutyl ether beta-cyclodextrin (SBECD), which may accumulate in renal insufficiency. Infusion-related reactions may occur with intravenous dosing. Consider discontinuation of infusion if reaction is severe.

Use caution in patients with an increased risk of arrhythmia (concurrent QT_c-prolonging drugs, hypokalemia, cardiomyopathy, or prior cardiotoxic therapy). Use caution in patients receiving concurrent non-nucleoside reverse transcriptase inhibitors (efavirenz is contraindicated).

Avoid use in pregnancy, unless an evaluation of the potential benefit justifies possible risk to the fetus. Safety and efficacy have not been established in children <12 years of age.

Adverse Reactions Note: Includes adverse reactions reported from all trials, including trials conducted in immunocompromised patients; cause:effect relationship not established for many reactions

>10%: Ocular: Visual changes (photophobia, color changes, increased or decreased visual acuity, or blurred vision occur in ~30%)

1% to 10%:

- Cardiovascular: Tachycardia (3%), hyper-/hypotension (2%), vasodilation (2%), peripheral edema (1%)
- Central nervous system: Fever (6%), chills (4%), headache (3%), hallucinations (3%), dizziness (1%)
- Dermatologic: Rash (6%), pruritus (1%)
- Endocrine & metabolic: Hypokalemia (2%), hypomagnesemia (1%)
- Gastrointestinal: Nausea (6%), vomiting (5%), abdominal pain (2%), diarrhea (1%), xerostomia (1%)
- Hematologic: Thrombocytopenia (1%)
- Hepatic: Alkaline phosphatase increased (4%), transaminases increased (2%), AST increased (2%), ALT increased (2%), cholestatic jaundice (1%)
- Renal: Acute renal failure (1%)

<1% (Limited to important or life-threatening): Acute tubular necrosis, adrenal cortical insufficiency, agranulocytosis, allergic reaction, anaphylactoid reaction, anemia (aplastic), anemia (macrocytic, megaloblastic, or microcytic), angioedema, aplastic anemia, ataxia, atrial arrhythmia, atrial fibrillation, AV block, bigeminy, bone marrow depression, bone necrosis, bradycardia, brain edema, bundle branch block, cardiac arrest, cerebral hemorrhage, cholecystitis, cholelithiasis, color blindness, coma, CHF, convulsion, delirium, dementia, depersonalization, depression, DIC, discoid lupus erythematosus, duodenal ulcer perforation, dyspnea, encephalopathy, enlarged liver, enlarged spleen, eosinophilia, erythema multiforme, exfoliative dermatitis, extrapyramidal symptoms, fixed drug eruption, gastrointestinal hemorrhage, grand mal seizure, Guillain-Barré syndrome, hematemesis, hemolytic anemia, hepatic coma, hepatic failure, hepatitis, intestinal perforation, intracranial hypertension, leukopenia, lung edema, myasthenia, MI, neuropathy, night blindness, optic atrophy, optic neuritis, pancreatitis, pancytopenia, papilledema, paresthesia, photosensitivity, psychosis, pulmonary embolus, QT interval prolongation, respiratory distress syndrome, sepsis, Stevens-Johnson syndrome, suicidal ideation, supraventricular tachycardia, syncope, thrombotic thrombocytopenic purpura, toxic epidermal necrolysis, ventricular arrhythmia, ventricular fibrillation, ventricular tachycardia, torsade de pointes, vertigo, visual field defect

Drug Interactions

Cytochrome P450 Effect: Substrate of CYP2C8/9 (major), 2C19 (major), 3A4 (minor); **Inhibits** CYP2C8/9 (weak), 2C19 (weak), 3A4 (moderate)

Increased Effect/Toxicity: Voriconazole may increase the serum concentrations of cisapride, pimozide leading to malignant arrhythmias; use is contraindicated. Concurrent use of QT_c-prolonging agents (including class Ia and III antiarrhythmics) may increase risk of arrhythmias. Serum levels of ergot alkaloids may be increased by voriconazole, leading to ergot toxicity; concurrent use is contraindicated. Rifabutin serum levels are increased by voriconazole; concurrent use is contraindicated. Serum concentrations of busulfan, docetaxel, and dofetilide may be increased; avoid concurrent use.

Serum concentrations of immunosuppressants (cyclosporine, sirolimus, and tacrolimus) may be increased; concurrent use of sirolimus is contraindicated. Decrease cyclosporine dosage by 50% when initiating voriconazole, decreased tacrolimus dosage by 66% when initiating voriconazole.

Serum levels of voriconazole may be increased by delavirdine. Indinavir did not appear to alter voriconazole serum concentrations during concurrent treatment; other protease inhibitors may result in increased voriconazole concentrations.

Voriconazole may increase the serum concentrations of buspirone, methylprednisolone, quinidine, sulfonylureas, trimetrexate, vinca alkaloids, or zolpidem. Methadone serum concentrations and duration/effects may be increased significantly (monitor and reduce methadone dose if necessary). Voriconazole may increase the levels/effects of benzodiazepines, calcium channel blockers, selected HMG-CoA reductase inhibitors mirtazapine, nateglinide, nefazodone, sildenafil (and other PDE-5 inhibitors), tacrolimus, venlafaxine, and other CYP3A4 substrates. In addition, the anticoagulant effect of warfarin may be increased.

Changes in gastric acidity (due to H_2 antagonists or proton pump inhibitors) do not appear to significantly affect voriconazole absorption. However, voriconazole may significantly increase serum levels of omeprazole. For omeprazole dosages >40 mg/day, reduce omeprazole dosage by 50%. Serum levels of other proton pump inhibitors may also be increased.

Decreased Effect: The levels/effects of voriconazole may be decreased by aminoglutethimide, carbamazepine, efavirenz, nevirapine, phenytoin, phenobarbital, secobarbital, rifampin, ritonavir, and other CYP2C8/9 or 2C19 inducers. Rifampin decreases voriconazole's serum concentration to levels which are no longer effective; avoid concurrent use. When used with phenytoin, prospective adjustment of voriconazole dosage is recommended. Serum levels of voriconazole may be decreased by efavirenz or nevirapine.

Ethanol/Nutrition/Herb Interactions

Food: May decrease voriconazole absorption. Voriconazole should be taken 1 hour before or 1 hour after a meal. Avoid grapefruit juice (may increase voriconazole serum levels).

Herb/Nutraceutical: St John's wort may decrease voriconazole levels.

Stability

Powder for injection: Store at 15°C to 30°C (59°F to 86°F). Reconstitute 200 mg vial with 19 mL of sterile water for injection (use of automated syringe is not recommended). Resultant solution (20 mL) has a concentration of 10 mg/mL. Must dilute to 0.5-5 mg/mL prior to infusion. Reconstituted solutions are stable for up to 24 hours under refrigeration at 2°C to 8°C (36°F to 46°F).

Powder for oral suspension: Store at 2°C to 8°C (36°F to 46°F). Add 46 mL of water to the bottle to make 40 mg/mL suspension. Reconstituted oral suspension may be stored at 15°C to 30°C (59°F to 86°F). Discard after 14 days.

Tablets: Store at 15°C to 30°C (59°F to 86°F).

Mechanism of Action Interferes with fungal cytochrome P450 activity, decreasing ergosterol synthesis (principal sterol in fungal cell membrane) and inhibiting fungal cell membrane formation.

Pharmacodynamics/Kinetics

Absorption: Well absorbed after oral administration

Distribution: V_d: 4.6 L/kg

Protein binding: 58%

Metabolism: Hepatic, via CYP2C19 (major pathway) and CYP2C9 and CYP3A4 (less significant); saturable (may demonstrate nonlinearity)

Bioavailability: 96%

Half-life elimination: Variable, dose-dependent

Time to peak: 1-2 hours

Excretion: Urine (as inactive metabolites)

Dosage

Children <12 years: No data available

Children ≥12 years and Adults:

- Invasive aspergillosis and other serious fungal infections: I.V.: Initial: Loading dose: 6 mg/kg every 12 hours for 2 doses; followed by maintenance dose of 4 mg/kg every 12 hours
- Candidemia and other deep tissue *Candida* infections: I.V.: Initial: Loading dose 6 mg/kg every 12 hours for 2 doses; followed by maintenance dose of 3-4 mg/kg every 12 hours
- **Note:** Conversion to oral dosing:
  - Patients <40 kg: 100 mg every 12 hours; increase to 150 mg every 12 hours in patients who fail to respond adequately
  - Patients ≥40 kg: 200 mg every 12 hours; increase to 300 mg every 12 hours in patients who fail to respond adequately
- Esophageal candidiasis: Oral:
  - Patients <40 kg: 100 mg every 12 hours
  - Patients ≥40 kg: 200 mg every 12 hours
  - **Note:** Treatment should continue for a minimum of 14 days, and for at least 7 days following resolution of symptoms.

Dosage adjustment in patients unable to tolerate treatment:

I.V.: Dose may be reduced to 3 mg/kg every 12 hours

(Continued)

Voriconazole *(Continued)*

Oral: Dose may be reduced in 50 mg increments to a minimum dosage of 200 mg every 12 hours in patients weighing ≥40 kg (100 mg every 12 hours in patients <40 kg)

Dosage adjustment in patients receiving concomitant phenytoin:

I.V.: Increase maintenance dosage to 5 mg/kg every 12 hours

Oral: Increase dose from 200 mg to 400 mg every 12 hours in patients ≥40 kg (100 mg to 200 mg every 12 hours in patients <40 kg)

Dosage adjustment in renal impairment: In patients with Cl_{cr} <50 mL/minute, accumulation of the intravenous vehicle (SBECD) occurs. After initial loading dose, oral voriconazole should be administered to these patients, unless an assessment of the benefit:risk to the patient justifies the use of I.V. voriconazole. Monitor serum creatinine and change to oral voriconazole therapy when possible.

Dosage adjustment in hepatic impairment:

Mild-to-moderate hepatic dysfunction (Child-Pugh Class A and B): Following standard loading dose, reduce maintenance dosage by 50%

Severe hepatic impairment: Should only be used if benefit outweighs risk; monitor closely for toxicity

Dietary Considerations Oral: Should be taken 1 hour before or 1 hour after a meal. Voriconazole tablets contain lactose; avoid administration in hereditary galactose intolerance, Lapp lactase deficiency, or glucose-galactose malabsorption. Suspension contains sucrose; use caution with fructose intolerance, sucrose-isomaltase deficiency, or glucose-galactose malabsorption.

Administration

Oral: Administer 1 hour before or 1 hour after a meal.

I.V.: Infuse over 1-2 hours (rate not to exceed 3 mg/kg/hour)

Monitoring Parameters Hepatic function, visual function, renal function

Dosage Forms

Injection, powder for reconstitution: 200 mg [contains SBECD 3200 mg]

Powder for oral suspension: 200 mg/5 mL (70 mL) [contains sodium benzoate and sucrose; orange flavor]

Tablet: 50 mg, 200 mg [contains lactose]

VoSol® HC *see* Acetic Acid, Propylene Glycol Diacetate, and Hydrocortisone *on page 629*

V.V.S.® *see* Sulfabenzamide, Sulfacetamide, and Sulfathiazole *on page 1080*

Vytone® *see* Iodoquinol and Hydrocortisone *on page 892*

VZIG *see* Varicella-Zoster Immune Globulin (Human) *on page 1149*

WinRho SDF® *see* Rh_o(D) Immune Globulin *on page 1038*

Wycillin® (Can) *see* Penicillin G Procaine *on page 995*

Xifaxan™ *see* Rifaximin *on page 1053*

Xigris® *see* Drotrecogin Alfa *on page 793*

Yellow Fever Vaccine (YEL oh FEE ver vak SEEN)

Related Information

Immunization Recommendations *on page 1249*

U.S. Brand Names YF-VAX®

Canadian Brand Names YF-VAX®

Generic Available No

Use Induction of active immunity against yellow fever virus, primarily among persons traveling or living in areas where yellow fever infection exists

Pregnancy Risk Factor C

Pregnancy Implications Animal reproduction studies have not been conducted. Adverse effects to the mother or fetus have not been noted in case reports, however, safety and efficacy for use during pregnancy have not been established. Vaccine should be administered if travel to an endemic area is unavoidable and the infant should be monitored after birth. Seroconversion after vaccination is reduced during pregnancy. Tests to verify immune response should be considered. If a pregnant woman is to be vaccinated only to satisfy an international requirement (as opposed to decreasing risk of infection), efforts should be made to obtain a waiver letter.

Contraindications Hypersensitivity to egg or chick embryo protein, or any component of the formulation; children <9 months of age unless in high risk area; children <6 months of age; immunosuppressed patients

Warnings/Precautions Do not use in immunodeficient persons (including patients <24 months after hematopoietic stem cell transplant) or patients receiving immunosuppressants (eg, steroids, radiation). Patients who are immunosuppressed have a theoretical risk of encephalitis with yellow fever vaccine administration; consider

delaying travel or obtaining a waiver letter. Patients on low-dose or short-term corticosteroids, or with asymptomatic HIV infection are not considered immunosuppressed and may receive the vaccine. Chicken embryos are used in the manufacture of this vaccine; have epinephrine available in persons with previous history of egg allergy if the vaccine must be used. The vial stopper contains latex. Avoid use in infants <9 months and pregnant women unless travel to high-risk areas are unavoidable; use in infants <6 months of age is contraindicated due to risk of encephalitis.

Adverse Reactions All serious adverse reactions must be reported to the U.S. Department of Health and Human Services (DHHS) Vaccine Adverse Event Reporting System (VAERS) 1-800-822-7967.

Frequency not defined (adverse reactions may be increased in patients <9 months or ≥65 years of age)

Central nervous system: Headache, myalgia, fever (incidence of these reactions have been reported to be as low as <5% and as high as 10% to 30% depending on the study)

Local: Injection site reactions (edema, hypersensitivity, mass, pain)

Neuromuscular & skeletal: Weakness

Miscellaneous: Hypersensitivity (immediate), vaccine-associated neurotropic disease (rare), viscerotropic disease (rare)

Drug Interactions

Decreased Effect: Decreased effect of live vaccines may occur; use of yellow fever vaccine in immunosuppressed patients is contraindicated due to possible risk of encephalitis or other serious adverse reactions.

Stability Yellow fever vaccine is shipped with dry ice; do not use vaccine unless shipping case contains some dry ice on arrival; maintain vaccine continuously at a temperature between 0°C to 5°C (32°F to 41°F). Do not freeze. Reconstitute only with diluent provided. Inject diluent slowly into vial and allow to stand for 1-2 minutes. Gently swirl until a uniform suspension forms; swirl well before withdrawing dose. Avoid vigorous shaking to prevent foaming of suspension. Vaccine must be used within 60 minutes of reconstitution; keep suspension refrigerated until used.

Pharmacodynamics/Kinetics

Onset: Seroconversion: 10-14 days

Duration: ≥30 years

Dosage Children ≥9 months and Adults: SubQ: One dose (0.5 mL) ≥10 days before travel; Booster: Every 10 years

Administration For SubQ injection only. Do not administer I.M. or I.V.

Monitoring Parameters Monitor for adverse effects up to 10 days after vaccination.

Patient Information Immunity develops by the tenth day and **WHO** requires revaccination every 10 years to maintain travelers' vaccination certificates

Additional Information Federal law requires that the date of administration, the vaccine manufacturer, lot number of vaccine, and the administering person's name, title, and address be entered into the patient's permanent medical record. A desensitization procedure is available for persons with severe egg sensitivity. Consult manufacturer's labeling for details. Some countries require a valid international Certification of Vaccination showing receipt of vaccine. The WHO requires revaccination every 10 years to maintain traveler's vaccination certificate.

The following CDC agencies may be contacted if serologic testing is needed or for advice when administering yellow fever vaccine to pregnant women, children < 9 months or patients with altered immune status:

Division of Vector-Borne Infectious Diseases: 970-221-6400

Division of Global Migration and Quarantine: 404-498-1600

Dosage Forms Injection, powder for reconstitution [17D-204 strain]: ≥4.74 Log_{10} plaque-forming units (PFU) per 0.5 mL dose [single-dose or 5-dose vial; produced in chicken embryos; packaged with diluent; vial stopper contains latex]

YF-VAX® *see* Yellow Fever Vaccine *on page 1154*

Yodoxin® *see* Iodoquinol *on page 891*

Zagam® [DSC] *see* Sparfloxacin *on page 1073*

Zalcitabine (zal SITE a been)

Related Information

Antiretroviral Agents *on page 1206*

Antiretroviral Therapy for HIV Infection *on page 1219*

U.S. Brand Names Hivid®

Canadian Brand Names Hivid®

Synonyms ddC; Dideoxycytidine

Generic Available No

Use In combination with at least two other antiretrovirals in the treatment of patients with HIV infection; it is not recommended that zalcitabine be given in combination with

(Continued)

Zalcitabine *(Continued)*

didanosine, stavudine, or lamivudine due to overlapping toxicities, virologic interactions, or lack of clinical data

Drug of Choice or Alternative for Organism(s):

Human Immunodeficiency Virus *on page 181*

Pregnancy Risk Factor C

Pregnancy Implications It is not known if zalcitabine crosses the human placenta. Animal studies have shown zalcitabine to be teratogenic, developmental toxicities were also observed. Cases of lactic acidosis/hepatic steatosis syndrome have been reported in pregnant women receiving nucleoside analogue drugs. It is not known if pregnancy itself potentiates this known side effect; however, pregnant women may be at increased risk of lactic acidosis and liver damage. Hepatic enzymes and electrolytes should be monitored frequently during the 3rd trimester of pregnancy in women receiving nucleoside analogues. Health professionals are encouraged to contact the antiretroviral pregnancy registry to monitor outcomes of pregnant women exposed to antiretroviral medications (1-800-258-4263 or www.APRegistry.com).

Contraindications Hypersensitivity to zalcitabine or any component of the formulation

Warnings/Precautions Careful monitoring of pancreatic enzymes and liver function tests in patients with a history of pancreatitis, increased amylase, those on parenteral nutrition or with a history of ethanol abuse; discontinue use immediately if pancreatitis is suspected; lactic acidosis and severe hepatomegaly and failure have rarely occurred with zalcitabine resulting in fatality (stop treatment if lactic acidosis or hepatotoxicity occur); some cases may possibly be related to underlying hepatitis B; use with caution in patients on digitalis, or with CHF, renal failure, or hyperphosphatemia; zalcitabine can cause severe peripheral neuropathy; avoid use, if possible, in patients with pre-existing neuropathy or at risk of developing neuropathy. Risk factors include CD4 counts <50 cells/mm^3, diabetes mellitus, weight loss, other drugs known to cause peripheral neuropathy.

Adverse Reactions

>10%:

- Central nervous system: Fever (5% to 17%), malaise (2% to 13%)
- Neuromuscular & skeletal: Peripheral neuropathy (28%)

1% to 10%:

- Central nervous system: Headache (2%), dizziness (1%), fatigue (4%), seizure (1.3%)
- Dermatologic: Rash (2% to 11%), pruritus (3% to 5%)
- Endocrine & metabolic: Hypoglycemia (2% to 6%), hyponatremia (4%), hyperglycemia (1% to 6%)
- Gastrointestinal: Nausea (3%), dysphagia (1% to 4%), anorexia (4%), abdominal pain (3% to 8%), vomiting (1% to 3%), diarrhea (<1% to 10%), weight loss, oral ulcers (3% to 7%), increased amylase (3% to 8%)
- Hematologic: Anemia (occurs as early as 2-4 weeks), granulocytopenia (usually after 6-8 weeks)
- Hepatic: Abnormal hepatic function (9%), hyperbilirubinemia (2% to 5%)
- Neuromuscular & skeletal: Myalgia (1% to 6%), foot pain
- Respiratory: Pharyngitis (2%), cough (6%), nasal discharge (4%)

<1% (Limited to important or life-threatening): Atrial fibrillation, chest pain, constipation, edema, epistaxis, heart racing, hepatic failure, hepatitis, hepatomegaly, hypersensitivity (including anaphylaxis), hypertension, hypocalcemia, jaundice, lactic acidosis, myositis, night sweats, pain, palpitation, pancreatitis, redistribution/accumulation of body fat, syncope, tachycardia, weakness

Overdosage/Toxicology Symptoms include delayed peripheral neurotoxicity. Following oral decontamination, treatment is supportive.

Drug Interactions

Increased Effect/Toxicity: Amphotericin, foscarnet, and aminoglycosides may potentiate the risk of developing peripheral neuropathy or other toxicities associated with zalcitabine by interfering with the renal elimination of zalcitabine. Other drugs associated with peripheral neuropathy include chloramphenicol, cisplatin, dapsone, disulfiram, ethionamide, glutethimide, gold, hydralazine, iodoquinol, isoniazid, metronidazole, nitrofurantoin, phenytoin, ribavirin, and vincristine. Concomitant use with zalcitabine may increase risk of peripheral neuropathy. Concomitant use of zalcitabine with didanosine is not recommended. Concomitant use of ribavirin and nucleoside analogues may increase the risk of developing lactic acidosis (includes adefovir, didanosine, lamivudine, stavudine, zalcitabine, zidovudine).

Decreased Effect: It is not recommended that zalcitabine be given in combination with didanosine, stavudine, or lamivudine due to overlapping toxicities, virologic interactions, or lack of clinical data. Doxorubicin and lamivudine have been shown

in vitro to decrease zalcitabine phosphorylation. Magnesium/aluminum-containing antacids and metoclopramide may decrease the absorption of zalcitabine.

Ethanol/Nutrition/Herb Interactions Food: Food decreases peak plasma concentrations by 39%. Extent and rate of absorption may be decreased with food.

Stability Tablets should be stored in tightly closed bottles at 59°F to 86°F

Mechanism of Action Purine nucleoside (cytosine) analog, zalcitabine or 2',3'-dideoxycytidine (ddC) is converted to active metabolite ddCTP; lack the presence of the 3'-hydroxyl group necessary for phosphodiester linkages during DNA replication. As a result viral replication is prematurely terminated. ddCTP acts as a competitor for binding sites on the HIV-RNA dependent DNA polymerase (reverse transcriptase) to further contribute to inhibition of viral replication.

Pharmacodynamics/Kinetics

Absorption: Well, but variable; decreased 39% with food

Distribution: Minimal data available; variable CSF penetration

Protein binding: <4%

Metabolism: Intracellularly to active triphosphorylated agent

Bioavailability: >80%

Half-life elimination: 2.9 hours; Renal impairment: ≤8.5 hours

Excretion: Urine (>70% as unchanged drug)

Dosage Oral:

Neonates: Dose unknown

Infants and Children <13 years: Safety and efficacy have not been established; suggested usual dose: 0.01 mg/kg every 8 hours; range: 0.005-0.01 mg/kg every 8 hours

Adolescents and Adults: 0.75 mg 3 times/day

Dosing adjustment in renal impairment: Adults:

Cl_{cr} 10-40 mL/minute: 0.75 mg every 12 hours

Cl_{cr} <10 mL/minute: 0.75 mg every 24 hours

Moderately dialyzable (20% to 50%)

Administration Food decreases absorption; take on an empty stomach. Administer around-the-clock. Do not take at the same time with dapsone.

Monitoring Parameters Renal function, viral load, liver function tests, CD4 counts, CBC, serum amylase, triglycerides, calcium

Patient Information Zalcitabine is not a cure; if numbness or tingling occurs, or if persistent, severe abdominal pain, nausea, or vomiting occur, notify prescriber. Women of childbearing age should use effective contraception while on zalcitabine; take on an empty stomach, if possible.

Additional Information Potential compliance problems, frequency of administration and adverse effects should be discussed with patients before initiating therapy to help prevent the emergence of resistance.

Dosage Forms Tablet: 0.375 mg, 0.75 mg

Selected Readings

"Drugs for AIDS and Associated Infections," *Med Lett Drugs Ther*, 1993, 35(904):79-86.

Hirsch MS and D'Aquila RT, "Therapy for Human Immunodeficiency Virus Infection," *N Engl J Med*, 1993, 328(23):1686-95.

Shelton MJ, O'Donnell AM, and Morse GD, "Zalcitabine," *Ann Pharmacother*, 1993, 27(4):480-9.

Skowron G, Bozzette SA, Lim L, et al, "Alternating and Intermittent Regimens of Zidovudine and Dideoxycytidine in Patients With AIDS or AIDS-Related Complex," *Ann Intern Med*, 1993, 118(5):321-30.

Zanamivir (za NA mi veer)

U.S. Brand Names Relenza®

Canadian Brand Names Relenza®

Generic Available No

Use Treatment of uncomplicated acute illness due to influenza virus A and B in adults and children ≥7 years of age; should not be used in patients with underlying airway disease. Treatment should only be initiated in patients who have been symptomatic for no more than 2 days.

Unlabeled/Investigational Use Investigational: Prophylaxis against influenza A/B infections

Drug of Choice or Alternative for Organism(s):

Influenza Virus *on page 193*

Pregnancy Risk Factor C

Pregnancy Implications Zanamivir has been shown to cross the placenta in animal models, however, no evidence of fetal malformations has been demonstrated.

Contraindications Hypersensitivity to zanamivir or any component of the formulation

Warnings/Precautions Patients must be instructed in the use of the delivery system. No data are available to support the use of this drug in patients who begin treatment after 48 hours of symptoms, as a prophylactic treatment for influenza, or in patients with significant underlying medical conditions. Not recommended for use in patients

(Continued)

Zanamivir *(Continued)*

with underlying respiratory disease, such as asthma or COPD, due to lack of efficacy and risk of serious adverse effects. Bronchospasm, decreased lung function, and other serious adverse reactions, including those with fatal outcomes, have been reported. For a patient with an underlying airway disease where a medical decision has been made to use zanamivir, a fast-acting bronchodilator should be made available, and used prior to each dose. Not a substitute for the flu shot. Consider primary or concomitant bacterial infections. Powder for oral inhalation contains lactose.

Adverse Reactions Most adverse reactions occurred at a frequency which was equal to the control (lactose vehicle).

>1.5%:

- Central nervous system: Headache (2%), dizziness (2%)
- Gastrointestinal: Nausea (3%), diarrhea (3% adults, 2% children), vomiting (1% adults, 2% children)
- Respiratory: Sinusitis (3%), bronchitis (2%), cough (2%), other nasal signs and symptoms (2%), infection (ear, nose, and throat; 2% adults, 5% children)

<1.5%: Malaise, fatigue, fever, abdominal pain, myalgia, arthralgia, and urticaria

Postmarketing and/or case reports: Allergic or allergic-like reaction (including oropharyngeal edema), arrhythmia, syncope, seizure, bronchospasm, dyspnea, facial edema, rash (including serious cutaneous reactions)

Overdosage/Toxicology Information is limited, and symptoms appear similar to reported adverse events from clinical studies.

Drug Interactions

Increased Effect/Toxicity: No clinically significant pharmacokinetic interactions are predicted.

Decreased Effect: No clinically significant pharmacokinetic interactions are predicted.

Stability Store at room temperature (25°C) 77°F; do not puncture blister until taking a dose using the Diskhaler®

Mechanism of Action Zanamivir inhibits influenza virus neuraminidase enzymes, potentially altering virus particle aggregation and release.

Pharmacodynamics/Kinetics

Absorption: Inhalation: 4% to 17%
Protein binding, plasma: <10%
Metabolism: None
Half-life elimination, serum: 2.5-5.1 hours
Excretion: Urine (as unchanged drug); feces (unabsorbed drug)

Dosage Children ≥7 years and Adults: 2 inhalations (10 mg total) twice daily for 5 days. Two doses should be taken on the first day of dosing, regardless of interval, while doses should be spaced by approximately 12 hours on subsequent days.

Prophylaxis (investigational use): 2 inhalations (10 mg) once daily for duration of exposure period (6 weeks has been used in clinical trial)

Administration Inhalation: Must be used with Diskhaler® delivery device. Patients who are scheduled to use an inhaled bronchodilator should use their bronchodilator prior to zanamivir.

Patient Information Use delivery device exactly as directed; complete full 5-day regimen, even if symptoms improve sooner. If you have asthma or COPD you may be at risk for bronchospasm; see prescriber for appropriate bronchodilator before using zanamivir. Stop using this medication and contact your prescriber if you experience shortness of breath, increased wheezing, or other signs of bronchospasm. You may experience dizziness or headache (use caution when driving or engaging in hazardous tasks until response to drug is known). Report unresolved diarrhea, vomiting, or nausea; acute fever or muscle pain; or other acute and persistent adverse effects.

Additional Information Majority of patients included in clinical trials were infected with influenza A, however, a number of patients with influenza B infections were also enrolled. Patients with lower temperature or less severe symptoms appeared to derive less benefit from therapy. No consistent treatment benefit was demonstrated in patients with chronic underlying medical conditions.

Dosage Forms Powder for oral inhalation: 5 mg/blister (20s) [4 blisters per Rotadisk® foil pack, 5 Rotadisk® per package; packaged with Diskhaler® inhalation device; contains lactose]

Selected Readings

Anonymous, "Neuraminidase Inhibitors for Treatment of Influenza A and B Infections," *MMWR*, 1999, 48(RR-14):1-9.

Cheer SM and Wagstaff AJ, "Zanamivir: An Update of Its Use in Influenza," *Drugs*, 2002, 62(1):71-106.

Hayden FG, Osterhaus AD, Treanor JJ, et al, "Efficacy and Safety of the Neuroaminidase Inhibitor Zanamivir in the Treatment of Influenza Virus Infections. GG167 Influenza Study Group," *N Engl J Med*, 1997, 337(13):874-80.

McNicholl IR and McNicholl JJ, "Neuraminidase Inhibitors: Zanamivir and Oseltamivir," *Ann Pharmacother*, 2001, 35(1):57-70.
Monto AS, Robinson DP, Herlocher ML, et al, "Zanamivir in the Prevention of Influenza Among Healthy Adults: A Randomized Controlled Trial," *JAMA*, 1999, 282:31-5.
Waghorn SL and Goa KL, "Zanamivir," *Drugs*, 1998, 55(5):721-5.

ZDV *see* Zidovudine *on page 1159*
ZDV, Abacavir, and Lamivudine *see* Abacavir, Lamivudine, and Zidovudine *on page 627*
Zeasorb®-AF [OTC] *see* Miconazole *on page 945*
Zerit® *see* Stavudine *on page 1076*
Ziagen® *see* Abacavir *on page 624*

Zidovudine (zye DOE vyoo deen)

Related Information

Antiretroviral Agents *on page 1206*
Antiretroviral Therapy for HIV Infection *on page 1219*
Management of Healthcare Worker Exposures to HBV, HCV, and HIV *on page 1227*
Prevention of Perinatal HIV-1 Transmission *on page 1235*

U.S. Brand Names Retrovir®

Canadian Brand Names Apo-Zidovudine®; AZT™; Novo-AZT; Retrovir®

Synonyms Azidothymidine; AZT (error-prone abbreviation); Compound S; ZDV

Generic Available No

Use Management of patients with HIV infections in combination with at least two other antiretroviral agents; for prevention of maternal/fetal HIV transmission as monotherapy

Unlabeled/Investigational Use Postexposure prophylaxis for HIV exposure as part of a multidrug regimen

Drug of Choice or Alternative for Organism(s):

Human Immunodeficiency Virus *on page 181*

Pregnancy Risk Factor C

Pregnancy Implications Zidovudine crosses the placenta. The use of zidovudine reduces the maternal-fetal transmission of HIV by ~70% and should be considered for antenatal and intrapartum therapy whenever possible. The Perinatal HIV Guidelines Working Group considers zidovudine the preferred NRTI for use in combination regimens during pregnancy. In HIV infected mothers not previously on antiretroviral therapy, treatment may be delayed until after 10-12 weeks gestation. Cases of lactic acidosis/hepatic steatosis syndrome have been reported in pregnant women receiving nucleoside analogues. It is not known if pregnancy itself potentiates this known side effect; however, pregnant women may be at increased risk of lactic acidosis and liver damage. Hepatic enzymes and electrolytes should be monitored frequently during the 3rd trimester of pregnancy in women receiving nucleoside analogues. Health professionals are encouraged to contact the antiretroviral pregnancy registry to monitor outcomes of pregnant women exposed to antiretroviral medications (1-800-258-4263 or www.APRegistry.com).

Contraindications Life-threatening hypersensitivity to zidovudine or any component of the formulation

Warnings/Precautions Often associated with hematologic toxicity including granulocytopenia, severe anemia requiring transfusions, or (rarely) pancytopenia. Use with caution in patients with bone marrow compromise (granulocytes <1000 cells/mm^3 or hemoglobin <9.5 mg/dL); dosage adjustment may be required in patients who develop anemia or neutropenia. Lactic acidosis and severe hepatomegaly with steatosis have been reported, including fatal cases; use with caution in patients with risk factors for liver disease (risk may be increased in obese patients or prolonged exposure) and suspend treatment with zidovudine in any patient who develops clinical or laboratory findings suggestive of lactic acidosis (transaminase elevation may/may not accompany hepatomegaly and steatosis). Prolonged use has been associated with symptomatic myopathy. Reduce dose in patients with renal impairment. Zidovudine has been shown to be carcinogenic in rats and mice.

Adverse Reactions

>10%:

Central nervous system: Severe headache (42%), fever (16%)

Dermatologic: Rash (17%)

Gastrointestinal: Nausea (46% to 61%), anorexia (11%), diarrhea (17%), pain (20%), vomiting (6% to 25%)

Hematologic: Anemia (23% in children), leukopenia, granulocytopenia (39% in children)

Neuromuscular & skeletal: Weakness (19%)

(Continued)

Zidovudine *(Continued)*

1% to 10%:

Central nervous system: Malaise (8%), dizziness (6%), insomnia (5%), somnolence (8%)

Dermatologic: Hyperpigmentation of nails (bluish-brown)

Gastrointestinal: Dyspepsia (5%)

Hematologic: Changes in platelet count

Neuromuscular & skeletal: Paresthesia (6%)

<1%, postmarketing and/or case reports: Amblyopia, anaphylaxis, angioedema, anxiety, aplastic anemia, back pain, cardiomyopathy, chest pain, confusion, constipation, cough, CPK increased, depression, diaphoresis, dizziness, dysphagia, dyspnea, flatulence, flu-like syndrome, generalized pain, gynecomastia, hearing loss, hemolytic anemia, hepatitis, hepatomegaly with steatosis, jaundice, lactic acidosis, LDH increased, leukopenia, loss of mental acuity, lymphadenopathy, macular edema, mania, mouth ulcer, muscle spasm, myopathy and myositis with pathological changes (similar to that produced by HIV disease), oral mucosal pigmentation, pancreatitis, pancytopenia with marrow hypoplasia, paresthesia, photophobia, pruritus, pure red cell aplasia, rash, rhabdomyolysis, rhinitis, seizure, sensitization reactions, sinusitis, skin and nail pigmentation changes, somnolence, Stevens-Johnson syndrome, syncope, taste perversion, toxic epidermal necrolysis, tremor, urinary frequency, urinary hesitancy, urticaria, vasculitis, vertigo

Overdosage/Toxicology Symptoms include nausea, vomiting, ataxia, and granulocytopenia. Erythropoietin, thymidine, and cyanocobalamin have been used experimentally to treat zidovudine-induced hematopoietic toxicity, yet none are presently specified as the agent of choice. Treatment is supportive.

Drug Interactions

Cytochrome P450 Effect: Substrate (minor) of CYP2A6, 2C8/9, 2C19, 3A4

Increased Effect/Toxicity: Coadministration of zidovudine with drugs that are nephrotoxic (amphotericin B), cytotoxic (flucytosine, vincristine, vinblastine, doxorubicin, interferon), inhibit glucuronidation or excretion (acetaminophen, cimetidine, indomethacin, lorazepam, probenecid, aspirin), or interfere with RBC/WBC number or function (acyclovir, ganciclovir, pentamidine, dapsone). Clarithromycin may increase blood levels of zidovudine (although total body exposure was unaffected, peak plasma concentrations were increased). Valproic acid significantly increases zidovudine's blood levels (believed due to inhibition first pass metabolism). Concomitant use of ribavirin and nucleoside analogues may increase the risk of developing lactic acidosis (includes adefovir, didanosine, lamivudine, stavudine, zalcitabine, zidovudine).

Decreased Effect: *In vitro* evidence suggests zidovudine's antiretroviral activity may be antagonized by doxorubicin and ribavirin; avoid concurrent use. Zidovudine may decrease the antiviral activity of stavudine (based on *in vitro* data); avoid concurrent use.

Stability Solution for injection should be diluted with D_5W to a concentration of ≤4 mg/mL; the solution is physically and chemically stable for 24 hours at room temperature and 48 hours if refrigerated; attempt to administer diluted solution within 8 hours, if stored at room temperature or 24 hours if refrigerated to minimize potential for microbially contaminated solutions; store undiluted vials at room temperature and protect from light

Mechanism of Action Zidovudine is a thymidine analog which interferes with the HIV viral RNA dependent DNA polymerase resulting in inhibition of viral replication; nucleoside reverse transcriptase inhibitor

Pharmacodynamics/Kinetics

Absorption: Oral: 66% to 70%

Distribution: Significant penetration into the CSF; crosses placenta

Relative diffusion from blood into CSF: Adequate with or without inflammation (exceeds usual MICs)

CSF:blood level ratio: Normal meninges: ~60%

Protein binding: 25% to 38%

Metabolism: Hepatic via glucuronidation to inactive metabolites; extensive first-pass effect

Half-life elimination: Terminal: 60 minutes

Time to peak, serum: 30-90 minutes

Excretion:

Oral: Urine (72% to 74% as metabolites, 14% to 18% as unchanged drug)

I.V.: Urine (45% to 60% as metabolites, 18% to 29% as unchanged drug)

Dosage

Prevention of maternal-fetal HIV transmission:

Neonatal: **Note:** Dosing should begin 8-12 hours after birth and continue for the first 6 weeks of life.

Oral:
Full-term infants: 2 mg/kg/dose every 6 hours
Infants ≥30 weeks and <35 weeks gestation at birth: 2 mg/kg/dose every 12 hours; at 2 weeks of age, advance to 2 mg/kg/dose every 8 hours
Infants <30 weeks gestation at birth: 2 mg/kg/dose every 12 hours; at 4 weeks of age, advance to 2 mg/kg/dose every 8 hours
I.V.: Infants unable to receive oral dosing:
Full term: 1.5 mg/kg/dose every 6 hours
Infants ≥30 weeks and <35 weeks gestation at birth: 1.5 mg/kg/dose every 12 hours; at 2 weeks of age, advance to 1.5 mg/kg/dose every 8 hours
Infants <30 weeks gestation at birth: 1.5 mg/kg/dose every 12 hours; at 4 weeks of age, advance to 1.5 mg/kg/dose every 8 hours
Maternal: Oral (per AIDSinfo guidelines): 100 mg 5 times/day **or** 200 mg 3 times/day **or** 300 mg twice daily. Begin at 14-34 weeks gestation and continue until start of labor.
During labor and delivery, administer zidovudine I.V. at 2 mg/kg over 1 hour followed by a continuous I.V. infusion of 1 mg/kg/hour until the umbilical cord is clamped

Treatment of HIV infection:
Children 3 months to 12 years:
Oral: 160 mg/m²/dose every 8 hours; dosage range: 90 mg/m²/dose to 180 mg/m²/dose every 6-8 hours; some Working Group members use a dose of 180 mg/m² to 240 mg/m² every 12 hours when using in drug combinations with other antiretroviral compounds, but data on this dosing in children is limited
I.V. continuous infusion: 20 mg/m²/hour
I.V. intermittent infusion: 120 mg/m²/dose every 6 hours
Adults:
Oral: 300 mg twice daily or 200 mg 3 times/day
I.V.: 1-2 mg/kg/dose (infused over 1 hour) administered every 4 hours around-the-clock (6 doses/day)

Prevention of HIV following needlesticks (unlabeled use): Oral: Adults: 200 mg 3 times/day plus lamivudine 150 mg twice daily; a protease inhibitor (eg, indinavir) may be added for high risk exposures; begin therapy within 2 hours of exposure if possible

Patients should receive I.V. therapy only until oral therapy can be administered

Dosing interval in renal impairment: Cl_{cr} <10 mL/minute: May require minor dose adjustment

Hemodialysis: At least partially removed by hemo- and peritoneal dialysis; administer dose after hemodialysis or administer 100 mg supplemental dose; during CAPD, dose as for Cl_{cr} <10 mL/minute

Continuous arteriovenous or venovenous hemodiafiltration effects: Administer 100 mg every 8 hours

Dosing adjustment in hepatic impairment: Reduce dose by 50% or double dosing interval in patients with cirrhosis

Dietary Considerations May be taken without regard to food.

Administration

Oral: Administer around-the-clock to promote less variation in peak and trough serum levels; may be administered without regard to food
I.M.: Do not administer I.M.
I.V.: Avoid rapid infusion or bolus injection
Neonates: Infuse over 30 minutes
Adults: Infuse over 1 hour

Monitoring Parameters Monitor CBC and platelet count at least every 2 weeks, MCV, serum creatinine kinase, viral load, and CD4 count; observe for appearance of opportunistic infections

Patient Information Zidovudine is not a cure for AIDS. Take as directed; may be taken without regard to food. Take around-the-clock; do not take with other medications. Take precautions to avoid transmission to others. You may experience headache or insomnia; if these persist notify prescriber. Report unresolved nausea or vomiting; signs of infection (eg, fever, chills, sore throat, burning urination, flu-like symptoms, fatigue); unusual bleeding (eg, tarry stools, easy bruising, or blood in stool, urine, or mouth); pain, tingling, or numbness of toes or fingers; skin rash or irritation; or muscles weakness or tremors.

Additional Information Potential compliance problems, frequency of administration and adverse effects should be discussed with patients before initiating therapy to help prevent the emergence of resistance.

Dosage Forms

Capsule: 100 mg
Injection, solution [preservative free]: 10 mg/mL (20 mL)
(Continued)

Zidovudine *(Continued)*

Syrup: 50 mg/5 mL (240 mL) [contains sodium benzoate; strawberry flavor]
Tablet: 300 mg

Selected Readings

"Drugs for AIDS and Associated Infections," *Med Lett Drugs Ther*, 1993, 35(904):79-86.
Hirsch MS and D'Aquila RT, "Therapy for Human Immunodeficiency Virus Infection," *N Engl J Med*, 1993, 328(23):1686-95.
McLeod GX and Hammer SM, "Zidovudine: Five Years Later," *Ann Intern Med*, 1992, 117(6):487-501.
Skowron G, Bozzette SA, Lim L, et al, "Alternating and Intermittent Regimens of Zidovudine and Dideoxycytidine in Patients With AIDS or AIDS-Related Complex," *Ann Intern Med*, 1993, 118(5):321-30.

Zidovudine, Abacavir, and Lamivudine *see* Abacavir, Lamivudine, and Zidovudine *on page 627*

Zidovudine and Lamivudine (zye DOE vyoo deen & la MI vyoo deen)

Related Information

Antiretroviral Agents *on page 1206*
Antiretroviral Therapy for HIV Infection *on page 1219*

U.S. Brand Names Combivir®

Canadian Brand Names Combivir®

Synonyms AZT + 3TC (error-prone abbreviation); Lamivudine and Zidovudine

Generic Available No

Use Treatment of HIV infection when therapy is warranted based on clinical and/or immunological evidence of disease progression. Combivir® given twice daily, provides an alternative regimen to lamivudine 150 mg twice daily plus zidovudine 600 mg/day in divided doses; this drug form reduces capsule/tablet intake for these two drugs to 2 per day instead of up to 8.

Drug of Choice or Alternative for Organism(s):

Human Immunodeficiency Virus *on page 181*

Pregnancy Risk Factor C

Pregnancy Implications See individual agents.

Adverse Reactions See individual agents.

Drug Interactions

Cytochrome P450 Effect: Zidovudine: **Substrate** (minor) of CYP2A6, 2C8/9, 2C19, 3A4

Increased Effect/Toxicity: See individual agents.

Decreased Effect: See individual agents.

Mechanism of Action The combination of zidovudine and lamivudine are believed to act synergistically to inhibit reverse transcriptase via DNA chain termination after incorporation of the nucleoside analogue as well as to delay the emergence of mutations conferring resistance

Pharmacodynamics/Kinetics See individual agents.

Dosage Children >12 years and Adults: Oral: One tablet twice daily

Note: Because this is a fixed-dose combination product, avoid use in patients requiring dosage reduction including children <12 years of age, renally impaired patients with a creatinine clearance ≤50 mL/minute, patients with low body weight (<50 kg or 110 pounds), or those experiencing dose-limiting adverse effects.

Dosage Forms Tablet: Zidovudine 300 mg and lamivudine 150 mg

Zinacef® *see* Cefuroxime *on page 725*
Zinc Undecylenate *see* Undecylenic Acid and Derivatives *on page 1139*
Zithromax® *see* Azithromycin *on page 674*
Zithromax® TRI-PAK™ *see* Azithromycin *on page 674*
Zithromax® Z-PAK® *see* Azithromycin *on page 674*
Zmax™ *see* Azithromycin *on page 674*
Zorbtive™ *see* Somatropin *on page 1069*
Zosyn® *see* Piperacillin and Tazobactam Sodium *on page 1003*
Zovirax® *see* Acyclovir *on page 629*
Zymar™ *see* Gatifloxacin *on page 837*
Zyvox™ *see* Linezolid *on page 914*
Zyvoxam® (Can) *see* Linezolid *on page 914*

APPENDIX TABLE OF CONTENTS

ANTIMICROBIAL ACTIVITY AGAINST SELECTED ORGANISMS

KEY TO TABLE

- A — Recommended drug therapy
- B — Alternate drug therapy
- C — Organism is usually or always sensitive to this agent
- D — Organism portrays variable sensitivity to this agent
- (Blank) This drug should not be used for this organism or insufficient data is available

		GRAM-POSITIVE AEROBES												
		Bacilli			Cocci									
		Listeria monocytogenes	*Corynebacterium jeikeium*	*Corynebacterium sp*	*Streptococcus*, Viridans Group	*Streptococcus pneumoniae*	*Streptococcus bovis* (Group D)	*Enterococcus sp*	*Streptococcus agalactiae* (Group B)	*Streptococcus pyogenes* (Group A)	*Staphylococcus epidermidis*: Methicillin-Resistant	*Staphylococcus epidermidis*: Methicillin-Susceptible	*Staphylococcus aureus*: Methicillin-Resistant	*Staphylococcus aureus*: Methicillin-Susceptible
Penicillins	Amoxicillin				C	C	C		C	C				
Penicillins	Ampicillin	A			C	C	C	A	C	C				
Penicillins	Penicillin G	A	B	B	A	A	A	A	A	A				
Penicillins	Penicillin V			C	C	C	C	C	C	C				
Penicillins	Azlocillin													
Penicillins	Mezlocillin				D	C	D	D	C	C				
Penicillins	Piperacillin				D	C	D	C	C	C				
Penicillins	Ticarcillin				D	C	D		C	C				
Penicillins	Cloxacillin				D					D		A		A
Penicillins	Dicloxacillin				D					D		A		A
Penicillins	Methicillin				D					D		A		A
Penicillins	Nafcillin				D					D		A		A
Penicillins	Oxacillin				D					D		A		A
Penicillin-Related Antibiotics	Amoxicillin/Clavulanate	C			C	C	C	C	C	C		C		C
Penicillin-Related Antibiotics	Ampicillin/Sulbactam	C			C	C	C	C	C	C		C		C
Penicillin-Related Antibiotics	Ticarcillin/Clavulanate				C	C	C	D	C	C		C		C
Penicillin-Related Antibiotics	Aztreonam													
Penicillin-Related Antibiotics	Imipenem/Cilastatin				C	C	C	D	C	C		C		C
Penicillin-Related Antibiotics	Meropenem				C	C	C		C	C		C		C
Penicillin-Related Antibiotics	Piperacillin/Tazobactam				C	C	C	C	C	C		C		C
Other Antibiotics	Chloramphenicol	C				B		D						
Other Antibiotics	Clindamycin			D	D	C			C	C		B		B
Other Antibiotics	Co-trimoxazole	B				C					B	C	B	C
Other Antibiotics	Daptomycin				C	C	D	C	C	C	C	C	C	C
Other Antibiotics	Linezolid				C	C		C	C	C	C	C	C	C
Other Antibiotics	Metronidazole													
Other Antibiotics	Quinupristin/Dalfopristin							D	C	C	C	C	C	C
Other Antibiotics	Rifampin			D							A	C	A	C
Other Antibiotics	Sulfonamides													
Other Antibiotics	Tetracyclines	C			C	C			C				A	D
Other Antibiotics	Tigecycline				C	C		C	C	C	C	C	C	C
Other Antibiotics	Vancomycin	D	A		B	B	B	B	B	B	A	B	A	B
UTI Agents	Indanyl Carbenicillin							D						
UTI Agents	Nitrofurantoin							D						

ANTIMICROBIAL ACTIVITY AGAINST SELECTED ORGANISMS *(Continued)*

KEY TO TABLE

- **A** Recommended drug therapy
- **B** Alternate drug therapy
- **C** Organism is usually or always sensitive to this agent
- **D** Organism portrays variable sensitivity to this agent
- (Blank) This drug should not be used for this organism or insufficient data is available

		GRAM-POSITIVE AEROBES												
		Bacilli			Cocci									
		Listeria monocytogenes	*Corynebacterium jeikeium*	*Corynebacterium sp.*	*Streptococcus*, Viridans Group	*Streptococcus pneumoniae*	*Streptococcus bovis* (Group D)	*Enterococcus sp.* (Group D)	*Streptococcus agalactiae* (Group B)	*Streptococcus pyogenes* (Group A)	*Staphylococcus epidermidis*: Methicillin-Resistant	*Staphylococcus epidermidis*: Methicillin-Susceptible	*Staphylococcus aureus*: Methicillin-Resistant	*Staphylococcus aureus*: Methicillin-Susceptible
1st Generation	Cefadroxil				B	B	C		B	B		B		B
	Cefazolin				B	B	C		B	B		B		B
	Cephalexin				B	B	C		B	B		B		B
	Cephalothin				B	B	C		B	B		B		B
	Cephapirin				B	B	C		B	B		B		B
	Cephradine				B	B	C		B	B		B		B
2nd Generation and others	Cefaclor				C	C	C		C	C		D		D
	Cefamandole				C	C	C		C	C		C		C
	Cefmetazole				C	C	C		C	C		D		D
	Cefonicid				C	C	C		C	C		D		D
	Cefotetan				C	C	C		C	C		D		D
	Cefoxitin				C	C	C		C	C		D		D
	Cefpodoxime Proxetil				C	C	C		C	C		D		D
	Cefprozil				C	C	D		C	C				D
	Ceftibuten					D			C	C				
	Cefuroxime				C	C	C		C	C		D		D
	Cefuroxime Axetil				C	C			C	C		C		C
	Loracarbef				C	C	D		C	C		C		C
3rd Generation	Cefepime				C	C			C	C		C		C
	Cefixime				D	D			C	C				
	Cefoperazone				D	D	C		C	C		D		D
	Cefotaxime				D	D	C		C	C		D		D
	Ceftazidime				D		D		D	D				
	Ceftizoxime				D	D	C		C	C		D		D
	Ceftriaxone				C	C	C		C	C		D		D
Aminoglycosides	Amikacin	C	C				D	D						
	Gentamicin	A	B		A		D	A			A	D	A	D
	Netilmicin	C	C					C						
	Streptomycin						D	C						
	Tobramycin	C	C				D							D
Macrolides	Azithromycin	C			C	C			C	C				C
	Clarithromycin	C			C	C			C	C				C
	Dirithromycin	C			C	C			C	C				C
	Erythromycin	C	C	A	C	B			B	B				C
Quinolones	Ciprofloxacin		D		D	D	D	D	D	D	D	D	D	D
	Gatifloxacin				C	C	C	D	C	C		C		C
	Levofloxacin				C	C	C	D	C	C	D	C	D	C
	Lomefloxacin		D		D	D	D	D	D	D	D	D	D	D
	Moxifloxacin				C	C	C	D	C	C		C		C
	Norfloxacin							D	D					
	Ofloxacin		D		D	D	D	D	D	D	D	D	D	D
	Sparfloxacin		D				C	D	C	C				
	Trovafloxacin				C	C	C	D	C	C	D	C	D	C

KEY TO TABLE

- A — Recommended drug therapy
- B — Alternate drug therapy
- C — Organism is usually or always sensitive to this agent
- D — Organism portrays variable sensitivity to this agent
- (Blank) This drug should not be used for this organism or insufficient data is available

		GRAM-NEGATIVE AEROBES													
		Enteric bacilli											Cocci		
		Yersinia enterocolitica	*Shigella sp*	*Serratia sp*	*Salmonella sp*	*Providencia sp*	*Proteus sp*	*Proteus mirabilis*	*Klebsiella pneumoniae*	*Escherichia coli*	*Enterobacter sp* [1]	*Citrobacter sp* [1]	*Neisseria meningitidis*	*Neisseria gonorrhoeae*	*Moraxella (Branhamella) catarrhalis*
Penicillin	Amoxicillin				B			A		C			C	D	
Penicillin	Ampicillin		A		B			A		A			C	D	
Penicillin	Penicillin G												A	D	
Penicillin	Penicillin V													D	
Penicillin	Azlocillin														
Penicillin	Mezlocillin			A		B	B	C	B	C	A	A		D	
Penicillin	Piperacillin			A		B	B	C	B	C	A	A		D	
Penicillin	Ticarcillin			A		B	B	C	D	C	A	A		D	
Penicillin	Cloxacillin														
Penicillin	Dicloxacillin														
Penicillin	Methicillin														
Penicillin	Nafcillin														
Penicillin	Oxacillin														
Penicillin-Related Antibiotics	Amoxicillin/Clavulanate				C			C	C	C			C	C	A
Penicillin-Related Antibiotics	Ampicillin/Sulbactam		C		C			C	C	C			C	C	C
Penicillin-Related Antibiotics	Ticarcillin/Clavulanate			A	C	C	B	C	B	C	A	A	C	C	C
Penicillin-Related Antibiotics	Aztreonam			B	C	C	C	C	B	C	A	C		C	C
Penicillin-Related Antibiotics	Imipenem/Cilastatin			B	C	B	B	B	B	C	B	B	D	C	C
Penicillin-Related Antibiotics	Meropenem		C	B	C	B	B	B	B	C	B	B	C	C	C
Penicillin-Related Antibiotics	Piperacillin/Tazobactam		C	A	C	B	B	B	B	C	A	A	C	C	C
Other Antibiotics	Chloramphenicol		C		B					C			B		
Other Antibiotics	Clindamycin														
Other Antibiotics	Co-trimoxazole	C	A	C	B	A	C	B	C	A	C	C			A
Other Antibiotics	Daptomycin														
Other Antibiotics	Linezolid														
Other Antibiotics	Metronidazole														
Other Antibiotics	Quinupristin/Dalfopristin														
Other Antibiotics	Rifampin												D		
Other Antibiotics	Sulfonamides		C		C			C	C	C			D		
Other Antibiotics	Tetracyclines	C	C				C	C		D			C	B	C
Other Antibiotics	Tigecycline		C	C	C				C	C	C	C		C	
Other Antibiotics	Vancomycin														
UTI Agents	Indanyl Carbenicillin			C		C	C	C	C	C	C	C			
UTI Agents	Nitrofurantoin								C	C	C	C			

[1] *Citrobacter freundii*, *Citrobacter diversus*, *Enterobacter cloacae* and *Enterobacter aerogenes* often have significantly different antibiotic sensitivity patterns. Speciation and susceptibility testing are particularly important.

ANTIMICROBIAL ACTIVITY AGAINST SELECTED ORGANISMS *(Continued)*

KEY TO TABLE

- A — Recommended drug therapy
- B — Alternate drug therapy
- C — Organism is usually or always sensitive to this agent
- D — Organism portrays variable sensitivity to this agent
- (Blank) This drug should not be used for this organism or insufficient data is available

		GRAM-NEGATIVE AEROBES													
		Enteric bacilli											Cocci		
		Yersinia enterocolitica	*Shigella* sp.	*Serratia* sp.	*Salmonella* sp.	*Providencia* sp.	*Proteus* sp.	*Proteus mirabilis*	*Klebsiella pneumoniae*	*Escherichia coli*	*Enterobacter* sp.[1]	*Citrobacter* sp.[1]	*Neisseria meningitidis*	*Neisseria gonorrhoeae*	*Moraxella (Branhamella) catarrhalis*
1st Generation	Cefadroxil							A	A	B					D
	Cefazolin							A	A	B					D
	Cephalexin							A	A	B					D
	Cephalothin							A	A	B					D
	Cephapirin							A	A	B					D
	Cephradine							A	A	B					D
2nd Generation and others	Cefaclor							C	A	B				C	B
	Cefamandole						D	C	A	B				C	B
	Cefmetazole	D	C	C		C	D	C	A	B				C	B
	Cefonicid							C	A	B				C	B
	Cefotetan	C	C	C		C	D	C	A	B				C	B
	Cefoxitin			D		C	D	C	A	B				C	B
	Cefpodoxime Proxetil							C	A	B				C	B
	Cefprozil		C					C	D	B				C	B
	Ceftibuten														
	Cefuroxime	C	C				D	C	A	B				C	B
	Cefuroxime Axetil							C	A	B			C	C	B
	Loracarbef							C	C	B				C	B
3rd Generation	Cefepime			C	C	C	C	C	C	C	B	B			C
	Cefixime		C	C			C	C	A	A				C	B
	Cefoperazone		B	A	A	A	A	C	A	A	B	B			B
	Cefotaxime	A	B	A	A	A	A	C	A	A	B	B	B	C	B
	Ceftazidime		B	A		A	A	C	A	A	B	B			B
	Ceftizoxime	A	B	A	A	A	A	C	A	A	B	B	B	C	B
	Ceftriaxone	A	B	A	A	A	A	C	A	A	B	B	B	C	B
Aminoglycosides	Amikacin	A		C		C	C	C	C	C	C	C			
	Gentamicin	A	D	C	D	D	C	C	C	C	C	C			
	Netilmicin	A	D	C	D	D	C	C	C	C	C	C			
	Streptomycin					D									
	Tobramycin	A		C	D	D	C	C	C	C	C	C			
Macrolides	Azithromycin													C	C
	Clarithromycin													C	C
	Dirithromycin														
	Erythromycin													D	C
Quinolones	Ciprofloxacin	C	B	C	B	C	C	C	C	C	B	B	C	A	C
	Gatifloxacin								C	C	B	B			C
	Levofloxacin	C	C	C	C	C	C	C	C	C	B	D	C	C	C
	Lomefloxacin		C	C	C	C	C	C	C	C	B	B	C	C	C
	Moxifloxacin								C	C	B	B			C
	Norfloxacin	C	C	C	C	C	C	C	C	C	B	B		C	
	Ofloxacin	C	C	C	C	C	C	C	C	C	B	B	C	A	C
	Sparfloxacin						C	C	C	C	B	B	C	C	C
	Trovafloxacin		C	C	C	C	C	C	C	C	B	B	C	C	C

[1] *Citrobacter freundii, Citrobacter diversus, Enterobacter cloacae* and *Enterobacter aerogenes* often have significantly different antibiotic sensitivity patterns. Speciation and susceptibility testing are particularly important

KEY TO TABLE

- A — Recommended drug therapy
- B — Alternate drug therapy
- C — Organism is usually or always sensitive to this agent
- D — Organism portrays variable sensitivity to this agent
- (Blank) This drug should not be used for this organism or insufficient data is available

GRAM-NEGATIVE AEROBES — Other bacilli

		Vibrio cholerae	*Stenotrophomonas maltophilia*	*Pseudomonas aeruginosa*	*Pasteurella multocida*	*Legionella pneumophila*	*Haemophilus influenzae*	*Haemophilus ducreyi*	*Gardnerella vaginalis*	*Francisella tularensis*	*Campylobacter jejuni*	*Brucella* sp.	*Bordetella pertussis*	*Alcaligenes*	*Acinetobacter* sp.
Penicillin	Amoxicillin				C		B		C						
	Ampicillin				C		B		B		D				
	Penicillin G				A										
	Penicillin V				C										
	Azlocillin														
	Mezlocillin			A	C		D								A
	Piperacillin			A	C		D								A
	Ticarcillin			A	C		D								A
	Cloxacillin														
	Dicloxacillin														
	Methicillin														
	Nafcillin														
	Oxacillin														
Penicillin-Related Antibiotics	Amoxicillin/Clavulanate				B		B	B	C						C
	Ampicillin/Sulbactam				B		C	C	C						C
	Ticarcillin/Clavulanate		B	A	C		C								A
	Aztreonam			C			C								B
	Imipenem/Cilastatin			B			C								B
	Meropenem			B	C		C				C				B
	Piperacillin/Tazobactam			A	C		C								A
Other Antibiotics	Chloramphenicol		C		C		B			A	C	C			
	Clindamycin								C		C				
	Co-trimoxazole	A	A				A	B				B	A		
	Daptomycin														
	Linezolid				C										
	Metronidazole								A						
	Quinupristin/Dalfopristin														
	Rifampin					A	D			D		A			
	Sulfonamides				C			C				C			
	Tetracyclines	A			C		C	C		B		A	C		
	Tigecycline		C		C	C	C								C
	Vancomycin														
UTI Agents	Indanyl Carbenicillin			D											C
	Nitrofurantoin														

ANTIMICROBIAL ACTIVITY AGAINST SELECTED ORGANISMS *(Continued)*

KEY TO TABLE

- A Recommended drug therapy
- B Alternate drug therapy
- C Organism is usually or always sensitive to this agent
- D Organism portrays variable sensitivity to this agent
- (Blank) This drug should not be used for this organism or insufficient data is available

		GRAM-NEGATIVE AEROBES													
		Other bacilli													
		Vibrio cholerae	*Stenotrophomonas maltophilia*	*Pseudomonas aeruginosa*	*Pasteurella multocida*	*Legionella pneumophila*	*Haemophilus influenzae*	*Haemophilus ducreyi*	*Gardnerella vaginalis*	*Francisella tularensis*	*Campylobacter jejuni*	*Brucella sp.*	*Bordetella pertussis*	*Alcaligenes*	*Acinetobacter sp.*
1st Generation	Cefadroxil						D								
	Cefazolin						D								
	Cephalexin						D								
	Cephalothin						D								
	Cephapirin						D								
	Cephradine						D								
2nd Generation and others	Cefaclor						B								
	Cefamandole				C		B								
	Cefmetazole				D		C								
	Cefonicid						C								
	Cefotetan				D		C								
	Cefoxitin				D		C			D					
	Cefpodoxime Proxetil						B								
	Cefprozil						B								
	Ceftibuten														
	Cefuroxime						B								
	Cefuroxime Axetil				D		B								
	Loracarbef						B								
3rd Generation	Cefepime			A			C								C
	Cefixime						A								D
	Cefoperazone		D	D	C		A	C							D
	Cefotaxime		D		C			C		C					A
	Ceftazidime		D	A				C		C					A
	Ceftizoxime		D		C			C							A
	Ceftriaxone		D		C			A		D					A
Aminoglycosides	Amikacin		C	A				C			C				C
	Gentamicin		C	A				C		A	C	C			C
	Netilmicin		C	A				C			C				C
	Streptomycin									A		C			
	Tobramycin		C	A				C			C				C
Macrolides	Azithromycin				D	B	C	C			C		C		
	Clarithromycin				D	B	C				C		C		
	Dirithromycin														
	Erythromycin				D	A		C		C	A		A		
Quinolones	Ciprofloxacin	C	B	B	C	B	C	B	C	C	B	C			C
	Gatifloxacin					C	C								
	Levofloxacin		C			C	C								
	Lomefloxacin	C	C	D	C		C	C	D		B	C			D
	Moxifloxacin						C								
	Norfloxacin			C							B				D
	Ofloxacin	C	B	D	C	C	C	C	C	C	B	C			C
	Sparfloxacin		C			C	C								
	Trovafloxacin		C			C	C								

KEY TO TABLE

- **A** Recommended drug therapy
- **B** Alternate drug therapy
- **C** Organism is usually or always sensitive to this agent
- **D** Organism portrays variable sensitivity to this agent
- (Blank) This drug should not be used for this organism or insufficient data is available

		OTHERS									ANAEROBES			
											Gram -	Gram +		
		Treponema pallidum	*Leptospira sp.*	*Borrelia burgdorferi* (Lyme disease)	*Rickettsia sp.*	*Ureaplasma urealyticum*	*Mycoplasma pneumoniae*	*Chlamydia trachomatis*	*Chlamydia pneumoniae* (TWAR)	*Chlamydia psittaci*	*Bacteroides sp.*	*Streptococcus*, anaerobic	*Clostridium perfringens*	*Clostridium difficile*[2]
Penicillin	Amoxicillin			B							D	C	D	
	Ampicillin			B							C	C	D	
	Penicillin G	A	A	B							C	A	A	
	Penicillin V	C	C	B							C	C	C	
	Azlocillin													
	Mezlocillin										C	C	C	
	Piperacillin										C	C	C	
	Ticarcillin										C	C	C	
	Cloxacillin													
	Dicloxacillin													
	Methicillin													
	Nafcillin													
	Oxacillin													
Penicillin-Related Antibiotics	Amoxicillin/Clavulanate										C	C	C	
	Ampicillin/Sulbactam										C	C	C	
	Ticarcillin/Clavulanate										C	C	C	
	Aztreonam													
	Imipenem/Cilastatin										B	C	B	
	Meropenem										B	C	B	
	Piperacillin/Tazobactam										B	C	C	
Other Antibiotics	Chloramphenicol				A						C	C	C	D
	Clindamycin										A	B	B	
	Co-trimoxazole													
	Daptomycin													
	Linezolid													
	Metronidazole										A	D	A	A
	Quinupristin/Dalfopristin													
	Rifampin													
	Sulfonamides							D						
	Tetracyclines	B	B	A	A	A	A	A	B	B	D	C	C	
	Tigecycline						C	C	C		C	C	C	C
	Vancomycin											B		B
UTI Agents	Indanyl Carbenicillin													
	Nitrofurantoin													

[2]Vancomycin is effective orally only.

ANTIMICROBIAL ACTIVITY AGAINST SELECTED ORGANISMS *(Continued)*

KEY TO TABLE

- A Recommended drug therapy
- B Alternate drug therapy
- C Organism is usually or always sensitive to this agent
- D Organism portrays variable sensitivity to this agent
- (Blank) This drug should not be used for this organism or insufficient data is available

		Others: *Treponema pallidum*	Others: *Leptospira* sp.	Others: *Borrelia burgdorferi* (Lyme disease)	Others: *Rickettsia* sp.	Others: *Ureaplasma urealyticum*	Others: *Mycoplasma pneumoniae*	Others: *Chlamydia trachomatis*	Others: *Chlamydia pneumoniae* (TWAR)	Others: *Chlamydia psittaci*	Anaerobes Gram -: *Bacteroides* sp.	Anaerobes Gram +: *Streptococcus*, anaerobic	Anaerobes Gram +: *Clostridium perfringens*	Anaerobes Gram +: *Clostridium difficile* [2]
1st Generation	Cefadroxil											B		
	Cefazolin											B		
	Cephalexin											B		
	Cephalothin											B		
	Cephapirin											B		
	Cephradine											B		
2nd Generation and others	Cefaclor													
	Cefamandole													
	Cefmetazole										C	C	C	
	Cefonicid													
	Cefotetan										B	C	C	
	Cefoxitin										B	C	C	
	Cefpodoxime Proxetil													
	Cefprozil													
	Ceftibuten													
	Cefuroxime											C	C	
	Cefuroxime Axetil													
	Loracarbef													
3rd Generation	Cefepime													
	Cefixime													
	Cefoperazone												D	
	Cefotaxime			C							D	C	C	
	Ceftazidime												D	
	Ceftizoxime			C							D	C	C	
	Ceftriaxone	C		A								C		
Aminoglycosides	Amikacin													
	Gentamicin													
	Netilmicin													
	Streptomycin													
	Tobramycin													
Macrolides	Azithromycin	D		C		B	C	C	C	C		D	D	
	Clarithromycin	D		D		B	C	C	C	C		D	D	
	Dirithromycin					C	C	C	C	C		D	D	
	Erythromycin	D		C		A	A	A	A	A		D	D	
Quinolones	Ciprofloxacin				D	D	D	D						
	Gatifloxacin						C					C		
	Levofloxacin						C	C	C					
	Lomefloxacin					D	D	D						
	Moxifloxacin						C					C		
	Norfloxacin													
	Ofloxacin				D	D	D	C						
	Sparfloxacin						C	C			D	D	D	D
	Trovafloxacin						C	C	C		C	C	C	

[2] Vancomycin is effective orally only.

BODY SURFACE AREA OF ADULTS AND CHILDREN

Calculating Body Surface Area in Children

In a child of average size, find weight and corresponding surface area on the boxed scale to the left; or, use the nomogram to the right. Lay a straightedge on the correct height and weight points for the child, then read the intersecting point on the surface area scale. (**Note:** 2.2 lb = 1 kg)

FOR CHILDREN OF NORMAL HEIGHT AND WEIGHT

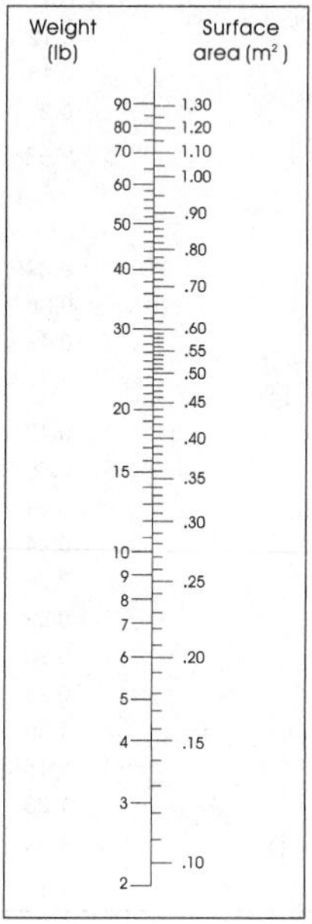

NOMOGRAM

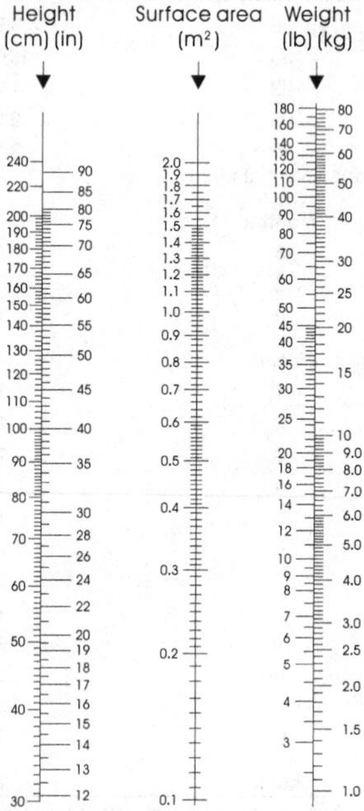

BODY SURFACE AREA FORMULA
(Adult and Pediatric)

$$BSA\ (m^2) = \sqrt{\frac{\text{ht (in)} \times \text{wt (lb)}}{3131}}$$ or, in metric: $$BSA\ (m^2) = \sqrt{\frac{\text{ht (cm)} \times \text{wt (kg)}}{3600}}$$

References

Lam TK and Leung DT, "More on Simplified Calculation of Body Surface Area," *N Engl J Med*, 1988, 318(17):1130 (letter).
Mosteller RD, "Simplified Calculation of Body Surface Area," *N Engl J Med*, 1987, 317(17):1098 (letter).

AVERAGE WEIGHTS AND SURFACE AREAS

Average Weight and Surface Area of Preterm Infants, Term Infants, and Children

Age	Average Weight (kg)*	Approximate Surface Area (m^2)
Weeks Gestation		
26	0.9-1	0.1
30	1.3-1.5	0.12
32	1.6-2	0.15
38	2.9-3	0.2
40 (term infant at birth)	3.1-4	0.25
Months		
3	5	0.29
6	7	0.38
9	8	0.42
Year		
1	10	0.49
2	12	0.55
3	15	0.64
4	17	0.74
5	18	0.76
6	20	0.82
7	23	0.90
8	25	0.95
9	28	1.06
10	33	1.18
11	35	1.23
12	40	1.34
Adult	70	1.73

*Weights from age 3 months and over are rounded off to the nearest kilogram.

IDEAL BODY WEIGHT CALCULATION

Adults (18 years and older) (IBW is in kg)

IBW (male) = 50 + (2.3 x height in inches over 5 feet)

IBW (female) = 45.5 + (2.3 x height in inches over 5 feet)

Children (IBW is in kg; height is in cm)

a. 1-18 years

$$IBW = \frac{(height^2 \times 1.65)}{1000}$$

b. 5 feet and taller

IBW (male) = 39 + (2.27 x height in inches over 5 feet)

IBW (female) = 42.2 + (2.27 x height in inches over 5 feet)

LIVER DISEASE

Pugh's Modification of Child's Classification for Severity

Parameter	Points for Increasing Abnormality 1	2	3
Encephalopathy	None	1 or 2	3 or 4
Ascites	Absent	Slight	Moderate
Bilirubin (mg/dL)	<2.9	2.9-5.8	>5.8
Albumin (g/dL)	>3.5	2.8-3.5	<2.8
Prothrombin time (seconds over control)	1-4	4-6	>6

Scores:

Mild hepatic impairment = <6 points.
Moderate hepatic impairment = 6-10 points.
Severe hepatic impairment = >10 points.

Considerations for Drug Dose Adjustment

Extent of Change in Drug Dose	Conditions or Requirements to Be Satisfied
None or minor change	Mild liver disease
	Extensive elimination of drug by kidneys and no renal dysfunction
	Elimination by pathways of metabolism spared by liver disease
	Drug is enzyme-limited and given acutely
	Drug is flow/enzyme-sensitive and only given acutely by I.V. route
	No alteration in drug sensitivity
Decrease in dose up to 25%	Elimination by the liver does not exceed 40% of the dose; no renal dysfunction
	Drug is flow-limited and given by I.V. route, with no large change in protein binding
	Drug is flow/enzyme-limited and given acutely by oral route
	Drug has a large therapeutic ratio
>25% decrease in dose	Drug metabolism is affected by liver disease; drug administered chronically
	Drug has a narrow therapeutic range; protein binding altered significantly
	Drug is flow-limited and given orally
	Drug is eliminated by kidneys and renal function severely affected
	Altered sensitivity to drug due to liver disease

Reference

Arns PA, Wedlund PJ, and Branch RA, "Adjustment of Medications in Liver Failure," *The Pharmacologic Approach to the Critically Ill Patient*, 2nd ed, Chernow B, ed, Baltimore, MD: Williams & Wilkins, 1988, 85-111.

CREATININE CLEARANCE ESTIMATING METHODS IN PATIENTS WITH STABLE RENAL FUNCTION

These formulas provide an acceptable estimate of the patient's creatinine clearance **except** in the following instances.

- Patient's serum creatinine is changing rapidly (either up or down).
- Patients are markedly emaciated.

In above situations, certain assumptions have to be made.

- In patients with rapidly rising serum creatinine (ie, >0.5-0.7 mg/dL/day), it is best to assume that the patient's creatinine clearance is probably <10 mL/minute.
- In emaciated patients, although their actual creatinine clearance is less than their calculated creatinine clearance (because of decreased creatinine production), it is not possible to easily predict how much less.

Infants

Estimation of creatinine clearance using serum creatinine and body length (to be used when an adequate timed specimen cannot be obtained). **Note:** This formula may not provide an accurate estimation of creatinine clearance for infants younger than 6 months of age and for patients with severe starvation or muscle wasting.

$$Cl_{cr} = K \times L/S_{cr}$$

where:

Cl_{cr} = creatinine clearance in mL/minute/1.73 m^2
K = constant of proportionality that is age specific

Age	K
Low birth weight ≤1 y	0.33
Full-term ≤1 y	0.45
2-12 y	0.55
13-21 y female	0.55
13-21 y male	0.70

L = length in cm
S_{cr} = serum creatinine concentration in mg/dL

Reference

Schwartz GJ, Brion LP, and Spitzer A, "The Use of Plasma Creatinine Concentration for Estimating Glomerular Filtration Rate in Infants, Children and Adolescents," *Pediatr Clin North Am*, 1987, 34(3):571-90.

Children (1-18 years)

Method 1: (Traub SL and Johnson CE, *Am J Hosp Pharm*, 1980, 37(2):195-201)

$$Cl_{cr} = \frac{0.48 \times (\text{height})}{S_{cr}}$$

where:

Cl_{cr} = creatinine clearance in mL/min/1.73 m^2
S_{cr} = serum creatinine in mg/dL
Height = height in cm

Method 2: Nomogram (Traub SL and Johnson CE, *Am J Hosp Pharm*, 1980, 37(2):195-201)

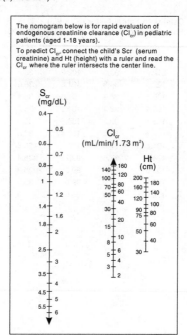

The nomogram below is for rapid evaluation of endogenous creatinine clearance (Cl_{cr}) in pediatric patients (aged 1-18 years).

To predict Cl_{cr}, connect the child's Scr (serum creatinine) and Ht (height) with a ruler and read the Cl_{cr} where the ruler intersects the center line.

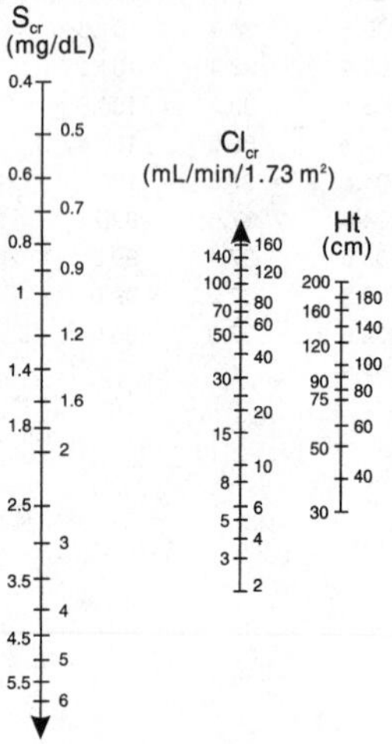

Adults (18 years and older)

Method 1: (Cockroft DW and Gault MH, *Nephron*, 1976, 16:31-41)

Estimated creatinine clearance (Cl_{cr}) (mL/min):

$$\text{Male} = \frac{(140 - \text{age}) \times \text{BW (kg)}}{72 \times S_{cr}}$$

$$\text{Female} = \text{male} \times 0.85$$

Note: Use of actual body weight (BW) in obese patients (and possibly patients with ascites) may significantly overestimate creatinine clearance. Some clinicians prefer to use an adjusted ideal body weight (IBW) in such cases [eg, IBW + 0.4(ABW-IBW)], especially when calculating dosages for aminoglycoside antibiotics.

Method 2: (Jelliffe RW, *Ann Intern Med*, 1973, 79:604)

Estimated creatinine clearance (Cl_{cr}) (mL/min/1.73 m^2):

$$\text{Male} = \frac{98 - 0.8\,(\text{age} - 20)}{S_{cr}}$$

$$\text{Female} = \text{male} \times 0.90$$

TEMPERATURE CONVERSION

Celsius to Fahrenheit = (°C x 9/5) + 32 = °F
Fahrenheit to Celsius = (°F - 32) x 5/9 = °C

°C	= °F	°C	= °F	°C	= °F
100.0	212.0	39.0	102.2	36.8	98.2
50.0	122.0	38.8	101.8	36.6	97.9
41.0	105.8	38.6	101.5	36.4	97.5
40.8	105.4	38.4	101.1	36.2	97.2
40.6	105.1	38.2	100.8	36.0	96.8
40.4	104.7	38.0	100.4	35.8	96.4
40.2	104.4	37.8	100.1	35.6	96.1
40.0	104.0	37.6	99.7	35.4	95.7
39.8	103.6	37.4	99.3	35.2	95.4
39.6	103.3	37.2	99.0	35.0	95.0
39.4	102.9	37.0	98.6	0	32.0
39.2	102.6				

DESENSITIZATION PROTOCOLS

PENICILLIN DESENSITIZATION PROTOCOL: MUST BE DONE BY PHYSICIAN!

Acute penicillin desensitization should only be performed in an intensive care setting. Any remedial risk factor should be corrected. All β-adrenergic antagonists such as propranolol or even timolol ophthalmic drops should be discontinued. Asthmatic patients should be under optimal control. An intravenous line should be established, baseline electrocardiogram (ECG) and spirometry should be performed, and continuous ECG monitoring should be instituted. Premedication with antihistamines or steroids is not recommended, as these drugs have not proven effective in suppressing severe reactions but may mask early signs of reactivity that would otherwise result in a modification of the protocol.

Protocols have been developed for penicillin desensitization using both the oral and parenteral route. As of 1987 there were 93 reported cases of oral desensitization, 74 of which were done by Sullivan and his collaborators. Of these 74 patients, 32% experienced a transient allergic reaction either during desensitization (one-third) or during penicillin treatment after desensitization (two-thirds). These reactions were usually mild and self-limited in nature. Only one IgE-mediated reaction (wheezing and bronchospasm) required discontinuation of the procedure before desensitization could be completed. It has been argued that oral desensitization may be safer than parenteral desensitization, but most patients can also be safely desensitized by parenteral route.

During desensitization any dose that causes mild systemic reactions such as pruritus, fleeting urticaria, rhinitis, or mild wheezing should be repeated until the patient tolerates the dose without systemic symptoms or signs. More serious reactions such as hypotension, laryngeal edema, or asthma require appropriate treatment, and if desensitization is continued, the dose should be decreased by at least 10-fold and withheld until the patient is stable.

Once desensitized, the patient's treatment with penicillin must not lapse or the risk of an allergic reaction increases. If the patient requires a β-lactam antibiotic in the future and still remains skin test-positive to penicillin reagents, desensitization would be required again.

Several patients have been maintained on long-term, low-dose penicillin therapy (usually bid-tid) to sustain a chronic state of desensitization. Such individuals usually require chronic desensitization because of continuous occupationally related exposure to β-lactam drugs.

Order for placement/availability at the bedside in the event of a hypersensitivity reaction during scratch/skin testing and desensitization:

Hydrocortisone: 100 mg IVP
Diphenhydramine: 50 mg IVP
Epinephrine: 1:1000 SubQ

Several investigators have demonstrated that penicillin can be administered to history positive, skin test positive patients if initially small but gradually increasing doses are given. However, patients with a history of exfoliative dermatitis secondary to penicillin should not be re-exposed to the drug, even by desensitization.

Desensitization is a potentially dangerous procedure and should be only performed in an area where immediate access to emergency drugs and equipment can be assured.

Begin between 8-10 AM in the morning.

Follow desensitization as indicated for penicillin G or ampicillin.

DESENSITIZATION PROTOCOLS *(Continued)*

AMPICILLIN
Oral Desensitization Protocol

1. Begin 0.03 mg of ampicillin
2. Double the dose administered every 30 minutes until complete
3. Example of oral dosing regimen:

Dose #	Ampicillin (mg)
1	0.03
2	0.06
3	0.12
4	0.23
5	0.47
6	0.94
7	1.87
8	3.75
9	7.5
10	15
11	30
12	60
13	125
14	250
15	500

PENICILLIN G
Parenteral Desensitization Protocol: Typical Schedule

Injection No.	Benzylpenicillin Concentration (units/mL)	Volume and Route (mL)[1]
1[2]	100	0.1 I.D.
2	↓	0.2 SubQ
3		0.4 SubQ
4		0.8 SubQ
5[2]	1000	0.1 I.D.
6	↓	0.3 SubQ
7		0.6 SubQ
8[2]	10,000	0.1 I.D.
9	↓	0.2 SubQ
10		0.4 SubQ
11		0.8 SubQ
12[2]	100,000	0.1 I.D.
13	↓	0.3 SubQ
14		0.6 SubQ
15[2]	1,000,000	0.1 I.D.
16	↓	0.2 SubQ
17		0.2 I.M.
18		0.4 I.M.
19	Continuous I.V. infusion (1,000,000 units/h)	

[1]Administer progressive doses at intervals of not less than 20 minutes.

[2]Observe and record skin wheal and flare response to intradermal dose.

Abbreviations: I.D. = intradermal, SubQ = subcutaneous, I.M. = intramuscular, I.V. = intravenous.

PENICILLIN
Oral Desensitization Protocol

Step[1]	Phenoxymethyl Penicillin (units/mL)	Amount (mL)	Dose (units)	Cumulative Dosage (units)
1	1000	0.1	100	100
2	1000	0.2	200	300
3	1000	0.4	400	700
4	1000	0.8	800	1500
5	1000	1.6	1600	3100
6	1000	3.2	3200	6300
7	1000	6.4	6400	12,700
8	10,000	1.2	12,000	24,700
9	10,000	2.4	24,000	48,700
10	10,000	4.8	48,000	96,700
11	80,000	1	80,000	176,700
12	80,000	2	160,000	336,700
13	80,000	4	320,000	656,700
14	80,000	8	640,000	1,296,700
	Observe patient for 30 minutes			
Change to benzylpenicillin G I.V.				
15	500,000	0.25	125,000	
16	500,000	0.50	250,000	
17	500,000	1	500,000	
18	500,000	2.25	1,125,000	

[1]Interval between steps, 15 min

ALLOPURINOL
Successful Desensitization for Treatment of a Fixed Drug Eruption

	Oral Dose of Allopurinol
Days 1-3	50 mcg/day
Days 4-6	100 mcg/day
Days 7-9	200 mcg/day
Days 10-12	500 mcg/day
Days 13-15	1 mg/day
Days 16-18	5 mg/day
Days 19-21	10 mg/day
Days 22-24	25 mg/day
Days 25-27	50 mg/day
Day 28	100 mg/day

Prednisone 10 mg/day through desensitization and 1 month after reaching dose of 100 mg allopurinol

Modified from *J Allergy Clin Immunol*, 1996, 97:1171-2.

DESENSITIZATION PROTOCOLS *(Continued)*

AMPHOTERICIN B

Challenge and Desensitization Protocol

1. Procedure supervised by physician
2. Epinephrine, 1:1000 wt/vol, multidose vial at bedside
3. Premixed albuterol solution at bedside for nebulization
4. Endotracheal intubation supplies at bedside with anesthesiologist on standby
5. Continuous cardiac telemetry with electronic monitoring of blood pressure
6. Continuous pulse oximetry
7. Premedication with methylprednisolone, 60 mg, I.V. and diphenhydramine, 25 mg I.V.
8. Amphotericin B (Fungizone®)[1] administration schedule
   a. 10^{-6} dilution, infused over 10 minutes
   b. 10^{-5} dilution, infused over 10 minutes
   c. 10^{-4} dilution, infused over 10 minutes
   d. 10^{-3} dilution, infused over 10 minutes
   e. 10^{-2} dilution, infused over 10 minutes
   f. 10^{-1} dilution (1 mg), infused over 30 minutes
   g. 30 mg in 250 mL 5% dextrose, infused over 4 hours

[1]Mixtures were prepared in 10 mL 5% dextrose by hospital intensive care unit pharmacy, unless otherwise noted.

From Kemp SF and Lockey RF, "Amphotericin B: Emergency Challenge in a Neutropenic, Asthmatic Patient With Fungal Sepsis," *J Allergy Clin Immunol*, 1995, 96(3):425-7.

BACTRIM™ ORAL DESENSITIZATION PROTOCOL

(Adapted from Gluckstein D and Ruskin J, "Rapid Oral Desensitization to Trimethoprim-Sulfamethoxazole (TMP-SMZ): Use in Prophylaxis for *Pneumocystis carinii* Pneumonia in Patients With AIDS Who Were Previously Intolerant to TMP-SMZ," *Clin Infect Dis*, 1995, 20:849-53.)

Please read the directions carefully before starting the protocol!

1. There must be a clear cut need for a sulfa drug or a sulfa drug combination product such as Bactrim™. The decision to use sulfa must be made prior to skin testing.
2. Informed consent from the patient or an appropriate relative must have been obtained.
3. A trained individual, physician, nurse, or aide, **must be with the patient** at all times.
4. A physician **must** be on the floor at all times.
5. Injectable epinephrine 0.3 mL 1:1000, diphenhydramine (Benadryl®) 50 mg, corticosteroids and oral ibuprofen 400 mg solution should be drawn up and available at the bedside.
6. Appropriate resuscitative equipment must be available.
7. All dilution of oral Bactrim™ should be made up prior to beginning procedure.
8. Patient should drink 180 mL of water after each Bactrim™ dose.

Dilution for Bactrim™ Desensitization

Final Concentration	Bottle #	Procedure
Oral Bactrim™ 40/200 mg/5 mL	A	Conventional oral Bactrim™ suspension 5 mL = 40/200 mg
Oral Bactrim™ 0.4/2 mg/mL	B	1. Add 5 mL conventional oral Bactrim™ suspension or A (concentration = 40/200 mg/5 mL) to 95 mL of sterile water 2. Shake well. This will give 100 mL of 40/200 mg Bactrim™; each mL = 0.4/2 mg Bactrim™. 3. Dispense 20 mL for use
Oral Bactrim™ 0.004/0.02 mg/mL	C	1. Add 1 mL of the 0.4/2 mg/mL Bactrim™ or B to 99 mL of sterile water 2. Shake well. This will give 100 mL of 0.4/2 mg Bactrim™; each mL = 0.004/0.02 mg Bactrim™. 3. Dispense 20 mL for use

Adverse Reactions and Response During the Protocol

Types of Reactions	Alteration of Protocol
Mild reactions (rash, fever, nausea)	I.V. diphenhydramine (Benadryl®) 50 mg and oral ibuprofen suspension 400 mg
Urticaria, dyspnea, severe vomiting, or hypotension	**STOP** the protocol IMMEDIATELY

- If patient tolerates up to Bactrim™ DS, he/she is desensitized.
- Assuming that there were no complications, the procedure will take up to 6 hours.

DESENSITIZATION PROTOCOLS *(Continued)*

Sample Bactrim™ Desensitization Flow Sheet

Patient Name ______________________ Age _____ Gender __________ Hospital # ______________________

Diagnosis ______________ Physician ______________________ Pager ________ History of sulfa reaction ______________________

# Hour	Actual Time	Suggested Dose	Form	Suggested Volume	Actual Dose	Form	Actual Volume	Reaction/ Notes	Initial
0		Bactrim™ 0.004/0.02 mg (use **0.004/0.02 mg/mL** bottle or bottle C)	Susp (C)	1 mL					
1		Bactrim™ 0.04/0.2 mg (use 0.004/0.02 mg/mL bottle or bottle C)	Susp (C)	10 mL					
2		Bactrim™ 0.4/2 mg (use **0.4/2 mg/mL bottle** or bottle B)	Susp (B)	1 mL					
3		Bactrim™ 4/20 mg (use 0.4/2 mg/mL bottle or bottle B)	Susp (B)	10 mL					
4		Bactrim™ 40/200 mg (use **40/200 mg/5 mL unit dose** Bactrim™ or A)	Susp (A)	5 mL					
5		Bactrim™ 80/400 mg (use 40/200 mg/5 mL unit dose Bactrim™ or A)	Susp (A)	10 mL					
6		Bactrim™ DS tablet	Tablet	1 DS pill					

Note: Drink 180 mL of water after each Bactrim™ dose.

ALTERNATIVE BACTRIM™ PROTOCOL

Adapted from Leoung GS, Stanford JF, Giordano MF, et al, "Trimethoprim-Sulfamethoxazole (TMP-SMZ) Dose Escalation Versus Direct Rechallenge for *Pneumocystis carinii* Pneumonia, Prophylaxis in Human Immunodeficiency Virus-Infected Patients With Previous Adverse Reaction to TMP-SMZ," *J Infect Dis*, 2001, 184(8):992-7.

Trimethoprim-Sulfamethoxazole (TMP-SMZ) Dose-Escalation Regimen in Human Immunodeficiency Virus-Infected Patients With Previous Mild-to-Moderate Treatment-Limiting Rash and/or Fever

Dosing Level	Portion of Single-Strength TMP-SMZ (%)	Amount (Frequency) of Pediatric Suspension (mL)	Total TMP Dose (mg)	Total SMZ Dose (mg)
1	12.5	1.25 qd	10	50
2	25	1.25 bid	20	100
3	37.5	1.25 tid	30	150
4	50	2.5 bid	40	200
5	75	2.5 tid	60	300
6	100	1 single-strength tablet	80	400

Note: Each dosing level is a daily dose. For successful completion of the reintroduction phase, patients must have taken each dose level at least once. Patients were permitted to repeat dose levels once; dose levels were completed in increasing increments, and the level 6 dose was taken no later than day 13 of the reintroduction phase. Patients were permitted to withhold study drug for 2 days during the reintroduction phase (withholding study drug for >2 days during reintroduction resulted in permanent discontinuation). Patients were required to take an antihistamine during dose escalation.

VANCOMYCIN DESENSITIZATION PROTOCOL

(Adapted from Wong JT, Ripple RE, MacLean JA, et al, "Vancomycin Hypersensitivity: Synergism with Narcotics and Desensitization by a Rapid Continuous Intravenous Protocol," *J Allergy Clin Immunol*, 1994, 94(2 Pt 1):189-94.)

Please read the directions carefully before starting the protocol!

1. Vancomycin desensitization is indicated only for cases with a definitive need for vancomycin and persistent allergic reaction despite slowing of infusion rate and the addition of Benadryl® or cases with reported vancomycin anaphylactic reactions.
2. Informed consent from the patient or an appropriate relative must have been obtained.
3. A trained individual, physician, nurse, or aide, **must be with the patient** at all times.
4. A physician **must** be on the floor at all times.
5. Injectable epinephrine 0.3 mL 1:1000, diphenhydramine (Benadryl®) 50 mg, corticosteroids and oral ibuprofen 400 mg solution should be drawn up and available at the bedside.
6. Appropriate resuscitative equipment must be available.
7. All dilution of I.V. vancomycin should be made up prior to beginning procedure.
8. All patients are pretreated with 25-50 mg Benadryl®.
9. Infusion rates are to be tightly regulated with **syringe pump**.

DESENSITIZATION PROTOCOLS *(Continued)*

Dilution for Vancomycin Desensitization

Final Concentration	Bottle #	Procedure
10 mg/mL	A	1. Dilute 1 g of vancomycin in 10 mL of sterile water 2. Shake well until the drug is completely dissolved 3. Add 2 mL of solution to 18 mL of 0.9% normal saline 4. Mix well 5. This will give 20 mL of 10 mg/mL concentration of vancomycin or (Bottle A) 6. Dispense 10-15 mL in a syringe for syringe pump. Label the syringe as "SYR A: conc = 10 mg/mL" with patient's name, ID, room number, date, and dispensor's initial/pharmacist's initial.
1 mg/mL	B	1. Add 2 mL of bottle A vancomycin (10 mg/mL) to 18 mL of 0.9% normal saline 2. Mix well 3. This will give 20 mL of 1 mg/mL concentration vancomycin or (Bottle B) 4. Dispense 10-15 mL in a syringe for syringe pump. Label the syringe as "SYR B: conc = 1 mg/mL" with patient's name, ID, room number, date, and dispensor's initial/pharmacist's initial.
0.1 mg/mL	C	1. Add 2 mL of Bottle B vancomycin (1 mg/mL) to 18 mL of 0.9% normal saline 2. Mix well 3. This will give 20 mL of 0.1 mg/mL concentration vancomycin or (Bottle C) 4. Dispense 10-15 mL in a syringe for syringe pump. Label the syringe as "SYR C: conc = 0.1 mg/mL" with patient's name, ID, room number, date, and dispensor's initial/pharmacist's initial.
0.01 mg/mL	D	1. Add 2 mL of Bottle C vancomycin (0.1 mg/mL) to 18 mL of 0.9% normal saline 2. Mix well 3. This will give 20 mL of 0.01 mg/mL concentration vancomycin or (Bottle D) 4. Dispense 10-15 mL in a syringe for syringe pump. Label the syringe as "SYR D: conc = 0.01 mg/mL" with patient's name, ID, room number, date, and dispensor's initial/pharmacist's initial.
0.001 mg/mL	E	1. Add 2 mL of Bottle D vancomycin (0.01 mg/mL) to 18 mL of 0.9% normal saline 2. Mix well 3. This will give 20 mL of 0.001 mg/mL concentration vancomycin or (Bottle E) 4. Dispense 10-15 mL in a syringe for syringe pump. Label the syringe as "SYR E: conc = 0.001 mg/mL" with patient's name, ID, room number, date, and dispensor's initial/pharmacist's initial.
0.0001 mg/mL	F	1. Add 2 mL of Bottle E vancomycin (0.001 mg/mL) to 18 mL of 0.9% normal saline 2. Mix well 3. This will give 20 mL of 0.0001 mg/mL concentration vancomycin or (Bottle F) 4. Dispense 10-15 mL in a syringe for syringe pump. Label the syringe as "SYR F: conc = 0.0001 mg/mL" with patient's name, ID, room number, date, and dispensor's initial/pharmacist's initial.

Sample Vancomycin Desensitization Flow Sheet

Patient Name ____________________ Age ________ Gender ____________ Hospital # ____________________

Diagnosis ______________ Physician ________________ Pager _______ History of vancomycin reaction ______________

Time (h/min)	Actual Time	Vancomycin Concentration (mg/mL)	Syr #	Fluid Infusion Rate (mL/min)	VIR (mg/min)	Actual Concentration (mg/mL)	Syr #	Infusion Rate (mL/min)	Reaction/ Notes	Initial
0:00		0.0001	F	1	0.0001					
0:10		0.001	E	0.33	0.00033					
0:20		0.001	E	1.0	0.001					
0:30		0.01	D	0.33	0.0033					
0:40		0.01	D	1.0	0.010					
0:50		0.1	C	0.33	0.033					
1:00		0.1	C	0.33	0.033					
1:10		1.0	B	0.33	0.33					
1:20		1.0	B	1	1					
1:30		10.0	A	0.22	2.2[1]					
1:30		10.0	A	0.44	4.4[1]					

[1]After a VIR of 2.2-4.4 mg/min is achieved, full dose of vancomycin can be administered at the VIR for the first day. The rate can be gradually advanced over the next few days as tolerated.

Patients in whom a VIR of 2.2-4.4 mg/min can**not** be achieved, continue to receive vancomycin at the highest tolerated infusion rate for the first day. The rate is to be gradually advanced over the next few days as tolerated.

DESENSITIZATION PROTOCOLS *(Continued)*

ALTERNATIVE VANCOMYCIN PROTOCOL

Adapted from Wazny LD and Daghigh B, "Desensitization Protocols for Vancomycin Hypersensitivity," *Ann Pharmacother*, 2001, 35(11):1458-64.

Rapid Vancomycin Desensitization Protocol (Lerner and Dwyer)

Premedication

Diphenhydramine 50 mg I.V. and hydrocortisone 100 mg I.V. 15 minutes prior to initiation of protocol, then q6h throughout protocol.

Infusion No.	Dilution	Vancomycin Dose (mg)	Concentration (mg/mL)
1	1:10,000	0.02	0.0002
2	1:1000	0.20	0.002
3	1:100	2	0.02
4	1:10	20	0.2
5	Standard	500	2

Preparation

1. Prepare a standard bag of 500 mg vancomycin in 250 mL NS or D_5W; label as infusion no. 5, vancomycin 2 mg/mL.
2. Draw up 10 mL of the standard vancomycin 2 mg/mL preparation and place in 100 mL bag of NS or D_5W; label as infusion no. 4, vancomycin 0.2 mg/mL.
3. Draw up 10 mL of the 0.2 mg/mL solution and place in a 100 mL bag of NS or D_5W; label as infusion no. 3, vancomycin 0.02 mg/mL.
4. Draw up 10 mL of the 0.02 mg/mL solution and place in a 100 mL bag of NS or D_5W; label as infusion no. 2, vancomycin 0.002 mg/mL.
5. Draw up 10 mL of the 0.002 mg/mL solution and place in a 100 mL bag of NS or D_5W; label as infusion no. 1, vancomycin 0.0002 mg/mL.

Infusion Rate Directions

Initiate infusion rate at 0.5 mL/min (30 mL/h) and increase by 0.5 mL/min (30 mL/h) as tolerated every 5 minutes to a maximum rate of 5 mL/min (300 mL/h). If pruritus, hypotension, rash, or difficulty breathing occurs, stop infusion and reinfuse the previously tolerated infusion at the highest tolerated rate. This step may be repeated up to three times for any given concentration.

Upon completion of infusion no. 5, immediately administer the required dose of vancomycin in the usual dilution of NS or D_5W over 2 hours. Decrease rate if patient becomes symptomatic or, alternatively, increase rate if patient tolerates dose. Administer diphenhydramine 50 mg P.O. 60 minutes prior to each dose.

CEFTRIAXONE DESENSITIZATION PROTOCOL

Dose	Concentration (mg/mL)	Volume (mL)	Dose (mg)
Subcutaneous Route: 15-minute intervals between all doses			
1	0.2	0.5	0.1
2	0.2	1	0.2
3	2	0.25	0.5
4	2	0.5	1
5	2	1	2
6	16	0.25	4
7	16	0.5	8
8	16	1	16
Intravenous Route: Infuse over 20-30 minutes; 15 minutes between doses			
9	20	1.5 mL qs to 50 mL	30 mg/50 mL
10	20	3 mL qs to 50 mL	60 mg/50 mL
11	20	6 mL qs to 50 mL	120 mg/50 mL
12	20	12.5 mL qs to 50 mL	250 mg/50 mL
13	–	–	1 g/50 mL

Pharmacy Admixture Instructions

1. Mix ceftriaxone 1 g/50 mL NS (concentration 20 mg/mL); label **Bag A**.
2. Remove 1 mL from Bag A and add 99 mL NS (concentration 0.2 mg/mL); label **Bag B**.
3. Use **Bag B** to make doses 1 and 2.
4. Remove 1 mL from Bag A and add 9 mL NS (concentration 2 mg/mL); label **Bag C**.
5. Use Bag C to make doses 3, 4, and 5.
6. Remove 1 mL from Bag A and add 0.25 mL NS (concentration 16 mg/mL); label **Bag D**.
7. Use Bag D to make doses 6 and 7.
8. Repeat step 6 to make dose 8 (step 6 only makes 1.25 mL; therefore need to repeat to make dose 8).
9. Take a 50 mL bag of NS and remove overfill plus 1.5 mL; add 1.5 mL from Bag A to NS bag (30 mg/50 mL); this is dose 9.
10. Take a 50 mL bag of NS and remove overfill plus 3 mL; add 3 mL from Bag A to NS bag (60 mg/50 mL); this is dose 10.
11. Take a 50 mL bag of NS and remove overfill plus 6 mL; add 6 mL from Bag A to NS bag (120 mg/50 mL); this is dose 11.
12. Take a 50 mL bag of NS and remove overfill plus 12.5 mL; add 12.5 mL from Bag A to NS bag (250 mg/50 mL); this is dose 12.
13. Dispense 1 g/50 mL for dose 13.

DESENSITIZATION PROTOCOLS *(Continued)*

CIPROFLOXACIN

Modified from *J Allergy Clin Immunol*, 1996, 97:1426-7.

Premedicated with diphenhydramine hydrochloride, ranitidine, and prednisone 1 hour before the desensitization.

The individual doses were administered at 15-minute intervals. Because the patient was intubated in the intensive care unit, vital signs were continually monitored. The patient's skin was inspected for development of urticaria, and his chest was auscultated for wheezing every 10 minutes. No rash, hypotension, or wheezing developed during desensitization. The procedure took 4 hours, and once finished, the patient had received an equivalent to his first scheduled dose (400 mg twice daily). The second dose was given 4 hours later, followed by routine administration of 400 mg every 12 hours, with a small dose (25 mg intravenously) between therapeutic doses to maintain a drug level in the blood. The patient subsequently received 4 weeks of ciprofloxacin treatment without difficulty.

Desensitization Regimen for Ciprofloxacin

Ciprofloxacin Concentration (mg/mL)	Volume Given (mL)	Absolute Amount (mg)	Cumulative Total Dose (mg)
0.1	0.1	0.01	0.01
0.1	0.2	0.02	0.03
0.1	0.4	0.04	0.07
0.1	0.8	0.08	0.15
1	0.16	0.16	0.31
1	0.32	0.32	0.63
1	0.64	0.64	1.27
2	0.6	1.2	2.47
2	1.2	2.4	4.87
2	2.4	4.8	9.67
2	5	10	19.67
2	10	20	39.67
2	20	40	79.67
2	40	80	159.67
2	120	240	399.67

Drug volumes <1 mL were mixed with normal saline solution to a final volume of 3 mL and then slowly infused; the other doses were administered over 10 minutes, except the last dose (240 mg in 120 mL), which was given with an infusion pump over 20 minutes.

IMIPENEM DESENSITIZATION PROTOCOL

Adapted from Saxon A, Adelman DC, Patel A, et al, "Imipenem Cross-Reactivity With Penicillin in Humans," *J Allergy Clin Immunol*, 1988, 82(2):213-7.

Indication: Need for imipenem in the setting of anaphylactic potential to penicillin. Cross-reactivity between imipenem and penicillin is high.

Subcutaneous Route: 15-minute intervals between all doses

Dose	Solution No.	Concentration (mg/mL)	SubQ Injections q15min Volume (mL)	SubQ Injections q15min Dosage (mg)
1	3	0.05	0.5	0.025
2		0.05	1	0.05
3	2	0.5	0.2	0.1
4		0.5	0.4	0.2
5		0.5	0.8	0.4
6	1	5	0.12	0.6
7		5	0.25	1.25
8		5	0.5	2.5
9		5	1	5

------------------- Wait 30 minutes -------------------

Intravenous Route: Infuse over 20-30 minutes; 15 minutes between doses

Dose	Solution No.	I.V. Imipenem Dose (using 50 mL NSS)	Concentration (mg/mL)	Total Dosage (mg)
10	1	2 mL in 50 mL NSS	10 mg/50 mL	10
11		4 mL in 50 mL NSS	20 mg/50 mL	20
12		8 mL in 50 mL NSS	40 mg/50 mL	40
13		12 mL in 50 mL NSS	60 mg/50 mL	60
	Add 10 mL NSS to 500 mg vial Primaxin®			
14		2.5 mL in 50 mL NSS	125 mg/50 mL	125
15		5 mL in 50 mL NSS	250 mg/50 mL	250

DESENSITIZATION PROTOCOLS *(Continued)*

INSULIN

Lilly's appropriate diluting fluid, sterile saline, or distilled water, to which 1 mL of the patient's blood or the addition of 1 mL of 1% serum albumin (making a 0.1% solution) for each 10 mL of stock diluent, is a satisfactory diluent. The albumin in the blood or serum albumin solution is necessary to retain the integrity of the higher dilutions by preventing adsorption to glass or plastic. Dilution is stable 30 days under refrigeration or room temperature, but should be used within 24 hours due to a lack of preservative.

1. Make a 1:1 dilution of single species (beef, pork, or human) insulin (50 units/mL).
2. Add 0.5 mL of the above dilution to 4.5 mL of diluent (5 units/mL).
3. Add 0.5 mL of the 5 units/mL dilution to 4.5 mL of diluent (0.5 unit/mL).
4. Add 0.5 mL of the 0.5 unit/mL dilution to 4.5 mL of diluent (0.05 unit/mL).
5. Add 0.5 mL of the 0.05 unit/mL dilution to 4.5 mL of diluent (0.005 unit/mL).

The 5 vials containing 50, 5, 0.5, 0.05, and 0.005 unit/mL are ready for skin testing or desensitization procedures.

One may start desensitization by giving 0.02 mL of 0.05 unit/mL concentration (1/1000 unit) intradermally. If no reaction occurs, administer 0.04 and 0.08 mL of the same concentration at 30-minute intervals.

The procedure continues proceeding to the next greater concentration (0.5 unit/mL) and giving 0.02, 0.04, and 0.08 mL at 30-minute intervals.

In the same manner proceed through the 5 units/mL and 50 units/mL concentrations with the exception that these injections should be given subcutaneously.

Note: If a reaction is noted, back up 2 steps and try to proceed forward again.

If the patient reacts to the initial injection, it will be necessary to utilize the lower concentration (0.005 unit/mL) to initiate the procedure.

It is essential that manifestations of allergic reactions not be obscured. Therefore, antihistamines or steroids should not be used during desensitization except to treat severe allergic reactions. The use of these agents may obscure mild to moderate reactions to the lower doses and result in more severe reactions as doses increase, leading to failure of the desensitization program.

NELFINAVIR DESENSITIZATION PROTOCOL

Adapted from Abraham PE, Sorensen SJ, Baker WH, et al, "Nelfinavir Desensitization," *Ann Pharmacother*, 2001, 35(5):553-6.

Step	Time (min)	Nelfinavir Dose (mg) q30min	Nelfinavir Dose (mg) Total
1	0	0.5	0.5
2	30	1	1.5
3	60	2	3.5
4	90	5	8.5
5	120	10	18.5
6	150	20	38.5
7	180	40	78.5
8	210	80	158.5
9	240	160	318.5
10	270	250	568.5
11	300	500	1068.5
12	330	750	1818.5

Observe patient in ICU for 2 hours before discharge

RIFAMPIN and ETHAMBUTOL
Oral Desensitization in Mycobacterial Disease

Time from Start (h:min)	Rifampin (mg)	Ethambutol (mg)
0	0.1	0.1
00:45	0.5	0.5
01:30	1	1
02:15	2	2
03:00	4	4
03:45	8	8
04:30	16	16
05:15	32	32
06:00	50	50
06:45	100	100
07:30	150	200
11:00	300	400
Next day		
6:30 AM	300 mg twice daily	400 mg 3 times/day

From *Am J Respir Crit Care Med*, 1994, 149:815-7.

SKIN TESTS

Penicillin Allergy

The recommended battery of major and minor determinants used in penicillin skin testing will disclose those individuals with circulating IgE antibodies. This procedure is therefore useful to identify patients at risk for immediate or accelerated reactions. Skin tests are of no value in predicting the occurrence of non-IgE-mediated hypersensitivity reactions to penicillin such as delayed exanthem, drug fever, hemolytic anemia, interstitial nephritis, or exfoliative dermatitis. Based on large scale trials, skin testing solutions have been standardized.

Antihistamines, tricyclic antidepressants, and adrenergic drugs, all of which may inhibit skin test results, should be discontinued at least 24 hours prior to skin testing. Antihistamines with long half-lives (hydroxyzine, terfenadine, astemizole, etc) may attenuate skin test results up to a week, or longer after discontinuation.

When properly performed with due consideration for preliminary scratch tests and appropriate dilutions, skin testing with penicillin reagents can almost always be safely accomplished. Systemic reactions accompany about 1% of positive skin tests; these are usually mild but can be serious. **Therefore skin tests should be done in the presence of a physician and with immediate access to medications and equipment needed to treat anaphylaxis.**

History of Penicillin Allergy

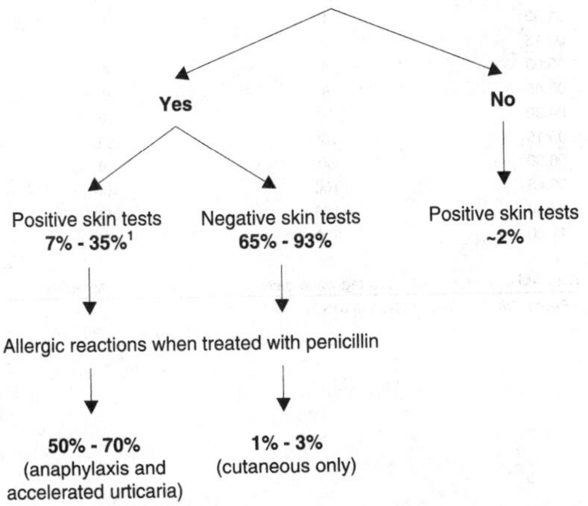

[1]One study found 65% positive.

Prevalence of positive and negative skin tests and subsequent allergic reactions in patients treated with penicilin (based on studies using both penicilloyl-polylysine and minor determinant mixture as skin test reagents).

Penicillin Skin Testing Protocol

Skin tests evaluate the patient for the presence of penicillin IgE — sensitive mast cells which are responsible for anaphylaxis and other immediate hypersensitivity reactions. Local or systemic allergic reactions rarely occur due to skin testing, therefore, a tourniquet, I.V., and epinephrine should be at the bedside. The breakdown products of penicillin provide the antigen which is responsible for the allergy. Testing is performed with benzylpenicilloyl-polylysine (Pre-Pen®), the major determinant, penicillin G which provides the minor determinants and the actual penicillin which will be administered.

Controls are important if the patient is extremely ill or is taking antihistamines, codeine, or morphine. Normal saline is the negative control. Morphine sulfate, a mast cell degranulator, can be used as a positive control, if the patient is not on morphine or codeine. Histamine is the preferred positive control, however, is not manufactured in a pharmaceutical formulation anymore. A false-positive or false-negative will make further skin testing invalid.

Control Solutions

Normal saline = negative control
Morphine sulfate (10 mg/100 mL 0.9% NaCl, 0.1 mg/mL) = positive control

Test Solutions

Order the necessary solutions as 0.5 mL in a tuberculin syringe. **Note:** May need to order 2 syringes of each — one for scratch testing and one for intradermal skin testing.

I. **Pre-Pen®: Benzylpenicilloyl-polylysine (0.25 mL ampul) = MAJOR DETERMINANT**
   A. Undiluted Pre-Pen®
   B. 1:100 concentration
      To make: Dilute 0.1 mL of Pre-Pen® in 10 mL of 0.9% NaCl
   C. 1:10,000 concentration
      (**Only necessary in patients with a history of anaphylaxis**)
      To make: Dilute 1 mL of the 1:100 solution in 100 mL of 0.9% NaCl

II. **Penicillin G sodium/potassium = MINOR DETERMINANT**
   A. 5000 units/mL concentration
   B. 5 units/mL concentration
      (**Only necessary in patients with a history of anaphylaxis**)
      To make: Dilute 0.1 mL of a 5000 units/mL solution in 100 mL of 0.9% NaCl

III. **Penicillin product to be administered — if not penicillin G**
   A. **Ampicillin** 2.5 mg/mL concentration
      To make: Dilute 250 mg in 100 mL of 0.9% NaCl
   B. **Nafcillin** 2.5 mg/mL concentration
      To make: Dilute 250 mg in 100 mL of 0.9% NaCl

Order for placement/availability at the bedside in the event of a hypersensitivity reaction during scratch/skin testing and desensitization:

Hydrocortisone: 100 mg IVP
Diphenhydramine: 50 mg IVP
Epinephrine: 1:1000 SubQ

Scratch / Skin Testing Protocol: Must Be Done by Physician!

1. Begin with the control solutions (ie, normal saline and morphine).
2. Administer **scratch tests** in the following order (beginning with the most dilute solution):

Pre-Pen®	Syringes: C,B,A
Penicillin G	Syringes: E,D
Ampicillin/Nafcillin	Syringe: F

   The inner volar surface of the forearm is usually used.

   A nonbleeding scratch of 3-5 mm in length is made in the epidermis with a 20-gauge needle.

   If bleeding occurs, another site should be selected and another scratch made using less pressure.

SKIN TESTS *(Continued)*

A small drop of the test solution is then applied and rubbed gently into the scratch using an applicator, toothpick, or the side of the needle.

The scratch test site should be observed for the appearance of a wheal, erythema, and pruritis.

A positive reaction is signified by the appearance within 15 minutes of a pale wheal (usually with pseudopods) ranging from 5-15 mm or more in diameter.

As soon as a positive response is elicited, or 15 minutes has elapsed, the solution should be wiped off the scratch.

If the scratch test is negative or equivocal (ie, a wheal of <5 mm in diameter with little or no erythema or itching appears), an intradermal test may be performed.

If significant reaction, treat and proceed to desensitization.

3. Administer **intradermal tests** in the following order (beginning with the most dilute solution):

Pre-Pen®	Syringes: C,B,A
Penicillin G	Syringes: E,D
Ampicillin/Nafcillin	Syringe: F

Intradermal tests are usually performed on a sterilized area of the upper outer arm at a sufficient distance below the deltoid muscle to permit proximal application of a tourniquet if a severe reaction occurs.

Using a tuberculin syringe with a $^{3}/_{8}$-$^{5}/_{8}$ inch 26- to 30-gauge needle, an amount of each test solution sufficient to raise the smallest perceptible bleb (usually 0.01-0.02 mL) is injected immediately under the surface of the skin.

A separate needle and syringe must be used for each solution.

Each test and control site should be at least 15 cm apart.

Positive reactions are manifested as a wheal at the test site with a diameter at least 5 mm larger than the saline control, often accompanied by itching and a marked increase in the size of the bleb.

Skin responses to penicillin testing will develop within 15 minutes.

If no significant reaction, may challenge patient with reduced dosage of the penicillin to be administered.

Physician should be at the bedside during this challenge dose!

If significant reaction, treat and begin desensitization.

Delayed Hypersensitivity (Anergy)

Delayed cutaneous hypersensitivity (DCH) is a cell-mediated immunological response which has been used diagnostically to assess previous infection (eg, purified protein derivative (PPD) and coccidioidin) or as an indicator of the status of the immune system by using mumps, *Candida*, tetanus toxoid, or trichophyton to test for anergy. Anergy is a defect in cell-mediated immunity that is characterized by an impaired response, or lack of a response to DCH testing with injected antigens. Anergy has been associated with several disease states, malnutrition, and immunosuppressive therapy, and has been correlated with increased risk of infection, morbidity, and mortality.

Many of the skin test antigens have not been approved by the FDA as tests for anergy, and so the directions for use and interpretation of reactions to these products may differ from that of the product labeling. There is also disagreement in the published literature as to the selection and interpretation of these tests for anergy assessment, leading to different recommendations for use of these products.

General Guidelines

Read these guidelines before using any skin test.

Administration

1. Use a separate sterile TB syringe for each antigen. Immediately after the antigen is drawn up, make the injection intradermally in the flexor surface of the forearm.

2. A small bleb 6-10 mm in diameter will form if the injection is made at the correct depth. If a bleb does not form or if the antigen solution leaks from the site, the injection must be repeated.
3. When applying more than one skin test, make the injections at least 5 cm apart.
4. Do any serologic blood tests before testing or wait 48-96 hours.

Reading

1. Read all tests at 24, 48, and 72 hours. Reactions occurring before 24 hours are indicative of an immediate rather than a delayed hypersensitivity.
2. Measure the diameter of the induration in two directions (at right angles) with a ruler and record each diameter in millimeters. Ballpoint pen method of measurement is the most accurate.
3. Test results should be recorded by the nurse in the Physician's Progress Notes section of the chart, and should include the millimeters of induration present, and a picture of the arm showing the location of the test(s).

Factors Causing False-Negative Reactions

1. Improper administration, interpretation, or use of outdated antigen
2. Test is applied too soon after exposure to the antigen (DCH takes 2-20 weeks to develop)
3. Concurrent viral illnesses (eg, rubeola, influenza, mumps, and probably others) or recent administration of live attenuated virus vaccines (eg, measles)
4. Anergy may be associated with:
   a. Immune suppressing chronic illnesses such as diabetes, uremia, sarcoidosis, metastatic carcinomas, Hodgkin's, acute lymphocytic leukemia, hypothyroidism, chronic hepatitis, and cirrhosis.
   b. Some antineoplastic agents, radiation therapy, and corticosteroids. If possible, discontinue steroids at least 48 hours prior to DCH skin testing.
   c. Congenital immune deficiencies.
   d. Malnutrition, shock, severe burns, and trauma.
   e. Severe disseminated infections (miliary or cavitary TB, cocci granuloma, and other disseminated mycotic infections, gram-negative bacillary septicemia).
   f. Leukocytosis (>15,000 cells/mm^3).

SKIN TESTS *(Continued)*

Factors Causing False-Positive Reactions

1. Improper interpretation
2. Patient sensitivity to minor ingredients in the antigen solutions such as the phenol or thimerosal preservatives
3. Cross-reactions between similar antigens

Candida **1:1000**

Dose = 0.1 mL intradermally (30% of children <18 months of age and 50% >18 months of age respond)

Can be used as a control antigen

Coccidioidin 1:1000

Dose = 0.1 mL intradermally (apply with PPD **and** a control antigen)
Mercury derivative used as a preservative for spherulin.

Multitest CMI (*Candida*, diphtheria toxoid, tetanus toxoid, *Streptococcus*, old tuberculin, *Trichophyton, Proteus* antigen, and negative control)

Press loaded unit into the skin with sufficient pressure to puncture the skin and allow adequate penetration of all points.

Mumps 40 cfu/mL

Dose = 0.1 mL intradermally (contraindicated in patients allergic to eggs, egg products, or thimerosal)

Dosage as Part of Disease Diagnosis

Tuberculin Testing

Purified Protein Derivative (PPD)

Preparation	Dilution	Units/0.1 mL
First strength	1:10,000	1
Intermediate strength	1:2000	5
Second strength	1:100	250

The usual initial dose is 0.1 mL of the intermediate strength. The first strength should be used in the individuals suspected of being highly sensitive. The second strength is used only for individuals who fail to respond to a previous injection of the first or intermediate strengths.

A positive reaction is ≥10 mm induration except in HIV-infected individuals where a positive reaction is ≥5 mm of induration.

Adverse Reactions

In patients who are highly sensitive, or when higher than recommended doses are used, exaggerated local reactions may occur, including erythema, pain, blisters, necrosis, and scarring. Although systemic reactions are rare, a few cases of lymph node enlargement, fever, malaise, and fatigue have been reported.

To prevent severe local reactions, never use second test strengths as the initial agent. Use diluted first strengths in patients with known or suspected hypersensitivity to the antigen.

Have epinephrine and antihistamines on hand to treat severe allergic reactions that may occur.

Treatment of Adverse Reactions

Severe reactions to intradermal skin tests are rare and treatment consists of symptomatic care.

Skin Testing

All skin tests are given intradermally into the flexor surface of one arm.

Purified protein derivative (PPD) is used most often in the diagnosis of tuberculosis. *Candida, Trichophyton*, and mumps skin tests are used most often as controls for anergy.

Dose: The usual skin test dose is as follows:

Antigen		Standard Dose	Concentration
PPD	1 TU	0.1 mL	1 TU — highly sensitive patients
	5 TU	0.1 mL	5 TU — standard dose
	250 TU	0.1 mL	250 TU — anergic patients in whom TB is suspected
Candida		0.02 mL	
Mumps		0.1 mL	
Trichophyton		0.02 mL	

Interpretation:

Skin Test	Reading Time	Positive Reaction
PPD	48-72 h	**≥5 mm considered positive for:** • close contacts to an infectious case • persons with abnormal chest x-ray indicating old healed TB • persons with known or suspected HIV infection **≥10 mm considered positive for:** • other medical risk factors • foreign born from high prevalence areas • medically underserved, low income populations • alcoholics and intravenous drug users • residents of long-term care facilities (including correctional facilities and nursing homes) • staff in settings where disease would pose a hazard to large number of susceptible persons **≥15 mm considered positive for:** • persons without risk factors for TB
Candida	24-72 h	≥5 mm induration
Mumps	24-36 h	≥5 mm
Trichophyton	24-72 h	≥5 mm induration

SKIN TESTS *(Continued)*

Recommended Interpretation of Skin Test Reactions

Reaction	Local Reaction	
	After Intradermal Injections of Antigens	After Dinitrochlorobenzene
1+	Erythema >10 mm and/or induration >1-5 mm	Erythema and/or induration covering <½ area of dose site
2+	Induration 6-10 mm	Induration covering >½ area of dose site
3+	Induration 11-20 mm	Vesiculation and induration at dose site or spontaneous flare at days 7-14 at the site
4+	Induration >20 mm	Bulla or ulceration at dose site or spontaneous flare at days 7-14 at the site

HEPATITIS LABORATORY DIAGNOSIS AND MANAGEMENT

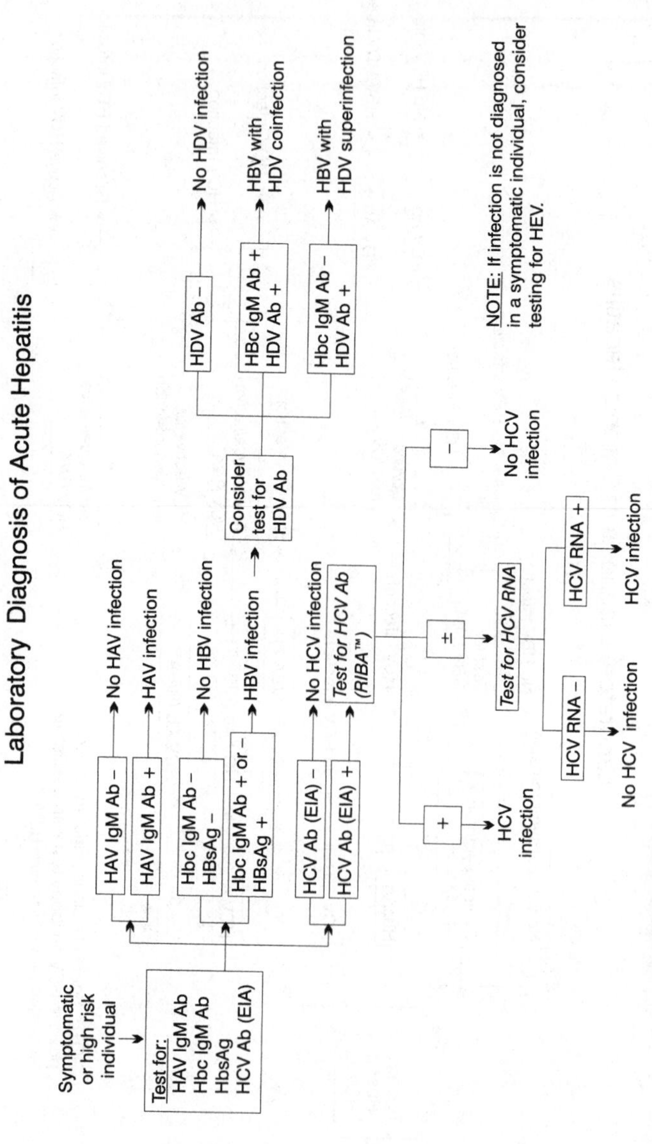

HEPATITIS LABORATORY DIAGNOSIS AND MANAGEMENT
(Continued)

Laboratory Diagnosis of Chronic Hepatitis

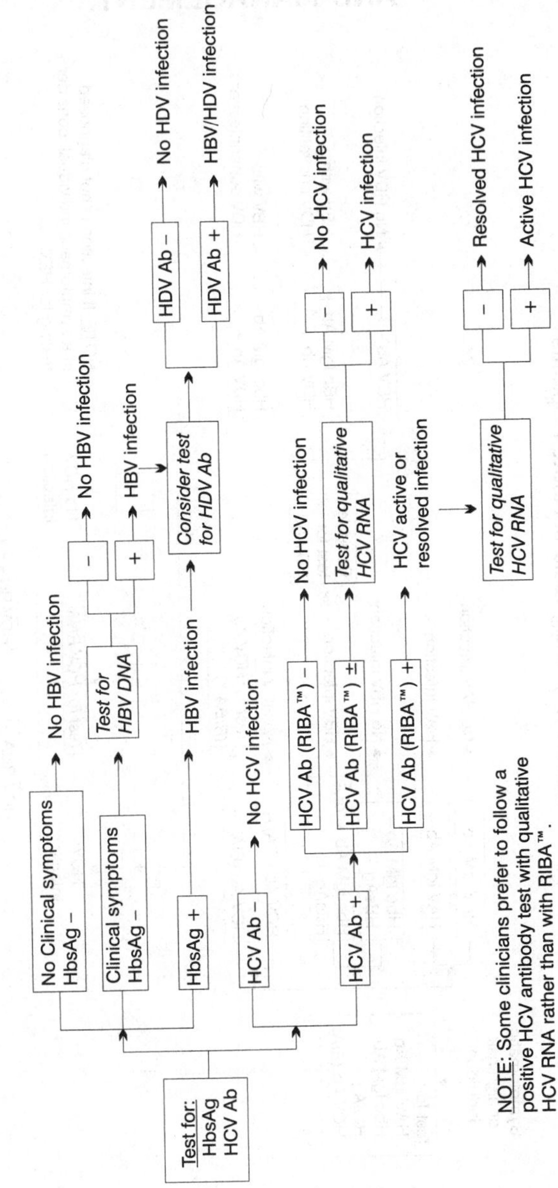

NOTE: Some clinicians prefer to follow a positive HCV antibody test with qualitative HCV RNA rather than with RIBA™.

Laboratory Management of Patients With Hepatitis

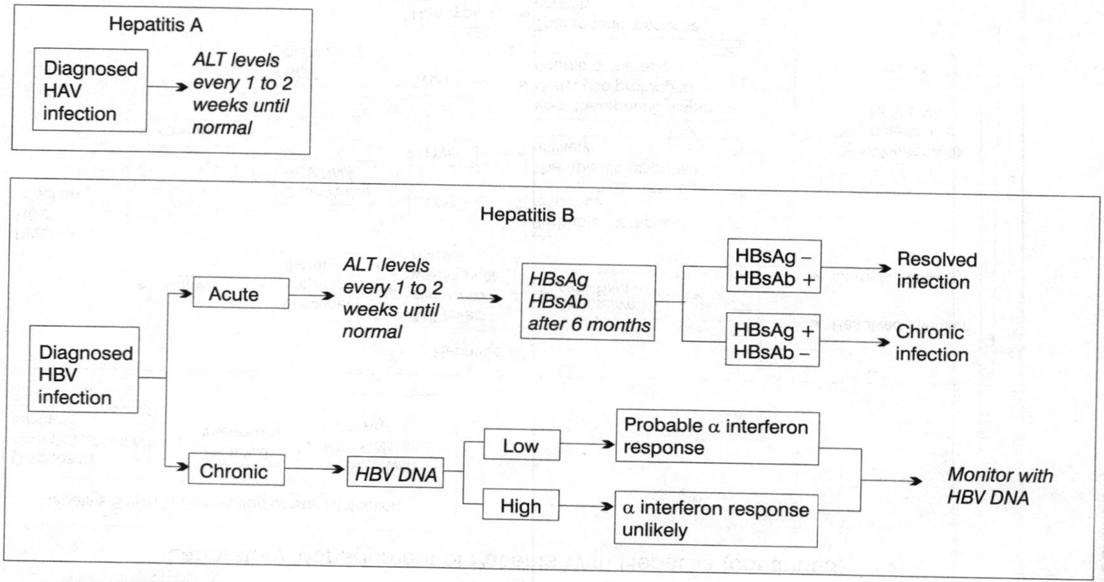

HEPATITIS LABORATORY DIAGNOSIS AND MANAGEMENT
(Continued)

Laboratory Management of Patients With Hepatitis (continued)

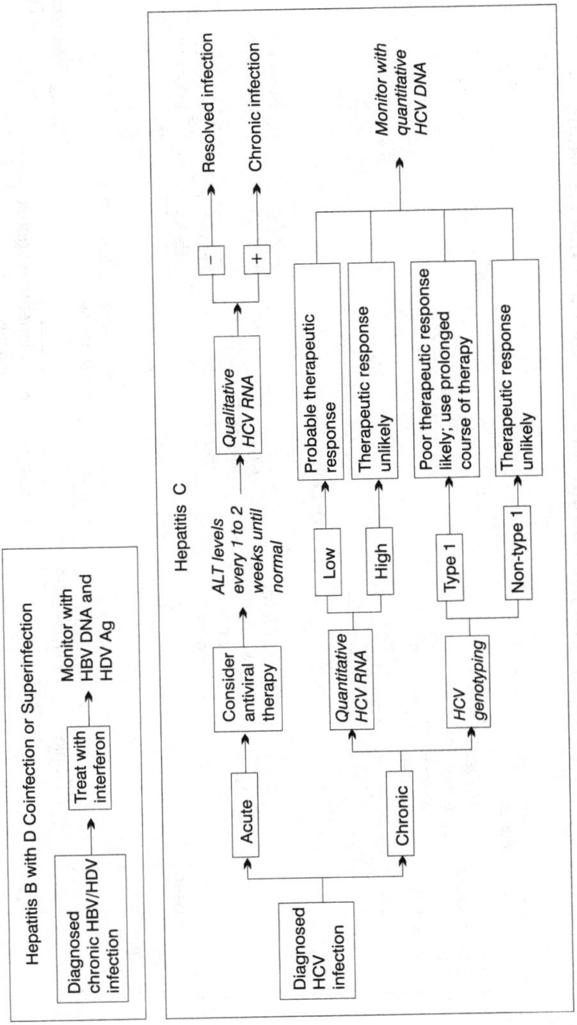

Adapted from Quest Diagnostics Nichols Institute, 2000, with permission.

AIDS WASTING TREATMENT

Drug	Adult Dose	Available Dosage Forms
Dronabinol (Marinol®)	Initial: 2.5 mg twice daily (before lunch and dinner); titrate up to a maximum of 20 mg/d	Capsule: 2.5 mg, 5 mg, 10 mg
Fluoxymesterone (Halotestin®)	10 mg twice daily	Tablet: 2 mg, 5 mg, 10 mg
Megesterol (Megace®)	Initial: 800 mg/d; daily doses of 400 and 800 mg/d were found to be clinically effective	Suspension, oral: 40 mg/mL with alcohol 0.06% Tablet: 20 mg, 40 mg
Nandrolone (Deca-Durabolin®, Durabolin®)	100 mg/week; up to 600 mg/week may be used	Injection: In oil, as phenproprionate: 25 mg/mL 50 mg/mL In oil, as decanoate: 50 mg/mL 100 mg/mL 200 mg/mL Respiratory, as decanoate: 50 mg/mL 100 mg/mL 200 mg/mL
Oxandrolone (Oxandrin®)	10 mg twice daily	Tablet: 2.5 mg
Oxymetholone (Anadrol®)	50 mg 3 times/d	Tablet: 50 mg
Somatropin (r-DNA origin for injection) (Serostim®)	SubQ: >55 kg: 6 mg/d; 45-55 kg: 5 mg/d; 35-45 kg: 4 mg/d	Injection: 4 mg, 5 mg, 6 mg
Testosterone (various)	I.M.: 200-400 mg every 2 weeks	Injection: Aqueous suspension: 25 mg/mL, 50 mg/mL, 100 mg/mL In oil, as cypionate: 100 mg/mL, 200 mg/mL In oil, as enanthate: 100 mg/mL, 200 mg/mL In oil, as propionate: 50 mg/mL, 100 mg/mL
Thalidomide	300 mg/d	Tablet: 50 mg

ANTIRETROVIRAL AGENTS

Table 1. Single Agent Nucleoside Reverse Transcriptase Inhibitors

Generic Name (Brand Name)	Dosage Form	Normal Dosing	Renal Dosing Adjustment	Hepatic Dosing Adjustment	Selected Adverse Reactions
Single Agent NRTIs (Nucleoside Reverse Transcriptase Inhibitors)					
Abacavir (Ziagen®)	Tablet: 300 mg Solution, oral: 20 mg/mL (240 mL)	300 mg bid or 600 mg daily	None necessary	No recommendation	Hypersensitivity syndrome (fever, fatigue, GI symptoms, ± rash); **do not restart abacavir in patients who have experienced this**; GI symptoms
Didanosine (ddl) (Videx®)	Tablet, chewable: 25 mg, 50 mg, 100 mg, 150 mg, 200 mg Capsule, sustained release: 125 mg, 200 mg, 250 mg, 400 mg	≥60 kg: 200 mg bid or 400 mg daily <60 kg: 125 mg bid or 250 mg daily (Take on empty stomach)	≥60 kg: 100-200 mg/day <60 kg: 75-150 mg/day (adjust for Cl_{cr} <60) Renal adjustment varies by dosage form and renal function. Consult additional references/product labeling.	No recommendation	Peripheral neuropathy, pancreatitis, abdominal pain, nausea, diarrhea, retinal depigmentation, anxiety, insomnia
Emtricitabine (Emtriva™)	Capsule: 200 mg	200 mg daily	Cl_{cr} 30-49: 200 mg q48h Cl_{cr} 15-29: 200 q72h Cl_{cr} <15 (including hemodialysis patients): 200 mg q96h	No recommendation	Headache, dizziness, insomnia, diarrhea, rash, hyperpigmentation of palms/soles
Lamivudine (3TC) (Epivir®)	Tablet: 150 mg, 300 mg Solution, oral: 5 mg/mL (240 mL); 10 mg/mL (240 mL)	150 mg bid or 300 mg daily	Cl_{cr} 30-49: 150 mg qd Cl_{cr} 15-29: 150 mg first dose, then 100 mg qd Cl_{cr} 5-14: 150 mg first dose, then 50 mg qd Cl_{cr} <5: 50 mg first dose, then 25 mg qd	No recommendation	Headache, insomnia, nausea, vomiting, diarrhea, abdominal pain, myalgia, arthralgia, pancreatitis in children
Stavudine (d4T) (Zerit®)	Capsule: 15 mg, 20 mg, 30 mg, 40 mg Solution, oral: 1 mg/mL (200 mL)	≥60 kg: 40 mg bid <60 kg: 30 mg bid	≥60 kg: Cl_{cr} 26-50: 20 mg bid Cl_{cr} 10-25: 20 mg daily <60 kg: Cl_{cr} 26-50: 15 mg bid Cl_{cr} 10-25: 15 mg daily	No recommendation	Peripheral neuropathy, headache, abdominal or back pain, asthenia, nausea, vomiting, diarrhea, myalgia, anxiety, depression, pancreatitis, lipodystrophy, hyperlipidemia, less frequently hepatotoxicity

Table 1. Single Agent Nucleoside Reverse Transcriptase Inhibitors *(continued)*

Generic Name (Brand Name)	Dosage Form	Normal Dosing	Renal Dosing Adjustment	Hepatic Dosing Adjustment	Selected Adverse Reactions
Tenofovir (Viread™)	Tablet: 300 mg	300 mg daily	Cl_{cr} 30-49: 300 mg q48h Cl_{cr} 10-29: 300 mg twice a week ESRD: 300 mg once a week	No recommendation	Nausea, vomiting, diarrhea
Zalcitabine (ddC) (Hivid®)	Tablet: 0.375 mg, 0.75 mg	0.75 mg q8h	Cl_{cr} 10-40: 0.75 mg bid Cl_{cr} <10: 0.75 mg qd	No recommendation	Peripheral neuropathy, oral/esophageal ulceration, rash, nausea, vomiting, diarrhea, abdominal pain, myalgia, pancreatitis
Zidovudine (AZT) (Retrovir®)	Tablet: 300 mg Capsule: 100 mg Syrup: 50 mg/5 mL (240 mL) Injection: 10 mg/mL (20 mL)	300 mg bid or 200 mg tid	ESRD: 100 mg q6-8h	No recommendation	Anemia, neutropenia, thrombocytopenia, headache, nausea, vomiting, myopathy, hepatitis, hyperpigmentation of nails

ANTIRETROVIRAL AGENTS *(Continued)*

Table 2. Combination Nucleoside Reverse Transcriptase Inhibitors

Generic Name (Brand Name)	Dosage Form	Normal Dosing	Renal / Hepatic Dosing / Adverse Reactions
Combination NRTIs (Nucleoside Reverse Transcriptase Inhibitors)			
Abacavir + lamivudine (Epzicom™)	Tablet: 600 mg abacavir + 300 mg lamivudine	1 tablet daily	See individual agents
Abacavir + lamivudine + zidovudine (Trizivir®)	Tablet: 300 mg abacavir + 150 mg lamivudine + 300 mg zidovudine	1 tablet bid	
Emtricitabine + tenofovir (Truvada™)	Tablet: 200 mg emtricitabine and 300 mg tenofovir	1 tablet daily	
Zidovudine + lamivudine (Combivir®)	Tablet: 300 mg zidovudine and 150 mg lamivudine	1 tablet bid (see lamivudine for dose adjustment)	

Table 3. Non-nucleoside Reverse Transcriptase Inhibitors

Generic Name (Brand Name)	Dosage Form	Normal Dosing	Renal Dosing Adjustment	Hepatic Dosing Adjustment	Selected Adverse Reactions
NNRTIs (Non-nucleoside Reverse Transcriptase Inhibitors)					
Delavirdine (Rescriptor®)	Tablet: 100 mg, 200 mg	400 mg tid	None necessary	No recommendation; use caution	Rash, abnormal liver function tests
Efavirenz (Sustiva™)	Capsule: 50 mg, 100 mg, 200 mg Tablet: 600 mg	600 mg qd (Take on empty stomach)	None necessary	No recommendation; use caution	Dizziness, psychiatric symptoms (hallucinations, confusion, depersonalization, others), agitation, vivid dreams, rash, GI intolerance
Nevirapine (Viramune®)	Tablet: 200 mg Suspension, oral: 50 mg/5 mL (240 mL)	200 mg qd for 14 days, then 200 mg bid	None necessary	Avoid use in mild to moderate hepatic impairment	Rash (severe), abnormal liver function tests, fever, nausea, headache

ANTIRETROVIRAL AGENTS *(Continued)*

Table 4. Protease Inhibitors

Generic Name (Brand Name)	Dosage Form	Normal Dosing	Renal Dosing Adjustment	Hepatic Dosing[1] Adjustment	Selected Adverse Reactions
PIs (Protease Inhibitors)					
Amprenavir (Agenerase™)	Capsule: 50 mg, 150 mg Solution, oral: 15 mg/mL (240 mL)	Capsule: 1200 mg bid Solution: 1400 mg bid (Avoid high fat meal)	Capsule: None necessary Solution: Contraindicated	C-P 5-8: 450 mg bid C-P 9-12: 300 mg bid	Rash (life-threatening), paresthesias (perioral), depression, nausea, diarrhea, vomiting, hyperglycemia (and sometimes diabetes), dyslipidemia including fat redistribution ("buffalo hump," "protease paunch"), hyperlipidemia, hypercholesterolemia
Atazanavir (Reyataz™)	Capsule: 100 mg, 150 mg, 200 mg	400 mg daily (Take with food)	None necessary	C-P 7-9: 300 mg daily C-P >9: Not recommended	Headache, nausea, increased bilirubin, lipodystrophy, hyperglycemia, increased P-R interval
Fosamprenavir (Lexiva™)	Tablet: 700 mg	1400 mg bid (1400 mg/day with ritonavir)	None necessary	C-P 5-8: 700 mg bid C-P 9-12: Not recommended	Rash, increased LFTs
Indinavir (Crixivan®)	Capsule: 100 mg, 200 mg, 333 mg, 400 mg	800 mg q8h with water	None necessary	Mild to moderate hepatic insufficiency due to cirrhosis: 600 mg q8h	Hyperbilirubinemia, nephrolithiasis, elevated AST/ALT, abdominal pain, nausea, vomiting, diarrhea, taste perversion, hyperglycemia (and sometimes diabetes), dyslipidemia including fat redistribution ("buffalo hump," "protease paunch"), hyperlipidemia, hypercholesterolemia

Table 4. Protease Inhibitors *(continued)*

Generic Name (Brand Name)	Dosage Form	Normal Dosing	Renal Dosing Adjustment	Hepatic Dosing[1] Adjustment	Selected Adverse Reactions
Lopinavir and ritonavir (Kaletra™)	Capsule: Lopinavir 133.3 mg and ritonavir 33.3 mg Solution, oral: Lopinavir 80 mg and ritonavir 20 mg/mL	3 capsules or 5 mL bid (Take with food)	None necessary	No recommendation; use caution	Asthenia, nausea, diarrhea, vomiting, anorexia, abdominal pain, circumoral and peripheral paresthesia, taste perversion, headache, hyperglycemia (and sometimes diabetes), dyslipidemia including fat redistribution ("buffalo hump," "protease paunch"), hyperlipidemia, hypercholesterolemia
Nelfinavir (Viracept®)	Tablet: 250 mg, 625 mg Powder, oral: 50 mg/g	750 mg tid or 1250 mg bid (Take with food)	None necessary	No recommendation; use caution	Diarrhea, nausea, hyperglycemia (and sometimes diabetes), dyslipidemia including fat redistribution ("buffalo hump," "protease paunch"), hyperlipidemia, hypercholesterolemia
Ritonavir (Norvir®)	Capsule: 100 mg Solution, oral: 80 mg/mL (240 mL)	600 mg bid (Take with food)	None necessary	No adjustment for mild impairment; use caution in moderate to severe impairment	Asthenia, nausea, diarrhea, vomiting, anorexia, abdominal pain, circumoral and peripheral paresthesia, taste perversion, headache, hyperglycemia (and sometimes diabetes), dyslipidemia including fat redistribution ("buffalo hump," "protease paunch"), hyperlipidemia, hypercholesterolemia

ANTIRETROVIRAL AGENTS *(Continued)*

Table 4. Protease Inhibitors *(continued)*

Generic Name (Brand Name)	Dosage Form	Normal Dosing	Renal Dosing Adjustment	Hepatic Dosing[1] Adjustment	Selected Adverse Reactions
Saquinavir (Invirase®, Fortovase®)	Hard gelatin capsule (hgc): 200 mg Tablet: 500 mg Soft gelatin capsule: 200 mg	1200 mg tid (hgc only) or 1000 mg bid (with ritonavir) (Take with food)	None necessary	No recommendation; use caution	Diarrhea, abdominal discomfort, nausea, headache, hyperglycemia (and sometimes diabetes), dyslipidemia including fat redistribution ("buffalo hump," "protease paunch"), hyperlipidemia, hypercholesterolemia

[1]Hepatic impairment as defined by the Child-Pugh (C-P) classification.

Table 5. Fusion Inhibitor

Generic Name (Brand Name)	Dosage Form	Normal Dosing	Renal Dosing Adjustment	Hepatic Dosing Adjustment	Selected Adverse Reactions
Enfuvirtide (Fuzeon™)	Injection (lyophilized powder): 90 mg/mL	90 mg SubQ bid	None necessary	No recommendation; use caution	Injection site reaction, bacterial pneumonia, hypersensitivity

ANTIRETROVIRAL AGENTS *(Continued)*

Antiretroviral Drug Interactions

Antiretroviral Agent	Interacting Agent	Severity[1]	Additional Comments
Abacavir	Ethanol	3	Increased abacavir AUC.
Amprenavir	Astemizole, rifampin, midazolam, bepridil, dihydroergotamine, ergotamine, cisapride	1	Contraindicated. Avoid concomitant use.
	Abacavir, clarithromycin, indinavir, ritonavir, cimetidine	2	Increased amprenavir C_{max} and AUC.
	Saquinavir	1	Decreased amprenavir AUC and C_{max}.
	Rifabutin	1	Increased rifabutin AUC by 193%; administer one-half usual rifabutin dose.
	Amiodarone, lidocaine, quinidine, warfarin, tricyclic antidepressants	1	Increased toxic effect of these agents; must have concentration monitoring.
	HMGCoA reductase inhibitors, diltiazem, nicardipine, nifedipine, nimodipine, alprazolam, clorazepate, diazepam, flurazepam, itraconazole, dapsone, erythromycin, loratadine, sildenafil, carbamazepine, pimozide	2	Increased serum concentrations of these agents, potential for increased toxic effects.
	Oral contraceptives	1	Decreased oral contraceptive concentrations.
Atazanavir	Bepridil, cisapride, ergot derivatives (dihydroergotamine, ergonovine, ergotamine, methylergonovine), irinotecan, lovastatin, midazolam, pimozide, simvastatin, triazolam	1	Atazanavir may increase serum concentrations leading to severe toxicity.
	Antiarrhythmics (amiodarone, lidocaine, quinidine), calcium channel blockers, immunosuppressants (cyclosporine, sirolimus, tacrolimus), tricyclic antidepressants	2	Serum concentrations may be increased by atazanavir.
	Proton pump inhibitors (esomeprazole, lansoprazole, omeprazole)	1	Serum concentrations of atazanavir may be decreased.
	Ritonavir	1	Specific dosing adjustment of atazanavir in combination with ritonavir and efavirenz has been established.
	Saquinavir	1	Serum concentrations may be increased by atazanavir. Dosing recommendations for the combination have not been established.
	Sildenafil	2	Serum concentration may be substantially increased by atazanavir. Do not exceed single doses of sildenafil 25 mg in 48 hours.
	Indinavir	1	May increase the risk of hyperbilirubinemia. Concurrent administration is not recommended.
	Clarithromycin	1	Atazanavir may increase serum concentrations of clarithromycin increasing the risk of QT_c prolongation. Reduce clarithromycin dose (50%) or select alternative agent (except in *Mycobacterium avium* complex infections).
	Rifabutin	1	Increase in rifabutin AUC (>200%) when coadministered with atazanavir (decrease rifabutin's dose by up to 75%).

Antiretroviral Drug Interactions *(continued)*

Antiretroviral Agent	Interacting Agent	Severity[1]	Additional Comments
Atazanavir *(continued)*	Antacids and buffered formulations (ie, didanosine buffered tablets)	2	Reduce serum concentrations of atazanavir. Administer atazanavir 2 hours before or 1 hour after these medications.
	H_2 antagonists	2	May reduce the absorption of atazanavir. Avoid concurrent use or administer at least 12 hours apart.
	Carbamazepine, phenobarbital, and rifampin	1	May decrease serum levels and result in a loss of virologic response and resistance.
Delavirdine	Protease inhibitors	2	Increased levels of protease inhibitors; start indinavir at 600 mg every 8 hours; nelfinavir may decrease delavirdine levels by 50%.
	Astemizole, cisapride, alprazolam, midazolam, triazolam	1	Delavirdine may significantly increase concentrations of these drugs.
	Dihydropyridine calcium channel blockers, ergot derivatives, quinidine	2	Delavirdine may increase concentrations of these drugs.
	Warfarin	2	Delavirdine may increase warfarin concentrations.
	Rifampin/rifabutin, phenytoin, carbamazepine	1	Avoid concomitant use; decreased delavirdine concentration.
	Antacids, H_2-antagonists, didanosine	2	Decreased delavirdine absorption. Administer antacids or didanosine at least 1 hour apart from delavirdine.
	Clarithromycin, dapsone	2	Delavirdine may increase levels of these drugs; clarithromycin may increase delavirdine levels.
	Ketoconazole, fluoxetine	3	May increase delavirdine concentration by 50%.
Didanosine	Tetracycline, itraconazole, ketoconazole, indinavir	2	Decreased absorption with didanosine.
	Dapsone	3	Administer 2 hours before didanosine.
	Ciprofloxacin/norfloxacin (quinolones)	2	Administer didanosine 6 hours before or 2 hours after quinolone.
	Tenofovir	1	Didanosine concentrations may be significantly increased by tenofovir. Separate doses by 2 hours.
Emtricitabine	Ribavirin	2	May increase the risk of lactic acidosis.
Efavirenz	Astemizole, cisapride, ergot derivatives, midazolam, triazolam	1	Contraindicated. Avoid concomitant use.
	Indinavir	2	Decreased indinavir AUC by 31% and Cp_{max} by 16%. Increase indinavir dose to 1000 mg every 8 hours.
	Ritonavir	3	Increased AUC by ~20% for each drug.
	Saquinavir	2	Decreased saquinavir AUC by 62% and Cp_{max} by 50%. Not recommended as sole protease inhibitor with efavirenz.
	Rifampin	2	Decreased efavirenz AUC by 26% and Cp_{max} by 20%.
	Clarithromycin	2	Decreased clarithromycin AUC by 39% and Cp_{max} by 49%; increased hydroxy metabolite of clarithromycin AUC by 34% and Cp_{max} by 49%.
	Ethinyl estradiol	2	Increased ethinyl estradiol AUC by 37%.
	Warfarin	2	Decreased or increased warfarin effects.

ANTIRETROVIRAL AGENTS *(Continued)*

Antiretroviral Drug Interactions *(continued)*

Antiretroviral Agent	Interacting Agent	Severity[1]	Additional Comments
Indinavir	Rifabutin	1	Increased rifabutin AUC by 204%; decrease rifabutin dose to one-half.
	Ketoconazole	2	Increased indinavir AUC by 68%; decrease indinavir dose to 600 mg every 8 hours.
	Didanosine	2	Decreased indinavir absorption; administer 1 hour apart on an empty stomach.
	Rifampin	1	Avoid concomitant use due to decreased indinavir concentration.
	Astemizole, cisapride, triazolam/ midazolam	1	Indinavir may increase toxicity of these drugs. Avoid concomitant use.
Lamivudine	Trimethoprim/sulfamethoxazole	3	Increased lamivudine AUC by 44%.
	Zidovudine	3	Increased zidovudine C_{max} by 39%.
Nelfinavir	Astemizole, cisapride, midazolam, rifampin, triazolam	1	Contraindicated. Avoid concomitant use.
	Rifabutin	2	Increased rifabutin concentrations; reduce rifabutin dose.
	Anticonvulsants	1	May decrease nelfinavir concentrations.
	Oral contraceptives	1	Decreased oral contraceptive concentrations.
	Delavirdine	2	Nelfinavir concentration doubled; delavirdine level decreased by 50%.
Nevirapine	Oral contraceptives	1	Decreased oral contraceptives concentration.
	Protease inhibitors	1	Decreased concentrations of protease inhibitors; avoid concomitant use.
	Rifabutin/rifampin	2	Decreased nevirapine concentrations.

Antiretroviral Drug Interactions *(continued)*

Antiretroviral Agent	Interacting Agent	Severity[1]	Additional Comments
Ritonavir, lopinavir, and ritonavir	Meperidine	2	Increased levels of metabolite.
	Piroxicam	1	Contraindicated. Alternative: Aspirin.
	Propoxyphene	1	Contraindicated. Alternative: Oxycodone.
	Amiodarone, encainide, flecainide, propafenone, quinidine/quinine	1	Contraindicated.
	Rifabutin	1	Contraindicated. Alternatives: Clarithromycin, ethambutol.
	Bepridil	1	Contraindicated.
	Astemizole	1	Contraindicated. Alternatives: Loratadine.
	Cisapride	1	Contraindicated.
	Bupropion	1	Contraindicated. Alternative: Fluoxetine, desipramine.
	Clozapine	1	Contraindicated.
	Alprazolam, clorazepate, diazepam, estazolam, flurazepam, midazolam, triazolam, zolpidem	1	Contraindicated. Alternatives: Temazepam, lorazepam.
	Clarithromycin	2	Increased clarithromycin AUC by 77%; decrease dose of clarithromycin by 50% if Cl_{cr} is 30-60 mL/minute and by 75% if Cl_{cr} is <30 mL/minute.
	Erythromycin	2	>3 times increase in AUC of erythromycin.
	Desipramine	2	Increased desipramine AUC by 145%.
	Disulfiram/metronidazole	2	Disulfiram-like reaction.
	Oral contraceptives	1	Decreased ethinyl estradiol AUC by 40%.
	Theophylline	2	Decreased theophylline AUC by 43%.
	Antiarrhythmics, anticoagulants, anticonvulsants, tricyclic antidepressants, neuroleptics	2	1.5 to >3 times increase in AUC of interacting drug.
	Phenytoin, phenobarbital, rifampin/rifabutin	2	May decrease ritonavir levels.
Saquinavir	Carbamazepine, dexamethasone, phenobarbital, phenytoin	2	May decrease saquinavir levels.
	Rifampin	1	Decreased saquinavir level by 80%.
	Rifabutin	2	Decreased saquinavir level by 40%.
Stavudine	None		
Tenofovir	Didanosine	1	Didanosine concentrations may be significantly increased by tenofovir. Separate doses by 2 hours.
	Protease inhibitors	2	Tenofovir may decrease protease inhibitor concentrations.
Zalcitabine	Antacids (aluminum-, magnesium-containing)	2	Decreased zalcitabine absorption by 25%; do not administer simultaneously.
	Pentamidine	2	Increased risk of pancreatitis; avoid concomitant use.
Zidovudine	Ganciclovir	1	Increased toxicity (hematologic).
	Interferon	2	Dose reduction or interruption may be necessary or change to foscarnet.
	Probenecid	2	Increased zidovudine levels.

[1]Severity: 1 = major; 2 = moderate; 3 = minor.

ANTIRETROVIRAL AGENTS *(Continued)*

Drugs That Should Not Be Used With Protease Inhibitors

Drug Category	Indinavir	Ritonavir[1]	Saquinavir[2]	Nelfinavir	Alternatives
Analgesics	None	Piroxicam, propoxyphene	None	None	ASA, oxycodone, acetaminophen
Cardiac	None	Amiodarone, encainide, flecainide, propafenone, quinidine	None	None	Limited experience
Antimycobacterial	Rifampin	Rifabutin[3]	Rifampin, rifabutin	Rifampin	For rifabutin (as alternative for MAI treatment): clarithromycin, ethambutol (treatment, not prophylaxis), or azithromycin
Calcium channel blocker	None	Bepridil	None	None	Limited experience
Antihistamine	Astemizole	Astemizole	Astemizole	Astemizole	Loratadine
Gastrointestinal	Cisapride	Cisapride	Cisapride	Cisapride	Limited experience
Antidepressant	None	Bupropion	None	None	Fluoxetine, desipramine
Neuroleptic	None	Clozapine, pimozide	None	None	Limited experience
Psychotropic	Midazolam, triazolam	Clorazepate, diazepam, estazolam, flurazepam, midazolam, triazolam, zolpidem	Midazolam, triazolam	Midazolam, triazolam	Temazepam, lorazepam
Ergot alkaloid (vasoconstrictor)		Dihydroergotamine (D.H.E. 45), ergotamine[4] (various forms)		Dihydroergotamine (D.H.E. 45), ergotamine[4] (various forms)	

[1]The contraindicated drugs listed are based on theoretical considerations. Thus, drugs with low therapeutic indices yet with suspected major metabolic contribution from CYP3A, CYP2D6, or unknown pathways are included in this table. Actual interactions may or may not occur in patients.

[2]Given as Invirase® or Fortovase™.

[3]Reduce rifabutin dose to one-fourth of the standard dose.

[4]This is likely a class effect.

ANTIRETROVIRAL THERAPY FOR HIV INFECTION

Adapted from the "Guidelines for the Use of Antiretroviral Agents in HIV-1-Infected Adults and Adolescents," developed by the Panel on Clinical Practices for Treatment of HIV Infection, Department of Health and Human Services, updated April 7, 2005; available at www.aidsinfo.nih.gov.

GOALS OF THERAPY

Goals of Therapy

- Maximal and durable suppression of viral load
- Restoration and/or preservation of immunologic function
- Improvement of quality of life
- Reduction of HIV-related morbidity and mortality

Tools to Achieve Goals of Therapy

- Maximize adherence to the antiretroviral regimen
- Rational selection and sequencing of drugs
- Preservation of future treatment options
- Use of resistance testing and therapeutic drug monitoring in selected clinical settings

WHEN TO TREAT

Indications for Viral Load Assessment

Indications for Plasma HIV RNA Testing[1]

Clinical Indication	Information	Use
Syndrome consistent with acute HIV infection	Establishes diagnosis when HIV antibody test is negative or indeterminate	Diagnosis[2]
Initial evaluation of newly diagnosed HIV infection	Baseline viral load "set point"	Decision to start or defer therapy (in conjunction with CD4+ T-cell counts)
Every 3-4 months in patients not on therapy	Changes in viral load	Decision to start therapy (in conjunction with CD4+ T-cell counts)
2-8 weeks after initiation or change in antiretroviral therapy	Initial assessment of drug efficacy	Decision to continue or change therapy
3-4 months after start of therapy	Virologic effect of therapy	Decision to continue or change therapy
Every 3-4 months in patients on therapy	Durability of antiretroviral effect	Decision to continue or change therapy
Clinical event or significant decline in CD4+ T cells	Association with changing or stable viral load	Decision to continue, initiate, or change therapy

[1]Acute illness (eg, bacterial pneumonia, tuberculosis, HSV, PCP) and immunizations can cause increases in plasma HIV RNA for 2-4 weeks; viral load testing should not be performed during this time. Plasma HIV RNA results should usually be verified with a repeat determination before starting or making changes in therapy.

[2]Diagnosis of HIV infection determined by HIV RNA testing should be confirmed by standard methods (eg, Western blot serology) performed 2-4 months after the initial indeterminate or negative test.

ANTIRETROVIRAL THERAPY FOR HIV INFECTION
(Continued)

Criteria for Initiating Treatment

The optimal time to initiate therapy in asymptomatic individuals with >200 CD4+ T cells is not known. This table provides general guidance rather than absolute recommendations for an individual patient. Recent literature suggests that a CD4+ cell count may be a more important prognostic indicator than viral load and that a significantly increased risk of progression occurs when viral load exceeds 100,000 copies/mL. All decisions to initiate therapy should be based on prognosis as determined by the CD4+ T-cell count and viral load, the potential benefits and risks of therapy, and the willingness of the patient to accept therapy.

Indications for the Initiation of Antiretroviral Therapy in the Chronically HIV-1 Infected Patient

Clinical Category	CD4+ T-Cell Count	Plasma HIV RNA	Recommendation
AIDS-defining illness or severe symptoms[1]	Any value	Any value	Treat
Asymptomatic[2]	CD4+ T cells <200/mm³	Any value	Treat
Asymptomatic	CD4+ T cells >200/mm³ but ≤350/mm³	Any value	Treatment should be offered following full discussion of pros and cons with each patient
Asymptomatic	CD4+ T cells >350/mm³	≥100,000 copies/mL	Most clinicians recommend deferring therapy, but some clinicians will treat
Asymptomatic	CD4+ T cells >350/mm³	<100,000 copies/mL	Defer therapy

[1]AIDS-defining illness per Centers for Disease Control, 1993. Severe symptoms include unexplained fever or diarrhea >2-4 weeks, oral candidiasis, or >10% unexplained weight loss.

[2]Clinical benefit has been demonstrated in controlled trials only for patients with CD4+ T cells <200/mm³; however, the majority of clinicians would offer therapy at a CD4+ T-cell threshold <350/mm³. A collaborative analysis of data from 13 cohort studies from Europe and North America found that lower CD4 count, higher HIV viral load, injection drug use, and age >50 were all predictors of progression to AIDS or death in antiretroviral naive patients beginning combination antiretroviral therapy. These data indicate that the prognosis is better for patients who initiate therapy at >200 cells/mm³, but risk after initiation of therapy does not vary considerably at >200 cells/mm³.

Early vs Delayed Treatment

Benefits and Risks of Delayed Initiation of Therapy in the Asymptomatic HIV-Infected Patient[1]

Benefits	Risks
• Avoid treatment-related negative quality of life effects (ie, inconvenience) • Avoid drug-related adverse events • Delay development of drug resistance • Preserve maximum number of available and future drug options • More time for patient to understand treatment demands	• Possibly irreversible immune system depletion • Possibly greater difficulty in suppressing viral replication • Possibly increased risk of HIV transmission[2] • Control of viral replication more difficult to achieve and maintain

[1]See table, "Indications for the Initiation of Antiretroviral Therapy in the Chronically HIV-1 Infected Patient," for consensus recommendations regarding when to initiate therapy.

[2]Antiretroviral therapy cannot substitute for primary HIV prevention measures (eg, use of condoms and safer sex practices).

TREATMENT OPTIONS

Recommended Antiretroviral Agents for Initial Treatment of Established HIV Infection

The following tables provide a guide to treatment regimens for patients who have no previous experience with HIV therapy. Regimens should be individualized based on the advantages and disadvantages of each combination such as pill burden, dosing frequency, toxicities, drug-drug interactions, patient variables (such as pregnancy), comorbid conditions, and level of plasma HIV-RNA. Regimens are designated as "preferred" for use in treatment-naive patients when clinical trial data suggest optimal efficacy and durability with acceptable tolerability and ease of use. Alternative regimens are those in which clinical trial data show efficacy, but may be disadvantageous compared to the preferred regimens in terms of antiviral activity, demonstrated durable effect, tolerability, or ease of use. Based on individual patient characteristics, a regimen listed as an alternative may actually be the preferred regimen for a selected patient. Of note, the designation of preferred or alternative regimens may change as new safety and efficacy data emerge, which, in the opinion of the Panel, warrants reassignment of regimens in these categories. Revisions will be updated on an ongoing basis. Clinicians initiating antiretroviral regimens in pregnant women or pediatric patients should refer to the specific guidelines found at http://www.aidsinfo.nih.gov/guidelines. Additional guidelines are available for postexposure prophylaxis (occupational and nonoccupational) as well as management of opportunistic infections.

NNRTI-Based Regimens

Preferred Regimens	**Efavirenz + (lamivudine or emtricitabine) + (zidovudine or tenofovir) – except in 1st trimester pregnancy or women with child-bearing potential**
Alternative Regimens	Efavirenz + (lamivudine or emtricitabine) + (abacavir or didanosine or stavudine[1]) – except in 1st trimester pregnancy or women with child-bearing potential[2]
	Nevirapine[3] + (lamivudine or emtricitabine) + (zidovudine or stavudine[1] or didanosine or abacavir or tenofovir). **Note:** Nevirapine should only be used if $CD4^+$ T-cell counts are ≤250 cells/mm^3 in women or ≤400 cells/mm^3 in men.

[1]Higher incidence of lipoatrophy, hyperlipidemia, and mitochondrial toxicities reported with stavudine than with other NRTIs.

[2]Women with child-bearing potential implies women who want to conceive or those who are not using effective contraception.

[3]High incidence (11%) of hepatotoxicity and skin reactions; close clinical monitoring advised, especially during 1st 18 months of therapy. Do not use if $CD4^+$ T-cell counts are >250 cells/mm^3 in women or >400 cells/mm^3 in men.

ANTIRETROVIRAL THERAPY FOR HIV INFECTION
(Continued)

PI-Based Regimens

Preferred Regimens	**Lopinavir / ritonavir (coformulated as Kaletra®) + (lamivudine or emtricitabine) + (zidovudine)**
Alternative Regimens	Fosamprenavir / ritonavir[1] + (lamivudine or emtricitabine) + (zidovudine or abacavir or tenofovir or didanosine or stavudine[2])
	Fosamprenavir + (lamivudine or emtricitabine) + (zidovudine or abacavir or tenofovir or didanosine or stavudine[2])
	Atazanavir + (lamivudine or emtricitabine) + (zidovudine or stavudine[2] or abacavir or didanosine) or (tenofovir + ritanovir 100 mg/day)
	Indinavir / ritonavir[1] + (lamivudine or emtricitabine) + (zidovudine or stavudine[2] or abacavir or tenofovir or didanosine)
	Lopinavir / ritonavir (coformulated as Kaletra®) + (emtricitabine or lamivudine) + (stavudine[2] or abacavir or tenofovir or didanosine)
	Nelfinavir + (lamivudine or emtricitabine) + (zidovudine or stavudine[2] or abacavir or tenofovir or didanosine)
	Saquinavir (soft or hard gel capsule) / ritonavir[1] + (lamivudine or emtricitabine) + (zidovudine or stavudine[2] or abacavir or tenofovir or didanosine)

[1]Low-dose (100-400 mg) ritonavir.
[2]Higher incidence of lipoatrophy, hyperlipidemia, and mitochondrial toxicities reported with stavudine than with other NRTIs.

Triple NRTI Regimen

Only as alternative to NNRTI- or PI-based regimen – should not be used first-line	Abacavir + lamivudine + zidovudine

TREATMENT LIMITATIONS

Antiretroviral Drugs Not Recommended as Initial Therapy

Drugs	Reasons for Not Recommending as Initial Therapy
Amprenavir (unboosted or ritonavir boosted)	• High pill burden
Delavirdine	• Inferior virologic efficacy • Inconvenient dosing (3 times/day)
Enfuvirtide	• No clinical trial experience in treatment-naive patients • Requires twice daily subcutaneous injections
Nevirapine	• High incidence of serious or fatal hepatic events
Indinavir (unboosted)	• Inconvenient dosing (3 times/day with meal restrictions)
Ritonavir as sole PI	• High pill burden • Gastrointestinal intolerance
Saquinavir (hard or soft) gel capsule (unboosted)	• High pill burden • Inferior virologic efficacy
Zalcitabine + zidovudine	• Inferior virologic efficacy • Higher rate of adverse effects than other 2-NRTI alternatives

Antiretroviral Regimens or Components That Should Not Be Offered at Any Time

	Rationale	Exception
Antiretroviral Regimens Not Recommended		
Monotherapy	• Rapid development of resistance • Inferior antiretroviral activity when compared to combination with three or more antiretrovirals	Pregnant women with HIV-RNA <1000 copies/mL using zidovudine monotherapy for prevention of perinatal HIV transmission[1] and not for HIV treatment for the mother
Two-NRTI drug combinations	• Rapid development of resistance • Inferior antiretroviral activity when compared to combination with three or more antiretrovirals	For patients currently on this treatment, it is reasonable to continue if virologic goals are achieved
Triple NRTI combination: abacavir + tenofovir + (lamivudine or emtricitabine)	High rate of early virologic nonresponse seen when this triple NRTI combination was used as initial regimen in treatment-naive patients	No exception
Triple NRTI combination: tenofovir + didanosine + (lamivudine or emtricitabine	High rate of early virologic nonresponse seen when this triple NRTI combination was used as initial regimen in treatment-naive patients	No exception
Antiretroviral Components Not Recommended as Part of Antiretroviral Regimen		
Amprenavir oral solution in: • pregnant women • children <4 y • patients with renal or hepatic failure • patients treated with metronidazole or disulfiram	Oral liquid contains large amount of the excipient propylene glycol, which may be toxic in the patients at risk	No exception
Amprenavir oral solution + ritanovir oral solution	Propylene glycol in amprenavir may compete metabolically with ethanol (vehicle in ritonavir) leading to accumulation of either vehicle	No exception
Atazanavir + indinavir	Potential additive hyperbilirubinemia	No exception
Didanosine + zalcitabine	Additive peripheral neuropathy	No exception
Efavirenz in 1st trimester pregnancy or in women with significant child-bearing potential[2]	Teratogenic in nonhuman primates	When no other antiretroviral options are available and potential benefits outweigh the risks[1]
Emtricitabine + lamivudine	• Similar resistance profile • No potential benefit	No exception
Fosamprenavir + amprenavir	Fosamprenavir is a prodrug for amprenavir, so no additional benefit	No exception
Lamivudine + zalcitabine	*In vitro* antagonism demonstrated	No exception
Nevirapine initiation with $CD4^+$ T-cell count >250 cells/mm^3 in women or >400 cells/mm^3 in men	Higher incidence of symptomatic (including serious or fatal) hepatic events	Only if benefit clearly outweighs risk

ANTIRETROVIRAL THERAPY FOR HIV INFECTION
(Continued)

Antiretroviral Regimens or Components That Should Not Be Offered at Any Time *(continued)*

	Rationale	Exception
Saquinavir hard gel capsule (Invirase®) as **single** protease inhibitor	• Poor oral bioavailability (4%) • Inferior antiretroviral activity when compared to other protease inhibitors	No exception
Stavudine + didanosine	• High incidence of toxicities – peripheral neuropathy, pancreatitis, and hyperlactatemia • Reports of serious, even fatal cases of lactic acidosis with hepatic steatosis with or without pancreatitis in pregnant women	When no other antiretroviral options are available and potential benefits outweigh the risks[1]
Stavudine + zidovudine	Antagonistic	No exception
Stavudine + zalcitabine	Additive peripheral neuropathy	No exception

[1]When constructing an antiretroviral regimen for an HIV-infected pregnant woman, please consult "Public Health Service Task Force Recommendations for the Use of Antiretroviral Drugs in Pregnant HIV-1-Infected Women for Maternal Health and Interventions to Reduce Perinatal HIV-1 Transmission in the United States" in http://www.aidsinfo.nih.gov/guidelines.

[2]Women with child-bearing potential implies women who want to conceive or those who are not using effective contraception.

SPECIAL CONSIDERATIONS

Resistance Testing

Viral drug resistance is generally determined by one of two methods: genotypic assays or phenotypic assays. Genotypic assays involve sequencing techniques to identify the presence of specific drug-resistant genes. While these assays produce relatively rapid results (1-2 weeks) they require knowledge of specific drug-resistance mutations for appropriate interpretation. Alternatively, phenotypic assays measure the ability of the patient's virus (as monitored by recombination with a reporter gene) to replicate in the presence of antiretroviral drugs. These assays can be more time-consuming and costly, and also suffer from the drawback that resistance level breakpoints are unknown.

Despite these methodological limitations, resistance testing can assist in designing an appropriate therapeutic regimen, by identifying, and thus avoiding less effective antiretroviral drugs in the setting of virologic failure. In addition, prior knowledge of specific drug-resistant viral phenotypes can guide selection of initial therapy which offers a greater likelihood of success.

The following table identifies the appropriate settings for the use of resistance testing.

Clinical Setting	Drug-Resistance Assay Recommendation	Rationale
Virologic failure during combination antiretroviral therapy	Recommended	Determine the role of resistance in drug failure and maximize selection of active drugs.
Suboptimal suppression of viral load after antiretroviral therapy initiation	Recommended	Determine the role of resistance and maximize selection of active drugs.
Acute HIV infection, if initiating therapy	Recommended	Determine if drug-resistant virus was transmitted to assist in designing initial regimen.
Chronic HIV infection before initiation of therapy	Should be considered	Assays may not detect minor drug-resistant species. Should consider if patient infected by person receiving antiretroviral therapy.
After discontinuation of drugs	Not usually recommended	Assays may not detect minor drug-resistant species which may occur in the absence of selective drug pressure.
Plasma viral load <1000 HIV RNA copies/mL	Not usually recommended	Assays may not reliably detect low numbers of viral RNA.

ANTIRETROVIRAL THERAPY FOR HIV INFECTION
(Continued)

Therapeutic Drug Monitoring

As with other notable drug classes (eg, antibiotics, anticonvulsants), the goal of therapeutic drug monitoring (TDM) is to maximize therapeutic efficacy and minimize drug-related toxicities. The utility of TDM in the setting of antiretroviral drug therapy is supported by data showing considerable interpatient variability with respect to drug concentrations among patients taking similar doses, as well as data demonstrating concentration/effect and concentration/toxicity correlations. The optimal plasma concentrations of many antiretroviral drugs have yet to be determined (eg, NRTIs). Those drugs for which target trough levels are defined are shown below.

Suggested Minimum Target Trough Concentrations for Persons With Wild-Type HIV-1

Drug	Concentration (ng/mL)
Amprenavir	400
Indinavir	100
Lopinavir / ritonavir (Kaletra®)	1000
Nelfinavir[1]	800
Ritonavir[2]	2100
Saquinavir	100-250
Efavirenz	1000
Nevirapine	3400

[1]Measurable active M8 metabolite.

[2]Ritonavir given as a single PI.

MANAGEMENT OF HEALTHCARE WORKER EXPOSURES TO HBV, HCV, AND HIV

Adapted from "U.S. Public Health Service Guidelines for the Management of Occupational Exposures to HBV, HCV, and HIV and Recommendations for Postexposure Prophylaxis," *MMWR Morb Mortal Wkly Rep*, 2001, 50(RR-11).

Factors to Consider in Assessing the Need for Follow-up of Occupational Exposures

- **Type of exposure**
  - Percutaneous injury
  - Mucous membrane exposure
  - Nonintact skin exposure
  - Bites resulting in blood exposure to either person involved
- **Type and amount of fluid/tissue**
  - Blood
  - Fluids containing blood
  - Potentially infectious fluid or tissue (semen; vaginal secretions; and cerebrospinal, synovial, pleural, peritoneal, pericardial, and amniotic fluids)
  - Direct contact with concentrated virus
- **Infectious status of source**
  - Presence of HB_sAg
  - Presence of HCV antibody
  - Presence of HIV antibody
- **Susceptibility of exposed person**
  - Hepatitis B vaccine and vaccine response status
  - HBV, HCV, HIV immune status

Evaluation of Occupational Exposure Sources

Known sources

- Test known sources for HB_sAg, anti-HCV, and HIV antibody
  - Direct virus assays for routine screening of source patients are **not** recommended
  - Consider using a rapid HIV-antibody test
  - If the source person is **not** infected with a bloodborne pathogen, baseline testing or further follow-up of the exposed person is **not** necessary
- For sources whose infection status remains unknown (eg, the source person refuses testing), consider medical diagnoses, clinical symptoms, and history of risk behaviors
- Do not test discarded needles for bloodborne pathogens

Unknown sources

- For unknown sources, evaluate the likelihood of exposure to a source at high risk for infection
  - Consider the likelihood of bloodborne pathogen infection among patients in the exposure setting

MANAGEMENT OF HEALTHCARE WORKER EXPOSURES TO HBV, HCV, AND HIV *(Continued)*

Recommended Postexposure Prophylaxis for Exposure to Hepatitis B Virus

Vaccination and Antibody Response Status of Exposed Workers[1]	Treatment		
	Source HB_sAg[2]-Positive	**Source HB_sAg[2] -Negative**	**Source Unknown or Not Available for Testing**
Unvaccinated	HBIG[3] x 1 and initiate HB vaccine series[4]	Initiate HB vaccine series	Initiate HB vaccine series
Previously vaccinated			
Known responder[5]	No treatment	No treatment	No treatment
Known nonresponder[6]	HBIG x 1 and initiate revaccination or HBIG x 2[7]	No treatment	If known high risk source, treat as if source was HB_sAg-positive
Antibody response unknown	Test exposed person for anti-HB_s[8] 1. If adequate,[5] no treatment is necessary 2. If inadequate,[6] administer HBIG x 1 and vaccine booster	No treatment	Test exposed person for anti-HB_s 1. If adequate,[4] no treatment is necessary 2. If inadequate,[4] administer vaccine booster and recheck titer in 1-2 months

[1]Persons who have previously been infected with HBV are immune to reinfection and do not require postexposure prophylaxis.

[2]Hepatitis B surface antigen.

[3]Hepatitis B immune globulin; dose is 0.06 mL/kg intramuscularly.

[4]Hepatitis B vaccine.

[5]A responder is a person with adequate levels of serum antibody to HB_sAg (ie, anti-HB_s ≥10 mIU/mL).

[6]A nonresponder is a person with inadequate response to vaccination (ie, serum anti-HB_s <10 mIU/mL).

[7]The option of giving one dose of HBIG and reinitiating the vaccine series is preferred for nonresponders who have not completed a second 3-dose vaccine series. For persons who previously completed a second vaccine series but failed to respond, two doses of HBIG are preferred.

[8]Antibody to HB_sAg.

Recommended HIV Postexposure Prophylaxis for Percutaneous Injuries

Exposure Type	Infection Status of Source				
	HIV-Positive Class 1[1]	HIV-Positive Class 2[1]	Unknown HIV Status[2]	Unknown Source[3]	HIV-Negative
Less severe[4]	Recommend basic 2-drug PEP	Recommend expanded 3-drug PEP	Generally, no PEP warranted; however, consider basic 2-drug PEP[5] for source with HIV risk factors[6]	Generally, no PEP warranted; however, consider basic 2 drug PEP[5] in settings where exposure to HIV-infected persons is likely	No PEP warranted
More severe[7]	Recommend expanded 3-drug PEP	Recommend expanded 3-drug PEP	Generally, no PEP warranted; however consider basic 2-drug PEP[5] for source with HIV risk factors[6]	Generally, no PEP warranted; however, consider basic 2 drug PEP[5] in settings where exposure to HIV-infected persons is likely	No PEP warranted

[1]HIV-Positive, Class 1 – asymptomatic HIV infection or known low viral load (eg, <1500 RNA copies/mL). HIV-Positive Class 2 – symptomatic HIV infection, AIDS, acute seroconversion, or known high viral load. If drug resistance is a concern, obtain expert consultation. Initiation of postexposure prophylaxis (PEP) should not be delayed pending expert consultation, and, because expert consultation alone cannot substitute for face-to-face counseling, resources should be available to provide immediate evaluation and follow-up care for all exposures.

[2]Source of unknown HIV status (eg, deceased source person with no samples available for HIV testing).

[3]Unknown source (eg, a needle from a sharps disposal container).

[4]Less severe (eg, solid needle and superficial injury).

[5]The designation "consider PEP" indicates the PEP is optional and should be based on an individualized decision between the exposed person and the treating clinician.

[6]If PEP is offered and taken and the source is later determined to be HIV-negative, PEP should be discontinued.

[7]More severe (eg, large-bore hollow needle, deep puncture, visible blood on device, or needle used in patient's artery or vein).

MANAGEMENT OF HEALTHCARE WORKER EXPOSURES TO HBV, HCV, AND HIV *(Continued)*

Recommended HIV Postexposure Prophylaxis for Mucous Membrane Exposures and Nonintact Skin[1] Exposures

	Infection Status of Source				
Exposure Type	**HIV-Positive Class 1**[2]	**HIV-Positive Class 2**[2]	**Unknown HIV Status**[3]	**Unknown Source**[4]	**HIV-Negative**
Small volume[5]	Consider basic 2-drug PEP[6]	Recommend basic 2-drug PEP	Generally, no PEP warranted; however, consider basic 2-drug PEP[6] for source with HIV risk factors[7]	Generally, no PEP warranted; however, consider basic 2-drug PEP[6] in settings where exposure to HIV-infected persons is likely	No PEP warranted
Large volume[8]	Recommend basic 2-drug PE	Recommend expanded 3-drug PEP	Generally, no PEP warranted; however consider basic 2-drug PEP[6] for source with HIV risk factors[7]	Generally, no PEP warranted; however, consider basic 2-drug PEP[6] in settings where exposure to HIV-infected persons is likely	No PEP warranted

[1]For skin exposures, follow-up is indicated only if there is evidence of compromised skin integrity (eg, dermatitis, abrasion, or open wound).

[2]HIV-Positive, Class 1 – asymptomatic HIV infection or known low viral load (eg, <1500 RNA copies/mL). HIV-Positive Class 2 – symptomatic HIV infection, AIDS, acute seroconversion, or known high viral load. If drug resistance is a concern, obtain expert consultation. Initiation of postexposure prophylaxis (PEP) should not be delayed pending expert consultation, and, because expert consultation alone cannot substitute for face-to-face counseling, resources should be available to provide immediate evaluation and follow-up care for all exposures.

[3]Source of unknown HIV status (eg, deceased source person with no samples available for HIV testing).

[4]Unknown source (eg, splash from inappropriately disposed blood).

[5]Small volume (eg, a few drops).

[6]The designation "consider PEP" indicates the PEP is optional and should be based on an individualized decision between the exposed person and the treating clinician.

[7]If PEP is offered and taken and the source is later determined to be HIV-negative, PEP should be discontinued.

[8]Large volume (eg, major blood splash).

Situations for Which Expert[1] Consultation for HIV Postexposure Prophylaxis Is Advised

- **Delayed (ie, later than 24-36 hours) exposure report**
  - The interval after which there is no benefit from postexposure prophylaxis (PEP) is undefined
- **Unknown source (eg, needle in sharps disposal container or laundry)**
  - Decide use of PEP on a case-by-case basis
  - Consider the severity of the exposure and the epidemiologic likelihood of HIV exposure
  - Do not test needles or sharp instruments for HIV
- **Known or suspected pregnancy in the exposed person**
  - Does not preclude the use of optimal PEP regimens
  - Do not deny PEP solely on the basis of pregnancy
- **Resistance of the source virus to antiretroviral agents**
  - Influence of drug resistance on transmission risk is unknown
  - Selection of drugs to which the source person's virus is unlikely to be resistant is recommended, if the source person's virus is unknown or suspected to be resistant to ≥1 of the drugs considered for the PEP regimen
  - Resistance testing of the source person's virus at the time of the exposure is not recommended
- **Toxicity of the initial PEP regimen**
  - Adverse symptoms, such as nausea and diarrhea, are common with PEP
  - Symptoms can often be managed without changing the PEP regimen by prescribing antimotility and/or antiemetic agents
  - Modification of dose intervals (ie, administering a lower dose of drug more frequently throughout the day, as recommended by the manufacturer), in other situations, might help alleviate symptoms

[1]Local experts and/or the National Clinicians' Postexposure Prophylaxis Hotline (PEPline 1-888-448-4911).

MANAGEMENT OF HEALTHCARE WORKER EXPOSURES TO HBV, HCV, AND HIV *(Continued)*

Occupational Exposure Management Resources

National Clinicians' Postexposure Prophylaxis Hotline (PEPline) Run by University of California-San Francisco/San Francisco General Hospital staff; supported by the Health Resources and Services Administration Ryan White CARE Act, HIV/AIDS Bureau, AIDS Education and Training Centers, and CDC	Phone: (888) 448-4911 Internet: http://www.ucsf.edu/hivcntr
Needlestick! A website to help clinicians manage and document occupational blood and body fluid exposures. Developed and maintained by the University of California, Los Angeles (UCLA), Emergency Medicine Center, UCLA School of Medicine, and funded in part by CDC and the Agency for Healthcare Research and Quality.	Internet: http:// www.needlestick.mednet.ucla.edu
Hepatitis Hotline	Phone: (888) 443-7232 Internet: http://www.cdc.gov/hepatitis
Reporting to CDC: Occupationally acquired HIV infections and failures of PEP	Phone: (800) 893-0485
HIV Antiretroviral Pregnancy Registry	Phone: (800) 258-4263 Fax: (800) 800-1052 Address: 1410 Commonwealth Drive, Suite 215 Wilmington, NC 28405 Internet: http://www.glaxowellcome.com/preg_reg/antiretroviral
Food and Drug Administration Report unusual or severe toxicity to antiretroviral agents	Phone: (800) 332-1088 Address: MedWatch HF-2, FDA 5600 Fishers Lane Rockville, MD 20857 Internet: http://www.fda.gov/medwatch
HIV/AIDS Treatment Information Service	Internet: http://www.aidsinfo.nih.gov

Management of Occupational Blood Exposures

Provide immediate care to the exposure site

- Wash wounds and skin with soap and water
- Flush mucous membranes with water

Determine risk associated with exposure by:

- Type of fluid (eg, blood, visibly bloody fluid, other potentially infectious fluid or tissue, and concentrated virus)
- Type of exposure (ie, percutaneous injury, mucous membrane or nonintact skin exposure, and bites resulting in blood exposure)

Evaluate exposure source

- Assess the risk of infection using available information
- Test known sources for HB_sAg, anti-HCV, and HIV antibody (consider using rapid testing)
- For unknown sources, assess risk of exposure to HBV, HCV, or HIV infection
- Do not test discarded needle or syringes for virus contamination

Evaluate the exposed person

- Assess immune status for HBV infection (ie, by history of hepatitis B vaccination and vaccine response)

Give PEP for exposures posing risk of infection transmission

- HBV: See Recommended Postexposure Prophylaxis for Exposure to Hepatitis B Virus Table
- HCV: PEP not recommended
- HIV: See Recommended HIV Postexposure Prophylaxis for Percutaneous Injuries Table and Recommended HIV Postexposure Prophylaxis for Mucous Membrane Exposures and Nonintact Skin Exposures Table
  - Initiate PEP as soon as possible, preferably within hours of exposure
  - Offer pregnancy testing to all women of childbearing age not known to be pregnant
  - Seek expert consultation if viral resistance is suspected
  - Administer PEP for 4 weeks if tolerated

Perform follow-up testing and provide counseling

- Advise exposed persons to seek medical evaluation for any acute illness occurring during follow-up

HBV exposures

- Perform follow-up anti-HB_s testing in persons who receive hepatitis B vaccine
  - Test for anti-HB_s 1-2 months after last dose of vaccine
  - Anti-HB_s response to vaccine cannot be ascertained if HBIG was received in the previous 3-4 months

HCV exposures

- Perform baseline and follow-up testing for anti-HCV and alanine amino-transferase (ALT) 4-6 months after exposures
- Perform HCV RNA at 4-6 months if earlier diagnosis of HCV infection is desired
- Confirm repeatedly reactive anti-HCV enzyme immunoassays (EIAs) with supplemental tests

HIV exposures

- Perform HIV antibody testing for at least 6 months postexposure (eg, at baseline, 6 weeks, 3 months, and 6 months)
- Perform HIV antibody testing if illness compatible with an acute retroviral syndrome occurs
- Advise exposed persons to use precautions to prevent secondary transmission during the follow-up period
- Evaluate exposed persons taking PEP within 72 hours after exposure and monitor for drug toxicity for at least 2 weeks

MANAGEMENT OF HEALTHCARE WORKER EXPOSURES TO HBV, HCV, AND HIV *(Continued)*

Basic and Expanded HIV Postexposure Prophylaxis Regimens

Basic Regimens

- Zidovudine (Retrovir™; ZDV; AZT) + Lamivudine (Epivir™; 3TC); available as Combivir™
  - ZDV: 600 mg daily, in two or three divided doses, and
  - 3TC: 150 mg twice daily

Alternative Basic Regimens

- Lamivudine (3TC) + Stavudine (Zerit™; d4T)
  - 3TC: 150 mg twice daily, and
  - d4T: 40 mg twice daily (if body weight is <60 kg, 30 mg twice daily)
- Didanosine (Videx™, chewable/dispersible buffered tablet; Videx™ EC, delayed-release capsule; ddI) + Stavudine (d4T)
  - ddI: 400 mg daily on an empty stomach (if body weight is <60 kg, 125 mg twice daily)
  - d4T: 40 mg twice daily (if body weight is <60 kg, 30 mg twice daily)

Expanded Regimen

Basic regimen plus one of the following:

- Indinavir (Crixivan™; IDV)
  - 800 mg every 8 hours, on an empty stomach
- Nelfinavir (Viracept™; NFV)
  - 750 mg three times daily, with meals or snack, or
  - 1250 mg twice daily, with meals or snack
- Efavirenz (Sustiva™; EFV)
  - 600 mg daily, at bedtime
  - Should not be used during pregnancy because of concerns about teratogenicity
- Abacavir (Ziagen™; ABC); available at Trizivir™, a combination of ZDV, 3TC, and ABC
  - 300 mg twice daily

Antiretroviral Agents for Use at PEP Only With Expert Consultation

- Ritonavir (Norvir™; RTV)
- Amprenavir (Agenerase™; AMP)
- Delavirdine (Rescriptor™; DLV)
- Lopinavir/Ritonavir (Kaletra™)
  - 400/100 mg twice daily

Antiretroviral Agents Generally Not Recommended for Use as PEP

- Nevirapine (Viramune™; NVP)
  - 200 mg daily for 2 weeks, then 200 mg twice daily

PREVENTION OF PERINATAL HIV-1 TRANSMISSION

Adapted from "U.S. Public Health Service Task Force Recommendations for Use of Antiretroviral Drugs in Pregnant Women Infected With HIV-1 for Maternal Health and for Reducing Perinatal HIV-1 Transmission in the United States." (http://AIDSinfo.nih.gov)

Pediatric AIDS Clinical Trials Group (PACTG) 076 Zidovudine (ZDV) Regimen

Time of ZDV Administration	Regimen
Antepartum	Oral administration of 100 mg ZDV 5 times/day,[1] initiated at 14-34 weeks gestation and continued throughout the pregnancy
Intrapartum	During labor, intravenous administration of ZDV in a 1-hour initial dose of 2 mg/kg body weight, followed by a continuous infusion of 1 mg/kg body weight/hour until delivery
Postpartum	Oral administration of ZDV to the newborn (ZDV syrup at 2 mg/kg body weight/dose every 6 hours) for the first 6 weeks of life, beginning at 8-12 hours after birth.[2]

[1]Oral ZDV administered as 200 mg 3 times/day or 300 mg bid is currently used in general clinical practice and is an acceptable alternative regimen to 100 mg orally 5 times/day.

[2]Intravenous dosage for full-term infants who cannot tolerate oral intake is 1.5 mg/kg body weight intravenously every 6 hours. ZDV dosing for infants <35 weeks gestation at birth is 1.5 mg/kg/dose intravenously, or 2 mg/kg/dose orally, every 12 hours, advancing to every 8 hours at 2 weeks of age if >30 weeks gestation at birth or at 4 weeks of age if <30 weeks gestation at birth.

Clinical Scenarios and Recommendations for the Use of Antiretroviral Drugs to Reduce Perinatal Human Immunodeficiency Virus (HIV-1) Transmission

SCENARIO #1
HIV-1-infected pregnant women who have not received prior antiretroviral therapy

- Pregnant women with HIV-1 infection must receive standard clinical, immunologic, and virologic evaluation. Recommendations for initiation and choice of antiretroviral therapy should be based on the same parameters used for persons who are not pregnant, although the known and unknown risks and benefits of such therapy during pregnancy must be considered and discussed.
- The three-part ZDV chemoprophylaxis regimen, initiated after the first trimester, is recommended for all HIV-1-infected pregnant women regardless of antenatal HIV-1 RNA copy number to reduce the risk for perinatal transmission.
- The combination of ZDV chemoprophylaxis with additional antiretroviral drugs for treatment of HIV-1 infection is recommended for infected women whose clinical, immunologic, or virologic status requires treatment or who have HIV-1 RNA over 1000 copies/mL regardless of clinical or immunologic status, and can be considered for women with HIV-1 RNA <1000 copies/mL.
- Women who are in the first trimester of pregnancy may consider delaying initiation of therapy until after 10-12 weeks gestation.

SCENARIO #2
HIV-1-infected women receiving antiretroviral therapy during the current pregnancy

- HIV-1-infected women receiving antiretroviral therapy in whom pregnancy is identified after the first trimester should continue therapy. ZDV should be a component of the antenatal antiretroviral treatment regimen after the first trimester whenever possible, although this may not always be feasible.
- For women receiving antiretroviral therapy in whom pregnancy is recognized during the first trimester, the woman should be counseled regarding the benefits and potential risks of antiretroviral administration during this period, and continuation of therapy should be considered. If therapy is discontinued during

PREVENTION OF PERINATAL HIV-1 TRANSMISSION
(Continued)

the first trimester, all drugs should be stopped and reintroduced simultaneously to avoid the development of drug resistance.

- Regardless of the antepartum antiretroviral regimen, ZDV administration is recommended during the intrapartum period and for the newborn.

SCENARIO #3
HIV-1-infected women in labor who have had no prior therapy

Several effective regimens are available. These include:

- single-dose nevirapine at the onset of labor followed by a single dose of nevirapine for the newborn at age 48 hours
- oral ZDV and 3TC during labor, followed by 1 week of oral ZDV/3TC for the newborn
- intrapartum intravenous ZDV followed by 6 weeks of ZDV for the newborn
- two-dose nevirapine regimen combined with intrapartum intravenous ZDV and 6-week ZDV for the newborn

In the immediate postpartum period, the woman should have appropriate assessments (eg, CD4+ count and HIV-1 RNA copy number) to determine whether antiretroviral therapy is recommended for her own health.

SCENARIO #4
Infants born to mothers who have received no antiretroviral therapy during pregnancy or intrapartum

- The 6-week neonatal ZDV component of the ZDV chemoprophylactic regimen should be discussed with the mother and offered for the newborn.
- ZDV should be initiated as soon as possible after delivery – preferably within 6-12 hours of birth.
- Some clinicians may choose to use ZDV in combination with other antiretroviral drugs, particularly if the mother is known or suspected to have ZDV-resistant virus. However, the efficacy of this approach for prevention of transmission has not been proven in clinical trials, and appropriate dosing regimens for neonates are incompletely defined for many drugs.
- In the immediate postpartum period, the woman should undergo appropriate assessments (eg, CD4+ count and HIV-1 RNA copy number) to determine whether antiretroviral therapy is required for her own health. The infant should undergo early diagnostic testing so that if HIV-1-infected, treatment can be initiated as soon as possible.

Note: Discussion of treatment options and recommendations should be noncoercive, and the final decision regarding the use of antiretroviral drugs is the responsibility of the woman. A decision to not accept treatment with ZDV or other drugs should not result in punitive action or denial of care. Use of ZDV should not be denied to a woman who wishes to minimize exposure of the fetus to other antiretroviral drugs and who, therefore, chooses to receive only ZDV during pregnancy to reduce the risk for perinatal transmission.

USPHS / IDSA GUIDELINES FOR THE PREVENTION OF OPPORTUNISTIC INFECTIONS IN PERSONS INFECTED WITH HIV

Adapted from "2001 USPHS/IDSA Guidelines for the Prevention of Opportunistic Infections in Persons Infected With Human Immunodeficiency Virus. USPHS/IDSA Prevention of Opportunistic Infections Working Group" (www.aidsinfo.nih.gov)

DRUG REGIMENS FOR ADULTS AND ADOLESCENTS

Prophylaxis to Prevent First Episode of Opportunistic Disease in HIV-Infected Adults and Adolescents

Pathogen	Indication	Preventive Regimens: First Choice	Preventive Regimens: Alternatives
I. Strongly Recommended as Standard of Care			
Pneumocystis carinii[1]	CD4+ count <200/μL or oropharyngeal candidiasis	TMP-SMZ, 1 DS P.O. every day; TMP-SMZ, 1 SS P.O. every day	Dapsone, 50 mg P.O. twice daily *or* 100 mg P.O. every day; dapsone, 50 mg P.O. every day *plus* pyrimethamine, 50 mg P.O. weekly *plus* leucovorin, 25 mg P.O. weekly; dapsone, 200 mg P.O. *plus* pyrimethamine, 75 mg P.O. *plus* leucovorin, 25 mg P.O. weekly; aerosolized pentamidine, 300 mg monthly via Respirgard II™ nebulizer; atovaquone, 1500 mg P.O. every day; TMP-SMZ, 1 DS P.O. 3 times/week
Mycobacterium tuberculosis			
Isoniazid-sensitive[2]	TST reaction ≥5 mm *or* prior positive TST result without treatment or contact with case of active tuberculosis **regardless of TST result**	Isoniazid, 300 mg P.O. *plus* pyridoxine, 50 mg P.O. every day x 9 months or isoniazid, 900 mg P.O. *plus* pyridoxine, 100 mg P.O. twice a week x 9 months	Rifampin, 600 mg P.O. every day x 4 months or rifabutin, 300 mg P.O. every day x 4 months Pyrazinamide, 15-20 mg/kg P.O. every day x 2 months *plus* either rifampin, 600 mg P.O. every day x 2 months or rifabutin, 300 mg P.O. every day x 2 months
Isoniazid-resistant	Same as above; high probability of exposure to isoniazid-resistant tuberculosis	Rifampin, 600 mg P.O. or rifabutin, 300 mg P.O. every day x 4 months	Pyrazinamide, 15-20 mg/kg P.O. every day *plus* either rifampin, 600 mg P.O. or rifabutin, 300 mg P.O. every day x 2 months
Multidrug (isoniazid and rifampin)-resistant	Same as above; high probability of exposure to multidrug-resistant tuberculosis	Choice of drugs requires consultation with public health authorities. **Depends on susceptibility of isolate from source patient.**	None

USPHS / IDSA GUIDELINES FOR THE PREVENTION OF OPPORTUNISTIC INFECTIONS IN PERSONS INFECTED WITH HIV *(Continued)*

Prophylaxis to Prevent First Episode of Opportunistic Disease in HIV-Infected Adults and Adolescents *(continued)*

Pathogen	Indication	Preventive Regimens	
		First Choice	Alternatives
Toxoplasma gondii[3]	IgG antibody to *Toxoplasma* and CD4⁺ count <100/µL	TMP-SMZ, 1 DS P.O. every day	TMP-SMZ, 1 SS P.O. every day; dapsone, 50 mg P.O. every day *plus* pyrimethamine, 50 mg P.O. once weekly *plus* leucovorin, 25 mg P.O. weekly; dapsone, 200 mg P.O. *plus* pyrimethamine, 75 mg P.O. *plus* leucovorin, 25 mg P.O. weekly; atovaquone, 1500 mg P.O. every day with or without pyrimethamine, 25 mg P.O. every day *plus* leucovorin, 10 mg P.O. every day
Mycobacterium avium complex	CD4⁺ count <50/µL	Azithromycin, 1200 mg P.O. weekly or clarithromycin,[4] 500 mg P.O. twice daily	Rifabutin, 300 mg P.O. every day; azithromycin, 1200 mg P.O. weekly *plus* rifabutin, 300 mg P.O. every day
Varicella zoster virus (VZV)	Significant exposure to chickenpox or shingles for patients who have no history of either condition or, if available, negative antibody to VZV	Varicella zoster immune globulin (VZIG), 5 vials (1.25 mL each) I.M., administered ≤96 hours after exposure, ideally within 48 hours	
II. Generally Recommended			
Streptococcus pneumoniae[5]	CD4⁺ count ≥200/µL	23 valent polysaccharide vaccine, 0.5 mL I.M.	None
Hepatitis B virus[6,7]	All susceptible (anti-HB_c-negative) patients	Hepatitis B vaccine: 3 doses	None
Influenza virus[6,8]	All patients (annually, before influenza season)	Inactivated trivalent influenza virus vaccine: One annual dose (0.5 mL) I.M.	Oseltamivir, 75 mg P.O. every day (influenza A or B); rimantadine, 100 mg P.O. twice daily, or amantadine, 100 mg P.O. twice daily (influenza A only)
Hepatitis A virus[6,7]	All susceptible (anti-HAV-negative) patients at increased risk for HAV infection (eg, illicit drug users, men who have sex with men, hemophiliacs) or with chronic liver disease, including chronic hepatitis B or hepatitis C	Hepatitis A vaccine: 2 doses	None

Prophylaxis to Prevent First Episode of Opportunistic Disease in HIV-Infected Adults and Adolescents *(continued)*

Pathogen	Indication	Preventive Regimens	
		First Choice	Alternatives
III. Evidence for Efficacy but Not Routinely Indicated			
Bacteria	Neutropenia	Granulocyte-colony-stimulating factor (G-CSF), 5-10 mcg/kg SubQ every day x 2-4 weeks or granulocyte-macrophage colony-stimulating factor (GM-CSF), 250 mcg/m² SubQ, I.V. x 2-4 weeks	None
Cryptococcus neoformans	CD4⁺ count <50/µL	Fluconazole, 100-200 mg P.O. every day	Itraconazole capsule, 200 mg P.O. every day
Histoplasma capsulatum[9]	CD4⁺ count <100/µL, endemic geographic area	Itraconazole capsule, 200 mg P.O. every day	None
Cytomegalovirus (CMV)[10]	CD4⁺ count <50/µL and CMV antibody positivity	Oral ganciclovir, 1 g P.O. 3 times/day	None

Note: Information included in these guidelines may not represent Food and Drug Administration (FDA) approval or approved labeling for the particular products or indications in question. Specifically, the terms "safe" and "effective" may not be synonymous with the FDA-defined legal standards for product approval.

Abbreviations: Anti-HB_c = antibody to hepatitis B core antigen; CMV = cytomegalovirus; DS = double-strength tablet; HAART = highly active antiretroviral therapy; HAV = hepatitis A virus; SS = single-strength tablet; TMP-SMZ = trimethoprim-sulfamethoxazole; and TST = tuberculin skin test. The Respirgard II™ nebulizer is manufactured by Marquest, Englewood, CO.

[1]Prophylaxis should also be considered for persons with a CD4⁺ percentage <14%, for persons with a history of an AIDS-defining illness, and possibly for those with CD4⁺ count >200 but <250 cells/µL. TMP-SMZ also reduces the frequency of toxoplasmosis and some bacterial infections. Patients receiving dapsone should be tested for glucose-6-phosphate dehydrogenase deficiency. A dosage of 50 mg every day is probably less effective than 100 mg every day. The efficacy of parenteral pentamidine (eg, 4 mg/kg/month) is uncertain. Fansidar® (sulfadoxine-pyrimethamine) is rarely used because of severe hypersensitivity reactions. Patients who are being administered therapy for toxoplasmosis with sulfadiazine-pyrimethamine are protected against *Pneumocystis carinii* pneumonia and do not need additional prophylaxis against PCP.

[2]Directly observed therapy is recommended for isoniazid (eg, 900 mg twice weekly); INH regimens should include pyridoxine to prevent peripheral neuropathy. If rifampin or rifabutin are administered concurrently with protease inhibitors or non-nucleoside reverse transcriptase inhibitors, careful consideration should be given to potential pharmacokinetic interactions. There have been reports of fatal and severe liver injury associated with the treatment of latent TB infection in HIV-uninfected persons treated with the 2 month regimen of daily rifampin and pyrazinamide; therefore it may be prudent to use regimens that do not contain pyrazinamide in HIV-infected persons whose completion of treatment can be assured (CDC. "Update: Fatal and Severe Liver Injuries Associated with Rifampin and Pyrazinamide for Latent Tuberculosis Infection and Revisions in American Thoracic Society/CDC Recommendations, United States 2001," *MMWR*, 2001, 50(34). Exposure to multidrug-resistant tuberculosis might require prophylaxis with two drugs; consult public health authorities. Possible regimens include pyrazinamide plus either ethambutol or a fluoroquinolone.

[3]Protection against toxoplasmosis is provided by TMP-SMZ, dapsone plus pyrimethamine, and possibly by atovaquone. Atovaquone may be used with or without pyrimethamine. Pyrimethamine alone probably provides little, if any, protection.

[4]**During pregnancy, azithromycin is preferred over clarithromycin because of the teratogenicity in animals of clarithromycin.**

[5]Vaccination **may** be offered to persons who have a CD4⁺ T-lymphocyte count <200 cells/µL, although the efficacy **is likely to** be diminished. Revaccination 5 years after the first dose or sooner if the initial immunization was given when the CD4⁺ count was <200 cells/µL and if the CD4⁺ count has increased to >200 cells/µL on HAART is considered optional. Some authorities are concerned that immunizations may stimulate the replication of HIV.

[6]Although data demonstrating clinical benefit of these vaccines in HIV-infected persons are not available, it is logical to assume that those patients who develop antibody responses will derive some protection. Some authorities are concerned that immunizations may stimulate HIV replication, although for influenza vaccination, a large observational study of HIV-infected persons in clinical care showed no adverse effect of this vaccine, including multiple doses, on patient survival (J. Ward, CDC, personal communication). Also, this concern may be less relevant in the setting of HAART. However, because of the theoretical concern that increases in HIV plasma RNA following vaccination during pregnancy might increase the risk of perinatal transmission of HIV, providers may wish to defer vaccination for such patients until after HAART is initiated.

[7]Hepatitis B vaccine has been recommended for all children and adolescents and for all adults with risk factors for hepatitis B virus (HBV). For persons requiring vaccination against both hepatitis A and hepatitis B, a combination vaccine is now available. For additional information regarding vaccination against hepatitis A and B, see CDC, "Hepatitis B Virus: A Comprehensive Strategy for Eliminating

USPHS / IDSA GUIDELINES FOR THE PREVENTION OF OPPORTUNISTIC INFECTIONS IN PERSONS INFECTED WITH HIV *(Continued)*

Transmission in the United States Through Universal Childhood Vaccination. Recommendations of the Advisory Committee on Immunization Practices (ACIP)," *MMWR Morb Mortal Wkly Rep*, 1991, 40(RR13).

[8]Oseltamivir is appropriate during outbreaks of either influenza A or influenza B. Rimantadine or amantadine are appropriate during outbreaks of influenza A (although neither rimantadine nor amantadine is recommended during pregnancy). Dosage reduction for antiviral chemoprophylaxis against influenza might be indicated for decreased renal or hepatic function, and for persons with seizure disorders. Physicians should consult the drug package inserts and the annual CDC influenza guidelines for more specific information about adverse effects and dosage adjustments. For additional information about vaccinations, antiviral chemoprophylaxis, and therapy against influenza, see CDC, "Prevention and Control of Influenza: Recommendations of the Advisory Committee on Immunization Practices (ACIP)," *MMWR Morb Mortal Wkly Rep*, 2001, 50(RR-4).

[9]In a few unusual occupational or other circumstances, prophylaxis should be considered; consult a specialist.

[10]Acyclovir is not protective against CMV. Valacyclovir is not recommended because of an unexplained trend toward increased mortality observed in persons with AIDS who were being administered this drug for prevention of CMV disease.

Prophylaxis to Prevent Recurrence of Opportunistic Disease (After Chemotherapy for Acute Disease) in HIV-Infected Adults and Adolescents

Pathogen	Indication	Preventive Regimens	
		First Choice	Alternatives
I. Recommended as Standard of Care			
Pneumocystis carinii	Prior *P. carinii* pneumonia	TMP-SMZ, 1 DS P.O. every day; TMP-SMZ, 1 SS P.O. every day	Dapsone, 50 mg P.O. twice daily or 100 mg P.O. every day; dapsone, 50 mg P.O. every day *plus* pyrimethamine, 50 mg P.O. weekly *plus* leucovorin, 25 mg P.O. weekly; dapsone, 200 mg P.O. *plus* pyrimethamine, 75 mg P.O. *plus* leucovorin, 25 mg P.O. weekly; aerosolized pentamidine, 300 mg monthly via Respirgard II™ nebulizer; atovaquone, 1500 mg P.O. every day; TMP-SMZ, 1 DS P.O. 3 times/week
Toxoplasma gondii[1]	Prior toxoplasmic encephalitis	Sulfadiazine, 500-1000 mg P.O. 4 times/day *plus* pyrimethamine 25-50 mg P.O. every day *plus* leucovorin, 10-25 mg P.O. every day	Clindamycin, 300-450 mg P.O. every 6-8 hours *plus* pyrimethamine, 25-50 mg P.O. every day *plus* leucovorin, 10-25 mg P.O. every day; atovaquone, 750 mg P.O. every 6-12 hours with or without pyrimethamine, 25 mg P.O. every day *plus* leucovorin 10 mg P.O. every day
Mycobacterium avium complex[2]	Documented disseminated disease	Clarithromycin,[2] 500 mg P.O. twice daily *plus* ethambutol, 15 mg/kg P.O. every day; with or without rifabutin, 300 mg P.O. every day	Azithromycin, 500 mg P.O. every day *plus* ethambutol, 15 mg/kg P.O. every day; with or without rifabutin, 300 mg P.O. every day
Cytomegalovirus	Prior end-organ disease	Ganciclovir, 5-6 mg/kg I.V. 5-7 days/week or 1000 mg P.O. 3 times/day; or foscarnet, 90-120 mg/kg I.V. every day; or (for retinitis) ganciclovir sustained-release implant, every 6-9 months *plus* ganciclovir, 1-1.5 g P.O. 3 times/day	Cidofovir, 5 mg/kg I.V. every other week with probenecid 2 g P.O. 3 hours before the dose followed by 1 g P.O. given 2 hours after the dose, and 1 g P.O. 8 hours after the dose (total of 4 g); fomivirsen, 1 vial (330 mcg) injected into the vitreous, then repeated every 2-4 weeks; valganciclovir 900 mg P.O. every day
Cryptococcus neoformans	Documented disease	Fluconazole, 200 mg P.O. every day	Amphotericin B, 0.6-1 mg/kg I.V. weekly to 3 times/week; itraconazole capsule, 200 mg P.O. every day
Histoplasma capsulatum	Documented disease	Itraconazole capsule, 200 mg P.O. twice daily	Amphotericin B, 1 mg/kg I.V. weekly
Coccidioides immitis	Documented disease	Fluconazole, 400 mg P.O. every day	Amphotericin B, 1 mg/kg I.V. weekly; itraconazole capsule, 200 mg P.O. twice daily
Salmonella species (non-*typhi*)[3]	Bacteremia	Ciprofloxacin, 500 mg P.O. twice daily for several months	Antibiotic chemoprophylaxis with another active agent
II. Recommended Only if Subsequent Episodes Are Frequent or Severe			
Herpes simplex virus	Frequent/severe recurrences	Acyclovir, 200 mg P.O. 3 times/day or 400 mg P.O. twice daily; famciclovir, 250 mg P.O. twice daily	Valacyclovir, 500 mg P.O. twice daily
Candida (oropharyngeal or vaginal)	Frequent/severe recurrences	Fluconazole, 100-200 mg P.O. every day	Itraconazole solution, 200 mg P.O. every day

USPHS / IDSA GUIDELINES FOR THE PREVENTION OF OPPORTUNISTIC INFECTIONS IN PERSONS INFECTED WITH HIV *(Continued)*

Prophylaxis to Prevent Recurrence of Opportunistic Disease (After Chemotherapy for Acute Disease) in HIV-Infected Adults and Adolescents *(continued)*

Pathogen	Indication	Preventive Regimens	
		First Choice	Alternatives
Candida (esophageal)	Frequent/ severe recurrences	Fluconazole, 100-200 mg P.O. every day	Itraconazole solution, 200 mg P.O. every day

Note: Information included in these guidelines may not represent Food and Drug Administration (FDA) approval or approved labeling for the particular products or indications in question. Specifically, the terms "safe" and "effective" may not be synonymous with the FDA-defined legal standards for product approval.

DS = double-strength tablet; SS = single-strength tablet; and TMP-SMZ = trimethoprim-sulfamethoxazole. The Respirgard II™ nebulizer is manufactured by Marquest, Englewood, CO.

[1]Pyrimethamine/sulfadiazine confers protection against PCP as well as toxoplasmosis; clindamycin-pyrimethamine does **not offer protection against PCP**.

[2]Many multiple-drug regimens are poorly tolerated. Drug interactions (eg, those seen with clarithromycin/rifabutin) can be problematic; rifabutin has been associated with uveitis, especially when administered at daily doses of >300 mg or concurrently with fluconazole or clarithromycin. **During pregnancy, azithromycin is recommended instead of clarithromycin because clarithromycin is teratogenic in animals.**

[3]Efficacy of eradication of *Salmonella* has been demonstrated only for ciprofloxacin.

Effects of Food on Drugs Used to Prevent Opportunistic Infections

Drug	Food Effect	Recommendation
Atovaquone	Bioavailability increased up to threefold with high-fat meal	Administer with food
Ganciclovir (capsules)	High-fat meal results in 22% (GCV) or 30% (VGCV) increase in AUC	High fat meal may increase toxicity of valganciclovir
Itraconazole	Grapefruit juice results in 30% decrease in AUC	Avoid concurrent grapefruit juice
Itraconazole (capsules)	Significant increase in bioavailability when taken with a full meal	Administer with food
Itraconazole (solution)	31% increase in AUC when taken under fasting conditions	Take without food if possible

Criteria for Starting, Discontinuing, and Restarting Opportunistic Infection Prophylaxis for Adult Patients With HIV Infection[1]

Opportunistic Illness	Criteria for Initiating Primary Prophylaxis	Criteria for Discontinuing Primary Prophylaxis	Criteria for Restarting Primary Prophylaxis	Criteria for Initiating Secondary Prophylaxis	Criteria for Discontinuing Secondary Prophylaxis	Criteria for Restarting Secondary Prophylaxis
Pneumocystis carinii pneumonia	$CD4^+$ >200 cells/µL or oropharyngeal candidiasis	$CD4^+$ >200 cells/µL for ≥3 months	$CD4^+$ <200 cells/µL	Prior *Pneumocystis carinii* pneumonia	$CD4^+$ >200 cells/µL for ≥3 months	$CD4^+$ <200 cells/µL
Toxoplasmosis	IgG antibody to *Toxoplasma* and $CD4^+$ <100 cells/µL	$CD4^+$ >200 cells/µL for ≥3 months	$CD4^+$ <100-200 cells/µL	Prior toxoplasmic encephalitis	$CD4^+$ >200 cells/µL sustained (eg, ≥6 months) and completed initial therapy, and asymptomatic for toxoplasmosis	$CD4^+$ <200 cells/µL
Disseminated *Mycobacterium avium* complex	$CD4^+$ <50 cells/µL	$CD4^+$ >100 cells/µL for ≥3 months	$CD4^+$ <50-100 cells/µL	Documented disseminated disease	$CD4^+$ >100 cells/µL sustained (eg, ≥6 months) and completed 12 months of MAC therapy, and asymptomatic for MAC	$CD4^+$ <100 cells/µL
Cryptococcosis	None	Not applicable	Not applicable	Documented disease	$CD4^+$ >100-200 cells/µL sustained (eg, ≥6 months) and completed initial therapy, and asymptomatic for cryptococcosis	$CD4^+$ <100-200 cells/µL
Histoplasmosis	None	Not applicable	Not applicable	Documented disease	No criteria recommended for stopping	Not applicable
Coccidioidomycosis	None	Not applicable	Not applicable	Documented disease	No criteria recommended for stopping	Not applicable

USPHS / IDSA GUIDELINES FOR THE PREVENTION OF OPPORTUNISTIC INFECTIONS IN PERSONS INFECTED WITH HIV *(Continued)*

Criteria for Starting, Discontinuing, and Restarting Opportunistic Infection Prophylaxis for Adult Patients With HIV Infection[1] *(continued)*

Opportunistic Illness	Criteria for Initiating Primary Prophylaxis	Criteria for Discontinuing Primary Prophylaxis	Criteria for Restarting Primary Prophylaxis	Criteria for Initiating Secondary Prophylaxis	Criteria for Discontinuing Secondary Prophylaxis	Criteria for Restarting Secondary Prophylaxis
Cytomegalovirus retinitis	None	Not applicable	Not applicable	Documented end-organ disease	$CD4^+$ >100-150 cells/µL sustained (eg, ≥6 months) and no evidence of active disease, and regular ophthalmic examination	$CD4^+$ <100-150 cells/µL

[1]The safety of discontinuing prophylaxis in children whose $CD4^+$ counts have increased in response to HAART has not been studied.

DRUG REGIMENS FOR INFANTS AND CHILDREN

Prophylaxis to Prevent First Episode of Opportunistic Disease in HIV-Infected Infants and Children

Pathogen	Indication	Preventive Regimens: First Choice	Preventive Regimens: Alternatives
I. Strongly Recommended as Standard of Care			
Pneumocystis carinii[1]	HIV-infected or HIV-indeterminate infants 1-12 mo of age HIV-infected children 1-5 y of age with CD4+ count <500/µL or CD4+ percentage <15% HIV-infected children 6-12 y of age with CD4+ count <200/µL or CD4+ percentage <15%	TMP-SMZ, 150/750 mg/m²/day in 2 divided doses P.O. 3 times/week on consecutive days Acceptable alternative dosage schedules: • Single dose P.O. 3 times/week on consecutive days • 2 divided doses P.O. every day; 2 divided doses P.O. 3 times/week on alternate days	Dapsone (children ≥1 mo), 2 mg/kg (max: 100 mg) P.O. every day or 4 mg/kg (max: 200 mg) P.O. once weekly) Aerosolized pentamidine (children ≥5 y), 300 mg/mo via Respirgard II™ nebulizer Atovaquone (1-3 mo and >24 mo, 30 mg/kg P.O. every day; 4-24 mo, 45 mg/kg P.O. every day)
Mycobacterium tuberculosis[2]			
Isoniazid-sensitive	TST reaction, ≥5 mm *or* prior positive TST result without treatment **or contact** with any case of active tuberculosis **regardless of TST result**	Isoniazid, 10-15 mg/kg (max: 300 mg) P.O. every day x 9 mo or 20-30 mg/kg (max: 900 mg) P.O. twice weekly x 9 mo	Rifampin, 10-20 mg/kg (max: 600 mg) P.O. every day x 4-6 mo
Isoniazid-resistant	Same as above; high probability of exposure to isoniazid-resistant tuberculosis	Rifampin, 10-20 mg/kg (max: 600 mg) P.O. every day x 4-6 mo	Uncertain
Multidrug (isoniazid and rifampin)-resistant	Same as above; high probability of exposure to multidrug-resistant tuberculosis	Choice of drug requires consultation with public health authorities and depends on susceptibility of isolate from source patient	
Mycobacterium avium complex[2]	For children ≥6 y, CD4+ count <50/µL; 2-6 y, CD4+ count <75/µL; 1-2 y, CD4+ count <500/µL; <1 y, CD4+ count <750/µL	Clarithromycin, 7.5 mg/kg (max: 500 mg) P.O. twice daily, or azithromycin, 20 mg/kg (max: 1200 mg) P.O. weekly	Azithromycin, 5 mg/kg (max: 250 mg) P.O. every day; children ≥6 y, rifabutin, 300 mg P.O. every day
Varicella zoster virus[3]	Significant exposure to varicella or shingles with no history of chickenpox or shingles	Varicella zoster immune globulin (VZIG), 1 vial (1.25 mL)/10 kg (max: 5 vials) I.M., administered ≤96 hours after exposure, ideally within 48 hours	None
Vaccine-preventable pathogens[4]	HIV exposure/infection	Routine immunizations	None
II. Generally Recommended			
Influenza virus	All patients (annually, before influenza season)	Inactivated split trivalent influenza vaccine	Oseltamivir (during outbreaks of influenza A or B) for children ≥13 y, 75 mg P.O. every day; rimantadine or amantadine (during outbreaks of influenza A); 1-9 y, 5 mg/kg/day P.O. in 2 divided doses (max: 150 mg/day); ≥10 y, use adult doses
Varicella zoster virus	HIV-infected children who are asymptomatic and not immunosuppressed	Varicella zoster vaccine	None

USPHS / IDSA GUIDELINES FOR THE PREVENTION OF OPPORTUNISTIC INFECTIONS IN PERSONS INFECTED WITH HIV *(Continued)*

Prophylaxis to Prevent First Episode of Opportunistic Disease in HIV-Infected Infants and Children *(continued)*

Pathogen	Indication	Preventive Regimens	
		First Choice	Alternatives
Toxoplasma gondii[5]	IgG antibody to *Toxoplasma* and severe immunosuppression	TMP-SMZ, 150/750 mg/m^2/d in 2 divided doses P.O. every day	Dapsone (≥1 mo of age), 2 mg/kg or 15 mg/m^2 (max: 25 mg) P.O. every day *plus* pyrimethamine, 1 mg/kg P.O. every day *plus* leucovorin, 5 mg P.O. every 3 days Atovaquone (aged 1-3 mo and >24 mo, 30 mg/kg P.O. every day; aged 14-24 mo, 45 mg/kg P.O. every day)
III. Not Recommended for Most Children; Indicated for Use Only in Unusual Circumstances			
Invasive bacterial infections[6]	Hypogammaglobulinemia (ie, IgG <400 mg/dL)	IVIG (400 mg/kg every 2-4 weeks)	None
Cryptococcus neoformans	Severe immunosuppression	Fluconazole, 3-6 mg/kg P.O. every day	Itraconazole, 2-5 mg/kg P.O. every 12-24 hours
Histoplasma capsulatum	Severe immunosuppression, endemic geographic area	Itraconazole, 2-5 mg/kg P.O. every 12-24 hours	None
Cytomegalovirus (CMV)[7]	CMV antibody positivity and severe immunosuppression	Oral ganciclovir 30 mg/kg P.O. 3 times/day	None

Note: Information included in these guidelines may not represent FDA approval or approved labeling for the particular products or indications in question. Specifically, the terms "safe" and "effective" may not be synonymous with the FDA-defined legal standards for product approval. CMV = cytomegalovirus; IVIG = intravenous immune globulin; TMP-SMZ = trimethoprim-sulfamethoxazole; and VZIG = varicella zoster immune globulin. The Respirgard II™ nebulizer is manufactured by Marquest, Englewood, CO.

[1]Daily TMP-SMZ reduces frequency of some bacterial infections. TMP-SMZ, dapsone-pyrimethamine, and possibly atovaquone (with or without pyrimethamine) appear to protect against toxoplasmosis, although data have not been prospectively collected. When compared with weekly dapsone, daily dapsone is associated with lower incidence of *Pneumocystis carinii* pneumonia (PCP) but higher hematologic toxicity and mortality (McIntosh K, Cooper E, Xu J, et al, "Toxicity and Efficacy of Daily vs Weekly Dapsone for Prevention of *Pneumocystis carinii* Pneumonia in Children Infected With HIV," *Ped Infect Dis J* 1999, 18:432-9.). Efficacy of parenteral pentamidine (eg, 4 mg/kg/every 2-4 weeks) is controversial. Patients receiving therapy for toxoplasmosis with sulfadiazine-pyrimethamine are protected against PCP and do not need TMP-SMZ.

[2]Significant drug interactions may occur between rifamycins (rifampin and rifabutin) and protease inhibitors, and non-nucleoside reverse transcriptase inhibitors. Consult a specialist.

[3]Children routinely being administered intravenous immune globulin (IVIG) should receive VZIG if the last dose of IVIG was administered >21 days before exposure.

[4]HIV-infected and HIV-exposed children should be immunized according to the childhood immunization schedule, which has been adapted from the January-December 2001 schedule recommended for immunocompetent children by the Advisory Committee on Immunization Practices, the American Academy of Pediatrics, and the American Academy of Family Physicians. This schedule differs from that for immunocompetent children in that both the conjugate pneumococcal vaccine (PCV-7) and the pneumococcal polysaccharide vaccine (PPV-23) are recommended and vaccination against influenza should be offered. MMR should not be administered to severely immunocompromised children. Vaccination against varicella is indicated only for asymptomatic nonimmunosuppressed children. Once an HIV-exposed child is determined not to be HIV infected, the schedule for immunocompetent children applies.

[5]Protection against toxoplasmosis is provided by the preferred antipneumocystis regimens and possibly by atovaquone. Atovaquone may be used with or without pyrimethamine. Pyrimethamine alone probably provides little, if any, protection.

[6]If available, respiratory syncytial virus (RSV) IVIG (750 mg/kg), not monoclonal RSV antibody, may be substituted for IVIG during RSV season to provide broad anti-infective protection.

[7]Oral ganciclovir and perhaps valganciclovir results in reduced CMV shedding in CMV-infected children. Acyclovir is not protective against CMV.

Prophylaxis to Prevent Recurrence of Opportunistic Disease (After Chemotherapy for Acute Disease) in HIV-Infected Infants and Children

Pathogen	Indication	Preventive Regimens: First Choice	Preventive Regimens: Alternatives
I. Recommended for Life as Standard of Care			
Pneumocystis carinii	Prior *P. carinii* pneumonia	TMP-SMZ, 150/750 mg/m²/d in 2 divided doses P.O. 3 times/week on consecutive days Acceptable alternative schedules for same dosage Single dose P.O. 3 times/week on consecutive days; 2 divided doses P.O. daily; 2 divided doses P.O. 3 times/week on alternate days	Dapsone (children ≥1 mo of age), 2 mg/kg (max: 100 mg) P.O. once daily *or* 4 mg/kg (max: 200 mg) P.O. weekly; aerosolized pentamidine (children ≥5 y of age), 300 mg monthly via Respirgard II™ nebulizer; atovaquone (children 1-3 mo and >24 mo of age, 30 mg/kg P.O. every day; children 4-24 mo, 45 mg/kg P.O. every day)
Toxoplasma gondii[1]	Prior toxoplasmic encephalitis	Sulfadiazine, 85-120 mg/kg/d in 2-4 divided doses P.O. daily *plus* pyrimethamine, 1 mg/kg *or* 15 mg/m² (max: 25 mg) P.O. every day *plus* leucovorin, 5 mg P.O. every 3 days	Clindamycin, 20-30 mg/kg/d in 4 divided doses P.O. every day *plus* pyrimethamine, 1 mg/kg P.O. every day *plus* leucovorin, 5 mg P.O. every 3 days
Mycobacterium avium complex[2]	Prior disease	Clarithromycin, 7.5 mg/kg (max: 500 mg) P.O. twice daily *plus* ethambutol, 15 mg/kg (max: 900 mg) P.O. every day; with or without rifabutin, 5 mg/kg (max: 300 mg) P.O. once daily	Azithromycin, 5 mg/kg (max: 250 mg) P.O. every day *plus* ethambutol, 15 mg/kg (max: 900 mg) P.O. every day; with or without rifabutin, 5 mg/kg (max: 300 mg) P.O. once daily
Cryptococcus neoformans	Documented disease	Fluconazole, 3-6 mg/kg P.O. every day	Amphotericin B, 0.5-1 mg/kg I.V. 1-3 times/week; itraconazole, 2-5 mg/kg P.O. every 12-24 hours
Histoplasma capsulatum	Documented disease	Itraconazole, 2-5 mg/kg P.O. every 12-48 hours	Amphotericin B, 1 mg/kg I.V. weekly
Coccidioides immitis	Documented disease	Fluconazole, 6 mg/kg P.O. every day	Amphotericin B, 1 mg/kg I.V. weekly; itraconazole, 2-5 mg/kg P.O. every 12-48 hours
Cytomegalovirus	Prior end-organ disease	Ganciclovir, 5 mg/kg I.V. every day, *or* foscarnet, 90-120 mg/kg I.V. every day	(For retinitis) — ganciclovir sustained-release implant, every 6-9 mo *plus* ganciclovir, 30 mg/kg P.O. 3 times/d
Salmonella species (non-*typhi*)[3]	Bacteremia	TMP-SMZ, 150/750 mg/m² in 2 divided doses P.O. every day for several months	Antibiotic chemoprophylaxis with another active agent
II. Recommended Only if Subsequent Episodes Are Frequent or Severe			
Invasive bacterial infections[4]	>2 infections in 1-year period	TMP-SMZ, 150/750 mg/m² in 2 divided doses P.O. every day; *or* IVIG, 400 mg/kg every 2-4 weeks	Antibiotic chemoprophylaxis with another active agent
Herpes simplex virus	Frequent/severe recurrences	Acyclovir, 80 mg/kg/d in 3-4 divided doses P.O. daily	

USPHS / IDSA GUIDELINES FOR THE PREVENTION OF OPPORTUNISTIC INFECTIONS IN PERSONS INFECTED WITH HIV *(Continued)*

Prophylaxis to Prevent Recurrence of Opportunistic Disease (After Chemotherapy for Acute Disease) in HIV-Infected Infants and Children *(continued)*

Pathogen	Indication	Preventive Regimens: First Choice	Preventive Regimens: Alternatives
Candida (oropharyngeal)	Frequent/ severe recurrences	Fluconazole, 3-6 mg/kg P.O. every day	
Candida (esophageal)	Frequent/ severe recurrences	Fluconazole, 3-6 mg/kg P.O. every day	Itraconazole solution, 5 mg/kg P.O. every day; ketoconazole, 5-10 mg/kg P.O. every 12-24 hours

Note: Information included in these guidelines may not represent Food and Drug Administration (FDA) approval or approved labeling for the particular products or indications in question. Specifically, the terms "safe" and "effective" may not be synonymous with the FDA-defined legal standards for product approval. IVIG = intravenous immune globulin and TMP-SMZ = trimethoprim-sulfamethoxazole. The Respirgard II™ nebulizer is manufactured by Marquest, Englewood, CO.

[1]Only pyrimethamine plus sulfadiazine confers protection against PCP as well as toxoplasmosis. Although the clindamycin plus pyrimethamine regimen is the preferred alternative in adults, it has not been tested in children. However, these drugs are safe and are used for other infections.

[2]Significant drug interactions may occur between rifabutin and protease inhibitors and non-nucleoside reverse transcriptase inhibitors. Consult an expert.

[3]Drug should be determined by susceptibilities of the organism isolated. Alternatives to TMP-SMZ include ampicillin, chloramphenicol, or ciprofloxacin. However, ciprofloxacin is not approved for use in persons aged <18 years; therefore, it should be used in children with caution and only if no alternatives exist.

[4]Antimicrobial prophylaxis should be chosen based on the microorganism and antibiotic sensitivities. TMP-SMZ, if used, should be administered daily. Providers should be cautious about using antibiotics solely for this purpose because of the potential for development of drug-resistant microorganisms. IVIG may not provide additional benefit to children receiving daily TMP-SMZ, but may be considered for children who have recurrent bacterial infections despite TMP-SMZ prophylaxis. Choice of antibiotic prophylaxis vs IVIG should also involve consideration of adherence, ease of intravenous access, and cost. If IVIG is used, RSV-IVIG (750 mg/kg), not monoclonal RSV antibody, may be substituted for IVIG during the RSV season to provide broad anti-infective protection, if this product is available.

IMMUNIZATION RECOMMENDATIONS

Standards for Pediatric Immunization Practices

Standard 1.	Immunization services are readily available.
Standard 2.	There are no barriers or unnecessary prerequisites to the receipt of vaccines.
Standard 3.	Immunization services are available free or for a minimal fee.
Standard 4.	Providers utilize all clinical encounters to screen and, when indicated, immunize children.
Standard 5.	Providers educate parents and guardians about immunizations in general terms.
Standard 6.	Providers question parents or guardians about contraindications and, before immunizing a child, inform them in specific terms about the risks and benefits of the immunizations their child is to receive.
Standard 7.	Providers follow only true contraindications.
Standard 8.	Providers administer simultaneously all vaccine doses for which a child is eligible at the time of each visit.
Standard 9.	Providers use accurate and complete recording procedures.
Standard 10.	Providers co-schedule immunization appointments in conjunction with appointments for other child health services.
Standard 11.	Providers report adverse events following immunization promptly, accurately, and completely.
Standard 12.	Providers operate a tracking system.
Standard 13.	Providers adhere to appropriate procedures for vaccine management.
Standard 14.	Providers conduct semiannual audits to assess immunization coverage levels and to review immunization records in the patient populations they serve.
Standard 15.	Providers maintain up-to-date, easily retrievable medical protocols at all locations where vaccines are administered.
Standard 16.	Providers operate with patient-oriented and community-based approaches.
Standard 17.	Vaccines are administered by properly trained individuals.
Standard 18.	Providers receive ongoing education and training on current immunization recommendations.

Recommended by the National Vaccine Advisory Committee, April 1992.

Approved by the United States Public Health Service, May 1992.

Endorsed by the American Academy of Pediatrics, May 1992.

The Standards represent the consensus of the National Vaccine Advisory Committee (NVAC) and of a broad group of medical and public health experts about what constitutes the most desirable immunization practices. It is recognized by the NVAC that not all of the current immunization practices of public and private providers are in compliance with the Standards. Nevertheless, the Standards are expected to be useful as a means of helping providers to identify needed changes, to obtain resources if necessary, and to actually implement the desirable immunization practices in the future.

IMMUNIZATION RECOMMENDATIONS *(Continued)*

Recommended Childhood and Adolescent Immunization Schedule United States, 2005

Vaccine ▼ / Age ▶	Birth	1 mo	2 mo	4 mo	6 mo	12 mo	15 mo	18 mo	24 mo	4-6 y	11-12 y	13-18 y
Hepatitis B[1]	HepB #1	only if mother $HB_sAg(-)$ HepB #2			HepB #3				HepB series			
Diphtheria, tetanus, pertussis[2]			DTaP	DTaP	DTaP		DTaP			DTaP	Td	Td
Haemophilus influenzae type b[3]			Hib	Hib	Hib	Hib						
Inactivated poliovirus			IPV	IPV	IPV					IPV		
Measles, mumps, rubella[4]						MMR #1				MMR #2	MMR #2	
Varicella[5]						Varicella			Varicella			
Pneumococcal[6]			PCV	PCV	PCV	PCV			PCV	PPV		
Influenza[7]					Influenza (yearly)				Influenza (yearly)			
Vaccines below this line are for selected populations												
Hepatitis A[8]									Hepatitis A series			

Range of recommended ages   Preadolescent assessment   Catch-up immunization

This schedule indicates the recommended ages for routine administration of currently licensed childhood vaccines, as of December 1, 2004, for children through age 18 years. Any dose not given at the recommended age should be given at any subsequent visit when indicated and feasible. Indicates age groups that warrant special effort to administer those vaccines not given previously. Additional vaccines may be licensed and recommended during the year. Licensed combination vaccines may be used whenever any components of the combination are indicated and the vaccine's other components are not contraindicated. Providers should consult the manufacturers' package inserts for detailed recommendations. Clinically significant adverse events that follow immunization should be reported to the Vaccine Adverse Event Reporting System (VAERS). Guidance about how to obtain and complete a VAERS form can be found on the Internet: http://**www.vaers.org** or by calling **800-822-7967**.

1 **Hepatitis B (HepB) vaccine**. All infants should receive the first dose of hepatitis B vaccine soon after birth and before hospital discharge; the first dose may also be given by age 2 months if the infant's mother is HB_sAg-negative. Only monovalent HepB can be used for the birth dose. Monovalent or combination vaccine containing HepB may be used to complete the series. Four doses of vaccine may be administered when a birth dose is given. The second dose should be given at least 4 weeks after the first dose, except for combination vaccines, which cannot be administered before age 6 weeks. The third dose should be given at least 16 weeks after the first dose and at least 8 weeks after the second dose. The last dose in the vaccination series (third or fourth dose) should not be administered before age 24 weeks.

Infants born to HB_sAg-positive mothers should receive HepB vaccine and 0.5 mL hepatitis B immune globulin (HBIG) within 12 hours of birth at separate sites. The second dose is recommended at age 1-2 months. The last dose in the vaccination series should not be administered before age 24 weeks. These infants should be tested for HB_sAg and anti-HB_s at 9-15 months of age.

Infants born to mothers whose HB_sAg status is unknown should receive the first dose of the HepB vaccine series within 12 hours of birth. Maternal blood should be drawn as soon as possible to determine the mother's HB_sAg status; if the HB_sAg test is positive, the infant should receive HBIG as soon as possible (no later than age 1 week). The second dose is recommended at age 1-2 months. The last dose in the vaccination series should not be administered before age 24 weeks.

2 **Diphtheria, tetanus toxoids, and acellular pertussis (DTaP) vaccine**. The fourth dose of DTaP may be administered as early as age 12 months, provided that 6 months have elapsed since the third dose and the child is unlikely to return at age 15-18 months. The final dose in the series should be given at age ≥4 years. **Tetanus and diphtheria toxoids (Td)** is recommended at age 11-12 years if at least 5 years have elapsed since the last dose of tetanus and diphtheria toxoid-containing vaccine. Subsequent routine Td boosters are recommended every 10 years.

3 ***Haemophilus influenzae* type b (Hib) conjugate vaccine**. Three Hib conjugate vaccines are licensed for infant use. If PRP-OMP (PedvaxHIB® or ComVax® [Merck]) is administered at ages 2 and 4 months, a dose at age 6 months is not required. DTaP/Hib combination products should not be used for primary immunization in infants at ages 2, 4, or 6 months, but can be used as boosters following any Hib vaccine. The final dose in the series should be given at age ≥12 months.

4 **Measles, mumps, and rubella vaccine (MMR)**. The second dose of MMR is recommended routinely at age 4-6 years but may be administered during any visit, provided at least 4 weeks have elapsed since the first dose and both doses are administered beginning at or after age 12 months. Those who have not previously received the second dose should complete the schedule by the visit at age 11-12-years.

5 **Varicella vaccine** is recommended at any visit at or after age 12 months for susceptible children (ie, those who lack a reliable history of chickenpox). Susceptible persons age ≥13 years should receive 2 doses, given at least 4 weeks apart.

6 **Pneumococcal vaccine**. The heptavalent **pneumococcal conjugate vaccine (PCV)** is recommended for all children age 2-23 months. It is also recommended for certain children age 24-59 months. The final dose in the series should be given at age ≥12 months. **Pneumococcal polysaccharide vaccine (PPV)** is recommended in addition to PCV for certain high-risk groups. See *MMWR*, 2000, 49(RR-9):1-35.

7 **Influenza vaccine** is recommended annually for children age ≥6 months with certain risk factors (including but not limited to asthma, cardiac disease, sickle cell disease, HIV, and diabetes), healthcare workers, and other persons (including household members) in close contact with persons in groups at high risk (see *MMWR*, 2004, 53(RR-6):1-40), and can be administered to all others wishing to obtain immunity. In addition, healthy children age 6-23 months and close contacts of healthy children age 0-23 months are recommended to receive influenza vaccine, because children in this age group are at substantially increased risk for influenza-related hospitalizations. For healthy persons age 5-49 years, the intranasally administered live, attenuated influenza vaccine (LAIV) is an acceptable alternative to the intramuscular trivalent inactivated influenza vacine (TIV). See *MMWR*, 2004, 53(RR-6):1-40. Children receiving TIV should be administered a dosage appropriate for their age (0.25 mL if 6-35 months or 0.5 mL if ≥3 years). Children age ≤8 years who are receiving influenza vaccine for the first time should receive two doses (separated by at least 4 weeks for TIV and at least 6 weeks for LAIV).

8 **Hepatitis A vaccine** is recommended for children and adolescents in selected states and regions, and for certain high-risk groups; consult your local public health authority. Children and adolescents in these states, regions, and high-risk groups who have not been immunized against hepatitis A can begin the hepatitis A vaccination series during any visit. The two doses in the series should be administered at least 6 months apart. See *MMWR*, 1999, 48(RR-12):1-37

Additional information about vaccines, including precautions and contraindications for vaccination and vaccine shortages is available at http://www.cdc.gov.nip or from the National Immunization Information Hotline, 800-232-2522 (English) or 800-232-0233 (Spanish). Approved by the Advisory Committee on Immunization Practices (http://www.cdc.gov/nip/acip), the American Academy of Pediatrics (http://www.aap.org), and the American Academy of Family Physicians (http://www.aafp.org).

Reference:
"Recommended Childhood and Adolescent Immunization Schedule — United States, 2005," *MMWR* , 2005, 53(51 & 52):Q1-3.

CATCH-UP SCHEDULE FOR CHILDREN AND ADOLESCENTS WHO START LATE OR WHO ARE >1 MONTH BEHIND

Tables 1 and 2 give catch-up schedules and minimum intervals between doses for children who have delayed immunizations. There is no need to restart a vaccine series regardless of the time that has elapsed between doses. Use the chart appropriate for the child's age.

Table 1. Catch-up Schedule for Children Age 4 Months - 6 Years

Vaccine (Minimum Age for Dose 1)	Minimum Interval Between Doses			
	Dose 1 to Dose 2	Dose 2 to Dose 3	Dose 3 to Dose 4	Dose 4 to Dose 5
DTaP (6 wk)	4 weeks	4 weeks	6 months	6 months[1]
IPV (6 wk)	4 weeks	4 weeks	4 weeks[2]	
HepB[3] (birth)	4 weeks	8 weeks (and 16 weeks after 1st dose)		
MMR (12 mo)	4 weeks[4]			
VAR (12 mo)				
Hib[5] (6 wk)	**4 weeks:** If 1st dose given at age <12 months **8 weeks (as final dose):** If 1st dose given at age 12-14 months **No further doses needed:** If 1st dose given at age ≥15 months	**4 weeks**[6]: If current age <12 months **8 weeks (as final dose)**[6]: If current age ≥12 months and 2nd dose given at age <15 months **No further doses needed** if previous dose given at age ≥15 months	**8 weeks (as final dose):** This dose only necessary for children age 12 months - 5 years who received 3 doses before age 12 months	
PCV[7] (6 wk)	**4 weeks:** If 1st dose given at age <12 months and current age <24 months **8 weeks (as final dose):** If 1st dose given at age ≥12 months or current age 24-59 months **No further doses needed** for healthy children if 1st dose given at age ≥24 months	**4 weeks**: If current age <12 months **8 weeks (as final dose):** If current age ≥12 months **No further doses needed** for healthy children if previous dose given at age ≥24 months	**8 weeks (as final dose):** This dose only necessary for children age 12 months - 5 years who received 3 doses before age 12 months	

IMMUNIZATION RECOMMENDATIONS *(Continued)*

Table 2. Catch-up Schedule for Children Age 7-18 Years

Vaccine	Minimum Interval Between Doses		
	Dose 1 to Dose 2	Dose 2 to Dose 3	Dose 3 to Booster Dose
Td	4 weeks	6 months	**6 months[8]**: If first dose given at age <12 months and current age <11 years **5 years[8]**: If first dose given at age ≥12 months and third dose given at age <7 years and current age ≥11 years **10 years[8]**: If third dose given at age ≥7 years
IPV[9]	4 weeks	4 weeks	IPV[2,9]
HepB	4 weeks	8 weeks (and 16 weeks after first dose)	
MMR	4 weeks		
Varicella[10]	4 weeks		

Footnotes to Table 1 and Table 2

[1]**DTaP (diphtheria, tetanus toxoids, and acellular pertussis):** The fifth dose is not necessary if the fourth dose was given after the fourth birthday.

[2]**IPV (inactivated poliovirus):** For children who received an all-IPV or all-oral poliovirus (OPV) series, a fourth dose is not necessary if third dose was given at age ≥4 years. If both OPV and IPV were given as part of a series, a total of four doses should be given, regardless of the child's current age.

[3]**HepB (hepatitis B):** All children and adolescents who have not been immunized against hepatitis B should begin the HepB immunization series during any visit. Providers should make special efforts to immunize children who were born in, or whose parents were born in, areas of the world where hepatitis B virus infection is moderately or highly endemic.

[4]**MMR (measles, mumps, and rubella):** The second dose of MMR is recommended routinely at age 4-6 years, but may be given earlier if desired.

[5]**Hib *(Haemophilus influenzae* type b):** Vaccine is not generally recommended for children age ≥5 years.

[6]**Hib:** If current age <12 months and the first 2 doses were PRP-OMP (PedvaxHIB® or ComVax® [Merck]), the third (and final) dose should be given at age 12-15 months and at least 8 weeks after the second dose.

[7]**PCV (pneumococcal conjugate vaccine):** Vaccine is not generally recommended for children age ≥5 years.

[8]**Td (tetanus and diphtheria):** For children age 7-10 years, the interval between the third and booster dose is determined by the age when the first dose was given. For adolescents age 11-18 years, the interval is determined by the age when the third dose was given.

[9]**IPV (inactivated poliovirus):** Vaccine is not generally recommended for persons age ≥18 years.

[10]**Varicella:** Give 2-dose series to all susceptible adolescents age ≥13 years.

Reporting Adverse Reactions

Report adverse reactions to vaccines through the federal Vaccine Adverse Event Reporting System. For information on reporting reactions following immunization, please visit **www.vaers.org** or call the 24-hour national toll-free information line **800-822-7967**. Report suspected cases of vaccine-preventable diseases to your state or local health department.

For additional information about vaccines, including precautions and contraindications for immunization and vaccine shortages, please visit the National Immunization Program web site at **www.cdc.gov/nip** or call the National Immunization Information Hotline at **800-232-2522 (English)** or **800-232-0233 (Spanish)**.

Recommended Adult Immunization Schedule, by Vaccine and Age Group United States, October 2004 - September 2005

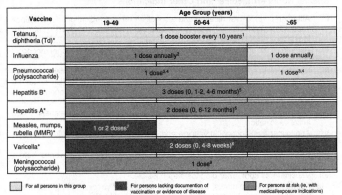

Vaccine	Age Group (years)		
	19-49	50-64	≥65
Tetanus, diphtheria (Td)*	1 dose booster every 10 years[1]		
Influenza	1 dose annually[2]		1 dose annually
Pneumococcal (polysaccharide)	1 dose[3,4]		1 dose[3,4]
Hepatitis B*	3 doses (0, 1-2, 4-6 months)[5]		
Hepatitis A*	2 doses (0, 6-12 months)[6]		
Measles, mumps, rubella (MMR)*	1 or 2 doses[7]		
Varicella*	2 doses (0, 4-8 weeks)[8]		
Meningococcal (polysaccharide)	1 dose[9]		

For all persons in this group — For persons lacking documention of vaccination or evidence of disease — For persons at risk (ie, with medical/exposure indications)

*Covered by the Vaccine Injury Compensation Program.

Recommended Adult Immunization Schedule, by Vaccine and Medical and Other Indications — United States, October 2004 - September 2005

Vaccine	Indication						
	Pregnancy	Diabetes, heart disease, chronic pulmonary disease, chronic liver disease (including chronic alcoholism)	Congenital immunodeficiency, cochlear implants, leukemia, lymphoma, generalized malignancy, therapy with alkylating agents, antimetabolites, CSF† leaks, radiation, or large amounts of corticosteroids	Renal failure/ end-stage renal disease, recipients of hemodialysis or clotting factor concentrates	Asplenia (including elective splenectomy and terminal complement component deficiencies)	HIV‡ infection	Healthcare workers
Tetanus, diphtheria (Td)*,1							
Influenza2		A, B			C		
Pneumococcal (polysaccharide)3,4		B	D	D	D, E, F	D, G	
Hepatitis B*,5				H			
Hepatitis A*,6		I					
Measles, mumps, rubella (MMR)*,7						J	
Varicella*,8			K				

For all persons in this group — For persons lacking documention of vaccination or evidence of disease — For persons at risk (ie, with medical/exposure indications) — Contraindicated

*Covered by the Vaccine Injury Compensation Program.
†Cerebrospinal fluid.
‡Human immunodeficiency virus.

IMMUNIZATION RECOMMENDATIONS *(Continued)*

Special Notes for Medical and Other Indications

I. Although chronic liver disease and alcoholism are not indications for influenza vaccination, administer 1 dose annually if the patient is ≤50 years, has other indications for influenza vaccine, or requests vaccination.

II. Asthma is an indication for influenza vaccination but not for pneumococcal vaccination.

III. No data exist specifically on the risk for severe or complicated influenza infections among persons with asplenia. However, influenza is a risk factor for secondary bacterial infections that can cause severe disease among persons with asplenia.

IV. For persons <65 years, revaccinate once after ≥5 years have elapsed since initial vaccination.

V. Administer meningococcal vaccine and consider *Haemophilus influenzae* type b vaccine.

VI. For persons undergoing elective splenectomy, vaccinate ≥2 weeks before surgery.

VII. Vaccinate as soon after diagnosis as possible.

VIII. For hemodialysis patients, use special formulation of vaccine (40 µg/mL) or two 20 µg/mL doses administered at one body site. Vaccinate early in the course of renal disease. Assess antibody titers to hepatitis B surface antigen (anti-HB) levels annually. Administer additional doses if anti-HB levels decline to <10 mIU/mL.

IX. For all persons with chronic liver disease.

X. Withhold MMR or other measles-containing vaccines from HIV-infected persons with evidence of severe immunosuppression (see *MMWR*, 1998, 47[RR-8]:21-2 and *MMWR*, 2002, 51[RR-2]:22-4).

XI. Persons with impaired humoral immunity but intact cellular immunity may be vaccinated (see *MMWR*, 1999, 48[RR-6]).

Footnotes to Recommended Adult Immunization Schedule

[1]**Tetanus and diphtheria (Td).** Adults, including pregnant women with uncertain history of a complete primary vaccination series, should receive a primary series of Td. A primary series for adults is 3 doses; administer the first 2 doses at least 4 weeks apart and the 3rd dose 6-12 months after the second. Administer 1 dose if the person received the primary series and if the last vaccination was received ≥10 years previously. Consult recommendations for administering Td as prophylaxis in wound management (see *MMWR*, 1991, 40[RR-10]). The American College of Physicians Task Force on Adult Immunization supports a second option for Td use in adults: a single Td booster at age 50 years for persons who have completed the full pediatric series, including the teenage/young adult booster.

[2]**Influenza vaccination.** The Advisory Committee on Immunization Practices (ACIP) recommends inactivated influenza vaccination for the following indications, when vaccine is available. *Medical indications:* Chronic disorders of the cardiovascular or pulmonary systems, including asthma; chronic metabolic diseases, including diabetes mellitus, renal dysfunction, hemoglobinopathies, or immunosuppression (including immunosuppression caused by medications or by human immunodeficiency virus [HIV]); and pregnancy during the influenza season. *Occupational indications:* Healthcare workers and employees of long-term care and assisted living facilities. *Other indications:* Residents of nursing homes and other long-term care facilities; persons likely to transmit influenza to persons at high risk (ie, in-home caregivers to persons with medical indications, household/close contacts and out-of-home caregivers of children 0-23 months, household members and caregivers of elderly persons and adults with high-risk conditions); and anyone who wishes to be vaccinated. For healthy persons 5-49 years without high-risk conditions who are not contacts of severely immunocompromised persons in special care units, either the inactivated vaccine or the intranasally administered influenza vaccine (FluMist®) may be administered (see *MMWR*, 2004, 53[RR-6]). **Note:** Because of the vaccine shortage for the 2004-5 influenza season, CDC has recommended that vaccination be restricted to the following priority groups, which are considered to be of equal importance: all children 6-23 months; adults ≥65 years; persons 2-64 years with underlying chronic medical conditions; all women who will be pregnant during the influenza season; residents of nursing homes and long-term care facilities; children 6 months to 18 years on chronic aspirin therapy; healthcare workers involved in direct patient care; and out-of-home caregivers and household contacts of children <6 months. For the 2004-5 season, intranasally administered, live, attenuated influenza vaccine, if available, should be encouraged for healthy persons who are 5-49 years and are not pregnant, including healthcare workers (except those who care for severely immunocompromised patients in special care units) and persons caring for children <6 months (see *MMWR*, 2004, 53:923-4).

[3]**Pneumococcal polysaccharide vaccination.** *Medical indications:* Chronic disorders of the pulmonary system (excluding asthma); cardiovascular diseases; diabetes mellitus; chronic liver diseases, including liver disease as a result of alcohol abuse (eg, cirrhosis); chronic renal failure or nephrotic syndrome; functional or anatomic asplenia (eg, sickle cell disease or splenectomy); immunosuppressive conditions (eg, congenital immunodeficiency, HIV infection, leukemia, lymphoma,

multiple myeloma, Hodgkins disease, generalized malignancy, or organ or bone marrow transplantation); chemotherapy with alkylating agents, antimetabolites, or long-term systemic corticosteroids; or cochlear implants. *Geographic/other indications:* Alaska natives and certain American Indian populations. *Other indications:* Residents of nursing homes and other long-term care facilities (see *MMWR*, 1997, 46[RR-8] and *MMWR*, 2003, 52:739-40).

[4]**Revaccination with pneumococcal polysaccharide vaccine.** One-time revaccination after 5 years for persons with chronic renal failure or nephrotic syndrome; functional or anatomic asplenia (eg, sickle cell disease or splenectomy); immunosuppressive conditions (eg, congenital immunodeficiency, HIV infection, leukemia, lymphoma, multiple myeloma, Hodgkins disease, generalized malignancy, or organ or bone marrow transplantation); or chemotherapy with alkylating agents, antimetabolites, or long-term systemic corticosteroids. For persons ≥65 years, one-time revaccination if they were vaccinated ≥5 years previously and were <65 years at the time of primary vaccination (see *MMWR*, 1997, 46[RR-8]).

[5]**Hepatitis B vaccination.** *Medical indications:* Hemodialysis patients or patients who receive clotting factor concentrates. *Occupational indications:* Healthcare workers and public-safety workers who have exposure to blood in the workplace; and persons in training in schools of medicine, dentistry, nursing, laboratory technology, and other allied health professions. *Behavioral indications:* Injection-drug users; persons with more than one sex partner during the previous 6 months; persons with a recently acquired sexually transmitted disease (STD); all clients in STD clinics; and men who have sex with men. *Other indications:* Household contacts and sex partners of persons with chronic hepatitis B virus (HBV) infection; clients and staff members of institutions for the developmentally disabled; inmates of correctional facilities; or international travelers who will be in countries with high or intermediate prevalence of chronic HBV infection for >6 months (http://www.cdc.gov/travel/diseases/hbv.htm) (see *MMWR*, 1991, 40[RR-13]).

[6]**Hepatitis A vaccination.** *Medical indications:* Persons with clotting factor disorders or chronic liver disease. *Behavioral indications:* Men who have sex with men or users of illegal drugs. *Occupational indications:* Persons working with hepatitis A virus (HAV)-infected primates or with HAV in a research laboratory setting. *Other indications:* Persons traveling to or working in countries that have high or intermediate endemicity of hepatitis A. If the combined hepatitis A and hepatitis B vaccine is used, administer 3 doses at 0, 1, and 6 months (http://www.cdc.gov/travel/diseases/hav.htm) (see *MMWR*, 1999, 48[RR-12]).

[7]**Measles, mumps, rubella (MMR) vaccination.** *Measles component:* Adults born before 1957 can be considered immune to measles. Adults born during or after 1957 should receive ≥1 dose of MMR unless they have a medical contraindication, documentation of ≥1 dose, or other acceptable evidence of immunity. A second dose of MMR is recommended for adults who 1) were recently exposed to measles or in an outbreak setting, 2) were previously vaccinated with killed measles vaccine, 3) were vaccinated with an unknown vaccine during 1963-1967, 4) are students in postsecondary educational institutions, 5) work in healthcare facilities, or 6) plan to travel internationally. *Mumps component:* 1 dose of MMR vaccine should be adequate for protection. *Rubella component:* Administer 1 dose of MMR vaccine to women whose rubella vaccination history is unreliable and counsel women to avoid becoming pregnant for 4 weeks after vaccination. For women of childbearing age, regardless of birth year, routinely determine rubella immunity and counsel women regarding congenital rubella syndrome. Do not vaccinate pregnant women or those planning to become pregnant during the next 4 weeks. For women who are pregnant and susceptible, vaccinate as early in the postpartum period as possible (see *MMWR*, 1998, 47[RR-8] and *MMWR*, 2001, 50:1117).

[8]**Varicella vaccination.** Recommended for all persons lacking a reliable clinical history of varicella infection or serologic evidence of varicella zoster virus (VZV) infection who might be at high risk for exposure or transmission. This includes healthcare workers and family contacts of immunocompromised persons; persons who live or work in environments where transmission is likely (eg, teachers of young children, child care employees, and residents and staff members in institutional settings); persons who live or work in environments where VZV transmission can occur (eg, college students, inmates, and staff members of correctional institutions, and military personnel); adolescents 11-18 years and adults living in households with children; women who are not pregnant but who might become pregnant; and international travelers who are not immune to infection. **Note:** Approximately 95% of U.S.-born adults are immune to VZV. Do not vaccinate pregnant women or those planning to become pregnant during the next 4 weeks. For women who are pregnant and susceptible, vaccinate as early in the postpartum period as possible (see *MMWR*, 1999, 48[RR-6]).

[9]**Meningococcal vaccine (quadrivalent polysaccharide for serogroups A, C, Y, and W 135).** *Medical indications:* Adults with terminal complement component deficiencies or those with anatomic or functional asplenia. *Other indications:* Travelers to countries in which meningococcal disease is hyperendemic or epidemic (eg, the "meningitis belt" of sub-Saharan Africa and Mecca, Saudi Arabia). Revaccination after 3-5 years might be indicated for persons at high risk for infection (eg, persons residing in areas where disease is epidemic). Counsel college freshmen, especially those who live in dormitories, regarding meningococcal disease and availability of the vaccine to enable them to make an educated decision about receiving the vaccination (see *MMWR*, 2000, 49[RR-7]). The American Academy of Family Physicians recommends that colleges should take the lead on providing education on meningococcal infection and availability of vaccination and offer it to students who are interested. Physicians need not initiate discussion of meningococcal quadrivalent polysaccharide vaccine as part of routine medical care.

Adapted from "Recommended Adult Immunization Schedule – United States, October 2004-September 2005," *MMWR*, 2004, 53(45)Q1-4.

IMMUNIZATION RECOMMENDATIONS *(Continued)*

The Recommended Adult Immunization Schedule has been approved by the Advisory Committee on Immunization Practices (ACIP), the American College of Obstetricians and Gynecologists (ACOG), and the American Academy of Family Physicians (AAFP).

This schedule indicates the recommended age groups for routine administration of currently licensed vaccines for persons ≥19 years of age. Licensed combination vaccines may be used whenever any components of the combination are indicated and when the vaccine's other components are not contraindicated. Providers should consult manufacturers' package inserts for detailed recommendations.

Additional information about the vaccines listed above and contraindications for immunization is available at http://www.cdc.gov/nip or from the National Immunization Hotline, 800-232-2522 (English) or 800-232-0233 (Spanish).

RECOMMENDATIONS OF THE ADVISORY COMMITTEE ON IMMUNIZATION PRACTICES (ACIP)

Recommendations for Measles Immunization

Category	Recommendations
Unimmunized, no history of measles (12-15 mo)	A 2-dose schedule (with MMR) is recommended. The first dose is recommended at 12-15 mo; the second is recommended at 4-6 y
Children 6-11 mo in epidemic situations	Immunize (with monovalent measles vaccine or, if not available, MMR); reimmunization (with MMR) at 12-15 mo is necessary, and a third dose is indicated at 4-6 y
Children 4-12 y who have received 1 dose of measles vaccine at ≥12 mo	Reimmunize (1 dose)
Students in college and other post-high school institutions who have received 1 dose of measles vaccine at ≥12 mo	Reimmunize (1 dose)
History of vaccination before the first birthday	Consider susceptible and immunize (2 doses)
History of receipt of inactivated measles vaccine or unknown type of vaccine, 1963-1967	Consider susceptible and immunize (2 doses)
Further attenuated or unknown vaccine given with IG	Consider susceptible and immunize (2 doses)
Allergy to eggs	Immunize; no reactions likely
Neomycin allergy, nonanaphylactic	Immunize; no reactions likely
Severe hypersensitivity (anaphylaxis) to neomycin or gelatin	Avoid immunization
Tuberculosis	Immunize; vaccine does not exacerbate infection
Measles exposure	Immunize and/or give IG, depending on circumstances
HIV-infected	Immunize (2 doses) unless severely immunocompromised
Personal or family history of seizures	Immunize; advise parents of slightly increased risk of seizures
Immunoglobulin or blood recipient	Immunize at the appropriate interval

MMR = measles-mumps-rubella vaccine; IG = immune globulin; HIV = human immunodeficiency virus.

Adapted from "Report of the Committee on Infectious Diseases," *2003 Red Book®*, 26th ed.

IMMUNIZATION RECOMMENDATIONS *(Continued)*

Immunization in HIV-Infected Persons

Vaccination of immunocompromised patients depends on the characteristics of the vaccine and the patient. Vaccines are typically divided into two broad categories: those which contain live virus/bacteria or those which are derived from a component of the organism (or an inactivated organism). Live virus or live bacterial vaccines have been associated with severe complications in immunocompromised patients, and should generally be avoided [(except in selected circumstances (noted below)]. Inactivated, recombinant, subunit, polysaccharide, and conjugate vaccines and toxoids can be administered to all immunocompromised patients. However, it should be recognized that the response to these vaccines may be suboptimal. If indicated, all inactivated vaccines are recommended in usual doses and according to prescribed schedules. Pneumococcal, meningococcal, and Hib vaccines are recommended only for specific subpopulations, including functional or anatomic asplenia.

Special consideration must be given to immunization with measles and/or varicella vaccines. Persons with HIV are at a higher risk for severe complications from measles infection. In patients without severe immunocompromise, measles vaccination in HIV-infected persons has not been reported to cause severe and/or unusual adverse events. MMR vaccination is recommended for all HIV-infected persons who do not have evidence of severe immunocompromise (defined as a low age-specific total $CD4^+$ T-lymphocyte count or a low $CD4^+$ T-lymphocyte count as a percentage of total lymphocytes).

Varicella and/or herpes zoster infections are also associated with an increased risk of severe complications in children with HIV infection. Asymptomatic or mildly symptomatic HIV-infected children receiving varicella vaccination have demonstrated adequate response to the vaccine without evidence of severe and/or unusual events. However, experience has been limited. Varicella vaccine should be considered for children who are classified as CDC class N1 or A1 with age-specific $CD4^+$ T-lymphocyte percentages ≥25%.

HIV-infected persons who are receiving IVIG may not respond to MMR or varicella vaccines (or an individual component) due to the presence of a passively acquired antibody. Measles vaccine should be considered approximately 2 weeks before the next scheduled dose of IVIG (unless otherwise contraindicated). Unless serologic testing confirms the production of specific antibodies, the vaccination should be repeated at the recommended interval. In patients receiving maintenance IVIG therapy, an additional dose of IVIG should be considered if the exposure to measles occurs ≥3 weeks following a standard dose. Persons with cellular immunodeficiency should not receive varicella vaccine; however, persons with humoral immunodeficiency should be vaccinated (including persons with dysgammaglobulinemia or hypogammaglobulinemia).

Summarized/adapted from Atkinson WL, Pickering LK, Schwartz B, et al, "General Recommendations on Immunization. Recommendations of the Advisory Committee on Immunization Practices (ACIP) and the American Academy of Family Physicians (AAFP)," *MMWR Recomm Rep*, 2002, 51(RR-2):1-35.

Recommendations for Pneumococcal Conjugate Vaccine Use Among Healthy Children During Moderate and Severe Shortages

Age at First Vaccination (mo)	No Shortage[1]	Moderate Shortage	Severe Shortage
<6	2, 4, 6, and 12-15 months	2, 4, and 6 months (defer fourth dose)	2 doses at 2-month interval in first 6 months of life (defer third and fourth doses)
7-11	2 doses at 2-month interval; 12-15 month dose	2 doses at 2-month interval; 12-15-month dose	2 doses at 2-month interval (defer third dose)
12-23	2 doses at 2-month interval	2 doses at 2-month interval	1 dose (defer second dose)
>24	1 dose should be considered	No vaccination	No vaccination
Reduction in vaccine doses used[2]		21%	46%

[1]The vaccine schedule for no shortage is included as a reference. Providers should not use the no shortage schedule regardless of their vaccine supply until the national shortage is resolved.

[2]Assumes that approximately 85% of vaccine is administered to healthy infants beginning at age <7 months; approximately 5% is administered to high-risk infants beginning at age <7 months; and approximately 10% is administered to healthy children beginning at age 7-24 months. Actual vaccine savings will depend on a provider's vaccine use.

Adapted from the Advisory Committee on Immunization Practices, "Updated Recommendations on Use of Pneumococcal Conjugate Vaccine in a Setting of Vaccine Shortage," *MMWR Morb Mortal Wkly Rep*, 2001, 50(50):1140-2.

Recommended Regimens for Pneumococcal Conjugate Vaccine Among Children With a Late Start or Lapse in Vaccine Administration

Age at Examination (mo)	Previous Pneumococcal Conjugate Vaccination History	Recommended Regimen[1]
2-6	0 doses	3 doses 2 months apart, 4th dose at 12-15 months
	1 dose	2 doses 2 months apart, 4th dose at 12-15 months
	2 doses	1 dose, 4th dose at 12-15 months
7-11	0 doses	2 doses 2 months apart, 3rd dose at 12-15 months
	1 or 2 doses before age 7 months	1 dose at 7-11 months, with another dose at 12-15 months (≥2 months later)
12-23	0 doses	2 doses ≥2 months apart
	1 dose before age 12 months	2 doses ≥2 months apart
	1 dose at ≥12 months	1 dose ≥2 months after the most recent dose
	2 or 3 doses before age 12 months	1 dose ≥2 months after the most recent dose
24-59		
Healthy children[2]	Any incomplete schedule	Consider 1 dose ≥2 months after the most recent dose
High risk[3]	<3 doses	1 dose ≥2 months after the most recent dose and another dose ≥2 months later
	3 doses	1 dose ≥2 months after the most recent dose

IMMUNIZATION RECOMMENDATIONS *(Continued)*

[1]For children vaccinated at age <1 year, the minimum interval between doses is 4 weeks. Doses administered at ≥12 months should be at least 8 weeks apart.

[2]Providers should consider 1 dose for healthy children 24-59 months, with priority to children 24-35 months, American Indian/Alaska native and black children, and those who attend group child care centers.

[3]Children with sickle cell disease, asplenia, human immunodeficiency virus infection, chronic illness, cochlear implant, or immunocompromising condition.

Adapted from "CDC. Notice to Readers: Pneumococcal Conjugate Vaccine Shortage Resolved," *MMWR Morb Mortal Wkly Rep*, 2003, 52(19):446-7.

POSTEXPOSURE PROPHYLAXIS FOR HEPATITIS B[1]

Exposure	Hepatitis B Immune Globulin	Hepatitis B Vaccine
Perinatal	0.5 mL I.M. within 12 h of birth	0.5 mL[2] I.M. within 12 h of birth (no later than 7 d), and at 1 and 6 mo[3]; test for HB_sAg and anti-HB_s at 12-15 mo
Sexual	0.06 mL/kg I.M. within 14 d of sexual contact; a second dose should be given if the index patient remains HB_sAg-positive after 3 mo and hepatitis B vaccine was not given initially	1 mL I.M. at 0, 1, and 6 mo for homosexual and bisexual men and regular sexual contacts of persons with acute and chronic hepatitis B
Percutaneous; exposed person unvaccinated		
Source known HB_sAg-positive	0.06 mL/kg I.M. within 24 h	1 mL I.M. within 7 d, and at 1 and 6 mo[4]
Source known, HB_sAg status not known	Test source for HB_sAg; if source is positive, give exposed person 0.06 mL/kg I.M. once within 7 d	1 mL I.M. within 7 d, and at 1 and 6 mo[4]
Source not tested or unknown	Nothing required	1 mL I.M. within 7 d, and at 1 and 6 mo
Percutaneous; exposed person vaccinated		
Source known HB_sAg-positive	Test exposed person for anti-HB_s.[5] If titer is protective, nothing is required; if titer is not protective, give 0.06 mL/kg within 24 h.	Review vaccination status[6]
Source known, HB_sAg status not known	Test source for HB_sAg and exposed person for anti-HB_s. If source is HB_sAg-negative, or if source is HB_sAg-positive but anti-HB_s titer is protective, nothing is required. If source is HB_sAg-positive and anti-HB_s titer is not protective or if exposed person is a known nonresponder, give 0.06 mL/kg I.M. within 24 h. A second dose of hepatitis B immune globulin can be given 1 mo later if a booster dose of hepatitis B vaccine is not given.	Review vaccination status[6]

POSTEXPOSURE PROPHYLAXIS FOR HEPATITIS B[1] *(continued)*

Exposure	Hepatitis B Immune Globulin	Hepatitis B Vaccine
Source not tested or unknown	Test exposed person for anti-HB_s. If anti-HB_s titer is protective, nothing is required. If anti-HB_s titer is not protective, 0.06 mL/kg may be given along with a booster dose of hepatitis B vaccine.	Review vaccination status[6]

[1]HB_sAg = hepatitis B surface antigen; anti-HB_s = antibody to hepatitis B surface antigen; I.M. = intramuscularly; SRU = standard ratio units.
[2]Each 0.5 mL dose of plasma-derived hepatitis B vaccine contains 10 mcg of HB_sAg; each 0.5 mL dose of recombinant hepatitis B vaccine contains 5 mcg (Merck Sharp & Dohme) or 10 mcg (SmithKline Beecham) of HB_sAg.
[3]If hepatitis B immune globulin and hepatitis B vaccine are given simultaneously, they should be given at separate sites.
[4]If hepatitis B vaccine is not given, a second dose of hepatitis B immune globulin should be given 1 month later.
[5]Anti-HB_s titers <10 SRU by radioimmunoassay or negative by enzyme immunoassay indicate lack of protection. Testing the exposed person for anti-HB_s is not necessary if a protective level of antibody has been shown within the previous 24 months.
[6]If the exposed person has not completed a three-dose series of hepatitis B vaccine, the series should be completed. Test the exposed person for anti-HB_s. If the antibody level is protective, nothing is required. If an adequate antibody response in the past is shown on retesting to have declined to an inadequate level, a booster dose (1 mL) of hepatitis B vaccine should be given. If the exposed person has inadequate antibody or is a known nonresponder to vaccination, a booster dose can be given along with one dose of hepatitis B immune globulin.

IMMUNIZATION RECOMMENDATIONS *(Continued)*

PREVENTION OF HEPATITIS A THROUGH ACTIVE OR PASSIVE IMMUNIZATION: RECOMMENDATIONS OF THE ADVISORY COMMITTEE ON IMMUNIZATION PRACTICES (ACIP)

PROPHYLAXIS AGAINST HEPATITIS A VIRUS INFECTION

Recommended Doses of Immune Globulin (IG) for Hepatitis A Pre-exposure and Postexposure Prophylaxis[1]

Setting	Duration of Coverage	IG Dose[2]
Pre-exposure	Short-term (1-2 months)	0.02 mL/kg
	Long-term (3-5 months)	0.06 mL/kg[3]
Postexposure	—	0.02 mL/kg

[1]Infants and pregnant women should receive a preparation that does not include thimerosal.

[2]IG should be administered by intramuscular injection into either the deltoid or gluteal muscle. For children <24 months of age, IG can be administered in the anterolateral thigh muscle.

[3]Repeat every 5 months if continued exposure to HAV occurs.

Recommended Dosages of Havrix®[1]

Vaccinee's Age (y)	Dose (EL.U.)[2]	Volume (mL)	No. Doses	Schedule (mo)[3]
2-18	720	0.5	2	0, 6-12
>18	1440	1.0	2	0, 6-12

[1]Hepatitis A vaccine, inactivated, SmithKline Beecham Biologicals.

[2]Enzyme-linked immunosorbent assay (ELISA) units.

[3]0 months represents timing of the initial dose; subsequent numbers represent months after the initial dose.

Recommended Dosages of VAQTA®[1]

Vaccinee's Age (y)	Dose (units)	Volume (mL)	No. Doses	Schedule (mo)[2]
2-17	25	0.5	2	0, 6-18
>17	50	1.0	2	0, 6

[1]Hepatitis A vaccine, inactivated, Merck & Company, Inc.

[2]0 months represents timing of the initial dose; subsequent numbers represent months after the initial dose.

Adapted from "Prevention of Hepatitis A Through Active or Passive Immunization: Recommendations of the Advisory Committee on Immunization Practices (ACIP)," *MMWR Recomm Rep*, 1999, 48(RR-12):1-37.

RECOMMENDATIONS FOR TRAVELERS

Recommended Immunizations for Travelers to Developing Countries[1]

Immunizations	Length of Travel		
	Brief, <2 wk	Intermediate, 2 wk - 3 mo	Long-term Residential, >3 mo
Review and complete age-appropriate childhood schedule	+	+	+
• DTaP; poliovirus vaccine, and *H. influenzae* type b vaccine may be given at 4-wk intervals if necessary to complete the recommended schedule before departure			
• Measles: 2 additional doses given if younger than 12 mo of age at first dose			
• Varicella			
• Hepatitis B[2]			
Yellow fever[3]	+	+	+
Hepatitis A[4]	+	+	+
Typhoid fever[4]	±	+	+
Meningococcal disease[5]	±	±	±
Rabies[6]	±	+	+
Japanese encephalitis[3]	±	±	+

[1]+ = recommended; ± = consider.

[2]If insufficient time to complete 6-month primary series, accelerated series can be given.

[3]For endemic regions, see *Health Information for International Travel* in *Red Book®*. For high-risk activities in areas experiencing outbreaks, vaccine is recommended even for brief travel.

[4]Indicated for travelers who will consume food and liquids in areas of poor sanitation.

[5]For endemic regions of Africa, during local epidemics, and travel to Saudi Arabia for the Hajj.

[6]Indicated for person with high risk of animal exposure, and for travelers to endemic countries.

Adapted from "Report of the Committee on Infectious Diseases," *2003 Red Book®*, 26th ed, 94.

Recommendations for Pre-exposure Immunoprophylaxis of Hepatitis A Virus Infection for Travelers[1]

Age (y)	Likely Exposure (mo)	Recommended Prophylaxis
<2	<3	IG, 0.02 mL/kg[2]
	3-5	IG, 0.06 mL/kg[2]
	Long-term	IG, 0.06 mL/kg at departure and every 5 mo if exposure to HAV continues[2]
≥2	<3[3]	HAV vaccine[4,5] or IG, 0.02 mL/kg[2]
	3-5[3]	HAV vaccine[4,5] or IG, 0.06 mL/kg[2]
	Long-term	HAV vaccine[4,5]

[1]IG = immune globulin; HAV = hepatitis A virus.

[2]IG should be administered deep into a large muscle mass. Ordinarily, no more than 5 mL should be administered in one site in an adult or large child; lesser amounts (maximum 3 mL) should be given to small children and infants.

[3]Vaccine is preferable, but IG is an acceptable alternative.

[4]To ensure protection in travelers whose departure is imminent, IG also may be given.

[5]Dose and schedule of hepatitis A vaccine as recommended according to age.

Adapted from "Report of the Committee on Infectious Diseases," *2003 Red Book®*, 26th ed, 312.

IMMUNIZATION RECOMMENDATIONS *(Continued)*

Prevention of Malaria[1]

Drug	Adult Dosage	Pediatric Dosage
	Chloroquine-Sensitive Areas[2]	
Chloroquine phosphate[3,4]	500 mg (300 mg base), once/week[5]	5 mg/kg base once/week, up to adult dose of 300 mg base[5]
	Chloroquine-Resistant Areas[2]	
Mefloquine[4,6,7]	250 mg once/week[5]	<15 kg: 5 mg/kg[5] 15-19 kg: 1/4 tablet[5] 20-30 kg: 1/2 tablet[5] 31-45 kg: 3/4 tablet[5] >45 kg: 1 tablet[5]
or		
Doxycycline[4,8]	100 mg/d[9]	2 mg/kg/d, up to 100 mg/d[9]
or		
Atovaquone/proguanil[4,10]	250 mg/100 mg (1 tablet) daily[11]	11-20 kg: 62.5 mg/25 mg[10,11] 21-30 kg: 125 mg/50 mg[10,11] 31-40 kg: 187.5 mg/75 mg[10,11] >40 kg: 250 mg/100 mg[10,11]
Alternative:		
Primaquine[8,12,13]	30 mg base daily	0.5 mg/kg base daily
Chloroquine phosphate[3]	500 mg (300 mg base) once/week[5]	5 mg/kg base once/week, up to adult dose of 300 mg base[5]
plus		
Proguanil[14]	200 mg once/day	<2 y: 50 mg once/day 2-6 y: 100 mg once/day 7-10 y: 150 mg once/day >10 y: 200 mg once/day

[1]No drug regimen guarantees protection against malaria. If fever develops within a year (particularly within the first 2 months) after travel to malarious areas, travelers should be advised to seek medical attention. Insect repellents, insecticide-impregnated bed nets, and proper clothing are important adjuncts for malaria prophylaxis.

[2]Chloroquine-resistant *P. falciparum* occurs in all malarious areas except Central America west of the Panama Canal Zone, Mexico, Haiti, the Dominican Republic, and most of the Middle East (chloroquine resistance has been reported in Yemen, Oman, Saudi Arabia, and Iran).

[3]In pregnancy, chloroquine prophylaxis has been used extensively and safely.

[4]For prevention of attack after departure from areas where *P. vivax* and *P. ovale* are endemic, which includes almost all areas where malaria is found (except Haiti), some experts prescribe in addition primaquine phosphate 26.3 mg (15 mg base)/day or, for children, 0.3 mg base/kg/day during the last 2 weeks of prophylaxis. Others prefer to avoid the toxicity of primaquine and rely on surveillance to detect cases when they occur; particularly when exposure was limited or doubtful.

[5]Beginning 1-2 weeks before travel and continuing weekly for the duration of stay and for 4 weeks after leaving.

[6]In the U.S., a 250 mg tablet of mefloquine contains 228 mg mefloquine base. Outside the U.S., each 275 mg tablet contains 250 mg base.

[7]The pediatric dosage has not been approved by the FDA, and the drug has not been approved for use during pregnancy. However, it has been reported to be safe for prophylactic use during the second or third trimester of pregnancy and possibly during early pregnancy as well (CDC Health Information for International Travel, 2001-2003, 113; BL Smoak, Writer JV, Keep LW, et al, "The Effects of Inadvertent Exposure of Mefloquine Chemoprophylaxis on Pregnancy Outcomes and Infants of US Army Servicewomen," *J Infect Dis*, 1997, 176(3):831-3). Mefloquine is not recommended for patients with cardiac conduction abnormalities. Patients with a history of seizures or psychiatric disorders should avoid mefloquine (*Medical Letter*, 1990, 32:13). Resistance to mefloquine has been reported in some areas, such as Thailand; in these areas, doxycycline should be used for prophylaxis. In children <8 years of age, proguanil plus sulfisoxazole has been used (KN Suh and JS Keystone, *Infect Dis Clin Pract*, 1996, 5:541).

[8]An approved drug, but considered investigational for this condition by the U.S. Food and Drug Administration.

[9]Beginning 1-2 days before travel and continuing for the duration of stay and for 4 weeks after leaving. Use of tetracyclines is contraindicated in pregnancy and in children <8 years of age. Doxycycline can cause gastrointestinal disturbances, vaginal moniliasis, and photosensitivity reactions.

[10]Atovaquone plus proguanil is available as a fixed-dose combination tablet: adult tablets (250 mg atovaquone/100 mg proguanil, *Malarone*) and pediatric tablets (62.5 mg atovaquone/25 mg proguanil, *Malarone Pediatric*). To enhance absorption, it should be taken within 45 minutes after eating (Looareesuwan S, Chulay JD, Canfield CJ, et al, "Malarone (Atovaquone and Proguanil Hydrochloride): A Review of Its Clinical Development for Treatment of Malaria. Malarone Clinical Trials Study Group," *Am J Trop Med Hyg*, 1999, 60(4):533-41). Although approved for once daily dosing, to decrease nausea and vomiting the dose for treatment is usually divided in two.

[11]Shanks GE et al, *Clin Infect Dis*, 1998, 27:494; Lell B, Luckner D, Ndjave M, et al, "Randomised Placebo-Controlled Study of Atovaquone Plus Proguanil for Malaria Prophylaxis in Children," *Lancet*, 1998, 351(9104):709-13. Beginning 1-2 days before travel and continuing for the duration of stay and for 1 week after leaving. In one study of malaria prophylaxis, atovaquone/proguanil was better tolerated than mefloquine in nonimmune travelers (Overbosch D, Schilthuis H, Bienzle U, et al, "Atovaquone-Proguanil Versus Mefloquine for Malaria Prophylaxis in Nonimmune Travelers: Results From a Randomized, Double-Blind Study," *Clin Infect Dis*, 2001, 33(7):1015-21).

[12]Primaquine phosphate can cause hemolytic anemia, especially in patients whose red cells are deficient in glucose-6-phosphate dehydrogenase. This deficiency is most common in African, Asian, and Mediterranean peoples. Patients should be screened for G6PD deficiency before treatment. Primaquine should not be used during pregnancy.

[13]Several studies have shown that daily primaquine, beginning 1 day before departure and continued until 7 days after leaving the malaria area, provides effective prophylaxis against chloroquine-resistant *P. falciparum* (Baird JK, Lacy MD, Basri H, et al, "Randomized, Parallel Placebo-Controlled Trial of Primaquine for Malaria Prophylaxis in Papua, Indonesia," *Clin Infect Dis*, 2001, 33(12):1990-7). Some studies have shown less efficacy against *P. vivax*. Nausea and abdominal pain can be diminished by taking with food.

[14]Proguanil (Paludrine – Wyeth Ayerst, Canada; AstraZeneca, United Kingdom), which is not available alone in the U.S.A. but is widely available in Canada and Europe, is recommended mainly for use in Africa south of the Sahara. Prophylaxis is recommended during exposure and for 4 weeks afterwards. Proguanil has been used in pregnancy without evidence of toxicity (Phillips-Howard PA and Wood D, "The Safety of Antimalarial Drugs in Pregnancy," *Drug Saf*, 1996, 14(3):131-45).

Adapted from "Report of the Committee on Infectious Diseases," *2003 Red Book®*, 26th ed, 760-1.

IMMUNIZATION RECOMMENDATIONS *(Continued)*

ADVERSE EVENTS AND VACCINATION

Reportable Events Following Vaccination[1]

Vaccine / Toxoid		Event	Onset Interval
Tetanus in any combination; DTaP, DTP, DTP-Hib, DT, Td, TT	A.	Anaphylaxis or anaphylactic shock	7 days
	B.	Brachial neuritis	28 days
	C.	Any sequela (including death) of above events	Not applicable
	D.	Events described in manufacturer's package insert as contraindications to additional doses of vaccine	See package insert
Pertussis in any combination; DTaP, DTP, DTP-Hib, P	A.	Anaphylaxis or anaphylactic shock	7 days
	B.	Encephalopathy (or encephalitis)	7 days
	C.	Any sequela (including death) of above events	Not applicable
	D.	Events described in manufacturer's package insert as contraindications to additional doses of vaccine	See package insert
Measles, mumps, and rubella in any combination; MMR, MR, M, R	A.	Anaphylaxis or anaphylactic shock	7 days
	B.	Encephalopathy (or encephalitis)	15 days
	C.	Any sequela (including death) of above events	Not applicable
	D.	Events described in manufacturer's package insert as contraindications to additional doses of vaccine	See package insert
Rubella in any combination; MMR, MR, R	A.	Chronic arthritis	42 days
	B.	Any sequela (including death) of above events	Not applicable
	C.	Events described in manufacturer's package insert as contraindications to additional doses of vaccine	See package insert
Measles in any combination; MMR, MR, M	A.	Thrombocytopenic purpura	7-30 days
	B.	Vaccine-strain measles viral infection in an immunodeficient recipient	6 months
	C.	Any sequela (including death) of above events	Not applicable
	D.	Events described in manufacturer's package insert as contraindications to additional doses of vaccine	See package insert
Inactivated polio (IPV)	A.	Anaphylaxis or anaphylactic shock	7 days
	B.	Any sequela (including death) of above events	Not applicable
	C.	Events described in manufacturer's package insert as contraindications to additional doses of vaccine	See package insert
Hepatitis B	A.	Anaphylaxis or anaphylactic shock	7 days
	B.	Any sequela (including death) of above events	Not applicable
	C.	Events described in manufacturer's package insert as contraindications to additional doses of vaccine	See package insert
Haemophilus influenzae type b (conjugate)	A.	Events described in manufacturer's package insert as contraindications to additional doses of vaccine	See package insert
Varicella	A.	Events described in manufacturer's package insert as contraindications to additional doses of vaccine	See package insert
Rotavirus	A.	Intussusception	30 days
	B.	Any sequela (including death) of above events	Not applicable
	C.	Events described in manufacturer's package insert as contraindications to additional doses of vaccine	See package insert
Pneumococcal conjugate	A.	Events described in manufacturer's package insert as contraindications to additional doses of vaccine	See package insert

[1]Effective date: August 26, 2002.

The Reportable Events Table (RET) reflects what is reportable by law (42 USC 300aa-25) to the Vaccine Adverse Event Reporting System (VAERS), including conditions found in the manufacturer's package insert. In addition, individuals are encouraged to report **any** clinically significant or unexpected events (even if you are not certain the vaccine caused the event) for **any** vaccine, whether or not it is listed on the RET. Manufacturers are also required by regulation (21CFR 600.80) to report to the VAERS program all adverse events made known to them for any vaccine.

Adapted from the website http://www.vaers.org/reportable.htm. For further information, contact VAERS at 1-800-822-7967.

AMINOGLYCOSIDE DOSING AND MONITORING

All aminoglycoside therapy should be individualized for specific patients in specific clinical situation. The following are guidelines for initiating therapy.

1. Loading dose based on estimated ideal body weight (IBW). **All patients require a loading dose independent of renal function.**

Agent	Dose
Gentamicin	2 mg/kg
Tobramycin	2 mg/kg
Amikacin	7.5 mg/kg

   Significantly higher loading doses may be required in severely ill intensive care unit patients.

2. Initial maintenance doses as a percent of loading dose according to desired dosing interval and creatinine clearance (Cl_{cr}):

$$\text{Male } Cl_{cr} \text{ (mL/min)} = \frac{(140 - \text{age}) \times \text{IBW}}{72 \times \text{serum creatinine}}$$

$$\text{Female} = 0.85 \times Cl_{cr} \text{ males}$$

Cl_{cr} (mL/min)	Dosing Interval (h) 8	12	24
90	84%	—	—
80	80%	—	—
70	76%	88%	—
60	—	84%	—
50	—	79%	—
40	—	72%	92%
30	—	—	86%
25	—	—	81%
20	—	—	75%

   Patients >65 years of age should not receive initial aminoglycoside maintenance dosing more often than every 12 hours.

3. Serum concentration monitoring

   a. Serum concentration monitoring is necessary for **safe** and **effective** therapy, particularly in patients with serious infections and those with risk factors for toxicity.

   b. Peak serum concentrations should be drawn 30 minutes after the completion of a 30-minute infusion. Trough serum concentrations should be drawn within 30 minutes prior to the administered dose.

   c. Serum concentrations should be drawn after 5 half-lives, usually around the third dose or thereafter.

AMINOGLYCOSIDE DOSING AND MONITORING *(Continued)*

4. Desired measured serum concentrations

	Peak (mcg/mL)	Trough (mcg/mL)
Gentamicin	6-10	0.5-2.0
Tobramycin	6-10	0.5-2.0
Amikacin	20-30	<5

5. For patients receiving hemodialysis:
   - administer the **same** loading dose
   - administer $^{2}/_{3}$ of the loading dose after each dialysis
   - **serum concentrations must be monitored**
   - watch for ototoxicity from accumulation of drug
6. For individual clinical situations the prescribing physician should feel free to consult Infectious Disease, the Pharmacology Service, or the Pharmacy.

"Once Daily" Aminoglycosides

High dose, "once daily" aminoglycoside therapy for treatment of gram-negative bacterial infections has been studied and remains controversial. The pharmacodynamics of aminoglycosides reveal dose-dependent killing which suggests an efficacy advantage of "high" peak serum concentrations. It is also suggested that allowing troughs to fall to unmeasurable levels decreases the risk of nephrotoxicity without detriment to efficacy. Because of a theoretical saturation of tubular cell uptake of aminoglycosides, decreasing the number of times the drug is administered in a particular time period may play a role in minimizing the risk of nephrotoxicity. Ototoxicity has not been sufficiently formally evaluated through audiometry or vestibular testing comparing "once daily" to standard therapy. Over 100 letters, commentaries, studies and reviews have been published on the topic of "once daily" aminoglycosides with varying dosing regimens, monitoring parameters, inclusion and exclusion criteria, and results (most of which have been favorable for the "once daily" regimens). The caveats of this simplified method of dosing are several, including assurance that creatinine clearances be calculated, that all patients are not candidates and should not be considered for this regimen, and that "once daily" is a semantic misnomer.

Because of the controversial nature of this method, it is beyond the scope of this book to present significant detail and dosing regimen recommendations. Considerable experience with two methods warrants mention. The Hartford Hospital has experience with over 2000 patients utilizing a 7 mg/kg dose, a dosing scheme for various creatinine clearance estimates, and a serum concentration monitoring nomogram.[1] Providence Medical Center utilizes a 5 mg/kg dosing regimen but only in patients with excellent renal function; serum concentrations are monitored 4-6 hours prior to the dose administered.[2] Two excellent reviews discuss the majority of studies and controversies regarding these dosing techniques.[3,4] An editorial accompanies one of the reviews and is worth examination.[5]

"Once daily" dosing may be a safe and effective method of providing aminoglycoside therapy to a large number of patients who require these efficacious yet toxic agents. As with any method of aminoglycoside administration, dosing must be individualized and the caveats of the method considered.

Footnotes

1. Nicolau DP, Freeman CD, Belliveau PP, et al, "Experience With a Once-Daily Aminoglycoside Program Administered to 2,184 Patients," *Antimicrob Agents Chemother*, 1995, 39:650-5.
2. Gilbert DN, "Once-Daily Aminoglycoside Therapy," *Antimicrob Agents Chemother*, 1991, 35:399-405.
3. Preston SL and Briceland LL, "Single Daily Dosing of Aminoglycosides," *Pharmacotherapy*, 1995, 15:297-316.
4. Bates RD and Nahata MC, "Once-Daily Administration of Aminoglycosides," *Ann Pharmacother*, 1994, 28:757-66.
5. Rotschafer JC and Rybak MJ, "Single Daily Dosing of Aminoglycosides: A Commentary," *Ann Pharmacother*, 1994, 28:797-801.

Aminoglycoside Penetration Into Various Tissues

Site	Extent of Distribution
Eye	Poor
CNS	Poor (<25%)
Pleural	Excellent
Bronchial secretions	Poor
Sputum	Fair (10%-50%)
Pulmonary tissue	Excellent
Ascitic fluid	Variable (43%-132%)
Peritoneal fluid	Poor
Bile	Variable (25%-90%)
Bile with obstruction	Poor
Synovial fluid	Excellent
Bone	Poor
Prostate	Poor
Urine	Excellent
Renal tissue	Excellent

Adapted from Neu HC, "Pharmacology of Aminoglycosides," *The Aminoglycosides*, Whelton E and Neu HC, eds, New York, NY: Marcel Dekker, Inc, 1981.

ANIMAL AND HUMAN BITES

Bite Wound Antibiotic Regimens

	Dog Bite	Cat Bite	Human Bite
Prophylactic Antibiotics			
Prophylaxis	No routine prophylaxis, consider if involves face or hand, or immunosuppressed or asplenic patients	Routine prophylaxis	Routine prophylaxis
Prophylactic antibiotic	Amoxicillin	Amoxicillin	Amoxicillin
Penicillin allergy	Doxycycline if >10 y or co-trimoxazole	Doxycycline if >10 y or co-trimoxazole	Doxycycline if >10 y or erythromycin and cephalexin[1]
Outpatient Oral Antibiotic Treatment (mild to moderate infection)			
Established infection	Amoxicillin and clavulanic acid	Amoxicillin and clavulanic acid	Amoxicillin and clavulanic acid
Penicillin allergy (mild infection only)	Doxycycline if >10 y	Doxycycline if >10 y	Cephalexin[1] or clindamycin
Outpatient Parenteral Antibiotic Treatment (moderate infections – single drug regimens)			
	Ceftriaxone	Ceftriaxone	Cefotetan
Inpatient Parenteral Antibiotic Treatment			
Established infection	Ampicillin + cefazolin	Ampicillin + cefazolin	Ampicillin + clindamycin
Penicillin allergy	Cefazolin[1]	Ceftriaxone[1]	Cefotetan[1] or imipenem
Duration of Prophylactic and Treatment Regimens			
Prophylaxis: 5 days			
Treatment: 10-14 days			

[1]Contraindicated if history of immediate hypersensitivity reaction (anaphylaxis) to penicillin.

ANTIBIOTIC TREATMENT OF ADULTS WITH INFECTIVE ENDOCARDITIS

Table 1. Suggested Regimens for Therapy of Native Valve Endocarditis Due to Penicillin-Susceptible Viridans Streptococci and *Streptococcus bovis* (Minimum Inhibitory Concentration ≤0.1 mcg/mL)[1]

Antibiotic	Dosage and Route	Duration (wk)	Comments
Aqueous crystalline penicillin G sodium	12-18 million units/24 h I.V. either continuously or in 6 equally divided doses	4	Preferred in most patients older than 65 y and in those with impairment of the eighth nerve or renal function
or			
Ceftriaxone sodium	2 g once daily I.V. or I.M.[2]	4	
Aqueous crystalline penicillin G sodium	12-18 million units/24 h I.V. either continuously or in 6 equally divided doses	2	When obtained 1 hour after a 20- to 30-minute I.V. infusion or I.M. injection, serum concentration of gentamicin of approximately 3 mcg/mL is desirable; trough concentration should be <1 mcg/mL
With gentamicin sulfate[3]	1 mg/kg I.M. or I.V. every 8 hours	2	
Vancomycin hydrochloride[4]	30 mg/kg/24 h I.V. in 2 equally divided doses, not to exceed 2 g/24 h unless serum levels are monitored	4	Vancomycin therapy is recommended for patients allergic to β-lactams; peak serum concentrations of vancomycin should be obtained 1 h after completion of the infusion and should be in the range of 30-45 mcg/mL for twice-daily dosing

[1]Dosages recommended are for patients with normal renal function. For nutritionally variant streptococci, see Table 3. I.V. indicates intravenous; I.M., intramuscular.

[2]Patients should be informed that I.M. injection of ceftriaxone is painful.

[3]Dosing of gentamicin on a mg/kg basis will produce higher serum concentrations in obese patients that in lean patients. Therefore, in obese patients, dosing should be based on ideal body weight. (Ideal body weight for men is 50 kg + 2.3 kg per inch over 5 feet, and ideal body weight for women is 45.5 kg + 2.3 kg per inch over 5 feet.) Relative contraindications to the use of gentamicin are age >65 years, renal impairment, or impairment of the eighth nerve. Other potentially nephrotoxic agents (eg, nonsteroidal anti-inflammatory drugs) should be used cautiously in patients receiving gentamicin.

[4]Vancomycin dosage should be reduced in patients with impaired renal function. Vancomycin given on a mg/kg basis will produce higher serum concentrations in obese patients than in lean patients. Therefore, in obese patients, dosing should be based on ideal body weight. Each dose of vancomycin should be infused over at least 1 hour to reduce the risk of the histamine-release "red man" syndrome.

ANTIBIOTIC TREATMENT OF ADULTS WITH INFECTIVE ENDOCARDITIS *(Continued)*

Table 2. Therapy for Native Valve Endocarditis Due to Strains of Viridans Streptococci and *Streptococcus bovis* Relatively Resistant to Penicillin G (Minimum Inhibitory Concentration >0.1 mcg/mL and <0.5 mcg/mL)[1]

Antibiotic	Dosage and Route	Duration (wk)	Comments
Aqueous crystalline penicillin G sodium	18 million units/24 h I.V. either continuously or in 6 equally divided doses	4	Cefazolin or other first-generation cephalosporins may be substituted for penicillin in patients whose penicillin hypersensitivity is not of the immediate type.
With gentamicin sulfate[2]	1 mg/kg I.M. or I.V. every 8 h	2	
Vancomycin hydrochloride[3]	30 mg/kg/24 h I.V. in 2 equally divided doses, not to exceed 2 g/24 h unless serum levels are monitored	4	Vancomycin therapy is recommended for patients allergic to β-lactams

[1]Dosages recommended are for patients with normal renal function. I.V. indicates intravenous; I.M., intramuscular.

[2]For specific dosing adjustment and issues concerning gentamicin (obese patients, relative contraindications), see Table 1 footnotes.

[3]For specific dosing adjustment and issues concerning vancomycin (obese patients, length of infusion), see Table 1 footnotes.

Table 3. Standard Therapy for Endocarditis Due to Enterococci[1]

Antibiotic	Dosage and Route	Duration (wk)	Comments
Aqueous crystalline penicillin G sodium	18-30 million units/24 h I.V. either continuously or in 6 equally divided doses	4-6	4-week therapy recommended for patients with symptoms <3 months in duration; 6-week therapy recommended for patients with symptoms >3 months in duration.
With gentamicin sulfate[2]	1 mg/kg I.M. or I.V. every 8 h	4-6	
Ampicillin sodium	12 g/24 h I.V. either continuously or in 6 equally divided doses	4-6	
With gentamicin sulfate[2]	1 mg/kg I.M. or I.V. every 8 hours	4-6	
Vancomycin hydrochloride[2,3]	30 mg/kg/24 h I.V. in 2 equally divided doses, not to exceed 2 g/24 h unless serum levels are monitored	4-6	Vancomycin therapy is recommended for patients allergic to β-lactams; cephalosporins are not acceptable alternatives for patients allergic to penicillin
With gentamicin sulfate[2]	1 mg/kg I.M. or I.V. every 8 h	4-6	

[1]All enterococci causing endocarditis must be tested for antimicrobial susceptibility in order to select optimal therapy. This table is for endocarditis due to gentamicin- or vancomycin-susceptible enterococci, viridans streptococci with a minimum inhibitory concentration of >0.5 mcg/mL, nutritionally variant viridans streptococci, or prosthetic valve endocarditis caused by viridans streptococci or *Streptococcus bovis*. Antibiotic dosages are for patients with normal renal function. I.V. indicates intravenous; I.M., intramuscular.

[2]For specific dosing adjustment and issues concerning gentamicin (obese patients, relative contraindications), see Table 1 footnotes.

[3]For specific dosing adjustment and issues concerning vancomycin (obese patients, length of infusion), see Table 1 footnotes.

Table 4. Therapy for Endocarditis Due to *Staphylococcus* in the Absence of Prosthetic Material[1]

Antibiotic	Dosage and Route	Duration	Comments
Methicillin-Susceptible Staphylococci			
Regimens for non-β-lactam-allergic patients			
Nafcillin sodium or oxacillin sodium	2 g I.V. every 4 h	4-6 wk	Benefit of additional aminoglycosides has not been established
With optional addition of gentamicin sulfate[2]	1 mg/kg I.M. or I.V. every 8 h	3-5 d	
Regimens for β-lactam-allergic patients			
Cefazolin (or other first-generation cephalosporins in equivalent dosages)	2 g I.V. every 8 h	4-6 wk	Cephalosporins should be avoided in patients with immediate-type hypersensitivity to penicillin
With optional addition of gentamicin[2]	1 mg/kg I.M. or I.V. every 8 hours	3-5 d	
Vancomycin hydrochloride[3]	30 mg/kg/24 h I.V. in 2 equally divided doses, not to exceed 2 g/24 h unless serum levels are monitored	4-6 wk	Recommended for patients allergic to penicillin
Methicillin-Resistant Staphylococci			
Vancomycin hydrochloride[3]	30 mg/kg/24 h I.V. in 2 equally divided doses; not to exceed 2 g/24 h unless serum levels are monitored	4-6 wk	

[1]For treatment of endocarditis due to penicillin-susceptible staphylococci (minimum inhibitory concentration ≤0.1 mcg/mL), aqueous crystalline penicillin G sodium (Table 1, first regimen) can be used for 4-6 weeks instead of nafcillin or oxacillin. Shorter antibiotic courses have been effective in some drug addicts with right-sided endocarditis due to *Staphylococcus aureus*. I.V. indicates intravenous; I.M., intramuscular.

[2]For specific dosing adjustment and issues concerning gentamicin (obese patients, relative contraindications), see Table 1 footnotes.

[3]For specific dosing adjustment and issues concerning vancomycin (obese patients, length of infusion), see Table 1 footnotes.

ANTIBIOTIC TREATMENT OF ADULTS WITH INFECTIVE ENDOCARDITIS *(Continued)*

Table 5. Treatment of Staphylococcal Endocarditis in the Presence of a Prosthetic Valve or Other Prosthetic Material[1]

Antibiotic	Dosage and Route	Duration (wk)	Comments
Regimen for Methicillin-Resistant Staphylococci			
Vancomycin hydrochloride[2]	30 mg/kg/24 h I.V. in 2 or 4 equally divided doses, not to exceed 2 g/24 h unless serum levels are monitored	≥6	
With rifampin[3]	300 mg orally every 8 h	≥6	Rifampin increases the amount of warfarin sodium required for antithrombotic therapy.
And with gentamicin sulfate[4,5]	1 mg/kg I.M. or I.V. every 8 h	2	
Regimen for Methicillin-Susceptible Staphylococci			
Nafcillin sodium or oxacillin sodium	2 g I.V. every 4 h	≥6	First-generation cephalosporins or vancomycin should be used in patients allergic to β-lactam. Cephalosporins should be avoided in patients with immediate-type hypersensitivity to penicillin or with methicillin-resistant staphylococci.
With rifampin[3]	300 mg orally every 8 h	≥6	
And with gentamicin sulfate[4,5]	1 mg/kg I.M. or I.V. every 8 h	2	

[1]Dosages recommended are for patients with normal renal function. I.V. indicates intravenous; I.M., intramuscular.

[2]For specific dosing adjustment and issues concerning vancomycin (obese patients, relative contraindications), see Table 1 footnotes.

[3]Rifampin plays a unique role in the eradication of staphylococcal infection involving prosthetic material; combination therapy is essential to prevent emergence of rifampin resistance.

[4]For a specific dosing adjustment and issues concerning gentamicin (obese patients, relative contraindications), see Table 1 footnotes.

[5]Use during initial 2 weeks.

Table 6. Therapy for Endocarditis Due to HACEK Microorganisms (*Haemophilus parainfluenzae, Haemophilus aphrophilus, Actinobacillus actinomycetemcomitans, Cardiobacterium hominus, Eikenella corrodens,* and *Kingella kingae*)[1]

Antibiotic	Dosage and Route	Duration (wk)	Comments
Ceftriaxone sodium[2]	2 g once daily I.V. or I.M.[2]	4	Cefotaxime sodium or other third-generation cephalosporins may be substituted
Ampicillin sodium[3]	12 g/24 h I.V. either continuously or in 6 equally divided doses	4	
With gentamicin sulfate[4]	1 mg/kg I.M. or I.V. every 6 h	4	

[1]Antibiotic dosages are for patients with normal renal function. I.V. indicates intravenous; I.M. intramuscular.

[2]Patients should be informed that I.M. injection of ceftriaxone is painful.

[3]Ampicillin should not be used if laboratory tests show β-lactamase production.

[4]For specific dosing adjustment and issues concerning gentamicin (obese patients, relative contraindications), see Table 1 footnotes.

Note: Tables 1-6 are from Wilson WR, Karchmer AW, Dajani AS, et al, "Antibiotic Treatment of Adults With Infective Endocarditis Due to Streptococci, Enterococci, Staphylococci, and HACEK Microorganisms," *JAMA*, 1995, 274(21):1706-13, with permission.

CLINICAL SYNDROMES ASSOCIATED WITH FOOD-BORNE DISEASES

Clinical Syndromes	Incubation Period (h)	Causes	Commonly Associated Vehicles
Nausea and vomiting	<1-6	*Staphylococcus aureus* (preformed toxins, A, B, C, D, E)	Ham, poultry, cream-filled pastries, potato and egg salad, mushrooms
		Bacillus cereus (emetic toxin)	Fried rice, pork
		Heavy metals (copper, tin, cadmium, zinc)	Acidic beverages
Histamine response and gastrointestinal (GI) tract	<1	Histamine (scombroid)	Fish (bluefish, bonito, mackerel, mahi-mahi, tuna)
Neurologic, including paresthesia and GI tract	0-6	Tetrodotoxin, ciguatera	Puffer fish Fish (amberjack, barracuda, grouper, snapper)
		Paralytic compounds	Shellfish (clams, mussels, oysters, scallops, other mollusks)
		Neurotoxic compounds	Shellfish
		Domoic acid	Mussels
		Monosodium glutamate	Chinese food
Neurologic and GI tract manifestations	0-2	Mushroom toxins (early onset)	Mushrooms
Moderate-to-severe abdominal cramps and watery diarrhea	8-16	*B. cereus* enterotoxin	Beef, pork, chicken, vanilla sauce
		Clostridium perfringens enterotoxin	Beef, poultry, gravy
	16-48	Caliciviruses	Shellfish, salads, ice
		Enterotoxigenic *Escherichia coli*	Fruits, vegetables
		Vibrio cholerae 01 and 0139	Shellfish
		V. cholerae non-01	Shellfish
Diarrhea, fever, abdominal cramps, blood and mucus in stools	16-72	*Salmonella*	Poultry, pork, eggs, dairy products, including ice cream, vegetables, fruit
		Shigella	Egg salad, vegetables
		Campylobacter jejuni	Poultry, raw milk
		Invasive *E. coli*	
		Yersinia enterocolitica	Pork chitterlings, tofu, raw milk
		Vibrio parahaemolyticus	Fish, shellfish
Bloody diarrhea, abdominal cramps	72-120	Enterohemorrhagic *E. coli*	Beef (hamburger), raw milk, roast beef, salami, salad dressings
Methemoglobin poisoning	6-12	Mushrooms (late onset)	Mushrooms
Hepatorenal failure	6-24	Mushrooms (late onset)	Mushrooms
Gastrointestinal then blurred vision, dry mouth, dysarthria, diplopia, descending paralysis	18-36	*Clostridium botulinum*	Canned vegetables, fruits and fish, salted fish, bottled garlic

Clinical Syndromes	Incubation Period (h)	Causes	Commonly Associated Vehicles
Extraintestinal manifestations	Varied	Brainerd disease	Unpasteurized milk
		Brucella	Cheese, raw milk
		Group A *Streptococcus*	Egg and potato salad
		Listeria monocytogenes	Cheese, raw milk, hot dogs, cole slaw, cold cuts
		Trichinella spiralis	Pork
		Vibrio vulnificus	Shellfish

Adapted from "Report of the Committee on Infectious Diseases," *1997 Red Book®*, 24th ed.

COMMUNITY-ACQUIRED PNEUMONIA IN ADULTS

The initial site of treatment should be based on a 3-step process:

1. assessment of pre-existing conditions that compromise safety of home care
2. calculation of the pneumonia PORT (Pneumonia Outcome Research Team) Severity Index with recommendation for home care for risk classes I, II, and III, and
3. clinical judgment

Algorithm

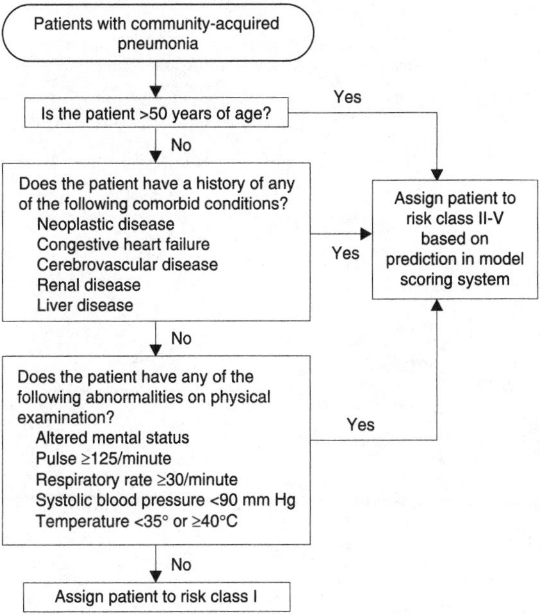

Stratification of Risk Score

Risk	Risk Class	Based on
	I	Algorithm
Low	II	≤70 total points
	III	71-90 total points
Moderate	IV	91-130 total points
High	V	>130 total points

Risk-Class Mortality Rates for Patients With Pneumonia

		Validation Cohort		
Risk Class	No. of Points	No. of Patients	Mortality (%)	Recommended Site of Care
I	No predictors	3034	0.1	Outpatient
II	≤70	5778	0.6	Outpatient
III	71-90	6790	2.8	Outpatient or brief inpatient
IV	91-130	13,104	8.2	Inpatient
V	>130	9333	29.2	Inpatient

Epidemiological Conditions Related to Specific Pathogens in Patients With Selected Community-Acquired Pneumonia

Condition	Commonly Encountered Pathogens
Alcoholism	*Streptococcus pneumoniae*, anaerobes
COPD and/or smoker	*S. pneumoniae, Haemophilus influenzae, Moraxella catarrhalis, Legionella* species
Nursing home residency	*S. pneumoniae*, gram-negative bacilli, *H. influenzae, Staphylococcus aureus*, anaerobes, *Chlamydia pneumoniae*
Poor dental hygiene	Anaerobes
Epidemic Legionnaires' disease	*Legionella* species
Exposure to bats or soil enriched with bird droppings	*Histoplasma capsulatum*
Exposure to birds	*Chlamydia psittaci*
Exposure to rabbits	*Francisella tularensis*
HIV infection (early stage)	*S. pneumoniae, H. influenzae, Mycobacterium tuberculosis*
HIV infection (late stage)	Above plus *P. carinii, Cryptococcus, Histoplasma* species
Travel to southwestern United States	*Coccidioides* species
Exposure to farm animals or parturient cats	*Coxiella burnetii* (Q fever)
Influenza active in community	Influenza, *S. pneumoniae, S. aureus, Streptococcus pyogenes, H. influenzae*
Suspected large-volume aspiration	Anaerobes (chemical pneumonitis, obstruction)
Structural disease of the lung (bronchiectasis, cystic fibrosis, etc)	*Pseudomonas aeruginosa, Burkholderia (Pseudomonas) cepacia, S. aureus*
Injection drug use	*S. aureus*, anaerobes, *M. tuberculosis, S. pneumoniae*
Airway obstruction	Anaerobes, *S. pneumoniae, H. influenzae, S. aureus*

COPD = chronic obstructive pulmonary disease.

COMMUNITY-ACQUIRED PNEUMONIA IN ADULTS
(Continued)

Scoring System: Assignment to Risk Classes II-V

Patient Characteristic	Points Assigned[1]
Demographic factors	
Age	
Male	No. of years
Female	No. of years -10
Nursing home resident	+10
Comorbid illnesses	
Neoplastic disease[2]	+30
Liver disease[3]	+20
Congestive heart failure[4]	+10
Cerebrovascular disease[5]	+10
Renal disease[6]	+10
Physical examination findings	
Altered mental status[7]	+20
Respiratory rate >30 breaths/minute	+20
Systolic blood pressure <90 mm Hg	+20
Temperature <35°C or >40°C	+15
Pulse >125 beats/minute	+10
Laboratory or radiographic findings	
Arterial pH <7.35	+30
BUN >30 mg/dL	+20
Sodium <130 mEq/L	+20
Glucose >250 mg/dL	+10
Hematocrit <30%	+10
pO_2 <60 mm Hg[8]	+10
Pleural effusion	+10

[1]A total point score for a given patient is obtained by adding the patient's age in years (age -10, for females) and the points for each applicable patient characteristic.

[2]Any cancer, except basal or squamous cell cancer of the skin, that was active at the time of presentation or diagnosed within 1 year of presentation.

[3]A clinical or histologic diagnosis of cirrhosis or other form of chronic liver disease such as chronic active hepatitis.

[4]Systolic or diastolic ventricular dysfunction documented by history and physical examination, as well as chest radiography, echocardiography, Muga scanning, or left ventriculography.

[5]A clinical diagnosis of stroke, transient ischemic attack, or stroke documented by MRI or computed axial tomography.

[6]A history of chronic renal disease or abnormal blood urea nitrogen (BUN) and creatinine values documented in the medical record.

[7]Disorientation (to person, place, or time; not known to be chronic), stupor, or coma.

[8]In the Pneumonia Patient Outcome Research Team cohort study, an oxygen saturation value <90% on pulse oximetry or intubation before admission was also considered abnormal.

Table 1. Initial Empiric Therapy for Suspected Bacterial Community-Acquired Pneumonia (CAP) in Immunocompetent Adults

Patient Variable	Preferred Treatment Options
	Outpatient
Previously healthy	
No recent antibiotic therapy	A macrolide[1] or doxycycline
Recent antibiotic therapy[2]	A respiratory fluoroquinolone[3] alone, an advanced macrolide[4] plus high-dose amoxicillin,[5] or an advanced macrolide plus high-dose amoxicillin-clavulanate[6]
Comorbidities (COPD, diabetes, renal or congestive heart failure, or malignancy)	
No recent antibiotic therapy	An advanced macrolide[4] or a respiratory fluoroquinolone
Recent antibiotic therapy	A respiratory fluoroquinolone[3] alone or an advanced macrolide plus a β-lactam[7]
Suspected aspiration with infection	Amoxicillin-clavulanate or clindamycin
Influenza with bacterial superinfection	A β-lactam[7] or a respiratory fluoroquinolone
	Inpatient
Medical ward	
No recent antibiotic therapy	A respiratory fluoroquinolone alone or an advanced macrolide plus a β-lactam[8]
Recent antibiotic therapy	An advanced macrolide plus a β-lactam or a respiratory fluoroquinolone alone (regimen selected will depend on nature of recent antibiotic therapy)
ICU	
Pseudomonas infection is not an issue	A β-lactam[8] plus either an advanced macrolide or a respiratory fluoroquinolone
Pseudomonas infection is not an issue but patient has a β-lactam allergy	A respiratory fluoroquinolone, with or without clindamycin
Pseudomonas infection is an issue[9]	Either (1) an antipseudomonal agent[10] plus ciprofloxacin, or (2) an antipseudomonal agent plus an aminoglycoside[11] plus a respiratory fluoroquinolone or a macrolide
Pseudomonas infection is an issue but the patient has a β-lactam allergy	Either (1) aztreonam plus levofloxacin,[12] or (2) aztreonam plus moxifloxacin or gatifloxacin, with or without an aminoglycoside
Nursing home	
Receiving treatment in nursing home	A respiratory fluoroquinolone alone or amoxicillin-clavulanate plus an advanced macrolide
Hospitalized	Same as for medical ward and ICU

COPD = chronic obstructive pulmonary disease; ICU = intensive care unit.

[1]Erythromycin, azithromycin, or clarithromycin.

[2]That is, the patient was given a course of antibiotic(s) for treatment of any infection within the past 3 months, excluding the current episode of infection. Such treatment is a risk factor for drug-resistant *Streptococcus pneumoniae* and possibly for infection with gram-negative bacilli. Depending on the class of antibiotics recently given, one or other of the suggested options may be selected. Recent use of a fluoroquinolone should dictate selection of a nonfluoroquinolone regimen, and vice versa.

[3]Moxifloxacin, gatifloxacin, levofloxacin, or gemifloxacin (oral gemifloxacin only, which was approved by the U.S. Food and Drug Administration on April 4, 2003 and which is the only fluoroquinolone approved for multidrug-resistant *S. pneumoniae*; not yet marketed).

[4]Azithromycin or clarithromycin.

[5]Dosage, 1 g P.O. 3 times/day.

[6]Dosage, 2 g P.O. twice daily.

[7]High-dose amoxicillin, high-dose amoxicillin-clavulanate, cefpodoxime, cefprozil, or cefuroxime.

[8]Cefotaxime, ceftriaxone, ampicillin-sulbactam, or ertapenem; ertapenem was recently approved for such use (in once-daily parenteral treatment), but there is little experience thus far.

[9]The antipseudomonal agents chosen reflect this concern. Risk factors for *Pseudomonas* infection include severe structural lung disease (eg, bronchiectasis), and recent antibiotic therapy or stay in hospital (especially in the ICU). For patients with CAP in the ICU, coverage for *S. pneumoniae* and *Legionella* species must always be assured. Piperacillin-tazobactam, imipenem, meropenem, and cefepime are excellent β-lactams and are adequate for most *S. pneumoniae* and *Haemophilus influenzae* infections. They may be preferred when there is concern for relatively unusual CAP pathogens, such as *Pseudomonas aeruginosa*, *Klebsiella* species, and other gram-negative bacteria.

[10]Piperacillin, piperacillin-tazobactam, imipenem, meropenem, or cefepime.

[11]Data suggest that elderly patients receiving aminoglycosides have worse outcomes.

[12]Dosage for hospitalized patients, 750 mg daily.

COMMUNITY-ACQUIRED PNEUMONIA IN ADULTS
(Continued)

Table 2. Empiric Antibacterial Selection for Community-Acquired Pneumonia (CAP): Advantages and Disadvantages

Patient Group, Drug(s)	Advantages	Disadvantages
	Outpatients	
Macrolides (azithromycin, clarithromycin, and erythromycin)	Active against most common pathogen, including atypical agents.	Macrolide resistance is reported for 20% to 30% of *Streptococcus pneumoniae*, and *in vitro* resistance has emerged during therapy.
	S. pneumoniae resistance *in vitro* may be deceptive, because the M phenotype may not be clinically relevant, and alveolar lining fluid or intracellular levels may be more important than serum levels used to determine *in vitro* activity.	Breakthrough pneumococcal bacteria with macrolide-resistant strains appear to be more common than with β-lactams or fluoroquinolones.
	Clinical trial data have shown consistently good results, including activity against strains resistant *in vitro*.	Erythromycin is poorly tolerated and is less effective against *Haemophilus influenzae*.
	Azithromycin and clarithromycin have the advantage of once-daily therapy and are well tolerated.	
Amoxicillin	Amoxicillin is the preferred drug for oral treatment of susceptible strains of *S. pneumoniae*.	Lacks activity against atypical agents and β-lactamase producing bacteria.
	Active against 90% to 95% of *S. pneumoniae* strains when used at a dosage of 3-4 g/day.	High dosages (3-4 g/day) required to achieve activity against >90% of *S. pneumoniae*
	Standard in many European CAP guidelines for empiric treatment of outpatients, as well as CDC guidelines.	The number of recent publications documenting efficacy is modest.
Amoxicillin-clavulanate	Compared with amoxicillin, spectrum *in vitro* includes β-lactamase producing bacteria, such as most *H. influenzae*, methicillin-susceptible *Staphylococcus aureus*, and anaerobes.	Lacks activity against atypical agents.
	Clinical trials reported to document efficacy.	More expensive and more gastrointestinal intolerance, compared with amoxicillin.
	Standard in many European CAP guidelines for empiric treatment of outpatients, as well as CDC guidelines.	The number of recent publications documenting efficacy is relatively modest.
Oral cephalosporins (cefpodoxime, cefprozil and cefuroxime axetil)	Active against 75% to 85% of *S. pneumoniae* and virtually all *H. influenzae*	All cephalosporins (and all β-lactams) are inactive against atypical agents.
	Clinical trial data support efficacy in outpatients with CAP.	Amoxicillin is more predictably active against *S. pneumoniae* (cefprozil and cefpodoxime are more active than cefuroxime).
Doxycycline	Active against 90% to 95% of strains of *S. pneumoniae*; also active against *H. influenzae*, atypical agents, and category A bacterial agents of bioterrorism.	Very limited recent published clinical data on CAP, and few clinicians use it.
	At least 1 recent report showing good outcomes in hospitalized patients with CAP.	
	Generally well tolerated and inexpensive.	

Table 2. Empiric Antibacterial Selection for Community-Acquired Pneumonia (CAP): Advantages and Disadvantages *(continued)*

Patient Group, Drug(s)	Advantages	Disadvantages
Fluoroquinolones (gatifloxacin, levofloxacin, moxifloxacin, and gemifloxacin)	Active against >98% of *S. pneumoniae* strains in United States, including penicillin-resistant strains.	Concern for abuse with risk of increasing resistance by *S. pneumoniae*; this includes clinical failures attributed to emergence of resistance during therapy and selection of resistant strains such as 23F that may be prevalent in selected areas and are usually resistant to macrolides and β-lactams as well.
	Substantial comparative clinical trial data to confirm equivalence or superiority to alternative commonly used regimens, and a meta-analysis of trials showed significantly better outcomes than for β-lactams or macrolides.	Expensive compared with some alternatives, such as doxycycline or erythromycin.
	Active against *H. influenzae*, atypical agents, methicillin-susceptible *S. aureus*, and category A bacterial agents of bioterrorism.	
	Regimens have advantage of once-daily administration and are well tolerated.	
Clindamycin	Active against 90% of *S. pneumoniae*.	Not active against *H. influenzae* or atypical agents.
	Good *in vitro* activity and established efficacy in anaerobic bacterial infections and favored for toxic shock associated with pneumonia due to group A streptococci.	Limited published data on use for CAP.
		High rates of diarrhea and *Clostridium difficile* associated colitis.
Macrolide plus amoxicillin-clavulanate	Macrolide adds activity against atypical agents to spectrum of amoxicillin-clavulanate (described above).	Limited published data for outpatients.
		Requires high dosages of amoxicillin-clavulanate (4 g/day).
		High rates of gastrointestinal intolerance anticipated.
		Unlikely to be effective against fluoroquinolone-resistant strains of *S. pneumoniae*.
		Escalating rates of resistance to both macrolides and penicillin by *S. pneumoniae*.
	Hospitalized Patients	
Fluoroquinolones (gatifloxacin, levofloxacin, moxifloxacin, and gemifloxacin)	Broad spectrum of activity against likely agents of CAP (summarized above).	Concern for increasing resistance, as summarized above.
	Extensive published data, including retrospective analysis of hospitalized Medicare patients, showing significantly lower mortality than for macrolides alone or cephalosporins alone.	Clinical failures attributed to resistant strains reported.
	Efficacy in serious infections, including bacteremic pneumococcal pneumonia, established.	

COMMUNITY-ACQUIRED PNEUMONIA IN ADULTS
(Continued)

Table 2. Empiric Antibacterial Selection for Community-Acquired Pneumonia (CAP): Advantages and Disadvantages *(continued)*

Patient Group, Drug(s)	Advantages	Disadvantages
	Available in oral and parenteral formulations (except for gemifloxacin, for which only oral formulations are available), facilitating intravenous-to-oral switch.	
Macrolides (azithromycin and erythromycin)	*In vitro* spectrum summarized above.	Retrospective analysis of 14,000 hospitalized Medicare recipients for 1998-1999 shows mortality rate for macrolide alone was significantly greater than that for cephalosporin plus a macrolide or a fluoroquinolone alone.
	Extensive clinical trial data and clinical experience to document efficacy for CAP.	Increasing *in vitro* resistance by *S. pneumoniae*, as summarized above.
	Azithromycin is included as an appropriate choice in many current CAP guidelines, including the guidelines of the American Thoracic Society.	Breakthrough bacteremia due to resistant strains of *S. pneumoniae* is unusual but appears to be more common with macrolides than with other agents.
Cephalosporins (ceftriaxone and cefotaxime)	Considered the parenteral drugs of choice (as well as penicillin G) for CAP caused by susceptible strains of *S. pneumoniae*.	Not active against atypical agents or category A agents of bioterrorism.
	Active *in vitro* against 90% to 95% of *S. pneumoniae*; also active against *H. influenzae* and methicillin-susceptible *S. aureus*.	Retrospective analysis of 14,000 Medicare patients showed higher mortality for cephalosporins alone than for cephalosporins plus macrolides or fluoroquinolones alone.
	Extensive clinical trial experience to document efficacy.	Increasing resistance by *S. pneumoniae*.
Fluoroquinolone plus cephalosporin	May increase antimicrobial activity against *S. pneumoniae*.	No documented benefit, compared with fluoroquinolone alone.
Macrolide plus cephalosporin	Cephalosporin provides better *in vitro* activity against *S. pneumoniae*, and macrolide adds activity against atypical agents.	Data suggesting that the macrolide-cephalosporin combination is superior to monotherapy in pneumococcal bacteremia are uncontrolled and inconsistent (P. Houck, personal communication).
	Retrospective analyses show reduced mortality for this combination, compared with single-agent therapy, in patients with pneumococcal bacteremia and for empiric treatment of pneumonia.	
Penicillin G	Preferred agent (along with ceftriaxone, cefotaxime, and amoxicillin) for proven penicillin-susceptible strains of *S. pneumoniae*.	Limited spectrum of activity against common pulmonary pathogens other than *S. pneumoniae*.
	Published experience to document clinical efficacy is extensive.	

Table 2. Empiric Antibacterial Selection for Community-Acquired Pneumonia (CAP): Advantages and Disadvantages *(continued)*

Patient Group, Drug(s)	Advantages	Disadvantages
	New Agents	
Telithromycin	Active *in vitro* against most *S. pneumoniae*, including macrolide-resistant strains; also active against *H. influenzae* and atypical agents.	Available only in oral formulation.
	Favorable pharmacokinetics.	Clinical trial data are considered preliminary.
	Clinical trials in CAP show equivalence to high-dose amoxicillin, macrolides, and trovafloxacin, including CAP caused by β-lactam resistant strains of *S. pneumoniae*.	
Gemifloxacin	Most active of the "respiratory fluoroquinolone" against *S. pneumoniae in vitro*.	High rate of rash, especially in women aged <40 years and with use for >10 days.
	Clinical trial data for CAP show good results.	Available only in oral formulation.
Ertapenem	Clinical efficacy for empiric treatment of CAP comparable to ceftriaxone.	Parenteral formulation only.
	Once-daily parenteral dosing.	Inactive against atypical agents and less active than imipenem against *Pseudomonas aeruginosa*.
	In vitro activity against *S. pneumoniae* is similar to ceftriaxone and cefotaxime.	
Linezolid	Active *in vitro* against most gram-positive bacteria, including multidrug resistant *S. pneumoniae* and *S. aureus*.	Lacks established activity against atypical agents.
	Efficacy comparable to ceftriaxone for treatment of pneumococcal pneumonia.	Alternative antimicrobials have more established role in CAP.
	Oral and parenteral formulations.	Concern about abuse, expense, drug-drug interaction, and toxicity.

Note: Durations of therapy are as follows: *S. pneumoniae*, until afebrile for 72 hours; *M. pneumoniae*, duration of therapy for newer agents is not well established; *C. pneumoniae*, numerous clinical trials indicate good clinical response with 7-14 days of treatment; *Legionella*, 10-21 days; pathogens that potentially cause pulmonary necrosis (*S. aureus, P. aeruginosa, Klebsiella* species, or anaerobes), ≥2 weeks. CDC, Centers for Disease Control and Prevention.

COMMUNITY-ACQUIRED PNEUMONIA IN ADULTS
(Continued)

ANTIMICROBIAL TREATMENT

Pathogen-Specific Therapy

S. pneumoniae: Susceptibility of *S. pneumoniae* isolates to cefotaxime and ceftriaxone in nonmeningeal infections should be defined as an MIC of ≤1 mcg/mL, intermediate should be defined as an MIC of 2 mcg/mL, and resistant should be defined as an MIC of ≥4 mcg/mL. Cefotaxime or ceftriaxone are the preferred parenteral agents for treatment of pneumococcal pneumonia without meningitis for strains with reduced susceptibility to penicillin but with MICs of cefotaxime or ceftriaxone of <2 mcg/mL. Amoxicillin is the preferred antibiotic for oral treatment of pneumococcal pneumonia involving susceptible strains.

Initial empiric therapy prior to availability of culture data for a patient ill enough to require admission to a hospital ward can be with a β-lactam plus macrolide combination or a respiratory fluoroquinolone alone. If sufficiently ill to need ICU management and if *Pseudomonas* infection is not a concern, a combination of a β-lactam plus either a macrolide or a respiratory fluoroquinolone should be used. Once culture data are available and it is known that the patient has pneumococcal pneumonia with bacteremia without evidence to support infection with a copathogen, treatment will depend upon *in vitro* susceptibility results. If the isolate is penicillin susceptible, a β-lactam (penicillin G or amoxicillin) alone may be used. If the isolate is penicillin resistant, cefotaxime, ceftriaxone, or a respiratory fluoroquinolone or other agent indicated by *in vitro* testing may be used.

Legionella: Treatment for legionnaires' disease is appropriate when there is epidemiologic evidence of this disease, despite negative diagnostic test results. The preferred treatment for legionnaires' disease for hospitalized patients is azithromycin or a fluoroquinolone (moxifloxacin, gatifloxacin, and levofloxacin; gemifloxacin is only available as an oral formulation). For patients who do not require hospitalization, acceptable antibiotics include erythromycin, doxycycline, azithromycin, clarithromycin, or a fluoroquinolone. Treatment should be initiated as rapidly as is feasible.

Influenza: Early treatment (within 48 hours after onset of symptoms) is effective in the treatment of influenza A using amantadine, rimantadine, oseltamivir, or zanamivir and is effective in the treatment influenza B using oseltamivir and zanamivir. Use of these drugs is not recommended for uncomplicated influenza with a duration of symptoms of >48 hours, but these drugs may be used to reduce viral shedding in hospitalized patients or for influenza pneumonia.

Herpes viruses: Pneumonia caused by varicella zoster virus or herpes simplex virus should be treated with parenteral acyclovir.

Other viruses: There is no antiviral agent with established efficacy for the treatment of adults with pulmonary infections involving parainfluenza virus, respiratory syncytial virus, adenovirus, metapneumovirus, the SARS agent, or Hantavirus.

Empiric Therapy

See Table 1 and Table 2.

Empiric treatment of suspected bacterial superinfection of influenza should provide activity against *S. pneumoniae, Staphylococcus aureus*, and *Haemophilus influenzae* with antibiotics such as amoxicillin-clavulanate, cefpodoxime, cefprozil, cefuroxime, or a respiratory fluoroquinolone.

Fluoroquinolones (gatifloxacin, gemifloxacin, levofloxacin, and moxifloxacin) are recommended for initial empiric therapy of selected outpatients with CAP. Other options (macrolides and doxycycline) are generally preferred for uncomplicated infections in outpatients. Fluoroquinolones (gatifloxacin, gemifloxacin, levofloxacin, and moxifloxacin) may be used as monotherapy for patients with CAP who are admitted to a hospital ward. With the exception of gemifloxacin (no intravenous formulation), they may be used as part of a combination for patients with CAP admitted to an ICU.

A macrolide is recommended as monotherapy for selected outpatients, such as those who were previously well and not recently treated with antibiotics. A macrolide plus a β-lactam is recommended for initial empiric treatment of outpatients in whom resistance is an issue and for hospitalized patients.

Telithromycin may have a role as an alternative to macrolides for treatment of patients with CAP.

Special Populations and Circumstances

SARS: Health care workers must be vigilant in recognizing SARS because of important epidemiologic implications, which include the potential for rapid spread to close contacts, including health care workers and household contacts. The major therapeutic intervention is supportive care. Preventive efforts include proper precautions in patients with suspected or established SARS. These include standard precautions (hand hygiene), contact precautions (use of gowns, goggles, and gloves), and airborne precautions (use of negative-pressure rooms and fit-tested N95 respirators).

Elderly patients: Antimicrobial selection for elderly patients with CAP is the same as for all adults with CAP.

Bioterrorism: Physicians should know the clues to bioterrorism and the appropriate mechanisms to alert public health officials in cases of suspected bioterrorism. Recommended diagnostic tests and management guidelines are those of the Johns Hopkins Center for Biodefense Strategies and of the CDC, as modified for the specific outbreak.

References

Bartlett JG, Breiman RF, Mandell LA, et al, "Community-Acquired Pneumonia in Adults: Guidelines for Management. The Infectious Diseases Society of America," *Clin Infect Dis*, 1998, 26(4):811-38.

Mandell LA, Bartlett JG, Dowell SF, et al, "Update of Practice Guidelines for the Management of Community-Acquired Pneumonia in Immunocompetent Adults," *Clin Infect Dis*, 2003, 37(11):1405-33.

HELICOBACTER PYLORI TREATMENT

Multiple Drug Regimens for the Treatment of *H. pylori* Infection

Drug	Dosages	Duration of Therapy
H_2-receptor antagonist[1]	Any one given at appropriate dose	4 weeks
plus		
Bismuth subsalicylate	525 mg 4 times/day	2 weeks
plus		
Metronidazole	250 mg 4 times/day	2 weeks
plus		
Tetracycline	500 mg 4 times/day	2 weeks
Proton pump inhibitor[1]	Esomeprazole 40 mg once daily	10 days
plus		
Clarithromycin	500 mg twice daily	10 days
plus		
Amoxicillin	1000 mg twice daily	10 days
Proton pump inhibitor[1]	Lansoprazole 30 mg twice daily or Omeprazole 20 mg twice daily	10-14 days
plus		
Clarithromycin	500 mg twice daily	10-14 days
plus		
Amoxicillin	1000 mg twice daily	10-14 days
Proton pump inhibitor[1]	Rabeprazole 20 mg twice daily	7 days
plus		
Clarithromycin	500 mg twice daily	7 days
plus		
Amoxicillin	1000 mg twice daily	7 days
Proton pump inhibitor	Lansoprazole 30 mg twice daily or Omeprazole 20 mg twice daily	2 weeks
plus		
Clarithromycin	500 mg twice daily	2 weeks
plus		
Metronidazole	500 mg twice daily	2 weeks
Proton pump inhibitor	Lansoprazole 30 mg once daily or Omeprazole 20 mg once daily	2 weeks
plus		
Bismuth	525 mg 4 times/day	2 weeks
plus		
Metronidazole	500 mg 3 times/day	2 weeks
plus		
Tetracycline	500 mg 4 times/day	2 weeks

[1]FDA-approved regimen.

Modified from Howden CS and Hunt RH, "Guidelines for the Management of *Helicobacter pylori* Infection," *AJG*, 1998, 93:2336.

INTERPRETATION OF GRAM STAIN RESULTS GUIDELINES

These guidelines are not definitive but presumptive for the identification of organisms on Gram stain. Treatment will depend on the quality of the specimen and appropriate clinical evaluation.

Gram-Negative Bacilli (GNB)	**Example**
Enterobacteriaceae	*Citrobacter* sp *Enterobacter* sp *Escherichia coli* *Klebsiella* sp *Serratia* sp
Nonfermentative GNB	*Bacteroides fragilis* group *Pseudomonas aeruginosa* *Stenotrophomonas maltophilia*
If fusiform (long and pointed)	*Capnocytophaga* sp *Fusobacterium* sp
Gram-Negative Cocci (GNC)	
Diplococci, pairs	*Moraxella (Branhamella) catarrhalis* *Neisseria gonorrhoeae* *Neisseria meningitidis*
Coccobacilli	*Acinetobacter* sp *Haemophilus influenzae*
Gram-Positive Bacilli (GPB)	
Diphtheroids (small pleomorphic)	*Corynebacterium* sp *Propionibacterium*
Large, with spores	*Bacillus* sp *Clostridium* sp
Branching, beaded, rods	*Actinomyces* sp *Nocardia* sp
Other	*Lactobacillus* sp *Listeria* sp
Gram-Positive Cocci (GPC)	
Pairs, chains, clusters	*Enterococcus* sp *Staphylococcus* sp *Streptococcus* sp
Pairs, lancet-shaped	*Streptococcus pneumoniae*

KEY CHARACTERISTICS OF SELECTED BACTERIA

Gram-Negative Bacilli (GNB)	Example
Lactose-positive	*Citrobacter* sp[1] (Enterobacteriaceae) *Enterobacter* sp[1] (Enterobacteriaceae) *Escherichia coli* (Enterobacteriaceae) *Klebsiella pneumoniae* (Enterobacteriaceae)
Lactose-negative/oxidase-negative	*Acinetobacter* sp *Morganella morganii* *Proteus mirabilis*: indole-negative *Proteus vulgaris*: indole-positive *Providencia* sp *Salmonella* sp *Serratia* sp[2] (Enterobacteriaceae) *Shigella* sp *Xanthomonas maltophilia*
Lactose-negative/oxidase-positive	*Aeromonas hydrophila* (may be lactose positive) *Alcaligenes* sp *Flavobacterium* sp *Moraxella* sp[3] *Pseudomonas aeruginosa* Other *Pseudomonas* sp
Anaerobes	*Bacteroides* sp (*B. fragilis*) *Fusobacterium* sp
Other	*Haemophilus influenzae* (coccobacillus)
Gram-Positive Bacilli (GPB)	
Anaerobes	*Lactobacillus* sp *Eubacterium* sp *Clostridium* sp (spores) *Bifidobacterium* sp *Actinomyces* sp (branching, filamentous) *Propionibacterium acnes*
Bacillus sp	*B. cereus, B. subtilis* (large with spores)
Branching, beaded; partial acid-fast positive	*Nocardia* sp
CSF, blood	*Listeria monocytogenes*
Rapidly growing mycobacteria	*M. fortuitum* *M. chelonei*
Vaginal flora, rarely blood	*Lactobacillus* sp
Often blood culture contaminants	Diphtheroids (may be *Corynebacterium* sp)
Resistant to many agents except vancomycin	*C. jeikeium*
Other	*Actinomyces* sp (branching, beaded)
Gram-Negative Cocci (GNC)	
Diplococci, pairs	*Capnocytophaga* sp *Fusobacterium* sp (fusiform) *Moraxella catarrhalis* *Neisseria meningitidis* *Neisseria gonorrhoeae*
Coccobacilli	*Acinetobacter* sp
Anaerobes	*Veillonella* sp
Gram-Positive Cocci (GPC)	
Catalase-negative	*Streptococcus* sp (chains) *Micrococcus* sp (usually insignificant)
Catalase-positive	*Staphylococcus* sp (pairs, chains, clusters)
Coagulase-negative	Coagulase-negative staphylococci (CNS)
Bloods	*S. epidermidis* or CNS
Urine	*S. saprophyticus* (CNS)
Coagulase-positive	*S. aureus*
Anaerobes	*Peptostreptococcus* sp

Fungi	
Molds	
Sparsely septate hyphae	Zygomycetes (eg, *Rhizopus* sp and *Mucor*)
Septate hyphae brown pigment	Phaeohyphomycetes, for example, *Alternaria* sp *Bipolaris* sp *Curvularia* sp *Exserohilum* sp
Nonpigmented (hyaline)	Hyalophomycetes, for example *Aspergillus* sp (*A. fumigatus, A. flavus*) Dermatophytes *Fusarium* sp *Paecilomyces* sp *Penicillium* sp
Thermally dimorphic (yeast in tissue; mold *in vitro*)	*Blastomyces dermatitidis* *Coccidioides immitis* *Histoplasma capsulatum* (slow growing) *Paracoccidioides brasiliensis* *Sporothrix schenckii*
Yeast	*Candida* sp (germ tube positive = *C. albicans* *Cryptococcus* sp (no pseudohyphae) *C. neoformans* *Rhodotorula, Saccharomyces* sp *Torulopsis glabrata* *Trichosporon* sp
Virus	Influenza Hepatitis A, B, C, D Human immunodeficiency virus Rubella Herpes Cytomegalovirus Respiratory syncytial virus Epstein-Barr
Chlamydiae	*Chlamydia trachomatis* *Chlamydia pneumoniae* (TWAR) *Chlamydia psittaci*
Rickettsiae	
Ureaplasma	
Mycoplasma	*Mycoplasma pneumoniae* *Mycoplasma hominis*
Spirochetes	*Treponema pallidum* *Borrelia burgdorferi*
Mycobacteria	*Mycobacterium tuberculosis* *Mycobacterium intracellulare*

Most Common Blood Culture Contaminants

Alpha-hemolytic streptococci

Bacillus sp

Coagulase-negative staphylococci

Diphtheroids

Lactobacilli

Micrococcus sp

Propionibacterium sp

[1]May be lactose-negative.

[2]May produce red pigment and appear lactose-positive initially.

[3]May be either bacillary or coccoid.

MALARIA TREATMENT

Drug of Choice	Adult Dosage	Pediatric Dosage
Chloroquine-Resistance *Plasmodium falciparum*[1]		
ORAL		
Quinine sulfate	650 mg q8h x 3-7 d[2]	25 mg/kg/d in 3 doses x 3-7 d[2]
plus doxycycline[3,4]	100 mg bid x 7 d	2 mg/kg/d x 7 d
or plus tetracycline[3,4]	250 mg qid x 7 d	6.25 mg/kg qid x 7 d
or plus pyrimethamine-sulfadoxine[5]	3 tablets at once on last day of quinine	<1 y: 1/4 tablet 1-3 y: 1/2 tablet 4-8 y: 1 tablet 9-14 y: 2 tablets
or plus clindamycin[3,6]	900 mg tid x 5 d	20-40 mg/kg/d in 3 doses x 5 d
OR		
Atovaquone/proguanil[7]	2 adult tablets bid x 3 d	11-20 kg: 1 adult tablet/day x 3 d 21-30 kg: 2 adult tablets/day x 3 d 31-40 kg: 3 adult tablets/day x 3 d >40 kg: 2 adult tablets bid x 3 d
***Alternatives:*[8]**		
Mefloquine[9,10]	750 mg followed by 500 mg 12 h later	<45 kg: 15 mg/kg P.O. followed by 10 mg/kg P.O. 8-12 h later
Halofantrine[11]	500 mg q6h x 3 doses; repeat in 1 week[12]	<40 kg: 8 mg/kg q6h x 3 doses; repeat in 1 week[12]
OR		
Artesunate[13]*	4 mg/kg/d x 3 d	
plus mefloquine[9,10]	750 mg followed by 500 mg 12 h later	15 mg/kg followed 8-12 h later by 10 mg/kg
Chloroquine-Resistant *P. vivax*[14]		
Quinine sulfate	650 mg q8h x 3-7 d[2]	25 mg/kg/d in 3 doses x 3-7 d[2]
plus doxycycline[3,4]	100 mg bid x 7 d	2 mg/kg/d x 7 d
OR		
Mefloquine[9,10]	750 mg followed by 500 mg 12 h later	15 mg/kg followed 8-12 h later by 10 mg/kg
Alternatives:		
Halofantrine[11,15]*	500 mg q6h x 3 doses	8 mg/kg q6h x 3 doses
Chloroquine	25 mg base/kg in 3 doses over 48 h	
plus primaquine[16]	2.5 mg base/kg in 3 doses over 48 h	
All *Plasmodium* Except Chloroquine-Resistant *P. falciparum*[1] and Chloroquine-Resistant *P. vivax*[14]		
ORAL		
Chloroquine phosphate[17]	1 g (600 mg base), then 500 mg (300 mg base) 6 h later, then 500 mg (300 mg base) at 24 and 48 h	10 mg base/kg (max 600 mg base), then 5 mg base/kg 6 h later, then 5 mg base/kg at 24 and 48 h
All *Plasmodium*[18]		
PARENTERAL		
Quinidine gluconate[19]	10 mg/kg loading dose (max 600 mg) in normal saline slowly over 1-2 h, followed by continuous infusion of 0.02 mg/kg/min until oral therapy can be started	Same as adult dose
OR		
Quinine dihydrochloride[19]	20 mg/kg loading dose I.V. in 5% dextrose over 4 h, followed by 10 mg/kg over 2-4 h q8h (max: 1800 mg/d) until oral therapy can be started	Same as adult dose
Alternative		
Artemether[20]*	3.2 mg/kg I.M., then 1.6 mg/kg daily x 5-7 d	Same as adult dose

Drug of Choice	Adult Dosage	Pediatric Dosage
Prevention of Relapses: *P. vivax* and *P. ovale* Only		
Primaquine phosphate[16,21]	26.3 mg (15 mg base)/d x 14 d **or** 79 mg (45 mg base)/wk x 8 wk	0.3 mg base/kg/d x 14 d

*Availability problems.

[1]Chloroquine-resistant *P. falciparum* occur in all malarious areas except Central America west of the Panama Canal Zone, Mexico, Haiti, the Dominican Republic, and most of the Middle East (chloroquine resistance has been reported in Yemen, Oman, Saudi Arabia, and Iran).

[2]In Southeast Asia, relative resistance to quinine has increased and the treatment should be continued for 7 days.

[3]An approved drug, but considered investigational for this condition by the U.S. Food and Drug Administration.

[4]Use of tetracyclines is contraindicated in pregnancy and in children <8 years of age.

[5]Fansidar® tablets contain 25 mg pyrimethamine and 500 mg sulfadoxine. Resistance to pyrimethamine-sulfadoxine has been reported from Southeast Asia, the Amazon Basin, sub-Saharan Africa, Bangladesh, and Oceania.

[6]For use in pregnancy.

[7]Atovaquone plus proguanil is available as a fixed-dose combination tablet: adult tablets (250 mg atovaquone/100 mg proguanil, Malarone™) and pediatric tablets (62.5 mg atovaquone/25 mg proguanil, Malarone™ Pediatric). To enhance absorption, it should be taken within 45 minutes after eating (Looareesuwan S, Chulay JD, Canfield CJ, "Malarone™ (Atovaquone and Proguanil Hydrochloride): A Review of Its Clinical Development for Treatment of Malaria, Malarone Clinical Trials Study Group," *Am J Trop Med Hyg*, 1999, 60(4):533-41). Although approved for once daily dosing, to decrease nausea and vomiting the dose for treatment is usually divided in two.

[8]For treatment of multiple-drug-resistant *P. falciparum* in Southeast Asia, especially Thailand, where resistance to mefloquine and halofantrine is frequent, a 7-day course of quinine and tetracycline is recommended (Watt G, Loesuttivibool L, Shanks GD, et al, "Quinine With Tetracycline for the Treatment of Drug-Resistant *Falciparum malariae* in Thailand," *Am J Trop Med Hyg*, 1992, 47(1):108-11). Artesunate plus mefloquine (Luxemburger C, ter Kuile FO, Nosten F, et al, "Single Day Mefloquine-Artesunate Combination in the Treatment of Multi-drug Resistant *Falciparum malariae*," *Trans R Soc Trop Med Hyg*, 1994, 88(2):213-7), artemether plus mefloquine (Karbwang J et al, *Trans R Soc Trop Med Hyg*, 1995, 89:296), mefloquine plus doxycycline or atovaquone/proguanil may also be used to treat multiple-drug-resistant *P. falciparum*.

[9]At this dosage, adverse effects including nausea, vomiting, diarrhea, dizziness, disturbed sense of balance, toxic psychosis, and seizures can occur. Mefloquine is teratogenic in animals and should not be used for treatment of malaria in pregnancy. It should not be given together with quinine, quinidine, or halofantrine, and caution is required in using quinine, quinidine, or halofantrine to treat patients with malaria who have taken mefloquine for prophylaxis. The pediatric dosage has not been approved by the FDA. Resistance to mefloquine has been reported in some areas, such as the Thailand-Myanmar and Cambodia borders and in the Amazon basin, where 25 mg/kg should be used.

[10]In the U.S.A., a 250 mg tablet of mefloquine contains 228 mg mefloquine base. Outside the U.S.A., each 275 mg tablet contains 250 mg base.

[11]May be effective in multiple-drug-resistant *P. falciparum* malaria, but treatment failures and resistance have been reported, and the drug has caused lengthening of the PR and QTc intervals and fatal cardiac arrhythmias. It should not be used for patients with cardiac conduction defects or with other drugs that may affect the QT interval, such as quinine, quinidine, and mefloquine. Cardiac monitoring is recommended. Variability in absorption is a problem; halofantrine should not be taken 1 hour before to 2 hours after meals because food increases its absorption. It should not be used in pregnancy.

[12]A single 250 mg dose can be used for repeat treatment in mild to moderate infections (Touze JE, Perret JL, Nicolas X, et al, "Efficacy of Low-Dose Halofantrine for Second Treatment of Uncomplicated *P. falciparum* malaria," *Lancet*, 1997, 349(9047):255-6.

[13]Na-Bangchang K, Tippanangkosol P, Ubalee R, et al, "Comparative Clinical Trial of Four Regimens of Dihydroartemisinin-Mefloquine in Multidrug-Resistant *Falciparum malaria*," *Trop Med Int Health*, 1999, 4(9):602-10.

[14]*P. vivax* with decreased susceptibility to chloroquine is a significant problem in Papua-New Guinea and Indonesia. There are also a few reports of resistance from Myanmar, India, Thailand, the Solomon Islands, Vanuatu, Guyana, Brazil, Colombia, and Peru.

[15]Baird JK, Basri H, Subianto B, et al, "Treatment of Chloroquine-Resistant *Plasmodium vivax* With Chloroquine and Primaquine or Halofantrine," *J Infect Dis*, 1995, 171(6):1678-82.

[16]Primaquine phosphate can cause hemolytic anemia, especially in patients whose red cells are deficient in glucose-6-phosphate dehydrogenase. This deficiency is most common in African, Asian, and Mediterranean peoples. Patients should be screened for G-6-PD deficiency before treatment. Primaquine should not be used during pregnancy.

[17]If chloroquine phosphate is not available, hydroxychloroquine sulfate is as effective; 400 mg of hydroxychloroquine sulfate is equivalent to 500 mg of chloroquine phosphate.

[18]Exchange transfusion has been helpful for some patients with high-density (>10%) parasitemia, altered mental status, pulmonary edema, or renal complications (Miller KD, Greenberg AE, and Campbell CC, "Treatment of Severe Malaria in the United States With a Continuous Infusion of Quinidine Gluconate and Exchange Transfusion," *N Engl J Med*, 1989, 321(2):65-7).

[19]Continuous ECG, blood pressure and glucose monitoring are recommended, especially in pregnant women and young children. For problems with quinidine availability, call the manufacturer (Eli Lilly, 800-821-0538) or the CDC Malaria Hotline (770-488-7788). Quinidine may have greater antimalarial activity than quinine. The loading dose should be decreased or omitted in those patients who have

MALARIA TREATMENT *(Continued)*

received quinine or mefloquine. If >48 hours of parenteral treatment is required, the quinine or quinidine dose should be reduced by 1/3 to 1/2.

[20]Artemether-Quinine Meta-Analysis Study Group, "A Meta-Analysis Using Individual Patient Data of Trials Comparing Artemether With Quinine in the Treatment of Severe *Falciparum* Malaria," *Trans R Soc Trop Med Hyg*, 2001, 95(6):637-50. Not available in the United States.

[21]Relapses have been reported with this regimen, and should be treated with a second 14-day course of 30 mg base/day. In Southeast Asia and Somalia the higher dose (30 mg base/day) should be used initially.

Adapted from "Report of the Committee on Infectious Diseases," *2003, Red Book*®, 26th ed, 756-9.

NEUTROPENIC FEVER GUIDELINES

From Hughes WT, Armstrong D, Bodey GP, et al, "2002 Guidelines for the Use of Antimicrobial Agents in Neutropenic Patients With Cancer," *Clin Infect Dis*, 2002, 34(6):730-51.

2002 GUIDELINES FOR THE USE OF ANTIMICROBIAL AGENTS IN NEUTROPENIC PATIENTS WITH CANCER

EXECUTIVE SUMMARY

Fever: A single oral temperature of ≥38.3°C (101°F) or ≥38.0°C (100.4°F) over at least 1 hour.

Neutropenia: Neutrophil count <500/mm^3 or <1000/mm^3 with predicted decline to <500/mm^3.

Evaluation: Cultures of blood (peripheral and catheter), lesions, and diarrheal stools; chest radiograph; complete blood count; determination of levels of transaminases, sodium, potassium, creatinine, and blood urea nitrogen. Other tests as indicated.

Initial Antibiotic Therapy

Oral therapy (low risk only): Ciprofloxacin **plus** amoxicillin-clavulanate

If vancomycin is **not** needed:

Monotherapy: Cefepime, ceftazidime, imipenem, or meropenem)

or

Duotherapy: Aminoglycoside **plus** antipseudomonal penicillin, cefepime, ceftazidime, imipenem, or meropenem

If vancomycin **is** needed (high risk):

Vancomycin

plus

Ceftazidime or cefepime ± aminoglycoside

or

Antipseudomonal penicillin + aminoglycoside

or

Imipenem or meropenem ± aminoglycoside

Modification During the First Week of Treatment

If afebrile within first 3-5 days of treatment:

- Etiologic agent identified: Adjust to most appropriate therapy.
- Etiologic agent not identified:
  - Low initial risk: Continue oral therapy or change to oral ciprofloxacin plus amoxicillin-clavulanate after 48 hours in patients initiated on intravenous therapy.
  - High initial risk: Continue intravenous regimen.

Persistent fever throughout first 3-5 days:

- Reassess therapy on day 3.
  - If no worsening, continue initial antibiotic regimen; discontinue vancomycin if cultures do not indicate organisms.
  - Change antibiotic regimen if there is clinical deterioration.
- If fever persists to day 5, consider antifungal therapy, with or without a change in initial antibiotic regimen.

NEUTROPENIC FEVER GUIDELINES *(Continued)*

Duration of Antibiotic Therapy

Afebrile by day 3:

- If neutrophil count ≥500/mm^3 for 2 consecutive days:
  - If there is no definite source of infection and cultures negative, stop when patient has been afebrile for ≥48 hours.
- If neutrophil count <500/mm^3 by day 7:
  - Low risk and no subsequent complications: Stop therapy when patient is afebrile for 5-7 days.
  - High risk and no subsequent complications: Continue antibiotics.

Persistent fever on day 3:

- If neutrophil count ≥500/mm^3: Stop therapy 4-5 days after the neutrophil count is ≥500/mm^3.
- If neutrophil count <500/mm^3 by day 7: Reassess and continue antibiotic therapy for 2 more weeks. Then reassess and consider stopping therapy if no disease site found.

Use of antivirals: Not routine

Use of colony-stimulating factors: Not routine; consider in certain cases with predicted worsening of course (defined).

Antibiotic prophylaxis in afebrile neutropenic patients: Not routine, except for *Pneumocystis carinii* pneumonitis prophylaxis.

OCCUPATIONAL EXPOSURE TO BLOODBORNE PATHOGENS (UNIVERSAL PRECAUTIONS)

Overview and Regulatory Considerations

Every healthcare employee, from nurse to housekeeper, has some (albeit small) risk of exposure to HIV and other viral agents such as hepatitis B and Jakob-Creutzfeldt agent. The incidence of HIV-1 transmission associated with a percutaneous exposure to blood from an HIV-1 infected patient is approximately 0.3% per exposure.[1] In 1989, it was estimated that 12,000 United States healthcare workers acquired hepatitis B annually.[2] An understanding of the appropriate procedures, responsibilities, and risks inherent in the collection and handling of patient specimens is necessary for safe practice and is required by Occupational Safety and Health Administration (OSHA) regulations.

The Occupational Safety and Health Administration published its "Final Rule on Occupational Exposure to Bloodborne Pathogens" in the Federal Register on December 6, 1991. OSHA has chosen to follow the Center for Disease Control (CDC) definition of universal precautions. The Final Rule provides full legal force to universal precautions and requires employers and employees to treat blood and certain body fluids as if they were infectious. The Final Rule mandates that healthcare workers must avoid parenteral contact and must avoid splattering blood or other potentially infectious material on their skin, hair, eyes, mouth, mucous membranes, or on their personal clothing. Hazard abatement strategies must be used to protect the workers. Such plans typically include, but are not limited to, the following:

- safe handling of sharp items ("sharps") and disposal of such into puncture resistant containers
- gloves required for employees handling items soiled with blood or equipment contaminated by blood or other body fluids
- provisions of protective clothing when more extensive contact with blood or body fluids may be anticipated (eg, surgery, autopsy, or deliveries)
- resuscitation equipment to reduce necessity for mouth to mouth resuscitation
- restriction of HIV- or hepatitis B-exposed employees to noninvasive procedures

OSHA has specifically defined the following terms: **Occupational exposure** means reasonably anticipated skin, eye mucous membrane, or parenteral contact with blood or other potentially infectious materials that may result from the performance of an employee's duties. **Other potentially infectious materials** are human body fluids including semen, vaginal secretions, cerebrospinal fluid, synovial fluid, pleural fluid, pericardial fluid, peritoneal fluid, amniotic fluid, saliva in dental procedures, and body fluids that are visibly contaminated with blood, and all body fluids in situations where it is difficult or impossible to differentiate between body fluids; any unfixed tissue or organ (other than intact skin) from a human (living or dead); and HIV-containing cell or tissue cultures, organ cultures, and HIV- or HBV-containing culture medium or other solutions, and blood, organs, or other tissues from experimental animals infected with HIV or HBV. An **exposure incident** involves specific eye, mouth, other mucous membrane, nonintact skin, or parenteral contact with blood or other potentially infectious materials that results from the performance of an employee's duties.[3] It is important to understand that some exposures may go unrecognized despite the strictest precautions.

A written Exposure Control Plan is required. Employers must provide copies of the plan to employees and to OSHA upon request. Compliance with OSHA rules may be accomplished by the following methods.

- **Universal precautions (UPs)** means that all human blood and certain body fluids are treated as if known to be infectious for HIV, HBV, and other bloodborne pathogens. UPs do not apply to feces, nasal secretions, saliva, sputum, sweat, tears, urine, or vomitus unless they contain visible blood.
- **Engineering controls (ECs)** are physical devices which reduce or remove hazards from the workplace by eliminating or minimizing hazards or by isolating the worker from exposure. Engineering control devices include sharps disposal containers, self-resheathing syringes, etc.
- **Work practice controls (WPCs)** are practices and procedures that reduce the likelihood of exposure to hazards by altering the way in which a task is performed. Specific examples are the prohibition of two-handed recapping of needles, prohibition of storing food alongside potentially contaminated material, discouragement of pipetting fluids by mouth, encouraging handwashing after removal of gloves, safe handling of contaminated sharps, and appropriate use of sharps containers.

OCCUPATIONAL EXPOSURE TO BLOODBORNE PATHOGENS (UNIVERSAL PRECAUTIONS) *(Continued)*

- **Personal protective equipment (PPE)** is specialized clothing or equipment worn to provide protection from occupational exposure. PPE includes gloves, gowns, laboratory coats (the type and characteristics will depend upon the task and degree of exposure anticipated), face shields or masks, and eye protection. Surgical caps or hoods and/or shoe covers or boots are required in instances in which gross contamination can reasonably be anticipated (eg, autopsies, orthopedic surgery). If PPE is penetrated by blood or any contaminated material, the item must be removed immediately or as soon as feasible. **The employer must provide and launder or dispose of all PPE at no cost to the employee.** Gloves must be worn when there is a reasonable anticipation of hand contact with potentially infectious material, including a patient's mucous membranes or nonintact skin. Disposable gloves must be changed as soon as possible after they become torn or punctured. Hands must be washed after gloves are removed. OSHA has revised the PPE standards, effective July 5, 1994, to include the requirement that the employer certify in writing that it has conducted a hazard assessment of the workplace to determine whether hazards are present that will necessitate the use of PPE. Also, verification that the employee has received and understood the PPE training is required.[4]

Housekeeping protocols: OSHA requires that all bins, cans, and similar receptacles, intended for reuse which have a reasonable likelihood for becoming contaminated, be inspected and decontaminated immediately or as soon as feasible upon visible contamination and on a regularly scheduled basis. Broken glass that may be contaminated must not be picked up directly with the hands. Mechanical means (eg, brush, dust pan, tongs, or forceps) must be used. Broken glass must be placed in a proper sharps container.

Employers are responsible for teaching appropriate clean-up procedures for the work area and personal protective equipment. A 1:10 dilution of household bleach is a popular and effective disinfectant. It is prudent for employers to maintain signatures or initials of employees who have been properly educated. If one does not have written proof of education of universal precautions teaching, then by OSHA standards, such education never happened.

Pre-exposure and postexposure protocols: OSHA's Final Rule includes the provision that employees, who are exposed to contamination, be offered the hepatitis B vaccine at no cost to the employee. Employees may decline; however, a declination form must be signed. The employee must be offered free vaccine if he/she changes his/her mind. Vaccination to prevent the transmission of hepatitis B in the healthcare setting is widely regarded as sound practice.[5] In the event of exposure, a confidential medical evaluation and follow-up must be offered at no cost to the employee. Follow-up must include collection and testing of blood from the source individual for HBV and HIV if permitted by state law if a blood sample is available. If a postexposure specimen must be specially drawn, the individual's consent is usually required. Some states may not require consent for testing of patient blood after accidental exposure. One must refer to state and/or local guidelines for proper guidance.

The employee follow-up must also include appropriate postexposure prophylaxis, counseling, and evaluation of reported illnesses. The employee has the right to decline baseline blood collection and/or testing. If the employee gives consent for the collection but not the testing, the sample must be preserved for 90 days in the event that the employee changes his/her mind within that time. Confidentiality related to blood testing must be ensured. **The employer does not have the right to know the results** of the testing of either the source individual or the exposed employee.[3]

The Management of Occupational Exposure to HIV in the Workplace[6]

1. Likelihood of transmission of HIV-1 from occupational exposure is 0.2% per parenteral exposure (eg, needlestick) to blood from HIV-infected patients.

2. Factors that increase risk for occupational transmission include advanced stages of HIV in source patient, hollow bore needle puncture, a poor state of health, or inexperience of healthcare worker (HCW).

3. Immediate actions an exposed healthcare worker should take include aggressive first aid at the puncture site (eg, scrubbing site with povodone-iodine solution for 10 minutes) or at mucus membrane site (eg, saline irrigation of eye for 15 minutes), then immediate reporting to the hospital's occupational medical service. The authors indicate that there is no direct evidence for the efficacy of their recommendations. Other institutions suggest rigorous scrubbing with soap.

4. After first aid is initiated, the healthcare worker should report exposure to a supervisor and to the institution's occupational medical service for evaluation.
5. Occupational medicine should perform a thorough investigation including identifying the HIV and hepatitis B status of the source, type of exposure, volume of inoculum, timing of exposure, extent of injury, appropriateness of first aid, as well as psychological status of the healthcare worker. HIV serologies should be performed on the healthcare worker. HIV risk counselling should begin at this point.
6. All parenteral exposures should be treated equally until they can be evaluated by the occupational medicine service, who will then determine the actual risk of exposure. Follow-up counselling sessions may be necessary.
7. Although the data are not clear, antiviral prophylaxis may be offered to healthcare workers who are parenterally or mucous membrane exposed. If used, antiretroviral prophylaxis should be initiated within 1-2 hours after exposure.
8. Counselling regarding risk of exposure, antiviral prophylaxis, plans for follow up, exposure prevention, sexual activity, and providing emotional support and response to concerns are necessary to support the exposed healthcare worker. Follow-up should consist of periodic serologic evaluation and blood chemistries and counts if antiretroviral prophylaxis is initiated. Additional information should be provided to healthcare workers who are pregnant or planning to become pregnant.

See also Postexposure Prophylaxis for Hepatitis B in the Appendix.

Hazardous Communication

Communication regarding the dangers of bloodborne infections through the use of labels, signs, information, and education is required. Storage locations (eg, refrigerators and freezers, waste containers) that are used to store, dispose of, transport, or ship blood or other potentially infectious materials require labels. The label background must be red or bright orange with the biohazard design and the word biohazard in a contrasting color. The label must be part of the container or affixed to the container by permanent means.

Education provided by a qualified and knowledgeable instructor is mandated. The sessions for employees must include:[4]

- accessible copies of the regulation
- general epidemiology of bloodborne diseases
- modes of bloodborne pathogen transmission
- an explanation of the exposure control plan and a means to obtain copies of the written plan
- an explanation of the tasks and activities that may involve exposure
- the use of exposure prevention methods and their limitations (eg, engineering controls, work practices, personal protective equipment)
- information on the types, proper use, location, removal, handling, decontamination, and disposal of personal protective equipment)
- an explanation of the basis for selection of personal protective equipment
- information on the HBV vaccine, including information on its efficacy, safety, and method of administration and the benefits of being vaccinated (ie, the employee must understand that the vaccine and vaccination will be offered free of charge)
- information on the appropriate actions to take and persons to contact in an emergency involving exposure to blood or other potentially infectious materials
- an explanation of the procedure to follow if an exposure incident occurs, including the method of reporting the incident
- information on the postexposure evaluation and follow-up that the employer is required to provide for the employee following an exposure incident
- an explanation of the signs, labels, and color coding
- an interactive question-and-answer period

Record Keeping

The OSHA Final Rule requires that the employer maintain both education and medical records. The medical records must be kept confidential and be maintained for the duration of employment plus 30 years. They must contain a copy of the employee's HBV vaccination status and postexposure incident information. Education records must be maintained for 3 years from the date the program was given.

OCCUPATIONAL EXPOSURE TO BLOODBORNE PATHOGENS (UNIVERSAL PRECAUTIONS) *(Continued)*

OSHA has the authority to conduct inspections without notice. Penalties for cited violation may be assessed as follows.

Serious violations. In this situation, there is a substantial probability of death or serious physical harm, and the employer knew, or should have known, of the hazard. A violation of this type carries a mandatory penalty of up to $7000 for each violation.

Other-than-serious violations. The violation is unlikely to result in death or serious physical harm. This type of violation carries a discretionary penalty of up to $7000 for each violation.

Willful violations. These are violations committed knowingly or intentionally by the employer and have penalties of up to $70,000 per violation with a minimum of $5000 per violation. If an employee dies as a result of a willful violation, the responsible party, if convicted, may receive a personal fine of up to $250,000 and/or a 6-month jail term. A corporation may be fined $500,000.

Large fines frequently follow visits to laboratories, physicians' offices, and healthcare facilities by OSHA Compliance Safety and Health Offices (CSHOS). Regulations are vigorously enforced. A working knowledge of the final rule and implementation of appropriate policies and practices is imperative for all those involved in the collection and analysis of medical specimens.

Effectiveness of universal precautions in averting exposure to potentially infectious materials has been documented.[7] Compliance with appropriate rules, procedures, and policies, including reporting exposure incidents, is a matter of personal professionalism and prudent self-preservation.

Footnotes

1. Henderson DK, Fahey BJ, Willy M, et al, "Risk for Occupational Transmission of Human Immunodeficiency Virus Type 1 (HIV-1) Associated With Clinical Exposures. A Prospective Evaluation," *Ann Intern Med,* 1990, 113(10):740-6.
2. Niu MT and Margolis HS, "Moving Into a New Era of Government Regulation: Provisions for Hepatitis B Vaccine in the Workplace, *Clin Lab Manage Rev,* 1989, 3:336-40.
3. Bruning LM, "The Bloodborne Pathogens Final Rule — Understanding the Regulation," *AORN Journal,* 1993, 57(2):439-40.
4. "Rules and Regulations," *Federal Register,* 1994, 59(66):16360-3.
5. Schaffner W, Gardner P, and Gross PA, "Hepatitis B Immunization Strategies: Expanding the Target," *Ann Intern Med,* 1993, 118(4):308-9.
6. Fahey BJ, Beekmann SE, Schmitt JM, et al, "Managing Occupational Exposures to HIV-1 in the Healthcare Workplace," *Infect Control Hosp Epidemiol,* 1993, 14(7):405-12.
7. Wong ES, Stotka JL, Chinchilli VM, et al, "Are Universal Precautions Effective in Reducing the Number of Occupational Exposures Among Healthcare Workers?" *JAMA,* 1991, 265:1123-8.

References

Buehler JW and Ward JW, "A New Definition for AIDS Surveillance," *Ann Intern Med,* 1993, 118(5):390-2.

Brown JW and Blackwell H, "Complying With the New OSHA Regs, Part 1: Teaching Your Staff About Biosafety," *MLO,* 1992, 24(4)24-8. Part 2: "Safety Protocols No Lab Can Ignore," 1992, 24(5):27-9. Part 3: "Compiling Employee Safety Records That Will Satisfy OSHA," 1992, 24(6):45-8.

Department of Labor, Occupational Safety and Health Administration, "Occupational Exposure to Bloodborne Pathogens; Final Rule (29 CFR Part 1910.1030),"*Federal Register,* December 6, 1991, 64004-182.

Gold JW, "HIV-1 Infection: Diagnosis and Management," *Med Clin North Am,* 1992, 76(1):1-18.

"Hepatitis B Virus: A Comprehensive Strategy for Eliminating Transmission in the United States Through Universal Childhood Vaccination," *MMWR Morb Mortal Wkly Rep,* 1991, 40(RR-13):1-25.

"Mortality Attributable to HIV Infection/AIDS — United States", *MMWR Morb Mortal Wkly Rep,* 1991, 40(3):41-4.

National Committee for Clinical Laboratory Standards, "Protection of Laboratory Workers From Infectious Disease Transmitted by Blood, Body Fluids, and Tissue," NCCLS Document M29-T, Villanova, PA: NCCLS, 1989, 9(1).

"Nosocomial Transmission of Hepatitis B Virus Associated With a Spring-Loaded Fingerstick Device — California," *MMWR Morb Mortal Wkly Rep*, 1990, 39(35):610-3.

Polish LB, Shapiro CN, Bauer F, et al, "Nosocomial Transmission of Hepatitis B Virus Associated With the Use of a Spring-Loaded Fingerstick Device," *N Engl J Med*, 1992, 326(11):721-5.

"Recommendations for Preventing Transmission of Human Immunodeficiency Virus and Hepatitis B Virus to Patients During Exposure-Prone Invasive Procedures," *MMWR Morb Mortal Wkly Rep*, 1991, 40(RR-8):1-9.

"Update: Acquired Immunodeficiency Syndrome — United States," *MMWR Morb Mortal Wkly Rep*, 1992, 41(26):463-8.

"Update: Transmission of HIV Infection During an Invasive Dental Procedure — Florida," *MMWR Morb Mortal Wkly Rep*, 1991, 40(2):21-7, 33.

"Update: Universal Precautions for Prevention of Transmission of Human Immunodeficiency Virus, Hepatitis B Virus, and Other Bloodborne Pathogens in Healthcare Settings," *MMWR Morb Mortal Wkly Rep*, 1988, 37(24):377-82, 387-8.

PREVENTION OF BACTERIAL ENDOCARDITIS

Recommendations by the American Heart Association (*JAMA*, 1997, 277:1794-801)

Consensus Process – The recommendations were formulated by the writing group after specific therapeutic regimens were discussed. The consensus statement was subsequently reviewed by outside experts not affiliated with the writing group and by the Science Advisory and Coordinating Committee of the American Heart Association. These guidelines are meant to aid practitioners but are not intended as the standard of care or as a substitute for clinical judgment.

Table 1. Cardiac Conditions[1]

Endocarditis Prophylaxis Recommended

High-Risk Category

- Prosthetic cardiac valves, including bioprosthetic and homograft valves
- Previous bacterial endocarditis
- Complex cyanotic congenital heart disease (eg, single ventricle states, transposition of the great arteries, tetralogy of Fallot)
- Surgically constructed systemic pulmonary shunts or conduits

Moderate-Risk Category

- Most other congenital cardiac malformations (other than above and below)
- Acquired valvar dysfunction (eg, rheumatic heart disease)
- Hypertrophic cardiomyopathy
- Mitral valve prolapse with valvar regurgitation and/or thickened leaflets

Endocarditis Prophylaxis Not Recommended

Negligible-Risk Category (no greater risk than the general population)

- Isolated secundum atrial septal defect
- Surgical repair of atrial septal defect, ventricular septal defect, or patent ductus arteriosus (without residua beyond 6 months)
- Previous coronary artery bypass graft surgery
- Mitral valve prolapse without valvar regurgitation
- Physiologic, functional, or innocent heart murmurs
- Previous Kawasaki disease without valvar dysfunction
- Previous rheumatic fever without valvar dysfunction
- Cardiac pacemakers (intravascular and epicardial) and implanted defibrillators

[1]This table lists selected conditions but is not meant to be all-inclusive.

Patient With Suspected Mitral Valve Prolapse

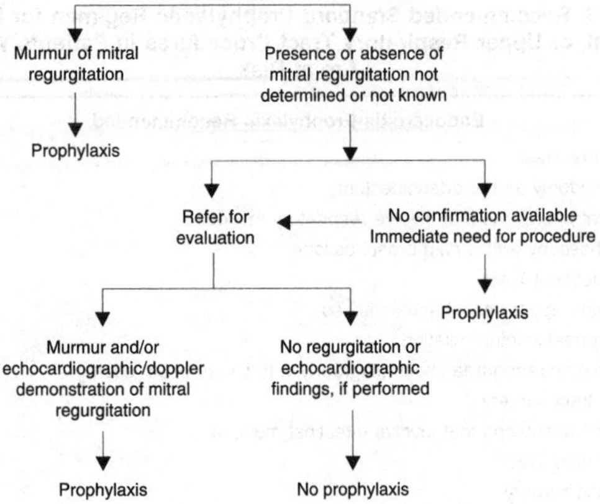

Table 2. Dental Procedures and Endocarditis Prophylaxis

Endocarditis Prophylaxis Recommended[1]
Dental extractions
Periodontal procedures including surgery, scaling and root planing, probing, and recall maintenance
Dental implant placement and reimplantation of avulsed teeth
Endodontic (root canal) instrumentation or surgery only beyond the apex
Subgingival placement of antibiotic fibers or strips
Initial placement of orthodontic bands but not brackets
Intraligamentary local anesthetic injections
Prophylactic cleaning of teeth or implants where bleeding is anticipated
Endocarditis Prophylaxis Not Recommended
Restorative dentistry[2] (operative and prosthodontic) with or without retraction cord[3]
Local anesthetic injections (nonintraligamentary)
Intracanal endodontic treatment; post placement and buildup[3]
Placement of rubber dams[3]
Postoperative suture removal
Placement of removable prosthodontic or orthodontic appliances
Taking of oral impressions[3]
Fluoride treatments
Taking of oral radiographs
Orthodontic appliance adjustment
Shedding of primary teeth

[1]Prophylaxis is recommended for patients with high- and moderate-risk cardiac conditions.

[2]This includes restoration of decayed teeth (filling cavities) and replacement of missing teeth.

[3]Clinical judgment may indicate antibiotic use in selected circumstances that may create significant bleeding.

PREVENTION OF BACTERIAL ENDOCARDITIS *(Continued)*

Table 3. Recommended Standard Prophylactic Regimen for Dental, Oral, or Upper Respiratory Tract Procedures in Patients Who Are at Risk

Endocarditis Prophylaxis Recommended

- Respiratory Tract
  - Tonsillectomy and/or adenoidectomy
  - Surgical operations that involve respiratory mucosa
  - Bronchoscopy with a rigid bronchoscope
- Gastrointestinal Tract[1]
  - Sclerotherapy for esophageal varices
  - Esophageal stricture dilation
  - Endoscopic retrograde cholangiography with biliary obstruction
  - Biliary tract surgery
  - Surgical operations that involve intestinal mucosa
- Genitourinary Tract
  - Prostatic surgery
  - Cystoscopy
  - Urethral dilation

Endocarditis Prophylaxis Not Recommended

- Respiratory Tract
  - Endotracheal intubation
  - Bronchoscopy with a flexible bronchoscope, with or without biopsy[2]
  - Tympanostomy tube insertion
- Gastrointestinal Tract
  - Transesophageal echocardiography[2]
  - Endoscopy with or without gastrointestinal biopsy[2]
- Genitourinary Tract
  - Vaginal hysterectomy[2]
  - Vaginal delivery[2]
  - Cesarean section
  - In uninfected tissues:
    - Urethral catheterization
    - Uterine dilatation and curettage
    - Therapeutic abortion
    - Sterilization procedures
    - Insertion or removal of intrauterine devices
- Other
  - Cardiac catheterization, including balloon angioplasty
  - Implanted cardiac pacemakers, implanted defibrillators, and coronary stents
  - Incision or biopsy or surgically scrubbed skin
  - Circumcision

[1]Prophylaxis is recommended for high-risk patients, optional for medium-risk patients.
[2]Prophylaxis is optional for high-risk patients.

Table 4. Prophylactic Regimens for Dental, Oral, Respiratory Tract, or Esophageal Procedures

Situation	Agent	Regimen[1]	
		Adults	Children
Standard general prophylaxis	Amoxicillin	2 g P.O. 1 h before procedure	50 mg/kg P.O. 1 h before procedure
Unable to take oral medications	Ampicillin	2 g I.M./I.V. within 30 min before procedure	50 mg/kg I.M./I.V. within 30 min before procedure
Allergic to penicillin	Clindamycin or	600 mg P.O. 1 h before procedure	20 mg/kg P.O. 1 h before procedure
	Cephalexin[2] or cefadroxil[2] or	2 g P.O 1 h before procedure	50 mg/kg P.O. 1 h before procedure
	Azithromycin or clarithromycin	500 mg P.O. 1 h before procedure	15 mg/kg P.O. 1 h before procedure
Allergic to penicillin and unable to take oral medications	Clindamycin or	600 mg I.V. within 30 min before procedure	20 mg/kg I.V. within 30 min before procedure
	Cefazolin[2]	1 g I.M./I.V. within 30 min before procedure	25 mg/kg I.M./I.V. within 30 min before procedure

[1]Total children's dose should not exceed adult dose.

[2]Cephalosporins should not be used in individuals with immediate-type hypersensitivity reaction (urticaria, angioedema, or anaphylaxis) to penicillins.

PREVENTION OF BACTERIAL ENDOCARDITIS *(Continued)*

Table 5. Prophylactic Regimens for Genitourinary / Gastrointestinal (Excluding Esophageal) Procedures

Situation	Agents	Regimen[1,2]	
		Adults	Children
High-risk[3] patients	Ampicillin plus gentamicin	Ampicillin 2 g I.M. or I.V. plus gentamicin 1.5 mg/kg (not to exceed 120 mg) within 30 min of starting the procedure; 6 h later, ampicillin 1 g I.M./I.V. or amoxicillin 1 g orally	Ampicillin 50 mg/kg I.M./I.V. (not to exceed 2 g) plus gentamicin 1.5 mg/kg within 30 min of starting the procedure; 6 h later, ampicillin 25 mg/kg I.M./I.V. or amoxicillin 25 mg/kg orally
High-risk[3] patients allergic to ampicillin/ amoxicillin	Vancomycin plus gentamicin	Vancomycin 1 g I.V. over 1-2 h plus gentamicin 1.5 mg/kg I.M./I.V. (not to exceed 120 mg); complete injection/ infusion within 30 min of starting the procedure	Vancomycin 20 mg/kg I.V. over 1-2 h plus gentamicin 1.5 mg/kg I.M./I.V.; complete injection/infusion within 30 min of starting the procedure
Moderate-risk[4] patients	Amoxicillin or ampicillin	Amoxicillin 2 g orally 1 h before procedure, or ampicillin 2 g I.M./ I.V within 30 min of starting the procedure	Amoxicillin 50 mg/kg orally 1 h before procedure, or ampicillin 50 mg/kg I.M./I.V. within 30 min of starting the procedure
Moderate-risk[4] patients allergic to ampicillin/amoxicillin	Vancomycin	Vancomycin 1 g I.V. over 1-2 h; complete infusion within 30 min of starting the procedure	Vancomycin 20 mg/kg I.V. over 1-2 h; complete infusion within 30 min of starting the procedure

[1]Total children's dose should not exceed adult dose.

[2]No second dose of vancomycin or gentamicin is recommended.

[3]High-risk: Patients are those who have prosthetic valves, a previous history of endocarditis (even in the absence of other heart disease, complex cyanotic congenital heart disease, or surgically constructed systemic pulmonary shunts or conduits).

[4]Moderate-risk: Individuals with certain other underlying cardiac defects. Congenital cardiac conditions include the following uncorrected conditions: Patent ductus arteriosus, ventricular septal defect, ostium primum atrial septal defect, coarctation of the aorta, and bicuspid aortic valve. Acquired valvar dysfunction and hypertrophic cardiomyopathy are also moderate risk conditions.

PREVENTION OF WOUND INFECTION AND SEPSIS IN SURGICAL PATIENTS

Nature of Operation	Likely Pathogens	Recommended Drugs	Adult Dosage Before Surgery[1]
Cardiac	*S. aureus*, *S. epidermidis*	Cefazolin or cefuroxime OR vancomycin[3]	1-2 g I.V.[2] 1.5 g I.V.[2] 1 g I.V.
Gastrointestinal			
Esophageal, gastroduodenal	Enteric gram-negative bacilli, gram-positive cocci	*High risk[4] only:* Cefazolin[5]	1-2 g I.V.
Biliary tract	Enteric gram-negative bacilli, enterococci, clostridia	*High risk[6] only:* Cefazolin[5]	1-2 g I.V.
Colorectal	Enteric gram-negative bacilli, anaerobes, enterococci	*Oral:* Neomycin + erythromycin base[7] OR neomycin + metronidazole[7]	
		Parenteral:	
		Cefotetan or cefoxitin OR cefazolin + metronidazole[5]	1-2 g I.V. 1-2 g I.V. 1-2 g I.V. 0.5-1 g I.V.
Appendectomy, nonperforated	Enteric gram-negative bacilli, anaerobes, enterococci	Cefoxitin or cefotetan OR cefazolin + metronidazole[5]	1-2 g I.V. 1-2 g I.V. 1-2 g I.V. 0.5-1 g I.V.
Ruptured viscus	Enteric gram-negative bacilli, anaerobes, enterococci	Cefoxitin or cefotetan ± gentamicin[5,8]	1-2 g I.V. q6h 1-2 g I.V. q12h 1.5 mg/kg I.V. q8h
Genitourinary	Enteric gram-negative bacilli, enterococci	*High risk[9] only:* Ciprofloxacin	500 mg P.O. or 400 mg I.V.
Gynecologic and Obstetric			
Vaginal, abdominal, or laparoscopic hysterectomy	Enteric gram-negative bacilli, anaerobes, group B streptococci, enterococci	Cefotetan or cefoxitin or cefazolin[5]	1-2 g I.V. 1-2 g I.V 1-2 g I.V
Cesarean section	Same as for hysterectomy	Cefazolin	1-2 g I.V. after cord clamping
Abortion	Same as for hysterectomy	*First trimester, high-risk[10]:*	
		Aqueous penicillin G OR doxycycline	2 mill units I.V. 300 mg P.O.[11]
		Second trimester:	
		Cefazolin	1-2 g I.V.
Head and Neck			
Incisions through oral or pharyngeal mucosa	Anaerobes, enteric gram-negative bacilli, *S. aureus*	Clindamycin + gentamicin OR cefazolin	600-900 mg I.V. 1.5 mg/kg I.V. 1-2 g I.V.
Neurosurgery	*S. aureus*, *S. epidermidis*	Cefazolin OR vancomycin[3]	1-2 g I.V. 1 g I.V.
Ophthalmic	*S. epidermidis*, *S. aureus*, streptococci, enteric gram-negative bacilli, *Pseudomonas*	Gentamicin, tobramycin, ciprofloxacin, gatifloxacin, levofloxacin, moxifloxacin, ofloxacin, or neomycin-gramicidin-polymyxin B	Multiple drops topically over 2-24 hours
		Cefazolin	100 mg subconjunctivally

PREVENTION OF WOUND INFECTION AND SEPSIS IN SURGICAL PATIENTS *(Continued)*

Nature of Operation	Likely Pathogens	Recommended Drugs	Adult Dosage Before Surgery[1]
Orthopedic			
Total joint replacement, internal fixation of fractures	*S. aureus*, *S. epidermidis*	Cefazolin[12] OR vancomycin[3,12]	1-2 g I.V. 1 g I.V.
Thoracic (Noncardiac)	*S. aureus*, *S. epidermidis*, streptococci, enteric gram-negative bacilli	Cefazolin or cefuroxime OR vancomycin[3]	1-2 g I.V. 1.5 g I.V. 1 g I.V.
Vascular			
Arterial surgery involving a prosthesis, the abdominal aorta, or a groin incision	*S. aureus*, *S. epidermidis*, enteric gram-negative bacilli	Cefazolin OR vancomycin[3]	1-2 g I.V. 1 g I.V.
Lower extremity amputation for ischemia	*S. aureus*, *S. epidermidis*, enteric gram-negative bacilli, clostridia	Cefazolin OR vancomycin[3]	1-2 g I.V. 1 g I.V.

[1]Parenteral prophylactic antimicrobials can be given as a single I.V. dose begun 60 minutes or less before the operation. For prolonged operations, additional intraoperative doses should be given at intervals 1-2 times the half-life of the drug for the duration of the procedure. If vancomycin or a fluoroquinolone is used, the infusion should be started 60-120 minutes before incision in order to minimize the possibility of an infusion reaction close to the time of induction of anesthesia and to have adequate tissue levels at the time of incision.

[2]Some consultants recommend an additional dose when patients are removed from bypass during open-heart surgery.

[3]For hospitals in which methicillin-resistant *S. aureus* and *S. epidermidis* are a frequent cause of postoperative wound infection, for patients previously colonized with MRSA, or for patients allergic to penicillins or cephalosporin. Rapid I.V. administration may cause hypotension, which could be especially dangerous during induction of anesthesia. Even if the drug is given over 60 minutes, hypotension may occur; treatment with diphenhydramine (Benadryl® and others) and further slowing of the infusion rate may be helpful. For procedures in which enteric gram-negative bacilli are likely pathogens, such as vascular surgery involving a groin incision, cefazolin or cefuroxime should be included in the prophylaxis regimen for patients not allergic to cephalosporins; ciprofloxacin, levofloxacin (750 mg), gentamicin, or aztreonam, each one in combination with vancomycin, can be used in patients who cannot tolerate a cephalosporin.

[4]Morbid obesity, esophageal obstruction, decreased gastric acidity, or gastrointestinal motility.

[5]For patients allergic to cephalosporins, clindamycin with either gentamicin, ciprofloxacin, levofloxacin (750 mg), or aztreonam is a reasonable alternative.

[6]Age >70 years, acute cholecystitis, nonfunctioning gallbladder, obstructive jaundice, or common duct stones.

[7]After appropriate diet and catharsis, 1 g of neomycin plus 1 g of erythromycin at 1 PM, 2 PM, and 11 PM or 2 g of neomycin plus 2 g of metronidazole at 7 PM and 11 PM the day before an 8 AM operation.

[8]Therapy is often continued for about 5 days. Ruptured viscus in postoperative setting (dehiscence) requires antibacterials to include coverage of nosocomial pathogens.

[9]Urine culture positive or unavailable, preoperative catheter, transrectal prostatic biopsy, placement of prosthetic material.

[10]Patients with previous pelvic inflammatory disease, previous gonorrhea, or multiple sex partners.

[11]Divided into 100 mg 1 hour before the abortion and 200 mg 30 minutes after.

[12]If a tourniquet is to be used in the procedure, the entire dose of antibiotic must be infused prior to its inflation.

Adapted with permission from "Antimicrobial Prophylaxis for Surgery," *Treatment Guidelines*, 2004, 2(20):28-9.

PROPHYLAXIS FOR PATIENTS EXPOSED TO COMMON COMMUNICABLE DISEASES

Disease	Exposure	Prophylaxis/Management
Anthrax	Postexposure inhalational	Doxycycline and ciprofloxacin; 60-day (oral and intravenous) regimens have been recommended.
Invasive *Haemophilus influenzae* disease	Close contact with an infected child for more than 4 hours	Give rifampin 20 mg/kg orally once daily for 4 days (600 mg maximum daily dose) to entire family with at least one household contact less than 48 months old. Contraindication: Pregnant contacts.
Hepatitis A	Direct contact with an infected child, or sharing of food or utensils	Give 0.02 mL/kg immune globulin (IG) within 7 days of exposure.
Hepatitis B	Needlestick (used needle) Mucous membrane exposure with blood or body fluid Direct inoculation of blood or body fluid into open cut, lesion, or laceration	**Known source and employee status unknown: Test patient for HB_sAg and employee for anti-HB_s.** If patient is HB_sAg negative and the patient does not have non-A, non-B hepatitis, do nothing. If patient is HB_sAg negative and has non-A, non-B hepatitis, **offer** ISG (optional). If patient is HB_sAg positive, give HBIG and hepatitis B vaccine within 48 hours of exposure. Employee antibody status may not be available for up to a week, so the above should be given as soon as patient's antigen status is known. Occasionally, the patient's antigen status will be unavailable for more than 24 hours. In these cases, HBIG should be given if the patient is high risk (ie, Asian immigrants, institutionalized patients, homosexuals, intravenous drug abusers, hemodialysis patients, patients with a history of hepatitis). If the employee is anti-HB_s negative, give the second and third doses of hepatitis B vaccine. **Known source and employee documented anti-HB_s positive:** If source has non-A, non-B hepatitis, offer ISG (optional). If employee is believed to be anti-HB_s positive due to vaccination, has received 3 doses of vaccine, and has not had an anti-HB_s test done, draw serum for anti-HB_s.
Measles	15 minutes or more in the same room with a child with measles from 2 days before the onset of symptoms to 4 days after the appearance of the rash	Children who have not been vaccinated and have not had natural infection should be isolated from the 7th through the 18th day after exposure and/or for 4 days after the rash appears. Those who have not been vaccinated should be vaccinated within 72 hours of exposure if no contraindication exists, or receive immune globulin (IG) 0.25 mL/kg I.M. for immunocompetent individuals and 0.5 mL/kg (maximum: 15 mL) for immunosuppressed individuals. Children who are younger than 15 months of age should be revaccinated at 15 months of age but at least 3 months after receipt of vaccine or IG. Older individuals who have received IG should be vaccinated 3 months later.
Meningococcal disease	Household contact or direct contact with secretions	Household, day care center, and nursery school children should receive rifampin prophylaxis for 2 days. Dosages are given every 12 hours for a total of 4 doses. Dosage is 10 mg/kg/dose for children ages 1 month to 12 years (maximum: 600 mg/dose), 5 mg/kg/dose for infants less than 1 month of age, and 600 mg/dose for adults. Alternatively, ciprofloxacin 750 mg as a single dose may be used. Contraindication: Pregnant contacts. **Because prophylaxis is not always effective, exposed children should be monitored for symptoms.** **Employee exposure: Anyone who develops a febrile illness should receive prompt medical evaluation. If indicated, antimicrobial therapy should be administered.**

PROPHYLAXIS FOR PATIENTS EXPOSED TO COMMON COMMUNICABLE DISEASES *(Continued)*

Disease	Exposure	Prophylaxis/Management
Pertussis	Housed in the same room with an infected child or spent 15 minutes in the playroom with the infected child	**Prophylaxis:** Contacts less than 7 years old who have had at least 4 doses of pertussis vaccine should receive a booster dose of DTP, unless a dose has been given within the past 3 years, and should receive erythromycin 40-50 mg/kg/day orally for 14 days. Contacts less than 7 years old who are not immunized or who have received less than 4 doses of DTP should have DTP immunization initiated or continued according to the recommended schedule. Children who have received their third dose 6 months or more before exposure should be given their fourth dose at this time. Erythromycin should also be given for 14 days. Contacts 7 years of age and above should receive prophylactic erythromycin (maximum: 1 g/day) for 10-14 days. All exposed patients should be watched closely for respiratory symptoms for 14 days after exposure has stopped because immunity conferred by the vaccine is not absolute and the efficacy of erythromycin in prophylaxis has not been established.
Tuberculosis	Housed in the same room with a child with contagious tuberculosis (tuberculosis is contagious if the child has a cough plus AFB seen on smear plus cavitation on CXR)	Administer PPD immediately and 10 weeks after exposure. Start on INH. Consult Infectious Diseases if seroconversion occurs.
Varicella-zoster	1 hour or more in the same room with a contagious child from 24 hours before vesicles appear to when all vesicles are crusted, which is usually 5 to 7 days after vesicles appear. In household exposure, communicability is 48 hours before vesicles appear.	**Immunocompetent** children who have not been vaccinated or had natural infection, should have titers drawn only if they will still be hospitalized for more than 10 days after exposure. If titers are negative, they should be isolated from 10-21 days after exposure and/or until all lesions are crusted and dry. If VZIG (varicella-zoster immune globulin) was given the child should be isolated from 10-28 days after exposure. **Immunocompromised** children who have not been vaccinated or had natural infection should first have titers drawn, and then receive VZIG **1 vial/10 kg I.M.** up to a maximum of 5 vials as soon as possible but at most 96 hours after exposure. Fractional doses are not recommended. If titers are positive, nothing further need be done. If titers are negative, the child should be isolated from 10-28 days after exposure and should be monitored very carefully for the appearance of vesicles so that treatment can be initiated. VZIG is available from the Blood Bank.

TREATMENT OF SEXUALLY TRANSMITTED INFECTIONS

Type or Stage	Drugs of Choice / Dosage	Alternatives
CHLAMYDIAL INFECTION AND RELATED CLINICAL SYNDROMES[1]		
Urethritis, cervicitis, conjunctivitis, or proctitis (except lymphogranuloma venereum)		
	Azithromycin 1 g oral once **or** Doxycycline[2,3] 100 mg oral bid x 7 d	Ofloxacin[3] 300 mg oral bid x 7 d **or** Levofloxacin[3] 500 mg oral once/d x 7 d **or** Erythromycin[4] 500 mg oral qid x 7 d
Infection in pregnancy		
	Azithromycin 1 g oral once **or** Amoxicillin 500 mg oral tid x 7 d	Erythromycin[4] 500 mg oral qid x 7 d
Neonatal ophthalmia or pneumonia		
	Azithromycin 20 mg/kg oral once daily x 3 d	Erythromycin 12.5 mg/kg oral qid x 14 d[5]
Lymphogranuloma venereum		
	Doxycycline[2,3] 100 mg oral bid x 21 d	Erythromycin[4] 500 mg oral qid x 21 d
EPIDIDYMITIS		
	Ofloxacin 300 mg bid x 10 d **or** Levofloxacin 500 mg oral once daily x 10 d	Ceftriaxone 250 mg I.M. once **followed by** doxycycline[2] 100 mg oral bid x 10 d
GONORRHEA[6]		
Disseminated gonococcal infection		
	Ceftriaxone 1 g I.M. or I.V. q24h	Cefotaxime 1 g I.V. q8h **or** Ceftizoxime 1 g I.V. q8h **or** **For persons allergic to β-lactam drugs:** Ciprofloxacin 400 mg I.V. q12h **or** Levofloxacin 250 mg I.V. once daily **or** Ofloxacin 400 mg I.V. q12h **or** Spectinomycin 2 g I.M. q12h All regimens should be continued for 24-48 hours after improvement begins, at which time therapy may be switched to one of the following regimens to complete a full week of antimicrobial therapy: Cefixime 400 mg oral bid **or** Ciprofloxacin 500 mg oral bid **or** Levofloxacin 500 mg oral once daily **or** Ofloxacin 400 mg oral bid
Gonococcal meningitis and endocarditis		
	Ceftriaxone 1-2 g I.V. q12h	
Urethral, cervical, rectal, or pharyngeal		
	Cefixime 400 mg oral once **or** Ceftriaxone 125 mg I.M. once	Cefpodoxime 400 mg oral once **or** Ciprofloxacin[3,7] 500 mg oral once **or** Ofloxacin[3,7] 400 mg oral once **or** Levofloxacin[3,7] 250 mg oral once **or** Spectinomycin 2 g I.M. once[8]

TREATMENT OF SEXUALLY TRANSMITTED INFECTIONS *(Continued)*

Type or Stage	Drugs of Choice / Dosage	Alternatives
PELVIC INFLAMMATORY DISEASE		
– parenteral	Cefotetan 2 g I.V. q12h **or** cefoxitin 2 g I.V. q6h **plus** doxycycline[3] 100 mg oral or I.V. q12h, until improved **followed by** doxycycline[3] 100 mg oral bid to complete 14 d[10] **or** Clindamycin 900 mg I.V. q8h **plus** gentamicin 2 mg/kg I.V. once, then 1.5 mg/kg I.V. q8h,[11] until improved **followed by** doxycycline[3] 100 mg oral bid to complete 14 d[10]	Ofloxacin[3] 400 mg I.V. q12h **or** levofloxacin[3] 500 mg I.V. once daily **plus** metronidazole 500 mg I.V. q8h[9] **or** Ampicillin/sulbactam 3 g I.V. q6h **plus** doxycycline[3] 100 mg oral or I.V. q12h **All continued until improved, then followed by** doxycycline[3] 100 mg oral bid to complete 14 d[10]
– oral	Ofloxacin[3] 400 mg bid x 14 d **or** Levofloxacin[3] 500 mg once daily x 14 d ± metronidazole[9] 500 mg bid x 14 d **or** Ceftriaxone 250 mg I.M. once **followed by** doxycycline[3,12] 100 mg bid x 14 d	Cefoxitin 2 g once **plus** probenecid 1 g oral once **followed by** doxycycline[3,12] 100 mg bid x 14 d
TRICHOMONIASIS		
	Metronidazole 2 g oral once **or** Tinidazole 2 g oral once	Metronidazole 375 or 500 mg oral bid x 7 d
BACTERIAL VAGINOSIS		
	Metronidazole 500 mg oral bid x 7 d **or** Metronidazole gel 0.75%[14] 5 g intravaginally once or twice daily x 5 d **or** Clindamycin 2% cream[14] 5 g intravaginally qhs x 3-7 d	Metronidazole 2 g oral once[13] or Flagyl ER® 750 mg once daily x 7 d **or** Clindamycin 300 mg oral bid x 7 d **or** Clindamycin ovules[14] 100 mg intravaginally once daily x 3 d
VULVOVAGINAL CANDIDIASIS		
	Intravaginal butoconazole, clotrimazole, miconazole, terconazole, or tioconazole[15] **or** Fluconazole 150 mg oral once	Nystatin 100,000 unit vaginal tablet once daily x 14 d
SYPHILIS		
Early (primary, secondary, or latent <1 y)		
	Penicillin G benzathine 2.4 million units I.M. once[16]	Doxycycline[3] 100 mg oral bid x 14 d
Late (>1 year's duration, cardiovascular, gumma, late-latent)		
	Penicillin G benzathine 2.4 million units I.M. weekly x 3 wk	Doxycycline[3] 100 mg oral bid x 4 wk
Neurosyphilis[17]		
	Penicillin G 3-4 million units I.V. q4h or 24 million units continuous I.V. infusion x 10-14 d	Penicillin G procaine 2.4 million units I.M. daily **plus** probenecid 500 mg qid oral, both x 10-14 d **or** Ceftriaxone 2 g I.V. once daily x 10-14 d
Congenital		
	Penicillin G 50,000 units/kg I.V. q8-12h for 10-14 d **or** Penicillin G procaine 50,000 units/kg I.M. daily for 10-14 d	
CHANCROID[18]		
	Azithromycin 1 g oral once **or** Ceftriaxone 250 mg I.M. once	Ciprofloxacin[3] 500 mg oral bid x 3 d **or** Erythromycin[4] 500 mg oral qid x 7 d

Type or Stage	Drugs of Choice / Dosage	Alternatives
GENITAL WARTS[19]		
	Trichloroacetic or bichloroacetic acid, or podophyllin[3] or liquid nitrogen 1-2 times/wk until resolved	Surgical removal
	or	**or**
	Imiquimod 5% 3 times/wk x 16 wk	Laser surgery
	or	**or**
	Podofilox 0.5% bid x 3 d, 4 days rest, then repeated up to 4 times	Intralesional interferon
GENITAL HERPES		
First episode		
	Acyclovir 400 mg oral tid x 7-10 d	Acyclovir 200 mg oral 5 times/d x 7-10 d
	or	
	Famciclovir 250 mg oral tid x 7-10 d	
	or	
	Valacyclovir 1 g oral bid x 7-10 d	
Severe (hospitalized patients)		
	Acyclovir 5-10 mg/kg I.V. q8h x 5-7 d	
Suppression of recurrences[20]		
	Acyclovir 400 mg oral bid	Acyclovir 200 mg oral, 2-5 times/d
	or	
	Famciclovir 250 mg oral bid	
	or	
	Valacyclovir 500 mg - 1 g once daily[21]	
Episodic treatment of recurrences[22]		
	Acyclovir 800 mg oral tid x 2 d or 400 mg oral tid x 3-5 d[23]	
	or	
	Famciclovir 125 mg oral bid x 3-5 d[23]	
	or	
	Valacyclovir 500 mg oral bid x 3 d	
GRANULOMA INGUINALE		
	TMP-SMZ 1 double-strength tablet oral bid for a minimum of 3 wk	Ciprofloxacin 750 mg oral bid for a minimum of 3 wk
	or	**or**
	Doxycycline 100 oral bid for a minimum of 3 wk	Erythromycin base 500 mg oral qid for a minimum of 3 wk
		or
		Azithromycin 1 g oral once per week for a minimum of 3 weeks

[1] Related clinical syndromes include nonchlamydial nongonococcal urethritis and cervicitis.

[2] Or oral tetracycline 500 mg qid.

[3] Not recommended in pregnancy.

[4] Erythromycin ethylsuccinate 800 mg may be substituted for erythromycin base 500 mg; erythromycin estolate is contraindicated in pregnancy.

[5] Pyloric stenosis has been associated with use of erythromycin in newborns.

[6] All patients should also receive a course of treatment effective for *Chlamydia*.

[7] Fluoroquinolones should not be used to treat gonorrhea acquired in Asia, Hawaii, Israel, or other areas where fluoroquinolone-resistant strains of *N. gonorrhoeae* are common.

[8] Recommended only for use during pregnancy in patients allergic to β-lactams. Not effective for pharyngeal infection.

[9] Some clinicians believe the addition of metronidazole is not required.

[10] Or clindamycin 450 mg oral qid to complete 14 days.

[11] A single daily dose of 3 mg/kg is likely to be effective, but has not been studied in pelvic inflammatory disease.

[12] Some experts would add metronidazole 500 mg bid.

[13] Higher relapse rate with single dose, but useful for patients who may not comply with multiple-dose therapy.

[14] In pregnancy, topical preparations have not been effective in preventing premature delivery; oral metronidazole has been effective in some studies.

[15] For preparations and dosage of topical products, see *Med Lett Drugs Ther*, 1994, 36:81; single-dose therapy is not recommended.

[16] Some experts recommend a repeat dose after 7 days, especially in patients with HIV infection or pregnant women.

[17] Patients allergic to penicillin should be desensitized and treated with penicillin.

[18] All regimens, especially single-dose ceftriaxone, are less effective in HIV-infected patients.

[19] Recommendations for external genital warts. Liquid nitrogen can also be used for vaginal, urethral, and oral warts. Podofilox or imiquimod can be used for urethral meatus warts. Trichloroacetic or bichloroacetic acid can be used for anal warts.

TREATMENT OF SEXUALLY TRANSMITTED INFECTIONS *(Continued)*

[20]Some Medical Letter consultants discontinue preventive treatment for 1-2 months once a year to reassess the frequency of recurrence.

[21]Use 500 mg once daily in patients with <10 recurrences per year and 500 mg bid or 1 g daily in patients with <10 recurrences per year.

[22]Antiviral therapy is variably effective for episodic treatment of recurrences; only effective if started early.

[23]No published data are available to support 3 days' use.

Adapted from "Sexually Transmitted Diseases Treatment Guidelines 2002," *MMWR Morb Mortal Wkly Rep*, 2002, 51(RR-6).

Adapted from "Drugs for Sexually Transmitted Infections," *Treatment Guidelines From The Medical Letter®*, 2004, 2(26):70-2.

TUBERCULOSIS

Tuberculin Skin Test Recommendations[1]

Children for whom immediate skin testing is indicated:

- Contacts of persons with confirmed or suspected infectious tuberculosis (contact investigation); this includes children identified as contacts of family members or associates in jail or prison in the last 5 years
- Children with radiographic or clinical findings suggesting tuberculosis
- Children immigrating from endemic countries (eg, Asia, Middle East, Africa, Latin America)
- Children with travel histories to endemic countries and/or significant contact with indigenous persons from such countries

Children who should be tested annually for tuberculosis[2]:

- Children infected with HIV or living in household with HIV-infected persons
- Incarcerated adolescents

Children who should be tested every 2-3 years[2]:

- Children exposed to the following individuals: HIV-infected, homeless, residents of nursing homes, institutionalized adolescents or adults, users of illicit drugs, incarcerated adolescents or adults, and migrant farm workers. Foster children with exposure to adults in the preceding high-risk groups are included.

Children who should be considered for tuberculin skin testing at ages 4-6 and 11-16 years:

- Children whose parents immigrated (with unknown tuberculin skin test status) from regions of the world with high prevalence of tuberculosis; continued potential exposure by travel to the endemic areas and/or household contact with persons from the endemic areas (with unknown tuberculin skin test status) should be an indication for repeat tuberculin skin testing
- Children without specific risk factors who reside in high-prevalence areas; in general, a high-risk neighborhood or community does not mean an entire city is at high risk; rates in any area of the city may vary by neighborhood, or even from block to block; physicians should be aware of these patterns in determining the likelihood of exposure; public health officials or local tuberculosis experts should help clinicians identify areas that have appreciable tuberculosis rates

Children at increased risk of progression of infection to disease: Those with other medical risk factors, including diabetes mellitus, chronic renal failure, malnutrition, and congenital or acquired immunodeficiencies deserve special consideration. Without recent exposure, these persons are not at increased risk of acquiring tuberculosis infection. Underlying immune deficiencies associated with these conditions theoretically would enhance the possibility for progression to severe disease. Initial histories of potential exposure to tuberculosis should be included on all of these patients. If these histories or local epidemiologic factors suggest a possibility of exposure, immediate and periodic tuberculin skin testing should be considered. An initial Mantoux tuberculin skin test should be performed before initiation of immunosuppressive therapy in any child with an underlying condition that necessitates immunosuppressive therapy.

---

[1]BCG immunization is not a contraindication to tuberculin skin testing.

[2]Initial tuberculin skin testing is at the time of diagnosis or circumstance, beginning as early as at age 3 months.

Adapted from "Report of the Committee on Infectious Diseases," *2003 Red Book*®, 26th ed, 646.

TUBERCULOSIS *(Continued)*

Table 1. Tuberculosis Prophylaxis
Infection Without Disease (Positive Tuberculin Test)[1]

Specific Circumstances/ Organism	Comments	Regimen
Regardless of age (see INH Preventive Therapy)	Rx indicated	INH (5 mg/kg/d, maximum: 300 mg/d for adults, 10 mg/kg/d not to exceed 300 mg/d for children). Results with 6 months of treatment are nearly as effective as 12 months (65% vs 75% reduction in disease). *Am Thoracic Society* (6 months), *Am Acad Pediatrics*, 1991 (9 months). If CXR is abnormal, treat for 12 months. In HIV-positive patient, treatment for a minimum of 12 months, some suggest longer. Monitor transaminases monthly (*MMWR Morb Mortal Wkly Rep* 1989, 38:247).
Age <35 y	Rx indicated	Reanalysis of earlier studies favors INH prophylaxis for 6 months (if INH-related hepatitis case fatality rate is <1% and TB case fatality is ≥6.7%, which appears to be the case, monitor transaminases monthly (*Arch Int Med*, 1990, 150:2517).
INH-resistant organisms likely	Rx indicated	Data on efficacy of alternative regimens is currently lacking. Regimens include ETB + RIF daily for 6 months. PZA + RIF daily for 2 months, then INH + RIF daily until sensitivities from index case (if available) known, then if INH-CR, discontinue INH and continue RIF for 9 months, otherwise INH + RIF for 9 months (this latter is *Am Acad Pediatrics*, 1991 recommendation).
INH + RIF resistant organisms likely	Rx indicated	Efficacy of alternative regimens is unknown; PZA (25-30 mg/kg/d P.O.) + ETB (15-25 mg/kg/d P.O.) (at 25 mg/kg ETB, monitoring for retrobulbar neuritis required), for 6 months unless HIV-positive, then 12 months; PZA + ciprofloxacin (750 mg P.O. bid) or ofloxacin (400 mg P.O. bid) x 6-12 months *(MMWR Morb Mortal Wkly Rep*, 1992, 41(RR11):68).

INH = isoniazid; RIF = rifampin; KM = kanamycin; ETB = ethambutol

SM = streptomycin; CXR = chest x-ray; Rx = treatment

See also guidelines for interpreting PPD in "Skin Testing for Delayed Hypersensitivity."

[1]Tuberculin test (TBnT). The standard is the Mantoux test, 5 TU PPD in 0.1 mL diluent stabilized with Tween 80. Read at 48-72 hours measuring maximum diameter of induration. A reaction ≥5 mm is defined as positive in the following: positive HIV or risk factors, recent close case contacts, CXR consistent with healed TBc. ≥10 mm is positive in foreign-born in countries of high prevalence, injection drug users, low income populations, nursing home residents, patients with medical conditions which increase risk (see above, preventive treatment). ≥15 mm is positive in all others (*Am Rev Resp Dis*, 1990, 142:725). Two-stage TBnT: Use in individuals to be tested regularly (ie, healthcare workers). TBn reactivity may decrease over time but be boosted by skin testing. If unrecognized, individual may be incorrectly diagnosed as recent converter. If first TBnT is reactive but <10 mm, repeat 5 TU in 1 week, if then ≥10 mm = positive, not recent conversion (*Am Rev Resp Dis*, 1979, 119:587).

Changes From Prior Recommendations on Tuberculin Testing and Treatment of Latent Tuberculosis Infection (LTBI)

Tuberculin Testing

- Emphasis on targeted tuberculin testing among persons at high risk for recent LTBI or with clinical conditions that increase the risk for tuberculosis (TB), regardless of age; testing is discouraged among persons at lower risk
- For patients with organ transplants and other immunosuppressed patients (eg, persons receiving the equivalent of ≥15 mg/day prednisone for 1 month or more), 5 mm of induration rather than 10 mm of induration rather than 10 mm of induration as a cut-off level for tuberculin positivity
- A tuberculin skin test conversion is defined as in increase of ≥10 mm of induration within a 2-year period, regardless of age

Treatment of Latent Tuberculosis Infection

- For human immunodeficiency virus (HIV)-negative persons, isoniazid given for 9 months is preferred over 6-month regimens
- For HIV-positive persons and those with fibrotic lesions on chest x-ray consistent with previous TB, isoniazid should be given for 9 months instead of 12 months
- For HIV-negative and HIV-positive persons, rifampin and pyrazinamide should be given for 2 months
- For HIV-negative and HIV-positive persons, rifampin should be given for 4 months

Clinical and Laboratory Monitoring

- Routine baseline and follow-up laboratory monitoring can be eliminated in most persons with LTBI, except for those with HIV infection, pregnant women (or those in the immediate postpartum period), and persons with chronic liver disease or those who use alcohol regularly
- Emphasis on clinical monitoring for signs and symptoms of possible adverse effects, with prompt evaluation and changes in treatment, as indicated

Adapted from *MMWR*, 2000, 49(RR-6).

TUBERCULOSIS *(Continued)*

Table 2. Recommended Treatment Regimens for Drug-Susceptible Tuberculosis in Infants, Children, and Adolescents

Infection or Disease Category	Regimen	Remarks
Latent tuberculosis infection (positive tuberculin skin test, no disease):		
• Isoniazid-susceptible	9 months of isoniazid once a day	If daily therapy is not possible, directly observed therapy twice a week may be used for 9 months.
• Isoniazid-resistant	6 months of rifampin once a day	
• Isoniazid-rifampin-resistant[1]	Consult a tuberculosis specialist	
Pulmonary and extrapulmonary (except meningitis)	2 months of isoniazid, rifampin, and pyrazinamide daily, followed by 4 months of isoniazid and rifampin[2]	If possible drug resistance is a concern, another drug (ethambutol or aminoglycoside) is added to the initial 3-drug therapy until drug susceptibilities are determined. Directly observed therapy is highly desirable. If hilar adenopathy only, a 6-month course of isoniazid and rifampin is sufficient. Drugs can be given 2 or 3 times/week under directly observed therapy in the initial phase if nonadherence is likely.
Meningitis	2 months of isoniazid, rifampin, pyrazinamide, and aminoglycoside or ethionamide, once a day, followed by 7-10 months of isoniazid and rifampin once a day or twice a week (9-12 months total)	A fourth drug, usually an aminoglycoside, is given with initial therapy until drug susceptibility is known. For patients who may have acquired tuberculosis in geographic areas where resistance to streptomycin is common, capreomycin, kanamycin, or amikacin may be used instead of streptomycin.

[1]Duration of therapy is longer for human immunodeficiency virus (HIV)-infected people, and additional drugs may be indicated.

[2]Medications should be administered daily for the first 2 weeks to 2 months of treatment and then can be administered 2-3 times/week by directly observed therapy.

Adapted from "Report of the Committee on Infectious Diseases," *2003 Red Book®*, 26th ed, 649.

Table 3. Recommended Drug Regimens for Treatment of Latent Tuberculosis Infection in Children

Drug	Interval and Duration	Comments
Isoniazid	Daily for 9 mo Twice weekly for 9 mo	This includes treatment for any child <5 years old who is exposed to household members or other close contacts who are potentially infectious even if skin test is negative
Rifampin	Daily for 4-9 mo	No controlled trials; only to be used in INH intolerant or resistant
Rifampin-pyrazinamide	Daily for 3 mo	No controlled trials; only to be used in INH intolerant or resistant

Modified from *MMWR*, 2000, 14(RR-6).

TUBERCULOSIS *(Continued)*

Table 4. Recommended Drug Regimens for Treatment of Latent Tuberculosis Infection in Adults

Drug	Interval and Duration	Comments	Rating[1] (Evidence)[2] HIV⁻	Rating[1] (Evidence)[2] HIV⁺
Isoniazid	Daily for 9 months[3,4]	In HIV-infected patients, isoniazid may be administered concurrently with nucleoside reverse transcriptase inhibitors (NRTIs), protease inhibitors, or non-nucleoside reverse transcriptase inhibitors (NNRTIs)	A (II)	A (II)
	Twice weekly for 9 months[3,4]	Directly observed therapy (DOT) must be used with twice-weekly dosing	B (II)	B (II)
Isoniazid	Daily for 6 months[4]	Not indicated for HIV-infected persons, those with fibrotic lesions on chest radiographs, or children	B (I)	C (I)
	Twice weekly for 6 months[4]	DOT must be used with twice-weekly dosing	B (II)	C (I)
Rifampin	Daily for 4 months	For persons who cannot tolerate pyrazinamide	B (II)	B (III)
		For persons who are contacts of patients with isoniazid-resistant, rifampin-susceptible TB who cannot tolerate pyrazinamide		
Rifampin plus pyrazinamide	Daily for 2 months	May also be offered to persons who are contacts of pyrazinamide patients with isoniazid-resistant, rifampin-susceptible TB	B (II)	A (I)
		In HIV-infected patients, protease inhibitors or NNRTIs should generally not be administered concurrently with rifampin. Rifabutin can be used as an alternative for patients treated with indinavir, nelfinavir, amprenavir, ritonavir, or efavirenz, and possibly with nevirapine or soft-gel saquinavir[5]		
	Twice weekly for 2-3 months	DOT must be used with twice-weekly dosing	C (II)	C (I)

[1]Strength of recommendation: A = preferred; B = acceptable alternative; C = offer when A and B cannot be given.

[2]Quality of evidence: I = randomized clinical trial data; II = data from clinical trials that are not randomized or were conducted in other populations; III = expert opinion.

[3]Recommended regimen for children <18 years of age.

[4]Recommended regimens for pregnant women. Some experts would use rifampin and pyrazinamide for 2 months as an alternative regimen in HIV-infected pregnant women, although pyrazinamide should be avoided during the first trimester.

[5]Rifabutin should not be used with hard-gel saquinavir or delavirdine. When used with other protease inhibitors or NNRTIs, dose adjustment of rifabutin may be required.

Adapted from *MMWR Recomm Rep*, 2000, 49(RR6).

Table 5. TB Drugs in Special Situations

Drug	Pregnancy[1]	CNS TB Disease	Renal Insufficiency
Isoniazid	Safe	Good penetration	Normal clearance
Rifampin	Safe	Fair penetration Penetrates inflamed meninges (10% to 20%)	Normal clearance
Pyrazinamide	Avoid	Good penetration	Clearance reduced Decrease dose or prolong interval
Ethambutol	Safe	Penetrates inflamed meninges only (4% to 64%)	Clearance reduced Decrease dose or prolong interval
Streptomycin	Avoid	Penetrates inflamed meninges only	Clearance reduced Decrease dose or prolong interval
Capreomycin	Avoid	Penetrates inflamed meninges only	Clearance reduced Decrease dose or prolong interval
Kanamycin	Avoid	Penetrates inflamed meninges only	Clearance reduced Decrease dose or prolong interval
Ethionamide	Do not use	Good penetration	Normal clearance
Para-amino-salicylic acid	Safe	Penetrates inflamed meninges only (10% to 50%)	Incomplete data on clearance
Cycloserine	Avoid	Good penetration	Clearance reduced Decrease dose or prolong interval
Ciprofloxacin	Do not use	Fair penetration (5% to 10%) Penetrates inflamed meninges (50% to 90%)	Clearance reduced Decrease dose or prolong interval
Ofloxacin	Do not use	Fair penetration (5% to 10%) Penetrates inflamed meninges (50% to 90%)	Clearance reduced Decrease dose or prolong interval
Amikacin	Avoid	Penetrates inflamed meninges only	Clearance reduced Decrease dose or prolong interval
Clofazimine	Avoid	Penetration unknown	Clearance probably normal

[1]Safe = the drug has not been demonstrated to have teratogenic effects.

Avoid = data on the drug's safety are limited, or the drug is associated with mild malformations (as in the aminoglycosides).

Do not use = studies show an association between the drug and premature labor, congenital malformations, or teratogenicity.

TUBERCULOSIS *(Continued)*

Table 6. Recommendations for Coadministering Different Antiretroviral Drugs With the Antimycobacterial Drugs Rifabutin and Rifampin

Antiretroviral	Use in Combination with Rifabutin	Use in Combination with Rifampin	Comments
Saquinavir[1]			
Hard-gel capsules (HGC)	Possibly[2], if antiretroviral regimen also includes ritonavir	Possibly, if antiretroviral regimen also includes ritonavir	Coadministration of saquinavir SGC with usual-dose rifabutin (300 mg/day or 2-3 times/week) is a possibility. However, the pharmacokinetic data and clinical experience for this combination are limited.
Soft-gel capsules (SGC)	Probably[3]	Possibly, if antiretroviral regimen also includes ritonavir	The combination of saquinavir SGC or saquinavir HGC and ritonavir, coadministered with 1) usual-dose rifampin (600 mg/day or 2-3 times/week), or 2) reduced-dose rifabutin (150 mg 2-3 times/week) is a possibility. However, the pharmacokinetic data and clinical experience for these combinations are limited. Coadministration of saquinavir or saquinavir SGC with rifampin is not recommended because rifampin markedly decreases concentrations of saquinavir.
Ritonavir	Probably	Probably	If the combination of ritonavir and rifabutin is used, then a substantially reduced-dose rifabutin regimen (150 mg 2-3 times/week) is recommended. Coadministration of ritonavir with usual-dose rifampin (600 mg/day or 2-3 times/week) is a possibility, though pharmacokinetic data and clinical experience are limited.
Indinavir	Yes	No	There is limited, but favorable, clinical experience with coadministration of indinavir[4] with a reduced daily dose of rifabutin (150 mg) or with the usual dose of rifabutin (300 mg 2-3 times/week). Coadministration of indinavir with rifampin is not recommended because rifampin markedly decreases concentrations of indinavir.
Nelfinavir	Yes	No	There is limited, but favorable, clinical experience with coadministration of nelfinavir[5] with a reduced daily dose of rifabutin (150 mg) or with the usual dose of rifabutin (300 mg 2-3 times/week). Coadministration of nelfinavir with rifampin is not recommended because rifampin markedly decreases concentrations of nelfinavir.
Amprenavir	Yes	No	Coadministration of amprenavir with a reduced daily dose of rifabutin (150 mg) or with the usual dose of rifabutin (300 mg 2-3 times/week) is a possibility, but there is no published clinical experience. Coadministration of amprenavir with rifampin is not recommended because rifampin markedly decreases concentrations of amprenavir.

Table 6. Recommendations for Coadministering Different Antiretroviral Drugs With the Antimycobacterial Drugs Rifabutin and Rifampin *(continued)*

Antiretroviral	Use in Combination with Rifabutin	Use in Combination with Rifampin	Comments
Nevirapine	Yes	Possibly	Coadministration of nevirapine with usual-dose rifabutin (300 mg/day or 2-3 times/week) is a possibility based on pharmacokinetic study data. However, there is no published clinical experience for this combination. Data are insufficient to assess whether dose adjustments are necessary when rifampin is coadministered with nevirapine. Therefore, rifampin and nevirapine should be used only in combination if clearly indicated and with careful monitoring.
Delavirdine	No	No	Contraindicated because of the marked decrease in concentrations of delavirdine when administered with either rifabutin or rifampin.
Efavirenz	Probably	Probably	Coadministration of efavirenz with increased-dose rifabutin (450 mg/day or 600 mg/day, or 600 mg 2-3 times/week) is a possibility, though there is no published clinical experience. Coadministration of efavirenz[6] with usual-dose rifampin (600 mg/day or 2-3 times/week) is a possibility, though there is no published clinical experience.

[1]Usual recommended doses are 400 mg twice daily for each of these protease inhibitors and 400 mg of ritonavir.

[2]Despite limited data and clinical experience, the use of this combination is potentially successful.

[3]Based on available data and clinical experience, the successful use of this combination is likely.

[4] Usual recommended dose is 800 mg every 8 hours; some experts recommend increasing the indinavir dose to 1000 mg every 8 hours if indinavir is used in combination with rifabutin.

[5]Usual recommended dose is 750 mg 3 times/day or 1250 mg twice daily; some experts recommend increasing the nelfinavir dose to 1000 mg if the 3-times/day dosing is used and nelfinavir is used in combination with rifabutin.

[6]Usual recommended dose is 600 mg/day; some experts recommend increasing the efavirenz dose to 800 mg/day if efavirenz is used in combination with rifampin.

Updated March 2000 from www.aidsinfo.nih.gov -"Updated Guidelines for the Use of Rifabutin or Rifampin for the Treatment and Prevention of Tuberculosis Among HIV-Infected Patients Taking Protease Inhibitors or Non-nucleoside Reverse Transcriptase Inhibitors," *MMWR,* March 10, 2000, 49(09):185-9.

TUBERCULOSIS *(Continued)*

Table 7. Criteria for Tuberculin Positivity, by Risk Group

Reaction ≥5 mm of Induration	Reaction ≥10 mm of Induration	Reaction ≥15 mm of Induration
HIV-positive persons	Recent immigrants (ie, within the last 5 years) from high prevalence countries	Persons with no risk factors for TB
Recent contacts of tuberculosis (TB) case patients	Injection drug users	
Fibrotic changes on chest radiograph consistent with prior TB	Residents and employees[1] of the following high risk congregate settings: prisons and jails, nursing homes and other long-term facilities for the elderly, hospitals and other healthcare facilities, residential facilities for patients with AIDS, and homeless shelters	
Patients with organ transplant and other immunosuppressed patients (receiving the equivalent of ≥15 mg/day of prednisone for 1 month)[2]	Mycobacteriology laboratory personnel Persons with the following clinical conditions that place them at high risk: silicosis, diabetes mellitus, chronic renal failure, some hematologic disorders (eg, leukemias and lymphomas), other specific malignancies (eg, carcinoma of the head or neck and lung), weight loss of ≥10% of ideal body weight, gastrectomy, and jejunoileal bypass Children <4 years of age or infants, children, and adolescents exposed to adults at high-risk	

[1]For persons who are otherwise at low risk and are tested at the start of employment, a reaction of ≥15 mm induration is considered positive.

[2]Risk of TB in patients treated with corticosteroids increases with higher dose and longer duration.

Modified from *MMWR Morb Mortal Wkly Rep*, 2000, 49(RR-6).

Table 8. Recommendations, Rankings, and Performance Indicators for Treatment of Patients With Tuberculosis (TB)

Recommendation	Ranking[1] (Evidence)[2]	Performance Indicator
Obtain bacteriologic confirmation and susceptibility testing for patients with TB or suspected of having TB	A (II)	90% of adults with or suspected of having TB have 3 cultures for mycobacteria obtained before initiation of antituberculosis therapy (50% of children 0-12 y)
Place persons with suspected or confirmed smear-positive pulmonary or laryngeal TB in respiratory isolation until noninfectious	A (II)	90% of persons with sputum smear-positive TB remain in respiratory isolation until smear converts to negative
Begin treatment of patients with confirmed or suspected TB disease with one of the following drug combinations, depending on local resistance patterns: INH + RIF + PZA **or** INH + RIF + PZA + EMB **or** INH + RIF + PZA + SM	A (III)	90% of all patients with TB are started on INH + RIF + PZA + EMB or SM in geographic areas where >4% of TB isolates are resistant to INH
Report each case of TB promptly to the local public health department	A (III)	100% of persons with active TB are reported to the local public health department within 1 week of diagnosis
Perform HIV testing for all patients with TB	A (III)	80% of all patients with TB have HIV status determined within 2 months of a diagnosis of TB
Treat patients with TB caused by a susceptible organism for 6 months, using an ATS/CDC-approved regimen	A (I)	90% of all patients with TB complete 6 months of therapy with 12 months of beginning treatment
Re-evaluate patients with TB who are smear positive at 3 months for possible nonadherence or infection with drug-resistant bacilli	A (III)	90% of all patients with TB who are smear positive at 3 months have sputum culture/susceptibility testing performed within 1 month of the 3-month visit
Add ≥2 new antituberculosis agents when TB treatment failure is suspected	A (II)	100% of patients with TB with suspected treatment failure are prescribed ≥2 new antituberculosis agents
Perform tuberculin skin testing on all patients with a history of ≥1 of the following: HIV infection, I.V. drug use, homelessness, incarceration, or contact with a person with pulmonary TB	A (II)	80% of persons in the indicated population groups receive tuberculin skin test and return for reading
Administer treatment for latent TB infection to all persons with latent TB infection, unless it can be documented that they received such treatment previously	A (I)	75% of patients with positive tuberculin skin tests who are candidates for treatment for latent TB infection complete a course of therapy within 12 months of initiation

Note: ATS/CDC = American Thoracic Society and Centers for Disease Control and Prevention; EMB = ethambutol; INH = isoniazid; PZA = pyrazinamide; RIF = rifampin; SM = streptomycin.

[1]Strength of recommendation: A = preferred; B = acceptable alternative; C = offer when A and B cannot be given.

[2]Quality of evidence: I = randomized clinical trial data; II = data from clinical trials that are not randomized or were conducted in other populations; III = expert opinion.

Adapted from the Infectious Diseases Society of America, *Clinical Infectious Diseases,* 2000, 31:633-9.

TUBERCULOSIS *(Continued)*

Table 9. Drug Regimens for Culture-Positive Pulmonary Tuberculosis Caused by Drug-Susceptible Organisms

Initial Phase			Continuation Phase			Range of Total Doses (minimal duration)	Rating[1] (Evidence)[2]	
Regimen	Drugs	Interval and Doses[3] (minimal duration)	Regimen	Drugs	Interval and Doses[3,4] (minimal duration)		HIV⁻	HIV⁺
1	INH RIF PZA EMB	Seven days per week for 56 doses (8 wk) or 5 d/wk for 40 doses (8 wk)[5]	1a	INH/RIF	Seven days per week for 126 doses (18 wk) or 5 d/wk for 90 doses (18 wk)[5]	182-130 (26 wk)	A (I)	A (II)
			1b	INH/RIF	Twice weekly for 36 doses (18 wk)	92-76 (26 wk)	A (I)	A (II)[6]
			1c[7]	INH/RPT	Once weekly for 18 doses (18 wk)	74-58 (26 wk)	B (I)	E (I)
2	INH RIF PZA EMB	Seven days per week for 14 doses (2 wk), then twice weekly for 12 doses (6 wk) or 5 d/wk for 10 doses (2 wk)[5], then twice weekly for 12 doses (6 wk)	2a	INH/RIF	Twice weekly for 36 doses (18 wk)	62-58 (26 wk)	A (II)	B (II)[6]
			2b[7]	INH/RPT	Once weekly for 18 doses (18 wk)	44-40 (26 wk)	B (I)	E (I)
3	INH RIF PZA EMB	Three times weekly for 24 doses (8 wk)	3a	INH/RIF	Three times weekly for 54 doses (18 wk)	78 (26 wk)	B (I)	B (II)

Table 9. Drug Regimens for Culture-Positive Pulmonary Tuberculosis Caused by Drug-Susceptible Organisms *(continued)*

Initial Phase			Continuation Phase			Range of Total Doses (minimal duration)	Rating[1] (Evidence)[2]	
Regimen	Drugs	Interval and Doses[3] (minimal duration)	Regimen	Drugs	Interval and Doses[3,4] (minimal duration)		HIV⁻	HIV⁺
4	INH RIF EMB	Seven days per week for 56 doses (8 wk) or 5 d/wk for 40 doses (8 wk)[5]	4a	INH/RIF	Seven days per week for 217 doses (31 wk) or 5 d/wk for 155 doses (31 wk)[5]	273-195 (39 wk)	C (I)	C (II)
			4b	INH/RIF	Twice weekly for 62 doses (31 wk)	118-102 (39 wk)	C (I)	C (II)

Definition of abbreviations: EMB = ethambutol; INH = isoniazid; PZA = pyrazinamide; RIF = rifampin; RPT = rifapentine.

[1]Definitions of evidence ratings: A = preferred; B = acceptable alternative; C = offer when A and B cannot be given; E = should never be given.

[2]Definitions of evidence ratings: I = randomized clinical trial; II = data from clinical trials that were not randomized or were conducted in other populations; III = expert opinion.

[3]When directly observed therapy (DOT) is used, drugs may be given 5 days/week and the necessary number of doses adjusted accordingly. Although there are no studies that compare five with seven daily doses, extensive experience indicates this would be an effective practice.

[4]Patients with cavitation on initial chest radiograph and positive cultures at completion of 2 months of therapy should receive a 7-month (31-week; either 217 doses daily] or 62 doses [twice weekly]) continuation phase.

[5]Five-day/week administration is always given by DOT. Rating for 5 day/week regimens is AIII.

[6]Not recommended for HIV-infected patients with CD4⁺ cell counts <100 cells/µL.

[7]Options 1c and 2b should be used only in HIV-negative patients who have negative sputum smears at the time of completion of 2 months of therapy and who do not have cavitation on initial chest radiograph. For patients started on this regimen and found to have a positive culture from the 2-month specimen, treatment should be extended an extra 3 months.

Adapted from *MMWR*, 2003, 52(RR11).

TUBERCULOSIS *(Continued)*

Table 10. Doses[1] of Antituberculosis Drugs for Adults and Children

Drug	Preparation	Adults / Children	Doses			
			Daily	1x	2x	3x
First-Line Drugs						
Isoniazid	Tablets (50 mg, 100 mg, 300 mg); elixir (50 mg/5 mL); aqueous solution (100 mg/mL) for I.V. or I.M injection	Adults (max.)	5 mg/kg (300 mg)	15 mg/kg (900 mg)	15 mg/kg (900 mg)	15 mg/kg (900 mg)
		Children (max.)	10-15 mg/kg (300 mg)	–	20-30 mg/kg (900 mg)	–
Rifampin	Capsule (150 mg, 300 mg) powder may be suspended for oral administration; aqueous solution for I.V. injection	Adults[3] (max.)	10 mg/kg (600 mg)	–	10 mg/kg (600 mg)	10 mg/kg (600 mg)
		Children (max.)	10-20 mg/kg (600 mg)	–	10-20 mg/kg (600 mg)	–
Rifabutin	Capsule (150 mg)	Adults[3] (max.)	5 mg/kg (300 mg)	–	5 mg/kg (300 mg)	5 mg/kg (300 mg)
		Children	Appropriate dosing for children is unknown			
Rifapentine	Tablet (150 mg, film coated)	Adults	–	10 mg/kg (continuation phase) (600 mg)	–	–
		Children	The drug is not approved for use in children			
Pyrazinamide	Tablet (500 mg, scored)	Adults	See table 11	–	See table 11	See table 11
		Children (max.)	15-30 mg/kg (2 g)	–	50 mg/kg (2 g)	–
Ethambutol	Tablet (100 mg 400 mg)	Adults	See table 12	–	See table 12	See table 12
		Children[4] (max.)	15-20 mg/kg daily (1 g)	–	50 mg/kg (2.5 g)	–
Second-Line Drugs						
Cycloserine	Capsule (250 mg)	Adults (max.)	10-15 mg/kg/d (1 g in two doses), usually 500-750 mg/d in two doses[5]	There are no data to support intermittent administration		
		Children (max.)	10-15 mg/kg/d (1 g/d)	–	–	–

Table 10. Doses[1] of Antituberculosis Drugs for Adults and Children *(continued)*

Drug	Preparation	Adults / Children	Doses: Daily	1x	2x	3x
Ethionamide	Tablet (250 mg)	Adults[6] (max.)	15-20 mg/kg/d (1 g/d), usually, 500-750 mg/d in a single daily dose or two divided doses[6]	There are no data to support intermittent administration		
		Children (max.)	15-20 mg/kg/d (1 g/d)	There are no data to support intermittent administration		
Streptomycin	Aqueous solution (1 g vials) for I.M. or I.V. administration	Adults (max.)	See footnote 7			
		Children (max.)	20-40 mg/kg/d (1 g)	–	20 mg/kg	–
Amikacin/ Kanamycin	Aqueous solution (500 mg and 1 g vials) for I.V. or I.M. administration	Adults (max.)	See footnote 7			
		Children (max.)	15-30 mg/kg/d (1 g) I.V. or I.M. as a single daily dose	–	15-30 mg/kg	–
Capreomycin	Aqueous solution (1 g vials) for I.M. or I.V. administration	Adults (max.)	See footnote 7			
		Children (max.)	15-30 mg/kg/d (1 g) as a single daily dose	–	15-30 mg/kg	–
p-Aminosalicylic acid (PAS)	Granules (4 g packets) can be mixed with food; tablets (500 mg) are still available in some countries, but not in the United States; a solution for I.V. administration is available in Europe	Adults	8-12 g/d in 2 or 3 doses	There are no data to support intermittent administration		
		Children	200-300 mg/kg/d in 2-4 divided doses (10 g)	There are no data to support intermittent administration		
Levofloxacin	Tablets (250 mg, 500 mg, 750 mg); aqueous solution (500 mg vials) for I.V. injection	Adults	500-1000 mg daily	There are no data to support intermittent administration		
		Children	See footnote 8			

TUBERCULOSIS *(Continued)*

Table 10. Doses[1] of Antituberculosis Drugs for Adults and Children *(continued)*

Drug	Preparation	Adults / Children	Doses			
			Daily	1x	2x	3x
Moxifloxacin	Tablets (400 mg); aqueous solution (400 mg/250 mL) for I.V. injection	Adults	400 mg daily	There are no data to support intermittent administration		
		Children	See footnote 9			
Gatifloxacin	Tablets (400 mg); aqueous solution (200 mg/20 mL; 400 mg/40 mL) for I.V. injection	Adults	400 mg daily	There are no data to support intermittent administration		
		Children	See footnote 10			

[1]Dose per weight is based on ideal body weight. Children weighing >40 kg should be dosed as adults.

[2]For purposes of this document adult dosing begins at age 15 years.

[3]Dose may need to be adjusted when there is concomitant use of protease inhibitors or non-nucleoside reverse transcriptase inhibitors.

[4]The drug can likely be used safely in older children but should be used with caution in children less than 5 years of age, in whom visual acuity cannot be monitored. In younger children EMB at the dose of 15 mg/kg per day can be used if there is suspected or proven resistance to INH or RIF.

[5]It should be noted that, although this is the dose recommended generally, most clinicians with experience using cycloserine indicate that it is unusual for patients to be able to tolerate this amount. Serum concentration measurements are often useful in determining the optimal dose for a given patient.

[6]The single daily dose can be given at bedtime or with the main meal.

[7]Dose: 15 mg/kg per day (1 g), and 10 mg/kg in persons more than 59 years of age (750 mg). Usual dose: 750-1000 mg administered intramuscularly or intravenously, given as a single dose 5-7 days/week and reduced to two or three times per week after the first 2-4 months or after culture conversion, depending on the efficacy of the other drugs in the regimen.

[8]The long-term (more than several weeks) use of levofloxacin in children and adolescents has not been approved because of concerns about effects on bone and cartilage growth. However, most experts agree that the drug should be considered for children with tuberculosis caused by organisms resistant to both INH and RIF. The optimal dose is not known.

[9]The long-term (more than several weeks) use of moxifloxacin in children and adolescents has not been approved because of concerns about effects on bone and cartilage growth. The optimal dose is not known.

[10]The long-term (more than several weeks) use of gatifloxacin in children and adolescents has not been approved because of concerns about effects on bone and cartilage growth. The optimal dose is not known.

Table 11. Suggested Pyrazinamide Doses, Using Whole Tablets, for Adults Weighing 40-90 kg

	Weight (kg)[1]		
	40-55	56-75	76-90
Daily, mg (mg/kg)	1000 (18.2-25)	1500 (20-26.8)	2000[2] (22.2-26.3)
Thrice weekly, mg (mg/kg)	1500 (27.3-37.5)	2500 (33.3-44.6)	3000[2] (33.3-39.5)
Twice weekly, mg (mg/kg)	2000 (36.4-50)	3000 (40-53.6)	4000[2] (44.4-52.6)

[1]Based on estimated lean body weight

[2]Maximum dose regardless of weight.

Table 12. Suggested Ethambutol Doses, Using Whole Tablets, for Adults Weighing 40-90 kg

	Weight (kg)[1]		
	40-55	56-75	76-90
Daily, mg (mg/kg)	800 (14.5-20)	1200 (16-21.4)	1600[2] (17.8-21.1)
Thrice weekly, mg (mg/kg)	1200 (21.8-30)	2000 (26.7-35.7)	2400[2] (26.7-31.6)
Twice weekly, mg (mg/kg)	2000 (36.4-50)	2800 (37.3-50)	4000[2] (44.4-52.6)

[1]Based on estimated lean body weight

[2]Maximum dose regardless of weight.

CLASSIFICATION OF ORGANISMS

Anaerobes

Chlamydia

DNA Viruses

Fungi

Gram-Negative Bacilli

Gram-Negative Cocci

(Continued)

RNA Viruses *(Continued)*

Spirochetes

ALPHABETICAL INDEX

INTERNATIONAL BRAND NAME INDEX

The following countries are included in this index and are abbreviated as follows:

Argentina (AR)
Australia (AU)
Austria (AT)
Bangladesh (BD)
Belgium (BE)
Brazil (BR)
Bulgaria (BG)
Canada (CA)
Chile (CL)
China (CN)
Colombia (CO)
Costa Rica (CR)
Croatia / Hrvatska (HR)
Cypress (CY)
Czech Republic (CZ)
Denmark (DK)
Dominican Republic (DO)
Ecuador (EC)
Egypt (EG)
El Salvador (SV)
Finland (FI)
France (FR)
Germany (DE)
Great Britain [UK] (GB)
Greece (GR)
Guatemala (GT)
Honduras (HN)
Hong Kong (HK)
Hungary (HU)
Iceland (IS)
India (IN)
Indonesia (ID)
Ireland (IE)
Israel (IL)
Italy (IT)
Japan (JP)
Jordan (JO)
Korea [South] (KR)
Kuwait (KW)
Lebanon (LB)
Lithuania (LT)
Luxemborg (LU)
Malta (MT)
Malaysia (MY)
Mexico (MX)
Monaco (MC)
Morocco (MA)
Netherlands (NL)
New Zealand (NZ)
Norway (NO)
Panama (PA)
Peru (PE)
Phillipines (PH)
Poland (PL)
Portugal (PT)
Puerto Rico (PR)
Romania (RO)
Russian Federation (RU)
Singapore (SG)
Slovak Republic (SK)
Slovenia (SI)
South Africa (ZA)
Spain (ES)
Sri Lanka (LK)
Sweden (SE)
Switzerland (CH)
Syria (SY)
Taiwan (TW)
Thailand (TH)
Turkey (TR)
Ukraine (UA)
United States (US)
Uruguay (UY)
Venezuela (VE)
Viet Nam (VN)
Yugoslavia (YU)

NOTES

NOTES

NOTES

NOTES

NOTES

NOTES

Complementary Products Offered by LEXI-COMP®

CLINICIAN'S GUIDE TO LABORATORY MEDICINE

—A Practical Approach by Samir P. Desai, MD and Sana Isa-Pratt, MD

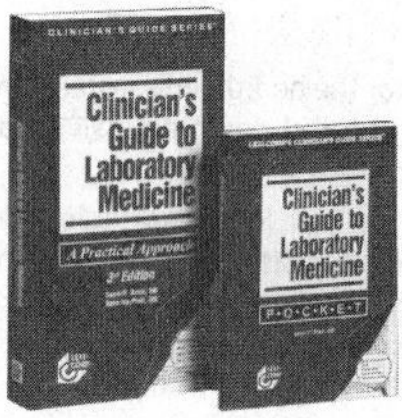

When faced with the patient presenting with abnormal laboratory tests, the clinician can now turn to the Clinician's Guide to Laboratory Medicine: A Practical Approach. This source is unique in its ability to lead the clinician from laboratory test abnormality to clinical diagnosis. Written for the busy clinician, this concise handbook will provide rapid answers to the questions that busy clinicians face in the care of their patients. No longer does the clinician have to struggle in an effort to find this information - it's all here.

Included is a **FREE** copy of Clinician's Guide to Laboratory Medicine - Pocket. Great to carry in your pocket! Perfect for use "in the trenches."

CLINICIAN'S GUIDE TO INTERNAL MEDICINE

—A Practical Approach by Samir P. Desai, MD

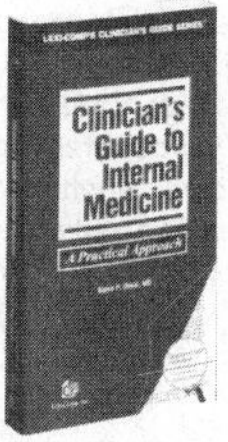

Provides quick access to essential information covering diagnosis, treatment, and management of commonly encountered patient problems in Internal Medicine. Contains up-to-date, clinically-relevant information in an easy-to-read format and is easily accessible. Contains practical approaches that are not readily available in standard textbooks. Contains algorithms to help you establish the diagnosis and select the appropriate therapy. There are numerous tables and boxes that summarize diagnostic and therapeutic strategies. It is an ideal reference for use at the point-of-care. This is a reference companion that will provide you with the tools necessary to tackle even the most challenging problems in Internal Medicine.

CLINICIAN'S GUIDE TO DIAGNOSIS

—A Practical Approach by Samir P. Desai, MD

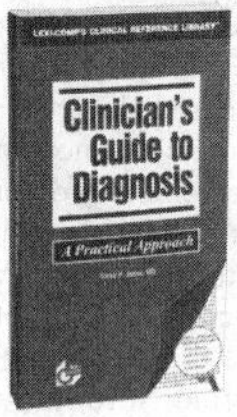

Symptoms are what prompt patients to seek medical care. In the evaluation of a patient's symptom, it is not unusual for healthcare professionals to ask "What do I do next?" This is precisely the question for which the Clinician's Guide to Diagnosis: A Practical Approach provides the answer. It will lead you from symptom to diagnosis through a series of steps designed to mimic the logical thought processes of seasoned clinicians. For the young clinician, this is an ideal book to help bridge the gap between the classroom and actual patient care. For the experienced clinician, this concise handbook offers rapid answers to the questions that are commonly encountered on a day-to-day basis. Let this guide become your companion, providing you with the tools necessary to tackle even the most challenging symptoms.

To order call toll free anywhere in the U.S.: 1-866-397-3433 or go to www.lexi.com

Outside of the U.S. call: 330-650-6506 or online at www.lexi.com

Other Products Offered by LEXI-COMP®

DRUG INFORMATION SERIES™

Anesthesiology & Critical Care Drug Handbook
Drug Information Handbook for Advanced Practice Nursing
Drug Information Handbook for Dentistry
Drug Information Handbook for Nursing
Drug Information Handbook for Oncology
Drug Information Handbook for the Allied Health Professional
Drug Information Handbook for the Criminal Justice Professional
Drug Interactions Handbook
Geriatric Dosage Handbook
Natural Therapeutics Pocket Guide
Pediatric Dosage Handbook
Pediatric Pharmacology Companion Guide
Pharmacology Companion Guide
Pharmacogenomics Handbook

DIAGNOSTIC MEDICINE SERIES™

Infectious Diseases Handbook
Poisoning & Toxicology Handbook

MENTAL HEALTH SERIES™

Drug Information Handbook for Psychiatry
Psychotropic Drug Information Handbook
Rating Scales in Mental Health
A Patient Guide to Mental Health Issues - Flip chart

DENTAL REFERENCE LIBRARY™

Clinician's Endodontic Handbook
Dental Insurance And Reimbursement
Dental Office Medical Emergencies
Employee Embezzlement and Fraud in the Dental Office
Illustrated Handbook of Clinical Dentistry
Little Dental Drug Booklet
Manual of Clinical Periodontics
Manual of Dental Implants
Oral Hard Tissue Diseases
Oral Soft Tissue Diseases
Patient Guide to Dental Implants - Flip chart & Booklet
Patient Guide to Periodontal Disease - Flip chart
Patient Guide to Root Canal Therapy - Flip chart
Your Roadmap To Financial Integrity In The Dental Office

OTHER

Medical Abbreviations by Neil Davis

For detailed information on any of these titles go to www.lexi.com

To order call toll free anywhere in the U.S.: 1-866-397-3433 or go to www.lexi.com
Outside of the U.S. call: 330-650-6506 or online at www.lexi.com

LEXI-C

MW00527375

Infectious Diseases Handbook

including

Antimicrobial Therapy & Diagnostic Tests/Procedures

6th Edition

LEXI-COMP

APhA